CASARETT AND DOULL'S
TOXICOLOGY

The Basic Science of Poisons

All substances are poisons; there is none which is not a poison. The right dose differentiates a poison and a remedy.

PARACELSUS
(1493–1541)

NOTICE

Medicine is an ever-changing science. As new research
and clinical experience broaden our knowledge, changes
in treatment and drug therapy are required. The editors
and the publisher of this work have checked with sources
believed to be reliable in their efforts to provide information
that is complete and generally in accord with the standards
accepted at the time of publication. However, in view of
the possibility of human error or changes in medical
sciences, neither the editors, nor the publisher, nor any
other party who has been involved in the preparation or
publication of this work warrants that the information
contained herein is in every respect accurate or complete,
and they are not responsible for any errors or omissions
or for the results obtained from use of such information.
Readers are encouraged to confirm the information contained herein with other sources. For example and in
particular, readers are advised to check the product information sheet included in the package of each drug they
plan to administer to be certain that the information
contained in this book is accurate and that changes have
not been made in the recommended dose or in the contraindications for administration. This recommendation is of
particular importance in connection with new or infrequently used drugs.

CASARETT AND DOULL'S
TOXICOLOGY

The Basic Science of Poisons

FOURTH EDITION

Editors:

Mary O. Amdur, Ph.D.

Research Professor
Institute of Environmental Medicine
New York University Medical Center
Tuxedo, New York

John Doull, Ph.D., M.D.

Professor
Department of Pharmacology and Toxicology
University of Kansas School of Medicine
Kansas City, Kansas

Curtis D. Klaassen, Ph.D.

Professor
Department of Pharmacology and Toxicology
University of Kansas School of Medicine
Kansas City, Kansas

McGRAW-HILL, INC.
Health Professions Division

New York St. Louis San Francisco Auckland Bogotá Caracas
Lisbon London Madrid Mexico Milan Montreal New Delhi Paris
San Juan Singapore Sydney Tokyo Toronto

Casarett and Doull's Toxicology: The Basic Science of Poisons

34567890 DOWDOW 987654

ISBN 0-07-105239-9

Previous edition © 1991 Pergamon Press, Inc.

Earlier editions: *Toxicology: The Basic Science of Poisons,* edited by Louis J. Casarett and John Doull, copyright © 1975 by Macmillan Publishing Company. *Casarett and Doull's Toxicology: The Basic Science of Poisons, Second Edition,* edited by John Doull, Curtis D. Klaassen, and Mary O. Amdur, copyright © 1980 by Macmillan Publishing Company. *Casarett and Doull's Toxicology: The Basic Science of Poisons, Third Edition,* edited by Curtis D. Klaassen, Mary O. Amdur, and John Doull, copyright © 1986, Macmillan Publishing Company.

Library of Congress Cataloging-in-Publication Data

Casarett and Doull's toxicology : the basic science of poisons /
    editors, Mary O. Amdur, John Doull, Curtis D. Klaassen. -- 4th ed.
        p.   cm.
    Earlier ed. entered under uniform title: Toxicology (Macmillan
Publishing Company)
    Includes bibliographical references.
    Includes index.
    ISBN 0-07-105239-9
    1. Toxicology. I. Casarett, Louis J. II. Doull, John, 1923-
III. Amdur, Mary O. IV. Klaassen, Curtis D. V. Title: Toxicology.
    [DNLM 1. Poisoning. 2. Poisons. QV 600 C335]
RA1211.C296 1991
615.9--dc20
DNLM/DLC
for Library of Congress   90-14324
                                                              CIP

Preface to the Fourth Edition

THE PHILOSOPHY AND DESIGN of the fourth edition of this textbook remain those set forth in the preface of the first edition fifteen years ago. It is meant to serve primarily as a text for, or an adjunct to, graduate courses in toxicology. We have attempted to retain those aspects that have made previous editions useful as a reference for students and scientists in broad areas of environmental health. The fourth edition again provides information on the many facets of toxicology and on the principles, concepts, and modes of thought that are the foundations of the discipline. Research toxicologists who have used previous editions as a reference source will find updated treatment of material in their areas of special or peripheral interests.

As in past editions, the book is divided into major sections covering General Principles of Toxicology (Unit 1), Systemic Toxicology (Unit II), Toxic Agents (Unit III), Environmental Toxicology (Unit IV), and Applications of Toxicology (Unit V). We have continued the policy of changing authorship of one-third of the chapters to broaden input and provide new coverage of the many aspects of toxicology.

The editors are grateful to our colleagues in academia, industry, and government as well as to graduate students who have made useful suggestions on ways to improve the fourth edition in its dual role as textbook and reference source. We are especially grateful to the contributors whose combined expertise made possible the breadth of coverage of a multifaceted discipline. We appreciate their efforts to limit chapters to lengths that would keep the fourth edition from becoming unwieldy in size and prohibitive in price.

M.O.A.
J.D.
C.D.K.

Preface to the First Edition

THIS VOLUME has been designed primarily as a textbook for, or adjunct to, courses in toxicology. However, it should also be of interest to those not directly involved in toxicologic education. For example, the research scientist in toxicology will find sections containing current reports on the status of circumscribed areas of special interest. Those concerned with community health, agriculture, food technology, pharmacy, veterinary medicine, and related disciplines will discover the contents to be most useful as a source of concepts and modes of thought that are applicable to other types of investigative and applied sciences. For those further removed from the field of toxicology or for those who have not entered a specific field of endeavor, this book attempts to present a selectively representative view of the many facets of the subject.

Toxicology: The Basic Science of Poisons has been organized to facilitate its use by these different types of users. The first section (Unit I) describes the elements of method and approach that identify toxicology. It includes those principles most frequently invoked in a full understanding of toxicologic events, such as dose-response, and is primarily mechanistically oriented. Mechanisms are also stressed in the subsequent sections of the book, particularly when these are well identified and extend across classic forms of chemicals and systems. However, the major focus in the second section (Unit II) is on the systemic site of action of toxins. The intent therein is to provide answers to two questions: What kinds of injury are produced in specific organs or systems by toxic agents? What are the agents that produce these effects?

A more conventional approach to toxicology has been utilized in the third section (Unit III), in which the toxic agents are grouped by chemical or use characteristics. In the final section (Unit IV) an attempt has been made to illustrate the ramifications of toxicology into all areas of the health sciences and even beyond. This unit is intended to provide perspective for the nontoxicologist in the application of the results of toxicologic studies and a better understanding of the activities of those engaged in the various aspects of the discipline of toxicology.

It will be obvious to the reader that the contents of this book represent a compromise between the basic, fundamental, mechanistic approach to toxicology and the desire to give a view of the broad horizons presented by the subject. While it is certain that the editors' selectivity might have been more severe, it is equally certain that it could have been less so, and we hope that the balance struck will prove to be appropriate for both toxicologic training and the scientific interest of our colleagues.

L.J.C.
J.D.

Although the philosophy and design of this book evolved over a long period of friendship and mutual respect between the editors, the effort needed to convert ideas into reality was undertaken primarily by Louis J. Casarett. Thus, his death at a time when completion of the manuscript was in sight was particularly tragic. With the help and encouragement of his wife, Margaret G. Casarett, and the other contributors, we have finished Lou's task. This volume is a fitting embodiment of Louis J. Casarett's dedication to toxicology and to toxicologic education.

J.D.

Contributors

Amdur, Mary O., Ph.D. Research Professor, Institute of Environmental Medicine, NYU Medical Center, Tuxedo, New York

Andrews, Larry S., Ph.D. Advisor in Toxicology, ARCO Chemical Company, Newton Square, Pennsylvania

Anthony, Douglas C., M.D., Ph.D. Assistant Professor of Pathology, Duke University School of Medicine, Durham, North Carolina

Blanke, Robert V., Ph.D. Professor of Pathology and Affiliate Professor of Pharmacology and Toxicology, Department of Pathology, Medical College of Virginia, Richmond, Virginia

Dart, Richard C., M.D. Section of Emergency Medicine, University of Arizona, Tucson, Arizona

Dean, Jack H., Ph.D. Vice President of Drug Safety Assessment, Sterling Research Group, Rensselaer, New York

Doull, John, Ph.D., M.D. Professor of Pharmacology and Toxicology, University of Kansas, School of Medicine, Kansas City, Kansas

Eaton, David L., Ph.D. Associate Professor and Toxicology, Program Director, Department of Environmental Health and Institute for Environmental Studies, University of Washington, Seattle, Washington

Ecobichon, Donald J., Ph.D. Professor, Department of Pharmacology and Therapeutics, McGill University, Montreal, Quebec, Canada

Emmett, Edward A., M.D. National Occupational Health and Safety Commission, Sydney, Australia

Gallo, Michael A., Ph.D. Department of Environmental and Community Medicine, UMDNJ—Robert Wood Johnson Medical School, Piscataway, New Jersey

Gandolfi, A. Jay, Ph.D. Professor, Anesthesiology, Pharmacology and Toxicology, University of Arizona, College of Medicine, Tucson, Arizona

Goldstein, Robin S., Ph.D. Department of Investigative Toxicology, Smith Kline Beecham Pharmaceuticals, King of Prussia, Pennsylvania

Gordon, Terry, Ph.D. Assistant Professor, Institute of Environmental Medicine, NYU Medical Center, Tuxedo, New York

Goyer, Robert A., M.D. Chairman and Professor, Department of Pathology, University of Western Ontario, Health Sciences Centre, London, Ontario, Canada

Graham, Doyle G., M.D., Ph.D. Professor of Pathology, Duke University Medical Center, Durham, North Carolina

Hanig, Joseph P., Ph.D. Division of Research and Testing, Center for Drug Evaluation and Research, U.S. Food and Drug Administration, Washington, D.C.

Harley, Naomi H., Ph.D. Research Professor, Institute of Environmental Medicine, NYU Medical Center, New York, New York

Herman, Eugene H., Ph.D. Division of Research and Testing, Center for Drug Evaluation and Research, U.S. Food and Drug Administration, Washington, D.C.

Hewitt, William R., Ph.D. Director, Development Project Management, Smith Kline Beecham Pharmaceuticals, R & D Division, King of Prussia, Pennsylvania

Hoffmann, George R., Ph.D. Professor and Chair, Department of Biology, College of the Holy Cross, Worcester, Massachusetts

Hook, Jerry B., Ph.D. Senior Vice President and Director, Research and Development, Smith Kline Beecham Pharmaceuticals, King of Prussia, Pennsylvania

Klaassen, Curtis D., Ph.D. Professor of Pharmacology and Toxicology, University of Kansas, School of Medicine, Kansas City, Kansas

Lampe, Kenneth F., Ph.D. (Deceased) Director, Department of Toxicology, Division of Drugs, American Medical Association, Chicago, Illinois

Lauwerys, Robert R., M.D., D.Sc. Professor, Industrial Toxicology and Occupational Medicine Unit, Catholic University of Louvain, Brussels, Belgium

Lovejoy, Frederick H., Jr., M.D. Associate Physician-in-Chief, The Children's Hospital, William Berenberg Professor of Pediatrics, Harvard Medical School, Boston, Massachusetts

Manson, Jeanne M., Ph.D. Director, Developmental and Reproductive Toxicology, Department of Safety Assessment, Merck, Sharp & Dohme Research Laboratories, West Point, Pennsylvania

Menzer, Robert E., Ph.D. Environmental Research Laboratory, United States Environmental Protection Agency, Sabine Island, Gulf Breeze, Florida

Merrill, Richard A., L.L.B., M.A. Dean, University of Virginia, School of Law, Charlottesville, Virginia

Miller, Sanford A., M.D. Graduate School of Biomedical Sciences, University of Texas, Health Science Center, San Antonio, Texas

Murray, Michael J., Ph.D. Research Toxicologist, Human and Environmental Safety Division, Research and Development Department, The Proctor and Gamble Company, Miami Valley Laboratories, Cincinnati, Ohio

Plaa, Gabriel L., Ph.D. Department of Pharmacology, Faculty of Medicine, University of Montreal, Montreal, Quebec, Canada

Poklis, Alphonse, Ph.D. Director, MCV Hospital Toxicology Laboratory, Richmond, Virginia

Potts, Albert M., M.D., Ph.D. 6751 N. Camino Abbey, Tucson, Arizona

Rozman, Karl, Ph.D. Professor of Pharmacology and Toxicology and Therapeutics, University of Kansas, Medical Center, Kansas City, Kansas; Head, Section of Environmental Toxicology, GSF—Institute of Toxicology, Neuherberg, Germany

Rumack, Barry H., M.D. Professor of Pediatrics, University of Colorado Health Sciences Center; Director, Rocky Mountain Poison and Drug Center, Denver, Colorado

Russell, Findlay E., M.D., Ph.D. University of Arizona, College of Pharmacy, Tucson, Arizona

Scala, Robert A., Ph.D. Senior Scientific Advisor, Exxon Biomedical Sciences, Inc., Mettlers Road, East Millstone, New Jersey

Sipes, I. Glenn, Ph.D. Professor and Head, Department of Pharmacology and Toxicology, University of Arizona, College of Pharmacy, Tucson, Arizona

Smith, Roger P., Ph.D. Professor of Pharmacology and Toxicology, Department of Pharmacology and Toxicology, Dartmouth Medical School, Hanover, New Hampshire

Snyder, Robert, Ph.D. Graduate Program in Toxicology, Rutgers University, College of Pharmacy, Piscataway, New Jersey

Thomas, John A., Ph.D. Professor, Department of Pharmacology (Division of Toxicology), Health Science Center, University of Texas, San Antonio, Texas

Weisburger, John H., Ph.D., M.D. Senior Member and Director Emeritus, American Health Foundation, Valhalla, New York

Williams, Gary M., M.D. Director of Medical Science, American Health Foundation, Valhalla, New York

Wise, L. David, Ph.D. Senior Research Fellow, Department of Safety Assessment, Merck, Sharp & Dohme Research Laboratories, West Point, Pennsylvania

Contents

UNIT III
Toxic Agents

UNIT IV
Environmental Toxicology

UNIT V
Applications of Toxicology

CASARETT AND DOULL'S
TOXICOLOGY

The Basic Science of Poisons

UNIT I

GENERAL PRINCIPLES
OF TOXICOLOGY

Chapter 1

HISTORY AND SCOPE OF TOXICOLOGY

Michael A. Gallo and *John Doull*

INTRODUCTION

Modern toxicology, which is defined as the study of the adverse effects of xenobiotics, is a borrowing science that evolved from the ancient poisoners. Historically, toxicology formed the basis of therapeutics and experimental medicine. The modern era of toxicology (1900 to present) continues to develop and expand by assimilating knowledge and techniques from most branches of biology, chemistry, mathematics, and physics. A recent addition to the field of toxicology is the application of the discipline to safety evaluation and risk assessment.

The contributions and activities of toxicologists are diverse and widespread. In the biomedical area, toxicologists are concerned with the mechanism(s) of action and exposure to chemical agents as a cause of both acute and chronic illness. Toxicologists contribute markedly to physiology and pharmacology by using toxic agents to understand physiological phenomena. They are involved in the recognition, identification, and quantitation of hazards resulting from occupational exposure to chemicals and the public health aspects of chemicals in air, water, food, drugs, and other parts of the environment. Traditionally, toxicologists have been intimately involved in the discovery and development of new drugs and pesticides. Toxicologists also participate in the development of standards and regulations designed to protect human health and the environment from the adverse effects of chemicals. Environmental toxicologists (a relatively new subset of the discipline) have expanded toxicology to study the effects of chemicals in flora and fauna. In all branches of toxicology, scientists explore the mechanisms by which chemicals produce adverse effects in biologic systems. Clinical toxicologists develop antidotes and treatment regimes for ameliorating poisonings and xenobiotic injury. Toxicologists carry out some or all of these activities as members of academic, industrial, and governmental organizations. In doing so, they share common methodologies for obtaining data on the toxicity of materials and the responsibility for using this information to make reasonable predictions regarding the hazards of the material to people and to their environment. These different but complementary activities characterize the discipline of toxicology.

Toxicology, like medicine, is both a science and an art. The science of toxicology is defined as the observational and data-gathering phase, whereas the art of toxicology is the predictive phase of the discipline. In most cases, these phases are linked since the "facts" generated by the science of toxicology are used to develop the extrapolations and hypotheses for the adverse effects of chemical agents in situations where there is little or no information. For example, the observation that administration of 2,3,7,8-tetrachlorodibenzo-*p*-dioxin (TCDD) to female (Sprague Dawley) rats induces hepatocellular carcinoma is fact. However, the conclusion that it will also do so in man is a prediction or hypothesis.

It is important to distinguish the facts from the predictions. When we fail to distinguish the science from the art, we confuse facts with predictions and argue that they have equal validity, which they clearly do not. In toxicology, as in all sciences, theories have a higher level of certainty than hypotheses, which in turn are more certain than speculations, opinions, conjectures, and guesses.

Some insight into modern toxicology and the roles, points of view, and activities of the toxicologist can be obtained by an examination of the historic evolution of the discipline.

HISTORY OF TOXICOLOGY

Antiquity

Toxicology dates to earliest man, who used animal venoms and plant extracts for hunting, waging war, and assassinations. The Ebers papyrus (circa 1500 B.C.) contains information pertaining to many recognized poisons: hemlock (the state poison of the Greeks); aconite (a Chinese arrow poison); opium (used as both poison and antidote); and such metals as lead, copper, and antimony. There is also an indication that plants containing substances akin to digitalis and belladonna alkaloids were known. Hippocrates (circa 400 B.C.) added a number of poisons and clinical toxicology principles pertaining to bioavailability in therapy and overdosage.

In the literature of ancient Greece, there are several references to poisons and their use. Theophrastus (370–286 B.C.), a student of Aristotle, included numerous references to poisonous plants in *De Historia Plantarum*. Dioscorides, a Greek physician in the court of Emperor Nero, made the first attempt at a classification of poisons, which was accompanied by descriptions and drawings. His separation into plant, animal, and mineral poisons not only remained a standard for 16 centuries but is still a convenient classification today (*see* Gunther, 1934). Dioscorides also dabbled in therapy, recognizing the use of emetics in poisoning and the use of caustic agents or cupping glasses in snakebite.

Poisoning with plant and animal toxins was quite common. Perhaps the best-known recipient of a poison used as a state method of execution was Socrates (470–399 B.C.). Expeditious suicide on a voluntary basis also made use of toxicologic knowledge. Demosthenes (385–322 B.C.), who took poison hidden in his pen, was only one of many examples. The mode of suicide calling for one to fall on his sword, although manly and noble, carried little appeal and less significance for ladies of the day. Cleopatra's (69–30 B.C.) knowledge of natural, primitive toxicology permitted her the more genteel method of falling on her asp instead.

The Romans, too, made considerable use of poisons in politics. One legend tells of King Mithridates VI of Pontus whose numerous acute toxicity experiments on unfortunate criminals led to his eventual claim that he had discovered "an antidote for every venomous reptile and every poisonous substance" (Guthrie, 1946). He himself was so fearful of poisons that he regularly ingested a mixture of 36 ingredients (Galen reports 54) as protection against assassination. On the occasion of his imminent capture by enemies, his attempts to kill himself with poison failed because of his successful concoction, and he was forced to use his own sword held by a servant. From this tale comes the term "mithridatic," referring to an antidotal or protective mixture. The term "theriac" also has become synonymous with "antidote," although the word

comes from the poetic treatise "Theriaca" by Nicander of Colophon (204–135 B.C.), which dealt with poisonous animals; his poem "Alexipharmaca" was about antidotes.

Poisonings in Rome took on epidemic proportions during the fourth century B.C. (Livy). It was during this period that a conspiracy of women to remove the men from whose death they might profit was uncovered. Similar large-scale poisoning continued until Sulla issued the *Lex Cornelia* (circa 82 B.C.). This appears to be the first law against poisoning, and it later became a regulatory statute directed at careless dispensers of drugs.

Middle Ages

Come bitter pilot, now at once run on
The dashing rocks thy seasick weary bark!
Here's to my love! O true apothecary!
Thy drugs are quick. Thus with a kiss I die.
          Romeo and Juliet, act 5, sc. 3

Prior to the Renaissance, the writings of Maimonides (Moses ben Maimon, A.D. 1135–1204) presented a treatise on treatment of poisonings from insects, snakes, and mad dogs (*Poisons and Their Antidotes,* 1198). He, like Hippocrates before him, wrote on the subject of bioavailability, noting that milk, butter, and cream could delay gut absorption. Maimonides also refuted many of the popular remedies of the day and stated his doubts about others.

From the early Renaissance, the Italians, with characteristic pragmatism, brought the art of poisoning to its zenith. The poisoner became an integral part of the political scene. The records of the city councils of Florence, and particularly the infamous Council of Ten of Venice, contain ample testimony of the political use of poisons. Victims were named, prices set, contracts recorded, and when the deed was accomplished, payment made.

An infamous figure of the time was a lady named Toffana, who peddled specially prepared arsenic-containing cosmetics *(Agua Toffana)*. Accompanying the product were appropriate instructions for use. Toffana was succeeded by an imitator with organizational genius, a certain Hieronyma Spara, who provided a new fillip by directing her activity toward specific marital and monetary objectives. A local club was formed of young, wealthy, married women, which soon became a club of eligible young, wealthy widows, reminiscent of the matronly conspiracy of Rome centuries earlier.

Among the prominent families engaged in poisoning, the Borgias are the most notorious. However, many deaths that were attributed to poisoning are now recognized as having occurred from infectious diseases such as malaria. It appears true, however, that Alexander VI, his son Cesare, and Lucretia Borgia were quite active. The deft applications of poisons to men of stature in the Church swelled the holdings of the Papacy, which was the prime heir.

A paragon of the distaff set of the period was Catherine de Medici. She exported her skills from Italy to France, where the prime targets of the ladies were their husbands. However, unlike others of an earlier period, the circle represented by Catherine (and epitomized by the notorious Marchioness de Brinvillers) depended on developing direct evidence to arrive at the most effective compounds for their purposes. Under guise of delivering provender to the sick and the poor, Catherine tested toxic concoctions, carefully noting the rapidity of the toxic response (onset of action), the effectiveness of the compound (potency), the degree of response of the parts of the body (specificity, site of action), and the complaints of the victim (clinical signs and symptoms).

Culmination of the practice in France is represented by the commercialization of the service by Catherine Deshayes, who earned thc title *La Voisine*. Her business was dissolved by her execution. Her trial was one of the most famous of those held by the Chambre Ardente, a special judicial commission established by Louis XIV to try such cases without regard to age, sex, or national origin. La Voisine was convicted of many poisonings, including over 2000 infants among the victims.

Age of Enlightenment

> All substances are poisons; there is none which is not a poison. The right dose differentiates a poison from a remedy.
>
> *Paracelsus*

A significant figure in the history of science and medicine in the late Middle Ages was the renaissance man Philippus Aureolus Theophrastus Bombastus von Hohenheim-Paracelsus (1493–1541). Between the time of Aristotle and the age of Paracelsus, there was little substantial change in the biomedical sciences. In the sixteenth century, the revolt against the authority of the Church was accompanied by a parallel attack on the godlike authority exercised by the followers of Hippocrates and Galen. Paracelsus, personally and professionally, embodied the qualities that forced numerous changes in this period. He and his age were pivotal, standing between the philosophy and magic of classic antiquity and the philosophy and science willed to us by figures of the seventeenth and eighteenth centuries. Clearly, one can identify in Paracelsus's

approach, his point of view, and his breadth of interest numerous similarities to the discipline we now call toxicology.

Paracelsus formulated many then-revolutionary views that remain an integral part of the present structure of toxicology. He promoted a focus on the "toxicon," the toxic agent, as a chemical entity. A view initiated by Paracelsus that became a lasting contribution held, as corollaries, that (1) experimentation is essential in examination of responses to chemicals; (2) one should make a distinction between therapeutic and toxic properties of chemicals: (3) these properties are sometimes, but not always, indistinguishable except by dose; and (4) one can ascertain a degree of specificity of chemicals and their therapeutic or toxic effects. The latter view presaged the "magic bullet" of Paul Ehrlich and the introduction of the therapeutic index. Further, in a very real sense, this was the first sound articulation of the dose-response relation, which is a bulwark of toxicology (Pachter, 1961).

The tradition of the poisoners spread throughout Europe, and their deeds played a major role in the distribution of political power through the Middle Ages. Pharmacology, as we know it today, had its beginning during the Middle Ages and early Renaissance. Concurrently, the study of the toxicity and the dose-response relationship of therapeutic agents was commencing (Paracelsus, 1493–1541). The developments of thc Industrial Revolution stimulated a rise in occupational diseases and, from these, Percival Pott's (1775) recognition of the role of xenobiotics in human disease. It should be noted that Paracelsus described Miners' disease approximately 240 years earlier in his treatise entitled *Bergsucht* (circa 1533–1534). These findings led to improved medical practices, but it was not until the nineteenth century and the classical works of Magendie (1783–1885), Orfila (1787–1853), and Bernard (1813–1878) that truly seminal research in experimental toxicology was carried out.

Orfila, a Spanish physician in the French court, was the first toxicologist to use autopsy material and chemical analysis systematically as legal proof of poisonings. His introduction of this detailed type analysis survives today as the underpinning of forensic toxicology. Magendie, a physician and experimental physiologist, studied the mechanisms of action of emetine, strychnine, and "arrow poisons." His research into the absorption and distribution of these compounds in the body remains a classic in toxicology and pharmacology. One of Magendie's more famous students, Claude Bernard, continued the studies on arrow poisons but also added works on the mechanism of action of carbon monoxide. Bernard's treatise entitled *An Introduction to the Study of Experimental Medicine* (translated by Greene in 1949) is a classic in the development of toxicology. Many German scientists contributed greatly to the growth of toxicology in the late nineteenth and early twentieth centuries. Among the giants of the field are Oswald Schmeideberg (1838–1921) and Louis Lewin (1850–1929).

Modern Toxicology

Modern toxicology has evolved rapidly during the past 100 years, but the exponential growth of the discipline can be traced to the World War II era and the marked increase in the production of such organic molecules as drugs, pesticides, and industrial chemicals. The history of many sciences is an orderly transition based on the theory, hypothesis testing, and synthesis of new ideas. Toxicology, as a borrowing science, has,

on the other hand, developed in fits and starts. Toxicology calls on almost all the basic sciences to test its hypotheses. This fact, coupled with the health regulations that have driven toxicology research since 1900, has made the discipline exceptional in the history of science. The differentiation of toxicology as an art and a science, though arbitrary, permits the presentation of historical highlights along two major lines.

Modern toxicology can be viewed as a continuation of the development of the biological and physical sciences in the late nineteenth and twentieth centuries (Table 1–1). During the latter half of the nineteenth century, the world witnessed an explosion in science that produced the beginning of the modern era of medicine, synthetic chemistry, physics, and biology. Toxicology has drawn its strength and diversity from its proclivity to borrow. With the advent of anesthetics and disinfectants in the late 1850s and the

Table 1–1. SELECTION OF DEVELOPMENTS IN TOXICOLOGY

Development of Early Advances in Analytic Methods
  Marsh, 1836: development of method for arsenic analysis
  Reinsh, 1841: combined method for separation and analysis of As and Hg
  Fresenius, 1845: von Babo, 1847: development of screening method for general poisons
  Stas-Otto, 1851: extraction and separation of alkaloids
  Mitscherlich, 1855: detection and identification of phosphorus

Early Mechanistic Studies
  F. Magendie, 1809: study of "arrow poisons," mechanism of action of emetine and
    strychnine
  C. Bernard, 1850: carbon monoxide combination with hemoglobin, study of mechanism
    of action of strychnine, site of action of curare
  R. Bohm, ca. 1890: active anthelmintics from fern, action of croton oil catharsis,
    poisonous mushrooms

Introduction of New Toxicants, Antidotes
  R. A. Peters, L. A. Stocken, and R. H. S. Thompson, 1945: development of British Anti
    Lewisite (BAL) as a relatively specific antidote for arsenic, toxicity of monofluoro-
    carbon compounds
  K. K. Chen, 1934: introduction of modern antidotes (nitrite and thiosulfate) for cyanide
    toxicity
  C. Voegtlin, 1923: mechanism of action of As and other metals on the SH groups
  P. Müller, 1944–1946: introduction and study of DDT (dichlorodiphenyltrichloroethane)
    and related insecticide compounds
  G. Schrader, 1952: introduction and study of organophosphorus compounds
  R. N. Chopra, 1933: indigenous drugs of India

Miscellaneous Toxicologic Studies
  R. T. Williams: study of detoxication mechanisms and species variation
  A. Rothstein: effects of uranium ion on cell membrane transport
  R. A. Kehoe: investigation of acute and chronic effects of lead
  A. Vorwald: studies of chronic respiratory disease (beryllium)
  H. Hardy: community and industrial poisoning (beryllium)
  A. Hamilton: introduction of modern industrial toxicology
  H. C. Hodge: toxicology of uranium, fluorides; standards of toxicity
  A. Hoffman: introduction of lysergic acid and derivatives; psychotomimetics
  R. A. Peters: biochemical lesions, lethal synthesis
  A. E. Garrod: inborn errors of metabolism
  T. T. Litchfield and F. Wilcoxon: simplified dose-response evaluation
  C. J. Bliss: method of probits, calculation of dosage-mortality curves

advancement of experimental pharmacology during the same period, toxicology, as currently understood, got its start. The introduction of ether, chloroform, and carbonic acid led to several iatrogenic deaths. These unfortunate outcomes spurred research into the causes of the deaths and also into early experiments on the physiological mechanisms by which the compounds caused both their beneficial and adverse effects. By the late nineteenth century, the use of organic chemicals was becoming more widespread, and benzene, toluene, and the xylenes went into larger-scale commercial production. During this same time period, the use of "patent" medicines was prevalent, and there were several incidents of poisonings from these medicaments. The adverse reactions to the patent medicines, coupled with the responses to Upton Sinclair's exposé of the meat-packing industry in his book *The Jungle,* culminated in the passage of the Wiley Bill (1906), the first of many U.S. pure food and drug laws (*see* Hutt and Hutt, 1984, for regulatory history).

A working hypothesis about the development of toxicology is that the discipline expands in response to legislation, which itself is a response to a real or perceived tragedy. The Wiley Bill was the first such reaction. A corollary to this hypothesis might be that the founding of scientific journals and/or societies also is sparked by legislation.

During the 1890s and early 1900s, the French scientists Becquerel and the Curies were to report on the discovery of "radioactivity." This opened up for exploration a very large area in physics, biology, and medicine, but it would not actively affect the science of toxicology for another 40 years. However, another discovery, that of vitamins or "vital amines," was to lead to the use of the first large-scale bioassays (multiple animal studies) to determine if these "new" chemicals were beneficial or harmful to laboratory animals. The initial work in this area took place around the time of World War I in the laboratory of Philip B. Hawk in Philadelphia. Hawk and a young associate, Bernard L. Oser, were responsible for the development and verification of many of the early toxicological assays, which in a slightly amended form are currently used. Oser's contributions to food and regulatory toxicology have been extraordinary. These early bioassays were possible because of a major advancement in toxicology—the availability of developed and refined strains of inbred laboratory rodents (*see* Donaldson, 1912).

The 1920s saw many events that began to mold the fledgling field of toxicology. The use of arsenicals for the treatment of such diseases as syphilis (arsenicals had been used in agriculture since the mid-nineteenth century) resulted in acute and chronic toxicity. Prohibition of alcoholic beverages in the United States opened the door for the early studies of neurotoxicology with the discoveries that triorthocresyl phosphate (TOCP), methanol, and lead (all products of "bootleg" liquor) were all neurotoxicants. TOCP, which is a modern gasoline additive, caused a syndrome that became known as "Ginger-Jake" walk, a spastic gait resulting from drinking adulterated ginger beer. Müller's discovery of dichlorodiphenyltrichloroethane (DDT) and several other organohalides during the late 1920s resulted in wider use of insecticidal agents. Other scientists were hard at work attempting to elucidate the structures of the estrogens and androgens. Work on the steroid hormones led to the use of several assays for the determination of biological activity of organ extracts and synthetic compounds. The efforts to synthesize steroidallike chemicals were spearheaded by E. C. Dodds and his coworkers, one of whom was a young organic chemist named Leon Golberg. Dodds's work on the bioactivity of the estrogenic compounds resulted in the synthesis of diethylstilbestrol (DES) and the discovery of the strong estrogenic activity of substituted stilbenes. Golberg's intimate involvement in this work stimulated his interest in biology, leading to degrees in biochemistry and medicine and a career in toxicology in which he oversaw the creation of the laboratories of the British Industrial Biological Research Association (BIBRA) and the Chemical Industry Institute of Toxicology (CIIT). Interestingly, the initial observations that led to the discovery of DES were the findings of feminization of animals treated with the experimental carcinogen 7,12-dimethylbenz[a]anthracene (DMBA).

The 1930s saw the world preparing for World War II and also a major effort by the pharmaceutical industry in Germany and the United States to manufacture the first mass-produced antibiotics. The first journal expressly dedicated to experimental toxicology, *Archiv für Toxikologie,* started publication in Europe in 1930, and Herbert Hoover signed the act that established the National Institutes of Health (NIH). The discovery of sulfanilamide had been heralded as a major event in combating bacterial diseases. However, for a drug to be effective, there must be a reasonable delivery system, and sulfanilamide is highly insoluble in an aqueous medium. Therefore, it was originally prepared in ethanol (elixir). But it was soon discovered that the drug was more soluble in ethylene glycol, which is a dihydroxy rather than a monohydroxy ethane. The drug was sold in the glycol solutions but labeled as an elixir, and several patients died of acute kidney failure resulting from the metabolism of the glycol to oxalic and glycolic acid and the acids crystallizing in the kidney tubules. This tragic event led to the passage of the Copeland Bill in 1938, the second major bill involving the formation of the U.S. Food and Drug Administration (FDA). The sulfanilamide disaster played a critical role in the further development of toxicology. It resulted in work by Eugene Maximillian Geiling in Chicago that elucidated the mechanism of toxicity of this chemical. The group of scientists associated with Geiling were to become the leaders of modern toxicology for the next 40 years. With few exceptions, toxicology in this country owes its immediate heritage to Geiling's innovativeness and ability to stimulate and direct young scientists. Because of his reputation, the U.S. government turned to this group for help in the war effort. There were three main areas in which the Chicago group took part during World War II: the toxicology and pharmacology of organophosphate chemicals, antimalarial drugs, and radionuclides. Each of these areas produced teams of toxicologists who became academic, governmental, and industrial leaders in the field. It was also during this time that DDT and the phenoxy herbicides were being developed for increased food production and, in the case of DDT, for control of insect-borne diseases. All these efforts between 1940 and 1946 led to an explosion in toxicology. Thus, in line with the hypothesis advanced above, the crisis of World War II caused the next major leap in the development of toxicology.

If one traces the history of the toxicity of metals over the past 40 years, the role of the Chicago group is quite visible. This engaging story commences with the use of uranium for the "bomb" and continues today with research on the role of metals in their interactions with deoxyribonucleic acid (DNA). Indeed, the "Manhattan Project" created a fertile environment resulting in the initiation of quantitative biology, radiotracer technology, and inhalation toxicology. These innovations have revolutionized modern biology, chemistry, therapeutics, and toxicology. Inhalation toxicology began at the University of Rochester under the direction of Stafford Warren, who headed the Department of Radiology. He developed a program with such colleagues as Harold Hodge (pharmacologist), Herb Stokinger (chemist), Sid Laskin (inhalation toxicologist), and Lou and George Casarett. These young scientists were to go on to become giants in the field.

The other sites for the study of radionuclides were Chicago, for the "internal" effects of radioactivity, and Oak Ridge, Tennessee, for the effects of "external" radiation. The work of scientists on these teams gave the scientific community the data for the early understanding of macromolecular binding of xenobiotics, cellular mutational events, methods for inhalation toxicology and therapy, toxicologic properties of trace metals, and a better appreciation for the complexities of the dose-response curve.

Another seminal event occurring at the same time was the discovery of organophosphate cholinesterase inhibitors. This class of chemicals, discovered by Willy Lange and Gerhard Schrader, was destined to become a driving force in the study of neurophysiology and toxicology for several decades. Again, the scientists in Chicago played major roles in elucidating the mechanisms of action of this new class of compounds. Geiling's group, and Kenneth Dubois in particular, were leaders in this area of toxicology and pharmacology. Dubois's students and their students are still in the forefront of this special area. The importance of the early research on the organophosphates takes on special meaning in later years (after 1960) when these compounds were destined to replace DDT and the organochlorines as insecticides of choice.

Early in the twentieth century, it was demonstrated that quinine had a marked effect on the malaria parasite. This discovery led to the development of quinine derivatives for the treatment of the disease and to the formulation of the early principles of chemotherapy. The pharmacology department at Chicago was charged with the development of antimalarials for the war effort. The original protocols called for testing of efficacy and toxicity in rodents and perhaps dogs, then to go directly to testing of efficacy in human volunteers. One of the investigators charged with generating the data to move a candidate drug from animals to humans was Fredrick Coulston. This young parasitologist and his colleagues, working under Geiling, were to evaluate potential drugs in the animal models and then establish the human clinical trials. It was during these experiments that the use of nonhuman primates came into vogue for toxicology testing. It had been noted by Russian scientists that some antimalarial compounds caused retinopathies in humans but did not apparently have the same adverse effect in rodents or dogs. This finding led Coulston to add one more step in the development process—that of toxicity testing in Rhesus monkeys just prior to efficacy studies in people. This addition resulted in the prevention of blindness in untold numbers of volunteers and perhaps some of the troops in the field. It also led to the school of thought that nonhuman primates may be one of the better models for man and the establishment of monkey colonies for the study of toxicity. Coulston pioneered this area of toxicology and remains committed to it today.

One other area not traditionally thought of as toxicology but one that evolved during the 1940s as an exciting and innovative field is experimental pathology. This branch of experimental biology developed from the bioassays of the estrogens and the early experiments in chemical and radiation-induced carcinogenesis. It is from these early studies that the hypotheses on tumor promotion and cancer progression have evolved.

Toxicologists of today owe a great deal to the researchers of chemical carcinogenesis of the 1940s. Much of today's work can be traced to Elizabeth and James Miller at Wisconsin. This husband and wife team started under the mentorship of Professor Rusch, the director of the newly formed McArdle Laboratory for Cancer Research, and Professor Baumann. The seminal research of the Millers led to the discovery of the role of reactive intermediates in carcinogenicity and to the discovery of mixed-function oxidases in the endoplasmic reticulum. These findings, which initiated the great works on the cytochrome P-450 family of proteins, were aided by two other major discoveries for which toxicologists (and all other biological scientists) are deeply indebted: paper chromatography in 1944 and the first use of radiolabeled dibenzanthracene in 1948. Other major events of note in drug metabolism included the work of Bernard Brodie on the metabolism of methyl orange (1947). This piece of seminal research led to the examination of blood and urine for chemical and drug metabolites. It became the tool by which one could study the relationship between blood levels and biological action. The classic treatise of R. T. Williams entitled *Detoxication Mechanisms* was first published in 1947. This text described the many pathways and possible mechanisms of detoxication and opened the field to several new areas of study.

The decade after World War II was not quiescent but certainly was not as boisterous as the period from 1935 to 1945. The first pesticide act was signed into law in 1947. The significance of the initial Federal Insecticide, Fungicide, and Rodenticide Act was that for the first time in U.S. history a substance that was neither drug nor food had to be shown as safe and efficacious. This decade, which coincided with the Eisenhower years, saw the dispersion of the groups from Chicago, Rochester, and Oak Ridge and the establishment of new centers of research and excellence. Adrian Albert's classic work *Selective Toxicity* was first published in 1951. This treatise, which has appeared in several editions, presented a concise documentation of the principles of site-specific action of chemicals.

Post World War II

You too can be a toxicologist
in two easy lessons, each of ten years.
Arnold Lehman (circa 1955)

The mid-1950s witnessed the strengthening of the U.S. Food and Drug Administration's commitment to toxicology under the guidance of another giant in the field, Arnold Lehman. Lehman's tutelage and influence are still felt today. The adage "You too can be a toxicologist" is as important a summation of toxicology as the oft-quoted statement of Paracelsus: "The dose makes the poison." The period from 1955 to 1958 produced two major events that would have long-lasting impacts on toxicology as a science and as a professional discipline. Lehman, Fitzhugh, and their coworkers formalized the experimental program for the appraisal of food, drug, and cosmetic safety, 1955; updated by the U.S. FDA in 1982, and the Gordon Research Conferences saw fit to establish a conference on Toxicology and Safety Evaluation, with Bernard L. Oser as its initial chairman. These two events led to close relationships among toxicologists from several groups and brought the field to its gestational phase. At about the same time, the U.S. Congress passed, and the president signed, the Additives Amendments to the Food, Drug, and Cosmetic Act. The Delaney clause of these amendments stated broadly that any chemical found to be carcinogenic in laboratory animals or humans could not be added to the U.S. food supply. The impact of this legislation cannot be overstated. Delaney became a battlecry for many groups, and it resulted in the inclusion, at a new level, of biostatisticians and mathematical modelers in the field of toxicology. It fostered the expansion of quantitative methods in toxicology and led to innumerable arguments about the "one-hit" theory of carcinogenesis. Regardless of one's view of Delaney, it has served as an excellent starting point in helping to understand the complexity of such a biological phenomenon as carcinogenicity and in the development of risk assessment models. One must remember that at the time of Delaney, the analytical detection level for most chemicals was 20 to 100 ppm (today, parts per quadrillion). Interestingly, the Delaney clause has only been invoked on a few occasions, and it has been stated that Congress added little to the food and drug law with this clause (*see* Hutt and Hutt, 1984).

Shortly after the Delaney amendment, and after three successful Gordon Conferences, the first American journal dedicated to toxicology was launched by Coulston, Lehman, and Hayes. *Toxicology and Applied Pharmacology* has been the flagship journal of toxicology ever since. The founding of the Society of Toxicology followed shortly thereafter, and the journal became its official publication. The society's founding members were: Fredrick Coulston, William Deichmann, Kenneth DuBois, Victor Drill, Harry Hayes, Harold Hodge, Paul Larson, Arnold Lehman, and C. Boyd Shaffer. These learned gentlemen deserve a great deal of credit for the growth of toxicology. DuBois and Geiling published their *Textbook of Toxicology* in 1959.

The 1960s were tumultuous times for society, and toxicology found itself swept up in the tide. Starting with the tragic thalidomide incident, in which several thousand children were born with serious birth defects, and the publishing of Rachel Carson's *Silent Spring* (1962), the field of toxicology developed at a feverish pitch. Attempts to understand the effects of chemicals on the embryo and fetus, and on the environment as a whole, gained momentum. New legislation was passed, and new journals were founded. The education of toxicologists spread from the deep traditions at Chicago and Rochester to Harvard, Miami, Albany, Iowa, Jefferson, and beyond. Many new fields were influencing and being assimilated into the broad scope of toxicology: environmental sciences, aquatic and avian biology, cell biology, analytical chemistry, and genetics.

During the 1960s, particularly the latter half of the decade, the analytical tools used in toxicology were developed to a level of sophistication that allowed detection of chemicals in tissues and other substrates at part per billion concentrations (today, part per quadrillion may be detected). The pioneering work of Bruce Ames (1983) in the development of point mutation assays that were replicable, quick, and inexpensive led to a better understanding of the genetic mechanisms of carcinogenicity. The combined work of Ames and the Millers (Elizabeth C. and James A.) at McArdle Laboratory allowed the toxicology community to make major contributions to the understanding of the carcinogenic process.

These levels of detection created several problems and opportunities for toxicologists and risk assessors that stemmed from interpretation of the Delaney amendment. This same period saw the growth and diversification of the science of toxicology and society. The establishment of the National Center for Toxicologic Research (NCTR), the expansion of the role of the U.S. Food and Drug Administration, and the establishment of the U.S. Environmental Protection Agency (EPA) and the National Institute of Environmental Health Sciences (NIEHS) all were considered as clear messages that the government had taken a strong interest in toxicology. Several new journals appeared during the 1960s, and new legislation was written quickly after *Silent Spring* and thalidomide. The end of the decade witnessed the "discovery" of TCDD as a contaminant in the herbicide Agent Orange. The research on the toxicity of this compound has produced some very good and some very poor research in the field of toxicology. The discovery of a high-affinity cellular binding protein (designated the *Ah* receptor) by A. Poland at McArdle and work on the genetics of the receptor by D. Nebert (*see* Nebert and Gonzalez, 1987) at NIH have revolutionized the field of toxicology. The importance of TCDD to toxicology is that it forced researchers, regulators, and the legal community, in a broad sense, to look at the role of mechanisms of toxic action in a fashion much differently than before.

At least one other event precipitated a great deal of legislation during the 1970s: Love Canal. The "discovery" of Love Canal led to major concerns regarding hazardous wastes, chemical dump sites, and disclosure of information regarding these sites. Soon after Love Canal, the EPA listed several equally contaminated sites in the United States, and the agency was given the responsibility to develop risk assessments for exposure to the effluents and to attempt to remediate these sites. These combined efforts supported ongoing research into mechanisms of action of chemicals in the body. Love Canal and similar issues created the legislative environment leading to the Toxic Substances Control Act and eventually to the Superfund bill. These omnibus bills were created to cover the toxicology of chemicals from initial synthesis to disposal.

The expansion of legislation, journals, and new societies involved with toxicology was exponential during the 1970s and 1980s and shows no signs of slowing down in the 1990s. Currently, in the United States there are dozens of professional, governmental, and other scientific organizations with thousands of members and over 120 journals dedicated to toxicology and related disciplines.

The history of toxicology has been interesting and varied but never dull. Perhaps as a borrowing science, it has suffered from an absence of a single goal, but its diversification has allowed for the interspersion of ideas and concepts from academe, industry, and government. As an example of this diversification, one now finds toxicology graduate programs in medical schools and schools of public health and pharmacy, as well as programs in environmental science and undergraduate programs in toxicology at several institutions. Surprisingly, courses in toxicology are now being offered in several liberal arts undergraduate schools as part of biology and chemistry curricula. This complex mixture has resulted in an exciting, innovative, and diversified field that is serving science and the community at large. Few disciplines can point to both basic sciences and direct application at the same time. Toxicology, the study of the adverse effects of xenobiotics, is unique in this regard.

REFERENCES

Albert, A.: *Selective Toxicity*. Methuen & Co., London, 1951.

Ames, B. N.: Dietary carcinogens and anticarcinogens. *Scence*, **221**:1249–1264, 1983.

Bernard, C.: Action du curare et de la nicotine sur le système nerveux et sur le système musculaire. *C. R. Séances Soc. Biol.*, **2**:195, 1850.

———: *An Introduction to the Study of Experimental Medicine*, translated by H. C. Greene, H. Schuman, New York, 1949.

Carson, R.: *Silent Spring*. Houghton Mifflin, Boston, 1962.

Christison, R.: *A Treatise on Poisons*, 4th ed. Barrington & Howell, Philadelphia, 1845.

Doll, R., and Peto, R.: *The Causes of Cancer*. Oxford University Press, New York, 1981.

Donaldson, H. H.: *J. Acad. Natl. Sci. Phila.*, **15**:365, 1912.

DuBois, K., and Geiling, E. M. K.: *Textbook of Toxicology*. Oxford University Press, New York, 1959.

Gunther, R. T.: *The Greek Herbal of Dioscorides*. Oxford University Press, New York, 1934.

Guthrie, D. A.: *A History of Medicine*. J. B. Lippincott Co., Philadelphia, 1946.

Handler, P.: Some comments on risk assessment. In *The National Research Council in 1979: Current Issues and Studies*. NAS, Washington, D. C., 1979.

Hutt, P. B., and Hutt, P. B. II: A history of government regulation of adulteration and misbranding of food. *Food Drug Cosmetic J.*, **39**:2–73, 1984.

Levey, M.: Medieval arabic toxicology. The book on poisons of Ibn Wahshiya and its relation to early Indian and Greek texts. *Trans. Am. Philos. Soc.*, **56**:Part 7, 1966.

Lewin, L.: *Die Gifte in der Weltgeschichte. Toxikologische, allgemeinverständliche Untersuchungen der historischen Quellen*. Springer, Berlin, 1920.

———: *Gifte und Vergiftungen*. Stilke, Berlin, 1929.

Loomis, T. A.: *Essentials of Toxicology*, 3rd ed. Lea & Febiger, Philadelphia, 1978.

Macht, D. J.: Louis Lewin: pharmacologist, toxicologist, medical historian. *Ann. Med. Hist.*, **3**:179–194, 1931.

Meek, W. J.: *The Gentle Art of Poisoning*. Medico-Historical Papers. University of Wisconsin, Madison, 1954; reprinted from *Phi Beta Pi Quarterly*, May 1928.

Müller, P.: Über zusammenhange zwischen Konstitution und insektizider Wirkung. I. *Helv. Chim. Acta*, **29**:1560–1580, 1946.

Munter, S. (ed.).: *Treatise on Poisons and Their Antidotes*. Vol. II of the *Medical Writings of Moses Maimonides*. J. B. Lippincott Co., Philadelphia, 1966.

Nebert, D., and Gonzalez, F. J.: P450 genes: structure, evolution and regulation. *Annu. Rev. Biochem*, **56**:945–993, 1987.

Olmsted, J. M. D.: *François Magendie. Pioneer in Experimental Physiology and Scientific Medicine in XIX Century France*. Schuman, New York, 1944.

Orfila, M. J. B.: *Traité des Poisons Tirés des Règnes Minéral, Végétal et Animal, ou, Toxicologie Générale Considérée sous les Rapports de la Physiologie, de la Pathologie et de la Médecine Légale*. Crochard, Paris, 1814–1815.

———: *Secours à Donner aux Personnes Empoisonées et Asphyxiées*. Feugeroy, Paris, 1818.

Pachter, H. M.: *Paracelsus: Magic into Science*. Collier Books, New York, 1961.

Pagel, W.: *Paracelsus: An Introduction to Philosophical Medicine in the Era of the Renaissance*. S. Karger, New York, 1958.

Paracelsus (Theophrastus ex Hohenheim Eremita): *Von der Besucht*. Dillingen, 1567.

Poland, A., and Knutson, J. C.: 2,3,7,8-Tetrachlorodibenzo-p-dioxin and related halogenated aromatic hydrocarbons, examination of the mechanism of toxicity. *Annu. Rev. Pharmacol. Toxicol.*, **22**:517–554, 1982.

Ramazzini, B.: *De Morbis Artificum Diatriba*. Modena, 1700.

Robert, R.: *Lehrbuch der Intoxikationen*. Enke, Stuttgart, 1893.

Schmiedeberg, O., and Koppe, R.: *Das Muscarin das giftige Alkaloid des Fliegenpilzes*. Vogel, Leipzig, 1869.

Thompson, C. J. S.: *Poisons and Poisoners. With Historical Accounts of Some Famous Mysteries in Ancient and Modern Times*. H. Shaylor, London, 1931.

U.S. FDA: *Toxicologic Principles for the Safety Assessment of Direct Food Additives and Color Additives Used in Food*. U.S. Food and Drug Administration, Bureau of Foods, Washington, D.C., 1982.

Voegtlin, C.; Dyer, H. A.; and Leonard, C. S.: On the mechanism of the action of arsenic upon protoplasm. *Public Health Rep.*, **38**:1882–1912, 1923.

Willams, R. T.: *Detoxication Mechanisms*, 2nd ed. Wiley & Sons, Inc., New York, 1959.

Supplemental Reading

Adams, F. (trans.): *The Genuine Works of Hippocrates*. Williams & Wilkins Co., Baltimore, 1939.

Beeson, B. B.: Orfila—pioneer toxicologist. *Ann. Med. Hist.* **2**:68–70, 1930.

Bernard, C.: Analyse physiologique des propriétés des systèmes musculaire et nerveux au moyen du curare. *C. R. Acad. Sci. (Paris)*, **43**:325–329, 1856.

Bryan, C. P.: *The Papyrus Ebers*. Geoffrey Bales, London, 1930.

Clendening, L.: *Source Book of Medical History*. Dover, New York, 1942.

Gaddum, J. H.: *Pharmacology*, 5th ed. Oxford University Press, New York, 1959.

Garrison, F. H.: *An Introduction to the History of Medicine*, 4th ed. W. B. Saunders Co., Philadelphia, 1929.

Hamilton, A.: *Exploring the Dangerous Trades*. Little, Brown & Co., Boston, 1943. (Reprinted by Northeastern University Press, Boston, 1985.)

Hays, H. W.: *Society of Toxicology History*, 1961–1986. Society of Toxicology, Washington, D.C., 1986.

Holmstedt, B., and Liljestrand, G.: *Readings in Pharmacology*. Raven Press, New York, 1981.

Chapter 2

PRINCIPLES OF TOXICOLOGY

Curtis D. Klaassen and *David L. Eaton*

INTRODUCTION TO TOXICOLOGY

Toxicology is the study of the adverse effects of chemicals on living organisms. The *toxicologist* is specially trained to examine the nature of these adverse effects (including their cellular, biochemical, and molecular mechanisms of action) and to assess the probability of their occurrence. The variety of potential adverse effects and the diversity of chemicals present in our environment combine to make toxicology a very broad science. Therefore, toxicologists are usually specialized to work in one area of toxicology.

Different Areas of Toxicology

The professional activities of toxicologists fall into three main categories: descriptive, mechanistic, and regulatory. The *descriptive toxicologist* is concerned directly with toxicity testing, which provides necessary information for safety evaluation and regulatory requirements. The appropriate toxicity tests (as described later in this chapter) in experimental animals are designed to yield information that can be used to evaluate the risk posed to humans and the environment by exposure to specific chemicals. The concern may be limited to effects on humans, as in the case of drugs or food additives. Toxicologists in the chemical industry, however, must be concerned not only with risk posed by the company's chemicals (insecticides, herbicides, solvents, etc.) to humans but also with potential effects on fish, birds, plants, and other factors that might disturb the balance of the ecosystem.

The *mechanistic toxicologist* is concerned with elucidating the mechanisms by which chemicals exert their toxic effects on living organisms. Results of these studies often lead to the development of sensitive predictive tests useful in risk assessment, design, and production of safer alternative chemicals and in rational therapy for chemical poisoning and treatment of diseases. In addition, an understanding of the mechanisms of toxic action contributes to the knowledge of basic physiology, pharmacology, cell biology, and biochemistry. For example, studies on the toxicity of fluoroorganic alcohols and acids contributed to the knowledge of basic carbohydrate and lipid metabolism; knowledge of regulation of ion gradients in nerve axonal membranes has been greatly aided by studies of natural and synthetic toxins such as tetrodotoxin and dichlorodiphenyltrichloroethane (DDT). Mechanistic toxicologists are active in universities, in research institutes supported by the government or by private sources, and in the pharmaceutical and chemical industries.

A *regulatory toxicologist* has the responsibility of deciding on the basis of data provided by the descriptive toxicologist if a drug or other chemical poses a sufficiently low risk to be marketed for a stated purpose. The Food and Drug Administration (FDA) is responsible for admitting drugs, cosmetics, and food additives onto the market according to the Federal Food, Drug and Cosmetic Act (FDCA). The Environmental Protection Agency (EPA) is responsible for regulating most other chemicals according to the Federal Insecticide, Fungicide and Rodenticide Act (FIFRA), the Toxic Substances Control Act (TSCA), the Resource Conservation and Recovery Act (RCRA), the Safe Drinking Water Act, and the Clean Air Act. The EPA is also responsible for enforcing the Comprehensive Environmental Response, Compensation and Liability Act (CERCLA), more commonly called "Superfund." This regulation provides direction and financial support for the clean-up of waste sites that contain toxic chemicals and may present a risk to human health or the environment. The Occupational Safety and Health Administration (OSHA) of the Department of Labor was established to ensure that safe and healthful conditions exist in the workplace. The Consumer Product Safety Commission has the responsibility of protecting the consumer from hazardous household substances, whereas the Department of Transportation (DOT) ensures that materials shipped in interstate commerce are labeled and packaged in a manner consistent with the degree of hazard they present. Regulatory toxicologists are also involved in the establishment of standards for the amount of chemicals permitted in ambient air, in industrial atmospheres, or in drinking water. Some of the philosophic and legal aspects of regulatory toxicology are discussed in Chapter 30.

Three specialized areas of toxicology are forensic, clinical, and environmental toxicology. *Forensic toxicology* is a hybrid of analytic chemistry and fundamental toxicologic principles. It is concerned primarily with the medicolegal aspects of the harmful effects of chemicals on humans and animals. The expertise of the forensic toxicologist is primarily invoked to aid in establishing the cause of death and elucidating its circumstances in a postmortem investigation (*see* Chapter 27). *Clinical toxicology* designates an area of professional emphasis within the realm of medical science concerned with disease caused by, or uniquely associated with, toxic substances (*see* Chapter 28). Generally, clinical toxicologists are physicians who receive specialized training in emergency medicine and poison management. Efforts are directed at treating patients poisoned with drugs or other chemicals and at development of new techniques to treat these intoxications. *Environmental toxicology* focuses on the impacts of chemical pollutants found in the environment on biological organisms. Although toxicologists concerned with the effects of environmental pollutants on human health fit within this definition, it is most commonly associated with studies on the impacts of chemicals on nonhuman organisms such as fish, birds, and other terrestrial animals. *Ecotoxicology* is a specialized area within environmental toxicology that focuses more specifically on the impacts of toxic substances on population dynamics within an ecosystem. The transport, fate, and interactions of chemicals in the environment constitute a critical component of both environmental toxicology and ecotoxicology.

Spectrum of Toxic Dose

One could define a *poison* as any agent capable of producing a deleterious response in a biologic system, seriously injuring function or producing death. This is not, however, a useful working definition for the very simple reason that virtually every known chemical has the potential to produce injury or death if present in a sufficient amount. Paracelsus (1493–1541) phrased this well when he noted, "All substances are poisons; there is none which is not a poison. The right dose differentiates a poison and a remedy."

Among chemicals there is a wide spectrum of

Table 2–1. APPROXIMATE ACUTE LD50s OF SOME REPRESENTATIVE CHEMICAL AGENTS

agent	LD50 (mg/kg)*
Ethyl alcohol	10,000
Sodium chloride	4,000
Ferrous sulfate	1,500
Morphine sulfate	900
Phenobarbital sodium	150
Picrotoxin	5
Strychnine sulfate	2
Nicotine	1
d-Tubocurarine	0.5
Hemicholinium-3	0.2
Tetrodotoxin	0.10
Dioxin (TCDD)	0.001
Botulinum toxin	0.00001

* LD50 is the dosage (mg/kg body weight) causing death in 50 percent of the exposed animals.

doses needed to produce deleterious effects, serious injury, or death. This is demonstrated in Table 2–1, which shows the dosage of chemical needed to produce death in 50 percent of the treated animals (LD50). Some chemicals will produce death in microgram doses and are commonly thought of as being extremely poisonous. Other chemicals may be relatively harmless following doses in excess of several grams. It should be noted, however, that measures of acute lethality such as the LD50 may not accurately reflect the full spectrum of toxicity, or hazard, associated with exposure to a chemical. For example, some chemicals with low acute toxicity may have carcinogenic or teratogenic effects at doses that produce no evidence of acute toxicity.

CLASSIFICATION OF TOXIC AGENTS

Toxic agents are classified in a variety of ways, depending on the interests and needs of the classifier. In this textbook, for example, toxic agents are discussed in terms of their target organ (liver, kidney, hematopoietic system, etc.), their use (pesticide, solvent, food additive, etc.), their source (animal and plant toxins), and their effects (cancer, mutation, liver injury, etc.). Toxic agents may also be classified in terms of their physical state (gas, dust, liquid), their labeling requirements (explosive, flammable, oxidizer), their chemistry (aromatic amine, halogenated hydrocarbon, etc.), or their poisoning potential (extremely toxic, very toxic, slightly toxic, etc.). Classification of toxic agents on the basis of their biochemical mechanism of action (sulfhydryl inhibitor, methemoglobin producer) is usually more informative than classification by general terms such as irritants and corrosives, but the more general classifications such as air pollutants, occupation-related agents, and acute and chronic poisons can provide a useful focus on a specific problem. It is evident from the above that no single classification will be applicable for the entire spectrum of toxic agents and that combinations of classification systems or classification based on other factors may be needed to provide the best rating system for a special purpose. Nevertheless, classification systems that take into consideration both the chemical and biologic properties of the agent and the exposure characteristics are most likely to be useful for legislative or control purposes and for toxicology in general.

CHARACTERISTICS OF EXPOSURE

Adverse or toxic effects in a biologic system are not produced by a chemical agent unless that agent or its biotransformation products reach appropriate sites in the body at a concentration and for a length of time sufficient to produce the toxic manifestation. Whether or not a toxic response occurs is dependent, therefore, on the chemical and physical properties of the agent, the exposure situation, and the susceptibility of the biologic system or subject. Thus, to characterize fully the potential hazard of a specific chemical agent, we need to know not only what type of effect it produces and the dose required to produce the effect but also information about the agent, the exposure, and the subject. The major factors that influence toxicity as it relates to the exposure situation for a specific chemical are the route of administration and the duration and frequency of exposure.

Route and Site of Exposure

The major routes by which toxic agents gain access to the body are through the gastrointestinal tract (ingestion), lungs (inhalation), skin (topical, percutaneous, or dermal), and other parenteral (other than intestinal canal) routes. Toxic agents generally elicit the greatest effect and produce the most rapid response when given by the intravenous route. An approximate descending order of effectiveness for the other routes would be: inhalation, intraperitoneal, subcutaneous, intramuscular, intradermal, oral, and dermal. The vehicle and other formulation factors can markedly alter the absorption following ingestion, inhalation, or topical exposure. In addition, the route of administration can influence the toxicity of agents. For example, an agent that is detoxified in the liver would be expected to be less toxic when given via the portal circulation (oral) than when given via the systemic circulation (inhalation).

Industrial exposure to toxic agents most frequently is the result of inhalation and dermal exposure, whereas accidental and suicidal poisoning occurs most frequently by oral ingestion. Comparison of the lethal dose of an agent by different routes of exposure often provides useful information concerning the absorption of the agent. In instances when the lethal dose after oral or dermal administration is similar to the lethal dose for intravenous administration, the assumption is that the toxic agent is absorbed readily and rapidly. Conversely, in those cases where the lethal dose by the dermal route is several orders of magnitude higher than the oral lethal dose, it is likely that the skin provides an effective barrier to absorption of the agent. Toxic effects by any route of exposure can also be influenced by the concentration of the agent in its vehicle, the total volume of the vehicle and the properties of the vehicle to which the biologic system is exposed, and the rate at which exposure occurs. Studies in which the concentration of the chemical in the blood is determined at various times after exposure are often needed to clarify the role of these and other factors on the toxicity of a compound. For more details on the absorption of toxicants, see Chapter 3.

Duration and Frequency of Exposure

Toxicologists usually divide the exposure of animals to chemicals into four categories: acute, subacute, subchronic, and chronic. Acute exposure is defined as exposure to a chemical for less than 24 hours, and examples of exposure routes are intraperitoneal, intravenous, and subcutaneous injection, oral intubation, and dermal application. While acute exposure usually refers to a single administration, repeated exposures may be given within a 24-hour period for some slightly toxic or practically nontoxic chemicals. Acute exposure by inhalation refers to continuous exposure for less than 24 hours, most frequently for 4 hours. Repeated exposure is divided into three categories: subacute, subchronic, and chronic. Subacute exposure refers to repeated exposure to a chemical for one month or less, subchronic for one to three months, and chronic for more than three months. These three categories of repeated exposure can be by any route, but most often it is by the oral route, with the chemical added directly to the diet.

For many agents, the toxic effects following a single exposure are quite different from those produced by repeated exposure. For example, the primary acute toxic manifestation of benzene is central nervous system depression, but repeated exposures can result in leukemia. Acute exposure to agents that are rapidly absorbed is likely to produce immediate toxic effects, but acute exposure can also produce delayed toxicity that may or may not be similar to the toxic effects of chronic exposure. Conversely, chronic exposure to a toxic agent may produce some immediate (acute) effects after each administration, in addition to the long-term, low-level, or chronic effects of the agent. In characterizing the toxicity of a specific chemical agent, it is evident that information is needed not only for the single-dose (acute) and long-term (chronic) effects, but also for exposures of intermediate duration.

The other time-related factor that is important in the temporal characterization of exposure is the frequency of administration. The relationship between elimination rate and frequency of exposure is shown in Figure 2-1. A single dose of a chemical that produces severe effects may have no effect if the same total dose is given in several intervals. For the chemical depicted by line B in Figure 2-1, in which the half-life for elimination (time necessary for 50 percent of the chemical to be removed from the bloodstream) is approximately equal to the dosing frequency, a theoretical toxic concentration of 2 units is not reached until the fourth dose of administration, whereas that same concentration is reached with two dosing intervals for chemical A, which has an elimination rate much slower than the dosing frequency. Conversely, for chemical C where the elimination rate is much shorter than the dosing interval, a toxic concentration at the site of toxic effect will never be reached regardless of how many doses are administered. Of course,

it is possible that residual cell or tissue damage could be occurring with each dose, even though the chemical itself is not accumulating. The important consideration then is whether the interval between doses is sufficient to allow for complete repair of tissue damage. It is evident that with any type of multiple dose the production of a toxic effect is not only influenced by the frequency of administration but may, in fact, be totally dependent on frequency rather than duration of exposure. Chronic toxic effects may occur, therefore, if the chemical accumulates in the biologic system (absorption exceeds biotransformation and/or excretion), if it produces irreversible toxic effects, or if there is insufficient time for the system to recover from the toxic damage within the exposure frequency interval. For additional discussion of these relationships, the reader should consult Chapter 3.

SPECTRUM OF UNDESIRED EFFECTS

The spectrum of undesired effects of chemicals is broad. Some are deleterious and others are not. In therapeutics, for example, each drug produces a number of effects, but usually only one of these is associated with the primary objective of the therapy; all other effects are referred to as undesirable or side effects of that drug for that therapeutic indication. However, some of these side effects might be desired for another therapeutic indication. For example, dryness of the mouth is a side effect of atropine when used to decrease gastric secretion in the treatment of peptic ulcer but is the desired effect when used for preanesthetic medication. Some side effects of drugs are never desirable and are deleterious to the well-being of humans. These are referred to as the *adverse, deleterious,* or *toxic* effects of the drug.

Allergic Reactions

Chemical allergy is an immunologically mediated adverse reaction to a chemical resulting from previous sensitization to that chemical or to a structurally similar one. The term *hypersensitivity* is most often used to describe this allergic state, but *allergic reaction* and *sensitization reaction* are also used to describe this situation where preexposure of the chemical is required to produce the toxic effect (Goldstein *et al.,* 1974; Loomis, 1978). *Once sensitization has occurred,* allergic reactions *may result from exposure* to low doses of chemicals, and therefore population-based dose-response curves for allergic reactions have seldom been obtained. Because of this omission, some people have assumed that allergic reactions are not dose related. Thus, they have not considered the aller-

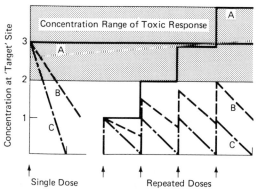

Figure 2-1. Diagrammatic view of the relationship between dose and concentration at the target site under different conditions of dose frequency and elimination rate. Line *A,* a chemical with very slow elimination (e.g., half-life of one year); *B,* a chemical with a rate of elimination equal to the frequency of dosing (e.g., one day); *C,* rate of elimination faster than the dosing frequency (e.g., five hours). *Shaded area* is representative of the concentration of chemical at the target site necessary to elicit a toxic response.

gic reaction to be a true toxic response. However, for a given allergic individual, allergic reactions are dose related. For example, it is well known that the allergic response to pollen in sensitized individuals is related to the concentration of pollen in the air. In addition, since the allergic response is an undesirable, adverse, deleterious effect, it obviously is also a toxic response. Sensitization reactions are sometimes very severe and may be fatal.

To produce an allergic reaction most chemicals or their metabolic products function immunologically as haptens and must combine with an endogenous protein to form an antigen (or immunogen). The antigen is then capable of eliciting the formation of antibodies, and usually at least one or two weeks are required for synthesis of significant amounts of antibodies. Subsequent exposure to the chemical will result in an antigen-antibody interaction, which provokes the typical manifestations of allergy. The manifestations of allergy are numerous. They involve various organ systems and range in severity from minor skin disturbance to fatal anaphylactic shock. The pattern of allergic response differs in various species. In humans, involvement of the skin (e.g., dermatitis, urticaria, and itching) and involvement of the eyes (e.g., conjunctivitis) are most common, whereas in guinea pigs bronchiolar constriction leading to asphyxia is common. Hypersensitivity reactions are discussed in more detail in Chapter 9.

Idiosyncratic Reactions

Chemical idiosyncrasy is a genetically determined abnormal reactivity to a chemical (Goldstein *et al.,* 1974; Levine, 1978). The response observed is usually qualitatively similar to that observed in all individuals but may take the form of extreme sensitivity to low doses or extreme insensitivity to high doses of the chemical. However, while some people use the term idiosyncratic as a catchall to refer to all reactions that occur with low frequency, it should not be used in this manner (Goldstein *et al.,* 1974).

An example of an idiosyncratic reaction is provided by patients who exhibit prolonged muscular relaxation and apnea, lasting several hours, after a standard dose of succinylcholine. Succinylcholine usually produces skeletal muscle relaxation of only a short duration because of its very rapid metabolic degradation by plasma pseudocholinesterase. Patients exhibiting this idiosyncratic reaction have an atypical pseudocholinesterase. Family pedigree studies have demonstrated that the presence of atypical cholinesterase is a genetically determined characteristic. Similarly, there is a group of people who

are abnormally sensitive to nitrites and other chemicals that produce methemoglobinemia. These individuals have a deficiency in NADH-methemoglobin reductase, which is inherited as an autosomal recessive trait.

Immediate versus Delayed Toxicity

Immediate toxicologic effects can be defined as those that occur or develop rapidly after a single administration of a substance, whereas delayed effects are those that occur after the lapse of some time. Carcinogenic effects of chemicals usually have a long latency period, often 20 to 30 years, before tumors are observed in humans. For example, the vaginal and uterine cancer produced by diethylstilbestrol in young women was due to their exposure *in utero* to diethylstilbestrol taken by their mothers to prevent miscarriages. Also, delayed neurotoxicity is observed after exposure to some organophosphorus anticholinesterase agents. The most notorious of the compounds that produce this type of neurotoxic effect is triorthocresylphosphate (TOCP). The effect is not observed until at least several days after exposure to the toxic compound. In contrast, most substances produce immediate toxic effects but fail to produce delayed effects.

Reversible versus Irreversible Toxic Effects

Some toxic effects of chemicals are reversible and others are irreversible. If a chemical produces pathologic injury to a tissue, the ability of the tissue to regenerate will largely determine whether the effect is reversible or irreversible. Thus, for a tissue such as liver, which has a high ability to regenerate, most injuries are reversible, whereas injury to the central nervous system is largely irreversible since differentiated cells of the central nervous system cannot divide and be replaced. Carcinogenic and teratogenic effects of chemicals, once they occur, are usually considered irreversible toxic effects.

Local versus Systemic Toxicity

Another distinction between types of effects is made on the general locus of action. Local effects refer to those that occur at the site of first contact between the biologic system and the toxicant. Local effects are produced by the ingestion of caustic substances or inhalation of irritant materials. The obverse of local effects is systemic effects that require absorption and distribution of the toxicant from its entry point to a distant site at which deleterious effects are produced. Most substances, except highly reactive materials, produce systemic effects. For some materials, both effects can be demonstrated. For example, tetraethyl lead produces effects on skin at the site of absorption and then is transported systemically to produce its typical effects on the central nervous system and other organs. If the local effect is marked, there may also be indirect systemic effects. For example, kidney damage following a severe acid burn is an indirect systemic effect because the toxicant does not reach the kidney.

Most chemicals that produce systemic toxicity do not cause a similar degree of toxicity in all organs but usually elicit the major toxicity in only one or two organs. These sites are referred to as the *target organs* of toxicity of a particular chemical. The target organ of toxicity is often not the site of highest concentration of the chemical. For example, lead is concentrated in bone, but its toxicity is due to the effects of lead in soft tissues. Likewise, DDT is concentrated in adipose tissue but produces no known toxic effects in this tissue.

The target organ of toxicity most frequently involved in systemic toxicity is the central nervous system. Even with many compounds having a prominent effect elsewhere, damage to the central nervous system, particularly the brain, can be demonstrated by the use of appropriate and sensitive methods. Next in order of frequency of involvement in systemic toxicity are the circulatory system; the blood and hematopoietic system; visceral organs, such as liver, kidney, and lung; and the skin. Muscle and bone are least often the target tissues for systemic effects. With substances having a predominantly local effect, the frequency with which tissues react depends largely on the portal of entry (skin, gastrointestinal tract, or respiratory tract).

INTERACTION OF CHEMICALS

In assessing the spectrum of responses, the accessibility of large numbers of toxicants creates an increasing necessity for consideration of interacting effects of toxicants. Interactions can occur in a variety of ways. Chemical interactions are known to occur by a number of mechanisms such as alterations in absorption, protein binding, and biotransformation or excretion of one or both of the interacting toxicants. In addition to these modes of interaction, the response of the organism to combinations of toxicants may be increased or decreased because of the toxicological responses at the site of action.

The effects of two chemicals given simultaneously will produce a response that may be simply additive of their individual responses or may be greater or less than that expected by addition of their individual responses. Study of these interactions often leads to a better understanding of the mechanism of toxicity of the chemicals involved. A number of terms have been used to describe pharmacologic and toxicologic interactions. An *additive* effect is the situation in which the combined effect of two chemicals is equal to the sum of the effect of each agent given alone (example: $2 + 3 = 5$). The effect most commonly observed when two chemicals are given together is an additive effect. For example, when two organophosphate insecticides are given together, the cholinesterase inhibition is usually additive. A *synergistic* effect is the situation in which the combined effect of two chemicals is much greater than the sum of the effect of each agent given alone (example: $2 + 2 = 20$). For example, both carbon tetrachloride and ethanol are hepatotoxic compounds, but together they produce much more liver injury than the mathematical sum of their individual effects on liver would suggest. *Potentiation* is the situation when one substance does not have a toxic effect on a certain organ or system, but when added to another chemical it makes the latter much more toxic (example: $0 + 2 = 10$). Isopropanol, for example, is not hepatotoxic, but when isopropanol is administered in addition to carbon tetrachloride, the hepatotoxicity of carbon tetrachloride is much greater than when given alone. *Antagonism* is the situation in which two chemicals, administered together, interfere with each other's actions or one interferes with the action of the other chemical (example: $4 + 6 = 8; 4 + (-4) = 0, 4 + 0 = 1$). Antagonistic effects of chemicals are often very desirable effects in toxicology and are the basis of many antidotes. There are four major types of antagonism: functional, chemical, dispositional, and receptor antagonism. *Functional antagonism* is the situation when two chemicals counterbalance each other by producing opposite effects on the same physiologic function. Advantage is taken of this principle in that the blood pressure can markedly fall during severe barbiturate intoxication, and it can be effectively antagonized by intravenous administration of a vasopressor agent, such as norepinephrine or metaraminol. Similarly, many chemicals, when given at toxic dose levels, produce convulsions and the convulsions can often be controlled by giving anticonvulsants, such as the benzodiazepines (e.g., diazepam). *Chemical antagonism* or *inactivation* is simply a chemical reaction between two compounds to produce a less toxic product. For example, dimercaprol (BAL) chelates with various metal ions such as arsenic, mercury, and lead, which decreases their toxicity. The use of antitoxins to treat various animal toxins is also an example of chemical antagonism. The use of the strongly basic low-molecular-weight protein protamine sulfate to form a stable complex with heparin, which abolishes its anticoagulant activity, is another example of chemical antagonism.

Dispositional antagonism is the situation in which the disposition, that is, the absorption, biotransformation, distribution, or excretion of the chemical, is altered such that the concentration and/or duration of the chemical at the target organ is diminished. Thus, prevention of absorption of a toxicant by ipecac or charcoal and the increased excretion of a chemical by administration of an osmotic diuretic or by alteration of the pH of the urine are examples of dispositional antagonism. If the parent compound is responsible for the toxicity of the chemical (such as the organophosphate insecticide paraoxon) and its metabolites are less toxic than the parent compound, then increasing the compound's biotransformation by a microsomal enzyme inducer (like phenobarbital) will decrease its toxicity. However, if the chemical's toxicity is largely due to a metabolic product (such as the organophosphate insecticide parathion), then inhibiting its biotransformation by an inhibitor of microsomal enzyme activity (SKF-525A or piperonyl butoxide) will decrease its toxicity. *Receptor antagonism* is when two chemicals that bind to the same receptor produce less of an effect when given together than the addition of their separate effects (example: 4 + 6 = 8) or when one chemical antagonizes the effect of the second chemical (example: 0 + 4 = 1). Receptor antagonists are often termed *blockers*. This concept is used to advantage in the clinical treatment of poisoning. For example, the receptor antagonist naloxone is used for treating the respiratory depressive effects of morphine and other morphine-like narcotics by competitive binding to the same receptor. The effect of oxygen in carbon monoxide poisoning is also an example of receptor antagonism. Treatment of organophosphate insecticide poisoning with atropine is an example not of the antidote competing with the poison for the receptor (cholinesterase) but rather blocking the receptor (cholinergic receptor) for the acetylcholine that accumulates by poisoning of the cholinesterase by the organophosphate.

TOLERANCE

Tolerance is a state of decreased responsiveness to a toxic effect of a chemical resulting from prior exposure to that chemical or to a structurally related chemical. Two major mechanisms are responsible for tolerance: one is due to a decreased amount of toxicant reaching the site where the toxic effect is produced *(dispositional tolerance),* and the other is due to a reduced responsiveness of a tissue to the chemical. Comparatively less is known about cellular mechanisms responsible for altering the responsiveness of a tissue to a toxic chemical than is known about dispositional tolerance. Two chemicals known to produce dispositional tolerance are carbon tetrachloride and cadmium. Carbon tetrachloride produces tolerance to itself by decreasing formation of the reactive metabolite (trichloromethyl radical) that produces liver injury *(see* Chapter 10). The mechanism of cadmium tolerance is explained by induction of a metal binding protein, metallothionein. Subsequent binding of cadmium to metallothionein rather than to critical macromolecules thereby decreases its toxicity (Goering and Klaassen, 1983).

DOSE-RESPONSE

The characteristics of exposure and the spectrum of effects come together in a correlative relationship customarily referred to as the *dose-response relationship.* This relationship is the most fundamental and pervasive concept in toxicology. Indeed, an understanding of this relationship is essential for the study of toxic materials.

From a practical perspective, there are two types of dose-response relationships: (1) that which describes the response of an *individual* to varying doses of a chemical, often referred to as "graded" responses because the measured effect is continuous over a range of doses, and (2) that which characterizes the distribution of responses to different doses in a *population* of individuals. Individual dose-response relationships are characterized by a dose-related increase in the severity of the response. The dose-relatedness of the response is often the result of an alteration of a specific biochemical process. For example, Figure 2–2 shows the dose-response relationship between different dietary doses of an organophosphate insecticide and the extent of inhibition of two different enzymes, acetylcholinesterase and carboxylesterase. The degree of inhibition of both enzymes is clearly dose related and spans a wide range, although the slopes of the curves are different. The toxicological response that results is directly related to the degree of cholinesterase enzyme inhibition, although the clinical expression (e.g., signs and symptoms) of the adverse response may vary with different doses because some organ systems will be relatively more sensitive to cholinesterase inhibition

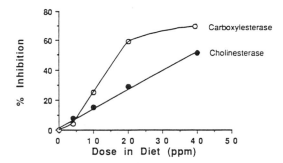

Figure 2–2. Dose-response relationship between different dietary doses of the organophosphate insecticide dioxathion, given for seven days, and enzyme inhibition (From Murphy, S. D., and Cheever, K. L.: Effects of feeding insecticides: inhibition of carboxylesterase and cholinesterase activities in rats. *Arch. Environ. Health,* **17:** 749–756, 1968).

than others. In general, the observed response to varying doses of a chemical in the whole organism is often complicated by the fact that most toxic substances have multiple sites or mechanisms of toxicity, each with its own "dose-response" relationship and subsequent adverse effect.

In the example shown in Figure 2–2, the dose expressed on an arithmetic scale yields the best fit for cholinesterase inhibition, whereas the data for inhibition of carboxylesterase fit best when dose is expressed on a logarithmic scale. Dose-response relationships are most often expressed as log-normal distributions, although the basis for this is largely empirical.

The dose-response relationships in a population are by definition quantal in nature—e.g., a specific end point is identified, and the dose required to produce that end point for each individual in the population is determined. Although these distinctions in "quantal population" and "graded individual" dose-response relationships are useful, the two types of responses are conceptually identical. The ordinate in both cases is simply labeled response, which may be the degree of response in an individual or system, or the fraction of a population responding, and the abscissa is the range in administered doses.

Assumptions

A number of assumptions must be considered before the dose-response relationships can be appropriately used. The first is that the response is due to the chemical administered. To describe the relationship between a toxic material and an observed effect or response, one must know with reasonable certainty that the relationship is indeed a causal one. For some data, it is not always apparent that the response is the result of chemical exposure. For example, an epidemiologic study might result in discovery of an "association" between a response (e.g., disease) and one or more variables. Frequently, the data are presented similarly to the "dose-response" in pharmacology and toxicology. Use of dose-response in this context is suspect, unless there is other convincing evidence supporting a causal connection between the estimated dose and the measured end point (response). Unfortunately, in nearly all retrospective and case control studies, and even many prospective studies, the dose, duration, frequency, and routes of exposure are seldom quantified, and other potential etiologic factors are frequently present with the chemical under study. In its most strict usage, then, the dose-response relationship is based on the knowledge that the effect is a result of a known toxic agent(s).

A second assumption seems simple and obvious, namely, that the response is, in fact, related to the dose. Perhaps because of its apparent simplicity, this assumption is often a source of misunderstanding. The assumption is really a composite of three others that will recur frequently.

1. There is a molecular or receptor site (or sites) with which the chemical interacts to produce the response.
2. The production of a response and the degree of response are related to the concentration of the agent at the reactive site.
3. The concentration at the site is, in turn, related to the dose administered.

The third assumption in using the dose-response relationship is that one has both a quantifiable method of measuring and a precise means of expressing the toxicity. A great variety of criteria or end points of toxicity could be used. The ideal criterion would be one closely associated with the molecular events resulting from exposure to the toxicant. Early in the assessment of toxicity, such an ideal is usually unapproachable; indeed, it might not be approachable at all even for well-known toxicants.

Failing in a mechanistic, molecular ideal criterion of toxicity, one looks to a measure of toxicity that is unequivocal and clearly relevant to the toxic effect. For example, with a new compound chemically related to the class of organophosphate insecticides, one might approach the measurement of toxicity by measuring inhibition of cholinesterase in blood. In this way, one would be measuring, in a readily accessible system by a technique that is convenient and reasonably precise, a prominent effect of the chemical and one that is usually pertinent to the mechanism by which toxicity is produced.

The selection of a toxic end point for measurement is not always so straightforward. Even the example cited above may be misleading as an organophosphate may produce a decrease in blood cholinesterase, but this change may not be directly related to its toxicity (DuBois, 1961). As additional data are gathered to suggest a mechanism of toxicity for any substance, other measures of toxicity might be selected. Although many end points are quantitative and precise, they are often indirect measures of toxicity. Changes in enzyme levels in blood can be indicative of tissue damage. For example, alanine aminotransferase (ALT or SGPT) and aspartate aminotransferase (AST or SGOT) are used to detect liver damage. Patterns of isozymes and their alteration may provide insight as to the organ or system that is the site of toxic effects. These measures may not be directly related to the mechanism of the toxic action.

Many direct measures of effects are also not necessarily related to the mechanism by which a substance produces its harm to the organism but have the advantage of permitting a causal relation to be drawn between the agent and its action. For example, measurement of the alteration of the tone of smooth or skeletal muscle for substances acting on muscles represents a rather fundamental approach to toxicologic assessment. Similarly, measures of heart rate, blood pressure, and electrical activity of heart muscle, nerve, or brain are examples of the use of physiologic functions as indices of toxicity. Measurement can also take the form of a still higher level of integration, such as the degree of motor activity or behavioral change.

The measurements used as examples all assume prior information about the toxicant, such as its target organ or site of action or a fundamental effect. Such information is usually available only after toxicologic screening and testing based on other measures of toxicity. With a new substance, the customary starting point in toxicologic evaluation utilizes lethality as an index. Determination of lethality is precise, quantal, and unequivocal and is, therefore, useful in its own right if only to suggest the level and magnitude of the potency of the substance. Lethality provides a measure of comparison among many substances whose mechanism and sites of action may be markedly different. Furthermore, from these studies clues to the direction to be taken in further studies are obtained. This comes about in two important ways. First, simply recording a death is not an adequate means of conducting a lethality study with a new substance. A key element must be a careful, disciplined, detailed observation of the intact animal extending from the time of administration of the toxicant to death of the animal. From properly conducted observations, immensely informative data can be gathered by the trained toxicologist. Second, a lethality study ordinarily is supported by histologic examination of major tissues and organs for abnormalities. From the latter observations, one can usually obtain more specific information about the events leading to the lethal effect, target organ(s) involved, and often a suggestion as to the possible mechanism of toxicity at a relatively fundamental level.

Calculations

Whatever response is selected for measurement, the relationship between the degree of response of the biologic system and the amount of toxicant administered assumes a form that occurs so consistently as to be considered classic and fundamental and is referred to as the dose-response relationship. This is the relationship that Trevan (1927) envisioned in his introduction of lethal dose as an index (LD50). The LD50 is the statistically derived single dosage of a substance that can be expected to cause death in 50 percent of the animals.

In toxicology the quantal dose-response is used extensively. Determination of the median lethal dose (LD50) is usually the first experiment performed with a new chemical. If a large number of doses is used with a large number of animals per dose, a sigmoid dose-response curve is observed, as depicted in the top panel of Figure 2–3. With the lowest dosage (6 mg/kg), 1 percent of the animals died. A normally distributed sigmoid curve, such as this one, approaches a response of 0 percent as the dose is decreased and approaches 100 percent as the dose is increased but theoretically never passes through 0 and 100 percent. However, the minimally effective dose of any chemical that evokes a stated all-or-none response is called the *threshold dose,* even though it cannot be determined experimentally.

The sigmoid curve has a relatively linear portion between 16 and 84 percent. These values represent the limits of 1 standard deviation (SD) of the mean (and the median) in a population with truly normal or gaussian distribution. However, it is usually not practical to describe the dose-response curve from this type of plot because one does not usually have large enough sample sizes to define adequately the sigmoid curve.

The middle panel of Figure 2–3 shows that quantal dose responses, such as lethality, exhibit a normal or gaussian distribution. The frequency histogram in this panel also shows the relationship between dose and effect. The data used to construct this histogram are the same as those

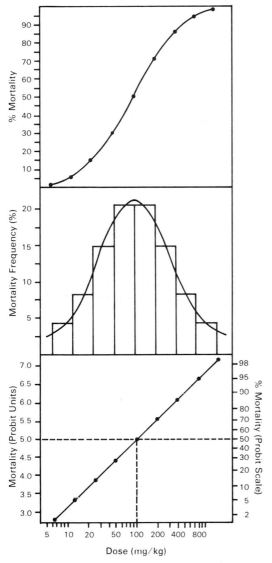

Figure 2–3. Diagram of quantal dose-response relationship. The abscissa is a log dosage of the chemical. In the top panel the ordinate is percent mortality; in the middle panel the ordinate is mortality frequency; and in the bottom panel the mortality is in probit units (see text).

tribution. The reason for this normal distribution is that there are differences in susceptibility among individuals to chemicals, which is known as biologic variation. Those animals responding at the left end of the curve are referred to as *hypersusceptible* and those at the right end of the curve as *resistant.*

In a normally distributed population, the mean ±1 SD represented 68.3 percent of the population, the mean ±2 SD represents 95.5 percent of the population, and the mean ±3 SD equals 99.7 percent of the population. Since quantal dose-response phenomena are usually normally distributed, one can convert the percent response to units of deviation from the mean or normal equivalent deviations (NEDs). Thus, the NED for a 50 percent response is 0; an NED of +1 is equated with 84.1 percent response. Later it was suggested (Bliss, 1957) that units of NED be converted by the addition of 5 to the value to avoid negative numbers and that these converted units be called probit units. The probit (from the contraction of probability unit), then, is an NED plus 5. In this transformation a 50 percent response becomes a probit of 5, +1 deviation becomes a probit of 6, and −1 deviation is a probit of 4.

PERCENT RESPONSE	NED	PROBIT
0.1	−3	2
2.3	−2	3
15.9	−1	4
50.0	0	5
84.1	+1	6
97.7	+2	7
99.9	+3	8

The data given in the top two panels of Figure 2–3 are replotted in the bottom panel with the mortality plotted in probit units. The data in the top panel (which was in the form of a sigmoid curve) and in the middle panel (a bell-shaped curve) form a straight line when transformed into probit units. In essence, what is accomplished in a probit transformation is an adjustment of mortality or other quantal data to an assumed normal population distribution, which results in a straight line. The LD50 is obtained by drawing a horizontal line from the probit unit 5, which is the 50 percent mortality point, to the dose-effect line. At the point of intersection, a vertical line is drawn, and this line intersects the abscissa at the LD50 point. It is evident from the line that information with respect to the lethal dose for 90 percent or for 10 percent of the population may also be derived by a similar procedure. Mathematically, it can be demonstrated that the range of values encompassed by the confidence limits is narrowest at the midpoint of the line (LD50) and is widest at both extremes (LD10 and LD90) of the dose-response curve (dotted lines in Figure 2–4). In addition to the LD50, the slope of

used in the top panel. The bars represent the percent of animals that died at each dose minus the percent that died at the immediately lower dose. One can clearly see that only a few animals responded to the lowest dose and also only a small number at the highest dose. Larger numbers of animals responded to doses intermediate between these two extremes, and the maximum frequency of response occurred in the middle portion of the dose range. Thus, we have a bell-shaped curve known as a *normal frequency dis-*

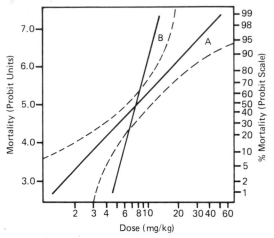

Figure 2-4. Diagram of dose-response relationships. Dose-response relationship is steeper for chemical B than chemical A. *Dotted lines* show the confidence limits for chemical A.

the dose-response curve can also be obtained. Figure 2-4 demonstrates the dose-response curves for mortality of two compounds. Compound A exhibits a "flat" dose-response curve showing that a large change in dosage is required before a significant change in response will be observed. However, compound B exhibits a "steep" dose-response curve where a relatively small change in dosage will cause a large change in response. It is evident that the LD50 for both compounds is the same (8 mg/kg). However, the slopes of the dose-response curves are quite different. At one-half of the LD50 of the compounds (4 mg/kg), less than 1 percent of the animals exposed to compound B would die, but 20 percent of the animals given compound A would die.

Determination of the LD50 has become a public issue because of increasing concern for the welfare and protection of laboratory animals. The LD50 is not a biological constant. There are many factors that influence toxicity and thus may alter the estimation of the LD50 in any particular study. Such factors as animal strain, age and weight, type of feed, caging, pretrial fasting time, and method of administration, volume and type of suspension medium, and duration of observation have all been shown to influence adverse responses to toxic substances. These and other factors have been discussed in detail in earlier editions of this textbook (*see* Doull, 1980). Because of this inherent variability in LD50 estimates, it is now recognized that for most purposes it is only necessary to characterize the LD50 within an order of magnitude range, e.g., 5-50 mg/kg, 50-500 mg/kg, and so on.

There are several traditional approaches to determining the LD50 and its 95 percent confidence limit as well as the slope of the probit line. The reader is referred to the classic works of Litchfield and Wilcoxon (1949), Bliss (1957), and Finney (1971) for a description of the mechanics of these procedures. A computer program in BASIC for determining probit and log-probit or logit correlations has been published (Abou-Setta *et al.*, 1986). These traditional methods for determining LD50s require a relatively large number of animals (40 to 50). Other statistical techniques that require fewer animals, such as the "moving averages" method of Thompson and Weill (1952; Weill, 1952), are available but do not provide confidence limits for the LD50 nor the slope of the probit line. Finney (1985) has succinctly summarized the advantages and deficiencies of many of the traditional methods. For most circumstances, an adequate estimate of the LD50 and an approximation of the 95 percent confidence intervals can be obtained with as few as six to nine animals, using the "up-and-down" method as modified by Bruce (1985). When this method was compared with traditional methods that typically utilize 40 to 50 animals, excellent agreement was obtained for all ten compounds tested (Bruce, 1987).

When animals are exposed to chemicals by the air they are breathing or the water they (fish) are living in, the dose the animals received is usually not known. For these situations, the lethal concentration 50 (LC50) is usually determined, that is, the concentration of chemical in the air or water that causes death to 50 percent of the animals. When reporting an LC50, it is imperative that the time of exposure be indicated.

Although by themselves the LD50 and LC50 are of limited value, acute lethality studies are essential for characterizing the toxic effects of chemicals and their hazard to humans. The most meaningful scientific information derived from acute lethality tests comes from the clinical observations and postmortem examination of the animals, rather than the specific LD50 value.

The quantal all-or-none response is not limited to lethality. Similar dose-effect curves can be constructed for cancer, liver injury, and other types of toxic responses, as well as for beneficial therapeutic responses, such as anesthesia. Figure 2-5 indicates the dose-response for three different chemical carcinogens. When higher doses were administered, higher percentages of the animals developed sarcomas. While some toxic and therapeutic responses, such as anesthesia, are all-or-none, other graded responses, such as blood pressure, can be transformed into quantal responses. This is usually performed by quantitating a particular parameter (e.g., blood pressure) in a large number of control animals and

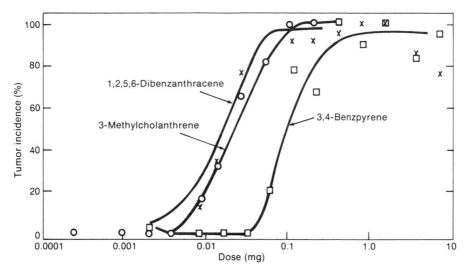

Figure 2–5. Dose-response relationship for carcinogens. Three carcinogenic polycyclic aromatic hydrocarbons were administered subcutaneously in a single dose, each to a group of 20 mice. The incidence of sarcomas at the site of injection was noted. (Modified from Bryan, W. R., and Shimkin, M. B.: Quantitative analysis of dose-response data obtained with three carcinogenic hydrocarbons in strain C3H male mice. *J. Natl. Cancer Inst.*, **3:** 503–531, 1943.)

determining its standard deviation, which is a measure of its variability. Because the mean ±3 SD represents 99.7 percent of the population, one can assign all animals that lie outside this range after treatment with a chemical as affected and those lying within this range as not being affected by the chemical. Using a series of doses of the chemical, one can thus construct a quantal dose-response curve similar to that described above for lethality.

In Figures 2–3 and 2–4, the dosage has been given on a log basis. Although the use of the log of the dosage is empiric, log-dosage plots usually provide a more nearly linear representation of the data. It must be remembered, however, that this is not universally the situation. Some radiation effects, for example, give a better probit fit when the dose is expressed arithmetically rather than logarithmically. There are other situations in which other functions (e.g., exponentials) of dosage provide a better fit to the data than the log function. It is also conventional to express the dosage in milligrams per kilogram. It might be argued that expression of dosage on a mole-per-kilogram basis would be better, particularly for making comparisons of a series of compounds. Although such an argument has considerable merit, dosage is usually expressed as milligrams per kilogram.

One might also view dosage on the basis of body weight as being less appropriate than other bases, such as surface area, which is approximately proportional to (body weight)$^{2/3}$. In Table 2–2 selected values are given to compare the differences in dosage by the two alternatives.

Given a dosage of 100 mg/kg, it can be seen that the dose (mg/animal), of course, is proportional to the dosage administered per body weight. Surface area is not proportional to weight: While the weight of a human is 3500 times greater than that of a mouse, the surface area of humans is only about 390 times greater than that of mice. Chemicals are usually administered in toxicologic studies as mg/kg. The same dosage given to humans and mice on a weight basis (mg/kg) would be approximately ten times greater in humans than mice if that dosage were expressed per surface area (mg/cm^2). Cancer chemotherapeutic agents are usually administered on a surface area basis.

Comparison of Dose-Responses

Figure 2–6 illustrates the quantal dose-response curve for a desirable effect of a chemical (ED), such as anesthesia, a toxic effect (TD), such as liver injury, and the lethal dose (LD). As depicted in Figure 2–6, a parallelism is apparent between the effective dose curve (ED) and the curve depicting mortality (LD). It is tempting to view the parallel dose-response curves as indicative of identity of mechanism, that is, to conclude that the lethality is a simple extension of the therapeutic effect. While this conclusion may ultimately prove to be correct in any particular case, it is not warranted solely on the basis of the two parallel lines. The same admonition applies to any pair of parallel "effect" curves or any other pair of toxicity or lethality curves.

Therapeutic Index. The hypothetical curves in Figure 2–6 illustrate two other in-

Table 2–2.   COMPARISON OF DOSAGE BY WEIGHT AND SURFACE AREA

	WEIGHT (g)	DOSAGE (mg/kg)	DOSE (mg/animal)	SURFACE AREA (cm^2)	DOSAGE (mg/cm^2)
Mouse	20	100	2	46	0.043
Rat	200	100	20	325	0.061
Guinea pig	400	100	40	565	0.071
Rabbit	1500	100	150	1270	0.118
Cat	2000	100	200	1380	0.145
Monkey	4000	100	400	2980	0.134
Dog	12000	100	1200	5770	0.207
Human	70000	100	7000	18000	0.388

terrelated points, namely, the importance of the selection of the toxic criterion and the interpretation of comparative effect. The concept of the "therapeutic index," introduced by Paul Ehrlich in 1913, can be used to illustrate this relationship. Although the therapeutic index is directed toward a comparison of the therapeutically effective dose to the toxic dose of a chemical, it is equally applicable to considerations of comparative toxicity. The *therapeutic index* (TI) in its broadest sense is defined as the ratio of the dose required to produce a toxic effect and the dose needed to elicit desired therapeutic response. Similarly, an index of comparative toxicity is obtained by either the ratio of doses of two different materials to produce identical response or the ratio of doses of the same material necessary to yield different toxic effects.

The most commonly used index of effect, whether beneficial or toxic, is the median dose, that is, the dose required to result in a response in 50 percent of a population (or to produce 50 percent of a maximal response). The therapeutic index of a drug is an approximate statement about the relative safety of a drug expressed as the ratio of the lethal or toxic dose to the therapeutic dose.

$$TI = \frac{LD50}{ED50}$$

From Figure 2–6 one can approximate a "therapeutic index" using these median doses. The larger the ratio, the greater the relative safety. The ED50 is approximately 20 and the LD50 about 200; thus, the therapeutic index is 10, a number indicative of a relatively safe drug. But the use of the median effective and median lethal doses is not without disadvantage, since median doses tell nothing about the slopes of the dose-response curves for therapeutic and toxic effects.

Margin of Safety.   One way to overcome this deficiency is to use the ED99 for the desired effect and the LD1 for the undesired effect. These parameters are used in the calculation of the margin of safety.

$$Margin\ of\ safety = \frac{LD1}{ED99}$$

The quantitative comparisons described above have been used mainly after a single administration of chemicals. However, for chemicals in which there is no beneficial or effective dose, and exposures are likely to occur repeatedly, the ratio of LD1 to ED99 has little relevance. Thus, for nondrug chemicals, the term "margin of safety" has found use in risk assessment procedures as an indicator of the magnitude of difference between an estimated exposed dose to a human population and the highest nontoxic dose determined in experimental animals.

A measure of the degree of accumulation of a chemical and/or its toxic effects can also be estimated from quantal toxicity data. The *chronicity index* (Hayes, 1975) of a chemical is a unitless value obtained by dividing its 1-dose LD50 by its 90-dose (90-day) LD50, where both are

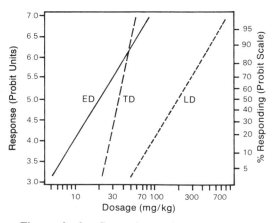

Figure 2–6.   Comparison of effective dose *(ED)*, toxic dose *(TD)*, and lethal dose *(LD)*. The plot is of log dosage versus percent of population responding in probit units.

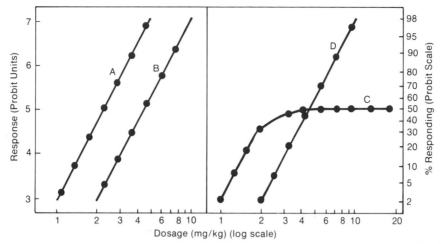

Figure 2–7. Schematic representation of the difference in the dose-response curves for four chemicals *(A–D)*, to illustrate the difference between potency and efficacy *(see* text).

expressed in milligrams per kilogram per day. Theoretically, if no cumulative effect occurs over the doses, the chronicity index would be 1. If a compound were absolutely cumulative, the chronicity index would be 90.

Similar statistical procedures that are used to calculate the LD50 can also be used to determine the lethal time 50 (LT50) or the time required for half the animals to die (Litchfield, 1949). The LT50 value for a chemical indicates the time course of the toxic effects but does not indicate whether one chemical is more toxic than another.

Potency versus Efficacy. To compare the toxic effects of two or more chemicals, first the dose-response to the toxic effects of each chemical needs to be established. One can then compare the potency and maximal efficacy of the two chemicals to produce a toxic effect. These two important terms can be explained by reference to Figure 2–7, which depicts dose-response curves to four different chemicals for the frequency of a particular toxic effect, such as the production of tumors. Chemical A is said to be more potent than chemical B because of their relative positions along the dosage axis. Potency thus refers to the range of doses over which a chemical produces increasing responses. Thus, A is more potent than B, and C is more potent than D. Maximal efficacy reflects the limit of the dose-response relationship on the response axis to a certain chemical. Chemicals A and B have equal maximal efficacy, whereas the maximal efficacy of C is less than that of D.

SELECTIVE TOXICITY

Selective toxicity means that a chemical produces injury to one kind of living matter without harming some other form of life, even though the two may exist in intimate contact (Albert, 1965, 1973). The living matter that is injured is termed the *uneconomic form* (or undesirable), and the matter protected is called the *economic form* (or desirable). They may be related to one another as parasite and host, or they may be two tissues in one organism. This biologic diversity interferes with the ability of the toxicologist to predict the toxic effects of a chemical in one species (humans) from experiments performed in another species (laboratory animals). However, by taking advantage of the biologic diversity, it is possible to develop agents that are lethal for an undesired species and harmless for other species. In agriculture, for example, there are fungi, insects, and even competitive plant life that injure the crop and thus selective pesticides are needed. Similarly, animal husbandry and human medicine require agents such as antibiotics that are selectively toxic to the undesirable form but do not produce damage to the desirable form.

Drugs and other chemical agents used for selective toxic purposes are selective for one of two reasons. Either (1) the chemical is equitoxic to both economic and uneconomic cells but is accumulated mainly by the uneconomic cells, or (2) it reacts fairly specifically with (a) a cytologic or (b) a biochemical feature that is absent from or does not play an important part in the economic form (Albert, 1965, 1973). Selectivity due to differences in distribution is usually the result of differences in absorption, biotransformation, or excretion of the toxicant. The selective toxicity of an insecticide spray may be partly due to a larger surface area per unit weight causing the insect to absorb a proportionally larger dose than the mammal being sprayed. The effectiveness of radioactive iodine in the treatment of hyperthyroidism is due to the selective ability of the thyroid gland to accumulate iodine. A major reason why chemicals are toxic to one but not to another type of tissue is that there are differences in accumulation of the ultimate toxic compound in various tissues. This, in turn, might be due to differences in the ability of various tissues to biotransform the chemical into the ultimate toxic product.

Selective toxicity due to differences in comparative cytology is exemplified by comparison of plant and animal cells. Plants differ from animals in many ways: for example, absence of a nervous system, an efficient circulatory system, and muscles and the presence of a photosynthetic mechanism and cell walls. The fact that bacteria contain cell walls and humans do not has been utilized in developing selective toxic chemotherapeutic agents, like penicillin and cephalosporins, that kill the bacteria but are relatively nontoxic to mammalian cells.

Selective toxicity can also be a result of a difference in biochemistry of the two types of cells. For example, bacteria do not absorb folic acid but synthesize it from *p*-aminobenzoic acid, glutamic acid, and pteridine, whereas mammals cannot synthesize folic acid but have to absorb it from their diet. Thus, sulfonamide drugs are selectively toxic to bacteria because the sulfonamides, which resemble *p*-aminobenzoic acid in both charge and dimensions, antagonize the incorporation of *p*-aminobenzoic acid into the folic acid molecule, a reaction that humans do not carry out.

Selectivity in response extends to chronic responses such as carcinogenicity. For example, mice are resistent to the hepatocarcinogenic effects of the fungal toxin aflatoxin B_1 largely because they express an isoenzyme of glutathione S-transferase that has a high affinity for the carcinogenic epoxide of aflatoxin B_1. Rats, which are less efficient at detoxifying the carcinogenic epoxide of aflatoxin, develop tumors at very low dietary doses of aflatoxin B_1.

GENERAL MECHANISMS OF TOXICITY

All chemicals produce their toxic effects via alterations in normal cellular biochemistry and physiology. A thorough understanding of the biochemical and molecular sites and modes of action of specific drugs and chemicals is an essential part of toxicology. Although cell death is one common outcome of chemical-induced injury, and can obviously have serious consequences, the extent of tissue damage necessary to elicit a life-threatening response is quite var-

ied depending on both the tissue type and the rate at which insult occurs. Some tissues, most notably epithelial tissues including liver, have some capacity to regenerate in response to a loss in tissue mass, whereas other tissues, such as neuronal cells, cannot regenerate once cells have died. It should also be recognized that most organs have a capacity for function that exceeds that required for normal homeostasis, sometimes referred to as *functional reserve capacity*. For example, it is well known that humans can function quite effectively with only one kidney, or with part of a lung removed, or only half their normal amount of hemoglobin. This excess function is a critical element in the ability of the body to survive severe toxic insults.

Although many toxic responses are ultimately a result of cell death and loss of critical organ function, other responses may be the result of biochemical and pharmacological imbalances in normal physiological processes that do not result in cell death. Other chemical effects may result in the expression of toxicity as a result of nonlethal genetic alterations in somatic cells. There are many ways in which chemicals can interfere with normal biochemistry and physiology, and a brief overview of some general sites of toxic action is useful in appreciating the diversity of biochemical and cellular processes that underlie toxic responses. The following general categories of sites of chemical actions are neither comprehensive nor mutually exclusive but represent the major mechanisms of action of many drugs and chemicals.

Receptor–Ligand Interactions and Stereoselective Actions of Chemicals

Receptors are macromolecular components of tissues with which a drug or chemical (ligand) interacts to produce its characteristic biological effects (Goldstein *et al.*, 1974). The binding between a receptor and ligand is usually reversible and can be described by the simple equilibrium expansion: $R + L \underset{k_2}{\overset{k_1}{\rightleftarrows}} RL$. The dissociation constant that describes this relationship is thus $K_d = k_1/k_2 = [L][R]/[LR]$, where [L], [R], and [LR] are the concentrations of ligand, unbound receptor, and ligand-bound receptor, respectively. The ligand may be an endogenous substance that interacts with the receptor to produce a normal physiological response, or it may be an exogenous substance that may either activate (agonist) or block (antagonist) the response. The total number of receptors available for binding is $[R]_T = [R] + [LR]$; therefore, $[R] = [R]_T - [LR]$, and substituting this into the equation that describes the dissociation constant and rearranging the expression yields the relationship:

$$\frac{[LR]}{[R]_T} \leftrightarrows \frac{[L]}{K_d + [L]}$$

$[LR]/[R]_T$ is the fraction of receptor that is occupied by ligand when it is present at concentration [L]. If the effect, E, that results from the interaction of ligand and receptor is dependent on the fraction of receptors occupied by the ligand, then the magnitude of the response is described by the relationship:

$$E = \frac{[S]}{K_d + [S]}$$

This equation expresses a hyperbolic function and is the basis of Michaelis-Menten kinetics described for enzyme-substrate interactions. Many of the linear transformations common to enzyme kinetics are applicable to other types of receptor-ligand interactions. The reader is referred to Goldstein *et al.* (1974) or other basic textbooks in pharmacology or enzymology for a more detailed discussion of the kinetics of receptor-ligand interactions.

Receptor-ligand interactions are generally highly stereospecific, and small changes in chemical structure can drastically reduce or eliminate the effect. The importance of stereoselectivity in pharmacologic and toxicologic responses cannot be overemphasized. Differences in activity extend not only to structurally distinct chemicals and geometric isomers but to those chemicals that have chirality and thus may be present as racemic mixtures of stereoisomers. Synthetic drugs and chemicals that have chiral centers generally contain both enantiomers, often at a 1:1 ratio, yet in many instances only one enantiomer is biologically active (eutomer). In pharmacologic or toxicologic studies, the inactive or poorly active enantiomer (distomer) should be viewed as an "impurity," which may confound the interpretation of results of studies obtained with the racemic mixture (Ariens *et al.,* 1988). In fact, in some instances the inactive isomer may contribute to the unwanted effects of a drug or chemical, while having little beneficial effect. For example, the 2R,3R-enantiomer of paclobutrazol has high fungicidal activity but little herbicidal activity, whereas the reverse is true for the 2S,3S-enantiomer (Ariens *et al.,* 1988). Because the enzymes responsible for biotransformation of xenobiotics also contain active sites with specific steric requirements, stereoisomers may be differentially metabolized, which can greatly alter the potency and efficacy of one enantiomer over another. Stereoselective differences in action among enantiomers should not be surprising if one considers that these

chemicals are mirror images, much as the right hand is of the left, and that receptors have a physical orientation that can be likened to a glove. Although the left-hand and right-hand gloves look remarkably similar, they do not fit the right hand equally well. However, as the chiral center of a stereoisomer is not necessarily involved with the active site of the receptor, chirality does not always confer differences in responsiveness among enantiomers.

The adverse effects of many chemicals are related directly to their ability to interfere with normal receptor-ligand interactions. This is especially true with neurotoxicants, as the function of the nervous system is highly dependent on a diverse array of receptor-ligand interactions. For example, the belladonna alkaloids atropine and scopolamine bind to and block the post-synaptic cholinergic receptors in the central and autonomic nervous system. However, not all cholinergic receptors are identical. The cholinergic receptors that are stimulated by muscarine as well as acetylcholine (muscarinic receptors principally in the postganglionic parasympathetic nervous system) are blocked by atropine, whereas other cholinergic receptors that respond to nicotine and acetylcholine, but not muscarine (nicotinic receptors, principally in autonomic ganglia and neuromuscular junctions), are not affected by atropine. Thus, toxic effects of atropine are largely related to inhibition of the parasympathetic nervous system. In contrast, *d*-tubocurarine binds to and selectively blocks postsynaptic nicotinic receptors at the neuromuscular junction, producing profound paralysis, but has little effect on parasympathetic nervous system function.

Interference with Excitable Membrane Functions

The maintenance and stability of excitable membranes are essential to normal physiology. Chemicals can perturb excitable membrane function in many ways. For example, the flux of ions across neuronal axons can be blocked by chemicals that act as ion channel blockers. The marine toxin, saxitoxin, produces its paralyzing effects by blocking sodium channels in excitable membranes. Tetrodotoxin, derived from the gonads and other organs of the puffer fish, is structurally quite different from saxitoxin yet acts in essentially the same manner. The insecticide DDT produces its neurotoxic action by interfering with the closing of sodium channels, thus altering the rate of repolarization of excitable membranes. Organic solvents appear to produce their CNS (central nervous system)-depressant effects via nonspecific alterations in membrane fluidity, largely as a property of their lipid solubility, rather than binding to specific macromolecular receptors.

Interference with Cellular Energy Production

Many chemicals produce their adverse effects by interfering with the oxidation of carbohydrates to produce adenosine triphosphate (ATP). This interference can occur by blocking effective delivery of oxygen to tissues. For example, chemical oxidation of the iron in hemoglobin (methemoglobin) by nitrites also interferes with oxygen delivery, as methemoglobin does not effectively bind oxygen. Utilization of oxygen in the tissues is blocked by cyanide, hydrogen sulfide, and azide because of their affinity for cytochrome oxidase. The ultimate formation of ATP via oxidation of carbohydrates can be blocked at other sites, as well. For example, rotenone and antimycin A interfere with specific enzymes in the electron transport chain, nitrophenols uncouple oxidative phosphorylation, and sodium fluoroacetate inhibits the tricarboxylic acid (Krebs) cycle. The consequences of ATP depletion are many and include effects noted above, such as interference with membrane integrity, ion pumps, and protein synthesis. Significant energy depletion will inevitably lead to loss of cell function and perhaps cell death.

Binding to Biomolecules

Proteins. Many toxic substances exert their effects via binding to the active sites of enzymes or proteins that are critical to cellular function. For example, hydrogen cyanide binds avidly to the ferric iron atom in cytochrome $a + a_3$ (cytochrome oxidase), which blocks the terminal event in electron transport. This single site of action is responsible for the rapid and often fatal toxic effects of cyanide, and the understanding of this mechanism led to the development of specific antidotes to cyanide poisoning (see Chapter 8). Carbon monoxide binds tightly to the reduced form of iron in hemoglobin, reducing the delivery of oxygen to tissues. Although this has for many years been thought to be the sole mechanism of toxicity of carbon monoxide, there is evidence to suggest that CO also binds to cytochrome $a + a_3$. Many toxic trace metals such as lead, mercury, cadmium, and arsenic bind to proteins with free sulfhydryl groups, which contribute to their toxicity. Chemical-induced porphyrias from lead, mercury, and other metals, as well as certain halogenated hydrocarbons (e.g., hexachlorobenzene) result, in part, from the inhibition of specific enzymes in the heme biosynthetic pathway.

Lipids. Although some of the processes discussed above are capable of producing adverse physiological responses without the actual death of cells in any tissue or organ (e.g., most receptor-ligand interactions), other of these processes will eventually lead to loss of organ function and cell death. This is especially true if exposure to the toxic substance occurs on a chronic basis, where tissue injury can accumulate from repeated cytotoxic episodes. The specific sequence of events leading to cell injury and death is complex and not fully understood (Boobis *et al.*, 1989). The most thorough understanding of the processes leading to chemical-induced cell death comes from studies on liver cells.

For most chemicals causing tissue necrosis, the initial step appears to be the formation of a reactive, electrophilic intermediate, often a free radical. Formation of free radicals may occur via enzyme-mediated one- or two-electron oxidations, as well as from the autoxidation of small molecules such as reduced flavines and thiols. Electron transfer from transition metals, such as iron, to oxygen-containing molecules can also initiate and propagate free radical reactions. The initiation of lipid peroxidation via interaction of free radicals with polyunsaturated fatty acids to form lipid peroxyradicals (ROO·), which then produce lipid hydroperoxides (ROOH) and further lipid peroxyradicals, has been proposed as one critical step leading to cell injury and death. Peroxidative damage to membrane lipids could then lead to a loss of membrane integrity and rupture of the cell membrane.

Intracellular Thiols. It is now recognized that lipid peroxidation by itself may not be sufficient to induce cell death. In addition to inducing lipid peroxidation, electrophilic intermediates may also covalently interact with other nucleophilic sites in the cell, including glutathione (GSH) and thiol-containing proteins, which results in "oxidative stress" to the cell. Depletion of intracellular stores of glutathione appears to be required before significant oxidative stress occurs. As many critical enzymes in the cell require one or more reduced thiols (SH-group) to maintain their activity, oxidative stress in excess of that necessary to deplete intracellular GSH can lead to oxidation of protein thiols to form disulfide linkages, thereby destroying enzymatic activity. Although the direct covalent interaction of electrophilic chemicals with protein thiols may contribute to enzyme inhibition, it appears that the majority of loss of activity of thiol-containing proteins is a result of reversible oxidation of the thiol group that occurs as a result of oxidative stress. One group of thiol-containing enzymes that may play a critical role in cell injury and death as a result of oxidative inactivation (oxidative stress) is the Ca^{2+}-transporting ATPases.

Nucleic Acids. There are numerous nucleophilic sites within DNA that may readily react with electrophilic chemicals. Alkylation of the O–6 position of guanine appears important in the mutagenicity and carcinogenicity of nitrosamines and other chemicals that readily form methyl carbonium ions. However, other sites, such as the N–7, N–2, and C–2 positions of guanine, may also be important sites of DNA adduct formation with other electrophilic chemicals. Adduction of DNA with exogenous chemicals may alter the expression of critical gene products necessary for the survival of the cell, and thus binding to DNA may lead to cell death. However, of perhaps more significance is the production of somatic mutations through chemical-DNA adduct formation that may serve as the initiating event in chemical carcinogenesis (see Chapter 5 for a detailed discussion). As with DNA, ribonucleic acid (RNA) also contains nucleophilic sites, and thus critical intracellular functions of RNA, e.g., protein synthesis, may be perturbed by covalent interaction of electrophilic chemicals with RNA.

Perturbation of Calcium Homeostasis

Interference with the normal process responsible for intracellular calcium homeostasis appears to play a critical role in chemical-mediated cell injury and death (Orrenius *et al.*, 1989). Calcium accumulates in tissues following necrotic injury, and Ca^{2+} accumulation has been associated with cell injury and death from ischemia, immunological responses, and a variety of toxic agents. Disruption of intracellular Ca^{2+} homeostasis can result from enhanced Ca^{2+} influx, release of Ca^{2+} from intracellular stores, and inhibition of Ca^{2+} extrusion at the plasma membrane. A wide variety of cytotoxic agents, including nitrophenols, quinones, peroxides, aldehydes, dioxins, halogenated alkanes and alkenes, and some metal ions, have been shown to disrupt Ca^{2+} homeostasis. Increased intracellular calcium has been associated with the development of membrane abnormalities (blebbing) in isolated cells, which appears to be a general phenomenon associated with toxic and ischemic cell injury and death. Ca^{2+} plays a key role as a second messenger in the regulation of many intracellular functions. For example, normal cytoskeletal organization is perturbed when intracellular Ca^{2+} increases, apparently as a result of a calcium-mediated dissociation of actin microfilaments and an activation of phospholipases and proteases. Although normally the Ca^{2+}-mediated activation of phospholipases plays a protective role by removing peroxidized phospholipids from damaged membranes, when activated by nonphysiologic changes in Ca^{2+} concentration phospholipases may enhance membrane phospholipid breakdown, which may lead to cell injury and death. It is also known that an increase in intracellular Ca^{2+} can activate nonlysosomal proteases. Although the endogenous substrates for these proteases have not been fully characterized, they appear to act on cytoskeletal proteins. The importance of these proteases in the process of cell death is demonstrated by the fact that inhibitors of Ca^{2+}-activated proteases delay or prevent the appearance of cytotoxic effects.

Ca^{2+} can also activate certain endonucleases, which results in DNA fragmentation and chromatin condensation. Although this process is important in the physiological "programmed" cell death that occurs naturally as a part of tissue growth and differentiation (apoptosis), chemically mediated premature activation of this enzyme system via a perturbation in Ca^{2+} homeostasis may contribute to the cytotoxic actions of some toxic substances.

Toxicity from Selective Cell Death

Selective cell loss within an organ or tissue may also result in toxicologic effects that are quite specific and in some instances may mimic other disease processes. For example, high doses of manganese, or the illicit street drug 1-methyl-4-phenyl-1,2,5,6-tetrahydropyridine (MPTP), cause selective damage to dopaminergic cells in the basal ganglia in the brain, producing a neurological condition nearly indistinguishable from Parkinson's disease. Some chemicals, both synthetic (e.g., Amitrole) and naturally occurring (e.g., 5-vinyloxazolidinethione from the rapeseed plant), stimulate the growth of the thyroid gland and production of excess thyroid hormone, resulting in a pathological condition indistinguishable from goiter. Conversely, other chemicals may selectively accumulate in the thyroid gland, where they reach toxic concentrations and destroy the thyroid cells (e.g., ^{125}I, propylthiouracil).

The developing embryo is also quite sensitive to many toxic substances. Because in the early stages of embryonic growth many cells may have pluripotent potential (can differentiate into a variety of mature cell types), loss of even a few cells can have major consequences, leading either to embryonic death (i.e., miscarriage) or some form of congenital malformation (birth defect). For example, the administration of the antinausea drug thalidomide to pregnant women at a specific stage of fetal development resulted in the cytotoxic loss of early limb bud cells, with the consequence that children were born with severely underdeveloped or missing legs and/or arms. (See Chapter 7 for a complete discussion of chemicals and birth defects.)

Nonlethal Genetic Alterations in Somatic Cells

As noted above, the covalent interaction of xenobiotics with DNA can result directly in the death of the cell but may also result in the initiation of a complex series of events that may ultimately result in cancer (*see* Chapter 5). Chemicals that can produce a carcinogenic response via somatic mutations are called *genotoxic carcinogens*. The vast majority of chemically induced lesions in DNA are repaired, but some may escape repair or be repaired incorrectly, leading to the introduction of a mutated gene that is "inherited" by all cells derived from the mutated cell. If the mutation occurs in a somatic cell, then the genetic lesion cannot be passed onto future generations but could serve as a precursor for the eventual development of cancer.

It is currently thought that genotoxic chemicals can induce cancer by activating cellular "proto-oncogenes." Proto-oncogenes, when aberrantly expressed, confer on a cell features of a cancerous phenotype. Many of the gene products from oncogenes determine a cell's response to growth-stimulating factors and/or differentiation. In normal cells, the expression of proto-oncogenes is tightly controlled for the specific requirement for growth and/or differentiation (Lutz and Maier, 1988). In addition to the direct, covalent interaction of a xenobiotic with DNA, proto-oncogenes may be activated via a number of genotoxic events, such as alterations in chromosome structure (e.g., rearrangements or deletions), interference with DNA replication, interference with DNA segregation, or interference with DNA repair (Lutz and Maier, 1988).

Although activation of proto-oncogenes via a genotoxic event is one mechanism by which chemicals can induce cancer, it has been recognized for decades that cancer is a multistep process and that some nongenotoxic chemicals may enhance the incidence of cancer, presumably through some mechanism other than by damaging DNA. Chemicals that are by themselves generally incapable of inducing cancer but enhance the development of tumors when given after an "initiator" are called *tumor promoters*. Tumor promoters act by enhancing the probability of an initiated cell developing into a tumor. Stimulation of an "initiated" cell into cell division and clonal expansion (e.g., mitogenic effect) appears to be a common feature of all tumor promoters (Lutz and Maier, 1988). There are a variety of mechanisms by which chemicals could act as tumor promoters: They could act directly as growth factors, or interact with modified growth factor receptors; they could stimulate the production and release of endogenous growth factors; they could shift differentiated cells from a resting state (G_0) to a cell cycle phase (G_1); they could induce normal repairative cell growth of neighboring cells via a cytotoxic effect; they could inhibit normal cellular differentiation, which is necessary to ensure that mature cells stop dividing; or they could interfere with normal cell-cell communication, which is important in regulation of normal cellular growth (Lutz and Maier, 1988).

Although birth defects are most commonly induced via cytotoxic events and are usually evident at birth, it is also possible to have "delayed" adverse effects develop in offspring that arise via genetic mutations induced *in utero*. For example, the synthetic estrogen diethylstibestrol (DES) has been claimed responsible for vaginal cancers in women who were exposed *in utero* because their mothers took DES to reduce the chance of miscarriage. Fortunately, there are very few examples of such "transplacental carcinogenesis."

Multiple Sites and Mechanisms of Action

It is obvious from the above survey that classification of the mechanism of action of a chemical to one specific process or site of action is difficult and not mutually exclusive. Cyanide binds to an enzyme with some described affinity and thus behaves like a receptor-ligand interaction. It also inhibits the enzyme activity, which depletes energy stores, which can induce oxidative stress and alter Ca^{2+} homeostasis. Lead has many different toxicologic effects, many of which may be mediated by binding to specific proteins, yet other effects are not easily traced to a specific enzyme or biochemical pathway. Although "target molecules" have been identified for many toxic substances, the specific mechanism and site(s) of action are poorly understood for the majority of hazardous chemicals.

Many other molecular, biochemical, and cellular sites of action of specific toxic agents have been identified, and examples of these will be found throughout this textbook (*see* Table 2–3). Research into the basic mechanisms of toxicity of both natural and synthetic chemicals is essential to the science of toxicology. The development of antidotes to poisonings, as well as rational preventive measures to avoid unwanted toxic effects, requires a thorough understanding of the mechanisms of action of chemicals and serves as a principal goal of scientists involved in both basic and applied research in toxicology.

Table 2–3. SOME GENERAL MECHANISMS OF TOXIC ACTION

Interference with Normal Receptor-Ligand Interactions
Neuroreceptors and neurotransmitters (e.g., atropine, strychnine, LSD, *d*-tubocurarine, organophosphates, antihistamines)
Hormone receptors (DES, TCDD, goitrogens)
Enzyme activity (organophosphates, cyanide, sodium fluoroacetate)
Transport proteins (carbon monoxide, nitrites)

Interference with Membrane Functions
Excitable membranes
Ion flux (saxitoxin, tetrodotoxin, DDT)
Membrane fluidity (organic solvents, ethanol, local anesthetics)
Membranes in organelles
Lysosomal membranes (carbon tetrachloride)
Mitochondrial membranes (organotins)

Interference with Cellular Energy Production
Oxygen delivery to tissues (CO, nitrite)
Uncoupling of oxidative phosphorylation (nitrophenols, organotins)
Inhibition of electron transport (rotenone, antimycin A)
Inhibition of carbohydrate metabolism (fluoroacetate)

Binding to Biomolecules
Interference with enzyme functions
Lipid peroxidation (CCl_4, paraquat, ozone)
Free radical generation
Formation of lipid hydroperoxides
Oxidative stress
Depletion of GSH (acetaminophen)
Oxidation of protein thiols
Nucleic acids
DNA
RNA

Perturbation in Calcium Homeostasis
Cytoskeletal alterations
Activation of phospholipases
Activation of proteases
Activation of endonucleases

Toxicity from Selective Cell Loss
Hormonal and physiological imbalances (e.g., loss of dopaminergic neurons; thyroid insufficiency)
Birth defects

Nonlethal Genetic Alterations in Somatic Cells
Cancer
Initiation
Promotion
Birth defects and transplacental carcinogenesis

DESCRIPTIVE ANIMAL TOXICITY TESTS

Two main principles underlie all descriptive animal toxicity testing. The first is that the effects produced by the compound in laboratory animals, when properly qualified, are applicable to humans. This premise applies to all of experimental biology and medicine. On the basis of dose per unit of body surface, toxic effects in humans are usually in the same range as those in experimental animals. On a body weight basis, humans are generally more vulnerable than ex-

perimental animals, probably by a factor of about 10. With an awareness of these quantitative differences, appropriate safety factors can be applied to calculate relatively safe dosages for humans. All known chemical carcinogens in humans, with the possible exception of arsenic, are carcinogenic in some species but not in all laboratory animals. Whether the converse is true—that all chemicals carcinogenic in animals are also carcinogenic in humans—is not known with certainty, but this assumption serves as the basis for carcinogenicity testing in animals. This species variation in carcinogenic response appears to be due in many instances to differences in biotransformation of the procarcinogen to the ultimate carcinogen.

The second main principle is that exposure of experimental animals to toxic agents in high doses is a necessary and valid method of discovering possible hazards in humans. This principle is based on the quantal dose-response concept that the incidence of an effect in a population is greater as the dose or exposure increases. Practical considerations in the design of experimental model systems require that the number of animals used in toxicology experiments will always be small compared with the size of human populations similarly at risk. To obtain statistically valid results from such small groups of animals requires the use of relatively large doses so that the effect will occur frequently enough to be detected. For example, an incidence of a serious toxic effect, such as cancer, as low as 0.01 percent would represent 20,000 people in a population of 200 million and would be considered unacceptably high. To detect such a low incidence in experimental animals directly would require a minimum of about 30,000 animals. For this reason, there is no choice but to give large doses to relatively small groups and then to use toxicologic principles in extrapolating the results to estimate risk at low doses.

Toxicity tests are not designed to demonstrate that a chemical is safe but rather to characterize what toxic effects a chemical can produce. There are no set toxicology tests that have to be performed on every chemical intended for commerce. Depending on the eventual use of the chemical, the toxic effects produced by structural analogs of the chemical, as well as the toxic effects produced by the chemical itself, all contribute to determine what toxicology tests should be performed. However, the FDA, EPA, and Organization for Economic Cooperation and Development (OECD) have written good laboratory practice (GLP) standards. These guidelines are expected to be followed when toxicity tests are conducted in support of the introduction of a chemical to the market.

Acute Lethality

The first toxicity test performed on a new chemical is acute toxicity. The LD50 and other acute toxic effects are determined after one or more routes of administration (one route being oral or the intended route of exposure), in one or more species. The species most often used are the mouse and rat, but sometimes the rabbit and dog are employed. In mice and rats, the LD50 is usually determined as described earlier in this chapter, but in the larger species only an approximation of the LD50 is obtained by in-

creasing the dose in the same animal until serious toxic effects of the chemical are demonstrated. Studies are performed in both adult male and female animals. Food is often withheld the night prior to dosing. The number of animals that die in a 14-day period after a single dosage is tabulated. In addition to mortality and weight, daily examination of test animals should be conducted for signs of intoxication, lethargy, behavioral modifications, morbidity, food consumption, and so on. The acute toxicity tests give (1) a quantitative estimate of acute toxicity (LD50) for comparison to other substances, (2) identify target organs and other clinical manifestations of acute toxicity, (3) establish the reversibility of the toxic response, and (4) give dose-ranging guidance for other studies.

If there is a reasonable likelihood of substantial exposure to the material by dermal or inhalation exposure, then acute dermal and acute inhalation studies are performed. The acute dermal toxicity test is usually performed in rabbits. The site of application is shaven. The test substance is kept in contact with the skin for 24 hours by wrapping with an impervious plastic material. At the end of the exposure period, the wrapping is removed and the skin wiped to remove any test substance still remaining. Animals are observed at various intervals for 14 days and the LD50 calculated. If no toxicity is evident at 2 g/kg, further acute dermal toxicity testing is usually not performed. Acute inhalation studies are performed similar to the other acute toxicity studies except the route of exposure is inhalation. Most often, the length of exposure is four hours.

Skin and Eye Irritations

The ability of the chemical to irritate the skin and eye after an acute exposure is usually determined in rabbits. For the dermal irritation test (Draize test), rabbits are prepared by removal of fur on a section of their backs by electric clippers. The chemical is applied to the skin (0.5 ml of liquid or 0.5 g of solid) under four covered gauze patches (1-inch square; one intact and two abraded skin sites on each animal) and usually kept in contact for a period of four hours. The nature of the covering patches depends on whether occlusive, semiocclusive, or nonocclusive tests are desired. For occlusive testing, the test material is covered with an impervious plastic sheet, whereas for semiocclusive tests, a gauze dressing may be used. Occasionally, studies may require that the material be applied to abraded skin. The degree of skin irritation is scored for erythema, eschar and edema formation, and corrosive action. These dermal irritation observations are repeated at various intervals after the covered patch is removed. To determine the degree of ocular irritation, the chemical is instilled into one eye (0.1 ml of liquid or 100 mg of solid) of each of the test rabbits. The contralateral eye is used as the control. The eyes of the rabbits are then examined at various times after application.

Controversy over this test has led to a reevaluation of the procedure. Based on reviews of this procedure and additional experimental data, a panel on eye irritancy of the National Academy of Sciences (NAS) recommended lowering the dose volume (NAS, 1977). More recent studies suggest that a volume of 0.01 ml is as sensitive a method for eye irritancy testing as the 0.1 ml test but causes less pain to the animals (Chan and Hayes, 1989).

Sensitization

Information about the potential of a chemical to sensitize skin is needed in addition to irritation testing for all materials that may repeatedly come into contact with the skin. There are numerous procedures developed to determine the potential of substances to induce a sensitization reaction in humans (delayed hypersensitivity reaction), including the Draize test, the open epicutaneous test, the Buehler test, Freund's complete adjuvant test, optimization test, split adjuvant test, and the guinea pig maximization test (Patrick and Maibach, 1989). Although they differ by route and frequency of duration, they all utilize the guinea pig as the preferred test species. In general, the test chemical is administered to the shaved skin topically, intradermally, or both and may include the use of adjuvants to enhance the sensitivity of the assay. Multiple administrations of the test substance are generally given over a period of two to four weeks. Depending on the specific protocol, the treated area may be occluded. Two to three weeks after the last treatment, the animals are challenged with a nonirritating concentration of the test substance, and the development of erythematous responses is evaluated.

Subacute (Repeated-Dose Study)

The subacute toxicity tests are performed to obtain information on the toxicity of the chemical after repeated administration and as an aid to establish the doses for the subchronic studies. A typical protocol is to give three to four different dosages of the chemicals to the animals by mixing it in the feed. For rats, ten animals per sex per dose are often used, whereas for dogs three dosages and three to four animals per sex are used. Clinical chemistry and histopathology are performed after 14 days' exposure, as described below in the subchronic toxicity testing section.

Subchronic

The toxicity of the chemical after subchronic exposure is then determined. Subchronic exposure can last for different periods of time, but 90 days is the most common test duration. The principal goals of the subchronic study are to establish a no-observable effect level and to further identify and characterize the specific organ(s) affected by the test compound after repeated administration. The subchronic study is usually conducted in two species (rat and dog) by the route of intended exposure (usually oral). At least three doses are employed (a high dose that produces toxicity but does not cause more than 10 percent fatalities, a low dose that produces no apparent toxic effects, and an intermediate dose) with 10 to 20 rats and 4 to 6 dogs of each sex per dose. Each animal should be uniquely identified with permanent markings such as ear tags or tattoos. Only healthy animals should be used, and each animal should be housed individually in an adequately controlled environment. Animals should be observed once or twice daily for signs of toxicity, including body weight changes, diet consumption, changes in fur color or texture, respiratory or cardiovascular distress, motor and behavioral abnormalities, and palpable masses. All premature deaths should be recorded and necropsied as soon as possible. Severely moribund animals should be terminated immediately to preserve tissues and reduce unnecessary suffering. At the end of the 90-day study, all remaining animals should be terminated and blood and tissues collected for further analysis. Gross and microscopic condition of the organs and tissues (about 15 to 20) and the weight of the major organs (about 12) are recorded and evaluated. Hematology and blood chemistry measurements are usually done prior to, in the middle of, and at the termination of exposure. Hematology measurements usually include hemoglobin concentration, hematocrit, erythrocyte counts, total and differential leukocyte counts, platelet count, clotting time, and prothrombin time. Clinical chemistry determinations commonly made include glucose, calcium, potassium, urea nitrogen, alanine aminotransferase (ALT, formerly SGPT), serum aspartate aminotransferase (AST, formerly SGOT), gamma-glutamyltranspeptidase (GGT), sorbitol dehydrogenase, lactic dehydrogenase, alkaline phosphatase, creatinine, bilirubin, triglycerides, cholesterol, albumin, globulin, and total protein. Urinalysis is usually performed in the middle and at the termination of the testing period and often includes determination of specific gravity or osmolarity, pH, glucose, ketones, bilirubin, and urobilinogen as well as microscopic examination of formed elements. If humans are likely to have significant exposure to the chemical by dermal contact or by inhalation, subchronic dermal and/or inhalation experiments might also be required. The subchronic toxicity studies not only characterize the dose-response relationship of a test substance following repeated administration but also provide data for a more reasonable prediction of appropriate doses for the chronic exposure studies.

For chemicals that are to be registered as drugs, acute and subchronic studies (and potentially additional special tests if the chemical has unusual toxic effects or therapeutic purposes) must be completed before the company can file an IND (Investigative New Drug) with the FDA. If the IND application is approved, clinical trials can commence. At the same time that phase I, phase II, and phase III clinical trials are being performed, chronic exposure of the animals to the test compound can be carried out in laboratory animals as well as additional specialized tests.

Chronic

Long-term or chronic exposure studies are performed similarly to the subchronic studies except the period of exposure is longer than 3 months. In rodents, chronic exposures are usually for 6 months to 2 years. Chronic studies in nonrodent species are usually for 1 year but may be longer. The length of exposure is somewhat dependent on the intended period of exposure in humans. If the agent is a drug planned to be used for short periods of time, such as an antimicrobial agent, a chronic exposure of six months might be sufficient, whereas if the agent is a food additive with the potential of lifetime exposure in humans, then a chronic study up to two years in duration is likely to be required.

Chronic toxicity tests are performed to assess the cumulative toxicity of chemicals, but the study design and evaluation often include a consideration of the carcinogenic potential of chemicals so that a separate lifetime feeding study to address carcinogenicity does not have to be performed. These studies are usually performed in rats and mice and extend over the average lifetime of the species (18 months to 2 years for mice; 2 to 2.5 years for rats). To ensure that 30 rats per dose survive the 2-year study, 60 rats per group per sex are often started in the study. Both gross and microscopic pathologic examinations are made, not only on those animals that survive the chronic exposure but also on those that die prematurely.

Dose selection is critical in these studies to ensure that premature mortality from chronic toxicity does not limit the number of animals surviving to normal life expectancy. Most regulatory guidelines require that the highest dose administered be the estimated maximum tolerable dose (MTD). This is generally derived from subchronic studies, but additional, longer studies (e.g., six months) may be necessary if delayed effects or extensive cumulative toxicity are indicated in the 90-day subchronic study. The MTD has found various definitions (Haseman, 1985). The National Toxicology Program's (NTP) Bioassay Program currently defines the MTD as the dose that suppresses body weight gain slightly (i.e., 10%) in a 90-day subchronic study, although the NTP and other testing programs are critically evaluating the use of parameters other than weight gain, such as physiologic and pharmacokinetic considerations and urinary metabolite profiles as indicators of an appropriate MTD. Generally, one or two additional doses, usually fractions of the MTD (e.g., ½ and ¼ MTD), and a control group are tested.

The use of the MTD in carcinogenicity has been the subject of much controversy. The premise that high doses are necessary for testing the carcinogenic potential of chemicals is derived from the statistical and experimental design limitations of chronic bioassays.

Consider that a 0.5 percent increase in cancer incidence in the United States would result in over 1 million additional cancer deaths each year—clearly an unacceptably high risk. However, to identify with statistical confidence a 0.5 percent incidence of cancer in a group of experimental animals would require a minimum of 1000 test animals, and this assumes that no tumors were present in the absence of exposure (zero background incidence).

Figure 2–8 shows the statistical relationship between minimum detectable tumor incidence and the number of test animals per group. This curve shows that in a chronic bioassay with 50 animals per test group a tumor incidence of about 8 percent could exist even though no animals in the test group had tumors. This example assumes that there were also no tumors in the control group. These statistical considerations illustrate why animals are tested at doses higher than that which will occur in human exposure. As it is impractical to use the large number of animals that would be required to test the potential carcinogenicity of a chemical at the doses usually encountered by people, the alternative is to assume that there is a relationship between administered dose and tumorigenic response and to give animals doses of the chemical that are high enough to produce a measurable tumor response in a reasonable size test group—e.g., 40 to 50

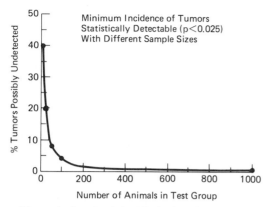

Figure 2–8. Statistical limitations in the power of experimental animal studies to detect tumorigenic effects.

animals per dose. The limitations of this approach will be discussed later in this chapter.

Developmental and Reproductive Toxicity

The effects of chemicals on reproduction and development also need to be determined. *Developmental toxicology* is the study of adverse effects on the developing organism occurring anytime during the life span of the organism that may result from exposure to chemical or physical agents prior to conception (either parent), during prenatal development, or postnatally until the time of puberty. *Teratology* is the study of defects induced during development between conception and birth. *Reproductive toxicology* is the study of the occurrence of adverse effects on the male or female reproductive system that may result from exposure to chemical or physical agents.

Four types of animal tests are utilized to examine the potential of an agent to alter development and reproduction. General fertility and reproductive performance (segment I or phase I) tests are usually performed in rats with two or three doses (20 rats per sex per dose) of the test chemical (neither produces maternal toxicity). Males are given the chemical 60 days and females 14 days prior to mating. The animals are given the chemical throughout gestation and lactation. Typical observations made are the percent of the females that become pregnant, the number of stillborn and live offspring, and the weight, growth, survival, and general condition of the offspring during the first 3 weeks of life.

Teratogenic potential of chemicals is also determined in laboratory animals (segment II). Teratogens are most effective when administered during the first trimester, the period of organogenesis. Thus, the animals (12 rabbits and 20 rats or mice per group) are usually exposed to one of three dosages during organogenesis (day 6 to 15 in rats and 6 to 18 in rabbits) and the fetuses removed by cesarean section a day prior to the estimated time of delivery (rabbit—day 31, rat—day 21). The uterus is excised and weighed, then examined for the number of live, dead, and resorbed fetuses. Live fetuses are weighed, and one-half of each litter is examined for skeletal abnormalities and the remaining one-half for soft tissue anomalies.

The perinatal and postnatal toxicities of chemicals are also often examined (segment III). This test is performed by administering the test compound to rats from the fifteenth day of gestation throughout delivery and lactation and determining its effect on birth weight, survival, and growth of the offspring during the first three weeks of life.

A multigeneration study is often carried out to determine the effects of chemicals on the reproductive system. At least three dosage levels are given to groups of 25 female and 25 male rats shortly after weaning (30 to 40 days of age). These rats are referred to as the F0 generation. Dosing continues throughout breeding (about 140 days of age), gestation, and lactation. The offspring (F1 generation) thus have been exposed to the chemical *in utero*, via lactation, and in the feed thereafter. When the F1 generation is about 140 days old, about 25 females and 25 males are bred to produce the F2 generation, and administration of the chemical is continued. The F2 generation is thus also exposed to the chemical *in utero* and via lactation. The F1 and F2 litters are examined as soon as possible after delivery. The percentage of F0 and F1 females that get pregnant, the number of pregnancies that go to full term, the litter size, number of stillborn, and number of live births are recorded. Viability counts and pup weights are recorded at birth, 4, 7, 14, and 21 days of age. The fertility index (percentage of mating resulting in pregnancy), gestation index (percentage of pregnancies resulting in live litters), viability index (percentage of animals that survive four days or longer), and lactation index (percentage of animals alive at four days that survived the 21-day lactation period) are then calculated. Gross necropsy and histopathology are performed on some of the parents (F0 and F1), with greatest attention being paid to the reproductive organs, and gross necropsy on all weanlings.

Numerous short-term tests for teratogenicity have been developed (Faustman, 1988). These tests utilize whole embryo culture, organ culture, and primary and established cell cultures to examine developmental processes and estimate potential teratogenic risks of chemicals. Many of these *in vitro* test systems are currently under evaluation for use in screening new chemicals for teratogenic effects. These systems vary in their ability to identify specific teratogenic events and alterations in cell growth and differentiation. In general, the assays available cannot identify functional or behavioral teratogens (Faustman, 1988).

Mutagenicity

Mutagenesis is the ability of chemicals to cause changes in the genetic material in the nucleus of cells in ways that can be transmitted during cell division. Mutations can occur in either of two cell types, with substantially different consequences. Germinal mutations damage DNA in sperm and ova, which can undergo meiotic division and therefore have the potential for transmission of mutations to future generations. If mutations are present at the time of fertilization in either the egg or sperm, the resulting combination of genetic material may not be viable, and death may occur in the early stages of embryonic cell division. Alternatively, the mutation in the genetic material may not affect early embryogenesis but may result in death of the fetus at a later developmental period, resulting in abortion. Congenital abnormalities may also result from mutations. Somatic mutations refer to mutations in all other cell types and are not heritable but may result in cell death or transmission of a genetic defect to other cells in the same tissue via mitotic division. Because the initiation event of chemical carcinogenesis is thought to be a mutagenic event, mutagenic tests are often used to screen for potential carcinogens.

Several *in vivo* and *in vitro* procedures have been devised for testing chemicals for their ability to cause mutations. Some genetic alterations are visible with the light microscope. In this case, cytogenetic analysis of bone marrow smears is used after the animals have been exposed to the test agent. Because some mutations are incompatible with normal development, the mutagenic potential of a chemical can also be measured by the dominant lethal test. This test is usually performed in rodents. The male is exposed to a single dose of the test compound and then mated with two untreated females weekly for eight weeks. The females are killed before term and the number of live embryos and the number of corpora lutea determined. The test for mutagens receiving the widest attention is the *Salmonella*/microsome test developed by Ames and colleagues (Ames *et al.*, 1975). This test uses several mutant strains of *Salmonella typhimurium* that lacks the enzyme phosphoribosyl ATP synthetase, which is required for histidine synthesis.

These strains are unable to grow in a histidine-deficient medium unless a reverse or back mutation to the wild type has occurred. Other mutations in these bacteria have been introduced to enhance the sensitivity of the strains to mutagenesis. The two most significant additional mutations enhance penetration of substances into the bacteria and decrease the ability of the bacteria to repair DNA damage. Since many chemicals are not mutagenic or carcinogenic unless they are biotransformed to a toxic product by the endoplasmic reticulum (microsomes), rat liver microsomes are usually added to the medium containing the mutant strain and the test chemical. The number of reverse mutations is then quantitated by the number of bacterial colonies that grow in a histidine-deficient medium. Mutagenicity is discussed in detail in Chapter 6.

Other Tests

Most of the tests described above will be included in a "standard" toxicity testing protocol because they are required by the various regulatory agencies. Additional tests may also be required or included in the protocol to provide information relating to a special route of exposure (inhalation) or to a special effect (behavior). Inhalation toxicity tests in animals are usually carried out in a dynamic (flowing) chamber rather than in static chambers, to avoid particulate settling and exhaled gas complications. Such studies usually require special dispersing and analytic methodologies depending on whether the agent to be tested is a gas, vapor, or aerosol; additional information on methods, concepts, and problems associated with inhalation toxicology is provided in Chapters 12 and 25 of this text. A discussion of behavioral toxicology can be found in Chapter 13 of this text. The duration of exposure for both inhalation and behavioral toxicity tests can be acute, subchronic, or chronic, but acute studies are more common with inhalation toxicology and chronic studies are more common with behavioral toxicology studies. Other special types of animal toxicity tests include immunotoxicology, toxicokinetics (absorption, distribution, biotransformation, and excretion), the development of appropriate antidotes and treatment regimes for poisoning, and the development of analytic techniques to detect residues of chemicals in tissues and other biologic materials. Approximate costs of some of the descriptive toxicity tests are given in Table 2–4.

PREDICTIVE TOXICOLOGY—RISK ASSESSMENT

In practical situations, the critical factor is not the intrinsic toxicity of a substance but the risk or hazard associated with its use. Risk is the probability that a substance will produce harm under

Table 2–4. TYPICAL COSTS OF DESCRIPTIVE TOXICITY TESTS

General Acute Toxicity	
Acute toxicity (rat; two routes)	$6,500
Acute dermal toxicity (rabbit)	3,000
Acute inhalation toxicity (rat)	6,500
Acute dermal irritation (rabbit)	900
Acute eye irritation (rabbit)	500
Skin sensitization (guinea pig)	700
Repeated Dose Toxicity	
14-day exposure (rat)	40,000
90-day exposure (rat)	100,000
1-year (diet; rat)	225,000
1-year (oral gavage; rat)	275,000
2-year (diet; rat)	625,000
2-year (oral gavage; rat)	800,000
Genetic Toxicology Tests	
Bacterial reverse mutation	1,850[a]–13,650[b]
Mammalian cell forward mutation	8,400[a]–13,650[b]
In vitro cytogenetics (CHO cells)	8,000[a]–19,000[b]
In vivo micronucleus (mouse)	10,775
In vivo chromosome aberration (rat)	26,500
Dominant lethal (mouse)	55,000
Drosophila sex-linked recessive lethal	35,000
Mammalian bone marrow cytogenetics (*in vivo;* rat)	26,500
Reproduction	
Segment I (rat)	95,000
Segment II (rat)	61,500
Segment II (rabbit)	66,500
Segment III (rat)	62,000
Acute toxicity in fish (LC50)	1,750
Daphnia reproduction study	1,750
Algae growth inhibition	1.750

[a] Minimum cost for U.S. registration.
[b] Worldwide registration.

specified conditions. Safety, the reciprocal of risk, is the probability that harm will not occur under specified conditions.

The term "hazard" is frequently used interchangeably with "intrinsic toxicity" in risk assessment guidelines (NAS, 1983), although some toxicologists have traditionally equated hazard with risk. Hazard has been defined as "the likelihood that injury will occur in a given situation or setting" (Plaa, 1989). Thus, hazard and risk are quite similar in meaning and include considerations of both intrinsic toxicity and the circumstances specific to exposure. Potentially highly toxic substances can be used safely pro-

vided one controls the environment to prevent exposure and/or absorption of sufficient quantities of the material to produce toxicity. In such a situation, although the chemical is highly toxic, it is not hazardous in the manner in which it is being used. Therefore, depending on the conditions under which it is used, a very toxic chemical may be less hazardous than a relatively nontoxic one.

Risk assessment is defined as "the characterization of the potential adverse health effects of human exposures to environmental hazards" (NAS, 1983). The process of risk assessment consists of several elements: (1) evaluation of the potential adverse health effects of a chemical, mixture of chemicals, or process, based on epidemiologic, clinical, toxicologic, and environmental research; (2) extrapolation from those results to predict the type and estimate the extent of health effects in humans under given conditions of exposure; (3) judgments as to the number and characteristics of persons exposed at various intensities and durations; (4) summary judgments on the existence and overall magnitude of the public health problem; and (5) characterization of the uncertainties inherent in the process of inferring risk (NAS, 1983).

Risk management, which should be distinct from *risk assessment,* is the process of weighing policy alternatives and selecting the most appropriate regulatory action, integrating the results of risk assessment with engineering data and with social, economic, and political concerns to reach a decision (NAS, 1983).

The process of risk assessment is commonly divided into four major steps: hazard identification, dose-response assessment, exposure assessment, and risk characterization (Figure 2–9). For a more comprehensive discussion, see Chapter 31.

The main purpose of the toxicity tests described in the preceding section of this chapter is to provide a data base that can be used to assess the risk (or evaluate the hazard) to humans associated with a situation in which the chemical agent, the subject, and the exposure conditions are defined. It is evident that the ideal situation is one in which the agent, the biologic system, and the exposure conditions used for the toxicity tests are identical to those for which risk assessment is desired. From the chronic toxicity studies in laboratory animals, one obtains a lowest-observed-effect level (LOEL), also referred to as the lowest-observed-adverse-effect level (LOAEL), as well as the no-observed-effect level (NOEL) for the species tested, also referred to as no-effect level (NEL) and no-observed-adverse-effect level (NOAEL). The NOEL is the highest dosage administered that does not pro-

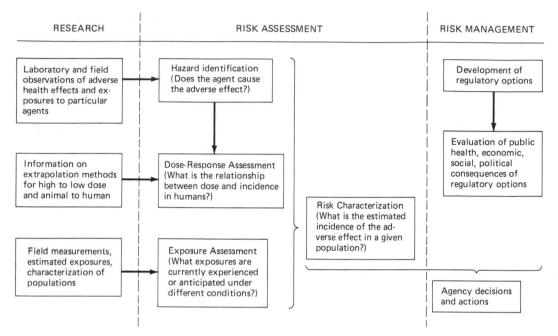

Figure 2–9. Elements of risk assessment and risk management. (From NAS: *Risk Assessment in the Federal Government*. National Academy Press, Washington, D.C., 1983.)

duce toxic effects. Thus, it is relatively easy to determine an approximate "safe" level of a compound for laboratory animals. However, the number obtained (NOEL) will depend on how closely the dosages are spaced (LOEL and NOEL) and the number of animals examined. The ultimate objective is usually to determine not the "safe" dosage in laboratory animals but the "safe" dosage for humans. Therefore, the extrapolation most often required of toxicologists is from high-dosage studies in laboratory animals to low doses in humans.

Thresholds

It has long been recognized that acute toxicological responses are associated with thresholds—that is, there is some dose below which the probability of an individual responding is zero. The biological basis of thresholds for acute responses is well founded and frequently can be demonstrated based on mechanistic information (Aldridge, 1986). The traditional approaches to establishing acceptable levels of exposure to chemicals are inherently different between threshold and nonthreshold responses. The existence of thresholds for chronic responses is less well defined, especially in the area of chemical carcinogenesis. It is, of course, impossible to scientifically prove the absence of a threshold, as one can never prove a negative. Nevertheless, for the identification of "safe" levels of exposure to a substance, the absence or

presence of a threshold is important for practical reasons.

"Safety" or Uncertainty Factors

Historically, the standard approach for establishing "acceptable" levels of exposure for chemicals that exhibit adverse effects in a "threshold" manner has been to reduce the NOEL by a safety or uncertainty factor that considers both intraspecies and interspecies differences. A safety factor of ten has been proposed for use in the rare instances where valid, chronic exposure data in humans are available. This factor of ten is often used to take into account the interindividual variability between humans, although it may be insufficient to protect the most susceptible individuals if idiosyncrasies are present. Most often, reliable chronic exposure data in humans are not available for the chemical in question, and one must extrapolate from chronic exposure studies in laboratory animals. A safety factor of 100 is often employed, with the justification of a factor of 10 for interindividual differences in the human population, and an additional factor of 10 for interspecies differences. When chemicals for which no reliable chronic exposure data in animals are available have to be regulated, an uncertainty factor of 1000 has been used. It should be emphasized that the primary purpose of safety factors is to establish exposure levels that are *protective* of human health; exposure levels derived from the use of safety factors are not intended to predict levels at which humans would respond. Thus, exposure of humans to a substance above the estimated "safe" level (animal NOEL/safety factor) does not imply that a toxic response is likely to occur.

The concept of safety factors and their application to the determination of "acceptable daily intakes," or ADIs, for many pesticides and food additives was established by the World Health Organization (WHO) in the early 1960s. The ADI was defined as "the daily intake of chemical which, during an entire lifetime, appears to be without appreciable risk on the basis of all known facts at the time" (WHO, 1962). A brief review of the history, use, and application of the ADI can be found in Lu (1988).

When a particular human exposure scenario is evaluated and compared with known toxicological data to determine the relative magnitude of the potential risk or hazard, "margins of safety" are often calculated. In this context, the margin of safety is the ratio of the NOEL determined in animals to the estimated daily dose to humans, in mg/kg/day, and thus is conceptually identical to a safety or uncertainty factor as described above. For example, a 70 kg individual who consumes 2 liters of water per day containing 1 ppm (1 mg/liter) of a chemical would ingest 2 mg of chemical each day, equivalent to a daily dose of 0.029 mg/kg/day. If the animal NOEL for this chemical was 100 mg/kg/day, then the margin of safety would be 3448 (100 divided by 0.029) for that chemical and that route of exposure. Margins of safety can be determined in this manner for a variety of exposure scenarios and for different toxicity end points, such as developmental, teratogenic, neurotoxic, or other tissue-specific effects. However, the estimated values determined in this manner do not consider the potential differences in sensitivity between humans and animals when dose is compared on a body weight basis, nor do they consider interindividual differences in sensitivity to chemicals that are likely to exist. Thus, a margin of safety of greater than 1 determined in this manner should not be construed as a "safe" level of exposure. Consistent with the "safety factor" approach discussed above, most regulatory agencies consider margins of safety calculated in this fashion as unacceptable unless they are at least greater than 100, or 1000 if the data upon which the NOEL was estimated are inadequate.

Because the terms "safety" and "acceptable" are value-laden and inherent in the ADI/safety factor approach to determining regulatory values for threshold responses, the EPA has modified the traditional procedure by explicitly standardizing "uncertainty factors" and including a

Table 2–5. MODELS USED IN RISK EXTRAPOLATION

Statistical or Distribution Models
  Log-probit
  Mantel-Bryan
  Logit
  Weibull

Mechanistic Models
  One-hit
  Gamma multihit (k-stage)
  Multistage (Armitage–Doll)
  Linearized multistage
  Stochastic two-stage (Moolgavkar-Venson-Knudson)

Model Enhancement
  Physiologically based pharmacokinetics (PB-PK)
  Time-to-tumor responses

"modifying factor," which is an additional uncertainty factor that allows for "professional judgment" in the estimation of allowable levels. Rather than referring to such regulatory values as acceptable, the term *reference dose,* or RfD, has been adopted (Barnes and Dourson, 1988). The procedure for calculating RfD values is obtained by dividing the NOEL determined in animal studies by the product of the uncertainty factors and the modifying factor. The difference between the traditional ADI approach and calculations of RfD is essentially semantic, although there is a more explicit process for estimating uncertainty factors than is present in the traditional ADI approach. The Food and Drug Administration also utilizes a similar approach to assess the relative safety of food additives in current use. A measure of relative concern, called an "R value," is determined as the ratio of the estimated human exposure to an additive to the lowest-observed-effect level (LOEL) in any tested species that shows a significant adverse effect in a suitable subchronic or chronic study (Rulis, 1987). The reciprocal of the R value (1/R) is referred to as a "safety assurance margin" and is similar to the margin of safety described above, except that a LOEL is used in place of a NOEL.

Quantitative Risk Extrapolation for "Nonthreshold" Effects

Numerous mathematical models have been developed for estimating the effects of exposure levels well below levels for which test data are available, with the goal that the risk will not be underestimated (i.e., they are conservative). The models commonly used in risk extrapolation are categorized in Table 2–5.

Statistical or Distribution Models. The distribution models are based on the assumption that every member of a population has a critical dosage below which the individual will not respond to the exposure in question (e.g., behaves in a threshold manner). These models also presume that the critical dosage varies among individuals and that this variability can be described in terms of a probability distribution. The log-probit model, as was discussed earlier in determination of the LD50, assumes that the distribution of log dose–responses is Gaussian (normal). It is therefore an extrapolation of the line obtained by plotting the experimental data on a probit versus $\log_{10}$ dosage scale to an "acceptable" level of lifetime risk such as 1×10^{-6} (e.g., one in a million). The log-probit model serves as the basis for the Mantel-Bryan extrapolation procedure (Mantel *et al.*, 1975). Rather than extend the slope of the observed log dose–probit response, this method uses a fixed slope of one (based on empirical knowledge or experimental carcinogenesis data that the slope is usually much greater than one) starting from the upper confidence limit of the observed proportion of animals with tumors at the experimental exposure level. The premise of this method is that the true dose-response curve lies somewhere below the extrapolation line passing through the upper confidence limit with a slope of one, thereby predicting a higher proportion of tumors than that which actually occurs at lower doses. The Logit model, like the probit model, leads to an S-shaped curve, symmetric about the 50 percent response point. However, it approaches zero response with decreasing dose more slowly than the log dose–probit curve. The Logit model thus results in a "virtually" safe dose that is about 25 times lower than that obtained with the probit model (Food Safety Council, 1980). The Weibull model (also called the "extreme value" model) was originally described as an empirical distribution that adequately modeled the strength of materials and has also been used to model time to failure of electrical and mechanical components. Its adaptation to dose-response data for carcinogens is also empirical and essentially assumes that each animal has its own tolerance to the carcinogen used in the experiment (Hanes and Wedel, 1985). In general, the Weibull model gives low dose extrapolation results between the multihit and multistage models (see below).

Mechanistic Models. Mechanistic models are based on a presumed mechanism of chemical carcinogenesis. As noted previously, the process of chemical carcinogenesis has widely been regarded as a nonthreshold phenomenon, in which a single and irreversible mutagenic event in a "normal" cell could give rise to a transformed cell, which then expands in a clonal fashion at a rate independent of the initial concentration or continued presence of the chemical. It has further been assumed that the probability of a single cell being transformed to a cancer cell is a linear function of the amount of carcinogen. These simplistic mechanistic assumptions about the process of chemical carcinogenesis form the basis of the so-called "one-hit" theory, in which even a single molecule of a genotoxic carcinogen would have some small but finite theoretical probability of causing cancer. However, it is now widely recognized that chemical carcinogenesis is likely to be a multistep process, and that the one-hit theory is overly simplistic as a biological model. Thus, additional models that attempt to consider this multistep process of carcinogenesis have been developed. A generalization of the one-hit model, called the gamma multihit model, assumes a Poisson distribution process where several "hits," or mutations, may be required before a single cell is transformed to a potentially cancerous one. At higher doses, this model is similar to a log normal distribution but behaves more like a Logit model at low doses. Because of the way in which this model treats background estimates, and the way it behaves if the dose-response curve is hyperlinear, the model may provide unrealistic "safe dose" estimates and thus is not considered "conservative," for example, is less likely to underestimate actual risk (Hanes and Wedel, 1985).

Armitage and Doll (1961) developed an alternative model that assumed that the production of a transformed cell was a multistep process requiring more than one change but still assumed that a malignant tumor could originate from a single transformed cell. This multistage model generally behaves in a linear fashion at low doses for direct carcinogenic processes in which the chemical or its metabolite produce irreversible and transmissible changes in a cell (Crump *et al.*, 1976). Thus, the slope of the dose-response curve in the low-dose region can provide an estimate of the carcinogenic potency of a chemical, with units of change in incidence per unit dose.

A mathematical procedure for estimating the slope of the one-hit model at doses well below the experimental range, referred to as β, has been described. This procedure generates a "maximum likelihood estimate" (MLE) slope of the extra risk predicted by the one-hit model when fitted to bioassay data. Crump *et al.* (1977) developed a procedure for estimating β that incorporates the multistage assumptions of Armitage and Doll but also includes a parameter that forces linearity of the model at low doses and utilizes the upper statistical confidence limits on risk, rather than the MLE. The MLE can be very sensitive to small changes in the experimental data (i.e., is unstable), whereas the upper bounds estimate of risk tends to be less influenced by small changes in the data set and is also more conservative (Park, 1989). This "linearized" multistage model, which was revised in 1984 (Crump, 1984), has been widely used in quantitative risk assessment procedures.

In addition to providing an estimate of the slope of the dose-response curve at low doses (e.g., carcinogenic potency), the linearized multistage and other similar models have been used to estimate a "virtually safe dose" (VSD) for a variety of chemical carcinogens. The VSD represents the daily lifetime dose that would yield a theoretical extra risk (above background) of some "acceptable" level. Just as the estimate of potency, β, utilizes the 95 percent upper bounds estimate of the slope, so does the VSD use the lower limits on dose and thus is also likely to be "conservative."

The EPA has utilized quantitative risk assessment procedures to establish a "unit risk" estimate for individual carcinogens. The unit risk is defined as the increased individual lifetime risk for a 70 kg individual breathing air containing 1 $\mu g/m^3$, or drinking 2 liters of water containing 1 mg/liter (ppm), of the chemicals for a 70-year life span (Anderson, 1983).

Although all the mechanistic models discussed above attempt to consider the biology of carcinogenesis by incorporating the notion of multiple steps or stages in the process, they remain rather simplistic and cannot account for differential effects on the rate of cell proliferation and other important considerations in the stepwise development of cancer that proceeds from the initiating molecular events.

Recently, new models for risk extrapolation have been proposed that attempt to consider more fully such biological processes in the extrapolation process. For example, the Moolgavkar-Venson-Knudson (MVK) model is based on a two-stage cell growth model that considers the birth and death rates of cells in the process of clonal expansion and offers a means to incorporate additional biological considerations into carcinogenicity modeling. It assumes that two specific, irreversible, and rate-limiting mutational events are necessary for a cancer to develop and provides for effects on cell proliferation that can increase the pool of initiated cells available for transformation (Moolgavkar, 1986). This model has been shown to be consistent with human epidemiological data for at least some types of cancers and is receiving increased attention for application to quantitative risk assessment procedures. The model is capable of addressing quantitatively such different phenomena as initiation/promotion, synergism/antagonism, and genetic predisposition to cancer. The major limitation of this model is that many of the important biological parameters that are allowed by the model, and thus make it biologically relevant, are often not readily available.

Model Enhancement.

Physiologically Based Pharmacokinetics. Although not required by the mathematical models, for the purposes of risk extrapolation it is generally assumed that the "exposed" dose is proportional to the "target" dose. However, if dose-dependent absorption, biotransformation, distribution, or excretion occurs, then the relationship between exposed dose and target dose will not be proportional at all doses.

It is known that many chemicals are only carcinogenic after they have been biotransformed. The amount of reactive metabolite formed might not be directly related to dosage because the enzyme that forms the reactive metabolite might become saturated at higher doses, or there may be depletion of cosubstrate. This is referred to as *nonlinear pharmacokinetics* (*see* Chapter 3). After the reactive metabolite is formed, it is often destroyed by a second enzyme, such as epoxide hydrolase or glutathione transferase (*see* Chapter 4). These enzymes can also be saturated. The reactive metabolites that are not destroyed by these detoxication pathways often bind to DNA. But the metabolites bound to DNA can be removed by various DNA repair systems. These systems also can be saturated. Figure 2–10 shows different dose-response curves that theoretically would result if there were no saturation (simple first-order kinetics), saturation of only the activation system, saturation of both the detoxication and repair systems, and saturation of activation, detoxication, and repair systems.

To account for such factors, physiologically based pharmacokinetic (PB-PK) models are finding increasing use in the process of risk assessment (Whitmore *et al.*, 1986; Bischoff, 1987; Menzel, 1987). The principal purpose of PB-PK modeling is to predict the concentration of carcinogen at the target site and describe the relationship between *exposed* dose and *target* dose over a range of concentrations. Once such a relationship is established and the important rate processes that cause a deviation from linearity between exposed dose and target dose are identified, this deviation can be corrected for species differences by incorporating the appropriate species-specific value. PB-PK models have been used in quantitative risk assessments for several halogenated hydrocarbons such as dichloromethane (Andersen *et al.*, 1987), trichloroethane

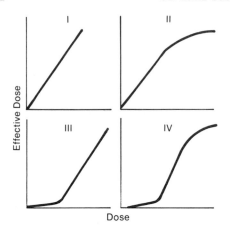

Figure 2–10. Possible relation between administered dose and effective dose for different kinetic models: *I*, simple first-order kinetics: *II*, saturation of the activation system: *III* and *IV*, combination of II and III. (*See* text for explanation; modified from Hoel, D. G.; Kaplan, N. L.; and Anderson, M. W.: Implications of nonlinear kinetics on risk estimation in carcinogenesis. *Science,* **219**, 1032–1037, 1983.)

(Bogen and Hall, 1989), and tetrachloroethylene (Travis, 1987). Such considerations can have a large influence on the predicted risk levels. For example, based on measured metabolic differences, Andersen *et al.* (1987) estimated that target tissue doses in humans exposed to low concentrations of dichloromethane in drinking water would be from 50- to 210-fold lower than would be expected from the linear extrapolation and body surface area factors used in covential risk assessment procedures. In many ways, PB-PK models are simply a specific means of determining the most appropriate "scaling factor" to use in cross species extrapolations (see below). The major disadvantage of the use of PB-PK modeling in quantitative risk assessment is that the measured parameters are often difficult to obtain and require knowledge of human metabolic processes that may be highly variable and difficult to assess. Nevertheless, the development of PB-PK models should provide a more scientific basis for quantitative risk assessment and may also help to improve the experimental design of chronic studies used for risk assessment procedures.

Biological Indicators of Target Dose. The use of biological markers as an index of target dose has been proposed as a means of enhancing the biological basis of quantitative risk assessment. For example, Hoel *et al.* (1983) presented a nonlinear kinetic model that predicts tumor response as a function of concentration of DNA adducts formed in the target organ. Their model is based on the assumption that for genotoxic agents the carcinogenic response in laboratory animals is related to the extent of DNA adduct formation in target tissues. Formation of chemical-hemoglobin adducts, excretion of DNA adducts in urine, and changes in lymphocyte chromosomal abnormalities (e.g., sister-chromatid exchange frequency) are all examples of potential biological markers that may prove useful in risk assessment procedures.

Time-to-Tumor. Time-to-tumor considerations stem from the realization that there is often an inverse relationship between carcinogenic potency and the time from first exposure necessary to produce detectable tumors. Thus, for potent carcinogens, tumors may become evident within several months after exposure, whereas tumors may not appear until the end of the animals' life span for weak carcinogens. Time-to-tumor considerations have been utilized in some mathematical models for risk assessment. For example, the Weibull function has been incorporated into the linearized multistage model to allow for consideration of time-to-tumor formation.

It is possible to make risk characterizations from animal tumor data without mathematical modeling of dose-response data by using time-to-tumor data and life table analysis (Sielkin, 1989). This approach considers the period of time in which animals remain tumor free, relative to control animals. Incorporation of time-to-tumor data with dose-response data often yields a more biologically meaningful interpretation of experimental data than dose-response data alone. For carcinogenic responses that increase tumor response only in the very late stages of life, the incorporation of time-to-tumor information can have a large effect on risk characterization. For example, human risk characterization of ethylene oxide exposure using time-to-tumor data from a rat bioassay indicates that the estimated human cancer risk for 0 to 50 years is 3000 times smaller than the estimated risk from 0 to 70 years, even when the same dose-response data and human exposure assumptions are used (Sielkin, 1989).

UNCERTAINTIES IN QUANTITATIVE RISK ASSESSMENT

The use of mathematical models to extrapolate animal data to estimate human risk is a controversial issue. Although the need to assess hazards of chemicals is clear, and the value of experimental animals studies to conduct scientifically sound appraisals of risk is widely accepted, the uncertainties and assumptions inherent in quantitative risk assessment are profound. Among the most controversial assumptions are selection of the appropriate mathematical model, relevance of high doses in experimental testing to low-dose human exposures, and selection of the appropriate means of dose conversion between animals and humans. These assumptions are discussed briefly below. There have been many published reviews of these and other controversial issues in quantitative risk assessment in recent years, which the reader is referred to for a more in-depth discussion (Food Safety Council, 1980; Krewski and Brown, 1981; Moolgavkar, 1986; Freedman and Zeisel, 1988; Haseman, 1989; Park, 1989).

Selection of Mathematical Model

The various models used in risk extrapolation usually fit the observed data equally well but can predict widely different potential risks at low doses. With the standard bioassay design of two, or at most three, experimental dose groups, the statistical determination of "goodness of fit" is of relatively little value in making decisions between models. Furthermore, even if the data fit well in the high-dose region, there is little biological justification to assume that the shape of the curve at high doses in test animals accurately reflects the shape at much lower doses in humans. Because of sometimes large differences in behavior of the various models in the low-dose region, model selection can be as important as the actual experimental data in the ultimate risk analysis.

To understand what is involved in the process of extrapolating carcinogenic responses obtained at high doses in experimental animals to the generally much lower human doses of potential environmental concern, the dose response curves for four carcinogens tested in animal bioassays are presented in Figure 2-11. To facilitate the comparison, the actual doses administered to the test animals, which are quite different among the different carcinogens shown, have been normalized to the lowest dose used that produced a detectable tumor response in each study. Thus, the relative dose ranges, rather than actual doses, are shown on the abscissa, and doses where no response occurred are not plotted. The lower panel shows the same data plotted on log-log scales that have been expanded to include both the dose range for estimated human exposures and response regions of regulatory concern (e.g., 1 additional cancer per million exposed, or 10^{-6}).

For each of these data sets, the daily human dose that would result in a theoretical excess (additive to background) risk of 1 in a million (virtually safe dose, VSD) was determined for four risk assessment models. To facilitate the comparison, the projected risk from the one-hit

model was set equal to 1 for each carcinogen, and the risk estimates derived for the other models are then expressed relative to the one-hit model (Table 2-6). Also shown in Table 2-6 is the relative "goodness of fit" of the experimental data to each mathematical model, expressed as a p value. It essentially represents the probability that another data set will fit the model more poorly. Thus, the higher the p value, the better the fit. It is evident from the results of this comparison that the selection of extrapolation model can have a substantial impact on the estimated VSD—up to eight orders of magnitude in one instance (vinyl chloride). Generally, the one-hit model provides the highest estimate of risk (lowest VSD), although it generally fits the data poorly. However, for vinyl chloride, where the data exhibit an unusual concave shape at higher doses, the opposite is true. The concave shape of this curve has been explained by pharmacokinetic effects that may result in a divergence of effective dose and administered dose at high exposure levels (Gehring et al., 1978). Utilization of only the four lowest doses results in much better concordance between models (Van Ryzin and Rai, 1980). Some of the experiments shown in Figure 2-11 and Table 2-6 are unusual in that four or five dose groups, in addition to a control, were available, which allow for some distinction in the goodness of fit of the models and thus could provide some statistical rationale for selection of one model over another. Unfortunately, for carcinogens tested in the standard two- or three-dose testing protocols, the data are generally too limited to obtain a meaningful estimate of goodness of fit (Food Safety Council, 1980). Even in those instances where the data fit the models equally well, there can be differences in risk estimates of several orders of magnitude. For example, with aflatoxin there is a 400-fold difference in estimated VSD between the multistage and multihit models.

Scaling Factors

Scaling factors are a means for correcting species differences in cross-species comparisons. From a mechanistic perspective, scaling factors implicitly consider two independent physiological processes: (1) differences in pharmacokinetics, which determine the actual dose delivered to target tissues, and (2) differences in tissue sensitivity between species to an identical delivered dose. In practice, scaling factors seldom incorporate such considerations explicitly but rather use dose adjustments across species based on some normalizing factor such as body weight or surface area. The most common form of scaling factor is body weight. This is largely empirical, as discussed previously (Table 2-2).

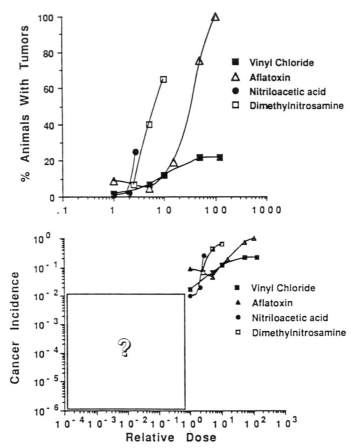

Figure 2–11. Illustration of the process of low-dose extrapolation. The *upper panel* represents a "traditional" log-dose–response plot of data from four carcinogenicity bioassays. The *lower panel* is the same data plotted on a log-log scale to demonstrate the range in dose extrapolation that is performed by the mathematical models. Doses have been normalized by setting the lowest dose group with a tumor response equal to 1. The actual dose ranges and routes of exposure for the four carcinogens are: vinyl chloride, 50–6000/ppm (inhalation); aflatoxin, 1–100 ppb (diet); nitriloacetic acid, 7,500–20,000 ppm (diet); dimethylnitrosamine, 5–20 ppm (diet). Only the data that had a positive response are shown. In these four studies, none of the animals in the control groups developed tumors. (Adapted from Food Safety Council: Quantitative risk assessment. *Food Cosmet. Toxicol.*, **18**: 711–734, 1980.)

Table 2–6.   DIFFERENCES IN MODEL-DERIVED ESTIMATES OF VIRTUALLY SAFE DOSES (VSDS) AT 10^{-6} RISK LEVEL, RELATIVE TO THE ONE-HIT MODEL.*

CARCINOGEN	ONE-HIT	LINEARIZED MULTISTAGE	WEIBULL	MULTIHIT
Vinyl chloride	1 (0.03)	1 (0.03)	1×10^{-7} (0.56)	2×10^{-8} (0.32)
Aflatoxin	1 (0.07)	20 (0.49)	1,000 (0.64)	8,000 (0.54)
Nitriloacetic acid	1 (< 0.001)	10 (0.09)	30,000 (0.48)	40,000 (0.48)
Dimethylnitrosamine	1 (0.04)	600 (0.57)	600 (0.63)	200 (0.72)

* The numbers shown represent the difference in VSD estimates compared with that obtained from the one-hit model. Values in parentheses represent the *p* value for goodness of fit of the data to the model. Data are derived from Food Safety Council: Quantitative risk assessment. *Food Cosmet. Toxicol.* **18**: 711–734, 1980.

The most appropriate scaling factor to use in interspecies extrapolations for carcinogenicity has been extensively debated. Surface area, which is roughly equivalent to (body weight) $^{2/3}$, may be a more accurate scaling factor between species than body weight directly (Davidson et al., 1986). Correlative data between measured human responses and animal responses support the use of the (body weight) $^{2/3}$ factor, although use of $3/4$ as the exponent provides a better fit of the data (Travis and White, 1988). However, the results of a comparison of human epidemiologic data with animal bioassay data for 23 known human carcinogens suggest that use of body weight directly may be more accurate (Allen et al., 1988). It is well recognized that no single scaling factor is going to be adequate in all circumstances and that incorporation of case-specific factors such as pharmacokinetics is required for the most scientifically defensible cross-species extrapolations (Brown et al., 1988).

Application of Quantitative Risk Assessment to Noncarcinogenic End Points

Although the procedures for quantitative extrapolation of laboratory animal data to estimated human exposures have largely focused on cancer risks, there have been some efforts to develop dose-response models for extrapolation of noncarcinogenic end points such as developmental toxicity. Rai and Van Ryzin (1985) described a model that characterizes dichotomous dose-response data from teratology studies using a conditional probability model. This has recently been more fully characterized, with results supporting the concept that such models may prove useful in risk assessment for developmental toxicity (Faustman et al., 1989).

Alternative Approaches to Quantitative Risk Assessment

Because of the many scientific uncertainties and assumptions present in the process of quantitative risk assessment, alternative approaches to the evaluation of carcinogenic risk have been proposed. As much of the uncertainty lies in the extrapolation from high doses to low, and from rodents to humans, Gold and colleagues have suggested a procedure to allow comparative evaluation of risks that is not dependent on either of these extrapolations (Gold et al., 1984, 1989; Ames et al., 1987). This approach involves an estimation of the TD50 in animals, which is defined as "the dose rate (in mg/kg/day) that, if administered chronically for a standard period—the 'standard lifespan' of the species—will halve the mortality-corrected estimate of the probability of remaining tumorless throughout that peri-

od" (Ames et al., 1987). This is similar in concept to the LD50 for acute toxicity but allows for consideration of background incidence of tumors and premature deaths that are unrelated to chemical exposure. As defined, the TD50 does not distinguish between fatal and incidental tumors. It can, however, be determined for specific tumor sites and/or types, as well as for total tumors. A data base of TD50s and their statistical upper and lower 95 percent confidence limits has been constructed for nearly 1000 chemicals tested for carcinogenicity in animal bioassays (Gold et al., 1984; a compilation of TD50 values for 492 chemicals that have tested positive for carcinogenicity can be found in Gold et al., 1989). By comparing the ratio of the estimated human exposed dose to the TD50 in rodents, a comparative index of possible carcinogenic hazard can be obtained that is not dependent on high- to low-dose extrapolation, or even cross-species differences (Ames et al., 1987). This procedure does not offer an indication of actual risk or tumor incidence in humans but rather provides a means of comparing one risk to another based on the carcinogenic potency of the chemical in rodents. Ames refers to this index of possible hazard as the "HERP" index (human exposed dose to rat potency dose) (Table 2–7). For example, the TD50 for chloroform-induced hepatomas in mice is estimated to be approximately 90 mg/kg/day, based on a combination of data from multiple studies (Gold et al., 1984). Drinking 1 liter of tap water containing 83 ppb of chloroform (83 μg) would then have an HERP value of 0.001 ([(0.083 mg/70 kg) /90 mg/kg] × 100)). While this value by itself is rather meaningless, when HERP values for other situations are calculated, a simple and convenient means of comparing risk results. This approach explicitly avoids a prediction of tumor incidence but does offer a convenient means of comparing one risk to another without relying on mathematical extrapolation well below the region of measured tumorigenic response in the experimental animals. This approach has been used to compare carcinogenic risks from pollutants to that from naturally occurring carcinogens (Ames et al., 1987), although the conclusions derived from such comparisons can be substantially influenced by the assumptions used to estimate human exposures (Perera and Boffetta, 1988).

QUALITATIVE RISK ASSESSMENT

Because of the numerous limitations and uncertainties associated with quantitative risk assessment procedures, it is essential that the assumptions and uncertainties utilized in quantitative risk estimates be explicitly noted. It

Table 2–7. COMPARISON OF RELATIVE CARCINOGENIC RISK USING THE TD50/HERP APPROACH[*]

CHEMICAL	SOURCE	ESTIMATED HUMAN DOSE	TD50 (mg/kg)	HERP (%)
Chloroform	Tap water (1 liter)	83 μg	90	0.001
Aflatoxin	Peanut butter (1 oz)	64 ng	0.003	0.03
Ethylene dibromide	Grain products	0.42 μg (U.S. avg)	1.5	0.0004
Polychlorinated biphenyls	Daily diet	0.2 μg (U.S. avg)	1.7	0.0003
Dimethylnitrosamine	Bacon (100 g)	0.3 μg	0.2	0.003

[*] Adapted from Ames, B. N.; Magaw, R.; and Gold, L. W.: Ranking possible carcinogenic hazards. *Science,* **236**: 271–280, 1987.

should be emphasized that in many instances where quantitative cancer risk estimates have been projected, the true value of risk is somewhere between zero and the projected upper bounds of risk. Thus, the potency factor derived from a quantitative risk assessment provides useful, but by itself insufficient, information to make informed judgments about the hazards of a chemical. In addition to the final results of a chronic bioassay, all other available and relevant scientific evidence should be considered when evaluating the potential human health and environmental hazards associated with a particular chemical or process. This approach, sometimes referred to as a "weight of evidence" determination of risk, entails consideration of all relevant scientific information about the chemical. In addition to a critical evaluation of the design and performance of the chronic bioassay, other available information such as mutagenicity assays, human epidemiology studies, metabolism and pharmacokinetics, mechanistic information, and structure-activity relationships should be considered in the final assessment.

Determining "Acceptable Risk"

Important factors often considered by regulatory agencies in establishing socially acceptable risk levels are shown in Table 2–8. The level of risk deemed acceptable is of course influenced by many factors in addition to the estimate of risk. Such decisions are multifaceted, complex, and highly value-laden and should involve a consideration of risks, benefits, and trade-offs. The elimination of a particular chemical or procedure seldom eliminates risk but rather substitutes one risk for another, as alternative chemicals or activities that themselves have some risk are usually invoked in place of the first. Although the acceptable level of risk is inherently chemical and situation-specific, regulatory agencies have seldom taken action when the estimated theoretical upper bounds of cancer risk is less than 1 in a

million (Rodricks *et al.,* 1987). This level has been proposed as a *de minimus,* or negligible, risk level.

Almost every aspect of modern living exposes people to health risks. Table 2–9 lists the estimated lifetime risks associated with a variety of activities. It should be noted that these estimates are based on actuarial data and thus represent best estimates of actual risk, rather than a theoretical upper bound estimate of risk. The lifetime

Table 2–8. SOME FACTORS CONSIDERED IN ESTABLISHING ACCEPTABLE RISK LEVELS

Beneficial Aspects of the Chemical
  Economic growth
  Employment
  Increased standard of living
  Increased quality of life
  Taxes generated

Detrimental Aspects of the Chemical
  Decreased quality of life
  Emotional difficulties
  Health effects
  Lawsuits
  Loss of environmental resources
  Loss of work
  Medical payments

Table 2–9. ESTIMATED LIFETIME RISKS FROM VARIOUS SOURCES[*]

CAUSES OF DEATH	LIFETIME RISK
Measles	1.5×10^{-6}
Smallpox vaccination	5.0×10^{-6}
Lightning	3.0×10^{-5}
Electrocution	3.0×10^{-4}
Drowning	2.5×10^{-3}
Falls	6.0×10^{-3}
Motor vehicles	1.5×10^{-2}

[*] These statistical estimates are based on actuarial data and thus represent best estimates of risk, rather than "upper bounds" on risk. Lifetime risk estimates are derived by multiplying annual deaths by 70 years, then dividing by the total U.S. population.

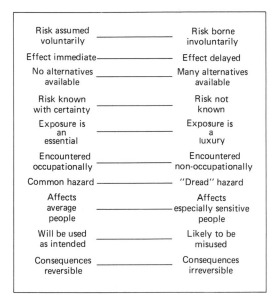

Risk assumed voluntarily	Risk borne involuntarily
Effect immediate	Effect delayed
No alternatives available	Many alternatives available
Risk known with certainty	Risk not known
Exposure is an essential	Exposure is a luxury
Encountered occupationally	Encountered non-occupationally
Common hazard	"Dread" hazard
Affects average people	Affects especially sensitive people
Will be used as intended	Likely to be misused
Consequences reversible	Consequences irreversible

Figure 2–12. Considerations that influence acceptability of risk. (From Lowrance, W. W.: *Of Acceptable Risk: Science and the Determination of Safety.* Kaufmann, Inc., Los Altos, Calif., 1976.)

risk estimates for activities shown in Table 2–9 are normalized to the population at large, rather than the population at risk. Obviously, the risks of dying in an auto accident are not the same for individuals who drive frequently, relative to those who seldom drive. Although risk comparisons are most meaningful when similar risk types are compared (e.g., one type of cancer risk with another; risk of one mode of transportation with another; *etc.*), it is sometimes useful to consider the universe of common risks to gain perspective on individual risks. When estimates of theoretical lifetime risk from exposure to carcinogenic chemicals obtained from quantitative risk assessment procedures are discussed, it is important to note that the denominator in the risk expression represents the population *at risk* (e.g., risk per million individuals *who meet all of the assumptions of the exposure scenario*) and *not* the population at large. This is very important when considering aggregate risk (e.g., the estimate of the number of individuals in a population who will be affected), because the population at risk and the population at large may be very different. The area of "risk communication" has become increasingly important in many areas of science and technology, including toxicology. A recent review of problems and approaches to risk communication has been published by the National Academy of Sciences (NAS, 1989).

Acceptability of individual risk is largely influenced by one's own perception of the risk. Figure 2–12 shows numerous factors that influence risk perception and acceptability of risk. Whether the risk is voluntary or is imposed involuntarily, the personal benefits derived from undertaking the risk, and the immediacy of the risk are all very important factors in acceptability of individual risk (Lowrance, 1976; NAS, 1989). Because those who reap the benefits are often different from those who bear the risks, when setting levels of acceptable risk, regulatory agencies must consider the aggregate social risks and benefits of their regulatory actions.

REFERENCES

Abou-Setta, M. M.; Sorrell, R. W.; and Childers, C. C.: A computer program in BASIC for determining probit and log-probit or Logit correlation for toxicology and biology. *Bull. Environ. Contam. Toxicol.,* **36**:242–249, 1986.

Albert, A.: Fundamental aspects of selective toxicity. *Ann. N.Y. Acad. Sci.,* **123**:5–18, 1965.

———: *Selective Toxicity.* Chapman and Hall, London, 1973.

Aldridge, W. N.: The biological basis and measurement of thresholds. *Annu. Rev. Pharmacol. Toxicol.,* **26**:39–58, 1986.

Allen, B. C.; Crump, K. S.; and Shipp, A. M.: Correlation between carcinogenic potency of chemicals in animals and humans. *Risk Anal.,* **8**:531–561, 1988.

Ames, B. N.; Magaw, R.; and Gold, L. W.: Ranking possible carcinogenic hazards. *Science,* **236**:271–280, 1987.

Ames, B.; McCann, J.; and Yamasaki, E.: Methods for detecting carcinogens and mutagens with the *Salmonella*/mammalian microsome mutagenicity test. *Mutat. Res.,* **31**:347–364, 1975.

Andersen, M. E.; Clewell, H. J., III; Gargas, M. L.; Smith, F. A.; and Reitz, R. H.: Physiologically based pharmacokinetics and the risk assessment process for methylene chloride. *Toxicol. Appl. Pharmacol.,* **87**:185–205, 1987.

Anderson, E. L., and Carcinogen Assessment Group (CAG) of the Environmental Protection Agency.: Quantitative approaches in use to assess cancer risk. *Risk Anal.,* **3**:277–295, 1983.

Ariens, E. J.; Wius, E. W.; and Veringa, E. J.: Stereoselectivity of bioactive xenobiotics. *Biochem. Pharmacol.* **37**:9–18, 1988.

Armitage, P. and Doll, R.: Stochastic model for carcinogenesis. In Lecam, W., and Heyman, J. (eds.): *Proceedings of the Fourth Berkeley Symposium on Mathematical Statistics and Probability,* Vol. 4. University of California Press, Berkeley, Calif., 1961, pp. 19–38.

Barnes, D. G., and Dourson, M.: Reference dose (RfD): description and use in health risk assessments. *Reg. Toxicol. Pharmacol.,* **8**:471–486, 1988.

Bischoff, K. B.: Physiologically based pharmacokinetic modeling. In *Pharmacokinetics in Risk Assessment.* National Academy Press, Washington D.C., 1987.

Bliss, C. L.: Some principles of bioassay. *Am. Sci.,* **45**:449–466, 1957.

Bogen, K. T., and Hall, L. C.: Pharmacokinetics for regulatory risk analysis: the case of 1,1,1-trichloroethane (methyl chloroform). *Reg. Toxicol. Pharmacol.,* **10**:26–50, 1989.

Boobis, A. R.; Fawthrop, D. J.; and Davis, D. S.: Mechanisms of cell death. *TiPS*, **10**:275–280, 1989.

Brown, S. L.; Brett, S. M.; Gough, M.; Rodericks, J. V.; Tardiff, R. G.; and Turnbull, D.: Review of interspecies risk comparisons. *Reg. Toxicol. Pharmacol.*, **8**:191–206, 1988.

Bruce, R. D.: An up-and-down procedure for acute toxicity testing. *Fundam. Appl. Toxicol.*, **5**:151–157, 1985.

———: A confirmatory study of the up-and-down method of acute oral toxicity testing. *Fundam. Appl. Toxicol.*, **8**:97–100, 1987.

Bryan, W. R., and Shimkin, M. B.: Quantitative analysis of dose-response data obtained with three carcinogenic hydrocarbons in strain C3H male mice. *J. Natl. Cancer Inst.*, **3**:503–531, 1943.

Chan, P. K., and Hayes, A. W.: Principles and methods for acute toxicity and eye irritancy. In Hayes, A. W. (ed.): *Principles and Methods of Toxicology*, 2nd ed. Raven Press, New York, 1989, pp. 169–220.

Covello, V. T.; Sandman, P. M.; and Slovic, P.: *Risk Communication, Risk Statistics, and Risk Comparisons: A Manual for Plant Managers*. Chemical Manufacturers Association, Washington, D.C., 1988.

Crump, K. S.: An improved procedure for low-dose carcinogenic risk assessment from animal data. *J. Environ. Pathol. Toxicol.*, **5**:339–348, 1984.

Crump, K. S.; Guess, H. A.; and Deal, K. L.: Confidence intervals and tests of hypotheses concerning dose-response relations inferred from animal carcinogenicity data. *Biometrics*, **33**:437–451, 1977.

Crump, K. S.; Hoel, D. C.; Langely, C. H.; and Peto, R.: Fundamental carcinogenic processes and their implication for low dose risk assessment. *Cancer Res.*, **36**:2973–2977, 1976.

Davidson, I. W. F.; Parker, J. C.; and Beliles, R. P.: Biological basis for extrapolation across mammalian species. *Reg. Toxicol. Pharmacol.*, **6**:211–237, 1986.

Doull, J.: Factors influencing toxicity. In Doull, J.; Klaassen, C. D.; and Amdur, M. O. (eds.): *Casarett and Doull's Toxicology: The Basic Science of Poisons*, 2nd ed. Macmillan Publishing Co., New York, 1980.

DuBois, K. P.: Potentiation of the toxicity of organophosphorus compounds. *Adv. Pest Control Res.*, **4**:117–151, 1961.

Faustman, E. M.: Short-term tests for teratogens. *Mutat. Res.*, **205**:355–384, 1988.

Faustman, E. M.; Wellington, D. G.; Smith, W. P.; and Kimmel, C. A.: Characterization of a developmental toxicity dose-response model. *Environ. Health Perspect.*, **79**:229–241, 1989.

Finney, D. J.: *Probit Analysis*. Cambridge University Press, Cambridge, 1971.

———: The median lethal dose and its estimation. *Arch. Toxicol.*, **56**:215–218, 1985.

Food Safety Council: Quantitative risk assessment. *Food Cosmet. Toxicol.*, **18**:711–734, 1980.

Freedman D. A., and Zeisel, H.: From mouse-to-man: quantitative assessment of cancer risks. *Stat. Sci.*, **3**:3–56, 1988.

Gehring, P. J.; Watanabe, P. G.; and Park, C. N.: Resolution of dose response toxicity data for chemicals requiring metabolic activation: example—vinyl chloride. *Toxicol. Appl. Pharmacol.*, **44**:581–591, 1978.

Goering, P. L., and Klaassen, C. D.: Altered subcellular distribution of cadmium following cadmium pretreatment: possible mechanism of tolerance to cadmium-induced lethality. *Toxicol. Appl. Pharmacol.*, **70**:195–203, 1983.

Gold, L. S.; Sawyer, C. B.; Magaw, R.; Backman, G. M.; de Veciana, M.; Levinson, R.; Hooper, N. K.; Havender, W. R.; Bernstein, L.; Peto, R.; Pike, M.; and Ames, B. N.: A carcinogenic potency database of the standardized results of animal bioassays published through December 1982. *Environ. Health Perspect.*, **67**:161–200, 1984.

Gold, L. S.; Slone, T. H.; and Bernstein, L.: Summary of carcinogenic potency and positivity for 492 rodent carcinogens in the carcinogenic potency database. *Environ. Health Perspect.*, **79**:259–272, 1989.

Goldstein, A.; Aronow, L; and Kalman, S. M.: *Principles of Drug Action*. John Wiley & Sons, Inc., New York, 1974.

Hanes, B., and Wedel, T.: A selected review of risk models: one hit, multihit, multistage, probit, Weibull and pharmacokinetic. *J. Am. Coll. Toxicol.*, **4**:271–278, 1985.

Haseman, J. K.: Issues in carcinogenicity testing: dose selection. *Fundam. Appl. Toxicol.*, **5**:66–78, 1985.

———: Sources of variability in rodent carcinogenicity studies. *Fundam. Appl. Toxicol.*, **12**:793–804, 1989.

Hayes, W. J., Jr.: *Toxicology of Pesticides*. Williams & Wilkins Co., Baltimore, 1975.

Hoel, D. G.; Kaplan, N. L.; and Anderson, M. W.: Implications of nonlinear kinetics on risk estimation in carcinogenesis. *Science*, **219**:1032–1037, 1983.

Krewski, D., and Brown, C.: Carcinogenic risk assessment: a guide to the literature. *Biometrics*, **37**:353–366, 1981.

Levine, R. R.: *Pharmacology: Drug Actions and Reactions*, 2nd ed. Little, Brown & Co., Boston, 1978.

Litchfield, J. T., Jr.: A method for rapid graphic solution of time-percent effective curve. *J. Pharmacol. Exp. Ther.*, **97**:399–408, 1949.

Litchfield, J. T., and Wilcoxon, F.: Simplified method of evaluating dose-effect experiments. *J. Pharmacol. Exp. Ther.*, **96**:99–113, 1949.

Loomis, T. A.: *Essentials of Toxicology*, 3rd ed. Lea & Febiger, Philadelphia, 1978.

Lowrance, W. W.: *Of Acceptable Risk: Science and the Determination of Safety*. Kaufmann, Inc., Los Altos, Calif., 1976.

Lu, F. C.: Acceptable daily intake: inception, evolution, and application. *Reg. Toxicol. Pharmacol.*, **8**:45–60, 1988.

Lutz, W. K., and Maier, P.: Genotoxic and epigenetic chemical carcinogenesis: one process, different mechanisms. *TiPS*, **9**:322–326, 1988.

Mantel, N.; Bohidar, N. R.; Brown, C. C.; Ciminera, J. L.; and Tukey, J. W.: An improved "Mantel Bryan" procedure for "safety testing" of carcinogens. *Cancer Res.*, **35**:865–872, 1975.

Menzel, D. B: Physiological pharmacokinetic modeling. *Environ. Sci. Technol.*, **21**:944–950, 1987.

Moolgavkar, S. H.: Carcinogenesis modeling: from molecular biology to epidemiology. *Annu. Rev. Public Health*, **7**:151–169, 1986.

Murphy, S. D., and Cheever, K. L.: Effects of feeding insecticides: inhibition of carboxylesterase and cholinesterase activities in rats. *Arch. Environ. Health*, **17**:749–756, 1968.

NAS, Committee for Revision of NAS Publication 1138: Dermal and eye toxicity tests. In *Principles and Procedures for Evaluating the Toxicity of Household Substances*. National Academy of Sciences, Washington, D.C., 1977, pp. 41–54.

NAS: *Improving Risk Communication*. National Academy Press, Washington D.C., 1989.

———: *Risk Assessment in the Federal Government: Managing the Process*. National Academy Press, Washington D.C., 1983.

Orrenius, S.; McConkey, D. J.; Bellomo, G.; and Nicotera, P.: Role of Ca^{2+} in toxic cell killing. *TiPS*, **10**:281–285, 1989.

Park, C. N.: Mathematical models in quantitative assessment of carcinogenic risk. *Reg. Toxicol. Pharmacol.*, **9**:236–243, 1989.

Patrick, E., and Maibach, H. I.: Dermatotoxicology. In Hayes, A. W. (ed.): *Principles and Methods of Toxicology*, 2nd ed. Raven Press, New York, 1989, pp. 383–406.

Perera, F., and Boffetta, P.: Perspective on comparing risk of environmental carcinogens. *J. Natl. Cancer Inst.*, **80**:1282–1293, 1988.

Plaa, G. L.: Introduction to toxicology: occupational & environmental toxicology. In Katzgun, B. G. (ed.): *Basic and Clinical Pharmacology*, 4th ed. Lang Publishers, Los Altos, Calif., 1989.

Rai, K., and Van Ryzin, J.: A dose response model for teratological experiments involving quantal responses. *Biometrics*, **41**:1–10, 1985.

Rodricks, J. V.; Brett, S. M.; and Wrenn, G. C.: Significant risk decisions in federal regulatory agencies. *Reg. Toxicol. Pharmacol.*, **7**:307–320, 1987.

Rulis, A. M.: Safety assurance margins for food additives currently in use. *Reg. Toxicol. Pharmacol.*, **7**:160–168, 1987.

Sielkin, R. L.: A time-to-response perspective on ethylene oxide's carcinogenicity. In Paustenbach, D. J. (ed.): *The Risk Assessment of Environmental Hazards*. Wiley Interscience, New York, 1989, chap. 4.

Thompson, W. R., and Weil, C. S.: On the construction of tables for moving average interpolation. *Biometrics*, **8**:51–54, 1952.

Travis, C. C.: Interspecies extrapolations in risk analysis. *Toxicology*, **9**:3–13, 1987.

Travis, C. C., and White, R. K.: Interspecific scaling of toxicity data. *Risk Anal.*, **8**:119–125, 1988.

Trevan, J. W.: The error of determination of toxicity. *Proc. R. Soc. Lond. (Biol.)*, **101**:483–514, 1927.

Van Ryzin, J., and Rai, K.: The use of quantal response data to make predictions. In Witschi, H. P. (ed.): *The Scientific Basis of Toxicity Assessment*. Elsevier/North Holland, New York, 1980, pp. 273–290.

Weil, C. S.: Tables for convenient calculation of median-effective dose (LD_{50} or ED_{50}) and instruction in their use. *Biometrics*, **8**:249–263, 1952.

Whitmore, A. S.; Grosser, S. C.; and Silvers, A.: Pharmacokinetics in low dose extrapolation using animal cancer data. *Fundam. Appl. Toxicol.*, **7**:183–190, 1986.

WHO: Principles governing consumer safety in relation to pesticide residues. *WHO Tech. Rep. Ser.* 240, 1962.

Wilson, R., and Crouch, E. A. C.: Risk assessment and comparisons: an introduction. *Science*, **236**:267–269, 1987.

Chapter 3

ABSORPTION, DISTRIBUTION, AND EXCRETION OF TOXICANTS

Curtis D. Klaassen and *Karl Rozman*

INTRODUCTION

As noted in the last chapter, the toxicity of any substance depends on the dose—that is, the higher the amount of a chemical taken up by an organism, the greater the toxic response. This concept, known as *dose-response*, requires further elaboration because ultimately it is not the dose but the concentration of a toxicant at the site(s) of action [target organ(s)] that determines toxicity. It should be noted that the words *toxicant, drug, xenobiotic* (= foreign compound), and *chemical* are used interchangeably throughout this text, since all chemical entities, endogenous or exogenous in origin, can cause toxicity at some dose. The concentration of any chemical at the site of action is proportional to the dose. But the same dose of two or more chemicals may lead to vastly different concentrations in a particular target organ of toxicity. This differential pattern is due to differences in the disposition of chemicals. Disposition may be conceptualized as consisting of absorption, distribution, biotransformation, and excretion. It should be noted, however, that these processes may occur simultaneously. The various factors affecting disposition are depicted in Figure 3–1. They will be discussed in detail in this chapter and Chapter 4. Any or all these factors may have a minor or major impact on the concentration and thus the toxicity of a chemical in a target organ. For example, (1) if the fraction absorbed or the rate of absorption is low, then a chemical may never attain sufficiently high concentrations at a potential site of action to cause toxicity; (2) the distribution of a toxicant may be such that it is concentrated in a tissue other than the target organ, thereby decreasing toxicity; (3) biotransformation of a chemical may result in the formation of less or more toxic metabolites at a fast or slow rate with obvious consequences for the concentration and thus toxicity at the target site; and (4) the more rapidly a chemical is eliminated from an organism, the lower will be its concentration and hence toxicity in (a) target

tissue(s). Furthermore, all these processes are interrelated and thus influence each other. For example, the rate of excretion of a chemical may depend to a large extent on its distribution and/or biotransformation. If a chemical is distributed to and stored in fat, its elimination is likely to be slow, because very low plasma levels preclude rapid renal or other clearances. Some lipid-soluble chemicals are very resistant to biotransformation. Their rate of excretion depends on biotransformation to water-soluble products and/or slow intestinal excretion of the parent compounds. As this brief introduction illustrates, disposition of xenobiotics is very important in determining the concentration and hence the toxicity of chemicals in organisms.

Quantitation and determination of the time course of absorption, distribution, biotransformation, and excretion of chemicals are referred to as *pharmacokinetics* or *toxicokinetics*. Mathematical models are used to describe parts or the whole process of disposition of a chemical. Calculations based on these models allow a numerical characterization of disposition (half-life, elimination rate constants, tissue profiles, *etc.*), which is essential for the assessment of the toxicity of a given compound. Examination of species differences combined with knowledge of species-specific pathways of handling chemicals often provides the tools for toxicologists to predict disposition and its role in the toxicity of a compound for human exposure.

The skin, lungs, and alimentary canal are the main barriers separating higher organisms from an environment that contains a large number of chemicals. Toxicants need to cross one or several of these incomplete barriers to exert their deleterious effects at one or several sites of the body. Exceptions are caustic and corrosive agents (acids, bases, salts, oxidizers), which act topically. A chemical absorbed through any of these three barriers into the bloodstream is distributed, at least to some extent, throughout the body, including the site where it produces damage. This site is often called the *target organ* or

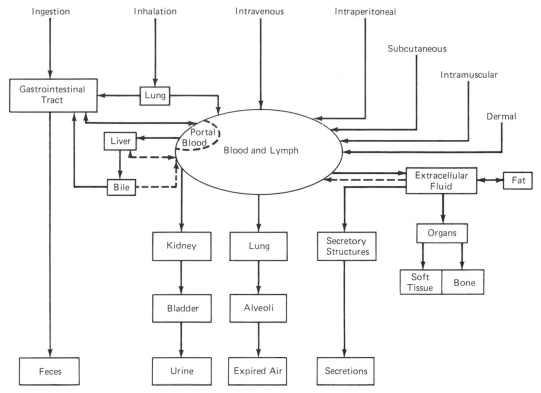

Figure 3–1. Routes of absorption, distribution, and excretion of toxicants in the body.

target tissue. A chemical may have one or several target organs, and in turn, several chemicals may have the same target organ(s). For example, benzene affects the hematopoietic system, and carbon tetrachloride the liver. Lead and mercury both damage the central nervous system, kidney, and the hematopoietic system. It is self-evident that in order to produce a direct toxic effect in an organ, a chemical must reach that organ. However, indirect toxic responses may be precipitated at distant sites if a toxicant alters regulatory functions. For example, cholestyramine, a nonabsorbable resin, may trap certain acidic vitamins in the intestinal lumen and cause systemic toxicity in the form of various vitamin deficiency syndromes. Several factors, other than the concentration, influence the susceptibility of organs to toxicants. Therefore, the organ or tissue with the highest concentration of a toxicant is not necessarily the site where toxicity is exerted. For example, chlorinated hydrocarbon insecticides (e.g., dichlorodiphenyltrichloroethane [DDT]) attain the highest concentrations in fat depots of the body but produce no known toxic effect in this tissue. A toxicant may also exert its adverse effect directly on the bloodstream, as is the case with arsine gas, which causes hemolysis.

Toxicants are removed from the systemic circulation by biotransformation, excretion, and storage at various sites of the body. The relative contribution of these processes to total elimination depends on the physical and chemical properties of the chemical. The kidney plays a major role in the elimination of most toxicants, but other organs may be of critical importance for some toxic agents. Examples include elimination of a volatile agent such as carbon monoxide by the lungs or that of lead in the bile. Although the liver is the most active organ in the biotransformation of toxicants, other organs or tissues (enzymes in plasma, kidney, lungs, gastrointestinal tract, etc.) may also contribute to overall biotransformation. Biotransformation often is a prerequisite for renal excretion, because many toxicants are lipid soluble and are therefore reabsorbed from the renal tubules after glomerular filtration. After a toxicant is biotransformed, its metabolites may be excreted preferentially into bile, as are the metabolites of DDT, or they may be excreted into urine, as are the metabolites of organophosphate insecticides.

In this chapter, qualitative and quantitative aspects of absorption, distribution, and excretion will be outlined. The fourth aspect of disposition, biotransformation of chemicals, will be dealt with in Chapter 4. As most toxic agents need to pass several membranes before exerting toxicity, we will start with a discussion of some general characteristics of this ubiquitous barrier in the body.

CELL MEMBRANES

Toxicants usually pass through a number of cells, such as the stratified epithelium of the skin, the thin cell layers of the lungs or of the gastrointestinal tract, the capillary endothelium, and the cells of the target organ(s) or tissue(s). The plasma membranes surrounding all these cells are remarkably similar. The thickness of the cell membrane is about 7 to 9 nm. Biochemical, physiological, and morphological (electron microscopy) studies provide strong evidence that membranes consist of a phospholipid bilayer with polar head groups (phosphatidyl choline, phosphatidyl ethanolamine) predominating on both outer and inner surfaces of the membrane and more or less perpendicularly directed fatty acids filling out the inner space. It is also quite well established that proteins are inserted in the bilayer, and some even cross it, allowing the formation of aqueous pores (Figure 3–2). Some cell membranes (eukaryotic) have an outer coat or glycocalyx consisting of glycoproteins and glycolipids. The fatty acids of the membrane do not have a rigid crystalline structure but are quasi fluid at physiological temperatures. The fluid character of membranes is largely determined by the structure and relative abundance of unsaturated fatty acids. The more unsaturated fatty acids membranes contain, the more fluidlike

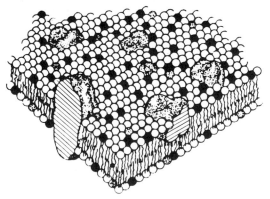

Figure 3–2. Schematic model of a biologic membrane. *Spheres* represent the ionic and polar head groups of the phospholipid molecules, different types being represented as black, white, or stippled. *Zigzag lines* represent the fatty acid chains. Proteins associated with the membrane are represented by the large bodies with *crosshatching.*

they are, facilitating more rapid active or passive transport.

A toxicant may pass through a membrane by one of two general processes: (1) passive transport (diffusion according to Fick's law) in which the cell expends no energy; and (2) specialized transport, in which the cell provides energy for translocating the toxicant across its membrane.

Passive Transport

Simple Diffusion. Most toxicants cross membranes by simple diffusion. Small hydrophilic molecules (up to a molecular weight of about 600 daltons) presumably permeate membranes through aqueous pores (Benz et al., 1980), whereas hydrophobic molecules diffuse across the lipid domain of membranes. The smaller a hydrophilic molecule, the more readily it traverses membranes by simple diffusion through aqueous pores. Consequently, ethanol is rapidly absorbed from the stomach and intestine and equally rapidly distributed throughout the body by simple diffusion from blood into all tissues. The majority of toxicants consist of larger organic molecules with differing degrees of lipid solubility. Their rate of transport across membranes correlates with their lipid solubility, which is frequently expressed as hexane/water or chloroform/water partition coefficients.

Many chemicals are weak organic acids or bases. In solution, they are ionized according to the theory of Arrhenius. The ionized form usually has low lipid solubility and hence does not readily permeate through the lipid domain of a membrane. Some transport of organic anions and cations (depending on molecular weight) may occur through the aqueous pores, but this is a slow process (except for very low molecular-weight compounds), as the total surface area of aqueous pores compared with the total surface area of the lipid domain of a membrane is small. In general, the nonionized form of weak organic acids and bases is to some extent lipid soluble, resulting in diffusion across the lipid domain of a membrane. The rate of transport of the nonionized form is proportional to its lipid solubility. The molar ratio of ionized to nonionized molecules of a weak organic acid or base in solution depends on the ionization constant. The ionization constant provides a measure for the weakness of organic acids and bases. The pH at which a weak organic acid or base is 50 percent ionized is called its pK_a or pK_b. Like the pH, the pK_a and pK_b are defined as the negative logarithm of the ionization constant of a weak organic acid or base. With the equation $pK_a = 14 - pK_b$, pK_a's can also be calculated for weak organic bases. An organic acid with a low pK_a is a relatively strong acid, and one with a high pK_a a weak acid. The opposite is true for bases. The numerical value of pK_a does not tell whether a chemical is an organic acid or a base. Knowledge of the chemical structure is required to distinguish between organic acids and bases.

The degree of ionization of a chemical depends on its pK_a and on the pH of the solution. The relationship between pK_a and pH is described by the Henderson-Hasselbalch equations:

$$\text{For acids: } pK_a - pH = \log\frac{[\text{nonionized}]}{[\text{ionized}]}$$

$$\text{For bases: } pK_a - pH = \log\frac{[\text{ionized}]}{[\text{nonionized}]}$$

The effect of pH on the degree of ionization of an organic acid (benzoic acid) and of an organic base (aniline) is shown in Figure 3–3. According to the Brönsted-Lowry acid-base theory, an acid is a proton (H^+) donor and a base is a proton acceptor. Thus, the ionized and the nonionized form of an organic acid represent an acid-base pair, the nonionized moiety being the acid, the ionized moiety the base. At a low pH, a weak organic acid, such as benzoic acid, is largely nonionized. At pH 4, exactly 50 percent of benzoic acid is ionized and 50 percent is nonionized, because this is the pK_a of the compound. As the pH increases, more and more protons are neutralized by hydroxyl groups, and benzoic acid continues to dissociate until almost all of it is in the ionized form. For an organic base like aniline, the obverse is true. At a low pH, when protons are abundant, almost all of aniline is protonated, viz., ionized. This form of aniline is an acid because it can donate protons. As the pH increases, anilinium ions continue to dissociate until almost all of aniline is in the nonionized form, which is the aniline base. As transmembrane passage is largely restricted to the nonionized form, benzoic acid will be more readily translocated through a membrane from an acidic environment, whereas more aniline will be transferred from an alkaline environment.

pH	Benzoic Acid	% Nonionized	Aniline	% Nonionized
1	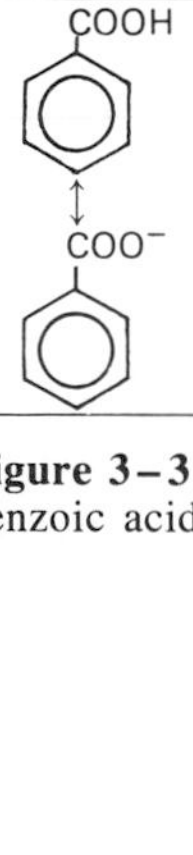 COOH	99.9	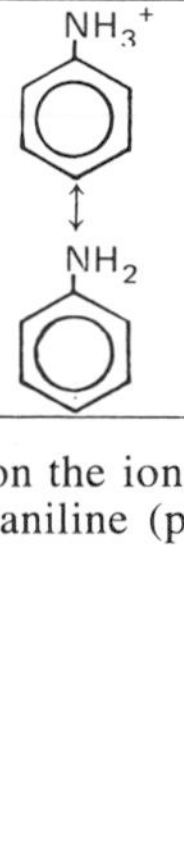 NH₃⁺	
2		99		0.1
3		90		1
4		50		10
5		10		50
6	COO⁻	1	NH₂	90
7		0.1		99

Figure 3–3. Effect of pH on the ionization of benzoic acid ($pK_a = 4$) and aniline ($pK_a = 5$).

Filtration. When water flows in bulk across a porous membrane, any solute that is small enough to pass through the pores flows with it. Passage through these channels is called *filtration,* as it involves bulk flow of water, owing to hydrostatic or osmotic force. One of the main differences between various membranes is the size of these channels. In the kidney glomeruli, these pores are relatively large (about 70 nm), allowing molecules smaller than albumin (molecular weight 60,000) to pass through. The channels in most cells are much smaller (<4 nm), permitting substantial passage of molecules with molecular weights of no more than a few hundred daltons (Schanker, 1961, 1962).

Special Transport

There are numerous examples of compounds whose movement across membranes cannot be explained by simple diffusion or filtration. Some compounds are too large to pass through aqueous pores or too insoluble in lipids to diffuse across the lipid domains of membranes. Nevertheless, they often are transported very rapidly across membranes, even against concentration gradients. To explain these phenomena, the existence of specialized transport systems has been postulated. These are responsible for the transport across cell membranes of many nutrients like sugars and amino and nucleic acids and also of some foreign compounds.

Active Transport. The following properties characterize an active transport system: (1) Chemicals are moved against electrochemical or concentration gradients; (2) the transport system is saturated at high substrate concentrations and thus exhibits a transport maximum (T_m); (3) the transport system is selective for certain structural features of chemicals and has the potential for competitive inhibition between compounds to be transported by the same transporter; and (4) the system requires expenditure of energy so that metabolic inhibitors block the transport process.

Substances actively transported across cell membranes presumably form a complex with a membrane-bound macromolecular carrier on one side of the membrane. The complex subsequently traverses to the other side of the membrane where the substance is released. Thereafter, the carrier returns to the original surface to repeat the transport cycle.

Active transport is particularly important to eliminate xenobiotics from the organism. The central nervous system has two transport systems at the choroid plexus to transport compounds out of the cerebrospinal fluid, one for organic acids and one for organic bases. The kidney also has two active transport systems, whereas the liver has at least four, two of which transport organic acids, one organic bases, and one neutral organic compounds.

Facilitated Diffusion. This term applies to carrier-mediated transport exhibiting the properties of active transport, except that the substrate is not moved against an electrochemical or concentration gradient, and the transport process does not require input of energy; viz. metabolic poisons do not interfere with this transport. The transport of glucose from the gastrointestinal tract across the basolateral membrane of the intestinal epithelium, from plasma into red blood cells and from blood into the central nervous system, occurs by facilitated diffusion.

Additional Transport Processes. Other forms of specialized transport have been proposed, but their overall importance is not as well established as that of active transport and of facilitated diffusion. Phagocytosis and pinocytosis are proposed mechanisms of cell membranes flowing around and engulfing particles. So far, this type of transfer has been shown to be important for removal of particulate matter from the alveoli by phagocytes and from blood by the reticuloendothelial system of liver and spleen.

ABSORPTION

The process whereby toxicants cross body membranes and enter the bloodstream is referred to as *absorption*. No specific systems or pathways exist for the sole purpose of absorbing toxicants. Xenobiotics penetrate membranes during absorption by the same processes as do biologically essential substances like oxygen, foodstuffs, and other nutrients. The main sites of absorption are the gastrointestinal tract, lungs, and the skin. However, absorption may also occur from other sites such as the subcutis, peritoneum, or muscle if a chemical is administered by special routes. Experimentalists and medical professionals often distinguish between parenteral and enteral administration of drugs and other xenobiotics. It is important to know that enteral administration includes all routes pertaining to the alimentary canal (sublingual, oral, and rectal), whereas parenteral administration depicts all other routes (intravenous, intraperitoneal, intramuscular, subcutaneous, etc.).

Absorption of Toxicants by the Gastrointestinal Tract

The gastrointestinal tract is one of the most important sites where toxicants are absorbed. Many environmental toxicants enter the food chain and are absorbed together with food from the gastrointestinal tract. This site of absorption is of particular interest to toxicologists because

suicide attempts frequently involve an overdose of an orally ingested drug. Oral intake is also the most common route by which children are accidentally exposed to poisons.

The gastrointestinal tract may be viewed as a tube traversing the body. Although within the body, its contents can be considered exterior to it. Therefore, poisons in the gastrointestinal tract usually do not produce systemic injury to an individual until absorbed, unless a noxious agent has caustic or irritating properties.

Absorption of toxicants can take place along the entire gastrointestinal tract, even in the mouth and rectum. Therefore, some drugs such as nitroglycerin are administered sublingually and others rectally, whereas the majority of drugs are given orally. If a toxicant is an organic acid or base, it will tend to be absorbed by simple diffusion in that part of the gastrointestinal tract in which it exists in the most lipid-soluble (nonionized) form. Because gastric juice is acidic, and the intestinal contents are nearly neutral, the lipid solubility of weak organic acids or bases can differ markedly in these two areas of the gastrointestinal tract. One can determine by the Henderson-Hasselbalch equations the fraction of a toxicant that is in the nonionized (lipid-soluble) form and estimate the rate of absorption from the stomach or the intestine. According to this equation, a weak organic acid is mainly

FOR WEAK ACIDS

$$pK_a - pH = \log \frac{[\text{nonionized}]}{[\text{ionized}]}$$

Benzoic acid $pK_a \approx 4$

Stomach pH ≈ 2

$$4 - 2 = \log \frac{[\text{nonionized}]}{[\text{ionized}]}$$

$$2 = \log \frac{[\text{nonionized}]}{[\text{ionized}]}$$

$$10^2 = \frac{[\text{nonionized}]}{[\text{ionized}]}$$

$$100 = \frac{[\text{nonionized}]}{[\text{ionized}]}$$

Ratio favors absorption

Intestine pH ≈ 6

$$4 - 6 = \log \frac{[\text{nonionized}]}{[\text{ionized}]}$$

$$-2 = \log \frac{[\text{nonionized}]}{[\text{ionized}]}$$

$$10^{-2} = \frac{[\text{nonionized}]}{[\text{ionized}]}$$

$$\frac{1}{100} = \frac{[\text{nonionized}]}{[\text{ionized}]}$$

present in the nonionized (lipid-soluble) form in the stomach and predominantly in the ionized form in the intestine. Therefore, one would expect that weak organic acids would be more readily absorbed from the stomach than from the intestine. In contrast, organic bases (unless a very weak organic base) are not in the lipid-soluble form in the stomach but are so in the intestine, suggesting that absorption of such compounds occurs predominantly in the intestine rather than in the stomach. However, the Henderson-Hasselbalch equations have to be interpreted with some qualifications, because other

FOR WEAK BASES

$$pK_a - pH = \log \frac{[\text{ionized}]}{[\text{nonionized}]}$$

Aniline $pK_a \approx 5$

Stomach pH ≈ 2

$$5 - 2 = \log \frac{[\text{ionized}]}{[\text{nonionized}]}$$

$$3 = \log \frac{[\text{ionized}]}{[\text{nonionized}]}$$

$$10^3 = \frac{[\text{ionized}]}{[\text{nonionized}]}$$

$$1000 = \frac{[\text{ionized}]}{[\text{nonionized}]}$$

Intestine pH ≈ 6

$$5 - 6 = \log \frac{[\text{ionized}]}{[\text{nonionized}]}$$

$$-1 = \log \frac{[\text{ionized}]}{[\text{nonionized}]}$$

$$10^{-1} = \frac{[\text{ionized}]}{[\text{nonionized}]}$$

$$\frac{1}{10} = \frac{[\text{ionized}]}{[\text{nonionized}]}$$

Ratio favors absorption

factors such as the mass action law, surface area, and blood flow rate also have to be taken into consideration when examining the absorption of weak organic acids or bases. For example, only 1 percent of benzoic acid is present in the lipid-soluble form in the intestine. Therefore, one might conclude that the intestine has little capacity to absorb this organic acid. However, absorption is a dynamic process. The blood keeps removing benzoic acid from the lamina propria of the intestine, and according to the mass action law, the equilibrium will always be maintained at 1 percent in the nonionized form, providing continuous availability of benzoic acid for absorption. Moreover, absorption by simple diffusion is also proportional to the surface area. Because the small intestine has a very large sur-

face (the villi and microvilli increase the surface area approximately 600-fold), the overall capacity of the intestine for absorption of benzoic acid is quite large. Similar considerations are valid for the absorption of all weak organic acids from the intestine.

The mammalian gastrointestinal tract has specialized transport systems (carrier-mediated) for the absorption of nutrients and electrolytes (Table 3–1). The absorption of some of these substances is complex and depends on a number of factors. The absorption of iron, for example, depends on the need for iron, and it takes place in two steps: Iron first enters the mucosal cells and then moves into the blood. The first step is a relatively rapid one, whereas the second is slow. Consequently, iron accumulates within the mucosal cells as a protein-iron complex termed *ferritin*. When the concentration of iron in blood drops below normal values, some of it is liberated from the mucosal stores of ferritin and transported into blood. As a consequence, absorption of more iron from the intestine is triggered to replenish these stores. Calcium is also absorbed by a two-step process—first, absorption from the lumen, then exudation into the interstitial fluid. The first step is faster than the second, and therefore intracellular calcium rises in mucosal cells during absorption. Vitamin D is required for both steps of calcium transport.

Some xenobiotics can be absorbed by these same specialized transport systems. For example, 5-fluorouracil is absorbed by the pyrimidine transport system (Schanker and Jeffrey, 1961), thallium by the system that normally absorbs iron (Leopold et al., 1969), and lead by the calcium transporter (Sobel et al., 1938). Cobalt and manganese compete for the iron transport system (Schade et al., 1970; Thomson et al., 1971a, 1971b).

The number of toxicants actively absorbed by the gastrointestinal tract is small; most enter the body by simple diffusion. Although lipid-soluble substances are more rapidly and extensively absorbed by this process than water-soluble substances, the latter may also be absorbed to some degree. After oral ingestion, about 10 percent of lead, 4 percent of manganese, 1.5 percent of cadmium, and 1 percent of chromium salts are absorbed. If the compound is very toxic, even small amounts of absorbed material will produce serious systemic effects. An organic compound not expected to be absorbed on the basis of the pH-partition hypothesis is the fully ionized quaternary ammonium compound, pralidoxime (2-PAM; molecular weight 137). Yet it is almost entirely absorbed from the gastrointestinal tract (Levine and Steinberg, 1966). The mechanism(s) by which some lipid-insoluble com-

Table 3–1.   SITE DISTRIBUTION OF SPECIALIZED TRANSPORT SYSTEMS IN THE INTESTINE OF MAN AND ANIMALS*

| | LOCATION OF ABSORPTIVE CAPACITY | | | |
| | Small Intestine | | | Colon |
SUBSTRATES	Upper	Mid	Lower	
Sugar (glucose, galactose, etc.)	++	+++	++	0
Neutral amino acids	++	+++	++	0
Basic amino acids	++	++	++	?
Gammaglobulin (newborn animals)	+	++	+++	?
Pyrimidines (thymine and uracil)	+	+	?	?
Triglycerides	++	++	+	?
Fatty acid absorption and conversion to triglyceride	+++	++	+	0
Bile salts	0	+	+++	
Vitamin B_{12}	0	+	+++	0
Na^+	+++	++	+++	+++
H^+ (and/or HCO_3^- secretion)	0	+	++	++
Ca^{2+}	+++	++	+	?
Fe^{2+}	+++	++	+	?
Cl^-	+++	++	+	0

*Adapted from Wilson, T. H.: *Mechanisms of Absorption.* W. B. Saunders, Philadelphia, (1962). pp. 40–68.

pounds are absorbed is (are) not entirely clear. It appears that organic ions of small molecular weight (122 to 188) can be transported across the mucosal barrier by paracellular transport, that is, passive penetration through aqueous pores at the tight junctions (see Aungst and Shen, 1986).

It is interesting that even particulate matter can be absorbed by the gastrointestinal epithelium. Particles of an azo dye, variable in size but averaging several thousand nm in diameter, have been shown to be taken up by the duodenum (R. J. Barnett, 1959). Emulsions of polystyrene latex particles of 22 μm in diameter have been demonstrated to be carried through the cytoplasm of the intestinal epithelium within intact vesicles and discharged into the interstices of the lamina propria, followed by absorption into the lymphatics of the mucosa (Sanders and Ashworth, 1961). Particles appear to enter intestinal cells by pinocytosis, a process much more prominent in the newborn than the adult (Williams and Beck, 1969). These examples demonstrate some of the principles and the variety of toxicants that can be absorbed at least to some extent by the gastrointestinal tract.

The resistance of chemicals, or the lack thereof to alteration by the acidic pH of the stomach, or by enzymes of the stomach or intestine, or by the intestinal flora, is of extreme importance. A toxicant may be hydrolyzed by stomach acid or biotransformed by enzymes of the microflora of the intestine to new compounds with greatly different toxicity than that of the parent compound. For example, snake venom is much less toxic

when administered orally than intravenously, because it is broken down by digestive enzymes of the gastrointestinal tract. Ingestion of well water with a high nitrate content has produced methemoglobinemia much more frequently in infants than in adults. This is due to higher pH of the gastrointestinal tract in newborns with the consequence of greater abundance of certain bacteria, especially *Escherichia coli (E. coli),* which convert nitrate into nitrite. Nitrite thus formed by bacterial action produces methemoglobinemia (Rosenfield and Huston, 1950). Nitrite is also often used as a food additive in meats and smoked fish. Some fish, vegetables, and fruit juices contain secondary amines. The acidic environment of the stomach facilitates a chemical reaction between nitrite and secondary amines, leading to the formation of carcinogenic nitrosamines (see Chapter 5). Also, the intestinal flora can reduce aromatic nitro groups to aromatic amines that may be goitrogenic or carcinogenic (Thompson *et al.,* 1954). Intestinal bacteria, more specifically *Aerobacter aerogenes,* have also been shown to degrade DDT to DDE (Mendel and Walton, 1966).

Many factors alter the gastrointestinal absorption of toxicants. For example, ethylenediaminetetraacetic acid (EDTA) increases the absorption of some toxicants by increasing intestinal permeability. Simple diffusion is not only proportional to surface area and permeability but also to residency time in various segments of the alimentary canal. Therefore, the rate of absorption of a toxicant remaining for longer periods of time in the intestine will increase, whereas that with a shorter residency time will decrease. The residency time of a chemical in the gut depends on intestinal motility. Some agents used as laxatives are known to exert such effects on the absorption of xenobiotics by altering intestinal motility (Levine, 1970).

Experiments have shown that oral toxicity of some chemicals is increased by diluting the dose (Ferguson, 1962; Borowitz et al., 1971). This phenomenon may be explained by more rapid stomach emptying induced by increased dosage volume, which in turn leads to more rapid absorption in the duodenum, because of the larger surface area there.

The absorption of a toxicant from the gastrointestinal tract also depends on the physical properties of a compound, such as lipid solubility, and dissolution rate. While it is often generalized that an increase in lipid solubility will increase the absorption of chemicals, an extremely lipid-soluble chemical will not dissolve in the gastrointestinal fluids, and absorption will be low (Houston et al., 1974). If the toxicant is a solid and relatively insoluble in gastrointestinal fluids, it will have limited contact with the gastrointestinal mucosa, and therefore, its rate of absorption will be low. Also, the larger the particle size, the less will be absorbed, as dissolution rate is proportional to particle size (Gorringe and Sproston, 1964; Bates and Gibaldi, 1970). This is the reason why metallic mercury is relatively nontoxic when ingested orally, and why finely powdered arsenic trioxide is significantly more toxic than a coarse, granular form of it (Schwartze, 1923).

The amount of a chemical entering the systemic circulation after oral administration depends on several factors. First, it depends on the amount absorbed into the gastrointestinal cells. Further, before a chemical enters the systemic circulation, it can be biotransformed by the gastrointestinal cells or extracted by the liver and excreted into bile with or without prior biotransformation. The lung can also contribute to biotransformation or elimination of chemicals prior to entrance into the systemic circulation, although its role is less well defined than that of the intestine and liver. This phenomenon of removal of chemicals before entrance to the systemic circulation is referred to as *presystemic elimination,* or *first-pass effect.*

A number of other factors have also been shown to alter absorption. For example, one ion can alter the absorption of another: Cadmium decreases the absorption of zinc and copper, and calcium that of cadmium; zinc decreases the absorption of copper, and magnesium that of fluoride (Pfeiffer, 1977). Milk has been found to increase lead absorption (Kelly and Kostial, 1973), and starvation enhances the absorption of dieldrin (Heath and Vandekar, 1964). The age of animals also appears to affect absorption: Newborn rats absorbed 12 percent of a dose of cadmium, whereas adult rats absorbed only 0.5 percent (Sasser and Jarboe, 1977). While lead and many other heavy metal ions are not readily absorbed from the gastrointestinal tract, EDTA and other chelators increase the lipid solubility and hence absorption of complexed ions. Thus, it is important not to give a chelator orally when excess metal is still present in the gastrointestinal tract after oral ingestion.

Absorption of Toxicants by the Lungs

It is well known that toxic responses to chemicals can result from their absorption after inhalation. The most frequent cause of death from poisoning, carbon monoxide, and probably the most important occupational disease, silicosis, are both due to the absorption or deposition of airborne poisons in the lungs. This site of absorption has been employed in chemical warfare (chlorine and phosgene gas, lewisite, mustard gas) and for executing criminals in gas chambers (hydrogen cyanide).

Toxicants absorbed by the lungs are usually gases (e.g., carbon monoxide, nitrogen dioxide, and sulfur dioxide), vapors of volatile or volatilizable liquids (e.g., benzene and carbon tetrachloride), and aerosols. Because the absorption of inhaled gases and vapor differs from that of aerosols, they will be discussed separately. However, the absorption of gases and vapors is governed by the same principles, and therefore the word *gas* will represent both in this section.

Gases and Vapors. Absorption of inhaled gases takes place mainly in the lungs. However, before a gas reaches the lungs, it passes through the nose with its turbinates, which increase the surface area. Because the mucosa of the nose is covered by a film of fluid, gas molecules can be retained by the nose and not reach the lungs if they are very water soluble or if they react with cell surface components. Therefore, the nose acts as a "scrubber" for water-soluble and for highly reactive gases, partially protecting the lungs from potentially injurious insults. A case in point is formaldehyde. The drawback of this protective mechanism for the lungs is that a typical nose breather like the rat develops tumors of the nasal turbinates when chronically exposed to high levels of formaldehyde by inhalation.

The absorption of gases in the lungs differs from intestinal and percutaneous absorption of compounds in that the dissociation of acids and bases and the lipid solubility of molecules are less important factors in pulmonary absorption because diffusion through cell membranes is not rate limiting in pulmonary absorption of gases. There are at least three reasons for that. First, ionized molecules are of very low volatility, and consequently their concentration in normal ambient air is insignificant. The second reason is that the epithelial cells lining the alveoli—that is, the type I pneumocytes—are very thin and the capillaries are in close contact with the pneumocytes, so that the distance for a chemical to diffuse is very short. The third reason is that chemicals absorbed by the lungs are rapidly removed by the blood, as it takes about three-fourths of a second for the blood to go through the extensive capillary network in the lungs.

When a gas is inhaled into the lungs, gas molecules diffuse from the alveolar space into the blood and dissolve. Except for some gases with a special affinity for certain body components (e.g., the binding of carbon monoxide to hemoglobin), the uptake of a gas by a tissue usually involves a simple physical process of dissolving. The end result is that gas molecules partition between the two media, air versus the blood during the absorptive phase and between blood and other tissues during the distribution phase. As the contact of the inspired gas with blood continues in the alveoli, more molecules dissolve in blood until gas molecules in blood are in equilibrium with gas molecules in the alveolar space. At equilibrium, the ratio of the concentration of chemical in the blood and in the gas phase is constant. This solubility ratio is called the *blood-to-gas partition coefficient*. This constant is unique for each gas. Note that only the ratio is constant, not the concentrations, as, according to Henry's law, the amount of gas dissolved in a liquid is proportional to the partial pressure of the gas in the gas phase at any given concentration prior to or at saturation. Thus, the higher the inhaled concentration of a gas (i.e., the higher the partial pressure), the higher will be the gas concentration in blood, but the ratio will not change unless saturation has occurred. When equilibrium is reached, the rate of transfer of gas molecules from the alveolar space to blood equals the rate of removal by the blood from the alveolar space. For example, chloroform has a high (15) and ethylene a low (0.14) blood/gas phase solubility ratio. For a substance with a low solubility ratio (e.g., ethylene), only a small percentage of the total gas in the lungs will be removed by blood during each circulation because blood is soon saturated with the gas. Therefore, an increase in the respiratory rate or minute volume does not change the transfer of such a gas to blood. In contrast, an increase in the rate of blood flow markedly increases the

rate of uptake of a low solubility ratio compound because of more rapid removal from the site of equilibrium, that is, the alveolar membranes. It has been calculated that the time to equilibrate between the blood and gas phase for a relatively insoluble gas is about 8 to 21 minutes.

Most of a gas with a high solubility ratio, such as chloroform, is transferred to blood during each respiratory cycle so that little, if any, remains in the alveoli just before the next inhalation. The more soluble a toxic agent is in blood, the more of it will be dissolved in blood by the time equilibrium is reached. Consequently, the time required to equilibrate with blood will be very much longer with high than with low solubility ratio gases. This has been calculated to take a minimum of one hour for high solubility ratio compounds, although it may be even longer if the gas also has a high tissue affinity (i.e., high fat solubility). With these highly soluble gases, the principal factor limiting the rate of absorption is respiration. Because the blood is already removing virtually all of a high solubility ratio gas from the lungs, increasing the blood flow rate does not substantially increase the rate of absorption. However, the rate can be greatly accelerated by increasing the rate of respiration, or the minute volume.

Thus, the rate of absorption of gases in the lungs is variable and depends on the toxicant's solubility ratio (concentration in blood/concentration in gas phase before or at saturation) at equilibrium. For gases with a very low solubility ratio, the rate of transfer depends mainly on blood flow through the lungs (perfusion limited), whereas for gases with a high solubility ratio, it is primarily a function of the rate and depth of respiration (ventilation limited). Of course, there is a wide spectrum of intermediate behavior between the two extremes, the median being a blood/gas concentration ratio of about 1.2.

The blood carries the dissolved gas molecules to the rest of the body. In each tissue, the gas molecules are transferred from the blood to the tissue until equilibrium is reached at a tissue concentration dictated by the tissue-to-blood partition coefficient. After releasing part of the gas to tissues, the blood returns to the lungs to take up more of the gas. The process continues until a gas reaches equilibrium between blood and each tissue, according to tissue-to-blood partition coefficients characteristic for each tissue. At this time, no net absorption of gas will take place as long as the exposure concentration remains constant, because steady state has been reached. Of course, if biotransformation and excretion occurs, alveolar absorption will continue until a corresponding steady state is established.

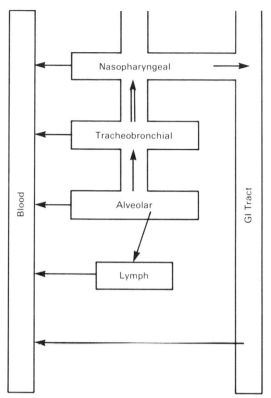

Figure 3-4. Schematic diagram of absorption and translocation of chemicals by lungs.

Aerosols and Particles. The degree of ionization and lipid solubility of chemicals are very important for oral and percutaneous exposures, whereas water solubility, tissue reactivity, and blood-to-gas phase partition coefficients are important after exposure to gases and vapors. The important characteristics affecting absorption after exposure to aerosols are aerosol size and water solubility of a chemical present in the aerosol.

The site of deposition of aerosols depends greatly on the size of the particles. This relationship is discussed in detail in Chapter 12. Particles of 5 μm or larger are usually deposited in the nasopharyngeal region (Figure 3-4). Those deposited on the unciliated anterior portion of the nose tend to remain at the site of deposition until they are removed by nose wiping, blowing, or sneezing. The mucous blanket of the ciliated nasal surface propels insoluble particles by the movement of the cilia. These particles as well as particles inhaled through the mouth are swallowed within minutes. Soluble particles may dissolve in the mucus and be carried to the pharynx or be absorbed through the nasal epithelium into blood.

Particles of 2 to 5 μm are mainly deposited in the tracheobronchiolar regions of the lungs, from where they are cleared by retrograde movement of the mucus layer in the ciliated portions of the respiratory tract. The rate of cilia-propelled movement of the mucus varies in different parts of the respiratory tract, although in general it is a rapid and efficient transport mechanism. Measurements have shown transport rates between 0.1 and 1 mm per minute, resulting in removal half-lives between 30 and 300 minutes. Coughing and sneezing increase greatly the movement of mucous and particulate matter toward the mouth. Particles may eventually be swallowed and absorbed from the gastrointestinal tract.

Particles 1 μm and smaller penetrate to the alveolar sacs of the lungs. They may be absorbed into blood, or they may be cleared through the lymphatics after being scavenged by alveolar macrophages.

In addition to gases, liquid aerosols as well as particles can be absorbed in the alveoli. Mechanisms responsible for the removal or absorption of particulate matter from the alveoli (usually less than 1 μm in diameter) are less clear than those responsible for removal of particles deposited in the tracheobronchial tree. Removal appears to occur by three major mechanisms. First, particles may be removed from the alveoli by a physical process. It is thought that particles deposited on the fluid layer of the alveoli are aspirated onto the mucociliary escalator of the tracheobronchial region. From there, they are transported to the mouth and may be swallowed as mentioned previously. The origin of the thin fluid layer in the alveoli is probably a transudation of lymph and secretions of lipids and other components by the alveolar epithelium. The alveolar fluid flows by some unknown mechanism to the terminal bronchioles. This flow seems to depend on lymph flow, capillary action, respiratory motion of the alveolar walls, the cohesive nature of the respiratory tract fluid blanket, and the propelling power of the ciliated bronchioles. Second, particles from the alveoli may be removed by phagocytosis. The principal cells responsible for engulfing alveolar debris are the mononuclear phagocytes, the macrophages. These cells are found in large quantities in normal lungs and contain many phagocytized particles of both exogenous and endogenous origin. They apparently migrate to the distal end of the mucociliary escalator and are cleared and eventually swallowed. Third, removal may occur via the lymphatics. The endothelial cells lining lymphatic capillaries are permeable for very large molecules (molecular weight $> 10^6$) and also for particles, although the rate of penetration is low above molecular weight 10,000 (Renkin, 1968). Nevertheless, the lymphatic system plays a prominent role in collecting large molecular weight proteins leaked from cells or blood capillaries and also particulate matter from the interstitium as well as from the alveolar spaces. Particulate matter may remain in lymphatic tissue for long periods of time and hence the name "dust store of the lungs."

For reasons discussed above, the overall removal of particles from the alveoli is relatively inefficient; within the first day only about 20 percent of particles are cleared, and the portion remaining longer than 24 hours is very slowly cleared. The rate of clearance by the lungs can be predicted by the compounds' solubility in lung fluids. The lower the solubility, the lower the removal rate. Thus, it appears that removal of particles from the lungs is still largely due to dissolution and vascular transport. Some particles may remain in the alveoli indefinitely. This may occur when proliferating, instead of desquamating, alveolar cells ingest dust particles and in association with a developing network of reticulin fibers form an alveolar dust plaque or nodule.

Absorption of Toxicants Through the Skin

Human skin comes into contact with many toxic agents. Fortunately, the skin is not very permeable. Therefore, it is a relatively good barrier separating organisms from their environment. However, some chemicals can be absorbed by the skin in sufficient quantities to produce systemic effects. For example, nerve gases, such as sarin, are readily absorbed by the intact skin. Also, carbon tetrachloride can be absorbed through the skin in sufficient quantities to bring about liver injury. Various insecticides have caused death in agricultural workers after absorption through the intact skin (see Chapter 15).

In order to be absorbed through the skin, a toxicant must pass either through the epidermis or through the appendages (sweat and sebaceous glands, and hair follicles). The sweat glands and hair follicles are scattered in varying density on the skin. Their total cross-sectional area is probably between 0.1 and 1.0 percent of the total skin surface. Although entry of small amounts of toxicants through the appendages may be rapid, chemicals are mainly absorbed through the epidermis, which constitutes the major surface area of the skin. Chemicals to be absorbed through the skin have to pass through several cell layers (a total of seven) before entering the small blood and lymph capillaries in the dermis (Figure 3–5). The rate-determining barrier in the dermal absorption of chemicals is the epidermis. More accurately, it is the stratum corneum

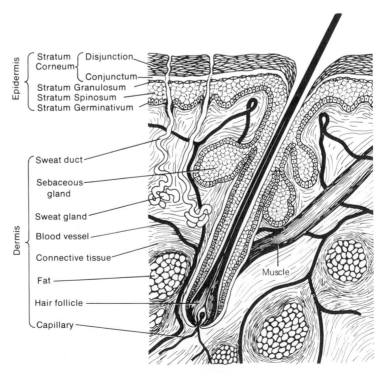

Figure 3–5. Diagram of a cross section of human skin.

(horny layer) that is the uppermost layer of the epidermis (Dugard, 1983). It is the outer horny layer of the skin consisting of densely packed, keratinized cells that have lost their nuclei and hence are biologically inactive. Passage through the six other cell layers is much more rapid than through the stratum corneum. Therefore, the most important considerations regarding dermal absorption of xenobiotics relate to the stratum corneum.

The first phase of percutaneous absorption is diffusion of xenobiotics through the rate-limiting barrier, the stratum corneum. Studies have shown that the stratum corneum is replenished about every three to four weeks in adults. This complex process includes a gross dehydration and polymerization of intracellular matrix, resulting in keratin-filled, dried cell layers. In the course of keratinization, the cell walls apparently double in thickness owing to inclusion or deposition of chemically resistant materials. This change in the physical state of the tissue causes a commensurate change in its diffusion barrier property. The transformation is from an aqueous fluid medium, characterized by liquid state, to a dry, keratinous semisolid state with much lower permeability for toxicants by diffusion (permeability by diffusion = diffusivity).

It appears that all toxicants move across the stratum corneum by passive diffusion and none by active transport. Kinetic measurements support the postulate that polar and nonpolar toxicants diffuse through the stratum corneum by different mechanisms. Polar substances appear to diffuse through the outer surface of protein filaments of the hydrated stratum corneum, whereas nonpolar molecules dissolve in and diffuse through the lipid matrix between the protein filaments (Blank and Scheuplein, 1969). The rate of diffusion of nonpolar toxicants is proportional to their lipid solubility and inversely related to the molecular weight (Marzulli *et al.*, 1965).

Human stratum corneum displays significant differences in structure and chemistry from one region of the body to another, which affect the permeability of the skin to chemicals. Skin from the plantar and palmar regions is much different from other areas of the body in that the stratum corneum of the palms and soles is adapted for weight bearing and friction. The stratum corneum of the rest of the body surface is adapted for flexibility and fine sensory discrimination. Permeability of the skin depends on both the diffusivity of the stratum corneum and its thickness. While the stratum corneum is much thicker on the palms and soles (being 400 to 600 μm in callous areas) than on the arms, back, legs, and abdomen (8 to 15 μm), it has much higher dif-

fusivity per unit thickness. Consequently, toxicants readily cross scrotum skin since it is extremely thin and has high diffusivity; they cross the abdominal skin less rapidly, as it is both thicker and exhibits less diffusivity; and they cross the sole with the greatest difficulty because the distance to traverse is great even though diffusivity here is highest.

The second phase of percutaneous absorption is diffusion of the toxicant through the lower layers of the epidermis (stratum granulosum, spinosum, germinativum) and the dermis. These cell layers are far inferior to the stratum corneum as diffusion barriers. In contrast to the stratum corneum, they contain a porous, nonselective, aqueous diffusion medium. Toxicants pass through this area also by diffusion and enter the systemic circulation through the large number of venous and lymphatic capillaries in the dermis. The rate of diffusion depends on blood flow, interstitial fluid movement, and perhaps other factors, including interactions with dermal constituents.

The absorption of toxicants through the skin varies depending on the condition of the skin. Because the stratum corneum plays a critical role in determining cutaneous permeability, removal of this layer causes a dramatic increase in the permeability of the epidermis for a variety of molecules, large or small, both lipid and water soluble (Malkinson, 1964). Injurious agents such as acids, alkalis, and mustard gases likewise will injure the stratum corneum and increase permeability. The most frequently encountered penetration enhancing damages to the skin are burns and various skin diseases. Water plays an extremely important role in skin permeability. Under normal conditions, the stratum corneum is partially hydrated, containing about 7 percent water by weight. This amount of water increases the permeability of the stratum corneum approximately tenfold over that when it is completely dry. Upon additional contact with water, the stratum corneum can increase its weight of tightly bound water up to three- to fivefold, which results in an additional two- to threefold increase in permeability. Studies on dermal absorption of toxicants often utilize the method of Draize and associates (1944), wrapping plastic around animals and placing the chemical between the plastic and the skin (occlusive application). This hydrates the stratum corneum and enhances the absorption of some toxicants.

Solvents such as dimethyl sulfoxide (DMSO) can also facilitate the penetration of toxicants through the skin. DMSO increases the permeability of the barrier layer of the skin, viz., of the stratum corneum. Little information is available concerning the mechanism by which DMSO enhances skin permeability. However, it has been suggested that DMSO (1) removes much of the lipid matrix of the stratum corneum, making holes or artificial shunts in the penetration barrier; (2) produces reversible configurational changes in protein structure brought about by substitution of integral water molecules; and (3) functions as a swelling agent (Allenby *et al.*, 1969; Dugard and Embery, 1969).

Various species have been employed in studying the dermal absorption of toxicants. Considerable species variation has been observed in cutaneous permeability. The skin of the rat and rabbit is for many chemicals more permeable, whereas the skin of the cat is usually less permeable, while the cutaneous permeability characteristics of the guinea pig, pig, and monkey are often similar to those observed in humans (Scala *et al.*, 1968; Coulston and Serrone, 1969; Wester and Maibach, 1977). Species differences in percutaneous absorption account for the differential toxicity of insecticides in insects and in humans. For example, the LD50 of DDT is approximately equal in insects and mammals when injected, but DDT is much less toxic to mammals than to insects when applied to the skin. This appears to be due to the fact that DDT is poorly absorbed through the skin of mammals but passes readily through the chitinous exoskeleton of insects. Furthermore, insects have a much greater body surface area relative to weight than do mammals (Winteringham, 1957; Albert, 1965; Hayes, 1965).

Absorption of Toxicants After Special Routes of Administration

Toxicants usually enter the bloodstream after absorption through the skin, lungs, or gastrointestinal tract. However, when studying chemical agents, toxicologists frequently administer these to laboratory animals by special routes. The most common of these are (1) intraperitoneal, (2) subcutaneous, (3) intramuscular, and (4) intravenous. The intravenous route of administration introduces the toxicant directly into the bloodstream, eliminating the process of absorption. Intraperitoneal injection of toxicants to laboratory animals is also a common procedure. It results in rapid absorption of xenobiotics because of the rich blood supply and the relative large surface area of the peritoneal cavity. In addition, this route of administration circumvents the delay and variability of gastric emptying. Compounds administered intraperitoneally are absorbed primarily through the portal circulation and therefore must pass through the liver before reaching other organs (Lukas *et al.*, 1971). Toxicants administered subcutaneously and intramuscularly are usually absorbed at slower rates, but they enter directly into the general circulation. The rate of absorption by these two routes can be altered by changing the blood flow to the injection site. For example, epinephrine causes vasoconstriction and will decrease the rate of absorption if coinjected intramuscularly with a toxicant. The formulation of a xenobiotic may also affect the rate of absorption; toxicants are absorbed more slowly from suspensions than from solutions.

The toxicity of a chemical may or may not depend on the route of administration. If a toxicant is injected intraperitoneally, most of the chemical will enter the liver via the portal circulation before reaching the general circulation. Therefore, an intraperitoneally administered compound might be completely extracted and biotransformed by the liver with subsequent excretion into the bile without gaining access to the systemic circulation. Propranolol (Shand and Rangno, 1972) and lidocaine (Boyes *et al.*, 1970) are two examples of drugs with efficient extraction during the first pass through the liver. Any toxicant, displaying first-pass effect with selective toxicity for an organ other than the liver and gastrointestinal tract is expected to be much less toxic when administered intraperitoneally than when injected intravenously, intramuscularly, or subcutaneously. For compounds with no appreciable biotransformation in the liver, toxicity ought to be independent of route of administration, provided rates of absorption are equal. This discussion indicates that it is possible to obtain some preliminary information on the biotransformation and excretion of xenobiotics by comparing their toxicity after administration by different routes.

DISTRIBUTION

After entering the blood (either by absorption or by intravenous administration), a toxicant is available for distribution (translocation) throughout the body. Distribution usually occurs rapidly. The rate of distribution to organs or tissues is primarily determined by blood flow and the rate of diffusion out of the capillary bed into the cells of a particular organ or tissue. The final distribution depends largely on the affinity of a xenobiotic for various tissues. In general, the initial phase of distribution is dominated by blood flow, whereas the eventual distribution is largely determined by affinity. The penetration of toxicants into cells occurs either by passive diffusion or special transport processes, as discussed previously. Small water-soluble molecules and ions apparently diffuse through aqueous channels or pores in the cell membrane. Lipid-soluble molecules readily permeate the membrane itself. Very polar molecules and ions of even moderate size (molecular weight 50 or more) cannot enter cells easily except by special transport mechanisms. The reason for this is probably that they are surrounded by a hydration shell, making their actual size much larger.

Volume of Distribution

The total body water may be divided into three distinct compartments: (1) plasma water, (2) interstitial water, and (3) intracellular water. Extracellular water is made up of plasma water plus interstitial water. The concentration of a toxicant in blood depends largely on its volume of distribution. For example, if 1 g of each of several chemicals were injected directly into the bloodstream of 70-kg humans, marked differences in their plasma concentrations would be observed depending on their distribution: A high concentration would be observed in the plasma if it distributed into plasma water only, and a much lower concentration would be reached if it distributed into a large pool, like total body water (see below).

The distribution of toxicants is usally quite complex and cannot be equated with distribution just into one of the water compartments of the body. Binding to and/or dissolution in various storage sites of the body such as fat, liver, or bone are usually more important factors in determining the distribution of chemicals.

Some toxicants do not readily cross cell membranes and therefore have restricted distribution, whereas other toxicants readily pass through cell membranes and distribute throughout the body. Some toxicants accumulate in certain parts of the body as a result of protein binding, active transport, or high solubility in fat. The site of accumulation of a toxicant may also be its site of major toxic action, but more often, it is not. If a toxicant accumulates at a site other than the target organ or tissue, the accumulation may be viewed as a protective process, in that plasma levels and consequently the concentration of a toxicant at the site of action are diminished. In this case, it is assumed that the chemical in the storage depot is toxicologically inactive. However, because any chemical in a storage depot is in equilibrium with the free fraction of toxicant

in plasma, it is released into the circulation as the unbound fraction of toxicant is eliminated, e.g., by biotransformation.

Storage of Toxicants in Tissues

As only the free fraction of a chemical is in equilibrium throughout the body, binding to or dissolving in certain body constituents greatly alters the distribution of a xenobiotic. Toxicants are often concentrated in a specific tissue. Some xenobiotics attain their highest concentration at their site of toxic action, such as carbon monoxide, which has a very high affinity for hemoglobin, and paraquat, which accumulates in the lungs. Other agents concentrate at sites other than their target organ. For example, lead is stored in bone, but manifestations of lead poisoning appear in soft tissues. The compartment where a toxicant is concentrated can be thought of as a storage depot. Toxicants in these depots are always in equilibrium with their free fraction in plasma. As a chemical is biotransformed or excreted from the body, more is released from the storage site. As a result, the biological half-life of stored compounds can be very long. The following discussion deals with the major storage sites of the body for xenobiotics.

Plasma Proteins as Storage Depot.   Several plasma proteins bind xenobiotics as well as some physiological constituents of the body. As depicted in Figure 3–6, albumin can bind a large number of different compounds. Transferrin, a β_1-globulin, is important for transport of iron in the body. The other main metal-binding protein in plasma is ceruloplasmin, which carries most of the copper. The α- and β-lipoproteins are very important for the transport of lipid-soluble compounds, such as vitamins, cholesterol, and steroid hormones as well as xenobiotics. The γ-globulins are antibodies that interact specifically with antigens. Compounds possessing basic characteristics often bind to α_1-acid glycoprotein (Wilkinson, 1983).

Many therapeutic agents have been examined with respect to plasma protein binding. The extent of plasma protein binding varies considerably among xenobiotics. Some, such as antipyrine, are not bound; others, such as secobarbital, are bound to about 50 percent; and some,

COMPARTMENT	PERCENT OF TOTAL	LITERS IN 70-kg HUMAN	PLASMA CONCENTRATION AFTER 1 g OF CHEMICAL
Plasma water	4.5	3	333 mg/liter
Total extracellular water	20	14	71 mg/liter
Total body water	55	38	26 mg/liter
Tissue binding	—	—	0–25 mg/liter

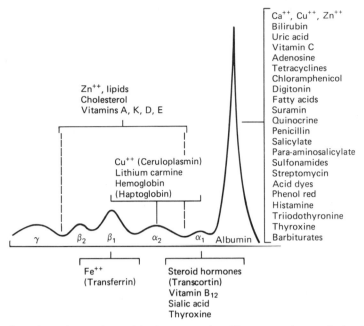

Figure 3–6. Ligand interactions with plasma proteins. Plasma proteins are depicted according to their relative amounts (y axis) and electrophoretic mobilities (x axis). Some representative interactions are listed. (From Goldstein, A.; Aronow, L.; and Kalman, S. M.: *Principles of Drug Action* [copyright © 1968, by Harper and Row; reprinted by permission of John Wiley & Sons, Inc., copyright proprietor]. Modified from Putman, F. W.: Structure and function of the plasma proteins. In Neurath, H. [ed.]: *The Proteins,* 2nd ed., Vol. III. Academic Press, Inc., New York, 1965.)

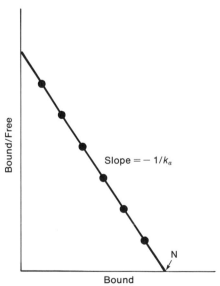

Figure 3–7. Schematic representation of the Scatchard plot for the analysis of the binding of small molecules to proteins.

like warfarin, are 99 percent bound. Plasma proteins can bind acidic compounds, like phenylbutazone, basic compounds, such as imipramine, and neutral compounds, like digitoxin.

Binding of toxicants to plasma proteins is usually determined by equilibrium dialysis or by ultrafiltration. The fraction that passes through the dialysis membrane or appears in the ultrafiltrate is the unbound or free fraction. The total concentration is the sum of the bound and free fraction. The bound fraction thus can be determined from the difference of the total and free fraction. The binding of toxicants to plasma proteins can be analyzed by Scatchard plots (Scatchard, 1949). In this analysis, the ratio of bound to free ligand (toxicant) is plotted on the ordinate and the concentration of bound ligand on the abscissa, as depicted in Figure 3–7. From this analysis, the number of ligand binding sites (N) per molecule of protein and the affinity constant of the protein-ligand complex can be determined. The Scatchard plot frequently exhibits nonlinearity, indicating the presence of two or more classes of binding sites with different affinity and capacity characteristics.

Most xenobiotics that are bound to plasma proteins bind to albumin. Albumin is the most abundant protein in plasma and serves as a depot and transport protein for numerous endogenous and exogenous compounds. Long-chain fatty acids and bilirubin are examples of endogenous ligands with affinity to albumin. There appear to be six binding regions on the protein (Kragh-Hansen, 1981). Protein-ligand interactions occur primarily as a result of hydrophobic forces, hydrogen bonding, and Van der Waals forces. Because of their high molecular weight, plasma proteins and toxicants bound to them cannot cross capillary walls. Consequently, the fraction of toxicant bound to plasma proteins is not immediately available for distribution into the extravascular space or for filtration by the kidneys. However, the interaction of a chemical with plasma proteins is a reversible process. As unbound chemical diffuses out of capillaries, bound chemical dissociates from the protein until the free fraction reaches equilibrium between the vascular and extravascular space. In turn, diffusion in the extravascular space away to more distant sites from the capillaries continues, and the resulting concentration gradient provides the thermodynamic force for continued dissociation of the bound fraction in plasma. Active transport processes are not limited by binding of chemicals to plasma proteins.

The binding of chemicals to plasma proteins is of special importance to toxicologists because severe toxic reactions can arise if a toxicant is displaced from plasma proteins by another agent, thereby increasing the free fraction of the former in plasma. This will result in increased equilibrium concentration of the toxicant in the target organ with the potential for toxicity. For example, if a strongly bound sulfonamide is given concurrently with an antidiabetic drug to a patient, the sulfonamide may displace the antidiabetic drug and induce hypoglycemic coma. Xenobiotics can also compete and displace endogenous compounds that are bound to plasma proteins. The importance of this phenomenon was demonstrated in a clinical trial comparing the efficacy of tetracycline and of a penicillin-sulfonamide mixture in the management of bacterial infections in premature infants (Silverman *et al.*, 1956). It was found that the penicillin-sulfonamide mixture led to much higher mortality than did tetracycline because the sulfonamide displaced a considerable amount of bilirubin from albumin. Bilirubin then diffused into brain through the not-fully-developed blood-brain barrier of the newborn, causing a severe brain damage termed *kernicterus*.

Most research on binding of xenobiotics to plasma proteins was conducted with drugs. However, other chemicals, such as the insecticide dieldrin, also bind avidly to plasma proteins (99 percent). Therefore, it is to be expected that such chemical-chemical interactions altering plasma protein binding will occur with many different xenobiotics.

Liver and Kidney as Storage Depots.
Liver and kidney have a high capacity to bind a multitude of chemicals. These two organs probably concentrate more toxicants than all other organs combined. Although all the mechanisms by which the liver and kidney remove toxicants from the blood have not yet been established, active transport or binding to tissue components seems to be involved in most cases.

A protein in the cytoplasm of the liver (ligandin) has been identified as having high affinity for many organic acids. It has been suggested that this protein may be important in the transfer of organic anions from plasma into liver (Levi *et al.*, 1969). This protein also binds azo dye carcinogens and corticosteroids (Litwack *et al.*, 1971). Another protein (metallothionein) has been found in the kidney and liver to bind cadmium and zinc with different affinities. Hepatic uptake of lead illustrates how rapidly liver binds foreign compounds: Just 30 minutes after a single dose, the concentration of lead in liver is 50 times higher than in plasma (Klaassen and Shoeman, 1974).

Fat as Storage Depot. Many organic compounds present in the environment are highly lipophilic. This characteristic permits rapid penetration of cell membranes and uptake by tissues. Therefore, it is not surprising that highly lipophilic toxicants distribute and concentrate in body fat. Such accumulation in adipose tissue has been demonstrated for a number of chemicals such as chlordane, DDT, and polychlorinated and polybrominated biphenyls.

Toxicants appear to accumulate in fat by physical dissolution in neutral fats, which constitute about 50 and 20 percent of the body weight of an obese and of a lean, athletic individual, respectively. Thus, large amounts of toxicants with a high lipid/water partition coefficient may be stored in body fat. Storage lowers the concentration of the toxicant in the target organ, and thus, the toxicity of such a compound could be expected to be less severe in an obese than in a lean individual. However, of more practical concern is the possibility of a sudden increase in the concentration of a chemical in the blood, and hence in the target organ of toxicity, when rapid mobilization of fat occurs. Several studies have shown that signs of intoxication can be produced by short-term starvation of experimental animals previously exposed to persistent organochlorine insecticides.

Bone as Storage Depot. Compounds like fluoride, lead, and strontium may be incorporated and thus stored in the bone matrix. For example, 90 percent of lead in the body is found in the skeleton.

The phenomenon of skeletal uptake of xenobiotics is essentially a surface chemistry phenomenon, exchange taking place between the bone surface and the fluid in contact with it. The fluid is the extracellular fluid, and the surface is that of the hydroxyapatite crystals of bone mineral. Many of these crystals are of such small dimensions that the surface is large in proportion to the mass. The extracellular fluid brings the toxicant into contact with the hydration shell of the hydroxyapatite, allowing diffusion through it and penetration of the crystal surface. By virtue of similarities in size and charge, F^- may readily displace OH^-, whereas lead or strontium may substitute for calcium in the hydroxyapatite lattice matrix by an exchange-absorption reaction.

Deposition and storage of toxicants in bone may or may not be detrimental. Lead is not toxic to bone, but the chronic effects of fluoride deposition (skeletal fluorosis) and radioactive strontium (osteosarcoma and other neoplasms) are well documented.

Foreign compounds deposited in bone are not irreversibly sequestered by this tissue. Toxicants can be released from the bone by ionic exchange at the crystal surface and by dissolution of bone crystals through osteoclastic activity. An increase in osteolytic activity, such as that seen after parathormone administration, leads to an enhanced mobilization of hydroxyapatite lattice, which can be reflected in increased plasma concentration of toxicants.

Blood-Brain Barrier

The blood-brain barrier is not an absolute barrier to the passage of toxic agents into the central nervous system (CNS). Rather, it represents a site that is less permeable than most other areas of the body. Nevertheless, many poisons do not enter the brain in appreciable quantities because of this barrier.

There are three major anatomical and physiological reasons why some toxicants do not readily enter the CNS. First, the capillary endothelial cells of the CNS are tightly joined, leaving few or no pores between the cells. Second, the capillaries of the CNS are to a large extent surrounded by glial cell processes (astrocytes). Third, the protein concentration in the interstitial fluid of the CNS is much lower than in other body fluids. For small- to medium-size water-soluble molecules, the tighter junctions of the capillary endothelium together with the lipid membranes of the glial cell processes represent the major barrier. Lipid-soluble compounds have to traverse not only membranes of the endothelial cells but also those of glial cell processes. More important perhaps, the low protein content of interstitial fluid of the brain greatly limits movement of water-insoluble compounds by paracellular transport, which is only possible for them when bound to proteins. These features together provide some protection against the distribution of toxicants to the CNS and thus against toxicity.

The effectiveness of the blood-brain barrier varies from one area of the brain to another. For example, the cortex, lateral nuclei of hypothalamus, area postrema, pineal body, and posterior lobe of the hypophysis are more permeable than are other areas of the brain. It is not clear whether this is due to the increased blood supply to these areas or to a more permeable barrier or to both.

In general, the entrance of toxicants into brain follows the same principle as does transfer across other cells in the body. Only the free fraction of a toxicant (i.e., not bound to plasma proteins) equilibrates rapidly with the brain. Lipid solubility plays an important role in determining the rate of a compound's entry into the CNS, as does the degree of ionization, discussed earlier. In general, increased lipid solubility enhances the rate of penetration of toxicants into the CNS, whereas ionization greatly diminishes it. For example, methylmercury is taken up by the brain much more readily than are inorganic mercury salts. Also, pralidoxime (2-PAM), a quaternary nitrogen derivative, does not readily penetrate the brain and is quite ineffective in reversing inhibition of brain cholinesterase caused by organophosphate insecticides. It is not clear why some very lipophilic chemicals such as 2,3,7,8-tetrachlorodibenzo-*p*-dioxin do not readily distribute into the brain, which in fact displays the lowest concentration among all tissues and body fluids. It is likely though, that strong binding to plasma proteins or lipoproteins may limit entry of very lipophilic compounds into the brain.

The blood-brain barrier is not fully developed at birth, and this is one reason why some chemicals are more toxic to newborns than to adults. Morphine, for example, is three to ten times more toxic to newborn than to adult rats because of the higher permeability of the brain of the newborn to morphine (Kupferberg and Way, 1963). Lead produces encephalomyelopathy in newborn rats but not in adults, also apparently because of differences in the stages of development of the blood-brain barrier (Pentschew and Garro, 1966).

Table 3–2. TISSUES SEPARATING FETAL AND MATERNAL BLOOD*

	MATERNAL TISSUE			FETAL TISSUE			
	Endo- thelium	Connective Tissue	Epithelium	Tropho- blast	Connective Tissue	Endo- thelium	Species
Epitheliochorial	+	+	+	+	+	+	Pig, horse, donkey
Syndesmochorial	+	+	–	+	+	+	Sheep, goat, cow
Endotheliochorial	+	–	–	+	+	+	Cat, dog
Hemochorial	–	–	–	+	+	+	Man, monkey
Hemoendothelial	–	–	–	–	–	+	Rat, rabbit, guinea pig

*Modified from Amaroso, E. C.: Placentation. In Parkes, A. S. (ed.): *Marshall's Physiology of Reproduction,* Vol. 2. Longmans, Green & Co., London, 1952.

Passage of Toxicants Across the Placenta

For years the term "placental barrier" typified the concept that the main function of the placenta was to protect the fetus against passage of noxious substances from the mother. However, the placenta has many functions: It provides nutrition for the conceptus, exchanges maternal and fetal blood gases, disposes of fetal excretory material, and maintains pregnancy by a complex hormonal regulation. Most of the vital nutrients necessary for the development of the fetus are transported by active transport systems. For example, vitamins, amino acids, essential sugars, and ions such as calcium and iron are transported from mother to fetus against a concentration gradient (Young, 1969; Ginsburg, 1971). In contrast, most toxic agents pass the placenta by simple diffusion. Exceptions are a few antimetabolites that are structurally similar to endogenous purines and pyrimidines, which are the physiological substrates for active transport from maternal to fetal circulation.

Many foreign substances can cross the placenta. In addition to chemicals, viruses (e.g., rubella virus), cellular pathogens (e.g., syphilis spirochete), globulin antibodies, and even erythrocytes (Goldstein *et al.,* 1974) can traverse the placenta.

Anatomically, the placental barrier consists of a number of cell layers interposed between fetal and maternal circulations. The number of layers varies with species and the state of gestation. Placentae in which the maximum number of cell layers is present, that is, all six layers, are called *epitheliochorial* (Table 3–2). Those in which the maternal epithelium is absent are depicted as *syndesmochorial.* When only the endothelial layer of the maternal tissue remains, it is termed *endotheliochorial;* when even the endothelium is gone, so that the chorionic villi bathe in the maternal blood, they are called hemochorial. In some species, some of the fetal layers are absent and then are called hemoendothelial (Dames, 1968). Within the same species, the placenta may also change its histologic classification during gestation (Amaroso, 1952). For example, at the beginning of gestation, the rabbit has a placenta with six major layers (epitheliochorial) and at the end only one layer (hemoendothelial). One might suspect that a relatively thin placenta like that of the rat would be more permeable to toxic agents than the placenta of humans, whereas a thicker placenta, such as that of the goat, would be less permeable. The exact relationship of the number of layers of the placenta to its permeability has not been investigated. Currently, it is not considered to be of primary importance in determining the distribution of chemicals to the fetus.

The same factors are important determinants of placental transfer of xenobiotics by passive diffusion (particularly lipid/water solubility), as discussed for passage of molecules across body membranes. It is uncertain if the placenta plays an active role in preventing the transfer of noxious substances from mother to fetus. However, the placenta has biotransformation capabilities that may prevent some toxic substances from reaching the fetus (Juchau, 1972). Among substances crossing the placenta by passive diffusion, more lipid-soluble substances attain more rapidly a maternal-fetal equilibrium. Under steady-state conditions, the concentrations of a toxic compound in the plasma of the mother and fetus are usually the same. The concentration in the various tissues of the fetus depends on the ability of fetal tissue to concentrate a toxicant. For example, the concentration of diphenylhydantoin in plasma of the fetal goat was about one-half of that found in the mother. This was due to differences in plasma protein concentration and binding affinity of diphenylhydantoin to plasma proteins (Shoeman *et al.*, 1972). Also, some organs such as the liver of the newborn (Klaassen, 1972) and fetus (Mirkin and Singh, 1972) do not concentrate some xenobiotics, and therefore lower levels are found in the liver of the fetus. In contrast, higher concentrations of some chemicals, like lead and methylmercury, are encountered in brain of the fetus because of a not fully developed blood-brain barrier.

Redistribution of Toxicants

As mentioned earlier, blood flow to and affinity of an organ or tissue are the two most critical factors affecting distribution of xenobiotics. Chemicals can have affinity to a binding site (e.g., intracellular protein or bone matrix) or to a cellular constituent (e.g., fat). The initial phase of distribution is primarily determined by blood flow to the various parts of the body. Therefore, a well-perfused organ like the liver may attain high initial concentrations of a xenobiotic. However, the affinity of less-well-perfused organs or tissues may be higher for a particular xenobiotic, causing redistribution with time. For example, two hours after administration, 50 percent of a dose of lead is found in the liver (Klaassen and Shoeman, 1974). However, one month after dosing, 90 percent of the dose remaining in the body is associated with the crystal lattice of bone. Similarly, five minutes after an intravenous dose of a lipophilic chemical, such as 2,3,7,8-tetrachlorodibenzo-*p*-dioxin, about 15 percent of the dose is localized in the lungs but only about 1 percent in adipose tissue. However, 24 hours later, only 0.3 percent of the remaining dose is found in the lungs but about 20 percent in adipose tissue.

EXCRETION

Toxicants are eliminated from the body by several routes. The kidney is perhaps the most important organ for excretion of xenobiotics, as more chemicals are eliminated from the body by this than by any other route (see Chapter 1). Many xenobiotics, though, have to be biotransformed first to more water-soluble products before they can be excreted into urine (see Chapter 4). The second important route of elimination of numerous xenobiotics is via feces, and the third, primarily for gases, is via the lungs. Biliary excretion of xenobiotics and/or their metabolites is most often the major source of fecal excretion, but a number of other sources can be significant for some compounds. All body secretions appear to have the ability to excrete chemicals; toxicants have been found in sweat, tears, and milk (Stowe and Plaa, 1968).

Urinary Excretion

The kidney is a very efficient organ for the elimination of toxicants from the body. Toxic compounds are excreted with urine by the same mechanisms the kidney uses to remove end products of intermediary metabolism from the body. These processes are glomerular filtration, tubular excretion by passive diffusion, and active tubular secretion.

The kidney receives about 25 percent of the cardiac output, and about 20 percent of this is filtered at the glomeruli. The glomerular capillaries have large pores (70 nm). Therefore, compounds will be filtered at the glomeruli up to a molecular weight of about 60,000 daltons (*e.g.*, proteins smaller than albumin). The degree of plasma protein binding affects the rate of filtration because protein-xenobiotic complexes are too large to pass through the pores of the glomeruli.

A toxicant filtered at the glomeruli may remain within the tubular lumen and be excreted with urine. Depending on the physicochemical properties of a compound, it may be reabsorbed across the tubular cells of the nephron back into the bloodstream. The principles governing reabsorption of toxicants across the kidney tubules are the same as discussed earlier for passive diffusion across cell membranes. Thus, toxicants with a high lipid/water partition coefficient will be reabsorbed efficiently, whereas polar compounds and ions will be excreted with urine. As can be deduced from the Henderson-Hasselbalch equations, bases will be excreted (i.e., not reabsorbed) to a greater extent at lower and acids at higher urinary pH values. A practical application of this knowledge may be illustrated by the treatment of phenobarbital poisoning with sodium bicarbonate. The percentage of ionization can be markedly increased within physiologically attainable pH ranges for a weak organic acid, such as phenobarbital (pK_a = 7.2). Consequently, alkalinization of urine by administration of sodium bicarbonate results in a significant increase in the excretion of phenobarbital (Weiner and Mudge, 1964). Similarly, acceleration of salicylate loss via the kidney can also be achieved by administration of sodium bicarbonate.

Toxic agents can also be excreted from plasma into urine by passive diffusion through the tubule. This process is probably of minor significance because filtration is much faster than excretion by passive diffusion through the tubules, providing a favorable concentration gradient for reabsorption rather than for excretion. Exceptions to this generalization may be some organic acids ($pK_a \approx 3-5$) and bases ($pK_a \approx 7-9$) that would be largely ionized and thus trapped at the pH of urine (pH $\approx$ 6). For renal excretion of such compounds, the flow of urine is likely to be important for the maintenance of a concentration gradient, favoring excretion. Thus, diuretics can hasten the elimination of weak organic acids and bases.

Toxic agents can also be excreted into urine by active secretion. There are two tubular secretory processes known—one for organic anions (acids) and the other for organic cations (bases). *p*-Aminohippurate is the prototype for the organic acid transport system, and *N*-methylnicotinamide for the organic base transporter. Specialized renal transport systems are located in the proximal tubules. In contrast to filtration, protein-bound toxicants are available for active transport. Active transport systems are located in the basolateral membranes, concentrating chemicals within the tubular epithelium. Often, xenobiotics are then excreted through the apical membrane of kidney tubule cells by facilitated diffusion. Like all active transport systems, renal secretion of xenobiotics also reveals competition. This fact was put to use during World War II when penicillin was in short supply. Penicillin is actively secreted by the organic acid system of the kidney. To lengthen its half-life and duration of action, another acid was sought to compete with penicillin for renal secretion. Probenecid was successfully introduced for this purpose. Uric acid is also secreted actively by renal tubules. It is of clinical relevance that toxicants transported by the organic acid transport system can increase plasma uric acid concentration and precipitate an attack of gout.

Because many functions of the kidney are incompletely developed at birth, some xenobiotics are eliminated more slowly in newborns than in adults. Therefore, they may be more toxic to newborns. For example, the clearance of penicillin by premature infants is only about 20 percent of that observed in older children (H. L. Barnett *et al.*, 1949). It has been demonstrated that development of this organic acid transport system in newborns can be stimulated by administration of substances normally excreted by this system (Hirsch and Hook, 1970). Some compounds such as cephaloridine are known to be nephrotoxic in adult animals but not in newborns. Because active uptake of cephaloridine by the kidneys is not well developed in newborns, it is not concentrated in the tubules and consequently is not nephrotoxic. If development of active transport in newborns is stimulated, the kidneys take up cephaloridine more readily, and nephrotoxicity is observed (Wold *et al.*, 1977).

Also, nephrotoxicity can be blocked by probenecid, which competitively inhibits the uptake of cephaloridine into kidneys (Tune *et al.*, 1977).

Species differences regarding urinary excretion of weak organic acids and bases are observed frequently, as the pH of urine varies widely among species. Differences in renal clearance can also occur for compounds filtered at the glomeruli, owing to differences in plasma protein binding. Interestingly, species variations can also arise as a result of differences in active renal secretion as was shown for captopril (Migdalof *et al.*, 1984).

Fecal Excretion

Fecal excretion is the other major pathway for the elimination of xenobiotics from the body. Fecal excretion of chemicals is a complex process not as well understood as urinary excretion. There are several important, and many more minor, sources contributing to the excretion of toxicants via the feces.

Nonabsorbed Ingesta. In addition to indigestible material, varying proportions of nutrients and xenobiotics present in the food or ingested voluntarily (drugs) pass through the alimentary canal unabsorbed, contributing to fecal excretion. Physicochemical properties of xenobiotics and biological characteristics facilitating absorption have been discussed earlier in this chapter. In general, most man-made chemicals are at least to some extent lipophilic and thus available for absorption. Exceptions include some macromolecules and some essentially completely ionized compounds of larger molecular weight. For example, absorption of polymers or quaternary ammonium bases is quite limited in the gut. Consequently, most of a dose of orally administered sucrose polyester, cholestyramine, or paraquat is found in feces. It is seldom that 100 percent of a compound is absorbed. Therefore, the nonabsorbed portion of xenobiotics contributes to fecal excretion of most chemicals to some extent.

Biliary Excretion. This route of elimination is perhaps the most important contributing source to fecal excretion of xenobiotics and even more important for the excretion of their metabolites. The liver is in a very advantageous position for removing toxic agents from blood after absorption from the gastrointestinal tract, because blood from the gastrointestinal tract passes through the liver before reaching the general circulation. Thus, liver can extract compounds from blood and thereby prevent their distribution to other parts of the body. Furthermore, the liver is the main site of biotransformation of toxicants, and the metabolites thus formed may be excreted directly into bile. Xenobiotics and/or their metabolites entering the intestine with bile may be excreted with feces, or when the physicochemical properties are favorable for reabsorption, an enterohepatic circulation may ensue.

Foreign compounds excreted into bile are often divided into three classes based on the ratio of their concentration in bile versus plasma. Class A substances have a ratio of nearly 1 and include sodium, potassium, glucose, mercury, thallium, cesium, and cobalt. Class B substances have a bile-to-plasma ratio greater than 1 (usually between 10 and 1000). Class B substances include bile acids, bilirubin, sulfobromophthalein, lcad, arsenic, manganese, and many other xenobiotics. Class C substances have a bile-to-plasma ratio less than 1 (e.g., inulin, albumin, zinc, iron, gold, and chromium). Compounds rapidly excreted into bile are most likely found among class B substances. However, a compound does not have to be highly concentrated in bile for biliary excretion to be of quantitative importance. For example, mercury is not concentrated in bile, yet bile is the main route of excretion for this slowly eliminated substance.

The mechanism of transport of foreign substances from plasma into liver and from liver into bile is not known with certainty. Especially little is known about the mechanism of transfer of class A and C compounds. However, it is thought that most class B compounds are actively transported across both sides of the hepatocyte. Liver has at least four transport systems for active excretion of organic compounds into bile. Two of these specifically transport organic acids, one organic bases and one neutral compounds. Biliary excretion of two organic acids, sulfobromophthalein (BSP) and indocyanine green (ICG), has been particularly well examined. The rate of removal of these two dyes has long been used in liver function tests. The test is performed by injecting either dye intravenously and determining the plasma disappearance profile of BSP or ICG. A lack of proper plasma clearance of BSP or ICG indicates reduced biliary excretion, suggesting liver injury. Bilirubin is also actively transported from plasma into bile. Therefore, jaundice is often observed after liver injury.

Like the kidneys, the liver also has an active transport system for the excretion of bases; procainamide ethyl bromide is the prototype for this transport system. There is an additional transport system in the liver for the excretion of neutral compounds such as ouabain. It appears that the liver has at least one more active transport sys-

tem for the excretion of metals (Klaassen, 1976). For example, lead is excreted into the bile against a large bile/plasma concentration ratio (100), with an apparent transport maximum. It is not known if other metals are also excreted into bile by the same or similar mechanisms.

As with renal tubular secretion, toxic agents bound to plasma proteins are fully available for active biliary excretion. The relative importance of biliary excretion depends on the substance and species concerned. It is not known what factors determine whether a chemical will be excreted into bile or into urine. However, low-molecular-weight compounds are poorly excreted into bile, but compounds (or their conjugates) with molecular weights exceeding about 325 can be excreted in appreciable quantities. Glutathione and glucuronide conjugates have a high predilection for excretion into bile. The percentage of a large number of compounds excreted into bile has been tabulated (Klaassen et al., 1981). Marked species variation in the biliary excretion of foreign compounds exists and can result in species difference regarding the biological half-life of a compound and its toxicity. This species variation in biliary excretion is compound specific. It is difficult, therefore, to categorize species into "good" or "poor" biliary excretors. However, in general, rats and mice tend to be better biliary excretors than other species (Klaassen and Watkins, 1984).

Once a compound is excreted into bile and enters the intestine, it can either be reabsorbed or eliminated with feces. Many organic compounds are conjugated before excretion into bile. Such polar metabolites are not sufficiently lipid soluble to be reabsorbed. However, intestinal microflora may hydrolyze glucuronide and sulfate conjugates, making the toxicant sufficiently lipophilic for reabsorption. Reabsorption of a xenobiotic completes an enterohepatic cycle. Repeated enterohepatic cycling may lead to very long half-lives of xenobiotics in the body. Therefore, it is often desirable to interrupt this cycle to hasten elimination of a toxicant from the body. This principle has been utilized in the treatment of methylmercury poisoning; ingestion of a polythiol resin binds the mercurial and thus prevents its reabsorption (Magos and Clarkson, 1976).

An increase in hepatic excretory function has also been observed after pretreatment with some drugs (Klaassen and Watkins, 1984). For example, it has been demonstrated that phenobarbital increases plasma disappearance by enhancing biliary excretion of BSP and a number of other compounds. The increase in bile flow caused by phenobarbital appears to be one important factor in increasing the biliary excretion of BSP. However, other factors such as induction of some phase II enzymes can also increase the conjugating capacity of the liver and thereby enhance plasma disappearance and biliary excretion of some compounds. Not all microsomal enzyme inducers increase bile flow and excretion; 3-methylcholanthrene and benzo[a]pyrene are relatively ineffective.

An increase in biliary excretion can decrease the toxicity of xenobiotics. Phenobarbital treatment of laboratory animals has been shown to enhance the biliary excretion and elimination of methylmercury from the body (Klaassen, 1975a; Magos and Clarkson, 1976). Two steroids known to induce microsomal enzymes, spironolactone and pregnenolone-16α-carbonitrile, have also been demonstrated to increase bile production and enhance biliary excretion of BSP (Zsigmond and Solymoss, 1972). These two steroids have also been shown to decrease the toxicity of several chemicals. (Selye, 1971), including cardiac glycosides (Selye, 1969), by increasing their biliary excretion. This in turn decreases concentration of cardiac glycosides in the heart, their target organ of toxicity (Castle and Lage, 1972, 1973; Klaassen, 1974a).

The toxicity of some compounds can be directly related to their biliary excretion. For example, indomethacin can cause intestinal lesions. The sensitivity of various species to this toxic response is directly related to the amount of indomethacin excreted into bile. The formation of intestinal lesions can be abolished by bile duct ligation (Duggan et al., 1975).

The hepatic excretory system is not fully developed in the newborn, which is another reason why some compounds are more toxic to newborns than to adults (Klaassen, 1972, 1973a). For example, ouabain is about 40 times more toxic in newborn than in adult rats. This is due to an almost complete inability of the newborn rat liver to remove ouabain from plasma. A decreased excretory function of newborn liver has also been demonstrated for other xenobiotics (Klaassen, 1973b). The development of hepatic excretory function can be promoted in newborns by administering microsomal enzyme inducers (Klaassen, 1974b).

Intestinal Excretion. It has been shown for a fairly large number of diverse chemicals (e.g., digitoxin, dinitrobenzamide, hexachlorobenzene, ochratoxin A, etc.) that their excretion into feces can be explained neither by the not-absorbed portion of an oral dosage nor by excretion into bile (Rozman, 1986). Experiments in bile duct–ligated animals and in animals provided with bile fistulae have revealed that the source of many chemicals in feces is a direct transfer from blood into the intestinal contents.

This transfer is thought to occur for most xenobiotics by passive diffusion. In some instances, rapid exfoliation of intestinal cells may also contribute to fecal excretion of some compounds. Intestinal excretion is a relatively slow process. Therefore, it is a major pathway of elimination only for compounds that have low rates of biotransformation and/or low renal or biliary clearance. The rate of intestinal excretion of some lipid-soluble compounds can be substantially enhanced by increasing the lipophilicity of the gastrointestinal contents, for example, adding mineral oil to the diet (Rozman, 1986). Active secretion of organic acids and bases has also been demonstrated in the gut (Lauterbach, 1977). The importance of active intestinal secretion for fecal elimination has been established only for a few chemicals.

Intestinal Wall and Flora. No systematic attempts have been undertaken to assess the role of biotransformation in the intestinal wall on the fecal excretion of xenobiotics. Nevertheless, evidence has accumulated in recent years that mucosal biotransformation and reexcretion into the intestinal lumen occur with many compounds. The significance of these findings for fecal excretion is difficult to judge because further interaction with the gut flora may still alter these compounds, making them more or less suitable for reabsorption or excretion (Rozman, 1986). More is known about the contribution of the intestinal flora to fecal excretion. It has been estimated that 30 to 42 percent of fecal dry matter originates from bacteria. Chemicals originating from the nonabsorbed portion of an oral dose, from the bile, or from the intestinal wall are taken up by these microorganisms according to the principles of membrane permeability. Therefore, a considerable proportion of fecally excreted xenobiotics is associated with the excreted bacteria. However, chemicals may be profoundly altered by bacteria prior to excretion with feces—particularly in the large intestine where intestinal flora is most abundant, and intestinal contents remain for 24 hours and longer. It seems that biotransformation by intestinal flora favors reabsorption rather than excretion. Nevertheless, there is evidence that in many instances xenobiotics found in feces derive from bacterial biotransformation. The importance of microbial biotransformation for fecal excretion can be studied by performing experiments in normal versus gnotobiotic animals (animals with no microflora).

Exhalation

Substances that exist predominantly in the gas phase at body temperature are eliminated mainly by the lungs. Because volatile liquids are in equilibrium with their gas phase in the alveoli, they may also be excreted via the lungs. The amount of a liquid eliminated via the lungs is proportional to its vapor pressure. A practical application of this principle is the breath analyzer test for determining the amount of ethanol in the body. Highly volatile liquids, such as diethyl ether, are almost exclusively excreted by the lungs.

No specialized transport systems have been described for excretion of toxic substances by the lungs. They seem to be eliminated by simple diffusion. Elimination of gases is roughly inversely proportional to the rate of their absorption. Therefore, gases with low solubility in blood, such as ethylene, are rapidly excreted, whereas chloroform, with a much higher solubility in blood, is eliminated very slowly by the lungs. Trace concentrations of highly lipid-soluble anesthetic gases, such as halothane and methoxyflurane, may be present in expired air for as long as two to three weeks after a few hours of anesthesia. Undoubtedly, this prolonged retention is due to deposition in and slow mobilization from adipose tissue of the highly lipid-soluble agents. The rate of elimination of a gas with low solubility in blood is perfusion limited, whereas that with a high solubility in blood is ventilation limited.

Other Routes of Elimination

Cerebrospinal Fluid. A specialized route of removal of toxic agents from a specific organ is represented by the cerebrospinal fluid. All compounds can leave the CNS with the bulk flow of cerebrospinal fluid through the arachnoid villi. In addition, lipid-soluble toxicants can also exit at the site of the blood-brain barrier. It is noteworthy that toxicants can also be removed from the cerebrospinal fluid by active transport similar to the transport system of the kidneys for the excretion of organic ions.

Milk. Secretion of toxic compounds into milk is extremely important because (1) a toxic material may be passed with milk from the mother to the nursing child, and (2) compounds can be passed from cows to people via dairy products. Toxic agents are excreted into milk by simple diffusion. Because milk is more acidic (pH $\approx$ 6.5) than plasma, basic compounds may be concentrated in milk, whereas acidic compounds may attain lower concentrations in milk than in plasma (Findlay, 1983; Wilson, 1983). More important, about 3 to 4 percent of milk consists of lipids, and lipid content of colostrum following parturition is even higher. Lipid-soluble xenobiotics diffuse along with fats from plasma into the mammary gland and are excreted with milk during lactation. Compounds like

DDT and polychlorinated and polybrominated biphenyls are known to occur in milk, and in fact milk can be a major route of their excretion. Species differences in excretion of xenobiotics with milk are to be expected, as the proportion of milk fat derived from the circulation versus that synthesized *de novo* in the mammary gland differs widely among species. Metals chemically similar to calcium, such as lead, and chelating agents that form complexes with calcium can also be excreted into milk to a considerable extent.

Sweat and Saliva. The excretion of toxic agents by these two routes is quantitatively of minor importance. Again, excretion depends on diffusion of the nonionized, lipid-soluble form of an agent. Toxic compounds excreted into sweat may produce dermatitis. Substances excreted in saliva enter the mouth, where they are usually swallowed and thus are available for gastrointestinal absorption.

TOXICOKINETICS

The study of the kinetics of chemicals was first initiated for drugs and consequently termed *pharmacokinetics*. However, toxicology is not limited to the study of adverse drug effects but entails investigation of deleterious effects of all chemicals. Therefore, the study of the kinetics of xenobiotics is more properly called *toxicokinetics*. Toxicokinetics are the modeling and mathematical description of the time course of disposition (absorption, distribution, biotransformation, and excretion) of xenobiotics in the whole organism. As will be shown later, it is also possible to model the individual steps of disposition (e.g., elimination alone) separately or even to describe the kinetics of xenobiotics in isolated organs (e.g., hepatic clearance). The most common way to characterize the kinetics of drugs in the past has been to represent the body as consisting of a number of compartments, even though these compartments have no apparent physiological or anatomical reality. More recently, physiologically based pharmacokinetic models have been advanced, where mass balance equations allow the modeling of each organ or tissue based on physiological considerations. It should be emphasized that there is no inherent contradiction between the classical and the physiologically based approach. Classical pharmacokinetics, as will be shown, require certain assumptions that the physiologically based models do not need. Under ideal conditions, physiological pharmacokinetic models are able to predict tissue concentrations, which classical models cannot do. However, the appropriate physiological (e.g., blood flow rate, tissue volume,

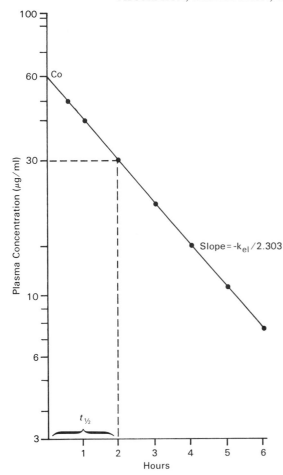

Plasma Concentration (μg/ml)

Hours

Figure 3–8. Schematic representation of the concentration of a chemical in the plasma as a function of time after intravenous injection if the body acts as a one-compartment system and elimination of the chemical obeys first-order kinetics with a rate constant (k_{el}).

etc.) and biochemical (e.g., rate of biotransformation in a particular tissue) parameters are often unknown or inexact, hampering a meaningful physiologically based pharmacokinetic modeling.

Classical Toxicokinetics

One-Compartment Model. The simplest case of a toxicokinetic modeling entails measurement of plasma concentrations of a xenobiotic at several time points after administration of a bolus intravenous injection. If the data obtained and plotted as the logarithms of plasma concentrations versus time yield a straight line, then the kinetics of such a compound can be described by a one-compartment model (Figure 3–8). Compounds whose toxicokinetics can be described by a one-compartment model rapidly equilibrate between blood and the various tissues. The one-compartment model depicts the body as a homogeneous unit. This does not mean that the concentration of a compound is the same throughout the body, but it does assume that changes occurring in plasma concentration reflect changes in tissue levels.

The elimination from the body of a chemical whose disposition is described by a one-compartment model occurs by a first-order process; that is, the rate of elimination at any time is proportional to the amount of chemical in the body at that time. Elimination includes all biotransformation and excretion routes. The rate constant k_{el} of this first-order elimination has units of reciprocal time (e.g., min^{-1} or hr^{-1}). Thus, if the elimination rate constant is, for example, $0.3\ \text{hr}^{-1}$, then 30 percent of the dose will be excreted within the first hour and 30 percent of the remaining dose in each subsequent hour. (See Table below.)

A mathematical expression of this first-order process is

$$\log C = \log C_0 - \frac{k_{el} \cdot t}{2.303}$$

and the antilogarithm yields $C = C_0 \cdot e^{-k_{el} \cdot t}$, a monoexponential equation where C is the plasma concentration; k_{el}, the first-order elimination rate constant; and t, the time of blood sampling. The logarithmic equation has the general form of an equation describing a straight line where $\log C_0$ represents the intercept, and $-k_{el}/2.303$ the slope of the line. Thus, the first-order elimination rate constant can be determined from the slope of the log C versus time plot.

Another important and frequently used parameter to characterize the time course of toxicants in an organism is the half-life ($t_{1/2}$). The half-life or elimination half-life $t_{1/2}$ is the time required for the plasma concentration of a chemical to decrease by one-half. Because of the relationship

TIME (hr)	0	1	2	3	4	5	6
Chemical remaining (mg)	60	42	29.4	20.6	14.4	10.1	7.0
Chemical eliminated (mg)		18	12.6	8.8	6.1	4.3	3.1	
Chemical eliminated (% of that remaining)		30	30	30	30	30	30	

$$t_{1/2} = \frac{0.693}{k_{el}}$$

the half-life of a compound can be calculated after k_{el} has been determined from the slope of the line. The $t_{1/2}$ can also be determined by visual inspection of the log C versus time plot, as shown in Figure 3–8. For compounds eliminated by first-order kinetics, the time required for the plasma concentration to decrease by one-half is constant. Therefore, toxicants eliminated from the body by first-order processes are theoretically never completely eliminated. However, during seven half-lives, 99.2 percent of a chemical is eliminated, which for practical purposes can be viewed as complete elimination.

Small laboratory animals may not have enough blood to support closely spaced sampling, required for a kinetic study, or often human subjects are unwilling to submit to repeated blood sampling. Fortunately, urinary excretion data can also be used to determine $t_{1/2}$. In practice, the concentration of the administered compound is measured in aliquots of urine samples collected at frequent time intervals. The amount is calculated by mutliplying the concentration with the total volume collected for that time period. The amounts, obtained for the various collection periods, are plotted semilogarithmically against the midpoints of the successive collection periods. The accuracy of this method greatly depends on how often, and how meticulously, continuous sampling of urine is carried out. A more precise method of determining the elimination half-life of a chemical from urine is to plot the logarithm of the amount yet to be excreted in the ordinate against time on the abscissa. It is necessary to collect urine for seven half-lives and not to lose any samples, in order to determine accurately the total amount to be excreted into urine. This method is called the Σ minus plot, because the amount remaining to be excreted is calculated by deducting the amount excreted for each collection period from the total amount excreted during seven half-lives. The Σ minus plot can also be employed to calculate half-lives in instances when the parent compound (administered drug or xenobiotic) is not excreted in urine (e.g., only metabolites) but in feces. The $t_{1/2}$ can be determined from the slope of the line obtained by either of these methods.

The half-life of a chemical obeying first-order elimination kinetics is independent of dose. This means that plotting the logarithm of concentration divided by dose as a function of time yields a single straight line (Figure 3–9). This is known as the *principle of superposition*. In a one-compartment open model (*open* indicating that the chemical is being eliminated from the

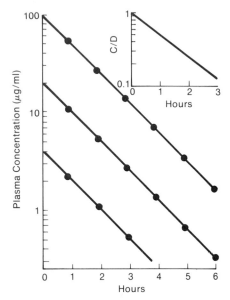

Figure 3–9. Schematic representation of the time course of elimination of different doses of a chemical after intravenous injection, assuming that the body acts as a one-compartment system and elimination obeys first-order kinetics. The *inset* is a semilogarithmic plot of plasma concentrations (C) divided by dose (D) as a function of time.

system), the concentration of a chemical in tissues is assumed to decrease with the same half-life as in the plasma (Figure 3–10). The ratio of tissue to plasma concentration is thus constant, and if known, tissue concentrations can be calculated from plasma concentrations.

In summary, important characteristics of first-order elimination according to a one-compartment model are: (1) the amount of chemical eliminated at any time is directly proportional to the amount of chemical in the body at that time; (2) a semilogarithmic plot of plasma concentration versus time yields a single straight line; (3) the half-life ($t_{1/2}$) is independent of dose; and (4) the concentration of chemical in plasma and other tissues decreases by some constant fraction per unit of time, referred to as elimination rate constant (k_{el}).

Toxicokinetic modeling of compounds administered by routes other than intravenously is slightly more complicated. Administration of xenobiotics by any other route will result in a distinct uptake phase with a lag period before peak concentration in plasma in reached. Figure 3–11 depicts a typical curve for a compound after oral administration. The elimination phase can be treated as an intravenous injection by extrapolating the terminal straight line of the log C versus time plot to intercept the ordinate at a

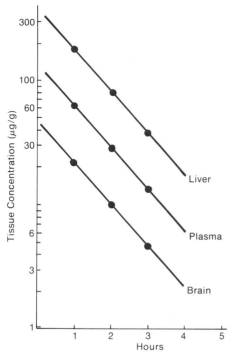

Figure 3–10. Schematic representation of the concentration of a chemical in plasma and various tissues as a function of time after intravenous injection if the body acts as a one-compartment system.

putative C_0. The first-order elimination rate constant (k_{el}) and $t_{1/2}$ can then be determined from the slope. The mathematical description of the uptake phase for first-order absorption is somewhat more complex because absorption and elimination overlap. The important fact is that a slope for the uptake phase can be determined by

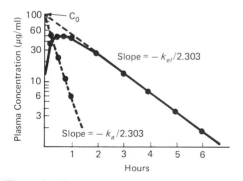

Figure 3–11. Semilogarithmic plot of concentration of chemical in plasma after oral administration of a chemical whose disposition can be described by a one-compartment open system. The rate constant for absorption (k_a) is determined by the method of residuals as discussed in the text.

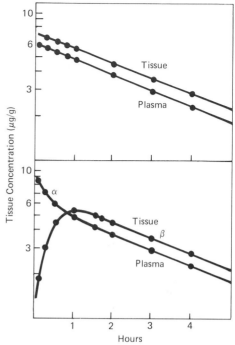

Figure 3–12. Schematic representation of the concentration of a toxicant in plasma and tissue with time in a one-compartment open model *(top panel)* and in a two-compartment open model *(bottom panel)*.

the method of residuals. This entails plotting of the difference between the above-described extrapolated portion of the slope and the experimentally determined early plasma concentrations. A plot of these calculated points yields a straight line with the slope of $k_a/2.303$, which permits determination of the first-order absorption rate constant (k_a) as well as of the absorption half-life.

Two-Component Model. If the semilogarithmic plot of plasma concentration versus time does not yield a straight line, but a curve after intravenous administration, then a multicompartmental analysis of the results is necessary. As noted earlier, a chemical whose toxicokinetics can be described by a one-compartment model rapidly distributes between the plasma and various tissues. However, some chemicals require longer time for their concentration in tissues to reach equilibrium with plasma, as depicted in the bottom panel of Figure 3–12. This results in a biexponential elimination of the toxicant from the plasma. The disposition of such a chemical is said to obey a two-compartment model.

In the simplest case, such a curve can be resolved into two monoexponential terms (two-compartment model) of the type $C = Ae^{-\alpha t} +$

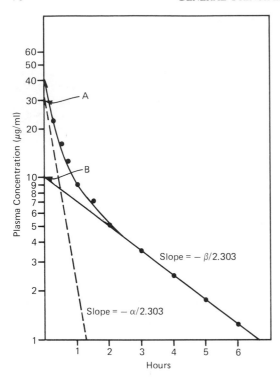

Figure 3–13. Semilogarithmic plot of concentration of chemical in plasma after intravenous injection when the body may be represented as a two-compartment open system. The *dashed line* is obtained by the method of residuals (see text).

$Be^{-\beta t}$, where A and B are proportionality constants, and α and β are rate constants with dimensions of reciprocal time (Figure 3–13). The logarithmic form of this equation yields terms for two straight lines according to

$$\log C = \log A - \frac{\alpha \cdot t}{2.303} + \log B - \frac{\beta \cdot t}{2.303}$$

The slope of the terminal straight line is $-\beta/2.303$. Extrapolation of this line to time zero yields B. The slope of the initial phase of the plasma concentration curve can be resolved by the method of residuals, also called "feathering" as depicted in Figure 3–13. By this method, the slope for the α-phase can be obtained by forming the difference between the observed points and the corresponding points of the extrapolated line. When the logarithms of these residuals are plotted against time, they give the line for the initial phase, with the slope $-\alpha/2.303$ and the intercept A. During the distribution or α-phase, concentrations of the chemical in the plasma will decrease more rapidly than in the postdistribution β-phase (also referred to as equilibrium or elimination phase) (Figure 3–13). The distribu-

tion phase may last for only a few minutes or for hours or days. Whether or not the distribution phase becomes apparent depends on the time when the first plasma samples are obtained.

A biexponential decline of a chemical from plasma is viewed pharmacokinetically as an open two-compartment system (Figure 3–14). The intercompartmental disposition rate constants between the two compartments can be calculated by the following equations:

$$k_{21} = \frac{\alpha B + \beta A}{A + B}$$

$$k_{12} = \alpha + \beta - k_{21} - k_{el}$$

The elimination rate constant from the central compartment is given by the equation

$$k_{el} = \frac{\alpha \beta}{k_{21}}$$

It should be noted that the elimination rate constant from the central compartment (k_{el}) in a two-compartment model is not a simple rate constant, as in a one-compartment model. The equivalent of k_{el} in a one-compartment model is β in a two-compartment model. Thus, half-life of a compound displaying characteristics of a two-compartment model can be calculated by the equation

$$\beta = \frac{0.693}{t_{1/2}}$$

Determination of the intercompartmental rate constants permits assessment of the relative contribution of distribution and elimination processes to the plasma disappearance profile of a chemical. For most chemicals, the valid assumption can be made that elimination occurs from

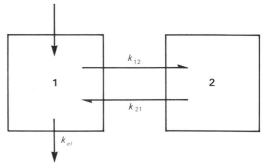

Figure 3–14. Schematic representation of the two-compartment system consisting of a central compartment (*1*) and a peripheral compartment (*2*). The numbering of the rate constants (*k*) indicates the originating compartment (first numeral) and the receiving compartment (second numeral).

the central or plasma compartment as depicted in Figure 3–14. The reason for this assumption is that the liver and kidney, the major sites of biotransformation and excretion, are well perfused with blood and thus are in essentially instantaneous equilibrium with plasma. Therefore, they are considered to belong to the central compartment. However, this assumption is not always correct. For example, it has been noted for some chemicals excreted by the intestinal tract, like hexachlorobenzene, that elimination occurs from the peripheral compartment. For such compounds, a different set of equations is required to yield data compatible with experimental results (Scheufler and Rozman, 1984).

The plasma concentration profile of many compounds cannot be satisfactorily described by an equation with two exponential terms. Sometimes three or four exponential terms are needed to fit a curve to the log C versus time plot. Such compounds are viewed as displaying characteristics of three- or four-compartment open models. The principles to deal with such models are the same as discussed for the two-compartment open model, but the mathematics are complex.

SATURATION OF ELIMINATION

The elimination of most chemicals occurs by first-order processes. However, as the dosage of a compound increases, its rate of elimination may decrease, as shown in Figure 3–15. This is usually referred to as to saturation or Michaelis-Menten kinetics. Biotransformation and active transport processes, as well as protein binding, have finite capacities and can be saturated. When the concentration of a chemical in the body is higher than its K_m, then the rate of elimination is not any more proportional to the dose. The transition from first-order to saturation kinetics is important in toxicology because it leads to prolonged residency time of a compound in the body, which can result in increased toxicity.

Some criteria that indicate nonlinear pharmacokinetics are the following: (1) Decline in the levels of the chemical in the body is not exponential; (2) $t_{1/2}$ increases with increasing dose; (3) the area under the plasma concentration versus time curve (AUC) is not proportional to the dose; (4) the composition of the excretory products may change both quantitatively and quali-

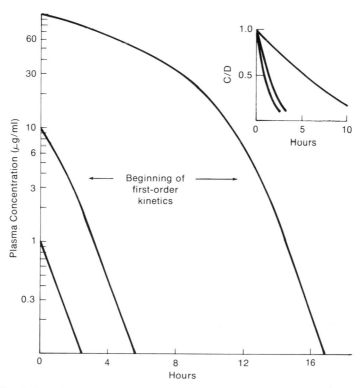

Figure 3–15. Schematic representation of the time course of elimination of different doses of a chemical after rapid intravenous administration of three different dosages, assuming the body acts as a one-compartment system and that it is easily saturated. The *inset* is a plot of the plasma concentrations (C) divided by dose (D).

tatively with dose; (5) competitive inhibition by other chemicals biotransformed or actively transported by the same enzyme system can occur; and (6) dose-response curves may show an unusually large increase in response to increasing dose, starting at the dose level where saturation effects become evident.

The elimination of some chemicals from the body is readily saturated. These compounds follow zero-order kinetics. Ethanol is an example of a chemical whose elimination follows zero-order kinetics, its biotransformation being the rate-limiting step in its elimination. As exemplified below, a constant amount is biotransformed per unit of time regardless of the amount of ethanol present in the body.

TIME (hr)	0	1	2	3	4	5
Ethanol remaining (ml)	50	40	30	20	10	0
Ethanol eliminated (ml)		10	10	10	10	10
Ethanol eliminated (% of that remaining)		20	25	33	50	100

Important characteristics of zero-order processes are: (1) an arithmetic plot of plasma concentration versus time yields a straight line; (2) the rate or amount of chemical eliminated at any time is constant and is independent of amount of chemical in the body; and (3) a true $t_{1/2}$ or k_{el} does not exist.

Apparent Volume of Distribution

The apparent volume of distribution (V_d) is a proportionality constant relating the concentration of a xenobiotic in plasma to the total amount of chemical in the body. V_d has no direct physiological meaning and usually does not refer to a real volume. This is the reason why it is correctly called the *apparent volume of distribution*. A chemical with high affinity for a tissue(s) will have a large volume of distribution. In fact, binding to tissues may be so avid that V_d of a chemical will be much larger than the actual body volume. The apparent volume of distribution of a chemical displaying characteristics of a one-compartment model is mathematically defined as the quotient between the amount of chemical in the body and its plasma concentration. Determination of V_d is analogous to adding a known amount of a dye to a container with an unknown volume of liquid. After the liquid has been well stirred, the volume of the liquid (i.e., the volume of distribution) can be determined by dividing the amount of dye added by the concentration measured in the container. Unlike the dye in the container, the concentration of a chemical in plasma declines owing to excretion, distribu-

tion, and biotransformation in tissues. Therefore, to estimate V_d, it is necessary to extrapolate the plasma disappearance curve after intravenous injection to the zero time point. This extrapolation yields the plasma concentration C_0 at the time zero, that is, before any elimination took place (Figure 3–8). The apparent volume of distribution (V_d) can be calculated by the following equation:

$$V_d = \frac{\text{Dose}_{iv}}{C_0}$$

where Dose_{iv} is the intravenous dose and C_0 the extrapolated plasma concentration at time zero. This equation is appropriate for chemicals displaying characteristics of a one-compartment model but is not valid for those that require two or more compartments for their modeling. For compounds displaying characteristics of a two-compartment model, not one but several V_d definitions are possible. For example, the volume of the central compartment may be defined as

$$V_c = \frac{\text{Dose}_{iv}}{A + B}$$

where A and B represent disposition constants of a two-compartment model (Figure 3–13). Or the volume of the peripheral compartment may be defined as

$$V_p = \frac{\text{Dose}_{iv}}{B}$$

where B is derived from the elimination or equilibrium phase of a two-compartment model.

A model independent method to determine V_d is to use the relationship

$$V_d = \frac{\text{Dose}_{iv}}{AUC_{0\to\infty} \cdot k_{el} \text{ (or } \beta)}$$

in which $AUC_{0\to\infty}$ is the total area under the plasma concentration versus time curve plotted on rectilinear graph paper, as depicted in Figure 3–16. This is usually determined by calculating the $AUC_{0\to\infty}$ from time zero to the last time point at which plasma has been collected by adding the area (A) of the trapezoids formed by each two successive plasma samples [$A = \frac{1}{2}(c_1 + c_2) \cdot (t_2 - t_1)$, where c_1 and c_2 are the plasma concentrations of the chemical at two consecutive time intervals, and $t_2 - t_1$ is the time interval between the two plasma samples] plus the area of the curve from the last plasma sample (t^*) to infinity, which is calculated by the following relationship:

Area from t^* to $\infty = C_t^*/k_{el}$

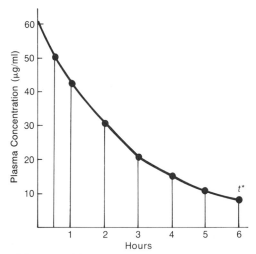

Figure 3–16. Schematic representation of the plasma concentration of a toxicant in plasma plotted on an arithmetic-arithmetic scale.

where C_t^* is the last plasma concentration data point. The elimination rate constant (k_{el}) can be obtained (Figure 3–8) from the slope of the semilogarithmic plasma disappearance line (slope = $-k_{el}/2.303$).

The apparent volume of distribution (V_d) of a chemical is also important for determining the body burden of a chemical. *Body burden* is the total amount of chemical in the body at a given time point. Because V_d is mathematically defined as the quotient of the amount of chemical in the body and its plasma concentration at time zero, it is evident that the body burden of a chemical equals the product of the plasma concentration of the chemical and V_d at any given time:

$$X = C \cdot V_d$$

where X is the amount; C, the concentration of a xenobiotic in plasma at a given time; and V_d, the apparent volume of distribution.

Clearance

Clearance is another important and frequently used toxicokinetic concept to characterize various compounds. Clearance is a proportionality constant relating a substance's rate of transfer or elimination to its concentration in an appropriate reference fluid, usually plasma. Clearance has the units of flow rate (ml/min). A clearance of 100 ml/min of a xenobiotic means that 100 ml of blood or plasma are completely cleared of the compound for each minute that passes. The overall efficiency of removal of a chemical from the body can be characterized by clearance. High values of clearance indicate efficient and gener-

ally rapid removal, whereas low clearance values indicate slow and less efficient removal of a xenobiotic from the body. Chemicals are cleared from the body by various routes, for example, via the kidneys, liver, or intestine. *Total body clearance* is defined as the sum of clearances by individual organs:

$$Cl = Cl_r + Cl_h + Cl_i + \ldots$$

whereby Cl_r depicts renal, Cl_h hepatic, and Cl_i intestinal clearance. It is important to note that the clearance of xenobiotics cannot be higher than blood flow to a particular organ. In the case of a xenobiotic being eliminated by hepatic biotransformation, clearance could not exceed hepatic blood flow rate. Total body clearance is defined mathematically by the equations

$$Cl = \frac{Dose_{iv}}{AUC_{0 \to \infty}}$$

or

$$Cl = V_d \cdot k_{el}$$

for a one-compartment model and

$$Cl = V_d \cdot \beta$$

for a two-compartment model. Clearance is an exceedingly important concept in toxicokinetics. It is the single most important index of a given organism's capacity to remove xenobiotics. Clearance is also the major determinant of the extent a xenobiotic accumulates during multiple dosing regimens. Often, it is more useful to define specific organ clearances because they may provide important information about the proper functioning or diseased state of an organ.

Hepatic Clearance. The general concept of organ clearance may be illustrated with the example of hepatic clearance. It is easiest to understand organ clearance by considering the situation in a well-perfused organ that is capable of elimination, such as the liver (Figure 3–17). Blood flow through the liver is designated as Q_h (ml/min); the concentration of the toxicant in arterial blood entering the organ is C_a and in the venous blood leaving the organ is C_v. If the liver biotransforms or excretes the compound, then $C_a > C_v$. The rate at which a chemical enters the liver is given by the product of C_a and Q_h, and the rate at which it leaves the liver by the product of C_v and Q_h. According to mass balance considerations, the rate of elimination by the liver equals the difference between rate *in* and rate *out*. Comparing the rate of elimination of a xenobiotic with the rate at which it enters the

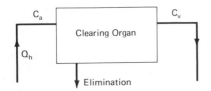

Figure 3–17. Flow model for clearance of xenobiotics by the liver. Q_h denotes blood flow rate through the liver, C_a and C_v the concentrations in arterial and venous blood, respectively.

organ yields a dimensionless quantity called the *extraction ratio* (E).

$$E_h = \frac{Q_h \cdot (C_a - C_v)}{Q_h \cdot C_a} = \frac{C_a - C_v}{C_a}$$

The extraction ratio is a quantitative measure for the efficiency of an organ (here the liver) to remove a chemical from blood under fixed conditions of blood flow. If an organ is incapable of extracting a xenobiotic, then $C_a = C_v$ and E will be zero. If it completely extracts it from blood, then $C_v \approx 0$ and E will approach unity. An extraction ratio of 0.8, for example, means that 80 percent of the blood flowing through the organ will be cleared of a toxicant. According to these considerations, clearance of a toxicant by the liver may be defined as the product of the flow and extraction ratio:

$$Cl_h = \frac{Q_h \cdot (C_a - C_v)}{C_a} = Q_h \cdot E_h$$

This direct proportionality indicates that changes in blood flow and altered extraction ratios will have an impact on hepatic clearance of xenobiotics. Numerous physiological conditions (supine posture, food) and pharmacological agents (glucagon, isoproterenol, phenobarbital) are known to alter hepatic blood flow. The extraction ratio may also be altered, for example, by increased rate of biotransformation due to enzyme induction. Because of the relationship of Cl_h to Q_h and E_h, it is apparent that the plasma disappearance profile (as indicative of hepatic clearance) will be more significantly altered for high than for low extraction ratio compounds, irrespective of route of administration. Therefore, the half-life of low extraction xenobiotics is minimally affected by, for example, decreased blood flow to the liver, whereas that of a high extraction ratio compound is greatly increased. In contrast, changes in Q_h will affect the plasma disappearance profile of compounds with a low extraction ratio significantly but that of high extraction ratio substances only minimally. It should be noted that the route of administration does affect the *AUC* (systemic availability) of high extraction ratio compounds because of the increased first-pass effect after oral as compared with intravenous administration. The difference between high and low extraction ratio xenobiotics can be best illustrated by defining the rate-determining step in their clearance. For substances exhibiting a high extraction ratio, the rate-limiting step is blood flow; for those with a low extraction ratio, it is extraction by the liver. If extraction is enhanced, for example, by increased biotransformation, then a reduced half-life results.

Renal Clearance. The renal excretory mechanisms (glomerular filtration, renal secretion, renal reabsorption, or any combination thereof) remove a constant fraction of a toxicant from the blood delivered to the kidneys. It is known that the polymeric carbohydrate inulin is neither bound to plasma proteins nor secreted into tubules nor reabsorbed from tubules but enters the urine by filtration only. Because inulin is not reabsorbed after being filtered, its clearance (Cl_{in}) is the same as the glomerular filtration rate (*GFR*).

Many substances are reabsorbed back into the circulation together with fluid after they have been filtered at the glomerulus. For these substances, the volume of plasma cleared is smaller than the filtered volume ($Cl_x < Cl_{in}$). For substances that are secreted actively by the kidney, the volume of plasma cleared of a substance can be greater than the *GFR* because theoretically all the chemical reaching the kidney can be cleared by active secretion ($Cl_x > Cl_{in}$). It must be remembered that renal plasma flow (660 ml/min) is much larger than the *GFR* (125 ml/min). Thus, by comparing the renal clearance of a toxicant to that of inulin, one can determine how substances are excreted by the kidney. However, after a chemical is filtered or secreted into renal tubules, it can be passively reabsorbed if present in the lipid-soluble form. For many toxicants, more than one process is responsible for their urinary excretion, and the use of competitive blockers of active transport systems and/or changes in acid-base balance may be necessary to elucidate fully the mechanisms of excretion. One must remember that only the unbound portion of a toxicant is available for filtration, whereas both bound and unbound toxicants are available for secretion. Because of these considerations, renal clearance is somewhat more complicated than the simple organ clearance concept developed for the liver. Renal clearance may be described by the following equation:

$$Cl_r = (Cl_{rf} + Cl_{rs}) (1 - F)$$

where Cl_{rf} is renal filtration clearance, CL_{rs} is renal secretion clearance, and F is that fraction of the filtered and secreted xenobiotic that is reabsorbed. The mathematical solution of this equation for blood flow dependence is complex, and interested readers are referred to specialty books (Gibaldi and Perrier, 1982). However, if urinary excretion is the sole or at least the predominant pathway of excretion, renal clearance will approximate total body clearance and may be determined by the equations shown for total body clearance.

Although renal clearance tells us the volume of plasma cleared per minute, it tells nothing about the rate of plasma disappearance of a xenobiotic. To determine this rate, it is necessary to know the apparent volume of distribution (V_d) of the toxicant. Clearly, the greater the V_d, the less of a chemical is present in plasma and thus the less of it is available for clearance. For example, if a toxicant is excreted solely by glomerular filtration (125 ml/min), its half-life would be about 16 minutes if it distributed into plasma water (3 liters) but would be about 200 minutes if it distributed into total body water (38 liters).

Intravenous Infusion

Intravenous infusion is seldom used in studying the toxicity of xenobiotics but is often used in drug therapy where toxic side effects may occur. More important, intravenous infusion is most suitable to illustrate another important concept of toxicokinetics, that of steady state. If a chemical is infused into a vein at a constant rate, then plasma concentrations will rise until the rate of infusion equals the rate of elimination by all routes (Figure 3–18). After an infusion time equaling four half-lives, the plasma concentration is within 10 percent; after seven half-lives, within 1 percent of plateau levels. This concentration is called the *steady-state plasma concentration* and is defined as

$$C_{ss} = \frac{k_0}{V_d \cdot k_{el}}$$

for a one-compartment model and as

$$C_{ss} = \frac{k_0}{V_d \cdot \beta}$$

for a two-compartment model. The steady-state concentration of a chemical is directly proportional to the rate of zero-order (constant) infusion (k_0) and inversely related to V_d and k_{el} for a one-compartment or to V_d and β for a two-compartment model. When infusion is stopped, without regard to having reached steady state or

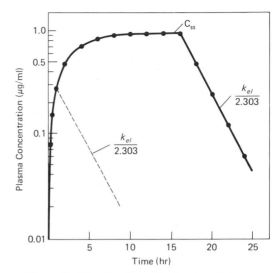

Figure 3–18. Semilogarithmic plot of plasma concentration as a function of time during and after stopping of a constant intravenous infusion of a chemical.

not, plasma concentration of a chemical declines according to the principles discussed for single intravenous injection. Exposure to chemicals by inhalation can also be modeled like intravenous infusion when equilibrium occurs very rapidly between the alveolar space and blood.

Kinetics of Repeated Exposure

Multiple dosing and intravenous infusion are related in that intravenous infusion may be viewed as repeated injections with infinitely small time intervals between consecutive injections. Therefore, there are similarities in the toxicokinetic treatment of these two models. However, additional considerations also have to be introduced when the dosing interval is finite. If the half-life of a xenobiotic is short in relation to the exposure interval, the substance may be almost completely eliminated by the time the next dose is given. In such instances, each consecutive dose can be dealt with as if it were a single dose. When the half-life is about the same or greater than the exposure interval, an appreciable amount of toxicant will still be present in the body before the second and subsequent exposures. In such cases, toxicants will accumulate until the steady state is reached (Figure 3–19). Unlike with intravenous infusion, the plasma concentration of a xenobiotic will fluctuate between two consecutive doses, depending on dosing interval and the inherent toxicokinetic characteristics of the chemical. The time required to attain about 90 and 99 percent of steady state is about four and seven biologic half-lives, as discussed for intravenous infusion.

The "average" steady-state concentration $\bar{C}_{ss}$ can be determined by the following equation for a one-compartment model:

$$\bar{C}_{ss} = \frac{\text{Dose}_{iv}}{V_d \cdot k_{el} \cdot \tau}$$

or

$$\bar{C}_{ss} = \frac{\text{Dose}_{iv}}{V_d \cdot \beta \cdot \tau}$$

for a two-compartment model, where τ depicts the constant dosing interval between two consecutive doses. A similar equation may be derived for oral administration:

$$\bar{C}_{ss} = \frac{f \cdot \text{Dose}_{oral}}{V_d \cdot k_{el} \cdot \tau}$$

where f is the fraction absorbed. Because $k_{el} = 0.693/t_{1/2}$, another useful equation to determine the average plasma concentration at steady state is

$$\bar{C}_{ss} = \frac{1.44 \cdot t_{1/2} \cdot f \cdot \text{Dose}_{oral}}{V_d \cdot \tau}$$

The preceding equations describe the average concentration of a chemical in plasma. When multiplied by V_d, the amount of chemical in the body is obtained. Thus, the average body burden at steady state ($\bar{X}_{ss}$) is described by the following relationship:

$$\bar{X}_{ss} = \bar{C}_{ss} \cdot V_d$$

Bioavailability

The extent of systemic absorption of a xenobiotic can be determined experimentally by comparing the plasma AUC after intravenous and oral dosing. The resulting index is called *bioavailability*. It is important to note that bioavailability can be determined by using different doses, provided that the compound does not display dose-dependent kinetics.

$$\text{Bioavailability} = \frac{\text{Dose}_{iv} \cdot AUC_{0 \to \infty, oral}}{\text{Dose}_{oral} \cdot AUC_{0 \to \infty, iv}}$$

This is an exceedingly important concept in pharmacokinetics and in toxicokinetics. As discussed earlier, the most critical factor in exerting toxicity is not necessarily the dose but the concentration of a toxicant at the site of action. Toxicants are delivered to most organs (other

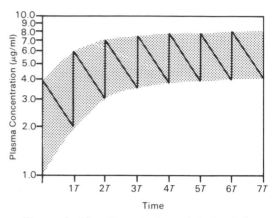

Figure 3–19. Concentration of toxicant in plasma as a function of time during repeated exposure to the toxicant at constant time intervals (τ).

than the alimentary canal and liver) by the systemic circulation. Therefore, the fraction of a chemical reaching the systemic circulation is of critical importance. Several factors can greatly alter this systemic availability: (1) limited absorption after oral dosing, (2) intestinal first-pass effect, (3) hepatic first-pass effect, and (4) mode of formulation, affecting, for example, dissolution rate or incorporation into micelles (for lipid-soluble compounds). However, not only the total amount of a xenobiotic reaching the systemic circulation is important but also the rate at which a xenobiotic becomes available systemically. A slowly absorbed chemical will not attain as high peak plasma concentrations (C_{max}) as rapidly absorbed one. Also, the time (t_{max}) to reach C_{max} will be longer for a slowly than for a rapidly absorbed compound. Because toxic effects occur only above a critical plasma/organ concentration, a slowly absorbed versus a rapidly absorbed chemical may not attain high enough levels in the target organ to cause toxicity. Therefore, C_{max} and t_{max} are two additional useful parameters to characterize the systemic availability of xenobiotics.

PHYSIOLOGICALLY BASED TOXICOKINETIC MODELING

A physiological toxicokinetic model is a mathematical description of the disposition of xenobiotics either in an entire organism or in a part of it (e.g., an organ) that is derived primarily from anatomical and physiological information. It does not require assumptions about fictitious compartments or first-order processes for elimination or absorption, as discussed for classical toxicokinetics. In principle, as many organs

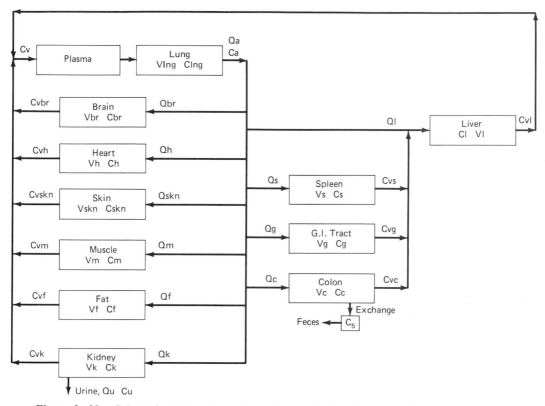

Figure 3–20. Schematic presentation of a physiologically based pharmacokinetic model.

and tissues can be modeled as desirable for a particular xenobiotic (Figure 3–20).

As a second step, it must be decided based on physiological and physicochemical considerations, or even better on experimental data, whether the distribution of a chemical into a particular compartment is perfusion rate (blood flow) or membrane transport limited. This is important because rigorous mathematical treatment is different for these two cases. Most xenobiotics are to some extent lipophilic, and the distribution of such compounds is often flow limited. Therefore, and for the sake of simplicity, we shall consider a flow-limited model for a particular tissue as an example for all tissues intended for modeling (Figure 3–21). The concentration of a chemical in the incoming arterial blood is C_a and in the outgoing venous blood C_v, blood flow to the tissue is Q_t, the volume of tissue is V_t, and the concentration of the xenobiotic in the tissue is assumed to be uniformly C_t. Based on these considerations, a mass balance equation may be written according to

$$\frac{d(V_t \cdot C_t)}{dt} = Q_t \cdot (C_v - C_a)$$

This simplified model presupposes that there is equilibrium between the vascular and interstitial space and cellular subcompartments. In addition, it also assumes that the organ modeled does not eliminate the compound by biotransformation or excretion. These and many other factors can be included in mass balance equations. However, the mathematics of such complex mass balance equations are increasingly difficult and not essential for toxicologists for understanding the principles of physiologically based toxicokinetic modeling. It is not practical to determine the concentration of a chemical in afferent arterial blood (C_a) and efferent venous blood (C_v). This is also not necessary because of the relationship

$$C_a = \frac{C_t}{R_t}$$

where R_t is the partition coefficient between blood and tissue at equilibrium. Thus, the usual form of a simple mass balance equation is

$$V_t \cdot \frac{dC_t}{dt} = Q_t \cdot \left(C_v - \frac{C_t}{R_t}\right)$$

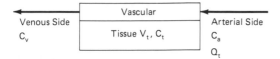

Figure 3–21. Tissue compartment model for writing a mass balance equation.

Blood flow to a tissue (Q_t) or organ and the volume of a tissue or organ (V_t) often can be obtained from the literature. Venous blood concentration (C_v) and the partition coefficient (R_t) have to be determined experimentally. Such differential equations may be written for any number of physiological compartments shown in Figure 3–21. In addition, algebraic equations accounting for growth rate of animals, changes in tissue weight ratios, and other physiological parameters may be also factored into the model. The set of differential equations thus generated is first-order and linear and can be solved numerically by using matrix algebra techniques. The last step in physiologically based toxicokinetic modeling is to identify critical compartments that account for most of the mass balance and/or organs of toxicological importance, in order to simplify subsequently the model by lumping other compartments.

Advantages of physiologically based over classical pharmacokinetics are that (1) they can provide time course of distribution of xenobiotics to any organ or tissue, (2) they allow estimation of effects of changing physiological parameters on tissue concentrations, and (3) the same model can predict toxicokinetics of chemicals across species by allometric scaling.

The disadvantages are that (1) accuracy is lacking for individual dosing, (2) mathematically complex equations are difficult for most toxicologists and clinicians to handle, and (3) physiological parameters are often ill defined in various species and strains, disease states, and the like, diminishing the accuracy of the predictions of this type of modeling. Nevertheless, physiologically based toxicokinetic models are conceptually sound, and they are potentially useful tools to gain insights into the kinetics of xenobiotics beyond what classical toxicokinetics can provide.

CONCLUSION

Humans are in continuous contact with toxic agents. Toxicants are in the food we eat, the water we drink, and the air we breathe. Depending on their physical and chemical properties, toxic agents may be absorbed by the gastrointestinal tract, lungs, and/or skin. Fortunately, the body has the ability to biotransform and to excrete these compounds into urine, feces, and air. However, when the rate of absorption exceeds the rate of elimination, toxic compounds may accumulate to a critical concentration at a certain target site, and toxicity may ensue (Figure 3–22). Whether a chemical elicits toxicity or not depends not only on its inherent potency and site specificity but also on how an organism can handle—viz., dispose of—a particular toxicant. Therefore, knowledge of disposition of chemicals is of great importance when judging the toxicity of xenobiotics. For example, for a potent CNS suppressant, displaying a strong hepatic first-pass effect, oral exposure will be of less concern than exposure by inhalation. Also, two equipotent gases—the absorption of one perfusion rate limited and that of the other ventilation rate limited—will exhibit completely different toxicity profiles at a distant site because of differences in the concentrations attained in the target organ.

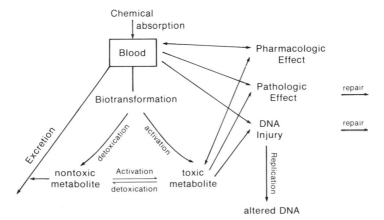

Figure 3–22. Schematic representation of the disposition and toxic effects produced by chemicals.

Many chemicals have very low inherent toxicity but have to be activated by biotransformation into toxic metabolites; the toxic response then depends on the rate of production of toxic metabolites. Alternatively, a very potent toxicant may be detoxified rapidly by biotransformation. Toxic effects are related to the concentration of the "toxic chemical" at the site of action (in the target organ) whether a chemical is administered or generated by biotransformation in the target tissue or at a distant site. Thus, the toxic response produced by chemicals is critically influenced by the rate of absorption, distribution, biotransformation, and excretion.

REFERENCES

Albert, A.: *Selective Toxicity*, 3rd ed. Meuthuen & Co., London, 1965.

Allenby, A. C.; Creasey, N. H.; Edginton, J. A. G.; Fletcher, J. A.; and Schock, C.: Mechanism of action of accelerants on skin penetration. *Br. J. Dermatol.*, **81** (Suppl. 4):47–55, 1969.

Amaroso, E. C.: Placentation. In Parks, A. S. (ed.): *Marshall's Physiology of Reproduction*, Vol. 2, 3rd ed. Longmans, Green & Co., London, 1952, pp. 127–311.

Aungst, B., and Shen, D. D.: Gastrointestinal absorption of toxic agents. In Rozman, K., and Hänninen, O. (eds.): *Gastrointestinal Toxicology*. Elsevier, Amsterdam/New York/Oxford, 1986, pp. 29–56.

Barnett, H. L.; McNamara, H.; Schultz, S.; and Tomposett, R.: Renal clearances of sodium penicillin G, procaine penicillin G, and inulin in infants and children. *Pediatrics*, **3**:418–422, 1949.

Barnett, R. J.: The demonstration with the electron microscope of the end-products of histochemical reactions in relation to the fine structure of cells. *Exp. Cell Res.* (Suppl. 7):65–89, 1959.

Bates, T. R., and Gibaldi, M.: Gastrointestinal absorption of drugs. In Swarbrick, J. (ed.): *Current Concepts in the Pharmaceutical Sciences: Biopharmaceutics*. Lea & Febiger, Philadelphia, 1970.

Benz, R.; Janko, K.; and Länger, P.: Pore formation by the matrix protein (porin) to *Escherichia coli* in planar bilayer membranes. *Ann. N.Y. Acad. Sci.*, **358**:13–24, 1980.

Blank, I. H., and Scheuplein, R. J.: Transport into and within the skin. *Br. J. Dermatol.*, **81** (Suppl. 4):4–10, 1969.

Borowitz, J. L.; Moore, P. F.; Him, G. K. W.; and Miya, T. S.: Mechanism of enhanced drug effects produced by dilution of the oral dose. *Toxicol. Appl. Pharmacol.*, **19**:164–168, 1971.

Boyes, R. N.; Adams, H. J.; and Duce, B. R.: Oral absorption and disposition kinetics of lidocaine hydrochloride in dogs. *J. Pharmacol. Exp. Ther.*, **174**:1–8, 1970.

Castle, M. C., and Lage, G. L.: Effect of pretreatment with spironolactone, phenobarbital or β-diethylaminoethyl diphenylpropylacetate (SKF 525-A) on tritium levels in blood, heart and liver of rats at various times after administration of [³H] digitoxin. *Biochem. Pharmacol.*, **21**:1149–1155, 1972.

————: Enhanced biliary excretion of digitoxin following spironolactone as it relates to the prevention of digitoxin toxicity. *Res. Commu. Chem. Pathol. Pharmacol.*, **5**:99–108, 1973.

Coulston, F., and Serrone, D. M.: The comparative approach to the role of nonhuman primates in evaluation of drug toxicity in man: a review. *Ann. N.Y. Acad. Sci.*, **162**:681–704, 1969.

Dames, G. S.: *Foetal and Neonatal Physiology: A Comparative Study of the Changes at Birth*. Year Book Medical Publishers, Inc., Chicago, 1968.

Dowling, R. H.: Compensatory changes in intestinal absorption. *Br. Med. Bull.*, **23**:275–278, 1967.

Draize, J. H.; Woodard, G.; and Calvery, H. O.: Methods for the study of irritation and toxicity of substances applied topically to the skin and mucous membranes. *J. Pharmacol. Exp. Ther.*, **82**:377–390, 1944.

Dugard, P. H.: Skin permeability theory in relation to measurements of percutaneous absorption in toxicology. In Marzulli, F. N., and Maibach, H. I. (eds.): *Dermatotoxicology*, 2nd ed, Hemisphere, Washington/New York/London, 1983, pp. 91–116.

Dugard, P. H., and Embery, G.: The influence of dimethylsulphoxide on the percutaneous migration of potassium butyl [³⁵S] sulphate, potassium methyl [³⁵S] sulphate and sodium [³⁵S] sulphate. *Br. J. Dermatol.*, **81** (Suppl. 4):69–74, 1969.

Duggan, D. E.; Hooke, K. F.; Noll, R. M.; and Kwan, K. C.: Enterohepatic circulation of indomethacin and its role in intestinal irritation. *Biochem. Pharmacol.*, **24**:1749–1754, 1975.

Ferguson, H. C.: Dilution of dose and acute oral toxicity. *Toxicol. Appl. Pharmacol.*, **4**:759–762, 1962.

Findlay, J. W. A.: The distribution of some commonly used drugs in human breast milk. *Drug Metab. Rev.*, **14**:653–686, 1983.

Gibaldi, M., and Perrier, D.: *Pharmacokinetics*, 2nd ed. Marcel Dekker, Inc., New York/Basel, 1982, pp. 1–494.

Ginsburg, J.: Placental drug transfer. *Annu. Rev. Pharmacol.*, **11**:387–408, 1971.

Goldstein, A.; Aronow, L.; and Kalman, S. M. (eds.): *Principles of Drug Action: The Basis of Pharmacology*, 2nd ed. John Wiley & Sons, Inc., New York, 1974.

Gorringe, J. A. L., and Sproston, E. M.: The influence of particle size upon the absorption of drugs from the gastrointestinal tract. In Binn, T. B. (ed.): *Absorption and Distribution of Drugs*. Williams & Wilkins Co., Baltimore, 1964, pp. 128–139.

Hayes, W. J., Jr.: Review of the metabolism of chlorinated hydrocarbon insecticides especially in mammals. *Annu. Rev. Pharmacol.*, **5**:27–52, 1965.

Heath, D. F., and Vandekar, M.: Toxicity and metabolism of dieldrin in rats. *Br. J. Ind. Med.*, **21**:269–279, 1964.

Hirsch, G. H., and Hook, J. B.: Maturation of renal organic acid transport: substrate stimulation by penicillin and *p*-aminohippurate (PAH). *J. Pharmacol. Exp. Ther.*, **171**:103–108, 1970.

Houston, J. B.; Upshall, D. G.; and Bridges, J. W.: A re-evaluation of the importance of partition coefficients in the gastrointestinal absorption of nutrients. *J. Pharmacol. Exp. Ther.*, **189**:244–254, 1974.

Juchau, M. R.: Mechanisms of drug biotransformation reactions in the placenta. *Fed. Proc.*, **31**:48–51, 1972.

Kelly, D., and Kostial, K.: The effect of milk diet on lead metabolism in rats. *Environ. Res.*, **6**:355–360, 1973.

Klaassen, C. D.: Immaturity of the newborn rat's hepatic excretory function for ouabain. *J. Pharmacol. Exp. Ther.*, **183**:520–526, 1972.

————: Comparison of the toxicity of chemicals in newborn rats to bile duct–ligated and sham-operated rats and mice. *Toxicol. Appl. Pharmacol.*, **24**:37–44, 1973a.

————: Hepatic excretory function in the newborn rat. *J. Pharmacol. Exp. Ther.*, **184**:721–728, 1973b.

————: Effect of microsomal enzyme inducers on the biliary excretion of cardiac glycosides. *J. Pharmacol. Exp. Ther.*, **191**:201–211, 1974a.

————: Stimulation of the development of the hepatic excretory mechanism for ouabain in newborn rats with microsomal enzyme inducers. *J. Pharmacol. Exp. Ther.*, **191**:212–218, 1974b.

————: Biliary excretion of mercury compounds. *Toxicol. Appl. Pharmacol.*, **33**:356–365, 1975a.

————: Effect of spironolactone on the distribution of mercury. *Toxicol. Appl. Pharmacol.*, **33**:366–375, 1975b.

————: Biliary excretion of metals. *Drug Metab. Rev.*, **5**:165–196, 1976.

Klaassen, C. D.; Eaton, D. L.; and Cagen, S. Z.: Hepatobiliary disposition of xenobiotics. In Bridges, J. W., and Chasseaud, L. F. (eds.): *Progress in Drug Metabolism.* John Wiley & Sons, Inc., New York, 1981, pp. 1–75.

Klaassen, C. D., and Shoeman, D. W.: Biliary excretion of lead in rats, rabbits and dogs. *Toxicol. Appl. Pharmacol.*, **29**:434–446, 1974.

Klaassen, C. D., and Watkins, J. B.: Mechanisms of bile formation, hepatic uptake, and biliary excretion. *Pharmacol. Rev.*, 36:1–67, 1984.

Kragh-Hansen, U.: Molecular aspects of ligand binding to serum albumin. *Pharmacol. Rev.*, **33**:17–53, 1981.

Kupferberg, H. J., and Way, E. L.: Pharmacologic basis for the increased sensitivity of the newborn rat to morphine. *J. Pharmacol. Exp. Ther.*, **141**:105–112, 1963.

Lauterbach, F.: Intestinal secretion of organic ions and drugs. In Kramer, M., and Lauterbach, F. (eds.): *Intestinal Permeation.* Excerpta Medica, Amsterdam/Oxford, 1977, pp. 173–195.

Leopold, G.; Furukawa, E.; Forth, W.; and Rummel, W.: Comparative studies of absorption of heavy metals in vivo and in vitro. *Arch. Pharmacol. Exp. Pathol.*, **263**:275–276, 1969.

Levi, A. J.; Gatmaitan, Z.; and Arias, I. M.: Two hepatic cytoplasmic protein fractions, Y and Z, and their possible role in the hepatic uptake of bilirubin, sulfobromophthalein, and other anions. *J. Clin. Invest.*, **48**:2156–2167, 1969.

Levine, R. R.: Factors affecting gastrointestinal absorption of drugs. *Am. J. Dig. Dis.*, **15**:171–188, 1970.

Levine, R. R., and Pelikan, E. W.: Mechanisms of drug absorption and excretion. Passage of drugs out of and into the gastrointestinal tract. *Annu. Rev. Pharmacol.*, **4**:69–84, 1964.

Levine, R. R., and Steinberg, G. M.: Intestinal absorption of pralidoxime and other aldoximes. *Nature (Lond.)*, **209**:269–271, 1966.

Litwack, G.; Ketterer, B.; and Arias, I. M.: Ligandin: a hepatic protein which binds steroids, bilirubin, carcinogens and a number of exogenous organic anions. *Nature (Lond.)*, **234**:466–467, 1971.

Lukas, G.; Brindle, S. D.; and Greengard, P.: The route of absorption of intraperitoneally administered compounds. *J. Pharmacol. Exp. Ther.*, **178**:562–566, 1971.

Magos, L., and Clarkson, T. W.: The effect of oral doses of a polythiol resin on the excretion of methylmercury in mice treated with cystein, D-penicillamine or phenobarbitone. *Chem.-Biol. Interactions*, **14**:325–335, 1976.

Malkinson, F. D.: Permeability of the stratus corneum. In Montagna, W., and Lobitz, W. C., Jr. (eds.): *The Epidermis.* Academic Press, Inc., New York, 1964.

Marzulli, F. N.; Callahan, J. F.; and Brown, D. W. C.: Chemical structure and skin penetrating capacity of a short series of organic phosphates and phosphoric acid. *J. Invest. Dermatol.*, **44**:339–344, 1965.

Mendel, J. L., and Walton, M. S.: Conversion of *p,p*-DDT to *p,p*-DDD by intestinal flora of the rat. *Science*, **151**:1527–1528, 1966.

Migdalof, B. H.; Antonaccio, M. J.; McKinstry, D. N.; Singhvi, S. M.; Lan, S. J.; Egli, P.; and Kripalani, K. J.: Captopril: pharmacology, metabolism, and disposition. *Drug Metab. Rev.*, **15**:841–869, 1984.

Mirkin, B. L., and Singh, S.: Placental transfer and pharmacokinetics of digoxin in the pregnant rat. *Proc. Fifth Int. Cong. Pharmacol.* (abstract), 949, 1972.

Pentschew, A., and Garro, F.: Lead encephalomyelopathy of the suckling rat and its implication on the porphyrinopathic nervous diseases. *Acta Neuropathol. (Berl.)*, **6**:266–278, 1966.

Pfeiffer, C. J.: Gastroenterologic response to environmental agents—absorption and interactions. In Lee, D. H. K. (ed.): *Handbook of Physiology. Section 9: Reactions to Environmental Agents.* American Physiological Society, Bethesda, Md., 1977, pp. 349–374.

Renkin, E. M.: Capillary permeability. In Mayerson, H. S. (ed.): *Lymph and the Lymphatic System.* Thomas, Springfield, Ill., 1968, pp. 76–88.

Rosenfield, A. B., and Huston, R.: Infant methemoglobinemia in Minnesota due to nitrates in well water. *Minn. Med.*, **33**:787–796, 1950.

Rozman, K.: Fecal excretion of toxic substances. In Rozman, K., and Hänninen, O. (eds.): *Gastrointestinal Toxicology.* Elsevier, Amsterdam/New York/Oxford, 1986, pp. 119–145.

Sanders, E., and Ashworth, C. T.: A study of particulate intestinal absorption of hepatocellular uptake. Use of polystyrene latex particles. *Exp. Cell Res.*, **22**:137–145, 1961.

Sasser, L. B., and Jarboe, G. E.: Intestinal absorption and retention of cadmium in neonatal rat. *Toxicol. Appl. Pharmacol.*, **41**:423–431, 1977.

Scala, J.; McOsker, D. E.; and Reller, H. H.: The percutaneous absorption of ionic surfactants. *J. Invest. Dermatol.*, **50**:371–379, 1968.

Scatchard, G.: The attraction of proteins for small molecules and ions. *Ann. N.Y. Acad. Sci.*, **51**:660–672, 1949.

Schade, S. G.; Felsher, B. F.; Glader, B. E.; and Conrad, M. E.: Effect of cobalt upon iron absorption. *Proc. Soc. Exp. Biol. Med.*, **134**:741–743, 1970.

Schanker, L. S.: Mechanisms of drug absorption and distribution. *Annu. Rev. Pharmacol.*, **1**:29–44, 1961.

————: Passage of drugs across body membranes. *Pharmacol. Rev.*, **14**:501–530, 1962.

Schanker, L. S., and Jeffrey, J.: Active transport of foreign pyrimidines across the intestinal epithelium. *Nature (Lond.)*, **190**:727–728, 1961.

Scheufler, E., and Rozman, K.: Effect of hexadecane on the pharmacokinetics of hexachlorobenzene. *Toxicol. Appl. Pharmacol.*, **75**:190–197, 1984.

Schwartze, E. W.: The so-called habituation to arsenic: variation in the toxicity of arsenious oxide. *J. Pharmacol. Exp. Ther.*, **20**:181–203, 1923.

Selye, H.; Krajny, M.; and Savoie, L.: Digitoxin poisoning: prevention by spironolactone. *Science*, **164**:842–843, 1969.

————: Mercury poisoning: prevention by spironolactone. *Science*, **169**:775–776, 1970.

————: Hormones and resistance. *J. Pharm. Sci.*, **60**:1–28, 1971.

Shand, D. G., and Rangno, R. E.: The deposition of propranolol. I. Elimination during oral absorption in man. *Pharmacology*, **7**:159–168, 1972.

Shoeman, D. W.; Kauffman, R. E.; Azarnoff, D. L.; and Boulos, B. M.: Placental transfer of diphenylhydantoin in the goat. *Biochem. Pharmacol.*, **21**:1237–1243, 1972.

Silverman, W. A.; Andersen, D. H.; Blanc, W. A.; and

Crozier, D. N.: A difference in mortality rate and incidence of kernicterus among premature infants allotted to two prophylactic antibacterial regimens. *Pediatrics,* **18**:614–625, 1956.

Sobel, A. E.; Gawron, O.; and Kramer, B.: Influence of vitamin D in experimental lead poisoning. *Proc. Soc. Exp. Biol. Med.,* **38**:433–435, 1938.

Stowe, C. M., and Plaa, G. L.: Extrarenal excretion of drugs and chemicals. *Annu. Rev. Pharmacol.,* **8**:337–356, 1968.

Thompson, R. Q.; Sturtevant, M.; Bird, O. D.; and Glazko, A. J.: The effect of metabolites of chloramphenicol (Chloromycetin) on the thyroid of the rat. *Endocrinology,* **55**:665–681, 1954.

Thomson, A. B. R.; Olatunbosun, D.; and Valberg, L. S.: Interrelation of intestinal transport system for manganese and iron. *J. Lab. Clin. Med.,* **78**:642–655, 1971a.

Thomson, A. B. R.; Valberg, L. S.; and Sinclair, D. G.: Competitive nature of the intestinal transport mechanism for cobalt and iron in the rat. *J. Clin. Invest.,* **50**:2384–2394, 1971b.

Tune, B. M.; Wu, K. Y.; and Kempson, R. L.: Inhibition of transport and prevention of toxicity of cephaloridine in the kidney. Dose-responsiveness of the rabbit and the guinea pig to probenecid. *J. Pharmacol. Exp. Ther.,* **202**:466–471, 1977.

Weiner, I. M., and Mudge, G. H.: Renal tubular mechanisms for excretion of organic acids and bases. *Am. J. Med.,* **36**:743–762, 1964.

Wester, R. C., and Maibach, H. I.: Percutaneous absorption in man and animal: a perspective. In Drill, V. A., and Lazar, P. (eds.): *Cutaneous Toxicity.* Academic Press, Inc., New York, 1977.

Wilkinson, G. R.: Plasma and tissue binding considerations in drug disposition. *Drug Metab. Rev.,* **14**:427–465, 1983.

Williams, R. M., and Beck, F.: A histochemical study of gut maturation. *J. Anat.,* **105**:487–501, 1969.

Wilson, J. T.: Determinants and consequences of drug excretion in breast milk. *Drug Metab. Rev.,* **14**:619–652, 1983.

Winteringham, F. P. W.: Comparative biochemical aspects of insecticidal action. *Chem. Ind. (Lond.),* 1195–1202, 1957.

Wold, J. S.; Joost, R. R.; and Owen, N. V.: Nephrotoxicity of cephaloridine in newborn rabbits: role of the renal anionic transport system. *J. Pharmacol. Exp. Ther.,* **201**:778–785, 1977.

Young, M.: Three topics in placental transport: amino transport; oxygen transfer; placental function during labour. In Klopper, A., and Diczfalusy, E. (eds.): *Foetus and Placenta.* Blackwell Scientific Publications, Oxford, 1969.

Zsigmond, G., and Solymoss, B.: Effect of spironolactone, pregnenolone-16α-carbonitrile and cortisol on the metabolism and biliary excretion of sulfobromophthalein and phenol-3,6-dibromophthalein disulfonate in rats. *J. Pharmacol. Exp. Ther.,* **183**:499–507, 1972.

Chapter 4

BIOTRANSFORMATION OF TOXICANTS

I. Glenn Sipes and *A. Jay Gandolfi*

INTRODUCTION

Humans and other animals are constantly exposed in their environment to a vast array of chemicals that are foreign to their bodies. These foreign chemicals, or *xenobiotics,* can be of natural origin or they can be man-made. In general, the more lipophilic compounds are readily absorbed through the skin, across the lungs, or through the gastrointestinal tract. Constant or even intermittent exposure to these lipophilic chemicals could result in their accumulation within the organism, unless effective means of elimination are present. Indeed, chemicals can be excreted unchanged into urine, bile, feces, expired air, and perspiration. Except for exhalation, the ease with which compounds are eliminated from the body largely depends on their water solubility. This is particularly true for nonvolatile chemicals that are eliminated in urine and feces, the predominant routes of elimination. Lipophilic compounds that are present in these excretory fluids tend to diffuse into cellular membranes and are reabsorbed, whereas water-soluble compounds are excreted. Therefore, it is apparent why lipophilic xenobiotics could accumulate within the body: They are readily absorbed but poorly excreted.

Fortunately, animal organisms have developed a number of biochemical processes that convert lipophilic compounds to more hydrophilic metabolites. These biochemical processes are termed *biotransformation* and are usually enzymatic in nature. It should be stressed that biotransformation is the sum of the processes by which a foreign chemical is subjected to chemical change by living organisms (Figure 4–1). This definition implies that a particular chemical may undergo a number of chemical changes. It may mean that the parent molecule is chemically modified at a number of positions or that a particular metabolite of the parent compound may undergo additional modification. The end result of the biotransformation reaction(s) is that the metabolites are chemically distinct from the parent compound. Metabolites are usually more hydrophilic than the parent compound. This enhanced water solubility reduces the ability of the metabolite to partition into biologic membranes and thus restricts the distribution of the metabolites to the various tissues, decreases the renal tubular and intestinal reabsorption of the metabolite(s), and ultimately promotes the excretion of the chemical by the urinary and biliary fecal routes.

Phase I and Phase II Biotransformation

A number of enzymes in animal organisms are capable of biotransforming lipid-soluble xenobiotics in such a way as to render them more water soluble. These enzymic reactions are of two types: phase I reactions, which involve oxidation, reduction, and hydrolysis; and phase II reactions, which consist of conjugation or synthetic reactions. Although phase I reactions generally convert foreign compounds to derivatives that are more water soluble than the parent molecule, a prime function of these reactions is to add or expose functional groups (e.g., —OH, —SH, —NH$_2$, —COOH). These functional groups then permit the compound to undergo phase II reactions. Phase II reactions are biosynthetic reactions where the foreign compound or a phase I–derived metabolite is covalently linked to an endogenous molecule, producing a conjugate. In these cases, the endogenous moieties (e.g., glucuronic acid, sulfate) usually confer upon the lipophilic xenobiotic or its metabolite increased water solubility and the ability to undergo significant ionization at physiologic pH. These conjugating moieties are normally added to endogenous products to promote their secretion or transfer across hepatic, renal, and intestinal membranes. The transport mechanisms that have developed recognize the conjugating moiety. Thus, the excretion of conjugated xenobiotics is enhanced by their ability to participate in transport systems that have evolved from the conjugated products of endogenous molecules.

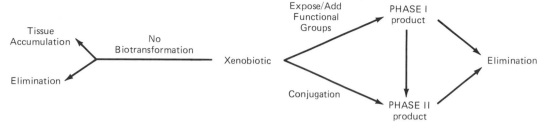

Figure 4–1.   Integration of phase I and phase II biotransformation reactions.

The relationship between phase I and phase II reactions is summarized in Figure 4–1. The fate of a particular chemical is determined by its physical/chemical products. Volatile organic compounds may be eliminated via the lungs with no biotransformation. Those with functional groups may be conjugated directly, whereas others undergo phase I reactions before conjugation. As implied, biotransformation is often integrated and can be complex. Because of this complexity, imbalances between phase I and phase II reactions or dose-related shifts in metabolic routes are often causes of chemical-induced tissue injury.

Organ and Cellular Location of Biotransformation

The enzymes or enzyme systems that catalyze the biotransformation of foreign compounds are localized mainly in the liver. This is not surprising, since a primary function of the liver is to receive and process chemicals absorbed from the gastrointestinal tract before they are distributed to other tissues. Liver receives all the blood that has perfused the splanchnic area, which contains nutrients and other foreign substances. Because of this, the liver has developed the capacity to extract these substances readily from the blood and to modify chemically many of these substances before they are stored, secreted into bile, or released into the general circulation. Other tissues can also biotransform foreign compounds. Nearly every tissue tested has shown activity toward some foreign chemicals (Figure 4–2). Extrahepatic tissues are limited with respect to the diversity of chemicals they can handle, and thus their contribution to the overall biotransformation of xenobiotics is limited. However, biotransformation of a chemical within an extrahepatic tissue may have an important toxicologic implication for that particular tissue.

Subcellular Localization of Biotransformation Enzymes

Biotransformation of foreign compounds within the liver is accomplished by several remarkable enzyme systems. These can chemically modify a wide variety of structurally diverse drugs and toxicants that enter the body through ingestion, inhalation, the skin, or injection. The phase I enzymes, those that add or expose functional groups, are located primarily in the endoplasmic reticulum, a network of interconnected channels present in the cytoplasm of most cells. These enzymes are membrane bound, since the endoplasmic reticulum is basically a contiguous membrane composed of lipids and proteins. The presence of enzymes within a lipoprotein matrix is critical, since the lipophilic substrates will preferentially partition into the lipid membranes, the site of biotransformation.

When liver is removed and homogenized, the tubular endoplasmic reticulum breaks up and fragments of the membrane are sealed off to form microvesicles. These are referred to as *microsomes*, which can be isolated by differential centrifugation of the liver homogenate. If the supernatant fraction that results from centrifugation of the homogenate at $9000 \times g$ (to remove nuclei, mitochondria, and lysosomes as well as unbroken cells and large membrane fragments) is subjected to centrifugation at $105,000 \times g$, a pellet highly enriched in microsomes is obtained. The resulting supernatant fraction, which contains a number of soluble enzymes, is referred to as the *cytosol*. This cytosol contains many of the enzymes of phase II biotransformation. Many of the important biotransformation enzymes are referred to as cytosolic or microsomal to indicate the subcellular location of the enzymes.

The microsomal enzymes that catalyze the phase I reactions were characterized primarily by their ability to metabolize drugs. Thus, much of the literature refers to these enzymes as the microsomal drug metabolizing enzymes. Indeed, the microsomal enzymes will convert drugs to more polar products, but they also act on in-

Capacity	Organ
High	Liver
Medium	Lung, kidney, intestine
Low	Skin, testis, placenta, adrenals

Figure 4–2.   Key organs involved in biotransformation.

numerous chemicals. Therefore, the word *biotransformation* is preferred to *drug metabolism,* since it conveys the more universal nature of the reactions. In addition, it delineates the normal process of metabolism of endogenous nutrients from that of biotransformation of foreign chemicals.

Detoxication–Toxication

Inasmuch as both phase I and phase II enzymes convert foreign chemicals to forms that can be more readily excreted, they are often referred to as *detoxication enzymes*. However, it should be emphasized that biotransformation is not strictly related to detoxication. In a number of cases, the metabolic products are more toxic than the parent compounds. This is particularly true for some chemical carcinogens, organophosphates, and a number of compounds that cause cell necrosis in the lung, liver, and kidney. In many instances, a toxic metabolite can be isolated and identified. In other cases, highly reactive intermediates are formed during the biotransformation of a chemical. The term *toxication* or *bioactivation* is often used to indicate the enzymatic formation of reactive intermediates. These reactive intermediates are thought to initiate the events that ultimately result in cell death, chemically induced cancer, teratogenesis, and a number of other toxicities.

Characterization of Biotransformation

The biphasic nature of biotransformation is best presented by considering phase I and phase II reactions separately. These will be discussed with emphasis on the nature of the reaction, the cofactors required, a general example of the type of reactions catalyzed, the mechanism of the reaction, the predominant tissue and subcellular localization of the enzymes, and the importance of each enzyme in detoxication/toxication. However, it must be remembered that each xenobiotic is presented to a variety of the enzymes at any given time; for this reason, the biotransformation of a foreign compound is one of an integrated approach.

The second consideration will focus on factors affecting biotransformation of xenobiotics. These include such factors as nutritional and disease status, age, route, dose, time of day/year, enzyme induction or inhibition, sex, and species differences as they relate to rates of biotransformation of foreign compounds and to toxicity.

Finally, the process of bioactivation will be discussed to explain its role in the toxicity of xenobiotics. Particular emphasis will be placed on the balance that exists between formation and detoxication of reactive intermediates.

PHASE I ENZYME REACTIONS

Characteristics of Microsomal Phase I Enzymes

Phase I is the predominant biotransformation pathway. These reactions may add functional groups by two oxidative enzyme systems: the cytochrome P-450 system (which is also referred to as the polysubstrate monooxygenase system or the mixed-function oxygenase [MFO] system) and the mixed-function amine oxidase (which is a flavin-monooxygenase). Basically, both enzyme systems add a hydroxyl moiety to the foreign substrate by mechanisms that will be outlined later.

Preexisting functional groups are exposed by a family of hydrolytic enzymes, esterases and amidases. The cleavage of the ester or amide bond, regardless of the remaining chemical structure, will produce two functional groups for further biotransformation, a carboxylic acid plus either an amine (from an amide) or an alcohol (from an ester).

Finally, a variety of oxidation-reduction systems can be considered part of the phase I enzymes since these are redox enzymes and often alter the oxidation state of a carbon to allow it to be more readily excreted or biotransformed by the phase II enzymes.

Cytochrome P-450

The most important enzyme systems involved in phase I reactions are the cytochrome P-450–containing monooxygenases. The cytochrome P-450 system is actually a coupled enzyme system composed of two enzymes: NADPH-cytochrome P-450 reductase, and a heme-containing enzyme, cytochrome P-450. These enzymes are embedded in the phospholipid matrix of the endoplasmic reticulum (Figure 4–3). The phospholipids play a crucial role in cytochrome P-450 reactions since they facilitate the interaction between the two enzymes. Accompanying this complex is another cytochrome called cytochrome b_5 and its associated reductase. The function of the cytochrome b_5 and cytochrome b_5 reductase in cytochrome P-450-mediated reactions is not clearly established.

The NADPH-cytochrome P-450 reductase has a preference for NADPH as its cofactor (Figure 4–4). It is a flavoprotein capable of transferring one or two electrons to cytochrome P-450. Cytochrome P-450 is actually a b-type cytochrome with a unique redox potential and spectral properties. It receives its name from the fact that when reduced cytochrome P-450 (Fe^{2+}) forms a ligand with carbon monoxide, the

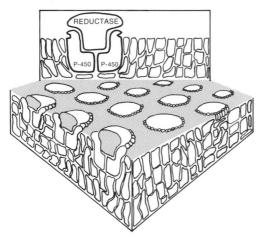

Figure 4–3. Schematic demonstration of the interaction of cytochrome P-450, reductase, and lipid. Note the low ratio of reductase to cytochrome P-450. (From Nebert, D. W.; Eisen, H. J.; Negishi, M.; Lang, M. A.; and Hjelmeland, L. M.: Genetic mechanisms controlling the induction of polysubstrate monooxygenase (P-450) activities. *Annu. Rev. Pharmacol. Toxicol.*, **21**:431–462, 1981.)

maximal absorbance of light occurs at 450 nm. This spectral property is present only when the cytochrome P-450 is intact and catalytically functional. When denatured, cytochrome P-450 loses its unique spectral peak at 450 nm and produces only a 420-nm absorbance maximum, similar to other hemoproteins.

Components of the Cytochrome P-450 System. In early studies, it was noted that treatment of rats and mice with certain chemicals produced a shift in the spectral maximum of cytochrome P-450. This shift was to 448 nm, and thus the cytochrome became known as cytochrome P-448. Other evidence for different forms came from the fact that cytochrome P-450 and cytochrome P-448 displayed different substrate specificity or they biotransformed similar substrates at different rates.

These differences prompted attempts to isolate and characterize the cytochrome P-450 components. Isolation was accomplished by solubilizing the microsomes with ionic and nonionic detergents and stabilizing the hemoproteins with sulfhydryl agents, glycerol, and metal chelators. The solubilized microsomes can then be resolved into their components by column chromatography. The resolved components are then characterized by electrophoresis, immunochemical analysis, peptide mapping, and amino acid analysis. When the cytochrome P-450 enzymes are recombined with NADPH-cytochrome P-450 reductase in the presence of the natural microsomal phospholipids or dilauroyl phosphatidyl choline, they reconstitute to form a complex capable of the biotransformation reactions observed with microsomes.

These studies provided evidence for multiple forms of cytochrome P-450. These differ in both the structure of the polypeptide chain and the specificity of the reactions they catalyze. The cytochrome P-450 composition of liver microsomes is altered by treatment of animals with different chemicals. In addition, the types and amounts of cytochrome P-450 vary with species, organ, age, health, sex, stress, and chemical exposure.

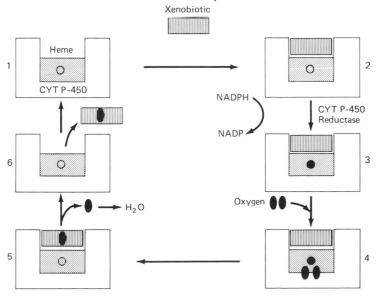

Figure 4–4. Cytochrome P-450 electron transport and oxidation of a xenobiotic.

Table 4–1. MAJOR MAMMALIAN CYTOCHROME P450 GENE FAMILIES

P450 GENE FAMILY/ SUBFAMILY	CHARACTERISTIC INDUCER	CHARACTERISTIC REACTION
IA	Polycyclic aromatic hydrocarbons	Benzo[a]pyrene hydroxylation
IIA		Steroid hydroxylation
IIB	Phenobarbital	Benzphetamine demethylation
IIC		Steroid hydroxylation
IID		Debrisoquine hydroxylation
IIE	Ethanol	Ethanol oxidation
IIIA	Steroids	Steroid hydroxylation
IVA	Hypolipidemic agents	Lauric acid hydroxylation
IVB		
XIA		Cholesterol side chain cleavage
XIB		Deoxycortisol 11β-hydroxylation
XVII		Pregnenolone 17α-hydroxylation
XIX		Androgen conversion to estrogens
XXI		Progesterone 21-hydroxylation

Classification of Cytochromes P-450. In the past few years, advances in recombinant DNA technology have allowed the identification of over 70 distinct cytochrome P-450 genes in various species. Sequence analysis of these genes and/or the corresponding cDNAs has enabled the development of a classification system for cytochromes P-450 based on the deduced amino acid sequences of the gene products. Cytochromes P-450 are grouped into families such that a cytochrome P-450 from one family exhibits $\leq$ 40 percent amino acid sequence identity to a cytochrome P-450 in any other gene family. Several of the gene families are further divided into subfamilies, the members of which are > 59 percent identical. This classification provides the basis for a unified nomenclature for cytochromes P-450.

To date, eight major mammalian gene families have been identified (Table 4–1). Gene families I, II, III, and IV consist of hepatic and extrahepatic cytochromes P-450 involved in phase I biotransformation reactions. Gene families XI, XVII, XIX, and XXI consist of specialized extrahepatic cytochromes P-450 involved in steroid hormone biosynthesis and will not be considered further here. The P450I gene family contains a single subfamily with two genes in humans, rats, mice, and rabbits. These genes are designated IA1 and IA2 and code for proteins inducible by polycyclic aromatic hydrocarbons and are often referred to in the older literature as P-448. The function of these two proteins tends to be conserved across species lines. Thus, P450IA1 is associated with benzo[a]pyrene hydroxylase activity and P450IA2 with arylamine metabolism. The P450II gene family is by far the largest, with five major subfamilies. The IIB subfamily contains the major phenobarbital-inducible cytochromes P-450 in the various species, whereas the IIE subfamily contains the major ethanol-inducible form. Members of the IIA, IIC, and IID subfamilies are in most cases constitutively expressed. The large number of genes in the P450II, in contrast to the P450I, gene family has made difficult the identification of orthologs (counterparts) in different species. The P450III gene family consists of a single subfamily, with multiple members in humans and rats but only a single member in rabbits. A number of these cytochromes P-450 are inducible by steroids and phenobarbital. Characteristic functions across species lines include steroid hydroxylation and macrolide antibiotic metabolism. Finally, the P450IV gene family consists of two subfamilies. A characteristic function of these enzymes is ω-hydroxylation of fatty acids and prostaglandins.

NADPH Cytochrome P-450 Reductase. In contrast to cytochrome P-450, only one NADPH cytochrome P-450 reductase has been isolated from a single source. Its concentration is usually one-tenth to one-thirtieth that of cytochrome P-450. Therefore, this enzyme must mediate the reduction of the many different forms of cytochrome P-450 (Figure 4–3). The composition of the phospholipids has received considerable attention. Dilauroylphosphatidylcholine can be substituted for the natural phospholipids.

Cytochrome P-450 Catalytic Cycle. In reactions catalyzed by cytochrome P-450, the substrate (RH) combines with the oxidized form of cytochrome P-450 (Fe^{3+}) to form a substrate-cytochrome P-450 complex. This complex then accepts an electron from NADPH (via NADPH-cytochrome P-450 reductase), which reduces the iron in the cytochrome P-450 heme moiety to the Fe^{2+} state. The reduced (Fe^{2+}) substrate-cytochrome P-450 complex combines with molecular oxygen, which then accepts an-

Table 4–2. EXAMPLE OF THE GENERAL TYPE OF OXIDATION REACTIONS CATALYZED BY THE CYTOCHROME P-450–CONTAINING MONOOXYGENASES*

REACTION	EXAMPLE
Aliphatic hydroxylation	$R-CH_2-CH_2-CH_2 \longrightarrow R-CH_2-CHOH-CH_3$
Aromatic hydroxylation	$R-\langle\bigcirc\rangle \longrightarrow R-\langle\bigcirc\rangle-OH$
Epoxidation	$R-CH=CH-R' \longrightarrow R-\overset{\displaystyle O}{\overset{\diagup\diagdown}{CH-CH}}-R'$
N-, *O*-, or *S*-dealkylation	$R-\overset{H}{(N, O, S)}-CH_3 \longrightarrow R-(NH_2, OH, SH) + CH_2O$
Deamination	$R-CH_2-NH_2 \longrightarrow R-\overset{\displaystyle O}{\overset{\|}{C}}-H + NH_3$
N-hydroxylation	$R-NH-\overset{\displaystyle O}{\overset{\|}{C}}-CH_3 \longrightarrow R-NOH-\overset{\displaystyle O}{\overset{\|}{C}}-CH_3$
Sulfoxidation	$R-S-R \longrightarrow R-\underset{\displaystyle O}{\overset{\|}{S}}-R'$
Desulfuration	$R_1R_2\overset{\displaystyle S}{\overset{\|}{P}}-X \longrightarrow R_1R_2\overset{\displaystyle O}{\overset{\|}{P}}-X + S$
Oxidative dehalogenation	$R-\overset{X}{\underset{H}{\overset{\|}{\underset{\|}{C}}}}-H \longrightarrow R-\overset{X}{\underset{H}{\overset{\|}{\underset{\|}{C}}}}-OH \longrightarrow R-\overset{\displaystyle O}{\overset{\|}{C}}-H + HX$

* X = halogen.

other electron from NADPH. In some instances, the second electron is donated by NADH via cytochrome b_5. In a series of steps that are not completely understood, both electrons are thought to be transferred to molecular oxygen. The resulting oxygen species is highly reactive and unstable. One atom of this reactive oxygen is introduced into the substrate, while the other is reduced to water. The oxygenated substrate then dissociates, regenerating the oxidized form of cytochrome P-450. Carbon monoxide is a strong inhibitor of cytochrome P-450–catalyzed reactions because it competes with oxygen for binding to the reduced cytochrome P-450.

Oxidative Reactions Catalyzed by the Cytochrome P-450 System. Examples of the reactions catalyzed by the microsomal cytochrome P-450 system are shown in Table 4–2. The participation of cytochrome P-450 in a reaction can be established by several criteria, some of which are outlined in Table 4–3. First, the *in vivo* and *in vitro* reaction rates can be altered by the use of inducing or inhibiting agents, which will be discussed later. Second, the demonstra-

tion that the substrates interact with the microsomal cytochrome P-450 to produce different spectra indicates a probable substrate. Finally, the use of isolated and reconstituted cytochrome P-450 systems to show that the reaction is specific for these components is essential.

Aliphatic hydroxylation of the ω-carbon (CH_3 group) or ω-1 (next-to-last carbon) occurs with compounds such as *n*-hexane, *n*-pentane, and compounds that contain aliphatic side chains (i.e., pentobarbital). The reaction occurs as a result of the insertion of an oxygen atom into a carbon-hydrogen bond, either directly or following hydrogen abstraction. *Aromatic hydroxylation* is also a common reaction. The hydroxyl is

Table 4–3. CRITERIA FOR CYTOCHROME P-450–MEDIATED BIOTRANSFORMATION

1. Enzymatic activity increased by induction
2. Enzymatic activity decreased by inhibitors
3. Carbon monoxide inhibits reaction
4. Enzymatic activity reconstituted with individual purified components

thought to be incorporated by one of two mechanisms: One mechanism involves direct insertion of an oxygen atom into the carbon-hydrogen bond. A more prevalent mechanism involves addition of the oxygen to the carbon-carbon double bond to produce an arene oxide intermediate, which then rearranges to form an aromatic hydroxyl compound. Depending on the ring substituents, the latter reaction leads to intramolecular migration and retention of groups attached to the two carbons being hydroxylated. These arene oxide intermediates are important in determining the possible toxicity of aromatic compounds. *Alkene epoxidation* proceeds via cytochrome P-450-mediated reaction analogous to arene oxide formation. The oxygen is added to the carbon-carbon double bond to produce an epoxide intermediate. Both the arene oxides and aliphatic epoxides are capable of being hydrolyzed by another microsomal enzyme, epoxide hydrolase to dihydrodiol products.

Oxidative dealkylation proceeds via a cytochrome P-450-mediated aliphatic hydroxylation. The alpha carbon of the alkyl group attached to an N, O, or S atom is hydroxylated by the insertion of an oxygen atom into its carbon-hydrogen bond. The resulting hydroxylalkyl moiety adjacent to the electronegative N, O, or S is unstable and decomposes into an aldehyde or ketone (the alkyl moiety) and a metabolite containing a free amino, hydroxyl, or sulfhydryl group.

Oxidative deamination can occur for xenobiotics that contain an aliphatic moiety with a primary amino group. The reaction is similar to that of *N*-dealkylation. In this case, the alpha carbon adjacent to the primary amine is hydroxylated, and the resulting unstable intermediate abstracts a hydride ion to form ammonia and the oxidized alpha carbon rearranges to an aldehyde or ketone.

Oxidation of sulfur and *nitrogen* or *desulfuration* also occur by the addition of oxygen via cytochrome P-450 to the unshared electron pair on the sulfur or nitrogen atom. In the case of nitrogen, the product often is a hydroxylamine that may be further oxidized. The addition of the oxygen to sulfur in a carbon-sulfur-carbon bond forms a stable sulfoxide metabolite. If the sulfur is in the form of a carbon-sulfur or phosphorus-sulfur double bond, the oxygen attaches to the double-bonded sulfur, which then converts to a resonance form in which the oxygen has a full negative charge. This oxygen atom then forms a three-component cyclic intermediate by attacking the carbon/phosphorus attached to the sulfur. The cyclic structure collapses to yield inorganic sulfur and a carbonyl or phosphoryl metabolite.

In total, the reaction is considered a substitution reaction.

In *oxidative dehalogenation,* the activated oxygen does not attack the carbon-halogen bond but inserts at the carbon-hydrogen bond. The resultant product is an unstable aliphatic halohydrin, which undergoes dehalogenation. Thus, the carbon-halogen bond is broken during the rearrangement phase of the reaction and is not the site of attack of the activated oxygen. If the carbon contained a single halogen, the resulting product would be an aldehyde. If it contained two halogens, the dihalohydrin moiety would rearrange to an acid halide. Both the aldehyde and acid halide are unstable and can react nonenzymatically with functional groups on biologic macromolecules.

Microsomal-Mediated Reductive Metabolism. Even though the microsomal cytochrome P-450 is classed as an oxygenase, it also catalyzes the *reductive biotransformation* of certain xenobiotics (Table 4–4). These reactions proceed most readily under conditions of low oxygen tension. Owing to the transfer to reducing equivalents in cytochrome P-450–catalyzed reactions, certain xenobiotic substrates may accept one or two of these electrons. In effect, the substrate rather than molecular oxygen accepts the electrons and is reduced. In fact, oxygen acts as an inhibitor of these reactions since it competes for the reducing equivalents. The classic inhibitors of the cytochrome P-450 system are also inhibitors of these reductive reactions since they either compete for the substrate binding sites or complex with the iron in the heme and thus stop electron flow.

The nitro or azo groups are reduced enzymatically in much the same manner as they would be reduced chemically. By accepting reducing equivalents (hydride ions), the oxidation state of the nitrogen is decreased. The nitro group progresses in sequential steps to a nitrone, a hydroxylamine, and finally an amine. The nitrogen-nitrogen double bond of azo compounds is progressively reduced until it is cleaved into two amine metabolites. Besides the reduction of azo and nitro compounds, other chemical groups are now known to be reduced by this system, such as arene oxides, *N*-oxides, and alkyl halides. Both the flavoprotein enzyme, NADPH-cytochrome P-450 reductase, and the terminal oxidase, cytochrome P-450, are involved in these reductions. The very low redox potential, broad substrate specificity, and strong ligand binding of these systems allow the donation of electrons to electron-accepting xenobiotics, which results in a reduction rather than the predominant oxidative biotransformation.

Table 4-4. REDUCTIVE BIOTRANSFORMATION BY THE CYTOCHROME P-450 SYSTEM

REACTION	EXAMPLE
Azo reduction	$R—N{=}N—R' \longrightarrow R—NH_2 + R'NH_2$
Aromatic nitro reduction	$R-\langle\bigcirc\rangle-NO_2 \longrightarrow R-\langle\bigcirc\rangle-NH_2$
Reductive dehalogenation	$R-\underset{X}{\overset{X}{C}}-X \longrightarrow R-\underset{X}{\overset{X}{C}}-H + HX$

This route of biotransformation may detoxify a xenobiotic, but it often results in more toxic products or reactive intermediates. For example, numerous nitro compounds undergo reduction to amino derivatives, which can then be oxidized to toxic N-hydroxyl metabolites. Polyhalogenated alkanes accept electrons to become radical anions that fragment into carbon-centered free radicals upon cleavage of the carbon-halogen bond. Carbon tetrachloride and halothane ($CF_3CHBrCl$) are two classic examples of cytochrome P-450–catalyzed reductive bioactivation to free radical intermediates.

Intestinal microflora are also known to mediate the reduction of a number of chemicals, particularly those with azo and nitro groups. These microbes have virtually all the enzymatic machinery to mimic the cytochrome P-450–mediated reactions observed in mammalian systems. Owing to the anaerobic environment and the high concentration of chemical seen upon ingestion or biliary excretion, these microbes can have a substantial effect on the *in vivo* biotransformation of xenobiotics. These microbes may also further modify metabolites of xenobiotics that were produced by hepatic cytochrome P-450. In some instances, a new reductive metabolite may be reabsorbed and further processed by hepatic enzymes.

Characterization of Human Liver Cytochromes P-450. Much of the basic knowledge about the structure, function, and regulation of cytochromes P-450 has been derived through studies with experimental animals. However, risk assessments based on extrapolation of the results of animal studies to humans clearly require a detailed understanding of human biotransformation enzymes. In recent years, major advances in the characterization of human liver cytochromes P-450 and their genes have been made. Essentially two approaches have been followed: (1) Human orthologs (counterparts) of animal cytochromes P-450 have been identified with antibody or nucleic acid probes; and (2) human cytochromes P-450 responsible for known *in vivo* polymorphisms of drug metabolism have been isolated through the use of highly selective *in vitro* assays. In some cases, the same human enzyme has been identified by both approaches.

Antibodies to rat liver cytochromes P-450 have been used to identify a number of human liver cytochromes P-450, including members of the IA, IIE, and IIIA gene subfamilies. The antibodies serve as specific reagents to detect the presence of the cross-reacting human protein in microsomal samples, as specific inhibitors for identifying a substrate for the human enzyme, and even as immunoaffinity reagents for isolating the human protein. Such studies have identified human IA2 as the major catalyst of phenacetin O-deethylation and documented the hepatic induction of this enzyme by cigarette smoking in humans. Similar studies have documented the role of ethanol-inducible human liver P450IIE1 in demethylation of the carcinogen N,N-dimethylnitrosamine. It should be emphasized, however, that the function of structurally related cytochromes P-450 is not always conserved across species lines and that the same function may be served by structurally unrelated cytochromes P-450. Therefore, an antibody to a rat liver cytochrome P-450 responsible for a particular reaction in that species may not recognize the cytochrome P-450 responsible for the same reaction in humans.

Human genetic polymorphisms in the metabolism of specific drugs have provided a unique method for identifying individual human liver cytochromes P-450. These polymorphisms are characterized by deficient metabolism of the compound in question by a certain segment of the population. These individuals are said to exhibit the poor metabolizer phenotype. The two best studied examples involve the drugs debrisoquine and mephenytoin.

In the case of the antihypertensive agent debrisoquine, approximately 3 to 10 percent of Caucasians are poor metabolizers. These individuals tend to accumulate the parent drug and are prone to exhibit an exaggerated hypotensive response to a normal dose of the compound. With debrisoquine 4-hydroxylation as a specific assay, human liver cytochrome P450IID1 was isolated and identified as the major catalyst of the *in vitro* metabolism of debrisoquine and at least 20 other basic drugs. Presumably, poor metabolizers of debrisoquine will also be poor metabolizers of these other compounds. In more than half of the poor metabolizers, a defect in the P450IID1 gene leads to the production of mRNAs of abnormal length, incapable of translation into stable proteins.

In the case of the antiepileptic drug mephenytoin, the poor metabolizer phenotype occurs with high frequency in the Japanese population (> 20 percent) compared with a frequency of 3 percent in Caucasians. With 6-mephenytoin 4'-hydroxylation as a specific assay, three related human liver cytochromes P-450 of the IIC subfamily were isolated, two of which catalyze this reaction. The presence of multiple proteins and genes associated with mephenytoin metabolism in humans has made the identification of the defect(s) responsible for the genetic polymorphism more difficult than with debrisoquine. However, the available evidence suggests that the poor metabolizers of mephenytoin produce a stable but catalytically defective protein.

Microsomal FAD-Containing Monooxygenase

Another oxidative enzyme involved in phase I biotransformation is an enzyme historically referred to as mixed-function amine oxidase. This FAD-flavoprotein is present in the endoplasmic reticulum and is capable of oxidizing nucleophilic nitrogen using NADPH and O_2. This enzyme activity is exceptionally high in humans and pigs, while low in rats. Flavin-containing monooxygenase competes with the cytochrome P-450 system in the oxidation of amines. It converts tertiary amines to amine oxides, secondary amines to hydroxyl amines and nitrones, and primary amines to hydroxylamines and oximes (Figure 4–5). The oxidation of nucleophilic divalent sulfur atoms by the flavin-containing monooxygenase is an interesting feature. This enzyme has a wider activity than previously believed. It also oxidizes sulfur compounds (sulfides, thioethers, thiols, thiocarbamates) and organophosphorus compounds.

It is believed that the endogenous substrate for the flavin-containing monooxygenase is cysteamine, which is oxidized to cystamine. The endogenous cystamine-cysteamine balance may then be controlled by this enzyme, and it thus may be involved in disulfide generation during peptide synthesis.

The flavin-containing monooxygenase is not under the same regulatory control as cytochrome P-450. In fact, it is repressed rather than induced by phenobarbital or 3-methylcholanthrene treatment. It appears the concentration of the enzyme is regulated by steroid sex hormones, with testosterone decreasing and progesterone increasing its concentration. The role the flavin-containing monooxygenase has in other biotransformation processes and the toxicity of xenobiotics is still being elucidated.

Peroxidase-Dependent Cooxidation

Most oxidative biotransformations share a common requirement for the reduced pyridine nucleotide cofactors NADPH and NADH and so are closely tied to the production of cellular reductants. An important exception is biotransformation by *peroxidases*, which couples the reduction of hydrogen peroxide and lipid hydroperoxides to the oxidation of other substrates. Peroxidase-dependent metabolism therefore requires a supply of hydroperoxides and is facilitated in tissues that can maintain an oxidizing environment. Metabolically active peroxidases are found in a variety of tissues and cell types. For example, urinary bladder epithelium, renal inner medulla, and skin contain prostaglandin synthetase-hydroperoxidase (PGS), mammary gland epithelium contains lactoperoxidase, and leukocytes contain myeloperoxidase. These enzymes catalyze a common generalized reaction in which the reduction of a hydroperoxide is coupled to the oxidation of a cosubstrate (equation 4.1).

$$ROOH + Substrate_{red} \rightarrow ROH + Substrate_{ox} \qquad (4.1)$$

The mechanism of the reaction is similar for each of the peroxidases described. Hydroperoxide reduction yields an oxidized enzyme intermediate, Compound I, which reacts with substrates by two sequential electron transfers to yield either two substrate radicals or a nonradical, two-electron oxidized product. Peroxidase-dependent metabolism is controlled by the availability of hydroperoxide substrates. Hydrogen peroxide is continuously generated by virtually all respiring cells, but its availability for peroxidase reactions depends on the efficiency of hydroperoxide scavenging by glutathione peroxidase and catalase. Hydrogen peroxide also may be produced by activated leukocytes, lymphocytes, and phagocytic cells, all of which contain peroxidases. PGS is unique among per-

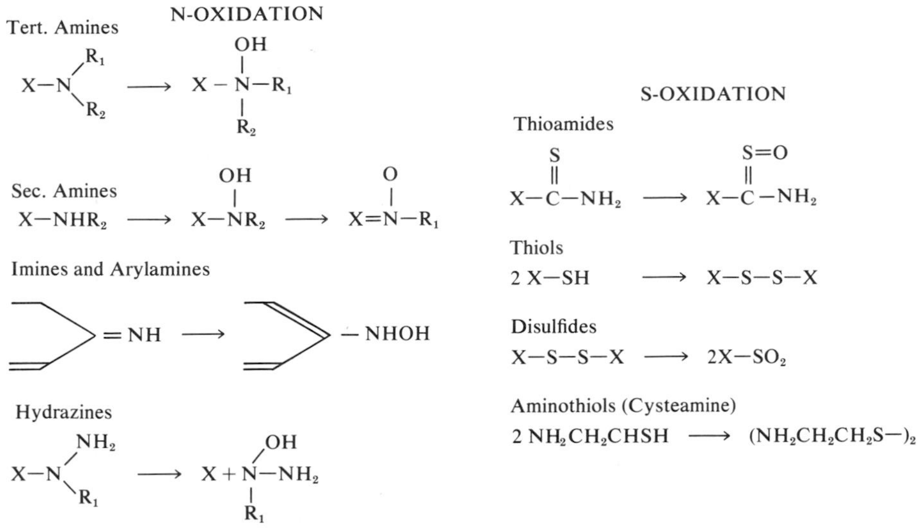

N-OXIDATION

Tert. Amines

$$X-N\begin{smallmatrix}R_1\\\\R_2\end{smallmatrix} \longrightarrow X-\underset{\underset{R_2}{|}}{\overset{\overset{OH}{|}}{N}}-R_1$$

Sec. Amines

$$X-NHR_2 \longrightarrow X-\underset{}{\overset{\overset{OH}{|}}{N}}R_2 \longrightarrow X=\underset{}{\overset{\overset{O}{|}}{N}}-R_1$$

Imines and Arylamines

$$\rangle = NH \longrightarrow \rangle -NHOH$$

Hydrazines

$$X-N\begin{smallmatrix}NH_2\\\\R_1\end{smallmatrix} \longrightarrow X + \underset{\underset{R_1}{|}}{N}\begin{smallmatrix}OH\\\\NH_2\end{smallmatrix}$$

S-OXIDATION

Thioamides

$$X-\overset{\overset{S}{||}}{C}-NH_2 \longrightarrow X-\overset{\overset{S=O}{||}}{C}-NH_2$$

Thiols

$$2\,X-SH \longrightarrow X-S-S-X$$

Disulfides

$$X-S-S-X \longrightarrow 2X-SO_2$$

Aminothiols (Cysteamine)

$$2\,NH_2CH_2CHSH \longrightarrow (NH_2CH_2CH_2S-)_2$$

Figure 4–5. Oxidations catalyzed by the flavin-containing monooxygenase.

oxidases because it can both generate hydroperoxides and catalyze peroxidase-dependent reactions. The hydroperoxides are generated by the cyclooxygenase reaction, which converts arachidonic acid to the hydroperoxide intermediate PGG_2 (equation 4.2).

$$\text{Arachidonic acid} + 2O_2 \rightarrow PGG_2\,(ROOH) \qquad (4.2)$$

PGG_2 then is reduced to the alcohol PGH_2 in the peroxidase reaction, in which a second substrate is oxidized (equation 4.3).

$$PGG_2 + \text{Substrate}_{red} \rightarrow PGH_2 + \text{Substrate}_{ox} \qquad (4.3)$$

The overall reaction in which arachidonic acid and another substrate are oxidized together to produce prostaglandins and other metabolites is termed *cooxidation*. Important classes of compounds known to undergo peroxidase-dependent metabolism include aromatic amines, phenols, hydroquinones, and polycyclic aromatic hydrocarbons. Many of the metabolites produced are reactive electrophiles. For example, polycyclic aromatic hydrocarbons, phenols, and hydroquinones are oxidized to electrophilic quinones. Aromatic amines yield cation radicals and reactive diimines. Peroxidase-dependent metabolism is apparently the principal bioactivation pathway for xenobiotics in certain tissues, particularly those with little mixed-function oxygenase activity. Examples include the urinary bladder epithelium, in which PGS bioactivation of benzidine and other aromatic amines yields reactive electrophiles that bind to DNA. Metabolism of acetaminophen, *p*-aminophenol, and phenacetin in the renal inner medulla yields semiquinone

radicals and reactive quinoneimines that bind to tissue macromolecules. Peroxidases also may complete biotransformation processes begun by other enzyme systems. For example, hepatic mixed-function oxidation of benzene yields phenol and hydroquinone metabolites that may be further bioactivated to reactive quinones by lymphocyte myeloperoxidase. This biotransformation sequence may account for the selective myelotoxicity of benzene. Although the carcinogenic polycyclic aromatic hydrocarbon benzo[a]pyrene is not completely metabolized to a reactive diol epoxide by PGS, the 7,8-dihydrodiol produced by cytochrome P-450 and epoxide hydrolase is readily metabolized to the corresponding 7,8-diol-9,10-epoxide by PGS.

Epoxide Hydrolase

An important hydrolytic enzyme thought to be located in close proximity to the microsomal cytochrome P-450 monooxygenases is epoxide hydrolase, formerly known as epoxide hydrase or epoxide hydratase. The enzyme catalyzes the hydration of arene oxides and aliphatic epoxides to their corresponding *trans*-1,2-dihydrodiols (Figure 4–6). An important toxicologic aspect of the reaction is that the corresponding diols are less electrophilic and, therefore, less chemically reactive than the epoxides. Arene oxides (epoxides of aromatic compounds) are generally unstable and rearrange to the corresponding phenol. The phenol is then available to participate in various phase II conjugation reactions.

Epoxide hydrolase has been found in a wide variety of tissues, including liver, testis, ovary, lung, kidney, skin, intestine, colon, spleen, thymus, brain, and heart. Its distribution among

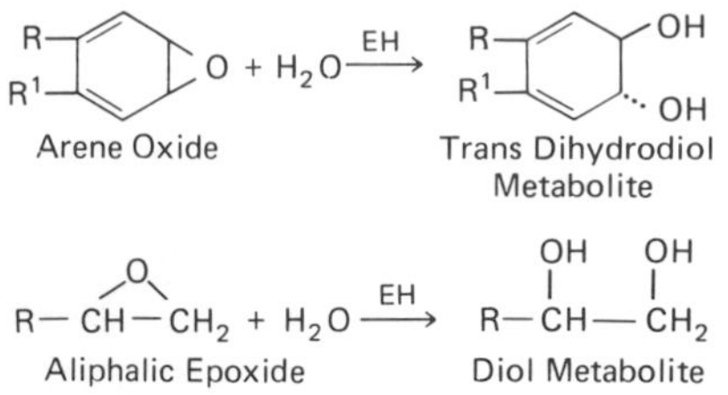

Figure 4-6. Dihydrodiol formation catalyzed by epoxide hydrolase (EH).

tissues with multiple cell types is heterogeneous. For example, the pulmonary clara cells possess three to four times more epoxide hydrolase activity than the alveolar type I cells. These are also the two cell types of the lung that contain the majority of the cytochrome P-450-dependent monooxygenase activity. From the nature of the reaction catalyzed by epoxide hydrolase, it is not surprising that the bulk of the activity is located in the endoplasmic reticulum of the various cell types that possess the enzyme. This close proximity to the site of formation of its substrates suggests that epoxide hydrolase may have evolved as an important means of detoxifying arene oxides and aliphatic epoxides.

A distinct cytosolic epoxide hydrolase exists in a number of animal tissues. This activity appears to be high in tissues from mice and rabbits but low in rats. The cytosolic and microsomal hydrolase enzymes are immunologically distinct and have different substrate specificities. Their role in detoxication of various epoxides is under investigation.

Available evidence indicates that epoxide hydrolase-catalyzed hydration of oxides occurs by activation of water to a nucleophilic species. The resulting nucleophilic species attacks the least hindered carbon atom from the side opposite to the oxide ring. Consequently, ring opening is directed away from the hydroxylation and the resulting diols have a *trans* configuration.

In general, epoxide hydrolase is considered a detoxication enzyme, since it inactivates a number of highly reactive oxides that have been implicated in tissue injury (bromobenzene 3,4-oxide) and mutagenicity (benzo[a]pyrene 4,5-oxide). However, the hydration of benzo[a]pyrene 7,8-oxide by epoxide hydrolase can be considered an activation reaction. The diol derivative (*trans*-7,8-dihydroxy-7,8-dihydrobenzo[a]pyrene) can be epoxidated by the cytochrome P-450 system to yield the highly reactive and carcinogenic species benzo[a]pyrene 7,8-dihydrodiol-9,10-oxide. This and other reactive diol epoxides of polycyclic aromatic hydrocarbons are poor substrates for epoxide hydrolase. Therefore, they cannot be readily deactivated and, thus, interact with critical tissue macromolecules.

Microsomal epoxide hydrolase activity is regulated by a number of factors. In rats, epoxide hydrolase activity in the liver becomes detectable at about four days before birth and then steadily increases to adult levels. Its activity in liver of male rats is about twice that in female rats. Inducers of the microsomal mixed-function oxygenases also induce epoxide hydrolase activity. No specific inducer has been identified. Several alcohols, ketones, and imidazoles stimulate microsomal epoxide hydrolase activity *in vitro*. Similarly, certain epoxides are known to inhibit the enzyme. The most widely used are 1,1,1-trichloropropane oxide and cyclohexene oxide.

Esterases and Amidases

Mammalian tissues contain a large number of nonspecific esterases and amidases that can hydrolyze ester and amide linkages in foreign compounds. This hydrolytic cleavage of ester and amide linkages liberates carboxyl groups and an alcohol function in the case of esters and an amine or NH_3 in the case of amides (Figure 4-7). These carboxyl, alcohol, and amine groups may undergo a variety of conjugations (phase II reactions). In certain cases, even thioesters can be hydrolyzed by this group of enzymes.

As summarized in Table 4-5, esterases may be broadly categorized into four main classes: (1) arylesterases, which preferentially hydrolyze aromatic esters (ArCOOR'); Ar = aromatic); (2) carboxylesterases, which hydrolyze aliphatic esters (RCH_2COOR'); (3) acetylesterases, in which the acid moiety of the ester is acetic acid (CH_3COOR'); and (4) cholinesterases, which hydrolyze esters in which the alcohol moiety is choline ($(CH_3)_3N^+{-}CH_2{-}CH_2{-}OOCR$). It should be noted that there is considerable overlap in substrate specificity among these classes

$$R{-}\overset{\displaystyle O}{\overset{\|}{C}}{-}O{-}R' + H_2O \rightarrow R{-}\overset{\displaystyle O}{\overset{\|}{C}}{-}OH + HOR'$$

Ester hydrolysis

$$R{-}\overset{\displaystyle O}{\overset{\|}{C}}{-}\underset{\displaystyle R}{\underset{|}{N}}{-}R' + H_2O \rightarrow R{-}\overset{\displaystyle O}{\overset{\|}{C}}{-}OH + HNR'R''$$

Amide hydrolysis

$$R{-}\overset{\displaystyle O}{\overset{\|}{C}}{-}S{-}R' + H_2O \rightarrow R{-}\overset{\displaystyle O}{\overset{\|}{C}}{-}OH + HSR'$$

Thioester hydrolysis

Figure 4-7. Hydrolytic biotransformation reactions.

Table 4–5. SIMPLIFIED CLASSIFICATION OF ESTERASES

ESTERASE	PREFERRED SUBSTRATES
A-esterases (arylesterases)	Aromatic ester
B-esterases (carboxylesterases)	Aliphatic ester
C-esterases (acetylesterases)	Acetyl ester
Cholinesterases	Choline esters

of esterases. For example, a carboxyl esterase may hydrolyze an aromatic ester at a detectable rate. Therefore, these classifications should not be considered to be absolute.

In general, enzymatic hydrolysis of amides occurs more slowly than with esters. Enzyme specificity for the various amides may be partially responsible for this slower rate of biotransformation. However, electronic factors are also important. Thus, substituent groups in primary, secondary, and tertiary amides that have electron-withdrawing properties will cause a weakening of the amide bond, making it more susceptible to enzymatic hydrolysis.

The esterases/amidases are both cytosolic and microsomal enzymes. The cytosolic esterases are usually associated with a specific reaction, such as acetyl cholinesterase and pseudocholinesterase, whereas the microsomal-associated esterases handle a diverse array of xenobiotic esters.

The esterases/amidases can be inhibited when substrates bind tightly to the active sites or when the resulting products are very reactive. This is the case with organophosphates, where metabolites bind to the active site following hydrolysis.

There is evidence for considerable genetic influence in certain of the esterase enzymes. For example, pseudocholinesterase detoxifies many of the aliphatic ester/amide muscle relaxants. However, the subunit makeup, enzymatic activity, and sensitivity to inhibition are under genetic control. Thus, extremes of high/low enzyme activity and resistance/susceptibility to inhibition are known.

Alcohol, Aldehyde, Ketone Oxidation-Reduction Systems

Aldehydes, ketones, and alcohols are functional groups that occur from the oxidation of carbon or the hydrolysis of ester linkages. In addition, they are frequent functional groups that appear in drugs and other xenobiotics. These functional groups are often further biotransformed in the body by oxidation or reduction. The principal enzymatic systems involved in this redox reaction, which are listed in Figure 4–8, are: alcohol dehydrogenase, aldehyde reductase, ketone reductase, and a variety of aldehyde oxidizing systems (such as aldehyde dehydrogenase and aldehyde oxidase). These soluble enzymes are present in a number of mammalian tissues. NAD^+ is frequently the cofactor for oxidation, and NADH or NADPH is the cofactor for reduction. Since alcohol, aldehyde, or ketone moieties often impart pharmacologic properties, the oxidation or reduction of these groups is a means of detoxication. However, in some cases more reactive functional groups may be produced that can lead to toxicity (i.e., oxidation of alcohols to reactive aldehydes).

One of the most important enzymes of this group is alcohol dehydrogenase, which oxidizes ethanol ($CH_3CH_2OH + NAD^+ \rightarrow CH_3CHO + NADH + H^+$). This cytosolic enzyme, located primarily in liver, is responsible for the biotransformation of ethanol. The resulting acetaldehyde is then oxidized to acetic acid by aldehyde dehydrogenase. Some alcohol dehydrogenase activity is associated with the endoplasmic reticulum. Other alcohols may also act as substrates for alcohol dehydrogenase, as may polyalcohols (methanol, ethylene glycol, and allyl alcohol).

While most of the alcohol dehydrogenase reactions detoxify the alcoholic substance, there are cases where the product is more toxic. Such is the case with the oxidation of methanol and ethylene glycol to their ultimate metabolic products formate and oxalate, respectively. In addition, the aldehyde products have also been found to react under physiologic conditions with primary amine groups to form Schiff's bases. Such interactions often alter the functional ability of that macromolecule. Pyrazole and certain of its derivatives inhibit alcohol dehydrogenase.

Aldehyde/Ketone Reductase(s)

Alcohol Dehydrogenase

Aldehyde Dehydrogenase

$R_1 = H$ or Organic Group

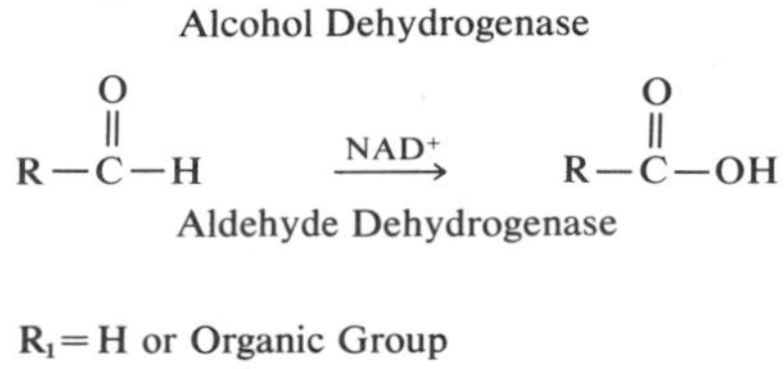

Figure 4–8. Alcohol, aldehyde, ketone oxidation-reduction systems.

Aldehyde dehydrogenase oxidizes aldehydes to carboxylic acids with NAD^+ as the cofactor. There are two major types of aldehyde dehydrogenases in mammals. One specifically oxidizes formaldehyde that is complexed with glutathione and is called formaldehyde dehydrogenase. The other oxidizes free aldehydes and has broad substrate specificity. This latter enzyme is the aldehyde dehydrogenase involved in most xenobiotic aldehyde oxidation. Isozymes of this enzyme are found in hepatic cytosol, mitochondria, and microsomes with characteristic specificities. For example, acetaldehyde is mainly oxidized by the mitochondrial enzyme, whereas xenobiotic aldehydes are oxidized mainly by the cytosolic and microsomal dehydrogenases. Genetic deficiencies in aldehyde dehydrogenase activity have been observed in many Japanese. Individuals with this deficiency accumulate acetaldehyde after ethanol ingestion.

It is the inhibition of the aldehyde dehydrogenase that usually results in toxicity of xenobiotics requiring this route of biotransformation. When *in vivo* inhibitors of aldehyde dehydrogenase activity (such as disulfiram and cyanamide) are present, the concentration of the aldehyde increases and, hence, is more likely to react with nucleophiles such as endogenous amines.

Aldehyde and ketones can be reduced to alcohols by aldehyde/ketone reductases. These are soluble enzymes that typically use NADPH as the source of reducing equivalents. Since cells typically have an overall potential for oxidation, with a high ratio of NAD^+ to NADH, the selective use of NADPH, which is present in excess of $NADP^+$, allows for the conversion of lipid-soluble carbonyls to less reactive and soluble alcohols in an oxidizing environment.

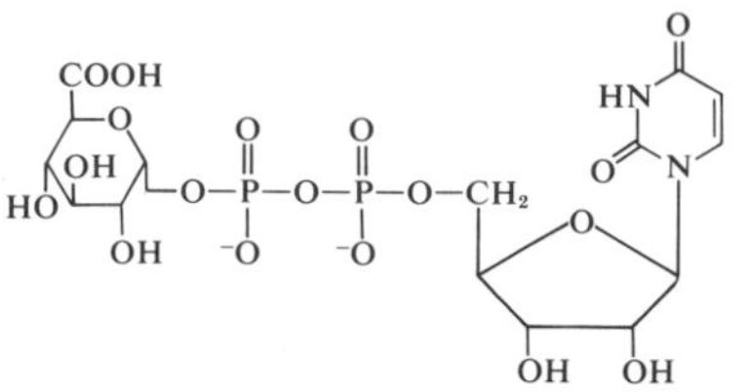

PHASE II ENZYME REACTIONS

The phase II biotransformation reactions are biosynthetic and thus require energy to drive the reaction. This is accomplished by activating the cofactors, or in one case the substrate, to high-energy intermediates. Since the cofactors are activated either directly or indirectly with ATP, the energy status of the organ is important in determining cofactor availability.

Glucuronosyltransferases

Glucuronidation represents one of the major conjugation phase II reactions in the conversion of both exogenous and endogenous compounds to polar, water-soluble compounds. The resulting glucuronides are eliminated from the body in the urine or bile. The widespread species occurrence, the broad range of substrates that are

Uridine-5'-diphospho-α-D-glucuronic acid (UDP-GA)

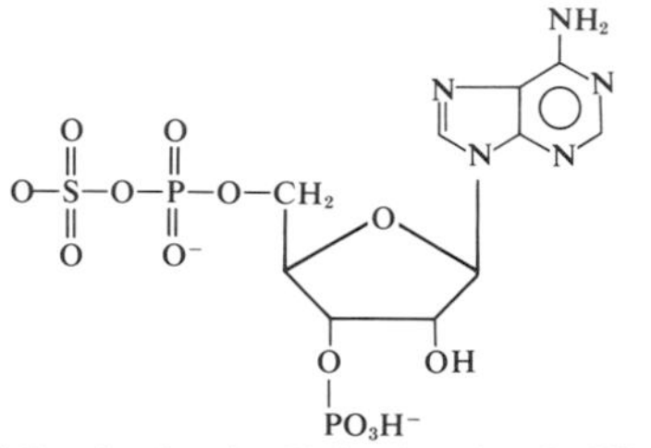

3'-Phosphoadenosine-5'-phosphosulfate (PAPS)

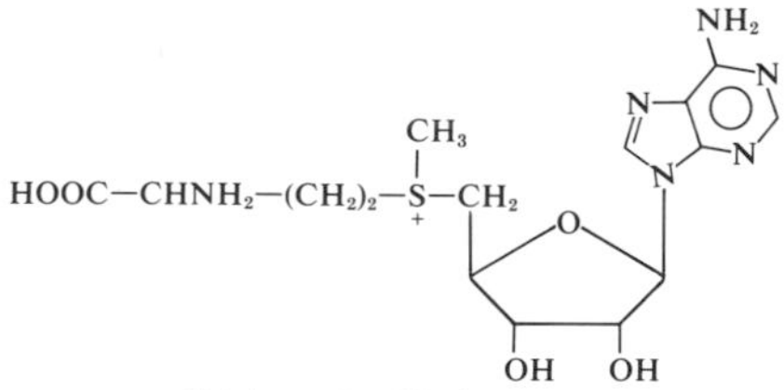

S-Adenosylmethionine (SAM)

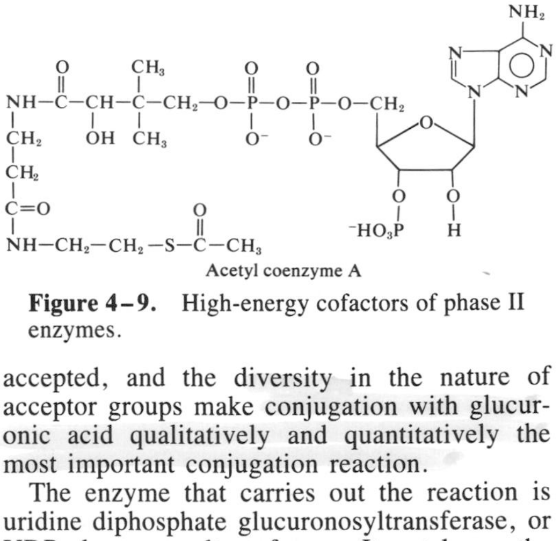

Acetyl coenzyme A

Figure 4–9. High-energy cofactors of phase II enzymes.

accepted, and the diversity in the nature of acceptor groups make conjugation with glucuronic acid qualitatively and quantitatively the most important conjugation reaction.

The enzyme that carries out the reaction is uridine diphosphate glucuronosyltransferase, or UDP-glucuronosyltransferase. It catalyzes the interaction between the high-energy nucleotide, UDP-glucuronic acid (UDP-GA, Figure 4–9), and the functional group on the acceptor molecule (the substrate or aglycone). Glucuronosyltransferase activity is localized in the endoplasmic reticulum of numerous tissues, whereas most phase II enzymes are cytosolic enzymes. Quantitatively, the liver is the most important tissue, but activity is also present in the kidney, intestine, skin, brain, and spleen. The location of glucuronosyltransferase in the microsomal membrane is important physiologically, since it may have direct access to the products formed by the action of microsomal cytochrome P-450. Thus, one can envision a highly integrated system within the microsomal membrane that results in the sequestration of highly lipophilic compounds, the addition or unmasking of a functional group, and the conjugation of this functional group with the highly polar glucuronic acid moiety.

There are several distinct forms of UDP-glucuronosyltransferase. Enzyme heterogeneity explains in part the differential increases in enzyme activities toward different aglycones following treatment with known microsomal enzyme inducing agents, differential decreases in activities with respect to inhibition, and species differences that lead to defects in glucuronidation of only certain classes of glucuronic acid acceptors.

The number of distinct forms of the enzyme is unknown at this time. Purification, chromatofocusing, and immunochemical studies provide evidence for a minimum of 11 forms. Four forms of UDP-glucuronyl-transferase have been cloned, sequenced, and expressed in cultured mammalian cells. These various forms respond to different inducing agents and show selectivity toward certain classes of substrates. For example, a form catalytically active toward 4-nitrophenol and 1-napthol showed little activity toward morphine, testosterone, bilirubin, and bile acids.

Numerous functional groups present in both foreign and endogenous compounds that undergo conjugation with glucuronic acid are listed in Table 4–6. These include aliphatic and aromatic alcohols, carboxyl acids, primary and secondary aromatic and aliphatic amines, and free sulfhydryl groups. These form O-, N-, and S-glucuronides, respectively. Certain nucleophilic carbon atoms have also been shown to form C-glucuronides.

During the conjugation reaction, the UDP-glucuronic acid cofactor, which is in the α configuration, undergoes inversion leading to glucuronides that have a β configuration. It is important to note that glucuronidation contributes a carboxyl group, which exists primarily in the ionized form at physiologic pH (Figure 4–10). This group promotes excretion not only because of the water solubility it confers but also because it can participate in biliary and renal organic anion transport systems that recognize this group.

Glucuronides are excreted from the body in either the bile or urine, depending on the size of the aglycone (parent compound or Phase I metabolite) (Table 4–7). In the rat, if the aglycone has a molecular weight below about 250, the glucuronide will be cleared by renal tubular

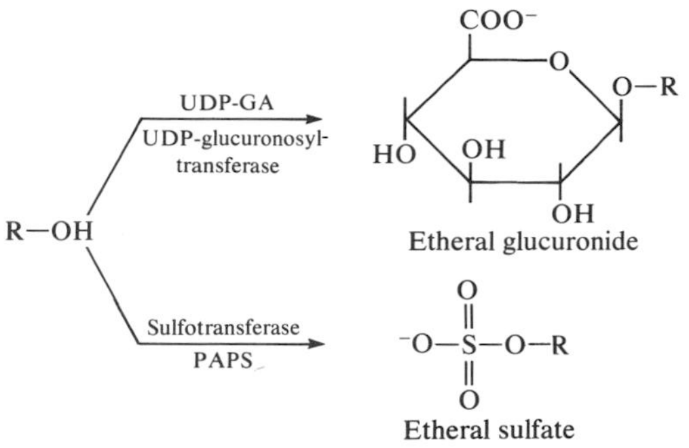

Figure 4–10. Glucuronidation and sulfation of a hydroxyl functional group.

organic acid secretion into urine. If the structure has a molecular weight greater than 350, the conjugate is often secreted into bile. From 250 to 350 molecular weight, the conjugate may be excreted by either pathway. Molecular weight cutoffs for the preferred route of excretion vary with the animal species.

Glucuronide conjugates of xenobiotics are substrates for β-glucuronidase. Although present in the lysozomes of some mammalian tissues, considerable β-glucuronidase activity is present in the intestinal microflora. Thus, this enzyme can release the aglycone, which can be reabsorbed and enter a cycle called the *enterohepatic recirculation*. Compounds involved in this cycle tend to have a longer lifetime in the body and may undergo more extensive biotransformation before being eliminated. N-Glucuronides are more slowly hydrolyzed by β-glucuronidase than O- or S-glucuronides. Glucuronides can also be hydrolyzed in the presence of acid or bases, an important point that must be considered when attempting to extract glucuronides from a biologic matrix.

Because of the susceptibility of certain glucuronides to enzymatic and chemical degradation, glucuronides may serve to transport potentially reactive compounds from the liver to the target tissue. The most widely cited examples are N-glucuronides of N-hydroxy-arylamines. These derivatives have been implicated in bladder cancer produced by 2-naphthylamine, 4-aminobiphenyl, and related compounds. It is proposed that these arylamines undergo N-hydroxylation in the liver, with the subsequent formation of the N-glucuronide of the N-hydroxyarylamine. The N-glucuronides, which accumulate in the urine of the bladder, are unstable in acidic pH and thus are hydrolyzed to the corresponding unstable carcinogenic N-hydroxylamine.

Sulfotransferase

In mammals, an important conjugation reaction for hydroxyl groups is sulfation. This reac-

Table 4–6. EXAMPLES OF THE DIFFERENT CLASSES OF GLUCURONIDE CONJUGATES*†

TYPES OF GLUCURONIDES*	ACCEPTOR	
	Functional Group	*Example*
O-Glucuronide		

⎪
—C—O—G
⎪
	Alcohol
	  Aliphatic
	  Alicyclic
	  Benzylic
	  Phenolic
		Trichloroethanol
		Hexobarbital
		Methylphenylcarbinol
		Estrone

—C—O—G
‖
O
	Carboxylic acid
	  Aliphatic
	  Aromatic
		α-Ethylhexanoic acid
		o-Aminobenzoic acid

—CH=C—O—G ⎪	α,β-Unsaturated ketone	Progesterone

—N—O—G
  ⎪
	N-Hydroxy	N-Acetyl-N-phenyl-
		  hydroxylamine

N-Glucuronide		

—O—C—N—G
   ‖ ⎪
   O H
	Carbamate	Meprobamate

Ar—N—G
   ⎪
   H
	Arylamine	2-Naphthylamine

(R)₃—N⁺—G	Aliphatic tertiary amine	Tripelennamine

R—SO₂—N—G
        ⎪
        H
	Sulfonamide	Sulfadimethoxine

S-Glucuronide Ar—S—G	Aryl thiol	Thiophenol
—C—S—G ‖ S	Dithiocarbamic acid	N,N-Diethyldithiocarbamic acid
C-Glucuronide		
⎪ —C—G ⎪	1,3-Dicarbonyl system	Phenylbutazone

* G = glucuronic acid.
† Modified from Jakoby, W. E. (ed.): *Enzymatic Basis of Detoxication,* Vol. 2. Academic Press, Inc., New York, 1980.

Table 4–7. PREFERRED ROUTE OF EXCRETION OF CONJUGATES OF XENOBIOTICS

Glucuronides	<250 M.W.—kidney >350 M.W.—bile
Sulfates	Kidney
Glutathione conjugates	Bile
Acetylated conjugates	Kidney
Amino acid conjugates	Kidney
Mercapturic acids	Kidney

tion is catalyzed by the sulfotransferases, a group of soluble enzymes found primarily in liver, kidney, intestinal tract, and lungs. Their primary function is to transfer inorganic sulfate to the hydroxyl group present on phenols and aliphatic alcohols. The resulting products are referred to as sulfate esters or ethereal sulfates (Figure 4–10). In addition, sulfation of aromatic amines and hydroxylamines to form the corresponding sulfamate and N-O-sulfates is occasionally seen.

As a detoxication process, sulfation is considered an effective means of decreasing the pharmacologic and toxicologic activity of com-

**Table 4–8. CLASSIFICATION OF
SULFOTRANSFERASES**

Aryl sulfotransferase	Phenols
	Catechols
	Hydroxylamines
Hydroxysteroid	Hydroxysteroids
sulfotransferase	Some primary/secondary
	alcohols
Estrone sulfotransferase	Phenolic steroids
Bile salt sulfotransferase	Bile acids

pounds. The products of this reaction are ionized organic sulfates and, therefore, are more readily excreted than the parent compound or hydroxylated metabolite. In addition, if the hydroxyl or amine function is important in expression of the toxicologic activity, sulfation would mask this functional group and prevent its interaction with some critical cellular component. Numerous low-molecular-weight endogenous compounds, such as catecholamines, hydroxy steroids, and bile acids, are known to undergo sulfation.

There are four classes of sulfotransferases involved in detoxication processes (Table 4–8). Aryl sulfotransferase conjugates phenols, catecholamines, and organic hydroxylamines. Hydroxysteroid sulfotransferase conjugates hydroxysteroids and certain primary and secondary alcohols. Estrone sulfotransferase is active with phenolic groups on the aromatic ring of steroids, and finally, bile salt sulfotransferases catalyze the sulfation of both conjugated and unconjugated bile acids. The activity of these enzymes is known to vary considerably with the sex and age of animals.

The sulfate donor for these reactions is 3'-phosphoadenosine-5'-phosphosulfate (PAPS, Figure 4–9). This cofactor is synthesized from inorganic sulfate and ATP. The major source of sulfate required for the synthesis of PAPS appears to be derived from cysteine through a complex oxidation sequence. Since the concentration of free cysteine is limited, an important determinant in the extent of sulfation of foreign chemicals is the availability of the cofactor, PAPS. In reactions catalyzed by the sulfotransferases, the SO_3^- group of PAPS is readily transferred in a reaction involving nucleophilic attack of the phenolic oxygen or the amine nitrogen on the sulfur atom with the subsequent displacement of adenosine-3',5'-diphosphate.

Sulfation seems to have a high affinity but low capacity for conjugation of phenols. The major alternative reaction for phenols, glucuronidation, has low affinity but a much higher capacity (Table 4–9, Figure 4–10). Therefore, following administration of low doses of phenols, the major phenolic conjugate may be the sulfate ester. However, as the dose of the phenol is increased,

the percent of dose and, occasionally, the absolute amount excreted as the sulfate may actually decrease, with a disproportionate increase in the amount excreted as the glucuronide. Although depletion of inorganic sulfate can explain a reduction in the percent of dose excreted as the sulfate with increasing doses of phenol, it does not explain the reduction in absolute amount. The most likely explanation for the reduced rate of sulfate conjugation is substrate inhibition of the transferase, as has been observed *in vitro* with preparations of purified acyl sulfotransferase. Because of the generally greater total activity of the glucuronosyltransferase reactions in most animal species, sulfate conjugation is considered to be of lesser importance in facilitating the excretion of hydrophobic alcohols and phenols. However, the preferred route of conjugation can be influenced by dose.

Although sulfate conjugation usually results in detoxication, examples exist where conjugation results in toxication. Certain sulfate conjugates are chemically unstable and degrade to form potent electrophilic species. The most notable example is the *N-O* sulfate esters of *N*-hydroxy-2-acetylaminofluorene, which will be discussed later.

Sulfate conjugates of xenobiotics are excreted mainly in urine (Table 4–7). Some of these conjugates can also be degraded enzymatically. Aryl sulfatases are present in gut microflora, but some activity is associated with the endoplasmic reticulum and lysozomes. Although these primarily degrade sulfates of endogenous compounds, they also possess activity toward sulfate conjugates of xenobiotics. Their role in the subsequent disposition of sulfate conjugates is poorly understood.

Methylation

Methylation is a common biochemical reaction for the metabolism of endogenous compounds but is not usually a quantitatively important pathway for xenobiotic biotransformation. Methylation differs from most other conjugation

**Table 4–9. RELATIVE CAPACITIES OF THE
CONJUGATION REACTIONS***

CAPACITY	REACTION
High	Glucuronidation
Medium	Amino acid conjugation
Low	Sulfation, glutathione
	conjugation
Variable	Acetylation

* From Caldwell, J. In Jenner, P., and Testa, B. (eds.): *Concepts in Drug Metabolism.* Marcel Dekker, Inc., New York, 1981. Reprinted by courtesy of the publisher.

Table 4–10. EXAMPLES OF PRODUCTS OF METHYLATION REACTIONS

SUBSTRATE	PRODUCT
1. Pyridine (pyridine ring with N)	Pyridine ring with N^+—CH$_3$
2. Catechol (benzene ring with —OH, —OH)	Benzene ring with —OCH$_3$, —OH
3. $(C_2H_5)_2N$—$\overset{\overset{\displaystyle S}{\|}}{C}$—SH Diethyldithiocarbamate	$(C_2H_5)_2N$—$\overset{\overset{\displaystyle S}{\|}}{C}$—S—CH$_3$

reactions in that it actually masks functional groups. This may reduce the water solubility of the chemical and/or impair its ability to participate in other conjugation reactions.

The functional groups involved in methylation reactions are aliphatic and aromatic amines, N-heterocyclics, mono- and polyhydric phenols, and sulfhydryl-containing compounds. In particular, methylthio metabolites or aromatic and aliphatic substances are being detected more routinely.

The nature of the methylation reaction is similar to that for the other conjugation processes in that the methyl group is transferred to the xenobiotic from a high-energy cofactor, S-adenosyl methionine (SAM, Figure 4–9). The methyl group bound to the sulfonium ion in SAM has the characteristics of a carbonium ion and is transferred by nucleophilic attack of the alcohol oxygen, the amine nitrogen, or the thiol sulfur on the methyl group, giving S-adenosylhomocysteine and the methylated substrate as products.

The O-methylation reaction of primary importance is catalyzed by catechol-O-methyl transferase (Table 4–10). This soluble enzyme is ubiquitous but concentrated in liver and kidney. It will catalyze this reaction only with catechols and will not methylate monohydric phenols.

Various specific (histamine and indole) and nonspecific N-methyl transferases have been described. The nonspecific N-methyl transferases are of most concern since these enzymes are capable of methylating a variety of primary, secondary, and tertiary exogenous and endogenous amines such as serotonin, benzylamine, amphetamine, and pyridine.

S-methyl transferases are believed to have evolved in the liver to handle the evolution and uptake of hydrogen sulfide produced by anaerobic bacteria in the intestinal tract. The hydrogen sulfide is methylated to methane thiol, which is further methylated to dimethylsulfide. Other free sulfhydryl compounds also appear to be handled by this system.

The largest source of substrates for this S-methyl transferase appears now to be the thio ethers of glutathione conjugates. Glutathione thio ethers are hydrolyzed to cysteine conjugates in the kidney prior to acetylation and excretion. Those conjugates escaping acetylation are substrates for cysteine conjugate β-lyase, an enzyme that cleaves cysteine thioethers. Owing to the large variety of xenobiotics proceeding through the glutathione conjugation pathway, a variety of organic sulfhydryl compounds can be produced that will ultimately be available for S-methylation.

N-Acetyl Transferases

A major route of biotransformation for arylamines found in most species is acetylation of the amine function. Examples of substrates for the N-acetyl transferases include aromatic primary amines, hydrazines, hydrazides, sulfonamides, and certain primary aliphatic amines (Table 4–11).

The enzymes that catalyze the acetylation of amines are designated as acetyl CoA: amine N-acetyl transferases. The cofactor for these reactions is acetyl coenzyme A (Figure 4–9). N-acetyl transferases are cytosolic enzymes found in many tissues of a number of species. It appears that multiple forms of the transferase occur in most tissues, but the number of different

Table 4–11. EXAMPLES OF PRODUCTS OF N-ACETYL TRANSFERASE REACTIONS

SUBSTRATE	PRODUCT
1. (aniline, C_6H_5–NH_2)	(acetanilide, C_6H_5–NH–$\overset{\displaystyle O}{\overset{\displaystyle \|}{C}}$–$CH_3$)
2. R—NH—NH$_2$ substituted hydrazine	R—NH—NH—$\overset{\displaystyle O}{\overset{\displaystyle \|}{C}}$—CH$_3$
3. R—SO—NH$_2$ aryl-substituted sulfonamide	R—SO—NH—$\overset{\displaystyle O}{\overset{\displaystyle \|}{C}}$—CH$_3$

enzymes that contribute to acetylation of foreign compounds is yet to be determined. The dog and related species are deficient in the major N-acetyl transferase and thus are unable to acetylate a wide number of substrates. Polymorphism of acetylation for selected substrates has been reported in humans, mice, rabbits, and squirrel monkeys. This polymorphism is of genetic origin. Subjects are classified as "rapid" or "slow" acetylators based on their ability to acetylate isoniazid. The existence of N-acetyl transferase polymorphism has been linked with chemical-induced toxicities, most notably the susceptibility of slow acetylators to isoniazid-induced peripheral nerve damage. In addition, susceptibility to cancer induced by aromatic amines may be dependent upon polymorphism in N-acetyl transferase activity. Both epidemiological and experimental studies have demonstrated that slow acetylators are more susceptible to benzidine-induced bladder cancer.

Data from a number of biochemical studies suggest that the transferases from rapid and slow acetylator rabbits are structurally different and that they possess different substrate specificity. Sulfanilamide and p-aminobenzoic acid are monomorphic substrates, since the capacity for N-acetylation of these amines displays a unimodal distribution, at least in the human population.

Acetylation of arylamines occurs in two sequential steps. Initially, the acetyl group from acetyl CoA is transferred to the N-acetyl transferase to form acetyl-N-acetyl transferase as an intermediate. The second step is acetylation of the amino group of the arylamine substrate with regeneration of the enzyme. The interaction between the amine and the acetyl group results in formation of an amide bond.

Although the amide bond is relatively stable, a number of deacetylases/amidases are present in the mitochondrial, microsomal, and soluble fractions. Thus, the overall production of N-acetyl conjugates in a particular species will depend on the relative rates of acetylation and deacetylation.

For N-acetylated amines that undergo N-hydroxylation, an arylhydroxamic acid:acyl transferase has been identified. This enzyme can remove the acetyl group from the aryl hydroxamic acid and transfer it to oxygen of the hydroxylamine. The resulting product is the highly unstable N-acyloxyarylamine, which degrades to the highly reactive arylnitrenium ion. The role of this enzyme in tumor induction of aromatic amines is currently being delineated. It is widely distributed throughout species and has been located in a number of tissues.

Acetylation is another example of a conjugation reaction that masks a functional group. Many N-acetyl derivatives are less water soluble than the parent compound. N-acetyl derivatives of certain sulfonamides have been reported to precipitate in the kidney tubules, an event that can result in kidney damage.

Amino Acid Conjugation

An important reaction for xenobiotics containing a carboxylic acid group is conjugation with one of a variety of amino acids. These reactions result in the formation of an amide (peptide) bond between the carboxylic acid group of the xenobiotic and the amino group of the amino acid. Substrates for conjugation include aromatic carboxylic acids, arylacetic acids, and aryl-substituted acrylic acids (Table 4–12). Although the most common reaction involves glycine, conjugation with glutamine is more prevalent in humans and certain monkeys, and conjugation with ornithine is seen in birds and reptiles. Taurine serves as an acyl acceptor for bile acid conjugation.

The formation of the peptide bond is a two-step coupled reaction catalyzed by different enzymes. The first reaction involves activation of the acid to a thioester derivative of coenzyme A. The energy for this reaction is supplied by ATP. The enzymes that catalyze this activation are called ATP-dependent acid:CoA ligases. The coenzyme A thioester then transfers its acyl moiety to the amino group of the acceptor amino acid. The ligase and the N-acyltransferase are soluble enzymes, but there is also activity within the matrix of hepatic and renal mitochondria. The number and specificity of the activating and

Table 4–12. EXAMPLES OF AMINO ACID CONJUGATES OF ORGANIC ACIDS*

ORGANIC ACID SUBSTRATE	AMINO ACID	PEPTIDE PRODUCT
(Aryl acid) Benzoate	Glycine	Hippurate
(Arylacetic acid) Phenylacetate	Glutamine	Phenylacetylglutamine
(Bile acid) Cholate	Taurine	Taurocholate

* Modified from Jakoby, W. E. (ed.): *Enzymatic Basis of Detoxication,* Vol. 2. Academic Press, Inc. New York, 1980.

acylating enzymes in all species are not known. In mammals, evidence exists for two acid:CoA ligases that can activate benzoic acid. Two different types of *N*-acyl transferases have been purified from mammalian hepatic mitochondria. One prefers benzoyl CoA as substrate, whereas the other prefers arylacetyl CoA.

The formation of amino acid conjugates of aromatic acids is quantitatively an important reaction in a number of animal species. Since carboxylic acids are also subjected to glucuronidation, competition between the glucuronosyltransferases and the amino acid transferases is expected. The degree to which glucuronide formation or amino acid conjugation predominates depends on both the animal species and the structure of the acid. For example, the major conjugate of phenylacetic acid in the rat, ferret, and monkey is the amino acid conjugate. However, diphenylacetic acid undergoes only glucuronidation in these three species. Other structure-activity comparisons also indicate the importance of structure in determining the degree of amino acid conjugation.

Amino acid conjugation can be classified as a system with high affinity and medium-to-low capacity (Table 4–9). As the dose increases, the pathway becomes readily saturated and other means of elimination predominate (*i.e.,* glucuronidation, or phase I reactions). Amino acid conjugates are eliminated primarily in urine. The addition of an endogenous amino acid to xenobiotics may facilitate this elimination by increasing their ability to interact with the tubular organic anion transport system (Table 4–7).

Glutathione S-Transferases

The glutathione *S*-transferases are a family of enzymes that catalyze the initial step in the formation of *N*-acetylcysteine (mercapturic acid) derivatives of a diverse group of foreign compounds. Glutathione *S*-transferases are localized in both the cytoplasm and the endoplasmic reticulum. However, the cytosolic glutathione transferase activities are usually 5 to 40 times greater than the microsomal activity. The enzymes are ubiquitous, with the greatest activity found in the testis, liver, intestine, kidney, and adrenal gland.

Elution chromatography of the transferases from rat liver cytosol has revealed numerous different isoforms, each species being a dimer differing in subunit composition. It is likely that molecular biological studies will reveal addition-

Table 4–13. GLUTATHIONE *S*-TRANSFERASE REACTIONS

Substitution Reaction	
Glutathione *S*-alkyltransferase:	CH_3I + GSH ⟶ CH_3-SG + HI Methyl iodide
Glutathione *S*-aryltransferase:	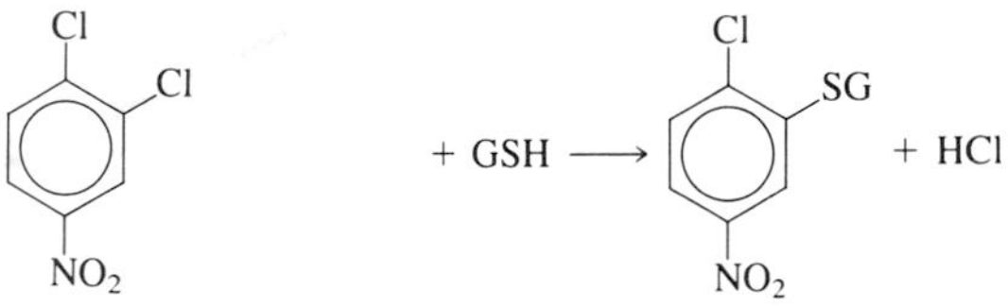 3,4-Dichloronitrobenzene
Glutathione *S*-aralkyltransferase:	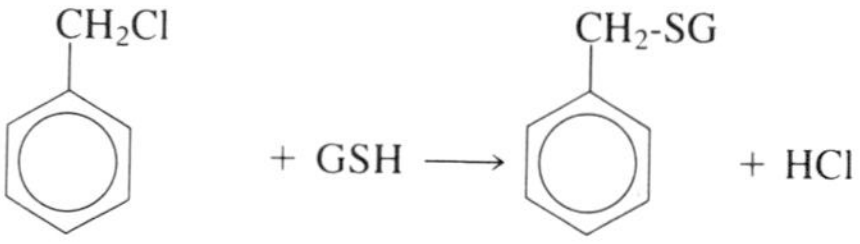 Benzyl chloride
Addition Reaction	
Glutathione *S*-alkenetransferase:	$CHCOOC_2H_5$ ‖ $CHCOOC_2H_5$ + GSH ⟶ $CH_2COOC_2H_5$ | GS-$CHCOOC_2H_5$ Diethyl maleate
Glutathione *S*-epoxidetransferase:	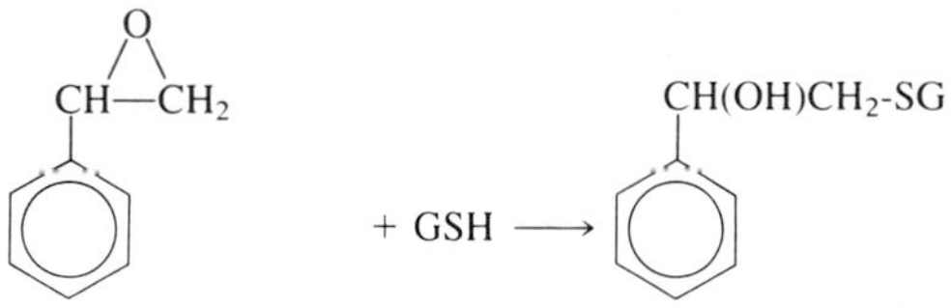 1,2-Epoxyethylbenzene
Glutathione *S*-aryl epoxidetransferase:	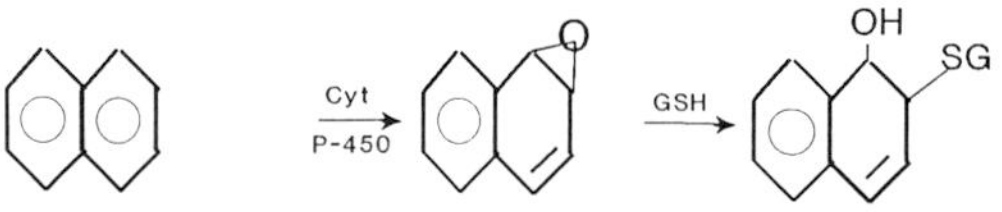 Naphthalene Naphthalene Oxide

al forms. A minimum of four gene families make up the glutathione *S*-transferase multi-gene family. As with most biotransformation enzymes, the various glutathione *S*-transferases demonstrate different but overlapping substrate selectivity. Examples of some reactions catalyzed by these enzymes are in Table 4–13.

The cofactor for reactions catalyzed by these enzymes is the tripeptide glutathione (GSH), which is composed of glycine, glutamic acid, and cysteine (Figure 4–11). The glutathione *S*-transferases catalyze the reaction of the nucleophilic sulfhydryl of glutathione with compounds containing electrophilic carbon atoms. The reaction of the glutathione thiolate anion (GS^-) results in formation of a thioether bond

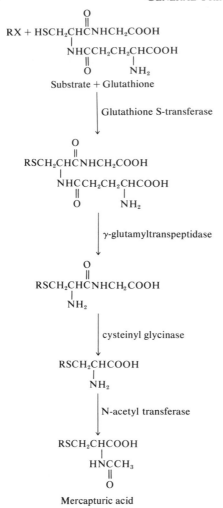

Figure 4–11. Glutathione conjugation and mercapturic acid biosynthesis.

between the carbon atom and the sulfhydryl group of glutathione (Figure 4–11).

Compounds that are substrates for the glutathione S-transferases share three common features: They must be hydrophobic to some degree, they must contain an electrophilic carbon atom, and they must react nonenzymatically with glutathione at some measurable rate. It is important to note that these transferases also serve as ligands for a number of compounds that are not substrates for the enzymic reactions. Lipophilic domains of the transferases serve as binding sites for a number of endogenous and exogenous chemicals. Thus, the glutathione S-transferases may serve as storage of transport proteins as well as enzymes.

The glutathione (GSH) conjugates are subsequently cleaved to cysteine derivatives, primarily by enzymes located in the kidney. These

derivatives are then acetylated to give the *N*-acetylcysteine (mercapturic acid) conjugates (Figure 4–11). Mercapturic conjugates are readily excreted into urine. The loss of glutamic acid from the glutathione conjugate is catalyzed by the enzyme γ-glutamyltranspeptidase, a membrane-associated enzyme found in high concentrations in cells that exhibit absorptive or excretory functions. Cysteinyl glycinase catalyzes the loss of glycine from the conjugate to yield the cysteine conjugate. Finally, *N*-acetyl transferase enzymes acetylate the amino group of cysteine to form the mercapturic acid derivative. The cofactor for the acetylation reaction is acetyl-CoA. In the rat, a microsomal acetyl transferase present in the kidney exhibited the highest activity toward *S*-substituted cysteines.

The importance of the nucleophilic reactions catalyzed by glutathione S-transferases has become increasingly apparent over the last few years. The glutathione S-transferase enzymes provide a means of reacting the diverse array of electrophilic xenobiotics with the endogenous nucleophile glutathione, thus preventing, to a degree, the reaction of these compounds with essential constituents of the cell. Considerable evidence indicates that glutathione S-transferases act to detoxify reactive intermediates produced by the cytochrome P-450 system. For example, bromobenzene, chloroform, and acetaminophen are biotransformed by the cytochrome P-450–containing monooxygenase enzyme system of the liver to highly reactive intermediates. These reactive intermediates may bind covalently to various macromolecule constituents in hepatocytes or react with GSH. The latter reaction prevents covalent binding of reactive intermediates to vital cellular constituents.

There is a delicate balance within cells between the rate of formation of the reactive metabolites and their inactivation by GSH. Thus, factors that affect this balance can dramatically alter the toxic potential of chemicals that produce toxicity via reactive intermediates. Reactive intermediates may also deplete cellular stores of GSH. Since GSH is a cofactor for glutathione peroxidase, its depletion can promote lipid peroxidation, a process that leads to deleterious results.

Rhodanese

An important reaction in the detoxication of cyanide is catalyzed primarily in the liver by the mitochondrial enzyme rhodanese (Figure 4–12). Thiosulfate can act as the donor of sulfur; however, it is unclear at this time which of the components of the sulfite pool is the true cofactor. Since the product of the reaction, thiocya-

$$CN^- + S_2O_3^{2-} \longrightarrow SCN^- + SO_3^{2-}$$

Cyanide Thiosulfate Thiocyanate Sulfite

Figure 4–12. Detoxication reaction of cyanide catalyzed by rhodanese.

nate, is far less toxic than cyanide, rhodanese catalyzes an unmistakable detoxication reaction.

EXTRAHEPATIC BIOTRANSFORMATION

Other Organs

Although biotransformation of xenobiotics occurs predominantly in the liver, biotransformation in extrahepatic tissues is important in regulating the fate of foreign compounds such as environmental pollutants in air and water, food additives and contaminants, industrial chemicals, or cigarette smoke. The major tissues of extrahepatic biotransformation are those involved in absorption or excretion of chemicals, such as lung, kidney, skin, and gastrointestinal mucosa. The rate of extrahepatic biotransformation may not be as high as in liver, and the total capacity is usually lower. However, humans are primarily exposed to low levels of environmental and occupational chemicals over long periods of time. Thus, biotransformation by these tissues may have a marked effect on the ultimate disposition of selected chemicals. Clearly, extrahepatic biotransformation has been implicated as a factor in toxicant-induced tissue injury.

Compared with extrahepatic tissues, the liver is a relatively homogenous mixture of cells, with all parenchymal cells having some biotransformation capacity. In most extrahepatic tissues, the biotransformation enzymes are usually concentrated within one or two cell types that comprise only a small percentage of the total cell population in an organ (Table 4–14). For example, the Clara and type II cells of the lung, the lining cells of the nasal turbinates and the S_3 segment of the renal proximal tubules are richest in cytochrome P-450 content in these tissues.

Table 4–14. MAJOR BIOTRANSFORMATION ENZYME-CONTAINING CELLS IN VARIOUS ORGANS

ORGAN	CELL(S)
Liver	Parenchymal cells (hepatocytes)
Kidney	Proximal tubular cells (S₃ segment)
Lung	Clara cells, type II cells, nasal cells
Intestine	Mucosa lining cells
Skin	Epithelial cells
Testes	Seminiferous tubules, Sertoli's cells

Phase II conjugation enzymes are more widely distributed among the tissues than is cytochrome P-450. In fact, certain phase II reactions are equivalent to or higher than cytochrome P-450 reactions in extrahepatic tissues.

Intestinal Microbial Biotransformation

An aspect of *in vivo* extrahepatic biotransformation of xenobiotics frequently overlooked is modification by intestinal microbes. It has been estimated that the gut microbes have the potential for biotransformation of xenobiotics equivalent to or greater than the liver. With over 400 bacterial species known to exist in the intestinal tract, differences in gut flora content as a result of species variation, age, diet, and disease states would be expected to influence xenobiotic modification.

Intestinal microbial biotransformation is of interest because bacterial reactions often produce less water-soluble metabolites and because the anaerobic state of the intestinal tract promotes reductive reactions. In addition, the presence of deconjugating enzymes (i.e., β-glucuronidases and arylsulfatases) leads to major modifications of metabolites produced in the liver and excreted in the bile. Such deconjugation usually promotes enterohepatic recycling.

FACTORS AFFECTING RATES OF BIOTRANSFORMATION OF FOREIGN COMPOUNDS

Intrinsic Factors Related to the Chemical

One of the important factors controlling the rate and/or route of enzymatic modification of foreign compounds is the concentration of the compound at the active center of enzymes involved in its biotransformation. The concentration at the active centers of these enzymes depends on the physicochemical properties of the compound as well as dose (Table 4–15).

Lipophilicity is an important property since it can govern the rate of absorption of a xenobiotic from its portal of entry (skin, intestine, lung). Lipophilic chemicals are more readily absorbed into the blood, whereas water-soluble substances are less rapidly absorbed. Similarly, the ease with which a compound crosses the cell membrane to reach the active sites of intracellular

Table 4–15. FACTORS AFFECTING INTRACELLULAR CONCENTRATION OF XENOBIOTICS

Lipophilicity
Protein binding
Dose
Route of administration

enzymes is governed by its lipid solubility. An important factor controlling the water solubility of foreign compounds is whether they contain ionizable groups in the molecule. Thus, compounds containing amine, carboxyl, phosphate, sulfate, phenolic hydroxyl, and other groups that are ionized at physiologic pH values are generally more water soluble and are less readily transferred across cell membranes than compounds not containing these groups.

Another factor controlling the absorption and penetration of xenobiotics to the intracellular biotransformation enzymes is protein binding. Intra- and extracellular proteins have the capacity to bind foreign compounds and to reduce the concentrations of these compounds at the active sites of enzymes involved in their biotransformation. This capacity to bind foreign compounds results from the presence in proteins of hydrophobic regions that will bind lipid-soluble compounds and hydrophilic regions that contain polar side chains of amino acids capable of forming hydrogen and electrostatic bonds with polar groups in water-soluble foreign compounds. Thus, proteins and particularly serum proteins (albumin) have a capacity for nonspecific binding of foreign compounds. This binding reduces the availability of these compounds for biotransformation and has a definite effect on the intrinsic clearance of a xenobiotic by the biotransformation enzymes.

Another important factor is the dose or exposure concentration. Dose often has an effect on the pathway of biotransformation. Certain enzymes have a high affinity but low capacity for xenobiotic biotransformation. These pathways will quickly become saturated as the does increases. Thus, the percentage of dose undergoing biotransformation by this pathway will decrease. However, low-affinity, high-capacity enzymatic pathways will now biotransform a larger percentage of the administered dose. Acetaminophen is an excellent example. At low doses (15 mg/kg in rats) over 90 percent of the dose is excreted as the sulfate conjugate. At high doses (300 mg/kg) only 43 percent is excreted as the sulfate, but larger amounts of parent compound, glucuronide, and mercapturic acids are now excreted in the urine.

Host Variables That Affect Xenobiotic Biotransformation

A number of physiologic, pharmacologic, and environmental factors affect rates of xenobiotic biotransformation (Table 4–16). Some of these factors are unique to laboratory animals but for the most part can be considered as broad factors that affect biotransformation in all species. Key factors to be addressed are induction and inhibi-

Table 4–16. VARIABLES AFFECTING XENOBIOTIC METABOLISM

Species	Enzyme induction
Strain	Enzyme inhibition
Age	Nutrition
Sex	Disease states
Time of day	

tion of the biotransformation enzymes, species-strain variations in xenobiotic metabolism, gender differences in biotransformation, alteration in metabolism with respect to age, role of genetics in biotransformation ability, nutritional status relative to biotransformation ability, and the effects of environment and disease states on xenobiotic disposition.

Induction of the Biotransformation Enzymes

A striking feature of the biotransformation enzymes is the fact that their activities can be enhanced following treatment of animals or humans with chemicals. These chemicals can be drugs, pesticides, industrial chemicals, natural products, and even ethanol. In general, this enhanced activity results from an increase in the rate of synthesis of the biotransformation enzymes. Therefore, this process has been termed *enzyme induction*, an event requiring *de novo* protein synthesis. Previously, induction was considered to be limited to cytochrome P-450-dependent monooxygenases, but certain conjugating enzymes can also be induced following exposure to selected chemicals. Literally hundreds of chemicals have been shown to induce monooxygenase activity and have been termed *microsomal-inducing agents*. Most of these chemicals have not been widely tested, and thus the extent of their inducing effects has not been well characterized.

The onset, magnitude, and duration of increases in monooxygenase activities are known to vary with the inducing agent and its dose, the substrates used to assay the activity of the enzymes, the species, strain, or sex of the animal, the duration of exposure, and the tissue in which enzyme activity is measured. When induction occurs in the liver, the net effect may be an increase in the rate of excretion of chemicals from the body. Although induction of monooxygenases can occur in extrahepatic tissues, the impact on the biologic half-lives of chemicals is generally much less pronounced.

Morphologic and Biochemical Results of Induction. The most widely studied inducing agents are phenobarbital and the polycyclic aromatic hydrocarbons (benzo[a]pyrene and 3-

**Table 4–17. CHARACTERISTICS OF THE HEPATIC EFFECTS
OF PHENOBARBITAL AND POLYCYCLIC AROMATIC
HYDROCARBONS**

CHARACTERISTICS	PHENOBARBITAL	POLYCYCLIC HYDROCARBONS
Onset of effects	8–12 hours	3–6 hours
Time of maximum effect	3–5 days	24–48 hours
Persistence of induction	5–7 days	5–12 days
Liver enlargement	Marked	Slight
Protein synthesis	Large increase	Small increase
Phospholipid synthesis	Marked increase	No effect
Liver blood flow	Increase	No effect
Biliary flow	Increase	No effect
Enzyme components		
Cytochrome P-450	Increase	No effect
Cytochrome P-448	No effect	Increase
NADPH-cytochrome c		
reductase	Increase	No effect
Substrate specificity		
N-Demethylation	Increase	No effect
Aliphatic hydroxylation	Increase	No effect
Polycyclic hydrocarbon		
hydroxylation	Small increase	Increase
Reductive dehalogena- tion	Increase	No effect
Glucuronidation	Increase	Small increase
Glutathione conjugation	Small increase	Small increase
Epoxide hydrolase	Increase	Small increase
Cytosolic receptor	None identified	Identified

methylcholanthrene). Although both classes of compounds induce certain monooxygenase activities, they produce different morphologic and biochemical effects in the liver. These are summarized in Table 4–17. Phenobarbital pretreatment results in marked hepatic hypertrophy, an increase in the concentration of microsomal protein (mg/g of liver), and a proliferation of the smooth endoplasmic reticulum. Accompanying these morphologic changes are increases in protein and phospholipid synthesis as well as induction of the synthesis of NADPH-cytochrome P-450 reductase (threefold) and selected cytochrome P-450 isozymes (up to 70-fold). The major cytochromal P-450 isozymes induced by phenobarbital are virtually absent from liver microsomes of untreated laboratory animals. Interestingly, these changes occur predominantly in hepatocytes located in the centrilobular region of the liver. The net effect of these morphologic and biochemical changes is enhanced biotransformation of a large number of chemicals. Those substrates with high affinity for the induced cytochrome P-450 isozymes show the greatest increase in rates of biotransformation. However, the increased liver size and proliferation of components of the smooth endoplasmic reticulum explain the smaller increases in the rates of

biotransformation of substrates with less affinity for the induced P-450 isozymes.

The pattern of induction in the liver following pretreatment with 3-methylcholanthrene or benzo[a]pyrene is dramatically different. The marked increase in liver weight, protein and phospholipid synthesis, and NADPH-cytochrome P-450 reductase does not occur (Table 4–17). Instead, there is a selective induction (up to 70-fold) of cytochrome P-450 isozymes with spectral and catalytic properties different than those from the phenobarbital-inducible cytochrome P-450 isozymes. As with phenobarbital, the 3-methylcholanthrene-inducible cytochrome P-450 isozymes are virtually absent from liver microsomes of untreated laboratory animals. One of the 3-methylcholanthrene-inducible forms of cytochrome P-450 has a high catalytic turnover for benzo[a]pyrene. This form of cytochrome P-450 has long been called cytochrome P-448, cytochrome P_1-450, or aryl hydrocarbon hydroxylase (AHH). Unlike phenobarbital, specificity of induction to a particular region of the liver lobule is not observed following administration of 3-methylcholanthrene or similar types of inducing agents.

Other major classes of inducing agents include halogenated pesticides (DDT, aldrin, hexachlorobenzene, lindane, chlordane); polychlorinated and polybrominated biphenyls; steroids and related compounds (testosterone, spironolactone, pregenolone-16α-carbonitrile); and chlorinated dioxins (2,3,7,8-tetrachlorodibenzo-p-dioxin, or TCDD). Certain of these produce a spectrum of induction similar to phenobarbital or the polycyclic aromatic hydrocarbons, whereas some induce the synthesis of other forms of cytochrome P-450. Selective induction of cytochrome P-450 may occur at low doses, whereas high doses may also result in liver hypertrophy.

Mechanism of Induction. In recent years, the actual mechanism of microsomal enzyme induction by the polycyclic aromatic hydrocarbons has become much clearer. Using TCDD, an extremely potent 3-methylcholanthrene-type inducer of AHH activity, Poland and his colleagues (1976) identified a high-affinity binding site for TCDD in the cytosol of liver and other tissues. This binding protein has the properties of a receptor in that it provides stereospecific recognition of the inducing compound. When the inducing agent (*i.e.*, TCDD) interacts with this receptor, the resulting receptor-ligand complex translocates to the nucleus. Following interaction of this complex with specific genomic recognition sites, transcription and translation of the specific genes that code for cytochrome P-448 activity are initiated. Benzo[a]pyrene, 3-methylcholanthrene, other polycyclic aromatic hydrocarbons, and 3,3',4,4'-tetrachlorobiphenyl were found to displace TCDD from this receptor. Therefore, these agents appear to interact with this common receptor and induce the synthesis of cytochrome P-448 by an identical mechanism. Critical requirements for interaction with the receptor include lipophilicity and a planar configuration. Other classes of inducers including phenobarbital and 2,2',4,4',5,5'-hexachlorobiphenyl will not displace TCDD from this receptor. To date, no analogous receptor for phenobarbital-type inducers has been identified, although the induction of specific cytochrome P-450 isozymes by phenobarbital is regulated at the transcriptional level and involves a dramatic increase in the mRNAs encoding these enzymes.

A number of small molecular weight compounds increase the hepatic concentration of cytochrome P-450IIE1 (P-450j). These include ethanol, acetone, and pyrazole. The mechanism of this increase may be a combination of induction as well as stabilization of the protein against degradation. Increased concentrations of this P-450 isoform have important toxicological implications, since it activates a number of environmental compounds (CCl_4; dimethylnitrosoamine) to toxic/carcinogenic metabolites. This isoform appears to be most active at low concentrations of substrate.

Time Course for Induction. Maximal induction following parenteral administration of hypnotic doses of phenobarbital occurs within three to five days. Induction following administration of 3-methylcholanthrene is more rapid, with maximal induction being achieved by 48 hours (Table 4–17). Induction is a reversible event. Withdrawal of the inducing agent results in a return to basal enzymic activity. Again, the duration of the induced state is a function of the dose and the inducing agent. Following withdrawal of phenobarbital, these induced activities return to basal level by seven to ten days. However, inducing agents that are highly lipophilic and poorly biotransformed (highly chlorinated biphenyls) will be retained by the body and lead to prolonged induction because of their continued presence.

Induction of Other Microsomal Biotransformation Enzymes. Microsomal UDP-glucuronosyltransferases and epoxide hydrolase are induced by phenobarbital, 3-methylcholanthrene, and related compounds. *Trans*-stilbene oxide, acetylaminofluorene, and certain polychlorinated biphenyls are good inducers of epoxide hydrolase. Antioxidants, such as butylated hydroxyanisole (BHA) and butylated hydroxytoluene (BHT), are potent inducers of epoxide hydrolase in mice but not in rats. Glucuronosyltransferase activities toward naphthol and p-nitrophenol are induced preferentially by 3-methylcholanthrene, whereas activities toward morphine and chloramphenicol are preferentially induced by phenobarbital. The major form(s) of cytochrome P-450 and UDP-glucuronosyltransferase inducible by pregnenolone-16α-carbonitrile are distinct from those induced by phenobarbital and 3-methylcholanthrene.

Induction of Extrahepatic Biotransformation Enzymes. Cytochrome P-450 enzymes in extrahepatic tissues are not readily induced by phenobarbital and compounds that produce a similar pattern of induction. However, the polycyclic aromatic hydrocarbons are known to be effective in such extrahepatic tissues as lung, kidney, intestinal tract, and skin. The cytosolic binding protein that complexes with polycyclic aromatic compounds is present in these tissues. It has been postulated that this rapidly inducible enzyme system at these portals of entry serves as a defense against noxious chemicals. In fact, this enzyme system, as measured by benzo[a]pyrene hydroxylation, can be decreased to undetectable levels in extrahepatic tissues if rats are maintained on highly purified diets and kept in isolated rooms that receive highly filtered air.

Induction of Cytosolic Enzymes. Except for the GSH-*S*-transferases, the major cytosolic conjugating enzymes are not readily induced. Specific inducers of the sulfotransferases, *N*-acetyltransferases, or amino acid conjugating enzymes are not known. In addition, these enzymes do not respond to the previously described inducers of the microsomal phase I and phase II enzymes. In rats, cytosolic glutathione-*S*-transferases are induced by 3-methylcholanthrene, phenobarbital, and *trans*-stilbene oxide. Depending on the isozyme, GSH-*S*-transferase induction may be as high as two- or threefold. Butylated hydroxyanisole (BHA) is the most effective inducer of cytosolic transferase activity in the mouse but is less effective in the rat.

Inhibition of the Biotransformation Enzymes

According to Testa and Jenner (1981), "inhibition of xenobiotic metabolism is said to occur when under *in vivo, ex vivo* or in *in vitro* conditions, a given factor (endogenous or exogenous) decreases the ability of an enzyme or enzyme system to metabolize an exogenous substrate relative to control activity. Such a broad and operational definition has the advantage of including all possible inhibitory mechanisms, such as competition for active sites or cofactors of the enzymes, inhibition of transport components in multienzymic systems, decreased biosynthesis or increased breakdown of enzymes or their cofactors" as well as allosteric changes in enzyme conformation and even loss of functional tissue (i.e., hepatic necrosis). Some of these mechanisms of inhibition are briefly discussed in order to familiarize the reader with the chemicals used to inhibit various biotransformation reactions.

Obviously, agents that affect *protein synthesis* will ultimately inhibit biotransformation reactions. This occurs because of reduced synthesis of the actual biotransformation enzymes as well as the enzymes necessary for the production of cofactors. However, certain chemicals are more specific in that they are not general inhibitors of protein synthesis. For example, 3-amino-1,2,3-triazole decreases cytochrome P-450 synthesis, probably via its inhibitory affect on porphyrin synthesis. Acute administration of cobalt chloride also decreases the hepatic concentration of cytochrome P-450 by its inhibitory effect on heme synthesis as well as its inductive effect on heme oxygenase, the enzyme that converts hemoproteins to biliverdin. Both chemicals have been shown to inhibit cytochrome P-450–catalyzed reactions.

Chemicals may also affect the tissue levels of necessary cofactors or conjugating species. For example, L-methionine-*S*-sulfoximine and buthionine sulfoximine inhibit the synthesis of glutathione, whereas diethylmaleate, glycidol, and selected other chemicals conjugate with and rapidly reduce tissue stores of glutathione. Similarly, galactosamine inhibits the synthesis of UDP-glucuronic acid by depleting hepatic stores of uridine, whereas borneol and salicylamide conjugate with and deplete UDP-glucuronic acid. The ultimate effect of treatment with these chemicals would be a reduction in the capacity to form glutathione or glucuronide conjugates of subsequently administered xenobiotics or their metabolites.

A number of chemicals have been shown to have inhibitory effects in the cytochrome P-450 system. These are illustrated in Figure 4–13. Carbon monoxide (CO) and ethylisocyanide act as ligands for the reduced heme moiety and thus compete with the endogenous ligand, molecular oxygen. These are potent inhibitors of oxidative reactions. CO also inhibits P-450–mediated reductive reactions. By far the most common type of inhibition is competition of two different substrates (xenobiotics) for the substrate binding site of cytochrome P-450. This competition will result in mutual metabolic inhibition. The degree of inhibition will depend on the relative affinities of the xenobiotics for the binding site. Individual forms of cytochrome P-450 show different sensitivities to the inhibitory action of selected chemicals. For example, 7,8-benzoflavone is a direct-acting, competitive inhibitor that is highly specific for cytochrome P-448, whereas SKF 525-A and metyrapone are more specific for the phenobarbital-inducible form of cytochrome P-450. SKF 525-A, piperonyl butoxide, and many other inhibitors produce a mixed type of inhibition. The parent molecule produces a competitive inhibition, while a metabolite forms a stable complex with cytochrome P-450 and results in noncompetitive inhibition.

Recently, several chemicals have been identified that act as suicide inhibitors of cytochrome P-450. Following activation of the chemical by the cytochrome P-450 system, reactive metabolites bind covalently to the pyrrole nitrogens present in the heme moiety. This interaction results in the destruction of heme and a loss of cytochrome P-450 activity. Various halogenated alkanes (CCl_4), alkenes (vinyl chloride, trichloroethylene), and compounds containing allylic (allylisopropylacetamide, secobarbital) and acetylenic (norethindrone acetate, acetylene) derivatives inhibit P-450–catalyzed reactions by suicide inactivation.

Inhibition of xenobiotic biotransformation *in vivo* is a complex situation. Many chemicals produce multiple effects, such as inhibition of

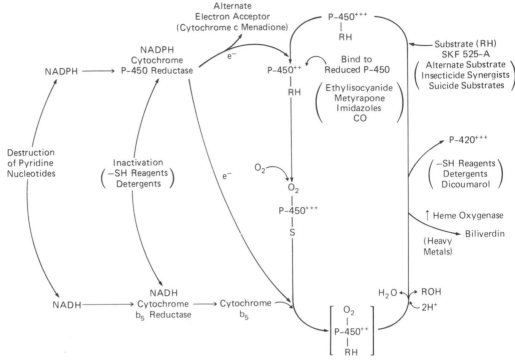

Figure 4–13. Inhibitors of the microsomal cytochrome P-450 system. (Modified and reprinted by permission of the publisher from Figure 8, page 117, Chapter 1 in *Extrahepatic Metabolism of Drugs and Other Foreign Compounds* by Theodore E. Gram (ed.). Copyright 1980, Spectrum Publications Inc., Jamaica, N.Y.)

both phase I and phase II reactions. Inhibitors may show pronounced effects on only certain cytochrome P-450 isozymes, and therefore, the degree of inhibition will vary in untreated animals versus those treated with inducing agents. The degree of inhibition is also time dependent. For example, many agents that initially inhibit cytochrome P-450 also result in its induction at later time points (e.g., SKF 525-A, piperonyl butoxide). Chronic treatment with metal ions may result in adaptive biochemical responses in heme synthesis and metal-binding proteins, such as metallothionein. Clearly, these factors must be considered when evaluating the effect of inhibitors on xenobiotic biotransformation.

Species, Strain, Genetic Variations

Variations in biotransformation between species may be readily divided into qualitative and quantitative differences. *Qualitative* differences involve metabolic routes and are due either to a species defect or to a reaction peculiar to a species. *Quantitative* variations may result from differences in enzymic levels or natural inhibitors, in the balance of reverse enzyme reactions, or in the extent of competing reactions (Table 4–18).

Species differences in phase I reactions are most readily explained by differences in the profile of cytochrome P-450 isozymes. Although these isozymes may have overlapping substrate specificity, they usually have a marked

Table 4–18. CHARACTERIZATION OF QUANTITATIVE AND QUALITATIVE DIFFERENCES OBSERVED IN BIOTRANSFORMATION AMONG SPECIES AND STRAINS

QUALITATIVE
Defective enzymes in certain species
Unique species reactions
Evolutionary
Some genetic aspects

QUANTITATIVE
Differences in enzyme concentration
Different cytochrome P-450 isozymes
Differences in regiospecific reactions
Genetic

regiospecificity. An excellent example of this is the observed species variation in the biotransformation of *N*-acetylaminofluorene. This carcinogenic amine undergoes several biotransformations. Two routes are *N*-hydroxylation and aromatic hydroxylation, which lead, respectively, to the hepatocarcinogenic *N*-hydroxy derivative and to the noncarcinogenic 7-hydroxy derivative. Marked species variations exist in the extent of these pathways. The guinea pig does not produce the *N*-hydroxy derivative *in vivo* or *in vitro,* and in this species the compound is not carcinogenic. On the other hand, the carcinogenic activity of 2-acetylaminofluorene is apparent in such species as mouse, rabbit, and dog, which generate the *N*-hydroxy metabolite. Since these two reactions are catalyzed by two different forms of cytochrome P-450 isozymes, the species differences can be explained by differences in the activity or amount of the particular enzyme.

Species variation in phase I biotransformation is also apparent with amphetamine and 2,2',4,4',5,5'-hexachlorobiphenyl. In rats, amphetamine is primarily biotransformed by aromatic hydroxylation, while in rabbits it is primarily deaminated. Of all species studied to date, only the dog can readily hydroxylate 2,2',4,4',5,5'-hexachlorobiphenyl, which explains why dogs can reduce their body burden of what in most species is an extremely persistent xenobiotic. This ability to biotransform 2,2',4,4',5,5'-hexachlorobiphenyl by dogs is the result of a unique isoform of cytochrome P-450 present in their livers.

Species variation in phase II reactions are more apparent and appear to be associated with evolutionary development. These variations can result from differences in the ability of an animal to synthesize and/or activate the necessary cofactor, the nature and amount of the transferase, the occurrence of the conjugating agent, and the nature of the xenobiotic involved. Certain species lack a widespread conjugative process or perform a peculiar reaction (Table 4–19). For example, conjugation with glucuronic acid is one of the most important conjugation reactions in mammals. However, the cat and a few closely related species have a defective glucuronide-forming system. Although they can conjugate bilirubin with glucuronic acid, they cannot form glucuronides of phenol, naphthol, and other phenolic derivatives.

The dog cannot acetylate aromatic amino compounds because it lacks the appropriate isozyme of *N*-acetyl transferase. Similarly, the pig is deficient in sulfate conjugation. Finally, conjugation with amino acids is phylogenetically determined. Primates utilize glycine and glutamine, whereas some birds utilize ornithine.

Strain differences in biotransformation are also under genetic control. These differences often account for variations in the observed biologic responses to xenobiotics. Unusual pharmacologic responses can result from genetic defects and may be associated with altered enzyme activity. These hereditary variations in biotransformation are apparent in humans as well as in animals and are referred to as *pharmacogenetics*.

Homozygous strains are routinely used in toxicological studies to avoid the added complications involved in the use of heterozygous animal groups. To ensure that an observed difference results from a genetic variation, care must be taken to eliminate environmental influences, which may produce greater or lesser degrees of enzyme induction or inhibition in one strain versus another.

Examples of strain variation in phase I biotransformation include the differences in the rates of oxidation of hexobarbital among Holtzman, Sprague-Dawley, and Wistar rats. The duration of sleep after hexobarbital is inversely related to these rates of biotransformation. Each

Table 4–19. SPECIES DEFECTS IN FOREIGN COMPOUND METABOLISM*

REACTION	DEFECTIVE SPECIES
Aliphatic amine *N*-hydroxylation	Rat, marmoset
Arylacetamide *N*-hydroxylation	Guinea pig
Arylamine *N*-acetylation	Dog
Glucuronidation	Cat, lion, lynx, Gunn rat
Sulfation	Pig, opossum, brachymorphic mice
Hippuric acid formation	African fruit bat
Mercapturic acid formation	Guinea pig

* Modified from Jakoby, W. E. (ed.): *Enzymatic Basis of Detoxication,* Vol. 1. Academic Press, Inc., New York, 1980.

strain can be further divided into short and long sleepers, and the activity of cytochrome P-450–mediated enzyme activities correlates with sleep time. Similar differences were found among inbred strains of mice. Marked strain differences in hepatic cytochrome P-450–related enzyme activities have been noted among various strains of rabbits. Genetically controlled polymorphism in the regiospecific hydroxylation of drugs is well established in humans. For example, 7 to 9 percent of British subjects are deficient in the 4-hydroxylation of debrisoquine. This same genetic polymorphism is apparently responsible for the interindividual variability observed in the biotransformation of propranolol, phenytoin, phenacetin, and other drugs. Studies that compared the plasma half-lives of drugs in identical versus fraternal twins found little or no differences between identical twins but large differences (two- to threefold) between fraternal twins. Even larger variations are observed among unrelated individuals. Much of these variations can be attributed to genetic differences.

Genetic differences in the ability of animals to respond to enzyme-inducing agents are well known. The most notable example is the difference in response to 3-methylcholanthrene between C57BL6J and DBA2 mice. The C57 mice respond with a marked induction of hepatic microsomal benzo[a]pyrene hydroxylase activity and are termed "responsive." The DBA2 mice are classified as "nonresponsive," since the induction in this species is minimal. The difference between the two strains is linked to the *Ah* locus, which codes for the cytosolic receptor that regulates certain cytochrome P-450 isozymes. This binding protein is defective in the nonresponsive DBA2 mice. These strain differences in enzyme induction can lead to strain differences in rates and routes of biotransformation following exposure to the inducing agent.

Individual or strain variations in phase II reactions are also known. The defect in glucuronide formation observed in the Gunn rat is similar to the inherited human metabolic disorder congenital familial nonhemolytic jaundice. This disorder is associated with reduced glucuronosyltransferase activity. Differences in glucuronide formation are considered to originate mainly from genetic deficiencies and affect only a few strains. On the other hand, differences in acetylation ability show a much wider distribution and are not associated with the concept of genetic deficiency or disorder but rather with genetic heterogeneity. In humans, large individual variations exist in the acetylation of the antituberculosis drug isoniazid. The population is generally considered to be bimodally distributed into rapid and slow acetylators. The inheritance of the rapid inactivator phenotype has been shown to be autosomal dominant. The incidence of slow and rapid activators is not the same in all racial groups. Among Caucasians, a slightly higher percentage of slow acetylators predominate (50 to 60 percent). In contrast, in Orientals rapid acetylators predominate.

Sex Differences in Biotransformation

A marked difference between male and female rats in the pharmacologic and toxicologic response to a number of xenobiotics has been noted. For example, female rats sleep considerably longer than male rats when treated with equivalent doses of hexobarbital. Similarly, the widely used organophosphate insecticide parathion is approximately twice as toxic to female rats as to males. These potentiated responses in female rats result from a reduced capacity of their livers to biotransform these as well as other chemicals. In these cases, the parent compound has a prolonged biologic half-life in females that leads to a prolonged response. If a metabolite or reactive intermediate produces the biologic response, then male rats will usually show the greater response. This is the reason male rats are more susceptible to hepatic injury produced by carbon tetrachloride and halothane. Male rats convert these chemicals to reactive intermediates at faster rates than female rats.

Sex differences in biotransformation also occur in extrahepatic tissues. Chloroform is converted to a reactive intermediate (phosgene) ten times faster by microsomes obtained from the kidneys of male mice than those from female mice. Male mice are susceptible to chloroform-induced nephrotoxicity, whereas female mice are resistant.

The balance between male and female sex hormones is important in determining the activity of cytochrome P-450 enzymes. Administration of testosterone to female rats increases their ability to biotransform a number of drugs and other xenobiotics. Following treatment, rates of biotransformation in female rats approach the activity observed in their male counterparts. Similarly, castration of male rats reduces their capacity to biotransform xenobiotics.

Measurements of cytochrome P-450 concentration and NADPH-cytochrome P-450 reductase activity in hepatic microsomes have shown preparations from male rats to contain 20 to 30 percent more of these components (Table 4–20). It is now established that the differences between the sexes reflect differences in the profile of cytochrome P-450 isozymes in liver microsomes from male and female rats. Both male-specific and female-specific forms of cytochrome P-450

Table 4–20. EFFECT OF SEX ON BIOTRANSFORMATION IN THE RAT

ANALYSIS	RATIO OF MALE/FEMALE
Cytochrome P-450	1.4
NADPH-cytochrome P-450 reductase	1.3
Benzphetamine N-demethylation	5.6
Aniline hydroxylation	5.5

have been identified. These forms may respond differently to chemical exposure, as in enzyme induction/inhibition. In rats, the expression of some forms changes during their lifetime, reflecting their regulation by growth and/or sex hormones.

Despite the large sex variations observed in the biotransformation of xenobiotics by rats and certain strains of mice, such variations are not so dramatic in humans. Differences in pharmacokinetic parameters for a variety of drugs have been reported between men and women. Although differences in bioavailability, protein binding, and volume of distribution can account, in part, for differences in pharmacokinetics, biotransformation capacity may play a role. The biotransformation ability of women can vary during menstrual cycle and by use of oral contraceptives. Further evaluations of differences in biotransformation between men and women and its implications are underway. If sex differences in a biologic response to a xenobiotic are observed, differences in rates of biotransformation should always be considered as a possible cause.

Effect of Age on Biotransformation

Fetal and newborn animals have been shown to be severely limited in their ability to biotransform xenobiotics, which provides a basis for the increased toxicity of xenobiotics in young animals. However, not all pathways of biotransformation are absent or limited in newborn animals.

In rats the low or negligible activity of cytochrome P-450–catalyzed reactions observed at birth develops rapidly and reaches maximal activity by 30 days of age. Enzyme activities then begin to decrease gradually with age. By 600 days of age, these activities are only 50 to 60 percent of maximum. In humans, cytochrome P-450 activities are 20 to 50 percent of adult activities by the second trimester of gestation. However, the isozyme pattern is qualitatively different from that observed in adults. This pattern of ontogenetic development appears to be

common to diverse species and has been characterized with several substrates.

The age-related changes observed in the activity of the biotransformation enzymes is correlated with biochemical differentiation of hepatocytes. Comparison of rat hepatic microsomal preparations from one- and three-day-old animals shows a marked increase in the quantity of both rough and smooth endoplasmic reticulum. The increase in smooth elements is far more pronounced and appears to arise from transformation of rough endoplasmic reticulum by loss of ribosomes. It is only at birth, however, that many of the constitutive membrane-bound enzymes appear, and it is unknown whether these enzymes are integrated into existing membranes or whether *de novo* synthesis occurs. The smooth endoplasmic reticulum appears in human hepatocytes around the third month of gestation, the time at which cytochrome P-450 activities appear.

Since a low level of biotransformation activity in neonates is due to an actual enzyme deficiency, activity can be increased by inducing agents. Polycyclic aromatic hydrocarbons and certain polychlorinated biphenyls are effective transplacental inducing agents. In humans, prolonged administration of phenytoin, phenobarbital, and perhaps alcohol leads to pharmacokinetic alterations in the newborn. These alterations have been related to the enzyme-inducing effects of these agents. Newborn animals also respond to enzyme inducers. Indeed, the increase in activity produced by inducing agents administered to immature animals is greater than that seen in adults.

A similar pattern of development in rats exists for some of the phase II conjugation enzymes. Both glutathione and glycine conjugation develop slowly after birth to adult levels by 30 days, while sulfation is almost at adult levels at birth. In the case of UDP-glucuronosyltransferase, activity toward bilirubin reaches adult levels by five to seven days, whereas 30 days are required for activity toward *ortho*-aminophenol to reach adult values.

Increased toxicity of xenobiotics often occurs in older animals and is often explained in terms of increased tissue sensitivity to the toxicant. Serum levels of some toxicants are known to reach higher values and to persist for longer periods in older rats (27 months) than in younger ones (six months). In addition, hepatic microsomes from older rats show decreased biotransformation capacity. Increased toxicologic activity of these xenobiotics with age parallels a decrease in *in vitro* biotransformation. Thus, compounds generating toxic metabolites will be associated with decreased toxicity in both the young and old. For example, inhibitors of cholinesterase are less effective in the elderly, whereas carbon tetrachloride is not hepatotoxic in newborn rats. Both these agents require biotransformation to exert these toxic effects.

Decreased capacity for biotransformation correlates with a reduction in the concentration of cytochrome P-450 and the activity of its associated reductase. It should be emphasized that in the elderly the observed increases in the biological half-lives of drugs may be related not only to decreased enzyme activities but also to decreased renal and hepatic blood flows, decreased liver size, decreased efficiency of urinary/biliary excretory systems, increased mass of adipose tissue, etc. Clearly, many biochemical and physiologic functions decrease in the elderly, and these changes can affect their response to xenobiotics.

Effect of Diet on Biotransformation

The nutritional status of experimental animals is an important factor influencing biotransformation. A number of examples are outlined in Table 4–21. Mineral deficiencies (calcium, copper, iron, magnesium, and zinc) decrease both cytochrome P-450–catalyzed oxidation and reduction reactions. Decreases in basal cytochrome P-450 concentrations can partly account for the lower biotransformation activity. A return to normal dietary mineral intake returns the enzyme activities to normal levels.

Vitamin deficiencies (C, E, and B complex) reduce the rates of xenobiotic biotransformation. These vitamins are directly or indirectly involved in the regulation of the cytochrome P-450 system. In addition, their deficiencies can alter the energy and redox state of the cells, thus

Table 4–21. DIETARY CONDITIONS AFFECTING BIOTRANSFORMATION

DIETARY ALTERATION	USUAL EFFECT
Mineral deficiencies	
Calcium	↓
Copper	↓
Iron	↓
Magnesium	↓
Zinc	↓
Vitamin deficiencies	
Ascorbic acid	↓
Tocopherol	↓
B complex	↓
Protein deficiencies	↓
Lipid composition	↑↓
Fasting (12 hours)	↑↓ *
Starvation (>48 hours)	↓
Natural substances	↑↓

* Certain phase II reactions.

hindering the production of the high-energy cofactors required for phase II biotransformation. Reintroduction of the vitamins to the diet will result in a return to basal enzyme activities.

Low-protein diets have been found to increase markedly the toxicity of a number of xenobiotics that are active as the parent compound but to reduce the toxicity of those that require biotransformation to express their toxicities. For example, the lethality and severity of hepatotoxicity produced by dimethylnitrosamine are markedly reduced in rats maintained on a low-protein diet. Correlated with these decreases in toxicity is a reduction in the N-demethylation of dimethylnitrosamine, the initial step in its conversion to an alkylating agent. Dietary lipids are important in determining the activity of biotransformation enzymes, particularly those enzymes that are membrane bound. In rats, diets high in polyunsaturated fats decrease the concentration of hepatic cytochrome P-450. This reduction results from the increased susceptibility of unsaturated fatty acids to undergo peroxidation. Thus, the microsomal membranes degrade with a concomitant loss of cytochrome P-450. The nature of the fatty acids present in the membrane may also affect its fluidity.

Overnight food deprivation is a common technique used in toxicologic studies. It decreases the volume of material present in the gut and thus promotes the absorption of orally administered chemicals. Since rodents are nocturnal feeders, they will have been deprived of food longer than the anticipated 12 to 16 hours. This procedure stimulates a number of biotransformation enzymes and can have a marked effect on toxicity. Food deprivation has been shown to increase the dealkylation of dimethylnitrosamine and to potentiate the liver injury it produces. Food deprivation can also reduce the concentration of cofactors and conjugating agents. The concentration of hepatic glutathione is reduced by 50 percent during an overnight fast, an event known to potentiate the hepatotoxicity of acetaminophen, bromobenzene, and other compounds that are detoxified by glutathione. If the animals are starved (i.e., without food for 48 hours), xenobiotic biotransformation is suppressed in vivo. However, until the starvation is severe, the biotransformation enzymes are present but not functioning appropriately, owing to the reduced energy state of the animals.

Natural substances present in the diets can also affect biotransformation enzymes. For example, the indoles in certain vegetables enhance the phase I biotransformation activity in the intestinal lining cells and the liver. Charcoal-broiled meat, because of the presence of polycyclic aromatic hydrocarbons, also induces enzymic activities in these tissues. Dietary chemicals that inhibit certain biotransformation reactions are also known. We are just beginning to understand how diet can affect xenobiotic biotransformation. Clearly, this is an important area that may explain the pronounced interindividual variation observed in the biologic response to xenobiotics.

Effect of Hepatic Injury on Biotransformation

Since the liver is the principal site of xenobiotic biotransformation, any disease state that severely interferes with the normal function of this organ can influence the processes of biotransformation. Similarly, chemically induced hepatic injury will decrease biotransformation.

Schistosomiasis, viral infections, carcinomas, obstructive jaundice, hepatitis, and cirrhosis compromise the liver and reduce hepatic biotransformation (Figure 4–14). In toxicologic studies, a toxicant can injure the liver or irreversibly inhibit the biotransformation enzymes. The impairment observed is related to the degree of damage. After such injuries, there will be a rapid regeneration phase, which often results in enzyme activities that are temporarily higher than the preinjury activities.

Conditions that decrease hepatic blood flow (i.e., delivery of the xenobiotic to the liver) suppress the biotransformation and clearance of a xenobiotic. These include cardiac complications, shock, and hypotension. Renal injury also reduces the clearance of xenobiotics. Such injury often leads to a decrease in hepatic function and a reduced biotransformation capacity.

Circadian Rhythms

An influence of the time of day on the rate of biotransformation of foreign compounds is often seen within a given animal species. This variation in the rate of biotransformation is often correlated with variations in endocrine functions as influenced by the light-dark cycle to which the animal is exposed. Thus, the *in vitro* biotransformation of aminopyrine and hexobarbital by the hepatic cytochrome P-450 monooxygenase system of rats is variable, depending on when during the day the animals are terminated. This variation in enzyme activity is thought to be largely the result of a variation in the activities of the cytochrome P-450 isozymes.

Concentrations of hepatic glutathione also exhibit circadian rhythmicity, with concentrations being highest at the end of the dark cycle. Thus, during the feeding period glutathione accumulates, but during the light period it declines. This circadian rhythmicity in glutathione can affect

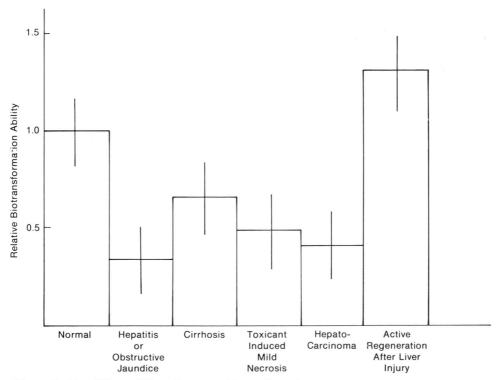

Figure 4–14.   Effects of liver disease on biotransformation.

the toxicity of xenobiotics that are detoxified by glutathione conjugation. The number of animals dying from acetaminophen and 1,1-dichloroethylene is greater when these toxicants are administered to animals at periods of low hepatic glutathione levels.

BIOACTIVATION

In the previous sections, it was emphasized that the biotransformation enzymes can produce reactive intermediates. These are defined as chemical species that are more reactive than the parent compound or its metabolites that are subsequently eliminated from the body. For convenience the enzymatic formation of reactive intermediates is termed bioactivation. It is important to emphasize that the nature of the reactive intermediate is dependent on the chemical and the biotransformation process. The insertion of an oxygen, addition of oxygen, acceptance of a reducing equivalent, or a conjugation process can produce a chemical structure that is a reactive intermediate or that rearranges to the unstable reactive intermediate. Thus, formation of reactive intermediates can be considered part of the overall biotransformation process. Reactive intermediates can interact with nucleophilic sites on tissue constituents, such as the sulfhydryl group of glutathione and cysteine, or the amino or hydroxyl groups present in DNA, RNA, or protein. This covalent interaction with tissue macromolecules is thought to be a key factor in the toxic effects produced by the xenobiotics. For many chemicals, these reactive intermediates can be detoxified. Provided there is a balance between rates of formation and rates of detoxication, the formation of reactive intermediates may not lead to adverse cellular events. When this balance is disturbed, either by enhanced production of reactive intermediates or diminished capacity for their detoxication, formation of reactive intermediates can be associated with cellular injury.

There are many conditions that can disturb balance between the rates of formation and detoxication of reactive intermediates. Enzyme induction can increase the overall rate of biotransformation of a chemical, which can in turn lead to an excess production of reactive intermediates. Large doses of a xenobiotic can rapidly deplete cellular defense mechanisms. Large doses can also lead to saturation of the major nontoxic biotransformation pathways. Minor pathways, which form reactive intermediates, may now become operative. Finally, conditions may exist in which detoxication pathways are compromised and nontoxic doses of a xenobiotic can now result in cellular injury.

The factors and variables that are known to affect normal biotransformation also affect the bioactivation of xenobiotics. These have been covered in detail earlier. It is important to emphasize that bioactivation is not limited to the liver. Extrahepatic bioactivation of xenobiotic explains why numerous toxic foreign compounds produce organ-specific toxicities.

Table 4–22 lists a few examples of chemicals that undergo bioactivation. Reactive intermediates have been implicated in the toxicities that they produce. From this table, it is apparent that epoxides, free radicals, acid chlorides, and N-hydroxy derivatives are often encountered as reactive intermediates. Certain of these examples will be discussed in greater detail to illustrate the nature of reactive intermediate formation and its role in xenobiotic-induced toxicities.

The cytochrome P-450 system produces reactive intermediates by either oxidative or reductive reactions. With polycyclic aromatic compounds, aromatic compounds, heterocyclic aromatic compounds, or olefinic compounds, the addition of an oxygen molecule to the carbon-carbon double bond can produce an epoxide. The epoxide may nonenzymatically react with macromolecular nucleophiles, resulting in an opening of the oxide and the formation of a covalent bond to the macromolecule. Numerous compounds with carbon-carbon double bonds proceed through arene oxide or epoxide intermediates during biotransformation. Not all, though, result in covalent binding. This, again, relates to the intrinsic reactivity of the specific epoxide and its steady-state concentration, since there are natural mechanisms that can defend against a certain quantity of these reactive intermediates.

The cytochrome P-450–mediated oxidative biotransformation of other xenobiotics can also produce reactive intermediates, primarily following a change in the resonance in the structure or a rearrangement of the initial metabolite. For example, the N-demethylation of dimethylnitrosamine is a common phase I biotransformation for secondary amines (Figure 4–15). Following loss of the alkyl group, the remaining unstable nitroso structure proceeds through resonance changes that result in an unstable intermediate. This decomposes and releases a reactive alkylating, carbonium ion. Similar examples exist for compounds undergoing O-dealkylation, N-hydroxylation, sulfur oxidation, etc. Cytochrome P-450–mediated reactions produce an entity that subsequently rearranges or degrades to an intermediate that covalently binds to tissue macromolecules.

Oxidative dehalogenation often leads to reactive chemical species. For example, when the

Table 4–22. EXAMPLES OF XENOBIOTICS KNOWN TO UNDERGO BIOACTIVATION

COMPOUND	REACTIVE PATHWAY OR INTERMEDIATE	ADDITIONAL FACTORS THAT ENHANCE TOXICITY
Acetaminophen	N-Hydroxylation	Sulfate and glutathione depletion
2-Acetylaminofluorene	N-Hydroxylation	Conjugation
Acetylhydrazine	N-Hydroxylation and subsequent rearrangement	
Aflatoxin B_1	Epoxidation	
Allyl alcohol	Oxidation to a reactive aldehyde	Glutathione depletion
Benzene	Epoxidation and further metabolism	
Benzo[a]pyrene and related compounds	Epoxidation, and other pathways	Secondary biotransformation of diol to diol epoxide
Bromobenzene	Epoxidation	Glutathione depletion
Bromotrichloromethane	Free radical formation	
Carbon disulfide	Oxidation with release of sulfur	
Carbon tetrachloride	Free radical formation	Reductive metabolism
Chloramphenicol	Formation of oxamyl chloride intermediate	
Chloroform	Carbonylchloride (phosgene) formation	Glutathione depletion
Cyclophosphamide	4-Hydroxylation and subsequent rearrangement	
Dimethylnitrosamine	α-Hydroxylation; rearrangement to yield a carbonium ion—CH^+_3	
Furosemide	Epoxidation of furan ring	
Halothane	Free radical formation	Reductive metabolism
4-Ipomeanol	Oxidation of furan ring	
Isoniazide	Acetylation, N-hydroxylation	Fast/slow acetyletor
Parathion	Oxidation with release of sulfur	
Polychlorinated and polybrominated biphenyls	Epoxidation and ring hydroxylation with subsequent oxidation of catechol nucleus	Glutathione depletion
Thioacetamide	S-Oxidation and subsequent further metabolism	
Trichloroethylene	Epoxidation	
Vinyl chloride	Epoxidation and other pathways	

carbon undergoing oxidation contains two halogens (usually chlorines or bromines), the product of oxygen insertion is a dihalohydrin, which undergoes dehydrohalogenation to a carbonyl halide entity (Figure 4–16). These acid halides are reactive and acylate macromolecules. A similar reaction is known to occur for chloroform. The initial reactive intermediate is phosgene, which can act as a bifunctional alkylating agent. Thus, in almost all cases where a xenobiotic has a terminal carbon with two halides attached, side chain oxidation mediated by cytochrome P-450 will produce a toxic, reactive intermediate.

Biotransformation of xenobiotics by the flavin-containing monooxygenase also produces reactive intermediates. Oxidation of amines to N-hydroxides produces, in some cases, metabolites that rearrange to reactive nitrogen centers or aryl imines. These reactive intermediates behave similarly to those produced by cytochrome P-450–mediated oxidative metabolism and result in covalent binding to cellular macromolecules.

Reductive metabolism of xenobiotics by the cytochrome P-450 enzymes also produces reactive intermediates. The reductive dehalogenation of specific halogenated aliphatics results in production of free radical intermediates owing to the uptake of the reducing equivalent (electron). Carbon tetrachloride ($CCl_4 \xrightarrow{e^-} \cdot CCl_3 + Cl^-$),

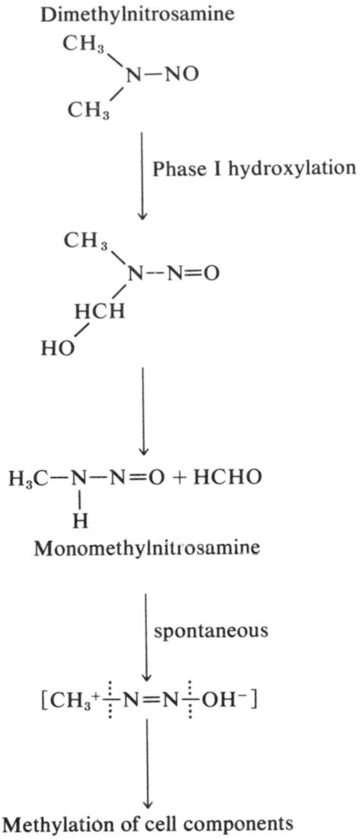

Dimethylnitrosamine

$$\begin{array}{c} CH_3 \\ \diagdown \\ N-NO \\ \diagup \\ CH_3 \end{array}$$

↓ Phase I hydroxylation

$$\begin{array}{c} CH_3 \\ \diagdown \\ N--N=O \\ \diagup \\ HCH \\ HO \end{array}$$

↓

$$H_3C-\underset{\underset{H}{|}}{N}-N=O + HCHO$$

Monomethylnitrosamine

↓ spontaneous

$$[CH_3^+ \vdots N=N \vdots OH^-]$$

↓

Methylation of cell components

Figure 4–15. Bioactivation of dimethylnitrosamine.

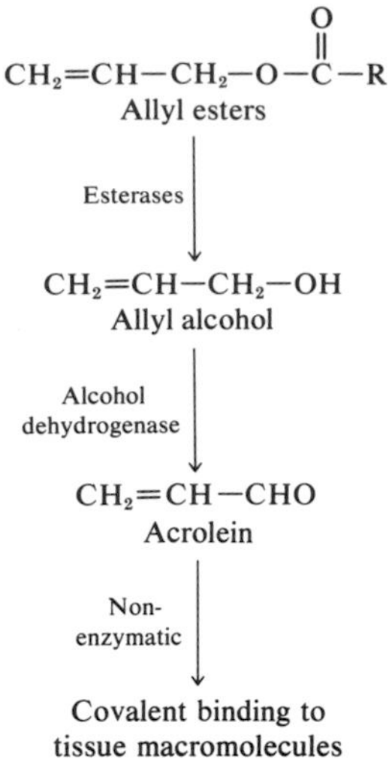

$$CH_2=CH-CH_2-O-\overset{\overset{\textstyle O}{\|}}{C}-R$$
Allyl esters

↓ Esterases

$$CH_2=CH-CH_2-OH$$
Allyl alcohol

↓ Alcohol dehydrogenase

$$CH_2=CH-CHO$$
Acrolein

↓ Non-enzymatic

Covalent binding to tissue macromolecules

Figure 4–17. Bioactivation of allyl esters. (Modified from Jenner, P., and Testa, B. [eds.]: *Concepts in Drug Metabolism,* Part B. Marcel Dekker, Inc., New York, 1981.)

bromotrichloromethane, and halothane are examples of chemicals that undergo reductive cleavage to toxic intermediates.

Often the product of one reaction can lead to a substrate for another enzyme that produces a toxic product. Biotransformation of allyl esters is a good example (Figure 4–17). These esters are cleaved by nonspecific esterases to allyl alcohol, which is then oxidized by alcohol dehydrogenases to the reactive allyl aldehyde. This aldehyde reacts with macromolecules or may be detoxified by glutathione conjugation. The rapid reactions catalyzed by the esterase and alcohol dehydrogenase produce a concentration of the aldehyde that overwhelms the detoxication path-

$$R-\underset{\underset{H}{|}}{\overset{\overset{Cl}{|}}{C}}-Cl \xrightarrow[\substack{Cytochrome \\ P\text{-}450}]{[O]} R-\underset{\underset{OH}{|}}{\overset{\overset{Cl}{|}}{C}}-Cl \longrightarrow R-\underset{}{\overset{\overset{Cl}{|}}{C}}=O$$

↓

Covalent Binding to Macromolecules

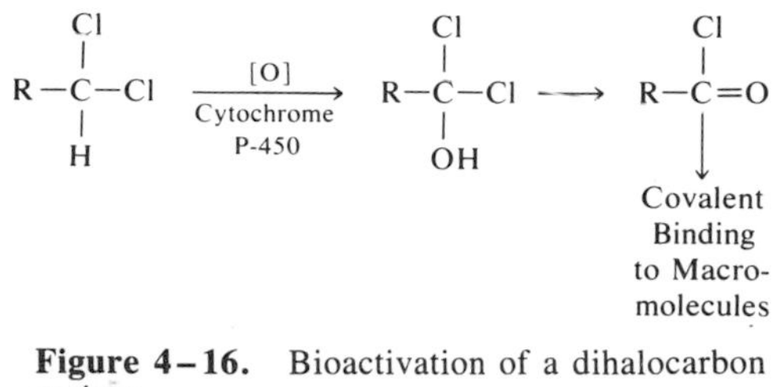

Figure 4–16. Bioactivation of a dihalocarbon moiety.

ways and results in the observed toxicities with these compounds.

The phase II biotransformation enzymes can also produce reactive intermediates. These usually result from rearrangement of unstable conjugates. When the unstable conjugate rearranges, the fragments are often reactive moieties that covalently bind to macromolecules. For example, conjugates of the phase I metabolite of 2-acetylaminofluorene are mutagenic and carcinogenic (Figure 4–18). The phase I–derived metabolite, N-hydroxy-2-acetylaminofluorene, can be converted via sulfate conjugation to a highly reactive electrophilic N-O-sulfate ester. This sulfate ester rearranges and fragments into a reactive intermediate that covalently binds to nucleic acids and proteins. The N-hydroxyl metabolite can form a glucuronide, which is also unstable and reactive. Acetyl transferases form an unstable O-acetyl conjugate (i.e., an N-acetoxy-2-aminofluorene), which results in a toxic reactive intermediate. Thus, conjugation of the N-hydroxy metabolite of 2-acetylaminofluorene with three separate conjugating species can lead to a reactive, potentially carcinogenic product.

Acetylation of drugs and xenobiotics can lead to toxic reactive products. A classic example is the acetylation of isoniazid (Figure 4–19) to form acetylisoniazid. This unstable metabolite rearranges to produce acetylhydrazine, which is oxidized by cytochrome P-450 to N-hydroxyl-acetyl hydrazine. This unstable derivative fragments to an acetyl radical or carbonium ion, which can acylate tissue macromolecules. Thus,

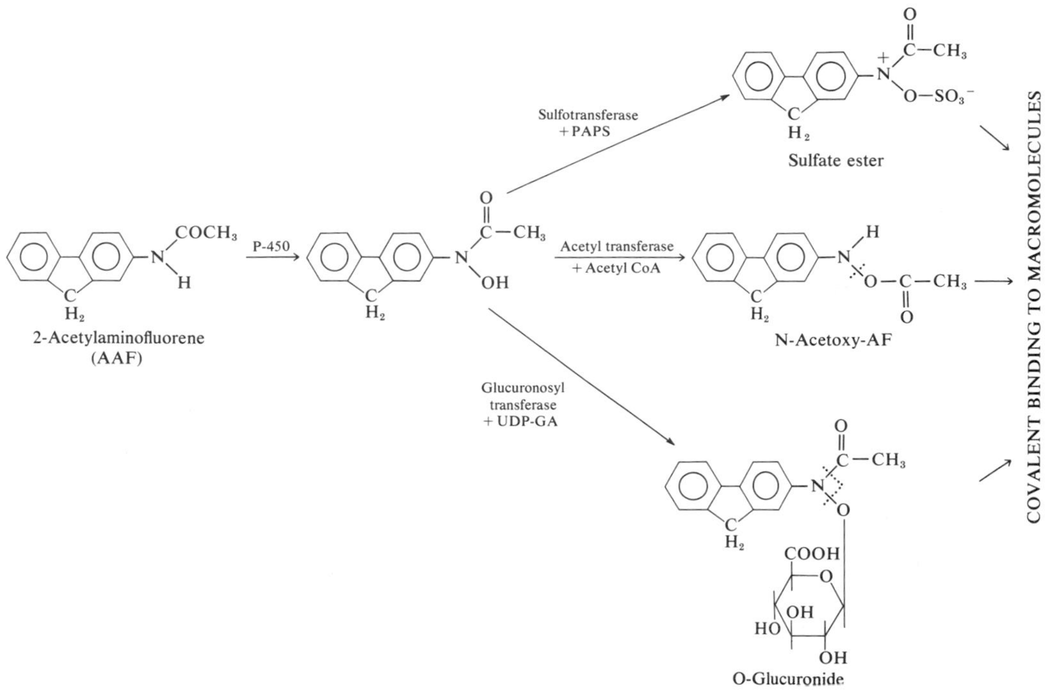

Figure 4–18. Bioactivation of 2-acetylaminofluorene.

the acetylation reaction produces a product that subsequently degrades and, in conjunction with cytochrome P-450–mediated N-hydroxylation, produces a toxic covalent-binding species.

Even the glutathione S-transferases can produce conjugates that can rearrange to reactive intermediates. For example, glutathione S-transferases can mediate the conjugation of 1,2-dihaloethanes with glutathione (Figure 4–20). In this reaction, a halogen (usually chloride or bromide) is displaced and S-(2-haloethyl)-glutathione is formed. Since the sulfur is still nucleophilic, it can displace the halogen on the adjacent carbon to form a highly strained, three-membered-ring intermediate called an episulfonium or thiiranium ion. This electrophilic species has been shown to alkylate nucleic acids, an event associated with mutagenicity and carcinogenicity.

Some glutathione conjugates that are hydrolyzed to cysteine conjugates by the kidney are then bioactivated by a cysteine β-lyase. The cleavage of the β-carbon-sulfur bond by this enzyme produces a sulfhydryl-containing moiety that can react with kidney macromolecules or be conjugated by methylation. Hexachlorobutadiene and various fluorinated ethylenes are toxic by this pathway (Figure 4–21).

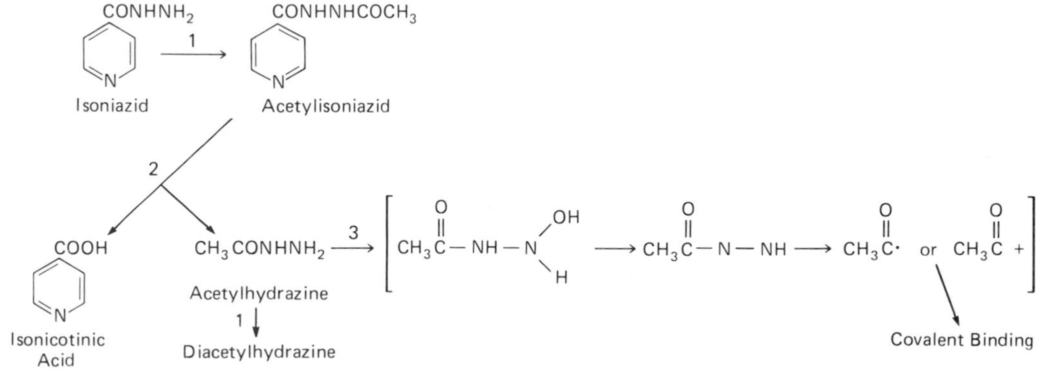

Figure 4–19. Bioactivation of isoniazid. *1*, N-acetyltransferase; *2*, hydrolysis; *3*, cytochrome P-450.

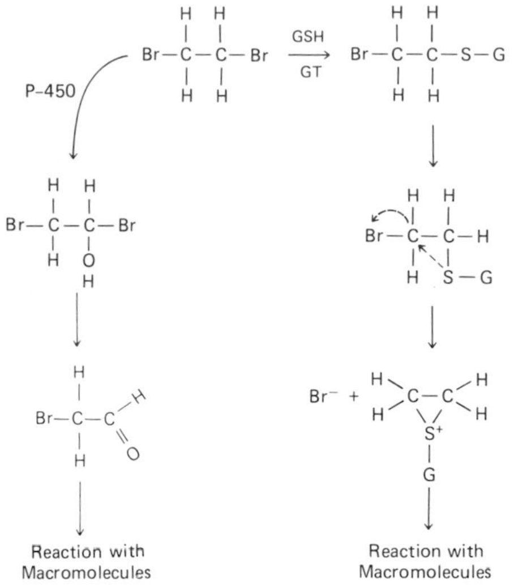

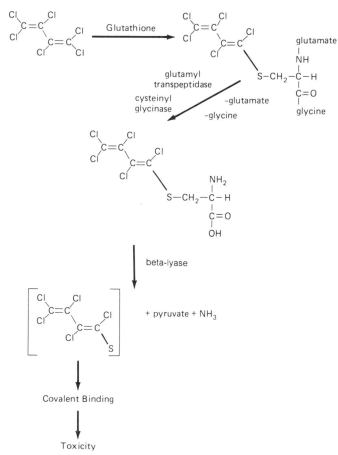

Figure 4–20. Bioactivation of 1,2-dibromo-ethane via glutathione transferase (*GT*) and cytochrome P-450.

The biotransformation of acetaminophen is a good example of how a minor metabolic pathway can result in tissue injury. This analgesic is quite safe, and only under abnormal conditions does acetaminophen administration result in hepatotoxicity. Acetaminophen (*N*-acetyl-4-aminophenol) is readily conjugated with sulfate and glucuronic acid (Figure 4–22). Following large doses, the sulfate pool becomes exhausted before much of the compound is biotransformed. Since the glucuronidation pathway is rate limited, more of the parent compound is available for biotransformation by the cytochrome P-450 system. This minor pathway produces *N*-hydroxy-acetaminophen, which converts to a quinoneimine resonance form. The carbon atom ortho to the phenolic group is electrophilic and reacts with the nucleophilic sulfhydryl of glutathione. As long as sufficient glutathione is available, this reactive intermediate can be detoxified. However, the pool of glutathione is limited and is depleted. When this occurs, the electrophilic intermediate reacts covalently with

Figure 4–21. Bioactivation of hexachlorobutadiene.

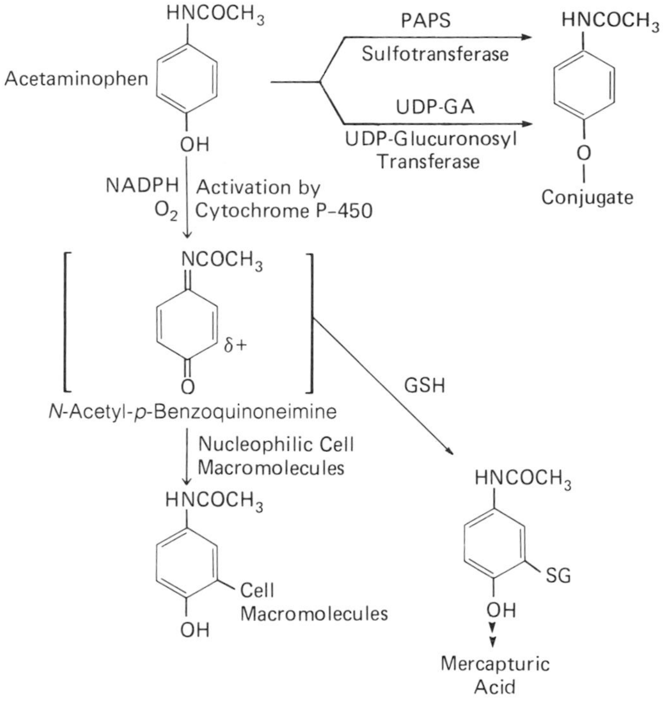

Figure 4–22. Bioactivation of acetaminophen.

nucleophilic substituents present on macromolecules, an event associated with hepatotoxicity. If the cytochrome P-450 pathway is enhanced by previous induction or if the sulfate and/or glutathione pools are depleted by a previous stress (fasting, another xenobiotic, etc.), the toxicity of a given dose of acetaminophen will be enhanced. Early administration of compounds containing a sulfhydryl group, such as cysteamine, cysteine, N-acetylcysteine, and methionine, can decrease the severity of liver injury.

In summary, the toxicity of acetaminophen requires a dose or doses such that there is a depletion of the sulfate pool, overwhelming of glucuronidation, increased biotransformation by the cytochrome P-450 system, and ultimately depletion of glutathione. Only this combination of events results in an overwhelming of defense mechanisms and increased covalent binding of toxic intermediates to cellular macromolecules. Acetaminophen is not a unique example. Most chemicals follow a similar sequence of events in that some critical pathway becomes overwhelmed by continued production of reactive intermediates.

Figure 4–23 summarizes the proposed relationship between biotransformation, bioactivation, and toxicity of a xenobiotic. It is seen that the parent compound or its metabolite may be converted to a reactive intermediate. Reactive intermediates can be detoxified and thus become metabolites that are eliminated. Indeed, only a small portion of these reactive intermediates may become covalently bound to tissue macromolecules. In some cases, covalent binding may be viewed as a detoxification of a reactive metabolite. However, if such binding results in inactivation of a critical enzyme, depletion of important cellular antioxidants (i.e., GSH), formation of an antigenic determinate, cross

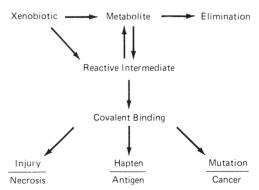

Figure 4–23. Proposed relationship between biotransformation, bioactivation, and toxicity of a xenobiotic. (Modified from Plaa, G. L., and Hewitt, W. R. [eds.]: *Toxicology of the Liver.* Raven Press, New York, 1982.)

linking of neurofilaments, and so on, toxicity may result. The relationship between covalent binding of xenobiotics to cellular components and tissue injuries remains to be established.

REFERENCES

Anders, M. W. (ed.): *Bioactivation of Foreign Compounds.* Academic Press, Inc., New York, 1985.

Anderson, D., and Conning, D. M. (eds.): *Experimental Toxicology.* Royal Society of Chemistry, London, 1988.

Caldwell, J., and Jakoby, W. B.: *Biological Basis of Detoxification.* Academic Press, Inc., New York, 1983.

Dutton, G. J.: *Glucuronidation of Drugs and Other Compounds.* CRC Press, Inc., Boca Raton, Fla., 1980.

Gonzalez, F. J.: The molecular biology of cytochromes P450s. *Pharmacol. Rev.,* **40**:243–288, 1989.

Gram, T. E. (ed.): *Extrahepatic Metabolism of Drugs and Other Foreign Compounds.* Spectrum Publications Inc., Jamaica, N.Y., 1980.

Gram, T. E., and Gillette, J. R.: Biotransformation of drugs. In Bacq., Z. M. (ed.): *Fundamentals of Biochemical Pharmacology.* Pergamon Press, Ltd., New York, 1971, pp. 571–609.

Guengerich, F. P.: *Mammalian Cytochromes P-450.* CRC Press, Inc., Boca Raton, Fla., 1987.

Guengerich, F. P., and Liebler, D. C.: Enzymatic activation of chemicals to toxic metabolites. *CRC Crit. Rev. Toxicol.,* **14**:259–307, 1985.

Hawkins, D. R. (ed.): *Biotransformations. Vol. 1: A Survey of the Biotransformations of Drugs and Chemicals in Animals.* Royal Society of Chemistry, London, 1988.

Hutson, D. H.; Caldwell, J.; and Paulson, G. D. (eds.): *Intermediary Xenobiotic Metabolism in Animals.* Taylor and Francis, London, 1989.

Jakoby, W. B. (ed.): *Enzymatic Basis of Detoxication.* Vols. 1–2. Academic Press, Inc., New York, 1980.

Jakoby, W. B.; Bend, J. R.; and Caldwell, J.: *Metabolic Basis of Detoxification: Metabolism of Functional Groups.* Academic Press, Inc., New York, 1982.

Jenner, P., and Testa, B. (eds.): *Concepts in Drug Metabolism,* Parts A–B. Marcel Dekker, Inc., New York, 1981.

Kato, R.; Estabrook, R. W.; and Cayen, M. N. (eds.): *Xenobiotic Metabolism and Disposition.* Taylor and Francis, London, 1989.

La Du, B. N.; Mandel, H. G.; and Way, E. L.: *Fundamentals of Drug Metabolism and Drug Disposition.* Williams & Wilkins Co., Baltimore, 1971.

Larsson, A.; Orrenius, S.; Holmgren, A.; and Mannervik, B. (eds.): *Functions of Glutathione.* Raven Press, New York, 1983.

Mantle, T. J.; Pickett, C. B.; and Hayes, J. D. (eds.): *Glutathione S-Transferases and Carcinogenesis.* Taylor and Francis, London, 1987.

Marnett, L. J., and Eling, T. E.: Cooxidation during prostaglandin biosynthesis: a pathway for the metabolic activation of xenobiotics. In Hodgson, E.; Bend, J. R.; and Philpot, R. M. (eds.): *Reviews in Biochemical Toxicology,* Vol. 5. Elsevier, New York, 1983, pp. 135–172.

Mulder, G. J. (ed.): *Sulfation of Drugs and Related Compounds.* CRC Press, Inc., Boca Raton, Fla., 1981.

Nebert, D. W.; Eisen, H. J.; Negishi, M.; Lang, M. A.; and Hjelmeland, L. M.: Genetic mechanisms controlling the induction of polysubstrate monooxygenase (P-450) activities. *Annu. Rev. Pharmacol. Toxicol.,* **21**:431–462, 1981.

O'Brien, P. J.: Radical formation during the peroxidase catalyzed metabolism of carcinogens and xenobiotics: the reactivity of these radicals with GSH, DNA and unsaturated lipid. *Free Rad. Biol. Med.,* **4**:169–183, 1988.

Plaa, G. L., and Hewitt, W. R. (eds.): *Toxicology of the Liver.* Raven Press, New York, 1982.

Poland, A.; Glover, E.; and Kende, A. S.: Stereospecific, high affinity binding of 2,3,7,8-tetrachlorodibenzo-*p*-dioxin by hepatic cytosol. Evidence that the binding species is the receptor for the induction of aryl hydrocarbon hydroxylase. *J. Biol. Chem.,* **251**:4936–4946, 1976.

Schenkman, J. B., and Kupfer, D. (eds.): *Hepatic Cytochrome P-450 Monooxygenase System.* Pergamon Press, Ltd., New York, 1982.

Sies, H., and Ketterer, B. (eds.): *Glutathione Conjugation Mechanisms and Biological Significance.* Academic Press, Inc., London, 1988.

Siest, G.; Magdalou, J.; and Burchell, B. (eds.): *Molecular and Cellular Aspects of Glucuronidation.* John Libbey Eurotex, London, 1989.

Sotaniemi, E. A., and Pelkonen, R. O. (eds.): *Enzyme Induction in Man.* Taylor and Francis, London, 1987.

Testa, B., and Jenner, P.: *Drug Metabolism: Chemical and Biochemical Aspects.* Marcel Dekker, Inc., New York, 1976.

Testa, B., and Jenner, P.: Inhibitors of cytochrome P-450s and their mechanism of action. *Drug Metab. Rev.,* **12**:1–117, 1981.

Weber, W. W.: *The Acetylator Genes and Drug Response.* Oxford University Press, New York, 1987.

Weber, W. W., and Hein, D. W.: *N*-Acetylation pharmacogenetics. *Pharmacol. Rev.,* **37**:25–79, 1985.

Ziegler, D. M.: Flavin-containing monooxygenase: catalytic mechanisms and substrate specificities. *Drug Metab. Rev.,* **19**:1–32, 1988.

Chapter 5

CHEMICAL CARCINOGENESIS

Gary M. Williams and John H. Weisburger

INTRODUCTION

Chemical carcinogens elicit as their specific, defining adverse effects the production of cancer in animals or humans. In many respects, carcinogenic chemicals are similar to other toxic agents or drugs. For example, carcinogens in a given experimental setting and in humans, where such data are available, show dose-response relationships. They undergo biotransformation, as would any similarly structured xenobiotic. In addition, the response to chemical carcinogens varies with the species, strain, and sex of the experimental animal, as is the case with other chemicals. Carcinogens interact with other environmental agents; their effect is sometimes enhanced and sometimes decreased, as occurs with drugs. Yet, some very important differences render chemical carcinogenesis a specialized field of toxicology. Chemical carcinogens of the type that have the ability to react with DNA differ from most other kinds of toxins in that (1) their biologic effect is persistent, cumulative, and delayed; (2) divided doses are in some cases more effective than an individual large dose; and (3) the underlying mechanisms, particularly in respect to interaction and alteration of genetic elements and other macromolecules, are distinct.

Early Discoveries in Chemical Carcinogenesis

Several types of chemicals were discovered to be carcinogenic in experimental animals after having first been suspected of causing cancer in humans. The association between exposure to soot and coal tars and cancer was identified in the late eighteenth century by the English physician Percival Pott, who observed that many of his patients who had cancer of the scrotum were chimney sweeps. That coal tar could cause cancer at the point of application in rabbits was reported from Japan by Yamagiwa and Ichikawa in 1916. In the 1920s, investigators in the United Kingdom directed by Kennaway fractionated coal tar and discovered the carcinogenic potency of pure polynuclear aromatic hydrocarbons, including dibenz[a,h]anthracene and benzo[a]pyrene.

The aromatic amines are another type of chemical carcinogen whose study also stems from the discovery of cancer in humans exposed to them. In the late 1800s, the German physician Rehn noted a cluster of cases of cancer of the urinary bladder among workers in the dye industry. The experimental evidence for the carcinogenicity of amines to which these workers were exposed did not appear until 1937, when Hueper and associates in the United States found that 2-aminonaphthalene could cause bladder cancer in dogs, reproducing the lesions seen in humans.

A third historically important type of carcinogen, azo dyes, has not been implicated in human cancer. Ehrlich in Germany discovered that exposure to a bisazo dye, scarlet red or C. I. Solvent Red 24, led to a reversible proliferation of liver cells. It was not until 25 years later, between 1932 and 1934, that in pioneering studies in Japan, Kinosita and Yoshida independently discovered the carcinogenic effect of some azo dyes in rodents.

In the years since, many other classes and types of chemicals were found to be carcinogenic in animals. Some, such as vinyl chloride, were discovered after they were suspected of being involved in the development of cancer in humans. Some chemicals were found to be carcinogenic in the course of bioassays for the detection of adverse effects in chronic toxicity studies; this was the case with 2-acetylaminofluorene and dimethylnitrosamine. Some chemicals were also discovered to be carcinogenic during investigations that attempted to reproduce in laboratory animals adverse effects that had been observed in humans or domestic animals. A study dealing with the possible causative factors of amyotrophic lateral sclerosis prevalent on Pacific islands led to the finding that the plant product cycasin was a potent carcinogen. 1,2-Dimethylhydrazine was found carcinogenic as a result of its structural similarity to the aglycone

**Table 5–1. CHEMICALS AND MIXTURES JUDGED TO BE
CARCINOGENIC TO HUMANS BY THE INTERNATIONAL
AGENCY FOR RESEARCH ON CANCER**

DNA-Reactive

Aflatoxins	Coal tars
4-Aminobiphenyl	Cyclophosphamide
2-Aminonaphthalene	Melphalan
5-Azacytidine	MOPP (nitrogen mustard, vincristine, procarbazine, and prednisone)
Benzidine	Nickel and nickel compounds
Betel quid with tobacco	Phenacetin-containing analgesic mixtures
N, N-bis(2-Chloroethyl)-2-aminonaphthalene	Soot
bis(Chloromethyl)ether	Sulfur mustard
1,4-Butanediol dimethanesulfonate (Myleran)	Triethylenethiophosphoramide (thiotepa)
Chlorambucil	Tobacco smoke and products
1-(2-Chloroethyl)ether methylcyclohexyl)-1-nitrosourea	Treosulphan
Chromium compounds, hexavalent	Vinyl chloride

Epigenetic

Azathioprine	Estrogens, steroidal
Cyclosporin A	Oral contraceptives
Diethylstilbestrol	

Unclassified

Alcoholic beverages	Mineral oils, untreated and mildly treated
Arsenic and arsenic compounds	Shale oils
Benzene	

Data from International Agency for Research on Cancer (1987). The table does not include processes or fibers.

of cycasin, methylazoxymethanol. Other studies in the 1950s investigating the cause of turkey x disease, which was responsible for extensive losses of livestock, pinpointed aflatoxin B_1 and, later, other mycotoxins as hepatotoxins and potent carcinogens. The powerful carcinogenicity of bis(chloromethyl)ether was observed first in the laboratory, and a few years later, lung cancer was noted in individuals exposed occupationally. At present, new carcinogens are being disclosed largely in studies aimed at establishing structure/activity relationships and in studies undertaken with chemicals found to be genotoxic. Such carcinogens, as well as all those mentioned above, are of a type that possess the ability to react with DNA.

Routine safety testing undertaken for candidate commercial products and national testing programs, such as the bioassay programs of the United States National Cancer Institute/National Toxicology Program or the Japanese Cooperative Program on Long Term Assays for Carcinogenicity, are also yielding evidence for new cancer causing agents. Many of these, in contrast to "classic" carcinogens, lack the ability to react with DNA and instead exert their effect on the carcinogenic process through other effects, which have been designated as epigenetic. In the context of developing effective pro-

grams of cancer prevention, it is important to discover and classify specific types of chemical carcinogens and to acquire information on their mechanism of action and possible interactions. Such information, together with information on environmental quantitative occurrence, forms the basis for a reliable assessment of risk to humans, the eventual goal of investigations on the possible carcinogenic effects of chemicals.

Human Cancer

Cancer is one of the three leading causes of death in most countries, heart disease and stroke being the other two. Great progress has been made in developing an understanding of the usually complex causes of the major types of cancer. Approximately 35 specific chemicals or processes have been judged by working groups of the International Agency for Research on Cancer to have caused cancer in humans (Table 5–1). Most of these are industrial chemicals or drugs and the majority are of the DNA-reactive genotoxic type. Such agents, however, do not account for most human cancer. Based on epidemiologic studies and mechanistic research, present understanding implicates life style elements, particularly use of tobacco products, diet, and alcohol consumption, in the majority of cancers in the United States.

DEFINITION OF CHEMICAL CARCINOGENS

The term *carcinogen* literally means giving rise to carcinomas, i.e., epithelial malignancies. This definition, however, is not adhered to for several reasons. First, the suffix *gen* implies *ab initio* genesis, but in fact the responses to a chemical that are accepted as evidence of carcinogenesis include increases in the occurrence of cryptogenic neoplasms. Also, agents that produce sarcomas of mesenchymal origin are generally called carcinogens, although the term *sarcomagen* or *oncogen* would be more correct. In practice, carcinogen is used for any agent that induces malignancies. In this chapter, the term will be used in the general sense for all neoplasm-inducing agents.

Chemical carcinogens are defined operationally by their ability to induce neoplasms. Four types of response have generally been accepted as evidence of induction of neoplasms: (1) an increase in the incidence of the tumor types that occur in controls; (2) the development of tumors earlier than in controls: (3) the presence of types of tumors not seen in controls; and (4) an increased multiplicity of tumors. A controversial aspect in the application of these criteria is whether to accept only malignant or also benign neoplasms as the end point. In favor of accepting benign neoplasms is the fact that no chemical has yet been identified that produces exclusively a significant incidence of benign neoplasms in chronic tests. An argument against the use of benign neoplasms is the consideration that differentiation from nonneoplastic processes can be controversial. A current practice is to accept combinations of benign and malignant neoplasms when there is not a significant increase in malignancies. A key element in controversial cases is to consider the possible mechanisms of action. This chapter presents only agents documented to induce reproducibly malignant neoplasms.

Chemicals capable of inducing malignant neoplasms, and which are thereby classified as carcinogens, comprise a highly diverse collection, including organic and inorganic chemicals, with various biologic actions such as alteration of the endocrine system or immunosuppression. For some of these chemicals, such as neoplasm enhancers or promoters, the designation *carcinogen* is perhaps unfortunate, but necessary, because these chemicals in specific situations do increase the yield of cancers, albeit usually those that occur cryptogenically. Thus, the diverse agents that can be considered as carcinogens have different properties and appear to produce neoplasms through different modes of action. It is clear then that analysis as to the distinct mechanism of action is required for each carcinogen and that health risk analyses appropriate to each mechanism must be developed.

MODE OF ACTION OF CHEMICAL CARCINOGENS

The elucidation of the mechanism of action of a carcinogen entails establishing how the effects of the chemical on a cell or tissue lead to the evolution of cells with abnormalities essential to the neoplastic phenotype. Carcinogens interact with numerous tissue constituents and produce a number of effects. To identify actions that are necessary or contributory to the production of neoplasms, an understanding of the neoplastic process is required. Although this has not yet been completely achieved, current knowledge provides considerable insight, which points to certain effects of chemicals as being crucial to carcinogenicity.

The induction of cancer in humans and in animals by chemicals proceeds through a complex series of reactions and processes, subject to and controlled by a number of modifying factors. Essentially, the whole process can be viewed as the gradual escape of somatic cells from the complex controls that regulate their growth. The process consists of two distinct sequences, one in which the normal cell is converted to a neoplastic cell and a second in which the neoplastic cell develops into an overt neoplasm (Figure 5–1). Historically, these are often referred to as *initiation* and *promotion*, but there are many divergent views on the meaning of those terms. In the two sequences, chemicals are involved, in diverse ways, both to enhance and to retard the process. A mechanistic analysis of the key elements, with distinct intrinsic properties, is shown in Figure 5–1.

Neoplastic Conversion

Biotransformation by Host Enzyme Systems. Numerous distinct enzyme systems that are involved in the metabolism of endogenous substrates also carry out the detoxification and elimination of xenobiotics (see Chapter 4). As part of this biotransformation, some chemicals undergo enzymatic activation to a reactive ultimate carcinogen in the form of an electrophile or radical cation. The effectiveness of a carcinogen under given conditions is a function of the ratio of the reactive metabolite to the detoxified metabolites. A small number of chemicals, mostly industrial intermediates and chemotherapeutic drugs, are reactive in their parent form and, therefore, do not require activation to be carcinogenic. Yet, they can undergo detoxifica-

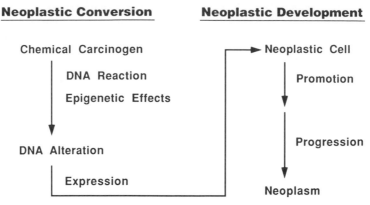

Figure 5 – 1. Main steps in the carcinogenic process.

tion through enzymic means. In addition, there seem to be carcinogens that, although not reactive themselves, generate reactive moieties intracellularly through specific enzymic activation processes.

Interaction of the Ultimate Carcinogen with Cellular Constituents. Carcinogens that form reactive species, electrophiles or free radicals, undergo covalent reactions with most cellular macromolecules containing nucleophilic sites, including DNA. The covalent addition products are called adducts. The damaged DNA is subject to removal and restoration by repair enzyme systems, whereas other altered macromolecules are disposed of and replaced. Thus, under these conditions, the cell can recover from most of the immediate effects of carcinogen interaction.

Fixation of Carcinogen Damage. If the cell replicates while DNA damage is present, permanent alterations in the genome can be produced in several possible ways, including the mispairing of bases leading to point mutations, errors in replication yielding frame shift mutations, transpositions resulting in genetic rearrangement, combinations of these alterations in sequential steps, and their amplification (see Chapter 6). Interactions with proteins that regulate gene expression or alteration of enzymatic methylation of DNA have also been suspected of being able to alter cell function permanently. In the case of interactions with the mitotic apparatus, chromosomal mutations and aneuploidy could result (Haluska *et al.*, 1987).

All these alterations can generate a permanently abnormal cell with altered genotype and phenotype. The abnormal cell may possess only some properties of neoplastic cells, or if the extent of the alterations is sufficient, may be fully neoplastic. The critical genetic alterations underlying neoplasia involve at least two types of genes, oncogenes and onco-suppressor (tumor suppressor) genes or anti-oncogenes. Cellular

oncogenes were first identified by the homology of their base sequences to genes in oncogenic viruses. More than 50 different oncogenes have been found to have transforming capabilites. Among these are *ras, myc, fos,* and *src* (Bos, 1989; Weinberg, 1989). They code for oncoproteins located in the nucleus or cytoplasm that are involved in growth control, as growth factors, factor recognition complexes, signal transduction elements, protein kinases, and DNA binding proteins (transcriptional activators). Oncogenes in their normal state, in which they are referred to as proto-oncogenes, are present in all cells. Activated oncogenes are defined by their ability to act dominantly to transform cells. Activation can occur through point mutations, chromosomal translocation, amplification, or retroviral insertion (insertional mutagenesis) (Würgler, 1989). Activated oncogenes are dominant over the corresponding proto-oncogene allele, suggesting that expression of at least two oncogenes may be required for full neoplastic conversion (Cooper and Grover, 1990).

Onco-suppressor genes are capable of suppressing neoplastic behavior in tumor cells in which they are present. Thus, they are recessive genes. The first onco-suppressor gene identified was the human retinoblastoma (Rb-1) gene. Recently gene p53, which encodes the cellular protein p53, (interestingly, the mutated p53 gene is an oncogene) and various chromosomal deletions have been identified as candidate onco-suppressor genes. Little is known about the structure or function of these genes. The predicted protein encoded by the ODC gene has a sequence similarity to neutral cell adhesion molecules and other related cell surface glycoproteins. There is some evidence that the products of onco-suppressor genes can be inactivated by oncoproteins. Thus, the lack of expression of onco-suppressor genes or inactivation of their products may lead to neoplastic conversion (Cavenee *et al.,* 1989; Weinberg, 1989).

Multiplication of Carcinogen Altered Cells. Abnormal cells that are fully neoplastic may be held in check by neighboring cells or tissue homeostatic factors that may be transmitted by cell-to-cell communication. If the conditions of carcinogen exposure or the abnormalities generated in the cells permit, they may undergo limited proliferation to form "preneoplastic" lesions. During these processes, further alterations of DNA as a result of transpositions and other error-prone processes are possible and would lead to the formation of a neoplastic cell (Bogen, 1989).

Neoplastic Development and Progression

Progressive Growth to Neoplasm Formation (Promotion). Cells that have undergone neoplastic conversion may remain dormant, presumably being controlled by tissue homeostatic factors. The regulatory factors are probably transmitted by one of several types of intercellular communication through gap junctions. Some neoplastic cells with the requisite abnormalities may be capable of progressive growth to form neoplasms. For suppressed neoplastic cells, their proliferation is facilitated by promoters, possibly by the interruption of tissue growth control, leading to neoplastic development. The growth of neoplasms is not "autonomous." In fact, some are highly dependent on permissive host conditions, for example, hormone-dependent neoplasms (Bulbrook, 1986; Henderson *et al.,* 1988). The factors underlying progressive growth are not fully understood, but increasingly appear to involve growth control elements coded for by oncogenes (Killion and Fidler, 1989).

Progression. Some neoplasms undergo qualitative changes in their phenotypic properties, possibly including transition from benign to malignant behavior. Benign neoplasms are progressively growing and expansive, but do not invade or metastasize to remote sites, as do malignancies.

Progression may reflect the selection during growth of a population with a genotype coding for advantageous phenotypic properties (Franks, 1988; Bogen, 1989). New genotypes could arise in neoplasms through additional changes in DNA produced by reactive carcinogens, errors in DNA replication, alterations in chromosome constitution, or hybridization of different cell types. The neoplasm that ultimately emerges is in most cases the progeny of a single cell; that is, it is a monoclonal population. Nevertheless, there is cellular heterogeneity in neoplasms, perhaps owing to lower fidelity in DNA replication, and they display abnormalities in expression of numerous gene products. This cellular diversity in solid neoplasms is a major obstacle in developing effective methods of chemotherapy.

Overall Mechanisms

Many of the specific steps in carcinogenesis are controlled and modified by numerous endogenous and exogenous factors. Thus, species, strain, sex, and age affect the processes in certain of these steps, particularly biotransformation and DNA repair. In addition, hormonal, immunologic, and other endogenous factors may enhance or diminish the extent and rate of the carcinogenic process. Cocarcinogens enhance neoplastic conversion, whereas promoters enhance neoplastic development. Among the exogenous elements, nutritional factors are heavily involved. Furthermore, many interactions occur between all of these elements as well as between synthetic and also naturally occurring chemicals which can augment or decrease the overall effectiveness of the administered agent in leading to cancer.

The neoplastic state is heritable at the cellular level (i.e., the progeny of the division of a neoplastic cell inherit the neoplastic potential), and thus theories on the mechanisms by which chemicals convert normal cells to malignant ones must ultimately explain how the effect becomes permanent. In the 1920s, Boveri advanced the suggestion that cancer arose from an imbalance of chromosomes. The important discovery that carcinogens interact with DNA provided a basis on which the permanent neoplastic state could be explained by alterations in the genotype. A number of considerations support the view that DNA is a critical target of carcinogens. These include the following: many carcinogens are or can be metabolized to electrophiles that react covalently with DNA; many carcinogens are mutagens; defects in DNA repair, such as in the human disease xeroderma pigmentosum, predispose to cancer development; several constitutional or chromosomal abnormalities (e.g., trisomy 21) predispose to cancer development; initiated dormant tumor cells are persistent, which is best explained by a change in DNA; cancer is heritable at the cellular level (i.e., the progeny of cancer cells are cancer cells) and, therefore, likely results from a permanent alteration of DNA; most, if not all, cancers display chromosomal abnormalities, including reciprocal translocation, deletions, or nonreciprocal rearrangements and duplication of whole chromosomes or chromosome segments; many cancers display aberrant gene expression; and cells from many cancers contain amplified oncogenes or deleted onco-suppressor genes.

Nevertheless, studies on the interactions of carcinogens with proteins and RNA have led to the alternate postulate that effects on these macromolecules could eventually be rendered permanent through epigenetic mechanisms on gene expression creating a new stable state of differentiation.

Although these two distinct mechanisms for neoplastic conversion, i.e., genetic and epigenetic, have often been thought of as alternatives for the action of carcinogens generally, the fact that carcinogens are an extremely diverse group of agents, both structurally and in terms of biologic effects, makes it likely that chemical carcinogens operate in a variety of different ways. The pioneering studies of Elizabeth and James Miller (1981) revealed that many structurally different types of carcinogens could give rise to electrophilic reactants that interacted with cellular macromolecules. Such carcinogens that interact with DNA are mutagenic, as revealed in the early studies of Auerbach, Tatum, and Demerec and firmly established by many investigators in the last decade (De Flora, 1988; Rosenkranz, 1988; Würgler, 1989). Nevertheless, a variety of carcinogens such as rodent-implanted plastics, asbestos, and hormones have structures that do not suggest an obvious reactive form (i.e., an electrophile), and have not been documented to alter DNA, or to be gene mutagens. Thus, it has been recognized that various modes of action seem to be involved in the overall carcinogenic effects of chemicals (Weinstein, 1988). Accordingly, several distinctions between different types of carcinogens have been proposed. In one of these, proposed by Williams and Weisburger in 1977 as a working hypothesis to call attention to possible differences in the properties of carcinogens, two major types, genotoxic and epigenetic, were described.

Carcinogens that interact with and alter DNA were categorized as genotoxic or DNA reactive. These carcinogens are, of course, mutagenic in appropriate test systems (see Chapter 6). DNA alteration leading to neoplastic conversion of cells in the first sequence in carcinogenesis is the likely basis for their carcinogenicity. Considering the variety of abnormalities in cancer cells, it seems that such carcinogens would have to produce multiple alterations of the gene mutation type, alterations in major regulatory genes, or changes in expression of large regions of the genome, as discussed above. Also, effects on tumor suppressor genes may be involved, leading to their inactivation.

Carcinogens designated as epigenetic were those for which no evidence of DNA reactivity had been found and for which there was evidence of another biologic effect that could be the basis for carcinogenicity. Possible mechanisms may involve cytotoxicity and chronic tissue injury, cell proliferation, specific intracellular generation of reactive species, hormonal imbalance, immunologic effects, or promotional activity. In some cases, these agents could indirectly cause genetic alterations and neoplastic conversion by means of the production of inaccurate DNA synthesis, reactive oxygen free radicals, aberrant methylation, and chromosomal abnormalities. Alternatively, they could produce neoplastic conversion by epigenetic effects on gene expression. Most likely some of these probably do not produce neoplastic conversion at all, but instead act in the sequence of neoplastic development to facilitate tumor development by cells that either already possess an altered genome, or have been independently changed by genotoxic carcinogens.

As will be detailed, it now seems likely that there is no single mode of action by which all carcinogens produce cancer. Nevertheless, the ultimate effect, the establishment of a neoplastic population with a permanently modified phenotype, is the same. Whether that comes about by totally diverse actions or actions that are initially diverse but that culminate in a final common step (e.g., oncogene activation) is not yet known. To elucidate completely the essential effects of any particular agent, it will be necessary to determine at what steps in the overall process of carcinogenesis and through what mechanism the agent functions.

CLASSES OF CHEMICAL CARCINOGENS

Carcinogens may be separated into classes based on their chemical or biologic properties. These in turn can be placed in the two general categories: DNA-reactive (genotoxic) and epigenetic (Table 5–2), where available information is sufficient. Otherwise, specific carcinogens or classes are left unassigned.

The scientific facts in support of mechanistically distinct types of carcinogens have increased greatly over the last 10 years and the concept has steadily achieved acceptance, although some remain unconvinced. Yet, the alternative to differentiating carcinogens according to their intrinsic properties is to maintain the assumptions of 40 years ago that all carcinogens are basically alike. This assumption allows simplistic approaches to risk assessment, but does not accommodate current scientific knowledge, and also is a poor if not erroneous basis for public health protection and effective cancer prevention.

The DNA-reactive (genotoxic) category com-

Table 5–2. CLASSIFICATION OF CARCINOGENIC CHEMICALS

CATEGORY AND CLASS	EXAMPLE
A. DNA-reactive (genotoxic) carcinogens	
1. Activation-independent organic	Alkylating agents
2. Activation-independent inorganic	Nickel, cadmium*
3. Activation-dependent	Polycyclic aromatic hydrocarbon, arylamine, nitrosamine
B. Epigenetic carcinogens	
1. Promoter	Organochlorine pesticides, saccharin
2. Hormone-modifying	Estrogen, amitrole
3. Peroxisome proliferators	Clofibrate, diethylhexylphthalate
4. Cytotoxic	Nitrilotriacetic acid
5. Immunosuppressor	Cyclosporin A, azathioprine
6. Solid state	Plastics, asbestos
C. Unclassified	
1. Miscellaneous	Ethanol, dioxane

* Some metals have yielded evidence of reaction with DNA; others may operate through epigenetic mechanisms such as alteration of fidelity of DNA polymerases.

prises carcinogens that chemically interact with DNA. The defining characteristic is a chemical property and, therefore, chemical assays of adduct formation are most definitive for identifying such agents (Williams, 1989; Wogan, 1989). Newer methods such as the ^{32}P-postlabeling assay developed by Randerath et al. (1989) provide sensitive and specific assays. Park et al. (1989) reported that high-performance liquid chromatography (HPLC) using electrochemical detection was an efficient means of determining DNA adducts. In the absence of such data, DNA reactivity can be indirectly assessed in short-term tests, but clearly the reliability of such evidence depends on the characteristics and performance of the tests. This category consists mainly of carcinogens that function as electrophilic reactants, as originally postulated by the Millers (1981). Also, because some metals have displayed genotoxic effects suggestive of DNA interaction, these have been tentatively placed in this category. However, the studies of Loeb and colleagues (1989) on effects of metals on the fidelity of DNA polymerases suggest that these might yield abnormal DNA by a mechanism distinct from the electrophilic DNA-damaging compounds. For an agent that has both DNA-reactive and epigenetic properties, assignment is made to the DNA-reactive category.

This category contains most of the "classic" organic carcinogens. This type of carcinogen was originally postulated by J. and E. Miller (1981) in the United States as being capable of forming electrophilic species. The underlying chemistry is now well understood and the structures of the reactive electrophiles can be recognized (Table 5–3). DNA-reactive carcinogens can be subdivided according to whether they are active in their parent form or require bioactivation.

DNA-reactive carcinogens often share a number of features. Some are active with a single dose, often subtoxic, and their effects are cumulative. They can act synergistically or additively with one another. Their effects are enhanced by promoters or cocarcinogens. Many have been shown to be active transplacentally. It is probably because of these features that most human carcinogens are of the DNA-reactive type (Table 5–1).

The second broad category, designated as epigenetic carcinogens, comprises those carcinogens for which there is evidence of an inability of the chemical to interact with genetic material and for which another biologic effect has been delineated that could be the basis for carcinogenicity. This category contains carcinogens characterized by their promoting activity, hormone-modifying activity, cytotoxicity, immunosuppressive action, or ability to induce peroxisome proliferation. Many of these agents increase DNA synthesis, mitosis, and cell duplication rates. Agents producing effects that might be indirectly genotoxic are grouped with epigenetic agents or left unclassified because of the fact that their genotoxicity (if ultimately established) still is secondary to an initial critical epigenetic biologic effect.

It is important to note that this scheme does not preclude genotoxic carcinogens as such, or in the form of their metabolites, from also having epigenetic effects. Indeed, the potency of some carcinogens may reside in their promoting as well as genotoxic actions.

The recognition of different types of carcinogens has major implications for human risk extrapolation from data on experimental carcinogenesis. Genotoxic carcinogens, because of their effects on genetic material, pose a clear qualitative hazard to humans. These carcinogens are occasionally effective after a single exposure, act in a cumulative manner, and act together with other genotoxic carcinogens having the same organotropism. Thus, the level of human exposure acceptable for "no risk" to ensue needs to be evaluated most stringently in the light of existing data and relevant mechanisms. Often, with powerful carcinogens, zero exposure is the goal, even though with some agents there is evidence for practical no-effect levels. Further discussion will deal with these quantitative aspects.

On the other hand, some classes of epigenetic carcinogens have carcinogenic effects occurring only with high and sustained levels of exposure that lead to prolonged physiologic abnormalities, hormonal imbalances, or tissue injury. Consequently, the risk from exposure may be of a purely quantitative nature. This is almost certainly the case with peroxisome proliferators, which are carcinogenic in animal studies at chronic exposure levels which induce peroxisome proliferation. Levels that do not produce the primary biologic effect, such as cytotoxicity or peroxisome proliferation, would not be expected to be carcinogenic, even when large groups of animals or humans are exposed. Thus, for epigenetic carcinogens, it is possible to establish a "safe" threshold of exposure, once their mechanism of action is elucidated.

The types of chemicals found in each of the nine major classes are reviewed at the end of this chapter. It will be noted that not all carcinogens can be precisely categorized, pointing to the need for additional data (unclassified group). Also, in some instances, structurally related chemicals (for example the large number of halogenated hydrocarbons) fall into different classes as a consequence of their differing biologic or toxicologic properties.

BIOTRANSFORMATION OF CHEMICAL CARCINOGENS

The biotransformation of carcinogens and other xenobiotics is performed by enzyme systems that have evolved for the biotransformation of endogenous substrates (Guengerich, 1988; Parke, 1990). Within the broad category of genotoxic carcinogens, the metabolism of activation-independent carcinogens invariably leads to less active, or inactive, products and hence represents detoxification. With activation-dependent carcinogens, the metabolism of most is likewise in the direction of detoxified products (except for nitrosamines). In this process, certain quantitatively minor biotransformation steps result in the generation of reactive species, which constitute the proximate carcinogen, sometimes via an intermediary step. The consequences of biotransformation can be elucidated by examining the mutagenicity of metabolic products. For example, an activation-independent compound would register positive in the Ames test without additional biochemical activation by the usual liver S-9 fraction, whereas an activation-dependent, or a proximate, carcinogen would require such a biochemical activation. Liver fractions are used most often for routine in vitro tests, but fractions of other tissues have permitted elucidation of metabolic factors bearing on organotropism.

The activated reactive species of carcinogens was established by J. Miller and E. Miller in the United States to be an electrophile or radical cation. An electrophile is a chemical entity that is deficient in electrons and is therefore capable of forming a covalent bond with a nucleophile that has electrons to share. Typical electrophilic species and cellular nucleophiles are shown in Table 5–3.

Activation-Independent Carcinogens

Metabolism leads to loss of activity in the case of the primary direct acting electrophilic carcinogens. In view of their reactive nature, such reactions can be straightforward chemical processes, involving an SN_1 or an SN_2 type of chemical interaction with cellular nucleophiles. Other reactions, which differ as a function of the structure of the carcinogen, can be enzyme mediated. The relative effectiveness of agents depends in part on the relative rates of interaction between the chemical and genetic material, DNA, versus competing reactions with other cellular nucleophiles. Thus, the relative activity in a given series of chemicals hinges principally on such competing interactions and also on metabolic detoxification reactions. Stability during transport, permeability across membranes, and similar factors also play a role.

Reactivity toward nucleophilic sites also controls hydrolytic destruction of lactone and similar structures built on strained ring systems. Thus, β-propiolactone is more carcinogenic than higher homologs because of its reactivity. Ethylene oxide likewise hydrolyzes readily in mammalian cells and is detoxified. Inhalation of

Table 5–3. STRUCTURES OF REACTIVE ELECTROPHILES

Some chemicals (A) are inherently electrophilic whereas others (B) require biotransformation to yield an electrophile, or radical cation.

A. Examples of Reactive Electrophiles

1. Carbonium ions

$$R—\overset{\overset{\displaystyle H}{|}}{\underset{\underset{\displaystyle R}{|}}{C}}\oplus$$

2. Nitrenium ions

$$R—\overset{}{\underset{\underset{\displaystyle H}{|}}{N}}\oplus$$

3. Free radicals

$$R—\overset{\overset{\displaystyle H}{|}}{\underset{\underset{\displaystyle R}{|}}{C}}\cdot$$

4. Diazonium ions

$$R\text{-}\overset{\oplus}{N}\equiv N\ ^{\ominus}OH$$

5. Epoxides

$$\begin{array}{c}R\\R\end{array}\!\!\!\!\triangleright\!\!O$$

6. Aziridinium ions

$$\triangleright\!\!\underset{\oplus}{N}\!\!\begin{array}{c}R\\R\end{array}$$

7. Episulfonium ions

$$\triangleright\!\!\overset{\oplus}{S}\text{-}R$$

8. Strained Lactones

(strained β-lactone structure with O and =O)

9. Sulfonates

$$RSO_2OCH_3$$

10. Halo ethers

$$ClCH_2OCH_2Cl$$

11. Enals

$$RCH=CHC\overset{\displaystyle O}{\underset{\displaystyle H}{}}$$

B. Examples of Compounds that Can be Converted to Electrophiles

1. To Carbonium ions

$$\underset{\underset{\displaystyle R_1}{|}}{\overset{\overset{\displaystyle N=O}{|}}{RCHNCHR_2}} \longrightarrow \underset{\underset{\displaystyle R_1\ \ OH}{|\ \ \ |}}{\overset{\overset{\displaystyle N=O}{|}}{RCHNCR_2}} \longrightarrow \underset{\underset{\displaystyle R_1}{|}}{RCH\text{-}N=NOH}$$

$$\underset{\underset{\displaystyle R_1\ \ O}{|\ \ \ ||}}{\overset{\overset{\displaystyle N=O}{|}}{RCHN\text{-}C\text{-}R}} \longrightarrow \underset{\underset{\displaystyle R_1}{|}}{RCH=NOH} \longrightarrow \underset{\underset{\displaystyle R_1}{|}}{\overset{\overset{\displaystyle H}{|}}{R\overset{}{C}\oplus}}$$

substantial quantities can overcome local hydrolytic capability and hence induce neoplasia in the nasal septum. In general, the rate of hydrolytic attack of these direct acting chemicals either by water in the host or mediated, in the case of esters, by enzymes affects carcinogenic potency. Such agents are also detoxified readily by chemical or enzyme-mediated reactions with

Table 5–3. *(Continued)*

Some chemicals (A) are inherently electrophilic whereas others (B) require biotransformation to yield an electrophile, or radical cation.

2. To Nitrenium ions

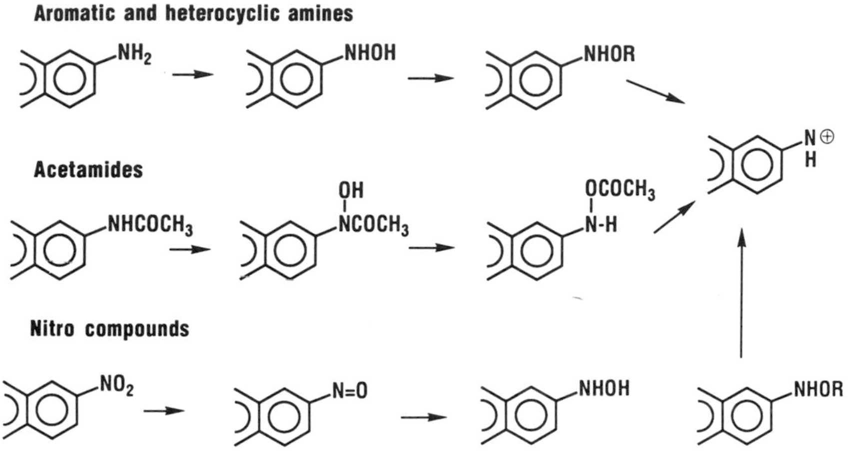

Aromatic and heterocyclic amines

$-NH_2 \rightarrow -NHOH \rightarrow -NHOR \rightarrow$

Acetamides

$$-NHCOCH_3 \rightarrow \overset{OH}{-NCOCH_3} \rightarrow \overset{OCOCH_3}{-N-H} \rightarrow \overset{N\oplus}{\underset{H}{}}$$

Nitro compounds

$-NO_2 \rightarrow -N=O \rightarrow -NHOH \quad -NHOR$

3. To free radicals

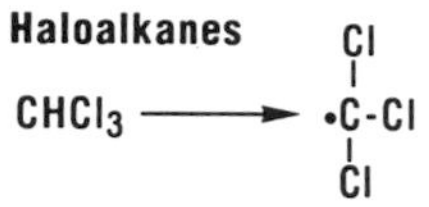

Haloalkanes

$$CHCl_3 \longrightarrow \overset{Cl}{\underset{Cl}{\cdot C\text{-}Cl}}$$

4. To diazonium ions

Nitroso compounds

$$\overset{O}{\overset{\|}{C}}CH_2CH_2CH_2N\overset{N=O}{\underset{CH_3}{}} \longrightarrow \overset{O}{\overset{\|}{C}}CH_2CH_2CHN\overset{N=O}{\underset{\overset{|}{OH}}{\underset{CH_3}{}}}$$

$$\overset{N=O}{\underset{\|}{CH_3N\text{-}C\text{-}NH_2}} \longrightarrow CH_3N\overset{\oplus}{\equiv}N \; {}^{\ominus}OH$$

Symmetrical hydrazines

$$CH_3NHNHCH_3 \longrightarrow CH_3N=NCH_3 \longrightarrow \underset{O^{\ominus}}{CH_3\overset{\oplus}{N}=NCH_3} \longrightarrow \underset{O^{\ominus}}{CH_3\overset{\oplus}{N}=NCH_2OH}$$

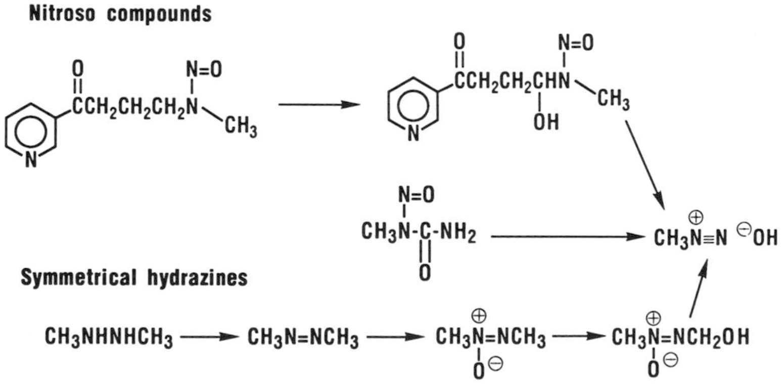

sulfur amino acids and peptides such as glutathione, yielding eventually the corresponding mercapturic acids. Reactions such as these produce compounds that appear more acutely toxic, because of their reaction with specific life supporting enzymes, and of lower carcinogenicity than might be expected from the reactive nature of this type of carcinogens.

Activation-Dependent Carcinogens

Most of the chemical carcinogens in the environment belong to this class. In contrast to

Table 5–3. (*Continued*)

5. To epoxides

Polycyclic aromatic hydrocarbons

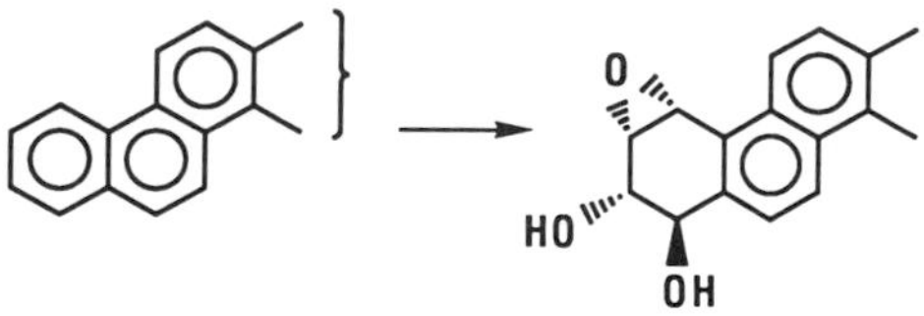
O
HO
OH

Aflatoxins

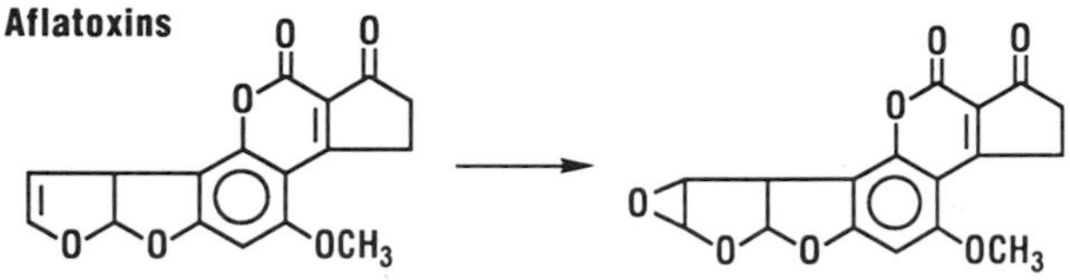
O O
O
O O
OCH3
O O
O
O
O O
OCH3

Alkenes

ClCH=CH2
O
ClCH-CH2

6. To aziridinium ions

Nitrogen mustards

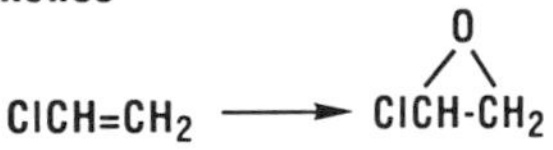

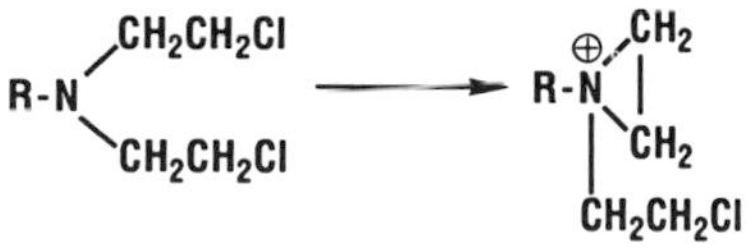
CH2CH2Cl
R-N
CH2CH2Cl
⊕ CH2
R-N
CH2
CH2CH2Cl

7. To episulfonium ions

Ethylene dibromide

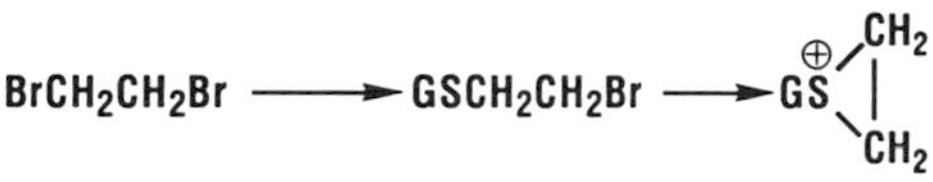

BrCH2CH2Br
GSCH2CH2Br
⊕ CH2
GS
CH2

GS= glutathione

---

activation-independent carcinogens, which are chemically reactive and therefore do not persist in the environment, activation-dependent carcinogens are often chemically stable entities. They are subject to a great variety of biotransformation reactions by mammalian as well as bacterial enzyme systems. Most of these biochemical reactions yield detoxified metabolites, but in the process toxication or activation reactions take place (Guengerich, 1988; Cooper and Grover, 1990). The activated metabolites usually account for only a small portion of a dose of most carcinogens, nitrosamines being a notable exception. A determination of the main metabolites, as is often performed in studies of drug, food additive, or pesticide metabolism, in part to fulfill regulatory requirements, would probably fail to identify the key active metabolites because of their small amount or transient nature.

A combination of the techniques of biochemical pharmacology and *in vivo* and *in vitro* studies of genetic toxicology testing constitutes a most useful approach to assess whether a given chemical is converted even in small yield to a potentially harmful DNA-reactive metabolite. If such a reactive product is detected, separation techniques can be directed toward isolating it for the purpose of structural identification. These procedures are useful not only for academic purposes but in general to assess whether or not under certain circumstances a potentially harmful product is present or has been generated through metabolism. As noted above, because the major metabolites of chemicals are often of little toxicologic consequence, this approach would permit a decision to be made as to possible adverse effects stemming from a given material. As will be discussed, not all such indications of electrophile characteristics necessarily imply hazard, and thus no immediate regulatory decision should be taken with materials that have apparent electrophile character. On the other hand, the presence of this property is a warning signal that cannot be ignored and must be investigated in detail.

It is outside the scope of this chapter to elaborate on all the known metabolic activation reactions for chemical carcinogens. Specific details have been provided for certain major and historically important classes, polycyclic aromatic hydrocarbons, aromatic amines, and nitrosamines. Here, only the general principles of these activation reactions will be discussed. Most of these reactions consist of biochemical oxidation or hydroxylation, performed by enzyme systems associated with the endoplasmic reticulum. The main enzymes, including the complex cytochromes, prostaglandin synthetases, and specific cofactors, exist in virtually all tissues in all species, but in differing amounts and often with a specificity for certain substrates (see Chapter 4). It is this feature that accounts in part for the organ-specific localization of the action of individual chemical carcinogens. Carcinogens are active at certain sites under specific conditions because of the presence of the necessary activation enzyme system. Liver is the organ with the greatest capacity for metabolizing chemical carcinogens because it contains the greatest concentration of the cytochrome P-450 system. Nevertheless, other organs, particularly kidney, lung, and the gastrointestinal tract have a definite specific capability. In addition, the metabolic fate of several carcinogens is dependent on, or affected by, the action of the bacterial flora in the gut. Cycasin, the β-glucoside of methylazoxymethanol, is split only by the mediation of bacterial enzymes. With other agents, such as simple azo dyes, the bacterial flora may assume mainly a detoxifying role, by virtue of its reducing capability. Inasmuch as diet and other conditions modify the gut microflora, the metabolism of carcinogens, drugs, and chemicals affected by the flora could be indirectly modulated. The activation of most carcinogens is mediated by mixed function oxidases which are part of the cytochrome P-450 system (see Chapter 4 for details on this system). Other oxidations may be performed by prostaglandin synthetases, peroxidases, xanthine oxidases, and the like. Such oxidations are designated as phase I reactions.

In some cases, reductive enzymes yield activated intermediates as, for example, the conversion of nitroaryl or nitroheterocyclic compounds to the corresponding hydroxylamino derivatives. This bacterial reduction accounts for the mutagenicity, without requiring biochemical activation, of these chemicals. The active intermediate of 4-nitroquinoline-*N*-oxide is the corresponding 4-hydroxylamino derivative, through the action of soluble xanthine oxidase. In other cases, the active intermediate is released from a transport form such as glucuronide conjugate by enzymic systems or a suitable pH in certain target organs, as for example the urinary bladder.

Some carcinogens require a series of activation steps that involves not only the cytochrome systems, but also other oxidative, reductive, or conjugative type I or type II enzymes. Examples discussed above are the aromatic amines and polycyclic aromatic hydrocarbons, or the specific action of halogenated hydrocarbon thioconjugates made in the liver and released for further activation by β-lyases in the kidneys.

When organic chemicals can be converted to electrophilic reagents within cells, they are almost certain to act as DNA-reactive carcinogens. However, administration of the same chemicals in their reactive form may be innocuous, for they can react with competing nucleophilic substrates such as water or select protein or peptide end groups, such as glutathione. Thus, the sulfate ester of N-hydroxy-N-2-acetylaminofluorene, although highly mutagenic, is not carcinogenic when administered to animals, simply because it undergoes rapid side reactions prior to reaching targets where it could be carcinogenic. Certain alkylating agents undergo similar reactions and are less carcinogenic than might be surmised on the basis of their structure. On the other hand, agents such as alkylnitrosoureas or alkylnitrosourethan which, because of their chemical configuration, can readily penetrate organ and cellular membranes and release the active alkyl carbonium ions inside cells by spontaneous or enzyme-mediated hydrolytic mechanisms, are among the most dangerous carcinogenic chemicals. Thus, intracellular activation is a major factor in the carcinogenicity of many chemicals.

REACTIONS OF CHEMICAL CARCINOGENS

Cellular Macromolecules

The study of the interaction of carcinogens with cellular constituents began with the observation by the Millers in 1947 of the detectable color produced in rat liver when carcinogens of the azo dye type reacted with liver proteins (Miller and Miller, 1981). The hues of the dyes bound to tissue proteins were pH dependent. As sensitive and specific techniques, mainly the use of carcinogens tagged with isotope, were established and as new knowledge on the function, isolation, and purification of other key cellular macromolecules such as various types of RNA and DNA became available, it was discovered that many chemical carcinogens associate with a variety of cellular and molecular entities.

Early work focused on the binding to proteins, leading to the recognition that there are two types of binding: reversible binding to acceptor proteins such as albumin or a specific globulin serving as transport carriers, and nonspecific irreversible covalent binding. Intracellular transport from cytoplasm or endoplasmic reticulum to nucleus may also involve a transport protein, sometimes a specific receptor.

The binding to acceptor proteins may be very important for certain of the biologic effects of carcinogens. For example, TCDD (2,3,7,8-tetracherodibenzo-p-dioxin) is a highly toxic material that has a high affinity for a receptor. This specific recognition step is probably required for the expression of the toxicity of TCDD, but does not account for all its effects.

As with protein, RNA is also a target for electrophilic reactants. Interactions have been demonstrated with transfer RNA, messenger RNA, and ribosomal RNA. Such interactions are very likely involved in the inhibition of protein synthesis which occurs with toxic doses of carcinogens, but have not been mechanistically linked to carcinogenesis.

DNA

Progressing from studies on protein and RNA binding of carcinogens, it was eventually established in the early 1960s, mainly by P. D. Lawley, P. Brookes, and P. N. Magee in the United Kingdom, that binding to DNA occurred, although at much lower levels than with other macromolecules. Subsequently, the nucleic acid bases to which carcinogens bind and the nature of the adducts formed have been extensively studied. Carcinogens that act as alkylating agents, for example nitrosamines, introduce a variety of lesions into DNA. Most monofunctional methylating agents, such as methyl methanesulfonate, produce primarily 7-methylguanine, an adduct that is believed to be innocuous due to its inability to block nucleic acid synthesis or cause misincorporation of bases in newly synthesized DNA. This altered base, however, has been postulated to be indirectly deleterious to cells due to the increased lability of the glycosidic bond, leading to the formation of noninstructive apurinic sites in the DNA template. Another abundant lesion formed is 3-methyladenine. This product has been shown to block nucleic acid synthesis, but direct evidence that it is a lethal moiety in mammalian cells is lacking. The primary promutagenic lesions formed by methylating agents are O^6-methylguanine and O-^{4}-methylthymine, both of which can cause base transitions in newly synthesized DNA (see Chapter 6). O^6-Methylguanine is formed to a higher extent than O-^{4}-methylthymine, and it has been demonstrated that guanines preceded at 5' by adenine are twice as likely to be methylated at the O^6 position as those preceded by thymine, indicating the existence of base sequence effects on adduct formation. Another lesion formed by methylating agents is the methylphosphotriester. This persistent adduct clearly slows nucleic acid synthesis in cell-free systems, but its effect on gene expression or mutagenesis in cells is not clear.

Longer chain alkylating agents produce similar spectra of damage, but the relative proportions of the adducts formed are significantly different. The lesions formed in the greatest quantities are the alkylphosphotriesters, which represent more than 50 percent of the total damage to the DNA. The promutagenic lesion that becomes increasingly important with these agents is O^4-alkylthymine. It is produced in amounts five- to tenfold greater than occur with methylating agents, and, although it is slowly removed from DNA, its half-life is significantly longer than that for O^6-alkylguanine, making it potentially more important in causing point mutations following DNA synthesis.

Bifunctional alkylating agents react with DNA to form mono-adducts as the initial damage followed by di-adduct formation (Barbin and Bartsch, 1989). The final lesions include DNA interstrand cross-links and DNA protein cross-links. The biologic consequences of these adducts are indeed quite serious. Covalent linkage of the DNA strands prevents dissociation of the helix during transcription and replication, impeding proper gene expression and cell growth. An example of a bifunctional alkylating agent is the antineoplastic drug chloroethylnitrosourea, which is carcinogenic.

Many agents that react with DNA form additional rings with the purine and pyrimidine constituents. These lesions fall into the broad category of cyclic nucleic acid adducts. Examples of compounds that produce cyclic derivatives are 1,2-dicarbonyls, aldehydes, vinyl halides, and alkyl carbamates. Most of these compounds are mutagenic and carcinogenic, but the specific mechanisms by which they initiate tumors are not well understood. Some of these cyclic adducts are the end products of more complex carcinogens such as the tobacco-specific nitrosamines (Hecht and Hoffmann, 1988). Many of the adducts formed interfere with the sites of hydrogen bonding in DNA and may exert their toxic and mutagenic actions by interfering with replication and transcription.

Carcinogens that yield reactive electrophilic species (see Table 5–3 for requisite structures) are capable of sharing electrons with nucleophiles and thereby forming covalent bonds. Nucleophilic sites in cellular macromolecules are principally carbon, nitrogen, oxygen, and sulfur. In proteins, the main reactive sites appear to be tryptophan, tyrosine, methionine, and perhaps histidine. In one instance, reaction with glycogen has been documented. These chemical interactions relate not only to the carcinogenic process but also to other toxic reactions.

The ability of carcinogens to interact with DNA was disputed in the early years when protein interactions were of principal interest. However, the demonstration of the interaction of polycyclic aromatic hydrocarbons with DNA by Brookes, Lawley, and Sims in the United Kingdom and Heidelberger and Gelboin in the United States opened this area of investigation. Subsequently, numerous carcinogens of the electro-

philic reactant type have been found to bind to DNA. This in turn led to the development of tests for genetic effects to detect such carcinogens (see Chapter 6).

Carcinogens that introduce bulkier adducts have also been studied in detail. With aflatoxin B_1, reaction of the bioactivated epoxide occurs at N-7 in guanine (Wogan, 1989). The metabolite derived from 2-acetylaminofluorene forms adducts on guanine at N-2 and C-8, as is true for a number of other arylamines (King et al., 1988; Weinstein, 1988; Howard et al., 1990). With the polycyclic aromatic hydrocarbon benzo[a]pyrene, through its activated form, the (R,S,S,R) isomer of the 7,8-dihydrodiol-9,10-epoxide, the reaction is through the 10 carbon of the benzo[a]pyrene metabolite to the 2-amino position in guanylic acid (Conney, 1982; Weinstein, 1988). In addition, there are also minor interactions with other purines and pyrimidines in DNA, as a function of the type of carcinogen and the tissue and cells affected.

As a result of interaction with DNA, DNA-reactive carcinogens generally exhibit genotoxicity in cellular systems (see Chapter 6), in which appropriate activation is provided. However, because of their high reactivity and electrophilic character, direct acting genotoxic carcinogens are often more active in the in vitro systems but less carcinogenic in animal biossays because of rapid detoxification in vivo.

Certain chemicals that can intercalate into the DNA strands in the absence of covalent binding are mutagenic to phage and bacteria. However, there is no documentation that carcinogenicity in mammalian systems arises from pure intercalation without covalent binding. On the other hand, it is clear that the molecular size and shape of covalently bound carcinogens can play a role in determining quantitative responses such as DNA repair or the events involved in mutagenesis and carcinogenesis. Thus, stereochemical molecular attractions are involved that facilitate the attachment of carcinogen to DNA mainly prior to and also after covalent bonds are formed. This is especially true with aromatic or heterocyclic compounds where potency increases with the number of rings up to an optimum of five or six benzene rings, or equivalent. Even here, specific stereoisomers of reactive molecules are the key active metabolites (Conney, 1982). Certain heterocyclic arylamines are among the most mutagenic chemicals known because of physical noncovalent attraction facilitating covalent binding.

Thus, considerable knowledge has accrued on the interaction with DNA of genotoxic carcinogens and a variety of techniques are available for detecting DNA adducts. However, few details are available on how the altered steric and chemical properties of DNA with covalent-bound carcinogen adducts affect transcription of the genetic code and its translation into phenotypic characteristics.

DNA Repair

Damaged DNA can be repaired by several distinct systems. The efficacy of repair bears on the organ specificity of the carcinogen. For example, methylnitrosourea reacts readily with DNA of the kidney, liver, and brain, but the damage is repaired in liver and somewhat less readily in kidney, and very slowly in brain. This accounts for the fact that under certain experimental conditions methylnitrosourea or ethylnitrosourea induces brain cancer in rodents. The three principal repair systems in mammalian cells are nucleotide excision, base excision, and O^6-alkylguanine transferase. In nucleotide excision, which often is elicited by chemicals that introduce bulky adducts, a stretch of DNA surrounding the lesion is removed. Base excision, which often occurs with small modifications of DNA such as alkylation, can involve removal of a single damaged base or a few adjacent bases. The O^6-alkylguanine transferase system specifically transfers alkyl groups from the O^6 of guanine to cysteine in protein, thus effecting repair of the alkylated site (Hanawalt, 1989).

Implications

DNA damage can lead to a number of serious consequences. Certain types of damage can activate genes. If damage persists when the cell enters the S phase of DNA replication cell death and mutation may occur. Mutations in certain critical genes appear to be the basis for the evolution of neoplastic cells.

A new primary tool to explore specific alterations in designated genes is the development of transgenic mice. The desired genetic elements is injected in a fertilized mouse embryo. Such genetically modified mice develop neoplasms derived from the injected gene element, and form excellent models for the determination of the molecular events associated with further genotoxic carcinogen or epigenetic agent exposures (Yuspa and Poirier, 1988).

INTERACTIVE CARCINOGENESIS

Types of Enhancement of Carcinogenesis

Syncarcinogenesis. A number of studies involving mixtures of chemical carcinogens of the type designated here as genotoxic have indicated that, when these agents act on the same target organ, the effects are additive and sometimes synergistic. For example, administration of a carcinogenic azo dye and diethylnitrosamine, both of which affect the liver, results in an increased incidence of liver tumors. On the other hand, agents that have distinct organ specificity often exert their carcinogenic effect independently. The tumor incidence in the various target organs is the same as when the two agents are administered separately. The latent period, too, is the same, provided it is similar for both agents. For example, a carcinogenic azo dye that affects the liver and 4-dimethylaminostilbene, which affects the ear duct, do not interact, because when given jointly, both types of neoplasms are seen in similar yields to what occurs when the carcinogens are administered individually.

The additive or synergistic effect of two carcinogens is designated as syncarcinogenesis. Two types may be distinguished: combination syncarcinogenesis in which the two carcinogens are given together and sequential syncarcinogenesis in which they are given one after another. It is important that initiation/promotion be distinguished from the latter, the sequential action of carcinogens. Two principal features distinguish these phenomena: (1) in syncarcinogenesis, both carcinogens are usually DNA reactive, whereas promoters are not; and (2) in syncarcinogenesis the sequence of compound administration can be reversed, and the effect maintained whereas promotion must follow initiation. Finally, promoters do not necessarily cause cancer themselves.

More detailed and realistic studies of such interactions between carcinogens are needed to shed light on possible interactions between agents in the complex environment in which humans live, or to which they are exposed with consequent real cancer risks, as to tobacco smoke, or certain nutritional traditions (Weisburger and Horn, 1991).

Distinction Between Cocarcinogenesis and Promotion. There are also noncarcinogenic chemicals that augment, sometimes very appreciably, the effect of a primary carcinogen. Originally, Berenblum (1974) defined all such agents as cocarcinogens. Thus, promoters were one type of cocarcinogen. However, more commonly a distinction has been made whereby cocarcinogens modify the effectiveness of a carcinogen present at the same time, whereas promotion occurs subsequent to the exposure to a carcinogen. According to this differentiation, cocarcinogens would enhance the first sequence of the carcinogenic process (Figure 5–1), neoplastic conversion, whereas promoters would produce their effects in the second sequence, neoplastic development. To maintain this mechanistic distinction, it must be recognized that cocarcinogens can also act after exposure to a DNA-reactive carcinogen at a time when DNA damage is still persistent, for example by increasing the rate of DNA replication, mitosis, and cell duplication. Also, promotion can take place during carcinogen administration if neoplastic conversion has occurred. Thus, to distinguish between these forms of enhancement requires detailed mechanistic studies.

Cocarcinogenesis. Cocarcinogens are agents that enhance the overall carcinogenic process initiated by a genotoxic carcinogen when administered before or together with the carcinogen or at a time when carcinogen damage to DNA is still persistent. Accordingly, cocarcinogenesis applies to events occurring during neoplastic conversion (Figure 5–1). The relevant mechanisms can be one or more of several possibilities: (1) increased uptake or availability of a carcinogen; (2) enhanced metabolic activation of a genotoxic carcinogen or decreased detoxification; (3) inhibition of DNA repair processes; and (4) increased proliferation of cells with DNA damage, thereby facilitating mutation, codon translocation, or amplification.

The demonstration of cocarcinogenesis was made over 40 years ago by Berenblum and Shubik, and by Shear (see Berenblum, 1974). Berenblum and Shubik noted that application of a carcinogenic polycyclic aromatic hydrocarbon to mouse skin together with croton oil, an oil extracted from the seed of a Euphorbiacea, *Croton tiglium L.*, induced a much higher incidence of skin cancer than in controls given the carcinogen alone. The cocarcinogenic action of croton oil was found to be species specific, not being demonstrable in the rabbit, rat, or guinea pig. The active constituents in croton oil eventually isolated and identified by Hecker and by Van Duuren (Schmidt and Hecker, 1989) were shown to be phorbol esters. The mechanisms of action of phorbol esters as enhancers when applied together with polycylic aromatic hydrocarbons to mouse skin depend on tissue damage, followed by regeneration, i.e., enhanced DNA synthesis and cell cycling. The molecular mechanisms involve induction of ornithine decarboxylase (ODC), and polyamine metabolism (Blumberg, 1988; Pegg, 1988). An antimetabolite, *d*-dimethylfluoroornithine, blocks ODC and promotion not only on mouse skin, but in other tissues, where ODC release is involved. Phorbol esters produced enhancement long after cessation of carcinogen exposure, which was interpreted to show that they promoted growth of dormant neoplastic cells into tumors. It could be that they act also as promoters even during concurrent administration of a carcinogen, if neoplastic conversion has occurred. In the mouse skin system not all cocarcinogens are promoters, catechol being an example. However, not many thorough studies have been done in other systems to distinguish mechanistically between cocarcinogenesis and promotion. Various forms of chemical or physical injury occurring before carcinogen exposure are cocarcinogenic by virtue of stimulating cell proliferation such that more cells are in DNA synthesis at the time of carcinogen damage to DNA and are, therefore, more susceptible to genetic alteration (Clayson *et al.*, 1989). Contemporary knowledge suggests that the levels of DNA replication and mitosis are significant parameters in the overall process of carcinogenesis (Lipkin, 1988). Lower DNA synthesis decreases promotion not only on mouse skin, but in other tissues, where ODC release is involved.

Cocarcinogens are important agents in human cancer. Tobacco smoke contains relatively small amounts of DNA-reactive carcinogens such as tobacco-specific nitrosamines, polycyclic aromatic hydrocarbons, and possibly certain pyrolysis products of proteins in the form of α- or β-carbolines and related materials. However, the enhancing factors such as catechols and other phenols, and also terpenes in tobacco smoke, play an essential role in the overall effect of the smoke in leading to human cancer. For that reason, removal of the pressure of the action of promoters on discontinuation of smoking progressively reduces the risk of cancer development, excellent evidence in a large population that promotion is reversible.

In addition, it has been shown that individuals who smoke and also drink alcoholic beverages regularly in appreciable amounts have a higher risk of head and neck cancers. It is likely that ethanol under these conditions functions as a cocarcinogen in augmenting the metabolic conversion of tobacco procarcinogens such as polycyclic aromatic hydrocarbons or nitrosamines to the reactive electrophilic products in the target organs (Seitz and Simanowski, 1988; Hoffmann and Hecht, in Cooper and Grover, 1990). Such a mechanism is demonstrated by the finding that the conversion of the model compound nitrosopyrrolidine to a mutagen is increased in rats concurrently given alcohol, and a higher yield of esophagus cancer is obtained. A greater conversion of benzo[*a*]pyrene to reactive carcinogenic metabolites occurred in rats on alcohol. Thus, cocarcinogenicity represents a major factor in determining human disease risk with the life style-associated important types of cancer.

Promotion. This phenomenon was first demonstrated in the laboratories of Rous, and of

Berenblum and Shubik in studies of skin carcinogenesis. In these experiments, croton oil was shown to have a highly specific and exquisite enhancing effect on cancer development in mouse skin when applied after a known carcinogen. In an impressive series of experiments it was shown that the genotoxic event, application of a polycyclic aromatic hydrocarbon, can be followed months later and, in fact, one year later by a promoting stimulus, such as the application of phorbol esters from croton oil, and still result in the production of skin tumors. From these observations developed the "two-stage" concept of carcinogenesis: initiation and promotion. In these studies, promotion was defined as the facilitation of growth of a latent neoplastic cell into a tumor. Conceptually then, promotion applies to events occurring after the completion of neoplastic conversion of the cell (Figure 5–1). However, in many other studies, particularly current ones, promotion has been used broadly to describe any situation yielding an increased development of neoplasms, through the action of a nongenotoxic agent. The active constituent of croton oil, certain phorbol esters, are true promoters. Sulfur, sulfur compounds, aldehydes, phenols, dodecane, and a number of natural products, discovered because they increased ODC, represent other examples of enhancers of the effect of polycyclic aromatic hydrocarbons and other carcinogens for mouse skin. In some of these instances, where the promoter was applied less than one week after the genotoxic carcinogen, it is not certain whether the increase in carcinogenicity results from a true promoting action, or from a more effective activity of the primary carcinogen as a result of effect on carcinogen damaged cells with persistent DNA adducts, a function that in contemporary terms would be better labelled cocarcinogenesis. Such sizable enhancing effects may account for the carcinogenicity of petroleum products, cutting oils, tobacco smoke, and the like, which is much greater than might be suspected from their content of carcinogenic polycyclic aromatic hydrocarbons and other genotoxic carcinogens. The same applies to roofing tar workers exposed to fumes of asphalt. To distinguish promotion from cocarcinogenesis, the agent must be tested at a sufficient interval after carcinogen application to allow for complete DNA repair.

Although phorbol esters remain a popular experimental model, a number of other promoters for different organ systems have been discovered (Fujiki et al., 1989). Hormones increase carcinogenicity through a mechanism of promotion when present in abnormal amounts (Bulbrook, 1986; Henderson et al., 1988). Bile acids and some other fatty acids are excellent promoters in colon carcinogenesis (American Health Foundation, 1987). In bladder carcinogenesis, high levels of saccharin or tryptophan are promoters (Cohen and Ellwein, 1990). Peraino and coworkers (Bannasch et al., 1989; Stevenson et al., 1990) observed that certain inducers of liver metabolic enzyme systems, such as phenobarbital, DDT (dichlorodiphenyltrichloroethane), and BHT (butylated hydroxytoluene) exerted enhancing effects when administered after small doses of 2-acetylaminofluorene, perhaps because they increase selectively cell duplication of transformed cells. In most instances, these same chemicals when administered together with hepatocarcinogens decrease the effect, because they induce type II enzymes, leading to conjugation, and thus inactivation, and elimination of the proximate carcinogenic metabolite (Weisburger, in Sontag, 1981).

The mechanism of the promoting effect of chemicals when administered after a primary carcinogen is complex and is not yet fully clear. Numerous studies have shown that phorbol esters exert various types of effects on cellular membranes and specifically bind to protein kinase C (Blumberg, 1988; Schmidt and Hecker, 1989). Phorbol esters can also produce gene derepression and repression.

Research in other systems has led to a concept of promotion, which is consistent with the original definition of Berenblum, and the mechanistic distinction developed above. Following neoplastic conversion of cells by a genotoxic carcinogen, these latent tumor cells in contact with normal can be visualized to be held in check by regulatory processes that maintain normal tissue homeostasis. Cells are able to interact with one another through specialized membrane structures known as gap junctions which permit the transfer of rather large molecular weight substances up to 1200 daltons having a growth regulatory function (Milman and Elmore, 1987). Possibly these gap junctions serve to transfer the factors that inhibit the growth of latent tumor cells. The groups of Trosko in the United States and Murray and Fitzgerald in Australia (Banbury Rept. 31, 1988; Stevenson et al., 1990) have shown in cell culture studies that tumor promoters are capable of inhibiting intercellular molecular exchange through gap junctions. Such inhibition in vivo, if it impeded transfer of regulatory factors, would serve to release dormant neoplastic cells for growth in tumors. It has been shown in the laboratories of Kitagawa, Pitot, and Williams that liver tumor promoters enhance the development of preneoplastic liver lesions. This action could reflect the release of abnormal cells from regulatory control.

Sound data now indicate that in humans cancer

of the larger bowel, pancreas, breast, prostate, ovary, and endometrium may depend to a very considerable extent not only on specific carcinogens but also on promoting phenomena and enhancing factors generally (American Health Foundation, 1987; Rogers and Longnecker, 1988; Weisburger and Horn, 1990). The evidence stems from a consideration of the diverse incidence of these diseases in various parts of the world as well as studies of the relevant mechanisms in animal models. Populations in a high-risk region for the types of neoplasms enumerated above, such as the United States, typically have a dietary intake high in fat, on the order of 40 percent of calories. On the other hand, the population of a country where the incidence is low usually consume diets low in fat, about 10 to 20 percent of calories. Simulation of such conditions in animal models shows that animals on a high-fat diet develop, for example, colon, pancreatic, or breast cancer in higher yield after doses of the appropriate carcinogens. In the case of colon cancer, a high-fat diet has been shown to lead to high flow of bile acids through the gut, and further that bile acids are good promoters in colon carcinogenesis. Humans on a high-fat diet also have higher intestinal levels of bile acids. Further evidence supporting this phenomenon comes from an explanation for the lower risk of Finnish people for colon cancer because of their simultaneous intake of a high-fiber wheat bran diet while consuming high levels of fat, in which the fiber, increasing stool bulk, acts as a nonspecific diluent and possibly specific absorbent of bile acids. In regard to the endocrine related cancers such as breast, endometrium, and prostate, current data show that dietary fat modulates hormonal balances which in turn may act as promoters. However, thus far, no synthetic chemical promoting agent, apart from hormones, has been implicated in human cancer, probably because exposure levels have been below thresholds.

A better understanding of the phenomenon of promotion may provide additional means to reduce cancer risk, complementing procedures to lower exposure to carcinogens. This is expected to be a fruitful approach insofar as animal experiments have indicated that with the same level of carcinogens, the incidence of cancer induced can be affected dramatically by changing the promotional stimulus. Humans who stop smoking have a progressively lower cancer risk. Current efforts to have people in the Western world lower total fat intake from 40 to 20 percent of total calories are designed on the principle that promotion, and hence cancer risk (American Health Foundation, 1987), would be appreciably reduced. In contrast, the risks of gastric cancer in migrants from high-incidence regions (Asia, Northern and Eastern Europe) to low-incidence situations (United States) retain risk, because gastric cancer induction involves mainly genotoxic carcinogens (in pickled, smoked fish or meat), a cocarcinogen (salt), but little promotion (Weisburger and Horn, 1991).

Chemical-Physical Interactions

Asbestos, which by itself produces pleural and peritoneal mesotheliomas, but infrequently yields lung cancer, contributes not additively but synergistically to the development of bronchogenic lung cancer in cigarette smokers who have occupational exposure. Asbestos and similar fibrous products thus have the properties of a cocarcinogen or promoter. In support of this point, asbestos has potentiated the effects of carcinogens in cell cultures. It is important, therefore, to control extensive exposure to asbestos and other mineral dusts. For those individuals who were unfortunately years or decades ago exposed to asbestos that cannot be removed from the respiratory tract, efforts to reduce their risk for lung cancer should involve smoking cessation programs.

Chemical-Radiation Interactions

In the United States alone there are about 500,000 cases per year of skin cancer. This disease carries a low mortality rate, about 1 percent, because it is detected early and cured. Skin cancer in humans and in parallel studies in hairless mice is induced by the ultraviolet (UV) component of sunlight. The molecular mechanism is the modification of DNA under the effect of light, mainly through the formation of thymine dimers. Individuals differ in repair capability. Highly sensitive to light are people with xeroderma pigmentosum, because of a genetically controlled defect in DNA-repair capability. Less prone, but still more sensitive than people from the Mediterranean, Asian, or African population, are individuals of Celtic origin. Some medications, e.g., the family of psoralenes, are activated by a component of UV radiation to yield DNA-reactive components, in turn leading to neoplasia.

In the United States, the incidence of malignant melanoma has risen. This condition is also associated with exposure to light. In the Nordic countries, melanoma had a low incidence 60 years ago, but has risen dramatically since then. The probable explanation is the greater mobility of Nordic people, who during the dark winters travel to southern areas. This sudden, although temporary, exposure to active sunlight appears sufficient to increase the risk of this malignancy.

Ultraviolet light is considered to be a cause of nonmelanocytic skin cancer and lip cancer in humans. Broad hard sources of UV radiation have been shown to induce skin cancers in numerous strains of mice. A variety of furocoumarins and psoralens have produced skin tumors in mice when administered with UV radiation, but not when given alone (Chambers *et al.*, 1988). These agents can be photoactivated to DNA-binding products.

Chemical-Viral Interactions

Several types of cancer in animals have a viral origin, e.g., certain leukemias, lymphomas, and mammary tumors in mice, leading to the suspicion that similar cancers in humans may have a viral etiology (Wyke and Weiss, 1984; Levine, 1988; Klein, 1989). An antecedent viral hepatitis has been postulated to account for the occurrence of human liver cancer in certain tropical countries (IARC Sci. Publ. 63, 1984; Yeh *et al.*, 1989), where this disease has a high incidence at a young age, especially in males. There is a replicate of this phenomenon in animals (De Flora *et al.*, 1989). In these areas of the world, consumption of foodstuffs contaminated with mycotoxins or Senecio alkaloids, which are liver carcinogens, also occurs, suggesting that both a virus and a chemical may be involved. Cervical cancer, a major neoplastic disease in the developing world and in the lower socioeconomic groups in the developed countries, has been associated with poor sexual hygiene, early age at onset of sexual intercourse, and multiplicity of partners. Human papilloma and herpes simplex viruses and smoking have been identified as causative factors (Banbury Rept. 21, 1986; IARC Sci. Publ. 94, 1989).

Carcinogens that are known to interact with DNA can also affect viral DNA sequences that are carried within mammalian cells. These sequences may be activated through either direct or indirect processes. A direct mechanism would involve interaction of the carcinogen with viral DNA, leading to alterations in the viral codon sequences, similar to those that occur in genomic DNA. Such alterations may affect the regulation of the viral transcription or replication, thereby leading to increased or decreased expression of viral proteins or overall viral sequences. An indirect process may involve changes in expression of cellular proteins that regulate the expression/replication of the viral sequences. The latter mechanism has been shown to occur with several DNA viruses (SV40, polyoma) that can be activated through protein factors that can act in *trans* (i.e., ability of proteins obtained from UV-damaged cells to induce replication of polyoma virus when the latter are tested in non-treated cells) on the viral sequences (Ronai *et al.*, 1990). These observations suggest that viral infection when combined with exposure to certain carcinogens may have a synergistic effect on the multistep carcinogenesis process (Weinstein, 1988).

It is also possible that viral infection, when combined with DNA damage caused by chemical carcinogens, may increase the susceptibility to tumor formation. This type of mechanism could be supported in one of the following mechanisms: (1) Effect on cell multiplication. Some viruses, on infection, increase rates of cell multiplication, which in the presence of a carcinogen may lead to enhanced changes at the genomic DNA level. (2) Viral reactivation of synchronous replication. Several types of DNA viruses, such as polyoma virus, SV40, herpes virus, hepatitis virus, and adeno-associated helper virus, respond to both chemical and physical carcinogens by synchronous DNA replication which leads to their excision from the genomic DNA and over-replication as free extrachromosomal elements (Ronai *et al.*, 1990). This phenomenon resembles the mechanism through which DNA amplification occurs (Amler and Schwab, 1989). (3) Gene amplification. An increase in the number of copies of specific genes has been observed in various tumor cells in the form of drug resistance as well as acquiring selective growth advantage (through amplification of genes that directly affect cell growth). The amplification of various genes has also been shown to increase following exposure to chemical or physical carcinogens. Thus, the combined effect of both carcinogens and viral infection may increase neoplastic conversion through a primary activation of viral sequences. (4) Effect on RNA tumor viruses. A somewhat different mechanism may play a role in RNA tumor viruses, mainly retroviruses. Retroviruses directly affect oncogenesis through three different routes: (1) expression of retroviral oncogenes, (2) activation of cellular proto-oncogenes in *cis* by insertional mutation, and (3) activation of proto-oncogenes in *trans* by viral transcription factors (Varmus and Brown, 1989). Recent studies have demonstrated that various retroviral sequences can be activated at the transcriptional level by chemical and physical carcinogens. Overall, the toxicity of certain chemicals may directly affect the expression of a specific subset of genes, thereby leading to changes at the level of gene expression, which can promote both directly and indirectly the reactivity of these compounds with DNA sequences. The combination of these two may lead to increased conversion of normal cells to neoplastic.

Inhibition of Carcinogenesis

In a variety of experimental situations, the effect of chemical carcinogens has been decreased by antagonistic effects (Troll *et al.*, 1987; De Flora, 1988; Ito and Hirose, 1989). Such observations have raised the possibility of chemoprevention of cancer (Greenwald *et al.*, 1986; McGinnis, 1988–1989). L. Wattenberg has categorized inhibitors into three groups: (1) inhibitors preventing formation of carcinogens, (2) blocking agents, and (3) suppressing agents.

An example of an inhibitor of carcinogen formation is the action of vitamin C in inhibiting nitrosation of amines in the stomach and thereby reducing formation of nitrosamines.

The joint administration of a chemical carcinogen and a structurally analogous noncarcinogenic chemical has sometimes resulted in inhibitory effects, especially if the noncarcinogenic analog was present in large excess. For example, non- or weakly carcinogenic, partially hydrogenated polycyclic hydrocarbons have reduced the carcinogenicity of the fully aromatic structure. A 20 molar excess of acetanilide reduced the carcinogenicity of 2-acetylaminofluorene on the liver and several other target organs in several species. The underlying mechanisms may be different in each case (E. K. Weisburger, in Sontag, 1981). These are examples of blocking effects.

The mechanisms of action of blocking agents could involve (1) competitive displacement at the level of the target, (2) variation in the effectiveness of an activating enzyme system, (3) a more general systemic effect leading to altered detoxification mechanisms or changed receptor ratios, or (4) reduction of replicative DNA synthesis, which is required to "fix" the carcinogen damage. The carcinogenic effect of a given chemical is dependent on the rate of metabolism of the chemical. This metabolic rate can be affected by environmental or host controlled factors, other carcinogens, or noncarcinogenic agents (Conney, 1982; Howard *et al.*, 1990). A variation in these factors will alter the ratio of activated metabolite over detoxified metabolites. Obviously, an increase in this ratio is likely to yield a picture of increased or synergistic effect, but a decrease, one of reduced or antagonistic action, may also occur. Most such studies have dealt with an evaluation of effects at the level of liver microsomal enzymes; others with effects on organs such as skin, lung, breast, and intestinal tract; and others yet with carcinogens in tissue culture.

In the last few years, the understanding of the operation of microsomal enzymes, the cytochrome P-450 systems, has increased considerably, in connection with the study not only of the metabolism of chemical carcinogens, but of drugs and exogenous chemicals generally. A number of recent reviews deal with these complex reaction systems (see Chapter 4). In general, agents that augment the effectiveness of type II microsomal enzymes lead to increased detoxification reactions and thus often, but not always, decrease carcinogenicity. An exception could be the case of certain halogenated hydrocarbons that seem to undergo activation by conjugation with glutathione in the liver, and then specifically are toxic and carcinogenic in the kidneys, as discussed herein (Dekant *et al.*, 1989).

The pioneering experiment of A. Conney, J. Miller, and E. Miller in the United States (Conney, 1982) demonstrated that dietary 3-methylcholanthrene increases the level of an enzyme system concerned with reduction of the azo bond in the carcinogenic dyestuff 4-dimethylaminoazobenzene yielding noncarcinogenic split products, and thus explained the inhibition of the dye's carcinogenicity by the hydrocarbon. Indeed, it is this experiment, which gave insight into the relationship between chemicals capable of increasing the levels of such enzyme systems and the subsequent physiologic effects, that laid the foundation for the entire field of enzyme induction in relation to drug metabolism and, in part, drug addiction.

Since that time, numerous other chemicals such as phenobarbital, DDT, benzoflavones, and synthetic antioxidants (Kahl, 1984) were found to induce enzymes and thus reduce the carcinogenicity not only of these azo dyes but of many types of carcinogens. These studies on interactions have been performed mainly in rats; experimentation with other species is needed because of species differences. For example, administration of 3-methylcholanthrene decreases the ratio of N-hydroxy-2-acetylaminofluorene, an activated carcinogenic intermediate derived from 2-acetylaminofluorene to detoxification metabolites in the rat, but increases the ratio in the hamster. Parallel to these findings are the biologic and toxicologic findings that in the rat 3-methylcholanthrene reduces the carcinogenicity of 2-acetylaminofluorene, but increases it in the hamster (E. K. Weisburger, in Sontag, 1981).

Less is known about the mode of action of suppressing agents. Candidates appear to be retinoic acid compounds which reduce cancer development when given after a carcinogen (Sporn and Roberts, 1983). Such agents may affect cellular differentiation or could enhance cell-to-cell communication, an effect opposite to that of promoters (Trosko *et al.*, 1983).

MODULATING FACTORS

Endogenous Factors

Species, Strain, and Organ Sensitivity. Human cancers were first found to relate to chronic exposure to considerable levels of specific chemical carcinogens at the work place. Even though, in time, a large fraction of those exposed developed a specific cancer, not all of those at risk were affected. Also, the latent period (the time to overt cancer presentation) differed widely from individual to individual. For cancers related to life style such as those due to cigarette smoking or nutrition, whether it is the high gastric cancer risk of the Japanese or Latin Americans, or the high colon or breast cancer risk seen in the Western world, it is fortunately true that not everyone in a given environment is affected to the same extent. In a specific setting, those genetically more sensitive will display an adverse effect such as cancer, but those more resistant will not, or do so at an older age. A bell-shaped curve describes this element, and most individuals fall in a very broad middle range, with average sensitivity. To be sure, there are competitive risks; someone on a high-fat diet might die of a heart attack and be withdrawn from the pool of those sensitive to colon or prostatic cancer. Another established example is the multiple disease risk in cigarette smokers, namely heart attacks, and cancer in the lung, pancreas, kidney, or urinary bladder. Deaths from any of those diseases will be recorded for that condition, and reduce the statistics for all the others. There are further external modulating factors. An individual on the traditional high-saturated-fat Western diet and a smoker has a higher risk of a heart attack. Another, on a high ω-6 polyunsaturated-fat diet and a smoker may have a lower risk of a heart attack, but have a greater likelihood of developing cancer of the pancreas. The cancer risk is modulated by the partially genetically controlled level of the specific cytochrome P-450 systems needed to convert the tobacco carcinogens to DNA-reactive metabolites. In turn, the carcinogens in tobacco smoke induce such enzymes. All of these elements need to be taken into account in studying the mechanisms of carcinogenesis. Likewise, in animal models utilizing random bred animals or highly inbred animals, variations in sensitivity or in target organs occur to a given carcinogenic challenge. Even a cryptogenic cancer seen in an aging, untreated population of animals occurs to different extents in different species and strains.

Among inbred strains of mice there are wide differences in the occurrence of cyptogenic neoplasms. Some, such as the strain A mouse, develop a high incidence of pulmonary neoplasms, and they are also very sensitive to the chemical induction of these tumors (Shimkin and Stoner, 1975). The C3H strain readily develops cyptogenic or induced neoplasms of the liver (Stevenson *et al.*, 1990). In contrast, the C57 black strain mouse is resistant to induced or spontaneous liver neoplasms, but cutaneous or subcutaneous cancer can be induced fairly readily by appropriate modes of compound application. Identical considerations apply to rat strains. The young female Sprague-Dawley rat is exquisitely sensitive to the development of mammary gland cancer by the use of specific carcinogens, whereas the Long-Evans strain is not; the latter develops leukemia. Within the class of broadly acting alkylnitrosamines, quantitative differences in response appear as regards tumor yield and latent period with a given amount of a specific nitrosamine. Distinct target organs are also affected. Thus, whereas in the rat diethylnitrosamine readily induces primary liver cancer, in the hamster a good yield of cancer in the esophagus is obtained. That does not mean that esophageal cancer is not induced in the rat with diethylnitrosamine, but simply reflects the fact that the liver is a much more sensitive target organ so that the animals die of primary liver cancer before they have a chance to develop cancer in the esophagus. If liver carcinogenesis is inhibited in the rat, then more cancer of the esophagus is seen. A conceptually important example is that of the tobacco specific nitrosamines, which at high dosages cause cancer in the lung, but at a lower chronic intake yield cancer in the pancreas, a secondary target organ in the human smoker. The same kind of differential sensitivity applies for 2-acetylaminofluorene, which usually causes primary liver cancer in male Wistar or Fischer strain rats, but in the presence of tryptophan, which delays liver carcinogenesis and promotes urinary bladder carcinogenesis, cancer in the urinary bladder is seen more frequently. For 1,2-dimethylhydrazine given as large doses orally or subcutaneously to rats or mice, the primary target organ is the large bowel. However, oral administration of lower dosages usually does not affect the large bowel, but leads to hemangioendotheliomas (Toth, 1988).

In animal models and in some human cases, it has been possible to delineate the complex mechanisms accounting in part for such species differences (IARC Sci. Publ. 51, 1983). A major factor accounting for the sensitivity or resistance resides in the biotransformation capability to convert procarcinogen to the reactive electrophilic, ultimate carcinogen. A well known example is the relative resistance of the guinea pig to the induction of any kind of cancer by a typical aromatic amine derivative, 2-acetyl-aminofluorene, because in the guinea pig the required metabolic activation to the proximate carcinogen, the *N*-hydroxy derivative, occurs to a minor extent, and the major *in vivo* metabolite is a detoxified 7-hydroxy derivative. As a first approximation to species- and strain-related differences in metabolic activation, the large differences found in rodents appear to be linked to the *Ah* locus, which, in turn, reflect the presence and/or inducibility of distinct forms of cytochrome P-450.

Similar considerations apply in regard to the organotropism of carcinogens in specific hosts, with the additional consideration that some proximate carcinogens have transport forms such as glucuronic acid conjugates, often generated in the liver, that release a reactive proximate carcinogen in a specific target organ such as urinary bladder or large bowel, where it is further converted to the reactive electrophile.

Both species differences and organotropism are also functions of the DNA-repair systems. For example, the hamster is more susceptible than the rat to liver cancer induced by dimethylnitrosamine because of its deficiency in repair of O^6 alkylation of guanine in DNA. In rats, a single large dose of dimethylnitrosamine induces kidney, but not liver, cancer because of the capability of liver repair enzymes to remove alkylated forms of DNA from the liver. Likewise, ethylnitrosourea initially forms DNA adducts in liver, kidney, and brain, but because of the limited repair capacity in brain tissue, the animals eventually develop cancer there, but do not develop liver, and rarely kidney, cancer.

In the nonhuman primates, such as the Rhesus monkey, some chemicals such as the food mutagen 2-amino-3-methylimidazo[4,5-*f*]quinoline or diethylnitrosamine lead to primary liver cancer extremely rapidly (in some instances in about one year), considering the greater longevity of this animal. On the other hand, following administration of the very powerful mycotoxin aflatoxin B_1, the first liver cancer was only seen after five years and usually required an average of ten years to develop. In rats or the sensitive rainbow trout, liver cancer is induced in a year. Powerful rodent carcinogens of the aromatic amine class have not yet led to any cancer, after about 15 years. In humans, aromatic amines usually lead to cancer in a high contamination occupational setting after 15, and more likely 25 to 40, years of exposure. In some instances, however, a larger dosage that might be found after intake of certain drugs such as chlornaphazine occasionally can induce cancer after five years, but in most instances, more than 10 to 15

years are needed. As has been noted elsewhere, most known human carcinogens can be detected by the appropriate high dosing in rodent models that have the required metabolic capability.

In light of the foregoing knowledge, it is clear that animal models cannot be assumed to represent quantitative indicators of human effects of carcinogens. Nevertheless, animal models are useful in hazard identification, especially when combined with collateral investigations on genetic or epigenetic properties, and in studies of mechanism of action of suspect hazards and of modulation of carcinogenesis.

Age. Age is an important variable in studies on carcinogenesis. Newborn animals exhibit higher sensitivity to certain carcinogens than older animals. Thus, injection of newborn mice with only a few doses of any one of a number of genotoxic chemical carcinogens results in tumors, primarily of the liver and lung, approximately a year after the administration of the carcinogen (IARC Sci. Publ. 96, 1989). Carcinogens may be effective when administered to young animals but ineffective when administered to older animals. For example, the polycyclic aromatic hydrocarbons do not usually induce liver cancer when administered to young adult mice or rats, but do so when given to newborn animals because of the then rapid growth of the liver. Likewise, aflatoxin B_1 fails to induce liver tumors in mice when administered after weaning, but does induce tumors when given at birth; hamsters, too, appear to be more sensitive to aflatoxin B_1 at birth than after weaning but the difference in sensitivity is not as great as that in rats. Cell duplication rates, in part, account for the increased sensitivity of newborn or young animals, or humans, to carcinogens. Populations where exposure to carcinogens in tobacco smoke occurs in the growth phase, such as boys or girls ages 12 to 16, are more likely to develop cancer than in populations (Japan) where tradition and family pressure lead to later initiation of smoking as grown adults. Puberty results in a prolonged rise in DNA synthesis and mitosis in endocrine-sensitive organs, increasing their sensitivity to carcinogens. Studies in migrants from Japan, an area with a low risk for breast and prostate cancer, to the high-risk Western world note an increased incidence only in the second generation, not in the migrants, because at the time of puberty they lived in a low-risk region. On the other hand, the risk for colon cancer is observed in the migrant generation, because the rate of DNA synthesis and cell duplication does occur at a given level, even on a lower fat Japanese diet.

Many investigators utilize weanling animals in experiments with chemical carcinogens. Such animals are quite sensitive, and with agents of low carcinogenicity requiring a long latent period for tumor development, it is useful to begin with animals as young as possible. However, in some instances weanling animals are considerably more sensitive to the toxic effect of an agent. Hence, failure to adjust dosages upward as the animal develops the capability of tolerating higher levels may result in fewer tumors and a longer experimental period. The greater susceptibility of young animals to carcinogenesis may also be seen in humans, as noted above.

Transplacental Exposure. Some carcinogens cross the placental barrier (IARC Sci. Publ. 96, 1989). In certain cases, the enzyme system necessary to produce activated metabolites is sufficiently developed in the fetus to give an adequate level of the required reactive intermediates. In other cases, the mother may generate the active intermediate in a transportable form, which is released in the fetus by select enzyme systems. Certain types of carcinogens that do not require enzymes to develop the reactive ultimate carcinogen, such as alkylnitrosoureas, are extremely powerful transplacentally. However, methylnitrosourea is less effective (DNA repair) than the ethyl homolog as a transplacental carcinogen. The method of experimental transplacental carcinogenesis has been developed by several investigators, including Druckrey, Napalkov, Tomatis, and Rice as a means of detecting possible environmental carcinogens (IARC Sci. Publ. 96, 1989). In addition, *in vivo–in vitro* systems, in which the agent is given to a pregnant female and tissues from the fetuses are explanted into tissue culture, can yield abnormal transformed tumor cells that are visualized after a short period of time.

It is quite probable that cancers occurring in childhood are the result of transplacental exposure. An important series of cases were discovered by Herbst *et al.* (see IARC Sci. Publ. 96, 1989) in young girls with a rare form of vaginal cancer that was traced to the fact that their mothers had been treated with high doses of the hormone diethylstilbestrol in attempts to maintain a successful pregnancy. The high level of this powerful estrogen imprinted the endocrine system, leading to abnormal differentiation, and expression at the time of puberty.

Sex and Endocrine Balance. Epidemiologic data show that some types of cancer occur more frequently in men than in women, and vice versa (American Cancer Society, 1990). In experimental animals, likewise, some chemical carcinogens induce cancer more frequently at specific target organs in one than the other sex, even when a nonendocrine organ is involved.

For example, 2-acetylaminofluorene induces liver cancer primarily in male rats, although females of certain strains are also sensitive, but usually less so (E. K. Weisburger, in Sontag, 1981). On the other hand, *o*-aminoazotoluene is somewhat more active in female mice than in males in causing liver cancer. Dimethyl- or diethylnitrosamine produces liver cancer often, but not always, with similar efficiency in males and females. On the other hand, a variety of carcinogens cause pulmonary tumors in male and female mice with equal frequency (Shimkin and Stoner, 1975). In nonendocrine target organs, the sex-linked effectiveness of a given carcinogen stems mostly from a sex-dependent activity of enzyme systems necessary for the conversion of a procarcinogen to the reactive ultimate carcinogen. For example, in the case of 2-acetylaminofluorene-induced liver cancer the key difference resides in the levels of the enzyme sulfotransferase giving rise to the reactive sulfate ester of *N*-hydroxy derivative (Lai *et al.*, 1985). Levels of enzyme are six to eight times higher in male than in female rats and some strains of mice. Alternatively, a sex difference in carcinogenic susceptibility may stem from varying ratios of detoxification enzymes. For example, for some substrates, glucuronic acid conjugation is higher in females than in males.

The endocrine system is important in relation to tumor growth in endocrine sensitive tissues such as the gonads, adrenals, thyroid, prostate, and breast. Also, alteration in the hormonal balance, e.g., by gonadectomy or hypophysectomy, may affect the carcinogenic process, even in nonendocrine organs if endocrine-sensitive enzyme systems are required for activation or detoxification of the carcinogen or for the growth and development of the tumor, as noted above. In any case, the situation is quite complex, for endocrine glands and their target organs are interconnected by delicately balanced feedback pathways. Alteration in one hormone level usually leads to repercussions in the entire system, yielding a new equilibrium. In mature females of most species, regular and periodic oscillations occur, corresponding to the normal estrus cycle. Age, in turn, plays a role in endocrine responsiveness. Thus, superimposition of an exogenous toxicant with an affinity for any of the endocrine-susceptible organs may also indirectly affect other organs in the body. Administration of a hormone or of a chemical affecting the endocrine system may have an even more complex action. Dietary restriction in animals and humans has a profound action on the endocrine system and on the rate of cell cycling in many organs. This in turn can have important effects. A dietary restriction of 10 to 20 percent of caloric intake severely lowers mammary gland carcinogenesis.

The long-term effect of chemicals on the endocrine balance and the periodicity of the system must also be considered. Chemicals such as BHT, PCB (polychlorinated biphenyls), DDT, or phenobarbital that at high chronic dosages induce specific components of the cytochrome P-450 system concerned with the metabolism of estrogens, or of thyroxine can alter the endocrine balances and "induce" cancer in organs such as the adrenals, uterus, or thyroid. Such chemicals, strictly speaking, may be thus labeled "carcinogen," but analysis of the underlying mechanism warrants the conclusion that such agents are not carcinogenicity risks to humans exposed to trace amounts that do not induce enzymes metabolizing endocrine-active substrates.

Hormones such as those contained in oral contraceptives may have an entirely different action in animals such as rodents or dogs with an estrus cycle quite unlike that of the human female. Continuous administration of hormonally active preparations to rodents often results in the development of tumors, especially in the mammary gland. This may not necessarily constitute a carcinogenic risk for sexually mature human females receiving the same preparation in low dosages on a rhythmic basis tailored to the normal menstrual cycle. In fact, such treatment serves to maintain the individual in hormonal balance and reduce the risk of cancer development in endocrine responsive organs. Nonetheless, a very small percentage of women on extended courses of oral contraceptives developed a benign liver neoplasm, sometimes fatal because of its hemorrhagic nature. The underlying mechanism is not known (WHO Collaborative Study, 1989). Exposure of newborn or immature animals, humans, or fetuses to an exogenous agent may permanently affect the differentiation of endocrine organs by leading to imprinting, and thus lead to cancer later in life due to either hormonal imbalance or aberrant tissue receptor response to prevailing hormone levels. Such processes have probably been involved in the etiology of vaginal cancer in young, pubertal girls, whose mothers were given large doses of the estrogenic drug diethylstilbestrol during pregnancy.

Immunologic Factors. Immunologic factors have been found in some instances to alter the rate and extent of tumor development (Penn, 1988). There are tumor-related antigens produced during transformation of normal to neoplastic cells that provide possible tools to detect and diagnose, and also specifically treat neoplasms (Goldenberg, 1990). Immunologic mechanisms have been thought to play a role in

the greater sensitivity of newborn animals to chemical carcinogens, for in some species and strains the immunologic competence in the newborn is either totally lacking or considerably less than that present in the adult animal. However, immunologic status is more relevant in the development of metastases than in the early effects in the carcinogenic process. Several carcinogens (apart from immunosuppressant agents) have been shown to suppress the immune system, but this has not been established to be critical to their carcinogenicity. In humans clinical drug-induced immunosuppression to maintain patency of organ transplants has sometimes caused lymphomas or leukemias. The severe immunosuppression associated with AIDS can lead to leukemias, lymphomas, or Kaposi's sarcoma.

Exogenous Factors

Diet. Developments in the area of azo dye carcinogenesis many years ago drew attention to the fact that diet can modify the effectiveness of chemical carcinogens. Rats fed a rice diet, low in protein and riboflavin, were highly sensitive to liver tumor formation when treated with 4-dimethylaminoazobenzene, but a diet containing adequate amounts of protein and riboflavin reduced and in some cases prevented the carcinogenic effect. Mueller and Miller (Conney, 1982) found that this diet-mediated change in carcinogenicity stemmed from an alteration in the level of a flavin adenine dinucleotide dependent azo dye reductase, which, in turn, altered the effective dosage of the carcinogen, through modulation of detoxification by reduction of the azo bond.

Other, more recent examples can be given in which diet exerted an effect on the outcome of the carcinogenic process by controlling the effectiveness of enzymes concerned with activation versus detoxification of the chemical carcinogens (Parke, 1990). For example, administration of the potent liver carcinogen dimethylnitrosamine to rats on a protein-free diet has virtually no toxic effect on the liver, mainly because of a severe decrease of microsomal enzymes in this organ. However, rats so treated exhibit tumors in the kidneys after a fairly long latent period. The acute toxicity of the mycotoxin aflatoxin B_1 is considerably reduced when rats are on a low-lipotrope diet, but the carcinogenicity to the liver is enhanced. Along those lines, lower availability of essential methyl donors such as methionine and choline can have major effects, especially in modifying hepatocarcinogenesis (Rogers and Longnecker, 1988).

Tumor induction in the mammary gland of rats is decreased when the animals are fed fat-restricted diets, but is augmented on high-fat diets (American Health Foundation, 1987). Skin tumor formation in mice is decreased when the food intake is restricted. In this instance the degree of tumor formation was dependent on the amount of food intake during the promoting phase. When the animals were placed on a restricted food intake during the application of the primary carcinogen, but were fed *ad libitum* during the promotion phase, the tumor incidence was identical to that seen in well-fed control animals. On the other hand, normal food intake during initiation by carcinogen, followed by dietary restriction during the promotion phase, reduced tumor incidence, pointing clearly to the fact that in this instance, the developmental phases of cancer cells are inhibited by lower food intake.

Restricted food intake, especially during the developmental phases, reduces the incidence of all neoplasms, but especially that in the endocrine-sensitive organs, and increases overall longevity. The underlying mechanism is a general decrease in the level of cell duplication rates (Clayson *et al.,* 1989). There is now an extensive literature on this subject indicating that diet exerts a major modifying role in many types of experimental and human cancers worldwide (U.S. Department of Health and Human Services, 1988; Committee on Diet and Health, 1989; Weisburger and Horn, 1991).

Specific Dietary Elements

Protein. Most rodent diets contain 18 to 25 percent protein. As the protein content increases above 50 percent, an unusually high level, a voluntary reduction in the number of total calories consumed takes place. Thus, in situations where caloric intake affects tumor induction, animals fed diets with elevated protein levels have been found to have fewer tumors. A diet restricted in protein, on the other hand, has a lesser effect. In fact, in the case of the carcinogenic azo dyes mentioned earlier, a protein-restricted (12%) diet appears to increase the relative efficiency of the carcinogen. However, this is a special case, probably because of lower levels of the detoxifying azo dye reductase and may not hold for other carcinogens. Diets completely devoid of protein, which can be administered only for limited periods of time, may decrease the effectiveness of certain carcinogens in specific target organs because of a reduction in the amount of specific cytochrome P-450 systems, and a consequent decrease in the biochemical activation of carcinogens. Also, such diets are a form of dietary restriction, with several underlying mechanisms.

Fats. For several types of chemical carcinogens, especially those affecting the endocrine-sensitive organs, the colon and pancreas, not all fats are equally good promoters. The ω-6-polyunsaturated oils are best, and saturated fats have lower promoting potential. The mainly monounsaturated oils such as olive oil have a neutral effect, and the ω-3-polyunsaturated oils are actually protective. Thus, the effectiveness of a carcinogen can for certain organs be increased appreciably by some high-fat diets. These considerations also appear to hold for humans (American Health Foundation, 1987; Weisburger and Horn, 1991). The relevant mechanisms are identical and depend on increased promotion. This factor appears most important in providing rational approaches to the prevention of important types of human cancer, through recommendation for a lower total fat calorie intake.

Carbohydrates and Starches. The starches contained in most commercial experimental diets exert relatively little effect on tumor induction. Semipurified diets, on the other hand, containing highly soluble carbohydrates such as glucose and sucrose, may enhance absorption of a carcinogen fed in the diet, thus enhancing toxicity. In humans, the risk of colon cancer has been related to low-residue, highly digestible foods, in contrast to diets high in starch, roughage, and residues, increasing stool bulk and diluting promoters such as fatty and bile acids (American Health Foundation, 1987). Animal experiments have confirmed that fibers such as bran or pectin reduce the carcinogenicity of certain colon carcinogens. For many other types of carcinogens, a difference is seen when animals are placed on a low-residue semipurified diet, compared to a diet composed of natural foodstuffs. In most instances, the carcinogen is somewhat less effective on the latter diet. There are exceptions for reasons that are not clear, but may involve the presence of enzyme inducers in a diet of natural foods, leading to better detoxification.

Micronutrients. A number of specific vitamins and minerals are essential cofactors for the effective operation of many key enzymes. Thus, a deficiency in these specific micronutrients would obviously have an effect on the physiology of the host and on the pharmacologic and toxicologic responses to exogenous agents, including carcinogens (Rogers and Longnecker, 1988; Weisburger, 1991). The effect of riboflavin on the carcinogenicity of azo dyes in the rat liver has already been discussed. In addition, riboflavin appears to be involved in tumor induction processes at other sites, such as the oral cavity, by a mechanism that has not yet been determined.

Vitamin A has been implicated in the differentiation of epithelial tissues. Beginning with Saffiotti and Sporn in the United States, a number of investigators have found that vitamin A levels affect the induction of pulmonary tumors in rodent systems and the incidence of lung cancer in human smokers or tobacco chewers (Stich *et al.*, 1989). Some other types of human cancer such as cancer of the cervix or bladder arise somewhat more frequently in people with low vitamin A intake. Vitamin A analogs or retinoic acid derivatives have been shown to inhibit carcinogenesis in several target organs, especially the mammary gland and the urinary bladder. One explanation is that they restore cell-to-cell communication, and thus reduce promotion.

Vitamin E and also several synthetic antioxidants, such as butylated hydroxytoluene, butylated hydroxyanisole, propyl gallate, and ethoxyquin, have modified tumor induction by certain carcinogens in a number of target organs. However, inhibition was achieved at high doses at which induction of biotransformation enzymes also occurs with the synthetics and, therefore, inhibition may not be due solely to antioxidant effects.

Selenium derivatives also decrease tumor incidence in specific experimental situations, but extrapolation to cancer in humans is not proven. Selenium salts and vitamin E are cofactors in glutathione peroxidase, accounting in part for the modifying actions. In some cases when high levels of the antioxidants were administered, the effect was traced directly to modification of enzyme levels, mainly in the liver, which led to changes in activation and detoxification of the metabolites of carcinogens. Dietary elements, particularly micronutrients such as vitamins A, E, and B_2, may provide some degree of protection against carcinogens through several distinct mechanisms. As was discussed above, vitamins C and E prevent the formation of nitrosamines and nitrosamides and thus reduce or eliminate cancer risk at various target organs such as the liver and upper gastrointestinal and respiratory tract (Mirvish, 1986). Further study of the mechanisms of action of dietary factors provides a sound base for means of reducing the prevalence of important human cancers (McGinnis, 1988–1989; Committee on Diet and Health, 1989; Weisburger, 1991).

QUANTITATIVE ASPECTS OF CARCINOGENESIS

DNA-Reactive Carcinogens

Extensive experimentation with a variety of chemical carcinogens has established the fact that, as is the case with other pharmacologic agents, the response to chemical carcinogens is dose dependent (Conning *et al.*, 1980). Chemical carcinogens of the electrophilic, reactive type, however, are quite distinct from ordinary pharmacologic agents in one way. Drugs and toxic chemicals generally exert their action rapidly, depending of course on mode of exposure. As the drug is metabolized and excreted, the effect diminishes to the vanishing point, and in most instances, no residual effect persists. In general, subsequent exposures act anew in the same manner without any long-lasting effects. In contrast, although the onset of the interaction between a reactive carcinogen and cells is fundamentally similar in that the chemical may undergo biotransformation, the key, often biochemically activated, ultimate carcinogen reacts with tissue macromolecules, of which DNA appears to be critical. During DNA synthesis and cell duplication, altered DNA can lead to gene or chromosomal mutations and thereby imprint a permanent effect in the cell.

Thus, with DNA-reactive (genotoxic) carcinogens, a given dose can result in permanent abnormalities of cells. Subsequent dosages can add to such a change. After a sufficient number of such alterations have been produced, the multiplication of abnormal cells results in a detectable lesion and eventually a neoplasm. Because the effects vary with the carcinogen and the tissue in which it exerts its action, the time required for a neoplasm to appear varies. Thus, time as well as dose is a factor in assessing the properties of chemical carcinogens. It is primarily in this way that DNA-reactive carcinogens differ from ordinary toxic agents; a number of small doses may give no immediate evidence of their action, but in time they can yield neoplasms within the life span of the host. Indeed, there are carcinogens of the DNA-reactive type that can induce cancer in animal models with a single dose. With toxins, comparable dosages for acute effects would likely be completely innocuous.

DNA-reactive carcinogens are further distinct from other types of toxins, insofar as the same total dose, when administered as smaller doses over a longer period of time, can actually be more effective than when given as larger, yet fewer individual doses in a shorter period of time. In the extreme, several chemicals that are potent carcinogens when administered chronically are not active at all when given as a single large dose. Also, administration of small single doses can be disproportionately effective compared to larger doses, especially when accompanied to promotion.

In quantifying carcinogenic effects from animal bioassays, the most superficial information is the overall incidence of neoplasms in exposed groups compared to the control group. This can be expressed as the dose that induces a 50 percent incidence in tumors, the TD_{50} (Gold *et al.*,

1989). More sensitivity is obtained if the parameters for evaluation include the latent period (time to tumor), often expressed as the time when the experimental group has reached a 50 percent incidence of neoplasms or the total time required for all animals to manifest neoplasms. Other relevent parameters of effect include the type of neoplasm, and the multiplicity of neoplasms, which, when considered in relationship to dosage, yields a more refined estimation of dose-response effects.

Also, the expression of the dose is important. Often, it is given only as the concentration in diet or drinking water. Better quantitation is obtained if it is expressed as the amount administered per unit body weight. Suggestions have been made to express dose per unit surface area of the animal, as is often done with cancer chemotherapeutic drugs, but this has not been demonstrated to provide better quantification. All of these measures, however, describe only the administered dose. A more refined expression would be the effective dose actually taken in by the animal, or, even better, that reaching the target site.

In numerous experiments using appropriate quantitative parameters, detailed dose-response relationships have been demonstrated. Two effects are usually observed with effective, often genotoxic carcinogens: with increasing dose (1) the percent yield and multiplicity of neoplasms increases and (2) time required for neoplasm appearance decreases. In most cases the overall neoplasm yield in any specific organ is proportional to the total dose, but the speed or rate of neoplasm appearance is related to the amount in an individual dose or dose rate.

A controversial issue in dose-response relationships is whether no effect or threshold levels exist for chemical carcinogens (Aldridge, 1986). In a classic study in 1943 by Bryan and Shimkin in the United States, 12 doses of each of three polycyclic aromatic hydrocarbons were injected subcutaneously in mice. There were 40 to 80 animals in the lower dose groups and 20 in the higher. The actual data show that two or three of the lower exposure levels yielded no evidence of tumor. Such observations, although clearly demonstrating thresholds within the context of the experiment, have not been accepted as evidence of thresholds for large numbers of subjects at risk because of statistical limitations. To develop some information on the actual shape of the dose-response curve at low levels of exposure, several relatively large-scale studies have been conducted. In one study conducted at the National Center for Toxicological Research (NCTR) mice were fed 2-acetylaminofluorene at seven doses ranging between 30 and 150 ppm (Staffa and Mehlman, 1980). The data were interpreted to demonstrate a linear dose-response for liver neoplasms, but yielded evidence of no effect levels at 45, 35, and 30 ppm for bladder cancer. Another large scale study performed at the British Industrial Biological Research Association (BIBRA) (IARC Sci. Publ. 57, 1984) involved administration of 15 dose levels of dimethylnitrosamine and diethylnitrosamine to rats, using doses as low as 0.033 ppm in the drinking water. This study also has been interpreted to show a linear response for liver neoplasms, but with a no-effect level for esophageal cancer. These studies, thus suggest carcinogenic effects at low-level exposures in liver, but not other tissues. Yet, in the NCTR study, the question arises as to findings had 3 ppm of carcinogen been used as the lowest dose. In the BIBRA experiments, the linear relationship was found only when combining all groups of males and females with the two nitrosamines used. Evaluation of the individual two to four lowest dose groups suggests, however, no excess of neoplasms compared to controls. In rats, aflatoxin B_1 causes liver cancer at 1 ppb, but in the United States peanuts and corn contain variable amounts, depending on weather. The Federal "action level" prohibiting human use is 20 ppb (Park and Stoloff, 1989). The incidence of liver cancer in the United States is low and has decreased for the last 40 years (American Cancer Society, 1990), suggesting that the prevailing exposures to such liver-specific mycotoxins has not led to cancer.

DNA-reactive carcinogens vary greatly in their potency. For example, among liver carcinogens, a greater than 50 percent incidence is produced by lifetime administration of aflatoxin B_1 at 1 ppb, of diethylnitrosamine at 5 ppm, of safrole at 1000 to 5000 ppm, and of acetamide (not a proven DNA-reactive liver carcinogen) at 12,500 ppm. Relatively few studies have been done on the effect of dose rate or even dose-response with the weaker DNA-reactive carcinogens. Shimkin (Shimkin and Stoner, 1975) examined the potential of alkylating drugs of diverse structures to induce pulmonary tumors in mice. They found that the strong carcinogens were active over a broad dose range, whereas weaker ones gave evidence of some carcinogenicity only at the highest, but not at lower dose levels. Safrole was fed in the diet to groups of 50 rats at levels of 100, 500, 1000, and 5000 ppm. Malignant liver cancers were obtained only at the highest dose level, and benign adenomas at the two highest, but not the lower doses. The underlying mechanism rests on a dose-related increasing biochemical formation of the proximate carcinogen, 1'-hydroxysafrole (Anthony *et al.,* 1987). Thus, available historic data show that a threshold or no-effect level can be observed even with DNA-reactive carcinogens under standard bioassay conditions. However, the question can always be raised whether such thresholds would be seen if larger numbers of animals were used, as in the two large-scale studies mentioned. Based on considerations of metabolism, the barriers to electrophiles in reaching critical targets in DNA, DNA repair processes, etc., it seems almost certain that for every carcinogen there must be a threshold. It may be very low for powerful carcinogens, as suggested by the two studies with 2-acetylaminofluorene and the nitrosamines, but seems to be correspondingly higher for weak carcinogens (Alridge, 1986).

These dose-response studies on DNA-reactive carcinogens have provided the data for mathematical modeling. A number of models have been proposed, and there is active debate on which of these is most appropriate. One that is widely used by regulatory agencies because it is "conservative" is a linear no-threshold extrapolation. As noted, proof has not been provided for any carcinogen that no threshold exists and, in fact, thresholds have been observed in many studies, particularly with weak carcinogens. The assumption of linearity at low doses is also not well founded. Indeed, even for the less complicated process of chemical mutagenesis *in vivo,* a drop below linearity at low doses has been demonstrated. Therefore, a "hockey stick"-shaped curve (Hoel *et al.,* 1988) would appear to best fit current data and concepts on carcinogenic mechanisms at low levels of exposure (Laska and Meisner, 1988; Farrar and Crump, 1990).

Dose-related carcinogenic effects have also been observed with human exposures to carcinogens. The most reliable quantitative data on human cancer resulting from exposure to specific carcinogens come from studies of occupational or therapeutic exposures (Sontag, 1981; Maltoni and Selikoff, 1988; Cooper and Grover, 1990). In these situations, adequate data exist with several carcinogens to show that human cancer incidence is proportional to dose, often measured by length of employment, because there are virtually no actual data on prevailing levels of any chemical in the industrial environment, especially in the past. The cancer incidence in workmen exposed to benzidine, vinyl chloride, or bis(chlormethyl)ether had a general relationship between exposure and disease occurrence. Workmen engaged in uranium or asbestos mining exhibited a risk of cancer broadly related to the length of time an individual was engaged in these particular occupations, especially if they

also smoked. Likewise, with the drug chlornaphazine, where intake was reasonably well established, the percentage of treated patients who subsequently developed bladder cancer was proportional to the amount of drug consumed. Many of the available dose-response relationships were observed in limited populations of people exposed iatrogenically (IARC Sci. Publ. 78, 1986).

As in experimental studies, the question of thresholds for human exposures to carcinogens is controversial (Aldridge, 1986). The issue has great contemporary importance in light of the capability of analytic chemists to measure accurately, at the parts-per-billion and even the parts-per-trillion level, the presence of several types of carcinogens in the food chain and in the environment generally. Several chemicals such as nitrosopyrrolidine, found in bacon, can induce liver cancer in several species with appropriate higher dosages, of the order of parts per million to parts per thousand. Primary liver cancer is rarely seen in populations that regularly consume fried bacon. Is this evidence for a no-effect level? Similar questions can be raised for the trace amounts of mycotoxins currently permitted in food. Such considerations are controversial; opinions abound and facts are few. It must be accepted that the issue is currently beyond the reach of exact science.

Nevertheless, several lines of evidence suggest that in the human context there are thresholds for DNA-reactive carcinogens. For example, hepatocellular carcinoma is relatively rare in much of the Western world even though unavoidable contamination of foods with the liver carcinogens aflatoxin and dimethylnitrosamine has occurred for decades and continues to be found. Thus, there may be practical no-effect levels even for strong carcinogens, in the absence of promoting factors. A recent, additional documentation on this point is an evaluation of the effect of the powerful pulmonary carcinogen bis(chloromethyl)ether. In one factory, evidence for a carcinogenic effect to workers was observed but in another it was not. Nonetheless, prudent policy dictates avoidance, wherever possible, of exposure to genotoxic carcinogens.

Epigenetic Carcinogens

In the case of carcinogens that are not DNA reactive and appear to operate by the production of other biologic effects, it would be expected that their carcinogenic effects would parallel dose-response relationships for their relevent biologic effects. Unfortunately, relatively few dose-response studies have been done with carcinogens of the epigenetic type and almost none with regard to underlying toxicologic or pharmacologic mechanisms. Reasonable data exist for the chelating agent nitrilotriacetic acid, showing that kidney and bladder tumors are produced by exposures to about 75 mmoles/kg diet and that this diminishes dramatically, in a nonlinear fashion, when the exposure is reduced below 50 mmoles/kg diet. A dose-response study in which saccharin was fed to large numbers of rats over two generations, using a highly sensitive bioassay system, shows that a 37 percent yield of bladder carcinoma plus papilloma was induced with 7.5 percent dietary saccharin, 20 percent with 6.25 percent, 15 percent with 5 percent, 12 percent with 4 percent, 8 percent with 3 percent, 5 percent with 1 percent, and 8 percent with 0 percent, the controls. Thus, the data show a two-thirds drop in neoplasm incidence with less than a one-half reduction of dose; 3 percent and 1 percent saccharin were no-effect levels. Saccharin is nongenotoxic, and the data are in agreement with a threshold effect (IARC Sci. Publ. 65, 1985; Gaylor et al., 1988).

For several types of epigenetic carcinogens, especially promoters, theoretical considerations as well as available data from experimental studies strongly support the existence of no-effect levels or thresholds. When agents such as DDT, phenobarbital, or butylated hydroxyanisole (BHA) were tested by themselves for carcinogenicity, an effect, meaning a low but statistically significant incidence of specific neoplasms, was evident only at the highest dose levels given in lifetime studies. These observations are supported by promoting studies with these agents where results can be obtained in shorter time with smaller numbers of animals. No-effect levels have been observed in promotion assays after exposures to the appropriate tissue-specific genotoxic carcinogens for saccharin in bladder cancer promotion and BHT and phenobarbital in liver cancer promotion.

These observations on dose-response for non-genotoxic agents apply also to the human setting (IARC Sci. Publ 65, 1985). Relatively few epigenetic agents have been carcinogenic to humans; examples are asbestos and diethylstilbestrol. Estrogens at high chronic dose are carcinogenic, but obviously not at the essential physiologic levels. There are no real dose-response data on the carcinogenic effects of these types of agents, although it is apparent that risk diminishes rapidly with reduction of exposures from the high levels associated with cancer causation.

Some data exist for dose-response of promoting agents. Bile acids are demonstrated promoters for colon cancer. In Western populations at high risk for colon cancer, the prevailing concentration of bile acids is 12 mg/g of feces. In Japan, with a low fat intake, or in Finland, with a high cereal fiber intake, the risk for colon cancer is low, and the concentration of fecal bile acids is about 4 mg/g, only one-third of the concentration associated with high risk (American Health Foundation, 1987). Complex tobacco smoke contains relatively small amounts of genotoxic polycyclic aromatic hydrocarbons, nicotine-derived nitrosamines, and certain heterocyclic amines. The major effect of tobacco stems from the promoting effect of the acidic fraction of the smoke. It is established that an individual chronically smoking 40 cigarettes per day is at high risk, but with 10 cigarettes per day the risk is much lower, and with four cigarettes per day the risk is most difficult to evaluate accurately. This represents evidence that enhancing factors have steep dose-response curves in humans, as in experimental animals. Also, individuals are encouraged to stop smoking based on the principle that removal of promotion progressively decreased the risk of cancer development. The action of promoters in reversible, that of strong DNA-reactive carcinogens is not.

Humans have been exposed to significant levels of a variety of epigenetic carcinogens such as organochlorine pesticides, phenobarbital, and natural estrogens without evidence of cancer causation (Clemmesen et al., 1981; IARC Sci. Publ. 65, 1985). Nevertheless, carcinogens that are not DNA reactive have produced cancer in humans, such as asbestos, through high-level occupational exposure with quasi-permanent retention of the product, and diethylstilbestrol at high pharmacologic levels in a transplacental mode with imprinting of the endocrine system of the fetus. The negative findings with other epigenetic agents, therefore, suggest that their exposure levels have been below the thresholds for cancer production.

In summary, carcinogens, both DNA-reactive and epigenetic, act in a dose-dependent fashion, although the dose-response relations appear to be different. There are observed thresholds for both types of carcinogens in experimental animals and humans. The thresholds for DNA-reactive carcinogens vary greatly and may be low. Those for epigenetic carcinogens, particularly of the promoter class, have been fairly high. In the latter case, there are some exceptions such as TPA (12-O-tetradecanoylphorbol-13-acetate) and TCDD, active at low levels in experimental systems, because of their affinity for specific receptors. These observations have implications regarding the type of carcinogen testing and regulation that should be done to delineate human risk and especially to prevent cancer.

BIOASSAY OF CHEMICAL CARCINOGENS

The testing of chemicals for possible carcinogenic effects has as its aim the detection of those that may be harmful to humans. Although the induction of cancer in animals defines a chemical as a carcinogen, evaluation of the basis for carcinogenicity cannot be based exclusively on chronic testing because chemical carcinogens exhibit varied modes of action (see above and Table 5–2), which are not necessarily revealed by chronic bioassay. Of prime importance, evidence of genotoxic versus epigenetic effects is not obtained in such chronic tests although inferences can sometimes be made from the nature of the carcinogenic effect, including the type of dose-response pattern.

Carcinogen testing involves many approaches. Some are based on traditional practices, others on regulatory requirements (IARC Sci. Publ. 83, 1986; Environmental Protection Agency, 1986; Office of Technology Assessment, 1989). Several of these have been previously discussed and will not be repeated here. Protocols are reviewed by Stevens and Gallo, and by Robins *et al.* in Hayes (1989). The essential information for a comprehensive risk extrapolation to humans can be obtained through a "decision point approach" to carcinogenicity evaluation (Williams and Weisburger, 1988), which is based entirely on established toxicologic methods applied in a systematic manner. In addition to providing a framework within which the information required for risk extrapolation can be obtained, this approach also offers a guide to the elimination of unnecessary procedures. It utilizes systems that yield definitive data with reduced animal usage, and thus is more economical and humane than routine large-scale bioassays. Based on established mechanisms of carcinogenesis, the Decision Point Approach takes the two main classes of genotoxic carcinogens, and nongenotoxic, epigenetic agents into account in two ways:

1. A battery of short-term tests is structured with the aim of identifying genotoxic carcinogens at an early stage. The battery also includes systems that may respond to epigenetic agents.
2. Test methods are offered with the realization that all types of subchronic testing may not detect some chemicals that can produce neoplasms in animals under specific conditions on chronic administration. Past history shows that virtually all known human carcinogens were genotoxic and were readily detected in limited animal bioassays.

Table 5–4. DECISION POINT APPROACH TO CARCINOGEN TESTING

A number of systematic, sequential tests must be undertaken in the evaluation of potential carcinogenicity of a chemical.

Stage A. Structure of chemical
Stage B. Short-term tests *in vitro*
    1. Mammalian cell DNA repair
    2. Bacterial mutagenesis
    3. Mammalian mutagenesis
    4. Chromosome integrity
    5. Cell transformation

Decision point 1: Evaluation of all tests conducted in stages A and B
Stage C. Tests for promoters
    1. *In vitro*
    2. *In vivo*

Decision point 2: Evaluation of results from stages A through C
Stage D. Limited *in vivo* bioassays
    1. Altered foci induction in rodent liver
    2. Skin neoplasm induction in mice
    3. Pulmonary neoplasm induction in mice
    4. Breast cancer induction in female Sprague-Dawley rats

Decision point 3: Evaluation of results from stages A, B, and C and the appropriate tests in stage D
Stage E. Long-term bioassay
Decision point 4: Final evaluation of all the results and application to health risk analysis. This evaluation must include data from stages A, B, and C to provide a basis for mechanistic considerations

THE DECISION POINT APPROACH

A series of sequential steps is followed in a stepwise progression (Table 5–4) and a critical evaluation of the information obtained and its significance in relation to the testing objective is performed at the end of each phase. A decision is made as to whether the data generated are sufficient to reach a definitive conclusion or whether a higher level of testing is required. There are four such decision points. Attention is paid to qualitative yes or no answers, and to quantitative high, medium, or low effects, in relation to known positive control compounds. Experimental procedures following, in general, the sequence of tests proposed have been detailed in Milman and Weisburger (1985).

Structure of Chemical

As detailed above, structure-activity studies have provided considerable information upon which predictions as to whether or not a given chemical might be carcinogenic can be made with fair success within certain classes of chemicals, particularly those that include known carcinogens (Arcos *et al.*, 1968–1988; Shahin, 1989). Rosenkranz and Klopman (1990) have developed a computer-based structure-activity analysis, CASE, that has been successfully applied to modeling of fragments of molecules with specific attributes, that predicts potential mutagenicity and carcinogenicity. Structure must always be evaluated in the light of known species differences in biotransformation, which can render a weak or a noncarcinogenic agent in one species a powerful carcinogen in another (such as aflatoxin B_1).

Information on structure and metabolism also provides a guide to the selection among limited bioassays at stage C and, as more information accrues, may eventually contribute to selection of specific short-term tests at stage B (Sobel, 1988; Zbinden, 1988).

In Vitro Short-Term Tests

The objective at this stage is to obtain information on the chemical reactivity of the test material. A crucial set of data needed is whether the chemical undergoes covalent reaction with DNA. If radiolabeled material is available, definitive determination of adduct formation can be made. Other biochemical and biophysical techniques are also available, but vary in specificity and sensitivity. Electrochemical detection combined with HPLC is a useful technique (Park *et al.*, 1989). Highly sensitive techniques for identifying adducts are direct pyrolysis-electron impact mass analyzed ion kinetic energy spectrometry or accelerator mass spectrometry, and biochemical ^{32}P-postlabeling techniques. In place of definitive chemical and biochemical determinations, short-term tests for genotoxicity can be used.

Short-term tests are discussed in detail in Chapter 6 but their application in that context is somewhat different than for carcinogen testing. Among *in vitro* assays, no individual test, which has been studied adequately, has detected all carcinogens tested. In many cases, as described, this is because the "carcinogens" are not all DNA reactive. Another important factor is the complexity of metabolism of chemical carcinogens. Known species differences in response to carcinogens can be related to a large extent (but not exclusively) to metabolism, and thus tests with different metabolic capabilities are extremely useful. Moreover, in addition to tests that identify genetic effects, newer procedures, still in the research stage, to detect epigenetic carcinogens are becoming available.

A number of reviews of aspects of short-term tests have appeared (Rosenkranz, 1988; Würgler, 1989; Quinto *et al.*, 1990). The two critical elements of a test are the end point and the metabolic parameters. The end point should be reliable and of definite biologic significance. The metabolic parameters of a test should be complementary to others in the battery and the battery should include some tests that mimic as closely as possible *in vivo* characteristics of biotransformation.

A screening battery must include microbial mutagenesis tests because these have been the most sensitive, effective, and readily performed screening tests

thus far. However, the bacterial mutagenesis tests require a mammalian enzyme preparation to provide for metabolism of procarcinogens, and hence other tests to be included should expand the metabolic capability of the battery because this factor is often the most limiting aspect of a test series. Among available short-term tests, several employing intact hepatocytes (Rauckman and Padilla, 1987) and other cell types have been developed. Because whole cell metabolism is closer to the *in vivo* condition, such systems are included. In particular, the hepatocyte primary culture/DNA repair test is useful because DNA repair is a specific response to DNA damage and, unlike other effects on DNA, cannot be attributed to toxicity (Hanawalt, 1989; Williams, 1989). Mutagenesis of mammalian cells is a definitive end point, as is bacterial mutagenesis, and is included to complement the latter end point in a eukaryotic system. Sister chromatid exchange is included to provide a measurement of effects at the highest level of genetic organization. Its sensitivity, ease, and objectivity of measurement exceeds that of clastogenicity, although in some instances its significance is not yet fully understood. Cell transformation is included because this alteration is potentially the most relevant to carcinogenesis. This test is considered optional because much more needs to be done to standardize systems and clarify the significance of the end point. Both sister chromatid exchange and transformation may have the potential to detect epigenetic agents.

Bacterial Mutagenesis. Widely used bacterial screening tests have been developed in the laboratories of Ames (1989). The Ames test measures back mutation to histidine independence of histidine mutants of *Salmonella typhimurium* and can be conducted with strains that are also repair deficient, possess abnormalities in the cell wall to make them permeable to carcinogens, and carry an R factor enhancing mutagenesis, or that are nitroreductase-deficient or responsive to oxidative mutagens. Hence, these organisms are highly susceptible to mutagenesis, making them sensitive indicators. Other bacterial and microbial mutagenicity systems are available. In a different type of test developed by Rosenkranz and associates, DNA-repair-deficient *Escherichia coli* are used to measure their enhanced susceptibility to cell killing by carcinogens. In this system a chemical that interacts with DNA is more toxic to the repair-deficient strain than to wild-type *E. coli*, because the mutant strain cannot repair the damage. Thus, by measurement of relative toxicity, an indication of DNA interaction is obtained. These tests are dependent on mammalian enzyme preparations for metabolism of carcinogens. The capability of the Ames test to detect many carcinogens has been enhanced significantly by preincubation of the compound and the activation system with the test organism or by a sensitive variant involving turbidity measurement, the flocculation test.

A limitation of the Ames test is that several chemicals not known to be carcinogenic, such as quercetin, or those not likely to be carcinogenic, such as glutathione and cystine, have been positive. For example, it is sensitive to chemicals that on metabolism produce H_2O_2 or active oxygen, which in most mammalian cells are neutralized through biochemical defense mechanisms. Thus, such chemicals are negative in *in vitro* bioassays using mammalian cells, and are usually not carcinogenic, if overloading doses are avoided.

Mammalian Mutagenesis. A variety of end points for mutational assays in mammalian cells are available, including resistance to bromodeoxyuridine, ouabain, or diphtheria toxin (Milman and Weisburger, 1985). Of these, purine analog and bromodeoxyuridine resistance are the most widely used. In purine analog resistance assays, mutants lacking the purine salvage pathway enzyme hypoxanthine guanine phosphoribosyl transferase are identified by their resistance to toxic purine analogs such as 8-azaguanine or 6-thioguanine which kill cells that utilize the analogs. This assay has the advantage over the measurement of thymidine kinase deficient mutants by resistance to bromodeoxyuridine in that the gene for the affected enzyme is on the X chromosome rather than a somatic chromosome, as with thymidine kinase, and consequently the gene is highly mutable without having to construct and maintain heterozygous mutants. The target cells used in purine analog resistance assays have almost all been fibroblast like, such as the V79 line, and have displayed little ability to activate carcinogens. This deficiency has been overcome by providing exogenous metabolism mediated by either cocultivated cells or enzyme preparations. The latter again offer no extension in metabolic capability over that used for bacterial systems. However, the use of freshly isolated hepatocytes as a feeder system offers additional possibilities because the metabolism of hepatocytes has been shown to be different from that of liver enzyme preparations as regards the presence of conjugating capability. Another interesting development is the finding that liver epithelial cultures can be mutated by activation-dependent carcinogens and may therefore provide another system with additional self-contained metabolic potential.

Hepatocyte Primary Culture DNA Repair Test. DNA repair synthesis is a specific response to various types of DNA damage and can be measured in a variety of ways (Hanawalt, 1989; Williams, 1989). Several of the definitive procedures are technically sufficiently demanding that they have not been widely used for screening purposes. Of the two procedures that have, autoradiographic measurement of repair synthesis has an advantage over liquid scintillation counting in that it excludes cells in replicative synthesis, whereas these are part of the background with liquid scintillation counting. In addition, with liquid scintillation counting, increases in incorporation can result from changes in uptake or the pool size of thymidine without any repair occurring. Furthermore, autoradiography affords a determination of the percentage of cells in the affected population that responds. Two features that complicated early repair assays were that they required suppression of replicative DNA synthesis because continuously dividing lines were used, and they were dependent on enzyme preparations for metabolic activation. Both of these complications were overcome with the introduction of the hepatocyte primary culture/DNA repair assay of

Williams (Williams *et al.*, 1989) which uses freshly isolated, nondividing liver cells that can metabolize carcinogens and respond with DNA repair synthesis measured autoradiographically. This assay has demonstrated substantial sensitivity and reliability with activation-dependent procarcinogens. It also offers the advantages of expanded metabolic capability in the battery and clear biologic significance of its end point. An *in vivo-in vitro* version of the test is available (Mirsalis *et al.*, 1985). This feature permits detection of agents that require biotransformation by enteric organisms. An alternative to this approach is simply to supplement the *in vitro* system with bacterial enzymes.

Sister Chromatid Exchange. Sister chromatid exchange is an exchange at one locus between the sister chromatids of a chromosome, which does not result in an alteration of overall chromosome morphology (Milman and Weisburger, 1985). The most widely used method for differentiating sister chromatids combines staining with a fluorescent dye plus Giemsa, the FPG or harlequin methods. Using this technique, the observation of sister chromatid exchanges induced by chemicals is one of the quickest, easiest, and most sensitive tests for genetic damage. Sister chromatid exchanges are suspected to be due to a recombination event that may occur at the DNA replication fork, but at present, the lesions responsible for exchanges are unknown. Thus far, this response has not been validated with a very extensive array of chemicals. Also, certain noncarcinogens or promoters have been positive. Nevertheless, this is still a useful complement to the other end points in the battery.

Cell Transformation. The first reliable system for transformation of cultured mammalian cells was introduced by Sachs and associates. This system utilizing hamster fibroblasts was subsequently developed into a colony assay for quantitative studies by DiPaolo and has been adapted as a screening test by Pienta and coworkers (Milman and Weisburger, 1985). In addition, a quantitative focus assay for transformation using mouse cells has been devised in the laboratory of the late C. Heidelberger (Sakai and Sato, 1989). The correlation between transformation and malignancy appears to be good in these systems (McCormick and Maher, 1989). Also, they provide an indication of the activity of chemicals, which could be due to either genotoxic or epigenetic mechanisms. Other approaches under development include the use of epithelial systems and cell systems carrying oncogenic viruses as a more sensitive means of detecting transforming chemicals (Weinstein, 1988).

Decision Point 1

The six steps (A, and B, 1–5) recommended thus far provide a basis for informative decision making at this stage. If clear-cut evidence of genotoxicity in more than one test has been obtained, the chemical is highly suspect. Positive results in both the bacterial mutagenicity test of Ames and the hepatocyte DNA repair test of Williams reflect likely carcinogenicity. Confirmation of carcinogenicity may be sought in the limited *in vivo* bioassays without the necessity of resorting to the more costly and time-consuming chronic bioassay.

Evidence of genotoxicity in only one test must be evaluated with caution. In particular, several types of chemicals such as intercalating agents are mutagenic to bacteria, but are not reliably carcinogenic. Positive results in bacterial tests also have been obtained with synthetic phenolic compounds or natural products with phenolic structures such as flavones. *In vivo,* such compounds are likely to be conjugated and readily excreted. Their carcinogenicity thus would depend on *in vivo* splitting of such conjugates, which may occur more readily in laboratory rodents than in humans. Also, some chemicals generate active oxygen, yielding a positive result in a bacterial test, but not in mammalian cells. Therefore, positive evidence of bacterial mutagenesis must be evaluated further with regard to chemical structure and metabolism.

If all the preceding test systems yield no indication of genotoxicity, the chemical should be evaluated according to two principal criteria: (1) the structure and known physiologic properties (e.g., hormone) of the material, and (2) the potential human exposure. If the chemical structure suggests a need for sequential bacterial mammalian cell metabolism, then an *in vitro* system supplemented with bacterial enzymes could be used, or an *in vivo–in vitro* assay. Where substantial human exposure is likely, careful consideration should be given to the necessity for additional testing with the likelihood of a standard chronic bioassay. The chemical structure and the properties of the material provide guidance on the appropriate course of action. Thus, organic chemicals with structures suggesting possible sites of activation may reveal their carcinogenicity in limited *in vivo* bioassays. On the other hand, substances such as solid-state materials, hormones, possibly some metal ions, and promoters that are negative in tests for genotoxicity operate by complex and as yet poorly understood mechanisms. For these, it is unlikely that the limited *in vivo* bioassays would yield any results when such materials are tested alone. The next step that is recommended for such chemicals is specific mechanistic studies, or assay for promoting activity, depending on structure.

Taking advantage of the concept proposed by Loeb (1989) that certain metal ions affect the fidelity of enzymes concerned with DNA synthesis, such ions may be tested in rapid bioassay. In addition, certain metal ions can be detected in tests for mutagenicity (Costa, 1989). It seems reasonable that the nature of the metal ion, of which there are only a limited number, would provide the necessary insight for further testing

in the type of assay most likely to reveal any adverse effects (IARC Sci. Publs. 53, 1984; 71, 1986).

Compounds other than the strictly androgen and estrogen type can nevertheless exert effects on endocrine glands, e.g., amitrole or ethylenethiourea, a breakdown product of a class of fungicides, the dithiocarbamates. Such chemicals cause cancer in animals mainly because they interfere with the normal, physiologic endocrine balances, when ingested chronically at high dose levels. More research is required on methods to test quickly for such properties. Standard clinical pathology and biochemistry techniques such as thyroid function tests may be useful. It is known, for example, that certain drugs lead to release of prolactin or other hormones from the pituitary gland. Chronic intake of such drugs causing a permanently higher serum and tissue peptide hormone level might, in turn, alter the relative ratio of other hormones. At this time, any substance with such properties needs to undergo a chronic bioassay with carefully and appropriately selected doses or an initiation promotion test with a suitable initiator so as to evaluate whether endocrine-sensitive tissues would be at higher risk. The interpretation of data needs to take into account the normal diurnal, monthly, and even seasonal cycles of the endocrine system and whether the test might have led to interference in this balanced, rhythmic system. Information on the relevant mechanisms is absolutely essential for a science-based, factual human risk assessment. Chemicals with such properties have been glibly labeled "carcinogen" with the implication of human risk, when in fact the environmental concentrations are such as to not interfere with the normal endocrine balances. Thus, objective review suggests no human hazard.

The implications of a positive response in specific chronic bioassays coupled with convincing data of the absence of genotoxicity are discussed under the final evaluation.

Tests for Promoting Agents

A major group of epigenetic agents are those that facilitate the development of neoplastic cells into tumors and are thus carcinogenic in animals with "spontaneously" or cryptogenically transformed cells, probably because of translocation and amplifications of certain oncogenes. A great variety of synthetic chemicals, certain drugs, immunosuppressants, and hormones belong to this group. Thus, tests for promoting activity are essential in the safety evaluation of chemicals. In determining the tumor enhancing activity of an agent, this is indicative of promotion only for nongenotoxic chemicals.

In Vitro Tests for Tumor Promoting Agents.

Much information has accumulated dealing with the mechanisms of action of the classic tumor promoters, the phorbol esters, in *in vitro* systems (Schmidt and Hecker, 1989). A variety of responses related to interactions with specific membrane receptors, especially protein kinase C, have been noted. Approaches to identification of promoters include the induction of plasminogen activator, ODC production, or sister chromatid exchange and aneuploidy. For most of these, effects have not been found with nonphorbol types of promoters. Nonetheless, many promoters can be detected by their ability to increase ODC, or their effect in increasing DNA synthesis (thymidine or bromodeoxyuridine incorporation). High levels of genotoxic carcinogens also increase DNA synthesis in some organs such as liver, and this fact requires consideration in data evaluation.

The transformation systems for genotoxic carcinogens can be modified and used to test for promoting substances if a limited amount of a carcinogen is used as initiator followed by, or even together with, another agent (cocarcinogenesis).

Based on the concept that important informational molecules are exchanged between cells in contact through gap junctions, the systems have been developed to detect promoting agents by their ability to block intercellular molecular exchange through gap junctions. A similar approach using liver cells has been devised by Williams (Stevenson *et al.*, 1990). This effect *in vitro* would cause cells with an abnormal genome to be isolated from the growth controlling elements provided by neighboring normal cells and thus released for progressive growth. These relatively new techniques for detecting promotion *in vitro* show considerable promise, but need extension and validation.

Another approach to the detection of some promoters depends on the appearance of cadmium-resistant cells as a result of amplification of metallothionein genes. The data so far suggest that promotion may involve gene amplification.

In Vivo Promoting Assays.

Promoters of neoplastic development often display a high degree of organ specificity. Consequently, *in vivo* assays involve the administration of a genotoxic initiating agent that affects the organ in which the promoting activity of the test substance is to be examined.

The most widely used system involves testing for promoting activity on mouse skin initiated with small doses of benzo [*a*]pyrene or 7,12-dimethylbenz[*a*]anthracene. Also, induction of ODC in the absence of initiation has been proposed and successfully used as an assay. New promoters have been discovered by this means (Fujiki *et al.*, 1989).

A material exhibiting hormonal properties or one affecting endocrine balances in general, or bile acids likewise may show an effect in modifying breast, colon, or endometrial cancer induction in animals given limited amounts of methylnitrosourea as an initiating dose (American Health Foundation, 1987), or utilizing mice with or without the mammary tumor virus (Highland *et al.*, 1977). Similarly, promoters for urinary bladder may be identified by specific enhancing effects subsequent to pretreatment with limited amounts of a .bladder carcinogen.

To test for promoting activity by a chemical in liver carcinogenesis, rapid *in vivo* bioassay tests have been designed by giving a few doses of a limited amount of an appropriate genotoxic hepatocarcinogen such as diethylnitrosamine or 2-acetylaminofluorene followed by the test chemical. An increase in number or size of carcinogen-induced altered foci can be identified as evidence of promotion with histochemical markers such as γ-glutamyl transpeptidase or iron exclusion.

Drugs or other chemicals that appear to be enzyme inducers that (1) in a chronic bioassay in rats and mice have given some evidence of liver tumor induction in mice but not in rats and (2) have been negative for genotoxicity in appropriate *in vitro* test batteries have shown promoting activity in such systems. Often, there is an increased rate of DNA synthesis. DNA of liver cells of certain mouse strains displays an abnormal genome, with activated and translocated oncogenes (Beer and Pitot, 1989; Stevenson *et al.*, 1990). Thus, promoters facilitate expression of this abnormal genome, resulting in the "induction" of liver neoplasms in chronic tests, such as those in the U.S. National Toxicology Program (Ashby *et al.*, 1989; Gold *et al.*, 1989). Products with such attributes are properly labeled "carcinogens," but of the promoter type; the implications need to be considered in the determination of human health risk of such chemicals (Roloff *et al.*, 1987; Williams and Weisburger, 1988).

These initiation-promotion schemes, when designed with a number of dose levels, including the possible prevailing environmental level, help provide the necessary background information for the establishment of a threshold level and for health risk analysis.

Decision Point 2

A positive response in the *in vitro* test for inhibition of intercellular communication is highly suggestive of a promoting potential. However, this test has not been sufficiently validated with known promoters of different types affecting distinct organs. Therefore, a positive response in this system indicates the advisability of an *in vivo* test for neoplasm promotion. A nongenotoxic chemical that is active in an *in vivo* test for neoplasm promotion must be regarded as a potential hazard, depending on dose or exposure rates. Therefore, the finding of a positive effect indicates the need for further safety testing. This should include a multidose administration following a short course of the appropriate genotoxic carcinogen, which may permit the determination of a relative no-effect level. Neoplasm promoters by themselves are almost certain to be negative in the limited *in vivo* bioassays (see below) for carcinogenicity. Therefore, no point is served by submitting the chemical to testing of this type; instead it should undergo chronic bioassay if the potential human exposure warrants it. Because a finding of promoting activity indicates a possible contribution to cancer risk, the chronic bioassay should be undertaken with a view to establishing a possible no-effect level by means of testing over a broad dose range. The finding of a no-effect level in chronic bioassay coupled with lack of genotoxicity and evidence for a promoting action would lead to a health risk assessment distinctly different from that of genotoxic carcinogens.

Limited Bioassays

This stage of evaluation employs tests that will provide further evidence of any potential hazard of chemicals giving limited evidence of genotoxicity without the necessity of undertaking a full-scale chronic bioassay. Also, certain of the tests can provide relative potency ratings, when the design includes positive controls.

Such *in vivo* tests will provide evidence of carcinogenicity (including cocarcinogenicity and promotion), in a relatively short period, i.e., 52 weeks or less. Studies of enhancing effects involve the use of a known initiating carcinogen for a specific target organ or organs to detect an unknown cocarcinogen or promoter. In a limited bioassay for carcinogenic potential, a known promoter for a specific organ can be used to enhance detection of an unknown initiator. The test chemical for such a study should have been positive in tests for genotoxicity.

Unlike the *in vitro* tests, limited bioassays are not applied as a battery, but rather selected according to the information available on the chemical. The types of chemicals that have been positive in the various tests are given for each test.

Altered Foci Induction in Rodent Liver. During liver carcinogenesis several distinct liver cell lesions precede the development of carcinomas. The earliest of these, the altered focus when sufficiently developed, can be demonstrated in routine histologic tissue sections. Also, foci are abnormal in a number of properties that permit their reliable and objective identification at early stages by more sensitive techniques. Altered foci in rat liver display abnormalities in the enzymes γ-glutamyl transpeptidase, glucose-6-phosphatase, and adenosine triphosphatase, which have been used for their histochemical detection (Bannasch *et al.*, 1989; Pitot *et al.*, 1989; Stevenson *et al.*, 1990). Another marker for foci that permits histochemical identification is their resistance to iron accumulation following iron loading (Williams, in Stevenson *et al.*, 1990). This latter property is sometimes more sensitive than the enzyme abnormalities and also, unlike the enzyme abnormalities, characterizes rat, mouse, and hamster liver lesions. Evaluation of the placental form of glutathione *S*-transferase using antibodies for immunostaining has proven useful in the rat (Hasegawa *et al.*, 1989) and, as with iron storage deficiency, can be done on fixed tissue.

Another approach to detecting altered foci employs their resistance to the cytotoxic effect of carcinogens.

In this approach, administration of the test chemical is followed by exposure to 2-acetylaminofluorene and partial hepatectomy or, instead of the latter, a necrogenic dose of CCl_4 (Ward *et al.*, 1989). The selective agent is biotransformed by normal liver cells and affects them so that they cannot proliferate in response to the partial hepatectomy; in contrast, the cells in altered foci proliferate and become extremely conspicuous. The current complexity of this carcinogen and surgical manipulation appears to be a disadvantage compared to the demonstration of foci resulting from repeated application of a free agent. However, future developments in this active field may lead to significant improvements in all these approaches.

With known carcinogens, foci have been detected within three weeks of carcinogen exposure and in high numbers by 12 to 16 weeks of exposure (Williams and Weisburger, 1988). Therefore, the recommended approach is that of exposure for 12 weeks to the test chemical with injection of subcutaneous iron during the last two weeks to produce the iron load that delineates the foci resistant to iron accumulation. Among the carcinogens that have been detected using foci induction are aromatic amines, nitrosamines, and amino azo compounds (Milman and Weisburger, 1985).

Pulmonary Neoplasm Induction in Mice. Andervont and Shimkin pioneered with the model involving the development of lung tumors in specific sensitive strains of mice, especially the A/Heston and related strains such as A/J. A singular advantage of this assay system is that, in addition to an end point that measures the percentage of animals with neoplasms compared to controls, the multiplicity of tumors is an additional parameter expressing the "potency" of any carcinogenic action. Most chemicals that are active in this system are also carcinogenic in other longer chronic animal tests. Another useful aspect of this assay is that significant results are obtained in as short a time as 30 to 35 weeks, and sometimes faster. Extension of the test for a longer period is not desirable because the incidence of pulmonary tumors in control animals increases rapidly after 35 weeks, and thus the test loses sensitivity. Positive results have been obtained with polycyclic aromatic hydrocarbons, certain nitrosamines and nitrosamides, aflatoxin B_1, ethyl carbamate, hydrazines, alkylating agents, and arylamines, the latter relatively weakly.

Skin Neoplasm Induction in Mice. The carcinogenicity of a limited number of chemicals and crude products can be revealed readily on continuous application to the skin of mice, producing papillomas or carcinomas, or on subcutaneous injection, yielding sarcomas. A highly sensitive strain, the SENCAR mouse, was developed as a specific tool to investigate the effect of genotoxic carcinogens and also of agents acting through epigenetic mechanisms in this selected tool, where the underlying molecular aspects begin to be understood (Robinson, 1986). Also, initiating activity can be rapidly determined by the concurrent or sequential application of a specific promoter, such as one of the phorbol esters, (Schmidt and Hecker, 1989). Tars from coal, petroleum, or tobaccos are active in such systems, as are the pure polycyclic aromatic hydrocarbons and congeners contained in such products. Mouse skin responds positively because it appears to have the necessary enzymes to yield the reactive metabolites leading to initiation, especially in the presence of cocarcinogens or promoters in the crude products. On the other hand, such mixtures rarely yield visceral neoplasms, mainly because the liver can detoxify these chemicals quickly. However, lung and lymphoid neoplasms in sensitive mouse strains can be a secondary tumor site.

Mouse skin is useful primarily, therefore, for chemicals such as polycyclic hydrocarbons, also direct acting chemical carcinogens such as sulfur or nitrogen mustard, bis(chloromethyl)ether, propiolactone, as well as alkylnitrosoureas. Arylamines and related carcinogens by themselves usually do not provide a positive response on mouse skin, although some exceptions are 2-anthramine and 3-methyl-2-naphthylamine, which are active in this system perhaps because these chemicals are converted to active epoxy intermediates, in the same manner as the polycyclic aromatic hydrocarbons. On the other hand, mouse skin does not appear to yield a positive result with a basic fraction of tobacco tar, even though this fraction is mutagenic and leads to cell transformation. Some arylamines and urethane, however, provide a positive indication even on oral or parenteral intake, but only on promotion with a phorbol ester.

Breast Cancer Induction in Female Sprague-Dawley Rats. This model is based on the original finding by Huggins that polycyclic hydrocarbons rapidly induce cancer in mammary gland of young, female, random-bred Wistar rats and still better in Sprague-Dawley rats (Milman and Weisburger, 1985). With powerful carcinogens, especially select polycyclic hydrocarbons, arylamines, certain chloroalkanes such as 1,2-dichloroethane, or nitrosoureas, positive results have been obtained rapidly, in less than nine months, sometimes after a single dose. As in the case of lung tumor induction in mice, the multiplicity of mammary tumors provides an additional quantitative criterion to denote relative strength of the carcinogenic stimulus. This system has been used in initiation-promotion schemes, especially in exploration of the fat-hormone-breast cancer sequence (American Health Foundation, 1987; Rogers and Longnecker, 1988).

Decision Point 3

Proven activity in more than one of the limited bioassays may be considered unequivocal qualitative evidence of carcinogenicity. A definite positive result in one of the limited *in vivo* bioassays, together with two positive results in a battery of rapid *in vitro* tests reliable for genotoxicity, also indicates potential carcinogenicity. This is true especially if the *in vivo* results were obtained with moderate dosages, and more so if there was evidence of a good dose-response, particularly as regards the multiplicity of the skin, lung, or mammary gland neoplasms, or of liver foci.

Positive results in one *in vivo* bioassay and in only one *in vitro* test makes the agent highly suspect, but further testing is indicated. A negative result in any of these assays does not constitute proof of noncarcinogenicity because they all have some limitations.

Chronic Bioassay

In the systematic approach described, chronic bioassay is used (1) for confirming questionable results in the more limited testing, or (2) for chemicals that are negative in the preceding stages of testing but where extensive human exposure is likely, or (3) for the acquisition of data on possible carcinogenicity through indirect epigenetic mechanisms. Of course, for a chemical subject to governmental regulations chronic bioassay may be required. Regardless, multispecies and dose-response data are most important if the data are to be applied to risk assessment. For chemicals found nongenotoxic in the *in vitro* tests (decision point 1), but some indication of promoting potential (decision point 2), it may be worthwhile and efficient to include an initiation promotion test using an initiating agent with broad tissue responses such as some of the nitrosamines, or especially nitrosamides such as *N*-nitrosomethylurea or *N*-nitrosoethylurea to secure solid data on promoting properties.

It is important to keep in mind that chronic rodent bioassays for carcinogenicity are extraordinarily expensive investments in time and money, and should not be conducted as theoretical exercises in estimations of response of animals to chemicals. Rather the deliberate aim and only goal of carcinogen test systems should be the acquisition of data that permit evaluation of the carcinogenic risk for humans (Clayson, 1987; Hayes, 1989). Therefore, a key issue regarding chronic bioassays is the degree to which data obtained in such systems actually reflect a human carcinogenic risk (Hoel *et al.*, 1988; Roloff *et al.*, 1987). As shown in Table 5–1 about 35 chemicals or mixtures have been found to be associated with cancer in humans (Tomatis *et al.*, 1989). Almost every one of these chemicals is also highly carcinogenic in several animal models. Therefore, the reverse may very likely be true, that is, a chemical that is reliably carcinogenic in animal models would also affect humans. The definition of "reliably carcinogenic" applies to chemicals that are active over several dose ranges in a number of species and that induce a high yield of neoplasms at a given site and possibly several select sites within a reasonably short latent period (15 months or shorter). Such chemicals are unquestionably human risks, especially if essential collateral data show them to be also genotoxic.

The known human carcinogens are typically endowed with such properties. An exception is arsenic in the form of inorganic arsenite, where animal models have failed to provide convincing evidence of carcinogenicity and where the underlying mechanisms are undefined. In this instance the evidence for carcinogenicity is based on epidemiologic studies in populations consuming water with elevated arsenic levels (Wu *et al.*, 1989). Perhaps the presence of confounding factors needs exploration.

Bioassay systems primarily use rats, mice, and for some specific purposes hamsters. Because younger animals are often more sensitive, exposure begins at weaning or shortly thereafter. Newborn mice, and in some cases newborn rats and hamsters, have been recommended because they appear to show even higher sensitivity to some carcinogens.

Certain bioassays have involved exposure of males and females of a parent generation that are mated during exposure, thus providing for possible transplacental exposure. The exposure of the offspring is then continued for a two-year period. Advantages and limitations of two-generation tests require definition (IARC Sci. Publ. 96, 1989). At this time, and in the framework of a systematic Decision Point Approach as described here, these two-generation tests are probably no more useful for delineating human cancer risk than is a standard bioassay.

All chemical carcinogens display dose-response effects, but the time factor needs to be considered because cancer induction under a variety of conditions, even with powerful carcinogens, requires a certain minimum period of time. This is because the entire process is very complicated, from the biochemical activation of the agent leading to transformation of cells in specific tissues, to the growth and development of abnormal cells to a visible neoplasm. This entire process has been thought to take at least one-eighth the life span of a species. Thus, mice, rats, and hamsters, with an average life of two to three years, usually develop detectable cancer in no less than three months after treatment with most carcinogens. With longer lived species, including primates, the process may be expected to take much longer. For example, diethylnitrosamine induces malignant liver cancer in rats in as little as three to five months, whereas in the Rhesus monkey the same point is reached in one to three years. The trend has been to use even shorter lived species as a means to decrease the time required for bioassays (Milman and Weisburger, 1985).

A high dose usually induces a greater yield of cancers in a given target organ more rapidly than a lower dose, even though the latter, given sufficient time, may eventually induce the same yield of tumors. In addition, varying the dosage may lead to shifts in target organs, mainly because of (1) early deaths due to faster cancer occurrence in a primary target organ, (2) alterations in metabolic pathways, and (3) possibly also tissue-related factors such as cell turnover times and repair mechanisms. For example, a few large doses of dimethylnitrosamine induce cancer of the kidneys after a fairly long latent period, whereas continuous low dosing with the same agent consistently results in a high incidence of liver cancer with a shorter latent period. The relevant mechanism involves DNA repair capability, which is expressed more in rat liver than in kidney tissue.

Potent carcinogens such as those with demonstrated activity in humans can be detected in mice or rats rather quickly, often in less than one year. Weaker agents take longer, even at high dose levels, and it may be necessary to observe the animals for their entire lifetime.

During studies of the pathogenesis of certain cancers induced by specific carcinogens, antecedent precancerous lesions have been discovered in some organs long before a definitive tumor was diagnosed. If this were true for all chemical carcinogens, their detection by early examination of tissues for such specific cellular alterations would be greatly facilitated. Indeed, the reliable detection of such lesions in the liver is the basis for a limited bioassay. Unfortunately, in some tests, autopsies performed even one year after the beginning of treatment have given no diagnostic signs, although neoplasms occurred after 18 months. Thus, in a study lasting less than two years, a negative finding would not necessarily mean that an agent was not carcinogenic, and in any case collateral data from other tests are important. On the other hand, the interpretation of the two-year and especially of lifetime tests can be difficult. As animals age, they die from causes unrelated to test chemical exposure and are thus lost to the experiment without necessarily exhibiting cancer. Also, they develop cryptogenic tumors, most often in the endocrine-sensitive organs, or lymphomas and leukemias, again not related to the treatment. The incidence of these crytogenic neoplasms is not constant and varies between studies and even groups in a study, sometimes substantially, as for example, with neoplasms in the pituitary or adrenal glands. Thus, it is necessary to compare the incidence in an experimental group not only to simultaneous controls, but also to historic controls.

Some investigators recommend lifetime studies, which, when animal colonies are carefully maintained, permit some strains of rats to live as long as three years and mice to live as long as two and one half years. Most current procedures, however, involve exposure of groups of male and female rats, mice, or hamsters in experiments that terminate after two years for rats and 21 to 24 months for mice and hamsters, depending on strain, thus allowing optimum survival time for nonexposed controls. An advantage of this scheme that we recommend is that 70 to 90 percent of the experimental animals live to the end of the test. Thus, under these conditions, tissues from scheduled necropsies are secured for microscopic study. In lifetime studies, it is sometimes difficult to avoid losses of valuable material due to autolysis when animals die between observations. Also, the variable increasing incidence of spontaneous tumors actually tends to decrease rather than improve the sensitivity of the test.

Furthermore, the question of the length of administration of the test compound requires consideration. With food additives and related materials, where humans are conceivably exposed by direct intake during their life span, it is useful to administer the compound throughout the test series. For industrial chemicals and other materials where the potential exposure may be intermittent, a period of 18 months might be more useful. This seems sufficiently long, because even with a weak carcinogen, it is logical to assume that the processes leading to tumor induction have been initiated, although no accurate comparative study to ascertain this point experimentally has been performed. Thus, discontinuing administration of the compound after 18 months and maintaining the animals for three to six additional months is actually useful to support the development of any tumor produced and lead to regression of many abnormal, yet noncancerous lesions. At the same time, the toxic stress of compound administration is removed, and thus a beneficial, more prolonged survival of the animals is actually facilitated.

Selection of Animal Types and Number. Within the numerous strains of mice, rats, and hamsters, strains should be selected that are readily available, have good breeding performance, are disease free, exhibit extended survival, and have good sensitivity to carcinogens. The availability of an extensive historical tumor data base is important. Some investigators prefer to use random-bred animals, others inbred animals. Because the variability is less and the reproducibility of tests is somewhat better in inbred animals, and also because certain transplantation experiments and related immunologic considerations are performed more readily or possibly exclusively in inbred animals, or F_1 hybrid descendants of two inbred strains, the trend has been toward the use of such inbred animals. Nevertheless, even with random-bred animals, properly conducted tests can be executed reproducibly. For example, the induction of mammary gland cancer is reliably and quickly performed in the random-bred Sprague-Dawley rat.

The Fisher (F344) rat was introduced in large-scale chronic bioassays by J. and E. K. Weisburger in the United States for tests carried out under the aegis of the U.S. National Cancer Institute, beginning in 1964. The advantage of this strain is that adults are of low body weight (about 500 g for males), compared to the Wistar or Sprague-Dawley strain (weight up to 1 kg). Thus, multiple housing is facilitated, a major economy. Also, the F344 rat is equally or more sensitive in a general bioassay than other strains, and requires less total amount of chemical, again a major saving. Yet, they display a low, reproducible incidence of spontaneous neoplasms, another advantage. A large-scale test of pesticides and agricultural chemicals carried out by Kotin, Falk, and Innes of the NCI uses two F_1 hybrid mouse strains, $C_{57}BL \times AKR$ and $C_{57}BL \times C3H$. In view of the satisfactory results obtained with the latter hybrid, the Weisburgers recommended its use for the NCI carcinogenicity tests. The large-scale use of the F344 rat and B6C3F$_1$ mouse strains by many laboratories in North America, Japan, and Europe has provided an impressive set of results relative to spontaneous neoplasms, survival records, and economy of use with these strains. These animals have also been utilized in pharmacologic, metabolic, and mechanistic investigations, providing additional background information in comparative toxicology.

The number of animals to be used depends on several factors, including the need to generate sufficient data for a dependable statistical evaluation. For a genotoxic carcinogen giving a high incidence of tumors in less than one year, the loss of animals due to treatment-unrelated causes may be minimal, and groups of 20 to 30 suffice. For an unknown agent or where the effect is weak, and therefore requires a lengthy experimental period, a larger number of animals is used to compensate for deaths unrelated to treatment. If the experiment calls for killing some of the animals prior to the termination of the main tests, for example, to delineate any early effects, the initial number would have to be increased, so as to take into account this reduction in the group size of the animals at risk in any set. Current practice is to use 50 or even more animals per group, or for specific tests such as dose-response studies. Such tests are best planned with the advice and continuing consultation of professional statisticians (Farrar and Crump, 1990; Hoel *et al.*, 1988; Laska and Meisner, 1988).

Dose Selection. This is a controversial aspect of bioassays. Some investigators advocate avoidance of any level of toxicity and accordingly use fractions of the LD_{50}. In the case of pharmacologically active substances, common general practice is to use the maximally tolerated dose (MTD) and a fraction or fractions thereof.

The MTD is established in preliminary assays, under the same conditions selected for the test series. The need for high level testing at the MTD has been discussed in detail. In brief, historic observations on occupational cancer in humans revealed that exposures were usually high and chronic. Reproduction in animal models of human cancer risks required high dosages, as with 2-naphthylamine or phenacetin. Acute LD_{50} determinations do not necessarily contribute information that will be useful in determining doses tolerated under chronic conditions. If a chemical leads to changes in the processing enzymes, the chronically tolerated dose could be higher or lower than an acute toxic dosage, depending on how the balance of activation or toxication over detoxification metabolites is altered.

With DNA-reactive carcinogens, the induction of tumors is often seen at several dose levels. Such studies have shown that even with powerful carcinogens there are doses at which no effect is obtained within the normal life span of the animals. The entire problem of revealing possible carcinogenicity in bioassays with small doses, approximately those prevailing in the general, not occupational, environment, is still unresolved. Analytic chemistry has advanced impressively, permitting accurate determinations of chemicals at parts-per-billion and even parts-per-trillion levels. Even with powerful carcinogens and with consideration of possibly synergistic interactions, the question remains whether levels in this range have any biologic significance, especially in defining human risk.

Even in simplified test series it is advisable to utilize at least one dose level below the MTD. The main reason is to ensure adequate survival of at least one of the groups of animals for the planned experimental period. If the preliminary toxicology leads to the selection of a high dose level that is tolerated for six to nine months but then results in the death of the experimental group without cancer or adverse effects, the entire study will have to be repeated. Thus, to save time, a similar group of animals is started simultaneously at a lower dose level; one-half or one-third of the MTD generally is adequate and usually permits survival of the animals for the necessary length of time. An active carcinogen would show a response, proportional to dose, at both dosages. If the MTD shortens life span, that group of test animals by dying sooner might actually exhibit a lower cancer incidence than those on the reduced dosage who live longer. However, in any case, the results of the battery of the short-term tests, and the limited *in vivo* bioassays will have yielded information essential for the design of the chronic tests. Often, a two-year bioassay will not be necessary because adequate information for decision making will have been obtained in the preceding set of short-term and limited bioassays. When the importance of the chemical mandates a chronic bioassay, in view of the possible extensive human contact this should be designed with three to five dose levels, from the MTD to one approximating the highest probable human exposure.

With weaker carcinogens, active when given at the MTD, it has been found that the second dose level fails to induce statistically significant rates of cancer in a chronic test with the usual number of animals at risk. Hence, careful selection of dosages is mandatory to detect relatively low degrees of carcinogenicity, unless, of course, larger numbers of animals are used. Such a pattern of activity is indicative not only of weaker genotoxic carcinogens, but even more so of nongenotoxic promoters that under some conditions at high dose levels can induce a low but significant yield of neoplasms in two-year or lifetime tests.

Modes of Administration. Activation-independent carcinogens will almost always cause cancer in any tissue to which they are directly applied. On the other hand, activation-dependent carcinogens, which require bioactivation, are rarely active at the site of application and, in contrast, exhibit sometimes quite specific organotropism, depending on the biochemical potential of a given tissue. Even so, the mode of administration can affect the tumor yield at a given site, because it dictates pathways of internal distribution and metabolism and hence the concentration in a tissue. For example, dibutylnitrosamine given subcutaneously to rats leads almost exclusively to tumors in the urinary bladder. After subcutaneous injection, absorption leads to direct passage via the blood into renal pathways. On the other hand, oral administration produces tumors in the liver, lung, and urinary bladder because these additional organs receive a sufficient concentration of the agent.

In general, the mode of administration should logically mimic the potential human exposure. Thus, food additives would normally be fed or given by gavage. Cosmetics would be applied to the skin. Drugs given by parenteral injection would be thus tested. However, if the only question asked is whether a given chemical structure has carcinogenic potential that, as discussed previously, is a highly specific, nonrandom property, then the route of administration may depend more on such mechanistic aspects. The mode used is the one that would most likely reveal a carcinogenic effect based on the chemical structure of the agent.

Certain commonly used techniques of administration are clearly in need of further study. For example, the daily administration of corn oil or other edible oil as a vehicle adds sizable fat calories and has specific metabolic effects and may, in turn, alter the action of a test compound. The induction of tumors in rodents at the site of single or repeated subcutaneous injection requires careful interpretation. With this proviso, this technique offers advantages. With direct acting carcinogens, tumors are formed at the site of injection, often quickly and with small amounts of chemical. Any systemic effects can also be observed. However, some chemicals induce local sarcomas, but this sole finding is not evidence of oncogenic potential. In fact, such materials may not be a hazard to the public, exposed to such chemicals by some way other than through the parenteral route. An example is the induction of sarcoma on subcutaneous injection or implantation of polymers or certain chemicals as in detergents, soaps, emulsifiers, or organic salts into rats or mice. This would normally not reflect a human oncogenic risk. Again, it is important to consider collateral data from tests for genotoxicity in judging risk from extrapolation of bioassays in rodents.

Study Conduct. Control groups are as important as experimental groups. In smaller studies evaluating the carcinogenicity of only one or two compounds, the control group must be of the same size as each experimental group. Some effort can be saved if a number of chemicals or drugs are studied simultaneously, for then one control group can serve as reference point for a number of contemporary experimental groups. The control group should involve a number of animals $x\sqrt{n}$, where x is the size of each group and n is the number of simultaneous experimental groups. If a vehicle is used, control groups treated with the vehicle alone, in addition to untreated control groups, are required to assess the possible effect of the treatment with the vehicle. In addition, it is desirable to give the positive control at two dose levels, one known to be effective quickly, as a means of assessing the responsiveness of the specific type of animals used. The other dose level could be lower to mimic any possible weaker effect of the unknown compounds.

An animal that has been part of a test series longer than a year becomes a valuable specimen. Every effort must be made not to lose it because of poor husbandry practices or inadequate professional supervision. Animals must be inspected every day, and toward the end of an experiment twice a day. Animals in poor health should be examined to establish whether survival is possible. If this is unlikely, proper necropsy procedures should be instituted immediately. After a substantial time on test, little is gained by maintaining an animal already in poor health for a few more days or weeks.

Autopsies must be performed by highly trained personnel, capable of detecting even minor grossly visible lesions. A complete autopsy includes opening of the skull and examination of the tissues of the nervous system, the brain, and the pituitary gland, as well as the other viscera. Proper fixation of tissues in suitable fluids, trimming of select tissues for histologic processing, and finally the microscopic study of stained sections should be supervised or performed by trained professionals. The entire assay hinges on the accurate execution of the total test series, but in particular it depends on the exact diagnosis and interpretation of the significance of any lesions noted. Again, individuals trained in experimental pathology should be part of the team designing and monitoring a test series. An experienced pathologist using correct diagnostic procedures will be in the best position to conclude the study successfully.

Final Evaluation

Chronic bioassays stemming from the systematic application of the decision point approach would be expected to yield definitive data on carcinogenicity. In any case, the results from biochemical studies and short-term tests must be considered for evaluation of possible mechanisms of action and risk extrapolation to humans (Hoel *et al.*, 1988; Williams and Weisburger, 1988; Salsburg, 1989). Convincing evidence of DNA reactivity or positive genotoxicity tests coupled with documented *in vivo* carcinogenicity permit classification of the chemical as a DNA-reactive carcinogen. It would, therefore, be anticipated that the chemical could display the properties characteristic of such carcinogens, which include the ability under some circumstances to be effective at a single dose, display cumulative effects, and act synergistically, or at least additively, with other DNA-reactive carcinogens that affect the same tissues. Such DNA-reactive carcinogens may vary in potency and demonstrate thresholds but in the absence of information to the contrary they must be regarded as qualitative hazards to humans. Accordingly, the level of human exposure permitted must be rigorously evaluated and controlled.

If appropriate studies yield no convincing evidence for DNA reactivity, but nonetheless the chemical displays carcinogenic effects in animal bioassays, there is a possibility or indeed likelihood that the agent is an epigenetic carcinogen. The strength of this conclusion depends on the relevance of the negative evidence for DNA reactivity and the degree to which an alternative mode of action has been established. For instance, the sensitive techniques of ^{32}P-postlabeling or direct measurement by pyrolysis electron impact analyzed ion kinetic energy or accelerator mass spectrometry can provide compelling chemical evidence for the absence of DNA adduct formation in the target organ of the carcinogen. A biologic approach is to assess for syncarcinogenesis between the agent in question and a DNA-reactive carcinogen with the same target organ.

The overall nature of epigenetic mechanisms is not completely understood at present, but they appear to be distinct for the different classes. They may involve chronic tissue injury and cell proliferation, generation of reactive species, immunosuppressive effects, hormonal imbalances, blocks in differentiation, breakage of gap junctions, promotion of preexisting genetically altered cells, or processes as yet unknown. In any event, many epigenetic carcinogens have displayed carcinogenicity only at the MTD in chronic bioassays. Detailed dose-response studies would be informative with such agents because it is probable that they represent only quantitative hazards to humans, and safe levels of exposure may be established by carrying out proper toxicologic and pharmacologic dose-response studies.

The extrapolation of animal carcinogenicity data to humans is a highly controversial topic. Humans, unlike many experimental species, are genetically heterogeneous. In addition, humans have wide variations in environment, diet, and life style. Thus, one would not expect a uniform response to exogenous agents such as carcinogens. In pharmacology and medicine, it is a well accepted fact that patients need to be considered as individuals when prescribing dosages of drugs. Animal systems, on the other hand, can be controlled much more effectively. Indeed, highly inbred strains of genetically uniform rodents, mice, rats, and hamsters are available. Animals can be housed under standard conditions, fed uniform purified diets, and, in essence, treated identically. Thus, it can be expected that the carcinogenic response would be more uniform in experimental animals than in humans. Nonetheless, cancer induction processes are very complex. They are strain and species dependent, and thus the response to a given chemical carcinogen is a function of the experimental system. Humans are not uniform, and it is probably true that some people will respond some of the time to a given carcinogenic challenge. One of the key elements in the response of any species, including humans, would appear to be the biochemical potential in activating or deactivating exogenous carcinogens. Promoting stimuli, stemming from elements such as dietary factors, the biosynthesis of cholesterol and bile acids, hormonal balances, immune competence, and endogenous viral profiles and intestinal flora, also are distinct as a function of species and strain. Nonetheless, with the curious exceptions of arsenic, all DNA-reactive carcinogens and promoting agents now known to play a role in human cancer causation have been reproduced rather well in animal models, provided the dose rate and time elements were taken into account. Thus, animal models do provide a basis for assessing human risk as to genotoxicity, promoting, or carcinogenic potential. The process, however, is complicated, and collateral mechanistic information is absolutely essential to determining which animal model is predictive.

EPILOGUE

During the last few decades, much progress has been made in the basic sciences underlying toxicology with specific reference to chronic effects, including carcinogenesis. Thus, we have come to realize that the great diversity of chemical structures capable of causing cancer depends for some on the specific property of such structures to be either electrophilic reactants or to become such after metabolic activation. At the same time, further insight into the molecular target of such carcinogens as electrophilic reactants implicates the genetic material in the cell—DNA. It has also been discovered that DNA with covalently bound carcinogens can be repaired and that some of the observed biologic effects, including that of organotropism, depend as much on such repair processes, or the lack thereof, as on the metabolic activation and interaction of intermediates with DNA. Of current interest is the role of tumor suppressor genes, and their neutralization, in the carcinogenic process.

The recognized interaction of some carcinogens with DNA has provided the necessary scientific background for relating mutagenicity to carcinogenicity. In turn, this connection has provided a sound basis for utilizing short-term tests measuring genotoxicity in prokaryotic and eukaryotic systems in the assessment of the carcinogenic potential of a chemical. In this chapter, we have organized chemical carcinogens as DNA-reactive agents, and as agents capable of inducing cancer through other mechanisms referred to as epigenetic. Inasmuch as current evidence shows that the carcinogenic properties of chemicals of these two broad categories differ, especially that most classes of epigenetic agents act in a reversible, highly dose-dependent fashion, attention needs to be directed toward developing distinct risk management procedures for different types of carcinogens. It is expected that further research on methods of detection in the light of the systematic classification described will provide a rational and scientific approach to the elimination of risk of potentially harmful substances. This is important inasmuch as there are sound data with respect to the causes of the main human cancers, that they are due as much to the presence of agents operating via epigenetic mechanisms as to genotoxic carcinogens. For example, epigenetic

agents play a major role in the development of cancer of the lung due to cigarette smoking, or of cancers of the colon, breast, prostate, and perhaps pancreas which involve certain dietary habits. Thus, some leads such as the lower risk of lung cancer after smoking cessation, or of endometrial cancer on reduction in body weight or lower use of estrogen, indicate that these major types of cancer can be controlled and indeed reversed by modifying the environment not only with respect to DNA-reactive carcinogens but also with respect to epigenetic carcinogens. In fact, public health programs (McGinnis, 1988–1989; U.S. Department of Health and Human Services, 1988, 1989; Greenwald et al., 1990) to decrease the habit of smoking, or to lower total dietary fat intake or increase bran fiber consumption, actually depend on the property of reversibility of promotion. Application of the classification of carcinogens to the analysis of the main causes of important types of cancer worldwide has provided insight into the mechanisms whereby they arise (Table 5–5). This approach has provided the basis for sound recommendations, often distinct for each kind of cancer, to reduce the risk of cancer development significantly. Because many types of cancer are the result of the presence and action of genotoxic carcinogens and epigenetic, promoting agents, risk reduction can be introduced successfully by several approaches. In Europe, the United States, and Japan, there are national plans for effective reduction of mortality from cancer by the year 2000 (McGinnis, 1988–1989; Greenwald et al., 1990). These efforts are realistic if current sound knowledge is applied expeditiously.

Nowadays the public is much more aware of environmental cancer risks, and their concern has led to legislation and regulation at many levels (Environmental Protection Agency, 1986; Office of Technology Assessment, 1989). The same public involvement has provided increased resources in toxicology from both private and public funds, which have contributed to the base of knowledge. At the same time, however, the public and the media, although concerned with cancer, are not at all well informed as to the actual risk factors. The facts and principles described in this chapter will hopefully not only assist professionals involved in toxicology and carcinogenesis, but can be translated into activities that will provide the public with reliable, science-based background and protection against avoidable cancer hazards. Worldwide, deliberate slight but specific changes in life style patterns, from childhood on, are major essential tools to lower significantly locally prevailing cancer risks (Weisburger and Horn, 1990).

Table 5-5. FACTORS AND POSSIBLE MECHANISMS IN MAIN EPITHELIAL CANCER CAUSATION AND PREVENTION

Application of knowledge derived from studies on the mechanisms of carcinogenesis and toxicology to an analysis of the genotoxic carcinogens, any enhancing or promoting factors, and any protective elements on an organ-site basis has provided insight into the causative elements of the main, important types of human cancer worldwide. This information in some instances has been the basis of public health activities, designed to lower the risk of developing a specific type of cancer, by eliminating or lowering the genotoxic carcinogens, or any promoting agents, or increasing any protective or inhibiting factors.

DISEASE	RISK FACTORS	MECHANISM	PROTECTIVE ELEMENTS	MECHANISM
Nasopharyngeal cancer	Salted, pickled fish	Contains specific nitrosamine?	Vegetables	Micronutrients
	Viral factors	Can increase cell cycling	Vaccination?	
	Wood and leather workers	Carcinogens/promoters		
Esophageal cancer	Salted, pickled food?	Specific nitrosamine	Yellow-green vegetables	Role of vegetables unknown if risk factor present in food
	Alcohol intake + smoking	Alcohol modifies esophageal metabolism of tobacco-specific carcinogens	Yellow-green vegetables	Carotene, vitamin A protective elements
	Tobacco chewing	Tobacco-specific carcinogens and promoters?	Vegetables?	β-carotene as antioxidant
Gastric cancer (glandular intestinal)	Salted, pickled food	Nitrosoindoles, phenolic diazotates	Green-yellow vegetables	Role of vegetables unknown if risk factor present in food, but may assist in differentiation
	Geochemical nitrate and salt	Carcinogens formed in the stomach	Green-yellow vegetables, fruits, vitamins C and E	Vitamin C and E prevent formation of carcinogen: vitamin increases cellular tissue defenses
Bladder cancer	Bilharzia: schistosomiasis	Carcinogens unknown; increased cell proliferation enhances risk	Yellow-green vegetables	Beneficial micronutrients
	Smoking	Unknown	Yellow-green vegetables	Retinoids
	Occupational	Chronic high exposure to some arylamines	—	—
Endocrine-related cancers: prostate, breast, ovary	Total dietary fat (saturated + ω-6 polyunsaturated lipids)	Complex multieffector elements: hormonal balances, membrane and intracellular effectors	Monounsaturated oil (olive)	Neutral action on hormone metabolism
			ω-3 polyunsaturated oils	Protective effect in hormone metabolism
			Medium chain triglycerides	Caloric equivalent to carbohydrate
			Cereal fiber and pectin	Affects enterohepatic cycling of hormones
			Yellow-green vegetables	Micronutrients

Cancer	Exposure	Mechanism	Prevention	Effect
	Fried/broiled meats	Heterocyclic aromatic amines (HAA)	Tryptophan and proline	Prevent formation of HAA
Endometrial cancer	Same as above; excessive body weight	Same as above; fat cells generate high levels of estrogen	Same as above; weight control/loss	Same as above; lowers excessive nonphysiologic estrogen levels
Pancreatic cancers	Same as endocrine cancer (total dietary fat)	High fat diets increase functional demands, increase cell duplication?	Vegetables	Micronutrients
	Cigarette smoking	Tobacco-specific nitrosamines		
	Fried/broiled meats	Heterocyclic aromatic amines (HAA)	Tryptophan and proline	Prevent formation of HAA
Colon cancer Proximal	?	?	?	?
Distal	Same as endocrine-related cancers	Biosynthesis of cholesterol, thence bile acids, and colon cancer promotion, including higher cell cycling rates	Cereal fiber, especially wheat	Increases stool bulk; dilutes promoters; lowers intestinal pH
Rectal cancer	Alcoholic beverages, especially beer	Increases cell cycling in rectum	Cereal fiber?	Dilutes effectors by increasing stool bulk
Liver cancer	Mold-contaminated foods	Mycotoxins	Avoid moldy foods; improve nutrition; more protein, fruits, and vegetables	Lower carcinogen intake
	Some plants	Pyrrolizidine alkaloids		
	Pickled foods	Nitrosamines	Avoid pickled foods	
	Chronic virus	Hepatitis B	Vaccination	
	High level of specific alcoholic beverages	Damages liver, risk of cirrhosis potentiates effect of carcinogens	Decrease intake of alcohol	
	Occupational, iatrogenic	Vinyl chloride; some oral contraceptives (infrequent occurrence)	Lower exposure	May lower cell duplication rates
	Cigarette smoking	Tobacco-specific nitrosamines		
	Fried/broiled meats	Heterocyclic aromatic amines (HAA)	Tryptophan and proline	Prevent formation of HAA

DNA-REACTIVE (GENOTOXIC) CARCINOGENS

Activation-Independent (Direct-Acting, Primary) Organic Carcinogens

Some types of activation-independent DNA-reactive carcinogens are listed in Table 5–6 together with typical examples of each type. Inherent in the chemical structure of these agents is the property of chemical reactivity, as shown in Table 5–3A; they are electrophilic reactants that can interact with nucleophilic targets, including DNA, usually but not always by an SN_1 mechanism. They alkylate at N^7 and O^6 of guanine and N^3 of adenine.

These agents are synthetic products used in chemical production and as cytostatic agents. The direct-acting carcinogens include strained lactones, such as propiolactone, propane sulfone, and unsaturated larger ring lactones, epoxides, imines, alkyl and other sulfate esters, and some active halogen derivatives, such as bis(chloromethyl)ether. Although such reactive chemicals might be thought to be carcinogenic under a variety of conditions, some agents, such as methyl methanesulfonate, are not highly carcinogenic in animals, mainly because they undergo secondary hydrolytic decomposition, or their reactive groupings provide ready targets for specific detoxification reactions. Nevertheless, these reagents can be potent carcinogens. Several, including ethylnitrosourea, produce cancer in the offspring of treated pregnant female animals (IARC Sci. Publ. 96, 1989). Dimethyl sulfate was reported to induce cancer in humans after laboratory handling without adequate precautions.

Halo Ethers and Other Active Halogen Compounds. Chemicals such as certain halo ethers in which the halogen carbon bond is chemically activated through electron transfer are extremely powerful alkylating agents and carcinogens. The most important example is bis(chloromethyl)ether, discovered first to be carcinogenic by Van Duuren, Laskin, and their associates in laboratory experiments (see Arcos et al., 1968–1988; Maltoni and Selikoff, 1988). It was subsequently found that this highly reactive alkylating agent, an important chemical intermediate in industry, led to cancer of the upper respiratory tract in humans exposed to apparently low levels of this chemical. In animal models, inhalation of as little as 0.1 ppm is carcinogenic.

The higher homologs appear to be less active.

Sulfuric Acid Esters. Dimethyl and diethyl sulfate are chemical reagents with powerful alkylating activity. They are mutagenic and carcinogenic in rodents. One case report noted that four laboratory workers handling dimethyl sulfate without adequate precautions (failure to use a well-vented exhaust hood) developed lung cancer. Drugs such as 1,4-butanediol dimethanesulfonate (Myleran®) are used in cancer therapy by virtue of their alkylating potential. They are carcinogenic in rodents. Methyl methanesulfonate, the simplest prototype of this class of chemicals, is mutagenic and carcinogenic.

Nitrosamides, Nitrosoureas, and Ethylenimines. Agents such as N-methylnitrosourea, N-methylnitrosourethane, and N-methyl-N'-nitro-N-nitrosoguanidine are chemically stable in the an-

hydrous state. However, in aqueous solutions at a pH above 7.0, they undergo hydrolytic decomposition, possibly enhanced by specific enzymes, to liberate an alkylating ethylenimonium ion (Table 5–3A). The cytostatic drug streptozocin is a substituted methylnitrosourea, which was first isolated as an antibiotic, that is carcinogenic in several species.

Ethylenimine derivatives have been developed as alkylating cytostatic drugs. One of these, triethylenethiophosphoramide (thiotepa), has caused cancer in treated patients.

Activation-Independent Inorganic Carcinogens

Radioactive Inorganic Compounds. The sources of exposure to radioactive materials and their toxicity are covered in detail in Chapter 21. Compounds of uranium, polonium, radium, and radon gas have demonstrated carcinogenicity attributed chiefly to their radioactive properties. Uranium, radium, and the derived radon gas have been implicated in the occurrence of lung cancer in individuals engaged in mining ores. Miners who smoke cigarettes are at higher risk, indicating a possible synergistic effect between ore dust, radiation, and cigarette smoking, as is true for the smoking-asbestos interaction.

The exposure of workers to radon in mines presents a given disease risk, compounded and increased by the presence of highly dusty atmospheres, themselves including radioactive particles that settle in the lung, and cigarette smoke (Lubin et al., 1990). This situation leads to a high risk of cancer in the respiratory tract. In the last few years, it was discovered in certain geographic regions of the United States and in Europe that the subsoil released radon gas to homes (Samet, 1989). Public concern has arisen that occupancy of radon-containing homes, particularly in the lower floor levels, might also be a cause of lung cancer. Estimates were made that of the total of 155,000 lung cancers, 101,000 in males and 54,000 in females, 20,000 might be associated with exposure to radon in the home in nonsmokers. Yet, this geologic emission of radon has been present for centuries, but lung cancer in males was low in the 1920s and did not rise until about 1930 in men and 1950 in women, associated wth the increasing smoking of cigarettes in that period. In smokers, the chronic presence of radon can augment the risk of lung cancer. As is true for all carcinogens, it is a matter of chronic high concentrations, as for example in the Reading Prong, a useful area for key pilot studies as to cancer risk of nonsmoking individuals living in homes with specific concentrations of radon. Thus, careful evaluation of the possible effect in nonsmokers of radon in homes is needed to provide proper toxicologic perspective and especially to establish a secure base for any recommendations for prevention, without unnecessarily alarming the public, as the media have done from time to time in relation to radon or low-level asbestos exposures (Mossman et al., 1990).

Deliberate or inadvertent intake of radioactive elements or their compounds that concentrate in certain organs or tissues may be a cancer risk. Thus, intake of labeled iodine and derivatives, concentrating in the

Table 5–6.　ACTIVATION-INDEPENDENT OR PRIMARY ORGANIC AND INORGANIC CARCINOGENS

These chemicals do not require biotransformation to yield the electrophiles shown in Table 5–3A that react with DNA. This class includes active halogen compounds, alkyl imines, alkylene epoxides, sulfates esters, nitrosamides, and nitorsoureas. Some of these are used as industrial intermediates and others as cytostatic drugs. Among the latter are the inorganic and organic platinum amine chelates. With these, the *cis* isomers are usually more active than the *trans* compounds.

Active Halogen Compounds

bis(Chloromethyl)ether　　　　$ClCH_2OCH_2Cl$

Chloroacetone (R-H); dichloroacetone　　　　$ClCH_2COCH_2R$
　(R-Cl)

Benzyl chloride　　　　$C_6H_5CH_2Cl$

Methyl iodide　　　　CH_3I

Dimethylcarbamyl chloride　　　　$(CH_3)_2NCOCl$

Alkyl Imines

Ethylene imine

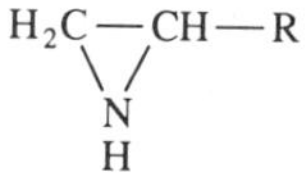

$$H_2C \underset{\underset{H}{\diagdown \ \diagup}{N}}{\overset{}{\longrightarrow}} CH \longrightarrow R$$

Alkylene Epoxides

1,2,3,4-Butadiene epoxide

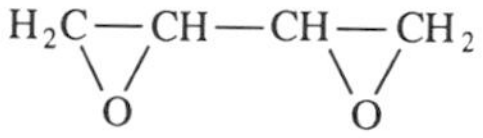

$$H_2C \underset{O}{\overset{}{-}} CH \longrightarrow CH \underset{O}{\overset{}{-}} CH_2$$

Small-Ring Lactones

β-Propiolactone

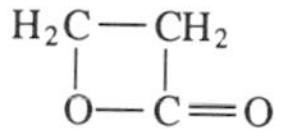

$$H_2C \longrightarrow CH_2 \\ | \qquad | \\ O \longrightarrow C = O$$

Propane sultone

$$CH_2 \longrightarrow CH_2 \\ | \qquad\qquad \searrow O \\ CH_2 \longrightarrow SO_2 \nearrow$$

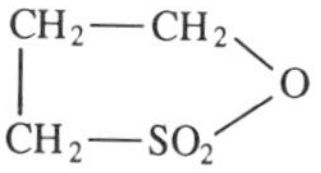

Sulfate Esters

Dimethyl sulfate　　　　$CH_3OSO_2OCH_3$

Methyl methanesulfonate　　　　$CH_3SO_2OCH_3$

1,4-Butanediol dimethanesulfonate　　　　$CH_3SO_2O(CH_2)_4OSO_2CH_3$
　(Myleran)

Nitrosamides and nitrosoureas

N-methyl-N-nitrosourea　　　　$CH_3N(NO)CONH_2$

N-methyl-N-nitrourethane　　　　$CH_3N(NO)COOCH_2CH_3$

N-methyl-N'-nitro-N-nitrosoguanidine　　　　$CH_3N(NO)C(NH)NHNO_2$

N-Ethyl-N-nitrosourea　　　　$CH_3CH_2N(NO)CONH_2$

Platinum amine chelates

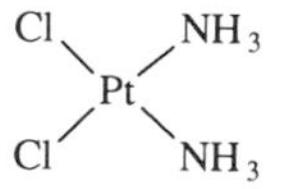

cis-Dichlorodiamine-
platinum (II) or DDP

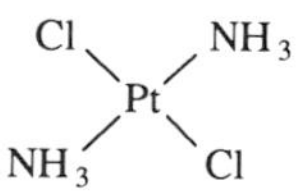

trans-DDP

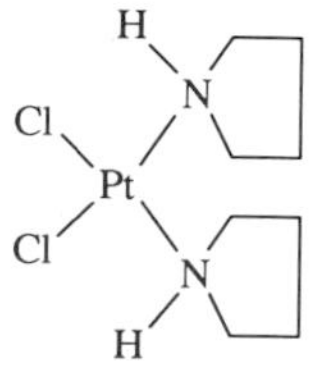

cis-Dichlorobis (pyrrolidine)-
platinum (III)

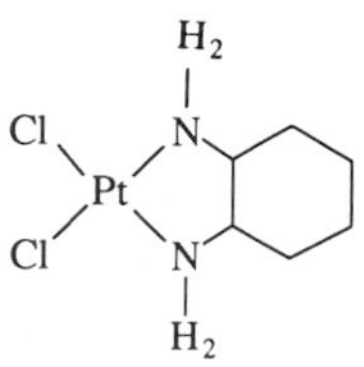

cis- or *trans*(-)-or *trans*(+)-
Dichloro-1,2-diaminocyclohexane-
platinum(II) complexes

thyroid gland, has been known to give rise to cancer in that organ. Chemicals that concentrate in bone, such as strontium derivatives, in their labeled forms, can induce osteosarcomas. These elements are the main contributors to the cancer hazard associated with radioactive fallout, consequent to the above ground use of nuclear weapons, a procedure no longer used, fortunately. The now abandoned medical use of thorotrast is known to induce liver cancer.

Metals and Metal Ions. Among the inorganic chemicals, the metals nickel, chromium, cobalt, lead, manganese, beryllium, and certain of their derivatives in specific valence states have been found carcinogenic under certain experimental conditions (Chambers *et al.*, 1989). Among these, salts of nickel appear to be the most powerful (Costa, 1989). Manganese antagonizes the effect of the nickel salts. In most instances, these chemicals lead to cancer formation at the point of application, as for example, the rapid formation of sarcoma after subcutaneous injection of nickel sulfide in rats. Nitrilotriacetate has a carcinogenic effect on kidney and bladder by virtue of cytotoxicity as a metal chelate. Oral intake of large amounts of lead acetate induces kidney cancer in rats. The mechanism may be deposition of lead salts, and thus depend on solid-state effects. Clearly, low levels would not have this adverse effect. Inhalation of beryllium salts or ores has induced pulmonary carcinoma in rats and Rhesus monkeys.

In humans, inorganic compounds have been shown definitely carcinogenic only in the case of nickel derivatives obtained by a process that was abandoned in the mid-1930s. Workmen on the job since that time do not appear to have appreciable risk, an impressive demonstration of prevention of occupational cancer by altering exposure conditions without detracting from commercial production.

In addition, human exposure to certain complex ores such as chromates, hematite, or nickel apparently has a high risk, particularly of cancer in the respiratory tract. The question of interaction with tobacco smoke needs consideration in interpreting these data. It is not certain whether the disease process is due to a direct carcinogenic reaction by the ore (likely for nickel ore, but perhaps not for hematite) or whether the neoplastic change is due more to a type of solid-state carcinogenesis, akin to that of asbestos discussed below.

Little is known about the mechanisms of the oncogenic action of inorganic chemicals. They do not seem to operate directly as electrophiles, as do the corresponding ultimate, organic molecule carcinogens. There are certain indications that they are active in rapid bioassay systems and thus may be genotoxic. However, a potentially important conceptual advance stems from the research of Loeb (1989), indicating that certain metal ions affect the fidelity of the polymerase involved in the biosynthesis of DNA, thus yielding abnormal DNA through this indirect mechanism.

Cis-Platinum(II) Coordination Complexes. This group of chemicals structurally represents a complex chelate of divalent platinum and an appropriate anion, which most of the time is chloride, with two residues possessing amino groups (Table 5–6). These structures can assume *cis* or *trans* configurations. The simplest compound in the series is the one where R is ammonia, namely *cis*-dichlorodiamineplatinum(II). This and related compounds have found use as drugs in cancer therapy. Other compounds of this series involve structures where the amine is pyrrolidine, cyclopentylamine, and 1,2-diaminocyclohexane. Several of these chemicals exist as *cis* and *trans* isomers and the cyclohexane compound as *cis, trans*(−), and *trans*(+). These chemicals are direct acting mutagens in the *Salmonella typhimurium* system of Ames, and they also exhibit activity in various other genetic tests such as inactivation of transforming DNA, which is typical of direct-acting genotoxic chemicals. In addition, they are powerfully carcinogenic as measured by a number of tests such as induction of lung tumors in mice, initiation of skin tumors when applied to the skin of mice followed by phorbol ester promotion, and induction of sarcomas on subcutaneous injection. The *cis* stereoisomer is more active than the *trans* compound. The reactive intermediate derived from the chloride derivatives appears to be an aquo species. The geometry of the stereoisomers of the *cis* compound is such that they chelate the 6 and the N positions of guanine, which may account for their mutagenic and carcinogenic effects.

Activation-Dependent (Procarcinogens, Secondary) Carcinogens

Most of the known chemical carcinogens are in the form of precursor compounds, often called parent, pre-, or procarcinogens. These activation-dependent carcinogens usually do not produce cancer at the site of application (except for certain mouse skin carcinogens such as the polycyclic aromatic hydrocarbons), but rather are carcinogenic to distant tissues where metabolic activation occurs. The capacity for biotransformation varies greatly between species and organs, accounting partially for the species differences and organotropism of these agents. The reactive electrophiles, capable of interacting with DNA and other nucleophilic molecules, are formed by biotransformation of these carcinogens, and their structure is known (Table 5–3B).

The large class of activation-dependent carcinogens includes both naturally occurring substances and synthetic chemicals, belonging to diverse chemical types, but all yield reactive products through metabolism.

Polycyclic or Heterocyclic Aromatic Hydrocarbons. These chemicals consist of annelated aromatic (benzene) rings (Table 5–7). These carcinogens occur in a number of environmental products such as soot, coal tar, tobacco smoke, petroleum, air pollutants, and cutting oils (Cooke and Dennis, 1988). The isolation of pure aromatic hydrocarbons from coal tar and the demonstration of their carcinogenicity by English investigators led by Kennaway in the 1930s was one of the milestones in studies on chemical carcinogenesis. There is good reason to suspect that these carcinogens are involved, for example, in lung cancer seen in cigarette smokers or tar roofing workers (U.S. Department of Health and Human Services, 1989). However, it is also clear that in complex mixtures such as tar and smoke, other agents, including promoters, contribute to overall carcinogenicity. Many rodent species are

Table 5–7. POLYCYCLIC AROMATIC HYDROCARBONS.

Many of these chemicals are derived from the anthracene (1) molecule. Anthracene (1) itself is not carcinogenic, but in some tests benz[a]anthracene (2) is carcinogenic and 7,12-dimethyl-benz[a]anthracene (3) is a potent carcinogen. 3-Methylcholanthrene (4), benzo[a]pyrene (5), and dibenz[a,h]anthracene (6) and other similar structures occur in products of incomplete combustion, including coal and petroleum tars, and exhausts of combustion engines. They are also important components of tobacco smoke.

1. Anthracene

2. Benz[a]anthracene

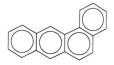

3. 7,12-Dimethylbenz[a]anthracene

4. 3-Methylcholanthrene

5. Benzo[a]pyrene

6. Dibenz[a,h]anthracene

exquisitely sensitive to chemical carcinogens of this type. In mice, skin application of the more powerful agents such as 3-methylcholanthrene, 7,12-dimethyl-benz[a]anthracene, and benzo[a]pyrene (Table 5–7) leads rather quickly to carcinoma formation. Subcutaneous injection produces sarcomas in rats or mice. Oral administration in sesame oil to 50-day-old female Sprague-Dawley rats results in the rapid induction of breast cancer, a model affected by endocrine control and diet, as is the disease in human females. However, administration of polycyclic aromatic hydrocarbons to Rhesus monkeys and other primates has so far not been highly successful in yielding tumors. On the other hand, application of a crude petroleum oil to monkeys has induced cancer.

Within the large class of polycyclic hydrocarbons, many structure-carcinogenicity studies have been done mostly in mice. Data so generated have led to theoretical developments relating chemical electronic structure to carcinogenic activity. For detailed historic and modern discussions of these aspects, the reader is referred to reviews by Arcos (1968–1988) and specialized monographs (T'so and DiPaolo, 1974; IARC Monograph series). Suffice it to say that many of the results obtained can be interpreted, in the light of contemporary concepts, in terms of chemical structure and susceptibility to biochemical activation and detoxification. In brief, the situation can be summarized as follows. Many of the carcinogenic polycyclic aromatic hydrocarbons are derived from an angular

benz[a]anthracene skeleton (Table 5–7). Anthracene itself is not carcinogenic, but benz[a]anthracene appears to have weak carcinogenicity. Addition of another benzene ring in select positions results in agents with powerful carcinogenicity such as dibenz-[a,h]anthracene or benzo[a]pyrene, which are "natural" products, resulting from incomplete combustion processes of carbonaceous materials. In addition, substitution of methyl groups on specific carbons of the ring also enhances carcinogenicity. Thus, 7,12-dimethylbenz[a]anthracene (DMBA) is one of the most powerful synthetic, polycyclic aromatic hydrocarbon carcinogens known.

As a result of the efforts of Lacassagne, Buu Hoi, Zajdela, and others who synthesized and tested many polynuclear heterocyclic compounds, a wide variety have been found to be carcinogenic, usually at the site of injection (T'so and DiPaolo, 1974; Woo and Arcos, in Sontag, 1981).

Biotransformation of Polycyclic Aromatic Hydrocarbons. Historically, on the basis of theoretic developments related to the electronic structure of these hydrocarbons, a certain area of the molecule, called the K region, was related specifically to the carcinogenic potential of a given compound. On the other hand, substitution of another portion of the molecule, the L region, such as the 7 and 12 carbons in benz[a]anthracene, increased carcinogenic potency. If these positions were free, there was a decrease in carcinogenicity. This simple scheme was a strong

Table 5–8. BIOACTIVATION OF POLYCYCLIC AROMATIC HYDROCARBONS

These hydrocarbons require a multistep metabolic activation by specific enzymes such as cytochrome P-450IIIA of the complex cytochrome P-450 enzyme system. The first reaction is an epoxidation. With benzo[*a*]pyrene (1), the product is the corresponding 7,8-epoxide (2) that, in turn, is subject to epoxide hydrolases (EHase) to form stereoisomeric diols (3). These are converted further to the 7,8-dihydrodiol-9,10-epoxide. The diol epoxide can exist in four stereoisomeric forms of which the key carcinogenic product is (+)-benzo[*a*]pyrene-7,8-diol-9,10-epoxide 2 (4).

1. Benzo[a]pyrene (BP)   2. BP-7,8-epoxide

3. BP-7,8-diol   4. BP-7,8-diol-9,10-epoxide

stimulus to research in structure-activity relationships between about 1945 and 1965. However, exceptions appeared for polycyclic aromatic hydrocarbons composed of other than five rings, and the scheme failed when chemicals with alkyl and, in particular, methyl substitution were involved. Boyland in England proposed as early as 1950 that an epoxide might be an active metabolite. In 1968, based on the fact noted by Gelboin in the United States, and independently by Sims in England, that binding to DNA of isotopes from a labeled polycyclic hydrocarbon is higher in the presence of a microsome fraction of liver, extensive research on the reactive metabolites from polycyclic hydrocarbons began (Conney, 1982). It was already known that with several other classes of carcinogens, especially the carcinogenic arylamines and nitrosamines, metabolism led to reactive intermediates. Sims proposed the now well-established concept that activation of polycyclic hydrocarbons was not likely to be on the K region, but rather stems from a two-step oxidation with the eventual formation of a dihydrodiol epoxide. Several groups in Europe and North America have rounded out this picture. Collaboration between the organic chemist Jerina and the pharmacologist Conney (1982) in the United States developed the actual sequence of steps for several polycyclic hydrocarbons leading to formation of the reactive epoxide in the part of the molecule called the bay region (Table 5–8). The adducts produced in DNA by covalent binding of these sites have been identified (Banbury Rept. 13, 1982; IARC Sci. Publ. 45, 1988).

Thus far, this activation process appears to be broadly applicable to many polycyclic hydrocarbons including benzofluoranthrenes and methyl-substituted

chemicals such as 11-methylcyclopenta[*a*]phenanthrenes, 5-methylchrysene, and 7,12-dimethylbenz[*a*]anthracene. The activated forms combine with hemoglobin, which provides a sensitive indicator to exposure (Gorelick *et al.*, 1989). Even a three-ring analog, 9,10-dimethylanthracene, and more so, the 1,2-epoxide, have shown mutagenic activity, thus reflecting a likely genotoxic intermediate. However, these simple epoxides are probably readily detoxified in mammalian cells through the action of epoxide hydrolase, and therefore are of low carcinogenic activity (Conney, 1982; Cooke and Dennis, 1988; Guengerich, 1988). It is possible that the metabolic conversion to other epoxides might also play a role and that there may be multiple active forms, especially with respect to distinct target organs. Nonetheless, the principal ultimate carcinogens of many polycyclic aromatic hydrocarbons are specific stereoisomers of diol epoxides, the *(S,R,R,S)* form. For any polycyclic aromatic hydrocarbon, however, the bulk of biotransformation leads to detoxified metabolites that are conjugated and rapidly excreted. Inhibition of the carcinogenicity of this class of compounds depends on increasing the level of detoxification reactions.

Monocyclic Aromatic Amines.   The prototype is aniline, a single aromatic ring compound with an amino substituent. Aniline was long considered to be noncarcinogenic, but in a bioassay, feeding at high doses over a long term resulted in a low yield of splenic sarcomas. The relevant mechanism has not yet been clarified but probably does not involve reaction with DNA. At high dose levels, aniline, through its metabolite, phenylhydroxylamine, is a powerful hematopoietic poison producing methemoglobinemia.

Most arylamines display this toxic effect, even in humans, especially at higher dosage. High chronic dosages cause chronic splenic congestion, and in turn sarcoma formation. Careful tests of the *N*-acetylated derivative, acetanilide, have not given any evidence of carcinogenicity, probably because the *N*-hydroxy metabolite is not formed in significant amounts. Likewise, the *para*-hydroxy derivative of acetanilide, the drug acetaminophen or paracetamol, is not carcinogenic, because it is detoxified easily by type II conjugation reactions. In contrast, phenacetin (4-ethoxyacetanilide) and *N*-hydroxyphenacetin are carcinogenic, producing kidney and nasal tumors and liver tumors, respectively, in rats (Dubach *et al.*, 1983).

The significance of the relatively weak carcinogenic effects in animal tests of single ring aromatic amines as regards human risk requires evaluation. In animals, a very high continuing dosage (8000 to 15,000 ppm in diet) is required to elicit a carcinogenic effect. However, even in situations of occupational exposure, monocyclic aromatic amines have not been associated with human cancer. Abuse, but not ordinary intermittent drug use, of phenacetin has led to human cancer in the bladder and renal pelvis (Dubach *et al.*, 1983). Likewise, most animal bioassays failed to reveal adverse effects, except one test, involving a chronic dietary intake of 25,000 ppm.

Polycyclic Aromatic Amines.   The prototype 2-annelated ring aromatic amine, 2-aminonaphthalene (2-naphthylamine) has demonstrated carcinogenicity in several species, including man, Rhesus monkey, dog, mouse, rat, and hamster (Maltoni and Selikoff, 1988; Tomatis *et al.*, 1989). The closely related 1-aminonaphthalene (1-naphthylamine), an important industrial intermediate, has been thought to cause human occupational cancer, but animal experimentation has not revealed carcinogenicity. Processes for the production of 1-aminonaphthalene can also generate the 2-isomer, as well as other possibly carcinogenic aromatic amines. Thus, the suspected carcinogenicity of 1-aminonaphthalene in humans may not in fact be due to the pure chemical, but relate to carcinogenic impurities. Polycyclic arylamines in which the amino group is in an α position to the adjoining ring are not usually carcinogenic because such compounds easily yield detoxified ring hydroxy metabolites, but undergo the activation reaction through *N*-hydroxylation only with difficulty, in contrast to arylamines with an amino group in other parts of the ring (King *et al.*, 1988). However, it appears that such inactive arylamines become weakly but definitely active if a methyl group is present in the *ortho* position as, for example, 1-amino-2-methylanthraquinone. The reason is not yet understood, but might hinge on an effect of this substitution in directing metabolic activation in a manner similar to that for larger polycyclic aromatic hydrocarbons. Thus, the active forms of such chemicals might be an epoxide or dihydrodiol epoxide. Small amounts are found in tobacco smoke and 4-aminobiphenyl has been used to establish factually smoking withdrawal (Maclure *et al.*, 1990). It is noteworthy, however, that arylamines bearing a substitution by an electron donating methyl group or by certain halogens in a position *ortho* to the amino group

appear to be more powerful carcinogens than the unsubstituted compounds.

The biphenyl series, which consists of two phenyl rings joined by a carbon-to-carbon bond and an exocyclic amino group, consists entirely of synthetic products used mainly as chemical intermediates in dyestuff and antioxidant production. The prototype, 4-aminobiphenyl (4-biphenylamine or xenylamine), is carcinogenic in humans and in a number of laboratory animals. It is no longer manufactured in most countries because of this hazard. Among the higher *para* substituted homologs, 4-aminoterphenyl is also carcinogenic, as would be expected.

The biphenyl derivative benzidine, which has a *para*-amino group on each ring, is an important industrial chemical intermediate. It is carcinogenic in several animal species and in humans under a variety of conditions. Substituted benzidines such as *o*-tolidine, the *ortho*-dimethyl derivative, and also the 3,3-dichloro compound are carcinogenic in laboratory animals and are suspected human carcinogens. In the same class are methylenedianiline (or 4,4-diaminodiphenylmethane) and its derivatives.

Among the tricyclic arylamine derivatives, a number of interesting structure-activity relationships have been found. 2-Aminofluorene (or 2-fluorenamine), a good but never used experimental insecticide, and its acetyl derivative were discovered to be carcinogenic in most species, except the guinea pig and the steppe lemming (King *et al.*, 1988). Tests in the Rhesus monkey are negative so far, even though exposures have been underway for more than 10 years.

In the anthracene and phenanthrene series, 1-anthramine and 1-phenanthrylamine are not carcinogenic, whereas the 2-isomers are highly active. 2-Anthramine, in addition to causing a variety of tumor types distant from the point of application, also induces skin cancer in rats on cutaneous application. 2-Phenanthrylamine is a good leukemogen and leads to a variety of other tumors in rats. Not many tests of the higher homologs have been conducted. However, 6-aminochrysene, a substituted arylamine, was carcinogenic to the liver when administered to newborn mice and induces skin tumors in mice after cutaneous application. This compound has been used in the chemotherapy of splenomegaly secondary to malaria and also of human cancer, particularly breast cancer. Chronic feeding to rats gave no evidence of carcinogenicity. The reason for the activity of 6-aminochrysene to mouse skin or newborn mice may be due to the fact that it yields reactive intermediates such as a substituted polycyclic hydrocarbon, rather than an aromatic amine (King *et al.*, 1988). 6-Nitrochrysene is also biotransformed to such reactive intermediates.

Heterocyclic Aromatic Amines.   Since 1978, new mutagenic heterocyclic chemicals have been found in "nature," as a result of the pyrolysis or cooking of protein-containing materials (King *et al.*, 1988). The pyrolysis of individual amino acids in model systems resulted in a series of pure products identified as heterocyclic amines that yielded mainly liver tumors in mice, although in rats several compounds exhibited carcinogenic action at select organs such as ear duct, small and large bowel, and bladder, similar to the action of the corresponding homocyclic compound 3,2'-dimethyl-4-aminobiphenyl. Among chemicals of the general class of aminoimidazoazaarenes or heterocyclic aromatic amines (HAA), obtained from the action of frying or broiling meat under realistic home cooking conditions, were several compounds based on an imidazoquinoline, -quinoxaline, or -pyridine ring system. Their formation can be inhibited by simple methods (Weisburger and Jones, 1990). These chemicals were among the most mutagenic chemicals found so far in the *Salmonella typhimurium* TA98 system and required metabolic activation by a liver S9 fraction. The carcinogenicity of several of these chemicals has been established. A key such compound, 2-amino-3-methylimidazo [4,5-*f*]quinoline, has induced primary liver cancer in nonhuman primates in three years, an extraordinarily rapid process. In rats, this compound specifically produces cancer in the liver, urinary bladder, and forestomach, not promoted by dietary fat levels, and in colon, breast, and pancreas, promoted by fat. It is postulated that this type of carcinogen, frequently ingested by humans eating cooked meats, might represent the agents associated with major human cancers such as cancer of breast, pancreas, and colon (King *et al.*, 1988; Weisburger, 1990; Weisburger and Horn, 1990). These chemicals have an exocyclic amino function, and it is likely that their mutagenicity and possible carcinogenicity stem from the biochemical conversion of the amino group to the corresponding hydroxylamino group, followed by appropriate target organ specific conversion to the alkylating intermediate (Yoshimi *et al.*, 1988).

Many, but not all, carcinogenic aromatic amines administered to rodents cause cancer of the liver or the urinary bladder, especially in male animals. In females, breast cancer is often the result. Depending on the specific structure of the aryl moiety, lesions at a number of other target sites are seen. The evidence thus far is that the urinary bladder is the site affected in humans exposed occupationally to high levels of certain of the carcinogenic aromatic amines (King *et al.*, 1988; Maltoni and Selikoff, 1988.

Biotransformation of Aromatic and Heterocyclic Amines. These chemicals, like polycyclic aromatic hydrocarbons, can be metabolized to ring epoxy derivatives, which, in turn, can be hydrated to dihydrodiols or can rearrange to phenols. For certain specific arylamines, ring epoxidation may play a role in carcinogenesis at certain target organs as, for example, mouse skin or mammary gland. This reaction seems to be involved even in liver carcinogenesis with certain chemicals such as quinoline, where epoxidation has been linked to activation. This kind of activation mechanism may also bear on the effect of certain polycyclic nitroaryl compounds such as 1-nitropyrene and 6-nitrochrysene (King *et al.*, 1988; Howard *et al.*, 1990).

Nevertheless, it seems clear that the major activation reaction of arylamines depends on *N*-hydroxylation, with the production of the corresponding hydroxylamine, or in the case of the *N*-acetyl derivative, of the *N*-hydroxy-*N*-acetyl compounds (Table 5-3B) (Miller and Miller, 1981; King *et al.*, 1988).

Most laboratory animals and humans have the necessary enzymes belonging to the cytochrome P-450 system, the IA1 or IA2 components, which can perform the *N*-oxidation reaction (Guengerich, 1988). However, in the steppe lemming and especially in the guinea pig, the cytochrome P-450 system isozymes tend to *C*-hydroxylate such compounds preferentially, and for that reason relatively small amounts of the reactive *N*-hydroxylation compound are formed. In turn, most studies have demonstrated that arylamine derivatives, including azo dyes, are not carcinogenic in the guinea pig or the steppe lemming. Humans have the ability to *N*-hydroxylate arylamines, but there are large quantitative differences between individuals (Rauckman and Padilla, 1987).

Once formed, arylhydroxylamines, under some conditions such as the acidic pH of urine or through enzymic oxidation, yield the reactive nitrenium ions that can combine with cellular macromolecules, especially with DNA, thus leading to toxicity and carcinogenicity. With the often used *N*-acyl and especially *N*-acetyl derivatives, the corresponding *N*-hydroxy-*N*-acetyl compounds require additional activation reactions (King *et al.*, 1988; Yamazoe *et al.*, 1989). In rodent liver, one such activation reaction is performed by the PAPS (3'-phosphoadenosine-5'-phosphosulfate)-linked sulfotransferase to yield the ultimate carcinogen, the *N*-hydroxy sulfate ester (King *et al.*, 1988).

Another important enzyme system in the disposition of aromatic amines is *N*-acetyltransferase and especially the arylhydroxylamine acyl transferase (King *et al.*, 1988). This activity has a polymorphic distribution in humans such that individuals are either rapid or slow acetylators. The rabbit also displays polymorphic expression whereas other species can be classified as rapid (e.g., hamster) or slow (e.g., dog, rat) acetylators. For many nitrogen-containing xenobiotics, acetylation is a detoxification reaction, but certain aromatic amines, through the *N*-hydroxy metabolite, appear to be directed toward activation in the liver or colon, by acetylation. Conversely, slow acetylation disposes some animals and humans to bladder cancer. This could stem from activation in other tissues, in which case aromatic amine target organs such as liver and breast might be at higher risk. Also, acetylation may block other activation reactions. There are sensitive and specific assays to measure the amount of circulating arylamines through the hemoglobin adducts (Maclure *et al.*, 1990; Sabbioni and Neumann, 1990).

In tissues other than liver, additional biotransformation processes seem to be involved in aromatic amine carcinogenicity. For example, a prostaglandin H synthetase that uses arachidonic acid as a cofactor (King *et al.*, 1988) appears to play a role in bladder activation. This system does not utilize acetylated aromatic amines very well, which may in part explain the higher risk of slow acetylator individuals to bladder cancer. In addition, there are deacetylases yielding the corresponding hydroxylamines. Although many tissues have an *N*-oxidation capability, most such biotransformation occurs in the liver (Bannasch *et al.*, 1989). These metabolites are converted by type II conjugation reactions to metabolites such as glucuronic acid derivatives that serve as transport forms and the occurrence of urinary bladder cancer has been traced to the enzymatic or acid-catalyzed splitting of conjugates in the bladder followed by additional specific activation reactions in this target tissue. Similar considerations may apply to processes of cancer induction in other target organs susceptible to carcinogenesis by certain of these aromatic amines.

Azo Compounds.   Simple azo dyes consist of two aromatic rings joined by an azo (N=N) bond whereas complex dyes are composed of benzidine or a congener linked to other polycyclics by one or more azo bonds. The simple azo dyes, of concern here, have an exocyclic amino group that is the key to any carcinogenicity, for this group undergoes biochemical N-oxidation and further conversion to reactive electrophiles similar to aromatic amines (Miller and Miller, 1981). The DNA adducts formed by covalent binding through the activated nitrogen have been identified.

Azo dyes are synthetic chemicals not found in nature. In the early 1930s, Yoshida and Kinosita, working in separate laboratories in Japan, discovered the carcinogenicity of some azo dye derivatives, including 4-dimethylaminoazobenzene (formerly commonly called butter yellow because it was used in the 1930s in some countries to color butter) and o-aminoazotoluene, which induced liver and bladder cancer after feeding. Many azo dyes were synthesized and examined for carcinogenic activity for the purpose of establishing structure-activity relationships. One of the salient conclusions drawn from these pioneering studies was that not all agents belonging to a given class of chemicals are carcinogenic or mutagenic. In fact, delicate alterations in structure modified the carcinogenic potential considerably.

In brief, some of the variations in activity as a function of structure stem from the susceptibility of the specific molecule to detoxification enzyme systems or, in reverse, to biochemical activation systems. An important detoxification process is splitting of the azo bond. This is readily performed by a bacterial and liver azo reductase. In fact, the activity of this enzyme system under adequate nutritional conditions initially resulted in a failure by Western researchers, who used a diet high in protein and riboflavin, to confirm the earlier studies of Japanese investigators, who fed rats a rice diet low in protein and riboflavin. This, in turn, led to the discovery by Kensler and coworkers in 1941 that riboflavin was involved in protecting against azo dye liver carcinogens, and by Mueller and Miller in 1950 that the underlying mechanisms depended on control of the detoxifying azo dye reductase by riboflavin, one of the first clear demonstrations of the role of nutrition in carcinogenesis, together with a definite mechanistic explanation. Mutagenicity and other tests for genotoxicity provide reasonable agreement with carcinogenicity, reflecting the potential of a given dye to yield a reactive metabolite (see Shahin, 1989; Williams et al., 1989). Most of the azo dyes studied are compounds with one azo link. All other things being equal, they are usually not carcinogenic if they contain polar substituents such as sulfonic acid residues. Thus, pure amaranth (FD & C Red Dye No. 2), with such a structure, is neither mutagenic nor carcinogenic, in spite of United States government regulatory actions banning this dye as a food additive. A related

dye, Allura Red, FD&C Red No. 40, with a similar structure, is likewise not carcinogenic.

Complex azo dyes consist of polycyclic structures linked by more than one azo group. Several dyestuffs in current commercial use have not yet been evaluated for chronic toxicity and possible carcinogenicity. Metabolic splitting of such compounds by reduction of the azo bonds has the opposite effect from splitting of a simple azo dyes, namely, the complexed carcinogenic aromatic amine, such as benzidine, is released. Because such dyestuffs can be metabolized not only by mammalian enzymes but also to a greater extent by bacterial enzymes in the gut, exposure to them is potentially harmful. Dyes such as direct blue 6, black 38, and brown 95 are potent rat liver carcinogens. With few exceptions, the carcinogenic complex azo dyes do not cause tumors at the point of injection. In rats, the usual end point is liver cancer, and in mice or hamsters, liver or urinary bladder tumors. Thus far, human cancer has not been traced to exposure to such dyes, albeit heavy occupational contact with arylamines, used as intermediates in dyestuff manufacture, has led to bladder cancer in the past when hygiene was poor (Maltoni and Selikoff, 1988).

Nitroaryl Compounds.   Nitro analogs of carcinogenic aromatic amines also lead to tumor formation. Better knowledge of the effects of this type of chemical is needed because nitro derivatives are used extensively as industrial chemical intermediates; they have been found in diesel engine exhausts and air pollution; and they exist in some commercial products in low concentrations, and one, aristolochic acid, occurs naturally (Howard et al., 1990). Nitro compounds can be reduced fairly readily to hydroxylamino derivatives and thence to the amines. The enzymatic systems performing such reductions are less stereospecific than those for the biochemical hydroxylation of amines. Hence, it may be that nitro derivatives would exhibit less stringent structure-activity relationships than the amines. In the few instances where this hypothesis was tested, arylhydroxylamines, except phenylhydroxylamine, have been found uniformly carcinogenic. For example, whereas 1-aminonaphthalene is inactive, 1-hydroxylaminonaphthalene is carcinogenic, in fact more so than the 2-isomer. Interestingly 1-nitronaphthalene has not been found active, which suggests that the rate of the in vivo reduction of the hydroxylamine to the inactive amine is much faster than its formation from the nitro compound. Likewise, in the fluorene series, N-acetyl-1-hydroxylamino and 3-hydroxylaminofluorene are carcinogenic, whereas the corresponding amines are not.

Technical dinitrotoluene fed to rats induced liver cancer, but the pure 2,4-dinitrotoluene was much less active. Attention was drawn to the 2,4-isomer, because of the known liver carcinogenicity of 2,4-diaminotoluene. However, examination of the potential to initiate hepatocellular altered foci showed that 2,6-dinitrotoluene, present in the technical product to about 20 percent, was much more active than the 2,4-isomer.

A number of analytical studies on the exhaust of functioning diesel engines have revealed that components of this mixture have mutagenic activity for *Salmonella typhimurium*. Among other chemicals, the compounds associated with the mutagenic activity were nitro derivatives of polycyclic aromatic hydrocarbons, such as 1-nitropyrene (IARC Monogr. 46, 1989). By analogy with tests of other nitro compounds, a hydrocarbon in which the nitro group is substituted in a position for which the corresponding amino compound would be carcinogenic (for example, 2-nitropyrene) can reasonably be assumed to be a carcinogenic nitro compound. For compounds such as 1-nitropyrene where the corresponding amine might not be carcinogenic, the effect would depend on the polycyclic aromatic hydrocarbon moiety, as discussed for 6-aminochrysene, and yield carcinogenicity at target organs in species under conditions appropriate for the substituted hydrocarbon (King *et al.*, 1988). And indeed, King's group (1988) found that 1-nitropyrene could induce mammary cancer in female rats. 1,6-Dinitropyrene was a more potent carcinogen than benzo[*a*]pyrene, when instilled into the lungs of rats (Iwagawa *et al.*, 1989). 2,4,7-Trinitrofluorenone, formerly used in some dry copying processes, is genotoxic (Rosenkranz in King *et al.*, 1988; Williams *et al.*, 1989). This chemical is related to the carcinogenic arylamine, 2-aminofluorene, and hence, these biologic properties are not unexpected, because the bacterial flora can reduce the nitro function to an amino group. The contribution of these chemicals at low levels in, for example, diesel exhaust or industrial products to human health risk remains to be defined. Nevertheless, at this time, they do not seem to represent the same degree of risk as do components of cigarette smoke, because of the great dilution of diesel exhaust, or low-level use of other nitro compounds, except at the place of manufacture, where humans should be protected.

N-Nitroso Compounds. This major class of important chemical carcinogens is characterized by chemicals derived from secondary amines or amides by nitrosation. Nitrosamines and nitrosamides are synthetic as well as naturally occurring substances. They were discovered to be carcinogenic only in the last 35 years beginning with the finding by Barnes and Magee in England that dimethylnitrosamine, an industrial solvent that caused jaundice and liver damage in workmen exposed to it, was highly hepatotoxic in rodents where it reproduced the lesions seen in humans. Subsequently, they demonstrated that this chemical was among the most carcinogenic chemicals then known. Some of the first studies on alteration of DNA by carcinogens were performed with nitrosamines and their patterns of alkylation of DNA have now been extensively documented. Because of extensive worldwide interest, regular international conferences on this topic are organized, and the proceedings published (IARC Sci. Publs. 84, 1987; 105, 1990).

The discovery of the carcinogenicity of dimethylnitrosamine led to an intensive effort to establish structure-activity relationships. The group headed by Druckrey in Germany, later that of Preussmann in Germany, those of Lijinsky, of Mirvish, and of Hoffmann and Hecht in the United States, and Okada in Japan studied many alkyl or alkylarylnitrosamines, cyclic nitrosamines, amides, and ureas. Many alkyl or alkylarylnitrosamines were found to be carcinogenic. Although most nitrosamines and nitrosamides are synthetic chemicals, some can be formed in nature through nitrosation reactions. For example, tobacco contains important carcinogens, the tobacco-specific nitrosamines produced by the nitrosation of nicotine during the curing process. Every smoker is inhaling considerable amounts of these potent carcinogens (Hecht and Hoffmann, 1988).

Dialkyl and Cyclic N-Nitroso Compounds. In rodents, the symmetric dialkyl compounds under some conditions exhibit delicate and yet specific organotropism; i.e., they preferentially cause cancer in a given organ, more so in rats than in mice, the latter showing mostly liver neoplasms. For example, dimethyl- and diethylnitrosamine usually cause liver cancer in rats whereas the dibutyl derivative causes cancer of the urinary bladder, and the diamyl compound cancer of the lung. The dose rate also plays a role. Dimethylnitrosamine administered to rats in moderate doses for a long time leads to cancer of the liver, whereas fewer high doses, or indeed, a single large dose results in renal carcinomas. The hamster, because it is characterized by a deficiency in liver activity of the alkyl acceptor protein involved in repair of O^6-alkylation of guanine, is extremely sensitive to liver carcinogenesis by dimethylnitrosamine.

The antibiotic streptozotocin has the structure of an *N*-methylnitrosamine. It was first isolated from *Streptozotocin achromogenes*. It is used mainly in cancer chemotherapy. Streptozotocin is carcinogenic, interestingly to the pancreas islet cells (IARC Monogr. 17, 1978). It is also diabetogenic, unless nicotinamide is administered at the same time. Similar in structure and probable mechanism of action are the alkyl and dialkylaryltriazeno derivatives. These materials, some of which are industrial products, have potent carcinogenic properties, including induction of brain, kidney, and mammary cancer in rats.

Tobacco-Specific Nitrosamines. Hoffmann, Hecht, and colleagues in the United States discovered that several carcinogenic nitrosamines derived from nicotine, in particular *N*-nitrosonornicotine (NNN) and 4-[methylnitrosamino-1(3-pyridyl)]-1-butanone (NNK), are found in tobacco, and are formed by bacterially mediated nitrosation of nicotine during the curing process (Hecht and Hoffmann, 1988). These and related nitrosamines are found also in tobacco smoke, and constitute a major source of carcinogenic nitrosamine exposure in smoking in humans, and to some extent also in nonsmoking humans through involuntary exposure to smokers (IARC Sci. Publ. 81, 1987).

In rats, the tobacco-derived nitrosamines cause cancer of the esophagus, lung, pancreas, and oral and nasal cavities and in hamsters, cancer of the upper respiratory tract (Hecht and Hoffmann, 1988). The contribution of these chemicals to carcinogenesis in humans who smoke cigarettes or chew tobacco products is likely to be important. In the United States, about 30 percent of all cancer deaths are seen in tobacco users (USDHHS, Surgeon General Report, 1989). Individuals who smoke and excessively drink alcoholic beverages (by definition more than six drinks per day) have a high risk of cancer of the oral cavity and esophagus. The relevant mechanism may be an induction by alcohol of enzymes capable of metabolizing nitrosamines such as nitrosonornicotine, or polycyclic aromatic hydrocarbons found in smoke, in the target tissues (Hecht and Hoffmann, 1988; Seitz and Simanowski, 1988).

The role of nitrosamines, other than those in tobacco, in human cancer has been under extensive study. The medical literature includes several case reports of individuals with acute intoxication to the point of overt hepatoxicity by certain nitrosamines, mostly dimethylnitrosamine. Yet, even though certain of these cases date to 1937, no reliable information exists that any of these individuals ever developed cancer due to exposure to this chemical. As noted above, the most likely carcinogens of this class that have an effect in humans are those found in tobacco and tobacco smoke. The properties of the smaller dialkylnitrosamines such as dimethyl- or diethylnitrosamine categorize them as very powerful, versatile carcinogens in animals. In the last 20 years, highly sensitive and specific techniques, such as those utilizing the thermal energy analyzer, have permitted the reliable determination of nitrosamines in the environment at levels down to the parts-per-trillion level (IARC Sci. Publ. 45, 1983). To induce cancer in rats and mice, continuing exposure to alkylnitrosamines at the parts-per-million level or infrequent exposure to amounts of parts per thousand are required. Rats possess a specific DNA repair activity, the alkyl acceptor protein system, for removing the alkyl group inserted in DNA by nitrosamines. Humans display a greater activity of this system than do rats. Thus, the biologic significance of concentrations of parts per billion or lower is obscure, yet these are the amounts found, for example, in certain foodstuffs, such as bacon. In fact, it is quite likely that larger amounts of such carcinogens were present in the food chain in previous years or decades, before the potential hazards due to such chemicals were known. Therefore, the cancer risks of such nitrosamines present in trace amounts seem to be quite minimal, compared to those inherent in other kinds of chronic exposures, as for example, nitrosonornicotine and analogs in tobacco products, where the concentration of these carcinogens is much higher.

Nitroso derivatives of alkylureas, alkylamides, and esters are some of the most remarkable carcinogens known. Many of these agents are chemically quite stable in the anhydrous state and do not require specific enzymic activation but spontaneously release a reactive intermediate in the presence of aqueous, preferably neutral to alkaline, systems; they are more stable at pH values of 2 to 5. Such materials are carcinogenic in virtually all living systems, even under *in vitro* conditions (IARC Sci. Publs. 84, 1987; 105, 1990). *N*-Butylnitrosourea causes leukemia, mainly the granulocytic type, similar to that seen in humans. Certain of these materials were actually used commercially in industry and in chemical laboratories because of their property to undergo alkali hydrolysis and yield reactive intermediates. For example, methylnitrosourea was the classic reagent for the laboratory preparation of diazomethane, itself utilized to esterify carboxylic acids. Since its carcinogenicity was demonstrated, methylnitrosourea has not been used for this purpose, but has been replaced by

methylnitrosotoluenesulfonamide, which is not carcinogenic. The gaseous diazomethane itself is a carcinogenic alkylating agent, yielding tumors in the respiratory tract, especially the lung, in rats and mice.

Given by oral administration, alkylnitrosoureas, such as methylnitrosourethan, and the closely related *N*-methyl-*N'*-nitro-*N*-nitrosoguanidine, nitrosobiuret, and *N*-methyl-*N*-nitroso-*N'*-acetylurea produced tumors in the gastrointestinal tract. In fact, these compounds are the chemicals of choice to induce experimental cancer of the glandular stomach, mimicking one of the most frequent human cancers in Japan, parts of Latin America, Iceland, Scandinavia, and certain other countries of Europe (Weisburger and Horn, 1991). Treatment of certain foods with nitrite, especially fish or beans frequently eaten in areas where stomach cancer is high, yields an extract with mutagenic activity, which in turn induces cancer of the glandular stomach in rats. Chemicals, like nitrosoindoles, or diazophenols appear to be the relevant mutagens and carcinogens. Foods eaten in areas such as China, where the risk for cancer in the upper respiratory and the upper gastrointestinal tract is high, also contain specific nitrosamines. Thus, there may be a relationship between nitrite, nitrosamines, nitrosoindoles, nitrosamides, or diazophenols, and certain human cancers highly prevalent in diverse parts of the world. High customary salt intake exerts an enhancing action, and also is a cause of hypertension and stroke.

Nitrosamines and related materials are synthesized by reaction of nitrous acid with a secondary amine. Sound evidence shows that in biologic systems, including humans, nitrosamines, nitrosoureas, and similar hazardous materials can be formed following oral administration of nitrite and the appropriate amine or amide.

In many places, nitrite is utilized as a food additive and it also occurs adventitiously in food supplies through reduction of nitrate. Nitrate is ubiquitous in the environment and is also used as a component of food preservatives. Under some conditions, nitrate is reduced to nitrite, particularly by microbiologic systems. This reduction is likely to occur in food stored at room temperature, a relatively common occurrence in less advanced countries where household refrigeration is uncommon (Weisburger and Horn, 1990). The reduction is also readily mediated by oral bacterial flora, in individuals having eaten foods, especially plants, high in nitrate (Banbury Rept. 12, 1982). Secondary amines and similar nitrosatable substrates likewise are widespread in the environment (food) and they also arise by digestive process. Potential exposure to exogenous nitrite or endogenous formation of nitrite can be assessed by the sensitive and specific procedure of Bartsch and coworkers (1990) which measures the presence of the noncarcinogenic nitrosoproline in the urine of individuals given a dose of proline.

These nitrosation reactions can be inhibited by preferential, competitive neutralization of nitrite with naturally occurring and synthetic materials such as vitamin C, vitamin E, sulfamate, and certain antioxidants such as butylated hydroxytoluene, butylated hydroxyanisole, gallic acid, and even amino acids or proteins (Machlin and Bendich, 1987; Ito and Hirose,

1989; Weisburger, 1990). Practical use has been made of these inhibitory reactions; for example, meats preserved with nitrite are at the same time treated with ascorbate or erythrobate, thereby appreciably lowering the amount of detectable dimethylnitrosamine, nitrosopyrrolidine, and other nitrosamines. In addition, this interaction may bear on the considerable decrease in the incidence of stomach cancer and hypertension in the United States during the last 40 years, traced to the replacement of salted and pickled foods by refrigerated foods (Weisburger, 1990). Concern has been expressed about the increasing concentration of nitrate in drinking water, owing to agriculture practices and fertilizer use. This is not a problem if people have daily intake of fruits and vegetables as sources of vitamins C and E which will destroy nitrite formed *in vivo* from nitrates. This propery of neutralization of nitrite by vitamin C is also being used in certain pharmaceutical preparations with potential nitrosatable substituents, by formulating such drugs with vitamin C or vitamin E.

Some of the alkylnitrosoureas, particularly the ethyl derivative, yield tumors of the brain on parenteral, especially intravenous, injection. These alkylnitrosoureas provide unique means of specifically inducing neurogenic tumors and related lesions. Chemicals of this type are also active transplacentally, yielding a high incidence of cancer in the offspring after a single dose to a pregnant female given in the last trimester (IARC Sci. Publs. 96, 1989). The question can be asked whether the relatively rare cancers of the human brain and nervous system occurring fairly early in life stem from a similar transplacental effect with as yet unknown compounds of this type. If so, optimal vitamin C and vitamin E intake might prevent this sequence of undesirable reactions (Weisburger, 1990).

Tertiary and quaternary amines, and in particular, dimethylamino derivatives, can react with nitrite under similar conditions, releasing dimethylnitrosamine (Banbury Rept. 12, 1982). Many drugs have a structure permitting nitrosation and this remains to be explored in regard to the possible human risk. Cimetidine, and related drugs used in the management of gastric or duodenal ulcers, can form a nitroso compound with a structure mimicking that of the alkylnitrosoureas. Although the compound is mutagenic, two tests for carcinogenicity have been totally negative, suggesting that under *in vivo* conditions this nitroso compound can be detoxified (Banbury Rept. 12, 1982).

Biotransformation of Nitrosamines. Nitrosamines as a class are converted to active electrophilic reactants through oxidation (IARC Sci. Publs. 84, 1987; 105, 1990). The active species alkylate DNA at specific sites, which have been determined for several nitrosamines. With the prototype dimethylnitrosamine, an active intermediate is the unstable oxymethyl compound, which is converted to a reactive electrophile, methyldiazohydroxide. Longer chain or cyclic nitrosamines are also metabolized by hydroxylation α or β to the N-nitroso function, but the key activation reaction is α-hydroxylation (Hecht and Hoffmann, 1988; Lee *et al.*, 1989). With an asymmetric nitrosamine such as the important tobacco specific N-nitrosonornicotine both α positions are attacked, de-

pending on the organ-specific enzymes, and thus distinct reactive intermediates are obtained that may account for the species, strain, and organ selectivity. Aliphatic longer chain nitrosamines such as dibutylnitrosamine can undergo α, β, or ω hydroxylation, and these yield specific products, including some derived from chain shortening oxidation. As is true for the polycyclic aromatic hydrocarbons, there is stereospecificity in the metabolic activation nitrosamines, as noted in the distinct carcinogenicity of two isomers of N-nitroso-2,6-dimethylmorpholine (Banbury Rept. 12, 1982).

Biochemical activation of nitrosamines takes place in all species so far studied. Whereas even the highly potent polycyclic hydrocarbons, such as 3-methylcholanthrene, have so far failed to reliably cause cancer in monkeys, a number of nitrosamines led to cancer relatively rapidly in Rhesus monkeys. For example, diethylnitrosamine induced liver cancer in less than two years, and in more recent experiments in less than one year. Species differences appear in relation to the tissue primarily affected. Diethylnitrosamine leads chiefly to liver cancer in rats or mice, but in the hamster, lung cancer is the main lesion, although liver and esophageal tumors also result. There is also a dramatic species difference in the capacity to repair the DNA damage produced by alkylating nitrosamines; in particular, the hamster is deficient in the removal of alkyl adducts in DNA.

Nitrogen Mustards, Cyclophosphamide, and Chloroethylnitrosoureas. Sulfur mustard was used as a war gas in World War I. The poisoning led to effects on the lymphoid system and leukopenia. There was a high incidence of respiratory tract cancers in exposed humans in a war gas factory in Japan. Early efforts in cancer chemotherapy rested on the synthesis of the analogous nitrogen mustards. The simplest compound in that series is mechlorethamine, which was useful in the management of lymphomas. Later, a whole variety of such compounds, including chlorambucil and cyclophosphamide, were found useful in the therapy of select neoplasms. Shimkin and associates developed systematic tests of these alkylating agents for carcinogenicity. As was expected, they showed carcinogenic potential and the effect was a function of specific chemical structure. In animals and later on in humans, it was found that cyclophosphamide caused bladder cancer. The target organ of other mustards in other animals is diverse. Several others have caused cancer in humans, after successful remission of the primary cancer, the main effect being leukemia. It is not yet known whether the leukemia observed is a direct effect of the drug, or secondary to severe immunosuppression, often associated with their use.

BCNU (N,N-Bis(2-chloroethyl)-N-nitrosourea) and CCNU (N-(2-chloroethyl)-N'-cyclohexyl-N-nitrosourea) are chloroethyl nitrosoureas, and as expected are carcinogenic in animal models. Yet, these drugs are useful in chemotherapy, and are frequent components of mixtures of drugs so used.

Dialkylhydrazines. Laqueur in the United States discovered that the flour made from the cycad nut led to a variety of cancers in the liver, kidney, and digestive tract of rats (Arcos *et. al.*, 1968–1988). Cycasin, the active ingredient, is the glucoside of methylazoxymethanol. It is a powerful carcinogen for the liver, kidney, and digestive tract on oral intake in conventional rats but is inactive both in germ-free rats and after intraperitoneal injection, because of the requirement for the bacterial enzyme glucosidase to hydrolyze the cycasin and release the active principle, methylazoxymethanol.

Methylazoxymethanol itself leads to cancer in various species of conventional and germ-free animals, irrespective of the mode of administration. Interestingly, in rodents, mainly colon cancer is induced, although duodenal, liver, kidney, and ear duct cancers also occur. Methylazoxymethanol is not entirely stable at physiologic pH, but its organospecificity suggested the need to search for enzymatically mediated activation mechanisms to yield the methyl carbonium ion. Thus, the natural product cycasin yields the same ultimate carcinogen as does synthetic dimethylnitrosamine after biochemical oxidation by host systems (Sohn et al., 1987). Yet, dimethylnitrosamine does not induce colon cancer because the organospecificity of each carcinogen depends on specific activation and repair enzyme systems in each tissue and cell type.

Based on the effects of cycasin, Druckrey in Germany examined the carcinogenic properties of 1,2-dimethylhydrazine, which was postulated and demonstrated to be oxidized to methylazoxymethanol via azomethane and azoxymethane (Sohn et al., 1987). 1,2-Dimethylhydrazine and azoxymethane, in fact, were found to be highly carcinogenic in many species and metabolized to methylazoxymethanol. In rodents these compounds cause a high incidence of cancer of the lower intestinal tract, colon, and rectum, and provide models to study prevalent types of human cancers (Lipkin, 1988; Weisburger and Horn, 1991). In monkeys, transplacental exposure to 1,2-dimethylhydrazine led to kidney cancer (Beniashvili, 1989). Curiously, the closely related 1,2-diethylhydrazine has an entirely different organotropism, yielding primarily cancer of the lung and liver. More information is required to understand the specific localization of the effect of this series of compounds. Among substituted methylhydrazine derivatives, the antitumor agent Natulan (procarbazine) is carcinogenic in several test systems. The mechanism may depend on the metabolic liberation of methylating agents, as is true for symmetric 1,2-dimethylhydrazine. The parent compound, 1-methyl-2-benzylhydrazine, has a similar pattern of carcinogenicity.

Some substituted hydrazines, including the important drug isoniazid, also lead to pulmonary tumors in specific strains of mice (Swiss or strain A), because of metabolic release of hydrazine. Tests of isoniazid in other strains of mice or in other rodent species have afforded dubious evidence of carcinogenicity. A number of other drugs and chemicals that possess this type of structure, potentially giving rise to hydrazine during metabolism, have induced pulmonary tumors in susceptible strains of mice (Shimkin and Stoner, 1975). 1,1-Dimethylhydrazine and similar unsymmetric hydrazines often induce vascular tumors in rodents (Toth, 1988). The acute toxicity of these compounds is antagonized by vitamin B_6, probably through its active product, pyridoxal phosphate. It is not yet known whether the carcinogenicity relates to such a reaction. However, pyridoxine-deficient monkeys developed liver cancer, perhaps as a result of endogenous carcinogen formation (Weisburger, 1990). Pyridoxine is a key cofactor for essential enzyme systems, such as transaminases. Two carcinogenic hydrazine derivatives, gyromitrum and agaratine, are natural products.

Nitro Alkyl Compounds. Nitro alkyl compounds have important industrial uses as solvents or intermediates. Nitromethane, nitroethane, and 1-nitropropane appear to be noncarcinogenic. However, inhalation or oral administration of 2-nitropropane caused liver cancer in rats. 2-Nitropropane is mutagenic (George et al., 1989) and induces unscheduled DNA synthesis in hepatocytes, thus having the attributes of genotoxicity. Hydrolysis of livers of rats given 2-nitropropane and isolation of the nucleosides gave evidence of the presence of 8-hydroxydeoxyguanosine from DNA and even more of 8-hydroxyguanosine from RNA, as well as some as yet unknown derivatives, perhaps produced by diverse mechanisms. 2-Nitropropane thus led to the biochemical formation of hydroxy radicals or reactive oxygen species (Fiala et al., 1989). Combustion products of gasoline type hydrocarbons contain nitroolefins with carcinogenic potential. Further exploration of this area would seem rewarding.

Aldehydes. In inhalation tests, formaldehyde, a widely used chemical in medicine as well as in industrial applications, induced tumors in the nasopharynx at two of three dose levels, 15 and 8 ppm, but not at 2 ppm in rats (Starr and Gibson, 1985; Bolt, 1987). Thus far tests in mice have been negative. Formaldehyde is genotoxic in a number of in vitro test systems. Also, higher but not lower levels stimulate DNA synthesis and mitosis, events favorable to carcinogenesis, accounting in part for the dose-response in the inhalation test. Even though formaldehyde has been used extensively for decades as a tissue fixative in pathology and in embalming practices, so far there appears to be no documented record of a higher incidence of respiratory tract neoplasia in the many humans exposed to it occupationally or generally (IARC Monogr. 29, 1982; Walrath and Fraumeni, 1983; Gerin et al., 1989; Purchase and Paddle, 1989). Nonetheless, there is a report of a single case (Halperin et al., 1983).

Hexamethylphosphoramide (HMPA). This chemical is a good solvent in various applications in the laboratory and in industry. It has a low acute toxicity but has a number of chronic effects including kidney damage and testicular atrophy. Inhalation of 50 to 4000 ppb leads to a dose-related incidence of nasal cancer of varied histologic types that begins to appear after approximately eight months. At the highest dose level of 4000 ppb, 83 percent of rats had nasal cancers; at 400, 82 percent; at 100, 38 percent; at 50 ppb 20 percent. Between 400 and 4000 ppb, the rats exhibited the same time trend in the occurrence of cancer, which suggests a saturation phenomenon (Lee and Trochimowicz, 1982). As with other N-methyl compounds, HMPA is oxidized by a cytochrome P-450 system, and the key intermediate, formaldehyde, may be produced in the nasal cavity, an observation further supporting the view that inhalation of formaldehyde, or of substances yielding formaldehyde by metabolism in the nasal cavity, would constitute a carcinogenic risk at that site. As is true for formaldehyde itself, the critical factor is the production of the carcinogenic intermediate versus its detoxification by reduction or oxidation. Thus, the presence of a rather low level of HMPA that yields cancer on continuing inhalation may be due to the production of the carcinogenic intermediate within the cell and this may be more effective than the exogenous administration of formaldehyde which is more likely to be detoxified further by cytoplasmic or microsomal enzymes. Similarly, other N-methyl or O-methyl compounds of sufficient volatility that could be inhaled might likewise show carcinogenicity in the nasal cavity.

Carbamates. These are synthetic chemicals comprised of esters or derivatives of carbamic acid. This class includes many important industrial chemicals, among which are pesticides and agricultural chemicals. Ethyl carbamate (urethan) was used as a veterinary anesthetic until its carcinogenicity was discovered in 1943. In mice, this agent readily induces pulmonary tumors, even with a single large dose (Shimkin and Stoner, 1975). Different strains of mice exhibit variable responsiveness. Most sensitive are strain A mice, whereas C57Bl mice are among the strains responding less readily. Depending on conditions and strain, other organs such as the liver and the hematopoietic system are also affected. Cutaneous application to mice or oral administration followed by a promoting skin treatment (see below) with croton oil or pure phorbol esters leads to skin tumors. In rats, urethan is also active as a multipotent carcinogen for several target organs. In hamsters this agent has produced melanotic lesions on the skin and also neoplasms in liver, forestomach, and lung. In monkeys, urethan caused neoplasms in several organs. In mice, urethan is active by the transplacental route and is passed to offspring in the milk. Thus administered, it leads to a variety of neoplasms in different organs.

In a series of related carbamates, the methyl ester, an industrial intermediate, is not carcinogenic and fails to inhibit the effect of the active ethyl ester. The propyl, isopropyl, and butyl esters are weakly active whereas the higher homologs are inactive. N-Hydroxyurethan exhibits the same degree of carcinogenicity as does urethan. The structure-activity relationships and the inactivity of the methyl derivative may relate to the fact that the metabolic activation pathway involves a dehydrogenation of the ethyl group, with formation of vinyl carbamate, a key proximate carcinogen, which can then further undergo epoxidation. Of course, this would not be possible for the methyl ester and hence accounts for its inactivity. Vinyl carbamate is more active than ethyl carbamate in several test systems, and hence is a good candidate for the metabolic intermediate (Miller and Miller, 1981). A series of diaryl acetylenic carbamates were synthesized as possible drugs, and a number were found highly carcinogenic (Arcos et al., 1968–1988). Thus, chemicals such as 1,1-bis(4-fluorophenyl)-2-propynyl N-cycloacetyl carbamate and the cycloheptyl or cyclohexyl esters induced leukemias rapidly, and

caused also neoplasms in the intestines, ear duct, mammary gland, liver, and even in the heart. Arcos et al. (1968–1988) provide a detailed review of carbamate pesticides, and reach the conclusion that although a few may be carcinogenic, most are not. In Japan, the group directed by Shirasu has performed extensive work on the mutagenicity of such compounds in S. typhimurium and note that some of the chemicals with $(CH_3)N\text{-}R$ structures are positive (Moriya et al., 1983).

Ethionine. This agent was synthesized as an antimetabolite to L-methionine and used in the study of transmethylation reactions in relation to the biochemistry of this essential amino acid. The hepatotoxic and carcinogenic effects of ethionine were discovered many years later by Farber (1986) in the United States. The mechanism underlying the chronic action of ethionine leading to liver tumors in rats has not yet been explained. Peroxisome proliferation may play a role (Chambers et al., 1988). Whereas ethionine is not mutagenic, the vinyl analog is highly mutagenic and binds to cellular macromolecules, including DNA (Leopold et al., 1982).

Vinyl chloride or monochloroethylene is an important intermediate in the production of useful end products made of polyvinylchloride. In 1970, vinyl chloride was found carcinogenic in animal models. The younger the animal at first exposure, the more sensitive it was, especially for hamsters (Drew et al., 1983). The reactive intermediate is the epoxide, or oxirane, that is mutagenic, and yields several metabolites, especially glutathione (GSH) conjugates and products derived therefrom, eventually excreted in the urine of exposed animals (Barbin and Bartsch, 1989).

Vinyl chloride was also identified as a human carcinogen when it was discovered that individuals charged with cleaning the reactor vessels in the polymerization plants, who presumably were exposed at that time to relatively large concentrations of vinyl chloride, developed angiosarcomas of the liver (Maltoni and Selikoff, 1988). There are some suggestions that such individuals might also be at higher risk for other cancers, including lung cancer, but the data for that target organ are not striking and are difficult to interpret because of the possible effect of cigarette smoking. It is significant that, thus far, only the reactor cleaners, who were exposed periodically over a long period of time to high concentrations, have exhibited disease, but not other individuals involved in the production or use of vinyl chloride.

1,2-Dichloroethane. 1,2-Dichloroethane is an important solvent, used also in the petroleum industry as a gasoline additive, as well as in agricultural applications as a fumigant. It is a powerful toxin for the liver and kidney and is also carcinogenic, leading to lung and liver tumors in mice, angiosarcomas in male rats, and interestingly, mammary adenocarcinoma in female rats, when the compound was administered in corn oil chronically by mouth. On the other hand, inhalation studies with rats or mice were negative. This suggests that there might be concentration and pulse dose effects and that lower levels such as might be absorbed chronically from inhaled air might not be adequate to induce neoplasia. This chemical is geno-

Table 5–9. CARCINOGENS PRODUCED IN NATURE

A wide variety of toxic and carcinogenic chemicals occur in nature. Human exposure to these chemicals is probably greater than that to synthetic carcinogens, and may be causes of several types of cancer. In animals some are carcinogens, others are promoters.

MICROORGANISMS	CLASSIFICATION	PLANTS	CLASSIFICATION
Actinomycins	D	Agaratine	D
Aflatoxins	D	Aplysiatoxin	E
Adriamycin	D	Aristolochic acid	U
Azaserine	D	β-Asarone (calamus oil)	U
Daunomycin	D	Betel nut	D
Elaiomycin	U	Bracken fern (ptaquiloside)	D
Ethionine	U	Cycasin	D
Griseofulvin	E	Coltsfoot	U
Islanditoxin	U	Debromoaplysiatoxin	E
Luteoskyrin	U	Gyromitrin	E
Mitomycin C	D	Okadaic acid	E
4-(Methylnitrosamino)- 1-(3-pyridyl-1-butanone	D	Phorbol esters	E
Nitrosonornicotine	D	Pyrrolizidine (Senecio) alkaloids	D
Ochratoxin A	D	Safrole	D
Sterigmatocystin	D	Teleocidin A and B	E
Streptozotocin	D	Thiourea, goitrogens	E

D = DNA-reactive; E = epigenetic; U = Unclassified.

toxic. Whereas with most chemicals and drugs, conjugation with GSH catalyzed by GSH transferase is a detoxication reaction, with dichloroethane, this conjugation leads to the production of a vinyl chloride S-conjugate. This appears to be an effective activation pathway to reactive metabolites specifically through a β-lyase enzyme present in the kidney but not the liver (Dekant *et al.,* 1989).

1,1-Dichloroethane. The asymmetric 1,1-dichloroethane or vinylidene chloride is toxic to liver and kidney in rodents as well as in dogs and monkeys. Vinylidene chloride was carcinogenic in mice, leading to kidney and liver tumors, particularly in males, as well as lung and liver angiosarcomas. However, tests in rats appeared to be negative. The closely related 1,1,1-trichloroethane or methylchloroform is not carcinogenic.

Acrylonitrile. Acrylonitrile or vinyl nitrile is a commercially important monomer in the plastics industry. It is also found in tobacco smoke. The structure of acrylonitrile is similar to that of vinyl chloride and its metabolism involves an epoxide intermediate that would constitute the genotoxic and mutagenic product (Chambers *et al.,* 1989). Inhalation tests have indicated carcinogenicity in rodents, and there are suggestions that some conditions of human exposure have led to cancer.

1,2-Dibromoethane and 1,2-Dibromo-3-Chloropropane. In general, 1,2-dibromoethane or ethylene dibromide has similar properties to 1,2-dichloroethane, but is more mutagenic and carcinogenic than the chloro analog. Oral administration induces squamous cell carcinoma of the stomach, in addition to a similar tumor pattern exhibited by the chloro compound. The latent period is shorter, testifying to its greater potency. Inhalation induces cancer in the nasal cavity. 1,2-

Dibromo-3-chloropropane exhibits an identical behavior, and appears more powerful. These dibromo compounds are also important industrially, although less so than the dichloro compounds, and find application in the agricultural industry. The dibromo compounds appear to undergo the same type of activation mechanisms as the dichloro compound (Kim and Guengerich, 1989). In addition, they appear to be able to react directly with important cellular receptors because they are mutagenic in assays without a liver S-9 fraction (Teramoto and Shirasu, 1989). These dibromo derivatives lead to sterility in rodents and also in men exposed during manufacture (Wong *et al.,* 1982). Considering their established carcinogenicity, already known for 15 years, and their definite genotoxicity in several tests, the extensive use of these two compounds is unwise without careful safety precautions.

Naturally Occurring Carcinogens. A number of toxins are formed in nature by plants or microorganisms (see Chapter 23). Compared to synthetics, relatively few of these have been tested for carcinogenicity, but nevertheless a wide variety has been found to induce cancer in test animals (Table 5–9) or in livestock consuming toxin-containing diets. Processed natural products, mainly tobacco and alcohol, are major causes of human cancer.

Many of these naturally occurring carcinogens clearly undergo metabolic activation to a DNA-reactive ultimate carcinogen, and these are discussed in the following sections. The mechanism of action of some is unknown, and others, such as phorbol esters, are nongenotoxic and are discussed with that category of carcinogens.

In addition to carcinogens that occur in nature, processing of natural products gives rise to carcinogens

Table 5–10.   CARCINOGENS IN PROCESSED NATURAL PRODUCTS

Important types of carcinogens, accounting for substantial portions of human cancers in many parts of the world, stem from the traditional use of specific processed natural products. Their genotoxicity, in most instances has been documented, as has their carcinogenicity, or cocarcinogenicity (alcohol).

PRODUCT	CARCINOGEN TYPE/ METABOLITE
Tobacco, snuff	Nicotine alkaloid-derived nitrosamines
Pickled/smoked food	Nitrosoindoles, phenol diazotates
Cooked foods	Heterocyclic aromatic amines
Alcoholic beverages	Acetaldehyde

(Table 5–10). Among these are important etiologic agents in human cancer.

Carcinogens from Plants.   A variety of different types of carcinogens are produced by plants. The best known of these, with a major impact as a cause of human cancer, accounting for at least 30 percent of all cancers in the United States, are the group of agents in the tobacco plant (U.S. Surgeon General Report, 1989). Tobacco contains certain carcinogens such as nitrosonornicotine and related agents even before burning and pyrolysis. Tobacco smoke is an exceedingly complex chemical mixture and contains diverse classes of carcinogens, cocarcinogens, accelerators, and promoters. The carcinogens include polycyclic aromatic hydrocarbons, heterocyclic compounds, phenolic derivatives, and so forth. The total worldwide increase in cancer in men, especially cancer of the respiratory tract in the United States and Western Europe, since 1930, and in women since 1960, can be accounted for by the increase in smoking of manufactured cigarettes by men since about 1915, and by women since about 1940. Newer low-tar products now on the market present a lower risk. Chewing tobacco and snuff are also hazardous, because they contain sizeable amounts of tobacco-specific nitrosamines, and cause cancer in the oral cavity and upper gastrointestinal tract. The reader is referred to specialized reviews for this important area of toxicology (IARC Monogrs. 37, 1985; 38, 1986), with great potential of truly successful preventive measures. Lung cancer in men in the United States has shown an encouraging beginning of a decline in 1984, because only about 30 percent of men are now regular smokers, compared to 65 percent around 1955. Unfortunately, there are now more women smokers, and lung cancer caused higher mortality than breast cancer. Also, the habit of smoking is increasing sharply in Africa, South America, and Asia, unquestionably leading to an epidemic increase in lung and other tobacco-related neoplasms, and also heart diseases.

In populations in India and Asia, betel chewing leads to cancer of the mouth and upper gastrointestinal tract, one of the major causes of death in that area. Current evidence on the carcinogenic constituents implicates both tobacco and certain constituents from the betel nut. Arecoline, the major alkaloid of the betel nut, for example, can be nitrosated to form a carcinogenic nitrosamine (IARC Monogr. 37, 1985; Hoffmann and Hecht, in Cooper and Grover, 1990).

Senecio Alkaloids.   These natural products, consisting mainly of monocrotaline, lasiocarpine, heliotrine, and the basic skeleton retronecine, are complex, aliphatic, hydroxylated fatty acid esters used extensively as teas or as drugs in some civilizations (Hirono, 1987). They have a distinct effect on the liver, namely hepatomegalocytosis, following prolonged administration of these agents (Moore *et al.*, 1989). They exert a pronounced antimitotic effect, but some of these alkaloids have a carcinogenic effect in rats. The intake of such alkaloids in some areas of the world, perhaps together with mycotoxins and in the presence of viral agents such as hepatitis B, may contribute to the liver cancer prevalent in these areas.

These chemicals require metabolic activation to pyrrole derivatives in which, on biochemical oxidation of the ring, the exocyclic ester as a leaving group splits to yield an electrophilic compound.

Bracken Fern.   In investigating the cause of hematuria and bladder cancers in cattle in Turkey and other regions, it was found that the consumption of bracken fern was etiologically related to the development of these lesions. In rats, administration of bracken fern has an effect not only on the urinary bladder but also on the upper intestinal tract. Human exposure to the carcinogen in bracken fern may occur through drinking the milk of cows that consumed the plant, or, in some areas of the world, eating the fern itself as part of traditional dietary patterns. A specific carcinogen in bracken fern is ptaquiloside, a norsesquiterpene glucoside (Hirono, 1987).

Mold Products.   These chemicals enter the human environment for a variety of uses, mainly as drugs. Several agents such as adriamycin, daunomycin, and dactinomycin are carcinogenic (Westendorf *et al.*, 1990). Adriamycin and daunomycin cause cancer at several target organs, including the mammary gland in rats, and give evidence of covalent binding. Streptozotocin, which is used as a drug for antineoplastic therapy, is a glucopyranose derivative of methylnitrosourea produced by *Streptomyces achromogenes*. Azaserine or serine diazoacetate, which is produced by *Streptomyces*, has been of interest as an antitumor agent. Azaserine was shown to produce primarily pancreatic and kidney cancer in rats. This organotropism correlates with localization of the agent. It inhibits purine biosynthesis through inhibition of the enzyme 2-formamido-*N*-ribosylacetamide 5'-phosphate: L-glutamine amidoligase. The enzyme inhibition is due to alkylation of the sulfhydryl group of a cysteine residue in the enzyme, and azaserine is mutagenic without metabolic activation. Thus, a genotoxic action seems probable.

Mycotoxins.   Investigations of the cause of an enormous loss of turkey poults with fulminating liver necrosis in the United Kingdom late in the 1950s led to the discovery of a mold toxin produced on feeds contaminated with a strain of *Aspergillus flavus* and related molds. The toxin accounted for the pronounced hepatotoxicity of such contaminated meals. The active components exhibit characteristic fluorescence patterns; they were isolated and their structure rapidly established, which was a significant achievement in the area of toxicologic studies. The key compound, named aflatoxin B_1, not only is highly hepatotoxic but is one of the most powerful carcinogens known, inducing liver tumors in several species after dietary intake of very low levels, of the order of parts per billion. The mold usually produces four types of aflatoxin: B_1, B_2, G_1, and G_2, so labeled because of a blue (B) or green (G) fluorescence. The B_2 and G_2 compounds are the dihydro derivatives of the B_1 and G_1 analogs, respectively. Among the four isomers found, aflatoxin B_1 is much more toxic and carcinogenic than the G_1 analog. The derivative is virtually not carcinogenic. Aflatoxin B_2, on the other hand, is definitely but slightly carcinogenic, probably because there is an enzyme that converts aflatoxin B_2 to B_1 to a small extent. All of the structural elements draw attention to the double bond in the furan portion of the molecule, where biochemical oxidation yields the ultimate carcinogenic metabolite, an epoxide, that reacts with DNA at N-7 of guanine, a marker of exposure (Wogan, 1989). Inasmuch as there are many other competing detoxifying biotransformation steps, including the production of ring hydroxylated metabolites and of the demethylated phenol, it would seem that the epoxide is indeed a highly active carcinogen.

Aflatoxin B_1 is highly hepatocarcinogenic in rats and is also appreciably carcinogenic in a number of other experimental species, including nonhuman primates, although mice are rather resistant. In highly sensitive species such as the rat, or the trout, aflatoxin B_1 exhibits carcinogenicity when fed in the diet at levels as low as 1 ppb. The major target organ is the liver, but under some conditions, low yields of kidney and colon tumors have been seen in rodents. The relatively low sensitivity of mice may relate to a high level of GSH transferase, providing a selective detoxification pathway for the reactive epoxide. Also, for the same reason, subcellular fractions from mouse liver activate aflatoxin to mutagenic metabolites less readily than fractions from rat liver.

In certain African and Asian countries, where staple foods have been contaminated by high levels of aflatoxins on the order of parts per million, primary liver cancer is one of the principal neoplastic diseases. In this region, hepatitis B antigen is also endemic, and it is thought that there might be a potentiating effect between this antigen and mycotoxicosis, accounting not only for the high incidence, but for the fact that the disease is seen at a young age, 20–30 years, especially in men (Yeh *et al.*, 1989). Sterigmatocystin is a related mycotoxin, which is likewise found in mold-contaminated food crops. It is also carcinogenic and may also play a role in human liver cancer.

Detection of Exposure to DNA-Reactive Compounds

DNA-reactive chemicals are either direct-acting alkylating agents, or are converted to such by host metabolism. These reactive intermediates react not only with DNA, but also with other nucleophiles, including proteins and specifically serum proteins

(Chambers *et al.*, 1989; Gorelick *et al.*, 1989). Thus, one means of measuring current and recent past exposure to a DNA-reactive chemical is to examine blood elements such as hemoglobin for the presence of adducts (Sabbioni and Newmann, 1990). Such components have been detected in individuals exposed to even small amounts of carcinogens occupationally. They have also been seen in smokers. Because of the relatively short half-life of the marker protein, this approach is best to visualize current or recent exposure. On cessation of smoking, for example, the level of a specific adduct with 4-aminobiphenyl declines (Maclure *et al.*, 1990).

The rate of turnover of cellular DNA is a function of the tissue. DNA adducts tend to be detectable longer than cellular protein adducts. Therefore, determination of DNA adducts is beginning to be introduced to assess current and even prior exposure to DNA reactive compounds (Wogan, 1989).

Breakdown products from modified DNA, such as 8-hydroxydeoxyguanosine, can be measured with great sensitivity by electrochemical detection in urine (Shigenaga *et al.*, 1989).

Current or short-term exposure to reactive carcinogens often leads to urinary excretion of a mutagenic metabolite that can be concentrated and measured quantitatively through specialized techniques (Doolittle *et al.*, 1988). For example, mutagenic activity was found in the urine of hospital personnel handling certain drugs used in cancer therapy, leading to the institution of preventive measures. Mutagenicity in urine was used as a marker for successful exposure prevention. Patients with primary liver cancers, particularly in some areas of Africa where this is a major cancer, reexpress fetal serum protein, α-fetoprotein, discovered in 1962 by Abelev in the USSR. The presence of this marker is noted early in hepatocarcinogenesis, and the relevant molecular events show an inverse association with albumin. The presence of α-fetoprotein is diagnostic for liver cancer and a few select other neoplasms. The carcinoembryonic antigen (CEA), first found by Gold in Canada, has been observed in humans with colon cancer, and several other cancers (Goldenberg, 1990).

EPIGENETIC CARCINOGENS

This category is by definition comprised of agents that have been reliably demonstrated not to react with DNA and that exert another kind of biologic effect that appears to be the basis for their carcinogenicity. Hence, a wide variety of types of agents are assigned to this category. The modes of action of different types of epigenetic carcinogens are quite different, some enhancing intrinsic carcinogenic processes and others exerting effects that appear to culminate indirectly in genetic alteration. These agents do not display the features of the carcinogenicity of DNA-reactive carcinogens. The main features of their carcinogenicity are that high doses and sustained exposure are usually required.

Promoters

Promoters, as originally defined by Berenblum (1974), are agents that facilitate the growth of dormant neoplastic cells into tumors. As such, promoters originally were not considered to be carcinogens. This assertion was initially questioned by Nakahara and others, who viewed "promotion" as merely representing the effect of a weak carcinogen in producing a synergistic effect when given in sequence after an initiating carcinogen. Indeed, skin tumor promoters of the phorbol ester type were found to induce low yields of skin tumors by themselves. Carcinogens are defined operationally by the production of tumors. Thus, a number of agents that have promoting activity are also "carcinogenic" by the operational definition.Tests demonstrating such an effect usually require chronic, high-dose administration. The chemicals discussed here are non-DNA-reactive carcinogens whose mode of action appears to be promotion.

Tetradecanoyl Phorbol Acetate (TPA). This naturally occurring component of croton oil, also known as phorbol myristate acetate, has been the classic "promoter" used in two-stage skin carcinogenesis experiments (Schmidt and Hecker, 1989). However, TPA by itself produces a low incidence of skin tumors even under conventional promoting conditions. TPA can produce chromosomal effects, possibly through generation of reactive oxygen (Larsson and Cerutti, 1989). Thus, TPA may be in fact an indirect genotoxin. The phorbol esters are distinct from other carcinogens of the promoting class by virtue of binding to a membrane receptor, involving protein kinase C and inducing ornithine decarboxylase (Blumberg, 1988; Pegg, 1988). A number of new potent promoters with such properties were discovered in plants and algae (Fujiki et al., 1989). TPA and other tumor-promoting phorbol esters were the first promoters found to inhibit intercellular communication in cultured cells in the laboratories of A. Murray in Australia and J. Trosko in the United States. This action is a property of tumor promoters and will be noted for other agents in this section.

Phenobarbital. The antiseizure drug phenobarbital, and other chemicals to be discussed next, increase the incidence of mouse liver tumors but cause cancer in the rat liver infrequently, if at all. By most measures, phenobarbital is nongenotoxic. Phenobarbital was first shown by Peraino in the United States to enhance the effects of hepatocarcinogens when administered after them. A major discovery by Kitagawa in Japan and Pitot and Williams in the United States was that phenobarbital enhanced the development of preneoplastic altered hepatocellular foci in rat liver. Based on this observation, Williams and Schulte-Hermann in Germany postulated that the carcinogenicity of phenobarbital and other similar agents occurs by a mechanism of promotion exerted on the preexisting abnormal liver cells, such as in foci, that eventually give rise to the cyptogenic liver lesions and neoplasms in old mice and rats (see Williams in Stevenson et al., 1990). Phenobarbital has been shown to inhibit intercellular communication in cultured liver cells (Williams in Stevenson et al., 1990). Ring hydrolysis of phenobarbital decreases its liver tumor promoting activity (Diwan et al., 1989).

The nature of the "inducing" agent yielding the abnormal cells may stem from a specific oncogene translocation in genetically sensitive strains of mice (Stevenson et al., 1990). The few liver cancers occasionally seen in chronic tests in rats given high levels of phenobarbital or DDT may likewise be due to a genetic factor, or could result from an intake of diets contaminated with mycotoxins or some nitrosamines.

Detailed epidemiologic studies on humans using phenobarbital have not revealed evidence of carcinogenicity (Clemmesen and Hjalgrim-Jensen, 1981; IARC Sci. Publ. 65, 1982).

Several other barbiturates have been shown to enhance liver carcinogenesis (Shinozuka et al., 1982) and would likely increase the yield of liver tumors in chronic tests.

Chlorinated Hydrocarbons. The class of chlorinated hydrocarbons includes, in addition to those that are genotoxic, a substantial number of chemicals for which genotoxicity has not been found (IARC Sci. Publ. 56, 1984; Banbury Rept. 25, 1987). Rather, many have been shown to inhibit cell-to-cell communication in culture and to liver neoplasia enhancing activity (Williams in Stevenson et al., 1990). Agents with these properties include DDT, chlordane, lindane, and polychlorinated and polybrominated biphenyls. It seems likely therefore that the chemicals are carcinogenic through promoting mechanisms on preexisting abnormal cells, as discussed above for phenobarbital.

DDT produced predominantly or exclusively liver cancer in rodents (IARC Monogr. Suppl. 7, 1987). Interestingly, DDT tested many times under widely different conditions has not been found carcinogenic in the hamster, in nonhuman primates, and indeed, despite the fact that the pesticide has been used extensively for almost 50 years, has given no evidence of cancer risk in humans (Austin et al., 1989). This includes not only the general public, where trace amounts of DDT have been found in body fat, but also individuals exposed to higher levels during its production or spraying. Although DDT is innocuous in hamsters, a lifetime test of the metabolite DDE induced a small number of neoplastic nodules (not cancer).

Polychlorinated and polybrominated biphenyls (PCBs and PBBs) are halogenated aromatic compounds that are comprised of a number of isomers containing up to 10 halogen atoms, depending on the technical production process (Safe, 1989; Kimbrough, 1990). These chemicals are toxic to the liver and kidney at high doses. The carcinogenicity of commerical PCB mixtures given at high lifetime doses may be positively correlated with the degree of chlorination (Lilienfeld and Gallo, 1989; Kimbrough, 1990). Liver tumor enhancing properties have been identified for PCBs and PBBs (Bannasch et al., 1989; Stevenson et al., 1990). Also, these chemicals inhibit intercellular communication in cultured cells (Williams in Stevenson et al., 1990).

Saccharin. The artificial sweetener saccharin has been extensively investigated for chronic toxicity and carcinogenicity (see Weisburger in Williams, 1988). In 1974, two studies reported a somewhat increased incidence of bladder tumors in the first-generation male offspring of rats fed 5 percent or 7.5 percent sodium saccharin throughout pregnancy, and continued on treatment for lifetime in the first generation.

These early studies were complicated by the presence of o-toluenesulfonamide in the saccharin and bladder parasites *trichosomoides crassicauda* and bladder stones in the test animals. A subsequent multigeneration experiment with Swiss mice in which saccharin was given at 0.5 percent in the diet for six generations did not reveal a carcinogenic effect. However, in a two-generation study in which rats were fed 5 percent saccharin, a small increase in bladder tumors in male rats was found even in the F_1 generation. Not every strain of rats responds positively. In fact, most tests involving chronic feeding of the high amount of 5 percent sodium saccharin failed to detect evidence of neoplasia in the bladder. In a study involving Sprague-Dawley, F344, Wistar, and ACI rats, results were negative, except for a 9 percent incidence of bladder cancer in the ACI strain. Yet, two-generation studies where 5 percent or more saccharin was administered to pregnant dams, and the offspring continued on 5 or 7.5 percent saccharin in the diet, usually resulted in a small but definite incidence of bladder papilloma or carcinoma in the F_2 generation. A major study, giving seven distinct dosages of sodium saccharin in the diet over two generations, showed that with 7.5 percent sodium saccharin, 23 percent of the male rats had urinary bladder cancer, and with 6.25, 5, and 4 percent sodium saccharin, the incidences were 13, 11, and 5.3 percent, respectively. However, in this intensive two-generation study, dosages of sodium saccharin of 3 and 1 percent had no effect. Another finding was that administration of 5 percent saccharin beginning with newborn rats gave the same yield of urinary bladder cancer as 5 percent fed in the two-generation study (Anderson *et al.*, 1988). Clearly, sodium saccharin in every study shows a no-effect level that is very high in relation to any human use. Even in experiments where animals were given a genotoxic urinary bladder carcinogen such as FANFT *N*-[4-(5-nitro-2-furyl)-2-thiazolyl]formamide and saccharin was used as a promoter, there were again clear indications of no-effect levels (see Weisburger in Williams, 1988). Thus, knowledge of the mechanism of action and the high dosages required to elicit an effect, and the fact that the sodium salt of saccharin may be the promoting agent, rather than saccharin as calcium salt or the free acid, suggest that human usage of this synthetic sweetener presents no risk. Gaylor *et al.* (1988) have provided a mechanistic and statistical overview for this concept.

Saccharin is not metabolized and has not been shown to be genotoxic, although some impurities have been noted to be mutagenic. Dietary saccharin produces a dose-related increase in the urinary excretion of indole metabolites as a result of altered metabolism of protein in the cecum. Because tryptophan and some of its metabolites such as indoles are known to be promoters for bladder carcinogenesis (see below), it is possible that the effect of saccharin on the bladder is an indirect one, resulting from its alteration of protein digestion in the intestine. In addition, saccharin itself, as the sodium salt, may have a direct action on bladder cell turnover rates because it was more effective than indoles (Anderson *et al.*, 1989). The sodium ion may play a major role in the enhancing effects seen with sodium saccharin, where saccharin may be a nontoxic carrier for the sodium ion. This would account for the high threshold effect (Shibata *et al.*, 1989). Sodium chloride is a potent promoter in the stomach through the induction of increased cell duplication rates, an effect counteracted by calcium chloride (Furihata *et al.*, 1989). Cohen and Ellwein (1989) have provided cogent arguments for the importance of considering cell growth in relation to cocarcinogenesis and especially as regards mechanistically based risk evaluation.

Butylated Hydroxyanisole (BHA) and Butylated Hydroxytoluene (BHT). These antioxidants have been utilized safely as food additives in many countries. Indeed, several tests of chronic toxicity have not revealed any adverse effects. Wattenberg discovered the chemopreventive action of BHA and BHT, administered together with several carcinogens affecting diverse target organs. The antioxidants increase detoxifying enzymes for carcinogens, and many act as free radical trapping agents. The structure of these agents does not suggest a likely electrophile and tests for genotoxicity have been uniformly negative. Both BHA and BHT have been shown to inhibit cell-to-cell communication in culture (Williams in Stevenson *et al.*, 1990).

BHA. Ito and Hirose (1989) found that dietary administration of the high dose of 20,000 ppm of BHA led to hyperplasia and neoplasia in the forestomach of Fischer strain rats in lifetime study, but 5000 ppm BHA had a much lower effect.

The mechanism of the effect of BHA in inducing cancer in the squamous stomach in rodents suggests that the effect may stem from an increased cell turnover rate caused by the high concentration of the antioxidant. Lower dosages have a much lower, or indeed no effect at 0.25 percent. Also, discontinuation of compound administration leads to a rapid decline of the effect (Nera *et al.*, 1988). During the metabolism of BHA, there may be generation of semiquinone radicals and also hydroxy radicals, which cannot be detoxified on high level intake. Thus clearly BHA and related compounds operate by a dose-related epigenetic action with no-effect levels. In a 12-week study in cynomolgous monkeys, gavage of up to 500 mg/kg BHA failed to reveal changes in the stomach and the esophagus, although the latter organ had an increased mitotic index. Liver size increased but little effect was seen on cytochrome P-450 and select microsomal enzymes. Thus, the rat forestomach is extraordinarily sensitive to the high level, 2 percent, of dietary BHA. BHA and BHT are classic anticarcinogens and antimutagens in systems using genotoxic liver carcinogens, because the antioxidants are effective inducers of detoxifying cytochrome P-450 and especially of type II conjugation enzyme systems (King *et al.*, 1988; Ito and Hirose, 1989).

Catechol, and to a lesser extent *p*-methylcatechol, interestingly induce cancer in the glandular stomach, whereas BHA does not affect that area of the stomach (Ito and Hirose, 1989). With catechol, high-dose levels are required and the mechanism of action appears to be also dependent on increasing cell duplication rates, ornithine decarboxylase induction, and on the generation of hydroxy radicals (Furihata *et al.*, 1989). Catechol and related compounds promote forestomach and significantly also glandular stomach carcinogenesis. Catechol is a component of tobacco smoke and may contribute to the adverse effects in the lung and possibly in the oral cavity as a cocarcinogen through this mechanism (Melikian *et al.*, 1989). In part, the protective effect of yellow-green vegetables, retinoids, and vitamin E in smokers might relate to the increased detoxification of hydroxy radicals derived from catechol and phenols generally, by these micronutrients in foods (Stich *et al.*, 1989).

BHT. The first generation of offspring in a two-generation study involving dietary intake of 250 mg/kg body weight BHT produced a small but significant yield of hepatocellular adenoma and carcinoma, more so in males than in females. BHT has also been found to increase the yield of liver neoplasms in mice (Inai *et al.*, 1988). When BHT is given following an initiating exposure to a carcinogen, enhancing effects were found in liver and bladder in rats (Williams 1984; Ito and Hirose, 1989) and in lungs in mice (Witschi and Morse, 1983). These findings are consistent with a promoting effect but more work needs to be done before assignment can be confidently made.

If the carcinogenic effects of BHA and BHT are due to a promoting action, dose-response studies will be important in assessing human risk. Indeed, a threshold for the liver neoplasm promoting effect of BHT was found at 1000 ppm BHT, and the forestomach promoting effect of BHA likewise had not only a threshold, but the effect was reversible (Nera *et al.*, 1988; Ito and Hirose, 1989). This follows logically for an epigenetic action based on the specific intrinsic effects observed, as on cell duplication rates, ornithine decarboxylase induction, and the like (Briggs *et al.*, 1989; Clayson *et al.*, 1989).

Hormone Modifiers

Over 50 years ago, it was shown that administration of sizeable amounts of hormones, especially of the estrogen type, would cause cancer in laboratory animals. Subsequently, it was found that agents or effects that perturb the physiology of endocrine organs or their circadian rhythms also lead to an increase in neoplasia in those organs in animals and in humans (Bulbrook, 1986; Henderson *et al.*, 1988).

Such actions are highly dose dependent, and the underlying mechanism rests on interference with the often complex, multifactorial homeostatic balances of the host. These activities are reversible on cessation of exposure, provided the imbalances have not lasted so long that stable endocrine-independent neoplasms have arisen. Also, transplacental exposure of a fetus by administration of an elevated dosage of an endocrine-active product can permanently bias differentiation of fetal organs. Later, during sexual maturation of the offspring, adverse effects such as sterility or neoplasia can result. Again, these actions are a function of dosage. Any dose of an agent that does not directly or indirectly affect homeostasis under conditions of actual use will be devoid of harmful effects. Human cancer in endocrine organs such as ovary, endometrium, breast, adrenal, thyroid, or prostate are attributed to life style traditions such as the high-fat nutritional habits in the Western world. Research has provided some mechanistic accounting for the effect of dietary fat in modulating the endocrine system, importantly during the developmental aspects at sexual maturation. These actions, in turn, lead to enhanced promotion in endocrine-sensitive organs.

Among the carcinogenic agents that operate through modification of hormonal systems are both hormones and agents that affect endocrine systems.

In animals and in humans, estrogenic hormone-mediated cancer development is most likely due to promoting action and not to a DNA adduct formation of the hormone. ^{32}P-Postlabeling techniques show that DNA in sensitive tissues such as the kidney is modified, but interestingly the same labeled spots were found with estradiol and DES-exposed rats (Liehr *et al.*, 1989). The conclusion is that the DNA does not yield specific adducts of the chemicals, but instead forms common, perhaps endogenous, reactive products. Vitamin C had an inhibiting effect, which may indicate production of active oxygen. The mechanism underlying neoplastic conversion of cells that develop into the neoplasms "induced" by excess estrogen is not known. It may be that activation of proto-oncogenes owing to increased cell turnover is involved in some situations. The mechanism of promotion by high levels of estrogen is no doubt complex and may involve systemic general hormonal imbalances, including pituitary hormones such as prolactin and growth hormone and possibly adrenal and thyroid hormones (Bulbrook, 1986; Henderson *et al.*, 1988). As a rule, hormones are required to be present in abnormal amounts for a long time to produce neoplasia in endocrine-sensitive tissues. Nutritional elements, particularly the type and amount of dietary fat, play a major role in the occurrence of cancer in the breast, ovary, or endometrium in the Western world, through such types of endocrine actions (American Health Foundation, 1987).

Estrogens. The mammalian hormone estradiol causes cancer in animals and in humans when administered chronically at high levels or when present in unphysiologic amounts for long periods of time because of disturbances in normal endocrine balances and receptor systems. In postmenopausal women maintained on estrogen, there is a higher risk of endometrial cancer, which disappears on removal of the medication (Austin and Roe, 1982). Mice harboring the mammary tumor virus displayed a hormone dose-related development of mammary tumors. Untreated mice had a 0 percent incidence of nodules, 0 percent with 100 ppb estradiol (E_2), 3 percent with 1000 ppb E_2, and 9 percent with 5000 ppb E_2. The corresponding adenocarcinoma rate was 4, 0, 8, and 7 percent for E_2 dosages of 0, 100, 1000, and 5000 ppb, respectively. There was a striking no-effect level of 100 ppb E_2.

Diethylstilbestrol (DES). The synthetic hormone DES has 10 times the estrogenic potency of estradiol. In the mammary tumor model this was reflected in a finding of 3 percent nodules and 0 percent mammary carcinoma with 10 ppb DES, and 14 and 7 percent with 500 ppb DES. Required doses of DES to produce effects were an order of magnitude lower than for estradiol. In the cervix there was a high incidence of adenosis, and in the uterine horns of glandular hyperplasia/adenomyosis at the high dosage of 5000 ppb E_2 of 500 ppb DES, but much less at the lower levels.

Importantly, in mice without mammary tumor virus, even the highest dosage of estradiol (5000 ppb) or of DES (500 ppb) failed to induce mammary tumors, evidence that promoting stimuli require antecedent neoplastic conversion of cells (Highland *et al.*, 1977).

Transplacental passage of high amounts of E_2 or of DES, stemming from abnormal levels of E_2 in the mother, or subsequent to elevated intake of DES used as drug, powerfully affects differentiation and imprinting of endocrine-sensitive organs in the fetus. At the time of sexual maturation, this produces abnormal hormonal balances, which in turn evoke neoplasia, and also sterility, the latter more in males. Such a mechanism most likely was operative in the young women, who were daughters of mothers treated with large amounts of DES during pregnancy and who developed clear cell adenoarcinoma of the vagina. In addition to these endocrine mechanisms, it has been proposed that DES can also act via a genetic mechanism through its metabolites (Metzler, 1986; Gladek and Liehr, 1989).

Oral Contraceptives. Among users of oral contraceptives, rare cases of liver neoplasms occur, considering the widespread use of these agents (Prentice and Thomas, 1987; WHO Collaborative Study, 1989; Stevenson *et al.*, 1990). In all of these situations, the hormones appear to have promoted the lesions, actually caused by unknown factors. On the other hand, most studies show that users of oral contraceptive have a lower risk of endocrine, breast, ovary, and endometrial cancers, perhaps because they stabilize the rhythmic function of the endocrine system.

Tamoxifen. This antiestrogen has as its main pharmacologic action the binding to estrogen receptors. Because of this action it has proven useful in the treatment of breast cancer. However, in animal studies conducted by the manufacturer, tamoxifen has induced liver tumors in rodents.

Zearalenone. This mycoestrogen has caused increases in pituitary and liver tumors in mice.

Androgens. Testosterone is carcinogenic to rats and mice, inducing cervical-uterine neoplasms in female mice and prostatic adenocarcinomas in male rats (IARC Monogr. Suppl. 7, 1987). However, in contrast to estrogens, the evidence for cancer induction in humans is limited. A few cases of liver cancer were reported in men taking large amounts of androgens as anabolic agents or as muscle builders for athletes.

Antithyroid Agents. As is true for the target organs of estrogenic hormones, where any deviation from the normal physiological balance can have pronounced adverse effects, including neoplasia, the same holds for the thyroid gland. In this instance, a main function of this gland is to biosynthesize thyroxin (T4, T3). This hormone circulates and provides essential signals for a number of important physiologic activities. One receptor for T4 is in the pituitary gland. One of the functions of that gland is to generate thyroid-stimulating hormone (TSH) which in turn reaches the thyroid gland and controls its function, namely the production of appropriate, necessary amounts of thyroxin. Thus, this is a well regulated feedback system. Any external chemical affecting the capability of the thyroid gland in synthesizing or releasing T4 will lead to a lower level of circulating T4, in turn increasing TSH production. Any persistent exogenous effect on T4 synthesis will lead to a continuing stimulation of thyroid gland growth by TSH. This condition in animals and humans has the attributes of goiter, but eventually leads to the occurrence of thyroid cancer. T4 is an iodinated compound. Deficiency of iodine intake can elicit this sequence of events leading to goiter and thyroid cancer. Fortification of salt or other foods in low iodine areas prevents goiter. Certain foods such as cabbage contain goitrogens, and frequent intake, especially in areas with low prevailing iodine, may produce goiter and thyroid cancer. The large family of thioureas blocks T4 synthesis. When given chronically and at high dosages, they induce thyroid neoplasia. Useful fungicides of the dithiocarbamate type yield ethylenethiourea. Bioassay of this chemical at high dose levels also causes thyroid cancer through these mechanisms. 3-Aminotriazole, an agricultural chemical, exerts such effects, as do certain sulfonamides. Clearly, an exogenous chemical, or iodine deficiency, or intake of foods containing goitrogens, leads to adverse effects, goiter and cancer, only at dosages that chronically suppress T4 formation. Low levels that do not affect T4 production clearly have no adverse effects. Thus all such chemicals display an S-shaped dose-response curve with a threshold. Also, there are certain species differences; for example, 3-aminotriazole affects the thyroid in rats but not in mice or hamsters.

Chemicals that do not directly act on T4 production, but rather induce enzymes in the liver that metabolize T4 and thus also lower the effective circulation level of this thyroid hormone, can also lead to thyroid neoplasia through such an indirect mechanism. This may be the case for phenobarbital (Diwan *et al.*, 1989).

Here also, the essential requirement is a chronic dose level of the enzyme inducer that decreases circulating T4. Any lower level of the enzyme inducer will have no effect. Thus, under most conditions, the general public will not be affected by the low prevailing levels of agents that are experimental thyroid carcinogens at high dose rates. Individuals potentially exposed to higher amounts, as may be true for those engaged in production of such chemicals, should be monitored regularly for circulating T4 and thyroid function.

Inhibitors of Gastric Secretion. Extremely useful drugs have been developed for treatment of peptic ulcers. These include cimetidine and ranitidine, which inhibit gastric secretion by blockade of the histamine H_2 receptor of gastric parietal cells, and omeprazole, which inhibits the K^+,H^+-ATPase of the parietal cells. Omeprazole was found to induce neoplasms of endocrine enterochromaffin-like cells (carcinoids) in the stomachs of rats, but not mice (Ekman *et al.*, 1985). The drug is not genotoxic, but rather a clear epigenetic mechanism has been elucidated. At high doses, omeprazole produces an almost complete inhibition of acid secretion and secondary hypergastrinemia results, leading to hyperplasia of enterochromaffin-like cells and the development of carcinoids. It is likely that comparable antisecretory activity by any agent would have the same effect (Hirth *et al.*, 1988).

Cytotoxins

Nitrilotriacetic Acid (NTA). This chelating agent is used for a number of industrial purposes and as an environment-friendly, noneutrophying replacement for phosphate in household detergents because it can be metabolized to harmless products in the soil. It causes kidney and urinary bladder neoplasms in rats and mice only when given as sodium salt at high levels in the diet (above 7500 ppm) or in drinking water. No neoplasms are observed at lower levels. There is a sharp no-effect level. NTA is not biotransformed and is excreted almost entirely in urine. It is not DNA reactive, and thus studies of its mode of action have focused on its toxic effects in kidney and bladder as a consequence of its chelating activity. In a series of studies, Anderson and coworkers have shown that NTA carries zinc into the renal tubular ultrafiltrate, where it is reabsorbed by the tubular epithelium. Zinc is toxic to these cells, producing cell injury and death leading to a hyperplastic and eventually neoplastic response. The NTA in urine chelates calcium, extracting it from the urothelium of the renal pelvis and bladder, thereby stimulating cellular proliferation, apparently leading to neoplasia. Ferric NTA injection increased 8-hydroxydeoxyguanosine in kidney DNA, evidence of the generation of ·OH radicals. NTA itself did not give that result (Umemura *et al.,* 1990). Thus, NTA at high doses may chelate specific metal ions, and indirectly lead to neoplasia.

$\alpha 2\mu$-Globulin Nephropathy and Kidney Tumors. Male rats are susceptible to chemically induced renal toxicity involving $\alpha 2\mu$-globulin, a protein of 162 amino acids that is synthesized in the liver and released into the blood. Like other low-molecular-weight proteins, the globulin is taken up by tubular epithelial cells and hydrolyzed in lysosomes. A large body of data shows that certain chemicals bind to the $\alpha 2\mu$ globulin and interfere with catabolism, leading to accumulation of chemical-$\alpha 2\mu$ complex in kidney cells and cell necrosis. The necrosis and consequent cell regeneration are believed to result in kidney tumorigenesis (Swenberg *et al.,* 1989). Chemicals that have caused kidney tumors in male rats by this mechanism include unleaded gasoline and petroleum hydrocarbons (Short *et al.,* 1987), trichloroethylene, perchloroethylene, and pentachloroethane (Goldsworthy *et al.,* 1988), decalin, isophorone, 1,4-dichlorobenzene, and *d*-limonene (Swenberg *et al.,* 1989).

Immunosuppressive Drugs

Immune processes can affect carcinogenesis in a variety of ways (IARC Monogrs. 26, 1981; IARC Sci. Publ. 78, 1986). Animals given immunosuppressive sera or drugs such as azathioprine or 6-mercaptopurine have developed leukemias and lymphomas (Sontag, 1981). Likewise, patients so treated developed cancers, usually leukemias or sarcomas but rarely solid tumors (Penn, 1988). Recently, cyclosporin A was found to be associated with an increase of lymphoma in treated organ transplant recipients and in mice it accelerated the development of cryptogenic or chemically induced leukemias (IARC Mongr. 50, 1990).

Some of these drugs may alter DNA synthesis or even be incorporated into DNA, but none react with DNA. Severely immunodeficient patients such as those with acquired immunodeficiency syndrome (AIDS) have a higher risk of Kaposi's sarcoma, lymphomas, and leukemias. In animal models, the underlying causative agent is often an oncogenic virus, and the same may be true in humans. Thus, it is thought that the carcinogenicity of immunosuppressants may stem from an epigenetic phenomenon, by which immunosuppression allows development of tumors initiated by a distinct genetic event (Wyke and Weiss, 1984; Levine, 1988; Klein, 1989).

Peroxisome Proliferators

A variety of agents that have produced liver tumors in rodents have the common property of increasing the numbers of peroxisomes in rodent liver which led J. Reddy and coworkers in the United States to propose that peroxisome proliferators as a class are carcinogenic. Hepatocarcinogenic peroxisome proliferators include the hypolipidemic drugs clofibrate, fenofibrate, gemfibozil, tibric acid; the plasticizer di(2-ethylhexyl)phthalate; the herbicide lactofen; and the organic solvent 1,1,2-trichloroethylene (Gibson, 1990). These agents were generally negative in assays for genotoxicity. Evidence has been adduced for a liver tumor-promoting effects with certain of these agents, but this has not been found for all agents of this type and at present cannot be asserted to be the mechanism of their carcinogenicity. Alternatively, it has been proposed by Reddy that, as a consequence of the increase in the numbers of peroxisomes, increased H_2O_2 could lead to the formation of reactive oxygen species that have the capability to damage DNA and initiate carcinogenesis (Reddy in Chambers *et al.,* 1989). In any case, such events should have theoretical and practical thresholds, which should be established in each case (Lock *et al.,* 1989; Nemali *et al.,* 1989).

Solid-State Materials

Plastics implanted subcutaneously in rodents can lead to sarcoma formation after a long latent period (see Brand, in Banbury Rept. 25, 1987). The chemical composition of the implanted material is relatively unimportant. Indeed, thin disks or sheets of metal (such as gold) were as effective as a variety of polymers. The important factors were the size and shape of the insert. Smooth materials were more effective than rough, perforated disks, and sheets were less effective than more solid types. Although the detailed mechanism is not yet known, it seems clear that the solid materials provide a substrate for proliferation of dermal fibroblasts, increased cell duplication rates, and possibly generation of active oxygen in an inflammatory field (Murrell *et al.,* 1990). There are a few reports of sarcomas occurring at the site of vascular grafts in humans, but the cases have in common the fact that the individuals involved were young at the time of implant, which may provide a clue to further epidemiologic investigations as well as laboratory studies.

Asbestos. Large amounts of inhaled asbestos alone, reaching the pleural cavity in animal models and in humans, lead to mesotheliomas, usually with a long expression period (IARC Sci. Publ. 90; 1988). Other fibers, such as fine fibrous glass, have a similar effect. The shape and size of fibers is important. Thus, the effect has features of solid-state carcinogenesis, especially because the lesion obtained is not epithelial, but mesenchymal. Apart from weak clastogenic effects at high concentrations, no firm evidence for DNA reactivity of asbestos has been developed.

Asbestos is not biotransformed and excreted but most of the inhaled fibers remain permanently in the body. It produces a fibroblastic pleural reaction, before the occurrence of mesothelioma. This may involve increased cell duplication rates, and inflammatory areas including cells generating reactive oxygen. As a consequence of its persistence, even limited exposure to high levels of asbestos, as used to be the case in occupational situations, leads to its continued presence in the body. Men exposed to asbestos during mining operations or in the large-scale shipbuilding effort in the United States in the 1940s and insulation workers are currently at high risk for this disease. This is apparent from the geographic "hot spots" of lung cancer in counties and areas in the United States, and in other countries where shipbuilding was a major industry, usually in individuals who were also chronic cigarette smokers.

In addition, a major health problem stems from the fact that asbestos particles, and other mineral ores, such as in uranium or hematite mining, potentiate the action of other carcinogens, such as cigarette smoke, reaching the same organ. Cases of disease have been seen even in relatives of workmen, who, through frequent indirect exposures such as laundering work clothing, inhaled this material, especially at young ages (IARC Sci. Publ. 90, 1988; Maltoni and Selikoff, 1988). Thus, this type of agent can be considered as dangerous (because of long, probably permanent retention in the respiratory tract and pleura) as organic carcinogens, although the latter are genotoxic. Yet, in spite of government-mandated removal of asbestos from schools in the United States, there are few sound data on effects of low level exposures in nonsmokers (Weill and Hughes, 1986; Mossman et al., 1990). Also, chrysotile fibers appear much less hazardous, because of their shape and dimensions compared to amphiboles.

Asbestos fibers ingested during high-level occupational exposure have been suggested to lead to cancer in the gastrointestinal tract. However, animal studies so far have not demonstrated any effects in the target organs when asbestos was fed at high levels alone or together with an appropriate carcinogen for the gastrointestinal tract.

Unclassified Carcinogens

There are a number of carcinogens that have not been demonstrated to react covalently with DNA, but whose mode of action is not sufficiently well understood to permit assignment to a specific class of epigenetic agents.

Ethanol. Ethanol in various types of frequently consumed beverages has been used for millennia around the world. Epidemiologic information has documented that individuals who smoke or chew tobacco and also consume appreciable amounts, usually considered to be six or more drinks per day of any kind of alcoholic beverage, have a higher risk of cancer of the oral cavity and esophagus (IARC Monogr. 44, 1990; Hoffmann and Hecht, in Cooper and Grover, 1990). Excessive use of alcohol without smoking may have an effect on the esophagus but the data are weak. Studies of the mechanism of alcohol in carcinogenesis of the esophagus and also oral cavity have suggested that ethanol modifies the biochemical activation in the oral cavity and esophagus of the tobacco-specific carcinogens (Seitz and Simanowski, 1988). If so, ethanol would be classified as cocarcinogenic.

Heavy intake of alcoholic beverages is toxic to the liver, where biotransformation occurs (Sohn et al., 1987). The toxicity is expressed as "alcoholic hepatitis" which leads to cirrhosis. Individuals with alcohol-induced cirrhosis also have a higher risk of hepatocellular carcinoma (Bannasch et al., 1989). It is not known whether the neoplastic change is due to alcohol or its reactive metabolite, acetaldehyde, or whether levels of hepatocarcinogens, as for example, aflatoxin B_1, at subthreshold dosages in healthy livers, lead to cancer in chronically damaged cirrhotic livers in which elevated levels of cell regeneration are present.

Alcoholic beverage intake has also been associated with an increased risk of rectal cancer, particularly in men. It has been demonstrated in humans and in rats that intake of alcohol increases cell duplication rates in the rectum, but not in the colon. Also, specialized analytical techniques have demonstrated increasing levels of acetaldehyde in the rectum (Seitz and Simanowski, 1988). Acetaldehyde is carcinogenic by inhalation.

Because alcoholic beverages are natural products with a long history of human use, there have been no legislative or regulatory actions anywhere in the world, except for the unsuccessful brief period of prohibition in the United States in the 1930s. Yet, objectively examined as a toxicant, with probable carcinogenic or cocarcinogenic properties, alcohol deserves more public attention as to the need of moderate use than some of the widely publicized actions by the government and the media in relation to synthetic agricultural chemicals, such as the recent noted episode with virtually nontoxic agents such as Alar. Classic animal bioassays on alcohol or alcoholic beverages have not demonstrated a carcinogenic effect. Rodents accept with difficulty fluids containing more than 15 percent ethanol. A special liquid diet developed by Lieber contains 35 percent and such solutions have displayed an enhancing effect with carcinogens such as nitrosopyrrolidone (Hoffmann and Hecht in Cooper and Grover, 1990).

Benzene. Occupational exposure to benzene under quantitatively ill-defined conditions has led to a number of cases of leukemia (Goldstein, 1988; Maltoni and Selikoff, 1988; Mehlman, 1989). The then prevailing hygienic conditions led to the suspicion that the air concentrations were high. The mechanism whereby benzene induces leukemia in humans is under intensive investigation. There is evidence of a dose-response relationship measured as concentration in air and years of exposure. Benzene, through its metabolites, affects the bone marrow and antecedent lesions are leukocytopenia and thrombocytopenia, which can serve as diagnostic indicators available through hematologic screening tests (Yager *et al.*, 1990).

Numerous attempts were made to document that benzene could induce leukemia in the conventional animal models. Although some of the antecedent lesions, evidence of bone marrow toxicity, were observed, there were only limited successes in reproducing the disease seen in humans, leukemia. However, in certain strains of mice, myelogenous tumors were observed on inhalation. Maltoni reported that ingestion or inhalation of benzene in several strains of rats and mice yielded several tumor types including ear duct, oral or nasal cavity, skin, squamous stomach, mammary gland, lung, angiosarcomas of the liver, and also lymphoreticular tumors (see Goldstein, 1988; Maltoni and Selikoff, 1988; Mehlman, 1989). These findings were confirmed and extended by the U.S. National Toxicology Program.

The mechanism of action of benzene as a carcinogen through studies on its metabolism has provided indication, not only of the expected metabolites, namely phenol, and dihydroxybenzenes, but also oxidation products such as benzoquinone, a candidate reactive product, or the open ring metabolites such as *trans*-muconic aldehyde. Tests of benzene for genotoxicity in the customary assays have been negative, perhaps because under the conditions of these tests, a volatile reactive product might be formed in low amounts. In industrial processes in the past where workers were exposed chronically to appreciable concentrations of benzene as high as 400 to 800 ppm, leukemias were often seen. Current regulations in the United States set a threshold limit at 1 ppm and based on its mode of action, it is probable that this level, especially if present intermittently, represents an amount that would lead to detoxified metabolites with minimal formation of a reactive product.

Thioamides. In connection with the determination of the safety of certain food additives, it was discovered that thiourea, thioacetamide, thiouracil, ethylene thiourea, and similar thioamides were carcinogenic. The usual target organ is the thyroid gland and in some instances the liver (Neal and Halpert, 1982). The action on the liver by specific agents such as thiouracil and thioacetamide has not yet been given a sound fundamental explanation. Metabolism studies suggest oxidation on the sulfur atom to thiono and sulfone derivatives might yield reactive compounds, involving a charge separation between the sulfur-oxygen and the carbon, the latter thus being electrophilic (Neal and Halpert, 1982).

Acetamide, a related chemical, when given to rats in doses as large as 1 to 5 percent in the diet, elicits hepatocellular carcinomas in 12 to 15 months. The mechanism of action of this chemical on the liver is quite different from that of the corresponding thioacetamide, the latter being effective in much lower dosages in a shorter span of time. Acetamide at such high concentrations may yield increased endogenous levels of ammonia, in turn affecting pyridoxal phosphate, the active component of vitamin B_6, and an essential component of transaminases. A chronic deficiency of this micronutrient produces liver neoplasms through unknown mechanisms (Weisburger, 1990).

Halogenated Hydrocarbons. Among this class of widely used industrial chemicals there are a number of agents whose mode of action remains unclear. Among these, carbon tetrachloride, chloroform, and several polychlorinated alkanes or alkenes yield negative or equivocal results in current test systems for genotoxicity. Furthermore, metabolism in mammalian systems *in vivo* or *in vitro* does not provide any evidence that they give risk to reactive electrophilic metabolites. These experiments include utilizing highly isotopically labeled chemicals in attempts to verify reaction with DNA.

On the other hand, one element that is quite clear is that these chlorinated hydrocarbons are cytotoxic after a single dose or on chronic intake. For the most part, the toxicity is expressed mainly in the liver and in the kidney of rodents. With some agents, where accidental or suicidal ingestion occurred, there was evidence of liver or kidney damage in humans.

There is no question but that halogenated hydrocarbons can be toxic and carcinogenic in the mouse liver (IACR Monogrs. 20, 1979; 41, 1986). The important finding was made that administration in an edible oil appeared to be more toxic than when equivalent amounts were administered in drinking water. Thus, the role of the vehicle will have to be defined. In addition, of course, this distinction is important in evaluating the possible effect of halogenated hydrocarbons present in small amounts in drinking water.

Methylene chloride, or dichloromethane, is a useful solvent and chemical with broad chemical application, especially because it is nonflammable, as are most of the halogenated hydrocarbons (IARC Monogr. 41, 1986). Methylene chloride is active in bacterial mutagenesis tests without requiring metabolic activation. However, it is inactive in most systems involving mammalian cells and has not been found to alkylate DNA. Therefore, methylene chloride may not justify classification as a genotoxin. The compound is metabolized to the toxic product phosgene ($COCl_2$), CO_2, and CO, the latter causing carboxyhemoglobin formation, a marker for intoxication. Chronic inhalation of methylene chloride by mice led to the development of neoplasms in lung and liver, but a similar test in rats led to equivocal results. Oral intake in an edible oil led to liver neoplasms in mice. On the other hand, administration in drinking water of rats and mice gave no evidence of carcinogenicity. The underlying reasons require clarification before sound human risk evaluations can be made.

Carbon Tetrachloride. This is a high-volume, nonflammable solvent. In virtually all species, it is severely hepatotoxic, and in mice of certain strains, it induces liver tumors (IARC Monogr. Suppl. 7, 1987). Metabolism yields a reactive Cl_3C radical (Knecht and Mason, 1988), that does not seem to bind to DNA, and also a number of other products. It has been proposed that during liver intoxication lipid peroxidative processes might play a role (Poli *et al.*, 1989). Plaa (1988) has noted potentiation of toxicity of carbon tetrachloride in rats by 1,3-butanediol and other alcohols and ketones. Even single doses lead to severe necrosis, followed by regeneration involving extensive cell duplication of parenchymal and nonparenchymal cells. Fibrosis and cirrhosis arise through complex mechanisms, including transforming growth factor B (Armendariz-Borunda *et al.*, 1990). The Solt-Farber protocol to detect liver carcinogens uses the extensive regeneration caused by CCl₄ to amplify any early carcinogenic effects by a test substance. The molecular events in liver cell duplication have been explored, and the findings are relevant to most types of carcinogens affecting the liver (Kalf *et al.*, 1987).

Chloroform. Chloroform was formerly used in human anesthesia and is an important industrial solvent (IARC Monogr. Suppl. 7, 1987). Sensitive chemical analytical procedures have revealed that chloroform is the main chlorinated hydrocarbon produced during chlorination of drinking water, and thus is present in small but definite amounts in water supplies. Similarly to carbon tetrachloride, chloroform at high doses causes liver and kidney damage, somewhat more in kidney and somewhat less in the liver, as compared to carbon tetrachloride. Chronic oral intake by gavage in an edible oil solution leads to liver tumors in mice. Lifetime administration to rats has induced a smaller yield of renal neoplasms, in addition to being severely nephrotoxic. The relevant mechanism may rest on the formation of GSH conjugates in the liver, which are toxic to the kidneys on further metabolism. Chloroform is not genotoxic in the appropriate tests (Rosenthal, 1987). Low levels of ingested chloroform are detoxified, and not likely cancer risks.

Trichloroethylene Trichloroethane, Tetrachloroethane Perchloroethylene. Administration of these chemicals to mice induces neoplasms in the liver, as is typical of virtually all chlorinated hydrocarbons (Bannash *et al.*, 1989; Stevenson *et al.*, 1990). These chemicals are highly toxic to kidneys in mice and even more so in rats.

Even though an epoxide is the critical genotoxic metabolite derived from vinyl chloride, it has been much more difficult to demonstrate the formation of a reactive epoxide from a halogenated ethene such as trichloroethylene. The properties of the synthetic epoxide are those expected of a reactive electrophile. However, formation of the epoxide in biologic systems may be difficult because of the steric highly hindered position of the ethylene bond due to the three neighboring chlorine atoms. It may be that the kinetics of the formation of the epoxide are slower than that of its reaction with a nucleophilic component in the cell other than DNA. No covalent binding of the reactive metabolite to DNA was observed. Importantly, the saturated trichloro- or tetrachloroethanes exhibit the same kind of toxicity and tumor spectrum as do the ethylene derivatives, so that the hindered double bond apparently is biochemically equivalent to the single bond in the polychlorinated ethanes. Trichloroethylene may act as a promoter, because it inhibits intercellular communication *in vitro* (Klaunig *et al.*, 1989). It is converted to trichloroacetic acid (TCA) in mice, but not much in rats (DeAngelo *et al.*, 1989; Lock *et al.*, 1989). TCA acts as a peroxisome proliferator, and the neoplasms in the liver of mice may arise through this mechanism. These chemicals are conjugated with GSH, yielding products that are converted to the reactive metabolites in the kidneys through the action of β-lyase (Dekant *et al.*, 1989). These steps occur to a greater extent in rats than in mice, and account for the pronounced nephrotoxicity,

involving α2μ-globulin accumulation, probably a key reaction. The nephorotoxicity expains the low but definite yield of kidney neoplasms.

2,3,7,8-Tetrachlorodibenzodioxin (TCDD).
TCDD arises during the heating or combustion of many polychlorophenols such as 2,4,5-trichlorophenol or 2,4,5-T, the latter being valuable agricultural products, especially herbicides (see Banbury Rept. 18, 1984; Lilienfield and Gallo, 1989; Kimbrough, 1990). Formerly, TCDD was present in low parts-per-million amounts in the commercial herbicide 2,4,5-T. Testing of the latter product displayed some adverse effects, particularly teratogenicity, which was ultimately traced not to 2,4,5-T, but to the trace contaminant TCDD. The production processes of 2,4,5,-T were improved to eliminate these polychlorinated aromatic contaminants. Tests of pure TCDD demonstrated that it was highly toxic at parts-per-billion levels, especially to the liver (see Chapter 10). Chronic administration of TCDD caused hepatocellular carcinoma and thyroid tumors in mice and rats (IARC Monogr. Suppl. 7, 1987). Also, in rats TCDD produced squamous cell carcinomas of the lung and tumors of the hard palate/nasal turbinates and tongue. Studies in a number of appropriate systems have failed to demonstrate genotoxicity. TCDD is bound to a high-affinity cellular receptor (the *Ah* receptor) that translocates to the nucleus, accounting in part for the high specificity at low dose levels (Lilienfield and Gallo, 1989). The situation may be analogous to that of the phorbol esters, which promote mouse skin cancer, and have a specific receptor. TCDD has been found to be an enhancer of liver carcinogenesis. Humans exposed to TCDD may exhibit the skin condition chloracne, but so far individuals with high exposures to TCDD have not displayed excess cancer in the liver or other organs (IARC Suppl. 7, 1987). The latent period to cancer, however, may be longer than the current period of observation.

Methapyrilene. This antihistaminic was widely used in sleep aids in the United States, until it was reported in 1980 that it produced liver tumors in rats (Lijinsky and Yamashita, 1988). Methapyrilene has also been shown to enhance liver tumor development when administered either before or after a genotoxic liver carcinogen (Williams, 1984). Methapyrilene is negative in most short-term tests for genotoxicity, but some positive results have been noted. It fails to show adduct formation with the sensitive ³²P-postlabeling technique. An unusual finding is a considerable increase in the number of mitochondria in liver cells of rats. This indicates the possibility of production of reactive oxygen species, as has been proposed for the peroxisome proliferators. Also, chronic intake increases the normally low rate of liver cell proliferation and increases methylation of DNA, as do high levels of hydrazine, an indication of an indirect effect through hepatotoxicity (Hernandez *et al.*, 1989).

Hydrazine. This inorganic compound (NH₂NH₂) induced pulmonary tumors in sensitive strains of mice at high dose levels, and a low incidence of liver tumors in rats (Shimkin and Stoner, 1975; Sontag, 1981). Under the effect of hydrazine, incorporation of one-carbon compounds to yield O^6-methylguanine and a 7-methylguanine in DNA was observed, where the methyl group stems from the metabolism of *S*-adenosylmethionine.

Potassium Bromate. This chemical is used in the baking industry and as a chemical reagent. It is directly mutagenic in salmonella typhimurium TA100, but not TA98. On intake in the drinking water it caused renal adenocarcinomas (Kurokawa *et al.*, 1983). There was also a small yield of peritoneal mesothelioma, and in females thyroid neoplasms. The underlying mechanism may involve generation of reactive oxygen in target organs with inadequate defensive enzyme levels.

Methylmercury Chloride. This neurotoxic agent has been found to induce renal toxicity and carcinogenicity administered at 10 ppm to mice chronically, but not at lower doses (Mitsumori *et al.*, 1990).

Arsenic. There seems to be an association between trivalent inorganic arsenic exposure of humans through drinking water or in certain occupations and the development of lung and skin cancer and lymphomas (IARC Monogr. Suppl 7, 1987). However, the exposure situation may not be to arsenic alone but to a complex environment containing excess arsenic, together with other materials. Some regions where water contains arsenic apparently have and others do not an excess of cancer (see Wu *et al.*, 1989). So far, animal tests of arsenic derivatives have not yielded firm evidence that inorganic arsenic compounds can cause cancer, a truly exceptional situation for a human carcinogen. Arsenic compounds can affect the fidelity of DNA biosynthesis (Rossman *et al.*, 1977).

REFERENCES

Continuing Series Source Material:

Advances in Cancer Research, Academic Press, New York

Banbury Reports, Cold Spring Harbor Laboratory, Cold Spring Harbor, NY.

Cancer Surveys, Oxford University Press, Oxford, U.K.

IARC Monograph series, vols. 1–46; and Suppl. 1–7: *Evaluation of the Carcinogenic Risk of Chemicals to Humans.* Internatl. Agency for Res. on Cancer (WHO), Lyon, France, 1972–1989.

IARC Scientific Publications, Vols., 1–99: Internatl. Agency for Res. on Cancer, Lyon, France, 1971–1990.

National Cancer Institute, Monograph series, Bethesda, MD.

Proceedings, Symposium of the Princess Takamatsu Cancer Research Fund, Tokyo

Recent Results in Cancer Research, Springer-Verlag, Berlin.

Aldridge, W. N.: The biological basis and measurements of thresholds. *Annu. Rev. Pharmacol. Toxicol.*, **26**:39–58, 1986.

American Cancer Society: *1990 Facts and Figures*. American Cancer Society, Inc., Atlanta, GA, 1990.

American Health Foundation. Workshop on new developments on dietary fat and fiber in carcinogenesis (optimal types and amounts of fat or fiber). *Prev. Med.*, **16**:449–595, 1987.

Amler, L. C., and Schwab, M.: Amplified N-*myc* in human neuroblastoma cells is often arranged as clustered tandem repeats of differentially recombined DNA. *Mol. Cell Biol.*, **9**:4903–4913, 1989.

Anderson, R. L.; Lefever, F. R.; and Maurer, J. K.: Comparison of the responses of male rats to dietary sodium saccharin exposure initiated during nursing with responses to exposure initiated at weaning. *Food Chem. Toxicol.*, **26**:899–907, 1988.

Anderson, R. L.; Lefever, F. R.; Miller, N. S.; and Maurer, J. K.: Comparison of the bladder response to indole and sodium saccharin ingestion by male rats. *Food Chem. Toxicol.*, **12**:777–7779, 1989.

Anthony, A.; Caldwell, J.; Hutt, A. J.; and Smith, R. L.: Metabolism of estragole in rat and mouse and influence of dose size on excretion of the proximate carcinogen 1'-hydroxyestragole. *Food Chem. Toxicol.*, **25**:799–806, 1987.

Arcos, J. C.; Woo, Y. T.; Argus, M. F.; and Lai, D. Y.: *Chemical Induction of Cancer*, Vols. I, IIA, IIB, IIIA, IIIB. Academic Press, New York, 1968–1988.

Armendariz-Borunda, J.; Seyer, J. M.; Kang, A. H.; and Raghow, R.: Regulation of TGFβ gene expression in rat liver intoxicated with carbon tetrachloride. *FASEB J.*, **4**:215–221, 1990.

Arnold, D. L.; Krewski, D. R.; Junkins, D. B.; McGuire, P. F., Moodie, C. A.; and Munro, I. C.: Reversibility of ethylenethiourea-induced thyroid lesions. *Toxicol. Appl. Pharmacol.*, **67**:264–273, 1983.

Ashby, J.; Tennant, R. W.; Zeiger, E.; and Stasiewicz, S.: Classification according to chemical structure, mutagenicity to *Salmonella* and level of carcinogenicity of a further 42 chemicals tested for carcinogenicity by the U.S. National Toxicology Program. *Mutat. Res.*, **223**:73–103, 1989.

Austin, D. F., and Roe, K. M.: The decreasing incidence of endometrial cancer: public health implications. *Am. J. Publ. Health*, **72**:65–68, 1982.

Austin, H.; Keil, J. E.; and Cole, P.: A prospective follow-up study of cancer mortality in relation to serum DDT. *Am. J. Publ. Health*, **79**:43–47, 1989.

Bannasch, P.; Keppler, D.; and Weber, G. (eds.): *Liver Cell Carcinoma*. Kluwer Academic Publishers, Dordrecht, Boston, London, 1989.

Barbin, A., and Bartsch, H.: Nucleophilic selectivity as a determinant of carcinogenic potency (TD_{50}) in rodents: a comparison of mono- and bifunctional alkylating agents and vinyl chloride metabolites. *Mutat. Res.*, **215**:95–106, 1989.

Barrett, J. C.; Lamb, P. W.; and Wiseman, R. W.: Multiple mechanisms for the carcinogenic effects of asbestos and other mineral fibers. *Environ. Health Perspect.*, **81**:81–89, 1989.

Bartsch, H.; Ohshima, H.; Shuker, D. E. G.; Pignatelli, B.; and Calmels, S.: Exposure of humans to endogenous *N*-nitroso compounds: implications in cancer etiology. *Mutat. Res.*, **238**:255–267, 1990.

Beniashvili, S.: Inductions of renal tumors in cynomolgus monkeys *(Macaca fascicularis)* by prenatal exposure to 1,2,-dimethylhydrazine.: *J. Natl. Cancer Inst.*, **81**:1325–1327, 1989.

Berenblum, I.: *Carcinogenesis as a Biological Problem*. North-Holland, Amsterdam, 1974.

Blumberg, P. M.: Protein kinase C as the receptor for the phorbol ester tumor promoters: *Cancer Res.*, **48**:1–8, 1988.

Bogen, K. T.: Cell proliferation kinetics and multistage cancer risk models. *J. Natl. Cancer Inst.*, **81**:267–277, 1989.

Bolt, H. M.: Experimental toxicology of formaldehyde. *J. Cancer Res. Clin. Oncol.*, **113**:305–309, 1987.

Bos, J. L.: Oncogenes in human cancer: a review. *Cancer Res.*, **49**:4682–4689, 1989.

Bredberg, A.; Brant, M.; Riesbeck, K.; Azou, Y.; and Forsgren, A.: 4-Quinolone antibiotics: positive genotoxic screening tests despite an apparent lack of mutation induction. *Mutat. Res.*, **211**:171–180, 1989.

Bridges, B. A. (ed.): Alcohol as a mutagenic agent. *Mutat. Res.*, **186**:173–277, 1987.

Briggs, D.; Lok, E.; Nera, E. A.; Karpinski, K.; and Clayson, D. B.: Short-term effects of butylated hydroxytoluene on the Wistar rat liver, urinary bladder and thyroid gland. *Cancer Lett.*, **46**:31–36, 1989.

Buffler, P. A.; Wood, S. M.; Suarez, L.; and Kilian, D. J.: Mortality follow-up of workers exposed to 1,4-dioxane. *J. Occup. Med.*, **20**:255–259, 1978.

Bulbrook, R. D., (ed.): Hormones and cancer: 90 years after Beatson. *Cancer Surv.*, **5**:435–687, 1986.

Cavenee, W. K.; Hastie, N. D.; and Stanbridge, E. J. (eds.): *Recessive Oncogenes and Tumor Suppression*. Cold Spring Harbor Laboratory Press, Cold Spring Harbor, New York, 1989.

Chambers, P. L.; Chambers, C. M.; and Dirheimer, G. (eds.): The target organ and the toxic process. *Arch. Toxicol.* (Suppl. 12), 1988.

Chambers, P. L.; Chambers, C. M.; and Greim, H. (eds.): Biological monitoring of exposure and the response at the subcellular level to toxic substances. *Arch. Toxicol.* (Suppl. 13), 1989.

Clayson, D. B.: The need for biological risk assessment in reaching decisions about carcinogens. *Mutat. Res.*, **185**:243–269, 1987.

Clayson, D. B.; Nera, E. A.; and Lok, E.: The potential for the use of cell proliferation studies in carcinogen risk assessment. *Regul. Toxicol. Pharmacol.*, **9**:284–295, 1989.

Clemmesen, J., and Hjalgrim-Jensen, S.: Does phenobarbital cause intracranial tumors? A follow-up through 35 years. *Ecotoxicol. Environ. Safety*, **5**:255–260, 1981.

Cohen, S. M., and Ellwein, L. B.: Cell proliferation in carcinogenesis. *Science*, **249**:1007–1011, 1990.

Committee on Diet and Health, Food and Nutrition Board.: *Diet and Health: Implications for Reducing Chronic Disease Risk*. National Academy Press, Washington, D.C., 1989.

Conney, A. H.: Induction of microsomal enzymes by foreign chemicals and carcinogenesis by polycyclic aromatic hydrocarbons. *Cancer Res.*, **42**:4875–4917, 1982.

Conning, D. M.; Magee, P.; Oesch, F.; and Clemmesen, J. (eds.): Quantitative aspects of risk assessment in chemical carcinogenesis. *Arch. Toxicol.* (Suppl. 3), 1980.

Cooper, C. S. and Grover, P. L. (eds.): *Chemical Carcinogenesis and Mutagenesis I*, Springer-Verlag, Berlin, Heidelberg, New York, 1990.

Cornfield, J.: Carcinogenic risk assessment. *Science*, **198**:693–99, 1977.

Cooke, M., and Dennis, A. J. (eds.).: *Polynuclear Aromatic Hydrocarbons: A Decade of Progress*. Battelle, Columbus, Ohio, 1988.

Costa, M.: Perspectives on the mechanism of nickel carcinogenesis gained from models of *in vitro* carcinogenesis. *Environ. Health Perspect.*, **81**:73–76, 1989.

DeAngelo, A. B.; Daniel, F. B.; McMillan, L.; Wernsing, P.; and Savage R. E., Jr.: Species and strain sensitivity to the induction of peroxisome proliferation by chloroacetic acids. *Toxicol. Appl. Pharmacol.*, **101**:285–298, 1989.

De Flora, S. (ed.): Role and mechanisms of inhibitors in prevention of mutation and cancer. *Mutat. Res.*, **202**:227–446, 1988.

De Flora, S.; Hietanen, E.; Bartsch, H.; Camoirano, A.; Izzotti, A.; Bagnasco, M.; and Millman, I.: Enhanced metabolic activation of chemical hepatocarcinogens in woodchucks infected with hepatitis B virus. *Carcinogenesis*, **10**:1099–1106, 1989.

Dekant, W.; Vamvakas, S.; and Anders, M. W.: Bioactivation of nephrotoxic haloalkenes by glutathione conjugation: formation of toxic and mutagenic intermediates by cysteine conjugate beta-lyase. *Drug Metabol. Rev.*, **20**:43–83, 1989.

Diwan, B. A.; Nims, R. W.; Ward, J. M.; Hu, H.; Lubet, R. A.; and Rice, J. M.: Tumor promoting activities of ethylphenylacetylurea and diethylacetylurea, the ring hydrolysis products of barbiturate tumor promoters phenobarbital and barbital, in rat liver and kidney initiated by *N*-nitrosodiethylamine. *Carcinogenesis*, **10**:189–194, 1989.

Doolittle, D. J.; Lee, D. A.; and Rahn, C. A.: The use of rat urine extracted on XAD-2 resin and assayed in a microsuspension-modified Ames test as an *in vivo* indicator of genotoxic exposure. *Mutat. Res.*, **206**:141–148, 1988.

Drew, R. T., Boorman, G. A.; Haseman, J. K.; McConnell, E. E.; Busey, W. M.; and Moore, J. A.: The effect of age and exposure duration on cancer induction by a known carcinogen in rats, mice, and hamsters. *Toxicol. Appl. Pharmacol.*, **68**:120–120, 1983.

Dubach, U. C.; Rosner, B.; and Pfister, E.: Epidemiologic study of abuse of analgesics containing phenacetin. *N. Engl. J. Med.*, **308**:357–362, 1983.

Ekman, L.; Hansson, E.; Havu, N.; Carlsson, E.; and Lundberg, C.: Toxicological studies on omeprazole. *Scand. J. Gastroenterol.*, **20**:53–79, 1985.

Environmental Protection Agency: Guidelines for carcinogen risk assessment. *Fed. Reg.* **51**:33992–34003, 1986.

Farber, E. (ed.): Experimental, epidemiological and clinical aspects of liver carcinogenesis. *Cancer Surv.*, **5**:695–819, 1986.

Farrar, D. B., and Crump, K. S.: Exact statistical tests for any carcinogenic effect in animal bioassays. *Fundam. Appl. Toxicol.*, **15**:710–721, 1990.

Fiala, E. S.; Conaway, C. C.; and Mathis, J. E.: Oxidative DNA and RNA damage in the livers of Sprague-Dawley rats treated with the hepatocarcinogen 2-nitropropane. *Cancer Res.*, **49**:5518–5522, 1989.

Franks, L. M.: Tumour progression and metastasis. *Cancer Surv.*, **7**:551–710, 1988.

Fujiki, H.; Suganuma, M.; and Sugimura, T.: Significance of new environmental tumor promoters. *Envir. Carcino. Revs.*, **C7(1)**:1–51, 1989.

Furihata, C.; Hatta, A.; and Matsushima, T.: Inductions of ornithine decarboxylase and replicative DNA synthesis but not DNA single strand scission or unscheduled DNA synthesis in the pyloric mucosa of rat stomach by catechol. *Jpn. J. Cancer Res.*, **80**:1052–1057, 1989a.

Furihata, C.; Sudo, K.; and Matsushima, T.: Calcium chloride inhibits stimulation of replicative DNA synthesis by sodium chloride in the pyloric mucosa of rat stomach. *Carcinogenesis*, **10**:2135–2137, 1989b.

Gaylor, D. W.; Kadlubar, F. F.; and West, R. W.: Estimates of the risk of bladder tumor promotion by saccharin in rats. *Regul. Toxicol. Pharmacol.*, **8**:467–470, 1988.

George, E.; Burlinson, B.; and Gatehouse, D.: Genotoxicity of 1- and 2-nitropropane in the rat. *Carcinogenesis*, **10**:2329–2334, 1989.

Gerin, M.; Siemiatycki, J.; Nadon, L.; Dewar, R.; and Krewski, D.: Cancer risks due to occupational exposure to formaldehyde: results of a multi-site case-control study in Montreal. *Int. J. Cancer*, **44**:53–58, 1989.

Gibson, G. G. (ed.): Peroxisome proliferation: mechanisms and biological consequences. *Biochem. Soc. Trans.*, **18**:85–99, 1990.

Gladek, A., and Liehr, J. G.: Mechanism of genotoxicity of diethylstilbestrol *in vivo*. *J. Biol. Chem.*, **264**:16847–16852, 1989.

Gold, L. S.; Slone, T. H.; and Bernstein, L.: Summary of carcinogenic potency and positivity for 492 rodent carcinogens in the carcinogenic potency database. *Environ. Health Perspect.*, **79**:259–272, 1989.

Goldenberg, D. M.: Second conference on radioimmunodetection and radioimmunotherapy of cancer. *Cancer Res.*, **50**(Suppl. 3), 778s–1058s, 1990.

Goldstein, B. D. (ed.): Benzene metabolism, toxicity and carcinogenesis. *Environ. Health Perspect.*, **82**:3–307, 1988.

Goldsworthy, T. L.; Lyght, O.; Burnett, V. L.; and Popp, J. A.: Potential role of α-2-μ globulin, protein droplet accumulation, and cell replication in the renal carcinogenicity of rats exposed to trichloroethylene, perchloroethylene, and pentachloroethane. *Toxicol. Appl. Pharmacol.*, **96**:367–379, 1988.

Gorelick, N. J.; Hutchins, D. A.; Tannenbaum, S. R.; and Wogan, G. N.: Formation of DNA and hemoglobin adducts of fluoranthene after single and multiple exposures. *Carcinogenesis*, **10**:1579–1587, 1989.

Greenwald, P.; Sondik, E.; and Lynch, B. S.: Diet and chemoprevention in NCI's research strategy to achieve national cancer control objectives. *Annu. Rev. Public Health*, 7:267–291, 1986.

Guengerich, F. P.: Roles of cytochrome P-450 enzymes in chemical carcinogenesis and cancer chemotherapy. *Cancer Res.*, **48**:2946–2954, 1988.

Halperin, W. E.; Goodman, M.; Stayner, L.; Elliott, L. J.; Keenlyside; and Landrigan, P. J.: Nasal cancer in a worker exposed to formaldehyde. *J.A.M.A.* **249**: 510–512, 1983.

Haluska, F. G.; Tsujimoto, Y.; and Croce, C. M.: Oncogene activation by chromosome translocation in human malignancy. *Annu. Rev. Genet.*, **21**:321–345, 1987.

Hanawalt, P. C.: Concepts and models for DNA repair; from *Escherichia coli* to mammalian cells. *Environ. Mol. Mutagen.*, **14**:90–99, 1989.

Hasegawa, R.; Mutai, M.; Imaida, K.; Tsuda, H.; Yamaguchi, S.; and Ito, N.: Synergistic effects of low-dose hepatocarcinogens in induction of glutathione S-transferase p-positive foci in the rat liver. *Jpn. J. Cancer Res.*, **80**:945–951, 1989.

Hayes, A. W. (ed.): *Principles and Methods of Toxicology*, 2nd ed. Raven Press, New York, 1989.

Hecht, S. S., and Hoffmann, D.: Tobacco-specific nitrosamines, an important group of carcinogens in tobacco and tobacco smoke. *Carcinogenesis*, **9**:875–884, 1988.

Henderson, B. E.; Ross, R.; and Bernstein, L.: Estrogens as a cause of human cancer. *Cancer Res.*, **48**:246–253, 1988.

Hernandez, L.; Patton, T. A.; Poirier, L. A.; and Lijinsky, W.: S-Adenosylmethionine, S-adenosylhomocysteine and DNA methylation levels in the liver of rats fed methapyrilene and analogs. *Carcinogenesis*, **10**:557–562, 1989.

Higginson, J.: Changing concepts in cancer prevention: limitations and implications for future research in environmental carcinogenesis. *Cancer Res.*, **48**:1381–1389, 1988.

Highland, B.; Norvell, M. J.; and Shellenberger, T.

E.: Pathological changes in female C3H mice continuously fed diets containing diethylstibestrol or 17β-estradiol. *J. Environ. Pathol. Toxicol.*, **1**:1–30, 1977.

Hirono, I. (ed.): *Naturally Occurring Carcinogens of Plant Origin*. Kodansha, Tokyo; Elsevier, Amsterdam, Oxford, New York, Tokyo, 1987.

Hirth, R. S.; Evans, L. D.; Buroker, R. A.; and Oleson, F. B.: Gastric enterochromaffin-like cell hyperplasia and neoplasia in the rat: an indirect effect of the histamine H_2-receptor antagonist, BL-6341. *Toxicol. Pathol.*, **16**:273–287, 1988.

Hoel, D. G.; Haseman, J. K.; Hogan, M. D.; Huff, J.; and McConnell, E. E.: The impact of toxicity on carcinogenicity studies: implications for risk assessment. *Carcinogenesis*, **9**:2045–2052, 1988.

Howard, P. C.; Hecht, S. S.; and Beland, F. A. (eds.): *The Occurrence, Metabolism and Biological Impact of Nitrated Polycyclic Aromatic Hydrocarbons*. Plenum Press, New York, 1990.

Inai, K.; Kobuke, T.; Nambu, S.; Takemoto, T.; Kou, E.; Nishina, H.; Fujihara, M.; Yonehara, S.; Suehiro, S.; Tsuya, T.; Horiuchi, K.; and Tokuoka, S.: Hepatocellular tumorigenicity of butylated hydroxytoluene administered orally to $B6C3F_1$ mice. *Jpn. J. Cancer Res.*, **79**:49–58, 1988.

Ip, C., and Ganther, H. E.: Activity of methylated forms of selenium in cancer prevention. *Cancer Res.*, **50**:1206–1211, 1990.

Ito, N., and Hirose, M.: Antioxidants—carcinogenic and chemopreventive properties. *Adv. Cancer Res.*, **53**:247–302, 1989.

Iwagawa, M.; Toshiharu, M.; Keisuke, I.; Otsuka, H.; Nishifuji, K.; Ohnishi, Y.; and Aoki, S.: Comparative dose-response study on the pulmonary carcinogenicity of 1,6-dinitropyrene and benzo[a]pyrene in F344 rats. *Carcinogenesis*, **10**:1285–1290, 1989.

Johnson, E. S.: Association between soft tissue sarcomas, malignant lymphomas, and phenoxy herbicides\ chlorophenols: evidence from occupational cohort studies. *Fundam. Appl. Toxicol.*, **14**:219–234, 1990.

Jones, P. A., and Buckley, J. D.: The role of DNA methylation in cancer. *Adv. Cancer Res.*, **54**:1–23, 1990.

Kahl, R.: Synthetic antioxidants: biochemical actions and interference with radiation, toxic compounds, chemical mutagens, and chemical carcinogens. *Toxicology*, **33**:185–228, 1984.

Kalf, G. F.; Post, G. B.; and Synder, R.: Solvent toxicology: recent advances in the toxicology of benzene, the glycol ethers, and carbon tetrachloride. *Annu. Rev. Pharmacol. Toxicol.*, **27**:399–427, 1987.

Killion, J. J., and Fidler, I. J.: The biology of tumor metastasis. *Semin. Oncol.*, **16**:106–115, 1989.

Kim, D., and Guengerich, F. P.: Excretion of the mercapturic acid S-[2-(N^7-Guanyl)ethyl]-N-acetylcysteine in urine following administration of ethylene dibromide to rats. *Cancer Res.*, **49**:5843–5847, 1989.

Kimbrough, R. D.: How toxic is 2,3,7,8,-tetrachlorodibenzodioxin to humans? *J. Toxicol. Environ. Health*, **30**(4):261–271, 1990.

King, C. M.; Romano, L. J.; and Schuetzle, D. (eds.): *Carcinogenic and Mutagenic Responses to Aromatic Amines and Nitroarenes*. Elsevier, New York, Amsterdam, and London, 1988.

Klaunig, J. W.; Ruch, R. J.; and Lin E. L. C.: Effects of trichloroethylene and its metabolites on rodent hepatocyte intercellular communication. *Toxicol. Appl. Pharmacol.*, **99**:454–465, 1989.

Klein, G.: Tumorigenic DNA viruses. *Adv. Viral Oncol.*, Vol. 8. Raven Press, New York, 1989.

Knecht, K. T., and Mason, R. P.: In vivo radical trapping and biliary secretion of radical adducts of carbon tetrachloride-derived free radical metabolites. *Drug Metabol. Dispos.*, **16**:813–817, 1988.

Kurokawa, Y.; Hayshi, Y., Maekawa, A.; Takahashi, M.; Kukubo, T.; and Odashima, S.: Carcinogenicity of potassium bromate administered orally to F344 rats. *J. Natl. Cancer Inst.*, **71**:965–972, 1983.

Lai, C.-C.; Miller, J. A.; Miller, E. C.; and Liem, A.: *N*-Sulfooxy-2-aminofluorene is the major ultimate electrophilic and carcinogenic metabolite of *N*-hydroxy-2-acetylaminofluorene in the livers of infant male C57BL/6J × C3H/HeJF$_1$ (B6C3F$_1$) mice. *Carcinogenesis*, **6**:1037–1045, 1985.

Larsson, R., and Cerutti, P.: Translocation and enhancement of phosphotransferase activity of protein kinase C following exposure in mouse epidermal cells to oxidants. *Cancer Res.*, **49**:5627–5632, 1989.

Laska, E. M., and Meisner, M. J.: Statistical methods and the application of bioassay. *Annu. Rev. Pharmacol. Toxicol.*, **27**:385–397, 1988.

Lee, K. P., and Trochimowicz, H. J.: Induction of nasal tumors in rats exposed to hexamethylphosphoramide by inhalation. *J. Natl. Cancer Inst.*, **68**:157–171, 1982.

Lee, M.; Ishizaki, H.; Brady, J. F.; and Yang, C. S.: Substrate specificity and alkyl group selectivity in the metabolism of *N*-nitrosodialkylamines. *Cancer Res.*, **49**:1470–1474, 1989.

Leonard, A., and Lauwerys, R. R.: Carcinogenicity, teratogenicity and mutagenicity of arsenic. *Mutat. Res.*, **75**:49–62, 1980.

Leopold, W. R.; Miller, J. A.; and Miller, E. C.: Comparison of some carcinogenic, mutagenic, and biochemical properties of *S*-vinylhomocysteine and ethionine. *Cancer Res.*, **42**:4364–4374, 1982.

Levine, A. J.: Oncogenes of DNA tumor viruses. *Cancer Res.*, **48**:493–496, 1988.

Liehr, J. G.; Roy, D.; and Gladek, A.: Mechanisms of inhibition of estrogen-induced renal carcinogenesis in male Syrian hamsters by vitamin C. *Carcinogenesis*, **10**:1983–88, 1989.

Lijinsky, W., and Yamashita, K.: Lack of binding of methapyrilene and similar antihistamines to rat liver DNA examined by ^{32}P-postlabeling. *Cancer Res.*, **48**:6475–6477, 1988.

Lilienfeld, D. E., and Gallo, M. A.: 2,4-D, 2,4,5-T, and 2,3,7,8-TCDD: an overview. *Epidemiol. Rev.*, **11**:28–58, 1989.

Lipkin, M.: Biomarkers of increased susceptibility to gastrointestinal cancer: new applications to studies of cancer prevention in human subjects. *Cancer. Res.*, **48**:235–245, 1988.

Lock, E. A.; Mitchell, A. M.; and Elcombe, C. R.: Biochemical mechanisms of induction of hepatic peroxisome proliferation. *Annu. Rev. Pharmacol. Toxicol.*, **29**:145–163, 1989.

Loeb, L. A.: Endogenous carcinogenesis: molecular oncology into the twenty-first century—Presidential Address. *Cancer Res.*, **49**:5489–96, 1989.

Lubin, J. H.; Qiao, Y.-L.; Taylor, P. R.; Yao, S.-X.; Schatzkin, A.; Mao, B.-L.; Rao, J.-Y.; Xuan, X.-Z.; and Li, J.-Y.: Quantitative evaluation of the radon and lung cancer association in a case control study of Chinese tin miners. *Cancer Res.*, **50**:174–180, 1990.

Machlin, L. J., and Bendich, A.: Free radical tissue damage: protective role of antioxidant nutrients. *FASEB J.*, **1**:441–45, 1987.

Maclure, M.; Bryant, M. S.; Skipper, P. L.; and Tannenbaum, S. R.: Decline of the hemoglobin adduct of 4-aminobiphenyl during withdrawal from smoking. *Cancer Res.*, **50**:181–184, 1990.

Maltoni, C., and Selikoff, I. J. (eds.): Living in a chemical world: occupational and environmental significance of industrial carcinogens. *Ann. NY Acad. Sci.*, **534**:1–1045, 1988.

McCormick, J. J., and Maher, V. M.: Maligant transformation of mammalian cells in culture, including human cells. *Environ. Mol. Mutagen.*, **14**:90–99, 1989.

McGinnis, J. M.: National priorities in disease prevention. *Issues Sci. Technol.*, **5**:46–92, Winter 1988–1989.

Mehlman, M. A. (ed.): *Benzene: Occupational and Environmental Hazards Scientific Update,* Princeton Scientific Publishing Co., Princeton, NJ, 1989.

Melikian, A. A.; Bagheri, K.; Goldin, B. F.; and Hoffmann, D.: Catechol-induced alterations in metabolic activation and binding of enantiomeric and racemic 7,8-dihydroxy-7,8-dihydrobenzo[*a*] pyrenes to DNA in mouse skin. *Carcinogenesis*, **10**:1863–1863, 1989.

Metzler, M.: DNA adducts of medicinal drugs: some selected examples. *J. Cancer Res. Clin. Oncol.*, **112**:210–215, 1986.

Miller, E. C., and Miller, J. A.: Mechanisms of chemical carcinogenesis. *Cancer*, **47**:1055–1064, 1981.

Miller, E. C., and Miller, J. A.: Carcinogens and mutagens that may occur in foods. *Cancer*, **58**:1795–1803, 1986.

Milman, H. A., and Elmore, E. (eds.): *Biochemical Mechanisms and Regulation of Intercellular Communication,* Princeton Scientific Publishing Co., Inc., Princeton, NJ, 1987.

Milman, H. A., and Weisburger, E. K. (eds.): *Handbook of Carcinogen Testing,* Noyes Publications, Park Ridge, NJ, 1985.

Mirsalis, J. C.; Tyson, C. K.; Loh, E. N.; Steinmetz, K. L.; Bakke, J. P.; Hamilton, C. M.; Spak, D. K.; and Spalding, J. W.: Induction of hepatic cell proliferation and unscheduled DNA synthesis in mouse hepatocytes following in vivo treatment. *Carcinogenesis*, **6**:1521–1524, 1985.

Mirvish, S. S.: Effects of vitamins C and E on *N*-nitroso compound formation, carcinogenesis, and cancer. *Cancer*, **58**:1842–1850, 1986.

Mitsumori, K.; Hirano, M.; Ueda, H.; Maita, K.; and Shirasu, Y.: Chronic toxicity and carcinogenicity of methylmercury chloride in B6C3F1 mice. *Fundam. Appl. Toxicol.*, **14**:179–190, 1990.

Moore, D. J.; Batts, K. P.; Zalkow, L. L.; Fortune, G. T., Jr.; and Powis, G.: Model systems for detecting the hepatic toxicity of pyrrolizidine alkaloids and pyrrolizidine alkaloid *N*-oxides. *Toxicol. Appl. Pharmacol.*, **101**:271–284, 1989.

Moriya, M.; Ohta, T.; Watanabe, K.; Miyazawa, T.; Kato, K.; and Shirasu, Y.: Further mutagenicity studies on pesticides in bacterial reversion assay systems. *Mutat. Res.*, **116**:185–216, 1983.

Mossman, B. T.; Bignon, J.; Corn, M.; Seaton, A.; and Gee, J. B. L.: Asbestos: scientific developments and implications for public policy. *Science*, **247**:294–301, 1990.

Murphy, E. D., and Beamer, W. G. (eds.): *Biology of Ovarian Neoplasia.* UICC Technical Report Series, International Union Against Cancer, Geneva, 1980.

Murrell, G. A. C.; Francis, M. J. O.; and Bromley, L.: Modulation of fibroblast proliferation by oxygen free radicals. *Biochem J.*, **265**:659–65, 1990.

Neal, R. A., and Halpert, J.: Toxicology of thionosulfur compounds. *Annu. Rev. Pharmacol. Toxicol.*, **22**:321–339, 1982.

Nemali, M. R.; Reddy M. K.; Usuda, N.; Reddy, P. G.; Comeau, L. D.; Rao, M. S.; and Reddy, J. K.: Differential induction and regulation of peroxisomal enzymes: predictive value of peroxisome proliferation in identifying certain nonmutagenic carcinogens. *Toxicol. Appl. Pharmacol.*, **97**:72–87, 1989.

Nera, E. A.; Iversen, F.; Lok, E.; Armstrong, C. L.; Karpinski, K.; and Clayson, D. B.: A carcinogenicity reversal study of butylated hydroxyanisole in the forestomach and urinary bladder of male Fischer F344 rats. *Toxicology*, **53**:251–268, 1988.

Office of Technology Assessment, Congress of the United States: *Identifying and Regulating Carcinogens*. Marcel Dekker, New York and Basel, 1989.

Park, D. L., and Stoloff, L.: Aflatoxin control-how a regulatory agency managed risk from an unavoidable natural toxicant in food and feed. *Regul. Toxicol. Pharmacol.*, **9**:109–130, 1989.

Park, J.; Cundy, K. C.; and Ames, B.: Detection of DNA adducts by high-performance liquid chromatography with electrochemical detection. *Carcinogenesis*, **10**:827–827, 1989.

Parke, D. V. (ed.): Development of mixed-function oxidases. *Biochem. Soc. Trans.*, **18**:7–36, 1990.

Pegg, A. E.: Polyamine metabolism and its importance in neoplastic growth and as a target for chemotherapy. *Cancer Res.*, **48**:759–774, 1988.

Penn, I.: Tumors of the immunocompromised patient. *Annu. Rev. Med.*, **39**:63–73, 1988.

Pitot, H. C.; Goodspeed, D.; Dunn, T.; Hendrich, S.; Maronpot, R. R.; and Moran, S.: Regulation of the expression of some genes for enzymes of glutathione metabolism in hepatoxicity and hepatocarcinogenesis. *Toxicol. Appl. Pharmacol.*, **97**:23–34, 1989.

Plaa, G. L.: Experimental evaluation of haloalkanes and liver injury. *Fundam. Appl. Toxicol.*, **10**:563–570, 1988.

Poli, G.; Cheeseman, K. H.; Biasi, F.; Chiarpotto, E.; Dianzani, M. U.; Esterbauer, H.; and Slater, T. F.: Promethazine inhibits the formation of aldehydic products of lipid peroxidation but not covalent binding resulting from the exposure of rat liver fractions to CCl_4. *Biochem J.*, **264**:527–532, 1989.

Prentice, R. L., and Thomas, D. B.: On the epidemiology of oral contraceptives and disease. *Adv. Cancer. Res.*, **49**:285–401, 1987.

Purchase, I. F. H., and Paddle, G. M.: Does formaldehyde cause nasopharyngeal cancer in man? *Cancer Lett.*, **46**:79–85, 1989.

Quinto, I.; Tenebaum, L.; and Radman, M.: Genotoxic potency of monofunctional alkylating agents in *E. coli:* comparisons with carcinogenic potency in rodents. *Mutat. Res.*, **228**:177–185, 1990.

Randerath, K.; Randerath, E.; Danna, T. F.; van Golen, K. L.; and Putman, K. L.: A new sensitive ^{32}P-postlabeling assay based on the specific enzymatic conversion of bulky DNA lesions to radiolabeld dinucleotides and nucleoside 5'-monophosphates. *Carcinogenesis*, **10**:1231–1239, 1989.

Rauckman, E. J., and Padilla, G. M. (eds.): *The Isolated Hepatocyte: Use in Toxicology and Xenobiotic Biotransformations*, Academic Press, Orlando and San Diego, 1987.

Robinson, M. (ed.): The SENCAR mouse in toxicological testing: *Environ. Health Perspect.*, **68**:3–151, 1986.

Rogers, A. E., and Longnecker, M. S.: Dietary and nutritional influences on cancer: a review of epidemiologic and experimental data. *Lab Invest.*, **59**:729–759, 1988.

Roloff, M. V.; Wilson, A. G. E.; Ribelin, W. E.; Ridley, W. P.; and Ruecker, F. A.: *Human Risk Assessment—The Role of Animal Selection and Extrapolation*. Taylor and Francis, New York, 1987.

Ronai, Z. A., and Weinstein, I. B.: Identification of a UV-induced transacting protein that stimulates polyoma DNA replication. *J. Virol.*, **62**:1057–1060, 1988.

Ronai, Z. A.; Lambert, M. E.; and Weinstein, I.

B.: Inducible cellular responses to ultraviolet light irradiation and other mediators of DNA damage in mammalian cells. *Environ. Occup. Cancer*, **17**:000–000, 1990.

Rosenkranz, H. S. (ed.): Strategies for the deployment of batteries of short-term tests. *Mutat. Res.*, **205**:1–424, 1988.

Rosenkranz, H. S., and Klopman, G.: Structural basis of carcinogenicity in rodents of genotoxicants and nongenotoxicants. *Mutat. Res.*, **228**:105–24, 1990.

Rosenthal, S. L.: A review of the mutagenicity of chloroform. *Environ. Mol. Mutagen.* **10**:211–226, 1987.

Rossman, T. G.; Meyn, M. S.; and Troll, W.: Effects of arsenite on DNA repair in *Escherichia coli*. *Environ. Health Perspect.*, **19**:229–233, 1977.

Sabbioni, G., and Neumann, H. G.: Biomonitoring of arylamines: hemoglobin adducts of urea and carbamate pesticides. *Carcinogenesis*, **11**:111–115, 1990.

Safe, S.: Polychlorinated biphenyls (PCBs): mutagenicity and carcinogenicity. *Mutat. Res.*, **220**:31–47, 1989.

Sakai, A., and Sato, M.: Improvement of carcinogen identification in BALB/3T3 cell transformation by application of a 2-stage method. *Mutat. Res.*, **214**:285–296, 1989.

Salsburg, D.: Does "everything" "cause" cancer: an alternative interpretation of the "carcinogenesis" bioassay. *Fundam. Appl. Toxicol.*, **13**:351–358, 1989.

Samet, J. M.: Radon and lung cancer. *J. Natl. Cancer. Inst.*, **10**:745–755, 1989.

Schmidt, R., and Hecker, E.: Biological assays for irritant, tumor-initiating and tumor-promoting activities. *J. Cancer Res. Clin. Oncol.*, **115**:516–524, 1989.

Seitz, H. K., and Simanowski, U. A.: Alcohol and carcinogenesis. *Annu. Rev. Nutr.*, **8**:99–119, 1988.

Shahin, M. M. (ed.): Structure-activity relationships in chemical mutagenesis. *Mutat. Res.*, **221**:163–286, 1989.

Shibata, M. A.; Tamano, S.; Kurata, Y.; Hagiwara, A.; and Fukushima, S.: Participation of urinary NA^+, K^+, pH, and 1-ascorbic acid in the proliferative response of the bladder epithelium after the oral administration of various salts and/or ascorbic acid to rats. *Food Chem. Toxicol.*, **27**:403–13, 1989.

Shigenaga, M. K.; Gimeno, C. J.; and Ames, B. N.: Urinary 8-hydroxy-2'-deoxyguanosine as a biological marker of in vivo oxidative DNA damage. *Proc. Natl. Acad. Sci. USA*, **86**:9697–9701, 1989.

Shimkin, M. B., and Stoner, G. D.: Lung tumors in mice: application to carcinogenesis bioassay. *Adv. Cancer Res.*, **21**:2–58, 1975.

Shinozuka, H.; Lombardi, B.; and Abanobi, S. E.: A comparative study of the efficacy of four barbiturates as promoters of the development of γ-glutamyltranspeptidase-positive foci in the liver of carcinogen treated rats. *Carcinogenesis*, **3**:1017–1020, 1982.

Short, B. G.; Burnett, V. L.; Cox, M. G.; Bus, J. S.; and Swenberg, J. A.: Site-specific renal cytotoxicity and cell proliferation in male rats exposed to petroleum hydrocarbons. *Lab. Invest.*, **57**:564–77, 1987.

Skipper, P. L., and Groopman, J. D.: *Molecular Dosimetry and Human Cancer*. The Telford Press, Caldwell, NJ, 1990.

Sobel, F. H. (ed.): Chemical, mutagenic and tumor-pattern characteristics of human and rodent carcinogens. *Mutat. Res.*, **204**:1–115, 1988.

Sohn, O. S.; Fiala, E. S.; Puz, C.; Hamilton, S. R.; and Williams, G. M.: Enhancement of rat liver microsmal metabolism of azoxymethane to methylazoxymethanol by chronic ethanol administration: similarity to the microsomal metabolism of *N*-nitrosodimethylamine. *Cancer. Res.*, **47**:3123–29, 1987.

Sontag, J. M. (ed.): *Carcinogens in Industry and the Environment*. Marcel Dekker, New York, 1981.

Sporn, M. B., and Roberts, A. B.: Role of retinoids in differentiation and carcinogenesis. *Cancer Res.* **43**:3034–40, 1983.

Staffa, J. A., and Mehlman, M. A.: Innovations in cancer risk assessment (Ed_{01} study). *J. Environ. Pathol. Toxicol.*, **3**:1–246, 1980.

Starr, T. B., and Gibson, J. E.: The mechanistic toxicology of formaldehyde and its implications for quantitative risk estimation. *Annu. Rev. Pharmacol. Toxicol.*, **25**:745–67, 1985.

Stein, B.; Rahmsdorf, H. J.; Steffen, A.; Liftin, M.; and Herrlich, P.: UV-induced DNA damage is an intermediate step in UV-induced expression of human immunodeficiency virus type 1, collagenase, c-*fos* and methallothionein. *Mol. Cell Biol.*, **9**:5169–5181, 1989.

Stevenson, D. E.; Popp, J. A.; Ward, J. M.; McClain, R. M.; Slaga, T. J.; and Pitot, H. C. (eds.): *Mouse Liver Carcinogenesis, Mechanisms and Species Comparisons*. Wiley-Liss, New York, 1990.

Stich, H. F.; Brunnemann, K. D.; Sankaranarayanan, R.; and Nair, M. K.: Chemopreventive trials with vitamin A and β-carotene: some unresolved issues. *Prev. Med.*, **18**:732–739, 1989.

Swenberg, J. A.; Short, B.; Borghoff, S.; Strasser, J.; and Charbonneau, M.: The comparative pathobiology of $\alpha_{2\mu}$-globulin nephropathy. *Toxicol. Appl. Pharmacol.*, **97**:35–46, 1989.

Takayama, S.; Hasegawa, H.; and Ohgaki, H.: Combination effects of forty carcinogens administered at low doses to male rats. *Jpn. J. Cancer Res.*, **80**:732–736, 1989.

Teramoto, S., and Shirasu, Y.: Genetic toxicology of 1,2-dibromo-3-chloropropane (DBCP). *Mutat. Res.*, **221**:1–9, 1989.

Tomatis, L.; Aitio, A.; Wilbourn, J.; and Shuker, L.: Human carcinogens so far identified. *Jpn J. Cancer Res.*, **80**:795–807, 1989.

Tornqvist, M.: Formation of reactive species that lead to hemoglobin adducts during storage of blood samples. *Carcinogenesis*, **11**:51–54, 1990.

Toth, B.: Actual new cancer-causing hydrazines, hydrazides, and hydrazones. *J. Cancer Res. Clin. Oncol.*, **97**:97–108, 1980.

Toth, B.: Toxicities of hydazines: a review. *In Vivo*, **2**:209–242, 1988.

T'so, P. O. P., and DiPaolo, J. A. (eds.): *Chemical Carcinogenesis*. Marcel Dekker, New York, 1974.

Troll, W.; Wiesner, R.; and Frenkel, K.: Anticarcinogenic action of protease inhibitors. *Adv. Cancer Res.*, **49**:265–283, 1987.

Trosko, J. E.; Chang, C.-C.; and Medcalf, A.: Mechanisms of tumor promotion: potential role of intercellular communication. *Cancer Invest.*, **1**:511–526, 1983.

Umemura, T.; Sai, K.; Takagi, A.; Hasegawa, R.; and Kurokawa, Y.: Formation of 8-hydroxydeoxyguanosine (8-OH-dG) in rat kidney DNA after intraperitoneal administration of ferric nitrilotriacetate (Fe-NTA). *Carcinogenesis*, **11**:345–347, 1990.

United States Department of Health and Human Services. *Reducing the health consequences of smoking: 25 years of progress: a report of the Surgeon General*. Public Health Service, DHHS Publication No. (CDC) 89-8411, Washington, D.C., 1989.

United States Department of Health and Human Services. *The Surgeon General's Report on Nutrition and Health*, Public Health Service, DHHS, Publication No. (PHS) 88-50210, Washington, D.C., 1988.

Varmus, H., and Brown, P.: Retroviruses. In Berg, D. E., and Howe, M. M. (eds.). *Mobile DNA*. American Society for Microbiology, Washington, D.C., 1989, pp. 54–108.

Walrath, J., and Fraumeni, J. F., Jr.: Mortality patterns among embalmers. *Int. J. Cancer*, **31**:407–411, 1983.

Ward, J. M.; Lynch, P.; and Riggs, C.: Rapid development of hepatocellular neoplasms in aging male C3H/HeNCr mice given phenobarbital. *Cancer Lett.*, **39**:9–18, 1988.

Ward, J. M.; Tsuda, H.; Tatematsu, M.; Hagiwara, A.; and Ito, N.: Hepatotoxicity of agents that enhance formation of focal hepatocellular proliferative lesions (putative preneoplastic foci) in a rapid rat liver bioassay. *Fundam. Appl. Toxicol.*, **12**:163–171, 1989.

Weill, H., and Hughes, J. M.: Asbestos as a public health risk: disease and policy. *Annu. Rev. Publ. Health*, **7**:171–192, 1986.

Weinberg, R. A.: Oncogenes, antioncogenes, and the molecular bases of multistep carcinogenesis. *Cancer Res.*, **49**:3713–3721, 1989.

Weinstein, I. B.: The origins of human cancer: molecular mechanisms of carcinogenesis and their implications for cancer prevention and treatment. *Cancer Res.*, **48**:4135–4143, 1988.

Weisburger, J. H.: Nutritional approach to cancer prevention with emphasis on vitamins, antioxidants and carotenoids. *Am. J. Clin. Nutr.*, **53**:226S–237S, 1991.

Weisburger, J. H. and Horn, C. L.: Causes of Cancer. In Holleb, A., and Fink, D. (eds.): *American Cancer Society Textbook on clinical Oncology*, 6th ed. American Cancer Society, Atlanta, GA, 1990, Chap. 7.

Weisburger, J. H., and Jones, R. C.: Prevention of formation of important mutagens/carcinogens in the human food chain. In Kuroda, Y.; Shankel, D. M.; and Waters, M. D. (eds.): *Antimutagenesis and Anticarcinogensis Mechanisms II*. Plenum Press, New York and London, 1990, pp. 105–118.

Westendorf, J.; Marquardt, H.; Poginsky, B.; Dominiak, M.; Schmidt, J.; and Marquardt, H.: Genotoxicity of naturally occurring hydroxyanthraquinones. *Mutat. Res.*, **240**:1–12, 1990.

WHO Collaborative Study of Neoplasias and Steroid Contraceptives: combined oral contraceptives and liver cancer. *Int. J. Cancer*, **43**:254–59, 1989.

Williams, G. M.: Modulation of chemical carcinogenesis by xenobiotics. *Fundam. Appl. Toxicol.*, **4**:325–344, 1984.

Williams, G. M. (ed.): *Sweeteners: Health Effects*, Princeton Scientific Publishing Co., Inc., Princeton, NJ, 1988.

Williams, G. M.: Methods for evaluating chemical genotoxicity. *Annu. Rev. Pharmacol. Toxicol.*, **29**:189–211, 1989.

Williams, G. M., and Weisburger, J. H.: Application of a cellular test battery in the decision point approach to carcinogen identification. *Mutat. Res.*, **205**:79–90, 1988.

Williams, G. M.; Mori, H.; and McQueen, C. A.: Structure-activity relationships in the rat hepatocyte DNA-repair test for 300 chemicals. *Mutat. Res.*, **221**:263–286, 1989.

Witschi, H. P., and Morse, C. C.: Enhancement of lung tumor formation in mice by dietary butylated hydroxytoluene: dose-time relationships and cell kinetics. *J. Natl. Cancer Inst.*, **71**:859–859, 1983.

Wogan, G. N.: Makers of exposure to carcinogens: methods for human biomonitoring. *J. Am. Col. Toxicol.*, **8**:871–881, 1989.

Wong, L. C. K.; Winston, J. M.; Hong, C. B.; and Plotnick, H.: Carcinogenicity and toxicity of 1,2-dibromoethane in the rat. *Toxicol. Appl. Pharmacol.*, **63**:155–165, 1982.

Wu, M.-M.; Kuo, T.-L.; Hwang, Y.-H; and Chen, C.-J.: Dose-response relation between arsenic concentration in well water and mortality from cancers and vascular diseases. *Am. J. Epidemiol.,* **130**:1123–1132, 1989.

Würgler, F. E. (ed.): Developments in genetic toxicology. *Mutat. Res.,* **213**:1–95, 1989.

Wyke, J., and Weiss, R. (eds): Viruses in human and animal cancers. *Cancer Surv.,* **3**:1–214, 1984.

Yager, J. W.; Eastmond, D. A.; Robertson, M. L.; Paradisin, W. M.; and Smith, M. T.: Characterization of micronuclei induced in human lymphocytes by benzene metabolites. *Adv. Cancer Res.,* **50**:393–399, 1990.

Yamazoe, Y.; Abu-Zeid, M.; Gong, D.; Staiano, N.; and Kato, R.: Enzymatic acetylation and sulfation of *N*-hydroxyarylamines in bacteria and rat livers. *Carcinogenesis* **10**:1675–1679, 1989.

Yeh, F.-S.; Yu, M. C.; Mo, C.-C.; Luo, S.; Tong, M. J.; and Henderson, B. E.: Hepatitis B virus, aflatoxins, and hepatocellular carcinoma in Southern Guangxi, China. *Cancer Res.,* **49**:2506–2509, 1989.

Yoshimi, N.; Sugie, S.; Iwata, H.; Mori, H.; and Williams, G. M.: Species and sex differences in genotoxicity of heterocyclic amine pryrolysis and cooking products in the hepatocyte primary culture/DNA repair test using rat, mouse, and hamster hepatocytes. *Environ. Mol. Mutagen.,* **12**:53–64, 1988.

Yuspa, S. H., and Poirier, M. C.: Chemical carcinogenesis: from animal models to molecular models in one decade. *Adv. Cancer Res.,* **50**:25–70, 1988.

Zbinden, G.: Biopharmaceutical studies, a key to better toxicology. *Xenobiotica,* **18**:9–14, 1988.

Chapter 6

GENETIC TOXICOLOGY

George R. Hoffmann

SCOPE OF GENETIC TOXICOLOGY

Genetic toxicology is concerned with effects of chemicals and radiation on DNA and on mechanisms of inheritance in cells and organisms. The focus is on the processes of mutagenesis. When defined broadly, mutagenesis includes the induction of DNA damage and all kinds of genetic alterations, ranging from changes in one or a few DNA base pairs (gene mutations) to gross changes in chromosome structure (chromosome aberrations) or in chromosome number. Any agent that causes mutation is a mutagen; the more specialized term clastogen is used for agents that cause chromosome aberrations.

Genetic toxicologists conduct research on mechanisms of mutagenesis, apply test systems for the detection and characterization of mutagens, and formulate means of assessing risks posed by mutagens. Mutagens are of concern because the induction of genetic damage may cause an increased incidence of genetic disease in future generations and contribute to somatic cell diseases, including cancer, in the present generation. Technical and political means of minimizing human mutagen exposures are therefore important issues in the application of genetic toxicology data.

This chapter introduces the historical development of genetic toxicology, the nature of genetic damage, implications of mutagenesis for human health, mechanisms of mutagenesis and DNA repair, tests used for mutagen testing, and the assessment of mutational hazards. For brevity, reviews and other syntheses of information are often cited instead of original research papers. Further information may be found in the literature cited in these reviews and in the three major specialty journals in the field: *Mutation Research, Environmental and Molecular Mutagenesis,* and *Mutagenesis.*

HISTORICAL DEVELOPMENT

The beginning of the modern era of mutation research is marked by Hermann J. Muller's dis-

covery in 1927 that X rays cause sex-linked recessive lethal mutations in the fruit fly *Drosophila melanogaster*. One year later, L. R. Stadler reported that X rays are mutagenic in plants. The mutagenicity of ultraviolet light (UV) was demonstrated shortly thereafter, and the search for chemical mutagens began. The first unequivocal evidence of chemical mutagenesis was obtained in Scotland in 1942 by Charlotte Auerbach and J. M. Robson, who found that mustard gas is mutagenic in *Drosophila*. The research of Auerbach and Robson was not reported until after World War II, when wartime censorship was lifted. Also during the war, Friedrich Oehlkers found in Germany that urethane causes chromosome aberrations. Shortly thereafter, I. A. Rapoport reported in the Soviet Union that ethylene oxide, ethylenimine, epichlorohydrin, diazomethane, diethyl sulfate, glycidol, and several other chemicals are mutagenic. By the end of the 1940s, chemical mutagenesis was a well established and growing area of interest in genetics.

The initial interest in mutagens concerned the process of mutation, the use of mutagens to obtain mutants for genetic studies, and the introduction of new genetic variations into organisms of agricultural and industrial importance. H. J. Muller had suggested in his 1927 article and during the 1930s that mutagenesis in somatic cells could cause cancer, but it was not until the late 1950s and early 1960s that the health hazard of mutagenesis was generally recognized. The primary focus was on germ-cell mutagenesis and genetic disease. The viewpoint that mutagenicity should be considered in the toxicologic evaluation of chemicals became widespread during this period.

A driving force in the newly evolving field of genetic toxicology in the 1960s was Alexander Hollaender, who led the founding of the Environmental Mutagen Society (EMS) in 1969. The EMS and related organizations now include hundreds of geneticists and toxicologists involved in research on mutation or in policy related to mutagenesis. The following decade gave rise to an extensive literature of basic mutation research and mutagenicity testing, and mutagenesis was gradually integrated into toxicology. The historical development of mutation research and genetic toxicology has been reviewed by Auerbach (1976) and by Wassom (1989).

KINDS OF GENETIC DAMAGE

Genetic toxicologists are principally concerned with three categories of genetic altera-tions: gene mutations, chromosome aberrations, and changes in chromosome number.

Gene Mutations

Gene mutations are changes in DNA sequence within a gene. Such mutations, restricted to a particular site in a chromosome, are also called point mutations. The two principal kinds of gene mutations are base-pair substitutions and frameshift mutations (Drake *et al.*, 1983; Hartl *et al.*, 1988). Gene mutations are illustrated in Figure 6–1.

In a base-pair substitution, one base pair in

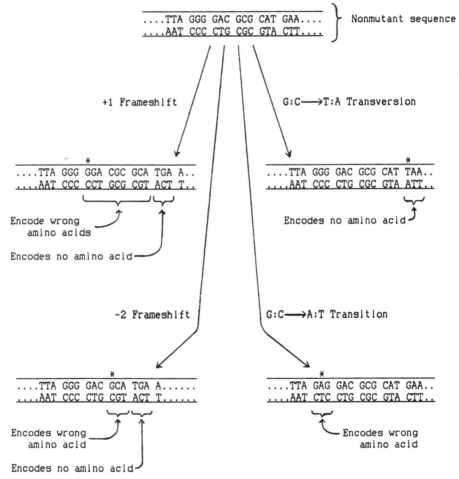

Figure 6–1. Frameshift mutations and base-pair substitutions. The figure shows the alteration of a DNA sequence by frameshift mutations and base-pair substitutions. The sites of the mutations are marked by asterisks, and the sequences are shown in units of three bases to indicate the reading frame of the mRNA codons that are specified by the DNA. The examples of frameshift mutations (on the left) are cases in which one base pair (G:C) has been added (the +1 frameshift) or two base pairs (G:C and C:G) have been deleted (the −2 frameshift). The examples of base-pair substitutions (on the right) are a transversion (G:C→T:A) and a transition (G:C→A:T). One of the base-pair substitutions (the transition) is a missense mutation, whereas the other is a nonsense mutation. In frameshift mutations, the reading frame of the genetic code is altered for all three-letter code words after the point of the mutation.

DNA (e.g., G:C) is replaced by another (e.g., A:T). Base-pair substitutions are called transitions if the purine:pyrimidine orientation of the base pair remains the same. This is the same as saying that one purine (e.g., G) is replaced by another purine (e.g., A) in a transition. In contrast, a base-pair substitution in which a purine is replaced by a pyrimidine (and vice versa) is called a transversion. Because of the specific pairing of adenine with thymine and guanine with cytosine, there are several possible transitions (G:C → A:T and A:T → G:C) and transversions (G:C → T:A, G:C → C:G, A:T → C:G, and A:T → T:A).

The consequences of a base-pair substitution depend on whether the mutation is a missense mutation or a nonsense mutation. In a missense mutation, there is a change from the code for one amino acid to that for another amino acid. The mutation can inactivate the gene product, have only a slight effect on function (i.e., a "leaky" mutation), or be virtually without effect, depending on the specific amino acid substitution and its specific position within the gene product. In a nonsense mutation, the gene product is incomplete and nonfunctional because of premature termination of protein synthesis. Another mechanism by which a mutation can prevent the formation of a functional gene product is prevention of transcription or normal splicing of RNA.

Mutations that alter the reading frame of the genetic code are called frameshift mutations. Most commonly, frameshift mutations involve the gain or loss of one or two base pairs in a gene. In a frameshift mutation, the gene product is grossly altered because of the change in reading frame. The gene product is also apt to be incomplete because the new reading frame is likely to include a nonsense codon (UAA, UAG, or UGA), which specifies no amino acid at all, somewhere in the altered message. Frameshift mutations therefore lead to nonfunctional gene products. The phenotypic effect of a frameshift mutation depends on how the lack of that specific gene function affects the viability and metabolism of the cell or organism.

Chromosome Aberrations

Chromosome aberrations are changes in chromosome structure. They involve gross alteration of the genetic material and are detected by light microscopy in appropriately prepared cells. Cytologically detected damage includes chromosome breakage and various chromosomal rearrangements that can result from broken chromosomes.

Aberrations may involve entire chromosomes (i.e., chromosome-type aberrations) or just one of the two chromatids of a replicated chromosome (i.e., chromatid-type aberrations). Ionizing radiation induces chromosome-type aberrations when cells are treated in the G_1 phase of the cell cycle (i.e., before DNA synthesis) and chromatid-type aberrations in G_2 (i.e., after DNA synthesis); in the S period (i.e., DNA replication period) both types are induced but chromatid aberrations predominate (Preston *et al.*, 1981; Carrano and Natarajan, 1988). Unlike radiation, most chemical clastogens induce primarily chromatid aberrations regardless of the cell-cycle stage during treatment. The preferential induction of chromatid aberrations apparently results from a requirement that chemically induced DNA lesions pass through DNA synthesis (i.e., the S period) to give rise to aberrations.

Some aberrations are stable, in that they can be transmitted through repeated cell divisions and therefore persist in the cell population. Major classes of chromosomal rearrangements that can be transmitted in populations of cells or organisms are deletions, duplications, inversions, and balanced translocations. Many of these rearrangements can be detected with staining techniques that reveal banding patterns on the chromosomes but cannot be detected with routine cytogenetic analysis of unbanded chromosomes. Banding techniques, however, are time-consuming and are more easily applied to a population of cells that all contain an identical aberration than to newly induced aberrations that are unique to the cells in which they occur (Preston, 1989). Cytogenetic analysis for chromosome damage therefore takes advantage of those aberrations that are readily detected on the basis of gross structural change.

Besides stable aberrations, chromosome breaks give rise to acentric fragments (i.e., broken pieces with no centromere), dicentric chromosomes, ring chromosomes, and various other asymmetrical rearrangements that are unstable, in that they usually bring about the death of the cell through loss of vital genetic material (Carrano and Natarajan, 1988). Although many of the aberrations routinely scored in cytogenetic analysis are unstable, they provide direct evidence of chromosome breakage and are representative of aberrations as a whole. Easily scored aberrations include chromatid breaks, chromatid exchanges, acentric fragments, dicentric chromosomes, ring chromosomes, and some reciprocal translocations (Bender *et al.*, 1988; Carrano and Natarajan, 1988).

Aneuploidy and Polyploidy

Aneuploid and polyploid cells have chromosome numbers that differ from the normal number for the species. In aneuploidy, the deviation in chromosome number involves one or a few chromosomes, whereas in polyploidy, the alteration involves complete sets of chromosomes. For example, in humans, where the normal diploid ($2n$) chromosome number is 46, cells with 45 or 47 chromosomes would be described as aneuploid, whereas cells with 69 chromosomes would be described as polyploid, in this case triploid ($3n$). Aneuploids with an extra chromosome are said to be trisomic, whereas those with a missing chromosome are called monosomic (Dellarco *et al.*, 1985). Aneuploidy and polyploidy are sometimes referred to as numerical chromosome aberrations, as opposed to the structural chromosome aberrations discussed earlier.

HEALTH IMPACT OF MUTATIONS

There are two main reasons for concern about human exposures to mutagens. First, an increase in the mutation rate in human germ cells (eggs, sperms, and their precursors) may cause an increased incidence of genetic disease in future generations. Second, mutations in somatic cells may contribute to various disorders, most notably cancer.

Mutations in Germ Cells

Gene mutations, chromosome aberrations, and aneuploidy all contribute to human genetic disease. The importance of gene mutations is evident from the many disorders that are inherited as simple Mendelian traits (McKusick, 1988). Gene mutations undoubtedly also contribute to human disease through the genetic component of diseases of complex etiology. It has been estimated that about 2 to 4 percent of newborns have serious abnormalities (National Academy of Sciences, 1983) and that about 10 percent of people are seriously affected by congenital abnormalities or constitutional and degenerative diseases, many of which have late onset (National Academy of Sciences, 1980). This total includes the roughly 1 percent of people who have defined autosomal dominant or X-linked diseases and the 0.1 percent with defined autosomal recessive diseases; the remainder have genetic disorders of complex etiology, including polygenic (multifactorial) inheritance. Such frequencies are necessarily approximate because of differences among surveys in the reporting and classification of disorders. A higher prevalence would be found if less severe disorders were included in the tabulation. Nevertheless, such estimates provide a sense of the heavy burden of genetic disease.

Chromosome banding and refined cytogenetic methods have led to the discovery of minor variations in chromosome structure that have no apparent effect. Nevertheless, other chromosome aberrations cause fetal deaths or serious abnormalities. Aneuploidy also contributes to fetal deaths and causes such disorders as Down syndrome, ascribable to trisomy for chromosome 21. Similarly, Turner syndrome is a monosomic condition in which there is a single X chromosome rather than the normal XX or XY, and Klinefelter syndrome is caused by the presence of two or more X chromosomes in males (e.g., XXY).

About 0.3 to 0.4 percent of infants have syndromes associated with chromosomal abnormalities (National Academy of Sciences, 1983). It has been estimated that cytogenetic abnormalities affect about 5 percent of all recognized pregnancies (Hook, 1983), causing many embryonic and perinatal deaths. About 6 percent of stillbirths and infant deaths and 30 percent of all spontaneous embryonic and fetal deaths involve chromosome abnormalities (Hook, 1983). Among the abnormalities detected, aneuploidy is most common, followed by polyploidy; structural aberrations comprise about 5 percent of the total (Hook, 1983).

Estimating human mutagen exposures and the increase in genetic disease that would result from a particular exposure is extremely complex and requires numerous assumptions. Therefore, estimates of genetic risk are imprecise (National Academy of Sciences, 1980, 1983), and the extent to which mutagens contribute to human genetic disease is unknown. Gene mutations, transmissible chromosome aberrations, and aneuploidy can all be induced in experimental organisms, but evidence for their induction in human germ cells is lacking.

Even though many genetic disorders are caused by the expression of recessive mutations (e.g., cystic fibrosis, phenylketonuria, Tay-Sachs disease), these mutations are mainly inherited from previous generations rather than being new mutations. New mutations undoubtedly make a larger contribution to the incidence of dominant genetic diseases, because dominant mutations with complete penetrance are expressed in the first generation after they occur. If the dominant disorder is severe, its transmission between generations is unlikely because of reduced fitness. For dominants with mild effect, reduced penetrance, or late age at onset, however, the contribution from previous generations is apt to be greater than that from new mutations.

The induction of dominant mutations is a greater concern for human welfare in the near future than is the induction of recessive mutations, because the latter would tend not to be expressed for many generations (National Academy of Sciences, 1983). Recessive mutations on the X chromosome, however, are like dominants in that they are subject to early expression in males. Another concern about recessives is that many of them may not be recessive in the strictest sense; rather, they may be expressed to a slight degree in heterozygotes (Simmons and Crow, 1977). For example, heterozygotes for the recessive disease ataxia telangiectasia do not have the high cancer incidence associated with the disease (about 10 percent in children and young adults), but they have a cancer incidence higher than that of the general population (Friedberg, 1985). Therefore, recessive mutations should not be dismissed as irrelevant for genetic risk, even though practical considerations call for emphasis on dominant and X-linked mutations when trying to quantify the impact of germ-cell mutagenesis on human health.

Mutations in Somatic Cells

An association between mutation and cancer causation has long been recognized (Straus, 1981). Many carcinogenic chemicals are mutagenic, and many mutagens are carcinogenic. Moreover, the sensitivity of particular animal strains or organs to carcinogenesis can sometimes be related to their capacity to metabolize carcinogens to their active forms or to repair the damage induced in DNA. Tumors typically arise as clones from individual transformed cells, and many cancers are closely associated with consistent chromosomal alterations. In addition, human chromosome instability syndromes and DNA repair deficiencies are associated with increased cancer risk (Straus, 1981; Friedberg, 1985).

Recent studies on oncogenes provide more direct support for the linkage between mutations and cancer (Bishop, 1987). Oncogenes are genes that cause normal cells to be converted into cancer cells. Oncogenes can be derived from proto-oncogenes, which have a role in normal cellular processes and development, by several genetic mechanisms. For example, proto-oncogene activation can be triggered by translocations that move the proto-oncogene to a new chromosomal location where it is expressed differently. Other genetic mechanisms that have been implicated in proto-oncogene activation include genetic amplification, insertion, and gene mutations (Bishop, 1987; Brusick, 1987). In addition to oncogenes that are genetically dominant, recessive mutant genes can cause cancers such as retinoblastoma and Wilm's tumor (Cavenee et al., 1986). Several genetic mechanisms, including chromosomal deletion, aneuploidy (chromosome loss), and mitotic recombination can lead to the expression of these recessive genes by eliminating the normal allele in the somatic cells of a heterozygote.

MECHANISMS OF MUTATION

Gene mutations, chromosome aberrations, aneuploidy, and polyploidy are all subject to induction by chemicals in experimental organisms. Although some mutagens may induce all these effects, most show some degree of specificity. It is useful to separate the induction of gene mutations and chromosome aberrations from the induction of aneuploidy and polyploidy, because the cellular targets tend to be different. Whereas the principal target for the induction of gene mutations and chromosome aberrations is DNA, the targets for inducing aneuploidy and polyploidy are often components of the cellular apparatus of mitosis and meiosis, most notably spindle fibers.

DNA Alterations and Mutagenesis

The underlying basis for mutagenesis is a chemical or physical alteration in the structure of DNA caused by a mutagen. For example, many electrophilic compounds react with DNA forming covalent addition products, called adducts. The position on the DNA bases at which adducts are formed can be quite specific for a given agent. For example, the aromatic amine acetylaminofluorene (AAF) binds specifically to the carbon at the 8-position of guanine, and the resultant adduct is an effective inducer of frameshift mutations (Koffel-Schwartz et al., 1984). Because mutagens differ with respect to the positions and properties of their adducts and the physical alterations that they cause in DNA, they also differ in the kinds of mutations that they induce.

Monofunctional alkylating agents, such as ethylnitrosourea (ENU) or diethyl sulfate (DES), cause the addition of alkyl groups to DNA (Figure 6–2). Alkylated bases may or may not exhibit the same pairing specificity as the normal bases. For example, guanine alkylated on the nitrogen at its 7-position pairs normally, but guanine alkylated on the oxygen at its 6-position is more apt than normal guanine to mispair with thymine (Hoffmann, 1980). The result of the mispairing of O^6-alkylguanine is a G:C $\rightarrow$ A:T transition. ENU, whose spectrum of alkylation products includes a relatively high proportion of O^6-ethylguanine, is a potent mutagen in microbial systems, *Drosophila,* and mammals. As one would expect for mutagenesis by mispairing, agents that alkylate the O^6 of guanine are effective inducers of base-pair substitutions (Pastink et al., 1989). Mispairing may be the simplest model for the mutagenicity of alkylating agents,

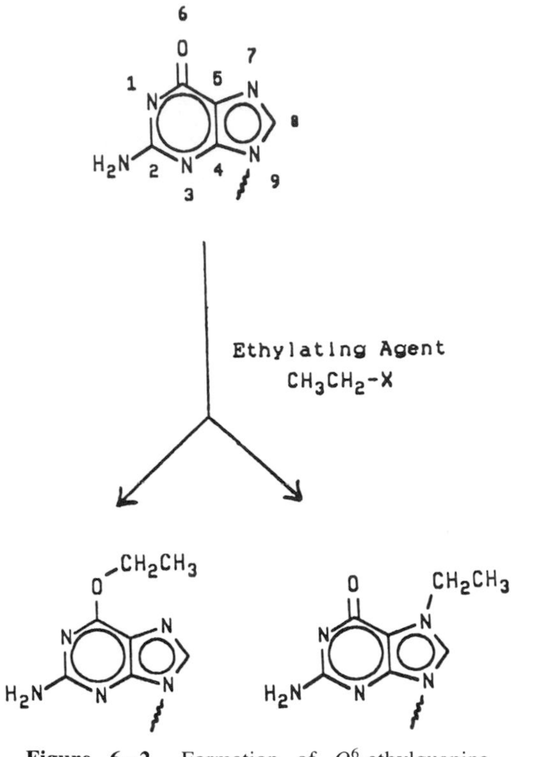

Figure 6–2. Formation of O^6-ethylguanine and N^7-ethylguanine by the reaction of a guanine residue with an alkylating agent.

but it is not the only model. Alkyl groups on some of the nitrogens in DNA are not apt to cause mispairing but may still contribute to mutagenesis by other routes, such as base-loss and errors in repair processes.

Not all mutagenesis requires covalent reaction of the mutagen with DNA. Rather, some planar molecules, such as 9-aminoacridine, intercalate between the base pairs of DNA. Such noncovalent interactions can apparently cause physical distortion that leads to the addition or deletion of base pairs when the DNA is replicated. Consequently, 9-aminoacridine is a frameshift mutagen. A widely accepted model that can explain the origins of some frameshift mutations involves slippage, or localized pairing out of register, at sites of repetitive bases in DNA (Drake *et al.*, 1983). Agents such as 9-aminoacridine are particularly effective mutagens in repetitive sequences and may operate by enhancing or stabilizing the slipped mispairing (Auerbach, 1976; Calos and Miller, 1981).

When cells or organisms are irradiated with ultraviolet light (UV), chemical alterations occur in DNA; major premutational lesions in UV-irradiated DNA are the cyclobutane pyrimidine dimer and the (6-4)-pyrimidine-pyrimidone photoproduct (Friedberg, 1985; Drobetsky *et*

al., 1989). These bulky lesions in DNA can block replication and cause death of the cell. Moreover, intracellular processing of the damaged DNA leads to mutations. The mutagenicity of UV therefore shows the complexity of mutation as a cellular process and is discussed further after DNA repair mechanisms are introduced.

DNA Repair

Agents that damage DNA and cause mutation occur naturally and have been present throughout the evolution of life. Therefore, one should not be surprised that living organisms have evolved a diversity of cellular mechanisms for coping with DNA damage. Such mechanisms fall into two broad categories—repair mechanisms and damage-tolerance mechanisms (Friedberg, 1985). Repair mechanisms remove premutational damage such as adducts in DNA, thereby restoring an intact DNA molecule with its normal nucleotide sequence. Tolerance mechanisms do not remove the damage but permit the cell to survive despite it.

Repair mechanisms may be classified into those that directly reverse DNA damage and those that remove damaged or incorrect bases and replace them with correct bases (Friedberg, 1985). Examples of direct reversal include the photorepair of UV damage, the removal of adducts from DNA bases, the insertion of purines into sites of base loss, and the sealing of single-strand breaks by a DNA ligase. Photorepair involves an enzyme that specifically cleaves pyrimidine dimers in DNA, thereby returning the two adjacent pyrimidines to their original configuration. The repair reaction involves the absorption of white light; such a photochemical system offers protection from dimers when it is needed, in that the sun is the source of natural UV exposure. In contrast, repair mechanisms that remove chemical adducts from DNA also operate in the dark. For example, an inducible repair system called the adaptive response removes potentially mutagenic methyl groups (and ethyl groups to a lesser extent) from the O^6 position of guanine by transferring them to the protein O^6-methylguanine-DNA methyltransferase (Volkert, 1988). Direct reversal of the premutational lesion thereby restores the normal base-pairing specificity.

Mechanisms that remove damaged bases, mispaired bases, or a segment of DNA containing damage are collectively called excision-repair mechanisms. Unlike photorepair and repair by a methyltransferase, excision mechanisms respond to a broad range of premutational lesions. They can repair the bulky photoproducts caused by UV, and diverse chemical adducts are suitable substrates for excision. Two major pathways of excision repair, called nucleotide excision and

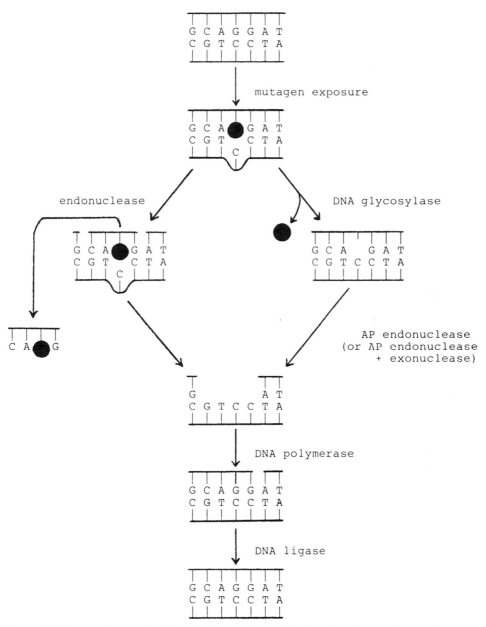

Figure 6–3. Excision repair of DNA damage. Chemical adducts or bulky photoproducts are formed in DNA as a consequence of exposure to a chemical mutagen or UV. The general repair pathways called nucleotide excision *(left)* and base excision *(right)* remove the damaged region and restore the intact DNA. The diagram shows a generalized scheme on which there are many variations.

base excision, are shown in Figure 6–3. Repair enzymes, lengths of the patches repaired, and variations in excision pathways have been reviewed by Friedberg (1985).

In nucleotide excision (Figure 6–3), the repair system recognizes the DNA damage, and an endonuclease (e.g., the *uvrABC* excinuclease of *E.*

coli) nicks the DNA backbone in its vicinity. Removal of the damaged region leaves a gap in the DNA. A repair polymerase (e.g., DNA polymerase I of *E. coli*) fills the gap with the correct bases, using the opposite strand as a template. The remaining break in the DNA strand is sealed by DNA ligase. The net result is restoration of the correct DNA sequence. Base excision involves some of the same enzyme activities as nucleotide excision and some different activities. The damage in DNA is recognized by a DNA glycosylase that releases the damaged base by cleaving the bond linking it to its sugar in the DNA backbone. The result is an "AP site," where "AP" denotes apurinic or apyrimidinic. An AP endonuclease then removes a section of DNA in the vicinity of the AP site. Polymerase and ligase steps complete the repair process in the same way as in nucleotide excision.

A special case of excision is the process of mismatch repair (Friedberg, 1985; Radman and Wagner, 1986) by which cells recognize and remove incorrect base pairs such as G:T or A:C. Such base pairs in DNA can arise by errors in replication, as intermediates in recombination, or by chemical modification of bases, such as the deamination of 5-methylcytosine, which occurs naturally in many species.

Damage-tolerance mechanisms allow cells to bypass a potentially lethal lesion in DNA. For example, an unrepaired pyrimidine dimer or other bulky lesion could block the replication of DNA. The replication mechanism, however, can bypass the lesion leaving a gap in the new strand opposite the damage. The gap can then be filled with the segment of DNA from the sister molecule by a recombinational process (Friedberg, 1985). An intact daughter strand is thereby made, and the cell survives. The damaged parental molecule may later be repaired.

An important approach in the study of DNA repair has been the isolation of repair-deficient mutants (Friedberg, 1985). Mutations that eliminate repair processes frequently confer high sensitivity to mutagen exposures. For example, bacteria carrying a *uvrA*, *uvrB*, or *uvrC* mutation are defective in their capacity for excision repair and are killed by smaller exposures to UV than are wild-type strains. Similarly *recA* mutants, which cannot carry out recombinational repair, are highly UV-sensitive. Repair deficiencies are also being characterized in eukaryotes, including fungi, *Drosophila*, and mammalian cells. The best known repair defect in humans is the genetic disease xeroderma pigmentosum (XP), which involves a deficiency for excision repair (Friedberg, 1985); patients with XP are extremely susceptible to the induction of skin cancer by UV. Bacterial repair deficiencies, XP cells, and other repair deficiencies in eukaryotes have played an important part in elucidating mechanisms by which organisms repair damage to their DNA. They have also found use in genetic toxicology testing, because they confer increased sensitivity to the effects of many mutagens.

Repair systems do not give complete protection against mutagenesis because repair processes can become saturated, some kinds of damage may be repaired inefficiently, and premutational lesions may be fixed as mutations prior to repair. Moreover, some repair processes are error-prone. Like the relatively error-free mechanisms of repair just described, error-prone repair enhances survival by producing a functional DNA molecule; however, the repaired DNA contains mutational errors rather than having the correct nucleotide sequence.

The best known case of error-prone repair is that of UV mutagenesis in the bacterium *E. coli* (Friedberg, 1985). UV mutagenesis had been studied for many years when the surprising discovery was made that UV is nonmutagenic in strains of bacteria that carry *recA* or *lexA* mutations. This observation led to the proposal that these genes are somehow involved in an error-prone response to DNA damage. It turned out that UV photoproducts in DNA stimulate (probably indirectly) the activation of a complex network of genetic functions, called the SOS system, in which the *recA*[+] and *lexA*[+] genes play a central role. Among the SOS functions is the error-prone processing of DNA damage that promotes survival at the expense of an elevated mutation frequency. Thus, bacterial cells participate in their own mutagenesis through error-prone repair processes. Although cellular responses to DNA damage have been most thoroughly characterized for UV mutagenesis in *E. coli*, such processes are now being explored for chemical mutagenesis and for eukaryotes (Rossman and Klein, 1988). It has become increasingly clear that DNA damage, repair, cellular metabolism, and the expression of mutations can no longer be considered in isolation, as mutagenesis is a complex cellular process involving diverse interactions among them.

Induction of Aneuploidy and Polyploidy

Cells with normal chromosome numbers can give rise to aneuploid cells by nondisjunction— the failure of homologous chromosomes in meiosis I or of sister chromatids in meiosis II or in mitosis to separate (i.e., disjoin) properly (Dellarco et al., 1985). The result of nondisjunction is that one pole of the spindle receives both homologues or chromatids while the other receives neither. Assuming that only one chromosome or pair of chromosomes is involved, the daughter nuclei will have one chromosome too many or one chromosome too few.

Unlike aneuploidy, polyploidy involves the entire set of chromosomes. For example, if there is chromosome duplication in interphase but no subsequent chromosome segregation to daughter cells, the chromosome number is doubled. Thus, a diploid cell can give rise to a tetraploid cell. Polyploid cells are commonly observed in some tissues and organs (e.g., mammalian liver and bronchial epithelium). Just as mitotic errors can give rise to polyploid cells, meiotic errors can give rise to gametes (or meiospores in plants) that are diploid rather than the normal haploid. If diploid gametes are involved in fertilization, the result is a polyploid zygote. An alternative mechanism by which polyploid individuals can arise is the fertilization of an egg by more than one sperm.

The induction of aneuploidy and polyploidy is distinct from other aspects of mutagenesis because it involves different targets (Dellarco *et al.*, 1985). For example, colchicine blocks the polymerization of tubulin, the principal protein of spindle fibers. Treatment of dividing cells with colchicine disrupts spindle formation and can cause polyploidy if there is complete blockage or aneuploidy in cases of lesser disruption. Agents that damage kinetochores, which are the structures by which the chromosomes attach to a spindle, can also cause aneuploidy.

Although some of the targets are common to mitosis and meiosis, others can be specific (Dellarco *et al.*, 1985). Agents that damage the synaptonemal complex can disrupt the pairing or segregation of homologous chromosomes in meiosis I. Cyclophosphamide, for example, has been reported to cause fragmentation of the synaptonemal complex and synaptic failure in mammalian germ cells; it induces aneuploidy, as well as other genetic effects by different mechanisms. In principle, any agent that increases the frequency of any of the following events can induce meiotic aneuploidy: extra chromosome replication, premature centromere division in meiosis I, improper pairing of homologous chromosomes in prophase I, and nondisjunction or chromosome loss in anaphase I or II. Besides structural components of the meiotic apparatus, the system of genetic recombination should be considered as a potential target for the induction of aneuploidy because crossing over and chiasma formation are involved in normal disjunction.

MUTAGEN TEST SYSTEMS

Mutagenicity testing has become a prominent part of toxicology during the last two decades. Genetic toxicology tests are used to identify germ-cell mutagens, somatic-cell mutagens, and potential carcinogens. Many compounds have now been tested for mutagenic effects in experimental organisms as diverse as bacteria and viruses, fungi, cultured mammalian cells, plants, insects, and mammals.

Survey of Test Systems

Table 6–1 lists test systems in genetic toxicology. It is hardly possible to include all methods that have been used to study mutagenesis. The table therefore selectively includes assays that have figured prominently in genetic toxicology testing or that illustrate the diversity of genetic end points and experimental organisms represented in mutagenicity tests. Methods that are used to elucidate mechanisms of mutagenesis but are not applied in testing are not included. Some of the most widely used tests in the table are the *Salmonella*/mammalian microsome test (i.e., the Ames test), tests for gene mutations in cultured mammalian cells, the sex-linked recessive lethal test in *Drosophila*, and cytogenetic tests in mammalian cell cultures and in rodents.

The tests in Table 6–1 range from inexpensive short-term tests that can be performed in a few days to involved tests for mutations in mammalian germ cells. Any agent that causes a reproducible positive response in any of these assays, or in other tests for DNA damage, gene mutations, clastogenic effects, recombinagenic effects, aneuploidy, or polyploidy, may be considered genotoxic. Because of time and expense, a large proportion of mutagenicity testing is done in microorganisms and cell cultures. Even in complex multicellular organisms, however, there has been an emphasis on designing tests that detect mutations with great efficiency. Nevertheless, there remains a gradation in which an increase in relevance for human risk entails more elaborate and costly tests. Because a great deal can be learned from the simpler tests, the most expensive mammalian tests are typically reserved for agents of special importance in basic research or risk assessment.

Design of Test Systems

Mutagenicity testing should detect the diverse kinds of mutation that are relevant for human health. Assays for gene mutations and chromosome aberrations are more highly developed than those for aneuploidy, but several promising assays for aneuploidy are now under development. Among gene mutations, both base-pair substitutions and frameshift mutations must be detected.

The most common means of detecting mutations in microorganisms is selecting for reversion in strains that have a specific nutritional requirement differing from wild-type members of the species; such strains are called auxotrophs. For example, in a widely used bacterial assay developed by Bruce Ames and his colleagues (Maron and Ames, 1983), one measures the frequency of histidine-independent

Table 6–1. TEST SYSTEMS IN GENETIC TOXICOLOGY

EFFECTS DETECTED	TESTS	REFERENCES*
I. Tests for Gene Mutations		
A. Bacterial tests		
1. Reversion of auxotrophs	*Salmonella*/mammalian microsome test (Ames test)	Maron and Ames, 1983; Kier *et al.*, 1986
	E. coli WP2 tryptophan reversion test	Green, 1984
2. Forward mutations conferring resistance	Arabinose resistance or azaguanine resistance in *Salmonella*	Dorado and Pueyo, 1988
B. Fungal tests		
1. Reversion of auxotrophs	Reversion of adenine mutations in *Neurospora*	Brockman *et al.*, 1984
	Reversion in various auxotrophs in yeast	Zimmermann *et al.*, 1984
2. Forward mutations and small deletions	Adenine mutants detected by red or white colonies in *Neurospora* or yeast	Brockman *et al.*, 1984; Zimmermann *et al.*, 1984
	Drug resistance in yeast	Zimmermann *et al.*, 1984
C. Mammalian cell culture tests		
1. Forward mutations	Thymidine kinase (TK) mutants selected by resistance to pyrimidine analogues in mouse lymphoma cells or human cells	DeMarini *et al.*, 1989
	Hypoxanthine-guanine phosphoribosyltransferase (HPRT) mutants selected by resistance to purine analogues in Chinese hamster or human cells	DeMarini *et al.*, 1989
D. Vascular plant tests		
1. Specific-locus mutations detected in endosperm, seedlings, pollen, or flowers	Forward mutations at the *yg-2* and *waxy* loci in corn and reversion of *waxy*	Plewa, 1982
	Stamen-hair color test in *Tradescantia*	Van't Hof and Schairer, 1982
2. Forward mutations at many unspecified loci	Chlorophyll-deficiency mutations in barley, corn, or other plants	Constantin and Nilan, 1982
E. *Drosophila* tests		
1. Gene mutations and small deletions in germ cells	Sex-linked recessive lethal test	Lee *et al.*, 1983
2. Mutations in somatic cells	Spot tests in eyes and wings	Würgler and Vogel, 1986
F. Mammalian tests		
1. Gene mutations and/or deletions in germ cells	Mouse specific locus test with visible markers	Russell and Shelby, 1985
	Mouse specific locus test with electrophoretic or immunological markers	Russell and Shelby, 1985
	Mouse skeletal mutations	Russell and Shelby, 1985
	Mouse cataract mutations	Russell and Shelby, 1985
2. Gene mutations in somatic cells	Mouse spot test (somatic cell specific locus test)	Styles and Penman, 1985
II. Tests for Chromosome Damage		
A. Mammalian cell culture tests		
1. Chromosome aberrations	Human or rodent cell cytogenetics	Ishidate *et al.*, 1988; Preston *et al.*, 1981
2. Sister chromatid exchanges	SCE in human cells or Chinese hamster cells	Latt *et al.*, 1981
B. Vascular plant tests		
1. Chromosome aberrations in mitotic cells	Cytogenetic analysis in root tips of *Vicia faba*, barley or onion or in *Tradescantia* pollen	Grant, 1982; Ma, 1982
2. Chromosome aberrations and micronuclei in meiotic cells	Chromosome damage in microsporocytes of *Tradescantia*	Ma, 1982
C. *Drosophila* tests		
1. Chromosome aberrations	Heritable translocation tests	Valencia *et al.*, 1984

Table 6–1.   (Continued)

EFFECTS DETECTED	TESTS	REFERENCES*
D. Mammalian tests		
1. Chromosome aberrations in somatic cells	Cytogenetic analysis of rodent bone marrow or lymphocytes	Preston *et al.*, 1981
2. Chromosome aberrations in germ cells	Cytogenetic analysis of spermatogonia, spermatocytes, or oocytes	Russell and Shelby, 1985; Preston *et al.*, 1981
3. Chromosome breakage in somatic cells	Micronucleus test in polychromatic erythrocytes	Mavournin *et al.*, 1990
4. Sister chromatid exchanges	SCE in rodent bone marrow, spleen, or spermatogonia	Latt *et al.*, 1981
5. Indirect evidence of chromosome damage in germ cells	Mouse or rat dominant lethal test	Green *et al.*, 1985; Russell and Shelby, 1985.
6. Heritable chromosome aberrations in germ cells	Mouse heritable translocation test	Russell and Shelby, 1985
III. Tests for Aneuploidy		
A. Fungal tests		
1. Mitotic aneuploidy	Genetic detection of chromosome loss and gain in yeast	Resnick *et al.*, 1986
2. Meiotic nondisjunction	Disomic ascospores in *Neurospora* or yeast	Griffiths *et al.*, 1986; Resnick *et al.*, 1986
B. Mammalian cell culture tests		
1. Mitotic chromosome gain	Hyperdiploid cells detected by chromosome counts	Galloway and Ivett, 1986
C. *Drosophila* tests		
1. Sex chromosome aneuploidy	Sex chromosome loss tests	Zimmering *et al.*, 1986; Valencia *et al.*, 1984
D. Mammalian tests		
1. Nondisjunction in germ cells	Aneuploidy detected by chromosome counts	Allen *et al.*, 1986
2. Sex chromosome loss by nondisjunction or chromosome breakage	Genetic detection of mice with a single X chromosome and no Y	Allen *et al.*, 1986; Russell and Shelby, 1985
IV. Other Indicators of Genetic Damage or Mutagen Exposure		
A. Bacterial tests		
1. Repairable DNA damage	Assays for differential killing of repair-proficient and repair-deficient strains of *E. coli* or *Bacillus*	Leifer *et al.*, 1981
2. SOS induction	Induction of phage lambda and other SOS functions by DNA damage in *E. coli*	Elespuru, 1984
B. Fungal tests		
1. Recombinagenicity	Mitotic crossing over tests in yeast	Zimmermann *et al.*, 1984
	Mitotic gene conversion tests in yeast	Zimmermann *et al.*, 1984
C. Mammalian cell culture tests		
1. Repairable DNA damage	Unscheduled DNA synthesis in human fibroblasts	Mitchell *et al.*, 1983
	Unscheduled DNA synthesis in rat hepatocytes	Mitchell *et al.*, 1983
2. DNA strand breaks	Direct detection of DNA damage by alkaline elution of DNA	Larsen *et al.*, 1982
D. *Drosophila* tests		
1. Recombinagenicity	Detection of mitotic recombination in eyes or wings	Würgler and Vogel, 1986
E. Mammalian tests		
1. Repairable DNA damage	Unscheduled DNA synthesis in mouse germ cells	Russell and Shelby, 1985
2. Adducts in germ cells	Molecular dosimetry with isotope-labeled mutagen	Russell and Shelby, 1985
3. Morphological sperm abnormalities	Sperm abnormality test for spermatotoxicity and possible genetic damage in mice	Russell and Shelby, 1985

* Table adapted from Hoffmann, 1982. The references provide an overview of the tests and guidance on controls, sample sizes, and other factors that are important for effective testing. Additional references may be found in the articles cited or in Hoffmann, 1982.

bacteria that arise in a histidine-requiring strain in the presence and absence of the chemical being tested. Revertants are selected by plating the bacteria on medium that is deficient in histidine. The assay is conducted in several different strains, so that reversion by base-pair substitutions and frameshift mutations in two DNA sequence contexts can be detected and distinguished. The mechanisms of reversion in the Ames tester strains have been known genetically for some time and are now being characterized by molecular methods (Hartman *et al.*, 1986; Cebula and Koch, 1990). Another commonly used means of detecting mutations in microorganisms is the selection of mutations that confer resistance to an inhibitory chemical (e.g., 8-azaguanine). Because of their speed and inexpensiveness, microbial assays have been widely used and offer an extensive data base.

Mutagenicity tests in cultured mammalian cells have some of the same advantages as microbial tests and use similar methods. The most common assays for gene mutations in mammalian cells involve the detection of forward mutations that confer resistance to a toxic chemical (DeMarini *et al.*, 1989). A forward mutation is a mutation that inactivates a wild-type gene; for example, mutations in the hypoxanthine-guanine phosphoribosyltransferase gene *(hprt)* confer resistance to the purine analogues 6-thioguanine or 8-azaguanine, and mutations in the thymidine kinase *(tk)* gene confer resistance to the pyrimidine analogue trifluorothymidine.

Forward-mutation assays can, in principle, respond to a broad spectrum of mutagens because any mutation that interferes with gene expression leads to the selected phenotype. In contrast, a back-mutation or reversion assay selects for mutations that correct or compensate for the mutational alteration in a mutant. In fact, some reversion assays respond to a broader spectrum of mutational changes than one might expect, because mutations at a site other than the original mutant site (i.e., a second-site mutation; a suppressor mutation) can sometimes confer the selected phenotype. Similarly, not all forward-mutation assays are responsive to diverse mechanisms of mutagenesis. For example, resistance to ouabain results from single-base changes that cause a specific alteration in a membrane-associated adenosine triphosphatase (ATPase); mutations that eliminate the ATPase activity are lethal (DeMarini *et al.*, 1989). Ouabain resistance is therefore not as useful as other drug resistances in screening for mutagens, because it permits the detection of only a small proportion of possible mutations.

In any application of mutagenicity tests, one must be aware of possible artifacts. For example, in the Ames assay one may see very small colonies arise in the petri dishes at highly toxic doses (Maron and Ames, 1983). Rather than being revertants, such colonies may be survivors that form small colonies by growing on the low concentration of histidine added to the plates. Were there millions of survivors, the amount of histidine would have been insufficient to allow any of them (except real revertants) to form colonies. To avoid this artifact, one should always observe that there is a faint lawn of bacterial growth in the plates; one can also confirm that colonies are revertants by streaking them on medium without histidine to be sure that they grow in its absence. Such pitfalls exist in all mutagenicity tests. Even though many of the short-term tests are simple in design and application, they can be performed incorrectly. Anyone performing mutagenicity tests must gain detailed familiarity with the laboratory application and literature of the assay and be observant about potential artifacts.

Assays for gene mutations are indirect, in that one observes a phenotype and reaches conclusions about genes. In contrast, cytogenetic tests involve the use of microscopy to observe the effect of interest directly. A key factor in the design of cytogenetic tests is obtaining appropriate cell populations for treatment and analysis (Preston *et al.*, 1981). Cells with a stable, well-defined karyotype, a short generation time, a low chromosome number, and relatively large chromosomes are ideal for cytogenetic analysis. For this reason, Chinese hamster ovary (CHO) cells have been used widely in cytogenetic testing. Other cell lines are also suitable, however, and cultured human leukocytes have been used extensively. In any case, it is important that the analysis includes cells treated at all stages of the cell cycle because of the stage-specificity of clastogens. Aberrations should be scored in the first mitotic division after treatment because unstable aberrations would have been lost in subsequent divisions, thereby reducing the sensitivity of the assay. Examples of chromosome aberrations are shown in Figure 6–4.

In vivo cytogenetic tests involve treating intact animals and later preparing cell samples for cytogenetic analysis (Preston *et al.*, 1981). *In vivo* tests offer the advantage that the mammalian metabolism and distribution of the test agent are part of the assay. Routes of exposure and dosages must be selected to assure adequate exposure of the target cell population. The target must be a tissue from which large numbers of dividing cells are easily prepared. The most widely used *in vivo* cytogenetic test involves analysis of mouse bone marrow cells.

Cytogenetic analysis is also conducted on

spermatogonia, spermatocytes, or oocytes because knowledge of the induction of aberrations in germ cells is important for assessing genetic risks to future generations. Besides cytological observation, indirect evidence for chromosome aberrations is used in some germ-cell assays. Specifically, the dominant lethal test measures embryonic and fetal deaths in the offspring of treated male mice or rats, and the mouse herita-

ble translocation test detects chromosomal rearrangements on the basis of reduced fertility of the offspring of treated males. Cytogenetic confirmation is possible in the heritable translocation test but not the dominant lethal test.

Data collection is a critical step in cytogenetic analysis. Results should be recorded for specific classes of aberrations, not just as an overall index of aberrations per cell (Preston *et al.*, 1981;

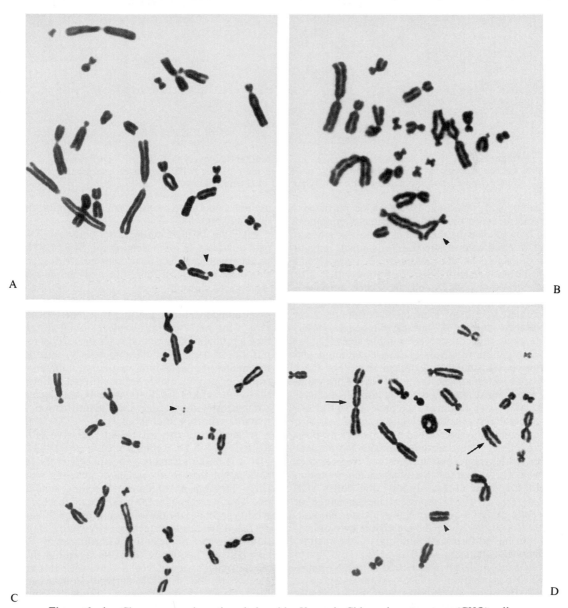

Figure 6–4. Chromosome aberrations induced by X rays in Chinese hamster ovary (CHO) cells. *A.* A chromatid deletion (▶) *B.* A chromatid exchange of the type commonly called a triradial (▶). *C.* A small interstitial deletion (▶) that resulted from chromosome breakage. *D.* A metaphase cell containing more than one aberration: a centric ring plus an acentric fragment (▶) and a dicentric chromosome plus an acentric fragment (→). (Courtesy of R. Julian Preston.)

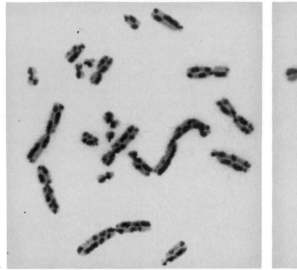 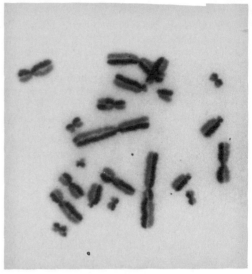

A   B

Figure 6–5.   Sister chromatid exchanges in Chinese hamster ovary (CHO) cells. Differentially stained chromatids permit the counting of SCE in cells treated with a mutagen (decarbamoyl mitomycin C) *(A)* and control cells *(B)*. (Courtesy of Sheila Galloway.)

Carrano and Natarajan, 1988). This is particularly true because there is not complete agreement on how to classify aberrations and on whether to count small achromatic (i.e., unstained) gaps in chromosomes as aberrations at all. Gaps should not be pooled with other aberrations. It is also essential that enough cells be scored because a negative result in a small sample is meaningless. A review by Preston *et al.* (1981) offers practical guidance on the design of cytogenetic tests, treatment procedures, and sample sizes.

Cytogenetic analysis is time-consuming and requires considerable technical skill. For these reasons, alternative cytological assays are widely used, most notably the detection of micronuclei and sister chromatid exchanges (SCE). The micronucleus assay (Mavournin *et al.,* 1990), most commonly performed in immature erythrocytes, detects chromosome damage as micronuclei, which represent chromosome fragments or whole chromosomes that escaped incorporation into the main nucleus in dividing cells. SCE (Latt *et al.,* 1981) represent the exchange of genetic material between the two sister chromatids of a chromosome and are visible cytologically through differential staining of chromatids. Many mutagens are active in SCE assays, but it is still incompletely understood how DNA damage or perturbations of DNA synthesis give rise to SCE. Figure 6–5 shows SCE in CHO cells. SCE and micronuclei are easier to score than chromosome aberrations, and the assays appear to be quite sensitive. The practical gains, however, entail some loss of information relative to complete cytogenetic analysis, and there is greater uncertainty with respect to underlying mechanisms.

Like the *in vivo* cytogenetic assays, *in vivo* genetic assays involve treating the target cells in intact animals. Selection of appropriate dosages, treatment procedures, controls, and sample sizes are critical elements in the conduct of all *in vivo* tests (Brusick, 1987). The design of the tests must compensate for the fact that mutation is a rare event, and even the simplest animal systems face a problem of numbers; one can easily screen millions of bacteria or cultured cells by selection techniques, but screening very large numbers of fruit flies or mice poses serious practical limitations. Therefore, assays in animals must offer a straightforward, unequivocal identification of mutants with minimal labor.

A strength of the sex-linked recessive lethal (SLRL) test in *Drosophila* (Lee *et al.,* 1983) is that it is based on many genes in relatively few flies rather than a few indicator genes in many flies. Through an ingenious breeding scheme, one simply screens for the presence or absence of wild-type males in the offspring of specifically designed crosses to detect recessive lethal mutations anywhere in the entire X chromosome. The spontaneous frequency of SLRL is about 0.20 percent, and a significant increase over this frequency in the lineages derived from treated males indicates mutagenesis. Although simple relative to most whole-animal tests, the SLRL test is still labor-intensive relative to microbial and cell culture tests. An adequate negative test, for example, requires about 7000 vials of fruit flies (Lee *et al.,* 1983). Nevertheless, the test yields information about mutagenesis in germ cells, which is lacking in all microbial and cell culture systems. Therefore, it is not surprising that the detection of SLRL, which was used as early as 1927 in H. J. Muller's classic demonstration that X rays are mutagenic, continues to be important in mutation research and genetic toxicology.

Despite the strengths of *Drosophila* assays, they do not provide sufficient basis for predicting human risks. Although metabolism and gametogenesis in *Drosophila* are analogous to the mammalian processes, they are not identical. Means of exposure and the measurement of dosages in flies also differ from mammalian toxicology. Therefore, mammalian tests have a central role in genetic toxicology despite their expense and complexity.

The specific-locus test in mice detects recessive mutations that produce easily scored phenotypes (e.g., coat color) conferred by seven defined genes (Russell and Shelby, 1985). This assay, developed by William L. Russell, has had a central place in assessing genetic risks of ionizing radiation and has been used to study various chemical mutagens including ethylnitrosourea, which is the most potent mutagen in mammalian spermatogonia yet discovered. Other gene-mutation assays in mouse germ cells detect recessive mutations that cause electrophoretic or immunological changes in proteins and dominant mutations that cause skeletal abnormalities or cataracts (Russell and Shelby, 1985). Together, these mammalian assays provide the best basis for quantitatively predicting genetic risks to human germ cells.

Metabolic Activation

Many compounds are not directly mutagenic or carcinogenic but can be converted into mutagens and carcinogens by mammalian metabolism. Such compounds are called promutagens and procarcinogens. Because microorganisms and mammalian cells in culture lack many of the metabolic capabilities of intact mammals, it is necessary to supply mammalian metabolism to short-term mutagenicity tests in order for them to detect promutagens.

Heinrich Malling first combined mammalian tissue homogenates for metabolic activation with a microbial test for mutation detection, demonstrating the activation of dimethylnitrosamine into a mutagen by mouse liver homogenates. Subsequently, many other compounds, including members of such important groups as polynuclear aromatic hydrocarbons and aromatic amines, have been shown to be activated into mutagens by *in vitro* metabolic activation systems, and metabolic activation has become a standard part of mutagenicity testing (Maron and Ames, 1983; Brusick, 1987).

The most common method for metabolic activation in microbial and mammalian cell assays is the addition of a postmitochondrial supernatant from a rat liver homogenate, along with appropriate buffers and cofactors (Maron and Ames, 1983; Brusick, 1987). The standard liver metabolic activation system is generally called an S9 mixture, to designate a supernatant from centrifugation at 9000 g. Variations based on other species or organs are sometimes also used. Unlike mutagenicity assays in intact animals, most of the short-term tests in Table 6–1 require exogenous metabolic activation for detecting promutagens. An exception is an assay for unscheduled DNA synthesis (an indication of repairable DNA damage) in cultured hepatocytes (Mitchell *et al.*, 1983). Yeast assays in which there is endogenous cytochrome P450 can also detect some promutagens (Zimmermann *et al.*, 1984).

Alternative metabolic activation systems that are sometimes used are metabolism by intact hepatocytes (Langenbach and Oglesby, 1983) and a metabolic system that includes a reduction step required for the mutagenicity of some azo dyes and nitro compounds (Dellarco and Prival, 1989). A method that uses *in vivo* metabolic activation is the host-mediated assay (Legator *et al.*, 1982), in which the test organisms (e.g., bacteria) are inserted in the animal (e.g., in the peritoneal cavity) before treatment of the animal; the test organisms are later recovered from the animal and assayed for mutagenicity, thereby detecting effects of the test chemical and those mammalian metabolites that reached the test organisms in the animal. The host-mediated assay tends to be a research tool rather than a routine testing method, and S9 remains the method of choice in screening for mutagens.

Despite their usefulness, metabolic activation systems do not mimic mammalian metabolism perfectly. There are differences among tissues in reactions that activate or inactivate foreign compounds, and organisms of the normal flora of the gut can contribute to metabolism in intact mammals. Agents that induce enzyme systems or otherwise alter the physiological state can also modify the metabolism of toxicants. Consequently, some metabolites that occur *in vitro* do not occur or are less prominent *in vivo,* and vice versa.

Validation and Predictiveness of Assays

Validating a short-term test consists of determining how well it performs with many compounds from diverse chemical classes in several laboratories. Thoroughly studied, potent mutagens offer an obvious reference point for test validation, but testing cannot be restricted to such agents because one must determine whether the assay can detect weak mutagens and whether it is nonresponsive to nonmutagens.

A common use of results from mutagenicity tests is attempting to predict which chemicals are carcinogens. The great majority of chemicals that are known to be carcinogenic in humans are active in one or more genetic toxicology tests (Brusick, 1987). In predicting carcinogenicity, however, one needs to consider both the sensitivity and the specificity of tests. Sensitivity refers to the proportion of carcinogens that are positive in the test, whereas specificity is the proportion of noncarcinogens that are negative in the test (Tennant et al., 1987). Both sensitivity and specificity contribute to the concordance of short-term tests with carcinogenicity, because concordance is simply the percentage of qualitative agreement (+ or −) between results in different assays. One should note that the word *sensitivity* is sometimes used to denote the ability of a test to detect a mutagen at low concentration or its ability to detect a small change in mutation rate, so alternative usages of *sensitivity* must be recognized from context.

The concordance of mutagenicity tests with carcinogenicity is usually evaluated by comparing results in short-term genetic tests to those in long-term carcinogenicity assays in rodents because the data base for humans is quite limited. A short-term test is said to exhibit high sensitivity if a large proportion of rodent carcinogens yield positive results in the test; it is said to exhibit high specificity if a large proportion of noncarcinogens yield negative results. A positive result in a short-term test is often called a false positive if the compound is found to be noncarcinogenic in a rodent cancer assay. Similarly, when a rodent carcinogen gives a negative result in a short-term test, the result is sometimes called a false negative for that test. Emphasis on sensitivity has sometimes led to underestimating the importance of specificity. Before arguing that sensitivity is more important than specificity because false negatives can pose a health risk, whereas false positives cannot, one must acknowledge that the sensitivity of a test that is always positive is 100%, and such a test would be useless. To be useful, a test must have reasonable predictive value for both carcinogens and noncarcinogens.

An article that has made a substantial impact in genetic toxicology testing is an evaluative study by Raymond Tennant and his colleagues on the ability of short-term genetic tests to predict the results of recent rodent carcinogenicity

tests in the National Toxicology Program (Tennant et al., 1987). Results from widely used genetic assays (the Ames test, mutations at the *tk* locus in mouse lymphoma cells, chromosome aberrations in CHO cells, and SCE in CHO cells) were compared with cancer bioassays of 73 chemicals in mice and rats. Each of the mutagenicity assays showed a concordance with the carcinogenicity assays of about 60 percent—a value much lower than early correlative studies would have anticipated.

Studies like that of Tennant et al. (1987) are essential because all toxicology tests should be subjected to critical, objective analysis. The implications of the result for the use of short-term genetic tests, however, are less clear. One possible interpretation is that short-term genetic assays are not especially useful in identifying carcinogens. Several reports (Brockman and DeMarini, 1988; Prival and Dunkel, 1989), however, have challenged the methods, assumptions, or interpretations of Tennant et al., and the central question of how much emphasis short-term genetic tests should receive in efforts to identify carcinogens is unresolved. Major points of uncertainty in evaluating whether these tests are effective predictors of carcinogenicity concern sampling issues and the reliability of the carcinogenesis assays (Brockman and DeMarini, 1988; Prival and Dunkel, 1989).

The discordance between short-term tests and rodent carcinogenicity may be interpreted as evidence that short-term tests produce many false positives and false negatives. Such an interpretation could be misleading, however, because it assumes that the carcinogenesis assay permits a correct classification of the chemical as a carcinogen or a noncarcinogen. In fact, many carcinogenesis tests are equivocal (Prival and Dunkel, 1989), and there is often discordance among species (Brockman and DeMarini, 1988). Such discordance raises troublesome questions; for example, if a compound is negative in both a bacterial mutagenicity test and a rat carcinogenicity test but positive in a mouse carcinogenicity test, should the bacterial assay be regarded as inadequate for failing to detect the mouse carcinogen?

Correspondence between mouse and rat, the two most commonly used species in carcinogenesis bioassays, is not especially high. For the 73 compounds evaluated by Tennant et al. (1987), the concordance between mouse and rat was 67 percent (Brockman and DeMarini, 1988). Moreover, in an evaluative study by Griesemer and Cueto (1980), only 44 of 98 agents that were carcinogenic in either rats or mice were carcinogenic in both species. Besides interspecific variation, factors that can complicate the interpretation of carcinogenesis assays include the high spontaneous incidence of some tumors in rodents, the lack of replicate experiments in expensive bioassays, equivocal results owing to lack of statistical power, and shortcomings in dosage regimens or other aspects of assay design (Brockman and De-Marini, 1988; Prival and Dunkel, 1989).

Although there are many compounds that are indisputably carcinogenic, the identification of noncarcinogens can be problematic (Prival and Dunkel, 1989). It is especially difficult to be confident of noncarcinogenicity of compounds in chemical classes in which structurally related compounds are carcinogenic. One must ask whether the compound is truly noncarcinogenic or whether its carcinogenicity was undetected because of the conditions of the assay (e.g., species, dosages, numbers of animals); if the latter, a positive short-term test may be regarded as a false positive when, in fact, it correctly identifies a carcinogen that was misclassified by the carcinogenesis bioassay.

It is commonly thought that deficiencies in the sensitivity or specificity of individual tests may be circumvented by using complementary tests in combinations called tiers or batteries. Recent evaluative studies, however, suggest that commonly used genetic toxicology tests tend to be consistent with one other, rather than complementing each other's strengths and weaknesses (Tennant *et al.*, 1987). Although this finding should provoke skepticism about the ability of tiers and batteries to perform better than individual tests, it gives reason for optimism about the ability of these tests to detect agents that are truly mutagenic. Rather than trying to assemble a battery of tests so as to compensate for perceived shortcomings in individual tests, it seems prudent to emphasize mechanistic considerations in selecting assays. One should test for both gene mutations and chromosomal alterations and should not overlook *in vivo* mammalian metabolism. Such considerations would give a well-validated mutagenicity assay, such as the Ames assay, and *in vivo* cytogenetics a central position in genetic toxicology testing.

Measuring a short-term test's ability to predict mammalian germ-cell mutagenesis is no simpler than measuring its ability to predict carcinogenicity, because too few compounds have been tested for mutagenicity in mammalian germ cells. However, a positive test for mutagenicity in a well-characterized mammalian germ-cell assay, such as the mouse specific-locus test, provides strong suggestion that the chemical is a human germ-cell mutagen. Unfortunately, nega-

tive results are more difficult to interpret because one must ask whether the assay conditions were optimal and whether the scale of the study was large enough to detect small increases in mutation frequencies.

Even without clear reference points for relating short-term tests to adverse health effects, a reproducible positive result in a short-term test indicates that a compound is a mutagen. The mechanistic evidence for an association of mutations and chromosome aberrations with cancer is strong. The existence of nonmutagenic carcinogens (sometimes called nongenotoxic or epigenetic carcinogens), such as some estrogens whose carcinogenicity undoubtedly occurs by nongenetic mechanisms (Brusick, 1987), does not undermine the importance of mutagenicity in the carcinogenicity of other chemicals. The demonstration of mutagenicity alone suggests that a compound may pose a hazard for humans—either for the individual through somatic-cell mutagenesis or for future generations through germ-cell mutagenesis. Any agent that causes a reproducible positive result in a short-term test warrants further molecular and toxicological study.

SCREENING FOR MUTAGENS

It is not feasible to conduct thorough tests of all chemicals to which people are exposed. There are more than 50,000 commercial chemicals in use in the United States, and hundreds of new chemicals are introduced each year (Hoffmann, 1982). Besides commercial chemicals, many compounds of environmental origin have significant toxicologic effects. The inability to test all compounds necessitates the setting of priorities for testing. Factors in deciding which compounds should be tested include production volumes, intended uses, the expected extent of human exposure, environmental distribution, and biological effects that may be anticipated on the basis of chemical structure or previous toxicologic tests. In setting priorities, one strives to ensure that compounds with the greatest potential for adverse effects receive the most thorough study. The massiveness of the problem, however, necessitates that rapid, inexpensive assays play a central role in screening for mutagens.

The most obvious use of genetic toxicology tests is the screening of pure compounds to detect mutagens. As of January, 1990, the data base of the Environmental Mutagen Information Center in Oak Ridge, Tennessee, included more than 71,000 publications concerning genetic effects of at least 21,000 chemicals (J. S. Wassom, personal communication). Screening data are used in setting priorities for further testing, and they contribute to decisions in the development of chemical products and in the regulatory process. An important consideration in screening is that laboratory practices meet a high standard with respect to procedures, safety, and data handling (Brusick, 1987).

Besides screening pure chemicals, the testing of environmental samples has received much attention in genetic toxicology because many mutagens exist in complex environmental mixtures (Hoffmann, 1982; Brusick, 1987). The Ames test has been used more than any other assay in tests of complex mixtures because its speed and simplicity allow the testing of large numbers of samples and fractions derived from them.

Complex mixtures that have been analyzed for mutagenicity are extremely diverse, including air; drinking water; other water sources; industrial emissions and effluents; municipal sewage; automotive emissions; emissions from burning wood, peat, coal, and oil; diverse oils and fuels; photocopy toners; typewriter ribbon; coal gasification and liquefaction products; coffee; tea; cooked meats; and tobacco smoke (Hoffmann, 1982). Testing environmental samples requires methods for collecting the samples and extracting or concentrating them (Hoffmann, 1982; Brusick, 1987). Such testing is most effective when combined with analytical chemistry, so that the components of the mixtures are characterized.

Testing complex mixtures poses difficult problems for several reasons: their composition is highly variable, there are many possible artifacts traceable to the collection and processing of samples, and effects of chemicals in mixtures need not be additive (Hoffmann, 1982). Synergistic and antagonistic effects among mutagens, as well as comutagenic and antimutagenic effects between mutagens and nonmutagens, are known to occur.

Besides evaluating environmental samples, mutagenicity tests can be used in quality control. For example, one can screen for the presence of mutagenic secondary products that may occur as contaminants in samples of nonmutagenic chemicals. Mutagenicity tests can also be used to monitor the effectiveness of pollution-control devices, containment facilities, and industrial processes (Hoffmann, 1982).

An alternative to controlled laboratory exposures is *in situ* monitoring for mutagens (Hoffmann, 1982). In *in situ* monitoring, one looks for mutagenic effects in test organisms that are grown in the environment of interest. Plant assays, such as the stamen hair test in *Trade-scantia* or the *waxy* locus test in corn, have frequently been used for this purpose. Natural populations of organisms can also be monitored for evidence of genetic damage, but doing so is prone to artifacts, and utmost precaution must be taken in defining appropriate control populations.

MOLECULAR ANALYSIS OF MUTATION

The methodology of molecular biology has added powerful new approaches for studying mutagenesis, and modern mutation research relies on a combination of genetic and molecular analysis. Some of the early systems for characterizing mutations through biochemical means involved comparing mutant proteins with wild-type proteins; conclusions were reached about changes in genes on the basis of the changes in their gene products (Auerbach, 1976; Ernst, 1985). Recent methodology, however, has made nucleic acids more amenable to direct analysis and is revolutionizing mutation research. Rather than relying exclusively on genetic analysis for characterizing mutations, several new mutation systems characterize mutations directly by DNA sequence analysis.

A key step in sequencing mutations is the isolation of a small fragment of DNA containing the mutation. Several strategies can be employed for this purpose. One can, for example, induce mutations randomly in the target DNA and then use a combination of genetic and molecular methods to localize and isolate the mutations. Alternatively, one can use methods that direct the mutagenesis to a predetermined, small, easily isolated region of DNA within a target gene. Once a mutation is isolated in a small DNA fragment, it can readily be sequenced by a variety of chemical and enzymatic methods.

DNA sequence analysis of mutations has been applied to various bacterial and bacteriophage genes, such as the *cI* repressor gene in phage lambda and the *rII* region in phage T4 (Ripley *et al.*, 1986). A powerful method for the genetic and molecular analysis of mutation in bacteria is the *lacI* system developed in *E. coli* by Jeffrey Miller and his colleagues. Mutations in the *lacI* gene, which encodes the repressor of the lactose operon, are easily identified on the basis of phenotype and characterized genetically. Molecular analysis in this system has been facilitated by transferring *lacI* mutations from the strain in which they originate to a multicopy plasmid (Calos and Miller, 1981) or a phage M13 cloning vector (Schaaper *et al.*, 1986) to obtain many copies of the mutant DNA (*i.e.*, cloning the mutation) for sequencing. For example, Calos and Miller (1981) induced *lacI* mutations with the acridine mustard ICR-191 and mapped them genetically to a small region of the gene. They transferred the mutation to a multicopy plasmid by genetic recombination. The plasmid was then cloned, isolated, and digested with restriction enzymes that cleave it near the site of the mutation. A small restriction fragment containing the mutation was isolated by electrophoresis and sequenced, thereby providing a direct determination of the changes in DNA sequence induced by ICR-191 (Calos and Miller, 1981).

The *lacI* system has been used to determine the spectra of both spontaneous (Schaaper *et al.*, 1986) and induced mutations (Calos and Miller, 1981). A mutation spectrum consists of the classes of nucleotide changes and their distribution within a gene. It therefore includes not only the specific base-pair substitutions, frameshifts, and complex mutations but also the sequence context in which they occur. Mutation spectra can reveal effects of neighboring sequences on the mutability of particular sites. For example, about 98 percent of the mutations induced by ICR-191 in the *lacI* system (Calos and Miller, 1981) are frameshift mutations in which a single G:C base pair has been gained or lost in a region of repetitive G:C base pairs; at some sites in the gene $+1$ frameshifts predominate, whereas at other sites -1 frameshifts predominate.

Highly mutable locations within a gene, called hotspots, have also been discovered in other mutation systems. For example, Robert Fuchs and his colleagues have developed a forward mutation system in which mutagenesis is directed to a small restriction fragment (276 base pairs) within the tetracycline-resistance gene of plasmid pBR322 in *E. coli*. Using this system, they found that mutations induced by adducts of N-2-acetylaminofluorene (AAF) are principally frameshift mutations that occur in two kinds of hotspots: repetitive sequences and the alternating G:C base pairs of the sequence GGCGCC (Koffel-Schwartz *et al.*, 1984).

Besides the chemical alteration of DNA caused by mutagens, physical alterations can be important in mutagenesis. For example, both AAF and the related aromatic amine, N-2-aminofluorene (AF), bind specifically to the C8 position of guanine, but their adducts have different effects on DNA conformation (Koffel-Schwartz *et al.*, 1984; Bichara and Fuchs, 1985). AAF adducts insert into the DNA, thereby extruding a guanine and causing localized denaturation of the double helix. In contrast, AF remains outside the helix and does not cause denaturation. Under the same assay conditions, AAF induces primarily frameshifts, and AF induces primarily transversions (Bichara and Fuchs, 1985). Studies of -2 frameshift muta-

tions in plasmids that have been constructed so as to contain single AAF adducts on one of the guanines of the sequence GGCGCC have provided support for speculation that the induction of -2 frameshifts in this hotspot involves a localized conformational shift from B-DNA to Z-DNA triggered by AAF (Burnouf *et al.*, 1989).

Other evidence for the importance of conformational changes in mutagenesis comes from analysis of the sequences involved in deletion mutations and in frameshifts that are not explainable by simple slipped mispairing (Ripley *et al.*, 1986). It seems that such mutations are often associated with palindromic (or nearly palindromic) DNA sequences that can form hairpin-like loops. An example is shown in Figure 6-6. Some complex mutations whose sequences would seem to entail the improbable event of a frameshift and a base-pair substitution occurring simultaneously can be explained by a single event in the metabolism of a nearly palindromic sequence (Drake *et al.*, 1983; Ripley *et al.*, 1986).

DNA sequence analysis of mutations has been extended to eukaryotes, including fungi (Ernst *et al.*, 1985) and *Drosophila* (Pastink *et al.*, 1989). A strategy that has proven effective for studying mechanisms by which DNA damage is processed into mutations in mammalian cells is the use of shuttle vectors (Dixon *et al.*, 1989). Shuttle vectors consist of a target gene for detecting mutations, such as the *E. coli supF* gene, incorporated into a plasmid or virus-based extrachromosomal element capable of replicating in mammalian cells. With a shuttle vector system, mutations can be induced in the target gene in a mammalian cell and then be recovered from the cells and transformed into bacteria for the detection and sequence analysis of the mutations. Shuttle vector systems thereby take advantage of refined analysis in microbial systems to obtain information on the processing of premutational lesions into mutations in mammalian cells. There has also been progress in the molecular analysis of endogenous genes in mammalian cells, and such analysis promises to complement the shuttle vector systems in the elucidation of molecular mechanisms of mutagenesis (Drobetsky *et al.*, 1989).

MONITORING HUMAN POPULATIONS

Screening people who have had known or suspected mutagen exposures can be useful in quantifying exposures and assessing risks. In some cases of human mutagen exposures, data collected from the same individuals prior to ex-

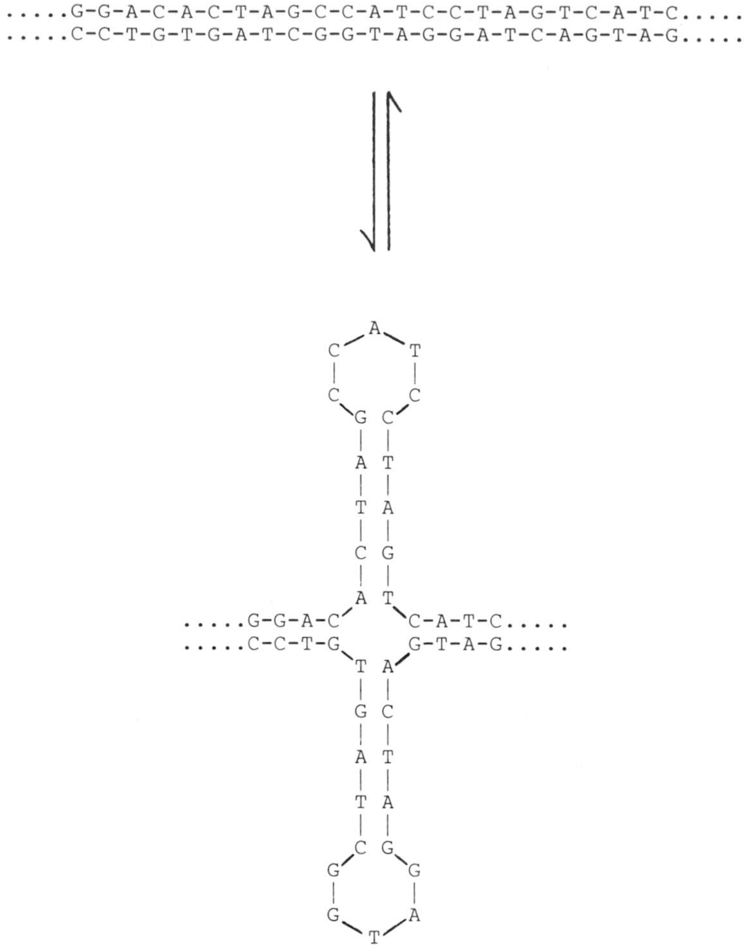

Figure 6-6. Formation of a hairpin-like secondary structure in a palindromic DNA sequence. Replication across the base of the hairpin can lead to deletion of the 15 base pairs in the hairpin.

posure can serve as a valuable baseline for comparison. Generally, however, the study population must be compared with an appropriate control population that is defined with cognizance of such factors as age, sex, smoking habits, and medical history.

Germ-Cell Mutagenesis

Monitoring for germ-cell mutagenesis involves looking for effects in the offspring of the study population. In principle, mutagenesis can be detected by monitoring for an increase in the frequency of sentinel phenotypes—characteristics that serve as indicators of new mutations—such as severe dominant genetic diseases. The requirements for serving as a sentinel phenotype are stringent and have been defined by Mulvihill and Czeizel (1983) as follows: "a clinical disorder or syndrome that occurs sporadical-

ly as a consequence of a single, highly penetrant mutant gene, that is a dominant or X-linked trait of considerable frequency and low fitness, and that is uniformly expressed and accurately diagnosable with minimal effort at or near birth." At least 36 autosomal dominant characteristics (e.g., Apert's syndrome, achondroplasia, aniridia) and five X-linked disorders are candidates for monitoring (Mulvihill and Czeizel, 1983).

The sentinel phenotypes approach is insensitive because the individual genetic diseases are rare, and large populations would be required to detect an increase in mutation rate. Moreover, the causes of disorders sometimes turn out to be more complex than had previously been thought (i.e., the new mutation of interest may not be the only cause of the phenotype) and diagnosis is not always unequivocal. There are also difficulties in study logistics that must be resolved, including the availability of appropriate medical records and confidentiality of data (Mulvihill and Czeizel, 1983). Monitoring for electrophoretic protein variants in blood samples of the offspring of a study population is an alternative to monitoring for diseases, but it similarly requires large populations.

Because of technical difficulties associated with mutation being a rare event, there is no clear evidence for the induction of heritable alterations in human germ cells. The sentinel phenotypes and electrophoretic methods may be appropriate in a few special instances of large mutagen exposures, such as survivors of childhood cancers who received large exposures to mutagenic chemotherapy or radiotherapy. They are not, however, suitable for monitoring small populations for evidence of mutagenesis, and they are not applicable to small exposures. For these reasons, a negative result in a population monitoring program for germ-cell mutagenesis may reflect the insensitivity of the method rather than the real absence of an effect (Hoffmann, 1983).

If one could detect mutations directly in spermatozoa, rather than in offspring of exposed individuals, one could collect useful data on human germ-cell mutagenesis from a small population, much as is done for somatic-cell mutagenesis. Various exposures cause morphological abnormalities in human sperm, including X rays, lead, and cigarette smoke. The mechanism underlying the formation of abnormal spermatozoa is uncertain, but the cause may be mutational in some cases. Nevertheless, because the origin is not necessarily genetic, morphological sperm abnormalities cannot be regarded as clear evidence of mutagenesis (Hoffmann, 1983).

Another alteration that has been studied in human spermatozoa is double fluorescent spots in quinacrine-stained preparations (Hoffmann, 1983; Allen *et al.*, 1986). Human Y chromosomes stained with quinacrine contain a fluorescent region, and it has been proposed that spermatozoa with two such spots (YFF) have two Y chromosomes. YFF sperm may therefore offer a means of detecting aneuploidy induced in human sperm. Increased frequencies of YFF sperm have been reported in men who have had exposures to X rays, the nematocide 1,2-dibromo-3-chloropropane, or the drugs Adriamycin or metronidazole. The YFF method, however, lacks genetic validation, and the fluorescent spots may occur by mechanisms other than nondisjunction and aneuploidy (Allen *et al.*, 1986). Consequently, evidence for the induction of aneuploidy in sperm based on the YFF method must be considered inconclusive (Hoffmann, 1983; Allen *et al.*, 1986).

The methods of molecular biology offer the possibility of novel strategies for measuring mutation rates in human populations. Approaches that have been considered include detecting alterations in restriction enzyme recognition sites in DNA, gradient electrophoresis of DNA heteroduplexes, RNAase digestion of RNA:DNA heteroduplexes, and hybridization with synthetic oligonucleotides (Delehanty *et al.*, 1986). These and other molecular approaches, however, are at an early stage of development and are not ready to be applied to monitoring for induced genetic changes. Moreover, they suffer from many of the same limitations as more traditional methods, notably that mutations occur at low frequencies, that many mutations are apt to be undetected by any single methodology, and that there are many confounding variables in studies of human populations. Nevertheless, there is room for optimism that refinements in molecular methodology will make human populations more amenable to mutational analysis in the future (Delehanty *et al.*, 1986).

Somatic-Cell Mutagenesis

Methods for detecting mutagenic effects in human somatic cells are more advanced than those in germ cells. Cytogenetics offers a direct link between mutagenicity tests in experimental organisms and effects in humans and is the most common means of detecting human mutagen exposures (Ashby and Richardson, 1985; Bender *et al.*, 1988; Carrano and Natarajan, 1988). Chromosome aberrations, including chromatid breaks, chromatid exchanges, acentric fragments, dicentric chromosomes, ring chromosomes, and some inversions and translocations can be scored in peripheral blood lymphocytes from people who have had mutagen exposures. Elevated frequencies of aberrations have been detected after exposures to ionizing radiation (Bender *et al.*, 1988) and diverse chemicals, including vinyl chloride, styrene, benzene, and ethylene oxide in occupational settings (Ashby and Richardson, 1985; Brusick, 1987). In the case of relatively large radiation exposures, one can estimate doses on the basis of frequencies of aberrations in promptly sampled lymphocytes (Bender *et al.*, 1988).

Like all toxicologic methods, cytogenetic monitoring has limitations. In instances of accidental and even medical exposures, preexposure aberration frequencies in the same individuals are often not known. It is therefore necessary to compare frequencies of aberrations to those of matched controls. Control frequencies, however, vary in different individuals and in different studies (Bender *et al.*, 1988). One reason for such variability is that many confounding variables affect the control and study populations (Carrano and Natarajan, 1988). The lack of baseline frequencies and variability in controls detract from the ability of cytogenetic methods to detect small increases in the frequency of aberrations. Another limitation is that aberrations in somatic cells cannot be interpreted clearly with respect to human health, and it is therefore difficult to tell a subject what his elevated frequency of aberrations means. Despite the limitations, elevated frequencies of aberrations in lymphocytes are a demonstrable genetic effect in human cells and provide evidence of mutagen exposure.

In addition to chromosome aberrations, sister chromatid exchanges (SCE) are readily monitored in people (Ashby and Richardson, 1985; Carrano and Natarajan, 1988). The mechanism of SCE is not well understood, but many mutagens are known to induce SCE, and SCE assays seem to be responsive to low doses. Moreover, the scoring of SCE is less subjective than the scoring of aberrations, and the assay is less costly. The problem of confounding variables in human populations remains, and the difficulty of explaining the result to subjects may be worse for SCE than for aberrations because of the lesser understanding of the alteration.

Gene mutations can be detected in human somatic cells *in vivo,* but methods for doing so are at an earlier stage of development than those for studying chromosomal alterations. Perhaps the most refined approach is a method developed by Richard Albertini and his colleagues for detecting lymphocytes that are resistant to 6-thioguanine because of a mutational alteration of HPRT activity (Nicklas *et al.,* 1989). This assay has permitted the detection of mutations in lymphocytes of patients receiving cancer chemotherapy or radiotherapy and is currently being used for the molecular analysis of mutations. Other methods that are under development for detecting mutations in human cells *in vivo* use fluorescent antibodies to detect mutant hemoglobins or mutant cell-surface glycoproteins in erythrocytes (Tates *et al.,* 1989).

Besides mutations and chromosomal alterations, other indicators of mutagen exposure have been applied in human monitoring (Brusick, 1987). The technique of ^{32}P-postlabeling is a sensitive method for detecting chemical adducts in DNA, and it may be applied in monitoring for exposure to various classes of mutagens and carcinogens. For example, it has been used to quantify adducts in DNA isolated from white blood cells of foundry workers who were occupationally exposed to polycyclic aromatic hydrocarbons (Phillips *et al.,* 1988). Similarly, the alkylation of amino acids in hemoglobin has been used as a quantitative indicator of occupational exposure to ethylene oxide (Ehrenberg, *et al.,* 1983). Testing concentrated urine for mutagenicity in short-term tests provides another indicator of mutagen exposures. Mutagenic substances have been detected in urine after exposures to cancer chemotherapy drugs, antiparasitic drugs, cigarette smoke, and several chemicals in occupational settings (Hoffmann, 1983).

ASSESSING MUTATIONAL HAZARDS

A troublesome aspect of human exposure to mutagens is that there is a long time between exposure and effect, whether it is the latency period in carcinogenesis or, even more so, the separation between germ-cell mutagenesis and effects in subsequent generations. Consequently, adverse effects in humans are not apt to be observed until after further exposures have occurred and, even then, the recognition of an effect and its cause may not be possible. Therefore, major goals in genetic toxicology are the identification of mutagens in experimental organisms, assessment of the risks that they pose, and prevention of unnecessary human exposures.

The fact that DNA is the hereditary material in all organisms provides a basis for extrapolating among species with respect to mutagenesis. Chemicals that are mutagens in one species are usually found to be mutagenic in others, and a positive result in any well-characterized mutagen assay therefore increases the likelihood that the agent is mutagenic in humans; such a test result calls for follow-up tests to characterize the nature of the mutagenic effect and evaluate its generality.

Despite the fact that DNA is the principal target for mutation induction, differences among species exist in mutagenesis, just as they exist in other areas of toxicology. Microorganisms and cultured mammalian cells differ from intact mammals in routes of exposure, dosimetry, distribution of toxicants, metabolism, and repair processes. Moreover, short-term tests cannot be related to mammalian germ cells, and even *Drosophila* does not parallel mammals perfectly in sensitivity of germ-cell stages to mutagenesis (National Academy of Sciences, 1983). The interpretation of test results with respect to human risk therefore requires extrapolation on many levels, and mammalian tests must have a central role. Genetic toxicology therefore relies on short-term tests for screening many chemicals and mammalian tests for the detailed study of selected model mutagens and for risk assessment.

Various strategies have been proposed for predicting risks to human germ cells on the basis of data from experimental organisms (National Academy of Sciences, 1983; Brusick, 1987; Sobels, 1989). These include direct extrapolation from nonmammalian species under various assumptions of proportionality among mutation rates; calculation of chemical mutagenic risks in terms of radiation equivalency; extrapolations based on ratios of molecular dosimetry data and mutation frequencies (i.e., the parallelogram approach); and the use of mouse data to estimate doses that would cause a proportional increase in frequencies of mutation or expected increases in human genetic diseases. Although not without shortcomings, estimations based on mouse germ-cell assays have received the greatest acceptance. Assays that have been prominent in risk assessment are the mouse specific-locus test (using visible genetic markers) and assays for dominant mutations that cause cataracts or skeletal abnormalities (National Academy of Sciences, 1980, 1983; Sobels, 1989).

Research and testing in genetic toxicology have brought progress in our ability to detect mutagens and understand the ways that they affect biological systems. However, the problems posed by environmental mutagens are complex, and our ability to assess mutational risks quantitatively is still rudimentary. A sustained effort in genetic toxicology will be required to discern which of the many environmental mutagens that have been identified pose significant risks and which pose negligible risks. Evaluating the impact of mutagenesis on humans must encompass gene mutations, chromosome aberrations, and aneuploidy and must consider effects in both somatic cells and germ cells.

ACKNOWLEDGMENTS

The author thanks Drs. S. Galloway and R. J. Preston for photographs of chromosomes; Drs. M. Bichara, D. M. DeMarini, H. Holden, K. Prestwich, and M. Shelby for helpful suggestions on the manuscript, and Mrs. Linda Hoffmann for her excellent secretarial assistance.

REFERENCES

Allen, J. W.; Liang, J. C.; Carrano, A. V.; and Preston, R. J.: Review of literature on chemical-induced aneuploidy in mammalian germ cells. *Mutat. Res.,* **167**:123–137, 1986.

Ashby, J., and Richardson, C. R.: Tabulation and assessment of 113 human surveillance cytogenetic studies conducted between 1965 and 1984. *Mutat. Res.,* **154**:111–133, 1985.

Auerbach, C.: *Mutation Research: Problems, Results, and Perspectives.* Chapman and Hall, London, 1976.

Bender, M. A.; Awa, A. A.; Brooks, A. L.; Evans, H. J.; Groer, P. G.; Littlefield, L. G.; Pereira, C.; Preston, R. J.; and Wachholz, B. W.: Current status of cytogenetic procedures to detect and quantify previous exposures to radiation. *Mutat. Res.,* **196**:103–159, 1988.

Bichara, M., and Fuchs, R. P. P.: DNA binding and mutation spectra of the carcinogen *N*-2-aminofluorene in *E. coli:* a correlation between the conformation of the premutagenic lesion and the mutation specificity. *J. Mol. Biol.,* **183**:341–351, 1985.

Bishop, J. M.: The molecular genetics of cancer. *Science,* **235**:305–311, 1987.

Brockman, H. E., and DeMarini, D. M.: Utility of short-term tests for genetic toxicity in the aftermath of the NTP's analysis of 73 chemicals. *Environ. Mol. Mutagen.,* **11**:421–435, 1988.

Brockman, H. E.; de Serres, F. J.; Ong, T.; DeMarini, D. M.; Katz, A. J.; Griffiths, A. J. F.; and Stafford, R. S.: Mutation tests in *Neurospora crassa:* a report of the U.S. Environmental Protection Agency Gene-Tox Program. *Mutat. Res.,* **133**:87–134, 1984.

Brusick, D.: *Principles of Genetic Toxicology,* 2nd ed. Plenum Press, New York, 1987.

Burnouf, D.; Koehl, P.; and Fuchs, R. P. P.: Single adduct mutagenesis: strong effect of the position of a single acetylaminofluorene adduct within a mutation hot spot. *Proc. Natl. Acad. Sci. USA,* **86**:4147–4151, 1989.

Calos, M. P., and Miller, J. H.: Genetic and sequence analysis of frameshift mutations induced by ICR-191. *J. Mol. Biol.,* **153**:39–66, 1981.

Carrano, A. V., and Natarajan, A. T.: Considerations for population monitoring using cytogenetic techniques. *Mutat. Res.,* **204**:379–406, 1988.

Cavenee, W. K.; Koufos, A.; and Hansen, M. F.: Recessive mutant genes predisposing to human cancer. *Mutat. Res.* **168**:3–14, 1986.

Cebula, T. A., and Koch, W. H.: Sequence analysis of *Salmonella typhimurium* revertants. In Mendelsohn, M. L. and Albertini, R. J. (eds.): *Mutation and the Environment, Part D: Carcinogenesis, Progress in Clinical and Biological Research,* Vol. 340D, Wiley-Liss, New York, 1990, pp. 367–377.

Constantin, M. J., and Nilan, R. A.: The chlorophyll-deficient mutant assay in barley *(Hordeum vulgaro):* a report of the U.S. Environmental Protection Agency Gene-Tox Program. *Mutat. Res.,* **99**:37–49, 1982.

Delehanty, J.; White, R. L.; and Mendelsohn, M. L.: Approaches to determining mutation rates in human DNA. *Mutat. Res.,* **167**:215–232, 1986.

Dellarco, V. L., and Prival, M. J.: Mutagenicity of nitro compounds in *Salmonella typhimurium* in the presence of flavin mononucleotide in a preincubation assay. *Environ. Mol. Mutagen.,* **13**:116–127, 1989.

Dellarco, V. L.; Voytek, P. E.; and Hollaender, A. (eds.): *Aneuploidy: Etiology and Mechanisms.* Plenum Press, New York, 1985.

DeMarini, D. M.; Brockman, H. E.; deSerres, F. J.; Evans, H. H.; Stankowski, L. F., Jr.; and Hsie, A. W.: Specific-locus mutations induced in eukaryotes (especially mammalian cells) by radiation and chemicals: a perspective. *Mutat. Res.,* **220**:11–29, 1989.

Dixon, K.; Roilides, E.; Hauser, J.; and Levine, A. S.: Studies on direct and indirect effects of DNA damage on mutagenesis in monkey cells using an SV40-based shuttle vector. *Mutat. Res.* **220**:73–82, 1989.

Dorado, G., and Pueyo, C.: L-Arabinose resistance test with *Salmonella typhimurium* as a primary tool for carcinogen screening. *Cancer Res.,* **48**:907–912, 1988.

Drake, J. W.; Glickman, B. W.; and Ripley, L.: Updating the theory of mutation. *Am. Scientist,* **71**:621–630, 1983.

Drobetsky, E. A.; Grosovsky, A. J.; and Glickman, B. W.: Perspectives on the use of an endogenous gene target in studies of mutational specificity. *Mutat. Res.*, **220**:235–240, 1989.

Ehrenberg, L.; Moustacchi, E.; and Osterman-Golkar, S.: Dosimetry of genotoxic agents and dose-response relationships of their effects. *Mutat. Res.*, **123**:121–182, 1983.

Elespuru, R.: Induction of bacteriophage lambda by DNA-interacting chemicals. In de Serres, F. J. (ed.): *Chemical Mutagens: Principles and Methods for Their Detection*, Vol. 9. Plenum Press, New York, 1984, pp. 213–231.

Ernst, J. F.; Hampsey, D. M.; and Sherman, F.: DNA sequences of frameshift and other mutations induced by ICR-170 in yeast. *Genetics*, **111**:233–241, 1985.

Friedberg, E. C.: *DNA Repair*. W. H. Freeman and Co., New York, 1985.

Galloway, S. M., and Ivett, J. L.: Chemically induced aneuploidy in mammalian cells in culture. *Mutat. Res.*, **167**:89–105, 1986.

Grant, W. F.: Chromosome aberration assays in *Allium*: a report of the U.S. Environmental Protection Agency Gene-Tox Program. *Mutat. Res.*, **99**:273–291, 1982.

Green, M. H. L.: Mutation testing using Trp$^+$ reversion in *Escherichia coli*. In Kilbey, B. J., Legator, M., Nichols, W., and Ramel, C. (eds.): *Handbook of Mutagenicity Test Procedures*, 2nd ed. Elsevier, Amsterdam, 1984, pp. 161–187.

Green, S.; Auletta, A.; Fabricant, J.; Kapp, R.; Manandhar, M.; Sheu, C.; Springer, J.; and Whitfield, B.: Current status of bioassays in genetic toxicology—the dominant lethal assay: a report of the U.S. Environmental Protection Agency Gene-Tox Program. *Mutat. Res.*, **154**:49–67, 1985.

Griesemer, R. A., and Cueto, C., Jr.: Toward a classification scheme for degrees of experimental evidence for the carcinogenicity of chemicals for animals. In Montesano, R.; Bartsch, H.; and Tomatis, L. (eds.): *Molecular and Cellular Aspects of Carcinogen Screening Tests*, IARC Scientific Publication 27. International Agency for Research on Cancer, Lyon, 1980, pp. 259–281.

Griffiths, A. J. F.; Brockman, H. E.; DeMarini, D. M.; and de Serres, F. J.: The efficacy of Neurospora in detecting agents that cause aneuploidy. *Mutat. Res.*, **167**:35–45, 1986.

Hartl, D. L.; Freifelder, D.; and Snyder, L. A.: *Basic Genetics*. Jones and Bartlett, Boston, 1988.

Hartman, P. E.; Ames, B. N.; Roth, J. R.; Barnes, W. M.; and Levin, D. E.: Target sequences for mutagenesis in *Salmonella* histidine-requiring mutants. *Environ. Mutagen.*, **8**:631–641, 1986.

Hoffmann, G. R.: Genetic effects of dimethyl sulfate, diethyl sulfate, and related compounds. *Mutat. Res.*, **75**:63–129, 1980.

————: Mutagenicity testing in environmental toxicology. *Environ. Sci. Technol.*, **16**:560A–574A, 1982.

————: Detection of effects of mutagens in human populations. In de Serres, F. J. (ed.): *Chemical Mutagens: Principles and Methods for Their Detection*, Vol. 8. Plenum Press, New York, 1983, pp. 1–53.

Hook, E. B.: Perspectives in mutation epidemiology: 3. Contribution of chromosome abnormalities to human morbidity and mortality and some comments upon surveillance of chromosome mutation rates. *Mutat. Res.*, **114**:389–423, 1983.

Ishidate, M., Jr.; Harnois, M. C.; and Sofuni, T.: A comparative analysis of data on the clastogenicity of 951 chemical substances tested in mammalian cell cultures. *Mutat. Res.*, **195**:151–213, 1988.

Kier, L. E.; Brusick, D. J.; Auletta, A. E.; Von Halle, E. S.; Brown, M. M.; Simmon, V. F.; Dunkel, V.; McCann, J.; Mortelmans, K.; Prival, M.; Rao, T. K.; and Ray, V.: The *Salmonella typhimurium*/mammalian microsomal assay: a report of the U.S. Environmental Protection Agency Gene-Tox Program. *Mutat. Res.*, **168**:69–240, 1986.

Koffel-Schwartz, N.; Verdier, J.-M.; Bichara, M.; Freund, A.-M.; Daune, M. P.; and Fuchs, R. P. P.: Carcinogen-induced mutation spectrum in wild-type, *uvrA* and *umuC* strains of *Escherichia coli*: strain specificity and mutation-prone sequences. *J. Mol. Biol.*, **177**:33–51, 1984.

Langenbach, R., and Oglesby, L.: The use of intact cellular activation systems in genetic toxicology assays. In de Serres, F. J. (ed.): *Chemical Mutagens: Principles and Methods for Their Detection*, Vol. 8. Plenum Press, New York, 1983, pp. 55–93.

Larsen, K. H.; Brash, D.; Cleaver, J. E.; Hart, R. W.; Maher, V. M.; Painter, R. B.; and Sega, G. A.: DNA repair assays as tests for environmental mutagens: a report of the U.S. EPA Gene-Tox Program. *Mutat. Res.*, **98**:287–318, 1982.

Latt, S. A.; Allen, J.; Bloom, S. E.; Carrano, A.; Falke, E.; Kram, D.; Schneider, E.; Schreck, R.; Tice, R.; Whitfield, B.; and Wolff, S.: Sister-chromatid exchanges: a report of the Gene-Tox Program. *Mutat. Res.*, **87**:17–62, 1981.

Lee, W. R.; Abrahamson, S.; Valencia, R.; von Halle, E. S.; Würgler, F. E.; and Zimmering, S.: The sex-linked recessive lethal test for mutagenesis in *Drosophila melanogaster*: a report of the U.S. Environmental Protection Agency Gene-Tox Program. *Mutat. Res.*, **123**:183–279, 1983.

Legator, M. S.; Bueding, E.; Batzinger, R.; Connor, T. H.; Eisenstadt, E.; Farrow, M. G.; Ficsor, G.; Hsie, A.; Seed, J.; and Stafford, R. S.: An evaluation of the host-mediated assay and body fluid analysis: a report of the U.S. Environmental Protection Agency Gene-Tox Program. *Mutat. Res.*, **98**:319–374, 1982.

Leifer, Z.; Kada, T.; Mandel, M.; Zeiger, E.; Stafford, R.; and Rosenkranz, H. S.: An evaluation of tests using DNA repair-deficient bacteria for predicting genotoxicity and carcinogenicity: a report of the U.S. EPA's Gene-Tox Program. *Mutat. Res.*, **87**:211–297, 1981.

Ma, T.: Tradescantia cytogenetic tests (root-tip mitosis, pollen mitosis, pollen mother-cell meiosis): a report of the U.S. Environmental Protection Agency Gene-Tox Program. *Mutat. Res.*, **99**:293–302, 1982.

Maron, D. M., and Ames, B. N.: Revised methods for the *Salmonella* mutagenicity test. *Mutat. Res.*, **113**:173–215, 1983.

Mavournin, K. H.; Blakey, D. H.; Cimino, M. C.; Salamone, M. F.; Heddle, J. C.: The in vivo micronucleus assay in mammalian bone marrow and peripheral blood: A report of the U. S. Environmental Protection Agency Gene-Tox Program. *Mutat. Res.* **239**:29–80, 1990.

McKusick, V. A.: *Mendelian Inheritance in Man: Catalogs of Autosomal Dominant, Autosomal Recessive, and X-Linked Phenotypes*, 8th ed. Johns Hopkins University Press, Baltimore, 1988.

Mitchell, A. D.; Casciano, D. A.; Meltz, M. L.; Robinson, D. E.; San, R. H. C.; Williams, G. M.; and Von Halle, E. S.: Unscheduled DNA synthesis tests: a report of the U.S. Environmental Protection Agency Gene-Tox Program. *Mutat. Res.*, **123**:363–410, 1983.

Mulvihill, J. J., and Czeizel, A.: Perspectives in mutation epidemiology, 6: a 1983 view of sentinel phenotypes. *Mutat. Res.*, **123**:345–361, 1983.

National Academy of Sciences, Committee on the Biological Effects of Ionizing Radiations: *The Effects on Populations of Exposure to Low Levels of Ionizing*

Radiation. National Academy Press, Washington, D.C., 1980.

National Academy of Sciences, Committee on Chemical Environmental Mutagens: *Identifying and Estimating the Genetic Impact of Chemical Mutagens*. National Academy Press, Washington, D.C., 1983.

Nicklas, J. A.; Hunter, T. C.; O'Neill, J. P.; and Albertini, R. J.: Molecular analyses of in vivo *hprt* mutations in human T-lymphocytes III. Longitudinal study of *hprt* gene structural alterations and T-cell clonal origins. *Mutat. Res., 215*:147–160, 1989.

Pastink, A.; Vreeken, C.; Nivard, M. J. M.; Searles, L. L.; and Vogel, E. W.: Sequence analysis of *N*-ethyl-*N*-nitrosourea-induced *vermilion* mutations in *Drosophila melanogaster. Genetics, 123*:123–129, 1989.

Phillips, D. H.; Hemminki, K.; Alhonen, A.; Hewer, A.; and Grover, P. L.: Monitoring occupational exposure to carcinogens: detection by ^{32}P-postlabeling of aromatic DNA adducts in white blood cells from iron foundry workers. *Mutat. Res., 204*:531–541, 1988.

Plewa, M. J.: Specific-locus mutation assays in *Zea mays:* A report of the U.S. Environmental Protection Agency Gene-Tox Program. *Mutat. Res., 99*:317–337, 1982.

Preston, R. J.: A short journey from classical to molecular cytogenetics. *Environ. Mol. Mutagen., 14*:126–132, 1989.

Preston, R. J.,; Au, W.: Bender, M. A.; Brewen, J. G.; Carrano, A. V.; Heddle, J. A.; Mc Fee, A.; Wolff, S.; and Wassom, J. S.: Mammalian in vivo and in vitro cytogenetic assays: a report of the U.S. EPA's Gene-Tox Program. *Mutat. Res., 87*:143–188, 1981.

Prival, M. J., and Dunkel, V. C.: Reevaluation of the mutagenicity and carcinogenicity of chemicals previously identified as "false positives" in the *Salmonella typhimurium* mutagenicity assay. *Environ. Mol. Mutagen., 13*:1–24, 1989.

Radman, M., and Wagner, R.: Mismatch repair in *Escherichia coli. Annu. Rev. Genet., 20*:523–538, 1986.

Resnick, M. A.; Mayer, V. W.; and Zimmermann, F. K.: The detection of chemically induced aneuploidy in *Saccharomyces cerevisiae:* an assessment of mitotic and meiotic systems. *Mutat. Res., 167*:47–60, 1986.

Ripley, L. S.; Clark, A.; and deBoer, J. G.: Spectrum of spontaneous frameshift mutations: Sequences of bacteriophage T4 *rII* gene frameshifts. *J. Mol. Biol., 191*:601–615, 1986.

Rossman, T. G., and Klein, C. B.: From DNA damage to mutation in mammalian cells: a review. *Environ. Mol. Mutagen., 11*:119–133, 1988.

Russell, L. B., and Shelby, M. D.: Tests for heritable genetic damage and for evidence of gonadal exposure in mammals. *Mutat. Res., 154*:69–84, 1985.

Schaaper, R. M.; Danforth, B. N.; and Glickman, B. W.: Mechanisms of spontaneous mutagenesis: An analysis of the spectrum of spontaneous mutation in the *Escherichia coli lacI* gene. *J. Mol. Biol., 189*:273–284, 1986.

Simmons, M. J., and Crow, J. F.: Mutations affecting fitness in *Drosophila* populations. *Annu. Rev. Genet., 11*:49–78, 1977.

Sobels, F. H.: Models and assumptions underlying genetic risk assessment. *Mutat. Res. 212*:77–89, 1989.

Straus, D. S.: Somatic mutation, cellular differentiation, and cancer causation. *J. Natl. Cancer Inst., 67*:233–241, 1981.

Styles, J. A., and Penman, M. G.: The mouse spot test: Evaluation of its performance in identifying chemical mutagens and carcinogens. *Mutat. Res., 154*:183–204, 1985.

Tates, A. D.; Bernini, L. F.; Natarajan, A. T.; Ploem, J. S.; Verwoerd, N. P.; Cole, J.; Green, M. H. L.; Arlett, C. F.; and Norris, P. N.: Detection of somatic mutants in man: HPRT mutations in lymphocytes and hemoglobin mutations in erythrocytes. *Mutat. Res., 213*:73–82, 1989.

Tennant, R. W.; Margolin, B. H.; Shelby, M. D.; Zeiger, E.; Haseman, J. K.; Spalding, J.; Caspary, W.; Resnick, M.; Stasiewicz, S.; Anderson, B.; and Minor, R.: Prediction of chemical carcinogenicity in rodents from in vitro genetic toxicity assays. *Science, 236*:933–941, 1987.

Valencia, R.; Abrahamson, S.; Lee, W. R.; Von Halle, E. S.; Woodruff, R. C.; Würgler, F. E.; and Zimmering, S.: Chromosome mutation tests for mutagenesis in *Drosophila melanogaster:* a report of the U.S. Environmental Protection Agency Gene-Tox Program. *Mutat. Res., 134*:61–88, 1984.

Van't Hof, J., and Schairer, L. A.: *Tradescantia* assay system for gaseous mutagens: a report of the U.S. Environmental Protection Agency Gene-Tox Program. *Mutat. Res., 99*:303–315, 1982.

Volkert, M. R.: Adaptive response of *Escherichia coli* to alkylation damage. *Environ. Mol. Mutagen., 11*:241–255, 1988.

Wassom, J. S.: Origins of genetic toxicology and the Environmental Mutagen Society. *Environ. Mol. Mutagen., 14*(Suppl. 16):1–6, 1989.

Würgler, F. E., and Vogel, E. W.: In vivo mutagenicity testing using somatic cells of *Drosophila melanogaster*. In de Serres, F. J. (ed.): *Chemical Mutagens: Principles and Methods for Their Detection*, Vol. 10. Plenum Press, New York. 1986, pp. 1–72.

Zimmering, S.; Mason, J. M.; and Osgood, C.: Current status of aneuploidy testing in Drosophila. *Mutat. Res., 167*:71–87, 1986.

Zimmermann, F. K.; von Borstel, R. C.; von Halle, E. S.; Parry, J. M.; Siebert, D.; Zetterberg, G.; Barale, R.; and Loprieno, N.: Testing of chemicals for genetic activity with *Saccharomyces cerevisiae:* a report of the U.S. Environmental Protection Agency Gene-Tox Program. *Mutat. Res., 133*:199–244, 1984.

Chapter 7

TERATOGENS

Jeanne M. Manson and *L. David Wise*

HISTORY

Teratology is concerned with the investigation of birth defects and is a field of study with roots going back to early primitive times. Abnormal births are events that have stimulated responses of awe, horror, and curiosity, and records of their occurrence have been transmitted in many forms. Legends, artistic renderings, and written descriptions of malformed infants can be found in cultural artifacts of many civilizations and provide a history of human perception of this event. It is believed that many mythologic figures originated with the birth of severely malformed infants (Thompson, 1930; Warkany, 1977). The similarities between some descriptions of mythologic beings and gods of antiquity to what we now recognize as patterns of human congenital malformations are remarkable. Births of abnormal infants have also been considered to be portents for events to come, and the word *monster* comes from a Latin root meaning *to warn* (Thompson, 1930). The most extensive early records of congenital malformations appear to have been kept for purposes of divination or foretelling the future, a practice that became so firmly established that a systematic record of congenital malformations was kept by many early civilizations (Warkany, 1977). Cross-breeding between humans and animals has been used as an explanation for abnormal births in offspring with hybrid features. An alternative belief, which still survives today in some parts of the world, is that the visual impressions and emotions of a woman during pregnancy can have a formative effect on fetal development. Unlike the situation in animals, which often cannibalize malformed offspring, the reaction of human populations to malformations has varied according to the belief of the culture. Responses have varied from practices of infanticide and withholding of life support to protective rearing and deification (Warkany, 1977). Today, scientific explanations are sought for the causes of birth defects, but there is no doubt that these strange, awe-some, and terrifying variations of human form are still a great mystery to us. Our reactions to them may not be so different from those of our ancestors, and profound ethical and legal questions remain concerning the causation and rearing of malformed children.

Experimental teratology first began in the late nineteenth century in studies of nonmammalian species. A variety of environmental conditions (temperature, microbial toxins, drugs) were found to perturb development in avian, reptile, fish, and amphibian species. Mammalian embryos were thought to be resistant to induction of malformations, and to be either killed outright or protected by the maternal system from adverse environmental conditions. The primary causal explanation for malformations in humans was genetic inheritance, and the terms *congenital* and *hereditary* were used interchangeably (Warkany, 1965). The first reports of induced birth defects in mammalian species came out in the 1930s to 1940s and were concerned with maternal nutritional deficiencies (i.e., vitamin A and riboflavin). These were followed by many other studies in which chemical and physical agents, i.e., nitrogen mustard, trypan blue, hormones, antimetabolites, alkylating agents, hypoxia, and X rays, to name a few (Warkany, 1965), were clearly shown to cause malformations in mammalian species.

The field of modern teratology has taken shape in the last 50 years with the development of animal models for producing birth defects, and with the occurrence of human epidemics of malformations induced by exogenous agents. The first such epidemic was reported by Gregg on rubella virus infections in pregnant women (Gregg, 1941). The eye, heart, and ear defects, as well as mental retardation, produced by rubella remained unrecognized until an epidemic of rubella infections in Austria elevated their incidence to the level where a clinical syndrome became apparent, and the etiology was identified. When rubella infection occurred during the first or second month of pregnancy, heart and eye defects predominated, whereas hearing defects were most commonly associated with infection in the third month. The risk of congenital anomalies associated with rubella infection in the first four weeks of pregnancy was estimated to be 61 percent; in weeks 5 to 8, 26 percent; and in weeks 9 to 12, 8 percent (Sever, 1967; Warkany, 1971b). Approximately 16 to 18 percent of pregnancies complicated by early rubella infections ended in miscarriage or stillbirth. Infections after the 14th week did not result in malformations but did carry risk for hearing and speech deficits, as well as mental retardation in the offspring (Warkany, 1971b). Rubella infections have not affected the overall incidence of malformations to a great extent, but their impact on pregnancy outcome has been severe at times of rubella epidemics. It has been estimated that in the United States alone approximately 20,000 children have been impaired as a consequence of prenatal rubella infections (Cooper and Krugman, 1966).

The embryos of mammals, including humans, were found to be susceptible to common external influences such as nutritional deficiencies and intrauterine infections. The full impact of these findings, however, was not brought to bear upon the public consciousness until 1961, when the association between thalidomide ingestion by pregnant women and the birth of severely malformed infants was established. In contrast to the situation with rubella, the teratogenicity of thalidomide in humans was recognized relatively quickly because a syndrome of severe and rare limb defects was produced. If only common malformations had been induced by thalidomide, it might have taken much longer to recognize the syndrome and to identify the cause.

Thalidomide was introduced in 1956 by the drug manufacturer Chemie Grunethal as a sedative/hypnotic, and was used throughout the world as a sleep aid and to ameliorate nausea and vomiting in pregnancy. It had no apparent toxicity or addictive properties in humans and adult animals at therapeutic exposure levels. The drug was widely prescribed under a variety of trade names (e.g., Contergan, Distaval, Kevadon), at an oral dose of 50 to 200 mg/day. There were a few reports of peripheral neuritis attributable to thalidomide, but only in patients with long-term use for up to 18 months (Fullerton and Kermer, 1961). In 1960, a large increase in newborns with rare limb malformations was recorded in West Germany. The affected children had amelia (absence of the limbs) or various degrees of phocomelia (preaxial reduction of the long bones of the limbs), usually affecting the arms more than the legs, and usually involving both left and right sides, although to different degrees. At the

University Pediatric Clinic in Hamburg, for example, no cases of phocomelia were seen in the decade 1949 to 1959. In 1959, there was a single case; in 1960, 30 cases; and in 1961, 154 cases (Taussig, 1962). Comparable increases in the frequency of these rare limb anomalies occurred in other parts of the world where thalidomide was in use. Congenital heart disease; ocular, intestinal, and renal anomalies; and malformations of the external ears were also involved, but the limb defects were the most characteristic element of the malformation pattern (Warkany, 1971a). In 1961, Lenz in Germany (Lenz, 1963) and McBride in Australia (McBride, 1961) independently identified thalidomide as the causative agent. The drug was withdrawn from the market at the end of 1961, and by August of 1962 the epidemic subsided. Subsequent studies indicated that 70 percent of mothers with characteristically affected children had taken thalidomide during the first three months of pregnancy, 14 percent had taken it without being able to identify accurately the time of ingestion, 8 percent had possibly taken it, and 8 percent had a definite negative history of thalidomide ingestion (Weicker, 1963).

The critical period for limb malformations was found to be the sixth and seventh weeks of pregnancy (35 to 50 days from the first day of the last menstrual period or 23 to 38 days after conception) (Nowack, 1965). Exposure beyond this period could result in minor defects such as hypoplastic thumbs and anorectal stenosis. The malformation rate was extremely high in infants exposed during the sensitive period, and some studies have suggested that every woman ingesting the drug during this period had an offspring with some type of malformation, ranging from major to minor defects (Knapp, 1963). No relationship has been established between the severity of the malformations and the amount of drug taken during the sensitive period (Schardein, 1976). Projections of the number of children deformed by thalidomide range upward to 10,000, but more conservative estimates place the number between 7000 and 8000 (Lenz, 1966). West Germany, England, Wales, and Japan were the countries most affected, whereas only a few cases were reported from the United States, where sale of thalidomide was delayed by Dr. Frances Kelsey of the Food and Drug Administration. Whereas malformations of the limbs were the most conspicuous element of thalidomide embryopathy, defects of the cardiovascular, intestinal, and urinary systems had most often been the cause of death in affected children (Warkany, 1971a).

After the discovery of the teratogenic effects of thalidomide in humans, experimental studies in animals were undertaken to reproduce the syndrome of malformations. An unexpected finding was that the mouse and rat were resistant, the rabbit and hamster variably responsive, and certain strains of primates were sensitive to thalidomide developmental toxicity. Different strains of the same species of animals were also found to have highly variable sensitivity to thalidomide. Factors such as differences in absorption, distribution, biotransformation, and placental transfer have been ruled out as causes of the variability in species and strain sensitivity. The New Zealand white rabbit had been the most widely used animal owing to its relatively consistent response, and thalidomide exposure during the sensitive period (days 8 to 10 of pregnancy) results in a wide spectrum of malformations, particularly of the limbs (reviewed in Fabro, 1981).

The chemical structure of thalidomide [(±)-3'-phthalimidoglutarimide] is shown in Figure 7–1. The compound is relatively insoluble and unstable in aqueous solutions. Primary hydrolysis products are formed by cleavage of the four amidic bonds, and these products then undergo additional nonenzymatic breakdown to form secondary, tertiary, and quarternary hydrolysis products (Schumacher et al., 1965). The relatively lipophilic parent compound is found at similar concentrations in maternal plasma and embryonic tissue and is believed to cross the

Thalidomide [(±)–3' phthalimidoglutarimide]

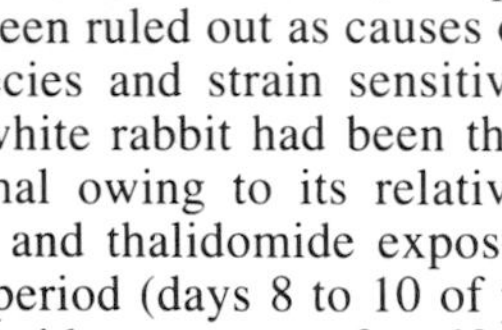

Teratogenic Analogs of Thalidomide

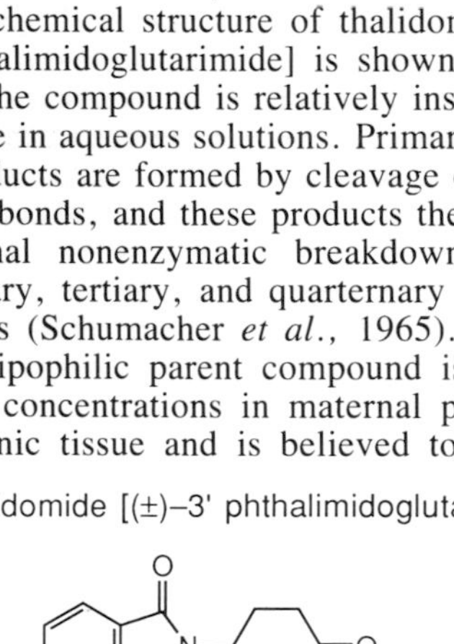

Figure 7–1. Chemical structures of thalidomide and analogs with teratogenic activity.

placenta by simple diffusion (Fabro et al., 1967). Several of the hydrolysis products are found at higher concentrations in the embryo than in the maternal plasma, a finding that has given rise to the "trapping" hypothesis. According to this hypothesis, the lipophilic parent compound crosses the placenta and enters the embryonic compartment where it undergoes spontaneous cleavage to the highly charged hydrolysis products. These products are then trapped in the embryonic compartment because they are too polar to pass back into the maternal circulation (Keberle et al., 1965). Even though bioaccumulation of the hydrolysis products in the embryo has been well established, the hydrolysis products themselves do not appear to possess significant teratogenic activity. Extensive structure-activity studies have been carried out with over 60 compounds stereochemically related to thalidomide (Schumacher, 1975). The structural requirements for teratogenicity appear to be quite strict insofar as only thalidomide itself and three other analogs (Figure 7–1) are clearly teratogenic in the rabbit. An intact phthalimide or phthalimidine group appears to be essential for teratogenic activity, and the glutarimide moiety can be replaced by a glutarimide ester group or a structure that can be converted into a glutarimide ring without loss of teratogenic activity.

A number of theories have been proposed to explain the biochemical and cellular mechanisms of thalidomide teratogenicity (reviewed in Schumacher, 1975; Fabro, 1981; Stephens, 1988). These have included interference with folic acid or glutamic acid metabolism, depurination of DNA through intercalation between base pairs, and acylation of polyamines. Potential sites of cellular toxicity that have been examined include direct toxic effects on limb mesenchyme tissue, inhibition of mesonephric-limb tissue interaction, and damage to the developing neural crest tissue leading to segmental sensory peripheral neuropathy. Despite intense effort made over the past 20 years, none of these hypotheses have been adequately substantiated, or definitively disproved, and the mode of action remains unknown. A more fundamental understanding of the mechanisms of normal morphogenesis will need to be achieved before there is an explanation for the teratogenic effects of thalidomide.

After the thalidomide episode and the recognition of species differences in response and sensitivity, the emphasis in the field of teratology shifted from genetic inheritance as a primary causal explanation for birth defects to xenobiotic exposures during pregnancy. There has been a tremendous increase in research on xenobiotic teratogens since the thalidomide episode, much of which has been influenced by the characteristic and perhaps unique events associated with the human response to this drug.

Another agent implicated in a spectrum of developmental toxicities in humans is diethylstilbestrol (DES). Between 1966 and 1969, seven young women between the ages of 15 and 22 were seen at the Massachusetts General Hospital with clear-cell adenocarcinoma of the vagina. This tumor had previously never been seen in patients below the age of 30, with a primary occurrence in women over 50. An epidemiologic case-control study was carried out to identify etiologic factors, and an association was found with maternal ingestion of DES in the first trimester of pregnancy (reviewed in Poskanzer and Herbst, 1977). DES was widely used from the mid-1940s to 1970 in the United States to prevent threatened miscarriage and was believed to stimulate the placenta to synthesize higher levels of estrogen and progesterone. A study of the therapeutic value of DES was carried out in 1953, and administration of DES in graduated amounts prior to the 20th week up to the 35th week of pregnancy was found to have no effect on the incidence of abortion, prematurity, postmaturity, perinatal mortality, or toxemia of pregnancy (Dieckmann *et al.*, 1953). Despite these findings, DES treatment continued, and in the 1960s a committee of the National Academy of Science rated the drug as "possibly effective" for the treatment of high-risk pregnancies.

After the association was made between maternal ingestion of DES during the first trimester and vaginal adenocarcinoma in female offspring, a registry of Clear Cell Adenocarcinoma of the Genital Tract in Young Females was established in 1971. Reports from this registry have indicated that treatment prior to the 18th week of pregnancy is necessary for genital tract abnormalities to occur. The incidence of genital cancer peaked in DES-exposed female offspring at age 19 and declined through age 22. The absolute risk for developing clear-cell adenocarcinoma of the vagina and cervix with prenatal exposure was low, in the range of 0.14 to 1.4/1000 through age 24 (Herbst *et al.*, 1977). A high proportion of DES-exposed female offspring had other disorders of the vagina and cervix, including vaginal adenosis, cervical erosion, transverse fibrous ridges of the vagina and cervix, and cervical pseudopolyps. In one study of approximately 100 female offspring per group, vaginal adenosis was found in 35 percent of exposed versus 1 percent of control subjects. Fibrous ridges of the vaginal and cervix were found in 22 percent of exposed and none in the

controls. Overall, abnormalities of a benign nature were found in about 75 percent of female offspring exposed to DES *in utero* (Poskanzer and Herbst, 1977).

Abnormal physical findings have also been identified in male offspring exposed *in utero* to DES (reviewed in Bibbo *et al.*, 1977). In one study with approximately 165 male offspring per group, epididymal cysts, hypotrophic testes, and capsular induration were found in 25 percent of exposed versus 6 percent of control males. Low ejaculate volume was found in 26 percent, and poor semen quality in 28 percent of exposed men and none in controls. Malignant lesions have not been observed in male offspring. The primary lesion induced in both sexes is believed to be persistence of Müllerian duct derivatives in the genital tract with DES exposure between 6 and 16 weeks of gestation in humans. The persistence of embryonic, columnar Müllerian epithelium is believed to occur in areas of the vagina that are normally transformed to squamous cells in female fetuses. In male fetuses, the Müllerian ducts normally regress, but derivatives participate in formation of the prostate and other accessory organs. Incomplete regression of Müllerian derivatives or abnormal participation of the derivatives in formation of the male genital tract may give rise to the genital lesions observed (McLachlan and Dixon, 1977).

Animal models have been developed to reproduce the human syndrome (reviewed in Schardein, 1985), and adenocarcinomas have been reported in mice at 18 months after exposure. In Wistar rats, vaginal adenocarcinoma and squamous cell carcinoma have been produced with DES in a dose-related manner. Although uterovaginal development is probably similar in rodents and humans, the timing is different with the critical periods occurring prenatally in humans and neonatally in rodents.

Chronic ingestion of alcohol during pregnancy has also been implicated in causing substantial risk to human pregnancy. It was not until 1973 that the embryotoxic effects of alcohol were placed into a category and termed fetal alcohol syndrome, or FAS. Chronic ingestion of alcohol produces variable and nonspecific embryotoxicity, most frequently manifested as intrauterine growth retardation, psychomotor dysfunction, and craniofacial anomalies (Jones and Smith, 1973). These features are not unique, and accurate diagnosis of FAS is often not possible without a prior knowledge of maternal alcohol consumption. It is estimated that full expression of FAS occurs in one or two live births/1000, and that partial expression is present in an additional three to five live births/1000 (Abel, 1980).

Intrauterine growth retardation is the most sensitive measure of prenatal alcohol exposure and is characterized by deficiencies in height and weight and a lack of postnatal catchup. Risk of intrauterine growth retardation increases with maternal consumption of at least 1 oz of absolute alcohol per day (Kaminski *et al.*, 1981). Heavy alcohol consumption, defined as consumption of five or more drinks per occasion and a consistent daily intake of more than 45 ml of absolute alcohol, is clearly associated with a threefold increase in small-for-gestation-age infants (Sokol *et al.*, 1980). The risk is significantly decreased if alcohol consumption is reduced during the third trimester (Rosett *et al.*, 1980).

Mental retardation characterized by IQ score more than 2 standard deviations below the mean has been found in 85 percent of FAS children. Learning disabilities are manifested as impulsiveness, restlessness, shortened attention span, distractability, and speech and language disorders (Streissguth *et al.*, 1978). Craniofacial anomalies include shortened palpebral fissure, epicanthal folds, broadened nasal bridge, upturned nose, and thinned upper lip. Additional and more severe neuropathologic effects are microcephaly, hydrocephaly, and cerebral and cerebellar disorganization. The risk for congenital anomalies is not as well defined as for intrauterine growth retardation. Consumption in excess of 2 oz of absolute alcohol/day is necessary to increase significantly the incidence of malformations (Sokol *et al.*, 1980). Consumption levels associated with these adverse outcomes have been obtained by self-reporting, and under-reporting of consumption by heavy drinkers is a likely source of bias. The potential synergistic effects of caffeine and cigarette smoking must also be taken into consideration.

Many species of laboratory animals have been treated with ethanol during pregnancy with varying degrees of success in reproducing human FAS. Attempts to develop a model of FAS in nonhuman primates have yielded equivocal results, and at present primates are not suitable for replicating the human syndrome (Scott and Fradkin, 1981). The most consistent findings in rats are intrauterine growth retardation, embryolethality, and behavioral deficits (Henderson *et al.*, 1979). The mouse appears to be the best species for producing birth defects with alcohol (Chernoff, 1980). The high exposure levels (4 to 8 g/kg) required to produce these developmental toxicities can cause prolonged maternal sedation. Consequently, the confounding role of food and water deprivation should be considered in animal models of FAS. Whether the human fetus is at risk from moderate social drinking or only from severe chronic alcoholism cannot be accurately determined at this time, leading to the recommendation that alcohol consumption be reduced to the greatest extent possible during pregnancy.

It is estimated that 25 million Americans used cocaine in 1986 and that 5 million are habitual users (NIDA, 1987). Increased cocaine use by people in their reproductive years is of particular concern because cocaine has been implicated as a potential human teratogen which can produce structural abnormalities and behavioral deficits in infants exposed *in utero*. The incidence of cocaine-induced birth defects is two to three times higher than the frequency observed in control populations. MacGregor *et al.* (1987) reported that 6 percent of the 70 cocaine-exposed infants in a case-controlled study had congenital malformations which included one case of the prune belly syndrome; one with jejunal atresia and bowel infarction; and one infarct with multiple malformations of the anus, kidney, and limbs. Similar abnormalities were observed by Bingol *et al.* (1987) in their study of 50 women who used cocaine only and 110 women who were polydrug users matched against 340 drug-free mothers for socioeconomic status and ethnicity. Chasnoff *et al.* (1988) observed nine infants with congenital defects in cocaine-complicated pregnancies; four had prune belly syndrome with limb defects, two had genital abnormalities (hypospadias), and three had renal defects. Thus, a broad spectrum of congenital defects has been observed, with the limbs and genitourinary systems being most frequently affected.

In addition to these malformations, there have been reports of sixfold to sevenfold elevations in the frequency of premature labor and abruptio placentae in cocaine-complicated pregnancies, and a significant difference in birth weights, lengths, and head circumference for infants who were delivered at term (Chasnoff, 1989). Cocaine acts peripherally to inhibit nerve conduction and prevent norepinephrine reuptake at nerve terminals, resulting in increased norepinephrine levels with subsequent vasoconstriction, tachycardia, and abrupt rise in blood pressure. Placental vasoconstriction also occurs which decreases blood flow to the fetus. Uterine contractility is also increased as a result of elevation in norepinephrine levels. The increased incidence of preterm labor and abruptio placentae is consistent with these pharmacologic actions of cocaine (reviewed in Chasnoff, 1989).

Newborn cocaine-exposed infants have been characterized as "fragile" and easily overloaded by environmental stimuli (reviewed in Chasnoff, 1989). Although significant improvement was shown by one month of age, the exposed infants still performed significantly poorer than controls in their management of stimulation and their ability to maintain alertness without becoming overloaded. The infants also displayed abnormal reflexes and hypertoxicity persisting through at least four months of age. Further research in this area is greatly needed and should focus on developmental disabilities of cocaine-exposed infants as well as the dynamics of maternal/infant interactions in a substance abusing mother.

Animal models for cocaine-induced developmental toxicity have been developed. Finnell *et al.* (1990) exposed mice on days 6 to 8 or 8 to 10 of gestation and observed dose-related increases in malformations without effects on resorption, maternal weight gain, or fetal weights. The types of malformations observed were similar to those reported in humans and included cardiovascular defects, limb abnormalities, and genitourinary malformations. The behavioral sequellae of neonatal cocaine administration have been examined in rats (Henderson and McMillen, 1990). The principal findings were that cocaine-exposed pups had delays in acquisition of righting reflex and were hyperactive at 30 days of age.

The greatest concern today over therapeutic drug usage during pregnancy centers around the synthetic retinoids. Isotretinoin (Accutane®) is a synthetic retinoid that is highly efficacious in treatment of recalcitrant cystic acne. Despite clear warnings against use during pregnancy on the label of this prescription drug, an extensive physician and patient education program, and restrictive requirements for prescription to women of child-bearing potential, an incidence of malformed babies attributed to isotretinoin exposure has been reported every year since 1983. In a prospective study of 57 pregnant women exposed during the first trimester, 9 had spontaneous abortion, 1 malformed stillbirth, 10 malformed live births, and 37 live births without evidence of major malformation (Lammer *et al.,* 1987). This represents a risk for malformation of 23 percent for fetuses that reach 20 weeks of gestation. Among 21 malformed infants reported in another study (Lammer *et al.,* 1985), 17 had craniofacial defects, 12 anomalies of the heart, 18 malformations of the CNS, and 7 thymus anomalies. A combination of defects was reported in 10 of the 21 infants. Follow-up of affected children is not complete, but preliminary findings indicate that neuropsychologic impairments are being found in 40 to 65 percent of prenatally exposed 5-year-old children without major malformations (Lammer and Adams, 1989).

Isotretinoin is teratogenic in all common laboratory animal species, as is excess of retinoic acid (vitamin A). The retinoids are so widely teratogenic in a consistently reproducible pattern that they are considered to be universal teratogens. A listing of the lowest doses of isotretinoin that malform organ systems in different species is given in Table 7–1. Of interest is the very high doses of isotretinoin needed to induce malformations in rats and mice, which are approximately an order of magnitude greater than for other laboratory animals and two orders of magnitude greater than for humans. The lack of potency in mice may be related to rapid elimination of isotretinoin from maternal plasma and a low level of placental transfer (Kraft *et al.,* 1987). A major metabolite of isotretinoin, 4-oxo-isotretinoin, has been found to possess teratogenic activity. *In vivo,* this metabolite is a more potent teratogen than the parent compound (Kochhar and Penner, 1987), whereas *in vitro* the two are of nearly equal potency (Webster *et al.,* 1986). However, in humans (Brazzell *et al.,* 1983), the level of 4-oxo-isotretinoin is two to five times higher than isotretinoin with repeated administration, and it is generally believed that teratogenicity occurs from exposure of the conceptus to isotretinoin, 4-oxo-isotretinoin as well as to retinoic acid derived by conversion from isotretinoin.

There is much controversy over regulation of isotretinoin exposure to women of child-bearing potential. Teenagers comprise a large segment of the patient population and it is recognized that this population can be sexually active without strict adherence to contraceptive measures. Stringent conditions have been placed on prescription of the drug to women of child-bearing potential which include mandatory contraceptive measures, oral and written warnings of hazards during pregnancy, serum pregnancy tests before and during therapy, and the necessity that the patient have severe disfiguring cystic acne that is recalcitrant to standard therapies. Despite these stringent conditions new cases of human malformations resulting from isotretinoin treatment continue to be reported. This tragedy has led some to demand withdrawal of the drug from the market and others to recommend restricted distribution in designated centers and physicians specifically trained in the criteria for prescribing isotretinoin. It is not clear how this therapeutically effective drug can be made available to those who will benefit from it while at the same time ensuring that exposure during early pregnancy does not occur. It is necessary that the manufacturer, the prescribing physician, and the patient must all play a role in resolution of this problem.

PROTOCOL TESTING

Following the thalidomide episode, a reexamination and expansion of testing procedures

Table 7–1. LOWEST EFFECT LEVEL OF ISOTRETINOIN IN LABORATORY ANIMALS AND HUMANS

SPECIES	DOSE (mg/kg/day)	TREATMENT PERIOD*	MALFORMATIONS	REFERENCE
Mouse	100	6–15	Craniofacial	Agnish, 1989
Rat	75	8–10	Craniofacial	Agnish, 1989
Rabbit	10	7–18	Skeletal, CNS, other visceral	Kamm et al., 1984
Monkey	5	70–84	Cleft palate	Kochhar and McBride, 1986
Human	0.4	Variable	Craniofacial, cardiovascular, CNS, thymus	Lammer et al., 1985

* Days of pregnancy.

for identification of developmental toxicity of drugs was carried out by the Food and Drug Administration. In 1966 the document *Guidelines for Reproduction Studies for Safety Evaluation of Drugs for Human Use* (FDA, 1966) was issued. Similar documents have been issued for evaluation of food additives, pesticides, and household products (FDA, 1970; CPSC, 1977). A brief description of these protocols will be given here, and additional information can be obtained from more comprehensive reviews (Adams and Buelke-Sam, 1981; Palmer, 1981; Manson and Kang, 1989).

In the multigeneration study, animals are continuously exposed to the test agent in the food or water throughout two to three generations. This test protocol was developed to assess chemical agents that are likely to accumulate in the body with long-term exposures, such as food additives and pesticides, and provides an overview of the reproductive process. Parental animals are first exposed shortly after weaning (30 to 40 days) and, when reproductively mature, are mated to produce the F_1 generation. F_1 offspring are selected to produce F_2 offspring, and the same procedure is followed for production of the F_3 generation, all of which are killed at weaning. Three treatment groups and one control group are employed, and a minimum of 20 pregnant females per group and per generation are included. Rodent species are most frequently used, allowing completion of the three-generation study within 20 months. The effect of the test agent on fertility, litter size, sex ratio, neonatal viability, and growth is monitored throughout each generation.

Testing procedures for evaluation of short-term exposures, particularly to drugs, are the three-segment single-generation studies. These consist of three segments: I, evaluation of fertility and general reproductive performance; II, assessment of developmental toxicity; and III, peri- and postnatal evaluation. Segment I tests include treatment of male rodents for 70 days and female rodents for 14 days, and treatment of females is continued during mating, pregnancy, and lactation. At term (days 20 to 21) half of the females are killed and uterine contents examined for preimplantation and postimplantation death, and fetuses for external, visceral, and skeletal morphogenesis. The other half are allowed to deliver and wean their offspring. Weanlings are killed and autopsied for gross visceral abnormalities. This study phase provides an overview of effects on fertility, conception rates, pre- and postimplantation survival, parturition, and lactation.

Segment II studies include the treatment of inseminated females during the organogenesis period alone. One day prior to birth, females are killed and fetuses are delivered by cesarean section. Developmental toxicity is assessed in terms of the occurrence of early or late embryo (fetal) deaths; reduced fetal body weight; and the presence of gross, visceral, and skeletal malformations. In Segment III studies, effects of perinatal and postnatal development are measured. Pregnant females are exposed during the last third of gestation and through weaning. The purpose of this study is to identify effects of the test agent on late fetal development, labor and delivery, lactation, neonatal viability, and growth of the offspring. Common variants of this test are to allow weanlings to survive to adulthood for assessment of neurobehavioral deficits, fertility, and the occurrence of perinatally induced cancer.

Much controversy exists today about the adequacy of these test protocols. They were based on the understanding of reproductive and developmental toxicology 25 years ago, which was strongly influenced by the thalidomide episode. As basic knowledge has improved, recommendations have been made for alterations of these protocols and for inclusion of *in vitro* tests. At best, these protocols have served as a "norm" for safety evaluation of chemicals for reproductive and developmental effects. They have provided a uniform format for compilation of extensive historical data. At worst, the protocols have inhibited development of new approaches for understanding reproductive and developmental toxicity. This is a topic of active consideration in academic, regulatory, and industrial sectors and one that should result in a reexamination of how to determine both safety and therapeutic efficacy of drugs intended for use by pregnant women, as well as the toxicity of environmental agents to which humans are inadvertently exposed.

DIMENSION OF THE PROBLEM

In the remainder of this chapter, the importance of xenobiotics as factors contributing to adverse pregnancy outcome is explored. Those outcomes associated with prenatal insult alone will be emphasized even though damage to the adolescent and adult reproductive and neuroendocrine systems can also result in reproductive dysfunction. These aspects are covered in Chapter 16 *(Toxic Responses of the Reproductive System)*. Extensive data are available on reproductive performance in the human population that provide useful information on the frequency but not the cause of reproductive failure. Although early spontaneous abortions often go unreported, particularly among pregnancies of less than 20 weeks' duration, their frequency has been estimated to be 15 percent of all recognized pregnancies (Warburton and Fraser, 1964). This figure is generally considered to be an underestimate insofar as most spontaneous abortions occur early in gestation, often before the pregnancy is recognized. Of approximately 3 million infants born alive each year, 13.1 per 1000 die within the first year (NCHS, 1980). Approximately 3 percent of liveborn infants have major congenital malformations recognized within the first year of life and birth defects account for 20% of postnatal deaths (National Foundation, 1981a). When defects that become apparent only later in life are included, the frequency of major and minor malformations increases to about 16 percent (Chung and Myrianthopoulos, 1975). Close to one-half of the children in hospital wards are there because of prenatally acquired malformations (Shepard, 1986). Approximately 7 percent of newborns are born prematurely (before the 37th week) and 7 percent of infants born at full term have low birth weights (2.5 kg or less) (USDHEW, 1972).

In very few cases has it been possible to separate the impact of a specific chemical exposure on human reproduction from the background rate of spontaneous defects or from other causes such as radiation, infection, nutritional deficiencies, or maternal diseases. Wilson (1973) has estimated that 23 to 35 percent of birth defects have an identifiable genetic component, and 7 to 11 percent have an identifiable external factor, such as radiation, drugs, environmental chemicals, infections, and maternal metabolic imbalances. For 55 to 70 percent of birth defects, no causal associations can be made at present. Correlation between exposure to a specific chemical agent and adverse pregnancy outcome is also complicated by the magnitude of chemical agents in the environment. The Chemical Abstract Service of the American Chemical Society listed 4,039,906 individual chemical entities as of November 1977, with an average growth rate of 6000 new entries per week (Maugh, 1978). In the NIOSH Registry of Toxic Substances (NIOSH, 1977), there were 37,860 entries of agents in common industrial use, of which 585 had notations of teratogenic activity. Schardein (1985) reported that a total of 2820 compounds had been tested for teratogenicity as of 1984, with 782 compounds showing positive effects and an additional 291 being possibly teratogenic. In the Catalog of Teratogenic Agents compiled by Thomas Shepard (1986), over 900 agents causing congenital anomalies in laboratory animals are listed, with only 30 known to cause defects in humans (see Table 7–2). Many gaps exist in our understanding of how to predict which chemicals among the thousands in the environment possess teratogenic activity, of the correlation between responses of laboratory animals and humans, and of the mechanisms of action of teratogens in any species. The following discussion of some well-established principles of teratology should indicate, however, that much progress has been made in these areas since the thalidomide episode.

PRINCIPLES OF TERATOLOGY

Definition of Terms

The term *developmental toxicity* covers any detrimental effect produced by exposures to developing organisms during embryonic stages of development. Such effects can be either irreversible or reversible. Embryolethal effects are incompatible with survival of the conceptus and result in resorption, spontaneous abortion, or stillbirth. Irreversible effects that are compatible with survival may result in structural or functional anomalies in live offspring, and these are called teratogenic. Persistent lesions that cause overall growth retardation or delayed growth of specific organ systems are generally referred to as embryotoxic. For a chemical to be labeled a teratogen, it must significantly increase the occurrence of structural or functional abnormalities in offspring after it is administered to either parent before conception, to the female during

Table 7–2.   KNOWN HUMAN TERATOGENS

Radiation	*Drugs/Chemicals*
Therapeutic	Androgenic hormones
Radioiodine	Aminopterin
Atomic weapons	Cyclophosphamide
	Busulfan
Infections	Thalidomide
Rubella virus	Mercury, organic
Cytomegalovirus	Chlorobiphenyls
Herpes simplex virus	Diethylstilbestrol
Toxoplasmosis	Diphenylhydantoin
Venezuelan equine encephalitis virus	Trimethadione
Syphilis	Coumarin anti-
	coagulants
Maternal Metabolic Imbalances	Valproic acid
Cretinism	Antithyroid drugs
Diabetes	Tetracyclines
Phenylketonuria	13-cis-retinoic acid
Virilizing tumors, metabolic conditions	Lithium
Alcoholism	Methimazole
Hyperthermia	
Rheumatic disease and congenital heart block	

Adapted from Shepard, 1986.

pregnancy, or directly to the developing organism.

Many teratologists believe that any xenobiotic administered under appropriate conditions of dose and time of development can cause some disturbances in embryonic development in some laboratory species (Karnofskey, 1965; Staples, 1975). For an agent to be classified as a developmental toxicant, it must produce adverse effects on the conceptus at exposure levels that do not induce severe toxicity in the mother (e.g., substantial reduction in weight gain, persistent emesis, hypo- or hyperactivity, or convulsions). Adverse effects on development under these conditions may be secondary to perturbations in the maternal system. The main reason for conducting developmental toxicity studies is to ascertain whether an agent causes specific or unique toxicity to pregnant animals or to the conceptus. If these studies are conducted under extreme conditions of maternal toxicity, then identification of exposures uniquely toxic to the conceptus or pregnant animal is not possible. Xenobiotics can be deliberately administered at maternally toxic doses to determine the threshold level for adverse effects on the offspring. In such cases conclusions can be qualified to indicate that adverse effects on the conceptus were obtained at maternally toxic exposure levels, and may not be indicative of selective or unique developmental toxicity.

Time of Exposure

Compared to adults, developing organisms undergo rapid and complex changes within a relatively short period. Consequently, the sus-

ceptibility of the conceptus to xenobiotic insult varies dramatically within the narrow time span of the major developmental stages, i.e., the preimplantation, embryonic, fetal, and neonatal periods. The embryologic characteristics of each of these stages and the types of spontaneous and chemically induced adverse outcomes associated with each stage will be described.

The major morphogenic events occurring during preimplantation development are formation of a compact mass of cells (the morula) and of the blastocyst. Development of the blastocyst involves differentiation of the trophectoderm, which is necessary for implantation, and the inner cell mass (ICM), which differentiates into primary endoderm and ectoderm before implantation. The ICM gives rise to the embryo and the extraembryonic membranes but cannot implant or survive in the uterus in the absence of trophectoderm.

As shown in Table 7–3, considerable similarity exists in the timing of preimplantation development across several mammalian species, regardless of the total length of gestation (Brinster, 1975). Shortly after fertilization, the mammalian embryo has a low oxygen consumption and metabolic capacity. From the time of fertilization to the two-cell stage, gene activity in the conceptus is based on expression of maternal mRNA present in the ovum. From the two-cell to the eight-cell stage, expression of the embryonic genome begins (Epstein, 1983). At the time of blastocyst formation, there is a dramatic increase in cell division and metabolic capacity. Both the total synthetic rate as well as the types of RNAs and proteins synthesized are

Table 7–3. TIMING OF KEY DEVELOPMENTAL EVENTS IN SOME MAMMALIAN SPECIES*

	RAT	RABBIT	MONKEY (RHESUS)	HUMAN
Blastocyst formation	3–4	3–4	5–7	5–8
Implantation	6	7	9	7
Organogenesis	6–17	6–18	20–45	21–56
Primitive streak	9	7	17–19	16–18
Neural plate	9	—	19–20	18–20
First somite	9–10	—	20–21	20–21
First pharyngeal arch	10	—	21–23	20
10 Somites	10–11	9	23–24	25–26
Upper limb buds	11	10–11	27–29	28
Lower limb buds	12	11	29–31	31–32
Forepaw rays	14	15	35–37	37
Testes differentiation	14–15	16–17	37–39	43–48
Heart septation	16	17	36	46–47
Palate closure	16–17	19–20	45–47	56–58
Length of gestation	22	32	165	267

* Developmental ages are days of gestation.

markedly increased. During the preimplantation period, biochemical changes in the uterine endometrium controlled by progesterone and estrogen result in the development of endometrial sensitivity to the blastocyst. It is now well established that the same basic hormonal sequence, *i.e.,* low levels of estrogen in a progesterone-primed uterus, initiates uterine receptivity. The blastocyst must implant within 24 hours after the progesterone-estrogen regimen when the uterus is in the peak receptive phase. One of the earliest signs of blastocyst implantation in all species investigated is a localized increase in endometrial vascular permeability, which is mediated by prostaglandins (Kennedy and Armstrong, 1981). Alterations in the hormonal milieu, as well as direct excretion of xenobiotics into uterine secretions during this period, can interfere with implantation and result in embryolethality. The preimplantation embryo appears to be susceptible to lethality but rarely to teratogenicity with chemical insult. In studies utilizing preimplantation embryo cultures, severe toxicity is manifested by rapid death of the embryo, whereas less severe effects are measured by decreases in cleavage rates and arrested development (Brinster, 1975). There have been few studies of the effects of sublethal exposures on preimplantation embryos, and the possibilities of persistent biochemical or morphologic alterations have not been adequately explored.

Following implantation, organogenesis takes place. The organogenesis period is characterized by the division, migration, and association of cells into primitive organ rudiments. The basic structural templates for organization of tissues and organs are established on the molecular, cellular, and morphologic levels. The most characteristic susceptibility of the embryo to xenobiotics during the organogenesis period is the induction of structural birth defects, although these are often accompanied by embryolethality. Within the organogenesis period, individual organ systems possess highly specific periods of vulnerability to teratogenic insult. Figure 7-2 depicts the sensitive periods of the major embryonic organ systems to teratogenic insult. Administration of a teratogen on day 10 of rat gestation would result in a high level of brain and eye defects, with the intermediate levels of heart and skeletal defects, and a low level of urogenital defects. If the same agent was administered on day 11, a different spectrum of malformations would be anticipated, with brain and palate malformations predominating. Consequently, the exact time of exposure has a strong effect on the final pattern of malformation. Figure 7–2 also illustrates that exposure to teratogens usually results in a spectrum of malformations involving a number of organ systems, reflecting the overlap of critical periods for individual organ systems. This situation is more evident in species with short gestation periods, such as rodents. Most human teratogens, however, have also been found to affect the development of several organ systems and induce syndromes of malformations rather than just single anomalies, as described for rubella and thalidomide.

The critical phase for inducing anomalies in individual organ systems may be as short as one day or may extend throughout organogenesis. Urogenital defects, for example, can result from

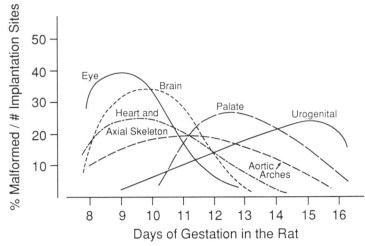

Figure 7–2. Pattern of susceptibility of embryonic organ rudiments to teratogenic insult. (Modified from Wilson, J. G.: *Environment and Birth Defects*. Academic Press, Inc., New York, 1973.)

drug treatment from the 9th to 18th days of gestation in the rat. This implies that development of the urogenital system is multiphasic, and that individual stages may have different sensitivities to chemical insult. Renal anomalies can be induced by irradiation on day 9 of rat gestation, for example, whereas the earliest primordium of the pronephric kidney is not present until day 10 (Wilson, 1973). Presumably, this is due to interference with molecular or cellular events preceding structural differentiation of the kidney. Xenobiotic insult on day 11.5 could interfere with formation of the mesonephric kidney, or on day 12 with entrance of the mesonephric duct into the urogenital sinus. On day 12.5, the metanephric kidney is first formed, and this is followed by formation of the definitive genital ducts and indifferent gonads from days 12 to 18 of gestation (Hoar and Monie, 1981). Depending on the mechanism of action of the agent and the time of administration, it is likely that only one or a few of these steps will be affected, but succeeding steps will be disrupted as a result of the original alteration. Processes governing embryonic differentiation are not well understood, yet most likely determine the intrinsic susceptibility of individual organs to teratogenic insult. The mechanism of action and the persistence of the toxic effect also affect the malformation pattern, as discussed in the next section.

Histogenesis, functional maturation, and growth are the major processes occurring during the fetal and neonatal (i.e., perinatal) periods. Insult at these late developmental stages leads to a broad spectrum of effects that can be generally manifested as growth retardation or more specifically manifested as functional disorders and transplacental carcinogenesis. The fetus is more resistant to lethal effects than is the embryo, but the incidence of stillbirths is measurable. The perinatal period of life is a time of high susceptibility to carcinogenesis. At least three factors contribute to this enhanced susceptibility: high cellular replication rates, ontogeny of xenobiotic biotransforming enzymes, and low immunocompetence. Several childhood tumors occur so early after birth that prenatal origin is considered likely. Among these are acute lymphocytic (but not myelogenous) leukemia, Wilms' tumor, neuroblastoma, primary carcinoma of the liver, and presacral teratoma (Miller, 1973). Cancer was the chief cause of death by disease in children under the age of 15 in the United States in 1976, accounting for 11.3 percent of all deaths. Leukemia and lymphoma account for approximately half of these deaths followed by cancers of the brain and central nervous system, soft tissues, kidney, and bone (ACS, 1980).

Studies with direct-acting transplacental carcinogens such as ethylnitrosourea (ENU) indicate that susceptibility to carcinogens begins after completion of the organogenesis period in rodents. Tumors in offspring occurred primarily when ENU was given during the fetal period, whereas birth defects and embryolethality predominated with exposures earlier in organogenesis (Ivankovic, 1979). This is not to imply that teratogenesis and carcinogenesis are mutually exclusive processes, however. Birth defects and neoplasias occur together in the same offspring with unusually high frequency, but not necessarily at the same site. Teratogenesis and carcinogenesis are viewed as graded responses of the embryo to injury, with teratogenesis representing the grosser response involving major tissue necrosis. Bolande (1977) has postulated that certain agents cause teratogenic damage in early relatively undifferentiated embryos, combined carcinogenic-teratogenic damage in older embryos, and finally, carcinogenic damage alone in the perinatal period. Alternatively, it has been suggested that embryotoxic insult may predispose the offspring to secondary tumor induction in later life.

Patterns of Dose-Response

Functional deficits and perinatally induced cancers are not manifested until adolescence or later. They are usually examined as end points in themselves without correlation to the outcomes observable at the time of birth. The major effects from prenatal exposure measured at the time of birth in developmental toxicity studies are embryolethality, malformations, and growth retardation. Embryolethality is reported as the ratio of resorptions and dead fetuses in the litter at term to the number of implantation sites. Growth retardation is measured by weighing and taking crown-rump measurements of live fetuses at term. The frequency and type of malformations are determined by gross inspection of fetuses and detailed skeletal and soft tissue analysis. The occurrence of embryolethality precludes measurements of growth retardation or malformation because the latter two events are observed in live fetuses only. The relationship between embryolethality, malformations, and growth retardation is quite complex and varies with the type of agent, the time of exposure, and the dose. To simplify the situation, conditions will be restricted to administration of agents at a single time point during organogenesis, and at exposure levels not severely toxic to the mother. Even under these strict conditions, diverse patterns of response for these major end points occur, three of which will be described.

Some developmental toxicants can cause malformations of the entire litter at exposure levels that do not cause embryolethality. A depiction of the dose-response pattern for such agents is given in Figure 7–3, A. If the dose is increased beyond that malforming the entire litter, embryolethality can occur, but often in conjunction with severe maternal toxicity. Malformed fetuses are often growth retarded, and the curve for growth retardation is often parallel to and slightly displaced from the curve for teratogenicity. Such a pattern of response is rare and is indicative of agents with high teratogenic potency.

A more common dose-response pattern involves embryolethality, malformations, and growth retardation of surviving fetuses (Figure

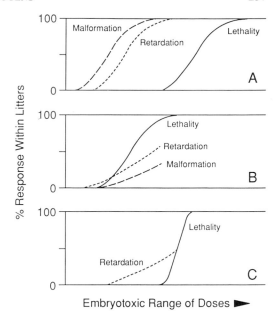

Figure 7–3. Dose-response patterns for different types of developmental toxicants. (Modified from Neubert, D.; Barrach, H. J.; and Merker, H. J.: Drug-induced damage to the embryo or fetus. *Curr. Top. Pathol.*, **69**:242–324, 1980.)

7–3, *B*). For agents producing this response pattern, exposure within the embryotoxic range of doses results in a combination of resorbed, malformed, growth-retarded, and "normal" fetuses within the litter. Depending on the teratogenic potency of the agent, lower doses may cause predominantly resorptions or malformations. As the dosage increases, however, embryolethality predominates until the entire litter is resorbed. Agents with high teratogenic potency would produce a pattern where the teratogenicity curve was to the left but still overlapping the embryolethality curve, whereas agents that were predominantly embryolethal would produce the pattern shown in Figure 7–3, *B*, where embryolethality was the most prominent outcome throughout the range of doses. Growth retardation can precede both these outcomes or parallel the teratogenicity curve.

A third dose-response pattern consists of growth retardation and embryolethality without malformations (Figure 7–3, *C*). The dose-response curve for embryolethality in this case is usually steep, implying the existence of a sharp threshold for survival of the embryo. Growth retardation of surviving fetuses usually precedes significant embryolethality. Agents producing this pattern of response would be considered embryotoxic or embryolethal, but not teratogenic. When such a pattern is observed, it is necessary to conduct additional studies with doses within the range causing growth retardation and embryolethality. Results obtained at these intermediary doses can indicate whether teratogenicity has been masked by embryolethality (Neubert *et al.*, 1980).

The existence of these three general patterns of response indicate that for some agents embryolethality and teratogenicity are different degrees of manifestations of the same primary insult (Figure 7–3, *B*). For other agents, there is a qualitative difference in response, and the primary insult leads to embryolethality alone (Figure 7–3, *C*) or teratogenicity alone (Figure 7–3, *A*). Separate evaluation of growth retardation, teratogenicity, and embryolethality with increasing dose must be carried out to arrive at conclusions about the primary mode of action of the agent.

With agents of unknown developmental toxicity, the sequence of testing begins with a dose range–finding study containing relatively small numbers of pregnant rodents (approximately eight per group). They are exposed on days 6 through 17 of gestation to the test agent at doses up to and including those causing limiting maternal toxicity and/or development toxicity (death, severe growth retardation). The purpose of the dose-range study is to obtain a qualitative yes/no signal about the potential developmental toxicity of the agent, and information on doses causing extreme maternal toxicity. At the next level of testing, larger numbers of animals (approximately 20 per group) are exposed on days 6 to 17 of gestation to obtain quantitative information on dose-response relationships. The highest dose should cause measurable but slight maternal toxicity (i.e., significant depression of weight gain) or developmental toxicity (i.e., significant depression of fetal body weight, increased embryolethality, and/or structural malformations), and the low dose should cause no observable effects. If evidence of selective developmental toxicity is obtained from this study, it is necessary to conduct a third study exposing dams on single days during organogenesis at doses that are not maternally toxic to obtain a clear definition of the dose-response pattern of developmental toxicity.

If an agent with selective developmental toxicity is administered throughout the organogenesis period (days 6 to 17 in the rat), it becomes difficult to identify the most sensitive target organs and to produce a consistent pattern of malformation. In addition, teratogenic effects induced by agents acting according to pattern B can be masked by embryolethality with repeated dosing during the organogenesis period. If the agent is administered at levels sufficiently toxic to the mother, then all responses can revert to pattern C, embryolethality or growth retardation, but rarely malformations.

It is generally accepted that developmental toxicity in the form of increased resorption and decreased fetal body weight can occur at maternally toxic dose levels. The role of maternal toxicity in causing congenital malformations, however, is not clear (for review see Chernoff *et al.*, 1989). Khera (1984) reviewed over 85 published studies in mice to examine the relationship between maternal toxicity, embryotoxicity, and birth defects. He noted that doses of test agents that caused maternal toxicity, as indicated by reduced maternal body weight, clinical signs of toxicity, or deaths, commonly caused reduction in fetal body weight, increased resorption, and, rarely, fetal deaths. He identified three patterns of association between maternal toxicity and malformations: (1) for some compounds, maternal toxicity was not associated with malformations; (2) for others, maternal toxicity was associated with a diverse pattern of malformations, which often included cleft palate; and (3) the maternal toxicity of still others was associated with a characteristic and unique pattern of malformation.

Compounds in the second category are the most difficult to classify in terms of teratogenic potential. Cleft palate has been reported as the principal malformation resulting from food and water deprivation during pregnancy in mice (Szabo and Brent, 1975); however, cleft palate is also a malformation specifically induced in mice by a number of teratogens, most notably the glucocorticoids, without apparent maternal toxicity. Complete ascertainment of food and water consumption, maternal body weights, and, occasionally, alterations in maternal homeostasis (i.e., organ histopathology, kidney or liver dysfunction, hematologic alterations, pharmacologic reactions, and stress-induced glucocorticoid elevations) are necessary to distinguish between cleft palate caused by a teratogenic effect of a chemical on the embryo and a systemic toxicity in the dam that secondarily affects embryonic development.

Compounds in the third category were those in which maternal toxicity was associated with a characteristic and unique pattern of malformation. The pattern of defects caused by these agents was exencephaly; open eyes; fused, missing, or supernumerary ribs; and fused or scrambled sternebrae. The severity and incidence of these defects could be directly related to the degree of maternal toxicity. They were absent or rare at doses that were nontoxic to the dam. Khera (1984) concluded that these defects resulted from maternal toxicity and did not reflect the teratogenic potential of the compounds.

Although most investigators accept that maternal toxicity can be the cause of minor variants in the ribs and sternebrae, it is not universally accepted as the cause of major malformations such as exencephaly and open eyes.

The timing of exposure and patterns of dose-response obtained in animal studies have important implications for extrapolating animal data to humans. The major implication is that a spectrum of end points can be produced, even under the controlled conditions of timing and exposure that can be achieved in animal studies. In some cases, the spectrum comprises a continuum of responses, with depressed birth weight or functional impairment occurring at low doses, birth defects at intermediate doses, and lethality at high doses. Less commonly, birth defects alone or lethality alone are produced. Consequently, in estimating human risk, all exposure-specific adverse outcomes must be taken into consideration, and not just birth defects.

A similar spectrum of response has been observed in humans after prenatal exposure to developmental toxicants. The spectrum of response is determined by the time and duration of exposure, magnitude of exposure, interindividual differences in sensitivity, and interactions among all these factors (Fraser, 1977). Consequently, manifestations of developmental toxicity cannot be presumed to be constant or specific across species; *i.e.*, an animal model cannot be expected to forecast exactly the human response to a given exposure. For instance, an agent that induces cleft palate in the mouse may elevate the frequency of spontaneous abortion or intrauterine growth retardation in humans. Any manifestation of exposure-related developmental toxicity in animal studies can be indicative of a spectrum of response in humans (Kimmel *et al.*, 1984).

Table 7–4 illustrates an important factor to be considered in extrapolation of animal data to humans. The most prevalent adverse pregnancy outcome in humans is spontaneous abortion or early fetal loss prior to 28 weeks of pregnancy, occurring in at least 10 to 20 percent of all recognized pregnancies. Estimates from prospective studies range even higher, on the order of 20 to 25 percent of conceptions (National Foundation, 1981b). The frequency of spontaneous abortion is highest in early pregnancy, especially during the first 12 weeks, and gradually decreases to 20 weeks, after which fetal loss is less uncommon. Approximately one-third of specimens obtained from spontaneous abortions occurring between 8 and 28 weeks of gestation contain chromosomal aberrations. The frequency of aberrations is at least 60-fold higher in spontaneous abortions than in term births. Of the remaining two-thirds of spontaneous abortions that do not have chromosomal aberrations, approximately half have structural malformations (National Foundation, 1981b). The occurrence of malformations in abortuses is not as well documented as that for chromosomal aberrations because of the difficulty in observing malformations in specimens that are often macerated or incomplete. The remaining one-third of specimens lack chromosomal and morphologic abnormalities, but the incidence of placental inflammations suggestive of uterine infections can be high in these "normal" abortuses (Ornoy *et al.*, 1981).

These figures suggest that the majority of human embryos bearing chromosomal and/or morphologic abnormalities are lost through early miscarriage, and that relatively few survive to term. Consequently, examination of adverse outcomes at the time of birth alone (malformations, stillbirths, low birthweight) is likely to result in a substantial underestimate of the true risk, insofar as the occurrence of embryolethality would be missed. It is possible that developmental toxicants operating according to pattern *A* in Figure

Table 7–4. FREQUENCY OF SELECTED ADVERSE PREGNANCY OUTCOMES IN HUMANS*

EVENT	FREQUENCY PER 100	UNIT
Spontaneous abortion, 8–28 weeks	10–20	Pregnancies or women
Chromosomal anomalies in spontaneous abortions, 8–28 weeks	30–40	Spontaneous abortions
Chromosomal anomalies from amniocentesis	2	Amniocentesis specimens
Stillbirths	2–4	Stillbirths and livebirths
Low birthweight <2500 g	7	Livebirths
Major malformations	2–3	Livebirths
Chromosomal anomalies	0.2	Livebirths
Severe mental retardation	0.4	Children to 15 years of age

* Modified from National Foundation/March of Dimes: Report of Panel II. Guidelines for reproductive studies in exposed human populations. In Bloom, A. D. (ed.): *Guidelines for Studies of Human Populations Exposed to Mutagenic and Reproductive Hazards*. The Foundation, New York, 1981, pp. 37–110.

Table 7–5. SENSITIVITY AND SPECIFICITY OF LABORATORY ANIMAL STUDIES FOR PREDICTING TERATOGENESIS

	NO.	PERCENT
SENSITIVITY		
Compounds with positive teratologic findings in humans	38	100
Positive in at least one laboratory animal test species	37	97
Positive in more than one laboratory animal test species	29	76
Positive in all laboratory animal species tested	8	21
SPECIFICITY		
Compounds studied in humans with no teratologic findings	165	100
"Negative" in at least one laboratory animal test species	130	79
"Negative" in more than one laboratory animal test species	84	51
"Negative" in all laboratory animal species tested	47	29
Positive in more than a single laboratory animal test species	68	41

Adapted from Frankos, V. H.: FDA perspectives on the use of teratology data for human risk assessment, *Fund. Appl. Toxicol.*, **5**:615–622, 1985.

7–3 could be picked up by monitoring malformations at the time of birth in humans, especially if the malformations were rare (thalidomide) or if the exposed population was large (rubella). Those agents operating according to patterns *B* and *C* would most likely be missed unless there was detailed examination of the frequency of early fetal loss and the presence of chromosomal and structural malformations in abortuses.

The sensitivity (ability to detect a true positive response in humans) and specificity (ability to detect a true negative response in humans) of laboratory animal studies have been evaluated (Frankos, 1985) and are presented in Table 7–5. Of 38 compounds having demonstrated or suspected teratogenic activity in humans, all except one (tobramycin, which causes otological deficits in humans) tested positive in at least one animal species. Over 80 percent of the compounds were positive in multiple species. A positive response was elicited 85 percent in the mouse, 80 percent in the rat, 60 percent in the rabbit, 45 percent in the hamster, and 30 percent in the monkey. Overall, these findings indicate that conventional laboratory animal species have high sensitivity for detecting human teratogens.

Evaluation of specificity has indicated that of 165 adequately tested compounds with no evidence of human teratogenic activity, 29 percent were negative in all species tested and 51 percent were negative in more than one species. However, 41 percent of the 165 compounds were positive in more than one animal species. The monkey and the rabbit had the highest specificity, testing negative for compounds reported to have no teratogenic activity in humans 80 percent and 70 percent of the time, respectively.

These findings indicate that laboratory animal species have high sensitivity but low specificity for predicting human teratogenesis. There are at least two possible explanations for this: the animal studies have yielded false-positive results because of test conditions and interpretation; or the true risk for adverse pregnancy outcome is underestimated in human studies that measure only outcomes from the time of birth onward. Human studies must be designed to measure all the manifestations of developmental toxicity and not just events measureable at the time of birth before adequate cross-species comparisons can be made.

Mechanism of Action

Despite the effect of time of exposure and the complex interaction between maternal toxicity and embryolethality on pregnancy outcome, developmental toxicity is not explained solely on the basis of these events. Agent specificity also occurs which encompasses the mechanism whereby classes of agents interact with differentiating tissues to produce specific patterns of developmental toxicity. Agent specificity is discussed in the framework of the three patterns of dose-response described in the previous section.

Cytotoxic Agents. The majority of well-known developmental toxicants produce pattern *B* of dose-response, i.e., both malformations and embryolethality. Such a pattern or response is typical of xenobiotics that are cytotoxic to replicating cells via alterations in replication, transcription, translation, or cell division. Examples of these xenobiotics include alkylating agents, antineoplastic agents, and many mutagens. The rationale for susceptibility of the embryo to these agents is that the rate of cell division is extremely high during the organogenesis period. Within days 8 to 11 of gestation in rats, the DNA content of the embryo increases 1000-fold (Neubert *et al.*, 1980). Therefore, it is not surprising that many agents known to interfere with cellular proliferation are embryotoxic. A characteristic, early response of embryonic tissues to these agents is the occurrence of excessive cell death in target organs destined to become malformed (Scott, 1977). Although cell death may not be the initial event in the cause of developmental toxicity, at some point it becomes an important intermediate or final manifestation of the primary insult. The increased necrosis must occur selectively and within a critical period of time for malformations to be found. Low doses of cytotoxic agents administered relatively early in the critical period may produce levels of cell death that can be replaced through compensatory hyperplasia of surviving cells, resulting in the formation of growth-retarded but morphologically normal fetuses at term. Higher doses administered later during the critical period may cause substantial depletion of cell number, leaving insufficient time for replacement prior to the occurrence of critical morphogenetic events. The resulting hypoplasia of the organ rudiments, as well as reduced proliferative rate of surviving cells, are important events related to the induction of malformations. High levels of exposure may damage too many cells and organ systems to be compatible with survival, and result in embryolethality (Ritter, 1977). A single exposure to a cytotoxic agent during organogenesis can result in all three outcomes both within and between litters. Some litters may be totally resorbed, others may contain only growth-retarded fetuses at term, whereas others may have a mixture of malformed and/or growth retarded fetuses and resorption sites at term. The variation in response has been ascribed to differences in pharmacokinetics of the agent in the maternal system, differential delivery of chemicals to individual embryos according to uterine position, as well as variations in developmental age of embryos within the litter (Neubert et al., 1980).

An example of an agent that produces this response is MNNG (N-methyl-N'-nitro-N-nitrosoguanidine), an alkylating agent that induces replication-dependent mutations and inhibition of DNA synthesis (Mandel, 1960). When administered on days 7 to 12 of gestation, a spectrum of malformations involving the brain, palate, vertebral column, ribs, and limbs is produced (Inouye and Murakami, 1978). Limb defects are prominent, but not unique, with exposure on day 10 or 11. Teratogenicity predominates under these exposure conditions, but embryolethality is elevated at all dose levels (Manson and Miller, 1983). When the types of limb malformations were examined, an unusual pattern was observed. Hindlimbs were more frequently malformed than forelimbs, and limbs on the left side were malformed more frequently than limbs on the right side (Table 7–6). The forelimb-hindlimb response is not unusual insofar as the hindlimbs (HL) develop a day behind the forelimbs (FL) with peak susceptibility for forelimb malformation on day 10, and for hindlimbs on day 11. The left-right (L-R) asymmetry is somewhat more unusual, although there are other xenobiotics known to cause asymmetric limb malformations in rodents (reviewed in Manson and Miller, 1983 and Collins et al., 1990).

The differential susceptibility of each of the four limb types to MNNG-induced malformations has been utilized to determine whether there was a correlation between the level and persistence of cell death in limb buds shortly after exposure and the frequency of malformations at term. Figure 7–4 contains results of this analysis, where the percentage of necrotic cells in the subridge mesenchyme of limb buds 1 to 72 hours after maternal exposure to MNNG on day 11 was measured. An increase in the number of necrotic cells in limb buds was first detected at four hours, was elevated at 18 hours, peaked at 24 hours, and began declining at 48 hours to reach the control baseline at 72 hours. The necrotic index values at 24 hours, when the level of cell death was the highest for all limb types, correlated with the pattern of limb malformations. The level of necrosis was highest in hindlimbs, and limbs on the left side had higher levels of necrosis than limbs on the right side. At all time points examined, left-sided limbs had higher levels of cell death than right-sided limbs. Thus, with MNNG, the level and persistence of cell death are quantitatively related to the fre-

Table 7–6. FREQUENCY OF MALFORMATION (POSTAXIAL ECTRODACTYLY) BY LIMB POSITION WITH MNNG EXPOSURE*†

	RFL	LFL	RHL	LHL
Control	0.0	0.0	0.0	0.0
Treated	8.6 ± 3.1	40.1 ± 4.2	23.5 ± 4.6	51.6 ± 4.5

* Results are presented as the mean litter frequency of fetuses with absence of digits 3 to 5 for each limb type.
† Modified from Manson, J. M., and Miller, M. L.: Contribution of mesenchymal cell death and mitotic alteration to assymmetric limb malformations induced by MNNG. *Teratogen. Carcinog. Mutagen.*, **3**:335–353, 1983.

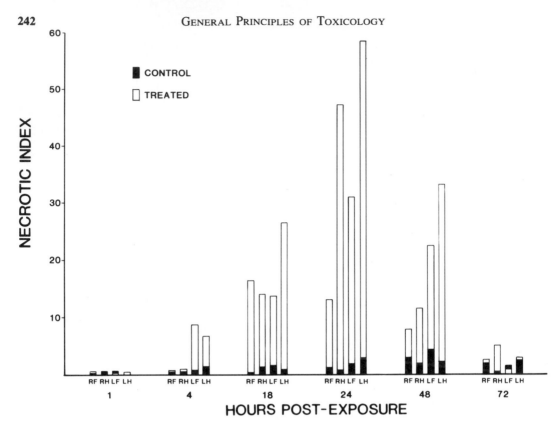

Figure 7–4. Necrotic index of control and MNNG-treated limbs. *RF,* right forelimb; *RH,* right hindlimb; *LF,* left forelimb; *LH,* left hindlimb. (From Manson, J. M., and Miller, M. L.: Contribution of mesenchymal cell death and mitotic alteration to asymmetric limb malformations induced by MNNG. *Teratogen. Carcinog. Mutagen.,* 3:335–353, 1983.)

quency of limb malformations. Additional studies have indicated that the asymmetry in limb malformation and necrosis observed with MNNG are not related to the uptake of the agent into each of the four limb types. Rather, it appears that the limb buds have different intrinsic susceptibility to MNNG, possibly based on the percentage of cells undergoing proliferation in each limb type.

Studies performed by Kochhar *et al.* (1978) with a different cytotoxic agent, cytosine arabinoside, have indicated that there is also a qualitative relationship between the location of necrotic areas in limb buds and the final morphologic pattern of malformation. The selective, regional susceptibility of limb mesenchyme cells to death after cytosine arabinoside exposure correlated with the proliferation rate; as proliferation zones moved from proximal to distal regions of the limb bud, so did the areas where cell death was the highest after exposure. A substantial body of literature exists (reviewed in Scott, 1977) indicating that sites of high proliferative activity in the embryo are susceptible to cell death after exposure to cytotoxic teratogens, and that the frequency and morphologic

pattern of the malformations are related to the localization and extent of necrosis in embryonic organ rudiments. Depression in DNA synthesis or DNA damage does not appear to be as important. The embryo can tolerate substantial depressions in DNA synthesis, which, unless accompanied by excessive necrosis, do not lead to malformations (Ritter, 1977; Kochhar *et al.,* 1978). Likewise, chromosomal aberrations have been observed in embryonic cells after exposure to a variety of alkylating agents during the organogenesis period (Adler, 1983; Meyne and Legator, 1983; Theiss *et al.,* 1983). Cells bearing chromosomal aberrations appear to be rapidly eliminated, usually within 24 hours after transplacental exposure, indicating that chromosomal aberrations may contribute to cell death but not to heritable mutations in surviving cells. Even stable chromosomal aberrations (i.e., small deletions, inversions, and reciprocal translocations) do not persist after several cell divisions with prenatal exposure to ENU (Theiss *et al.,* 1983). There may be insufficient time for repair of DNA damage with the rapid rate of cell division during organogensis. Depressions in DNA synthesis and cell death are more likely outcomes of DNA damage in embryonic tissues than are heritable mutations (Manson, 1981).

Snow (1983, 1985) has used the term *restorative growth* to describe the process whereby mammalian embryos replace cells lost through tissue damage or deficits. It is well recognized that some degree of restorative growth, or increased mitotic activity, occurs in embryonic tissue after cytotoxic insult. As demonstrated for MNNG (Figure 7–4), cell death is first apparent at 4 hours in treated limbs and increases in frequency and severity to peak at 24 hours. Mitotic activity of surviving cells is initially depressed at 24 hours after treatment, and exceeds control values up to 72 hours (Figure 7–5). Mitotic activity remains elevated long after the necrotic episode has subsided, especially in the left hindlimbs which have the highest level of cell death and malformation.

Restorative growth can contribute to either repair or exacerbation of cytotoxic insult. Differential cell death, most likely due to differences in cell cycle characteristics, is the necessary prerequisite and initial trigger to restorative growth. With the high variability in cell cycle times of embryonic tissues during organogenesis, a common strategy for restorative growth cannot be followed by all cells within a tissue. To repair teratogenic damage, each cell type would adopt a strategy that most rapidly restores the balance between different cell types in a tissue and between tissues and organs to maintain coordinated development. What is most often observed, however, is that restorative growth is a highly uncoordinated process. Each cell type undergoes restorative growth as quickly as possible and juxtaposed tissues independently restore tissue mass. This uncoordinated growth process exacerbates mis-timing of inductive interactions between tissues that are initially perturbed by differential cell death.

With cytotoxic agents, the embryo is usually more susceptible than is the mother, although rapidly proliferating maternal tissues (hematopoietic, epithelial) can be affected. A full spectrum of malformations can be induced by these agents, and site specificity is primarily determined by the time of exposure. Those organ rudiments undergoing rapid proliferation at the time of exposure are likely to be the sites of future malformation. Many of the resulting malformations involve reduction deformities, or missing elements, presumably because insufficient cells were available to form the organ rudiment. There is often a steep dose-response curve for teratogenicity with these agents because there is little difference in doses that will malform the embryo and those that kill the embryo. Malformations are often induced at doses that cause death in a significant portion of the litter.

Teratogens Affecting Specific Events in Differentiation. While necrosis is a common event in the developmental toxicity of cytotoxic agents, it is not a universal mechanism. There are agents that disrupt development by highly specific mechanisms of action not involving excessive necrosis or embryolethality. These are characterized by the dose-response patterns exhibited in Figure 7–3, *A*, where malformations occur without embryolethality. These specific teratogens usually induce a subset of all possible malformations at a given time of exposure, and usually at narrow time points within the organogenesis period. A well-defined structural anomaly or a distinct malformation syndrome occurs from prenatal exposure to these agents. It is not possible to make generalities about the mechanism of action of agents falling within this class. Rather, each agent appears to operate according to its own unique mechanism of action.

Glucocorticoids, both natural and synthetic, are a classic example of such a teratogen. Physiologic levels of glucocorticoids are required for normal growth and differentiation of embryonic tissue, whereas pharmacologic doses

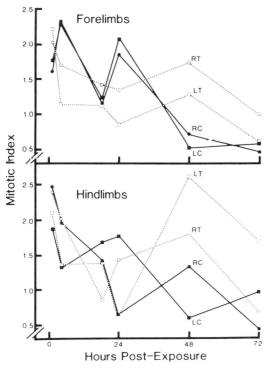

Figure 7–5. Mitotic index of control and MNNG-treated limbs. LT, left treated; RT, right treated; RC, right control, LC, left control.

administered at midgestation in laboratory animals induce malformations primarily of the palate, and less frequently of the limbs. Different strains of inbred mice exhibit different degrees of susceptibility to glucocorticoid-induced cleft palate. The level of cytoplasmic glucocorticoid receptors in the maxillary mesenchyme cells of embryo correlates with the strain susceptibility; i.e., higher receptor levels are found in responsive strains and lower levels in nonresponsive strains (Pratt and Salomon, 1981). High levels of glucocorticoids cause significant growth inhibition in maxillary mesenchyme cells and subsequent alteration in production of extracellular matrix. The target organ specificity of glucocorticoids is also related to the concentration of the receptor protein, which is higher in the craniofacial region than in other parts of the embryo (Pratt and Salomon, 1981). Glucocorticoid induction of cleft palate alone in the absence of embryolethality, extensive necrosis, and overall growth retardation is a good example of a teratogen operating through a specific mechanism of action involving receptor-mediated events.

Another example of a teratogen that produces a distinct malformation syndrome through what appears to be a specific mechanism of action is the diuretic acetazolamide (2-acetyl-amino-1,3,4-thiadiazole-5-sulfonamide). The first report of acetazolamide's teratogenic effects was by Layton and Hallesy (1965), who fed pregnant rats a diet containing 0.4 or 0.6 percent of the drug throughout gestation and obtained offspring with an unusual limb malformation. The limb defects were unusual in that they were primarily reductions of the distal postaxial portion of the right forelimb; usually digits 4 and 5 were missing. Since that first report many researchers have examined various aspects of acetazolamide's intriguing teratogenicity (reviewed by Hirsch and Scott, 1983). At low teratogenic doses of acetazolamide the incidence of embryolethality is not significantly increased and the effect on fetal body weight is relatively minor. With higher or continuous single oral doses other organ systems become affected and embryolethality increases.

Acetazolamide's primary pharmacological activity is the inhibition of the enzyme carbonic anhydrase. This enzyme (several isozymic forms exist), which is abundant in tissues involved in ion transport (primarily in erythrocytes and kidney), catalyzes the hydration of CO_2 and the dehydration of bicarbonate ions and is a major factor in the control of blood pH. Because other structurally diverse carbonic anhydrase inhibitors have also been shown to produce the same pattern of malformations, it is widely assumed that inhibition of the enzyme is the basis for the teratogenicity.

Even though teratogenic doses of acetazolamide produce severe metabolic acidosis, diuresis, and weight loss in the pregnant animal, several lines of evidence suggest that the changes in the extraembryonic membranes or the embryo are the important factors. Experiments by Scott (1970) with intrauterine injections of acetazolamide, and embryo transfer experiments by Biddle (1975) confirmed that the teratogenic action is initiated in the embryo or its immediate environment at a critical period in limb development when carbonic anhydrase is detectable (in the embryonic red cells but not the limb mesenchyme). A significant advancement was made when it was shown that exposing mice at the critical period to a high CO_2 environment, while producing a pronounced respiratory acidosis in the dams, produced the same limb defects as acetazolamide (Weaver and Scott, 1984a,b). In some respects the high CO_2 environment mimics the effects of acetazolamide. Acetazolamide produces both respiratory acidosis due to inhibition of carbonic anhydrase in the red blood cell and metabolic acidosis due to inhibition of HCO_3 reabsorption in the kidney; the former elevating plasma and tissue CO_2 tension (as does high CO_2 exposure alone). Further experiments that manipulated the metabolic acidosis led these workers to the hypothesis that acetazolamide-induced limb reduction defects are the products of a hypercapnic (high CO_2) embryonic environment resulting from carbonic anhydrase inhibition in the mother and the embryo. The increased CO_2 tension would inevitably result in a reduction of intracellular pH (pH_i). Changes in pH_i are linked to the regulation of various cell functions such as glycolysis, protein synthesis, and cell-cell coupling to name a few (reviewed by Busa, 1986). There is also a strong correlation between pH_i and cell proliferation in a number of different cell types such that reduced pH_i results in reduced proliferation. The observed absence of cell death in acetazolamide-exposed limbs (Holmes and Trelstad, 1979) suggests that the reductional defects are a result of reduced cell proliferation. In support of this hypothesis, Scott and coworkers (1990) have actually measured a pH_i decrease of 0.15 to 0.2 units in mouse embryos after acetezolamide exposure, as well as decreases of pH in embryo plasma and exocoelomic and amniotic fluids. The unique asymmetry of the acetazolamide-induced limb defects is yet to be explained. Perhaps there are blood flow differences between the right and left limb buds which makes the right more susceptible, and within the right limb bud the distal postaxial region may be more sensitive to reductions in pH_i.

The collaborative work of Nau and Scott (1986, 1987) measuring intracellular pH in rodent embryos has revealed an interesting phenomenon with potentially very significant implications. The pH_i of developing embryos is higher than the pH of maternal blood; the pH_i is highest in young embryos and decreases with developmental age. Because maternal blood pH remains relatively constant, there is a pH gradient between the mother and embryo during this critical period of development. This pH gradient would be expected to have a major impact on transplacental drug distribution. Evidence in support of the pH partition hypothesis has been collected for two weak acid teratogens, methoxyacetic acid and valproic acid, both of which accumulate in the embryo to higher concentrations than in the maternal plasma. When it is recognized that a number of human teratogens or their metabolites (valproic acid, isotretinoin, trimethadione, phenytoin, thalidomide, warfarin, aminopterin) are weak acids and none is a weak base, the degree of drug ionization may well be recognized as being of paramount importance in the ability of drugs to reach and accumulate in the embryo.

Nonspecific Developmental Toxins. The third pattern of response is one in which growth retardation and embryolethality occur without teratogenicity (Figure 7–3, *C*). Examples of agents that fall within this class are the mitochondrial protein synthesis inhibitors chloramphenicol and thiamphenicol (Neubert *et al.*, 1980). After treatment on days 10 and 11, the dose-response for embryolethality is steep, increasing from control levels to 100 precent mortality at doses between 100 and 125 mg/kg/day for thiamphenicol (Bass *et al.*, 1978). Dose-dependent inhibition of mitochondrial respiration, ATP content, and cytochrome oxidase activity in embryonic tissue correlated with growth retardation and death of embryos. Inhibition of cellular processes as fundamental as mitochondrial function is believed to result in nonspecific effects such as overall growth retardation and lethality. There is no basis for target organ susceptibility in the early embryo for perturbation of such a fundamental cellular process, and consequently all tissues appear to be affected to an equal extent. The early signs of perturbation are overall growth retardation progressing to complete lethality of the litter once a critical threshold for cellular energy depletion was crossed. These conditions are incompatible with teratogenicity in which some tissues are permanently damaged and others are spared, permitting survival of abnormal embryos to term.

Developmental Toxicity Mediated by Perturbations in Maternal and Placental Homeostasis. The agents discussed so far are believed to exert developmental toxicity through a direct effect on the conceptus, either by killing proliferating cells or by altering differentiative processes. There are examples of agents and conditions that are embryotoxic through indirect effects on the conceptus resulting from alterations in the maternal system. The best example of these are perturbations that lead to maternal nutritional deficiencies. Generalized malnutrition, caloric restriction, and protein deficiency during pregnancy lead to severe growth retardation, thyroid deficiencies, and delays in CNS maturation that are not reversible with augmentation of the food supply to the neonate (Shrader *et al.*, 1977). Deprivation of specific nutrients in the maternal diet, i.e., vitamin A (Warkany and Roth, 1948), zinc (Hurley *et al.*, 1971), and folic acid (Johnson and Chepenik, 1981), can lead to malformations, growth retardation, and embryolethality. Treatment of the mother with agents that reduce availability of essential nutrients to the embryo, i.e., EDTA for trace metals, aminopterin for folic acid, results in syndromes similar to those obtained with restriction in the maternal diet. Developmental toxicity studies in rabbits given oral antibiotics (Clark *et al.*, 1986) also demonstrate this point. Oral administration of norfloxacin produced maternal weight loss and reduced food intake, abortion, and decreased fetal weight. The degree of embryotoxicity appeared related to the severity of the maternal toxicity which was due to alterations in the animal's gut flora. Maternal food deprivation alone produced similar types of maternal and fetal effects.

Agents that reduce the transport of nutrients from the maternal to embryonic compartment through specific interference with placental function can have an indirect embryotoxic effect. Trypan blue is believed to be teratogenic through interference with histiotrophic nutrition of the embryo by the yolk sac placenta (Beck, 1981). This type of nutrition involves pinocytosis/phagocytosis of maternal macromolecules and hydrolytic breakdown by lysosomal enzymes in cells of the yolk sac placenta, followed by passage of soluble nutrients to the embryo. Trypan blue inhibits the process of pinocytosis and the lysosomal enzymes involved in the hydrolysis of macromolecules. Teratogenic activity of the dye ceases between days 10 to 11 of gestation in rats, which coincides with the transition from a yolk sac placenta to a chorioallantoic placenta. Hemotrophic nutrition, or the simple diffusion of nutrients between closely apposed maternal and embryonic circulations, is characteristic of the chorioallantoic placenta and is not affected by trypan blue. Demonstration that developmental toxicants do not penetrate into embryonic tissues is the usual approach taken to defining the "indirect" mode of action. This can prove to be difficult insofar as few analytic techniques are sufficiently sensitive to detect low levels of xenobiotics in the early embryo. A more accurate approach may be to utilize cultures of postimplantation rat embryos where test agents are either added directly to the culture medium, or control embryos are cultured in serum derived from treated mothers. This approach has been taken by Steele *et al.* (1983) to determine whether hypolipidemic agents that were embryotoxic *in vivo* were so due to maternal hypolipidemia or to direct effects on the embryo. Results indicated that the culture of embryos in hypolipidemic serum had no adverse effects, whereas direct exposure of embryos to the agents themselves in normal serum was embryotoxic.

Alteration of uteroplacental blood flow is an important factor in indirect effects of developmental toxicants. Uteroplacental blood flow is reduced in women with hypertension, a condition that is associated with the birth of growth-retarded infants. In rats, the effects of short-term but total arrest of circulation have been studied by uterine vascular clamping (Barr and Brent, 1978). When conducted prior to the sixth day of gestation, embryolethality in the clamped horn was high, but survivors were not growth retarded. Clamping during the organogenesis period for up to an hour produced a spectrum of malformations specific for the developmental age at the time of obstruction, but negligible lethality or growth retardation. Partial but permanent reduction in uteroplacental blood flow by uterine artery ligation is generally associated with growth retardation, especially when performed at later stages of gestation (Barr and Brent, 1978). Vasoactive drugs such as serotonin, epinephrine, and ergotamine have been shown to cause malformations, embryolethality, and growth retardation (Neubert *et al.*, 1980). Intravenous infusion of epinephrine into pregnant rabbits elevated maternal blood pressure and caused extensive uterine vasoconstriction, placental cyanosis, and functional cardiovascular alterations in the fetus. The placental cyanosis coincided with, or slightly preceded, the fetal hemodynamic changes (Dornhorst and Young, 1952).

Hydroxyurea, an agent whose teratogenicity has been attributed to inhibition of DNA synthesis and cytotoxicity, was found to have a dramatic effect on uteroplacental blood flow in pregnant rabbits. Within two to five minutes after maternal exposure, uteroplacental blood flow decreased 77 percent and uterine vascular resistance increased 400 percent compared to controls. (Millicovsky *et al.*, 1981). Immediately thereafter, craniofacial and cardiac hemorrhages were observed in rabbit embryos. The same effects were produced in rabbit embryos after clamping the uterine vessels for ten minutes. These findings indicate that the developmental toxicity of hydroxyurea may be partly attributed to alteration of maternal and uterine hemodynamics, which cause an immediate pathologic effect on the embryo. Inhibition of DNA synthesis and cell death may constitute secondary effects that compromise the recovery of the embryo from the initial vascular insult. This example indicates that developmental toxicity is a far more complex process than can be explained on the basis of mutagenicity or cytotoxicity of the test agent. Assumptions cannot be made that the mode of embryotoxic action is identical to the mode of cellular action, even for agents with well-defined cellular mechanisms of action such as hydroxyurea, given the complex interchange that occurs between maternal, placental, and embryonic systems.

DISTRIBUTION AND BIOTRANSFORMATION OF XENOBIOTICS DURING PREGNANCY

The manner in which chemicals are absorbed during pregnancy, whether or not they reach the conceptus, and in what form, are topics of highly specialized research in pharmacokinetics. It is now accepted that every aspect of xenobiotic disposition and biotransformation is modified by the physiologic changes associated with pregnancy. The maternal, placental, and fetal compartments comprise independent, yet interacting, systems that undergo profound changes throughout the course of pregnancy. Each of these components will first be considered separately, and then attempts will be made to describe their interactions at different stages of pregnancy, i.e., the organogenesis and fetal periods, to determine whether the balance is in favor of or against protection of the conceptus. More detailed information on xenobiotic disposition and biotransformation during pregnancy can be found in a number of reviews (Neims *et al.*, 1976; Juchau, 1981; Hytten, 1984; Metcalf *et al.*, 1988).

Physiologic Changes in Pregnancy That Alter the Pharmacokinetics of Xenobiotics

Several pregnancy-related physiologic alterations favor increased absorption of xenobiotics in humans. Gastric emptying and transport through the small intestine are delayed, leading to more complete absorption. Likewise, increased tidal volume and reduced residual lung volume favor increased absorption of volatile and soluble substances through the lung. The uptake of particles and aerosols is also increased with the elevation in airstream velocity. The skin and mucous membranes also have increased blood flow and xenobiotics applied to these sites are more likely to be rapidly absorbed. Early in pregnancy the cardiac output increases by about 30 percent owing to an elevation in both heart rate and stroke volume. This results in increased tissue concentrations of absorbed xenobiotics, especially in organs that are highly perfused, such as the placenta and uterus (reviewed in Hytten, 1984 and Metcalfe et al., 1988).

Pregnancy alters several factors that influence the distribution of xenobiotics. These include an increase in total body water and body fat, and a decrease in plasma binding proteins (reviewed in Hytten, 1984). Plasma volume is elevated by 50 percent, whereas the increase in red cell volume is only approximately 18 percent, leading to borderline anemia. The generalized edema characteristic of normal pregnancy is due to a 70 percent elevation of the extracellular fluid space, which represents an increased area for distribution of xenobiotics. The average pregnant woman stores 3 to 4 kg of body fat in subcutaneous depots. This fat is gained in the first six months of pregnancy and tends to be mobilized in the last trimester. The increase in body fat can act as a reservoir for fat-soluble compounds, which, when released during late pregnancy, can result in increased xenobiotic exposure to both mother and fetus.

Many xenobiotics are bound to plasma proteins, predominantly albumin. This binding is usually reversible, saturable, and relatively nonspecific. The concentration of plasma albumin declines in the first half of pregnancy by approximately 20 percent owing to an increase in maternal plasma volume and actual decrease in total plasma albumin content. For highly bound xenobiotics, the hypoalbuminemia of pregnancy results in a decrease in the bound and a corresponding increase in the free plasma fraction. The mobilization of fat stores in the last trimester and subsequent competition for albumin binding sites by free fatty acids enhances the fraction of unbound xenobiotic. As the maternal plasma albumin concentration falls during pregnancy, levels of albumin in fetal plasma gradually increase. Since the biologic activity of a xenobiotic is usually related to the concentration of the unbound molecule, i.e., the free fraction in the plasma, changes in the degree of maternal and fetal binding can influence toxicity. Thus, for a compound absorbed in early pregnancy, if lower fetal plasma albumin concentration is combined with a high free xenobiotic fraction in maternal plasma, a net accumulation of unbound compound in the fetal compartment will occur, even at lower-than-normal maternal plasma drug concentrations (Levy, 1984).

Although several studies have been published, little is known about the effect of pregnancy on the relative rates of activating and detoxifying reactions for any given substrate (Juchau, 1981). The human liver is not enlarged in pregnancy as it is in rats, which have a 40 percent increase in absolute liver weight during pregnancy. When expressed in units of hepatic microsomal protein or wet weight of hepatic tissue, rates of most oxidation and conjugation reactions were decreased during pregnancy in rats. The lowered specific activity of these reactions is counteracted by the increase in maternal liver weight, however, so that the total activity in the whole liver can be comparable to that in the nonpregnant female. The decreased level of monooxygenase activity in maternal liver has been attributed to decreased enzyme levels as well as to competitive inhibition by circulating steroids (Neims et al., 1976). Another factor that could contribute to the lower monooxygenase activities is that pregnant rats appear to be less responsive to induction of hepatic cytochrome monooxygenase systems by phenobarbital (but not 3-methylcholanthrene) than are nonpregnant females (Guenther and Mannering, 1977). Despite the absence of a comprehensive literature on this subject, there appears to be an overall decrease in hepatic xenobiotic biotransformation during pregnancy. There is not sufficient information on extrahepatic biotransformation during pregnancy to generalize about their contribution to maternal biotransformations.

Excretion by the kidneys accounts for a major portion of xenobiotic elimination, and during pregnancy renal function undergoes a greater change than any other maternal system. In humans, the renal plasma flow and the glomerular filtration rate double by the end of the second trimester and remain elevated until term. The effect of increased glomerular filtration rate on xenobiotic elimination depends on the concentration of free drug in plasma. It is likely that the increase in filtration has a major effect on elimination of those drugs excreted unchanged in urine and of conjugates. In summary, the physiologic changes that occur in the maternal system during pregnancy are increased absorption and distribution of xenobiotics, accompanied by decreased hepatic biotransformation. These alterations will tend to favor retention of xenobiotics, but may be offset by the increase in renal function (Hytten, 1984).

Transport and Biotransformation of Xenobiotics by the Placenta

The placenta should be viewed as a lipid membrane that permits bidirectional transfer of substances between maternal and fetal compartments rather than as a "barrier." The transfer depends on three major elements: the type of placentation, the physiochemical properties of the compound, and the placental biotransformation. There are two distinctly different placentas in most mammalian species during organogenesis. In rodents, the yolk sac placenta predominates during organogenesis, whereas in primate species including humans, the chorioallantoic placenta is dominant. Except for cases where the xenobiotic is selectively toxic to one type of placenta over another (i.e., trypan blue), few correlations have been made between anatomic classification of the placenta and transfer of chemicals between mother and fetus (Waddell and Marlowe, 1981). Although earlier work suggested that placental membrane thickness or the number of placental layers limited diffusion, it is now clear that the situation is more complex. For example, the observed decrease in tissue layers and thickness of the trophoblast does not predict the decrease in placental permeability between the 7th and 14th days of rodent pregnancy (Green et al., 1979). The fetal endothelium, which is not markedly altered during pregnancy, is believed to be the layer responsible for diffusional resistance to larger-molecular-weight substances in rabbits (Thornburg and Faber, 1976). For smaller polar molecules, diffusion through sheep and rabbit placentas has been associated with the presence of interstitial water-filled pores of fixed diameter. Species differences in this parameter are great, however, and the calculated pore radii are 0.4 nm for sheep and approximately 30 nm for rabbits (Morris and Boyd, 1988). Blood flow constitutes the major rate-limiting factor in placental transfer of the more lipid-soluble compounds. Placental blood flow progressively increases throughout pregnancy at a rate that is proportional to fetal size even though placental mass, relative to fetal mass, is reduced (Green et al., 1979).

The movement of xenobiotics from maternal to fetal circulation occurs primarily by diffusion.

Active transport, facilitated diffusion, and carrier-mediated transfer are important for endogenous molecules but seem to play a much more limited role for xenobiotics. Lipid solubility, ionic charge, molecular weight, and structural configuration affect transport. The most rapid transplacental passage occurs with compounds that are lipophilic and nonionized at physiologic pH, and their transfer is flow-limited. For very hydrophilic compounds passage is likely to depend on restricted diffusion through water-filled channels and is directly dependent on molecular size. In general water-soluble xenobiotics with molecular weights less than 800 daltons readily cross the human placenta. Passage of hydrophilic drugs is much lower in animals with small interstitial pore radius such as the sheep than in primates or rodents. Protein binding of a xenobiotic will affect molecular size and lipid solubility and have a major effect on placental transfer. Maternal and fetal plasma pH affect permeability by altering ionization and the lipid solubility of the compound (Morris and Boyd, 1988).

The different possibilities of xenobiotic transfer based on lipid solubility are illustrated in Figure 7–6. In panel A, the parent compound is lipid soluble and crosses the placenta without difficulty. Polar metabolites (i.e., conjugates) are formed in the mother, but do not cross the placenta and are excreted from the maternal compartment. Another possibility is illustrated in panel B, where nonpolar metabolites (i.e., products of phase I reactions) are formed in the mother and the parent compound, and stable, nonpolar metabolites cross the placenta. Additional biotransformation to polar metabolites and subsequent excretion occur primarily in the maternal compartment. A third possibility is that the lipid-soluble parent compound and nonpolar metabolites equilibrate across the placenta, and polar metabolites formed in either maternal or fetal compartments do not cross the placenta. Excretion occurs to a greater extent on the maternal side, and polar metabolites may accumulate on the fetal side (Figure 7–6, C). A fourth possibility is that the parent compound is so polar that it does not cross the placenta and is excreted unchanged from the maternal compartment (Figure 7–6, D).

The human placenta appears to contain the enzyme systems for classic xenobiotic biotransformation, i.e., oxidation, reduction, hydrolysis, and conjugations. Compared to hepatic tissues, the xenobiotic biotransforming capacity of the placenta is negligible unless the mother has been exposed to 3-methylcholanthrene-type inducing agents during pregnancy. Cigarette smoking, for example, is positively correlated

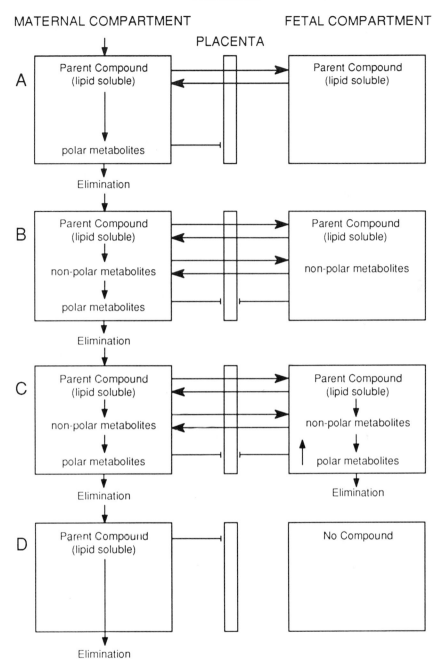

MATERNAL COMPARTMENT   PLACENTA   FETAL COMPARTMENT

Figure 7–6. Influence of lipid solubility on the distribution and accumulation of xenobiotics in maternal and fetal compartments. See text for explanation. (Modified from Krauer, B.; Krauer, F.; and Hytten, F. E.: Drug disposition and pharmacokinetics in the maternal-placental-fetal unit. *Pharmacol. Ther.*, **10**:301–328, 1980.)

with increased AHH (aryl hydrocarbon hydroxylase, now called cytochrome P-450IA1) activity in the placenta. A high, dose-related correlation ($r = 0.9$) between placental AHH activity and smoking of 1 to 40 cigarettes a day during pregnancy has been found (Gurtoo *et al.*, 1983).

Saturation of AHH induction occurred with smoking more than 20 to 25 cigarettes per day.

The genes that synthesize the cytochrome P-450s responsible for metabolism of polycyclic hydrocarbons (cytochrome P-450IA1) to reactive intermediates have been identified as

Cyp1a1 and *Cyp1a2*. The induction process of both genes requires the aromatic hydrocarbon receptor. Inducible *Cyp1a1* enzyme activity is detectable in the placenta of rats or mice receiving polycylic hydrocarbons and in the human placenta and embryo during the first trimester in smoking mothers. Using *in situ* hybridization, the localization of the genes and the timing of their expression have been examined in mice following induction with 3-methylcholanthrene. Between days 5.3 and 14.5 of gestation, inducible *Cyp1a1* mRNA was detected in extraembryonic tissues only and not in the embryo proper. *Cyp1a2* was not detected under any conditions and in the absence of induction *Cyp1a1* was also not detected (Dey *et al.*, 1989). Using polyclonal antibodies against cytochrome P-450IA1, Yang *et al.* (1989) came to a similar conclusion: inducibility of the cytochrome P-450IA1 was greatest in the visceral yolk sac of the rat but was barely detectable in the embryo proper during organogenesis.

Use of these molecular probes has permitted far more sensitive evaluation of the appearance, inducibility, and substrate specificity of the cytochrome P-450 enzymes during development than has previously been possible. Findings using these molecular approaches are likely to supplant the conventional wisdom that embryonic and placental tissues of laboratory animals are not inducible until late in gestation. Although signs of cytochrome P-450 activity have now been detected early in the organogenesis period, it is still not possible to determine if inducibility of this system protects or predisposes the conceptus to toxicity from xenobiotic exposure. With a primary localization in extraembryonic tissues, the cytochrome P-450 system could either prevent exposure of the conceptus or function in the generation of reactive intermediates that have a toxic effect on the conceptus.

Fetal Disposition and Biotransformation of Xenobiotics

Xenobiotics that have crossed the placenta enter the fetal circulation via the umbilical vein. The fetal liver is located between the umbilical vein and the inferior vena cava so that xenobiotics passing the placenta must traverse the fetal liver before entering the heart and the systemic circulation. The umbilical venous flow is diverted in the fetal liver so that substantial amounts of blood may enter the ductus venosus and bypass the liver, while the remainder flows into the portal vein and perfuses the hepatic parenchymal cells.

Amniotic fluid has the potential for being a slowly equilibrating reservoir for xenobiotics with the characteristics of a deep compartment

(Hytten, 1984). Up to 20 weeks of human development, the fetal epidermis is highly permeable and amniotic fluid has the same composition as fetal extracellular fluid. After 20 weeks the fetal skin becomes keratinized, limiting the exchange between amniotic fluid and extracellular fluid. The composition and volume of amniotic fluid then represent a balance between fetal urine production and fetal swallowing, and entry of xenobiotics into amniotic fluid is dependent on excretion via fetal urine. The major route of removal for xenobiotics in amniotic fluid is for the fluid to be swallowed by the fetus, filtered out by the fetal kidney, and returned to the maternal system via the umbilical artery.

SUMMARY AND CONCLUSIONS

The field of teratology has evolved from an experimental science concerned with anatomic description of malformations. As advances were made in the basic understanding of embryology, xenobiotics were used as tools for disrupting normal development to achieve a greater understanding of differentiation. This still constitutes the major underpinning of experimental research in teratology and is the critical factor in any advances made in the field. Today, additional demands are placed on teratologists to predict the risk of xenobiotic exposure on human pregnancy outcome. The necessity of evaluating risks to the conceptus from xenobiotic exposure has been forcefully demonstrated in epidemics of human birth defects induced by nutritional deficiencies, infectious agents, and xenobiotic exposure of the population. Consequently, the objectives of teratology research are increasingly oriented to an understanding of developmental toxicology, or how xenobiotics are taken up, distributed, accumulated, and biotransformed by pregnant mammals and their effects on the conceptus. The methodologies for carrying out this type of research are relatively well established and principles of general systemic toxicology in adult animals can be applied. Disciplined application of these principles will no doubt reveal that xenobiotics can interfere with the state of pregnancy and the process of development by unique and highly complex mechanisms. The key to understanding how some xenobiotics specifically interfere with the successful completion of pregnancy, however, ultimately depends on a more complete comprehension of the basic processes of development.

REFERENCES

Abel, E.: Fetal alcohol syndrome: behavioral teratology. *Psychol. Bull.*, **87**:29–50, 1980.

Adams, J., and Buelke-Sam, J.: Behavioral assessment for the postnatal animal: Testing and methods development. In Kimmel, C. A., and Buelke-Sam, J. (eds.): *Developmental Toxicology*. Raven Press, New York, 1981, pp. 233–258.

Adler, I-D.: New approaches to mutagenicity studies in animals for carcinogenic and mutagenic agents. II. Clastogenic effects determined in transplacentally treated mouse embryos. *Teratogen. Carcinog. Mutagen.*, 3:321–334, 1983.

Agnish, N.: Personal communication, 1989.

American Cancer Society (ACS): *Cancer Facts and Figures*. The Society, New York, 1980.

Barr, M., and Brent, R.: Uterine vascular interruption and combined radiation and surgical procedures. In Wilson, J. G., and Fraser, F. C. (eds.): *Handbook for Teratology*, Vol. 4. Plenum Press, New York, 1978, pp. 275–304.

Bass, R.; Oerter, D.; Krowke, R.; and Speilmann, H.: Embryonic development and mitochondrial function. III. Inhibition of respiration and ATP generation in rat embryos by thiamphenicol. *Teratology*, 18:93–102, 1978.

Beck, F.: Comparative placental morphology and function. In Kimmel, C. A., and Buelke-Sam, J. (eds.): *Developmental Toxicology*. Raven Press, New York, 1981, pp. 35–54.

Bibbo, M.; Gill, W.; Azizi, F.; Blough, R.; Fnag, V.; Rosenfield, R.; Schumacher, G.; Sleeper, K.; Sonek, M.; and Wied, G.: Follow-up study of male and female offspring of DES-exposed mothers. *Obstet. Gynecol.*, 49:1–8, 1977.

Biddle, F. G.: Teratogenesis of acetazolamide in the CBA/J and SWV strains of mice. II. Genetic control of the teratogenic response. *Teratology*, 11:37–46, 1975.

Bingol, N.; Fuchs, M.; Diaz, V.; Stone, R. K.; and Gromisch, D. S.: Teratogenicity of cocaine in humans. *J. Pediatr.*, 110:93–96, 1987.

Bolande, R. P.: Teratogenesis and oncogenesis. In Wilson, J. G., and Fraser, F. C. (eds.): *Handbook of Teratology*, Vol. 2. Plenum Press, New York, 1977, pp. 293–328.

Brazzell, R. K.; Vane, F. M.; Ehmann, C. W.; and Colburn, W. A.: Pharmacokinetics of isotretinoin during repetitive dosing to patients. *Eur. J. Clin. Pharmacol.*, 24:695–702, 1983.

Brinster, R. L.: Teratogen testing using preimplantation mammalian embryos. In Shepard, T. H.; Miller, J. R.; and Marois, M. (eds.) *Methods for Detection of Environmental Agents That Produce Congenital Defects*. American Elsevier, New York, 1975, pp. 113–124.

Busa, W.: Mechanisms and consequences of pH-mediated cell regulation. *Annu. Rev. Physiol.*, 48:389–402, 1986.

Chasnoff, I. J.: Cocaine, pregnancy and the neonate. *Women Health*, 15:23–35, 1989.

Chasnoff, I. J.; Chisum, G. M.: and Kaplan, W. E.: Maternal cocaine use and genitourinary tract malformations. *Teratology*, 37:201–204, 1988.

Chernoff, G.: The fetal alcohol syndrome in mice: maternal variables. *Teratology*, 22:71–75, 1980.

Chernoff, N.; Rogers, J. M.; and Kavlock, R. J.: An overview of maternal toxicity and prenatal development: considerations for developmental toxicity hazard assessments. *Toxicology*, 59:111–125, 1989.

Chung, C. S., and Myrianthopoulos, N. C.: Factors affecting risks of congenital malformations. *The National Foundation March of Dimes Original Articles Series*, Vol. XI, No. 10, 1975.

Clark, R. L.; Robertson, R. T.; Chennakatu, P. P.; Bland, J. A.; Nolan, T. E.; Oppenheimer, L.; and Bokelman, D. L.: Association between adverse maternal and embryo-fetal effects in Norfloxacin-treated and food-deprived rabbits. *Fund. Appl. Toxicol.*, 7:272–286, 1986.

Collins, M. D.; Fradkin, R.; and Scott, W. J.: Induction of postaxial forelimb ectrodactyly with anticonvulsant agents in A/J mice. *Teratology*, 41:61–70, 1990.

Consumer Product Safety Commission (CPSC): *Toxicity Testing of Household Products*. Document 1138. Washington, D.C., 1977.

Cooper, L. Z., and Krugman, S.: Diagnosis and management: congenital rubella. *Pediatrics*, 37:335–342, 1966.

Dey, A.; Westphal, H.; and Nebert, D.: Cell-specific induction of mouse Cyp1a1 mRNA during development. *Proc. Natl. Acad. Sci. USA*, 86:7446–7450, 1989.

Dieckmann, W. J.; Davis, M. E.; and Rynkiewicz, L. M.: Does administration of diethylstilbestrol during pregnancy have therapeutic value? *Am. J. Obstet. Gynecol.*, 66:1062–1081, 1953.

Dornhorst, A. C., and Young, M. I.: The action of adrenalin and noradrenaline on the placental and foetal circulations in the rabbit and guinea pig. *J. Physiol. (Lond.)*, 118:282–291, 1952.

Epstein, C. J.: Molecular and genetic aspects of early embryonic development. In Warshaw, J. B. (ed.) *The Biological Basis of Reproductive and Developmental Medicine*. Elsevier Biomedical, New York, 1983, pp. 43–60.

Fabro, S.: Biochemical basis of thalidomide teratogenicity. In Juchau, M. R. (ed.): *The Biochemical Basis of Chemical Teratogenesis*. Elsevier/North-Holland, New York, 1981, pp. 159–178.

Fabro, S.; Smith, R. L.; and Williams, R. T.: Fate of ^{14}C-thalidomide in the pregnant rabbit. *Biochem. J.*, 104:565–569, 1967.

Finnell, R.; Toloyan, S.; van Waes, M.; and Kalivas, P.: Preliminary evidence for cocaine-induced embryopathy in mice. *Toxicol. Appl. Pharmacol.* 103:228–238, 1990.

Food and Drug Administration (FDA): *Guidelines for Reproduction Studies for Safety Evaluation of Drugs for Human Use*. Washington, DC, 1966.

————: Advisory Committee on Protocols for Safety Evaluation, Panel on Reproduction: report on reproduction studies in the safety evaluation of food additives and pesticide residues. *Toxicol. Appl. Pharmacol.*, 16:264–296, 1970.

Frankos, V H.: FDA perspectives on the use of teratology data for human risk assessment. *Fund. Appl. Toxicol.*, 5:615–622, 1985.

Fraser, F. C.: Relation of animal studies to the problem in man. In Wilson, J. G., and Fraser, F. C. (eds.): *Handbook of Teratology*, Vol. 1. Plenum Press, New York, 1977, pp. 75–96.

Fullerton, P. M., and Kremer, M.: Neuropathy after intake of thalidomide (Distaval). *Br. Med. J.*, 2:855–858, 1961.

Green, T. P.; O'Dea, R. F.; and Mirkin, B. L.: Determinants of drug disposition and effect in the fetus. *Annu. Rev. Pharmacol. Toxicol.*, 19:285–322, 1979.

Gregg, N. M.: Congenital cataract following German measles in the mother. *Trans. Opthalmol. Soc. Aust.*, 3:35–46, 1941.

Guenther, T. M., and Mannering, G. T.: Induction of hepatic monooxygenase systems of pregnant rats with phenobarbital and 3-methylcholanthrene. *Biochem. Pharmacol.*, 26:577–584, 1977.

Gurtoo, H. L.; Williams, C. J.; Gottlieb, K.; Mulhern, A.; Caballes, L.; Vaught, J.; Marinello, A.; and Bansal S.: Population distribution of placental benzo(a)pyrene metabolism in smokers. *Int. J. Cancer*, 31:29–37, 1983.

Henderson, G.; Hoyumpa, A.; McClain, C.; and Shenker, S.: The effects of chronic and acute alcohol administration on fetal development in the rat. *Alcohol. Clin. Exp. Res.*, **3**:99–106, 1979.

Henderson, M., and McMillen, B.: Effects of prenatal exposure to cocaine or related drugs on rat developmental and neurological indices. *Brain Res. Bull.* **24**:207–212, 1990.

Herbst, A. L.; Cole, P.; Colton, T.; Robboy, S.; and Scully, R.: Age-incidence and risk of diethylstilbestrol-related clear cell adenocarcinoma of the vagina and cervix. *Am. J. Obstet. Gynecol.*, **128**:43–50, 1977.

Hirsch, K. S., and Scott, W. J.: Searching for the mechanism of acetazolamide teratogenesis. In Kalter, H. (ed.): *Issues and Reviews in Teratology* Vol. 1. Plenum Press, New York, 1983, pp. 309–347.

Hoar, R. M., and Monie, I. W.: Comparative development of specific organ systems. In Kimmel, C. A., and Buelke-Sam, J. (eds.): *Developmental Toxicology.* Raven Press, New York, 1981, pp. 13–33.

Holmes, L. B., and Trelstad, R. L.: The early limb deformity caused by acetazolamide. *Teratology*, **20**:289–296, 1979.

Hurley, L. S.; Gowan, J.; and Swenerton, H.: Teratogenic effects on short-term and transitory zinc deficiency in rats. *Teratology*, **4**:199–204, 1971.

Hytten, F. E.: Physiologic changes in the mother related to drug handling. In Krauer, B., Krauer, F., Hytten, F., and del Pozo, E. (eds.): *Drugs and Pregnancy.* Academic Press, New York, 1984, pp. 7–17.

Inouye, M., and Murakami, U.: Teratogenic effect on *N*-methyl-*N'*-nitronitrosoguanidine. *Teratology*, **18**:263–268, 1978.

Ivankovic, S.: Teratogenic and carcinogenic effects of some chemicals during prenatal life in rats, Syrian Golden hamsters and minipigs. In *Perinatal Carcinogenesis.* National Cancer Institute Monograph 51, DHEW Publication No. (NIH) 7a-1063, 1979, pp. 103–116.

Johnson, E. M., and Chepenik, K. P.: Teratogenicity of folate antagonists. In Juchau, M. R. (ed.): *The Biochemical Basis of Chemical Teratogenesis.* Elsevier/North Holland, New York, 1981, pp. 137–178.

Jones, K., and Smith, D.: Recognition of the fetal alcohol syndrome in early infancy. *Lancet*, **ii**:999–1001, 1973.

Juchau, M. R.: Enzymatic bioactivation and inactivation of chemical teratogens and transplacental carcinogens/mutagens. In Juchau, M. R. (ed.): *The Biochemical Basis of Chemical Teratogenesis.* Elsevier/North Holland, New York, 1981, pp. 63–94.

Kaminski, M.; Le Bouvier, F.; du Mazanbrun, C.: and Runzeau-Rouquette, C.: Moderate alcohol use and pregnancy outcome. *Neurobehav. Toxicol. Teratol.,* **3**:173–181, 1981.

Kamm, J. J.; Ashenfelter, K. O.; and Ehman, C. W.: Preclinical and clinical toxicology of selected retinoids. In Sporn, M.; Roberts, A. B.; and Goodman, D. S. (eds): *The Retinoids*, Vol. 2. Academic Press, New York, 1984, pp. 287–326.

Karnofskey, D. A.: Mechanism of action of certain growth-inhibiting drugs. In Wilson, J. G., and Warkany, J. (eds.): *Teratology: Principles and Techniques.* University of Chicago Press, Chicago, 1965, pp. 185–193.

Keberle, H.; Faigle, J. W.; Fritz, H.; Knuesel, F.; Loustalot, P.; and Schmid, K.: Theories on the mechanism of action of thalidomide. In Roberson, J. M.; Sullivan, F. M.; and Smith, R. L. (eds.): *Embryopathic Activity of Drugs.* Churchill Livingstone, London, 1965, pp. 210–233.

Kennedy, T. Q., and Armstrong, D. T.: The role of prostaglandins in endometrial vascular changes at implantation. In Glasser, S. R., and Bullock, D. W. (eds.): *Cellular and Molecular Aspects of Implantation.* Plenum Press, New York, 1981, pp. 349–361.

Khera, K. S.: Maternal toxicity—a possible factor in fetal malformations in mice. *Teratology*, **29**:411–416, 1984.

Kimmel, C. A.; Holson, J. F.; Hogue, C. J.; and Carlo, G. L.: Reliability of experimental studies for predicting hazards to human development. Final report NCTR Technical Report for Experiment No. 6015. National Center for Toxicological Research, Jefferson, Arkansas, 1984, p. 56.

Knapp, K.: Das thalidomid-syndrom. *Bull. Soc. Roy. Belge. Gynecol. Obstet.*, **33**:37–42, 1963.

Kochhar, D. M., and McBride, W.: Isotretinoin metabolism and its role in teratogenesis in mice and marmosets. *Teratology*, **33**:47C (abstract), 1986.

Kochhar, D. M., and Penner, J. D.: Developmental effects of isotretinoin and 4-oxo-isotretinoin: the role of metabolism in teratogenicity. *Teratology*, **36**:67–75, 1987.

Kochhar, D. M.; Penner, J. D.; and McDay, J. A.: Limb development in mouse embryos. II. Reduction defects, cytotoxicity and inhibition of DNA synthesis produced by cytosine arabinoside. *Teratology*, **18**:71–92, 1978.

Kraft, J. C.; Kochhar, D. M.; Scott, W. J.; and Nau, H.: Low teratogenicity of 13-cis retinoic acid (isotretinoin) in the mouse corresponds to low concentrations during organogenesis: comparison with the all-*trans* isomer. *Toxicol. Appl. Pharmacol.*, **87**:474–482, 1987.

Lammer, E. J., and Adams, J.: Dermatologic drugs advisory committee hearing, FDA, May, 1989.

Lammer, E. J.; Chen, D. T.; Hoar, R. M.; Agnish, N. D.; Benke, P. J.; Braun, J. T.; Curry, C. J.; Fernhoff, P. M.; Grix, A. W.; and Lott, I. T. Retinoic acid embryopathy. *N. Engl. J. Med.*, **313**:837–841, 1985.

Lammer, E. J.; Hayes, A. M.; Schunior, A.; and Holmes, L. B. Risk for major malformations among human fetuses exposed to isotretinoin (13-*cis*-retinoic acid). *Teratology*, **35**:68A, 1987.

Layton, W. M., and Hallesy, D. W.: Deformity of forelimb in rats; association with high doses of acetazolamine. *Science*, **149**:306–308, 1965.

Lenz, W.: Das Thalidomid-syndrom. *Fortschr. Med.,* **81**:148–153, 1963.

———: Malformations caused by drugs in pregnancy. *Am. J. Dis. Child.*, **112**:99–106, 1966.

Levy, G.: Protein binding of drugs in the maternal-fetal unit and its potential clinical significance. In Krauer, B., Krauer, F., Hytten, F. and del Pozo, E. (eds.): *Drugs in Pregnancy.* Academic Press, Orlando, 1984, pp. 29–45.

Lucier, G. W.; and Lamartiniere, C.: Metabolic activation/deactivation reactions during perinatal development. *Environ. Health Perspect.*, **29**:7–16, 1979.

MacGregor, S. N.; Keith, L. G.; Chasnoff, I. J.; Rosner, M. A.; Chisum, G. M.; Shaw, P.; and Minogue, J. P.: Cocaine use in pregnancy: adverse perinatal outcome. *Am. J. Obstet. Gynecol.*, **157**:686–690, 1987.

Mandel, J. D.: A new chemical mutagen for bacteria, 1-methyl-3-nitro-1-nitrosoguanidine. *Biochem. Biophys. Res. Commun.*, **3**:575–577, 1960.

Manson, J. M.: Developmental toxicity of alkylating agents: Mechanism of action. In Jachau, M. R. (ed.): *The Biochemical Basis of Chemical Teratogenesis.* Elsevier/North-Holland, New York, 1981, pp. 95–136.

Manson, J. M., and Kang, Y. J.: Test methods for assessing female reproductive and developmental toxicity. In Hayes, A. W. (ed.): *Principles and*

Methods of Toxicology. Raven Press, New York, 1989, pp. 311–360.

Manson, J. M., and Miller, M. L.: Contribution of mesenchymal cell death and mitotic alteration to asymmetric limb malformations induced by MNNG. *Teratogen. Carcinog. Mutagen.,* **3**:335–353, 1983.

Maugh, T. H.: Chemicals: how many are there? *Science,* **199**:162, 1978.

McBride, W. G.: Thalidomide and congenital anomalies. *Lancet,* **ii**:1358, 1961.

McLachlan, J., and Dixon, R.: Toxicologic comparisons of experimental and clinical exposure to diethylstilbestrol during gestation. *Adv. Sex Horm. Res.,* **3**:309–336, 1977.

Metcalfe, J.; Stock, M.; and Barron, D.: Maternal physiology during pregnancy. In Knobil, E. and Neill, J. (eds.): *The Physiology of Reproduction.* Raven Press, New York, 1988, pp. 2145–2177.

Meyne, J., and Legator, M.: Clastogenic effects of transplacental exposure of mouse embryos to nitrogen mustard or cyclophosphamide. *Teratogen. Carcinog. Mutagen.,* **3**:281–287, 1983.

Miller, R. W.: Prenatal origins of cancer in man: Epidemiological evidence. In Tomatis, L., and Mohr, E. (eds.): *Transplacental Carcinogenesis.* IARC Pub. No. 4, 1973, p. 175.

Millicovsky, G.; DeSesso, J.; Kleinman, L.; and Clark, K.: Effects of hydroxyurea on hemodynamics of pregnant rabbits: a maternally mediated mechanism of embryotoxicity. *Am. J. Obstet. Gynecol.,* **140**:747–752, 1981.

Morris, F., and Boyd, R.: Placental transport. In Knobil, E. and Neill, J. (eds.): *The Physiology of Pregnancy.* Raven Press, New York, 1988, pp. 2043–2085.

National Center for Health Statistics (NCHS): Births, marriages, divorces, and deaths for 1979. Monthly Vital Statistics Report. U.S. Department of Health, Education and Welfare, 1980.

National Foundation/March of Dimes: *Facts 1980.* The Foundation, New York, 1981a.

———: Report of Panel II. Guidelines for reproductive studies in exposed human populations. In Bloom, A. D. (ed.): *Guidelines for Studies of Human Populations Exposed to Mutagenic and Reproductive Hazards.* The Foundation, New York, 1981b, pp. 37–110.

National Institute on Drug Abuse (NIDA): Statistical series, Washington, D.C., 1987.

National Institute for Occupational Safety and Health (NIOSH): *Registry of Toxic Substances,* 1977.

Nau, H., and Scott, W. J.: Weak acids may act as teratogens by accumulating in the basic milieu of the early mammalian embryo. *Nature* **323**:276–287, 1986.

Nau, H., and Scott, W. J.: Teratogenicity of valproic acid and related substances in the mouse: drug accumulation and pH_i in the embryo during organogenesis and structure-activity considerations. *Arch. Toxicol., Suppl.* **11**:128–139, 1987.

Neims, A. H.; Warner, M.; Loughnan, P. M.; and Aranda, J. V.: Developmental aspects of the hepatic cytochrome P_{450} monooxygenase system. *Annu. Rev. Pharmacol. Toxicol.,* **16**:427–444, 1976.

Neubert, D.; Barrach, H. J.; and Merker, H. J.: Drug-induced damage to the embryo or fetus. *Curr. Top. Pathol.,* **69**:242–324, 1980.

Nowack, E.: Die sensible phase bei der thalidomid-embryopathie. *Humangenetik,* **1**:516–522, 1965.

Ornoy, A.; Salamon-Aron, J.; Ben-Zur, A.; and Kohn, G.: Placental findings in spontaneous abortions and stillbirths. *Teratology,* **24**:243–251, 1981.

Palmer, A. K.: Regulatory requirements for reproductive toxicology: Theory and practice. In Kimmel, C. A., and Buelke-Sam, J. (eds.): *Developmental Toxicology.* Raven Press, New York, 1981, pp. 259–287.

Pelkonen, O.: Transplacental transfer of foreign compounds and their metabolism by the foetus. In Bridges, J. W., and Chasseaund, L. F. (eds.): *Progress in Drug Metabolism,* Vol. 2. John Wiley & Sons, New York, 1977, pp. 119–161.

———: Biotransformation of xenobiotics in the fetus. *Pharmacol. Ther.,* **10**:261–281, 1980.

Poskanzer, D., and Herbst, A.: Epidemiology of vaginal adenosis and adenocarcinoma associated with exposure to stilbestrol in utero. *Cancer,* **39**:1892–1895, 1977.

Pratt, R. M., and Salomon, D. S.: Biochemical basis for the teratogenic effects of glucocorticoids. In Juchau, M. R. (ed.): *The Biochemical Basis of Chemical Teratogenesis.* Elsevier/North-Holland, New York, 1981, pp. 179–199.

Ritter, E. J.: Altered biosynthesis. In Wilson, J. G., and Fraser, F. C. (eds.): *Handbook of Teratology,* Vol. 2. Plenum Press, New York, 1977, pp. 99–116.

Rosett, H.; Weiner, L.; Zuckerman, B.; McKinlay, S.; and Edelin, K.: Reduction of alcohol consumption during pregnancy with benefits to the newborn. *Alcohol. Clin. Exp. Res.,* **4**:178–184, 1980.

Schardein, J.: Sedatives-hypnotics. In *Drugs as Teratogens.* CRC Press, Cleveland, 1976, pp. 145–153.

———: Hormones and hormone antagonists. In *Chemically Induced Birth Defects.* Marcel Dekker, New York, 1985, pp. 272–275.

———: Introduction. In *Chemically Induced Birth Defects.* Marcel Dekker, New York, 1985, pp. vii–x.

Schumacher, H. J.: Chemical structure and teratogenic properties. In Shepard, T.; Miller, R.; and Marois, M. (eds.): *Methods for Detection of Environmental Agents That Produce Congenital Defects.* American Elsevier, New York, 1975, pp. 65–77.

Schumacher, H. J.; Smith, R. L.; and Williams, T. T.: The metabolism of thalidomide: The spontaneous hydrolyses of thalidomide solutions. *Br. J. Pharmacol. Chemother.,* **25**:324–337, 1965.

Scott, W. J.: Effects of intrauterine administration of acetazolamide in rats. *Teratology,* **3**:261–268, 1970.

———: Cell death and reduced proliferative rate. In Wilson, J. G., and Fraser, F. C. (eds.): *Handbook of Teratology,* Vol. 2. Plenum Press, New York, 1977, pp. 81–98.

Scott, W. J., and Fradkin, R.: Effects of alcohol on non-human primate pregnancy. *Teratology,* **24**:31A, 1981.

Scott, W. J.; Duggan, C. A.; Schreiner, C. M.; and Collins, M. D.: Reduction of embryonic intracellular pH: a potential mechanism of acetazolamide-induced limb malformations. *Toxicol. Appl. Pharmacol.* **103**:238–254, 1990.

Sever, J. L.: Rubella as a teratogen. *Adv. Teratol.,* **2**:127–138, 1967.

Shepard, T. H.: *Catalog of Teratogenic Agents,* 5th ed. Johns Hopkins University Press, Baltimore, 1986.

Shrader, R. E.; Ferlatte, M. I.; Hastings-Roberts, M. H.; Schoenborne, B. M.; Hoernicke, C. A.; and Zeman, F. J.: Thyroid function in prenatally protein-deprived rats. *J. Nutr.,* **107**:221–229, 1977.

Snow, J.: Restorative growth and its problems for morphogenesis. In *Prevention of Physical and Mental Congenital Defects.* Alan R. Liss, New York, 1985, pp. 295–299.

Snow, M.: Restorative growth in mammalian embryos. In Kalter, H., (ed.): *Issues and Reviews in Teratology,* Vol. I. Plenum Press, New York, 1983, pp. 251–276.

Sokol, R.; Miller, S.; and Reed, G.: Alcohol abuse during pregnancy: an epidemiologic study. *Alcohol. Clin. Exp. Res.* **4**:178–184, 1980.

Staples, R. E.: Definition of teratogenesis and teratogens. In Shepard, T. H.; Miller, J. R.; and Marois, M. (eds.): *Methods for Detection of Environmental Agents That Produce Congenital Defects.* American Elsevier, New York, 1975, pp. 25–26.

Steele, C. E.; New, D. A. T.; Ashford, A.; and Copping, G. P.: Teratogenic action of hypolipidemic agents: an in vitro study with postimplantation embryos. *Teratology,* **28**:229–236, 1983.

Stephens, T. D.: Proposed mechanisms of action in thalidomide embryopathy. *Teratology,* **38**:229–239, 1988.

Streissguth, A.; Herman, C.; and Smith, D.: Intelligence, behavior, and dysmorphogenesis in the fetal alcohol syndrome: a report on 20 patients. *J. Pediatr.,* **92**:363–367, 1978.

Szabo, K., and Brent, R. L.: Reduction of drug-induced cleft palate in mice. *Lancet,* **i**:1296–1297, 1975.

Taussig, H. B.: A study of the German outbreak of phocomelia. The thalidomide syndrome. *JAMA,* **180**:1106, 1962.

Theiss, I.; Basler, A.; and Rohrborn, G.: Transplacental and direct exposure of mouse and marmoset to ethylnitrosourea: analysis of chromosomal aberrations. *Teratogen. Carcinog. Mutagen.,* **3**:219–230, 1983.

Thompson, C. J. S.: *The Mystery and Lore of Monsters.* Bell Publishing, New York, 1930.

Thornburg, K. C., and Faber, J.: The steady-state concentration gradients of an electron dense marker (ferritin) in the three-layered hemochorial placenta of the rabbit. *J. Clin. Invest.,* **58**:912–925, 1976.

U.S. Department of Health, Education and Welfare (USDHEW): The women and their pregnancies. The Collaborative Perinatal Study of the National Institute of Neurological Diseases and Strokes. DHEW Publication No. (NIH) 73–379, 1972.

Waddell, W. J., and Marlowe, C.: Biochemical regulation of the accessibility of teratogens to the developing embryo. In Juchau, M. R. (ed.): *The Biochemical Basis of Chemical Teratogenesis.* Elsevier/North Holland, New York, 1981, pp. 1–62.

Warburton, D., and Fraser, F. C.: Spontaneous abortion risks in man: data from reproductive histories collected in a medical genetics unit. *Hum. Genet.,* **16**:1–12, 1964.

Warkany, J.: Development of experimental mammalian teratology. In Wilson, J. G., and Warkany, J. (eds.): *Teratology: Principles and Techniques.* University of Chicago Press, Chicago, 1965, pp. 1–11.

———: Drugs. In *Congenital Malformation: Notes and Comments.* Year Book Medical Publishers, Chicago, 1971a, pp. 84–96.

———: Environmental factors, infection. In *Congenital Malformations: Notes and Comments.* Year Book Medical Publishers, Chicago, 1971b, pp. 62–70.

———: History of teratology. In Wilson, J. G., and Fraser, F. C., (eds.): *Handbook of Teratology,* Vol. I. Plenum Press, New York, 1977, pp. 3–46.

Warkany, J., and Roth, C. B.: Congenital malformations induced in rats by maternal vitamin A deficiency. II. Effect of varying the preparatory diet upon the yield of abnormal young. *J. Nutr.,* **35**:1–12, 1948.

Weaver, T. E., and Scott, W. J.: Acetazolamide teratogenesis: Association of maternal respiratory acidosis and ectrodactyly in C57BL/6J mice. *Teratology,* **30**:187–193, 1984a.

———: Acetazolamide teratogenesis: Interaction of maternal metabolic and respiratory acidosis in the induction of ectrodactyly in C57BL/6J mice. *Teratology,* **30**:195–202, 1984b.

Webster, W. S.; Johnson, M. C.; Lammer, E. J.; and Sulik, K. K.: Isotretinoin embryopathy and the cranial neural crest: an in vivo and in vitro study. *J. Craniofac. Genet. Dev. Biol.,* **6**:211–222, 1986.

Weicker, H.: Klinik und epidemiologie der thalidomid-embryopathie. *Bull. Soc. Roy. Belge. Gynecol. Obstet.,* **33**:21–32, 1963.

Wilson, J. G.: *Environment and Birth Defects.* Academic Press, New York, 1973, pp. 11–35.

Yang, H. Y.; Namkung, M.; and Juchau, M.: Immunodetection, immunoinhibition, immunoquantitation and biochemical analysis of cytochrome P-450Ial in tissues of the rat conceptus during the progression of organogenesis. *Biochem. Pharmacol.* **38**:4027–4036, 1989.

UNIT II

SYSTEMIC TOXICOLOGY

Chapter 8

TOXIC RESPONSES OF THE BLOOD

Roger P. Smith

INTRODUCTION

For many years, hematology was considered exclusively the study of the formed elements of the blood, namely, red cells, white cells, and platelets. An immense body of morphologic information has accrued from the microscopic study of smears of peripheral blood (Bessis, 1977). The formed elements constitute a complex organ with a total mass equivalent to that of the liver. Gradually, hematology expanded to include other parts of the system such as bone marrow, spleen, lymph nodes, and the reticuloendothelial tissue (phagocytic macrophages in the reticulum of various organs or lining some sinuses). Obviously, the formed elements have a functional relationship with the blood plasma and with the heart and lungs. Most of the biochemical and hematologic normal values used in this chapter apply to humans; Mitruka and Rawnsley (1977) have compiled an extensive anthology of biochemical and hematologic values for laboratory animals. Less elaborate compendia are also available (Burns and de Lannoy, 1966; Calsey and King, 1980) that include data on proteins, enzymes, electrolytes, and other constituents of plasma.

HEMATOPOIESIS

In the human fetus, several organs are sequentially involved in the production of blood cells. For a brief period, the yolk sac produces nucleated red cells containing an embryonic hemoglobin designated as $(\alpha^{2+}\epsilon^{2+})_2$. Subsequently, red cells are furnished by the liver, the spleen, and eventually the bone marrow. The liver is also the first organ to produce white cells and platelets. The hepatic red cells are not nucleated, but they contain fetal hemoglobin, $(\alpha^{2+}\gamma^{2+})_2$. The oxygen affinity of human fetal blood is higher than that of human adult blood, which helps the fetus extract oxygen from the maternal circulation (see also below).

At birth, only the marrow is producing red cells. A slow "switchover" from the synthesis of fetal to adult hemoglobin, $(\alpha^{2+}\beta^{2+})_2$, begins at that time; it is usually complete by the fourth to sixth month of age. Up to the age of about four years, hepatic and splenic red cell production can be reactivated in response to hypoxic demands associated with normal growth, but beyond that age, these extramedullary sites are activated only in pathophysiologic states. For example, the spleen is reactivated to serve as a reserve source of red cells in rats and mice exposed to high altitude (Ou *et al.*, 1980), but in most mammals it cannot support life in the event of bone marrow failure. Thus, bone marrow damage is always a grave threat to survival. It is also abnormal to find nucleated red cells in the systemic circulation of adult mammals. However, birds, fish, reptiles, and amphibians always have nucleated red cells in peripheral blood (Prankerd, 1961) because the cells are formed inside blood vessels instead of in bone marrow (see below).

The Bone Marrow

Bone marrow contains stem cells which are the immature precursors of the formed elements of the blood (Figure 8–1). This multipotential stem cell pool is stimulated to differentiate into unipotential or committed cells that eventually mature into red cells (erythrocytes), platelets (thrombocytes), or one of several series of white cells (leukocytes). Decreased numbers of these elements in peripheral blood as determined by actual counts usually with an electronic cell counter are referred to, respectively, as anemia, thrombocytopenia, and leukopenia. Stimulation of the stem cell pool is carried out by blood-borne factors called *poietins* or *colony stimulating factors*. It is likely that each circulating cell type has its own or more than one stimulating factor.

Erythropoiesis refers to the process by which red cells are produced. Control over the rate of erythropoiesis is exerted primarily through the activity of a plasma hormone, *erythropoietin*.

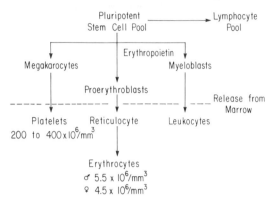

Figure 8-1. Bone marrow differentiation into the formed elements of peripheral blood. See also Figure 8-3 for further differentiation and classification of lymphocytes and leukocytes.

The kidney is critical in the production of erythropoietin after birth, but in the fetus, it is produced by the liver. Synthesis is stimulated by hypoxia, and it appears that the oxygen sensor is a heme protein. It is hypothesized that when kidney tissue oxygen tension decreases, the sensor is converted to its deoxy-conformation, which triggers increased expression of the erythropoietin gene. As the oxygen tension rises, the sensor binds oxygen, and the stimulus for erythropoietin synthesis is suppressed (Goldberg et al., 1988).

In the marrow, erythropoietin acts on the differentiation process at the stage in which a stem cell is converted to a proerythroblast (Figure 8-1). Therefore, erythropoietin may be thought of as regulating the size of the committed red cell pool. After several additional stages, the immature red cell is released from the marrow as a reticulocyte. This occurs in specialized marrow vessels (marrow sinuses) in which the walls are an attenuated epithelium. Oddly, the reticulocyte passes through the cytoplasm of a single epithelial cell instead of through the space between cells. If the cell has not already actively extruded its nucleus, it is pitted out during this process (Figure 8-2). This is the first of endless deformations that the cell must undergo during its life span. Thus, the endothelium forms a barrier that can exert considerable control over what enters the systemic circulation (bone marrow–blood barrier). The cell still possesses an endoplasmic reticulum (hence, its name), and it can synthesize small amounts of hemoglobin. Systems for aerobic metabolism are still functional in the reticulocyte, but all these are absent in the mature mammalian red cell. Maturation of reticulocytes into erythrocytes occurs over the first 24 to 36 hours in the systemic circulation.

The presence of an abnormally large number of reticulocytes in the peripheral blood (> 2 percent of the erythrocytes in adults or > 6 percent in infants) is called *reticulocytosis*, and it indicates an accelerated replacement function of the bone marrow such as might occur in chronic hemolytic disease, exposure to hypoxia, or following an acute episode of intravascular hemolysis. Reticulocytes are easily distinguished after supravital staining of peripheral blood smears. The absolute count of reticulocytes may be reported (normal is about 60,000/mm^3), or the absolute count may be corrected for abnormal changes in the hematocrit.

The presence of nucleated "blast" forms of immature red cells in peripheral blood may indicate an even greater demand for replacement. Megaloblastic, macrocytic anemia with large oval red cells (macroovalocytes) in peripheral blood is indicative of a defect in DNA synthesis in marrow. This so-called maturation block may be a sign of a deficiency of the essential cofactors, vitamin B_{12} or folic acid. Folic acid antagonist drugs used in cancer chemotherapy (methotrexate) or as antimalarials (pyrimethamine, chlorguanide) may induce megaloblastic anemia as a side effect because of their effects on DNA synthesis in marrow (Stebbins and Bertino, 1976).

In contrast, a microcytic, hypochromic anemia is seen in iron deficiency as it may occur in premature infants, infants and children during rapid growth spurts, blood loss, pregnancy or lactation, or malabsorption syndromes. Oral replacement as with enteric coated tablets of ferrous sulfate is effective in all these conditions except malabsorption where parenteral forms of iron may be required.

Bone marrow failure is characterized by inadequate production of red cells and/or other formed elements. Chemicals toxic to bone marrow can result in a decrease in the circulating numbers of all three major groups of formed elements, a condition called *pancytopenia*. A diagnosis of pancytopenia is based on actual cell counts in peripheral blood. Agents regularly associated with pancytopenia if the exposure is sufficiently intense include ionizing radiation, benzene, antimetabolites, lindane or chlordane, nitrogen mustards, arsenic, chloramphenicol, trinitrotoluene, gold salts, hydantoin derivatives, and phenylbutazone (Harris and Kellermeyer, 1970).

Damage to bone marrow may be so severe that it fails to proliferate normally, a condition described morphologically as *aplastic anemia*. This diagnosis is made after microscopic examination of bone marrow biopsy specimens. On the other hand, in some conditions the marrow

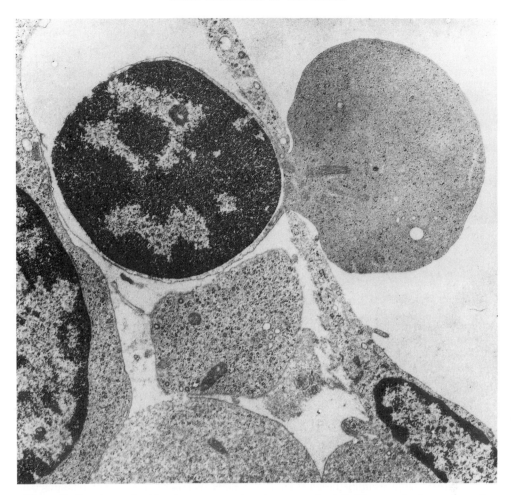

Figure 8–2.   An erythroblast in a marrow sinus is seen on the *left*. The vascular lumen is on the *right*. Between the two is a thin endothelial cell with an elongated nucleus *(bottom right)*. A mature but nucleated red cell is in the process of passing through the wall of the endothelial cell. The cytoplasm is completely within the lumen. The nucleus of the red cell, however, cannot pass through the aperture and must remain behind in the marrow sinus. ×8500. (From Tavassoli, M., and Crosby, W. H.: Fate of the nucleus of the marrow erythroblast. *Science,* **179**:912–913, 1973. Copyright 1973 by AAAS.)

can have a normal cellularity or even hypercellularity but still fail to deliver normal formed elements or normal numbers of formed elements. Ineffective erythropoiesis is a functional description of a normal-appearing but unresponsive marrow.

It has been known for almost a century that benzene exposure is associated with bone marrow toxicity, and since the mid-1970s benzene has been recognized as a human leukemogen. It is not clear whether the former is an absolute requirement for the latter. Most authorities agree that biotransformation is essential for benzene-induced bone marrow damage. The toxic metabolite(s) is (are) not known with certainty,

although some evidence suggests that benzoquinone plays an important role. There is disagreement about whether benzene is activated in the marrow or in other tissues such as the liver with transport of the toxic metabolite(s) to the marrow (Snyder, 1987). In addition to direct cytotoxic effects of chemicals like benzene on the marrow, which are usually mediated through disturbances in DNA function, bone marrow damage may have an immunologic basis, as sometimes appears to be the case with chloramphenicol (see Chapter 9).

Thrombocytes.   The process of differentiation into thrombocytes, the smallest of the formed elements of the blood, is unique. Large numbers of thrombocytes are batch-produced and released from a single megakaryocyte, the largest cell type in marrow. The spent form of this giant cell is then phagocytized.

Platelets are the first line of defense against accidental blood loss. They accumulate rapidly at sites where vascular injury has exposed collagen fibers. Within seconds, the normally non-sticky circulating platelets will adhere to these fibers (adhesion), undergo degranulation, and release ADP, which causes further adhesion but also causes platelets to stick to each other (aggregation). With the loss of individual membranes, the platelets form a viscous mass, the platelet plug, which quickly arrests bleeding, but the process is still reversible at this point. The process becomes irreversible when the intrinsic and extrinsic clotting systems are activated to generate insoluble fibrin to reinforce the platelet plug. Fibroblasts then infiltrate the area to complete the repair with scar formation.

Platelet aggregation *in vitro* can be studied by turbidimetric techniques in which aggregating agents are added to platelet-rich plasma; as the platelets aggregate, the optical density decreases (Born, 1962). If it is suspected that an active metabolite of a drug is involved, the drug can be given to a patient and its effects on platelet aggregation can be examined *ex vivo*. The primary aggregating agent *in vivo* is believed to be ADP, but aggregation can also be induced by epinephrine, thrombin, collagen, or other agents. Inhibition of platelet aggregation by drugs can be useful in preventing the thromboembolic complications of atherosclerosis. In 1986, the Food and Drug Administration (FDA) approved the labeling of aspirin to indicate that a single tablet taken daily may reduce the risks of death in patients who have already survived one myocardial infarction or who have unstable angina. The effects of aspirin on prostaglandin synthesis are unique among nonsteroidal anti-inflammatory drugs because it alone irreversibly acetylates cyclooxygenase in platelets; moreover, platelets lack the capacity to synthesize new enzyme. This irreversible effect on circulating platelets suppresses the synthesis of thrombaxane A_2, which promotes aggregation.

Platelet aggregation is also inhibited by the so-called nitric oxide vasodilator drugs including glyceryl trinitrate and its chemical relatives and sodium nitroprusside. Other xenobiotics in the group not used therapeutically as vasodilators include sodium azide, hydroxylamine hydrochloride, and sodium nitrite (Schwerin *et al.*, 1983). These drugs owe their ability to relax vascular smooth muscle and inhibit platelet aggregation by virtue of their conversion to nitric oxide. The nitric oxide is believed to activate guanylate cyclase to increase the synthesis of cGMP, which initiates a cascade of kinase or phosphorylase reactions to produce the effects.

Normal human blood contains several hundred million platelets per mm^3 (Figure 8–1). The minimal number thought be needed for normal hemostasis is about 50,000/mm^3. Thrombocytopenia is defined as a count of <20,000/mm^3, and it may be manifested by hemorrhagic disorders, the most common of which is leakage of blood from capillaries following minor injury (purpura). Petechiae, prolonged bleeding time, and impaired clot retraction are also consequences. Thrombocytopenia accompanies a bewildering array of congenital or acquired disorders, but drugs are the most common cause. The myelosuppressive anticancer drugs may cause thrombocytopenia as part of a generalized depression of bone marrow function. Quinidine and phenacetin are recognized as causes of autoimmune thromocytopenia, resulting in increased peripheral platelet destruction. An abnormally increased number of circulating platelets (thrombocytosis) has yet to be associated with chemical exposure.

Leukocytes. Leukocytes have the most complex organization of the formed elements. They differ from other blood cells in that they perform important functions outside the vascular compartment. Although each subtype seems to have some unique functions, the primary purpose for their existence appears to be to defend the body against "foreignness." Defense against foreign organisms or extraneous materials involves two mechanisms: (1) phagocytosis and (2) antibody production as carried out by the immunocytic series (Figure 8–3). The immunocytes are discussed at length in Chapter 9 and will not be referred to further here.

The phagocytes are subdivided into granulocytes (neutrophils, eosinophils, and basophils) and the monocyte/macrophages. Subdivision of the granulocytes is accomplished on the basis of their reactivity with Wright's stain (Figure 8-3), but these distinctions would be more valuable if their various functions were more clearly understood. Neutrophils are the most active phagocytes; eosinophils are less so. Eosinophilia occurs in some allergic diseases and infestations with large parasites. They may play a role in allergic inflammatory states. Basophils seem to be related to tissue mast cells and release histamine and other mediators in response to immunologic stimuli.

Granulocytes spend less than a day in the circulation before they become marginated (attached to blood vessel walls); they then pass between vascular endothelial cells by diapedesis

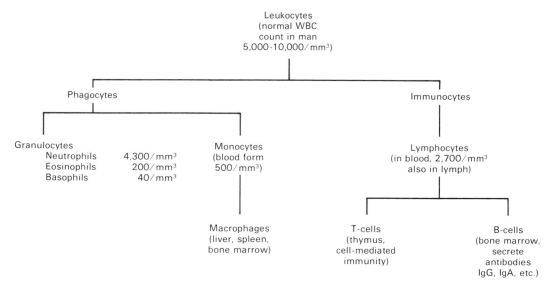

Figure 8–3. A classification of leukocytes and their normal values in man.

and are disposed of in various tissues. Mediators that increase capillary permeability are released from inflammatory lesions, and specific leukotactic factors (leukotrienes) attract granulocytes to the area of injury. Foreign particles or bacteria are phagocytized and destroyed by a "respiratory" burst that involves hydrogen peroxide and halide. In some cases, the destruction of bacterial membranes, release of lysosomal enzymes, and formation of pyrogens may temporarily exacerbate the local inflammatory response. Pharmacologic doses of glucocorticoids tend to decrease the numbers of granulocytes that will diapedese and enter an inflammatory exudate because of their inhibitory effect on the synthesis of leukotrienes as well as prostaglandins. Presumably, this phenomenon accounts for the well-known increased susceptibility of patients on steroids to infections since steroids do not decrease the rate of granulocyte production.

Monocytes circulate in the blood for three or four days. After they migrate into reticuloendothelial tissues like the liver, spleen, and bone marrow, they are called *macrophages,* and in these sites they survive for several months. Macrophages play a role in the phagocytic response to inflammation and infection, but they are also responsible for the ongoing destruction of senile blood cells and in the pinocytotic removal of denatured plasma proteins and lipoproteins. Macrophages are also involved in iron metabolism and possess inducible heme oxidase activity for the catabolism of hemoglobin.

The term *granulocytopenia* is used when the total granulocyte count falls to 3000/mm³ (*see* Figure 8-3). When the count reaches 1000/mm³, the patient becomes vulnerable to infection, and at 500/mm³, the risk is very serious. The confusing term *agranulocytosis* refers to a condition in which both the marginated pool and the bone marrow are devoid of neutrophils (also called *neutropenia*).

Granulocytopenia is the most common manifestation of chemically induced bone marrow damage. The reaction can also be induced by ionizing radiation. Alkylating agents and antimetabolites regularly cause granulocytopenia, and phenothiazines, nonsteroidal antiinflammatory drugs, antithyroid drugs, and some anticonvulsants sometimes elicit the reaction (Pisciotta, 1973). Peripheral destruction of granulocytes is a much less common reaction occurring by drug haptens after exposure to aminopyrine or phenylbutazone.

An excessive number of granulocytes in peripheral blood occurs transiently after the administration of epinephrine, cortisone, and some endotoxins, but it is not believed to be of physiologic significance. The term *granulocytosis* is used for counts > 10,000/mm³. Chronic granulocytosis has not been associated with exposure to specific chemicals except when it occurs as a preliminary phase of leukemia. Leukemia is associated with counts of > 30,000/mm³. In patients with far-advanced disease, the volume of leukocytes in blood may exceed the hematocrit, and the blood will appear pale. Chronic granulocytic leukemia has a better prognosis than the acute form of the disease. The chronic form more commonly occurs in middle age, and although chemicals are suspected as

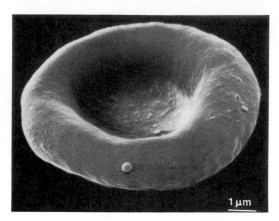

1 μm

Figure 8–4. Scanning electron micrograph of an unetched normal red blood cell. (From Stuart, P. R.; Osborn, J. S.; and Lewis, S. M.: The use of radio-frequency sputter ion etching and scanning electron microscopy to study the internal structure of biological material. *Proc. 2nd Annual Scanning Electron Microscope Symposium,* IIT Research Institute, Chicago, Ill., April 1969.)

etiologic agents, clear-cut associations have been difficult to make. The acute leukemias are rapidly fatal in the absence of effective chemotherapy. They are divided into two groups: (1) acute lymphocytic leukemia and (2) acute myelogenous leukemia, which lumps together all other marrow-derived leukocytes. Benzene is the only agent definitely linked to acute leukemia in man, but butadiene, ethylene oxide, and alkylating agents produce it in laboratory animals. Neither monocytosis nor monocytopenia appears to be induced specifically by chemical injury, but either can be part of a generalized syndrome of bone marrow damage.

Erythrocytes. No cell type in the human body has been studied as extensively as the red blood cell (Surgenor, 1974, 1975). This unique disk-shaped element (Figure 8–4) has a diameter of about 8 mm, and its biconcave sides make it more than twice as thick at the periphery (about 2.4 mm) as it is in the center. The reason for its shape is not known, but it would tend to decrease intracellular diffusional distances. Although devoid of intracellular organelles, special techniques in combination with scanning electron microscopy suggest that an internal structure may exist (*e.g.,* Figure 8–8). As much as 30 percent of the wet weight of red cells consists of hemoglobin, which is the most extensively studied protein in the body.

Erythrocytes perform the essential function of transporting oxygen from the alveoli of lungs to peripheral tissue, where it is used to support aerobic metabolism. On the return trip, red cells serve as a means for the transport of waste carbon dioxide for excretion via the lungs. A small amount of carbon dioxide is transported in simple solution within the cell, but the bulk (75 percent) is transported as bicarbonate by virtue of the activity of intracellular carbonic anhydrase. Another small fraction combines directly with free amino groups on hemoglobin to form carbaminohemoglobin (R-NH-COOH). An analogous reaction can occur with cyanate (*see* below). Hemoglobin can also accept hydrogen ions, and it accounts for about 85 percent of the buffer capacity of the blood.

Acute damage to red cells or their content of hemoglobin can result in an impairment of oxygen transport and secondary peripheral hypoxia. The signs and symptoms in such cases are mediated through the central nervous system, the organ most sensitive to oxygen lack. Normally, the human erythrocyte remains in the blood for an average of 120 days before its life is ended in the spleen. Common laboratory animals (rabbits, rats, and especially guinea pigs and mice) have much shorter red cell survival times than humans (Prankerd, 1961).

Anemia may arise if for any reason the rate of red cell destruction in the periphery exceeds the normal rate for their production in bone marrow. Some chemicals have acute and direct hemolytic effects *in vivo*—for example, saponin, phenylhydrazine, arsine, and naphthalene. Many other chemicals such as primaquine produce hemolysis only in red cells deficient in glucose-6-phosphate dehydrogenase (*see* below). In other cases, peripheral red cell destruction may involve an immunologic mechanism after sensitization by a drug such as acetanilid (*see also* Chapter 9).

Laboratory evidence for an accelerated rate of hemolysis includes decreases in red cell life span, plasma haptoglobin levels, hematocrit and red cell counts, and increases in plasma hemoglobin (hemoglobinemia) and bilirubin (Rifkind *et al.,* 1980). An unusual hematologic condition is a hemoglobinemia in the face of polycythemia (increased hematocrit or red cell count). This reaction has been demonstrated in several species of laboratory animals when exposed to chronic extreme hypoxia in the form of simulated altitude. Under these conditions, it appears that splenic, and perhaps hepatic, erythropoiesis is reactivated in an attempt to meet the demand for increased oxygen transport to peripheral tissues. At least part of this effort, however, appears to be ineffective in that the cells hemolyze shortly after or even before reaching the systemic circulation (Ou and Smith, 1978).

When hemoglobin is released into plasma, the

iron of its heme groups undergoes autoxidation, and the entire porphyrinic structure is labilized (*see* below) and may exchange with albumin, haptoglobin, or hemopexin (Müller-Eberhard, 1970). These transport the heme to reticuloendothelial tissues that have inducible heme oxidase activity, which helps to conserve the iron. If the rate of hemolysis is such as to saturate these carrier systems, free hemoglobin may be found in the urine, and hemoglobinuria is a sign of a severe hemolytic crisis that may eventually compromise renal function.

Polycythemia vera may be an acquired disease in which there is an overproduction of red cells in the absence of an appropriate stimulus (altitude, cardiopulmonary disease, anemic hypoxia). Perhaps it is caused by an unusual sensitivity of the stem cell pool to erythropoietin. A known inappropriate stimulus for erythropoiesis is cobalt ion. It was regularly seen along with other signs in the epidemics of beer drinker's cardiomyopathy in the 1960s. The onset of these epidemics coincided with the introduction of minute amounts of cobalt into some brands of beer to stabilize the foamy head (Gosselin *et al.*, 1984). The tissue sensor for hypoxia (above) also responds to cobalt ion to increase the synthesis of erythropoietin.

CHEMICALLY INDUCED HYPOXIA

Hypoxia refers to any condition in which there is a decreased supply of oxygen to peripheral tissues short of anoxia, but hypoxias can be subdivided into three classes with quite different root causes. *Arterial (anoxic) hypoxia* is characterized by a lower-than-normal P_{O_2} in arterial blood when the oxygen capacity and rate of blood flow are normal or even elevated. Among toxic insults, this type of hypoxia results from exposure to pulmonary irritants that produce airway obstruction ranging from spasm or edema of the glottis to pulmonary edema (adult respiratory distress syndrome). Opiod narcotics and other drugs that depress the respiration also produce arterial hypoxia. *Anemic hypoxia* is characterized by a lowered oxygen capacity when the arterial P_{O_2} and the rate of blood flow are normal or elevated. This type of hypoxia results from a decreased concentration of functional hemoglobin, a reduced number of red cells, or chemically induced alterations in hemoglobin. *Stagnant (hypokinetic) hypoxia* is characterized by a decreased rate of blood flow as in heart failure or uncorrected vasodilatation. Sometimes a fourth condition, *histotoxic hypoxia,* is included in the classification even though in this condition the peripheral tissue oxygen tension may be normal or even elevated, and the defect is in the ability of the cell to utilize molecular oxygen (below).

Oxygen Binding to Hemoglobin

Normal adult hemoglobin A is an oligomeric protein with a molecular weight of about 67,000 daltons containing four separate globin peptide chains: two alpha chains and two beta chains, $(\alpha^{2+}\beta^{2+})_2$. Each peptide chain has a noncovalently bound porphyrinic heme group (Figure 8–5). The globin chains have irregularly folded conformations that enclose the heme group in a hydrophobic pocket. Hemoglobin is one of the proteins for which the complete tertiary structure is known (Perutz *et al.*, 1968).

The structure of a single heme group may be represented as a square, planar complex with the four nitrogens of the porphyrin ring at the angles (Figure 8–5). The central iron atom has a hexavalent coordination shell analogous to the inorganic iron complexes, ferrocyanide, or nitroprusside. The two remaining coordination bonds are closely associated with imidazole (histidyl) residues from the particular globin chain to which the heme group is attached. One of these bonds is available for reversible combination with molecular oxygen, which binds between the iron and the histidyl. No ligand occupies this site in deoxyhemoglobin.

The reversible binding of oxygen by hemoglobin is called *oxygenation;* the tertiary structures of the oxygenated and deoxygenated forms of hemoglobin are known to differ. Since conformational changes do not occur on oxygenation of a single globin-heme unit such as myoglobin, it follows that there are interactions between the four subunits composing a hemoglobin molecule. These interactions are called *cooperativity.*

There are two physiological regulators of the affinity of hemoglobin for oxygen, which is

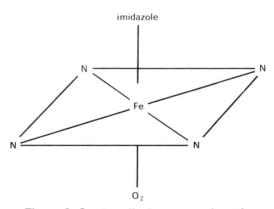

Figure 8–5. A stylized representation of a single heme group.

usually defined in terms of a P_{50}, or that partial pressure of oxygen necessary to half-saturate the hemoglobin. The two regulators are hydrogen ion, which is responsible for the Bohr effect, and 2,3-diphosphoglycerate (2,3-DPG). Increasing concentrations of either of these tends to decrease the affinity of hemoglobin for oxygen, whereas increasing concentrations have the opposite effect.

The red cell can both synthesize and degrade 2,3-DPG (Figure 8–6), and 2,3-DPG is normally present in red cells in about the same molar concentration as hemoglobin. One molecule of 2,3-DPG binds reversibly with one molecule of hemoglobin in the central cavity formed by the four subunits. This complex tends to stabilize hemoglobin in the deoxy form, so that 2,3-DPG and oxygen could be regarded as competitive ligands for hemoglobin, although they bind to different sites to exert allosteric effects. A decreased affinity of hemoglobin for oxygen shifts the oxygen dissociation curve (Figure 8–7) in a parallel fashion to the right (increases the P_{50}), whereas an increased affinity produces a left-shifted dissociation curve. A number of drugs, chemicals, and manipulations are known to result in shifts in either direction (Norton and Smith, 1981).

Normal adult human hemoglobin binds 2,3-DPG more tightly than does fetal hemoglobin, accounting for the higher oxygen affinity of fetal blood noted above. Sickle cell anemia is due to the inheritance of an abnormal hemoglobin with a single amino acid substitution on the β-globin chains. Hemolytic crises are triggered by hypoxia because only the deoxy form of hemoglobin S can form the polymeric structures that distort the shape of the red cell (Figure 8–8). Irreversible carbamylation of the terminal valine residues on the globin chains by cyanate (above) increases the oxygen affinity of both hemoglobins A and S. This makes hemoglobin S less likely to exist in the deoxy form at any one time, which decreases the incidence of hemolytic crises. Although cyanate was effective in limited clinical trials, it proved to be too neurotoxic for chronic use in human patients (Cerami and Manning, 1971). An alternative approach might be to devise some way of decreasing the red cell concentration of 2,3-DPG, which would also increase the affinity of hemoglobin S for oxygen. Finally, if a safe and reliable way of reactivating the synthesis of fetal hemoglobin could be devised, its higher oxygen affinity might benefit the patient with sickle cell trait. In this case, the γ-globin chains would substitute for the defective β-chains on hemoglobin S (Letvin et al., 1984).

Deoxygenation of hemoglobin occurs in four separate steps, each with a different dissociation constant because of cooperativity changes that accompany the release of each successive oxygen molecule:

$$\begin{array}{lll}
Hb(O_2)_4 \rightarrow Hb(O_2)_3 + O_2 & & K_1 \\
Hb(O_2)_3 \rightarrow Hb(O_2)_2 + O_2 & & K_2 \\
Hb(O_2)_2 \rightarrow Hb(O_2) \ \ + O_2 & & K_3 \\
Hb(O_2) \ \ \rightarrow Hb \ \ \ \ \ \ + O_2 & & K_4
\end{array}$$

The exact values for the individual dissociation constants above are unknown, but they represent equilibrium constants of the form:

$$K_1 = \frac{[Hb(O_2)_3]\,[O_2]}{[Hb(O_2)_4]}$$

with units of moles/liter. The comparable association constant would be the reciprocal expression with units of liters/mole. The smaller the dissociation constant, the more tightly the ligand is bound and the more stable is the complex.

When the hemoglobin molecule is fully saturated, all the oxygens may be thought of as equivalent since it is not known whether the two types of globin chains play a role in sequencing deoxygenation. A fall in the ambient P_{O_2} results in the release of one oxygen molecule. Its release triggers a cooperativity change that greatly facilitates the release of the second oxygen molecule; thus, K_1 is considerably smaller than K_2. Similarly, the release of the second oxygen facilitates the release of the third oxygen. Release of the fourth oxygen does not occur under normal physiological conditions.

The above sequence is responsible for the sigmoid shape of the normal oxygen dissociation curve (Figure 8–7). Since the total oxygen content of normal blood is about 20 ml/100 ml, the release of 5 ml O_2/100 ml blood could be considered as analogous to the release of one oxygen molecule from a single hemoglobin tetramer; in each case, it is one-fourth of the total load. That release requires a decrease in the P_{O_2} of about 60 mm Hg (from point a to point V). The release of an additional 5 ml O_2/100 ml blood (or the second molecule of O_2 from a tetramer) requires a further decrease in the P_{O_2} but only of about 15 mm Hg (from about 40 down to 25 mm Hg) because of cooperativity. The release of a third increment of oxygen can then be effected by a decrease in the P_{O_2} of only 10 mm Hg. Thus, cooperativity facilitates the loading and unloading of large amounts of oxygen over a physiologically critical range of P_{O_2}.

Carbon Monoxide Binding to Hemoglobin

Carbon monoxide is the best-studied example of a chemical agent that can produce anemic hypoxia. The elucidation of its mechanism of

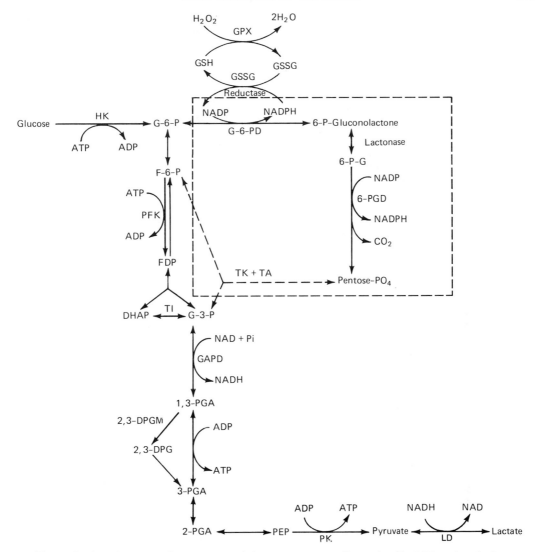

Figure 8–6. The metabolic resources of the mature mammalian red cell. *GSH*, reduced glutathione; *GSSG*, oxidized glutathione; *G-6-P*, glucose-6-phosphate; *F-6-P*, fructose-6-phosphate; *FDP*, fructose-1,6-diphosphate; *DHAP*, dihydroxyacetone phosphate; *G-3-P*, glyceraldehyde-3-phosphate; *LD*, lactic dehydrogenase; *NADP*, oxidized triphosphopyridine nucleotide; *NADPH*, reduced triphosphopyridine nucleotide; *NAD*, oxidized diphosphopyridine nucleotide; *NADH*, reduced diphosphopyridine nucleotide; *6-P-G*, 6-phosphogluconate; *G-6-PD*, glucose-6-phosphate dehydrogenase; *TK*, transketolase; *TA*, transaldolase; *Pi*, inorganic phosphate; *ADP*, adenosine diphosphate; *ATP*, adenosine triphosphate; *PEP*, phosphoenolpyruvate; *PK*, pyruvic kinase; *1,3-PGA*, 1,3-phosphoglyceric acid; *3-PGA*, 3-phosphoglyceric acid; *2-PGA*, 2-phosphoglyceric acid; *2,3-DPG*, 2,3-diphosphoglyceric acid; *6-PGD*, 6-phosphogluconate dehydrogenase; *PFK*, phosphofructokinase; *HK*, hexokinase; *TI*, trioseisomerase; *GPX*, glutathione peroxidase; *GAPD*, glyceraldehyde-3-phosphate dehydrogenase; *2,3-DPGM*, 2,3-diphosphoglycerate mutase. (Modified from Harris, J. W., and Kellermeyer, R. W.: *The Red Cell—Production, Metabolism, Destruction: Normal and Abnormal*, rev. ed. Harvard University Press, Cambridge, Mass., 1970.)

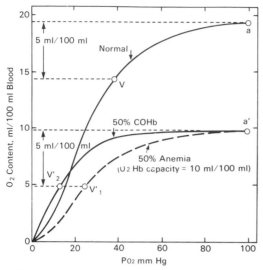

Figure 8–7. Normal oxyhemoglobin dissociation curve and curves for the case of a 50 percent anemia and the case of a 50 percent carboxyhemoglobinemia. The delivery of 25 percent of the total oxygen content of fully oxygenated arterial blood (5 ml/100 ml blood) requires a drop in the P_{O_2} of about 60 mm Hg (from point *a* to point *V* on the normal curve). Delivery of a comparable volume of oxygen in the case of a 50 percent anemia requires a drop in the P_{O_2} of more than 75 mm Hg (from point *a'* to point *V'$_1$*), but an even greater fall in the P_{O_2} is required to deliver the same volume of oxygen in the case of the curve distorted by the presence of carboxyhemoglobin (from point *a'* to point *V'$_2$*). See text for an explanation of this phenomenon. (From Bartlett, D., Jr.: Effects of carbon monoxide in human physiological processes. *Proceedings of the Conference on Health Effects of Air Pollutants.* U.S. Government Printing Office, Washington, D.C., Serial 93–15, November 1973, pp. 103–126.

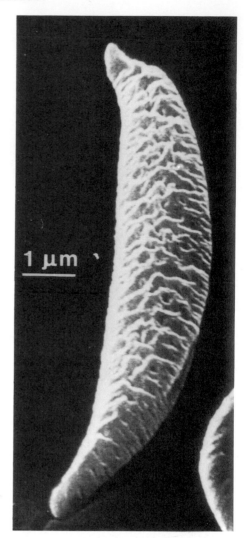

Figure 8–8. Scanning electron micrograph of a red blood cell from a patient with sickle cell disease after ion etching in oxygen for five minutes at 1 mtorr. The technique was carried out with equipment normally used for the study of metals and inorganic materials. (From Stuart, P. R.; Osborn, J. S.; and Lewis, S. M.: The use of radio-frequency sputter ion etching and scanning electron microscopy to study the internal structure of biological material. *Proc. 2nd Annual Scanning Electron Microscope Symposium,* IIT Research Institute, Chicago, Ill., April 1969.)

action by Claude Bernard in 1865 is a classic example of the successful application of the experimental method (Bernard, 1957). Bernard's original deductions were formalized (Douglas *et al.,* 1912) as the so-called Haldane equation, which defined quantitatively the competitive nature of oxygen and carbon monoxide for the same ferrous heme binding sites on hemoglobin:

$$\frac{[Hb(CO)_4]}{[Hb(O_2)_4]} = M\frac{[P_{CO}]}{[P_{O_2}]}$$

The constant, *M,* has the value of 245 at pH 7.4 for human blood. Therefore, if the $P_{CO} = 1/245 \ P_{O_2}$, the blood at equilibrium will be half-saturated with oxygen and half-saturated with carbon monoxide. Since air contains 21 percent oxygen by volume, exposure to a gas mixture of about 0.1 percent carbon monoxide in air would

result in a 50 percent carboxyhemoglobinemia at equilibrium and at sea level. For this reason, carbon monoxide is dangerous at very low concentrations. However, the rate at which the arterial blood approaches equilibrium with the inspired gas concentration depends on such factors as the diffusion capacity of the lungs and the alveolar ventilation, both of which in turn depend on the level of exercise of the subject.

Some species variation is recognized with respect to the value of M in the Haldane equation, but this is not necessarily the major determinant of the sensitivity of a given species to carbon monoxide. For example, the M value for canary blood is less than half of the value for human blood. The very rapid rate of breathing by canaries needed to support a higher rate of aerobic metabolism allows them to reach equilibrium between blood and inspired carbon monoxide more rapidly than humans. However, the canary brain appears to be less sensitive to hypoxia than the human brain. Because of these opposing factors, canaries are more sensitive than humans to short exposures at high concentrations of carbon monoxide, but with long exposures to low concentrations, the roles can be reversed (Spencer, 1962).

If instead of air or oxygen, hemoglobin is exposed to pure carbon monoxide, a gradual decrease in the P_{CO} would allow one to derive a carboxyhemoglobin dissociation curve of the same shape as the oxyhemoglobin dissociation curve. With adjustment of the values on the abscissa by a factor of 245, the two curves would even be superimposable. Thus, cooperativity is a property of the hemoglobin tetramer, and it is not influenced by the ligands occupying the ferrous heme binding sites; that is, the hemoglobin molecule has no intrinsic mechanism for distinguishing between oxygen and carbon monoxide.

When the ambient atmosphere contains both oxygen and carbon monoxide, another phenomenon is observed that has profound physiological significance (Figure 8-7). If the ambient P_{CO} is 1/245 of the ambient P_{O_2}, at equilibrium, half of the ferrous heme binding sites will be occupied by CO and half by O_2. The distribution of the two ligands among the four heme groups on any one tetramer, however, is random. Thus, the blood will contain a distribution of hybrid species in which most tetramers will contain both oxygen and carbon monoxide. Chance would dictate that the most common hybrid species would be a molecule with two oxygens and two carbon monoxides, for example, $Hb(O_2)_2(CO)_2$.

The effect of these hybrid species on the oxyhemoglobin dissociation curve in comparison with a simple 50 percent anemia is shown in Figure 8–7. Since half of the total number of ferrous heme binding sites are always going to be occupied by carbon monoxide, the total oxygen capacity is only half of normal, as in the simple anemia. However, the curve for a simple anemia retains its sigmoid shape because its hemoglobin is normal, so that for any given value for the P_{O_2} on the abscissa, the value for the oxygen content on the ordinate is half of that for the normal dissociation curve. In contrast, the curve for a 50 percent carboxyhemoglobinemia is shifted to the left, and it has lost its sigmoid shape.

The physiologic significance of this phenomenon can be grasped from Figure 8–7 where a change in the P_{O_2} of 75 mm Hg (from point a' to point V'_1) is required to deliver 5 ml $O_2/100$ ml of blood to peripheral tissues in the case of a 50 percent anemia, whereas in the case of a 50 percent carboxyhemoglobinemia, a change in the P_{O_2} of 85 mm Hg (from point a' to point V'_2) is required to deliver the same amount of oxygen to peripheral tissues. Obviously, the person with a 50 percent carboxyhemoglobinemia is more severely compromised than the person with a simple 50 percent anemia. As noted above, cooperativity remains normal in hybrid species in which both oxygen and carbon monoxide are bound to the same tetramer. Thus, the basis for the effect on the oxygen dissociation curve is simply a loss of the number of opportunities for cooperativity to facilitate the dissociation of oxygen. In the most common hybrid species above, which contains two oxygens and two carbon monoxides, cooperativity facilitates the unloading of the second oxygen, but thereafter there are no more oxygens left to unload. In contrast, in the 50 percent anemia, each tetramer has a full complement of four oxygens, and cooperativity could facilitate the unloading of the third and even the fourth oxygen in times of great demand. In effect, in a 50 percent carboxyhemoglobinemia, only the top half of the normal oxyhemoglobin dissociation curve is available for use.

Carbon Monoxide Poisoning. The above model illustrates the molecular mechanisms at work in terms of hemoglobin, but in intact humans and animals other factors play important roles in the pathophysiology of carbon monoxide poisoning. Changes are known to occur in cardiac output and regional blood flow. Changes in ventilation will influence the rate at which equilibrium between the inspired gas concentration and the blood content is achieved. Exposure to very high ambient concentrations can result in sufficient hemoglobin saturation to produce unconsciousness or death in minutes with few, if any, premonitory signs. At low ambient concentrations, however, considerable time may be required to reach equilibrium with the blood (for example, as long as four hours for a sedentary person exposed to 0.1 percent by volume. For these reasons, the correlation between blood carboxyhemoglobin levels and the signs and symptoms of poisoning sometimes shows surprising discrepancies.

Although the presence of carboxyhemoglobin can result in significant decreases in the oxygen content of blood, ambient concentrations are rarely high enough to cause a detectable decrease in the P_{O_2} of arterial blood. Therefore, it is uncommon for chemoreceptor mechanisms to be triggered, and the parameters of ventilation usually remain within normal limits. Peripheral vasodilation occurs in response to a slowly developing hypoxia, which necessitates an increase in cardiac output. This compensatory mechanism is limited, and fainting is more common than dyspnea in victims of carbon monoxide poisoning. Consciousness may be lost for long periods before death. Tachycardia and electrocardiogram (ECG) changes suggestive of hypoxia may be observed at 30 percent or greater carboxyhemoglobin saturation. Other symptoms include headache, weakness, nausea, dizziness, and dimness of vision. Lactic acidemia indicates a limitation on aerobic metabolism. Unconsciousness, coma, convulsions, and death are associated with 50 to 80 percent saturation.

Carbon monoxide is not a cumulative poison in the usual sense. Carboxyhemoglobin is fully dissociable, and once exposure has been terminated, the pigment will revert to oxyhemoglobin. Liberated carbon monoxide is eliminated via the lungs. Many individuals are occupationally exposed to carbon monoxide—for example, garage workers, traffic police—and may suffer acute, recurring intoxications. Without an adequate history, the unwary physician may be baffled by the symptomatology. Any hypoxic insult of sufficient severity, however, including carbon monoxide poisoning, may induce permanent neurologic sequelae if the victim survives.

Carboxyhemoglobin is a cherry-red color, and its presence in blood can be detected only by spectroscopic examination. Its presence in the venous return may impart an abnormal red coloration to skin and mucous membranes. Carbon monoxide combines *in vitro* with myoglobin and heme enzymes, but these reactions have little or no significance in acute poisonings. Considerable experimental effort has gone into attempts to show that factors other than simple hypoxia contribute to carbon monoxide poisoning (for example, Gosselin *et al.*, 1984). However, when mice were placed in a high concentration of carbon monoxide together with two atmospheres of oxygen, enough oxygen was carried in physical solution in blood to prevent signs of poisoning even when the hemoglobin was totally saturated with carbon monoxide (Haldane, 1895).

Management of Carbon Monoxide Poisoning. The obvious, specific antagonist to carbon monoxide is oxygen. After termination of the exposure, respirations must be supported by artificial means if necessary. Advantage can be taken of the mass law to accelerate the rate of conversion of carboxy- to oxyhemoglobin *in vivo* by increasing the ambient P_{O_2}. For example, the half-recovery time in terms of blood carboxyhemoglobin in resting adults breathing air at 1 atmosphere is 320 minutes. When oxygen is given instead, the time is decreased to 80 minutes. Further reductions can be effected through the use of hyperbaric chambers to deliver pure oxygen at greater-than-atmospheric pressures, but hyperbaric oxygen was no better than normobaric oxygen in a large series of victims who had not lost consciousness as a result of exposure (Raphael *et al.*, 1989). Exchange transfusion has also been used for the moribund victim, but the addition of 5 to 7 percent carbon dioxide to oxygen to serve as a respiratory stimulant may compound the risk of metabolic acidosis arising from tissue hypoxia (Gosselin *et al.*, 1984).

Endogenous and Environmental Carbon Monoxide. Nonsmoking human adults normally do not have more than 1 percent of their total circulating hemoglobin in the form of carboxyhemoglobin, but heavy smokers may show values as high as 5 to 10 percent saturation. Combustion of fossil fuels and automobile exhaust (4 to 7 percent carbon monoxide) are other key environmental sources of exposure. It is now known, however, that carbon monoxide is generated endogenously in normal humans (Coburn *et al.*, 1967). This carbon monoxide arises from the catabolism of heme proteins, principally hemoglobin, with heme enzymes contributing smaller amounts. The carbon monoxide comes from the α-methene bridge of porphyrins, and it is generated in amounts that are equimolar to the bile pigment produced. The average rate of production (0.4 ml/hour) is increased in hemolytic disease (National Academy of Sciences, 1977a).

Methemoglobinemia

As opposed to oxygenation, the heme irons of hemoglobin are susceptible to chemical oxidation through the loss of an electron with a valence change from 2^+ to 3^+. The resulting pigment is greenish-brown to black in color, it is called methemoglobin, and it can no longer combine reversibly with oxygen or carbon monoxide. Therefore, methemoglobinemia is another possible cause of anemic hypoxia. As in the oxidation of simple inorganic coordination complexes of iron, oxidation does not change the total number of bonds in the coordination shell (Figure 8–5). The additional positive charge on the heme iron is satisfied *in vivo* by hydroxyl or chloride anion. The ferric heme iron can also combine with a variety of nonphysiological anions, and this property has been exploited for therapeutic purposes (below).

No way has yet been devised to test the hypothesis that short of completely saturating concentrations, carboxyhemoglobin exists as hybrid species in which both oxygen and carbon monoxide are found on the same tetramer. In contrast, it is known with certainty that "methemoglobin" as generated either *in vivo* or *in vitro* by partial oxidation of hemoglobin or partial reduction of the totally oxidized pigment consists of a mixture of two hybrid species, $(\alpha^{2+}\beta^{3+})_2$ and $(\alpha^{3+}\beta^{2+})_2$. Complete oxidation of $(\alpha^{2+}\beta^{2+})_2$ to $(\alpha^{3+}\beta^{3+})_2$ can be forced with an excess of oxidant *in vitro*, but it would certainly be fatal *in vivo* (Tomoda and Yoneyama, 1981). Like carboxyhemoglobinemia, methemoglobinemia both decreases the oxygen content of blood and shifts the oxygen dissociation curve to the left with a distortion in its sigmoid shape. The explanation for the effect of methemoglobinemia on oxygen dissociation is also believed to rest with a decrease in the number of opportunities for cooperativity to facilitate oxygen unloading. The proof of hybrid species in the case of methemoglobin, however, lends credence to the hypothesis about carboxyhemoglobin.

Methemoglobin has an additional property that is of toxicological interest, namely, its ability to dissociate complete heme groups as units. Free hemoglobin in plasma rapidly undergoes autoxidation to methemoglobin, which is able to transfer heme groups to plasma albumin to form the pigment methemalbumin. Methemalbumin is associated with acute hemolytic crises such as transfusion reactions, severe malaria, paroxysmal nocturnal hemoglobinuria, and poisonings by such chemicals as chlorate salts. If a blood sample drawn under anaerobic conditions appears abnormally dark in color, inadequate oxygenation can be distinguished from oxidation by simply shaking in air. A change in color to bright red indicates the sample originally contained abnormally high concentrations of deoxyhemoglobin. Persistence of a dark color may indicate the presence of methemoglobin (an intraerythrocytic pigment) or methemalbumin (an extracellular pigment). Centrifugation often allows one to distinguish between these two.

Hemoglobin Autoxidation. A variety of chemicals greatly increase the rate of hemoglobin oxidation (below), but oxidation also occurs spontaneously in the presence of oxygen. This autoxidation presumably accounts for the low concentrations (< 2 percent) of methemoglobin normally found in circulating blood in humans and most other common mammals. As studied *in vitro*, autoxidation appears to be a first-order process with respect to the ferrous forms of either hemoglobin or myoglobin. The first-order rate constants, however, depend in a complex way on the P_{O_2}. The rate constant is maximal at a P_{O_2} that corresponds to half-saturation of the reduced pigment. Since a reaction mechanism in which a deoxygenated heme group interacts with an oxygenated one would not exhibit first-order kinetics, a multistep mechanism is inferred. The quasi–first-order kinetics can then be explained as arising from an algebraic artifact rather than any single intramolecular rate-determining step.

The complexity of these reactions is illustrated by studies on their stoichiometry. Both myoglobin and hemoglobin autoxidation consume many times more oxygen than can be accounted for on the basis of the reduction of an appropriate amount of oxygen to water (Smith and Olson, 1973). It has been suggested that the reduced heme may simply transfer an electron to molecular oxygen to form superoxide anion (Fridovich, 1983), but this mechanism does not account for the peculiarities above.

Methemoglobin-Generating Chemicals.
Some chemicals capable of mediating the oxidation of hemoglobin are active both *in vitro* and *in vivo*. Others are active only *in vivo*, and a third group are much more active in lysates or solutions of hemoglobin than in intact cells whether *in vitro* or *in vivo*. Sodium nitrite and hydroxylamine hydrochloride are active both *in vitro* and *in vivo*; both directly relax vascular smooth muscle; and both are converted to nitric oxide in red cell suspensions and in mice (Kruszyna *et al.*, 1988). Despite these similarities, they appear to oxidize hemoglobin by different mechanisms (Cranston and Smith, 1971).

Under strictly anaerobic conditions, 1 mole of nitrite yields 1 mole of ferric heme and 1 mole of the ferroheme-NO complex. Under physiologic conditions and in the presence of excess nitrite, complete oxidation of hemoglobin occurs, and the heme oxygen is largely consumed in the process. After a lag phase, the reaction proceeds with a pronounced autocatalytic phase that is not observed when hemoglobin reacts with deoxyhemoglobin. Nitrite is one of the nonphysiological anions that complex with ferric heme groups. Thus, excess nitrite can force complete oxidation with subsequent formation of a nitrite-methemoglobin complex. The phenomenon has no toxicological significance, but it can produce artifacts in the *in vitro* spectrophotometric determination of methemoglobin (van Assendelft and Zijlstra, 1965; R. P. Smith, 1967).

Organic compounds active both *in vivo* and *in vitro* include some aminophenols, certain *N*-hydroxylamines, amyl nitrite and other aliphatic esters of nitrous acid, and some aliphatic esters of nitric acid such as glyceryl trinitrate (Kiese, 1974). As tested in mice, phenylhydroxylamine and some simple homologues were all about equipotent in terms of peak levels of methemoglobin generated. At the same time, these were ten times more potent than nitrite, hydroxylamine, or simple aminophenols, (Smith *et al.*, 1967). Intraerythrocytic recycling must account for the high potency of N-hydroxylamines relative to the other compounds since phenylhydroxylamine is no more potent than nitrite in lysates. According to Kiese (1974), phenylhydroxylamine and related compounds react with hemoglobin to form methemoglobin and nitrosobenzene or homologues. In the normal red cell, mechanisms apparently exist for the reduction of nitrosobenzene to regenerate phenylhydroxylamine. A requirement for glucose in this system, as opposed to lactate, suggests that the pentose phosphate shunt is involved; perhaps the system needs NADPH (Figure 8–6).

Aromatic amino and nitro compounds such as aniline and nitrobenzene only generate methemoglobin *in vivo*. Obviously, these chemicals must be bioactivated, probably to aminophenols or to N-hydroxylamines, but the relative importance of these two possibilities is still not known for the two examples above. In contrast, the active metabolite of p-aminopropiophenone (PAPP), the most widely studied example of this type of agent, is known with certainty to be the N-hydroxyl metabolite in several laboratory animal species. This biotransformation is probably mediated by one of the isozymes of hepatic cytochrome P-450, but the bioactivation of nitrobenzene may be mediated by nitroreductases in the intestinal microflora of the rat (Reddy *et al.*, 1976). Prominent species differences in potency occur with this type of chemical because of differences in rates of activation and inactivation of the parent compound and its metabolites.

Some aromatic amines are human carcinogens, and there is considerable interest in adducts formed between amine metabolites and globin as a possible means for monitoring bioactivation or the exposure to cigarette smoke or other environmental carcinogens. Significant differences between smokers and nonsmokers were found for several adducts to amines known to be human bladder carcinogens (Bryant *et al.*, 1988). In rats, there seemed to be a correlation between the extent of amine adduct formation on globin and the ability of the compound to generate methemoglobin (Birner and Neumann, 1988). Whether or not this approach offers advantages over the older techniques for adduct formation with DNA (Chapter 5) remains to be evaluated.

Three unusual compounds are active largely or exclusively in lysates. The first of these, potassium ferricyanide, is unable to penetrate the intact red cell membrane. It is, however, the most widely used reagent for standardizing methemoglobin assays. One mole of ferricyanide mediates the oxidation of 1 mole of reduced heme whether oxygen is present or not. The ferricyanide reaction with oxyhemoglobin is unique in that it is the only methemoglobin-generating agent known that effects a quantitative release of the heme oxygen. This phenomenon has been exploited as a means for the laboratory determination of the oxygen content of hemoglobin. The ferrocyanide generated binds tenaciously to the globin chains of methemoglobin.

The second agent is molecular oxygen, which is probably equally active in intact red cells and lysates. In intact cells, however, its activity is masked because of the efficient mechanisms for reducing methemoglobin back to hemoglobin (below and Figure 8–9). For reasons that are not clearly understood, hemolysis virtually abolishes methemoglobin reductase activity, and the oxidized pigment accumulates until the reaction has gone to completion. The redox dye, methylene blue, is somewhat similar except that in intact cells it can activate a separate methemoglobin-reducing system that is additive to the effects of methemoglobin reductase (also below and Figure 8–9). Hemolysis abolishes the methemoglobin-reducing activity of methylene blue as well as the activity of methemoglobin reductase. In lysates, methylene blue actually generates methemoglobin and leucomethylene blue. The latter is susceptible to oxidation by molecular oxygen, so that a cyclic mechanism exists for hemoglobin oxidation in lysates where methylene blue can be as potent as is phenylhydroxylamine in intact cells, although the reaction proceeds much more slowly. It is presumed that this reaction also occurs in intact cells, but it is masked by the methemoglobin-reducing activity of methylene blue. Although methemoglobin never accumulates under these conditions, it is inferred that the rate of hemoglobin-methemoglobin turnover is accelerated. This may account for the weak anticyanide activity of methylene blue *in vivo* (below and Smith and Thron, 1972).

Susceptibility of Mammalian Hemoglobins to Oxidation. Small differences are recognized among mammalian hemoglobins in the rates of their oxidation by various chemicals (Bartels *et al.*, 1963). Such differences undoubtedly reflect conformational or structural variations, but this information has not yet provided insights into the

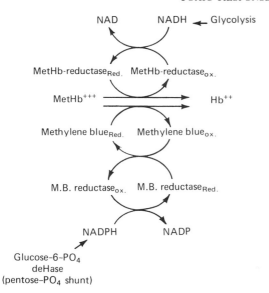

Figure 8–9. The spontaneous *(NADH)* and the dormant *(NADPH)* methemoglobin reductase systems. Methemoglobin *(MetHb)* reductase is active in intact red cells in the presence of substrates that can provide for NAD reduction. The NADPH system requires intact red cells, glucose or its metabolic equivalent, a functioning pentose phosphate shunt, and methylene blue *(M.B.)*. M.B.-reductase reduces M.B., which in turn nonenzymatically rduces MetHb.

molecular mechanisms of heme iron oxidation. J. E. Smith and Beutler (1966b) found that the conversion half-times in minutes for hemoglobin solutions exposed to the same concentration of nitrite to be about 2 for sheep, goat, and bovine hemoglobin; 3 for human hemoglobin; 4 for equine hemoglobin; and up to 7 for porcine hemoglobin. These values are small relative to the duration of a nitrite-methemoglobinemia induced in any of these species *in vivo*, which would be on the order of several hours.

Pathophysiology of Methemoglobine-mias. As an experimental tool for the study of the effects of peripheral hypoxia, methemoglobinemia is much less satisfactory than simulated altitude, oxygen replacement, or even exposure to carbon monoxide. Unless the methemoglobin-generating chemical is infused continuously, it is impossible to maintain stable circulating levels of the pigment for long periods of time. A variety of intraerythrocytic mechanisms are able to reduce methemoglobin back to hemoglobin. After a single dose of the agent, methemoglobin levels rise abruptly and then decline toward normal at rates that vary widely

with the species (Table 8–1) and result in wide variations in peripheral tissue oxygen tensions.

Moreover, the chemicals that produce acquired methemoglobinemias, unlike carbon monoxide, have additional effects that can make important contributions to the toxic syndrome. Nitrite, hydroxylamine, aliphatic esters of nitrous and nitric acid, and nitroprusside are all vasodilators by virtue of their conversion to nitric oxide *in vivo* (Kruszyna *et al.*, 1988). These may produce orthostatic hypotension, reflex tachycardia, circulatory inadequacy, and cardiovascular collapse so that the anemic hypoxia is compounded by a stagnant or hypokinetic hypoxia. The aromatic amino and nitro compounds seem to have complex central and cardiac effects that may be the proximal cause of death in humans and some animal species. Intravascular hemolysis is induced by chlorate salts, arsine, large doses of hydroxylamine (Cranston and Smith, 1971), and even PAPP. The "methemoglobinemia" may be largely extracellular and confounded by sulfhemoglobinemia and Heinz bodies (below). The methemoglobinemia induced by paraquat (Ng *et al.*, 1982) is almost trivial in comparison with its devastating effects on the lungs and other organ systems.

It is doubtful that any chemical produces a "pure" methemoglobinemia uncomplicated by effects on other organs or tissues, but PAPP in moderate doses has few, if any, "side effects." Large differences exist among various agents for the methemoglobin levels at death as measured in a single species (Smith and Olson, 1973). It is, therefore, inappropriate to suggest that there is a lethal level of methemoglobin without account to the particular agent and species involved.

Metabolic Resources of the Mature Mammalian Red Cell. The reversal of a carboxyhemoglobinemia is spontaneous and passive in accord with the ambient partial pressure of the gas and oxygen. In contrast, energy must be expended by the red cell to reverse an acquired methemoglobinemia. Indeed, much of the total energy expenditure of red cells is directed toward that end, the maintenance of the integrity of the membrane, and the restoration of the shape of the cell after deformation. The metabolic resources of the red cell, however, are rather meager. Only two anaerobic alternatives are available for glucose metabolism: the Embden-Myerhof glycolytic sequence and the pentose phosphate (hexosemonophosphate) shunt (Figure 8–6).

The enzyme, glucose-6-phosphate dehydro-

Table 8–1. SPONTANEOUS METHEMOGLOBIN REDUCTASE ACTIVITY OF MAMMALIAN ERYTHROCYTES*

SPECIES	(1)	(2)	(3)	(4)	(5)
			Activity in Species/Activity in Man		
Pig	0.37	0.37		0.09	
Horse	0.75	0.50		0.64	
Cat		0.50	0.85	1.2	1.0
Cow	0.80	0.75		1.1	
Goat	1.1	0.75			
Dog		0.88	1.4	1.3	1.0
Sheep	1.4	1.0		2.1	
Rat		1.4	1.3	1.9	5.0
Guinea pig		1.2	2.4	1.9	4.5
Rabbit		3.5	3.3	3.8	7.5
Mouse					9.5

*Data from various investigators using nitrited red cells with glucose as a substrate have been normalized by making a ratio of the activity of the species to the activity in human red cells. The indicated investigators are: (1) Smith and Beutler, 1966b; (2) Malz, 1962; (3) Kiese and Weis, 1943; (4) Robin and Harley, 1966; (5) Stolk and Smith, 1966; Smith *et al.*, 1967; Bolyai, *et al.*, 1972.

genase (G-6-PD), occupies a key position in red cell metabolism. It introduces the pentose phosphate shunt and mediates the reduction of NADP. Another mole of NADPH is generated in the next step mediated by 6-phosphogluconate dehydrogenase. These are the only sources of NADPH for the red cell. If lactate is substituted for glucose as a metabolic fuel, the cell can produce NADH through the activity of lactic dehydrogenase but not NADPH. In some mammalian red cells, stereospecificity of G-6-PD prevents the utilization of galactose by the pentose phosphate shunt, although it can be utilized by glycolysis (J. E. Smith and Beutler, 1966a).

Methemoglobin-Reducing Systems. *Spontaneous Methemoglobin Reduction.* The major system responsible for methemoglobin reduction in mammalian red cells is methemoglobin reductase, which has been identified as cytochrome b_5. This intracellular enzyme requires NADH as a cofactor.

Chronic, congenital methemoglobinemia has been recognized in rare individuals for more than a century. This condition is due to an inherited deficiency of methemoglobin reductase (Scott and Griffith, 1959). Such individuals may chronically have 10 to 50 percent of their circulating blood pigment in the form of methemoglobin. The deficit is primarily a cosmetic one, since they have a compensatory polycythemia and little in the way of pathophysiologic signs or symptoms. Since the methemoglobin levels are at a steady state short of complete oxidation, alternative mechanisms for methemoglobin reduction must exist in the red cell, but these individuals are particularly sensitive to methemoglobin-generating chemicals. Any additional acquired pigment persists for abnormally long periods of time. Newborns are also said to be unusually sensitive to methemoglobin-generating chemicals both because of a transient deficiency in methemoglobin reductase and because of a high concentration of fetal hemoglobin in their erythrocytes.

Congenital methemoglobinopathies due to abnormal amino acid substitutions in globin chains constitute separate disease entities. The abnormal hemoglobins M or H apparently have an enhanced ability to dissociate their heme groups, which makes the iron more susceptible to autoxidation. These people are also more sensitive to methemoglobin-generating chemicals in that higher peak concentrations are produced, but the methemoglobin reductase system functions normally.

The duration of a methemoglobinemia after an acute challenge with a chemical such as sodium nitrite depends both on the peak concentrations generated and the methemoglobin reductase activity in the red cells of the species involved. Some evidence, however, suggests that nitrite or a product of the nitrite-hemoglobin reaction may inhibit the reductase system in mice (Kruszyna *et al.*, 1982). Mouse red cells have unusually high rates of methemoglobin reductase activity (Table 8–1), but nitrite produces a uniquely prolonged methemoglobinemia in that species in comparison with all other agents tested. In human red cells, the reductase activity is so sluggish that the methemoglobinemia was of about the same duration with all agents tested.

Table 8–2. STIMULATION OF METHEMOGLOBIN REDUCTASE ACTIVITY OF MAMMALIAN ERYTHROCYTES BY METHYLENE BLUE*[†]

| SPECIES | INVESTIGATORS | | | | |
| | (1) | (2) | (3) | (4) | (5) |
	Increased Activity, Species/Increased Acivity, Man				
Pig	0.05	0.03		0.15	
Horse	0.10	0.06		0.25	
Goat	0.50	0.03			
Sheep	0.38	0.28		0.45	
Cow	0.42	0.34		1.0	
Cat		0.69	0.16	0.65	1.0
Dog		0.41	0.24	0.85	1.0
Rabbit		0.50	1.4	0.70	0.50
Mouse					1.1
Guinea pig		1.3	0.94	2.4	
Rat		2.1	1.0	2.2	1.9

*Data from various sources using nitrited red cells with glucose as a substrate have been normalized by the ratio:

$$\frac{\text{(activity M.B. and glucose—activity glucose)}_{species}}{\text{(activity M.B. and glucose—activity glucose)}_{human}}$$

[†]See footnote to Table 8–1 for literature citation.

As shown in Table 8–1, methemoglobin reductase activities differ over more than an order of magnitude among the red cells of the species tested. It is presumed that these differences reflect primarily differences in methemoglobin reductase activity, but possible contributions from alternative mechanisms were not evaluated. In each case, glucose was the substrate, and the data have been expressed as a ratio of the species activity to that in human red cells. In order to place the ratios is some perspective, estimates of the reduction half-time for 80 to 100 percent levels of methemoglobin in human red cells under the same conditions range from 6 to 24 hours (Bolyai *et al.*, 1972). The data are too crude to define precisely the elimination kinetic pattern, but in general rates of reduction seemed to decrease with decreasing methemoglobin levels.

Pig and horse red cells have considerably slower rates of reductase activity than human cells when glucose is the substrate (Table 8–1). *In vivo* both porcine and equine red cells seem to utilize plasma lactate in preference to glucose as a metabolic fuel for methemoglobin reduction (Rivkin and Simon, 1965; Robin and Harley, 1967). Rat, guinea pig, mouse, and rabbit have high rates of methemoglobin reductase activity in relation to humans, but the significance of these differences remains unknown.

The Dormant NADPH-Linked Reductase System. Human and most mammalian red cells have a second methemoglobin reductase system that can be activated by methylene blue and requires NADPH as a cofactor (Figure 8–9). Because of the requirement for NADPH, methylene blue will not increase the rate of methemoglobin reduction in G-6-PD–deficient cells. The physiological function of the enzyme capable of reducing methylene blue is unknown. In a very rare case of congenital deficiency of this enzyme, methylene blue also failed to accelerate the rate of methemoglobin reduction. However, the methemoglobin levels were normal, and the propositus had no other obvious pathophysiology (Sass *et al.*, 1967). Reduced or leuco-methylene blue transfers its acquired electron in normal subjects to reduce methemoglobin nonenzymatically (Sass *et al.*, 1969). The injection of methylene blue in severe acquired methemoglobinemias can be a life-saving intervention. It will also temporarily return levels to normal in subjects with methemoglobin reductase deficiency, but it should not be used chronically for that purpose. Large doses of ascorbic acid on a chronic basis are sometimes effective for this cosmetic purpose.

Species differences also exist in terms of the magnitude of the response to exogenous methylene blue (Table 8–2), but all species tested responded to 1 to 2×10^{-5} M dye with an increase in reductase activity over that observed with glucose alone. The data are again expressed as a ratio of the species increase to the increase observed in human cells under the same conditions. To place these data in perspective, estimates of the reduction half-time of 70 to 90 percent levels of methemoglobin in human red cells with methylene blue range from 45 to 90 minutes (Layne and Smith, 1969). The observations are too crude to establish the precise kinetics of the reduction, but the data were approximately linear with time.

A certain parallelism can be seen between Tables 8–1 and 8–2 in that species with high rates of spontaneous reductase activity respond more vigorously to methylene blue, with the possible exception of the rabbit. The nucleated red cells of birds, reptiles, and amphibians also have both NADH and NADPH reductase systems, but in these species the tricarboxylic acid cycle appears to be the source of the cofactors (Board *et al.*, 1977).

Minor Pathways for Methemoglobin Reduction. Red cells have several minor pathways for nonenzymatic methemoglobin reduction. Reduced glutathione slowly reduces methemoglobin, but it can account for only 12 percent of the total reductive capacity (Scott *et al.*, 1965). Ascorbic acid (vitamin C) is sometimes used in patients with methemoglobin reductase deficiency (above), but it normally accounts for only 16 percent of the total reductive effort. Scorbutic subjects (ascorbate-deficient) and G-6-PD–deficient subjects with decreased red cell levels of reduced glutathione do not have elevated levels of methemoglobin. Primates and guinea pigs are among the rare mammals that require exogenous ascorbate. Oddly, guinea pig red cells do not respond to ascorbate as do human cells (Bolyai *et al.*, 1972). Cysteine, ergothioneine, NADH, and NADPH also have limited capabilities for direct methemoglobin reduction.

Management of Acquired Methemoglobinemias. As already noted, methemoglobin-generating chemicals usually have additional toxic effects that contribute to the intoxication syndrome. Nevertheless, reductions in the circulating levels of methemoglobin in symptomatic patients is a desirable therapeutic goal. For agents that produce hemolysis as well, this can be accomplished only by exchange transfusion. If the methemoglobin is intracellular and the cells are normal, the intravenous administration of 1 to 2 mg/kg of methylene blue usually results in a dramatic response (Gosselin *et al.*, 1984). Although methylene blue is not equally efficacious against all chemically induced methemoglobinemias as tested *in vitro* in human red cell suspensions, it provides unequivocal protection against death in laboratory animals against all agents tested (Smith and Layne, 1969; Smith and Olson, 1973).

A possible alternative to methylene blue that would bypass the lesion in oxygen transport might be hyperbaric oxygen. Oxygen at 4 atmospheres decreased mortality and methemoglobin levels in rats given nitrite. After PAPP administration to rats, however, methemoglobin levels were actually increased (Goldstein and Doull, 1971, 1973). The mechanism of the effect on nitrite poisoning is not known, but hyperbaric oxygen seems to inhibit the acetylation of PAPP, which is an important mechanism for its detoxification. The same may be true for all related aromatic amino compounds that generate methemoglobin. In mice, methylene blue and hyperbaric oxygen seemed to have additive effects in preventing nitrite poisoning (Way and Sheehy, 1971).

Oxidative Hemolysis

Sulfhemoglobin. The term *sulfhemoglobin* was coined more than a century ago to describe a pigment generated *in vitro* by passing a stream of pure hydrogen sulfide through blood. This pigment plays no role in acute hydrogen sulfide poisoning (below). When generated in that way, the pigment seems to be unstable, but the solutions become so turbid that visible absorption spectra can only be derived indirectly (Drabkin and Austin, 1935–36).

Sulfhemoglobin may have a weak absorption maximum at about 620 nm, which overlaps to some extent the absorption maximum of methemoglobin at 630 nm. This coincidence may have contributed to confusion in the early literature. In contrast to methemoglobin, the absorption maximum at 620 nm for sulfhemoglobin is not abolished by cyanide. This difference is the basis for methods said to be suitable for the determination of both pigments in mixtures (Evelyn and Malloy, 1938; van Kampen and Zijlstra, 1965). So-called sulfhemoglobins of high purity have been generated *in vitro* with hydrogen sulfide under special conditions (e.g., Nichol *et al.*, 1968), but their relationship to the originally described pigment is unknown.

When the criterion of an absorption band at 620 nm, which is stable toward cyanide, was applied to large numbers of human blood samples in clinical laboratories, positive results were obtained in some patients (Evelyn and Malloy, 1938). These patients were said to be sulfhemoglobinemic even though no source of exposure to hydrogen sulfide or even to exogenous sulfur-containing xenobiotics could be documented. All attempts to find this pigment in laboratory animals exposed to hydrogen sulfide failed. In retrospect, it appears likely that two unrelated phenomena have been identified by the same name for many years because of a coincidence in the position of an absorption maximum and its stability toward cyanide (National Academy of Sciences, 1977b).

Over the years, sulfhemoglobin has come to

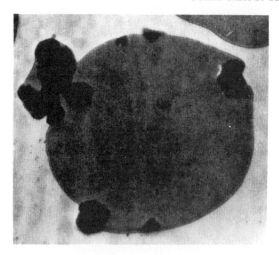

Figure 8–10. End-stage Heinz bodies lying under and distorting the plasma membrane of a mature erythrocyte. ×26,000. (From Rifkind, R. A., and Danon, D.: Heinz body anemia—an ultrastructural study. I. Heinz body formation. *Blood*, **25**:885–896, 1965.)

mean an abnormal blood pigment or pigments generated either *in vivo* or *in vitro* in the absence of exogenous sulfur. Perhaps this pigment might better be called pseudosulfhemoglobin, but it is associated with three clinical conditions: (1) the ingestion of "oxidant" drugs such as phenacetin, chlorate, or naphthalene, which may also generate low levels of methemoglobin in normal subjects; (2) the presence of an abnormal hemoglobin such as M or H (Tönz, 1968); and (3) the exposure of individuals with G-6-PD deficiency to certain drugs or chemicals such as primaquine, sulfonamides, or methylene blue (below).

It seems likely that as encountered in the circumstances above, sulfhemoglobin is a partially oxidized and denatured mixture of pigments arising as a result of nonspecific oxidative damage (Beutler, 1969). No mechanism exists in red cells for the reversal of sulfhemoglobinemia, but it has never been encountered in life-threatening concentrations. It either persists until the red cell containing it is replaced by erythropoiesis, or it is part of a broader and more serious hemolytic reaction (below).

Heinz Body Hemolytic Anemia. Heinz bodies are dark-staining, dense, refractile granules consisting of denatured hemoglobin, possibly sulfhemoglobin (Figure 8–10). They appear to be covalently bound to the interior surface of red cell membranes, perhaps through disulfide bridges (Jacob *et al.*, 1968). Gross distortions in the shape of the cell may occur, resulting in premature splenic phagocytosis, or impairment

of active or passive ion transport may cause changes in osmotic pressure, hyperpermeability, and intravascular hemolysis. Thus, sulfhemoglobinemia, Heinz body formation, and hemolysis represent a continuum of oxidative stress to the red cell.

Some authorities believe that the above triad is preceded by a transient methemoglobinemia (Jandl *et al.*, 1960), but others point to a poor (or even inverse) correlation between the ability of a given chemical to generate methemoglobin and its tendency to produce Heinz bodies (Rentsch, 1968). Methemoglobinemia *per se* does not lead to hemolysis (Beutler, 1969), although in some cases this may simply be a matter of dose or concentration. Oxygen is necessary for Heinz body formation but not for methemoglobin generation. Hydroxylamine reacts with deoxyhemoglobin to form methemoglobin, but the reaction with oxyhemoglobin results in both sulf- and methemoglobin formation (Cranston and Smith, 1971).

Mechanisms of Heinz Body Formation. Congenital Heinz bodies are found in individuals with certain types of abnormal hemoglobins that apparently facilitate dissociation of the heme group from the globin chains. Partial or total loss of heme groups results in decreased water solubility and an increased tendency for the pigment to precipitate. The heme group can be stabilized *in vitro* in such pigments by the addition of cyanide (below) or carbon monoxide (Jacob *et al.*, 1968; Rieder, 1970). Heme dissociation, however, has not been demonstrated in acquired Heinz body anemias as in the reaction of normal red cells with phenylhydrazine or the reaction of G-6-PD–deficient cells with primaquine. Heme loss did not occur during hemoglobin oxidation and denaturation by hydroxylamine (Cranston and Smith, 1971).

It is now thought that oxidant chemicals such as phenylhydrazine generate hydrogen peroxide within red cells either by direct reaction with molecular oxygen or by a coupled reaction with oxyhemoglobin. The peroxide can be detoxified by glutathione peroxidase (Figure 8–6), resulting in the oxidation of reduced glutathione. Oxidized glutathione is reduced by the activity of glutathione reductase, which also requires NADPH generated by G-6-PD. These three enzymes work in concert, and a deficiency in any one of them carries with it an increased sensitivity of the cell to oxidative stress. Red cells also contain catalase, but catalase-deficient red cells are not more sensitive to peroxide-induced damage. With the recent discovery that catalase also has a need for NADPH for maximum peroxide detoxification, it appears likely that G-6-PD deficiency compromises the activity of both glutathione peroxidase and catalase (Gaetani *et al.*, 1989). The extent of the involvement of other active oxygen species such as superoxide anion and superoxide dismutase, which is also present in red cells, is not clear. An early event in this reaction whether it is induced in normal red cells or in G-6-PD–deficient ones is a precipitous fall in the levels of glutathione. Oxidized glutathione may form mixed disulfides with free sulfhydryl groups on globin chains to contribute to instability and denaturation (Allen and Jandl, 1961).

Agents Producing Heinz Bodies. Aniline, nitrobenzene, and related homologues produce Heinz bodies in many species. Whether the active matabolites are the same as those that are responsible for methemoglobin formation is not known. Prominent species differences probably relate to differences in the rates of activation and inactivation of these chemicals *in vivo*. Nonnitrogenous compounds also generate Heinz bodies: phenols, propylene glycol, ascorbic acid, sulfite dichromate, arsine, and stibine are examples. Hydroxylamine and chlorate salts were among the earliest agents recognized as eliciting the response. Ingestion of crude oil has resulted in Heinz body hemolytic anemia in marine birds (Leighton *et al.*, 1983), and dimethyl disulfide produces the reaction in chickens (Maxwell, 1981). Perhaps Heinz body formation is a less specific oxidative process than methemoglobin formation.

Species Differences. Cat, mouse, dog, and human red cells are said to be particularly susceptible to Heinz body formation, whereas rabbit, monkey, chick, and guinea pig are relatively resistant. Unfortunately, these impressions are not based on systematic, quantitative investigations. Indeed, there is no general agreement about how to quantify the damage in such reactions. The morphology and ultrastructure of Heinz bodies also vary with species and with agents. Under certain conditions, large numbers of small bodies are seen. Perhaps these eventually coalesce into larger multibodied inclusions. In the nucleated turkey red cell, phenylhydrazine-induced Heinz bodies were smaller than those produced under identical conditions in dog or horse red cells, and they were seen in both the nucleoplasm and the cytoplasm. Extraerythrocytic Heinz bodies were observed with suspensions of horse red cells but not dog or turkey red cells (Simpson, 1971).

The Spleen. Although red cells normally end their life in the spleen after 120 days in the circulation, splenectomy in man does not result in an increase in red cell survival time. The function of senescent red cell destruction is quickly subsumed by other segments of the reticuloendothelial system such as the liver and bone marrow. The anatomic ultrastructure of the spleen, however, is particularly well suited for that task. Red cells enter the spleen via the Billroth cord from a terminal arteriole or capillary, percolate through the fine spaces formed by reticular fibers and macrophages, and then exit by gaining access to a splenic sinusoid. This is the moment of truth, for it now has to pass through fenestrations in the sinusoidal basement membrane that are smaller than its own diameter. The apertures are lined with macrophages. Cells with unusual shapes such as sickle cells, cells with Heinz bodies, or cells lacking the metabolic energy to resume their normal conformation after passage through capillaries are phagocytized, as also are cells flagged with immunoglobulin or complement (Weed *et al.*, 1969). After hemolysis, the hemoglobin is catabolized, and the heme groups are degraded to bilirubin. Splenic engorgement and increased heme oxidase activity are signs of hemolytic disease because of the increased demand for these functions.

HISTOTOXIC HYPOXIA

Semantic purists object to the term *histotoxic hypoxia* because in this condition the P_{O_2} in peripheral tissues is normal or even higher than normal. The lesion is one of an inability to utilize molecular oxygen at the cellular level. The chemicals known to have this action are the soluble salts or weak acids of sulfide and cyanide. The key features for the case of hydrogen cyanide are illustrated in Figure 8–11, but hydrogen sulfide is very similar. Some evidence suggests that it is the undissociated acids that actually interrupt electron transport down the chain by inhibiting at the cytochrome a–cytochrome a_3 step (L. Smith *et al.*, 1977). Since these cytochromes are isolated as a single unit, they are referred to as cytochrome aa_3 or cytochrome oxidase. As a result of cyanide inhibition, oxidative phosphorylation and metabolism are compromised. Electron transfer from cytochrome oxidase to molecular oxygen is blocked, peripheral tissue P_{O_2} begins to rise, and the unloading gradient for oxyhemoglobin is decreased. As a result, abnormally high concentrations of oxyhemoglobin are found in the venous return, imparting a flush to skin and mucous membranes not unlike that seen in carbon monoxide poisoning. The increased demand placed on glycolysis results in a profound lactic acidemia.

Cyanide and sulfide directly stimulate the chemoreceptors of the carotid and aortic bodies to produce a brief period of hyperpnea. Cardiac irregularities are often noted, but the heart invariably outlasts the respirations. Death is due to

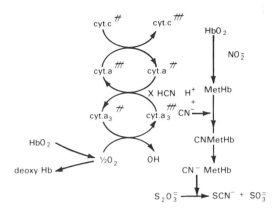

Figure 8–11. Principles of the therapeutic management of cyanide poisoning. Although the exact chemical details are still unknown, the undissociated form *(HCN)* appears to block electron transfer in the cytochrome a₃ complex, which is isolated *in vitro* as a single unit. As a consequence, oxygen utilization is decreased and oxidative metabolism may slow to the point that it cannot meet metabolic demands. At the level of the brainstem nuclei, this effect may result in central respiratory arrest and death. On injection of sodium nitrite, methemoglobin is generated, which can compete effectively with cytochrome aa₃ for free cyanide. Note that it is the ionic form that complexes with methemoglobin. The injection of thiosulfate provides subtrate for the enzyme rhodanese, which catalyzes the biotransformation of cyanide to thiocyanate.

central respiratory arrest, which can occur within seconds or minutes of the inhalation of high concentrations of hydrogen cyanide or sulfide gas. Because of slower absorption, death may be delayed after the ingestion of cyanide salts, but the critical events still occur within the first hour.

Other sources of cyanide have been responsible for human poisonings such as amygdalin, a cyanogenic glycoside found in sweet almonds and apricot, peach, and other fruit pits. Amygdalin is a complex of glucose, benzaldehyde, and cyanide; the latter is released by the action of β-glucosidase or emulsin. Such enzymes are not found in mammalian tissues, but they are present in normal human intestinal microflora. For this reason, amygdalin is about 40 times more toxic by mouth than by intravenous injection. Thus, the quack anticancer remedy Laetrile®, which consisted chiefly of amygdalin, could be given safely by parenteral routes but caused cyanide poisoning when accidentally ingested by children.

The antihypertensive drug sodium nitroprusside can cause cyanide poisoning in overdose. Its reaction with hemoglobin results in the direct

formation of cyanmethemoglobin, but most of the cyanide seems to be released by its reaction with the vascular endothelium or smooth muscle (R. P. Smith and Kruszyna, 1974; Devlin *et al.*, 1989b). Fortunately, the therapeutic index for nitroprusside is quite large. The acute toxic effects of a series of commercially important aliphatic nitriles also appears to be due to the metabolic release of free cyanide (Willhite and Smith, 1981; Doherty *et al.*, 1982).

Treatment of Cyanide Poisoning

Time is of the essence in treating cyanide poisoning, and traditionally three drugs are given. The most controversial of these is the amyl nitrite as given by inhalation. Amyl nitrite is a poor methemoglobin former in man, especially as given by the pulmonary route, but it seems to serve no other useful purpose (Klimmek and Krettek, 1988). This is followed by sodium nitrite given intravenously in an initial dose of 300 mg for an adult. At least the nitrite converts a tolerable fraction of the total circulating hemoglobin to methemoglobin (Figure 8–11). Ferric heme groups avidly bind ionic cyanide to form the stable complex cyanmethemoglobin. As the blood concentration of free cyanide falls, it effects a dissociation of the cyanide complex with cytochrome oxidase and a resumption of oxidative metabolism. Up to this point, the same basic principles hold for sulfide as well.

Although this approach can be rapidly efficacious, there are two undesirable results to this stopgap measure. Cyanmethemoglobin is inert in terms of oxygen transport, and although the cyanide is bound very tenaciously, it is still a fully reversible complex, which carries a risk of release of free cyanide and a recurrence of poisoning. In some species such as rabbits and mice, cyanmethemoglobin can apparently serve as a substrate for methemoglobin reductase. Late deaths may ensue as the cyanide is released from this biologically inert store (Kruszyna *et al.*, 1982). Permanent, irreversible detoxification of cyanide is accomplished by the intravenous injection of sodium thiosulfate. Thiosulfate contains a sulfane-sulfur, one bound only to another sulfur, which can be utilized by the widely distributed enzyme rhodanese (thiosulfate-cyanide sulfurtransferase) to convert cyanide to thiocyanate. This much less toxic product is excreted in the urine. After dissociation of its cyanide for biotransformation, methemoglobin is restored to functional blood pigment by the action of methemoglobin reductase (Figure 8–9).

It has long been believed that liver rhodanese plays the major role in cyanide detoxification, particularly when exogenous thiosulfate is provided, but rhodanese in skeletal muscle makes a significant contribution. Indeed, in the absence of thiosulfate, skeletal muscle clears more cyanide than the liver (Devlin et al., 1989a). This observation and an inferred large redundancy of the liver enzyme may explain why surgical removal of two-thirds of the liver or severe liver damage induced by carbon tetrachloride did not increase cyanide lethality in mice whether or not thiosulfate was also given (Rutkowski et al., 1986). Although oxygen can do no harm, from the principles summarized in Figure 8–11, it would seem to serve no useful purpose. Even hyperbaric oxygen alone had no effect on cyanide poisoning in mice (Way et al., 1972). However, oxygen further and significantly decreased mortality when it was used in combination with nitrite and thiosulfate in cyanide-poisoned mice (Way et al., 1966). Since rhodanese is not sensitive to oxygen, the mechanism for this potentiation is unknown.

Hydrogen Sulfide Poisoning

As noted above, hydrogen sulfide is also established as an in vitro inhibitor of cytochrome oxidase (L. Smith et al., 1977). Human poisonings are invariably a result of exposure to the gas, but soluble salts are used experimentally by the parenteral route in laboratory animals. In either case, the signs of poisoning are similar in almost all respects to those induced by cyanide. Sulfide, however, has a greater tendency to produce local tissue reactions such as conjunctivitis (gas eye) and pulmonary edema (Lopez et al., 1989).

As already noted, the hydrosulfide anion (HS^-) forms a complex with methemoglobin known as sulfmethemoglobin, which is analogous to cyanmethemoglobin. Sulfmethemoglobin is a well-characterized entity in contrast to the confusion (above) about the identity of sulfhemoglobin. The dissociation constant for sulfmethemoglobin is about 6×10^{-6} moles/liter, whereas the dissociation constant for cyanmethemoglobin is on the order of 2×10^{-8} moles/liter. Despite the lower binding affinity, a nitrite-induced methemoglobinemia provides unequivocal protection and has antidotal effects against sulfide poisoning in laboratory animals (Smith and Gosselin, 1964). The procedure has been used successfully in the resuscitation of several human victims of hydrogen sulfide poisoning (Stine et al., 1976; Peters, 1981). Neither thiosulfate nor oxygen has significant effects alone or in combination with nitrite (Smith et al., 1976), but oxygen would be indicated if the victim shows signs of adult respiratory distress syndrome. Sulfide reacts rapidly to split disulfide bridges under physiologic conditions; thus, oxidized glutathione and other simple disulfides have protective and possibly antidotal effects (Smith and Abbanat, 1966). Sulfide in vivo is metabolized to sulfite and sulfate.

Hydrogen sulfide can be encountered in high concentrations in natural and volcanic gases and petroleum deposits. Hydrothermal vents in certain locations on the ocean floor continuously release high concentrations, and vent tube worms thriving in the vicinity may have blood concentrations that would be lethal to mammalian species. A primitive form of hemoglobin in their blood binds sulfide by virtue of its ability to split disulfide bonds and transports it to an organ containing symbiotic bacteria that utilize it as an energy-producing substrate (Powell and Somero, 1983).

Sewer gas, a synonym, refers to its presence wherever organic matter undergoes putrefaction. It is found in the emissions from industrial paper plants using the Kraft process. The leather industry uses hydrosulfide to remove the hair from hides prior to tanning, and ton quantities have been employed in facilities for the production of heavy water for nuclear reactors (National Academy of Sciences, 1977). Carbonyl sulfide, a by-product of coal hydrogenation and gasification, is metabolized in vivo to hydrogen sulfide by carbonic anhydrase (Chengelis and Neal, 1980).

REFERENCES

Allen, D. W., and Jandl, J. H.: Oxidative hemolysis and precipitation of hemoglobin. II. Role of thiols in oxidant drug action. J. Clin. Invest., **40**:454–475. 1961.

Bartels, H.; Hilpert, P.; Barbey, K.; Betke, K.; Riegel, K.; Lang, E. M.; and Metcalfe, J.: Respiratory functions of blood of the yak, llama, camel, Dybowski deer and African elephant. Am. J. Physiol., **205**:331–336, 1963.

Bartlett, D., Jr.: Effects of carbon monoxide in human physiological processes. Proceedings of the Conference on Health Effects of Air Pollutants. U.S. Government Printing Office, Washington, D.C., Serial 93–15, November 1973, pp. 103–126.

Bernard, C.: An Introduction to the Study of Experimental Medicine (first published in 1865). Reprinted by Dover, New York, 1957.

Bessis, M.: Blood Smears Reinterpreted, translated by G. Brecher. Springer-Verlag, Berlin, 1977.

Beutler, E.: Drug-induced hemolytic anemia. Pharmacol. Rev., **21**:73–103, 1969.

Birner, G., and Neumann, H. -G.: Biomonitoring of aromatic amines II: hemoglobin binding of some monocyclic amines. Arch. Toxicol., **62**:110–115, 1988.

Board, P. G.; Agar, N. S.; Gruca, M.; and Shine, R.: Methaemoglobin and its reduction in nucleated erythrocytes from reptiles and birds. Comp. Biochem. Physiol., **57B**:265–267, 1977.

Bolyai, J. Z.; Smith, R. P.; and Gray, C. T.: Ascorbic acid and chemically induced methemoglobinemias. Toxicol. Appl. Pharmacol., **21**:176–185, 1972.

Born, G. V. R.: Aggregation of blood platelets by adenosine diphosphate and its reversal. *Nature,* **194**:927–929, 1962.

Bryant, M. S.; Vineis, P.; Skipper, P. L.; and Tannenbaum, S. R.: Hemoglobin adducts of aromatic amines: associations with smoking status and type of tobacco. *Proc. Natl. Acad. Sci. USA,* **85**:9788–9791, 1988.

Burns, K. F., and de Lannoy, C. W., Jr.: Compendia of normal blood values of laboratory animals, with indications of variations. I. Random-sexed populations of small animals. *Toxicol. Appl. Pharmacol.,* **8**:429–437, 1966.

Calsey, J. D., and King, D. J.: Clinical chemical values for some common laboratory animals. *Clin. Chem.,* **26**:1877–1879, 1980.

Cerami, A., and Manning, J. M.: Potassium cyanate as an inhibitor of the sickling of erythrocytes *in vitro. Proc. Natl. Acad. Sci. USA,* **68**:1180–1183, 1971.

Chengelis, C. P., and Neal, R. A.: Studies of carbonyl disulfide toxicity: metabolism by carbonic anhydrase. *Toxicol. Appl. Pharmacol.,* **55**:198–202, 1980.

Coburn, R. F.; Williams, W. J.; White, P.; and Kahn, S. B.: The production of carbon monoxide from hemoglobin *in vivo. J. Clin. Invest.,* **46**:346–356, 1967.

Cranston, R. D., and Smith, R. P.: Some aspects of the reactions between hydroxylamine and hemoglobin derivatives. *J. Pharmacol. Exp. Ther.,* **177**:440–446, 1971.

Devlin, D. J.; Smith, R. P.; and Thron, C. D.: Cyanide metabolism in the isolated, perfused, bloodless hindlimbs or liver of the rat. *Toxicol. Appl. Pharmacol.,* **98**:338–349, 1989a.

———: Cyanide release from nitroprusside in the isolated, perfused, bloodless liver and hindlimbs of the rat. *Toxicol. Appl. Pharmacol.* **99**:354–356, 1989b.

Doherty, P. A.; Smith, R. P.; and Ferm, V. H.: Tetramethyl substitution on succinonitrile confers pentylenetetrazole-like activity and blocks cyanide release in mice. *J. Pharmacol. Exp. Ther.,* **223**:635–641, 1982.

Douglas, C. G.; Haldane, J. S.; and Haldane, J. B. S.: The laws of combination of haemoglobin with carbon monoxide and oxygen. *J. Physiol. (Lond.),* **44**:275–304, 1912.

Drabkin, D. L., and Austin, J. H.: Spectrophotometric studies. II. Preparations from washed blood cells; nitric oxide hemoglobin and sulfhemoglobin. *J. Biol. Chem.,* **112**:51–65, 1935–36.

Evelyn, K. A., and Malloy, H. T.: Microdetermination of oxyhemoglobin, methemoglobin and sulfhemoglobin in a single sample of blood. *J. Biol. Chem.,* **126**:655–662, 1938.

Fridovich, I.: Superoxide radical, an endogenous toxicant. *Annu. Rev. Pharmacol. Toxicol.,* **23**:239–257, 1983.

Gaetani, G. F.; Galiano, S.; Canepa, L.; Ferraris, A. M.; and Kirkman, H. N.: Catalase and glutathione peroxidase are equally active in detoxification of hydrogen peroxide in human erythrocytes. *Blood,* **73**:334–339, 1989.

Goldberg, M. A.; Dunning, S. P.; and Bunn, H. F.: Regulation of the erythropoietin gene: evidence that the oxygen sensor is a heme protein. *Science,* **242**:1412–1415, 1988.

Goldstein, G. M., and Doull, J.: Treatment of nitrite-induced methemoglobinemia with hyperbaric oxygen. *Proc. Soc. Exp. Biol. Med.* **138**:137–139, 1971.

———: The use of hyperbaric oxygen in the treatment of *p*-aminopropiophenone-induced methemoglobinemia. *Toxicol. Appl. Pharmacol.,* **26**:247–252, 1973.

Gosselin, R. E.; Smith, R. P.; and Hodge, H. C.: *Clinical Toxicology of Commercial Products,* 5th ed. Williams & Wilkins Co., Baltimore, 1984.

Haldane, J.: The relation of the action of carbonic oxide to oxygen tension. *J. Physiol.,* **18**:201–217, 1895.

Harris, J. W., and Kellermeyer, R. W.: *The Red Cell—Production, Metabolism, Destruction: Normal and Abnormal,* rev. ed. Harvard University Press, Cambridge, Mass., 1970.

Jacob, H. S.; Brian, M. C.; and Dacie, J. V.: Altered sulfhydryl reactivity of hemoglobins and red blood cell membranes in congenital Heinz body hemolytic anemia. *J. Clin. Invest.,* **47**:2644–2677, 1968.

Jandl, J. H.; Engle, L. K.; and Allen, D. W.: Oxidative hemolysis and precipitation of hemoglobin. I. Heinz body anemias as an acceleration of red cell aging. *J. Clin. Invest.,* **39**:1818–1836, 1960.

Kiese, M.: *Methemoglobinemia: A Comprehensive Treatise.* CRC Press, Cleveland, Ohio, 1974.

Kiese, M., and Weis, B.: Die Reduktion des Hämiglobins in den Erythrocyten verschiedener Tiere. *Naunyn Schmiedebergs Arch. Pharmacol.,* **202**:493–501, 1943.

Klimmek, R., and Krettek, C.: Effects of amyl nitrite on circulation, respiration and blood hemostasis in cyanide poisoning. *Arch. Toxicol.,* **62**:161–166, 1988.

Kruszyna, R.; Kruszyna, H.; and Smith, R. P.: Comparison of hydroxylamine, 4-dimethylaminophenol and nitrite protection against cyanide poisoning in mice. *Arch. Toxicol.,* **49**:191–202, 1982.

Kruszyna, R.; Kruszyna, H.; Smith, R. P.; and Wilcox, D. E.: Generation of valency hybrids and nitrosylated species of hemoglobin in mice by nitric oxide vasodilators. *Toxicol. Appl. Pharmacol.,* **94**:458–465, 1988.

Layne, W. R., and Smith, R. P.: Methylene blue uptake and the reversal of chemically induced methemoglobinemias in human erythrocytes. *J. Pharmacol. Exp. Ther.,* **165**:36–44, 1969.

Leighton, F. A.; Peakall, D. B.; and Butler, R. G.: Heinz body hemolytic anemia from the ingestion of crude oil, a primary toxic effect in marine birds. *Science,* **220**:871–873, 1983.

Letvin, N. L.; Linch, D. C.; Beardsley, G. P.; McIntyre, K. W.; and Nathan, D. G.: Augmentation of fetal-hemoglobin production in anemic monkeys by hydroxyurea. *N. Engl. J. Med.,* **310**:869–873, 1984.

Lopez, A.; Prior, M. G.; Reiffenstein, R. J.; and Goodwin, L. R.: Peracute toxic effects of inhaled hydrogen sulfide and injected sodium hydrosulfide on the lungs of rats. *Fund. Appl. Toxicol.,* **12**:367–373, 1989.

Malz, E.: Vergleichende Untersuchungen über die Methämoglobinreduktion in kernhaltigen und kernlosen Erythrozyten. *Folia Haematol. (Leipz.),* **78**:510–515, 1962.

Maxwell, M. H.: Production of a Heinz body anemia in the domestic fowl after ingestion of dimethyl disulfide: a haematological and ultrastructural study. *Res. Vet Sci.,* **30**:233–238, 1981.

Mitruka, B. M., and Rawnsley, H. M.: *Clinical Biochemical and Hematological Reference Values in Normal Experimental Animals.* Masson Publishing USA, Inc., New York, 1977.

Müller-Eberhard, U.: Hemopexin. *N. Engl. J. Med.,* **238**:1090–1094, 1970.

National Academy of Sciences: *Carbon Monoxide.* Committee on Medical and Biological Effects of Environmental Pollutants, National Research Council, Washington, D.C., 1977a.

———: *Hydrogen Sulfide.* Committee on Medical and Biological Effects of Environmental Pollutants, National Research Council, Washington, D.C., 1977b.

Ng, L. L.; Naik, R. B.; and Polak, B.: Paraquat ingestion with methaemoglobinaemia treated with methylene blue. *Br. Med. J.*, **284**:1445, 1982.

Nichol, A. W.; Hendry, I.; and Morrell, D. B.: Mechanism of formation of sulfhaemoglobin. *Biochim. Biophys. Acta*, **156**:97–108, 1968.

Norton, J. M., and Smith, R. P.: Drugs affecting the oxygen transport function of hemoglobin. In *Respiratory Pharmacology, Section 104, International Encyclopedia of Pharmacology and Therapeutics* (section ed., J. Widdicombe). Pergamon Press, Oxford, 1981.

Ou, L. C.; Kim, D.; Layton, W. M., Jr.; and Smith, R. P.: Splenic erythropoiesis in polycythemic response of the rat to high altitude exposure. *J. Appl. Physiol.: Respirat., Environ., Exercise Physiol.*, **48**:857–861, 1980.

Ou, L. C., and Smith, R. P.: Hemoglobinuria in rats exposed to high altitude. *Exp. Hematol.*, **6**:473–478, 1978.

Perutz, M. F.; Muirhead, H.; Cox, J. M.; and Goaman, L. C. G.: Three-dimensional Fourier synthesis of horse oxyhaemoglobin at 2.8 Å resolution: the atomic model. *Nature*, **219**:131–139, 1968.

Peters, J. W.: Hydrogen sulfide poisoning in a hospital setting. *JAMA*, **246**:1588–1589, 1981.

Pisciotta, A. V.: Immune and toxic mechanisms in drug-induced agranulocytosis. *Semin. Hematol.*, **10**:279–310, 1973.

Powell, M. A., and Somero, G. N.: Blood components prevent sulfide poisoning of respiration of the hydrothermal vent tube worm *Rifitia pachytila*. *Science*, **219**:297–299, 1983.

Prankerd, T. A. J.: *The Red Cell. An Account of Its Clinical Physiology and Pathology*. Blackwell Scientific Publications, Oxford, England, 1961.

Raphael, J. -C.; Elkharrat, D.; Jars-Guincestre, M. -C.; Chastang, C.; Chasles, V.; Vercken, J. -B.; and Gajdos, P.: Trial of normobaric and hyperbaric oxygen for acute carbon monoxide intoxication. *Lancet*, **2**:414–419, 1989.

Reddy, B. G.; Pohl, L. R.; and Krishna, G.: The requirement of the gut flora in nitrobenzene-induced methemoglobinemia in rats. *Biochem. Pharmacol.*, **25**:119–122, 1976.

Rentsch, G.: Genesis of Heinz bodies and methemoglobin formation. *Biochem. Pharmacol.* **17**:423–427, 1968.

Rieder, R. F.: Hemoglobin stability: observations on the denaturation of normal and abnormal hemoglobins by oxidant dyes, heat and alkali. *J. Clin. Invest.*, **49**:2369–2376, 1970.

Rifkind, R. A.; Bank, A.; Marks, P. A.; Nossell, H. L.; Ellison, R. R.; and Lindenbaum, J.: *Fundamentals of Hematology*, 2nd ed. Yearbook Medical Publishers, Inc., Chicago, 1980.

Rifkind, R. A., and Danon, D.: Heinz body anemia— an ultrastructural study. I. Heinz body formation. *Blood*, **25**:885–896, 1965.

Rivkin, S. E., and Simon, E. R.: Comparative carbohydrate metabolism and methemoglobin reduction in pig and human erythrocytes. *J. Cell Comp. Physiol.*, **66**:49–56, 1965.

Robin, H., and Harley, J. D.: Factors influencing response of mammalian species to the methemoglobin reduction test. *Aust. J. Exp. Biol. Med. Sci.*, **44**:519–526, 1966.

————: Regulation of methaemoglobinemia in horse and human erythrocytes. *Aust. J. Exp. Biol. Med. Sci.*, **45**:77–88, 1967.

Rutkowski, J. V.; Roebuck, B. D.; and Smith, R. P.: Liver damage does not increase the sensitivity of mice to cyanide given acutely. *Toxicology*, **38**:305–314, 1986.

Sass, M. D.; Caruso, C. J.; and Axelrod, D. R.: Mech-

anism of the TPNH-linked reduction of methemoglobin by methylene blue. *Clin. Chim. Acta*, **24**:77–85, 1969.

Sass, M. D.; Caruso, C. J.; and Farhangi, M.: TPNH-methemoglobin reductase deficiency: a new red cell enzyme defect. *J. Lab. Clin. Med.*, **70**:760–767, 1967.

Schwerin, F. T.; Rosenstein, R.; and Smith, R. P.: Cyanide prevents the inhibition of platelet aggregation by nitroprusside, hydroxylamine and azide. *Thromb. Haemostas.* **50**:780–783, 1983.

Scott, E. M.; Duncan, I. W.; and Ekstrand, V.: The reduced pyridine nucleotide dehydrogenases of human erythrocytes. *J. Biol. Chem.*, **240**:481–485, 1965.

Scott, E. M., and Griffith, I. V.: Enzymatic defect of hereditary methemoglobinemia: the diaphorase. *Biochim. Biophys. Acta*, **34**:584–586, 1959.

Simpson, C. F.: The ultrastructure of Heinz bodies in horse, dog, and turkey erythrocytes. *Cornell Vet.*, **61**:228–238, 1971.

Smith, J. E., and Beutler, E.: Anomeric specificity of human erythrocyte glucose-6-phosphate dehydrogenase. *Proc. Soc. Exp. Biol. Med.*, **122**:671–673, 1966a.

————: Methemoglobin formation and reduction in man and various animal species. *Am. J. Physiol.*, **210**:347–350, 1966b.

Smith, L.; Kruszyna, H.; and Smith, R. P.: The effect of methemoglobin on the inhibition of cytochrome *c* oxidase by cyanide, sulfide and azide. *Biochem. Pharmacol.*, **26**:2247–2250, 1977.

Smith, R. P.: The nitrite-methemoglobin complex—its significance in methemoglobin analyses and its possible role in methemoglobinemia. *Biochem. Pharmacol.*, **16**:1655–1664, 1967.

Smith, R. P., and Abbanat, R. A.: Protective effect of oxidized glutathione in acute sulfide poisoning. *Toxicol. Appl. Pharmacol.*, **9**:209–217, 1966.

Smith, R. P.; Alkaitis, A. A.; and Shafer, P. R.: Chemically induced methemoglobinemias in the mouse. *Biochem. Pharmacol.*, **16**:317–328, 1967.

Smith, R. P., and Gosselin, R. E.: The influence of methemoglobinemia on the lethality of some toxic anions. II. Sulfide. *Toxicol. Appl. Pharmacol.*, **6**:584–592, 1964.

Smith, R. P., and Kruszyna, H.: Nitroprusside produces cyanide poisoning via a reaction with hemoglobin. *J. Pharmacol. Exp. Ther.*, **191**:557–563, 1974.

Smith, R. P.; Kruszyna, R.; and Kruszyna, H.: Management of acute sulfide poisoning. Effects of oxygen, thiosulfate, and nitrite. *Arch. Environ. Health*, **33**:166–169, 1976.

Smith, R. P., and Layne, W. R.: A comparison of the lethal effects of nitrite and hydroxylamine in the mouse. *J. Pharmacol. Exp. Ther.*, **165**:30–35, 1969.

Smith, R. P., and Olson, M. V.: Drug-induced methemoglobinemia. *Semin. Hematol.*, **10**:253–268, 1973.

Smith, R. P., and Thron, C. D.: Hemoglobin, methylene blue and oxygen interactions in human red cells. *J. Pharmacol. Exp. Ther.*, **183**:549–558, 1972.

Snyder, C. A.: Benzene. In Snyder, R. (ed.): *Ethel Browning's Toxicity and Metabolism of Industrial Solvents*, 2nd ed., Vol. 1: *Hydrocarbons*. Elsevier, Amsterdam, 1987.

Spencer, T. D.: Effect of carbon monoxide on man and canaries. *Ann. Occup. Hyg.*, **5**:231–240, 1962.

Stebbins, R., and Bertino, J. R.: Megaloblastic anemias produced by drugs. *Clin. Haematol.*, **5**:619–630, 1976.

Stine, R. J.; Slosberg, B.; and Beacham, B. E.: Hydrogen sulfide intoxication: a case report and discussion of treatment. *Ann. Intern. Med.*, **85**:756–758, 1976.

Stolk, J. M., and Smith, R. P.: Species differences in

methemoglobin reductase activity. *Biochem. Pharmacol.,* **15**:343–351, 1966.

Stuart, P. R.; Osborn, J. S.; and Lewis, S. M.: The use of radio-frequency sputter ion etching and scanning electron microscopy to study the internal structure of biological material. *Proc. 2nd Annual Scanning Electron Microscope Symposium,* IIT Research Institute, Chicago, Ill., April 1969.

Surgenor, D. M.: *The Red Blood Cell,* 2nd ed. Academic Press, Inc., New York, Vol. I, 1974; Vol. II, 1975.

Tavassoli, M., and Crosby, W. H.: Fate of the nucleus of the marrow erythroblast. *Science,* **179**:912–913, 1973.

Tomoda, A., and Yoneyama, Y.: A simple method for preparation of valency hybrid hemoglobins, $(\alpha^{3+}\beta^{2+})_2$ and $(\alpha^{2+}\beta^{3+})_2$. *Anal. Biochem.,* **110**:431–436, 1981.

Tönz, O.: *The Congenital Methemoglobinemias, Physiology and Pathophysiology of Hemoglobin Metabolism.* S. Karger, Basel, 1968. Published simultaneously as Bibliotheca Haematologica, No. 28.

van Assendelft, O. W., and Zijlstra, W. G.: The formation of haemoglobin using nitrites. *Clin. Chim. Acta,* **11**:571–577, 1965.

van Kampen, E. J., and Zijlstra, W. G.: Determination of hemoglobin and its derivatives. In Sobotka, H., and Stewart, C. P. (eds.): *Advances in Clinical Chemistry,* Vol. 8. Academic Press, Inc., New York, 1965.

Way, J. L.; End, E.; Sheehy, M.; de Miranda, P.; Feitknecht, U. F.; Bachand, R.; Gibbon, S. L.; and Burrows, G. E.: Effect of oxygen on cyanide intoxication. IV. Hyperbaric oxygen. *Toxicol. Appl. Pharmacol.,* **22**:415–421, 1972.

Way, J. L.; Gibbon, S. L.; and Sheehy, M.: Effect of oxygen on cyanide intoxication. I. Prophylactic protection. *J. Pharmacol. Exp. Ther.,* **153**:381–385, 1966.

Way, J. L., and Sheehy, M.: Antagonism of sodium nitrite intoxication. *Toxicol. Appl. Pharmacol.,* **19**:400–401, 1971.

Weed, R. I.; LaCelle, P. L.; and Merritt, E. W.: Metabolic dependence of red cell deformability. *J. Clin. Invest.,* **48**:795–809, 1969.

Willhite, C. C., and Smith, R. P.: The role of cyanide liberation in the acute toxicity of aliphatic nitriles. *Toxicol. Appl. Pharmacol.,* **59**:589–602, 1981.

Chapter 9

TOXIC RESPONSES OF THE IMMUNE SYSTEM*

Jack H. Dean and Michael J. Murray

INTRODUCTION

The immune system functions in resistance to infectious agents, homeostasis of leukocyte maturation, immunoglobulin production, and immune surveillance against arising neoplastic cells. Cells of the immune system providing these functions are termed leukocytes and arise from pluripotent stem cells within the bone marrow, where they undergo highly controlled proliferation and differentiation before giving rise to functionally mature cells. The functionally mature cells are divided into granulocytes, lymphocytes, and macrophages. Lymphocytes can be subdivided into thymus-derived (T lymphocytes) and bursa-equivalent (B lymphocytes) depending on the primary lymphoid tissue where maturation occurs. The interaction of environmental chemicals or drugs with lymphoid tissue may alter the delicate balance of the immune system and can result in five types of undesirable effects: (1) immunosuppression, (2) uncontrolled proliferation (i.e., leukemia and lymphoma), (3) alterations of host defense mechanisms against pathogens and neoplasia, (4) allergy, and (5) autoimmunity.

---

* A partial listing of abbreviations used in this chapter includes the following: AIDS = acquired immunodeficiency syndrome; Ab = antibody; ADCC = antibody-dependent cellular cytotoxicity; CMI = cell-mediated immunity; CF = chemotactic factor; C' = complement; con A = concanavalin A; Fc = constant portion of Ab molecule; Cy = cyclophosphamide; CYA = cyclosporin A; CTL = cytotoxic T lymphocyte; DTH = delayed-type hypersensitivity; ELISA = enzyme-linked immunosorbent assay; GALT = gut-associated lymphoid tissue; HMI = humoral-mediated immunity; Ig = immunoglobulin; IFN = interferon; IL-1 = interleukin-1; K cell = killer cell; LPS = lipopolysaccharide; MØ = macrophage; MAF = macrophage-activating factor; MIF = migration inhibition factor; MLC = mixed leukocyte culture; NC lymphocyte = natural cytotoxic lymphocyte; NK cell = natural killer cell; PHA = phytohemagglutinin; PFC = plaque-forming cell; PWM = pokeweed mitogen; PMN = polymorphonuclear leukocyte; PGs = prostaglandins; RAST = radioallergosorbent test; RBC = red blood cell; SLE = systemic lupus erythematosus; SRBC = sheep red blood cell; SRS-A = slow-reacting substance of anaphylaxis; TNF = tumor necrosis factor.

Traditional methods for toxicologic assessment have implicated the immune system as a target organ of toxic insult following chronic or subchronic exposure to some chemicals and drugs. Alterations in lymphoid organ weight or histology; quantitative changes in peripheral leukocyte counts and differentials; depressed cellularity of lymphoid tissues; and increased susceptibility to infections by opportunistic organisms may reflect potential immune alterations and have been observed in animals exposed to chemicals at doses where overt toxicity was not apparent. Also, an increased incidence of allergy and autoimmunity has been associated with exposure to certain chemicals and drugs in both animals and humans. It is becoming increasingly apparent that the immune system represents an important target organ for studying the toxicology of chemical exposure for the following reasons: Immunocompetent cells are required for host resistance, and thus exposure to immunotoxicants can result in increased susceptibility to disease; immunocompetent cells require continued proliferation and differentiation for self-renewal and are thus sensitive to agents that affect cell proliferation; chemicals and drugs have been shown to induce allergy and autoimmunity; the cellular physiology of the immune system is better understood than in many other target organ systems, and thus the mechanism(s) by which toxicants produce cytotoxicity can be determined; enumeration of leukocytes or functional assessment can be easily achieved using a small volume of blood or lymphoid tissue; and finally, observations obtained in experimental animals can be confirmed using human leukocytes to provide a basis for risk extrapolation. Now that sensitive, reproducible, and validated assays of immune function and host resistance are available (Luster *et al.*, 1988), attention has focused on the usefulness of immunotoxicity as an adjunct in the routine safety evaluations of chemicals and drugs under development.

This chapter will provide an overview of the current concepts regarding the organization and

Table 9–1.   DIFFERENCES BETWEEN NONSPECIFIC AND SPECIFIC MECHANISMS OF HOST RESISTANCE

PARAMETER	NONSPECIFIC	SPECIFIC
Exogenous stimulation	Not required	Required
Specificity of reaction	None	High degree
Cell types involved	Polymorphonuclear leukocytes Monocytes/macrophages (effector cells)	T lymphocytes B lymphocytes Monocytes/macrophages (accessory cells)

function of the cellular elements of the immune system; dysfunctions of the immune system; approaches and methods for assessing immunotoxicity; and a partial listing of chemicals, metals, and drugs that have been found to produce immunosuppression, allergy, or autoimmunity.

CELLS OF THE IMMUNE SYSTEM AND THEIR FUNCTION

The immune system is a highly evolved organ system involved in host defense against infectious agents, neoplastic cells, transplanted tissue grafts, and environmental agents. These functions are provided by two major mechanisms: a nonspecific or constitutive mechanism not requiring prior contact with the inducing agent and lacking specificity; and a specific or adaptive mechanism directed against and specific for the eliciting agent (Table 9–1). Mononuclear phagocytes (i.e., blood monocytes and tissue macrophages) and granulocytes are phagocytic cells involved with nonspecific resistance. Lymphoid cells, macrophages, and their cytokine products (e.g., lymphokines and monokines) are all involved in specific host resistance.

The circulating cellular elements of the immune system all have their origin with the pluripotent stem cells. Pluripotent stem cells comprise a unique group of cells that are unspecialized and have renewal capacity. During fetal development, pluripotent stem cells are found in the blood islands of the yolk sac in the embryo, in the liver of the fetus, and later in the bone marrow. The pluripotent stem cell differentiates along several different pathways, giving rise to erythrocytes, myeloid series cells (i.e., macrophages, and granulocytes or polymorphonuclear leukocytes [PMNs]), megakaryocytes (which produce platelets), or lymphocytes. Maturation generally occurs within the bone marrow. Lymphoid progenitor cells are, however, disseminated by the vasculature to the primary lymphoid organs where they differentiate

under the influence of the microenvironment of these organs (Figure 9–1).

Nonspecific and Specific Mechanisms of Immunity

Two categories of phagocytic leukocytes, the polymorphonuclear phagocyte or granulocyte and the mononuclear phagocyte or macrophage (MØ), are involved with nonspecific mechanisms of host resistance. Both cell types originate from the same myeloid progenitor in bone marrow, pass through several developmental stages, and enter the bloodstream where they circulate for one to three days. PMNs can traverse blood vessels and represent the primary line of defense against infectious agents. Both PMNs and MØs exhibit phagocytic activity toward foreign material, especially in the presence of specific opsonic antibodies and complement (see below for description), and can destroy most microorganisms. In the event that PMNs either cannot contain or are destroyed by the infectious agent, as is the case with certain bacteria such as Listeria monocytogenes, macrophages are recruited to the site. Macrophages can be activated to a state of enhanced bactericidal activity by soluble mediators (lymphokines) produced by T lymphocytes sensitized to a specific microbial antigen. Macrophages are unique since they can adhere to glass or plastic, can be recruited by sensitized T lymphocytes to a specific tissue location, can be activated to become more efficient killers of intracellular microorganisms and tumor cells, and produce cytokines (e.g., IL-1 [interleukin-1], TNF [tumor necrosis factor], CFU-GM, and others) active on other cells of the immune system.

The immune response involved with adaptive host resistance represents a series of complex events that occur after the introduction of a foreign material (i.e., antigen) into an immunocompetent host. There are two major types of immune responses: (1) cell-mediated immunity (CMI), which is a response by specifically sensitized, thymus-dependent lymphocytes and

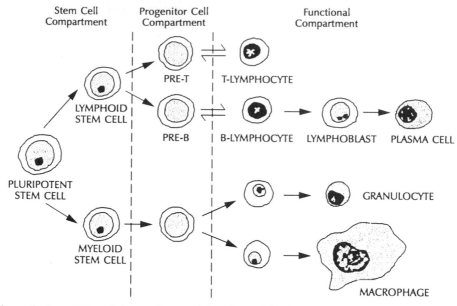

Figure 9–1. Differentiation pathways of lymphomyeloid pluripotent stem cells.

is generally associated with delayed-type hypersensitivity, graft rejection, and resistance to persistent infectious agents (e.g., certain viruses, bacteria, protozoa, and fungi); and (2) humoral-mediated immunity (HMI), which involves the production of specific antibodies (immunoglobulins) by bursa-equivalent lymphocytes or plasma cells following sensitization to a specific antigen.

Lymphocyte Differentiation

Replenishment and renewal of the cellular elements of the immune system constitute a major task of lymphoid tissue and occur in the primary lymphoid organs. The primary lymphoid organs include the bone marrow and thymus in all vertebrates and the bursa of Fabricius in avian species, or bursa-equivalent tissue in mammals. Primary lymphoid organs are generally lymphoepithelial in origin, derived from ectoendodermal junctional tissue in association with gut epithelium. During the second half of embryogenesis (days 12 to 13 in the mouse), lymphoid stem cells migrate into the epithelia of the thymus and bursa-equivalent areas and begin their differentiation into T cells and B cells, respectively (Figure 9–2). The maturation of lymphoctyes in the primary lymphoid organs is independent of antigenic stimulation.

The thymus, which is derived embryologically from the third and fourth pharyngeal pouches, is an organization of lymphoid tissue located in the chest (above the heart). Thymus development occurs during the sixth week of embryologic

development in humans and day 9 of gestation in the mouse. The thymus reaches its maximum size (approximately 0.27 percent of body weight) at birth or shortly thereafter in most mammals and then begins a gradual involution until at 5 to 15 years in humans it represents only 0.02 percent of body weight. Lymphocytes that differentiate from lymphoid stem cells in the thymus are termed thymus-dependent lymphocytes (T cells).

Histologically, the thymus consists of many lobules, each containing a cortex and medulla. Lymphocyte precursors from bone marrow proliferate in the cortex of the lobules and then migrate to the medulla, where they further differentiate under the influence of thymic epithelium into mature T lymphocytes before emigrating to secondary lymphoid tissues. The neonatal/postnatal thymus has an endocrine function associated with the nonlymphoid thymic epithelium cells. These cells produce hormones and growth factors essential for T-lymphocyte maturation and differentiation. A role for the adult thymus as an endocrine organ responsible for maintaining immune system homeostasis is also now speculated.

In birds, B-cell differentiation occurs in the bursa of Fabricius, a lymphoepithelial organ that develops from a diverticulum of the posterior wall of the cloaca. It is divided into a medullary region, containing lymphoid follicles, and a cortical region. Bursectomy in young birds results in impairment of germinal center formation in lymphoid tissue *(see below),* plasma cell forma-

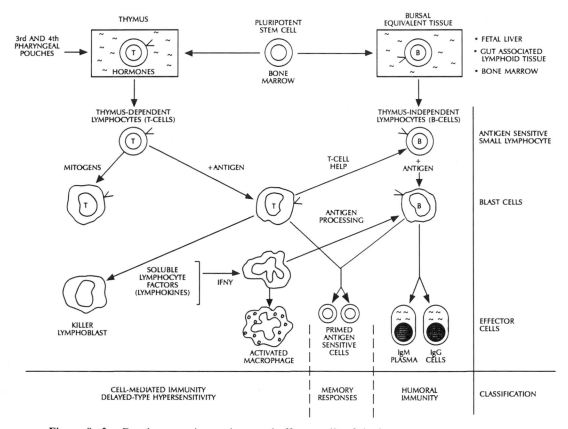

Figure 9–2. Development, interactions, and effector cells of the immune system.

tion, and immunoglobulin production. The mammalian bursa-equivalent is believed to be the fetal liver, the neonatal spleen, gut-associated lymphoid tissue, and adult bone marrow. Mature B lymphocytes (B cells) migrate from the bursa-equivalent tissue to populate the B-dependent areas of the secondary lymphoid tissues.

Neonatal removal or chemical destruction of primary lymphoid organs prior to the maturation of lymphocytes into T or B cells or prior to their population of secondary lymphoid tissue dramatically depresses the immunologic capacity of the host. However, removal of these same organs in adults has little influence on immunologic capacity. In addition, neonatal thymectomy in mammals dramatically impairs the development of CMI but does not generally influence the generation of immunoglobulin-producing cells involved in humoral antibody responses unless they require T-lymphocyte help for induction of antibody production. In contrast to the removal of primary lymphoid organs, removal of secondary lymphoid organs does not inhibit the development of immunocompetence, although it may suppress the magnitude or alter the

tissue localization of the responsive cells (Table 9–2).

Markers of Differentiation

T lymphocytes, B lymphocytes, and M∅s can be identified by a distinct pattern of cell surface–associated markers and receptors found on each of these cell types (Table 9–3). B cells, for example, have a high density of immunoglobulin on their surface, whereas T cells lack immunoglobulin. Conversely, B cells lack specific alloantigens that are found on T cells at different stages of differentiation. Macrophages, granulocytes, killer cells, and plasma cells possess a receptor for the Fc region of antibody molecules.

In contrast to T and B lymphocytes, macrophages and blood monocytes have the ability to phagocytose bacteria and other foreign particles. A group of mononuclear cells has been described that lack well-defined cell surface markers and are nonphagocytic. These cells possess a receptor for the Fc region of the immunoglobulin molecule and, when mixed with antibody and tumor target cells, are able to lyse the tumor target cells. They have been termed

Table 9–2. ORIGIN AND CHARACTERISTICS OF LYMPHOID ORGANS

PARAMETER	PRIMARY LYMPHOID ORGANS	SECONDARY LYMPHOID ORGANS
Lymphoid organs	Thymus Bursa of Fabricius (birds) Fetal liver (mammals) Adult bone marrow	Spleen Lymph nodes Mucosa
Embryonic origin and development	Ectoendodermal junction Thymus—day 9 to 10, mouse; week 6, man Bursa-equivalent—day 10 to 13, mouse; week 10, man	Mesoderm
Lymphoid cell proliferation	Independent of antigenic stimulation	Dependent on antigenic stimulation
Germinal center formation	Nonexistent	Occurs after antigenic stimulation
Cells repopulating after depletion	Stem cells only	Differentiated lymphocytes
Early surgical or drug removal	Depressed numbers of T and B cells, depressed immune responses	No significant effect on immune function

killer cells (K cells) and are believed to mediate cytolytic reactions against tumors and foreign tissue grafts in the presence of antibody, a process termed antibody-dependent cellular cytotoxicity (ADCC) (Perlmann *et al.*, 1975). Other subpopulations of lymphocytes have been described that possess spontaneous cytolytic activity toward neoplastic cells but not normal cells. These are termed natural killer (NK) cells (see the review by Herberman and Holden, 1978) and natural cytotoxic (NC) lymphocytes (Stutman and Cuttito, 1981).

Table 9–3. DIFFERENTIAL CHARACTERISTICS OF LYMPHOID CELLS

PARAMETER	T CELLS	B CELLS	MACROPHAGES
Phagocytosis	No	No	Yes
Adherence	No (blasts only)	No (plasma cells)	Yes
Surface receptors:			
Antigens	Yes	Yes	No
Fc region of Ig	Some	Yes	Yes
Complement	No	Yes	Yes
Common differentiation antigens:			
Mouse	Thy-1, CD5, CD8, CD4	Ig	CD11b
Man	CD3, CD4, CD8	Ig	—
Proliferation to:			
Phytohemagglutinin	Yes	No	No
Concanavalin A	Yes	No	No
Lipopolysaccharide of gram-negative bacteria	No	Yes (mouse only)	No
Allogeneic leukocyte antigens in mixed leukocyte culture	Yes	No	No
Effector functions:			
Immunologic memory	Yes	Yes	No
Tumor cell cytotoxicity	Yes	No	Yes
Bactericidal activity	No	No	Yes
Immunoglobulin production	No	Yes	No
Cytokine production	Yes (lymphokines)	No	Yes (monokines)

Organization of Secondary Lymphoid Organs

The organized areas of secondary lymphoid tissues consist of the lymph nodes, spleen, and gut-associated lymphoid tissue (Table 9–2). The anatomic organization of these tissues provides a microenvironment for functional development of lymphocytes, and histomorphologic alterations are often indicative of immunotoxicity or immune stimulation.

Lymph Nodes. Lymph nodes are discrete, organized secondary lymphoid organs and serve as filtering devices for lymphatic fluid. Lymph nodes are divided structurally into three areas: the cortex, paracortex, and medulla (Figure 9–3). Each lymph node is served by several afferent lymphatic vessels collecting lymphatic fluid from distal sites, and this fluid or lymph may contain foreign antigens. The efferent lymphatic vessel, which drains lymph from the node, contains antibodies, lymphokines, and lymphocytes produced in response to foreign antigenic stimulation. The cortex is located beneath the subcapsular sinus and receives the afferent lymph. It is the major site of B-lymphocyte localization. In the absence of antigenic stimulation, the cortex consists of a narrow rim of small lymphocytes. Also located in the cortex are aggregations of small lymphocytes, termed lymphoid follicles, which contain dendritic reticulum cells capable of retaining antigens on their plasma membranes. When the lymphocytes composing the lymphoid follicles are stimulated by antigen, they undergo proliferation, giving rise to dense aggregations of lymphocytes, termed germinal centers, which serve as sites for differentiation of B lymphocytes to plasma cells capable of antibody production. Following antigenic stimulation, germinal centers are easily detectable by histological methods as spherical or ovoid structures containing many large and medium-sized lymphocytes. Histologically, the germinal center is predominantly a B-lymphocyte area and contains three principal regions termed the densely populated, thinly populated, and lymphocyte cuff regions. In the densely populated region, the lymphocytes are actively mitotic, whereas in the thinly populated area one finds an accumulation of large to medium-sized lymphocytes. The cuff contains many small to medium-sized lymphocytes that are part of the recirculating B-lymphocyte memory cell pool.

The paracortex, lying between the cortex and the medulla, is predominantly a T-lymphocyte area (Figure 9–3) and is a major area of macrophage/T-cell interactions. Neonatal thymectomy or short-term lymphocyte depletion by thoracic duct cannulation reduces paracortical lymphocytes, leading to depressed immune capacity. In addition, the paracortex contains specialized blood vasculature, termed postcapillary venules, which serve as points of entry for recirculating lymphocytes from the bloodstream.

The medulla of the lymph node is primarily composed of networks of cords and sinuses. The

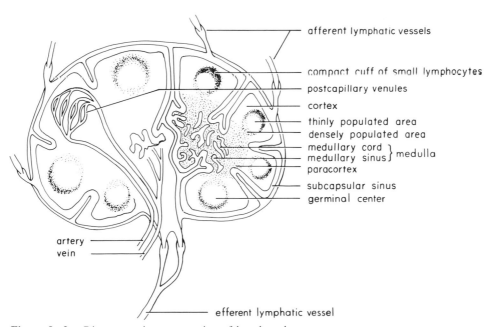

afferent lymphatic vessels

compact cuff of small lymphocytes

postcapillary venules

cortex

thinly populated area

densely populated area

medullary cord } medulla
medullary sinus }

paracortex

subcapsular sinus

germinal center

artery
vein

efferent lymphatic vessel

Figure 9–3. Diagrammatic cross section of lymph node.

sinuses are continuations of the subcapsular space passing through the cortex and medulla and are interspersed between the medullary cords. They ultimately merge in the hilus of the lymph node to form an efferent lymphatic vessel (Figure 9–3). The medullary cords consist of a structural network of dendritic cells surrounded by dense aggregations of lymphocytes. Together, this system of cords and sinuses serves as an effective filter for removing particulate material from lymphatic fluid. Following antigenic stimulation, a major portion of the antibody is produced by plasma cells found within these medullary cords.

Spleen. Lymph nodes serve as a major filter for lymph, whereas the spleen serves a similar function for blood. Since the spleen is the major filter of bloodborne antigens, it is also the major site of immunologic responses to these antigens. In addition, the spleen is a site of extramedullary erythropoiesis and removal of damaged blood cells. There are two major histologic regions within the spleen: the red and the white pulp (Figure 9–4). These areas have been named for their color in a freshly cut spleen. The white pulp consists of numerous white blood cell aggregates and lymphoid follicles. The red pulp contains cords and venous sinuses analogous to the medullary region of lymph nodes. The spleen has no afferent lymphatic vessels; thus, all antigenic material or cells enter the spleen through the blood vasculature. The marginal sinus in the spleen is structurally and functionally similar to the subcapsular sinus of the lymph node.

Gut-Associated Lymphoid Tissue (GALT). The lamina propria of the intestinal tract represents another secondary lymphoid tissue and, on a volume basis, is a major source of lymphoid tissue. Lymphocytes within the GALT are scattered in loose connective tissue or organized into lymphoid follicles (i.e., Peyer's patches) that contain germinal centers and diffuse concentrations of T lymphocytes analogous to the cortex and paracortex of the lymph node. As in all other lymphoid tissue, the lymphocyte cuff of the germinal center in the GALT is located nearest the source of antigenic stimulation (i.e., lumen of the intestine).

Antigen Recognition and Induction of Immunity

In 1959, Burnet proposed the clonal selection theory to describe the recognition of foreign antigens by lymphocytes, the induction of the immune response that followed, and the discrimination by the immune system between self and nonself. In this theory, a specific antigen was believed to be nonstimulatory to all but a few lymphocytes possessing receptors with a surface structure complementary to the configuration of the antigen. Following interaction with specific antigen, the receptor-bearing cell was stimulated to undergo proliferation and differentiation, producing a clone of progeny cells that were derived from a single ancestral cell. There is convincing evidence in support of Burnet's hypothesis. Immunoglobulin (Ig) molecules are thought to represent the primary cell

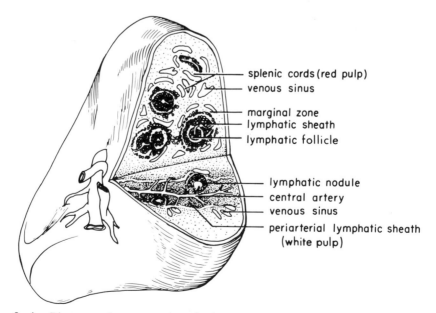

splenic cords (red pulp)
venous sinus

marginal zone
lymphatic sheath
lymphatic follicle

lymphatic nodule
central artery
venous sinus
periarterial lymphatic sheath
(white pulp)

Figure 9–4. Diagrammatic cross section of spleen.

membrane receptor on B lymphocytes. Likewise, T lymphocytes have unique cell membrane receptors involved with antigen recognition and subsequent differentiation.

Whether or not an antigen induces CMI, antibody production, or both presumably depends on a multitude of factors, including the physical and chemical nature of the antigen, the mode of presentation of the antigen to lymphocytes, the localization pattern of the antigen within lymphoid tissue, and the molecular configuration of the antigen. Those antigens generally found to elicit CMI include tissue antigens present on cells; chemical agents and drugs that conjugate with autologous proteins; and antigenic determinants on persistent intracellular microorganisms. In contrast, some antigens—for example, the pneumococcal polysaccharides—predominantly elicit antibodies. The route of exposure also plays a role in the type of response generated. Sheep erythrocytes, for example, will elicit antibodies when injected intravenously or will elicit both antibodies and CMI if injected intracutaneously. It is now established that intradermal presentation of antigen favors the development of CMI.

The induction of CMI proceeds by small lymphocytes differentiating into large pyroninophilic cells that do not contain rough endoplasmic reticulum and are thus distinct from plasma cells. These large lymphocytes ultimately divide, giving rise to cells responsible for immunologic memory and effector function. T cells can further differentiate into effector cells endowed with cytotoxic potential (i.e., cytotoxic T cells); helper cells (T_H), which facilitate antibody responses by B lymphocytes and aid in some T-lymphocyte responses; or T-suppressor cells (T_S) capable of inhibiting both T- and B-cell responses. The interleukins and their regulatory function on lymphoid cells are shown in Table 9–4. These lymphokines include interferons (IFN), and macrophage-activating factor (MAF), which represent nonspecific effectors of cell-mediated immunity and specific growth and differentiation factors (e.g., IL-1–6) that are responsible for amplification and regulation of the CMI response.

The main function of B lymphocytes is production of antibody molecules in response to antigenic stimulation. Antibody molecules are specific serum proteins synthesized in response to an antigen, which react specifically with that antigen. Based on chemical structure and biologic function, there are five major classes of antibody molecules: IgM, IgG, IgA, IgD, and IgE. Table 9–5 lists the principal physical and biologic characteristics of each of the classes.

Over a period of three to five days following the introduction of antigens into an immunocompetent host, B lymphocytes differentiate into lymphoblasts, immature plasma cells, and finally antibody-secreting plasma cells. There is an early rise in IgM antibody titer in the serum, followed several days later by the appearance of IgG antibodies. The production of IgM antibodies precedes that of IgG antibodies. Figure 9–5 depicts the time course of detectable serum antibody following immunization. During this differentiation process, lymphocytes are committed to immunologic memory so that when the same antigen is encountered a second time, an enhanced response is observed, characterized by a shorter latency to the appearance of serum IgG, increased production of Ig, and sustained production of IgG antibodies.

Figure 9–6 is a diagrammatic representation of an immunoglobulin molecule. It consists of four peptide chains, two light chains and two heavy chains, held together by disulfide bonds. Furthermore, each heavy and light chain is subdivided into a variable and constant region. It is the variable region that determines the molecular specificity for antigen, whereas the constant region of the heavy chains is responsible for the biologic activities of the molecule. For example, the constant region contains the sites that allow IgE to bind to mast cells or allow IgG to bind complement. All antibody molecules are variations of this basic structure and may occur as monomers or, in some instances, as dimers (some IgA molecules) or pentamers (IgM).

Antibody molecules exhibit four basic functions in protecting the host from infectious agents: (1) virus neutralization, whereby antibodies made to viral antigens may bind to the virus particles and prevent them from infecting target cells; (2) opsonization, whereby antibody molecules coat an infectious agent (i.e., bacteria or virus) and the antibody-antigen complex then binds to PMNs or macrophages via their Fc receptors, resulting in enhanced phagocytosis or elimination of the antibody-coated agent; (3) antibody-dependent cellular cytotoxicity (ADCC), which is mediated through leukocytes bearing receptors for the constant portion (Fc) of the molecule; following interaction of the antibody with antigens on target cells, the Fc portion binds to the leukocyte, which can then lyse the target cell; in this way, the antibody molecule provides the specificity for the action of the effector cell; and (4) complement (C')-mediated cell lysis; this C' system consists of 20 chemically and immunologically distinct serum proteins (see review by Muller-Eberhard, 1975) that can combine in a cascade with antibody following its interaction with antigen to generate

Table 9–4. INTERLEUKINS AND THEIR REGULATORY FUNCTIONS

LYMPHOKINE	SYNONYM	SOURCE	FUNCTION
IL-1	Lymphocyte activating factor, endogenous pyrogen, serum amyloid-A inducer	Monocytes, macrophages, and many other cell types	Promotes multiplication and activation of T and B cells; activates macrophages and NK cells; induces prostaglandin synthesis in many cell types; induces IL-6 production
IL-2	T-cell–derived growth factor	Helper T cells	Costimulates T-cell multiplication and effector functions; costimulates B-cell multiplication and differentiation
IL-3	Mast-cell growth factor and multiple colony stimulating factor	Helper T cells	Stimulates mast-cell multiplication; stimulates proliferation and differentiation of hemopoietic stem cells
IL-4	B-cell stimulatory factor I, B-cell growth factor II, T-cell growth factor II, and macrophage activating factor	Helper T cells, B cells	Costimulates B-cell multiplication and IgE and IgG_1 secretion; reduces IgG_{2a}, IgG_{2b}, IgG_3, and IgM secretion; enhances MHC class II expression on B cells and macrophages; T-cell growth factor; activates macrophages
IL-5	T-cell replacing factor, B-cell growth factor II, and eosinophil differentiation factor	Helper T cells	Costimulates B-cell multiplication and antibody secretion; stimulates eosinophil differentiation
IL-6	Hybridoma growth factor, B-cell differentiation factor, interferon-β_2, and B-cell stimulatory factor-2	T cells, monocytes, fibroblasts	Costimulates growth and differentiation of B cells; copromotes IL-2 production by mature T cells
IFN-α	Interferon-α	Leukocytes	Differentiation of B cells; increases IgM and IgG production; enhances MHC class I expression on lymphoid cells; potentiates IL-1 production by macrophages
IFN-β	Interferon-β_1	Fibroblasts, epithelial cells	Potentiates IL-1 production and decreases prostaglandin E production by macrophages
IFN-γ	Macrophage activating factor	Helper T cells, cytotoxic T cells	Enhances MHC class II expression on macrophages; activates macrophages; induces MHC class II expression on epithelial and endothelial cells; antagonizes IL-4 effects of B cells; stimulates B-cell multiplication and differentiation
Lymphotoxin	Tumor necrosis factor β	Lymphocytes, NK cells	Effector molecule of T-cell–mediated cytostasis and cytolysis
Tumor necrosis factor	Tumor necrosis factor α, cachectin	Monocytes/macrophages, and other cell types	Enhances IL-2 receptor expression of T cells; inhibits antibody secretion; activates macrophages; promotes MHC class I and II expression on various cells; induces IL-6

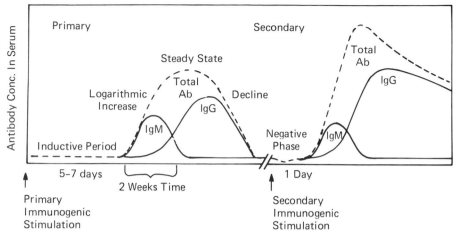

Figure 9–5. Kinetics of the antibody response.

biologic activities that result in lysis of red blood cells, foreign or transplanted cells, lymphocytes, platelets, bacteria, and certain enveloped viruses (Figure 9–7); many of the products of the complement activation pathway mediate inflammatory reactions (e.g., the C5 cleavage products); evidence for the biologic importance of the C' system comes from the markedly increased susceptibility to infections in individuals with congenital or acquired deficiencies in complement components.

Cellular Regulation of Immune Responses

Macrophages are required for activation of some antigen-specific T cells, in particular T-helper cells and T cells involved in delayed-type

Table 9–5. BIOLOGIC PROPERTIES OF IMMUNOGLOBULIN CLASSES

CLASS	MOLECULAR WEIGHT	HALF-LIFE (DAYS)	BIOLOGIC FUNCTION
IgG	150,000	23	Fix complement Cross placenta Heterocytotropic antibody
IgA	170,000	6	Secretory antibody Properdin pathway
IgM	890,000	5	Fix complement Efficient agglutination
IgD	150,000	2.8	Lymphocyte receptor?
IgE	196,000	1.5	Reaginic antibody Homocytotropic antibody

hypersensitivity (DTH), but not for activation of T-suppressor cells. The physical interaction between lymphocytes and macrophages has been well documented. In addition, T-helper cells are required for the induction of B cells to synthesize antibodies (Ab) to certain T-dependent antigens such as foreign red blood cells or serum proteins. In contrast, a variety of antigens do not require T-helper cells for induction of antibody synthesis and are termed T-independent antigens. It has been postulated that T-independent antigens can trigger B cells in the absence of T cells because their structure allows them to bind multivalently to the immunoglobulin receptor on the B-cell surface. T-dependent antigens are believed to lack this characteristic and can only bind to individual antigen recognition sites on B cells. Macrophages are required for triggering some T and B cells because the surface of the macrophage may act as a matrix to concentrate the relevant antigenic determinants (epitopes) in a manner similar to the multivalent antigens. T cells are also responsible for switching from IgM to IgG antibody expression. There is now ample data suggesting that certain T cells may exert a suppressive influence on immune responses and that these cells belong to a distinct subset of T cells with the Lyt-2,3 phenotype in mice and CD-5,8 phenotype in humans (i.e., suppressor T cell). In contrast, T-helper cells have the Lyt-2,3 phenotype in mice and CD-4 phenotype in humans. Helper and suppressor T cells exist in the circulation of humans and mice in a ratio of approximately 2 : 1 helper to suppressor cells. An imbalance in the ratio of helper to suppressor cells is observed in acquired immune deficiency syndrome (AIDS).

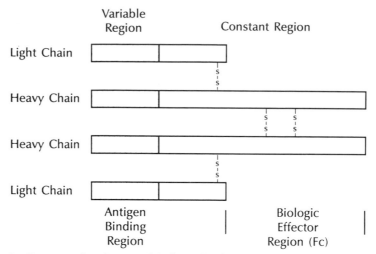

Figure 9–6. Structure of an immunoglobulin molecule.

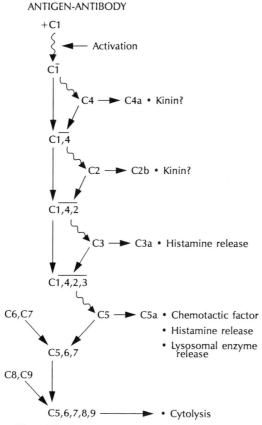

Figure 9–7. Schematic diagram of the classic complement activation cascade. (Modified from Cooper, N. R.: The complement system. In Stites, D. P.; Stobo, J. D.; Fudenberg, H. H.; and Wells, J. V. (eds.): *Basic and Clinical Immunology,* 4th ed. Lange Medical Publications, Los Altos, Calif., 1980, pp. 124–135.)

IMMUNE DYSFUNCTION

Hypersensitivity and Allergy

The function of the immune system is to recognize and eliminate agents that are harmful to the host. When the immune system is functioning properly, the foreign agents are eliminated quickly and efficiently. Occasionally, the immune system responds adversely to environmental agents, resulting in an allergic reaction. Coombs and Gell (1975) have divided allergic responses into four general categories based on the mechanism of immunologic involvement. These are summarized in Table 9–6 (for review, *see* Wells, 1982).

The type I or anaphylactic reactions are mediated by homocytotropic antibodies (IgE in man). The Fc portion of IgE antibodies can bind to receptors on mast cells and basophils. If the antibody molecule then binds antigen, pharmacologically active amines such as slow-reacting substance of anaphylaxis and histamine are released from the mediator cell (e.g., mast cell, basophil). These agents result in vasodilation, edema, and generation of an inflammatory response. The main targets of this type of reaction are the gastrointestinal tract (food allergies), the skin (urticaria and atopic dermatitis), the respiratory system (rhinitis and asthma), and the vasculature (anaphylactic shock). These responses tend to occur quickly after rechallenge with an antigen to which the individual has been sensitized and are termed immediate hypersensitivity.

The type II or cytolytic reactions are mediated by both IgG and IgM antibodies. These reactions are usually attributed to the antibody's ability to fix complement, opsonize particles, or function in an antibody-dependent cellular cytotoxicity

Table 9–6.   GELL AND COOMBS CLASSIFICATION SCHEME OF ALLERGY

CLASSIFICATION	EXAMPLES	MECHANISM
Type I Anaphylaxis or immediate hypersensitivity	Asthma, urticaria, rhinitis, atopic dermatitis	IgE bound to mast cell/basophil triggers release of soluble mediators (e.g., histamine)
Type II Cytolytic	Hemolytic anemia, Goodpasture's disease	IgG and/or IgM binds to cells and results in destruction via complement, opsonization, or ADCC
Type III Arthus	Systemic lupus erythematosus, glomerular nephritis, rheumatoid arthritis, serum sickness	Antigen-antibody complexes deposit in various tissues and may then fix complement
Type IV Delayed-type hypersensitivity	Contact dermatitis, tuberculosis	Sensitized T lymphocytes induce a DTH response

reaction. The major target is often tissues of the circulatory system including red and white blood cells and platelets. The interaction of cytolytic antibody with these cells or their progenitors results in their depletion and the production of hemolytic anemia, leukopenia, or thrombocytopenia. Additional target organs include the lungs and kidneys, as observed in Goodpasture's disease. In these type II reactions, an individual may develop antibodies to respiratory and glomerular basement membranes, resulting in glomerulonephritis and pulmonary hemorrhaging.

The type III or Arthus reactions are mainly mediated by IgG through a mechanism involving the generation of antigen-antibody complexes that subsequently fix complement. The complexes become deposited in the vascular endothelium, where a destructive inflammatory response occurs. This is contrasted to the type II reaction, where the inflammatory response is induced by antibodies directed against the tissue antigens. The main target tissues are the skin (lupus), the joints (rheumatoid arthritis), the kidneys (glomerulonephritis), the lungs (hypersensitivity pneumonitis), and the circulatory system (serum sickness). The antigens responsible for these types of reactions may be self-antigens, as is thought to occur in lupus and rheumatoid arthritis, or foreign antigens, as in serum sickness.

The type IV or delayed-hypersensitivity response is not mediated by antibodies but rather by macrophages and sensitized T lymphocytes. When sensitized T lymphocytes come in contact with the sensitizing antigen, an inflammatory reaction is generated: Lymphokines are produced, followed by an influx of granulocytes and macrophages. The target for this type of reaction can be almost any organ, the classic example being skin contact sensitivity.

Autoimmune Responses

For the immune system to function properly, it must be able to distinguish self-antigens from nonself-antigens. Occasionally, the delicate balance that prevents an individual from elaborating an immune response to self-antigens becomes perturbed, resulting in an inappropriate response to self. This phenomenon is known as autoimmunity and can be manifested by the production of antibodies to self- or modified self-antigens or by tissue destruction from T lymphocytes or macrophages (for a review of autoimmunity, see Theofilopoulos, 1982.)

Autoimmune responses can belong to any of the four Gell and Coombs classifications (see Table 9–6). There are several hypotheses to explain the pathogenesis of autoimmune responses. During embryonic development, it is thought that the immune system becomes tolerant to the tissues and antigens to which it is exposed either by eliminating those lymphocytes that react with self-antigens or by generating suppressor T cells that inhibit the production of an immune response to self-antigens. If effector cells arise that are specific for self-antigens, or specific suppressor T cells are lost or become nonfunctional, an immune response directed against self may occur, resulting in tissue destruction. Alternatively, during development of the immune system there are many sequestered self-antigens to which the immune system is not exposed and thus are not perceived as self-antigens. Some examples of these types of antigens are found in the tissue of the central nervous system, the lens of the eye, the thyroid gland, and the testes, as well as antigens such as DNA or RNA sequestered within cells. If these antigens become exposed, an autoimmune response may develop. Some examples of autoimmune diseases include systemic lupus erythematosus (SLE) (type III,

Table 9–7. EXAMPLES OF CONGENITAL IMMUNODEFICIENCY

TYPE	DEFECT	TREATMENT
Thymic hypoplasia (DiGeorge's syndrome)	T lymphocytes	Fetal thymus transplant thymosin?
Infantile X-linked agammaglobulinemia	B lymphocytes	γ-Globulin
Severe combined immunodeficiency	T and B lymphocytes	Bone marrow transplant Fetal liver transplant Fetal thymus transplant
Chronic granulomatous disease	Enzyme deficiency in granulocytes	Early and prolonged antibiotic therapy
C3 deficiency	Deficiency of C3 activator	Infusion of normal plasma

IV), rheumatoid arthritis (type III), Goodpasture's disease (type II), serum sickness (type III), and hemolytic anemia and thrombocytopenia (type II).

Autoimmune diseases are not necessarily the result of an immune response to self-components. Environmental agents may bind to tissue or serum proteins, and an immune response may be generated against these modified self-antigens, resulting in cell injury or death. Many drugs, chemicals, and metals have been implicated as causative agents in autoimmune diseases. For example, hydralazine and procainamide can induce an SLE-like syndrome, α-methyldopa and the pesticide dieldrin have been shown to cause an autoimmune-like hemolytic anemia, and metals (gold, mercury) have induced a glomerular nephritis similar to that seen in Goodpasture's disease.

Immunodeficiency

Pathogenic states of decreased immunoresponsiveness can be illustrated using examples of well-characterized, naturally occurring immunodeficiency disorders. These disorders may be subdivided according to etiology into primary and secondary deficiencies. Primary immunodeficiencies are genetic or congenitally acquired and can affect either specific or nonspecific components of the immune response. Patients with these disorders are subject to characteristic alterations in resistance to various types of infections, depending on the cell types or other lesions involved. In some instances, the study of immunodeficient patients has helped clarify many of the mechanisms involved in resistance to infectious agents. The majority of primary immunodeficiencies involve defects in either cellular or humoral immune responses, or both, subsequent to a loss of immune cell function or absence of a particular immune cell population (Table 9–7).

Secondary or acquired immunodeficiency dis-

orders are more common than primary immunodeficiencies and have varied etiologies (*see* Table 9–8). Viral infection, malnutrition, cancer, renal diseases, and aging are a few examples of potential causes of acquired immunodeficiency; however, in many instances, the underlying cause of the condition remains obscure. Acquired as well as primary immunodeficiencies can be life-threatening. Immunosuppressive drugs may also lead to immunodeficiency and are often clinically exploited for this characteristic.

Immunosuppression is of particular clinical importance in the prolongation of allograft survival and in the treatment of autoimmune disorders. In general, primary immune responses are amenable to suppression, and secondary responses are not. Drug-induced immunosuppression depends on the characteristics of the drug and the time of its administration relative to the generation of an immune response. In this regard, the immune response can be subdivided into two phases: the inductive phase, which follows antigen exposure and is characterized by

Table 9–8. CAUSATIVE AGENTS THAT MAY RESULT IN SECONDARY IMMUNODEFICIENCY

Drugs	Immunosuppressants, anticonvulsants, corticosteroids, chemotherapeutic agents
Infections	Acute viral, coccidioidomycosis, measles, tuberculosis, leprosy, HIV
Neoplasia	Acute leukemia, Hodgkin's disease, chronic leukemia, lymphosarcoma, thymoma, multiple myeloma, reticulum cell sarcoma
Autoimmune disease	Systemic lupus erythematosus, rheumatoid arthritis
Others	Aging, genetic disorders, malnutrition, radiation, nephrotic syndrome, chemical exposure

lymphoproliferation; and the productive or effector phase, characterized by antibody production and cell-mediated effector function. Most immunosuppressive agents are maximally active when administered during or just prior to the inductive phase of the immune response. An alternative classification of immunosuppressive drugs is based on their mode of action. In general, these drugs are effective because of their antiproliferative or lympholytic and lymphomodulatory actions. They usually function as general rather than specific immunosuppressants.

Many immunosuppressive drugs were originally developed as cytoreductive cancer chemotherapeutic agents because of their ability to interfere with cell growth and proliferation. Because of the high rate of proliferation in antigen-stimulated lymphocytes, these cells are sensitive to many of the same drugs as rapidly dividing tumor cells, and the use of antiproliferative drugs in transplant patients or patients with certain autoimmune diseases has become almost routine. Azathioprine is a commonly utilized antiproliferant whose active metabolite interferes with the synthesis of compounds required for cell metabolism, growth, and division. Therefore, this drug and other antiproliferatives are most effective when administered following antigen stimulation, during the inductive portion of the immune response.

Lympholytic or lymphomodulatory agents generally act by directly destroying the lymphocyte or lethally damaging its ability to undergo mitosis; thus, as immunosuppressants these agents are most successfully used when administered just prior to the introduction of antigen. Common examples include the corticosteroids, which cause massive lympholysis in some species and act primarily through modulation of lymphocyte trafficking and effector functions in other species, including man. In contrast, alkylating agents such as cyclophosphamide cross-link DNA, causing immediate cell death or cytolysis during mitosis. Since these effects are similar to radiation-induced cell injury, alkylating agents are often referred to as radiomimetic drugs. Cyclosporin A® is a relatively new immunosuppressant that appears to act by mechanisms dissimilar to those previously discussed (for review, see D. J. White, 1982). Although its mode of action is not completely understood, immunosuppression by Cyclosporin A may involve altered lymphokine release or blocking of lymphocyte membrane receptors for an interleukin (IL-2) required to stimulate lymphocyte proliferation. Its major benefit is its apparent specificity for T-helper cells and its minimal effects on other immunoresponsive cells.

Immunosuppression may also be achieved through methods other than drug administration. Common approaches involve the use of radiation, antilymphocyte serum, and antigen (e.g., allergic desensitization). Immunosuppression, as evidenced by depressed antibody-mediated immunity and/or cell-mediated immunity, has also been observed in rodents exposed to sublethal levels of several chemicals of environmental concern. Chemicals that have produced immune alterations in rodents include: 2,3,7,8-tetrachlorodibenzo-p-dioxin (TCDD); diethylstilbestrol (DES); polychlorinated biphenyls (PCBs); polybrominated biphenyls (PBBs); dimethyl vinyl chloride (DMVC); gallic acid; hexachlorobenzene (HCB); orthophenylphenol; organometals; and heavy metals. The observations that residents of Japan and China accidentally exposed to polychlorinated biphenyl exhibited immune alterations similar to those observed in rodent studies has increased concern over the effects of xenobiotic agents on suppression of the immune system (Chang *et al.*, 1980).

IMMUNOLOGIC MECHANISMS OF HOST RESISTANCE

The eradication and control of most bacterial agents that produce acute infections (e.g., *Staphylococcus, Streptococcus*) are facilitated by the production of specific antibodies. These antibodies enhance phagocytosis and killing of pathogenic microorganisms by granulocytes and macrophages through opsonization (Figure 9–8). In contrast, chronic bacterial infections are usually caused by organisms such as *Listeria monocytogenes* or *Mycobacterium tuberculosis*, which are facultative intracellular pathogens that can multiply within the phagocytic cell and thus escape antibody-mediated reactions. CMI enhances granulocyte phagocytosis or macrophage-mediated killing of such intracellular pathogens through the production of lymphokine (see Figure 9–8). Toxigenic infections, which result from the production of toxins by certain bacteria, require the production of specific antibody for toxin neutralization (e.g., tetanus toxin). CMI plays little, if any, role in managing toxigenic infections. Antibodies responsible for neutralization of bacterial toxins often prevent binding of the toxin to specific receptors, thus preventing their harmful effects.

Viral antigens expressed on the surface of infected cells may also serve as targets for cytotoxic T-lymphocyte–mediated cytolysis. CMI is also instrumental in eliminating viral infections through the production and release of the lymphokine interferon by lymphocytes. Interferon signals adjacent cells to produce an antiviral pro-

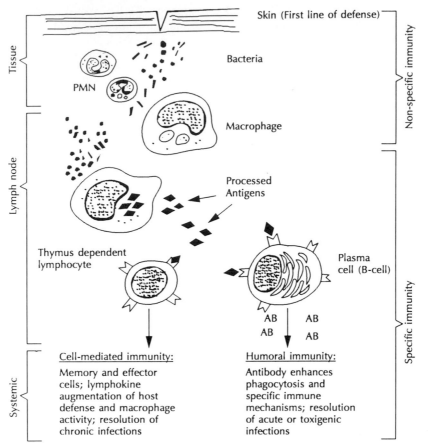

Figure 9–8. Diagrammatic representation of host resistance to bacteria indicating the roles of cell-mediated and humoral immunity.

tein that blocks virus replication. Interferon does not have direct antiviral activity but causes adjacent cells to manufacture antiviral proteins.

An increased incidence of infectious disease and neoplasia has been frequently associated with primary immunodeficiency diseases and immunosuppressive therapy. Gatti and Good (1971) observed a significant frequency of lymphoreticular neoplasia in patients with primary immunodeficiency diseases (Table 9–9) and suggested that the incidence would have been higher had not most of the patients died of bacterial or fungal infections before they developed neoplasia. Immunosuppressive therapy has been widely used to prevent rejection of transplanted organs and to treat certain autoimmune diseases, collagen-vascular diseases, and chronic inflammatory disorders. Nonspecific therapeutic depression of immunity has frequently caused serious complications with bacterial, viral, fun-

gal, and parasitic infections and, less frequently, has been associated with an increased incidence of certain malignancies. One important complication in transplant patients on immunosuppressive therapy is the inadvertent transplantation of malignant cells in an organ obtained from a cadaver or living donor suffering from cancer. Of 89 patients who received organs from donors who had been diagnosed for neoplasia within five years of donation, 42 percent of the recipients developed the transplanted neoplasia (Penn, 1978). Currently, transplantation of cancer is a rare event, as surgeons avoid using organs from donors with cancer.

A second and more important complication in immunosuppressed transplant patients has been the high frequency of *de novo* cancer. In a sampling of renal transplant patients (Table 9–9) who survived one year, 26 percent had developed cancer, whereas at ten years 47 percent

Table 9–9. EVIDENCE OF INCREASED CANCER INCIDENCE IN CONGENITALLY IMMUNODEFICIENT AND RENAL TRANSPLANT PATIENTS*

DISEASE	IMMUNE ALTERATION	% CANCER INCIDENCE	TUMOR TYPE
Congenital (Bruton's) agammaglobulinemia	B cells[†]	6 (10,000 × normal)	Acute lymphatic leukemia
Severe combined immunodeficiency	T and B cells	2	Lymphoreticular
Common variable immunodeficiency	B cells[†]	10	Lymphoreticular and carcinomas
Ataxia-telangiectasia	T cells	10	Lymphoreticular, sarcoma, and carcinomas
Renal transplant patients	T and B cells	26 (by 1 year) 47 (by 10 years)	Skin and lip cancer, non-Hodgkin's lymphoma, Kaposi's sarcoma, carcinoma of cervix

* Data from Gatti and Good (1971) and Penn (1985).
† Evidence of excessive suppressor cell activity.

were so affected (see Penn, 1985). The types of tumors observed included skin and lip cancer (21-fold increase over general population), non-Hodgkin's lymphomas (28- to 49-fold increase), and carcinomas of the cervix (14-fold increase) (Penn, 1985).

Cell-mediated immune responses are believed to be important in controlling spontaneously arising tumors and limiting the growth of established neoplasms. In this regard, an imbalance or transient dysfunction of the immune surveillance mechanism is thought to facilitate development of neoplastic disease. Most tumor cells have unique cell surface antigens that clearly distinguish them from normal cells, although immune responses to these antigens may vary considerably. In rodents, for example, chemically and virally induced tumors evoke strong anti-tumor immune responses, which may result in regression or elimination of the developing tumor, whereas spontaneously arising tumors are generally less immunogenic. The weight of the evidence, however, suggests that cell-mediated immune responses are important in recognition and destruction of arising neoplasms. Indeed, this hypothesis is the basis for the concept of immune surveillance, which views CMI as the effector mechanism for eliminating spontaneously arising neoplastic clones.

The principal methods of tumor cytolysis have been elucidated through *in vitro* studies and involve direct T-cell–mediated cytotoxicity, antibody-dependent cellular cytotoxicity (ADCC), and natural killer cell cytolysis of tumor cells. Cytotoxic T lymphocytes (CTLs) can be generated in response to specific membrane-associated antigens on tumor cells or foreign grafts. CTLs are capable of lysing the sensitizing tumor cells through direct cellular contact. *In vitro* studies with rodents have clearly shown the effector cell to be the T lymphocyte and have also demonstrated the tumor specificity of cytolysis.

In contrast, the macrophage can be considered as both an antigen-specific and nonspecific cellular mediator of tumor cytolysis. Macrophages may specifically lyse tumor targets following interactions with lymphokines or by serving as the effector cell in ADCC. In ADCC, specific antibodies to tumor membrane antigens serve to focus the effector cell on the tumor cell. Several cell types may participate as effectors of ADCC including killer (K) cells, which are lymphoid in origin but are devoid of the usual B- and T-cell surface markers, macrophages, and granulocytes. In addition, fully activated macrophages are capable of nonspecific tumoricidal activity without the requirement of an interposed antibody, through a nonphagocytic mechanism of cytolysis.

An additional subpopulation of lymphocytes with tumoricidal activity, called natural killer or NK cells, has been functionally characterized in humans and rodents (*see* reviews by Herberman and Holden, 1978; Herberman and Ortaldo, 1981). These blood cells have unique cell surface markers distinguishing them from other cytolytic effectors and are constitutively present in nonimmune animals. They are capable of spontaneously lysing tumor cells *in vitro* and respond to different immunomodulators than either T cells, B cells, or macrophages. NK cells are circulating lymphocytes whose activity may be potentiated by a variety of chemical and biologic agents including interferon and interferon inducers.

Table 9–10. SCREENING PANEL (TIER I) FOR DETECTING IMMUNE ALTERATION FOLLOWING CHEMICAL AND DRUG EXPOSURE IN RODENTS

PARAMETER	PROCEDURES PERFORMED
Immunopathology	Hematology—complete blood count and white blood cell differential Weights—body, spleen, thymus, kidney, adrenal Histology—spleen, thymus, bone marrow, lymph node, (local and distal to exposure site), adrenal Spleen and bone marrow cellularity
Cell-mediated immunity	Lymphocyte blastogenesis in response to allogeneic leukocytes (mixed leukocyte response) Natural killer cell activity
Humoral immunity	Antibody plaque-forming cell response to sheep erythrocytes (IgM) or antigen specific antibody level

THE TIER APPROACH TO ASSESSMENT OF IMMUNOLOGIC FUNCTION

Since a single immune function assay cannot be used to evaluate comprehensively deleterious effects on the immune system following exposure to chemicals or drugs, a flexible tier of sensitive *in vivo* and *in vitro* assays has been proposed to assess immunotoxicity in rodents (Dean *et al.*, 1979a) and has now been validated (Luster *et al.*, 1987). The tier approach to immunotoxicity assessment consists of a screening panel assessing three parameters (TIER I), which enables the identification of compounds that may produce immune alterations. Agents testing positive in TIER I assays can be further evaluated with assays selected from a more comprehensive panel (TIER II). TIER II assays allow

an in-depth evaluation of the underlying mechanism(s) of immunotoxicity. Since most immune function assays require a working knowledge of the complex interactions and functions of the immune system, it is recommended that a competent immunologist assist with any evaluation of immunotoxicity.

Immunocompetency assessment should include the evaluation of immunopathology, CMI function, humoral immunity, M∅ function, and host resistance. These parameters form the basis for the assays used in the TIER I screening panel (Table 9–10). If warranted by data obtained in the preliminary TIER I screen, additional immunologic tests can be selected from TIER II (Table 9–11) to examine the underlying mechanism(s) of a particular chemical or drug-induced immune alteration. If the pathophysiological mechanism responsible for the deleterious

Table 9–11. COMPREHENSIVE PANEL (TIER II) FOR FURTHER CHARACTERIZING IMMUNE ALTERATIONS FOLLOWING CHEMICAL OR DRUG EXPOSURE

PARAMETER	PROCEDURES PERFORMED
Immunopathology	Cell surface marker profile (% T, B, M∅; T-cell subsets)
Host resistance	*Listeria monocytogenes* challenge Susceptibility to transplantable syngeneic tumor (TD 10–20 of PYB6 sarcoma or B16F10 melanoma) *Streptococcus* challenge Influenza challenge
Cell-mediated immunity	Lymphokine quantitation (mitogen induced IL-2 production) Cytotoxic T-lymphocyte function Antibody-dependent cellular cytotoxicity
Humoral immunity	B-cell progenitor-cell quantitation Primary antibody response (IgM) to T-independent (LPS) antigen and secondary antibody response (IgG) to T-dependent antigen (SRBC) Mishell-Dutton assay
Macrophage function*	Quantitation of peritoneal macrophage cell number and phagocytic ability Cytolysis of tumor target cells or bactericidal activity Cytokine quantitation (IL-1)
Granulocyte function	NBT reduction or bacterial phagocytosis and killing
Bone marrow	Pluripotent stem cell quantitation Granulocyte/macrophage progenitor quantitation

* Utilizes both resident and activated peritoneal macrophages.

effect on the target cell can be defined, it may be possible to synthesize new analogues of the compound that produce the desirable effects but lack the immunoalterative effects.

The number of immunologic tests available or under development to study altered immune function is extensive. The procedures in general used to evaluate immune function following exposure to chemicals and drugs have been described in detail (Dean *et al.*, 1979a; Luster *et al.*, 1982b). Assays in TIER I represent a general immunologic screen and offer a means of assessing compounds for their immunotoxic potential. These methods in TIER I are well defined for both mice and rats and are frequently used in the clinical immunologic evaluation of humans. If the immune function data obtained from the TIER I panel are negative, there can be reasonable confidence regarding the safety of the drug or chemical for the immune system under the conditions and dosages defined in the screen. If conservative extrapolations are made using data from appropriate and clinically relevant immune function and host challenge assays, the most accurate estimate possible of chemical safety relative to the immune system will be obtained. The following is a brief description of the tests currently utilized to assess the immunomodulatory potential of a suspect agent in rodents.

Immunopathology

Lymphoid organ weight, cellularity, and histopathology are useful in initially screening the immunomodulatory potential of an environmental agent or drug in rodents. Thymic and splenic weights, which are best expressed as organ-to-body-weight ratios, may be indicators of immune dysfunction. Thymic atrophy occurs following exposure to many chemicals and appears to be a useful indicator of chemical insult to the immune system; however, thymic atrophy alone is not necessarily a specific indicator of immunosuppression since stress, severe weight loss, or general toxicity can also induce similar thymic lesions. Cellularity and histologic studies of bone marrow, spleen, and lymph nodes are also recommended. Splenic weights and cellularity may be decreased as a result of lymphoid depletion or markedly increased by extramedullary hematopoiesis since the spleen retains its hematopoietic potential during adult life. Histologic evaluation of the spleen is often helpful in determining the nature of a weight change. For example, following the introduction of an antibody-inducing antigen, there is a rapid increase in both the size and number of germinal centers. Lack of a germinal center reaction is a common finding following the administration of certain immunosuppressive drugs, chemicals, and radiation and is accompanied by a decreased ability of the animal to produce antibodies. In contrast, the induction of cell-mediated immunity by antigen results in a massive proliferation (i.e., 50- to 100-fold increase) in the cells within the paracortex of lymph nodes. Both proliferation and recruitment of new cells to the paracortex occur. The use of drugs that suppress CMI depresses this massive cellular expansion within the paracortical region.

Another potentially useful procedure in rodents is quantitation of lymphocyte subpopulations. Specific surface markers and receptors on macrophages and lymphocytes are well characterized in rodents and humans (see Table 9–3). One method for quantitating splenic leukocyte subpopulations in mice uses fluorochrome-conjugated antisera against specific cell surface antigens identifying B cells (Ig), T cells (Thy-1 and Lyt-1,2,3), and MØs (MAC-1).

Cell-Mediated Immunity

While the previously mentioned procedures allow quantitation of leukocyte populations, they do not allow an assessment of the functional capacity of these cells. Several assays are available to examine cell-mediated immunologic functions (for detailed methods, *see* Luster *et al.*, 1982b). These include both *in vivo* (e.g., delayed hypersensitivity, graft-versus-host reactions, or skin graft rejection) and *in vitro* techniques (e.g., lymphoproliferation and lymphokine production). Historically, CMI has been examined using delayed-type cutaneous hypersensitivity responses. Current approaches include measuring the *in vitro* lymphoproliferative responses to allogeneic leukocytes in mixed leukocyte cultures (MLCs). Values obtained from animals exposed to several doses of chemical are analyzed and compared with values from vehicle-treated controls.

Lymphoproliferative responses are widely used in assessing CMI. The lymphocyte proliferation assay utilizes leukocyte antigens to stimulate proliferation in selective lymphocyte populations. Proliferation is quantitated by incorporation of tritiated thymidine into lymphoblast DNA. In some instances, animals treated with immunosuppressants will exhibit depressed proliferative responses that can be seen when normal numbers of lymphocytes are present, thus indicating a failure of cell function. Studies have demonstrated that altered responsiveness may also occur through suppression by regulatory subpopulations of macrophages and T lymphocytes (Katz, 1977). Other factors may also cause depressed proliferative responses. These include chemically induced cytotoxicity of lymphocytes or accessory cells; redistribution of lymphocyte subpopulations (i.e., T, B, or null cells), and maturational defects in lymphocyte development. The lymphoproliferative assays are reliable predictors of immune alteration and are widely used in clinical medicine.

Assessment of Humoral Immunity

There are a variety of methods to quantitate immunoglobulins (Igs) and specific antibodies. A disadvantage of merely quantitating Ig levels is that the half-life of some immunoglobulins may exceed the subchronic (14-day) exposure period, thus rendering the method insensitive to change in short-term studies. However, quantitating immunoglobulin levels is an acceptable procedure for chronic dosing studies, although it may lack the predictive ability of methods that measure specific antibody responses following antigenic challenge.

Assessment of a specific immune response following challenge with a novel antigen such as sheep erythrocytes (sheep red blood cells [SRBCs]) or bovine gamma globulin has more commonly been used in immunotoxicity assessment in rodents. Antigenic challenge is usually performed following exposure to the chemical or drug. The immune response to the antigen can be quantitated either by measuring serum antibody titers or by determining the number of splenic lymphocytes producing antibody to the specific eliciting antigen. Both methods are acceptable, and the former methodology can be quantitated by hemagglutination, complement lysis, or antibody precipitin procedures. Enzyme-linked immunosorbent assays (ELISAs) and radioimmunoassay methodology provide even more sensitive methods for quantitating specific serum antibodies and, in addition, lend themselves to automation.

We prefer the method of quantitating numbers of splenic lymphocytes producing antibody to a specific eliciting antigen. In this procedure, single cell suspensions of splenocytes from animals previously exposed to sheep erythrocytes (SRBCs) are mixed with complement and SRBCs in a specialized hemocytometer. After incubation, plaques (clear areas) indicative of sheep erythrocyte lysis occur circumscribing the cells producing the specific antibody. If one adds an anti-IgG antisera to the mixtures described above, the number of cells producing IgG-type antibodies can be quantitated as well. These assays are sensitive, simple, and useful in characterizing a variety of chemical- and drug-induced lesions in the humoral immune response.

Macrophage Function Assays

Macrophages not only provide nonspecific phagocytic functions but are also specifically directed and regulated by lymphocytes through lymphokines. In addition, they are involved in cellular interactions and the elaboration of products (i.e., prostaglandins and monokines) that have feedback and regulatory roles in immune responses. Macrophage functions include phagocytosis, intracellular killing of infectious agents, antigen processing and presentation, interferon production, and cytostasis and cytolysis of virally infected or neoplastically transformed cells. Obviously, an evaluation of MØ function is essential in immune assessment. Chemical exposure may alter basal activity or the ability of MØ to respond to activation stimulants. Thus, macrophage function in chemical- or drug-exposed mice should be assessed in resident and activated macrophages. Assays quantitating phagocytosis and inhibition of tumor cell growth are preferred for TIER II analysis of MØ function. Assays defining MØ activation can be utilized to characterize impairment of MØ function further. Most of these functional tests can be readily quantitated and are described by Adams and Dean (1982).

Granulocyte Function

Granulocyte function can be assessed by measuring physiologic activities such as phagocytosis, chemotactic activity, bactericidal activity, or nitro blue tetrazolium (NBT) dye reduction. Perhaps the best single assay is the NBT dye reduction procedure, which has been extensively employed in the diagnosis of persons with chronic granulomatous disease. Failure of granulocytes to reduce NBT was found to correlate with an impaired enzymatic ability to kill phagocytosed bacteria. The number of granulocytes reducing dye can be easily quantitated histochemically. This procedure is included in the TIER II panel and can be utilized if altered bacterial resistance is observed in the presence of normal CMI, HMI, and macrophage function.

Bone Marrow Progenitors

Bone marrow hypoplasia is a significant complication of cancer chemotherapy and has also been implicated as a result of exposure to numerous drugs and environmental agents. The bone marrow contains pluripotent stem cells capable of differentiating along hematopoietic lines giving rise to lymphocytes, macrophages, or granulocytes. Chemical toxicity to progenitor cells, which ordinarily possess impressive proliferative capacity, can result in a magnification of chemically induced lesions, which may ultimately be expressed as altered host resistance. During the past decade, a variety of *in vitro* culture techniques have been developed for quantitating precursors for all the hematopoietic cell lines. Examination of colony formation by hematopoietic progenitor cells following exposure to various agents has proved to be a sensitive indicator of toxicity; therefore, bone marrow cellularity (TIER I) and progenitor cell assays (TIER II) are included as an integral part of the panels.

One method for quantitating murine pluripotent stem cells is by injecting bone marrow cells into irradiated recipients and subsequently counting the number of colonies forming in the spleen. *In vitro* assays quantitating progenitor cells are also available. Committed progenitor cells can be stimulated to form colonies in semisolid media by adding appropriate growth factors to the culture medium. Currently, clonal progenitor assays exist for quantitating B-lymphocyte, T-lymphocyte, macrophage-granulocyte, megakaryocyte, eosinophil, and erythroid precursors.

Challenge Models

A simple method for detecting immunosuppressive chemicals or drugs is to challenge the chemically exposed animal with an infectious agent. This procedure provides a general approach to determine whether the chemical interferes with host resistance to pathogens. Analysis of host susceptibility to carefully selected pathogens constitutes a holistic approach that can aid in characterizing immune dysfunctions. Challenge with *Salmonella typhimurium, Klebsiella pneumoniae, Escherichia coli, Streptococcus pneumoniae, or pyogenes,* and *Staphylococcus aureus;* with facultative intracellular organisms such as *Listeria monocytogenes* and *Candida albicans;* or with influenza or herpes virus allows assessment of humoral or cell-mediated immune resistance. Immune defense to extracellular organisms requires the interaction of T lymphocytes, B lymphocytes, and macrophages for the production of specific antibodies that may activate the complement system to aid in phagocytosis and/or lysis. Antibodies also can directly neutralize some bacteria and viruses. Resistance to intracellular organisms requires induction of CMI through T-lymphocyte and macrophage interactions, which results in the production of lymphokines and further facilitates the bactericidal activities of macrophages. A chemical- or drug-induced lesion in any of

these cells or a disruption of their activation or ability to interact with each other could result in an enhanced susceptibility to infection.

Resistance to transplantable syngeneic or semisyngeneic tumor cells is also a sensitive parameter for detecting altered host resistance following chemical exposure (Dean *et al.*, 1982). The tumor models used include PYB6 fibrosarcoma and B16F10 melanoma. Almost any tumor model in which resistance is dependent on T-cell immunity or natural cytotoxicity can be employed.

APPROACHES TO HYPERSENSITIVITY ASSESSMENT

Another consideration in immunotoxicity assessment involves evaluating the potential of chemicals and drugs to induce and elicit allergic (hypersensitivity) responses. These responses are classified into four types using a system devised by Gell and Coombs, which was described earlier in this chapter (see Table 9–6). Although examples of each type of chemical-induced hypersensitivity exist, there are two principal types of allergic responses distinguishable from each other on the basis of both mechanism and kinetics that occur most frequently in chemically hypersensitive individuals. Delayed-type (type IV) hypersensitivity is a cell-mediated (T-cell, macrophage) response, whereas immediate (type I) hypersensitivity is antibody-mediated (IgE in humans). Contact sensitivity represents an important subset of delayed-type hypersensitivity. Contact sensitizers are low-molecular-weight compounds that serve as haptens and conjugate with proteins following contact with the skin to form the allergen. Both delayed-type and immediate hypersensitivity responses require an initial exposure to an allergen to *induce* a response, followed by subsequent exposure to *elicit* clinical symptoms. Elicitation of immediate responses may occur within minutes following exposure to the allergen, whereas delayed-type responses require 24 to 48 hours following allergen exposure to develop.

Both types of hypersensitivity responses are of considerable importance from a health and safety standpoint. Immediate responses may be life-threatening in severe cases; contact hypersensitivity, although not life-threatening, is of considerable importance from an economic and occupational disease perspective. The principal laboratory animal models for predictive testing and evaluation of chemical-mediated hypersensitivity utilize the guinea pig.

For potential contact sensitizers, differences between testing methods in the guinea pig involve the use (or lack of use) of an adjuvant in conjunction with the test material, as well as variations in schedules and methods of application of the test compound. Commonly used methods are the open epicutaneous test, the Buehler occluded-patch test, and the Magnusson and Kligman guinea pig maximization test (for review of guinea pig contact sensitization testing methods, see Andersen and Maibach, 1985).

Briefly, in the open epicutaneous test, the material of interest is repeatedly applied to the skin and left uncovered during induction. Challenge with the test material is also by epicutaneous application, with the test site remaining uncovered. Allergic responses, indicated by erythema and edema at the challenge site, are scored, usually 24 to 48 hours following challenge. The Buehler occluded-patch test (Ritz and Buehler, 1980) is similar, except the test agent is applied by an occluded patch rather than by open epicutaneous application. A more rigorous method for experimentally determining the contact sensitization potential of a compound is the Magnusson and Kligman guinea pig maximization test (Magnusson and Kligman, 1969). Animals are induced with and without Freund's adjuvant, followed with further induction by occluded patch. Challenge is by topical application with occluded patch.

In contrast to predictive guinea pig tests for contact sensitizers, few laboratory animal models exist for predicting sensitizers resulting in immediate hypersensitivity responses. Two models currently being evaluated use guinea pigs as the test species and determine the sensitization potential of compounds following exposure by the respiratory tract. One model was developed for the evaluation of low-molecular-weight compounds following inhalation exposure (Karol, 1983, 1985); the other model was developed to evaluate the sensitization potential of proteinaceous compounds using an intratracheal route of exposure (McNeill et al., 1986; Ritz and Bond, 1986). In both models, following induction, guinea pigs are challenged with the test material and subsequently monitored either visually or by plethysmography for immediate respiratory responses. Serum titers of allergic antibody are also determined, usually by a passive cutaneous anaphylaxis assay.

Clinical methods for detecting chemically mediated hypersensitivity in humans commonly utilize skin testing (reviewed by Norman, 1976). Testing for immediate hypersensitivity is usually by intradermal injection of the suspect allergen or topical application of the test material on a patch of skin that is subsequently scratched or pricked through with the suspect allergen. For clinical evaluation of contact sensitivity, the test

material is applied to the skin by an occluded patch (reviewed by Hjorth, 1987; Marzulli and Maibach, 1987). Additionally, one patch test procedure, the human repeat insult patch test (HRIPT), also provides predictive data on the contact sensitization potential of chemicals in humans. By monitoring both the time course and appearance of the elicited response, these assays can be used to identify sensitized individuals and distinguish between type I and type IV allergic responses.

In addition, in humans, immediate hypersensitivity responses are mediated by IgE; thus, as an alternative to actual challenge with a suspected allergen, the individual can be evaluated for the presence of allergen-specific serum IgE antibodies in a radioallergosorbent test (RAST) (for review, see Gleich et al., 1983). In most (but not all) instances, there is a good correlation between positive RAST results, positive skin test results, and clinical symptoms of allergy (reviewed by Grammer et al., 1989).

AGENTS THAT ALTER THE IMMUNE RESPONSE

Allergy Induced by Chemicals and Metals

The problem of occupational and environmental chemical hypersensitivity is widely recognized. Industrial workers and consumers are exposed to many materials capable of inducing asthma and/or contact dermatitis. This section will provide an overview of sensitization to environmental and occupational chemical allergens followed by a discussion of some of the classes of compounds of most concern (Table 9–12).

Immunologic Lung Disease. One of the major types of hypersensitivity observed in an industrial setting is asthma. In the United States, the exact proportion of asthma cases with an occupational or environmental link is unknown. Estimates of the occurrence of occupational asthma in the adult population of Europe and the United States range from 0.2 to 6 percent (Davis et al., 1983). In the United States, 2 percent of all asthma cases are thought to be of occupational origin (Salvaggio, 1979). The Japanese have determined that 15 percent of asthma in men may be directly attributable to industrial exposure (Kobayashi, 1980). While there are no precise figures on the general incidence of occupational asthma, some data are available concerning asthma induction by industrial exposure to specific compounds (for review, see Luster and Dean, 1982; Chan-Yeung and Lam, 1986). For example, 5 to 10 percent of workers exposed to the chemical toluene diisocyanate (TDI) reportedly develop asthma. Studies among bakers

Table 9–12. EXAMPLES OF AGENTS THAT INDUCE ALLERGIC REACTIONS

COMPOUND	EXPOSURE	TYPE OF REACTION	REFERENCE
Formaldehyde	Disinfectants, cosmetics, deodorants, paper, dyes, photography, textiles, inks, wood products, resins	Type IV	Maibach, 1983
Phthalic anhydrides	Saccharin production	Type I	Bernstein et al., 1982
B. subtilis	Detergents	Type I	Luster and Dean, 1982
Pesticides	Food, exterminators, farm workers	Type I, IV	Ercegovich, 1973 P. T. Thomas et al., 1990a
Ethylenediamine	Plastic industry	Type I	Popa et al., 1969
Food additives (azodyes, BHT, BHA)	Ingestion of processed foods	Type I	Juhlin, 1980
Antimicrobials (e.g., parabene, EDTA, mercurials)	Cosmetics, shampoos, creams, lotions	Type IV	Schorr, 1971; Baer et al., 1973
Resins and plasticizers (toluene diisocyanate, trimellitic anhydride)	Plastics, glues, nail lacquers, wood products, resins	Type I, IV	Patterson et al., 1982 Bernstein et al., 1982
Platinum compounds	Metal refining	Type I	Luster and Dean, 1982
Nickel	Jewelry, garment fasteners	Type I, IV	Baer et al., 1973 Wahlberg, 1976
Chromium	Leather products, printing	Type IV	Peltonen and Fräki, 1980
Gold, mercury	Medicinal treatments, photography	Type II, III, IV	Druet et al., 1982 Baer et al., 1973
Beryllium	Manufacture of alloys	Type I, IV	Reeves and Preuss, 1985
Drugs (penicillin, quinidine, tetracycline)	Medicinal treatments	Type I, II, III, or IV	de Weck, 1978 Van Arsdel, 1981 Parker, 1982

in West Germany indicate approximately 20 percent develop allergic symptoms including rhinitis and asthma following exposure to flour. In addition, it has been found that direct industrial exposure in the workplace does not always appear to be necessary for development of allergic responses to some of these agents. Living near an industrial source of certain of these compounds may result in sufficient exposure to develop "bystander" allergy (e.g., castor bean allergy reported in individuals living near an industrial source of castor bean dust; Figley and Elrod, 1928; Small, 1952). Inhalation of certain chemicals may produce symptoms of disease that mimic immunological syndromes (Table 9–13) but are not immunologically mediated. Some chemicals produce a pseudoallergic reaction, which resembles immediate hypersensitivity including secretion of inflammatory mediators, although demonstrable antibody is not detectable. Irritation of mucosal surfaces may stimulate protective responses (e.g., sneezing, coughing, and tearing) that appear superficially to be immunological in nature but are related to the stimulation of epithelial irritant receptors by chemicals. This category of disease is common

with inhaled toxicants and may coexist with immunological syndromes.

Allergic Contact Dermatitis. Allergic contact dermatitis is another major type of allergic response that can occur following exposure to some occupational and environmental agents. It is a type IV response mediated by sensitized T lymphocytes and may result in rash, swelling, itching, and possibly blistering of the skin. A variety of substances may cause allergic contact dermatitis including poison ivy, drugs, cosmetics, certain metals, (e.g. nickel, chromium), and many chemicals (Table 9–13). In allergic contact dermatitis, sensitization can occur as early as seven to ten days following the initial exposure to the agent but more often develops over several years of continued low-level exposure. Once sensitized, contact with the offending agent will produce symptoms within 24 to 48 hours. Patch tests (see above) are the preferred method for diagnosing the specific causative agent(s).

Chemicals That Are Allergenic. *Plastics and Resins.* A common criterion of most agents inducing contact hypersensitivity is a low molecular weight, usually less than 500 to 1000

Table 9–13.   CLASSIFICATION SCHEME FOR ENVIRONMENTALLY PROVOKED ALLERGIES*

CLASSIFICATION	SYMPTOMS	MECHANISM	CHEMICAL AGENTS
Immediate (type I) hypersensitivity	Bronchial asthma, asthmatic bronchitis, urticaria, rhinitis, atopy	Reaginic cytotropic antibody bound to mast cell/basophil triggers release of soluble vasoactive amines (e.g., histamine)	Amino ethanolamine, beryllium, chloramine, copper-ammonia solutions, ethylenediamine, enzymes (subtilisin), ethylene oxide, formaldehyde, isocyanates (toluene, diphenylmethane, hexamethylene, diisocyanate), platinum salts, nickel salts, phthalic anhydrides, trimellitic anhydrides
Cytolytic (type II) hypersensitivity	Chemically induced hemolytic anemia, bone marrow depression, thrombocytopenia	Homocytotropic IgG or IgM binds to cells or haptenated cell constituents and results in destruction via complement, opsonization, or ADCC by lymphocytes, macrophages	Trimellitic anhydride, mercury
Arthus-immune complex (type III) hypersensitivity	Hypersensitivity pneumonitis, rheumatoid disease, sarcoidosis, vasculitis	Antigen-antibody complexes deposit in target tissues; complement-mediated damage	Trimellitic anhydride, mercury
Cell-mediated (type IV) hypersensitivity	Contact dermatitis, sarcoidosis, anergy, delayed hypersensitivity	Sensitized T lymphocytes induce a cell-mediated response after latent period	Beryllium, bismarck brown, butesin picrate, chromium, dichlorophene, ethylenediamine, formaldehyde, isocyanates, mercury bichloride, mercaptobenzothiazole, potassium dichromate, paraphenylenediamine, phthalic anhydride, trimellitic anhydride
Immunosuppression	Altered immune responses and host resistance following inhalation exposure	Direct injury to BALT cells or systemic effects due to immune dysregulation or extension of local effects	Asbestos, silica, metals, particles, oxidant gases, tobacco smoke, benzene, toluene
Irritancy or nonimmunological	Pseudoallergic symptoms of bronchial asthma and asthmatic bronchitis	Sensory irritancy, toxic injury; may involve direct stimulation of sensory receptors	Formaldehyde, trimellitic isocyanates, ethylenediamine, paraphenylenediamine

* Modified from review by Thurmond, L. M., and Dean, J. H.: Immunological exposure to chemical hazards. In Gardner, E. E.; Crapo, J. D.; and Massaro, E. J. (eds.): *Toxicology of the Lung*. Raven Press, New York, 1988, pp. 375–406.

MW. In most cases, the offending agent is not sufficient to induce the allergic reaction itself but must be conjugated to a protein (haptenization) to induce sensitization. Certain anhydrides (e.g., trimellitic anhydride) sensitize in this manner. Presumably, the sensitizing agent conjugates with self-proteins *in vivo,* and this antigenic complex results in the generation of an allergic immune response. Some chemicals may induce contact hypersensitivity only after interacting with sunlight (i.e., photoallergy). This topic has been recently reviewed by Epstein (1987). In photo-induced allergies, the immune response is thought to be directed against antigens that arise after the chemical, one of its metabolites, or an altered host molecule absorbs light energy. The prototype photoallergic chemical is tetrachlorosalicylanilide, an antibacterial agent once used in soaps.

Anhydrides. TRIMELLITIC ANHYDRIDE. Trimellitic anhydride (TMA) is widely used in the manufacture of plastics, epoxy resins, and paints. A number of clinical syndromes that encompass three different types of hypersensitivity are now recognized as being induced by the inhalation of TMA dust or fumes. The most common syndrome is an immediate type (type I) airway response (TMA-asthma) that requires a latent period of exposure for sensitization, with an immediate onset of symptoms after subsequent exposures. The syndrome has been found to be mediated by IgE antibodies directed against TMA human serum albumin conjugates. Studies by Patterson and coworkers (1982) have demonstrated that workers exposed during the manufacture of TMA may have IgM and IgG antibodies to TMA conjugated with human serum albumin (TMA-HSA) in addition to IgE antibodies. Antibodies of the IgE class directed against TMA are predictive of the development of immunologically mediated respiratory illness and can be used to monitor workers for removal from TMA exposure. The monitoring of reaginic antibodies to TMA-HSA has been used to identify asymptomatic workers who may be at future risk and in defining the degree of sensitization of the work force.

A syndrome tentatively associated with TMA exposure, termed pulmonary disease–anemia syndrome, is characterized by anemia, hemoptysis, dyspnea, pulmonary infiltrates, and restrictive lung disease (*see* review by Patterson *et al.*, 1982). This syndrome, although rarer than type I hypersensitivity, can occur after high-dose exposure to TMA fumes (e.g., following heating of metal surfaces sprayed with materials containing TMA for corrosion resistance). High titers of IgG, IgA, and IgM antibody to TMA-protein complex and TMA-erythrocytes have been identified in these patients and also in monkeys experimentally exposed to TMA.

Inhalation exposure to TMA as well as certain other chemicals (e.g., TDI, organic gold, or mercury compounds) may also result in an apparent type III hypersensitivity response expressed as hypersensitivity pneumonitis (Patterson *et al.*, 1982). The clinical syndrome occurring in some individuals 4 to 12 hours following occupational TMA exposure is sometimes referred to as TMA flu and is characterized by cough, mucus production, wheezing, dyspnea, malaise, chills, myalgia, and arthralgia. This syndrome resembles hypersensitivity pneumonitis, has a similar latent period of exposure before onset, and is accompanied by high levels of serum immunoglobulins directed against TMA-serum conjugates.

In addition, lymphocytes from TMA-exposed workers proliferate *in vitro* in response to TMA–

human serum albumin. This delayed-type hypersensitivity response (type IV) may occur simultaneously with late respiratory systemic syndrome (type III hypersensitivity) or anemia (type II hypersensitivity).

Isocyanates. TOLUENE DIISOCYANATE.
Toluene diisocyanate (TDI) is the most common, commercially used member of the highly reactive isocyanates. Occupations with potential risk of isocyanate exposure include diisocyanate workers, polyurethane foam makers, upholstery workers, spray painters, wire coating workers, plastic foam makers, plastic molders, and rubber workers. Both immunological and nonimmunological mechanisms appear to be operative in isocyanate-induced asthma (see review by Bernstein *et al.*, 1982).

TDI is highly reactive with amino groups and can readily haptenate self-proteins and produce allergic reactions. Both asthma and contact dermatitis have been demonstrated in workers exposed to TDI. In addition, allergic antibodies specific for isocyanates have been identified in exposed workers through radioallergosorbent testing (see review by Thurmond and Dean, 1988). TDI sensitization following both dermal and inhalation exposure has also been demonstrated in guinea pigs (Karol *et al.*, 1980). Guinea pig sensitization to TDI was dependent on exposure to a threshold concentration of TDI vapor for the induction of pulmonary sensitivity and reaginic antibody production. When animals were exposed to the same total amount of TDI as those developing hypersensitivity responses, but at a lower level for a longer period of time, no allergic responses were noted (Karol, 1983). This was consistent with human data where workers exposed to high levels of TDI (i.e., spills or splashes) developed a pulmonary response, whereas workers exposed to continuous low levels of TDI remained free from TDI-induced allergic reactions. Inhalation exposure did not appear to be mandatory for the induction of pulmonary hypersensitivity, since dermal exposure sensitized guinea pigs such that subsequent inhalation of TDI resulted in a pulmonary response (Karol *et al.*, 1981). Recent work (reviewed by Karol, 1988) supports the continued utility of the guinea pig as a model for isocyanate-induced hypersensitivity.

With most allergens, removal of the offending agent abrogates the allergic response. Interestingly, patients with TDI-induced asthma may continue to be symptomatic for months and even years after cessation of TDI exposure. The reason for this is unknown, but it is thought that TDI may cause the airways to become hyperreactive to many agents such as smoke and other air pollutants. This response may be due to a nonimmunologic condition known as reactive airways dysfunction syndrome (RADS), which can occur following exposure to toxic levels of highly irritating compounds (Brooks *et al.*, 1985). In addition, some individuals susceptible to TDI-induced asthma develop cross-reactivity to other diisocyanates (e.g., diphenylmethane diisocyanate) to which they have never been exposed.

Metals and Metal Salts. Metals have also been implicated in many hypersensitivity responses. Some individuals exposed to nickel in costume jewelry and metal garment fasteners have developed contact hypersensitivity to these compounds. It has been estimated that 5 percent of all eczema can be linked to contact with nickel-containing compounds. Other metals known to cause hypersensitivity responses include platinum, chromium (from the tanning of leather products and from the printing industry), mercury, and gold (usually from the medicinal use of gold salts). This subject has been reviewed by IARC (1981) and Chan-Yeung and Lam (1986).

PLATINUM SALTS. Sensitivity to inhaled complexes of platinum is encountered in some workers involved in platinum refining processes and usually manifests itself in rhinitis, conjunctivitis, and asthma. Conjugates of platinum salts with human serum albumin were found to give positive reactions by intracutaneous testing in passive transfer testing, in skin prick tests, and in RAST testing, which has demonstrated IgE antibodies specific to platinum chloride complexes in sensitized workers (Cromwell *et al.*, 1979).

BERYLLIUM. Beryllium was previously used to coat fluorescent lamps, which led to skin sensitization when shards of broken lamps became embedded under the skin. This use of beryllium has since been discontinued. Another reaction associated with beryllium exposure thought to involve immune hypersensitivity is the chronic pulmonary syndrome berylliosis. This disease is frequently fatal and involves cough, chest pain, and a chronic progressive pneumonitis. Berylliosis is an immune reaction to beryllium compounds and is expressed as granulomatous hypersensitivity resulting from small-crystalline beryllium oxide formed through atmospheric oxidation or *in situ* through the aging of beryllium hydroxide particles in buffered tissues. The proximate antigen is a protein conjugate. The cellular responses involved include phagocytosis by macrophages, leading to swelling and rupture of the lysosomes; the process is accompanied by the development of delayed cutaneous hypersensitivity as measured by a patch test, lymphocyte blastogenesis, and macrophage migration inhibition to beryllium oxide–protein conjugates. Sarcoidosis has been suggested to result from inhalation exposure to beryllium and causes bilateral hilar lymphadenopathy. Eventually, progressive pulmonary fibrosis develops and may extend to other organ systems (for review, see Reeves and Preuss, 1985).

Pesticides. Pesticides have been implicated as both immediate and contact sensitizers in laboratory animals and humans (reviewed by P. T. Thomas *et al.*, 1990a). Clinical symptoms consistent with pesticide-induced immediate hypersensitivity (e.g., rhinitis, asthma) have been reported in humans; however, it has been difficult to demonstrate allergic antibodies to pesticides in symptomatic individuals. Studies in laboratory animals also suggest some pesticides may act as immediate sensitizers, since conjugates of malathion or 2,4-dichlorophenoxyacetic acid have been demonstrated to induce allergic antibody production in mice following intraperitoneal exposure to the pesticide (Cushman and Street, 1982, 1983).

Considerable evidence exists associating certain pesticides with contact sensitivity. Although the overall incidence of confirmed cases of contact sensitization as a result of pesticide exposure is low, both laboratory animal and human data confirm the sensitization potential of some pesticides. Examples of pesticides characterized as being weak to extreme contact sensitizers can be identified, although human and laboratory animal data do not always agree along these lines. The pesticides malathion, captan, benomyl, maneb, and naleb have been reported as being strong to extreme sensitizers based on guinea pig maximization tests, although some tests in humans as well as the reported incidence of human sensitization to these pesticides as a result of occupational use might suggest otherwise (P. T. Thomas *et al.*, 1990a).

Cosmetics. Antimicrobials used in cosmetics comprise a group of chemicals that may result in hypersensitivity. These chemicals include paraben esters, sorbic acid, phenolics (e.g., hexachlorophene), organic mercurials, quaternary ammonium compounds, ethylenediamine tetraacetate (EDTA), and formaldehyde (for review, see Schorr, 1971). Cosmetics are topically applied; thus, the major type of hypersensitivity response observed is a contact dermatitis.

Textile Finishes. Another class of chemicals that has been demonstrated to induce allergy is the resin finishes used in the textile industry to improve the wrinkle resistance and durability of fabrics. Probably the most prevalent and best studied compound in this field has been formaldehyde, which has been implicated as both a contact and respiratory allergen. This highly reactive, low-molecular-weight compound is extremely soluble in water and haptenates human proteins quite easily (Maibach, 1983). When formaldehyde resins were first used in the garment industry to provide wrinkle-resistant finishes, many workers developed allergic reactions due to the free formaldehyde. Fabrics are now allowed time to "off-gas" the free formaldehyde or are washed prior to being used.

Sensitization with formaldehyde can induce type IV (contact dermatitis) reactions. In addition, occupational exposure to formaldehyde has been associated with the occurrence of asthma in certain instances, although it has been difficult to demonstrate allergic antibodies to formaldehyde in symptomatic individuals (Hendrick, et al., 1982). Those who are sensitive to formaldehyde may have difficulty avoiding formaldehyde exposure. There have been reports of individuals so sensitive that they will react to formaldehyde found in newsprint dyes (free formaldehyde of 0.02 percent) and photographic films and papers. When one considers the ubiquitous nature of formaldehyde and its increasing usage in everyday products (furniture, auto upholstery, cosmetics, resins), the magnitude of the problem becomes apparent (for review, see Cronin, 1980).

Other Chemicals. SILICA. Silicosis is a chronic fibrosing lung disease inititated by prolonged and extensive exposure to respirable free silica (uncombined forms of silicon dioxide). The disease is observed most frequently in individuals employed in mining, sandblasting, foundry work, and abrasive processing industries, where approximately one-half the workers may be at risk because of unrecognized dust hazards. Symptoms and pulmonary X-ray changes may require decades for development, or accelerated development of symptoms may occur within months to a few years after short-term acute exposures to silica. A substantial number of studies support an adjuvant effect of silica on specific antibody responses that may reflect B-lymphocyte hyperreactivity or an effect mediated through macrophage activation. The B-lymphocyte hyperreactivity seen in rodent studies has not been demonstrated in human clinical epidemiological studies. Although an abundance of antibody and cellular immunological abnormalities have been associated with silica exposure, the role of these changes in disease pathogenesis is uncertain at present (for review, see Stankus and Salvaggio, 1985).

Subtilisin. Inhalation exposure to subtilisin—a proteolytic enzyme produced by *Bacillus subtilis* and used in enzyme-fortified detergents—causes sensitization of guinea pigs and severe immediate hypersensitivity reactions on subsequent challenge (Karol et al., 1985). As many as 2 percent of workers exposed to this protein similarly exhibited hypersensitivity reactions (Luster and Dean, 1982). Antibody production to the enzyme in cynomolgus monkeys exposed to enzyme-detergent combinations was potentiated by the presence of detergent, which may suggest that irritants may contribute to development of the response.

Autoimmunity Induced by Chemicals and Metals

Autoimmune diseases are disorders of immune regulation involving autoreactive T cells and/or B cells producing autoreactive antibodies. These autoreactive cells and antibodies respond to "self" components in a manner that results in adverse tissue responses. Immune mechanisms mediating autoimmune responses and autoimmune disease can be classified according to the Gell and Coombs scheme (see earlier discussion). True autoimmune disease is of a multifactorial etiology. Age, nutritional status, environment, and importantly, genetic background are among those factors that may predispose to the development of autoimmune disease. As a result, animal models have been difficult to develop in this area of study. Consequently, the data base concerning chemically mediated autoimmunity is limited.

Many reports exist describing responses to chemicals and, in particular, drugs that result in autoimmune-like symptoms or exacerbate existing autoimmune disease (reviewed by Bigazzi, 1988; Kammuller et al., 1989). The classes of chemicals capable of causing these responses in predisposed individuals are diverse; however, quite often they are low-molecular-weight compounds that may conjugate with proteins. In the case of chemically mediated autoimmune responses, removal of the offending chemical usually abrogates the symptoms. In this regard, many chemical and drug-related autoimmune responses are similar to allergic responses to low-molecular-weight sensitizers. The different targets of toxicity observed between those agents resulting in sensitization and those resulting in autoimmune responses may result, in part, from the different routes of exposure to the chemicals.

Occupational exposure of humans to certain chemicals has been associated with occasional reports of autoimmune responses (for review, see Gleichmann et al., 1989, Kammuller et al., 1989). For example, an individual who had been exposed to the pesticide dieldrin reportedly developed immune hemolytic anemia (Hamilton et al., 1978). When blood from this person was analyzed, it was found to contain anti-dieldrin antibodies bound to the red blood cells (RBCs). Presumably, this subsequently led to the autoimmune destruction of the RBCs (Hamilton *et al.*, 1978).

Instances of workers exposed to such diverse agents as monomeric vinyl chloride, quartz, trichloroethylene, perchloroethylene, and epoxy resins have been associated with the occurrence of autoimmune scleroderma-like lesions. Similarly, a syndrome consistent with the autoimmune disease systemic lupus erythematosus has been observed in certain individuals exposed to hydrazine.

Heavy metals have often been implicated in autoimmune processes that may be classified as type II or type IV responses. For example, gold salts and mercury-containing compounds can induce an immune complex glomerulonephritis (Druet *et al.*, 1982), or they may induce antiglomerular basement membrane antibodies resulting in glomerulonephritis similar to that seen in Goodpasture's disease. The mechanism by which heavy metals produce autoimmune responses is unknown. One hypothesis views metals as haptens, whereas another hypothesis suggests that metals alter the antigenicity of cellular proteins, rendering them "foreign" to the host. However, in mercury-induced glomerulonephritis in rabbits and gold salt–induced glomerulonephritis in humans, metals have not been observed localized at the site of the lesion (Druet *et al.*, 1982). These observations have led to a third hypothesis, which suggests metals may interfere with immune regulatory cells, resulting in the generation of an anti-self response. There is experimental evidence supporting the latter hypothesis. Weening *et al.* (1981) found that mercury was able to significantly inhibit the generation of suppressor T lymphocytes in PVG/c rats. It is plausible that metals may decrease the suppressor T-lymphocyte balance necessary for preventing the formation of anti-self antibodies, thus leading to autoimmunity.

Associations between chemical exposure and subsequent autoimmune responses occurring in large human populations have also been made. Perhaps the best-studied example is the Spanish toxic oil syndrome, which, in its acute phase, affected approximately 20,000 people. This epidemic outbreak of individuals suffering from allergic and autoimmune symptoms was reported in Spain in 1981 (reviewed by Kammuller *et al.*, 1988). The toxicological responses observed were linked to consumption of aniline-adulterated rapeseed oil. It has been speculated that formation of hydantoin-related compounds in the adulterated oil may have played a role in the resultant autoimmune responses. The toxic oil syndrome has been linked to over 350 deaths.

Allergy and Autoimmunity Induced by Drugs

Clinically, it is difficult to distinguish between immunologic and nonimmunologic reactions to drugs. In clinical diagnosis of drug or chemical allergy, certain guidelines strongly suggest an immunologic basis for an adverse drug reaction. These have been summarized by de Weck (1978) as follows: The reaction should (1) not resemble the pharmacologic reaction of the drug; (2) be elicited by minute amounts of the drug; (3) occur only after an induction period of at least five to seven days following primary exposure to the drug; (4) include symptoms classic for allergic reactions to natural macromolecular antigens (e.g., anaphylaxis, urticaria, serum sickness syndrome, asthma); (5) reappear promptly on readministration of the drug in small amounts; and (6) be reproduced by drugs possessing similar and cross-reacting chemical structure. Immunologic testing can in some instances verify the existence of drug hypersensitivity through the detection of antibodies or sensitized lymphocytes specific for the suspected allergen. More commonly, however, the immunologic basis for the reactivity is difficult to establish since an appropriate test antigen or reactive metabolite may be difficult to identify.

Penicillin. The β-lactam antibiotics (penicillin, semisynthetic penicillin, and cephalosporins) share a common molecular structure and are responsible for the majority of allergic reactions to drugs (for reviews, see de Weck, 1978; Ahlstedt *et al.*, 1980). Penicillin allergy has been studied in detail, and much of our current knowledge on the induction and elicitation of drug hypersensitivity has been based on results obtained from studies of penicillin hypersensitivity.

There is a high frequency of anaphylactic reactions in patients demonstrating adverse reactions to penicillin, although these individuals do not usually have detectable serum antibody titers to penicillin itself. Instead, it appears that the biotransformation product of penicillin (e.g., the penicilloyl group) is capable of combining with self-proteins, which then act as effective inducers of an antibody response (Parker, 1982). Penicillin, itself, does not appear to be sufficiently immunogenic to elicit a response. Alternatively, commercially prepared penicillin solutions may contain high-molecular-weight contaminants that could serve as carriers for penicillin antigens, thereby increasing the immunogenicity of penicillin (Ahlstedt *et al.*, 1980). Additional sources of carrier molecules might include the gastrointestinal contents, bacteria or bacterial products, and autologous proteins. Route of administration also appears to be an important consideration in development of penicillin allergy. There is, for example, a higher frequency of allergic reaction following intramuscular compared with oral administration (Ahlstedt et al., 1980; Van Arsdel, 1981).

Penicillin allergy can be of either the immediate or delayed type (Saxon et al., 1987). Of these, the immediate type, particularly those involving anaphylaxis, can be life-threatening. Penicillin hypersensitivity is the most frequent cause of anaphylaxis in man. Therefore, it is of clinical importance to be able to identify those patients at risk for possible adverse reactions to penicillin. Usually a patient's history concerning drug allergy provides the major basis for this assessment; however skin testing and, more recently, radioallergosorbent tests (RASTs) and enzyme-linked immunosorbent assays (ELISAs) measuring serum IgE to penicilloyl-polylysine, penicillin, and penicilloic acid have been used to identify individuals at risk (Ahlstedt et al., 1980; Parker, 1982). In addition to anaphylaxis, penicillin and other β-lactams have been implicated in the clinical incidence of several types of hypersensitivity reactions including serum sickness, urticaria, allergic fever, hemolytic anemia, rashes, allergic contact dermatitis, and possible renal disease. Penicillin may, in fact, produce nephropathy in renal tubules suggestive of a drug-induced autoimmune reaction in which autoantibodies to tubular epithelial basement membranes can be demonstrated (Border et al., 1974; Parker, 1982).

Methyldopa. Methyldopa is extensively used in the treatment of essential hypertension. Allergic reactions may occur in patients receiving methyldopa over extended periods. Perhaps the most serious of these are a number of reported cases of hemolytic anemia. This drug-induced autoimmune reaction usually regresses upon discontinuation of the drug (Van Arsdel, 1981; Parker, 1982). In contrast to penicillin-induced hemolytic anemia, where penicillin acts as a hapten, methyldopa is not haptenic (Parker, 1982) but appears instead to modify erythrocyte surface antigens. IgG against modified erythrocyte surface antigens can be demonstrated in the blood of these patients. Although this autoantibody response is present in only about 1 percent of patients receiving chronic high dosages of methyldopa, other indications of immune reactivity have been more prevalent, in particular the development of positive direct antiglobulin Coombs reactivity. There have also been reports of positive tests for lupus and

rheumatoid factor (Parker, 1982) in patients receiving methyldopa.

Analgesics. Intolerance to analgesics is common in patients with bronchial asthma, nasal polyps, and urticaria (see review by Szczeklik, 1986). Symptoms of intolerance resemble those of allergy (e.g., pseudoallergy), but the events precipitating them can rarely be traced to reactions between the drug and a specific antibody or sensitized T lymphocytes (de Weck, 1978). Aspirin and several other analgesics provoke asthmatic attacks in 8 to 20 percent of adult asthmatics, probably through inhibition of the cyclooxygenase oxidative pathway for prostaglandin synthesis (Flower et al., 1980). The weight of the evidence clearly indicates a nonimmunological basis for aspirin intolerance since molecularly unrelated drugs produce responses similar to aspirin in aspirin-sensitive individuals, whereas molecularly similar drugs (e.g., sodium salicylate) do not (Settipane, 1981).

Immunosuppression

Benzene. Benzene exposure has frequently been associated with myelotoxicity expressed as leukopenia, pancytopenia, anemia, aplastic or hypoplastic bone marrow, lymphocytopenia, granulocytopenia, and thrombocytopenia (see review in IARC, 1982). In workers occupationally exposed to benzene, a strong correlation was noted between the most frequently cited symptom, lymphocytopenia, and abnormal immunologic parameters. Benzene exposure in rabbits, rats, and mice resulted in anemia, hypoplastic bone marrow, and dose-related lymphocytopenia. Myelotoxicity also correlated with the appearance of benzene metabolites in the bone marrow, and it is now evident that bone marrow can metabolize benzene (see review, IARC, 1982). Recent studies by Wierda and associates (King et al., 1987) suggest that benzene myelotoxicity may be due, in part, to altered differentiation of marrow lymphoid cells, since acute exposure of IgM^+ cell depleted marrow cell cultures to hydroquinone, an oxidative metabolite of benzene, blocked the final maturation stages of B-cell differentiation.

Studies in benzene-exposed rabbits have described increased susceptibility to tuberculosis and pneumonia as well as a reduced antibody response to bacterial antigens (IARC, 1982). Wierda et al. (1981) observed that exposure of C57B16 mice to benzene inhibited both antibody production and the mitogenic response of lymphocytes. Likewise, chronic inhalation exposure in rodents to as low as 30 ppm benzene resulted in impaired host resistance to Listeria monocytogenes (Rosenthal and Snyder, 1985). Thus, the altered immune parameters reported in experimental animals may explain why the terminal event in severe benzene toxicity is often an acute, overwhelming infection.

Evaluation of a large number of workers exposed to benzene revealed depressed levels of serum complement, IgG, and IgA but not IgM. Thus, benzene appears to be an immunotoxicant for humans, although the magnitude of this effect and the exposure threshold for immunotoxicity remain to be established.

Halogenated Aromatic Hydrocarbons. There is substantial evidence that a number of isomers of polyhalogenated aromatics are carcinogenic, teratogenic, neurotoxic, and immunotoxic (see review, Kimbrough, 1980). Both mixtures and individual isomers of halogenated aromatic hydrocarbons have been studied, and their immunologic effects are summarized in Table 9–14 and described in the following sections.

Polychlorinated Biphenyls. Polychlorinated biphenyls (PCBs) have been used for over a half-century in plasticizers and other industrial applications and as a heat transfer medium in transformers. PCB mixtures have been reported to suppress immune responses and alter host defense mechanisms (reviewed by Kerkvliet, 1984). The most common findings in laboratory animals exposed orally or cutaneously to sublethal levels of various PCB mixtures (e.g., Aroclors®) have been severe atrophy of primary and secondary lymphoid organs, lower circulating immunoglobulin levels, and decreased specific antibody responses following immunization with antigens (Loose *et al.*, 1978; P. J. Thomas and Hinsdill, 1978; Vos *et al.*, 1980).

Effects of PCBs on CMI are inconclusive; both augmentation and suppression have been reported. Perinatal and adult exposure to PCBs have been found to depress delayed-type cutaneous hypersensitivity (DTH) (P. T. Thomas and Hinsdill, 1980). However, graft-versus-host reactivity, T-lymphocyte responses to mitogens, and proliferation of leukocytes in mixed leukocyte cultures (Silkworth and Loose, 1978, 1979) have been enhanced after PCB exposure. The augmentation of selected CMI assays may reflect a relative increase in T-cell numbers due to selective depletion of B cells or, alternatively, alterations in immunoregulation through alteration of the helper/suppressor cell balance. A recent study in adult rhesus monkeys would support PCB-mediated changes in T-helper/T-suppressor cell balance and possibly immunoregulation. Oral exposure of monkeys to 80 g/kg of a PCB mixture (Aroclor 1254®) for 23 months resulted in a significantly lower T_H/T_S ratio based on both a decrease in T-helper cells and an increase in T-suppressor cells. A concomitant suppression of antigen-specific serum IgM and IgG antibodies following immunization with the T-dependent antigen, sheep red blood cells, was also observed in PCB-treated monkeys.

Studies in which PCB-exposed animals were challenged with infectious agents have indicated decreased resistance in ducks to hepatitis virus

Table 9–14.　EFFECT OF POLYHALOGENATED AROMATIC HYDROCARBONS ON HOST RESISTANCE AND IMMUNE FUNCTIONS IN RODENTS*

PARAMETER	CHEMICAL			
	PCB	*PBB*	*TCDD*	*TCDF*
Host resistance to challenge with				
Bacteria	D	NE	D	—
Endotoxin	D	NE	D	—
Virus	D	—	D	—
Parasite	D	NE	—	—
Tumor cells	D	—	D	—
Cell-mediated immunity				
DTH	D	—	D	D
Lymphocyte proliferation	I	D	D	D
Humoral immunity				
PFCs (T-dependent antigen)	D	D	D	—
Antibody titer or Ig levels	D	D	D	—
Macrophage function	—	NE	NE	—

* Modified from Dean, J. H.; Luster, M. I.; Boorman, G. A.; Luebke, R. W.; and Lauer, L. D.: Application of tumor, bacterial, and parasite susceptibility assays to study immune alterations induced by environmental chemicals. *Environ. Health Perspect.*, **43**:81–88, 1982.
I = increased; D = decreased; NE = no effect; — = not done; PBB = polybrominated biphenyls; PCB = polychlorinated biphenyls; TCDD = 2,3,7,8-tetrachlorodibenzo-*p*-dioxin; TCDF = tetrachlorodibenzofuran.

and in mice to challenge with herpes simplex virus, ectromelia virus, *Plasmodium berghei, Listeria monocytogenes,* or *Salmonella typhimurium* (see review, Dean *et al.*, 1985). The effect of PCB on tumor resistance in rodents is unclear since both augmentation and suppression have been reported (Kerkvliet and Kimeldorf, 1977; Lubet *et al.*, 1986).

Human exposure to PCB has been reported in Japan and China where PCB-contaminated rice oil was consumed. In Japan (Yusho accident), PCB-exposed individuals exhibited chloracne and were more susceptible to respiratory infections (Shigematsu *et al.*, 1978). Decreased serum Ig levels were also observed. In clinical studies of individuals exposed to PCB-contaminated rice oil in China (Chang *et al.*, 1980; Lee and Chang, 1985), decreased DTH responses to *Streptococcus* antigens, decreased serum IgM and IgA levels, and altered T-cell numbers and functions were observed. In addition, mean percentages of PMNs and monocytes bearing F_c and complement receptors were lower in PCB-exposed individuals relative to controls.

Polybrominated Biphenyls. Firemaster® BP-6 and FF-1 are commonly used flame retardants that consist of mixtures of polybrominated biphenyls (PBBs) containing primarily 2,4,5,2',4',5'-hexabromobiphenyl and 2,3,4,5,2',4'5'-heptabromobiphenyl. In Michigan, in 1973, Firemaster® BP-6 was accidentally substituted for a magnesium oxide food supplement for livestock (Dunckel, 1975), and widespread pollution of the food chain occurred over a period of several months. There was prolonged PBB contamination of meat and dairy products in the area. These contaminated products were widely consumed, and high levels of PBB were subsequently found in the serum and adipose tissues of many Michigan dairy farmers, chemical workers, and local residents (Bekesi *et al.*, 1978). A high percentage of Michigan dairy farm residents had abnormalities in a number of immune parameters that were not evident in Wisconsin control farm families (NIEHS, 1983). These included decreased peripheral T-cell numbers, increased numbers of lymphocytes without detectable membrane markers (i.e., so-called null cells), increased Ig levels, and hyperreactivity to recall antigens upon skin testing. Lymphoproliferative responses were depressed in some Michigan dairy farm residents. PBB plasma concentrations did not correlate with depressed immune responses in these individuals, although all had significantly elevated plasma PBB levels. Bekesi and associates (1987) have now confirmed their original observations in the 1978 study groups and have extended this analysis to include 333 Michigan farm residents.

A similar frequency of immunologic abnormalities was observed in the expanded population.

Animals experimentally exposed to PBB demonstrated depressed CMI and antibody responses to a wide variety of antigens. However, the CMI effects, which included suppression of lymphoproliferative responses and DTH, were not as severe as the suppression of antibody responses, since CMI effects occurred only at near toxic dosages (Luster *et al.*, 1978, 1980b), whereas antibody suppression occurred at lower concentrations. Host resistance to parasitic and bacterial challenge in PBB-exposed mice was not affected (see review, Dean *et al.*, 1982).

Dibenzodioxins. Rodents exposed to 2,3,7,8-tetrachlorodibenzo-*p*-dioxin (TCDD) (reviewed by McConnell, 1980; Vos *et al.*, 1980) demonstrated severe thymus atrophy. Histologic evaluation of the thymus revealed cortical lymphoid depletion similar to cortisone-induced thymus atrophy. Depressed antibody responses, DTH, graft-versus-host, and lymphoproliferative responses were observed at slightly higher dosages of TCDD (see review, P. T. Thomas and Faith, 1985). In addition, increased susceptibility to challenge with the bacteria *Salmonella bern,* but not *Listeria monocytogenes* or *Pseudorabies* virus, was noted at low dosages (Thigpen *et al.*, 1975). Depressed antibody responses and DTH were also observed in guinea pigs receiving cumulative dosages of TCDD as low as 0.32 µg/kg over an eight-week period (Vos *et al.*, 1973). Clark *et al.* (1983) observed depressed T-cell function following exposure of adult mice to TCDD, which was associated with an increase in suppressor T-lymphocyte expression and loss of T-lymphocyte cytotoxicity for tumor target cells. Dean and Lauer (1984) reported depressed antibody (PFC) responses and depressed lymphoproliferative responses to mitogens without alteration in cytotoxicity for tumor cells or susceptibility to bacterial or tumor cell challenge in mice exposed to TCDD. Similarly, House *et al.* (1990) have observed decreased antibody plaque responses with no effect on macrophage or NK cell function in TCDD-treated mice. These results were consistent with an increased susceptibility of TCDD-exposed mice to infection with influenza virus and a lack of effect on a *Listeria* bacterial challenge. TCDD, and other dioxin isomers, may also suppress serum complement levels in mice, resulting in an increased susceptibility to challenge with *Streptococcus pneumoniae* infection in these animals (White *et al.*, 1986).

Exposure to TCDD during thymic organogenesis in rodents has resulted in more severe CMI suppression than that occurring following adult exposure. In some species, *in utero* exposure (via maternal dosing) appears to be necessary to induce maximum immunosuppression. At higher dosages, antibody responses and bone marrow stem cell numbers are depressed in most species. Administration of TCDD *in utero* also results in decreased resistance of offspring to bacterial and tumor cell challenge, which correlates with altered CMI (Luster *et al.*, 1980b) in these mice.

In certain instances, the immunological consequences of human exposure to TCDD have been studied. In a recent case of 44 schoolchildren residing in the TCDD-contaminated area of Seveso, Italy (Reggiani, 1980), it was revealed that 20 children exhibited chloracne (a classic sign of TCDD toxicity), although their serum immunoglobulin levels and circulating complement levels were normal. Lymphoproliferative responses to T- and B-cell mitogens were significantly elevated, a finding frequently reported following low-level TCDD exposure in rodents. Other reports of TCDD-related immune alterations in humans include a study in which residents of a Missouri trailer park exposed to dirt and dust containing TCDD were reported to have depressed DTH responses relative to controls (Hoffman *et al.*, 1986). The Air Force has also recently completed the preliminary evaluation of the health and immune status of individuals involved in the aerosol use of Agent Orange in Vietnam (Ranch Hand II study) to establish or refute health effects of TCDD exposure in humans (Lathrop *et al.*, 1984). Immunologic abnormalities were not apparent in these studies.

Currently, it is believed that TCDD-induced immunosuppression is mediated through a cytosolic receptor for TCDD. The TCDD receptor was originally described by Poland and Glover (1976) in hepatic cytosol and subsequently in thymic cytosol (Poland and Glover, 1980). Both genetic and structure-activity data indicate that TCDD-induced thymic atrophy is mediated through the TCDD cytosolic receptor protein, since thymic atrophy segregates with the *Ah* locus; and halogenated congeners of TCDD that compete with [^{3}H]-TCDD for specific binding sites in thymic cytosol fractions produce thymic atrophy *in vivo* (Poland and Glover, 1980). The target for immunotoxicity is thought to principally be the thymic epithelial cells, as suggested by Clark *et al.* (1983) and Greenlee *et al.* (1985). TCDD receptor-mediated events in the thymus may include altered T-cell maturation and differentiation and may be the molecular basis for the thymic atrophy and immunotoxicity observed. Since the endocrine influence of thymic epithelium in adult animals and humans is poorly understood, immunosuppression observed in rodents following adult exposure to TCDD

may also involve toxicity to the thymic epithelium.

TCDBF (2,3,7,8-tetrachlorodibenzofuran), another dibenzodioxin, has been identified in various preparations of commercial Aroclors® (Vos et al., 1970). Its toxicity is of similar magnitude as that of TCDD. The similarity between TCDD and TCDBF in chemical structure suggests competition of these substances for the putative TCDD cytosol receptor. One might expect, therefore, that TCDBF would also be immunotoxic. In animal studies, TCDBF produced severe thymic atrophy in most species studied (Moore *et al.*, 1976) and suppressed lymphocyte responses to mitogens, DTH to novel antigens, and lymphokine (MIF) production in adult guinea pigs (Luster *et al.*, 1979a). Although immunotoxicity studies with TCDBF are more limited than those with TCDD, the immunotoxicological changes attributed to both compounds appear to be similar; however, when compared with TCDD, higher doses of TCDBF are required to produce the same magnitude of effect (reviewed by Vecchi, 1987).

Polycyclic Aromatic Hydrocarbons (PAHs). Polycyclic aromatic hydrocarbons are an ubiquitous class of chemicals produced during the combustion of fossil fuels. It is estimated in the United States that nearly 900 tons of one PAH alone, benzo[a]pyrene, are emitted into the air each year. As a class, PAHs consist of three or more benzene rings containing only carbon and hydrogen atoms. Exposure of mice to 3-methylcholanthrene (MCA), 1,2-benzanthrene, or 1,2,5,6-dibenzanthracene produces a marked depression in the serum antibody response to sheep erythrocytes (SRBCs) (Malmgren *et al.*, 1952). Subsequent studies have confirmed that MCA suppresses immune responses, resulting in long-lasting reductions in antibody-producing cells. A similar long-term reduction in the response to SRBCs was observed in mice exposed to 7,12-dimethylbenz[a]anthracene (DMBA) (Ward *et al.*, 1986) and benzo[a]pyrene (B[a]P); this depression persisted for more than 32 days after exposure (Stjernsward, 1966).

B[a]P-exposed mice have been observed to have depressed responses to T- and B-cell mitogens but not to alloantigenic stimulation (Dean *et al.*, 1983). Exposure to the noncarcinogenic congener, B[e]P, did not alter mitogen responses. Host susceptibility following challenge with syngeneic PYB6 tumor cells and the bacterium *Listeria monocytogenes* was also unaltered in B[a]P-exposed mice, as were DTH and allograft rejection following B[a]P exposure. These data suggest that T-cell immunocompetence was minimally affected. In contrast, the primary antibody plaque-forming cell responses to both T-dependent and T-independent antigens were severely depressed. Zwilling (1977) similarly noted unaltered skin graft rejection in hamsters following inhalation exposure to $B[a]P-Fe_2O_3$, despite severely depressed humoral antibody responses. *In utero* exposure to B[a]P resulted in a depressed anti-SRBC response, which persisted for up to eight weeks. Urso and Gengozian (1980) also found that exposure of pregnant mice to a single dose (100 to 150 $\mu g/g$ body weight) of B[a]P resulted in severe suppression of antibody responses in pups shortly after birth. This suppression persisted for at least 78 weeks and was accompanied by an increased frequency of tumors in these mice during adulthood.

Data suggest that 3-methylcholanthrene exposure in mice suppresses T-cell proliferative responses to mitogens and the generation of cytotoxic T lymphocytes (Wojdani and Alfred, 1983). Prolongation of skin graft survival, an additional measure of CMI, has also been reported following administration of MCA (Di-Marco *et al.*, 1971) but was only observed if the grafting occurred 11 or more weeks after exposure, a time that corresponded to the appearance of tumors. Thus, it was not possible to ascertain whether this was a tumor or chemical-related effect.

DMBA is among the best-studied PAHs relative to its immunotoxic properties. Neonatal exposure of mice to DMBA results in suppression of both the primary (IgM) and secondary (IgG) antibody response to SRBCs, whereas exposure of adult mice to DMBA has been reported to cause a kinetic shift in the IgM PFC response, although no change in magnitude of the response was observed (Ball, 1970). This observation conflicts with more recent studies in which murine exposure to DMBA suppressed the number of antibody-producing cells and CMI functions including NK and CTL cytotoxicity for up to two months (Ward *et al.*, 1986). Therefore, DMBA exposure appears to result in long-lasting immunosuppression of CMI, HMI, and tumor resistance mechanisms in mice. Suppression of immunological mechanisms of tumor resistance by PAHs tends to correlate with their carcinogenic properties and may contribute to their carcinogenicity. Immunosuppressive PAHs tend to be carcinogenic, whereas their nonimmunosuppressive congeners are not (Ward *et al.*, 1985).

The mechanism of PAH-mediated immunosuppression is unclear. Recent studies, however, suggest the T-helper cell represents at least one important target of DMBA-mediated immunotoxicity, since DMBA-induced suppression of certain *in vitro* cell-mediated immune functions could be at least partially restored by the exogenous addition of untreated T-helper cells or one of their principal soluble mediator products, IL-2 (House *et al.*, 1987). Further investigation has suggested faulty antigen recognition by the T cell as a possible mechanism of DMBA-induced immunosuppression of certain immune responses (House *et al.*, 1989).

Urethane. Urethane (ethyl carbamate) is a potent multipotential carcinogen in mice, rats, and hamsters, producing leukemia, lymphomas, lung adenomas, hepatomas, and melanomas (IARC, 1974). Exposure of mice to tumorigenic dosages of ethyl carbamate caused severe myelotoxicity, led to a marked suppression of natural killer cell activity, inhibited immune elimination of B16F10 melanoma cells, and increased metastatic tumor growth in the lungs (Luster *et al.*, 1982a). Exposure to the noncarcinogenic congener methyl carbamate did not alter immune parameters. Previous studies had demonstrated that exposure to aliphatic carcinogens, especially urethane, inhibited antibody responses to SRBCs (Malmgren *et al.*, 1952). Gorelik and Herberman (1981) found that exposure to urethane suppressed natural killer cell activity, which was accompanied by an increased frequency of spontaneous lung adenomas in susceptible mouse strains.

Pesticides. Pesticides studied for immunotoxicity in rodents can be grouped into four general classes: carbamates, including carbaryl (Sevin®) and aldicarb; organochlorines, which include DDT, mirex, and representatives of the chlorinated cyclodines, aldrin, and lindane; organophosphates, including parathion, methylparathion, dichlorophos, and malathion; and the organotins. Increasing evidence suggests that certain pesticides or formulation contaminants can alter immune function in rodents (*see* Table 9–15), although studies in humans are limited and ambiguous (see reviews by Street, 1981; P. T. Thomas *et al.*, 1990a).

Additionally, certain classes of pesticides (e.g., organochlorines) are stable and may persist in the environment, affording greater immunotoxic potential due to chronic adult and neonatal exposures. In general, the developing immune system is more sensitive to toxic chemical insult than the mature adult immune system. In this regard, *in utero* or neonatal exposure studies with pesticides have been limited and produced mixed results. However, preweanling rats exposed to tributyltin oxide had reversible immune alterations at a dose below that which altered immune parameters in adult rats (Smialowicz *et al.*, 1988). Similarly, mice exposed to chlordane *in utero* displayed a decreased DTH response and had increased survival and anti-

Table 9–15.   PESTICIDES MODULATING IMMUNITY IN EXPERIMENTAL ANIMALS AND HUMANS

PESTICIDE	SPECIES	OBSERVED EFFECTS	REFERENCE
A. *Carbamates*			
Aldicarb	Mouse	Decreased AFC response to sheep erythrocytes	Olson *et al.*, 1987
	Mouse	No alterations in AFC response, B or T lymphocyte mitogenesis, host resistance to influenza virus infection, CTL response or percentages of T cells, T cell subpopulations or B cells	P. T. Thomas *et al.*, 1987, 1990b
Carbofuran	Rabbit	Reduced DTH response	Street and Sharma, 1974
	Mouse	Decreased host resistance to *S. typhimurium* infection	Fan *et al.*, 1978
B. *Organochlorines*			
Chlordane	Mouse	Decreased contact hypersensitivity after *in utero* exposure	Barnett *et al.*, 1985b
	Mouse	Suppression of AFC responses and T-cell activity	Johnston *et al.*, 1986
DDT	Rabbit	Thymus atrophy and reduced DTH response	Street and Sharma, 1974
Dieldrin	Mouse	Decreased AFC response and increased susceptibility to viral infection	Bernier *et al.*, 1987; Krzystyniak *et al.*, 1985
Hexachlorobenzene	Mouse	Increased sensitivity to endotoxin and malaria challenge	Loose *et al.*, 1978
	Rat	Increased humoral immune responses to tetanus toxoid and DTH to ovalbumin	Vos *et al.*, 1983
Mirex	Chicken	Decreased IgG levels	Rao and Glick, 1977
Pentachlorophenol	Mouse	Altered immune function and decreased host resistance to virus-induced tumor	*See* review, Kerkvliet *et al.*, 1985
C. *Organophosphates*			
Malathion	Mouse	Suppression of CTL response *in vitro*	Rodgers *et al.*, 1986
Methylparathion	Rabbit	Thymus atrophy and reduced DTH response	Street and Sharma, 1974
	Mouse	Decreased host resistance to *Salmonella typhimurium* infection	Fan *et al.*, 1978; Street, 1981
Parathion	Mouse	Altered colony forming activities of bone marrow hematopoietic stem cells	Gallicchio *et al.*, 1987
D. *Organotin Compounds*			
Tributyltin oxide (TBTO)	Rat	Reduced T-cell, natural killer cell, and macrophage responses; decreased host resistance to *Trichinella spiralis* infection	Vos *et al.*, 1984a
Triphenyltin hydroxide (TPTH)	Rat	Reduced DTH response to tuberculin	Vos *et al.*, 1984b

body response to influenza challenge as adults (Barnett *et al.*, 1985a, 1985b; Menna *et al.*, 1985).

The carbamate insecticide carbaryl (Sevin®) has been frequently studied as an immunotoxicant. As early as 1971, Perelygin (see Street, 1981) observed that exposure of albino rats and rabbits to carbaryl at 20 mg/kg depressed antibody responses and phagocytosis by granulocytes. Subsequent studies in rats and chickens reported that orally administered Sevin® resulted in an acute, and sometimes prolonged, depression of splenic germinal center formation and antibody production (see Street, 1981). Pre-

viously reported effects of carbaryl on granulocyte phagocytosis were confirmed and found to be prolonged for up to nine months following exposure to the chemical. In contrast to studies from Soviet or eastern European laboratories, which have demonstrated that carbaryl is immunosuppressive, most studies performed in this country have found no consistent indication of immunosuppression except at near-lethal doses (Street and Sharma, 1974; Street, 1981).

Aldicarb, another carbamate pesticide, has recently been reported to alter immune function. Olson *et al.* (1987) reported an unusual inverse dose-related suppression of the antibody response in mice following exposure to aldicarb at concentrations as low as 1 ppb for 34 days in drinking water. In contrast, Thomas *et al.* (1987, 1990b), using similar exposure conditions that encompassed and exceeded earlier concentrations used by Olson *et al.*, a similar and additional mouse strain, and a more comprehensive testing battery, were unable to substantiate immune modulation or altered susceptibility to challenge with infectious agents in aldicarb-treated mice. To complicate this issue further, Fiore *et al.* (1986) observed that women chronically ingesting low levels of aldicarb-contaminated groundwater had altered numbers of T cells and an altered CD4/CD8 cell ratio.

Following an exothermic reaction and explosion in a methyl isocyanate (intermediate in carbamate pesticide production) storage tank at a pesticide production facility in Bhopal, India (1984), a variety of effects on immune parameters were reported in exposed individuals, including an increase in the number of T cells and T-helper cells and depressed lymphocyte mitogenesis responses (Deo *et al.*, 1987). Laboratory studies of mice exposed to methyl isocyanate by inhalation exposure failed to reveal significant immune alterations, and all changes observed were thought to be secondary to respiratory toxicity (Luster *et al.*, 1986). From the data developed to date with carbamate pesticides or their intermediates, there is insufficient evidence in humans (albeit under poorly documented exposure conditions) or experimental animals (under well-defined exposure conditions) to indicate a significant human immunological health risk from this class of pesticides.

In general, organophosphate insecticides have been shown to be immunosuppressive in certain animal species. Street and Sharma (1974) and Street (1981) observed that a 28-day oral exposure of rabbits to methylparathion (1.5 mg/kg/day) produced a marked reduction in splenic germinal centers following antigenic stimulation, as well as thymus cortical atrophy, and a reduced DTH response to tuberculin. Similarly, Fan (see Street, 1981) noted a dose-related increase in mortality following challenge with *Salmonella typhimurium* and a depressed lymphocyte response to mitogens following methylparathion exposure. In contrast, Wiltrout (see Street, 1981) observed that another member of this class of insecticides, parathion, produced depression of humoral immunity but only when administered at near-lethal levels. Studies by Desi *et al.* (1978) found that exposure to malathion depressed antibody responses to *Salmonella typhi*. Rodgers *et al.* (1986) observed

that O,O,S-trimethylphosphorothioate, a contaminant of malathion, altered immune function, suggesting that a contaminant may account for the previously reported immunotoxicity of this agent. Desi *et al.* (1980) found that rabbits exposed to dichlorophos had depressed humoral antibody responses and tuberculin skin test reactivity. The dosage utilized in this study was near the LD50, and no general toxicity data were provided; thus, it is difficult to separate the immunosuppression observed from general toxicity in these animals.

Impairment of neutrophil chemotaxis accompanied by an increase in upper respiratory tract infections was correlated with length of occupational exposure in 85 workers handling organophosphate pesticides (Hermanowicz and Kossman, 1984). In general, the evidence is quite good that organophosphate insecticides can suppress the immune response. It is therefore prudent to be concerned about their potential for immunotoxicity in man.

Accumulating data suggest that the organochlorine pesticides may also alter immune function (see review by Koller, 1979). Class representatives examined in rodents include DDT, mirex, aldrin, hexachlorobenzene, dieldrin, pentachlorophenol, and lindane. Depressed serum antibody titers against ovalbumin were observed in rats orally exposed to 200 ppm of DDT (see Street, 1981). In contrast, guinea pigs and rats fed DDT had normal levels of antitoxin antibody and gamma globulin and a reduced propensity to develop anaphylaxis, which correlated with a decreased number of mast cells (Gabliks *et al.*, 1975). Likewise, chickens exposed to DDT or mirex had significantly depressed levels of IgG and IgM, although specific antibody responses were normal (Street, 1981). In the studies of Street and Sharma (1974) and Street (1981), a four-week exposure to DDT resulted in a reduced number of germinal centers in lymph nodes, thymus cortical atrophy, and suppression of CMI. Studies by Rao and Glick (1977) of chickens exposed to DDT or mirex revealed a marked reduction in total antibody production and serum IgG level, although serum IgM levels were elevated. The alteration in IgG levels was thought to be related to altered T-cell function. Likewise, studies of rabbits exposed to lindane demonstrated a depressed antibody response to *Salmonella typhi* antigen (Desi *et al.*, 1978). Leukopenia and impaired leukocyte phagocytosis were also observed following the oral administration of lindane (Evdokimov, 1974). Most studies have focused on the effects of DDT on specific antibody responses. It appears that DDT produces slight to negligible CMI immunotoxicity. However, the effects of DDT on macrophage function, CMI, and host resistance have not been intensively investigated and appear to be an open question.

In a study of pesticide formulators in India by Kashyap (1986), 73 percent of the workers exposed to four pesticides (DDT, hexachlorocyclohexane, malathion, and parathion) had altered levels of serum immunoglobulins, although no increase in infections was noted. This observation is similar to that reported by Wysocki *et al.* (1985), who observed increased serum IgG and decreased serum IgM and C3 component of complement in the absence of altered host resistance to infections in 51 men exposed to chlorinated pesticides. This lack of correlation between altered host resistance and immune dysfunction reported in the two human studies described above may indicate that the "physiological threshold" known for immune function reserve (Dean *et al.*, 1987) was exceeded by the immunotoxicant exposure.

Airborne Pollutants. The defense of the lung against noxious gases, particulates, or infectious agents is dependent on both physical and immunological protective mechanisms. The former are largely represented by upper airway filtering mechanisms, whereas immunologic defense of the lung involves complex interactions between phagocytic cells (i.e., polymorphonuclear neutrophils (PMNs) and macrophages), cells secreting humoral factors (e.g., lymphokines and immunoglobulins), and immune effector cells. This secondary means of pulmonary defense is required when the physical mechanisms fail to provide complete protection against environmental agents.

Inhalation exposure to a large number of xenobiotics may adversely affect the pulmonary immune system, induce hypersensitivity (see earlier discussion), or produce other systemic immune alterations (see reviews by Gardner, 1982, 1984; Thurmond and Dean, 1988). The widespread distribution of some of these agents in the environment coupled with their known pulmonary effects in humans focuses concern that inhalation exposure to chemicals may play an even greater role than yet demonstrated in pulmonary disease causation. This section attempts to describe and categorize the impact of some of these agents on the pulmonary immune response (Table 9–16), particularly with regard to their immunosuppressive properties.

In vitro and *in vivo* methodology is now available to assess the effects of inhalation exposure to xenobiotics on the systemic immune response, on pulmonary alveolar leukocytes obtained by lavage or biopsy, and on host resistance to pulmonary challenge of rodents with infectious agents. Pulmonary alveolar lavage is an accepted and safe method in clinical and experimental studies for obtaining leukocytes or lavage fluids. Studies utilizing pulmonary lavage fluid and cells are useful in identifying possible adverse immunological effects at a cellular and molecular level resulting from inhalation of xenobiotics. Recent advances in our understanding of leukocyte activations, intercellular and intracellular regulatory networks, and the cytokine repertoire of macrophages and lymphocytes should facilitate a more precise understanding of their role in the etiology of pulmonary disease. Several studies implicate a central role for macrophages and their cytokines in lung injury after exposure to some pulmonary toxicants (see review by Adams *et al.*, 1988).

Increased fluid and serum components may be observed in certain disease states, originating from pulmonary exposure to irritant chemical hazards. Surfactant functions within alveoli to reduce tension on expiration, thereby preventing alveolar collapse. Pulmonary edema may result

Table 9–16. EXAMPLES OF IMMUNOMODULATION BY VARIOUS INHALANT HAZARDS STUDIED IN EXPERIMENTAL ANIMALS*

CHEMICAL	ASSAY[†]	SPECIES	TISSUE/ORGAN/ENDPOINT
Acrolein	HRC—*Staphylococcus aureus*	Swiss	Lung
Asbestos	Antibody PFC	BALB/c	Splenocytes
	HR—*Streptococcus*	Mice	Mortality
Benzene	B-lymphocyte numbers	BALB/c	Spleen, blood
	T-lymphocyte numbers		Spleen
	IgG antibody PFC		Spleen
	Type IV hypersensitivity		Skin
	HR—*Listeria* (transient)	C57Bl/6	Spleen
	Antibody PFC	C57Bl/6	Spleen
	Mitogenesis		
	B.T lymphocyte numbers		Bone marrow

Table 9–16. (*continued*)

CHEMICAL	ASSAY[†]	SPECIES	TISSUE/ORGAN/ENDPOINT
Beryllium	HR—*Streptococcus*	Mice	Mortality
	Type IV hypersensitivity	Guinea Pig	Lung, skin
Cadmium	Antibody PFC	Mice	Spleen
	Phagocytosis	Mice	PAM[‡]
	HR—*Streptococcus*	Mice	Mortality
Carbon monoxide	Antibody PFC	Guinea Pig	Spleen, lung
Cigarette smoke	Protein synthesis	Rabbit	PAM
	Increased oxidative metabolism	Hamsters	PAM
	Immunoglobulin titer	Rats	BAL fluid
	Lymphocyte mitogenesis	Rabbit	Blood
Chromium	Increased phagocytosis	Rabbit	PAM
	Antibody PFC	Rats	Spleen
	Increased antibody PFC (low dose)		
	Phagocytosis		PAM
	Increased phagocytosis (low dose)		
Coal dust	Protein synthesis	Guinea Pig	PAM
Cobalt	Increased phagocytosis		
	HR—*Streptococcus*	Mice	Mortality
Ethylenediamine	Type I hypersensitivity	Humans	—
Fly ash	Tumoricidal activity	Hamster	PAM
	ADCC		
	Antibody PFC	BALB/c	Spleen
Formaldehyde	Increased H$_2$O$_2$ production	B6C3F1	PEM§
	Increased HR—*Listeria*		Mortality
Manganese	HR—*Streptococcus*	CD-1	Mortality
Methyl isocyanate	MLR	B6C3F1	Spleen
Nickel	Enhanced phagocytosis	Rat	PAM
	Antibody PFC		Spleen
	Antibody PFC		Blood
	Antibody PFC	Mice	Spleen
Nitrogen dioxide	HR—*Streptococcus*	CF-1, CD$_2$F$_1$	Mortality
Ozone	Chemotaxis	Rhesus	PAM
	HR—*Streptococcus*	CD-1	Lung
	Chemotaxis	Rat	PAM
	HR—*Streptococcus*	Mice	Mortality
Paraphenylenediamine	Type IV hypersensitivity	Humans	—
Silica	Antibody PFC	BALB/c	Spleen
	CTL		
	Phagocytosis—*S. aureus*		PAM
	Type IV hypersensitivity (ADCC)	Hamsters	PAM
	Tumoricidal activity		PAM
Subtilisin	Type I hypersensitivity	Guinea Pig	Lung
	Increased IgG precipitins	Cynomolgus	Serum
Sulfuric acid	Immunoglobulin titer fluctuation	CD-1	Serum
	Antibody PFC		Spleen
	HR—*Klebsiella*		Mortality
	HR—*Influenza*		Mortality
Toluene	HR—*Streptococcus*	CD-1	Lung
	Microbicidal activity		
Toluene diisocyanate	Increased anti-TDI antibodies	Guinea Pig	Lung
	Increased anti-TDI antibodies	Guinea Pig	Serum
Trimellitic anhydride	Anti-TMA antibodies	Rhesus	Serum, BAL
	Anti-TMA antibodies	Humans	Serum
	Type I–IV hypersensitivities	Humans	Serum, lymphoctyes, skin

* Modified from Thurmond, L. M., and Dean, J. H.: Immunological responses following inhalation exposure to chemical hazards. In Gardner, E. E.; Crapo, J. D.; and Massaro, E. J. (eds.): *Toxicology of the Lung*. Raven Press, New York, 1988, pp. 375–406. See this reference for detailed references to table inserts.
† Unless specifically indicated as enhancement or increase, end points are immune suppression.
‡ HR indicates altered host resistance, expressed either as microbicidal activity within the lung or as mortality.
§ PEM = peritoneal exudate macrophages; PAM = pulmonary alveolar macrophages.

from local irritation of lung surface epithelium by a wide variety of chemical hazards (e.g., tobacco smoke, silica, asbestos, diesel exhaust) and is caused by the leakage of plasma into alveolar spaces. Brain (1986) observed altered macrophage phagocytic function associated with oxygen toxicity. It was speculated that the oxygen-induced progressive pulmonary edema produced overt cell damage by alteration of the microenvironment.

Chemicals such as isocyanates, trimellitic anhydride, formaldehyde, silica, ethylenediamine, and paraphenylenediamine have been classed as pulmonary or dermal irritants. Irritants may produce hypersensitivity-like symptoms. Hyperreactive airway syndrome is characterized by nonspecific irritability on exposure to a variety of airborne pollutants. Bronchial provocation with methacholine may be used to demonstrate preexisting airway hypersensitivity. Toxicant-induced changes in airway membranes in conjunction with mediator release from mast cells may induce this condition (see review, Thurmond and Dean, 1988).

Formaldehyde. Irritant tissue damage may be produced by macrophages from mice exposed to formaldehyde vapor. Dean *et al.* (1984) have shown increased synthesis of H_2O_2 by peritoneal macrophages from formaldehyde-exposed mice, which could contribute to enhanced bactericidal activity and the potential to damage local tissue.

Ozone. Exposure to O_3 causes infiltration of inflammatory polymorphonuclear leukocytes and pulmonary alveolar macrophages into the lungs, which may then secrete lysosomal acid hydrolases, neutral proteinase, lipids, peroxides, and oxygen free radicals into the extracellular environment of the lung. These potent inflammatory agents may contribute to O_3-induced lung edema, bronchial constriction, and pulmonary vascular changes (see review, Thurmond and Dean, 1988). Recent evidence suggests that arachidonic acid oxidation products generated by PMNs play a critical role in mediating hyperreactive airways after O_3 exposure in dogs. The mechanism of O_3-induced hyperresponsiveness has been shown in rats, dogs, and rhesus monkeys to be related to an influx of neutrophils and can be prevented through the induction of neutropenia or pretreatment with indomethacin.

Asbestos. Human exposure to asbestos is associated with several pulmonary diseases, including fibrosis, asbestosis, and mesothelioma. Immunological impairments, such as decreased delayed-type hypersensitivity responses, reduced numbers of circulating T cells, and depressed T-cell proliferation, are associated with pulmonary asbestosis (see review, Miller and Brown, 1985). In addition to suppressing CMI, increased levels of serum immunoglobulins and autoantibodies have been observed. The immunotoxic response to asbestos and silica inhalation appears not to be strictly dose-responsive, in that low dose may be stimulatory, whereas high exposure levels result in immunosuppression. There are data suggesting a direct effect of asbestos on T-cell function, which may account for asbestos-altered immunoregulation. The significance of these immunological changes and their causal role in the disease process are uncertain.

Altered alveolar macrophage activity has been implicated as playing a significant role in asbestos-induced immunological dysfunction. On reaching the alveoli, asbestos particles are phagocytized by macrophages, resulting in cell lysis and release of lysosomal enzymes and macrophage activation, with the production of an inflammatory product. Depressed T-dependent, macrophage-dependent antibody response was detected in mice exposed to asbestos. A cytotoxic effect of asbestos on alveolar and splenic macrophages has been demonstrated *in vitro,* as has impaired phagocytic activity.

Oxidant Gases. Numerous studies demonstrate that exposure to ozone (O_3) at levels as low as 0.1 ppm or O_3-sulfuric acid mixtures alter susceptibility of mice to challenge by pathogenic bacteria (Coffin and Gardner, 1972). Similarly, mice exposed to nitrogen dioxide (NO_2) for less than three hours and challenged with a *Streptococcus*-containing aerosol have a significantly increased mortality at doses of NO_2 above 2 ppm (Ehrlich *et al.,* 1977). The mortality was potentiated on continuous long-term exposure to NO_2. Although NO_2 and NO_3 have produced adverse effects on host resistance after aerosol challenge with bacteria, exposure to other gaseous pollutants, such as sulfur dioxide, has not altered host resistance, although suppression of splenic antibody PFCs has been reported (see review, Graham and Gardner, 1985). Decreased resistance is believed to be related to a decreased phagocytic and bactericidal activity of PAM after exposure to these oxidant gases.

Tobacco Smoke. Mice and guinea pigs exposed to cigarette smoke have reduced numbers of antibody PFCs in the spleen. Splenic lymphocytic mitogen-induced blastogenesis is also depressed in exposed mice. Macrophages exposed to cigarette smoke display a range of altered morphological and functional characteristics, including increased size, decreased phagocytic capacity, and pertubed oxygen metabolism. Acrolein, a major component of cigarette smoke, has been shown to impair resistance to aerosolized *Staphylococcus aureus.*

Agents Causing Nonimmunological Disease Syndromes. Chemically induced misdirection of a normal immune response may result in substantial tissue damage by nonspecific triggering of immunocyte metabolism. For example, local irritation of mucosal surfaces may self-amplify to cause changes in vascular permeability and cellular accumulation. Secretion of oxygen metabolites or enzymes normally produced in phagosomes may cause significant tissue damage. Inhaled particulates may activate complement, resulting in chemotaxis of phagocytes to the site. Generally, such syndromes fall into the categories either of irritancy or of elastin-collagen imbalances.

Airborne Metals. There is also evidence suggesting that a number of trace metals that alter the physiology or function of macrophages can cause a significant increase in susceptibility to infection. Animals exposed to airborne nickel, cadmium, zinc, magnesium, and lead have modified susceptibility to aerosol challenge with bacteria (Ehrlich, 1980). Increased susceptibility to challenge with pneumonia-producing bacteria in animals exposed to airborne metals was correlated with an alteration of phagocytic and enzymatic activity in alveolar macrophages (Aranyi *et al.*, 1979). Inhalation of airborne nickel and cadmium not only altered alveolar macrophage function but also depressed primary humoral immunity (Graham *et al.*, 1978, 1979). In addition, increased mortality has been observed in animals exposed to copper smelter fly ash samples but not in mice exposed to coal fly ash samples. These results correlated with the adverse effects of metals on alveolar macrophages (Aranyi *et al.*, 1981).

In summary, inhalation exposure to gaseous pollutants, airborne metals, and complex metallic mixtures has been shown to produce altered susceptibility to bacterial challenge in mice that correlates with impairment of phagocytic, enzy-matic, and bactericidal activity in alveolar macrophages. With some agents, systemic immune depression can also be observed.

Metals. Systemic metal exposure may also adversely affect the immune response and alter host resistance to infectious agents and tumors (Koller, 1979, 1980; Dean *et al.*, 1982; Lawrence, 1985). Suppression of host resistance to challenge with infectious agents is among the most consistently reported observations of metal-induced immunotoxity (Table 9–17). However, depending on conditions of dosing and route of exposure, as well as species, strain, and overall genetic constitution of the test animal, metals may sometimes enhance certain immune responses (Koller, 1980; Lawrence, 1985). Metal-induced enhancement of immune function is consistent with the known role some metals play in the induction of hypersensitivity and auto-immune responses. The multiplicity of possible outcomes (i.e., suppression, hypersensitivity responses, autoimmune responses) resulting from metal interactions with the immune system may provide an explanation for some of the seemingly contradictory data in the literature on this subject. In this section, immunotoxic effects of metal pollutants will be discussed using lead as the prototype, since metals may share a common mechanism of immunotoxicity and the interactions of lead with the immune system have been extensively studied.

Lead. Several studies assessing the influence of lead on susceptibility to infectious agents have consistently demonstrated lead impairment of both CMI and antibody-mediated host resistance (Table 9–17). Mice injected with lead nitrate intraperitoneally (ip) for 30 days and subsequently challenged with the bacterium *Salmonella typhimurium* had significantly higher mortality than controls (Hemphill *et al.*, 1971). Similar results were observed in rats exposed intravenously to lead and challenged with *Es-*

Table 9–17.   EXAMPLES OF METALS FOUND TO IMPAIR HOST RESISTANCE TO INFECTIOUS AGENTS

SPECIES	METAL	INFECTIOUS AGENT	REFERENCE
Mouse	Pb	*S. typhimurium*	Hemphill *et al.*, 1971
Mouse	Pb	EMC virus	Gainer 1977; Exon *et al.*, 1979
Mouse	Pb	Langat virus	Thind and Kahn, 1978
Mouse	Pb	*L. monocytogenes*	Lawrence, 1981a
Mouse	Pb	*S. aureus,* *L. monocytogenes,* *Candida*	Selski *et al.*, 1975
Rat	Pb	*E. coli, S. epidermidis*	Cook *et al.*, 1975
Mouse	Hg	EMC virus	Gainer, 1977
Rabbit	Hg	Pseudorabies virus	Koller, 1973

cherichia coli (see review, Cook *et al.*, 1975). In these two studies, lead may have interfered with the clearance or detoxication of endotoxin, resulting in death. In another study, mice exposed orally to lead for four weeks and challenged with *Listeria* were assayed for viable *Listeria* 48 and 72 hours following challenge (Lawrence, 1981a). The highest dose of lead caused significant inhibition of early bactericidal activity, and the medium and high doses produced 100 percent mortality from the bacteria challenge within ten days.

Lead exposure also increased host susceptibility to viral infections. Gainer (1977) observed that mice administered lead in drinking water for two weeks had a significantly increased mortality to encephalomyocarditis (EMC) viral challenge. It has been speculated that the enhanced susceptibility of lead-treated mice to viral challenge might be due to a decreased capacity of these animals to develop an immune response or to produce interferon (IFN). Studies by Gainer (1977) indicated that exposure of mice to lead did not inhibit the antiviral action of IFN *in vivo* or *in vitro*, although it appeared to suppress viral IFN production *in vivo*. Blakley *et al.* (1982) found that mice exposed to lead acetate in drinking water produced similar amounts of IFN as controls when both were given the viral IFN inducer tilorone. Similarly, the *in vitro* induction of immune IFN by the T-cell mitogens phytohemagglutinin, concanavalin A, and staphylococcal enterotoxin in lymphocytes from lead-exposed mice was unaltered compared with controls (Blakley and Archer, 1982). Thus, lead exposure does not appear to significantly alter the ability of lymphocytes to produce immune interferon.

There is evidence suggesting that host resistance in humans may be altered by lead exposure. It has been noted that children with persistently elevated blood lead levels and naturally infected with *Shigella enteritis* had prolonged diarrhea (Sachs, 1978). In addition, lead smelter workers have been reported to have more colds and influenza infections per year (Ewers *et al.*, 1982) than people not exposed to lead. Secretory IgA, a major factor in immune defense against respiratory and gastrointestinal infections, was found to be suppressed in lead workers with a median blood lead level of 52 μg/dl or greater.

Alterations in antibody-mediated immunity have also been reported in rodents following lead exposure. Reduced antibody titers in animals exposed to lead might explain the decreased host resistance to infectious agents observed, since specific antibodies can directly neutralize viruses, activate complement, and enhance opsonic phagocytosis. Lead has little effect on the serum immunoglobulin levels in rabbits, in children with >40 μg Pb/dl of blood (Reigart and Garber, 1976), or in individuals chronically exposed to lead (Ewers *et al.*, 1982; Kimber *et al.*, 1986).

Rats pre- and postnatally exposed to lead have significantly reduced numbers of IgM PFCs (Luster et al., 1978). In contrast, CBA/J mice exposed to lead for one to ten weeks had unaltered IgM PFC responses to SRBCs (Lawrence, 1981a). Acute oral lead exposure produces a decreased titer of specific antibodies in rabbits immunized with typhus vaccine or with pseudorabies virus. Likewise, lead-poisoned children had reduced specific antitoxoid antibody titers following booster immunizations with tetanus toxoid (Reigart and Garber, 1976). Tetraethyl lead (organic lead) also results in reduced specific antibody titers in mice and a significant reduction in IgM and IgG PFCs against sheep red blood cells (Blakley *et al.*, 1980). Although it appears likely that lead can affect antibody production, these variable data suggest that suppression may be genetically based.

The influence of inorganic lead exposure on the development of antibody responses has been further assessed by removal of splenic lymphocytes from lead-exposed mice for *in vitro* plasma cell development (Blakley and Archer, 1981). Lead exposure consistently inhibited plasma cell development. Through *in vitro* reconstitution experiments, it was concluded that inhibition of HMI by lead was caused by a macrophage defect. This finding was supported by studies where 2-mercaptoethanol (2-ME), a sulfhydryl reagent that substitutes for macrophage function, was found to reverse HMI inhibition by lead. These data may explain why results of studies following *in vivo* lead exposure have been variable, as some of the test systems utilized 2-ME in the *in vitro* assays of immune function. Recent studies by Burchiel *et al.* (1987) suggest lead may also impair macrophage differentiation. Lead treatment of mice resulted in a reduction of bone marrow cells expressing macrophage cell surface differentiation markers and also resulted in a shift toward more immature cells in the bone marrow. This was consistent with increased numbers of bone marrow granulocyte/macrophage precursors.

In summary, lead exposure appears to inhibit the development of antibody-producing cells and serum antibody titers. The adverse effects of lead on humoral immunity may be due to either interference with macrophage antigen processing or antigen presentation to lymphocytes, rather than to a direct effect of lead on B lymphocytes.

The effect of lead exposure on CMI is less clearly characterized. In a comprehensive study in Sprague-Dawley rats (Faith *et al.*, 1979), chronic low-level pre- and postnatal exposure suppressed several CMI parameters, including DTH and lymphoproliferation in response to mitogens. Gaworski and Sharma (1978) also noted that splenic lymphocytes from mice exposed orally to lead for 30 days, but not for 15 days, had significantly depressed proliferative responses to T- and B-cell mitogens. In contrast, several laboratories have reported that lead exposure does not suppress T-cell proliferation (Koller *et al.*, 1979; Lawrence, 1981b; Blakley and Archer, 1982). These differences are not easily reconciled since the lead dosages and exposure periods employed do not appear to account for the differences observed.

The mechanism of lead-induced toxicity to lymphoid cells is complex. Lead, like many metals, is a sulfhydryl alkylating agent with a high affinity for subcellular sulfhydryl groups. Thus, the immunomodulatory effects of lead on immune cells may involve its association with membrane and intracellular thiols, important in lymphocyte activation, proliferation, and differentiation. The study by Blakley and Archer (1982) supports this hypothesis because the inhibitory effects of lead were overcome by the addition of an exogenous thiol reagent.

Cadmium. Cadmium, like lead, is a widespread environmental pollutant producing alterations in host resistance and immune function in rodents similar to those produced by lead. Cadmium has been found to alter host susceptibility to bacterial endotoxins, *E. coli* challenge, and EMC viral challenge in mice (see review, Koller, 1980). Some groups, however, have reported cadmium-exposed mice to be more resistant to tumor and EMC virus challenges. Chronic cadmium exposure can result in decreased numbers of antibody-producing cells and depressed serum antibody titers in rabbits (Koller, 1973) and mice (Koller *et al.*, 1975), which is consistent with effects of other heavy metals on humoral immunity.

Gaworski and Sharma (1978) observed depressed lymphoproliferative responses to the mitogens PHA and PWM, no effect with con A, and an enhanced response to LPS in lymphocytes from mice exposed to cadmium. Koller *et al.* (1979) confirmed that cadmium produced no effect on con A or MLC-induced lymphoproliferation, although they observed enhanced proliferative responses to LPS stimulation. T-cell–mediated tumor cell cytotoxicity was found to be enhanced in cadmium-exposed mice (Kerkvliet *et al.*, 1979). The data regarding effects on T-cell and macrophage function following cadmium exposure are ambiguous owing to conflicting findings between different laboratories;

however, there is a consensus that humoral immune responses are depressed following cadmium exposure, results similar to those obtained with lead.

Organic and Inorganic Mercury. Several groups have reported altered host resistance in rodents following mercury exposure. Mice exposed for 84 days to 1 or 10 ppm of methyl mercury chloride in food had increased mortality following challenge with EMC virus (Koller, 1975). This observation was confirmed using inorganic mercury (Gainer, 1977).

Koller (1973) and Koller and associates (1977) examined humoral immunity in rabbits after inorganic mercury exposure and in mice following methyl mercury exposure. They found significantly depressed primary antibody (IgM) PFC responses. Likewise, Ohi *et al.* (1976) observed that methyl mercury suppressed both the IgM and IgG antibody PFC responses in rodents when it was administered pre- and postnatally but not when given at weaning or after. Studies by Blakley *et al.* (1980) have confirmed that subchronic, low-level mercury exposure in rodents results in thymic cortex and splenic follicular atrophy with concomitant depression of IgM as well as IgG antibody PFC responses.

The effect of mercury exposure on lymphocyte function and CMI has been less clearly defined. Gaworski and Sharma (1978) found that exposure of mice for 30 days to 10 ppm mercury in drinking water produced depressed lymphocyte responses to mitogens. Likewise, Hirokawa and Hayashi (1980) reported that acute exposure to nonlethal levels of methyl mercury (70 mg/kg) resulted in severely depressed lymphocyte responses to T-cell mitogens. Thus, methyl mercury exposure depresses polyclonal activation of lymphocytes by T-cell mitogens and antibody responses to specific antigenic stimulation.

Organotins. The biological activities as well as the immunotoxicity of organotin compounds have been extensively reviewed (Seinen and Penninks, 1979; Snoeij *et al.*, 1987; Boyer, 1989). These compounds are used primarily as heat stabilizers, catalytic agents, and antifungal/antimicrobials. In long-term subchronic feeding studies of triphenyltin acetate in guinea pigs, lymphoid depletion and antibody suppression were observed. Studies by Seinen and Penninks (1979) have demonstrated that di-*n*-octyltindichloride (DOTC) or di-*n*-butyltindichloride (DBTC) exposure can selectively depress thymus cellularity and weight as well as T-lymphocyte function in rats without causing myelotoxicity or nonlymphoid toxicity. A direct effect of DOTC and DBTC on the thymus resulting in cellular depletion of the thymus as well as peripheral lymphocyte depletion is consistent with the immunosuppression observed in these animals. Lymphocyte depletion cannot be explained solely due to altered corticosteroid levels. The finding by Snoeij et al. (see review 1987) that the immunotoxic action declined within the series of trialkyltin compounds from tributyltin to trioctyltin may be explained by a limited absorption or metabolism of the higher trialkyltin homologues.

Depressed CMI evidenced by increased skin graft rejection time, reduced DTH, reduced graft-versus-host responses, and decreased responses to T-cell mitogens (see review, Seinen and Penninks, 1979; Snoeij et al., 1987) was observed in rats exposed to DOTC and DBTC. These dialkytin compounds also suppressed resistance to Listeria challenge. Inhibition of HMI was also observed, expressed as reduced PFC numbers and antibody titers to sheep erythrocytes. The antibody response to E. coli was not affected in DOTC- and DBTC-exposed rats, suggesting that the dialkyltins do not directly affect B-lymphocyte function but that they may alter T-helper cell function. As with most immunotoxic chemicals, immunosuppression following DOTC or DBTC exposure is more pronounced in animals exposed immediately after birth rather than as adults.

Immune function is not impaired in mice or guinea pigs fed dialkyltins, which correlates with the absence of lymphoid tissue atrophy observed in these species following chemical exposure (Seinen and Penninks, 1979). That thymic atrophy can be demonstrated in mice following intravenous or intraperitoneal exposure to DBTC or DOTC suggests interspecies variability in this response may involve species differences in gastrointestinal absorption, metabolism, and/or elimination of these compounds. No species specificity is apparent following in vitro treatment, since DOTC or DBTC added to rat or human thymocytes causes decreases in cell survival, responses to mitogens, and E-rosette formation (Seinen et al., 1979) in cell cultures from both species. Histologic evaluation of dialkyltin-induced thymus atrophy does not support dysfunction of the thymic reticuloepithelial cells (Penninks et al., 1985a) but rather suggests a direct antiproliferative effect on thymocytes, which is supported by both in vivo and in vitro studies. Immunotoxic effects similar to those produced with the diorganotins have also been described for certain triorganotin compounds (reviewed by Vos et al., 1984). Some tributyltin compounds (e.g., tri-n-butyltin oxide and tri-n-butyltin chloride) can result in lymphocyte depletion similar to that described for DOTC and DBTC. Alterations in immune function parameters, including T-dependent immune responses,

as well as certain host resistance end points have also been reported. Recent studies propose that the thymic atrophy observed in rats following exposure to tributyltin does not result from the parent compound but rather from a dibutyltin metabolite (Snoeij et al., 1988).

Other Metals. Toyama and Kolmer (1918) reported over 60 years ago that feeding animals low concentrations of arsenic enhances antibody production, whereas antibody suppression occurs following high-level exposure. Similar observations have been reported in mice fed various arsenate compounds. While high levels of arsenicals increased susceptibility to viral infection and decreased interferon activity, low levels had the opposite effect, causing increased viral resistance and viral interferon production (Gainer, 1972; Gainer and Pry, 1972). General toxicity occurring at higher levels of arsenical exposure may be, in part, responsible for the increased viral susceptibility. It appears that further studies with arsenicals are warranted.

There is evidence in laboratory animals that nickel exposure results in altered resistance to virus and bacteria (Adkins et al., 1979). A direct effect on macrophage function has also been attributed to nickel (Graham et al., 1978), as has suppression of NK responses in both rats and mice. Altered macrophage and NK activity are consistent with a decreased resistance to tumor cell challenge observed in both species.

Drugs. The majority of drugs clinically utilized for immunosuppressive purposes were initially developed for alternative reasons. Suppression of the immune response, in many instances, was an undesirable side effect. Recently, certain abused drugs have also been shown to cause immune alterations. A partial listing of drugs that suppress the immune response is given in Table 9–18. A limited number of these agents will be discussed below to illustrate prototype agents having quite different mechanisms of immunosuppression.

Alkylating Agents. Alkylating agents are chemicals that form covalent linkages (alkylation) with biologically important molecules, including DNA, which result in disruption of cell functions, especially mitosis. Thus, these agents are particularly toxic to rapidly proliferating cells including neoplastic, lymphoid, bone marrow, intestinal mucosal, and germinal cells. The alkylating agents are effective at any part of the cell cycle, although cytotoxicity is usually expressed during S phase as the cell prepares to divide. Cyclophosphamide (Cytoxan®) is the prototype oxazaphosphorine, being a stable inactive compound that when transported into the cell is cleaved by phosphamidase in cells to phosphoramide mustard, a powerful alkylating

Table 9–18. IMMUNOSUPPRESSIVE DRUGS

Therapeutic Drugs
  Alkylating agents
    Nitrogen mustards: cyclophosphamide, L-phenylalanine mustard, chlorambucil
    Alkyl sulfonates: busulfan
    Nitrosoureas: carmustine (BCNU), lomustine (CCNU)
    Triazenes: dimethyltriazenoimidazolecarboxamide (DTIC)
  Antiinflammatory agents
    Aspirin, indomethacin, penicillamine, gold salts
    Adrenocorticosteroids—prednisone
  Antimetabolites
    Purine antagonists: 6-mercaptopurine, azathioprine, 6-thioguanine
    Pyrimidine antagonists: 5-fluorouracil, cytosine arabinoside, bromodeoxyuridine
    Folic acid antagonists: methotrexate (amethopterine)
  Natural products
    Vinca alkaloids: vinblastine, vincristine, procarbazine
    Antibiotics: actinomycin D, adriablastine, bleomycin, daunomycin, puromycin, mitomycin C, mithramycin
    Antifungal agents: griseofulvin
    Enzymes: L-asparaginase
  Cyclosporin A
  Estrogens—diethylstilbestrol, ethinyl estradiol

Abused Drugs
  Ethanol
  Cannabinoids
  Cocaine
  Opiates

---

agent at physiologic pH, and acrolein. Other members in this family include trofosfamide, ifosfamide, and sufosfamide. In general, these agents exert their immunosuppressive activity by inhibiting DNA replication through alkylation of N7 guanine in DNA, leading to miscoding, destruction of the purine ring structure of guanine (depurination), and DNA cross-linking, which block cell replication. Myelosuppression, hemorrhagic cystitis, alopecia, and gonadal damage are the main toxic side effects.

As a chemotherapeutic agent, cyclophosphamide alone or in combination with other drugs has been effective in treating Hodgkin's disease, lymphosarcoma, Burkitt's lymphoma, and acute lymphoblastic leukemia (Calabresi and Parks, 1985). As an immunosuppressant, cyclophosphamide is beneficial in reducing symptoms of certain autoimmune diseases (Calabresi and Parks, 1985), although its major use has been in pretreatment of bone marrow transplant recipients in an effort to prevent subsequent graft rejection (Shand, 1979).

Several reports indicate that there may be subpopulations of lymphocytes preferentially affected by cyclophosphamide treatment, at least in certain species (Shand, 1979; Webb and Winkelstein, 1982). B cells in guinea pigs, chickens, and mice, for example, have been demonstrated to be more sensitive than T cells to cyclophosphamide-induced toxicity (Shand,

1979). In contrast, higher dosages of cyclophosphamide can also suppress T-cell function in mice (Dean *et al.*, 1979b). Both T-helper and T-suppressor cells have at times been implicated as targets; however, recent evidence indicates that certain T-suppressor cell populations are extremely sensitive to cyclophosphamide (Shand, 1979). Thus, cyclophosphamide-induced immunosuppression is probably due to a direct cytotoxic effect of the drug on immunocompetent lymphocytes, particularly those that have undergone antigenic differentiation and division.

As is observed with other conventional immunosuppressants, treatment with cyclophosphamide can increase the risk of cancer and infection, which may relate to the lymphopenia and neutropenia seen following cyclophosphamide therapy (Webb and Winkelstein, 1982). In addition, exposure of experimental animals to cyclophosphamide increases host susceptibility to transplantable tumors (Dean *et al.*, 1979b).

Corticosteroids. Corticosteroids and their synthetic analogues can suppress both inflammatory and immune responses. The synthetic corticosteroids prednisone and methylprednisolone are common adjuncts in immunosuppressive therapy in transplant recipients and individuals with extreme hypersensitivity. Although the precise basis for their immunologic effects is unknown, corticosteroids cause a transient lymphopenia (Webb and Winkelstein, 1982), alter phagocytosis, and depress T- and B-lymphocyte function (Santiago-Delpin, 1979). In rodents, a dramatic lymphopenia due to lympholysis can be demonstrated following corticosteroid therapy; however, lymphocytes from humans are relatively resistant to lympholysis by corticosteroids (Webb and Winkelstein, 1982). Thus, suppression in humans may be due to other diverse corticosteroid-induced effects such as alterations in leukocyte mobility, production and/or responses to lymphokines, and immune cell interactions. Part of these effects, as well as many of the antiinflammatory properties of corticosteroids, might be attributed to their stabilization of biomembranes, including plasmalemmal and lysosomal membranes (Santiago-Delpin, 1979). At a molecular level, these changes may be mediated through steroid-receptor complexes capable of interacting with DNA, thereby modifying enzyme synthesis, and ultimately resulting in the immunomodulatory properties of this group of compounds (Santiago-Delpin, 1979).

Antimetabolites. The antimetabolites are frequently used clinically in transplant patients as immunosuppressive drugs and can be categorized as folate, purine, pyrimidine, and amino acid analogues. The most widely used antimetabolite is the purine antagonist azathioprine. It is a derivative of 6-mercaptopurine (6-MP) and was originally synthesized with the intent of preventing the rapid methylation and oxidation common to 6-MP, thus improving its therapeutic:toxic ratio. Azathioprine is more effective in cycling cells and is maximally active as an immunosuppressant when given following antigenic stimulation (Santos, 1974). Immunosuppression may result from azathioprine-induced inhibition of purine synthesis; however, other mechanisms have been suggested, including the binding of azathioprine to T lymphocytes and the subsequent inactivation of surface antigen receptors (Webb and Winkelstein, 1982).

Azathioprine can also act as an antiinflammatory agent and can reduce the numbers of neutrophils, monocytes, and large lymphocytes. The question of specificity of this drug remains unclear. Regarding lymphocytes, there is evidence that cell-mediated immunity and T-cell functions are the main target of azathioprine-mediated suppression, which is consistent with the clinical picture (Santiago-Delpin, 1979). However, recent *in vitro* studies demonstrate substantial toxicity of azathioprine for both T and B cells, although the drug concentrations used in these experiments were higher than plasma levels commonly obtained in therapeutic situations (Kazmers *et al.,* 1983).

The major clinical complication of azathioprine therapy is bone marrow toxicity and leukopenia, which may predispose to secondary infection. In addition, long-term administration of azathioprine may increase the risk of developing certain malignancies.

Cyclosporin. Cyclosporin A (CyA) is a cyclic peptide containing 11 amino acids isolated from fermentation products of two fungi, *Trichoderma polysporum* and *Cylindrocarpon lucidum,* and has a very narrow range of antibiotic activity against fungi and yeast. CyA was found to inhibit lymphocyte proliferation in early tests designed to detect nonspecific cellular toxicity, which further increased the doubt of its potential value as an antibiotic. Fortunately, its lymphostatic and immunologic properties were further characterized. The result has been the development of a family of cyclosporins. Cyclosporin A is the most widely known of these drugs; however, cyclosporins C and G have also been shown to be effective immunosuppressants.

An important characteristic of CyA is its relative lack of secondary toxicity at therapeutic dosages sufficient to maintain immunosuppression in transplant recipients (Calne *et al.,* 1981). For example, CyA does not appear to be myelotoxic, an important consideration, particularly in bone marrow transplant recipients, although some hepato- and nephrotoxicity have been reported in patients receiving CyA. The incidence of secondary infection is also less frequent in transplant patients receiving CyA compared with those receiving more conventional immunosuppressants.

Borel *et al.* (1976) demonstrated that cyclosporin A inhibited the proliferative response to mitogens, although it was not until the lymphokine cascade was proposed that one was able to determine that cyclosporin's effect on lymphocyte proliferation was mediated through the inhibition of the interleukin-2 receptor and IL-2 production by inhibiting the transcription of IL-2 mRNA. The identification of a cytoplasmic receptor for cyclosporin A on human lymphocytes (e.g., cyclophilin) greatly facilitated a detailed examination of the biochemical basis for its mechanism of action (Ryffel *et al.,* 1978). It has been suggested that cyclosporin competes with prolactin for binding to the prolactin receptor on lymphocytes, affects Ca^{2+} flux and membrane fluidity, and produces a marked and selective decrease in the transcription of mRNA for IL-2 (*see* review, Harding and Handschumacher, 1988). The widespread phytogenetic distribution of cyclophilin and the diverse actions of cyclosporin on cellular response other than T-cell activation suggest the receptor may play a pleiotropic role in cell growth and differentiation.

FK-506. FK-506 is a recently discovered immunosuppressive agent that is structurally distinct from cyclosporin A but shares many of its properties. It interferes with the production of IL-2 and other lymphokines, lacks myelotoxicity, and induces transplantation tolerance (*see* review, Thomson, 1989). It, too, is a product of a soil fungus, *Streptomyces tsukubaensis*, found in northern Japan. The minimum effect dose of FD-506 for inhibition of the T-lymphocyte function appears to be approximately one-tenth that of cyclosporin.

Estrogens. Diethylstilbestrol (DES) is a synthetic nonsteroidal compound possessing estrogenic activity that has widespread commercial usage. Mice exposed to DES during prenatal (Luster *et al.*, 1979b) or adult (Boorman *et al.*, 1980) life exhibited severe thymic cortical lymphoid depletion along with depressed MLC responses, DTH, and mitogen-induced lymphocyte blastogenesis (Kalland *et al.*, 1979; Luster *et al.*, 1979b; Luster *et al.*, 1980a). The usual ratios of T-cell subpopulations in neonatally DES-exposed mice were altered, suggesting a defect in maturation of T cells. A subsequent report has related the reduced proportion of T-helper cells to suppressed antibody PFC responses to T-dependent antigens (Kalland, 1980). Suppressed antibody responses following immunization with T-independent antigens also occur in rodents treated with DES and are consistent with the depressed *in vitro* proliferative response to LPS, a polyclonal B-cell mitogen (Kalland *et al.*, 1979; Luster *et al.*, 1979b; Luster *et al.*, 1980a). Macrophage functions, assessed by phagocytosis and tumor growth inhibition by adherent peritoneal cells, are potentiated by DES exposure (Boorman *et al.*, 1980), whereas macrophage suppressor cell activity is enhanced (Luster *et al.*, 1980a).

The effects of DES on immune surveillance and host resistance to disease are well characterized. Exposure of adult mice to DES resulted in increased mortality following challenge with the bacterium *Listeria monocytogenes*, the parasite *Trichinella spiralis*, and a transplantable syngeneic tumor, suggesting a lesion in CMI and/or macrophage function (Dean *et al.*, 1980).

DES probably exerts its immunosuppressive effects via estrogen receptors on lymphoid cells and thymic epithelial cells. The immunosuppressive effects of DES may be mediated through selective depletion or functional impairment of T lymphocytes and/or the induction of suppressor macrophages. The exact relationship between the putative thymic epithelial receptor for DES, DES-induced thymic atrophy, macrophage activation, and T-cell immunosuppression has yet to be clarified.

Drugs of Abuse. Chronic alcohol abuse in humans has been associated with impaired T-lymphocyte function (Berenyi *et al.*, 1975), myelosuppression, and a defective humoral immunity (Gluckman *et al.*, 1977) as well as with a higher and more severe incidence of infections (Tapper, 1980). In studies by Loose *et al.* (1975), the primary, but not secondary, humoral response was reduced in rats chronically dosed with ethanol. In another study, rats chronically fed ethanol exhibited suppressed DTH, thymic and splenic atrophy, and suppressed secondary HMI (Tennenbaum *et al.*, 1969).

Naturally occurring cannabinoids, unique to the plant *Cannabis sativa* and constituting 15 percent of the cannabis by weight, are also implicated as immunomodulatory (see review, Holsapple and Munson, 1985). The natural cannabinoids may be subdivided into psychoactive, with Δ9-tetrahydrocannabinol (Δ-9-THC) as the major constituent, and nonpsychoactive, of which there are five known constituents. Both psychoactive and nonpsychoactive cannabinoids have been examined to characterize their immunosuppressive properties, and several studies have shown that they suppress both humoral and cell-mediated immunity in experimental animals (for review, see Munson and Fehr, 1983).

The effective dose for 50 percent suppression (ED50) of the antibody plaque response to SRBCs in mice was 70, 14, 13, and 8 mg/kg for Δ-9-THC, Δ-8-THC, 1-methyl-Δ8-THC (nonpsychoactive), and abnormal Δ-8-THC (nonpsychoactive), respectively (Smith *et al.*, 1978). In the same studies, at a dose of 100 mg/kg the cannabinoids suppressed the DTH response 35 to 64 percent. Studies in humans have been less conclusive, although Δ-9-THC has been found to suppress CMI but not humoral immunity (see Munson and Fehr, 1983). Nonpsychoactive cannabinoids have also been synthesized in attempts to develop novel immunosuppressants.

FUTURE DIRECTIONS

The application of the discipline of immunology to the toxicologic assessment of drugs and chemicals is progressing rapidly, with methods development and selection, and validation stages completed. The preceding few years of research have provided new models; data on correlations of immune function and host resistance; a better understanding of the biologic relevance of certain immune function parameters; and a better standardized panel of methods for immunotoxicity assessment. Future research is needed to examine mechanisms of immunotoxicity at the cellular and molecular level, to develop better immunologic data on humans occupationally or environmentally exposed to chemicals shown to be immunotoxic in laboratory animals, and to better define risk using immunological data.

REFERENCES

Adams, D. O., and Dean, J. H.: Analysis of macrophage activation and biological response modifier effects by use of objective markers to characterize the stages of activation. In Herberman, R. (ed.): *Natural Cell-Mediated Immunity. II.* Academic Press, Inc., New York, 1982, pp. 511–518.

Adams, D. O.; Lewis, J. G.; and Dean, J. H.: *Activation of Mononuclear Phagocytes by Xenobiotics of Environmental Concern: Analysis and Host Effects.* In Gardner, D. E.; Crapo, J. D.; and Massaro, E. J. (eds.): *Toxicology of the Lung.* Raven Press, New York, 1988, pp. 351–373.

Adkins, B.; Richards, J. H.; and Gardner, D. E.: Enhancement of experimental respiratory infections following nickel-inhalation. *Environ. Res.,* 20:33–42, 1979.

Ahlstedt, S.; Ekstrom, B.; Svard, P. O.; Sjoberg, B.; Kristofferson, A.; and Ortengren, B.: New aspects on antigens in penicillin allergy. *CRC Crit. Rev. Toxicol.,* 7(3):219–277, 1980.

Andersen, K. E., and Maibach, H. I. (eds.): *Contact Allergy Predictive Tests in Guinea Pigs: Current Problems in Dermatology,* Vol. 14. Karger, Basel, 1985.

Aranyi, C.; Gardner, D.; and Huisingh, J. L.: In Dunham D. D. (ed.): *Evaluation of Potential Inhalation Hazard of Particulate Silicous Compounds by In Vitro Alveolar Macrophage Test. Application to Industrial Particulates Containing Hazardous Impurities.* American Society for Testing Materials, Philadelphia, 1981.

Aranyi, C.; Miller, F. J.; Andres, S.; Ehrlich, R.; Fenters, J.; Gardner, D.; and Waters, M.: Cytotoxicity to alveolar macrophages of trace metals absorbed on fly ash. *Environ. Res.,* 20:14–23, 1979.

Baer, R. L.; Ramsey, D. L.; and Bondi, E.: The most common contact allergens. *Arch. Dermatol.,* 108:74–78, 1973.

Ball, J. K.: Immunosuppression and carcinogenesis: contrasting effects with 7,12-dimethylbenz(a)anthracene, benz[a]pyrene, and 3-methylcholanthrene. *J. Natl. Cancer Inst.,* 44:1, 1970.

Barnett, J. B.; Holcomb, D.; Menna, J. H.; and Soderberg, L. S. F.: The effect of prenatal chlordane exposure on specific anti-influenza cell-mediated immunity. *Toxicol. Lett.,* 25:229–238, 1985a.

Barnett, J. B.; Soderberg, L. S. F.; and Menna, J. H.: The effect of prenatal chlordane exposure on the delayed hypersensitivity response of BALB/c mice. *Toxicol. Lett.,* 25:173–183, 1985b.

Bekesi, J. G.; Holland, J. F.; Anderson, H. A.; Fischbein, A. S.; Rom, W.; Wolff, M. S.; and Selikoff, I. J.: Lymphocyte function of Michigan dairy farmers exposed to polybrominated biphenyls. *Science,* 199:1207–1209, 1978.

Bekesi, J. G.; Roboz, J. P.; Fischbein, A.; and Selikoff, I. J.: Clinical immunology studies in individuals exposed to environmental chemicals. In Berlin, A.; Dean, J.; Draper, M. H.; Smith, E. M. B.; and Spreafico, F. (eds.): *Immunotoxicology.* Martinus Nijhoff Publishers, Dordrecht, 1987, pp. 347–361.

Berenyi, M. R.; Straus, B.; and Avila, L.: T-rosettes in alcoholic cirrhosis of the liver. *J.A.M.A.,* 232:44–46, 1975.

Bernier, J.; Hugo, P.; Krzystyniak, K.; and Fournier, M.: Suppression of humoral immunity in inbred mice by dieldrin. *Toxicol. Lett.,* 35:231–240, 1987.

Bernstein, D. I.; Patterson, R.; and Zeiss, C. R.: Clinical and immunologic evaluation of trimellitic anhydride- and phthalic anhydride-exposed workers using a questionnaire with comparative analysis enzyme-linked immunosorbent and radioimmunoassay studies. *J. Allergy Clin. Immunol.,* 69:311–318, 1982.

Bigazzi, P. E.: Autoimmunity induced by chemicals. *J. Clin. Toxicol.,* 26:125–156, 1988.

Blakley, B. R., and Archer, D. L.: The effect of lead acetate on the immune response in mice. *Toxicol. Appl. Pharmacol.,* 61:18–26, 1981.

———: Mitogen stimulation of lymphocytes exposed to lead. *Toxicol. Appl. Pharmacol.,* 62:183–189, 1982.

Blakley, B. R.; Archer, D. L.; and Osborne, L.: The effect of lead on immune and viral interferon production. *Can. J. Comp. Med.,* 46:43–46, 1982.

Blakley, B. R.; Sisodia, C. S.; and Mukkur, T. K.: The effect of methylmercury, tetraethyl lead, and sodium arsenite on the humoral immune response in mice. *Toxicol. Appl. Pharmacol.,* 52:245–254, 1980.

Boorman, G. A.; Luster, M. I.; Dean, J. H.; and Wilson, R. E.: The effect of adult exposure to diethylstilbestrol in the mouse on macrophage function. *J. Reticuloendothel. Soc.,* 28:547–559, 1980.

Border, W. A.; Lehmann, D. H.; Egan, J. D.; Sass, H. J.; Glode, J. E.; and Wilson, C. B.: Antitubular basement-membrane antibodies in methicillin associated interstitial nephritis. *N. Engl. J. Med.,* 291:381–382, 1974.

Borel, J. F.; Feurer, C.; Gobler, H. V.; and Stahelin, H.: Biological effects of cyclosporin A. *Agents Actions,* 6:468–475, 1976.

Boyer, I. J.: Toxicity of dibutyltin, tributyltin and other organotin compounds to humans and experimental animals. *Toxicology,* 55:253–298, 1989.

Brain, J. D.: Toxicological aspects of alterations of pulmonary macrophage function. *Annu. Rev. Pharmacol. Toxicol.,* 26:547–565, 1986.

Brooks, S. M.; Weiss, M. A.; and Bernstein, I. L.: Reactive airways dysfunction syndrome (RADS). Persistent asthma syndrome after high level irritant exposures. *Chest,* 88:376–384, 1985.

Burchiel, S. W.; Hadley, W. M.; Cameron, C. L.; Fincher, R. H.; Lim, T.; Elias, L.; and Stewart, C. C.: Analysis of heavy metal immunotoxicity by multiparameter flow cytometry: correlation of flow cytometry and immune function data in B6C371 mice. *Int. J. Immunopharmacol.,* 9:597–610, 1987.

Burnet, F. M.: *The Clonal Selection Theory of Acquired Immunity.* Cambridge University Press, London, 1959.

Calabresi, P., and Parks, R.: Antiproliferative agents and drugs used for immunosuppression. In Gilman, A. G.; Goodman, L. S.; Rall, T. W.; and Murad, F. (eds.): *Goodman and Gilman's The Pharmacological Basis of Therapeutics,* 7th ed. Macmillan Publishing Co., New York., 1985, pp. 1247–1306.

Calne, R. Y.; Rolles, K.; White, D. J.; Thiru, S.; Evans, D. B.; Henderson, R.; Hamilton, D. L.; Boone, N.; McMaster, P.; Gibby, O.; and Williams, R.: Cyclosporin A in clinical organ grafting. *Transplant. Proc.,* 13:349–358, 1981.

Chang, K. J.; Ching, J. S.; Huang, P. C.; and Tung, T. C.: Study of patients with PCB poisoning. *J. Formosan Med. Assoc.,* 79:304–312, 1980.

Chan-Yeung, M., and Lam, S.: Occupational asthma. *Am. Rev. Respir. Dis.,* 133:686–703, 1986.

Clark, D. A.; Sweeney, G.; Safe, S.; Hancock, E.; Kilburn, D. G.; and Gauldie, J.: Cellular and genetic basis for suppression of cytotoxic T-cell generation by haloaromatic hydrocarbons. *Immunopharmacology,* **6**: 143–153, 1983.

Coffin, D. L., and Gardner, D. E.: Interaction of biological agents and chemical air pollutants. *Ann. Occup. Hyg.,* **15**:219–235, 1972.

Cook, J. A.; DiLuzio, N. R.; and Hoffman, E. O.: Factors modifying susceptibility to bacterial endotoxin: the effect of lead and cadmium. *CRC Crit. Rev. Toxicol.,* **3**:201–229, 1975.

Coombs, R. R. A., and Gell, P. G. H.: Classification of allergic reactions responsible for clinical hypersensitivity and disease. In Gell, P. G. H.; Coombs, R. R. A.; and Lachman, P. J. (eds.): *Clinical Aspects of Immunology,* J. B. Lippincott, Philadelphia, 1975, p. 761.

Cooper, N. R.: The complement system. In Stites, D. P.; Stobo, J. D.; Fudenberg, H. H.; and Wells, J. V. (eds.): *Basic and Clinical Immunology,* 4th ed. Lange Medical Publications, Los Altos, Calif., 1980, pp. 124–135.

Cromwell, O.; Pepys, J.; Parish, W. E.; and Hughes, E. G.: Specific IgE antibodies to platinum salts in sensitized workers. *Clin. Allergy,* **9**:109–117, 1979.

Cronin, E.: *Contact Dermatitis.* Churchill Livingston, London, 1980.

Cushman, J. R., and Street, J. C.: Allergic hypersensitivity to the herbicide 2,4-D in BALB/c mice. *J. Toxicol. Environ. Health,* **10**:729–741, 1982.

———: Allergic hypersensitivity to the insecticide malathion in BALB/c mice. *Toxicol. Appl. Pharmacol.,* **70**:29–42, 1983.

Davis, R. J.; Blainey, A. D.; and Pepys, J.: Occupational asthma. In Middleton, E. Jr.; Reed, C. E.; and Ellis, E. F. (eds.): *Allergy: Principles and Practices.* C. V. Mosby Company, St. Louis, 1983, pp. 1037–1065.

Dean, J. H., and Lauer, L. D.: Immunological effects following exposure to 2,3,7,8-tetrachlorodibenzo-*p*-dioxin: a review. In Lowrance, W. W. (ed.): *Public Health Risk of the Dioxins.* William Kaufmann, Los Altos, Calif., 1984, pp. 275–294.

Dean, J. H.; Lauer, L. D.; House, R. V.; *et al.:* Studies of immune function and host resistance in B6C3F1 mice exposed to formaldehyde. *Toxicol. Appl. Pharmacol.,* **72**:519–529, 1984.

Dean, J. H.; Luster, M. I.; and Boorman, G. A.: Immunotoxicology. In Sirois, P., and Rola-Pleszgyski. M. (eds.): *Immunopharmacology.* Elsevier Biomedical Press, Amsterdam, 1985, pp. 349–397.

Dean, J. H.; Luster, M. I.; Boorman, G. A.; Lauer, L. D.; Luebke, R. W.; and Lawson, L. D.: Immune suppression following exposure of mice to the carcinogen benzo(a)pyrene but not the non-carcinogenic benzo(e)pyrene. *Clin. Exp. Immunol.,* **52**:199–206, 1983.

Dean, J. H.; Luster, M. I.; Boorman, G. A.; Luebke, R. W.; and Lauer, L. D.: The effect of adult exposure to diethylstilbestrol in the mouse: alterations in tumor susceptibility and host resistance parameters. *J. Reticuloendothel. Soc.,* **28**:571–583, 1980.

———: Application of tumor, bacterial, and parasite susceptibility assays to study immune alterations induced by environmental chemicals. *Environ. Health Perspect.,* **43**:81–88, 1982.

Dean, J. H.; Padarathsingh, M. L.; and Jerrells, T. R.: Assessment of immunobiological effects induced by chemicals, drugs, and food additives. I. Tier testing and screening approach. *Drug Chem. Toxicol.,* **2**:5–17, 1979a.

Dean, J. H.; Padarathsingh, M. L.; Jerrells, T. R.; Keys, L.; and Northing, J. W.: Assessment of immunobiological effects induced by chemicals, drugs, and food

additives. II. Studies with cyclophosphamide. *Drug Chem. Toxicol.,* **2**:133–153, 1979b.

Dean, J. H.; Thurmond, L. D.; Lauer, L. D.; and House, R. V.: Comparative toxicology and correlative immunotoxicology in rodents. In *Environmental Chemical Exposure and Immune Integrity, Advances in Modern Environmental Toxicology,* Vol. 13. Princeton Scientific Publishers, Princeton, N. J., 1987, pp. 85–102.

Deo, M. G.; Gangal, S.; Bhisey, A. N.; Somasundaram, R.; Balsara, B.; Gulwani, B.; Darbari, B. S.; Sumati, B; and Maru, G. B.: Immunological, mutagenic and genotoxic investigations in gas-exposed population of Bhopal. *Indian J. Med. Res.,* **86**:63–76, 1987.

Desi, I.; Varga, L.; and Farkas, I.: Studies on the immunosuppressive effect of organochlorine and organophosphoric pesticides in subacute experiments. *J. Hyg. Epidemiol. Microbiol. Immunol.,* **22**:115–122, 1978.

———: The effect of DDVP, an organophosphate pesticide, on the humoral and cell-mediated immunity of rabbits. *Arch. Toxicol. Suppl.,* **4**:171–174, 1980.

de Weck, A. L.: Drug reactions. In Samter, M. (ed.): *Immunological Diseases,* Vol. I. Little, Brown & Co., Boston, 1978, pp. 413–439.

DiMarco, A. T.; Franceschi, C.; Xerri, L.; and Prodi, G.: Depression of homograft rejection and graft-versus-host reactivity following 7,12-dimethylbenz(a)thracene exposure in the rat. *Cancer Res.,* **31**:1446–1450, 1971.

Druet, P.; Bernard, A.; Hirsch, F.; Weening, J. J.; Gengoux, P.; Mahieu, P.; and Brikeland, S.: Immunologically mediated glomerulonephritis by heavy metals. *Arch. Toxicol.,* **50**:187–194, 1982.

Dunckel, A. E.: An updating on the polybrominated biphenyl disaster in Michigan. *J. Am. Vet. Med. Assoc.,* **167**:838–843, 1975.

Ehrlich, R.: Interaction between environmental pollutants and respiratory infections. *Environ. Health Perspect.,* **35**:89–100, 1980.

Ehrlich, R.; Findlay, J. C.; Fenters, J. D.; and Gardner, D. E.: Health effects of short-term inhalation of nitrogen dioxide and ozone mixtures. *Environ. Res.,* **14**:223, 1977.

Epstein, J. H.: Photocontact allergy in humans. In Marzulli, F. N., and Maibach, H. I. (eds.): *Dermatotoxicity.* Hemisphere Publishing Corp., New York, 1987, pp. 441–456.

Ercegovich, C. D.: Relationship of pesticides to immune responses. *Fed. Proc.,* **32**(9):2010–2016, 1973.

Evdokimov, E. S.: Effect of organochlorine pesticides on animals. *Veterinariya,* **12**:94–95, 1974.

Ewers, U.; Stiller-Winkler, R.; and Idel, H.: Serum immunoglobulin complement C3, and salivary IgA levels in lead workers. *Environ. Res.,* **29**:351–357, 1982.

Exon, J. H.; Koller, L. K.; and Kerkvliet, N. I.: Lead-cadmium interaction: effects on viral-induced mortality and tissue residues in mice. *Arch. Environ. Health,* **34**:469–475, 1979.

Faith, R. E.; Luster, M. I.; and Kimmel, C. A.: Effect of chronic developmental lead exposure on cell mediated immune function. *Clin. Exp. Immunol.,* **35**:413–424, 1979.

Fan, A.; Street, J. C.; and Nelson, R. M.: Immunosuppression in mice administered methyl parathion and carbofuran by diet. *Toxicol. Appl. Pharmacol.* **45**:235, 1978.

Figley, K. O., and Elrod, R. M.: Endemic asthma due to castor bean dust. *J.A.M.A.,* **90**:79, 1928.

Fiore, M. C.; Anderson, H. A.; Hong, R.; Golubjatnikov, R.; Seiser, J. E.; Nordstrom, D.; Hanraham, L.; and Belluck, D.: Chronic exposure to aldicarb-contaminated groundwater and human immune function. *Environ. Res.*, **41**:633–645, 1986.

Flower, R. J.; Moncada, S.; and Vane, J. R.: Analgesic-antipyretics, anti-inflammatory agents; drugs employed in the therapy of gout. In Gilman, A. G.; Goodman, L. S.; and Gilman, A. (eds.): *Goodman and Gilman's The Pharmacological Basis of Therapeutics*, 6th ed. Macmillan Publishing Co., New York., 1980, pp. 682–728.

Gabliks, J.; Al-Zubaidy, T.; and Askari, E.: DDT and immunological responses. 3. Reduced anaphylaxis and mast cell population in rats fed DDT. *Arch. Environ. Health,* **30**:81–84, 1975.

Gainer, J. H.: Effects of arsenicals on interferon formation and action. *Am. J. Vet. Res.*, **33**:2579–2586, 1972.

————: Effects of heavy metals and of deficiency of zinc on mortality rates in mice infected with encephalomyocarditis virus. *Am. J. Vet. Res.*, **38**:869–873, 1977.

Gainer, J. H., and Pry, T. W.: Effects of arsenicals on viral infection in mice. *Am. J. Vet. Med. Res.*, **33**:2299–2309, 1972.

Gallicchio, V. S.; Casale, G.; Bartholomew, P.; and Watts, T. D.: Altered colony-forming activities of bone marrow hematopoietic stem cells in mice following short-term exposure to parathion. *Int. J. Cell Cloning,* **5**:231–241, 1987.

Gardner, D. E.: Effect of gases and airborne particles on lung infections. In McGrath, J. J., and Barnes, C. D. (eds.): *Air Pollution—Physiological Effects.* Academic Press, Inc., New York, 1982, pp. 47–79.

————: Alterations in macrophage function by environmental chemicals. *Environ. Health Perspect.*, **55**:343–358, 1984.

Gatti, R. A., and Good, R. A.: Occurrence of malignancy in immunodeficiency disease: a literature review. *Cancer*, **28**:89–98, 1971.

Gaworski, C. L., and Sharma, R. R.: The effects of heavy metals on 3H-thymidine uptake in lymphocytes. *Toxicol. Appl. Pharmacol.*, **46**:305–313, 1978.

Gleich, G. J.; Yunginger, J. W.; and Stobo, J. D.: Laboratory methods for studies of allergy. In Middleton, E. Jr.; Reed, C. E.; and Ellis, E. F. (eds.): *Allergy: Principles and Practices.* C. V. Mosby Company, St. Louis, 1983, pp. 271–293.

Gleichmann, E.; Kimber, I.; and Purchase, I. F. H.: Immunotoxicology: suppressive and stimulatory effects of drugs and environmental chemicals on the immune system. *Arch. Toxicol.*, **63**:257–273, 1989.

Gluckman, S. J.; Dvorak, V. C.; and MacGregor, R. R.: Host defenses during prolonged alcohol consumption in a controlled environment. *Arch. Intern. Med.*, **137**:1539–1543, 1977.

Gorelik, E., and Herberman, R.: Susceptibility of various strains of mice to urethane-induced lung tumors and depressed natural killer activity. *J. Natl. Cancer Inst.*, **67**:1317–1322, 1981.

Graham, J. A., and Gardner, D. E.: Immunotoxicity of air pollutants. In Dean, J. H.; Luster, M. I.; Munson, A. R.; and Amos, H. (eds.): *Immunotoxicology and Immunopharmacology.* Raven Press, New York, 1985, pp. 367–380.

Graham, J. A.; Gardner, D. E.; Waters, M. D.; and Coffin, D. L.: Effect of trace metals on phagocytosis by alveolar macrophages. *Infect. Immun.*, **11**:1278–1283, 1979.

Graham, J. A.; Miller, F. J.; Daniels, M. J.; Payne, E. A.; and Gardner, D. E.: Influence of cadmium, nickel, and chromium on primary immunity in mice. *Environ. Res.*, **16**:77–87, 1978.

Grammer, L. C.; Patterson, R.; and Zeiss, C. R.: Guidelines for the immunologic evaluation of occupational lung disease: report of the subcommittee on immunologic evaluation of occupational immunologic lung disease. *J. Allergy Clin. Immunol., Suppl.*, **84**:805–814, 1989.

Greenlee, W. F.; Dold, K. M.; Irons, R. D.; and Osborne, R.: Evidence for direct action of 2,3,7,8-tetrachlorodibenzo-p-dioxin (TCDD) on thymic epithelium. *Toxicol. Appl. Pharmacol.*, **79**:112–120, 1985.

Hamilton, H. E.; Morgan, D. P.; and Simmons, A.: A pesticide (dieldrin)-induced immunohemolytic anemia. *Environ. Res.*, **17**:155–164, 1978.

Harding, M. W., and Handschumacher, R. E.: Cyclosporin and its receptor, cyclophilin. In Lewis, A.; Ackerman, N.; and Otterness, I. (eds.): *Advances in Inflammation Research*, Vol. 12. Raven Press, New York, 1988.

Hemphill, R. E.; Kaeberle, M. L.; and Buck, W. B.: Lead suppression of mouse resistance to *Salmonella typhimurium. Science,* **172**:1031–1032, 1971.

Hendrick, D. J.; Rando, R. J.; Lane, D. J.; and Morris, M. J.: Formaldehyde asthma: challenge exposure levels and fate after five years. *J. Occup. Med.*, **24**:893–897, 1982.

Herberman, R. B., and Holden, H. T.: Natural cell-mediated immunity. *Adv. Cancer Res.*, **27**:305–372, 1978.

Herberman, R. B., and Ortaldo, J. R.: Natural killer cells: their role in defenses against disease. *Science,* **214**:24, 1981.

Hermanowicz, A., and Kossman, S.: Neutrophil function and infectious disease in workers occupationally exposed to phosphoorganic pesticides: role of mononuclear-derived chemotactic factor for neutrophils. *Clin. Immunol. Immunopathol.*, **33**:13–22, 1984.

Hirokawa, K., and Hayashi, Y.: Acute methyl mercury intoxication in mice. *Acta Pathol. Jpn.*, **30**:23–32, 1980.

Hjorth, N.: Diagnostic patch testing. In Marzulli, F. N., and Maibach, N. I. (eds.): *Dermatotoxicology.* Hemisphere Publishing Corp., New York, 1987, pp. 307–318.

Hoffman, R. E.; Stehr-Green, P. A.; Webb, K. B.; Evans, R. G.; Knutsen, A. P.; Schramm, W. F.; Staake, J. L.; Gibson, B. B.; and Steinberg, K. K.: Health effects of long-term exposure to 2,3,7,8-tetrachlorodibenzo-p-dioxin. *J.A.M.A.*, **255**:2031–2038, 1986.

Holsapple, M. P., and Munson, A. E.: Immunotoxicology of abused drugs. In Dean, J. H.; Luster, M. I.; Munson, A. E.; and Amos, H. E. (eds.): *Immunotoxicology and Immunopharmacology*. Raven Press, New York, 1985, pp. 381–392.

House, R. V.; Lauer, L. D.; Murray, M. J.; and Dean, J. H.: Suppression of T-helper cell function in mice following exposure to the carcinogen 7,12-dimethylbenz[a]anthracene and its restoration by interleukin-2. *Int. J. Immunopharmacol.*, **9**:89–97, 1987.

House, R. V.; Lauer, L. D.; Murray, M. J.; Thomas, P. T.; Ehrlich, J. P.; Burleson, G. R.; and Dean, J. H.: Examination of immune parameters and host resistance mechanisms in B6C3F1 mice following adult exposure to 2,3,7,8-tetrachlorodibenzo-p-dioxin. *J. Toxicol. Environ. Health*, **31**:203–215, 1990.

House, R. V.; Pallardy, M. J.; and Dean, J. H.: Suppression of murine cytotoxic T-lymphocyte induction following exposure to 7,12-dimethylbenz[a]anthracene: dysfunction of antigen recognition. *Int. J. Immunopharmacol.*, **11**:207–215, 1989.

IARC: Benzene. In *Monographs on the Evaluation of*

the Carcinogenic Risk of Chemicals to Humans, Vol. 29. International Agency for Research on Cancer, Lyons, France, 1982, pp. 93–148.

———: Some metals and metallic compounds. In Monographs on the Evaluation of the Carcinogenic Risk of Chemicals to Humans, Vol. 23. International Agency for Research on Cancer, Lyons, France, 1981, pp. 143–204.

———: Urethane. In Monographs on the Evaluation of the Carcinogenic Risk of Chemicals to Man, Vol. 7. International Agency for Research on Cancer, Lyons, France, 1974, p. 111.

Johnston, K. W.; Holsapple, M. P.; and Munson, A. E.: An immunotoxicological evaluation of gamma-chlorodane. Fund. Appl. Toxicol., 6:317–326, 1986.

Juhlin, L.: Incidence of intolerance to food additives. Int. J. Dermatol., 19:548–551, 1980.

Kalland, T.: Decreased and disproportionate T cell population in adult mice after neonatal exposure to diethylstilbestrol. Cell Immunol., 51:55–63, 1980.

Kalland, T.; Strand, O.; and Forsberg, J.: Long term effects of neonatal estrogen treatment on mitogen responsiveness of mouse spleen lymphocytes. J. Natl. Cancer Inst., 63:413–421, 1979.

Kammuller, M. E.; Bloksma, N.; and Seinen, W.: Chemical-induced autoimmune reactions and Spanish toxic oil syndrome. Focus on hydentoins and related compounds. J. Toxicol. Clin. Toxicol., 26:157–174, 1988.

———(ed.): Autoimmunity and Toxicology: Immune Disregulation Induced by Drugs and Chemicals. Elsevier, Amsterdam, 1989.

Karol, M. H.: Concentration-dependent immunologic responses to toluene diisocyanate (TDI) following inhalation exposure. Toxicol. Appl. Pharmacol., 68:229–241, 1983.

———: The development of an animal model for TKI asthma. Bull. Eur. Physiopathol. Respir., 23:571–576, 1988.

Karol, M. H.; Dixon, D.; Brady, M.; and Alarie, Y.: Immunologic sensitization and pulmonary hypersensitivity by repeated inhalation of aromatic isocyanates. Toxicol. Appl. Pharmacol., 53:260–270, 1980.

Karol, M. H.; Hauth, B. A.; Riley, E. J.; and Magreni, C. M.: Dermal contact with toluene di-isocyanate (TDI) produces respiratory tract hypersensitivity in guinea pigs. Toxicol. Appl. Pharmacol., 58:221–230, 1981.

Karol, M. H.; Stadler, J.; and Magreni, C.: Immunotoxicologic evaluation of the respiratory system: animal models for immediate- and delayed-onset pulmonary hypersensitivity. Fund. Appl. Toxicol., 5:459–472, 1985.

Kashyap, S. K.: Health surveillance and biological monitoring of pesticide formulators in India. Toxicol. Lett., 33:107–114, 1986.

Katz, D. H.: Lymphocyte differentiation, recognition and regulation. In Dixon, F. J., and Kunkel, H. G. (eds.): Immunology: An International Series of Monographs and Treatises. Academic Press, Inc., New York, 1977, pp. 40–69.

Kazmers, I. S.; Doddona, P. E.; Dalke, A. P.; and Kelley, W. H.: Effect of immunosuppressive agents on human T- and B-lymphocytes. Biochem. Pharmacol., 32:805–810, 1983.

Kerkvliet, N.: Halogenated aromatic hydrocarbons (HAH) as immunotoxicants. In Chemical Regulation of Immunity in Veterinary Medicine. A. R. Liss, New York, 1984, pp. 369–387.

Kerkvliet, N. I.; Brauner, J. A.; and Matlock, J. P.: Humoral immunotoxicity of polychlorinated diphenyl ethers, phenoxyphenols, dioxins and furans present as contaminants of technical grade pentachlorophenol. Toxicology, 36:307–324, 1985.

Kerkvliet, N. I., and Kimeldorf, D. J.: Antitumor activity of a polychlorinated biphenyl mixture, Aroclor 1254, in rats inoculated with Walker 256 carcinosarcoma cells. J. Natl. Cancer Inst., 59:951–955, 1977.

Kerkvliet, N. I.; Koller, L. D.; Beacher, L. G.; and Brauner, J. A.: Effect of cadmium exposure on primary tumor growth and cell-mediated cytotoxicity in mice bearing MSB-6 sarcomas. J. Natl. Cancer Inst., 63:479–486, 1979.

Kimber, I.; Stonard, M. D.; Gidlow, D. A.; and Niewola, Z.: Influence of chronic low-level exposure to lead on plasma immunoglobulin concentration and cellular immune function in man. Int. Arch. Occup. Environ. Health, 57:117–125, 1986.

Kimbrough, R. D.: Halogenated Biphenyls, Terphenyls, Naphthalenes, Dibenzodioxins and Related Products. Elsevier/North-Holland Biomedical Press, New York, 1980.

King, A. G.; Landreth, K. S.; and Wierda, D.: Hydroquinone inhibits bone marrow pre-B cell maturation in vitro. Mol. Pharmacol., 32:807–812, 1987.

Kobayashi, S.: Different aspects of occupational asthma in Japan. In Frazier, C. A. (ed.): Occupational Asthma. Van Nostrand Reinhold, New York, 1980, pp. 229–244.

Koller, L. D.: Immunosuppression produced by lead, cadmium and mercury. Am. J. Vet. Res., 34:1457–1458, 1973.

———: Methylmercury: effect on oncogenic and non-oncogenic viruses in mice. Am. J. Vet. Res., 36:1501–1504, 1975.

———: Effects of environmental contaminants on the immune system. Adv. Vet. Sci. Comp. Med., 23:267–295, 1979.

———: Immunotoxicology of heavy metals. Int. J. Immunopharmacol., 2:269–279, 1980.

Koller, L. D.; Exon, J. H.; and Arbogast, B.: Methylmercury: effect on serum enzymes and humoral antibody. J. Toxicol. Environ. Health, 2:1115–1123, 1977.

Koller, L. D.; Exon, J. H.; and Roan, J. G.: Antibody suppression by cadmium. Arch. Environ. Health, 30:598–601, 1975.

Koller, L. D.; Roan, J. G.; and Kerkvliet, N. I.: Mitogen stimulation of lymphocytes in CBA mice exposed to lead and cadmium. Environ. Res., 19:177–188, 1979.

Krzystyniak, K.; Hugo, P.; Flipo, D.; and Fournier, M.: Increased susceptibility to mouse hepatitis virus 3 of peritoneal macrophages exposed to dieldrin. Toxicol. Appl. Pharmacol., 80:397–408, 1985.

Lathrop, G. D.; Wolfe, W. H.; Albanese, R. A.; and Moynahan, P. M.: Airforce Health Study (Project Ranch Hand II). An Epidemiologic Investigation of Health Effects in Air Force Personnel Following Exposure to Herbicides, Baseline Morbidity Study Results. USAF School of Aerospace Medicine, Brooks Air Force Base, Texas, 1984, pp. XVI-2-1-2-12.

Lawrence, D. A.: Heavy metal modulation of lymphocyte activities—II. Lead, an in vitro mediator of B-cell activation. Int. J. Immunopharmacol., 3:153–161, 1981a.

———: In vivo and in vitro effects of lead on humoral and cell mediated immunity. Infect. Immun., 31:136–143, 1981b.

———: Immunotoxicity of heavy metals. In Dean, J. H.; Luster, M. I.; Munson, A. E.; and Amos, H. E. (eds.): Immunotoxicology and Immunopharmacology. Raven Press, New York, 1985, pp. 341–353.

Lee, T. P., and Chang, K. J.: Health effects of polychlorinated biphenyls. In Dean, J. H.; Luster, M. I.;

Munson, A. E.; and Amos, H. E. (eds.): *Immunotoxicology and Immunopharmacology*. Raven Press, New York, 1985, pp. 415–422.

Loose, L. D.; Silkworth, J. B.; Pittman, K. A.; Benitz, K. F.; and Mueller, W.: Impaired host resistance to endotoxin and malaria in polychlorinated biphenyl- and hexachlorobenzene-treated mice. *Infect. Immun.*, 20:30–35, 1978.

Loose, L. D.; Stege, T.; and DiLuzio, N. R.: The influence of acute and chronic ethanol or bourbon administration on phagocytic and immune responses in rats. *Exp. Mol. Pathol.*, 23:459–472, 1975.

Lubet, R. A.; Lemaire, B. N.; Avery, D.; and Kouri, R. E.: Induction of immunotoxicity in mice by polyhalogenated biphenyls. *Arch. Toxicol.*, 59:71–77, 1986.

Luster, M. I.; Boorman, G. A.; Dean, J. H.; Luebke, R. W.; and Lawson, L. D.: The effect of adult exposure to diethylstilbestrol in the mouse. Alterations in immunological function. *J. Reticuloendothel. Soc.*, 28:561–569, 1980a.

Luster, M. I.; Boorman, G. A.; Harris, M. W.; and Moore, J. A.: Laboratory studies on polybrominated biphenyl–induced immune alterations following low-level chronic or pre/postnatal exposure. *Int. J. Immunopharmacol.*, 2:69–80, 1980b.

Luster, M. I., and Dean, J. H.: Immunologic hypersensitivity resulting from environmental or occupational exposure to chemicals: a state-of-the-art workshop summary. *Fund. Appl. Toxicol.*, 2:327–330, 1982.

Luster, M. I.; Dean, J. H.; Boorman, G. A.; Lawson, L.; Lauer, L.; Hayes, T.; Rader, J.; and Dieter, M.: Host resistance and immune functions in methyl and ethyl carbamate treated mice. *Clin. Exp. Immunol.*, 50:223–230, 1982a.

Luster, M. I.; Dean, J. H.; and Moore, J. A.: Evaluation of immune functions in toxicology. In Hayes, W. (ed.): *Methods in Toxicology*. Raven Press, New York, 1982b, pp. 561–586.

Luster, M. I.; Faith, R. E.; and Kimmel, C. A.: Depression of humeral immunity in rats following chronic developmental lead exposure. *J. Environ. Pathol. Toxicol.*, 1:397–402, 1978.

Luster, M. I.; Faith, R. E.; and Lawson, L. D.: Effects of 2,3,7,8-tetrachlorodibenzofuran (TCDF) on the immune system in guinea pigs. *Drug Chem. Toxicol.*, 2:49–60, 1979a.

Luster, M. I.; Faith, R. E.; McLachlan, J. A.; and Clark, G. C.: Effect of *in utero* exposure to diethylstilbestrol on the immune system in mice. *Toxicol. Appl. Pharmacol.*, 47:287–293, 1979b.

Luster, M. I.; Faith, R. E.; and Moore, J. A.: Effects of polybrominated biphenyls (PBB) on immune response in rodents. *Environ. Health Perspect.*, 23:227–232, 1978.

Luster, M. I.; Munson, A. E.; Thomas, P. T.; Holsapple, M. P.; Fenters, J. D.; White, K. L.; Lauer, L. D.; Germolec, D. R.; Rosenthal, G. J.; and Dean, J. H.: Development of a testing battery to assess chemical-induced immunotoxicity: National Toxicology Program's guidelines for immunotoxicity evaluation in mice. *Fund. Appl. Toxicol.*, 10:2–19, 1988.

Luster, M. I.; Tucker, J. A.; Germolec, D. R.; Silver, M. T.; Thomas, P. T.; Vore, S. J.; and Bucher, J. R.: Immunotoxity studies in mice exposed to methyl isocyanate. *Toxicol. Appl. Pharmacol.*, 86:140–144, 1986.

Magnusson, B., and Kligman, A. M.: The identification of contact allergens by animal assay. The guinea pig maximization test. *J. Invest. Dermatol.*, 52:268, 1969.

Maibach, H.: Formaldehyde: effects on animal and human skin. In Gibson, J. (ed.): *Formaldehyde Toxicity*. Hemisphere Publishing Corp., New York, 1983, pp. 166–174.

Malmgren, R. A.; Bennison, B. E.; and McKinley, T. W., Jr.: Reduced antibody titers in mice treated with carcinogenic and cancer chemotherapeutic agents. *Proc. Soc. Exp. Biol. Med.*, 70:484–488, 1952.

Marzulli, F. N., and Maibach, H. I.: Contact allergy: predictive testing in humans. In Marzulli, F. N., and Maibach, H. I. (eds.): *Dermatoxicology*. Hemisphere Publishing Corp., New York, 1987, pp. 319–340.

McConnell, E. E.: *Acute and Chronic Toxicity, Carcinogenesis, Reproduction, Teratogenesis, and Mutagenesis in Animals*. Elsevier/North-Holland Biomedical Press, New York, 1980, pp. 241–266.

McNeill, D. A.; Ritz, H. L.; Evans, B. L. B.; Deskin, R.; Russell, J. L.; and Fisher, G. L.: Immunological responses of guinea pigs to subchronic inhalation of detergent dusts containing various levels of enzyme antigens. *Toxicologist*, 6:66, 1986.

Menna, J. H.; Barnett, J. B.; and Soderberg, L. S. F.: Influenza type A virus infection of mice exposed *in utero* to chlordane; survival and antibody studies. *Toxicol. Lett.*, 24:45–52, 1985.

Miller, K., and Brown, R. C.: The immune system and asbestos-associated disease. In Dean, J. H.; Luster, M. I.; Munson, A. E.; and Amos, H.: *Immunotoxicology and Immunopharmacology*. Raven Press, New York, 1985, pp. 429–440.

Moore, J. A.; Gupta, B. N.; and Vos, J. G.: Toxicity of 2,3,7,8-tetrachlorodibenzofuran—preliminary results. In *Proc. Natl. Conf. on Polychlorinated Biphenyls*. Environmental Protection Agency, Washington, D.C., 1976, pp. 77–79.

Muller-Eberhard, H. J.: Complement. *Annu. Rev. Biochem.*, 44:697, 1975.

Munson, A. E., and Fehr, K. O.: Immunological effects of cannabis. In Fehr, K. O., and Kalant, H. (eds.): *Adverse Health and Behavioral Consequences of Cannabis Use*. Working Papers for the ARS/WHO Scientific Meeting, Toronto, 1981; Addiction Research Foundation, Toronto, 1983, pp. 257–353.

NIEHS Contract NO1–ES90004: *Investigation of the Immunological, Toxicological Effects of PBB in Michigan Farmers and Chemical Workers, Progress Report*. 1983.

Norman, P. S.: Skin testing. In Rose, N. R., and Frailman, H. (eds.): *Manual of Clinical Immunology*. American Society for Microbiology, Washington, D.C., 1976, p. 585.

Ohi, G.; Fukunda, M.; Seta, H.; and Yagyu H.: Methylmercury on humoral immune responses in mice under conditions stimulated to practical situations. *Bull. Environ. Contam. Toxicol.*, 15:175–190, 1976.

Olson, L. J.; Erickson, B. J.; Hinsdill, R. D.; Wyman, J. A.; Porter, W. P.; Binning, L. K.; Bidgood, R. C.; and Nordheim, E. V.: Aldicarb immunomodulation in mice: an inverse dose-response to parts per billion levels in drinking water. *Arch. Environ. Contam. Toxicol.*, 16:433–439, 1987.

Parker, C. W.: Allergic reactions in man. *Pharmacol. Rev.*, 34(1):85–104, 1982.

Patterson, R.; Zeiss, C. R.; and Pruzansky, J. J.: Immunology and immunopathology of trimellitic anhydride inhalation reactions. *J. Allergy Clin. Immunol.*, 70:19–23, 1982.

Peltonen, L., and Fräki, J.: Prevalence of dichromate sensitivity. *Contact Dermatitis*, 9:190–194, 1980.

Penn, I.: Tumors occurring in organ transplant recipients. In Klein, G., and Weinhouse, S. (eds.): *Advances in Cancer Research*, Vol. 28. Academic Press, Inc., New York, 1978, pp. 31–61.

————: Neoplastic consequences of immunosuppression. In Dean, J. H.; Luster, M. I.; Munson, A. E.; and Amos, H. E. (eds.): *Immunotoxicology and Immunopharmacology.* Raven Press, New York, 1985, pp. 79–89.

Penninks, A. H.; Kuper, F.; Spit, B. J.; and Seinen, W.: On the mechanism of dialkyltin induced thymus involution. *Immunopharmacology,* **10**:1–10, 1985a.

————: Neoplastic consequences of immunosuppression. In Dean, J. H.; Luster, M. I.; Munson, A. E.; and Amos, H. E. (eds.): *Immunotoxicology and Immunopharmacology.* Raven Press, New York, 1985b, pp. 79–89.

Perlmann, P.; Perlmann, H.; Larsson, A.; and Wahlin, B.: Antibody-dependent cytolytic effector lymphocytes (K cells) in human blood. *J. Reticuloendothel. Soc.,* **17**:241, 1975.

Poland, A., and Glover, E.: Stereospecific, high affinity binding of 2,3,7,8-tetrachlorodibenzo-*p*-dioxin by hepatic cytosol. *J. Biol. Chem.,* **251**:4936–4945, 1976.

————: 2,3,7,8-Tetrachlorodibenzo-*p*-dioxin: segregation of toxicity with the *Ah* locus. *Mol. Pharmacol.,* **17**:86–94, 1980.

Popa, V.; Teculescu, D.; Stanescu, D.; and Gavrilescu, N.: Bronchial asthma and asthmatic bronchitis determined by simple chemicals. *Dis. Chest,* **56**(5):395–404, 1969.

Rao, D. S. V. S., and Glick, B.: Pesticide effects on the immune response and metabolic activity of chicken lymphocytes. *Proc. Soc. Exp. Biol. Med.,* **154**:27–29, 1977.

Reeves, A. L., and Preuss, O. P.: The immunotoxicity of beryllium. In Dean, J. H.; Luster, M. I.; Munson, A. E.; and Amos, H. E. (eds.): *Immunotoxicology and Immunopharmacology.* Raven Press, New York, 1985, pp. 441–455.

Reggiani, G.: Acute human exposure to TCDD in Seveso, Italy. *J. Toxicol. Environ. Health,* **6**:27–43, 1980.

Reigart, J. R., and Garber, C. D.: Evaluation of the humoral immune response of children with low level lead exposure. *Bull. Environ. Contam. Toxicol.,* **16**:112–117, 1976.

Ritz, H. L., and Bond, G. G.: Respiratory and immunological responses of guinea pigs to repeated intratracheal administration of enzyme-detergent solutions: a comparison of intratracheal and inhalation modes of exposure. *Toxicologist,* **6**:138, 1986.

Ritz, H. L., and Buehler, E. V.: Planning, conduct, and interpretation of guinea pig sensitization patch tests. In Drill, J. A., and Lazur, P. (eds.): *Concepts in Cutaneous Toxicity.* Academic Press, Inc., New York, 1980, pp. 25–40.

Rodgers, K. E.; Imamura, T.; and Devens, B. H.: Organophosphorus pesticide immunotoxicity: effects of *O,O,S*-trimethyl phosphorothioate on cellular and humoral immune response systems. *Immunopharmacology,* **12**:193–202, 1986.

Rosenthal, G. J., and Synder, C. A.: Modulation of the immune response to *Listeria monocytogenes* by benzene inhalation. *Toxicol. Appl. Pharmacol.,* **80**:502–510, 1985.

Ryffel, B., Gotz, U.; and Heuberger, B.: Cyclosporin receptors on human lymphocytes. *J. Immunol.,* **129**:1978–1982, 1978.

Sachs, H. K.: Intercurrent infections in lead poisoning. *Am. J. Dis. Child.,* **32**:315–316, 1978.

Salvaggio, J. (ed.): *Occupational and Environmental Respiratory Disease in NIAID Task Force Report: Asthma and Other Allergic Disease.* U.S. Department of Health, Education and Welfare, Washington, D.C., 1979. (NIH Publication #79–387)

Santiago-Delpin, E. A.: Principles of clinical immunosuppression. In Simmons, R. L. (ed.): *Surgical Clinics of North America,* Vol. 59. W. B. Saunders Co., Philadelphia, 1979, pp. 283–298.

Santos, G. W.: Immunological toxicity of cancer chemotherapy. In Mathe, G., and Oldham, R. K. (eds.): *Complications of Cancer Chemotherapy.* Springer-Verlag, New York, 1974, pp. 20–23.

Saxon, A.; Beall, G. N.; Rohr, A. S.; and Adelman, D. C.: Immediate hypersensitivity reactions to betalactam antibiotics. *Ann. Intern. Med.,* **107**:204–215, 1987.

Schorr, W. F.: Cosmetic allergy. A comprehensive study of the many groups of chemical antimicrobial agents. *Arch. Dermatol.,* **104**:459–465, 1971.

Seinen, W., and Penninks, A.: Immune suppression as a consequence of a selective cytotoxic activity of certain organometallic compounds on thymus and thymus-dependent lymphocytes. *Ann. N.Y. Acad. Sci.,* **320**: 499–517, 1979.

Seinen, W.; Vos, J. G.; Brands, R.; and Hooykaas, H.: Lymphocytotoxicity and immunosuppression by organotin compounds. Suppression of GVH reactivity, blast transformation and E. rosette formation by di-*n*-butyldichloride and di-*n*-octyldichloride. *Immunopharmacology,* **1**:343–353, 1979.

Selski, J.; Louria, D. B.; and Thind, I. S.: Influence of lead intoxication on experimental infections. *Clin. Res.,* **23**:417A, 1975.

Settipane, G. A.: Adverse reactions to aspirin and related drugs. *Arch. Intern. Med.,* **141**:328–332, 1981.

Shand, F. L.: Review/commentary: the immunopharmacology of cyclophosphamide. *Int. J. Immunopharmacol.,* **1**:165–171, 1979.

Shigematsu, N.; Ishmaru, S.; Saito, R.; Ikeda, T.; Matsuba, K.; Sugiyams, K.; and Masuda, Y.: Respiratory involvement in PCB poisoning. *Environ. Res.,* **16**:92–100, 1978.

Silkworth, J. B., and Loose, L. D.: Cell-mediated immunity in mice fed either Aroclor 1016 or hexachlorobenzene. *Toxicol. Appl. Pharmacol.,* **45**:326–327, 1978.

————: PCB and HCB induced alteration of lymphocyte blastogenesis. *Toxicol. Appl. Pharmacol.,* **49**:86, 1979.

Small, W.: Increasing castor bean allergy in southern California due to fertilizer. *J. Allergy,* **23**:406, 1952.

Smialowicz, R. J.; Riddle, M. M.; Rogers, R. R.; Luebke, R. W.; Copeland, C. B.; and Adams, R. C.: Immunotoxicity of tributyltin oxide in rats exposed as adults or preweanlings. *Toxicologist,* **8**:80, 1988.

Smith, S. H.; Sanders, V. M.; Barrett, B. A.; Borzelleca, J. E.; and Munson, A. E.: Immunotoxicology evaluation on mice exposed to polychlorinated biphenyls. *Toxicol. Appl. Pharmacol.,* **45**:A336, 1978.

Snoeij, N. J.; Penninks, A. H.; and Seinen, W.: Biological activity of organotin compounds—an overview. *Environ. Res.,* **44**:335–353, 1987.

————: Dibutyltin and tributyltin compounds induce thymic atrophy in rats due to a selective action on thymic lymphoblasts. *Int. J. Immunopharmacol.,* **10**:889–891, 1988.

Stankus, R. P., and Salvaggio, J. B.: The immunology of experimental and human silicosis. In Dean, J. H.; Luster, M. I.; Munson, A. H.; and Amos, H. (eds.): *Immunotoxicology and Immunopharmacology.* Raven Press, New York, 1985, pp. 423–428.

Stjernsward, J.: Effect of noncarcinogenic and carcinogenic hydrocarbons on antibody-forming cells measured at the cellular level *in vitro*. *J. Natl. Cancer Inst.,* **36**:1189–1195, 1966.

Street, J. C.: Pesticides and the immune system. In Sharma, R. P. (ed.): *Immunologic Considerations in Toxicology*. CRC Press, Inc., Boca Raton, Fla., 1981, pp. 46–66.

Street, J. C., and Sharma, R. P.: Quantitative aspects of immunosuppression by selected pesticides. *Toxicol. Appl. Pharmacol.*, **29**:135–136, 1974.

Stutman, O., and Cuttito, M. J.: Normal levels of natural cytotoxic cells against solid tumors in NK-deficient beige mice. *Nature*, **270**:254–257, 1981.

Szczeklik, A.: Analgesics, allergy and asthma. *Drugs*, **32**:148–163, 1986.

Tapper, M. L.: Infections complicating the alcoholic host. In Grieco, M. H. (ed.): *Infections in the Abnormal Host*. Yorke Medical Books, New York, 1980, p. 474.

Tennenbaum, J. I.; Ruppert, R. D.; St. Pierre, R. L.; and Greenberger, N. J.: The effect of chronic alcohol administration on the immune responsiveness of rats. *J. Allergy*, **44**:272–278, 1969.

Theofilopoulos, A. N.: Autoimmunity. In Sites, D. P.; Stobo, J. D.; Fudenberg, H. H.; and Wells, J. V. (eds.): *Basic and Clinical Immunology*. Lange Medical Pub., Los Altos, Calif., 1982, pp. 156–188.

Thigpen, J. E.; Faith, R. E.; McConnell, E. E.; and Moore, J. A.: Increased susceptibility to bacterial infection as a sequela of exposure to 2,3,7,-8-tetrachlorodibenzo-*p*-dioxin. *Infect. Immun.*, **12**:1319–1324, 1975.

Thind, I. S., and Kahn, M. Y.: Potentiation of the neurovirulence of Langat virus infection by lead intoxication in mice. *Exp. Mol. Pathol.*, **29**:342–347, 1978.

Thomas, P. T.; Busse, W. W.; Kerkvliet, N. I.; Luster, M. I.; Munson, A. E.; Murray, M.; Roberts, D.; Robinson, M.; Silkworth, J.; Sjoblad, R.; and Smialowicz, R.: Immunologic effects of pesticides. In Baker, S. R., and Wilkinson, C. F. (eds.): *The Effects of Pesticides on Human Health*, Vol. 18. Princeton Scientific Publishers, Inc., New York, 1990a, pp. 261–295.

Thomas, P. T., and Faith, R. E.: Adult and perinatal immunotoxicity induced by halogenated aromatic hydrocarbons. In Dean, J. H.; Luster, M. I.; Munson, A. E.; and Amos, H. E. (eds.): *Immunotoxicology and Immunopharmacology*. Raven Press, New York, 1985, pp. 305–313.

Thomas, P. T., and Hinsdill, R. D.: Effect of polychlorinated biphenyls on the immune responses of rhesus monkeys and mice. *Toxicol. Appl. Pharmacol.*, **44**:41–52, 1978.

———: Perinatal PCB exposure and its effects on the immune system of young rabbits. *Drug Chem. Toxicol.*, **3**:173–184, 1980.

Thomas, P. T.; Ratajczak, H. V.; Demetral, D.; Hagen, K.; and Baron, R.: Aldicarb immunotoxicology: functional analysis of cell mediated immunity and quantitation of lymphocyte subpopulations. *Fund. Appl. Toxicol.*, 1990b.

Thomas, P. T.; Ratajczak, H. V.; Eisenberg, W. C.; Furedi-Machacek, M.; Ketels, K. V.; and Barbera, P. W.: Evaluation of host resistance and immunity in mice exposed to the carbamate pesticide aldicarb. *Fund. Appl. Toxicol.*, **9**:82–89, 1987.

Thomson, A. W.: FK-506—how much potential? *Immunol. Today*, **10**:6–9, 1989.

Thurmond, L. M., and Dean, J. H.: Immunological responses following inhalation exposure to chemical hazards. In Gardner, E. E.; Crapo, J. D.; and Massaro, E. J. (eds.): *Toxicology of the Lung*. Raven Press, New York, 1988, pp. 375–406.

Toyama, I., and Kolmer, J. A.: The influence of arsphenamine and mercuric chloride upon complement and antibody production. *J. Immunol.*, **3**:301–316, 1981.

Urso, P., and Gengozian, N.: Depressed humoral immunity and increased tumor incidence in mice following *in utero* exposure to benzo(a)pyrene. *J. Toxicol. Environ. Health*, **6**:569–576, 1980.

Van Arsdel, P. P., Jr.: Drug allergy, an update. *Med. Clin. North Am.*, **65**(5):1089–1103, 1981.

Vecchi, A.: Some aspects of immune alterations induced by chloro-dibenzo-*p*-dioxin and chlorodibenzofurans. In Berlin, A.; Dean, J.; Draper, M. H.; Smith, E. M. B.; and Spreafico, F. (eds.): *Immunotoxicology*. Martinus Nijhoff Publishers, Dordrecht, 1987, pp. 308–316.

Vos, J. G.; Brouwer, G. M. J.; van Leenwen, F. X. R.; and Wagenaar, S. J.: Toxicity of hexachlorobenzene in the rat following combined pre- and post-natal exposure. Comparison of effects on immune system, liver and lung. In Gibson, G. G.; Hubbard, R.; and Parke, D. V. (eds.): *Immunotoxicology*, Academic Press, New York, 1983, pp. 219–230.

Vos, J. G.; de Klerk, A.; Krajno, E. I.; Kruizinga, W.; van Ommen, B.; and Rozing, J.: Toxicity of bis-(tributyltin) oxide in the rat. II. Suppression of thymus-dependent immune responses and of parameters of nonspecific resistance after short-term exposure. *Toxicol. Appl. Pharmacol.*, **75**:387–408, 1984a.

Vos, J. G.; Faith, R. E.; and Luster, M. I.: *Immune Alterations*. Elsevier/North-Holland Biomedical Press, New York, 1980, pp. 241–266.

Vos, J. G.; Koeman, J. H.; Van Der Maas, H. L.; Ten Noever De Braaw, M. C.; and De Vos, R. H.: Identification and toxicological evaluation of chlorinated dibenzofuran and chlorinated naphthalene in two commercial polychlorinated biphenyls. *Toxicology*, **8**:625–673, 1970.

Vos, J. G.; Moore, J. A.; and Zinkl, J. G.: Effects of 2,3,7,8-tetrachlorodibenzo-*p*-dioxin on the immune system of laboratory animals. *Environ. Health Perspect.*, **5**:149–162, 1973.

Vos, J. G.; van Logten, M. J.; Kreeftenberg, J. G.; and Kruizinga, W.: Effect of triphenyltin hydroxide on the immune system of the rat. *Toxicology*, **29**:325–336, 1984b.

Wahlberg, J. E.: Sensitization and testing of guinea pigs with nickel sulfate. *Dermatologica*, **152**:321–330, 1976.

Ward, E. C.; Murray, M. J.; and Dean, J. H.: Immunotoxicity of nonhalogenated polycyclic aromatic hydrocarbons. In Dean, J. H.; Luster, M. I.; Munson, A. E.; and Amos, H. (eds.): *Immunotoxicology and Immunopharmacology*. Raven Press, New York, 1985, pp. 291–304.

Ward, E. C.; Murray, M. J.; Lauer, L. D.; House, R. V.; and Dean, J. H.: Persistent suppression of humoral and cell-mediated immunity in mice following exposure to the polycyclic aromatic hydrocarbon, 7,12-dimethyl-benz[a]anthracene. *Int. J. Immunopharmacol.*, **8**:13–22, 1986.

Webb, D. R., and Winkelstein, A.: Immunosuppression, immunopotentiation and anti-inflammatory drugs. In Stites, D. P.; Stobo, J. D.; Fudenberg, H. H.; and Wells, J. V. (eds.): *Basic and Clinical Immunology*, 4th ed. Lange Medical Publications, Los Altos, Calif., 1982, pp. 277–292.

Weening, J. J.; Hoedemuekinr, P. J.; and Bukker, W. W.: Immunoregulation and antinuclear antibodies in mercury induced glomerulopathy in the rat. *Clin. Exp. Immunol.*, **45**:64–71, 1981.

Wells, J. V.: Immune mechanisms in tissue damage. In Stites, D. P.; Stobo, J. D.; Fudenberg, H. H.; and Wells, J. V. (eds.): *Basic and Clinical Immunology*.

Lange Medical Publications, Los Altos, Calif., 1982, pp. 136–150.

White, D. J.: *Cyclosporin A: Proc. Int. Conf.* Elsevier Biomedical, Amsterdam, 1982.

White, K. L.; Lysy, H. H.; McCay, J. A.; and Anderson, A. C.: Modulation of serum complement levels following exposure to polychlorinated dibenzo-*p*-dioxins. *Toxicol. Appl. Pharmacol.* **84**:209–219, 1986.

Wierda, D.; Irons, R. D.; and Greenlee, W. F.: Immunotoxicity in C57BL/6 mice exposed to benzene and Aroclor 1254. *Toxicol. Appl. Pharmacol.,* **60**:410–417, 1981.

Wojdani, A., and Alfred, L. J.: *In vitro* effects of certain polycyclic hydrocarbons on mitogen activation of mouse T-lymphocytes: action of histamine. *Cell. Immunol.,* **77**:132–142, 1983.

Wysocki, J.; Kalina, Z.; and Owczarzy, I.: Serum levels of immunoglobulins and C-3 component of complement in persons occupationally exposed to chlorinated pesticides. *Med. Prac.,* **36**:111–117, 1985.

Zeiss, C. R.; Wolkonsky, P.; Pruzansky, J. J.; and Patterson, R.: Clinical and immunologic evaluation of trimellitic anhydride workers in multiple industrial settings. *J. Allergy Clin. Immunol.,* **70**:15–18, 1982.

Zwilling, B. S.: The effect of respiratory carcinogenesis on systemic humoral and cell-mediated immunity of Syrian Golden hamsters. *Cancer Res.,* **37**:250–252, 1977.

Chapter 10

TOXIC RESPONSES OF THE LIVER

Gabriel L. Plaa

INTRODUCTION

Liver injury induced by chemicals has been recognized as a toxicologic problem for over 100 years (Zimmerman, 1978). Around 1880, scientists were concerned about the hepatic disposition of lipids following exposure to yellow phosphorus. Hepatic lesions produced by arsphenamine, carbon tetrachloride, and chloroform were also studied in laboratory animals over 50 years ago. During the same period, the association between excessive ethanol consumption and hepatic cirrhosis was established.

It was recognized early that "liver injury" is not a single entity; the lesion observed depends not only on the chemical agent involved but also on the duration of exposure. After acute exposure, one usually finds hepatocellular lipid accumulation *(steatosis)*, hepatocellular necrosis, or hepatobiliary dysfunction, whereas cirrhotic or neoplastic changes are usually considered to be the result of chronic exposures. No single mechanism seems to govern the appearance of degenerative hepatocellular changes or alterations in hepatic function. Some forms of liver injury are reversible, whereas others result in a permanently altered organ. The mortality associated with various forms of liver injury varies. The incidence of injury differs among animal species, and a relationship between dose and effect may not always be apparent. It is no wonder that today the phrase "produces liver injury" has little meaning to the toxicologist; the nature of the injury requires precision before its consequences can be assessed.

MORPHOLOGIC AND FUNCTIONAL CONSIDERATIONS

The classic manner of presenting the relationships between the hepatic cell, its vascular supply, and the biliary system has been the configuration of the hexagonal lobule (Figure 10–1), as introduced by Kiernan in 1833. In the center of this lobule, one finds the terminal hepatic venule (central vein) and at the periphery, the portal space, containing a branch of the portal vein, an hepatic arteriole, and a bile duct. Based on this configuration, zonal pathologic lesions of the hepatic parenchyma are classified as centrilobular (pericentral), midzonal, or periportal.

It is now clear that the hexagonal lobule configuration does not correspond to the functional unit of the liver. Injection of colored gelatin mixtures into the portal vein or the hepatic artery shows that terminal afferent vessels supply blood to only sectors of adjacent hepatic lobules. These sectors occur around terminal portal branches and extend from the central vein of one hexagon to the central vein of an adjacent hexagon. This led Rappaport and coworkers to define the parenchymal mass in terms of functional units called the *liver acini* (Rappaport, 1980). The simple liver acinus consists of a small parenchymal mass that is irregular in size and shape and is arranged around an axis consisting of a terminal portal venule, an hepatic arteriole, a bile ductule, lymph vessels, and nerves (Figure 10–2). This acinus lies between two or more terminal hepatic venules (central veins) with which its vascular and biliary axis interdigitates. There is no physical separation between two liver acini. The hepatic cells of the simple acini are in cellular and sinusoidal contact with the cells of adjacent or overlapping acini. Even with this extensive communication, the hepatic cells of one particular acinus are preferentially supplied by their parent vessels. There are circulatory zones within each acinus. Rappaport (1980) has divided these into three, depending on their distance from the supplying terminal vascular branch (Figure 10–2). Three or more simple acini can constitute what is called *complex acinus*. This unit consists of three simple units and a sleeve of parenchyma around the preterminal afferent vessels, the lymph vessels, and the nerves that eventually give origin to the terminal axial channels of the simple acini.

Although it was assumed for some time that the various hepatic parenchymal cells within the

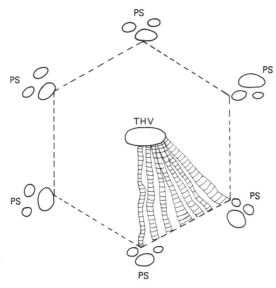

Figure 10–1. Schematic representation of the classic hexagonal lobule. *PS* is the portal space, consisting of a branch of the portal vein, an hepatic arteriole, and bile duct; *THV* is the terminal hepatic venule (central vein).

liver lobule have the same kind of functional specificity, it now appears that there are zonal differences in hepatic function within the liver acinus (Gumucio, 1989). Quantitative zonal differences in cytochrome P-450 monooxygenase, glucuronidation, sulfation, and glutathione-*S*-transferase activities have been observed. Hepatic metabolic and enzymic zonation has led to a reappraisal of the liver acinus concept (Lamers *et al.*, 1989). Recently, Zajicek and coworkers (Arber *et al.*, 1988) demonstrated that hepatocytes normally migrate from the portal space to the terminal hepatic vein *(cell streaming)* as they age (life span in the rat is about 200 days); thus, cells originally found in zone 1 eventually appear in zone 3. The functional characteristics of the cells at the various stages of zonal migration have yet to be determined. Nevertheless, the liver acinus is thought to be composed of two cellular compartments, one progenitor and the other functional; however, hepatocytes in the progenitor zone, which coincides with zone 1, also exhibit functional activity. The concept of heterogeneity in various hepatic cells and in various zones is only in a state of early development. The concept, however, may permit a better rationalization of differing mechanisms of action in the development of lesions associated with hepatotoxicants.

The classic descriptions of focal, midzonal, periportal, and centrilobular lesions are compatible with Rappaport's zonal acinar configuration (Rappaport, 1980). Centrilobular necrosis, for

instance, involves a region that corresponds to the distal acinar zone (zone 3 in Figure 10–2). Regeneration is thought to occur from cells located in the midzonal region of the classic representation; this would correspond to the acinar zone closest to the terminal afferent vessel (zone 1), a zone shown to be particularly high in cytogenic enzyme activity. Therefore, it would appear that the acinar circulatory visualization of the hepatic lobule does not come in conflict with earlier descriptions of pathologic lesions.

Morphologically, chemical-induced injury can manifest itself in different ways. The acute effects can consist of an accumulation of lipids (steatosis, fatty liver) and the appearance of degenerative processes leading to cell death (necrosis). The necrotic process can affect small groups of isolated parenchymal cells *(focal necrosis)*, groups of cells located in zones *(centrilobular, midzonal, or periportal necrosis)*, or virtually all the cells within an hepatic lobule *(massive necrosis)*. Steatosis can also be zonal or more widespread. While the acute injury caused by carbon tetrachloride and chloroform usually consists of both necrosis and steatosis, it is not necessary that both features be present to constitute liver injury. For example, tannic acid, when administered acutely, produces centrilobular necrosis, but extensive fat accumulation does not occur. Thioacetamide also produces centrilobular necrosis without a marked accumulation of lipids. Ethionine, on the other hand, produces

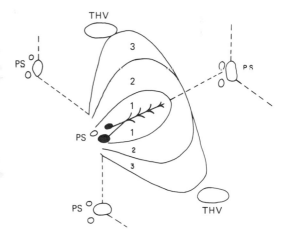

Figure 10–2. Schematic representation of a simple hepatic acinus. *PS* is the portal space, consisting of a branch of the portal vein, an hepatic arteriole, and a bile duct; *THV* is the terminal hepatic venule (central vein); *1, 2,* and *3* represent the various zones drifting off the terminal afferent vessel *(in black).* (Modified from Rappaport, A. M.: Anatomic considerations. In Schiff, L., (ed.): *Diseases of the Liver,* 3rd ed. J. B. Lippincott Co., Philadelphia, 1969.)

steatosis upon acute administration with little or no necrosis. Chemical-induced liver injury resulting from chronic exposure can produce marked alterations of the entire liver structure with degenerative and proliferative changes observed in the different forms of cirrhosis. Neoplastic changes may be another end point of chemical liver injury.

CLASSIFICATION OF CHEMICAL-INDUCED LIVER INJURY

There are a variety of ways of classifying hepatic lesions induced by various chemical substances. In addition to acute hepatic necrosis and steatosis (Table 10–1), there is cholestasis (Table 10–2). This latter lesion results in diminution or cessation of bile flow, with ensuing retention of bile salts and bilirubin. The retention of bilirubin leads to the presence of jaundice. Industrial chemicals are not usually associated with cholestasis, although a large number of drugs are (Table 10–2). Another hepatic lesion, a type of chemical-induced hepatitis resembling closely that produced by viral infections, can occur with certain drugs. The drugs associated with this lesion are less numerous (Table 10–2). Some drugs are also associated with a mixed type of lesion, that is, one that possesses both cholestatic and hepatocellular components (Zimmerman, 1978).

In 1979, the U.S. Public Health Service promulgated a set of guidelines for the detection of hepatotoxicity due to drugs and chemicals (Davidson *et al.*, 1979). A classification scheme for drug- and chemical-induced liver injury was formulated and the hepatic lesions were divided into two categories. *Type I lesions* are those that

Table 10–1. EXAMPLES OF ACUTE HEPATOTOXIC CHEMICALS

CHEMICAL	PRODUCES NECROSIS	PRODUCES STEATOSIS	REFERENCE*
Acetaminophen	X		1
Allyl alcohol	X		2
Allyl formate		X	3
Aflatoxin	X	X	4
Amanita phalloides	X	X	1
Azaserine	X	X	1
Beryllium	X		1
Bromobenzene	X		1
Bromotrichloromethane	X	X	1
Carbon tetrachloride	X	X	1
Cerium		X	5
Chloroform	X	X	1
Cycloheximide		X	1
Dimethylaminoazobenzene	X	X	2
Dimethylnitrosamine	X	X	1
Emetine		X	1
Ethanol		X	1
Ethionine		X	1
Furosemide	X		1
Galactosamine	X	X	1
Methotrexate		X	1
Mithramycin	X		1
Mitomycin C		X	1
Penicillum islandicum	X	X	6
Phosphorus	X	X	1
Puromycin		X	1
Pyrrolizidine alkaloids	X	X	1
Tannic acid	X	X	1
Tetrachloroethane	X	X	3
Tetracycline		X	1
Thioacetamide	X		1
Trichloroethylene	X	X	2
Urethane	X		1
Valproic acid		X	7

  * (1) Zimmerman, 1978; (2) Rouiller, 1964; (3) Rees and Tarlow, 1967; (4) Raisfeld, 1974; (5) Lombardi and Recknagel, 1962; (6) Uraguchi *et al.*, 1961; (7) Olson *et al.*, 1987.

Table 10–2. **EXAMPLES OF DRUG-ASSOCIATED LIVER INJURY**

DRUG	REFERENCE*	DRUG	REFERENCE*
Intrahepatic Cholestasis			
Ajmaline	1	Methyltestosterone	1
p-Aminobenzylcaffeine	1	Methylthiouracil	1
p-Aminosalicylic acid	2	Nitrofurantoin	1
Amitriptyline	3	Norethandrolone	1
Arsphenamine	1	Norethyndrol	1
Azathioprine	1	Oxacillin	1
Carbamazepine	1	Oxandrolone	1
Carbarsone	2	Oxymetholone	1
Carbimazole	1	Oxyphenisatin	1
Chlordiazepoxide	1	Penicillamine	1
Chlorpromazine	1	Perphenazine	1
Chlorpropamide	1	Phenindione	1
Chlorthiazide	2	Prochlorperazine	1
Diazepam	1	Promazine	1
Erythromycin estolate	1	Propoxyphene	1
Estradiol	1	Propylthiouracil	1
Ethacrynic acid	1	Quinethazone	1
Fluphenazine	1	Thiobendazol	1
Haloperidol	1	Thioridazine	1
Imipramine	1	Thiothixene	1
Mepazine	1	Thiouracil	1
Mestranol	1	Tolazamide	1
Methandrostenolone	1	Tolbutamide	1
Methimazole	1	Triacetyloleandomycin	1
17-Methylnortestosterone	1	Triflupromazine	1
Virallike Hepatitis			
Acetoheximide	3	Methoxyflurane	1
p-Aminosalicylic acid	4	α-Methyldopa	1
Carbamazepine	4	Nialamide	3
Cinchophen	1	Oxyphenisatin	1
Colchicine	4	Papaverine	1
Dantrolene	1	Phenelzine	3
Ethacrynic acid	4	Phenindione	4
Ethionamide	1	Phenylbutazone	1
Halothane	1	Phenylisopropylhydrazine	3
Ibufenac	1	Pyrazinamide	1
Indomethacin	1	Sulfamethoxazole	4
Imipramine	1	Sulfisoxazole	4
Iproniazid	1	Tranylcypromine	4
Isoniazid	1	Trimethobenzamide	4
6-Mercaptopurine	1	Zoxazolamine	1

* (1) Zimmerman, 1978; (2) Popper and Schaffner, 1959; (3) Schaffner and Raisfeld, 1969; (4) Perez *et al.*, 1972.

are "predictable, dose- and time-dependent, occurring in most, if not all, subjects exposed to appropriate doses of the causative substance; the lesions are usually readily reproducible in animals." *Type II lesions* are those that are "nonpredictable, dose- and time-independent, occurring sporadically and often becoming apparent only after monitoring a large number of exposed individuals; the lesions usually are not reproducible in animals." It is important to note that the distinction between a type I and a type II lesion is made on the basis of predictability, dose

and time dependency, frequency of appearance, and reproducibility in animals; the actual morphologic characteristics of the liver injury are not used for classification in this scheme.

For a morphologic classification, the five categories of reactions elaborated by Popper and Schaffner (1959) are still quite appropriate. The first is called "zonal hepatocellular alterations without inflammatory reaction." The substances included in this group all produce zonal changes, either necrosis or steatosis (Table 10–1). Because of its great reproducibility in several animal species, its dose dependence, and its predictable character, this type of lesion is probably the best understood type of hepatic injury (a type I lesion).

The second category is called "intrahepatic cholestasis." This group contains chemicals that are capable of producing, in a small percentage of the population, a jaundice resembling that produced by extrahepatic biliary obstruction (Table 10–2). The important histologic features associated with this response are presence of bile stasis, dilatation of the canaliculi with subsequent loss of the microvilli, and occurrence of focal necrosis. There appears to be little relationship between dose and effect, and production of the lesion in animals is not possible with most of these substances (a type II lesion).

The third category is called "hepatic necrosis with inflammatory reaction." The progression to a massive necrosis characteristic of viral hepatitis (Table 10–2) is a prominent feature. The incidence is usually extremely low, dose dependency does not seem to exist, and reproducibility of these lesions in animals is quite difficult (a type II lesion).

The fourth category is called an "unclassified group." This grouping contains a variety of hepatic injuries that do not fit into any type of scheme. The lesions can be associated with manifestations of pathology in several other organs.

The fifth category consists of those agents producing "hepatic cancer." A number of chemicals are now recognized as being hepatocarcinogens in animals.

CELLULAR SITES OF LIVER INJURY

For the last 50 years, many investigators have been interested in unraveling hepatotoxic mechanisms, particularly those involved in carbon tetrachloride–induced liver injury. Historically, the determination of biochemical mechanisms of action was limited by the methodology available at the time. Efforts centered around the evolution of biochemical approaches to the functioning of various structural components of the hepatocyte. The various organelles affected by different hepatotoxicants are summarized in Table 10–3. Some agents affect multiple cellular sites. The relative importance of these sites in hepatocellular degeneration or dysfunction has not been resolved (Popper, 1988). Studies relating biochemical changes to hepatocellular dysfunction represent a more fruitful approach to unraveling mechanisms of action. Mitochondria, the endoplasmic reticulum, and lysosomes have all received considerable attention, but interest in alterations in plasma membrane permeability is

now much greater than it was in the past. A number of biochemical parameters are now used for detecting liver dysfunction or injury in humans (Zimmerman, 1978) and laboratory animals (Plaa and Hewitt, 1989).

MECHANISMS OF LIVER INJURY

Accumulation of Lipids

A number of agents that produce liver injury also cause the accumulation of abnormal amounts of fat, predominantly triglyceride, in the parenchymal cells (Table 10–1). Triglyceride accumulation is the result of an imbalance between the rate of synthesis and the rate of release of triglyceride by the parenchymal cells into the systemic circulation.

A block in the secretion of hepatic triglyceride into plasma is the major mechanism underlying the steatosis induced in rats by carbon tetrachloride, ethionine, phosphorus, puromycin, tetracycline, or orotic acid (Lombardi, 1966; Dianzani, 1979; Deboyser et al., 1989). The accumulation of triglycerides in the hepatic cells is paralleled by a decrease in the concentration of plasma lipids and plasma lipoproteins. The plasma concentration of triglyceride in fasted rats can be diminished to almost one-half its normal value within 30 minutes after exposure to carbon tetrachloride. By two hours, triglycerides have begun to accumulate abnormally in the liver. Tetracycline induces steatosis and interferes with triglyceride secretion (Deboyser et al., 1989).

When hepatic triglyceride is released into the plasma, it is not released as such but is combined with a lipoprotein. Carbon tetrachloride and ethionine can lower the level of circulating lipoprotein. The very-low-density lipoproteins are principally affected. This fraction is involved in the transport of hepatic triglycerides to extrahepatic tissues. A decrease in the proportion of triglyceride combined with lipoprotein can occur if (1) synthesis of triglyceride and the other lipid moieties increases, (2) synthesis of the protein moiety is decreased, (3) the two moieties are formed but do not associate, and (4) the formed lipoprotein is normal but cannot be secreted by the cell. Carbon tetrachloride, ethionine, phosphorus, and puromycin can interfere with the synthesis of the protein moiety (Dianzani, 1979). Although there is evidence that all these substances can affect synthesis of lipoproteins, it is by no means clear that this is the only mechanism involved. With ethionine and phosphorus, this factor is most likely the key defect; however, Recknagel (1967) has pointed out that with carbon tetrachloride the coupling

Table 10–3. EXAMPLES OF HEPATOTOXICANTS AFFECTING VARIOUS ORGANELLES

ORGANELLES AFFECTED	COMPOUND	REFERENCE*
Plasma membrane	Acetaminophen	12
	Amanita phalloides	1
	Carbon tetrachloride	13
	Phalloidin	1
Endoplasmic reticulum	Allyl formate	2
	Carbon tetrachloride	3
	Dimethylaminoazobenzene	2
	Dimethylnitrosamine	4
	Ethionine	1
	Galactosamine	5
	Phosphorus	2
	Pyrrolizidine alkaloids	6
	Tannic acid	1
	Thioacetamide	1
Mitochondria	Acetaminophen	12
	Amanita phalloides	2
	Carbon tetrachloride	3
	1,1-Dichloroethylene	7
	Dimethylnitrosamine	2
	Ethionine	1
	Hydrazine	8
	Phosphorus	2
	Pyrrolizidine alkaloids	6
Lysosomes	*Amanita phalloides*	1
	Beryllium	9
	Carbon tetrachloride	1
	Ethionine	10
	Phosphorus	10
	Pyrrolizidine alkaloids	6
Nucleus	Aflatoxin	1
	Beryllium	11
	Dimethylnitrosamine	1
	Ethionine	10
	Galactosamine	5
	Hydrazine	8
	Pyrrolizidine alkaloids	6
	Tannic acid	1
	Thioacetamide	1
Cytoskeleton	Cytochalasin B	14
	Norethandrolone	14
	Phalloidin	14

* (1) Zimmerman, 1978; (2) Rouiller, 1964; (3) Recknagel, 1967; (4) Magee and Swann, 1969; (5) Decker and Keppler, 1974; (6) McLean, 1970; (7) Reynolds *et al.*, 1975; (8) Ganote and Rosenthal, 1968; (9) Witschi and Aldridge, 1968; (10) Dianzani, 1976; (11) Witschi, 1970; (12) Placke *et al.*, 1987; (13) Popper, 1988; (14) Phillips and Satir, 1988.

phase of triglyceride secretion is probably affected. With tetracycline, impaired release of very-low-density lipoprotein occurs, and it appears that the association between triglycerides and apoproteins may be the phase affected (Deboyser *et al.*, 1989).

The function of the lipoproteins seems to be one of a vehicle, containing protein, phospholipid, and cholesterol; a defect could thus occur in the synthesis of the phospholipid or cholesterol moieties. In choline-deficient animals, a situation that results in lipid accumulation, phospholipid synthesis is impaired. This effect of choline deficiency can result in impaired release of very-low-density lipoproteins (Lombardi and Oler, 1967). Orotic acid can produce fatty livers when fed to rats and also results in a block in the secretion of very-low-density lipoproteins (Windmueller and von Euler, 1971).

Since the rate of synthesis of triglycerides is

directly proportional to the concentration of the substrates present (fatty acids and glycerophosphate), it is theoretically possible that increased hepatic triglyceride synthesis could occur because of increased fatty acids or increased glycerophosphate. Little evidence supports the idea that altered fatty acid metabolism is involved in the development of steatosis following the administration of most hepatotoxicants. However, a microvesicular, zone-specific hepatic steatosis observed after valproic acid administration is thought to be due to inhibition of β-oxidation of fatty acids resulting from inhibited ketogenesis (Olson et al., 1987). Increased mobilization of free fatty acids from adipose tissue has also been proposed as a possible mechanism. In the case of carbon tetrachloride, Recknagel (1967) concluded that accelerated movement of fatty acids from peripheral stores is not a factor to be considered. The peripheral stores play a permissive rather than a controlling role.

Steatosis does not necessarily lead to death of the hepatocytes; ethionine, puromycin, and cycloheximide all cause fat accumulation without producing necrosis. Promethazine protects rats against the necrogenic effects of carbon tetrachloride but does not abolish the fatty liver (Rees et al., 1961). Following partial hepatectomy in rats, a largely hormone-mediated mobilization of fat from adipose tissue occurs; neutral fat accumulates in the remainder of the liver within 18 to 24 hours, reaching a value ten times that of normal livers and bringing about distortion of the normal lobular pattern (Bucher and Malt, 1971). The hepatic cells, in the presence of this fat, still function as well as normal.

Protein Synthesis

With many hepatotoxicants known to produce necrosis, relatively similar morphologic changes occur rapidly after the administration of the agent. Loss of cytoplasmic basophilic material occurs well before the appearance of hepatocellular damage. Cytoplasmic vacuoles appear within one hour after injection of carbon tetrachloride. At this time, the endoplasmic reticulum is also abnormal; the membranes are less well defined and dilated. Similar observations were reported when rats were administered dimethylnitrosamine, carcinogenic azo dyes, ethionine, and thioacetamide (Magee, 1966).

Magee (1966) doubts that these changes actually represent early changes leading to necrosis. He feels that they are merely related to the inhibitory effects of these substances on protein synthesis. Ethionine, dimethylnitrosamine, carbon tetrachloride, thioacetamide, and galactosamine inhibit incorporation of amino acids into liver proteins. Some investigators have

thought that inhibition of protein synthesis is the cause of liver necrosis, but this cannot be considered to be entirely correct, since ethionine and cycloheximide inhibit protein synthesis for many hours but do not result in liver necrosis (E. Farber, 1971).

Extensive work has been carried out to determine how various agents affect protein synthesis (Dianzani, 1976). Ethionine replaces methionine and forms S-adenosylethionine, which leads to a trapping of cellular adenine, a diminution in the rate of ATP synthesis, and inhibition of RNA synthesis. Dimethylnitrosamine probably acts by causing a loss of messenger RNA. Inhibition of protein synthesis in rat liver by carbon tetrachloride is thought to occur by an action on single unit ribosomes and not on polysomes (E. Farber, 1971); the damage induced by carbon tetrachloride appears to be irreversible in contrast to observations made with ethionine or puromycin.

Galactosamine also inhibits protein synthesis; reduced synthesis of RNA has been observed (Decker and Keppler, 1974). The depression is the result of a UTP deficiency induced by galactosamine; galactosamine-1-phosphate formed in the liver leads to the accumulation of UDP derivates of galactosamine; in turn, this results in depletions of hepatic UTP, UDP hexoses, and a depression of uracil nucleotide – dependent biosynthesis of macromolecules. This is believed to result in injury to cellular organelles. Galactosamine-induced liver injury passes through several stages, depending on the dosage schedule (reversible acute hepatitis, chronic progressive hepatitis, cirrhosis, production of liver tumors), but is highly specific to this amino sugar. In addition, morphologic studies indicate that all hepatocytes are affected to a varying degree, so that the result is an experimental model of diffuse liver cell injury (Medline et al., 1970).

Lipid Peroxidation

Slater (1966) and Recknagel (Recknagel and Ghoshal, 1966) independently proposed that homolytic cleavage of the carbon-chlorine bond in carbon tetrachloride yielded free radicals that could then interact with neighboring lipid-rich material, causing alterations in structure and function. Recknagel and Ghoshal (1966) hypothesized that free radicals attacked the methylene bridges of unsaturated fatty acid side chains of microsomal lipids, resulting in morphological alteration of the endoplasmic reticulum, loss of activity of drug-metabolizing enzymes, loss of glucose-6-phosphatase activity, loss of protein synthesis, and loss of the capacity of the liver to form and excrete low-density lipoproteins. They demonstrated the appearance of conjugated dienes, typical of peroxidized polyenoic fatty acids. In subsequent work, the appearance *in vivo* of conjugated dienes was observed in animals and in humans subjected to the intoxicating doses of carbon tetrachloride. In the rat, conjugated dienes, evidence of lipid peroxidation, appear within one hour after carbon tetrachloride administration. Extensive work carried out by a number of investigators has laid the foundation of the lipid peroxidation theory as it concerns carbon tetrachloride liver injury (Recknagel, 1967; Recknagel and Glende, 1973; Comporti, 1985).

Carbon tetrachloride–induced alterations in membrane lipids of the hepatic endoplasmic reticulum are observed shortly after treatment (Comporti, 1985). Both the simple addition of carbon tetrachloride free radicals to fatty acids and a chain termination addition reaction of carbon tetrachloride free radicals to fatty acid free radicals containing conjugated dienes are observed; the latter products possess abnormal physical characteristics. The binding of carbon tetrachloride free radicals to microsomal lipids occurs under aerobic and anaerobic environments. Lipids undergo peroxidation and depression of glucose-6-phosphatase—however, only in an aerobic environment. The peroxidative cleavage of unsaturated fatty acids can result in the release of carbonyl compounds or formation of carbonyl functions in the acyl residue; these products can move from their site of origin to other membrane sites. Some of them are toxicologically active and have been identified as 4-hydroxyalkenals (Comporti, 1985).

Alpers and coworkers (1968) studied the role of lipid peroxidation in the pathogenesis of carbon tetrachloride–induced inhibition of protein synthesis. They found *in vivo* that the administration of antioxidants prevents the appearance of steatosis and necrosis; however, protein synthesis does not appear to be altered by the administration of antioxidants. These authors concluded that the demonstration of lipid peroxidation *in vitro* may not always imply functional damage to the subcellular component affected. They raised the possibility that *in vivo* inhibition of protein synthesis may not have a direct relationship to the degree of lipid peroxidation. There is still some controversy regarding the relative importance of carbon tetrachloride–induced peroxidation in the subsequent pathologic changes, and there are inconsistent reports in the literature (Plaa and Witschi, 1976). It is clear that additional events are involved in the pathologic changes that result in fat accumulation, alteration of the cell membrane, and cellular necrosis (Recknagel *et al.*, 1982;

Recknagel, 1983). Lipid peroxidation, in itself, is unable to account for all these events.

Klaassen and Plaa (1969) found no evidence of the presence of conjugated dienes after administration of chloroform in rats with doses that resulted in steatosis and necrosis; furthermore, they found no depression of glucose-6-phosphatase. Brown and coworkers (1974) reported that rats pretreated with phenobarbital, but not untreated rats, produce conjugated dienes during chloroform anethesia; depression of glucose-6-phosphatase activity also occurs after chloroform only in phenobarbital-pretreated rats (Lavigne and Marchand, 1974). Since chloroform-induced liver injury is more severe in phenobarbital-pretreated rats, the possibility exists that the initial lesion induced by chloroform in these animals is only aggravated by the appearance of lipid peroxidation. These findings cast doubt on the general applicability of lipid peroxidation as a mechanism for necrogenic haloalkanes.

Lipid peroxidation along with elevated liver triglycerides is reported to occur after tetrachloroethane administration in mice (Tomokuni, 1970). Sell and Reynolds (1969) compared the lesions produced by iodoform and carbon tetrachloride. Morphologically, the lesions were quite comparable, and lipid peroxidation occurred within 30 minutes, being associated with a depression in glucose-6-phosphatase activity. Lipid peroxidation also occurs after phosphorus poisoning in rats (Ghoshal *et al.*, 1969). *In vitro*, lipid peroxidation is associated with the following halomethanes: bromotrichloromethane, carbon tetrabromide, bromoform, iodoform, and dibromochloromethane (de Groot and Noll, 1989).

Several other hepatotoxicants are known to produce acute liver necrosis in the absence of *in vivo* demonstration of lipid peroxidation (Plaa and Witschi, 1976; Cluet *et al.*, 1986): 1,1-dichloroethylene, trichloroethylene, ethylene dibromide, dimethylnitrosamine, and thioacetamide. With halothane and ethanol, some evidence of lipid peroxidation exists, but its importance in the pathogenesis of their hepatotoxic effects is still unresolved (Comporti, 1985; Knights *et al.*, 1988). While there is no doubt that lipid peroxidation does occur with some hepatotoxicants, it is evident that with others this component is either absent or of doubtful significance. Lipid peroxidation as a general mechanism of action for hepatotoxicants is less attractive than it was several years ago (Anders, 1988; Popper, 1988).

Calcium Homeostasis

The role of calcium as a mediator of toxicant-induced hepatocyte death has been a matter of conjecture for more than 30 years (J. L. Farber, 1982; Plaa and Hewitt, 1989); early alterations in calcium homeostasis were first reported with carbon tetrachloride–induced liver injury. Accumulation of calcium in the liver accompanies the cell death produced by a variety of other hepatotoxicants (acetaminophen, galactosamine, phalloidin, chloroform, carbon disulfide, and 1,1-dichloroethylene). These observations are consistent with the hypothesis that toxicant-induced hepatocellular injury results in the influx of Ca^{2+} into the cell, initiating a series of cytotoxic events common to various hepatotoxicants and resulting in cell death.

Intracellular distribution of calcium exerts a profound influence on cell metabolism, motility, and division. Thus, intracellular calcium homeostasis is of importance to cell viability. Disruption of Ca^{2+} homeostasis related to activation of molecular oxygen (oxidative stress) is gaining considerable interest (Thomas and Reed, 1989). Sites identified as being involved in Ca^{2+} transport and storage include the plasma membrane, endoplasmic reticulum, mitochondria, and cytosol. Of importance in terms of the role of calcium in the pathogenesis of cell injury is the fact that substantial calcium is obtained in the mitochondrial and endoplasmic reticular pools; the redistribution of calcium from these pools into the cytosol can elevate cytosolic free Ca^{2+} concentration to the point where initiation of cell injury may occur. Depletion of the endoplasmic reticular pool is preceded by the oxidation of cellular glutathione, suggesting that an alteration of the thiol redox status could be responsible for the sequence of events observed in oxidative stress. A role for extracellular Ca^{2+} in hepatocyte death is not universally accepted (Plaa and Hewitt, 1989; Thomas and Reed, 1989). Carbon tetrachloride, bromobenzene, cadmium, and adriamycin cytotoxicity to isolated hepatocytes are enhanced in calcium-free environments. Many conclusions are based on laboratory findings obtained with isolated hepatocytes or liver subcellular fractions. Thus, it is difficult to establish cause-and-effect relationships to the production of liver injury *in vivo*. Although the bulk of the evidence indicates that calcium plays an important role in hepatotoxicity, a multiplicity of pathways exists by which calcium may exert its effects. The relative importance of the participation of calcium in cell injury depends on the nature of the chemical insult.

Immunologic Reactions

Some forms of drug-induced liver injury can be attributed to hypersensitivity reactions (Zimmerman, 1978; Lewis and Zimmerman,

1989). Those associated with other clinical signs of hypersensitivity (fever, rash, eosinophilia), as well as histologic evidence of drug allergy (eosinophilic or granulomatous inflammation), include chlorpromazine, phenytoin, *p*-aminosalicylic acid, sulfonamides, and erythromycin estolate. Reappearance of clinical signs on rechallenge is characteristic with these agents. In these instances, the drug or its metabolite probably acts as a hapten. Other drugs may produce immunologically based reactions that are unaccompanied by other indications of hypersensitivity. These reactions may be the result of aberrant biotransformation leading to hepatotoxic metabolites. Some drugs suspected of such reactions include halothane, isoniazid, and valproic acid.

Evidence indicates that halothane-induced hepatotoxicity can be considered as two entities (Benjamin *et al.*, 1985; Hubbard *et al.*, 1988). A mild form of liver injury is seen shortly after anesthesia and can be reproduced in animals; the other form, delayed and severe, appears to be due to an immune-mediated mechanism. Patients with halothane-induced liver injury can generate liver antibodies that react with trifluoroacetyl-carrier proteins. There is also the suggestion that enflurane, as well as the trifluroracetyl halide metabolite of halothane, covalently binds to similar hepatic proteins and may become immunogens in susceptible individuals (Christ *et al.*, 1988; Pohl *et al.*, 1988).

Cholestasis

The mechanisms involved in drug-induced cholestasis are still poorly understood. One of the major reasons for this deficiency lies in the fact that, with the possible exception of some steroids, it is extremely difficult to reproduce in animals the drug-induced cholestatic syndrome seen in humans. It is possible, however, to produce cholestatic responses in animals with certain chemicals that have no therapeutic utility. The induction of intrahepatic cholestasis in animals following the administration of certain bile acids, α-naphthylisothiocyanate (ANIT), certain steroids, and manganese has provided important contributions to the understanding of the characteristics, and perhaps the causes, of the cholestatic syndrome (Plaa and Priestly, 1976; Tuchweber *et al.*, 1986).

Lithocholic acid is a naturally occurring monohydroxy bile acid that exhibits both choleretic and cholestatic properties. The taurine conjugate of lithocholic acid (taurolithocholic acid), when administered intravenously in the rat, results in a prompt diminution of bile flow. The cessation of bile flow is dose dependent, and bile flow usually returns to normal within six hours. Prolonged infusions result in hyperbilirubinemia. The canalicular microvilli are reduced in size and number; the Golgi apparatus is dilated and vacuolated. Taurocholate can compete with taurolithocholate and can antagonize the cholestatic response induced by the latter substance. Intracanalicular precipitates have been invoked to explain the cholestatic effects of some bile acids; with others, however, correlations are unclear (Tuchweber *et al.*, 1986). The structure and permeability of the membrane of the bile canaliculus can be affected by cholestatic bile acids. Taurolithocholate and lithocholate are associated with augmented cholesterol content of the membrane; interestingly, an unidentified hepatocellular cytosolic protein appears to be involved in this process and the ensuing cholestasis (Yousef *et al.*, 1984; Dahlström-King and Plaa, 1989). Evidence of increased canalicular permeability has been observed with lithocholate. Cholestasis in isolated rat livers perfused with lithocholic, chenodeoxycholic, glycolithocholic, or taurolithocholic acid has been reported. The three α-sulfate esters of taurolithocholic acid and glycolithocholic acid are less cholestatic than the nonsulfated conjugates. Chenodeoxycholate causes hepatocellular necrosis in rats. Lithocholate and chenodeoxycholate differ in the mechanisms by which they produce cholestasis (Plaa and Priestly, 1976). Chenodeoxycholate is cytotoxic, and cholestasis seems to result from a generalized hepatocellular dysfunction, whereas lithocholate seems to interact directly with the bile secretory function of the canalicular membrane.

A single oral dose of ANIT produces both bile stasis and hyperbilirubinemia in the rat; the cessation of bile flow occurs within 24 hours (Plaa and Priestly, 1976). Electron microscopic studies also indicate alterations of hepatocellular membranes. ANIT can affect several hepatocellular functions. In addition to the development of hyperbilirubinemia, sulfobromophthalein (BSP) retention and inhibition of microsomal drug-metabolizing activity have been demonstrated. The bilirubin retention induced by ANIT could be due to a number of defects in hepatic cell function. The maximal rate of biliary bilirubin excretion is diminished in ANIT-treated animals. ANIT can increase the synthesis of bilirubin from nonerythropoietic sources; this effect can be demonstrated two hours after its administration. While all these mechanisms could participate in the response, it is predominantly the decrease in biliary excretion of bilirubin that contributes to the hyperbilirubinemia observed.

There is a considerable amount of indirect evidence that indicates that the cholestatic properties of ANIT may be due to a metabolite. A marked species variation is observed; both the cholestatic and hyperbilirubinemic responses can be enhanced if the animals are pretreated with enzyme inducers; inhibitors of microsomal enzyme activity can diminish the ANIT response; temperature can also affect the response; inhibitors of protein synthesis are known to reduce markedly the cholestatic and hyperbilirubinemic responses to ANIT.

The cholestatic reaction associated with the clinical use of anabolic and contraceptive steroids has prompted experimental studies designed to characterize the response in animals. Imai and Hayashi (1970) reported that large doses of norethisterone produce jaundice consistently in mice. Canalicular bile plugs were observed after treatment with norethisterone, methyltestosterone, oxymetholone, mestranol, or norethandrolone. No plugs were observed when testosterone proprionate, progesterone, or 17β-estradiol was administered. Electron microscopy revealed dilatation of the bile canaliculi and a decrease in the appearance of microvilli. An important strain difference was observed. Anabolic steroids do cause BSP retention in rabbits (Plaa and Priestly, 1976). With ethinyl estradiol, reduced bile flow was observed in rats as well as altered membrane fluidity (Miccio *et al.*, 1989). Estrogens can affect the permeability of the biliary tree, reduce bile salt–independent bile flow, and decrease the clearance of infused bile salts; it is not clear which parameter is of major importance in producing the cholestatic reaction. With various oral contraceptive steroids, decreased bile flow and a decrease in biliary excretory maximum for bilirubin have been reported, but the mechanism has not been elucidated. Certain glucuronide conjugates of naturally occurring estrogens can produce a dose-dependent, reversible cholestasis in rats or monkeys (Meyers *et al.*, 1980, 1981; Slikker *et al.*, 1983); D-ring conjugates are active, whereas A-ring conjugates are not. The canalicular membrane appears to be the site of action; both bile salt–dependent and bile salt–independent bile flow are depressed. Whether during pregnancy these D-ring conjugates can attain concentrations sufficient to induce intrahepatic cholestasis remains to be determined.

Intrahepatic cholestasis can also be produced in rats by the administration of an intravenous load of manganese sulfate (Witzleben, 1972). Manganese ingestion has been associated with hepatotoxicity in humans (Lustig *et al.*, 1982). In the rat, this response is associated with the development of necrotic lesions, which varies from focal necrosis to subtotal midzonal necrosis. Widespread dilatation of bile canaliculi with loss of microvilli is observed 20 hours after treatment. Biliary excretion of bilirubin is markedly diminished in the manganese-loaded rats; there is no correlation between the extent of necrosis and the cholestatic response. Manganese treatment followed by bilirubin infusion can cause a more severe cholestasis; recovery of bile flow is partial at 24 hours and essentially complete at 48 hours. Small doses of manganese produce cholestasis only if followed by an injection of bilirubin; a close relationship exists between manganese and bilirubin in order to elicit the fully developed cholestatic response (de Lamirande and Plaa, 1979). The manganese-bilirubin model is particularly interesting, since the severity and duration of cholestasis are dose dependent on bilirubin, whereas the dose of manganese regulates the time period during which bilirubin can exert its effect (de Lamirande and Plaa, 1979). There are indications that the site of action of the manganese-bilirubin combination is the bile canalicular membrane (de Lamirande *et al.*, 1981; Plaa *et al.*, 1982). It is postulated (Ayotte and Plaa, 1985, 1986) that the incorporation of manganese and bilirubin may disrupt bile canalicular membrane fluidity and permeability.

There is still considerable controversy as to whether phenothiazines and tricyclic antidepressants cause cholestasis in humans because of a direct toxic effect or because of a hypersensitivity reaction. These compounds have been the subject of extensive investigation in animals (Plaa and Priestly, 1976; Plaa and Hewitt, 1982). An important species variation exists in chlorpromazine-induced hepatobiliary dysfunction. In the dog and Rhesus monkey, a reduction in bile flow occurs after its acute intravenous administration, whereas chronic administration does not result in cholestasis in rats. Chlorpromazine rapidly inhibits bile flow in a dose-dependent manner in isolated perfused rat livers. Phenothiazines, thioxanthenes, and tricyclic antidepressants are hepatocytotoxic. With chlorpromazine, demethylation, multiple ring hydroxylations, and free radical generation appreciably increase its toxicity. Sulfoxidation results in a striking reduction of toxicity. These observations appear to be more consistent with a direct hepatotoxic action rather than an indirect hypersensitivity response.

A number of mechanisms leading to cholestasis have been proposed based on various experimental results, but these are far from being definitive (Plaa and Priestly, 1976; Plaa and Hewitt, 1982; Schreiber and Simon, 1983; Tuchweber *et al.*, 1986). The mechanisms include impaired bile salt–independent canalicular bile flow (chlorpromazine, ethinylestradiol, ethacrynic acid), canalicular membrane function

(ANIT, taurolithocholate, cytochalasin B), altered ductular cell permeability (ANIT), hypertrophic hypoactive smooth endoplasmic reticulum (bile salts, ANIT), intracanalicular precipitation (taurolithocholate, chlorpromazine, erythyromycin lactobionate), and cytoskeletal modifications of microtubules and microfilaments (phalloidin, cytochalasin B, norethandrolone, manganese-bilirubin).

Cirrhosis

Cirrhosis is a chronic morphologic alteration of the liver that has received a great amount of attention. Histologically, cirrhosis is characterized by the presence of septae of collagen distributed throughout the major portion of the liver (Schinella and Becker, 1975). These appear to form fibrous sheaths in a three-dimensional network, which appear as bands in a two-dimensional histologic section; the circumscribed areas of aggregated liver cells appear as nodules. Invariably, the pattern of hepatic blood flow is altered. In the majority of cases, single-cell necrosis appears as the major element in its pathogenesis. This necrotic process is associated with a deficiency in the repair mechanism of the residual cells; this deficiency leads to fibroblastic activity and scar formation. The pathogenesis of cirrhosis is not at all clearly understood. Other factors, such as intrahepatic vascular alterations, may play a contributory role in the development of cirrhosis.

Cirrhosis can be induced in animals by chronic administration of carbon tetrachloride or aflatoxin or the administration of several chemical carcinogens. In humans, however, the single most important cause of cirrhosis is chronic ingestion of alcoholic beverages (Lelbach, 1975; Rankin *et al.*, 1975). In the usual laboratory animal, cirrhosis, as seen in humans, is not observed after the chronic feeding of ethanol alone (Schinella and Becker, 1975). However, precirrhotic changes (increased hydroxyproline, increased proline incorporation into collagen, and increased collagen proline hydroxylase activity) can be observed after ethanol ingestion. Lieber and DeCarli (1976) reported the production of cirrhosis in baboons after long-term feeding of ethanol.

For a number of decades, a controversy has existed whether ethanol itself causes cirrhosis in humans by a direct hepatotoxic effect or indirectly by a nutritional deficiency closely associated with alcoholism. The proponents of the nutritional theory (Hartroft, 1975) indicate that in dogs and rats the development of cirrhosis depends on the duration of the consumption of ethanol, the percentage of total calories provided by ethanol, and the composition of the accompanying diet; diets that are inadequate in choline, proteins, methionine, vitamin B_{12}, and folic acid favor the development of cirrhosis. Supplementation of the diets with these nutrients appears to abolish the effect of long-term feeding of ethanol. The proponents of the direct hepatotoxic theory (Lieber, 1975) emphasize the requirement of long-term ingestion of large quantities of ethanol by animals on nutritionally adequate diets and the demonstrated effects of precirrhotic changes in the various animal models. The development of cirrhosis in the baboon (Lieber and DeCarli, 1976) maintained on an otherwise nutritionally adequate diet lends considerable weight in favor of the direct hepatotoxic theory.

Carcinogenesis

Chemical carcinogenesis is covered elsewhere in detail (*see* Chapter 5). Consequently, only a brief view of hepatocarcinogenesis will be described in this section.

A wide variety of chemicals can elicit hepatocarcinogenic changes in laboratory animals (Pitot, 1988). Among naturally occurring substances that are liver carcinogens in animals, one finds aflatoxin B_1 and other mycotoxins, some pyrrolizidine alkaloids, cycasin, and safrol. Among synthetic substances, one finds some dialkylnitrosamines, some organochlorine pesticides, certain polychlorinated biphenyls, carbon tetrachloride, chloroform, vinyl chloride, dimethylaminoazobenzene, acetylaminofluorenc, thioacetamide, urethane, ethionine, dimethylbenzanthracene, and galactosamine.

Hepatocarcinogenesis is thought to be a multistage process, including initiation, promotion, and progression (E. Farber, 1982; Pitot, 1988). The initiating event may be a mutation, but perturbations in cell differentiation may also be involved. Acute inhibition of cell proliferation is suggested to be of importance; perhaps this leads to an altered cell population that can grow in the presence of a cytotoxic environment (cell selection). Organizationally, the hepatocytes are not arranged as in the normal adult liver but assume a "pseudofetal" configuration; this organizational difference also expresses itself in biochemical patterns (emergence of fetal isozymes, production of α-fetoprotein and fetal antigens). Each individual neoplasm is unique (pattern of enzymes, antigenic composition, morphologic appearance), and this property is consistent with the hypothesis of an origin from a single clone of cells. The promotion phase is reversible, and dose-dependent relationships, as well as thresholds, can be demonstrated for known promoters. E. Farber (1982) proposes that the histogenesis of hepatocellular carcinoma involves a series of altered or new hepatocytic populations that evolve into malignant neoplasia; each population develops from its immediate precursor by a process of selection.

Little is known about the selection process that favors the development of malignant hepatocytes. Perhaps resistance to necrosis occurs (selective cytotoxicity). Endogenous and exogenous modulating factors are known to affect the incidence and time of appearance of liver cancers; these include nutrients, hormones, drugs, and other chemicals. Their roles are poorly understood, as are immunological factors and the presence of cirrhosis. The absence of such knowledge greatly limits extrapolation of results obtained in animals under controlled conditions to humans exposed in undefined conditions.

FACTORS INVOLVED IN LIVER INJURY

Biotransformation of Toxicants

The phenomenon of biotransformation to a more active metabolite is well known in toxicology. Active metabolites are very important in chemically induced liver injury. The hepatotoxic properties of carbon tetrachloride are caused by cleavage of the carbon-chlorine bond and formation of reactive moieties (Recknagel and Glende, 1973; Sipes and Gandolfi, 1982; Cheeseman *et al.*, 1985). Studies reveal: The cleavage occurs in the endoplasmic reticulum and is mediated by cytochrome P-450; NADPH-dependent flavoproteins do not appear to be involved; both reductive and oxidative metabolism occur; some of the products are incorporated into microsomal lipids and proteins; free radical scavengers and lipid antioxidants protect against the liver injury; inducers of cytochrome P-450 can enhance carbon tetrachloride–induced liver injury. Noguchi and associates (1982) characterized a form of cytochrome P-450 (52,000 daltons) that exhibits high activity for the generation of the trimethyl radical from carbon tetrachloride.

Chloroform is also bioactivated by hepatic enzymes (Cheeseman *et al.*, 1985). Two groups of investigators (Mansuy *et al.*, 1977, Pohl *et al.*, 1977) demonstrated that *in vitro* microsomes derived from phenobarbital-treated rats were capable of converting chloroform to phosgene, a highly reactive electrophilic compound. They proposed that this activation proceeds through the hydroxylation of chloroform to trichloromethanol, which spontaneously dehydrochlorinates to produce phosgene; the site of activation is cytochrome P-450 rather than NADPH cytochrome *c* reductase. The hepatotoxicity of chloroform is augmented by inducers of cytochrome P-450; chloroform treatment also results in the depletion of hepatic glutathione and the alkylation of macromolecules.

A number of other haloalkanes are bioactivated by rat hepatic microsomes (Sipes and Gandolfi, 1982; Cheeseman *et al.*, 1985); some of these proceed to a greater degree under nitrogen than under oxygen (carbon tetrachloride, bromotrichloromethane, halothane). *In vivo*, hypoxia augments the liver injury produced by carbon tetrachloride and halothane. Furthermore, there are important differences among the haloalkanes regarding inducibility and covalent binding properties to microsomal proteins, microsomal lipids, or calf thymus DNA. Biotransformation is a key event in halothane-induced hepatotoxicity (de Groot and Noll, 1983; Pohl *et al.*, 1988).

Biotransformation is important in the case of hepatic lesions produced by bromobenzene (Lau and Monks, 1988). Brodie and coworkers (1971) postulated that the necrosis was produced by an active metabolite of bromobenzene, presumably an epoxide, capable of reacting covalently with macromolecules in liver cells. They showed that liver microsomes could convert bromobenzene to a compound that reacted covalently with glutathione. It was postulated that the epoxide formation is sufficiently great that normal amounts of glutathione cannot protect tissue proteins from alkylation. In this regard, diethyl maleate, which depletes hepatic glutathione, increases the incidence of hepatic lesions produced by low doses of bromobenzene. The toxic metabolite appears to be bromobenzene-3,4-oxide, but other reactive secondary metabolites may also be involved (Buben *et al.*, 1988; Lau and Monks, 1988; Narashimhan *et al.*, 1988).

Recently, an interesting interaction between α-adrenergic blocking agents and bromobenzene, which may be related to the glutathione-dependent detoxification of bromobenzene, has been described; adrenergic blocking agents antagonize bromobenzene hepatotoxicity in mice (Kerger *et al.*, 1988a, 1988b). Bromobenzene bioactivation and pharmacokinetics remain unaltered. The dose-effect characteristics of the protection, however, suggest that the adrenergic agents may block a catecholamine-mediated lowering of hepatic glutathione.

Acetaminophen-induced hepatotoxicity is also caused by a chemically reactive metabolite (Mitchell *et al.*, 1982), presumably *N*-acetyl-*p*-benzoquinone imine (Birge *et al.*, 1988; Koymans *et al.*, 1989). The formation of this metabolite can be followed by the irreversible binding of radiolabel, derived from the acetaminophen to liver protein. Little covalent binding occurs after subtoxic doses, but it increases as the dose approaches the toxic range. Inducers of

cytochrome P-450 enhance formation of the reactive metabolite and liver toxicity, whereas inhibitors reduce metabolite formation and toxicity. The reactive intermediate is further conjugated with glutathione and excreted as a mercapturic acid. Cytochrome P-450 isozymes capable of activating acetaminophen in humans were recently characterized (Raucy *et al.*, 1989).

The experimental work carried out to unravel acetaminophen- and bromobenzene-induced liver injury has led to some very important observations. One is that hepatotoxicity need not be correlated with the pharmacokinetics of the parent substance or even its major metabolites but may be correlated with the formation of quantitatively minor, highly reactive intermediates. A second concept is that a threshold tissue concentration must be attained before liver injury is elicited; if it is not attained, injury does not occur. Third, endogenous substances like glutathione play an essential role in protecting hepatocytes from injury by chemically reactive intermediates; this provides the cell with a means of preventing the reactive metabolite from attaining a critical, effective concentration. Finally, other enzymic pathways, like glutathione transferase and epoxide hydrolase, also play a role in protecting the hepatocyte by catalyzing the further degradation of toxic reactive intermediates. Furthermore, these studies have provided investigators relatively simple biochemical procedures for uncovering the possible existence of potentially toxic chemically reactive metabolites or intermediates in new compounds.

The production of reactive metabolites that bind irreversibly to hepatic proteins is observed in animals with furosemide and acetylisoniazid (Mitchell *et al.*, 1976a). With furosemide, a dose threshold exists for both necrosis and covalent binding, but the threshold in mice is not due to depletion of hepatic glutathione. At subthreshold doses, most of the furosemide is highly bound to plasma proteins and eventually eliminated unchanged, whereas with high doses, plasma binding becomes saturated and more furosemide becomes available for hepatic bioactivation. In the case of acetylisoniazid, the major metabolite of isoniazid, increased covalent binding to liver proteins and enhanced hepatotoxicity are observed in phenobarbital-pretreated rats; enhanced covalent binding also occurs with iproniazid. In both cases, the reactive metabolites are thought to be free radicals arising from monoalkyl diazenes (Mitchell *et al.*, 1976b).

Other hepatonecrogenic responses appear to be due to the production of toxic metabolites. The hepatotoxic effect of dimethylnitrosamine is linked to its biotransformation (Magee and

Swann, 1969). The pyrrolizidine alkaloids in "bush teas" made from *Crotalaria fulva* result in venoocclusive hepatic disease. These substances are said to be converted to toxic metabolites in the liver (Mattocks, 1968). Allyl alcohol and its precursor allyl formate produce periportal necrosis. Rees and Tarlow (1967) showed that allyl formate is converted to a highly reactive aldehyde, acrolein, by alcohol dehydrogenase. Hepatotoxic reactive metabolites have been proposed (Hunter *et al.*, 1977) for thioacetamide and thioacetamide sulfite, the major metabolite of thioacetamide, to account for their acute necrogenic effects. The formation of a reactive epoxide has been proposed to account for the acute focal necrosis seen in rats given aflatoxin B_1; the biochemical characteristics of this epoxide are said to be similar to those described for bromobenzene epoxide (Mgbodile *et al.*, 1975).

Biotransformation also appears to be involved in cholestatic reactions, although the evidence is less striking (Plaa and Hewitt, 1982). With α-naphthylisothiocyanate, the toxicity can be modified by inducers and inhibitors of mixed-function oxidase; the presence of reactive metabolites has been demonstrated, although no correlation with toxicity is apparent. Chlorpromazine metabolites vary in their hepatotoxic properties, as do those of the tricyclic antidepressants. Some estradiol conjugates possess cholestatic properties. Indirect evidence indicates that the cholestatic response elicited in rats by dantrolene is caused by a metabolic product.

Alteration of Hepatic Blood Flow

With some heptatoxicants, alterations in hepatic blood flow are observed as a result of the injury. These alterations manifest themselves 24 hours or more after the injury. Hemorrhagic necrosis occurs in rats after the administration of beryllium (Cheng, 1956). Dimethylnitrosamine produces hemorrhagic necrosis, where the center of the lobule becomes entirely occupied by blood; this "venoocclusive" lesion can be observed ten days after administration of the substance (Magee and Swann, 1969). Similar lesions have been observed in animals and children ingesting *Crotalaria*, a pyrrolizidine alkaloid (McLean, 1970). The lesion seems to be a characteristic of those substances that produce hemorrhagic necrosis and are not typically found after administration of carbon tetrachloride. Butler and Hard (1971) attribute this to the fact that carbon tetrachloride induces a coagulative necrosis of the hepatocytes that does not affect the sinusoid lining cells, permitting retention of an intact vascular pattern; however, dimethylnitrosamine affects both the parenchymal cells and the sinusoid lining cells, resulting in hemorrhage and a collapse of the trabecular reticulin framework around the central veins.

In 1960, Calvert and Brody proposed that hepatic vasoconstriction, due to the elaboration of catecholamines, was the primary effect of carbon tetrachloride. The hypothesis was based on indirect evidence. High spinal cord transection at the level of C6 or C7 protected rats against the necrotic effects of carbon tetrachloride. Larson and Plaa (1965) showed that cordotomy results in hypothermia. They also demonstrated that if cord-transected animals were placed in an incubator to maintain their body temperature, carbon tetrachloride produced its hepatic necrotic effects. Oxygen consumption of transected rats maintained at room temperature dropped markedly. It thus appears that in hypothermic rats metabolic activity of the liver is diminished, and this would explain the apparent protective effects of cervical cordotomy. Large infusions of norepinephrine, epinephrine, or mixtures of these substances do not result in lesions similar to those produced by carbon tetrachloride. In rats sympathectomized immunologically, the hepatic lesion induced by carbon tetrachloride was still present (Larson *et al.*, 1965). Finally, in cats, the data indicate that diminished hepatic blood flow is not a causative factor in the initial phase of carbon tetrachloride liver injury, and at later times increased hepatic arterial blood flow is observed (Lautt and Plaa, 1974). Therefore, it appears that the vascular role attributed to carbon tetrachloride via release of catecholamines can be rejected as a primary cause of hepatic injury.

Potentiation of Hepatotoxicity

Individuals recovering from an acute ingestion of ethanol are more susceptible to the liver-damaging properties of haloalkanes than are individuals not ingesting ethanol. Since the early investigators studying this phenomenon in animals used simultaneous administration of both agents, the explanation seemed to be that ethanol enhanced the absorption of the hydrocarbon. However, the ingestion of ethanol several hours before exposure to the hydrocarbons can cause enhanced toxic responses. The latter phenomenon is observed in mice, rats, and dogs. The haloalkanes shown to exert an enhanced hepatotoxic response after ethanol pretreatment include carbon tetrachloride, chloroform, trichloroethylene, and 1,1,2-trichloroethane (Klaassen and Plaa, 1967).

Cornish and Adefuin (1967) showed that several aliphatic alcohols, such as methanol, ethanol, isopropanol, *n*-butanol, *sec*-butanol, and tert-butanol, also exert a similar potentiating

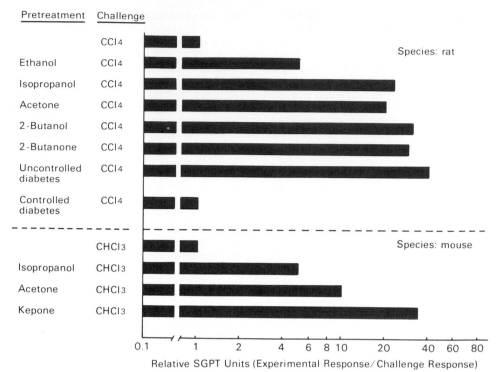

Figure 10–3. Potentiation of haloalkane-induced hepatotoxicity. Rats or mice were subjected to the specified various pretreatments before receiving a challenge dose of carbon tetrachloride or chloroform. Diabetes was produced by administering alloxan, either alone *(Uncontrolled)* or with insulin *(Controlled)*. The severity of the liver injury was assessed 24 hours after the haloalkane challenge using serum glutamic pyruvic transaminase (SGPT) activity. Relative SGPT units were obtained by dividing the activity in the experimenal group *(Pretreatment plus Challenge)* by the activity in the respective control group *(Challenge Alone)*. Details can be found in the following references: Hanasono *et al.*, 1975a; Plaa *et al.*, 1975; Traiger and Bruckner, 1976; W. R. Hewitt *et al.*, 1979, 1980.

effect on the acute inhalation toxicity of carbon tetrachloride. Several examples of potentiation are depicted in Figure 10–3. The remarkable potentiating effect of isopropanol has been studied in detail (Plaa *et al.*, 1975; Plaa, Hewitt, *et al.*, 1982), and the biotransformation of isopropanol to acetone plays a crucial role. Acetone itself can potentiate carbon tetrachloride hepatotoxicity, and the response can be correlated with blood acetone concentrations (Plaa, 1988). The interaction between isopropanol and carbon tetrachloride was documented in two industrial accidents, where workers exposed to both agents exhibited enhanced hepatotoxicity (Folland *et al.*, 1976; Deng *et al.*, 1987).

Isopropanol and acetone also cause enhanced hepatotoxicity with chloroform, trichloroethylene, 1,1,2-trichloroethane, or 1,1,1-trichloroethane (Plaa *et al.*, 1975). Acetone potentiates the responses to 1,1-dichloroethylene, bromodichloromethane, and dibromochloromethane; the subchronic administration of acetone and car-

bon tetrachloride accelerates the appearance of cirrhosis in rats (Plaa, 1988).

With ethanol, the potentiation seems to be due to the presence of the unmetabolized alcohol; however, with isopropanol the effect appears to be caused by the presence of both unmetabolized alcohol and acetone. The results obtained with *n*-butanol resemble those for ethanol, whereas with 2-butanol they resemble those of isopropanol; 2-butanol is also metabolized to a ketone (2-butanone) (Traiger and Bruckner, 1976). The mechanisms underlying the potentiations are not completely known. It appears, however, that the interactions involve cytochrome P-450 in the endoplasmic reticulum. With isopropanol and acetone, one could attempt to explain the potentiation on the basis of enhanced bioactivation of carbon tetrachloride (Sipes *et al.*, 1973), but other possible mechanisms require consideration (Plaa, 1988).

The potentiation of haloalkane hepatotoxicity occurs with a number of different ketonic solvents (W. R. Hewitt *et al.*, 1980; Plaa, 1988); experiments conducted with acetone, 2-butanone, 2-pentanone, 2-hexanone, and 2-heptanone indicate that the carbon skeleton chain length plays a role in determining the relative potentiating capacity of ketonic solvents (W. R. Hewitt *et al.*, 1983). *n*-Hexane, which is biotransformed to methyl *n*-butyl ketone (2-hexanone) and 2,5-hexanedione, also potentiates chloroform toxicity (W. R. Hewitt *et al.*, 1980). Chlordecone (Kepone®), a chlorocyclic pesticide containing a carbonyl group, exhibits remarkable potentiating properties with chloroform, carbon tetrachloride, bromodichloromethane, and dibromochloromethane (Curtis *et al.*, 1979; W. R. Hewitt *et al.*, 1979; Klingensmith and Mehendale, 1981; Plaa, 1988); mirex, the noncarbonyl analog of chlordecone, does not possess this property. 1,3-Butanediol, which is metabolized to the ketone bodies β-hydroxybutyrate and acetoacetate, also potentiates carbon tetrachloride hepatotoxicity in a dose-related manner (W. R. Hewitt *et al.*, 1980; Plaa, 1988), and the effect is associated with the development of the ketotic state (Pilon *et al.*, 1986). Thus, it appears that the potentiation phenomenon observed with these various substances is closely related to the presence of exogenous or endogenous ketones. The mechanisms involved are not completely known, but enhanced bioactivation of a toxic haloalkane metabolite appears to play a major role. With chlordecone potentiation, enhanced formation of haloalkane-derived reactive metabolites, as well as changes in their macromolecular binding in hepatic tissue, has been demonstrated (L. A. Hewitt *et al.*, 1986b); enhanced haloalkane bioactivation is also observed with acetone, 2-butanone, and 2-hexanone (L. A. Hewitt *et al.*, 1987). Nevertheless, there are indications that other mechanisms may be involved (Plaa, 1988; Rao *et al.*, 1989).

The diabetic state induced in rats by either alloxan or streptozotocin enhances the hepatotoxic properties of carbon tetrachloride (Figure 10–3); reversal of the diabetic state by insulin treatment can prevent the potentiated response (Hanasono *et al.*, 1975a; Villarruel *et al.*, 1982). Chemically induced diabetes can also enhance the response to chloroform, 1,1,2-trichloroethene, galactosamine, bromobenzene, or thioacetamide (Hanasono *et al.*, 1975b; El-hawari and Plaa, 1983; Watkins *et al.*, 1988). However, Price and Jollow (1982) observed no potentiation of acetaminophen liver injury in streptozotocin-diabetic rats; instead, an increased resistance to the hepatotoxicant was observed. The mechanisms involved have yet to be resolved, but increased bioactivation of

haloalkanes has been demonstrated (Villarruel *et al.*, 1982).

Potentiation of the liver injury is not limited to necrogenic hepatotoxicants. With cholestatic agents, such interactions are less frequent but are observed (Plaa, 1988). Inducers of mixed-function oxidase can enhance the acute cholestatic or hyperbilirubinemic response to α-naphthylisothiocyanate; isopropanol and acetone potentiate its hyperbilirubinemic effect. Rats maintained on 1,3-butanediol exhibit potentiated cholestatic responses to taurolithocholate or manganese-bilirubin injections; with α-naphthylisothiocyanate, the hyperbilirubinemia is enhanced but not the depression in bile flow (de Lamirande and Plaa, 1981). Methyl *n*-butyl ketone and methyl isobutyl ketone can aggravate taurolithocholate-induced cholestasis in rats (Plaa, 1988). Thus, ketones and a ketogenic chemical (1,3-butanediol) enhance some types of cholestatic reactions. The mechanisms involved are not known; some evidence suggests the bile canalicular membrane as a possible site of action (L. A. Hewitt *et al.*, 1986a). Some unpredictable cholestatic drug reactions in humans indicate that other associated predisposing conditions (altered metabolic state, interacting chemicals) may be involved. This concept warrants further investigation in light of the results obtained experimentally.

REFERENCES

Alpers, D. H.; Solin, M.; and Isselbacher, K. J.: The role of lipid peroxidation in the pathogenesis of carbon tetrachloride–induced liver injury. *Mol. Pharmacol.*, **4**: 566–573, 1968.

Anders, M. W.: Bioactivation mechanisms and hepatocellular damage. In Arias, I. M.; Jakoby, W. B.; Popper, H.; Schachter, D.; and Shafritzs, D. A. (eds.): *The Liver: Biology and Pathobiology*, 2nd ed. Raven Press, New York, 1988, pp. 389–400.

Arber, N.; Zajicek, G.; and Ariel, I.: The streaming liver II. Hepatocyte life history. *Liver*, **8**: 80–87, 1988.

Ayotte, P., and Plaa, G. L.: Hepatic subcellular distribution of manganese in manganese and manganese-bilirubin induced cholestasis. *Biochem. Pharmacol.*, **21**: 3857–3865, 1985.

———: Modification of biliary tree permeability in rats treated with a manganese-bilirubin combination. *Toxicol. Appl. Pharmacol.*, **84**: 295–303, 1986.

Benjamin, S. B.; Goodman, Z. D.; Ishak, K. G.; Zimmerman, H. J.; and Irey, N. S.: The morphologic spectrum of halothane-induced hepatic injury: analysis of 77 cases. *Hepatology*, **5**: 1163–1171, 1985.

Birge, R. B.; Bartolone, J. B.; Nishanian, E. V.; Bruno, M. K.; Mangold, J. B.; Cohen, S. D.; and Khairallah, E. A.: Dissociation of covalent binding from the oxidative effects of acetaminophen. Studies using dimethylated acetaminophen derivatives. *Biochem. Pharmacol.*, **37**: 3383–3393, 1988.

Brodie, B. B.; Reid, W. D.; Cho, A. K.; Sipes, I. G.; Krishna, G.; and Gillette, J. R.: Possible mechanism of liver necrosis caused by aromatic organic compounds. *Proc. Natl. Acad. Sci. USA*, **68**: 160–164, 1971.

Brown, B. R., Jr.; Sipes, I. G.; and Sagalyn, A. M.: Mechanisms of acute hepatic toxicity: chloroform, halothane, and glutathione. *Anesthesiology*, **41**: 554–561, 1974.

Buben, J. A.; Narasimhan, N.; and Hanzlik, R. P.: Effects of chemical and enzymic probes on microsomal covalent binding of bromobenzene and derivatives. Evidence for quinones as reactive metabolites. *Xenobiotica*, **18**: 501–510, 1988.

Bucher, N. L. R., and Malt, R. A.: *Regeneration of Liver and Kidney*. Little, Brown & Co., Boston, 1971.

Butler, W. H., and Hard, G. C.: Hepatotoxicity of dimethylnitrosamine in the rat with special reference to veno-occlusive disease. *Exp. Mol. Pathol.*, **15**: 209–219, 1971.

Calvert, D. N., and Brody, T. N.: Role of the sympathetic nervous system in CCl$_4$ hepatotoxicity. *Am. J. Physiol.*, **198**: 669–676, 1960.

Cheeseman, K. H.; Albano, E. F.; Tomasi, A.; and Slater, T. F.: Biochemical studies on the metabolic activation of halogenated alkanes. *Environ. Health Persp.*, **64**: 85–101, 1985.

Cheng, K. K.: Experimental studies on the mechanism of the zonal distribution of beryllium liver necrosis. *J. Pathol. Bacteriol.*, **71**: 265–276, 1956.

Christ, D. D.; Kenna, J. G.; Kammerer, W.; Satoh, H.; and Pohl, L. R.: Enflurane metabolism produces covalently bound liver adducts recognized by antibodies from patients with halothane hepatitis. *Anesthesiology*, **69**: 833–838, 1988.

Cluet, J. -L.; Boisset, M.; and Boudene, C.: Effect of pretreatment with cimetidine or phenobarbital on lipoperoxidation in carbon tetrachloride- and trichloroethylene-dosed rats. *Toxicology*, **38**: 91–102, 1986.

Comporti, M.: Lipid peroxidation and cellular damage in toxic liver injury. *Lab. Invest.*, **53**: 599–623, 1985.

Cornish, H. H., and Adefuin, J.: Potentiation of carbon tetrachloride toxicity by aliphatic alcohols. *Arch. Environ. Health*, **14**: 447–449, 1967.

Curtis, L. R.; Williams, W. L.; and Mehendale, H. M.: Potentiation of the hepatotoxicity of carbon tetrachloride following preexposure to chlordecone (Kepone) in the male rat. *Toxicol. Appl. Pharmacol.*, **51**: 283–293, 1979.

Dahlström-King, L., and Plaa, G. L.: Effect of inhibition of protein synthesis on cholestasis induced by taurolithocholate, lithocholate, and a manganese-bilirubin combination in the rat. *Biochem. Pharmacol.*, **38**: 2543–2549, 1989.

Davidson, C. S.; Leevy, C. M.; and Chamerlayne, E. C.: *Guidelines for Detection of Hepatotoxicity Due to Drugs and Chemicals. NIH Publication No. 79–313.* U.S. Department of Health, Education and Welfare, Washington, D.C., 1979.

Deboyser, D.; Goethals, F.; Krack, G.; and Roberfroid, M.: Investigation into the mechanism of tetracycline-induced steatosis: study in isolated hepatocytes. *Toxicol. Appl. Pharmacol.*, **97**: 473–479, 1989.

Decker, K., and Keppler, D.: Galactosamine hepatitis: key role of the nucleotide deficiency period in the pathogenesis of cell injury and cell death. *Pharmacol. Rev. Physiol. Biochem.*, **71**: 77–106, 1974.

de Groot, H., and Noll, T.: Halothane hepatotoxicity: relation between metabolic activation, hypoxia, covalent binding, lipid peroxidation and liver cell damage. *Hepatology*, **3**: 601–606, 1983.

———: Halomethane hepatotoxicity: induction of lipid peroxidation and inactivation of cytochrome P-450 in rat liver microsomes under low oxygen partial pressures. *Toxicol. Appl. Pharmacol.*, **97**: 530–537, 1989.

de Lamirande, E., and Plaa, G. L.: Dose and time relationships in manganese-bilirubin cholestasis. *Toxicol. Appl. Pharmacol.*, **59**: 467–475, 1979.

———: 1,3-Butanediol pretreatment on the cholestasis induced in rats by manganese-bilirubin combination, taurolithocholic acid, or α-naphthylisothiocyanate. *Toxicol. Appl. Pharmacol.*, **59**: 467–475, 1981.

de Lamirande, E.; Tuchweber, B.; and Plaa, G. L.: Hepatocellular membrane alterations as a possible cause of manganese-bilirubin–induced cholestasis. *Biochem. Pharmacol.*, **30**: 2305–2312, 1981.

Deng, J. -G.; Wang, J. -D.; Shih, T. -S.; and Lan, F. -L.: Outbreak of carbon tetrachloride poisoning in a color printing factory related to the use of isopropyl alcohol and an air conditioning system in Taiwan. *Am. J. Indust. Med.*, **12**: 11–19, 1987.

Dianzani, M. U.: Toxic liver injury by protein synthesis inhibitors. In Popper, H., and Schaffner, F. (eds.): *Progress in Liver Diseases*, Vol. 5. Grune & Stratton, New York, 1976, pp. 232–245.

———: Reactions of the liver to injury: fatty liver. In Farber, E., and Fisher, M. M. (eds.): *Toxic Injury of the Liver*, Part A. Marcel Dekker, Inc., New York, 1979, pp. 281–331.

El-hawari, A. M., and Plaa, G. L.: Potentiation of thioacetamide-induced hepatotoxicity in alloxan- and streptozotocin-diabetic rats. *Toxicol. Appl. Pharmacol.*, **17**: 293–300, 1983.

Farber, E.: Biochemical pathology. *Annu. Rev. Pharmacol.*, **11**: 71–96, 1971.

———: Chemical carcinogenesis: a biologic perspective. *Am. J. Pathol.*, **106**: 271–296, 1982.

Farber, J. L.: Calcium and the mechanisms of liver necrosis. In Popper, H., and Schaffner, F. (eds.): *Progress in Liver Diseases*, Vol. 7. Grune & Stratton, New York, 1982, pp. 347–360.

Folland, D. S.; Schaffner, W.; Grinn, H. E.; Crofford, O. B.; and McMurray, D. R.: Carbon tetrachloride toxicity potentiated by isopropyl alcohol. *JAMA*, **236**: 1853–1856, 1976.

Ganote, C. E., and Rosenthal, A. S.: Characteristic lesions of methylazoxymethanol-induced liver damage. *Lab. Invest.*, **19**: 382–398, 1968.

Ghoshal, A. K.; Porta, E. A.; and Hartroft, W. S.: The role of lipoperoxidation in the pathogenesis of fatty livers induced by phosphorus poisoning in rats. *Am. J. Pathol.*, **54**: 275–291, 1969.

Gumucio, J. J.: Hepatocyte heterogeneity: the coming of age from the description of a biological curiosity to a partial understanding of its physiological meaning and regulation. *Hepatology*, **9**: 154–160, 1989.

Hanasono, G. K.; Côté, M. G.; and Plaa, G. L.: Potentiation of carbon tetrachloride–induced hepatotoxicity in alloxan- or streptozotocin-diabetic rats. *J. Pharmacol. Exp. Ther.*, **192**: 592–604, 1975a.

Hanasono, G. K.; Witschi, H. P.; and Plaa, G. L.: Potentiation of the hepatotoxic responses to chemicals in alloxan-diabetic rats. *Proc. Soc. Exp. Biol. Med.*, **149**: 903–907, 1975b.

Hartroft, W. S.: On the etiology of alcoholic liver cirrhosis. In Khanna, J. M.; Israel, Y.; and Kalant, H. (eds.): *Alcoholic Liver Pathology*. Addiction Research Foundation, Toronto, 1975, pp. 189–197.

Hewitt, L. A.; Ayotte, P.; and Plaa, G. L.: Modifications in rat hepatobiliary function following treatment with acetone, 2-butanone, 2-hexanone, mirex or chlordecone and subsequently exposed to chloroform. *Toxicol. Appl. Pharmacol.*, **83**: 465–473, 1986a.

Hewitt, L. A.; Caillé, G.; and Plaa, G. L.: Temporal relationships between biotransformation, detoxication, and chlordecone potentiation of chloroform-induced hepatotoxicity. *Can. J. Physiol. Pharmacol.*, **64**: 477–482, 1986b.

Hewitt, L. A.; Valiquette, C.; and Plaa, G. L.: The role of biotransformation-detoxication in acetone-, 2-butanone-, and 2-hexanone-potentiated chloroform-induced hepatotoxicity. *Can. J. Physiol. Pharmacol.,* **65**: 2313–2318, 1987.

Hewitt, W. R.; Brown, E. M.; and Plaa, G. L.: Relationship between carbon skeleton length of ketonic solvents and potentiation of chloroform-induced hepatotoxicity in rats. *Toxicol. Lett.,* **16**: 297–304, 1983.

Hewitt, W. R.; Miyajima, H.; Côté, M. G.; and Plaa, G. L.: Acute alteration of chloroform-induced hepato- and nephrotoxicity by mirex and Kepone. *Toxicol. Appl. Pharmacol.,* **48**: 509–527, 1979.

———: Modification of haloalkane-induced hepatotoxicity by exogenous ketones and metabolic ketosis. *Fed. Proc.,* **13**: 3118–3123, 1980.

Hubbard, A. K.; Gandolfi, A. J.; and Brown, B. R., Jr.: Immunological basis of anesthetic-induced hepatotoxicity. *Anesthesiology,* **69**: 814–817, 1988.

Hunter, A. L.; Holscher, M. A.; and Neal, R. A.: Thioacetamide-induced hepatic necrosis. I. Involvement of the mixed-function oxidase enzyme system. *J. Pharmacol. Exp. Ther.,* **200**: 439–448, 1977.

Imai, K., and Hayashi, Y.: Steroid-induced intrahepatic cholestasis in mice. *Jpn. J. Pharmacol.,* **20**: 473–481, 1970.

Kerger, B. D.; Gandy, J. T.; Bucci, J.; Roberts, S. M.; Harbison, R. D.; and James, R. C.: Antagonism of bromobenzene-induced hepatotoxicity by the α-adrenergic blocking agents, phentolamine and idazoxan. *Toxicol. Appl. Pharmacol,* **95**: 12–23, 1988a.

Kerger, B. D.; Roberts, S. M.; Hinson, J. A.; Gandy, J.; Harbison, R. D.; and James, R. C.: Antagonism of bromobenzene-induced hepatotoxicity by phentolamine: evidence for a metabolism-independent intervention. *Toxicol. Appl. Pharmacol.,* **95**: 24–31, 1988b.

Klaassen, C. D., and Plaa, G. L.: Relative effects of various chlorinated hydrocarbons on liver and kidney function in dogs. *Toxicol. Appl. Pharmacol.,* **10**: 119–131, 1967.

———: Comparison of the biochemical alterations elicited in livers from rats treated with carbon tetrachloride, chloroform, 1,1,2-trichloroethane and 1,1,1-trichloroethane. *Biochem. Pharmacol.,* **18**: 2019–2027, 1969.

Klingensmith, J. S., and Mehendale, H. M.: Potentiation of brominated halomethane hepatotoxicity in the male rat. *Toxicol. Appl. Pharmacol.,* **61**: 378–384, 1981.

Knights, K. M.; Gourlay, G. K.; Gibson, R. A.; and Cousins, M. J.: Halothane induced hepatic necrosis in rats: the role of *in vivo* lipid peroxidation. *Pharmacol. Toxicol.,* **63**: 327–332, 1988.

Koymans, L.; van Lenthe, J. H.; van de Straat, R.; Donné-Op den Kelder, G. M.; and Vermeulen, N. P. E.: A theoretical study on the metabolic activation of paracetamol by cytochrome P-450: indications for a uniform oxidation mechanism. *Chem. Res. Toxicol.,* **2**: 60–66, 1989.

Lamers, W. H.; Hilberts, A.; Furt, E.; Smith, J.; Jonges, G. N.; and Moorman, A. F. M.: Hepatic enzymic zonation: a reevaluation of the concept of the liver acinus. *Hepatology,* **10**: 72–76, 1989.

Larson, R. E., and Plaa, G. L.: A correlation of the effects of cervical cordotomy, hypothermia, and catecholamines on carbon tetrachloride–induced hepatic necrosis. *J. Pharmacol. Exp. Ther.,* **147**: 103–111, 1965.

Larson, R. E.; Plaa, G. L.; and Brody, M. J: Immunological sympathectomy and CCl₄ hepatotoxicity. *Proc. Soc. Exp. Biol. Med.,* **116**: 557–560, 1965.

Lau, S. S., and Monks, T. J.: The contribution of bromobenzene to our current understanding of chemically-induced toxicities. *Life Sci.,* **42**: 1259–1269, 1988.

Lautt, W. W., and Plaa, G. L.: Hemodynamic effects of CCl₄ in the intact liver of the cat. *Can. J. Physiol. Pharmacol.,* **52**: 727–735, 1974.

Lavigne, J. G., and Marchand, C.: The role of metabolism in chloroform hepatotoxicity. *Toxicol. Appl. Pharmacol.,* **29**: 312–326, 1974.

Lelbach, W. K.: Quantitative aspects of drinking in alcoholic liver cirrhosis. In Khanna, J. M.; Israel, Y.; and Kalant, H. (eds.): *Alcoholic Liver Pathology.* Addiction Research Foundation, Toronto, 1975, pp. 1–18.

Lewis, J. H., and Zimmerman, H. J.: Drug-induced liver disease. *Med. Clin. North Am.,* **73**: 775–792, 1989.

Lieber, C. S.: Alcohol and the liver: transition from metabolic adaptation to tissue injury and cirrhosis. In Khanna, J. M.; Israel, Y.; and Kalant, H. (eds.): *Alcoholic Liver Pathology.* Addiction Research Foundation, Toronto, 1975, pp. 171–188.

Lieber, C. S., and DiCarli, L. M.: Animal models of ethanol dependence and liver injury in rats and baboons. *Fed. Proc.,* **35**: 1232–1236, 1976.

Lombardi, B.: Considerations on the pathogenesis of fatty liver. *Lab. Invest.,* **15**: 1–20, 1966.

Lombardi, B., and Oler, A.: Choline deficiency fatty liver. Protein synthesis and release. *Lab. Invest.,* **17**: 308–321, 1967.

Lombardi, B., and Recknagel, R. O.: Interference with secretion of triglycerides by the liver as a common factor in toxic liver injury. *Am. J. Pathol.,* **40**: 571–586, 1962.

Lustig, S.; Pitlik, S. D.; and Rosenfeld, J. B.: Liver damage in acute self-induced hypermanganemia. *Arch. Intern. Med.,* **142**: 405–406, 1982.

Magee, P. N.: Toxic liver necrosis. *Lab. Invest.,* **15**: 111–131, 1966.

Magee, P. N., and Swann, P. F.: Nitroso compounds. *Br. Med. Bull.,* **25**: 240–244, 1969.

Mansuy, D.; Beaune, P.; Cresteil, T.; Lange, M.; and Leroux, J. P.: Evidence for phosgene formation during liver microsomal oxidation of chloroform. *Biochem. Biophys. Res. Commun.,* **79**: 513–517, 1977.

Mattocks, A. R.: Toxicity of pyrrolizidine alkaloids. *Nature (Lond.),* **217**: 723–728, 1968.

McLean, E. K.: The toxic actions of pyrrolizidine (senecio) alkaloids. *Pharmacol. Rev.,* **22**: 429–483, 1970.

Medline, A.; Schaffner, F.; and Popper, H.: Ultrastructural features in galactosamine-induced hepatitis. *Exp. Mol. Pathol.,* **12**: 201–211, 1970.

Meyers, M.; Slikker, W.; Pascoe, G.; and Vore, M.: Characterization of cholestasis induced by estradiol-17βD-glucuronide in the rat. *J. Pharmacol. Exp. Ther.,* **214**: 87–93, 1980.

Meyers, M.; Slikker, W.; and Vore, M.: Steroid D-ring glucuronides: characterization of a new class of cholestatic agents in the rat. *J. Pharmacol. Exp. Ther.,* **218**: 63–73, 1981.

Mgbodile, M. U. K.; Holscher, M.; and Neal, R. A.: A possible protective role for reduced glutathione in aflatoxin B₁ toxicity: effect of pretreatment of rats with phenobarbital and 3-methylcholanthrene on aflatoxin toxicity. *Toxicol. Appl. Pharmacol.,* **34**: 128–142, 1975.

Miccio, M.; Orzes, N.; Lunazzi, G. C.; Gassin, B.; Corsi, R.; and Tiribelli, C.: Reversal of ethinyl estradiol-induced cholestasis by epomediol in rat. The role of liver plasma-membrane fluidity. *Biochem. Pharmacol.,* **38**: 3559–3563, 1989.

Mitchell, J. R.; Hughes, H.; Lauterberg, B. H.; and Smith, C. V.: Chemical nature of reactive intermediates as determinant of toxicologic responses. *Drug Metab. Rev.,* **13**: 539–553, 1982.

Mitchell, J. R.; Nelson, S. D.; Thorgeirsson, S. S.;

McMurty, R. J.; and Dubing, E.: Metabolic activation: biochemical basis for many drug-induced liver injuries. In Popper, H., and Schaffner, F. (eds.): *Progress in Liver Diseases,* Vol. 5. Grune & Stratton, New York, 1976a, pp. 259–279.

Mitchell, J. R.; Snodgrass, W. R.; and Gillette, J. R.: The role of biotransformation in chemical-induced liver injury. *Environ. Health Perspect.,* **15**: 27–38, 1976b.

Narashimban, N.; Weller, P. E.; Buben, J. A.; Wiley, R. A.; and Hanzlik, R. P.: Microsomal metabolism and covalent binding of [^{3}H/^{14}C]-bromobenzene. Evidence for quinones as reactive metabolites. *Xenobiotica,* **18**: 491–499, 1988.

Noguchi, T.; Fong, K. L.; Lai, E. K.; Alexander, S. S.; King, M. M.; Olson, L.; Poyer, J. L.; and McCay, P. B.: Specificity of a phenobarbital-induced cytochrome P-450 for metabolism of carbon tetrachloride to the trichloromethyl radical. *Biochem. Pharmacol.,* **31**: 615–624, 1982.

Olson, M. J.; Handler, J. F.; and Thurman, R. G.: Mechanism of zone-specific hepatic steatosis caused by valproate: inhibition of ketogenesis in periportal regions of liver lobule. *Mol. Pharmacol.,* **30**: 520–525, 1987.

Perez, V.; Schaffner, F.; and Popper, H.: Hepatic drug reactions. In Popper, H., and Schaffner, F. (eds.): *Progress in Liver Diseases,* Vol. 4. Grune & Stratton, New York, 1972, pp. 597–625.

Phillips, M. J., and Satir, P.: The cytoskeleton of the hepatocyte: organization, relationships, and pathology. In Arias, I. M.; Jakoby, W. B.; Popper, H.; Schachter, D.; and Shafritzs, D. A. (eds.): *The Liver: Biology and Pathobiology,* 2nd ed. Raven Press, New York, 1988, pp. 11–27.

Pilon, D.; Brodeur, J.; and Plaa, G. L.: 1,3-Butanediol-induced increases in ketone bodies and potentiation of CCl$_4$ hepatotoxicity. *Toxicology,* **40**: 165–180, 1986.

Pitot, H. C.: Hepatic neoplasia: chemical induction. In Arias, I. M.; Jakoby, W. B.; Popper, H.; Schachter, D.; and Shafritzs, D. A. (eds.): *The Liver: Biology and Pathobiology,* 2nd ed. Raven Press, New York, 1988, pp. 1125–1146.

Plaa, G. L.: Experimental evaluation of haloalkanes and liver injury. *Fundam. Appl. Toxicol.,* **10**: 563–570, 1988.

Plaa, G. L.; de Lamirande, E.; Lewittes, M.; and Yousef, I. M.: Liver cell plasma membrane lipids in manganese-bilirubin–induced intrahepatic cholestasis. *Biochem. Pharmacol.,* **31**: 3698–3701, 1982.

Plaa, G. L., and Hewitt, W. R.: Biotransformation products and cholestasis. In Popper, H., and Schaffner, F. (eds.): *Progress in Liver Diseases,* Vol. 7. Grune & Stratton, New York, 1982, pp. 179–194.

———: Detection and evaluation of chemically induced liver injury. In Hayes, A. W. (ed.): *Principles and Methods of Toxicology,* 2nd ed. Raven Press, New York, 1989, pp. 599–628.

Plaa, G. L.; Hewitt, W. R.; du Souich, P.; Caillé, G.; and Lock, S.: Isopropanol and acetone potentiation of carbon tetrachloride–induced hepatotoxicity: single versus repetitive pretreatment in rats. *J. Toxicol. Environ. Health,* **9**: 235–250, 1982.

Plaa, G. L., and Priestly, B. G.: Intrahepatic cholestasis induced by drugs and chemicals. *Pharmacol. Rev.,* **28**: 207–273, 1976.

Plaa, G. L.; Traiger, G. J.; Hanasono, G. K.; and Witschi, H. P.: Effect of alcohols on various forms of chemically induced liver injury. In Khanna, J. M.; Israel, Y.; and Kalant, H. (eds.): *Alcoholic Liver Pathology.* Addiction Research Foundation, Toronto, 1975, pp. 225–244.

Plaa, G. L., and Witschi, H. P.: Chemicals, drugs, and

lipid peroxidation. *Annu. Rev. Pharmacol. Toxicol.,* **16**: 125–141, 1976.

Placke, M. E.; Ginsberg, G. L.; Wyand, D. S.; and Cohen, S. D.: Ultrastructural changes during acute acetaminophen-induced hepatotoxicity in the mouse: a time and dose study. *Toxicol. Pathol.,* **15**: 431–438, 1987.

Pohl, L. R.; Bhooshan, B.; Whittaker, N. F.; and Krishna, G.: Phosgene: a metabolite of chloroform. *Biochem. Biophys. Res. Commun.,* **79**: 684–691, 1977.

Pohl, L. R.; Satoh, H.; Christ, D. D.; and Kenna, J. G.: The immunologic and metabolic basis of drug hypersensitivities. *Annu. Rev. Pharmacol. Toxicol.,* **28**: 367–387, 1988.

Popper, H.: Hepatocellular degeneration and death. In Arias, I. M.; Jakoby, W. B.; Popper, H.; Schachter, D.; and Shafritzs, D. A. (eds.): *The Liver: Biology and Pathobiology,* 2nd ed. Raven Press, New York, 1988, pp. 1087–1103.

Popper, H., and Schaffner, F.: Drug-induced hepatic injury. *Ann. Intern. Med.,* **51**: 1230–1252, 1959.

Price, V. F., and Jollow, D. J.: Increased resistance of diabetic rats to acetaminophen-induced hepatotoxicity. *J. Pharmacol. Exp. Ther.,* **220**: 504–513, 1982.

Raisfeld, I. H.: Models of liver injury: the effect of toxins on the liver. In Becker, F. F. (ed.): *The Liver: Normal and Abnormal Functions,* Part A. Marcel Dekker, Inc., New York, 1974, pp. 203–223.

Rankin, I. G.; Schmidt, W. P.; Popham, R. E.; and de Lint, J.: Epidemiology of alcoholic liver disease—insights and problems. In Khanna, J. M.; Israel, Y.; and Kalant, H. (eds.): *Alcoholic Liver Pathology.* Addiction Research Foundation, Toronto, 1975, pp. 31–41.

Rao, S. B.; Young, R. A.; and Mehendale, H. M.: Hepatic polyamines and related enzymes following chlordecone-potentiated carbon tetrachloride toxicity in rats. *J. Biochem. Toxicol.* **4**: 55–63, 1989.

Rappaport, A. M.: Anatomic considerations. In Schiff, L. (ed.): *Diseases of the Liver,* 3rd ed. J. B. Lippincott Co., Philadelphia, 1969.

———: Hepatic blood flow: morphologic aspects and physiologic regulation. *Int. Rev. Physiol.,* **21**: 1–63, 1980.

Raucy, J. L.; Lasker, J. M.; Lieber, C. S.; and Black, M.: Acetaminophen activation by human liver cytochromes P450IIE1 and P450IA2. *Arch. Biochem. Biophys.,* **271**: 270–283, 1989.

Recknagel, R. O.: Carbon tetrachloride hepatotoxicity. *Pharmacol. Rev.,* **19**: 145–208, 1967.

———: A new direction in the study of carbon tetrachloride hepatotoxicity. *Life Sci.,* **33**: 401–408, 1983.

Recknagel, R. O., and Ghoshal, A. K.: Lipoperoxidation as a vector in carbon tetrachloride hepatotoxicity. *Lab. Invest.,* **15**: 132–148, 1966.

Recknagel, R. O., and Glende, E. A., Jr.: Carbon tetrachloride hepatotoxicity: an example of lethal cleavage. *CRC Crit. Rev. Toxicol.,* **2**: 263–297, 1973.

Recknagel, R. O.; Glende, E. A., Jr.; Waller, R. L.; and Lowrey, K.: Lipid peroxidation: biochemistry, measurement, and significance in liver cell injury. In Plaa, G. L., and Hewitt, W. R. (eds.): *Toxicology of the Liver.* Raven Press, New York, 1982, pp. 213–241.

Rees, K. R.; Sinha, P.; and Spector, W. G.: The pathogenesis of liver injury in carbon tetrachloride and thioacetamide poisoning. *J. Pathol. Bacteriol.,* **81**: 107–118, 1961.

Rees, K. R., and Tarlow, M. J.: The hepatotoxic action of allyl formate. *Biochem. J.,* **104**: 757–761, 1967.

Reynolds, E. S.; Moslen, M. T.; Szabo, S.; Jaeger, R. J.; and Murphy, S. D.: Hepatotoxicity of vinyl chloride and 1,1-dichloroethylene. *Am. J. Pathol.*, **81**: 219–232, 1975.

Rouiller, C.: Experimental toxic injury of the liver. In Rouiller, C. (ed.): *The Liver*, Vol. 2. Academic Press, Inc., New York, 1964, pp. 335–476.

Schaffner, F., and Raisfeld, I. H.: Drugs and the liver: a review of metabolism and adverse reactions. *Adv. Intern. Med.*, **15**: 221–251, 1969.

Schinella, R. A., and Becker, F. F: Cirrhosis. In Becker, F. F. (ed.): *The Liver: Normal and Abnormal Functions*, Part B. Marcel Dekker, Inc., New York, 1975, pp. 711–723.

Schreiber, A. J., and Simon, F. R.: Estrogen-induced cholestasis: clues to pathogenesis and treatment. *Hepatology*, **3**: 607–613, 1983.

Sell, D. A., and Reynolds, E. A.: Liver parenchymal cell injury. VIII. Lesions of the membranous cellular components following iodoform. *J. Cell. Biol.*, **41**: 736–752, 1969.

Sipes, I. G., and Gandolfi, A. J.: Bioactivation of aliphatic organohalogens: formation, detection, and relevance. In Plaa, G. L., and Hewitt, W. R. (eds.): *Toxicology of the Liver*. Raven Press, New York, 1982, pp. 181–212.

Sipes, I. G.; Stripp, B.; Krishna, G.; Maling, H. M.; and Gillette, J. R.: Enhanced hepatic microsomal activity by pretreatment of rats with acetone or isopropanol. *Proc. Soc. Exp. Biol. Med.*, **142**: 237–240, 1973.

Slater, T. F.: Necrogenic action of carbon tetrachloride in the rat: a speculative mechanism based on activation. *Nature (Lond.).*, **209**: 36–40, 1966.

Slikker, W., Jr.; Vore, M.; Bailey, J. R.; Meyers, M.; and Montgomery, C.: Hepatotoxic effects of estradiol-17-D-glucuronide in the rat and monkey. *J. Pharmacol. Exp. Ther.*, **225**: 138–143, 1983.

Thomas, C. E., and Reed, D. J.: Current status of calcium in hepatocellular injury. *Hepatology*, **10**: 375–384, 1989.

Tomokuni, K.: Studies on hepatotoxicity induced by chlorinated hydrocarbons. II. Lipid metabolism and absorption spectrum of microsomal lipid in mice exposed to 1,1,2,2-tetrachloroethane. *Acta Med. Okayama*, **24**: 315–322, 1970.

Traiger, G. J., and Bruckner, J. V.: The participation of 2-butanone in 2-butanol–induced potentiation of carbon tetrachloride hepatotoxicity. *J. Pharmacol. Exp. Ther.*, **196**: 493–500, 1976.

Tuchweber, B.; Weber, A.; Roy, C. C.; and Yousef, I. M.: Mechanisms of experimentally induced cholestasis. In Popper, H., and Schaffner, F. (eds.): *Progress in Liver Diseases*, Vol. 8. Grune & Stratton, New York, 1986, pp. 161–178.

Uraguchi, K.; Sakai, F.; Tsukioka, M.; Noguchi, Y.; and Tatsuno, M.: Acute and chronic toxicity in mice and rats of the fungus mat of *Penicillum islandicium* sopp added to the diet. *Jpn. J. Exp. Med.*, **31**: 435–461, 1961.

Villarruel, M. C.; Fernández, G.; de Ferreyra, E. C.; de Fenos, O. M.; and Castro, J. A.: Studies on the mechanism of alloxan-diabetes potentiation of carbon tetrachloride–induced liver necrosis. *Br. J. Exp. Pathol.*, **63**: 388–393, 1982.

Watkins III, J. B.; Sanders, R. A.; and Beck, L. V.: The effect of long-term streptozotocin-induced diabetes on the hepatotoxicity of bromobenzene and carbon tetrachloride and hepatic biotransformation in rats. *Toxicol. Appl. Pharmacol.*, **93**: 329–338, 1988.

Windmueller, H. G., and von Euler, L. H.: Prevention of orotic acid–induced fatty liver with allopurinol. *Proc. Soc. Exp. Biol. Med.*, **136**: 98–101, 1971.

Witschi, H. P.: Effects of beryllium on deoxyribonucleic acid–synthesizing enzymes in regenerating rat liver. *Biochem. J.*, **120**: 623–634, 1970.

Witschi, H. P., and Aldridge, W. N.: Uptake, distribution and binding of beryllium to organelles of the rat liver cell. *Biochem. J.*, **106**: 811–820, 1968.

Witzleben, C. L.: Physiologic and morphologic natural history of a model of intrahepatic cholestasis (manganese-bilirubin overload). *Am. J. Pathol.*, **66**: 577–582, 1972.

Yousef, I. M.; Lewittes, M.; Tuchweber, B.; Roy, C. C.; and Weber, A.: Lithocholic acid–cholesterol interactions in rat liver plasma membrane fractions. *Biochim. Biophys. Acta*, **796**: 345–353, 1984.

Zimmerman, H. J.: *Hepatotoxicity*. Appleton-Century-Crofts, New York, 1978.

Chapter 11

TOXIC RESPONSES OF THE KIDNEY

William R. Hewitt, Robin S. Goldstein, and *Jerry B. Hook*

INTRODUCTION

The mammalian kidney is an extremely complex organ, both anatomically and functionally. In addition to the excretion of wastes, the kidney plays a significant role in the regulation of total body homeostasis; it is the predominant organ involved in regulation of extracellular fluid (ECF) volume and electrolyte composition. The kidney also is a major site of formation of hormones that influence systemic metabolic functions, including erythropoietin, 1,25-dihydroxy-vitamin D_3, renin, and several vasoactive prostanoids and kinins. A toxicologic insult to the kidney could affect any or all these functions. However, the effects usually reported following toxic insult reflect decreased elimination of wastes, that is, an increase in blood urea nitrogen (BUN) or an increase in plasma creatinine. This does not necessarily mean that excretory functions are primarily affected by nephrotoxicants; rather, these are renal functions that are measured rapidly and reliably. Thus, the use of BUN and plasma creatinine as clinical indices of nephrotoxicity reflects the state of technology, not necessarily the primary sites of nephrotoxicity.

RENAL PHYSIOLOGY AND PATHOPHYSIOLOGY

Functional Anatomy

Gross examination of a sagittal section of the kidney clearly demonstrates two major anatomic areas, the cortex and the medulla (Figure 11–1). The cortex constitutes the major portion of the kidney and consequently receives most of the nutrient blood flow to the organ. Thus, when a blood-borne toxicant is delivered to the kidney, a high percentage of the material will reach sites in the cortex. In a single pass through the kidney, most chemicals will have a greater opportunity to influence cortical, rather than medullary, function. A smaller percentage of the total chemical delivered to the kidney would reach the medulla. However, because of the low blood flow to the medulla and because of the anatomic arrangement of the vasa rectae and loops of Henle (Figure 11–1), a chemical may be trapped by the countercurrent mechanism. Thus, a foreign compound could remain in the medulla and achieve relatively high concentrations.

A discussion of the functional anatomy of this organ is most appropriately based on the functional unit of the kidney, the nephron (Figure 11–1). The nephron may be considered in three portions: the vascular element including the afferent and efferent arterioles, the glomerulus, and the tubular element. All nephrons have their primary vascular elements and glomeruli in the cortex. The proximal convoluted tubule is localized in the cortex and sends the pars recta (straight portion) of the proximal tubule and loops of Henle into the substance of the kidney. Those glomeruli close to the medulla (juxtamedullary glomeruli) are associated with nephrons that send their loops of Henle deep into the medulla. Other glomeruli closer to the surface of the kidney often form nephrons whose loops of Henle are contained within the cortex (Figure 11–1). The relative proportion of nephrons with long versus short loops varies with species.

Each element of the nephron has specific functions, all of which may be influenced by nephrotoxicants. The vascular element serves to: (1) deliver waste and other materials to the tubule for excretion; (2) return reabsorbed and synthesized materials to the systemic circulation; and (3) deliver oxygen and metabolic substrates to the nephron. It is within the afferent arteriole that renin is formed. The glomerulus is a specialized capillary bed; it is unique in that it is the only capillary bed in the body positioned between vasoactive arterioles. The glomerulus is a relatively porous capillary and acts as a selective filter of the plasma. Based on molecular size, net charge, and shape, certain materials will be filtered into the lumen of the tubule and others will be retained in the circulation (Figure 11–2). The tubular element of the nephron selectively reab-

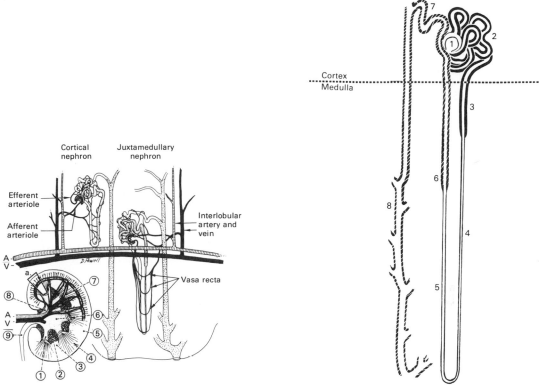

Figure 11–1. *A.* Sagittal section of a mammalian (human) kidney is illustrated in the *lower left*. *A* and *V* refer to renal artery and vein, respectively: (*1*) minor calix; (*2*) fat in sinus; (*3*) renal column of Bertin; (*4*) medullary ray; (*5*) cortex; (*6*) pelvis; (*7*) interlobar artery; (*8*) major calix; (*9*) ureter. Insert (*a*) from the upper pole of the kidney is enlarged to illustrate the relationships between the nephrons and the vasculature. (From Tisher, C. C., and Madsen, K. M.: Anatomy of the kidney. In Brenner, B. B., and Rector, F. C., Jr. [eds.]: *The Kidney.* W. B. Saunders Co., Philadelphia, 1976.)

B. Anatomy of a juxtamedullary nephron. Note the demarcation between cortex and medulla: (*1*) glomerulus; (*2*) proximal convoluted tubule; (*3*) proximal straight tubule (pars recta); (*4*) descending limb of the loop of Henle; (*5*) thin ascending limb of the loop of Henle; (*6*) thick ascending limb of the loop of Henle; (*7*) distal convoluted tubule; (*8*) collecting duct. (Modified from Gottschalk, C. W.: Osmotic concentration and dilution of the urine. *Am. J. Med., 36*:670–685, 1964.)

sorbs the bulk of the filtrate. Approximately 98 to 99 percent of the salts and water are reabsorbed; filtered sugars and amino acids are nearly completely reabsorbed. Furthermore, the tubular element, particularly the proximal tubule, actively secretes material into the urine. Secretory activity is primarily responsible for excretion of certain organic compounds and for elimination of hydrogen and potassium ions. The tubular element is also actively involved in the synthesis of ammonia and glucose and the activation of vitamin D.

The cellular response to a toxic insult may vary from an imperceptible biochemical aberration to cell death with resulting necrosis. Functionally, toxicity may be reflected as a minor alteration in transport capability (*e.g.,* transient glucosuria, aminoaciduria), as polyuria with decreased concentrating capacity, or as frank renal

failure with anuria and elevated BUN. Depending on the magnitude of the insult, these changes may be permanent and, ultimately, may be lethal. Theoretically, these effects may be brought about in one of several ways: (1) Vasoconstriction could decrease renal blood flow and glomerular filtration rate, reducing urine flow, eventually resulting in an increase in BUN. Vasoconstriction also can lead to tissue ischemia with resultant loss of function and, eventually, tissue destruction. (2) The nephrotoxicant could affect the glomerular element directly, altering permeability such that filtration is compromised. (3) Alternatively, or in combination with these other possibilities, administration of a nephrotoxicant could influence tubular function directly. Either specific reabsorptive or secretory mechanisms could be influenced by the toxicant, or the general permeability of the

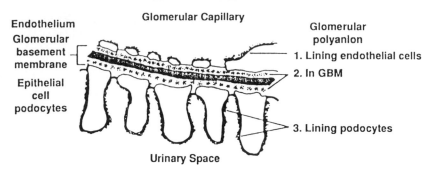

Figure 11–2. The glomerular barrier. The distribution of glomerular polyanion in the glomerular basement membrane and on the endothelial and epithelial cell layers is shown. (Modified from Schnaper, H. W., and Robsen, A. M.: Nephrotic syndrome: minimal change disease, focal glomerulosclerosis, and related disorders. In Schrier, R. W., and Gottschalk, C. W. (eds.): *Diseases of the Kidney,* Vol. 2. Little, Brown and Co., Boston, 1988, pp. 1945–2004.)

tubule could be influenced such that the normal ability of the tubule to act as a barrier to diffusion could be altered. (4) In addition, the nephrotoxicant could precipitate within the tubular lumen, blocking urine flow and decreasing glomerular filtration rate as intratubular pressure increased.

REASONS FOR SUSCEPTIBILITY OF THE KIDNEY

Concentrating Mechanisms

The unusual susceptibility of the mammalian kidney to the toxic effects of noxious chemicals often can be attributed to its unique physiologic and anatomic features. For example, the kidney regulates volume and composition of the extracellular fluid by filtering and reabsorbing large quantities of H_2O and electrolytes; approximately 99 percent of the filtered load of H_2O and electrolytes is reabsorbed. The work associated with such a complex system may appear inefficient. However, it does permit exquisite control over the volume and composition of the ECF and, secondarily, the intracellular fluid (ICF). For example, a decrease in H_2O reabsorption of only 1 percent can result in a doubling of the daily excretion of H_2O from ~ 1.5 liters to ~ 3.0 liters. Thus, fractional changes in reabsorption can produce substantial alterations in urinary excretion of fluid and electrolytes, and the ramifications of a toxicant-induced perturbation in normal renal function also are immediately apparent. For instance, if a 1 percent toxicant-induced depression of H_2O reabsorption resulted in the inappropriate excretion of 1.5 to 1.7 liters of H_2O, ECF volume could be reduced by approximately 9 percent (~ 4 percent of total body water). Alternatively, a reduction in H_2O (and electrolyte) excretion, subsequent to a tox-

icant-induced reduction in glomerular filtration rate (GFR) and filtered load, can result in rapid expansion of the ECF volume as well as aberrations in ECF electrolyte composition; serious abnormalities in organ function (e.g., cardiac function) can follow.

As water and electrolytes are reabsorbed from the glomerular filtrate, the materials remaining (including potential toxicants) in the urine may be concentrated (Figure 11–3). Thus, a nontoxic concentration of a chemical in the plasma could become toxic in the kidney subsequent to concentration within the urine. Furthermore, a chemical reaching the kidney might be concentrated in the cells in one or both of the following ways: If the material is actively secreted into the tubular urine, it will first be accumulated within the cells of the proximal tubule in concentrations higher than in plasma; this process will expose these cells to very high concentrations of the agent, which could produce toxicity. Similarly, a material that is reabsorbed (even by passive means) from the urine into the blood will pass through the cells of the nephron in a relatively high concentration, potentially leading to intracellular toxicity.

Renal Blood Flow

Maintenance of normal function requires delivery of large amounts of fluid, electrolytes, metabolic substrates, and oxygen to the kidney. Total renal blood flow in humans, rats, and dogs ranges from 3 to 5 ml/min/g of kidney (Brenner *et al.,* 1986). In a normal human male (total kidney weight: ~ 290 g), renal blood flow is about 1160 ml/min or about 20 to 25 percent of the cardiac output. Together the kidneys constitute only about 0.5 percent of total body mass; renal oxygen extraction is low—only about 10 to 15 percent—suggesting that the high rate of renal perfusion is not dictated by the oxygen de-

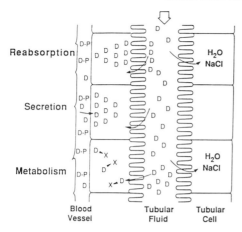

Figure 11–3. Schematic representation of nephron function. *D*, drug; *P*, protein; *X*, metabolite.

mand of the kidney but rather is a prerequisite for maintaining a high glomerular filtration rate. Because of the high blood flow, any drug or chemical in the systemic circulation will be delivered in relatively high amounts to this organ.

Intrarenal Xenobiotic Metabolism

Metabolism of xenobiotics, although traditionally considered a detoxication process, can result in the formation of toxic reactive metabolites, generally electrophiles or free radicals. These intermediates may bind covalently to cellular macromolecules and disrupt normal cell function. In addition to the extensively studied hepatic systems, xenobiotic metabolizing enzymes also are present in many extrahepatic organs including the kidney (Rush *et al.*, 1984b). Renal xenobiotic metabolism is quantitatively much less than hepatic metabolism and, with few exceptions, appears to make only a minor contribution to total body metabolism of most chemicals. However, in specific cases, intrarenal metabolism may play a crucial role in nephrotoxicity.

Extrarenal Factors

The kidney is sensitive to extrarenal factors that would decrease blood pressure or blood volume, as in shock or hemorrhage. Such changes may induce ischemia and functional deficit in this highly active metabolic organ. The kidney is under the influence of the sympathetic nervous system, and changes in neural activity can markedly influence renal function. Direct effects of the renal sympathetic nerves on renal vascular resistance and on renin secretion have been documented, and renal nerve activity might directly influence proximal tubular function as well. Therefore, any change in systemic ho-

meostasis that would alter sympathetic nerve activity also could influence the kidney. Similarly, dehydration may occur due to decreased water intake, due to elevated body temperature, or as a secondary effect of a chemical. This could lead to decreased plasma volume, which could decrease glomerular filtration. Probably of greater importance in this case is the fact that in the presence of antidiuretic hormone the urine would be maximally concentrated, and the possibility of a chemical reaching excessively high concentrations in the urine would be maximized.

SITES OF ACTION OF NEPHROTOXICANTS

The adult rat kidney contains approximately 30,000 to 34,000 nephrons, whereas the human kidney has been estimated to contain about 1 million (Tisher and Madsen, 1986). Each nephron consists of the renal corpuscle (glomerulus plus Bowman's capsule) and at least 12 morphologically and functionally distinct tubular segments; one or more cell types may be contained within each nephron segment (Burg, 1986; Tisher and Madsen, 1986). Thus, in one sense, the nephron consists of a group of organs linked in series with striking differences in structure, function, and enzymatic composition. Few data are available that define specific cellular or subcellular sites of action of nephrotoxicants. Only rarely have specific receptors (in the classic sense of the word) for specific nephrotoxicants been identified. Rather, in many cases it appears that several tissue constituents may be influenced by poisons. There are two interrelated reasons for this apparent lack of specificity: (1) In contrast to a specific pharmacologic effect of a chemical that requires activation or inhibition of a specific endogenous receptor, cell damage may follow interruption of one or several of the many required cellular functions; (2) certain renal cell types may be more susceptible to damage merely because they are exposed to concentrations of chemicals many times higher than are other cells of the body, leading to nonspecific cellular damage.

This is not to say, however, that there are not specific targets for certain nephrotoxicants in the kidney. Although the proximal tubule is often the primary target of nephrotoxicants, cell injury to areas other than the proximal tubule strongly argues for specific biochemical targets. For instance, the loop of Henle appears to be the site of damage produced by chronic administration of analgesic mixtures (aspirin and phenacetin) and other materials that act in the medulla, such as fluoride ion. The distal convoluted tubule is a relatively small part of the total nephron and does not appear to be a primary site of toxicant-induced damage. However, compounds such as amphotericin have been shown to influence the ability of the kidney to acidify the urine, which is probably a distal tubular event. The collecting duct also appears to be relatively insensitive to most nephrotoxicants. For example, following intoxication with analgesic mixtures, histologic evaluation of the medulla showed that most of the ascending limbs of the loops of Henle had been destroyed, whereas the collecting ducts appeared to be unaffected. Damage due to outdated tetracyclines also may occur in this area.

Glomerulus

As blood enters the glomerular capillary network, it is subjected to an ultrafiltration process. The glomerular capillary filtration barrier is a highly complex structure that permits a high rate of fluid filtration, with 20 to 40 percent of the plasma entering the glomeruli of each kidney being separated into a solution that is a nearly ideal ultrafiltrate of plasma. Despite the high rate of fluid flux, the glomerular capillary filtration barrier markedly restricts the transmural passage of macromolecules, predominantly proteins with an effective molecular radius of 20 Å or greater, such that the concentration of the majority of plasma proteins in the glomerular ultrafiltrate is normally quite low.

Within the glomerulus, there are three cell types, all of which are important for the constitution of the glomerular capillary filtration barrier: (1) the endothelial cells; (2) the mesangial cells; and (3) the epithelial cells of the visceral layer (also known as podocytes) (Figure 11–2). In addition to the cellular components, the basement membrane of the capillaries and the mesangial matrix are components of the glomerular filter. The glomerular basement membrane (GBM) is sandwiched between the endothelial and epithelial cells (Figure 11–2); both cell types contribute to its synthesis. The GBM has three layers of approximately equal size: the lamina rara interna (LRI), lamina densa (LD), and the lamina rara externa (LRE). The composition of the GBM is quite complex. It contains several highly anionic sialoglycoproteins along with anionic glycoproteins containing sulfated constituents. The anionic groups of the GBM coupled with the anionic coating (provided by sialoglycoprotein[s]) of the epithelial and endothelial cells provide the charge-selective properties of the glomerular filtration barrier (Kanwar, 1984; Dousa, 1985; Kriz and Kaissling, 1985; Tisher and Madsen, 1986).

The high rate of fluid flux through the glomerular capillary filtration barrier is due to the fact that water movement occurs primarily through extracellular paths. The major hydraulic barrier of the glomerulus is the slit diaphragm, largely because the aggregate area of the pores in the slit diaphragm is 2 to 3 percent of the total filtration area. The resistance of the endothelium to the movement of water is trivial because of the large fenestrae, whereas the GBM exerts some resistance to the movement of water (Kanwar, 1984; Kriz and Kaissling, 1985).

The forces driving the movement of fluid across the glomerular capillary wall can be summarized by the following equation (Arendshorst and Gottschalk, 1985; Dworkin and Brenner, 1985; Brenner et al., 1986):

$$SNGFR = K_f \cdot [(P_{GC} - P_T) - (\Pi_{GC} - \Pi_T)]$$

$$K_f = k \cdot S$$

where

$SNGFR$	=	Single nephron glomerular filtration rate
K_f	=	Ultrafiltration coefficient
P_{GC}	=	Glomerular capillary hydraulic pressure
P_T	=	Hydraulic pressure in Bowman's space
Π_{GC}	=	Oncotic pressure in the glomerular capillary
Π_T	=	Oncotic pressure in Bowman's space
k	=	Effective hydraulic permeability of the glomerular capillary wall
S	=	Total capillary surface area available for filtration

Alterations in K_f result in changes in $SNGFR$. The K_f of the glomerular capillary bed is one to two orders of magnitude greater than in other capillary beds. It is the high effective hydraulic permeability of the glomerular capillary bed that allows glomerular filtration to proceed rapidly. Reductions in K_f due to decreases in the hydraulic permeability of the filtration barrier (k) and/or the surface area available for filtration (S) reduce $SNGFR$. Infiltration of the interstitium by macrophages and lymphocytes often is observed in progressive glomerulosclerosis (Klahr et al., 1988). These cells may contribute to the functional and morphologic aberrations of glomerulosclerosis by altering the function of the mesangial cells. Macrophages, for example, can produce thromboxane A_2 (TxA$_2$) which decreases SNGFR, at least in part, by decreasing K_f as a result of mesangial-cell contraction; contraction of mesangial cells is believed to reduce S, the surface area available for filtration. TxA$_2$ also is released by platelets, and platelet-derived TxA$_2$ may be involved in the reduction of $SNGFR$ in

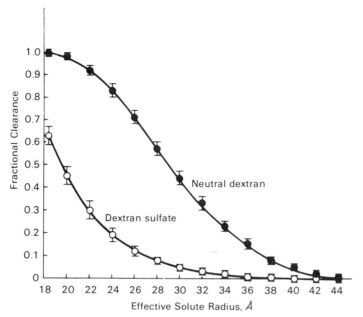

Figure 11–4. Fractional clearances (clearance compared with inulin clearance) of neutral dextran and dextran sulfate by rat kidney plotted as a function of effective molecular radius. As effective molecular radius increases, the fractional clearance, which reflects glomerular permeability, decreases. The permeability to neutral dextran is considerably greater than that of the charged dextran sulfate. (From Brenner, B. M.; Bohrer, M. P.; Baylis, C.; and Deen, W. M.: Determinants of glomerular permselectivity: insights derived from observations *in vivo. Kidney Int.*, **12**:229–237, 1977. Reprinted with permission.)

various chronic renal diseases (Klahr *et al.*, 1988). Inhibitors of thromboxane synthesis have been shown to increase renal plasma flow and GFR, decrease proteinuria, and prevent histologic damage in various experimental models of renal disease (Klahr *et al.*, 1988).

Macromolecules tend to be restricted at different levels of the filtration barrier based on their relative size and charge. Large circulating polyanionic molecules, such as albumin, likely are restricted by the endothelium and the LRI of the GBM. For uncharged macromolecules, the GBM is generally considered to provide the major restrictive influence. Cationic macromolecules appear to be hindered at the level of the slit diaphragm (Kanwar, 1984; Dworkin and Brenner, 1985; Skorecki *et al.*, 1986).

The glomerular filtration barrier discriminates between macromolecules on the basis of charge (Figure 11–4). Neutral dextran molecules of the same molecular radius as albumin pass the glomerular filtration barrier to a greater extent than albumin, a polyanionic macromolecule. When dextrans of various size and charge were examined, it was found that filtration of anionic dextrans (dextran sulfate) was retarded to a greater extent than filtration of neutral dextrans of comparable molecular radii; filtration of cationic dextrans (DEAE dextran) was actually enhanced compared with neutral dextrans of comparable molecular radii. It appears that the highly anionic coatings of the elements of the filtration barrier produce an electrostatic hindrance with circulating polyanionic macromolecules that markedly retards the passage of these molecules across the filtration barrier (Kanwar, 1984; Dworkin and Brenner, 1985; Skorecki *et al.*, 1986).

Various nephrotoxicants can reduce the number of fixed anionic charges on glomerular structural elements. This reduces the charge- and/or size-selective properties of the glomerular filtration barrier and allows large, circulating polyanions such as albumin to be excreted in the urine in excessive amounts. For example, a 45-minute infusion of the polycationic molecule hexadimethrine (HDM) to rats results in a heavy proteinuria; protein excretion (albumin and IgG) increases from about 8 μg/min to approximately 1525 μg/min (Hunsicker *et al.*, 1981; Bertolatus *et al.*, 1984). The HDM-induced proteinuria is associated with HDM binding to the LRE and LRI, reduction in the amount of glomerular polyanions, and morphologic abnormalities of the epithelial cell foot processes. Significantly, HDM increases the excretion of both albumin and IgG. Albuminuria is consistent with a loss in the charge-selective properties of the filtration barrier as would be expected following neutralization of glomerular polyanion. However, the increased IgG (molecular radius ~ 52 Å, small net charge) excretion suggests that the HDM-induced neutralization of glomerular polyanion also alters the size-selective properties of the filtration barrier (Hunsicker *et al.*, 1981; Bertolatus *et al.*, 1984). Chronic doxorubicin poisoning, which produces proteinuria in rats, also appears to alter both the charge- and size-selective properties of the filtration barrier (Bertolatus and Hunsicker, 1985). Similarly, the aminonucleoside of puromycin (PAN) damages the epithelial cell foot processes and produces defects in the charge- and size-selective properties of the filtration barrier secondary to a loss of glomerular polyanion; these aberrations account for the proteinuria produced by PAN (Elema *et al.*, 1988; Grond *et al.*, 1988). PAN-induced glomerular damage may be a model of minimal change glomerular disease in humans.

Proximal Tubule

Many nephrotoxicants appear to have their primary site of action on (in) the proximal tubule. This is reasonable, since most blood flow to the kidney is delivered to the cortex, which is predominantly proximal tubule. In addition, active secretion and reabsorption of compounds occur in the proximal tubule that can result in large, potentially toxic concentrations of a chemical within the proximal tubular cell.

Overall, the proximal tubule is the workhorse segment of the nephron. Approximately 60 to 80 percent of solute and water filtered at the glomerulus is reabsorbed within the various segments of the proximal tubule. In addition to active Na^+ reabsorption, the proximal tubule reabsorbs electrolytes such as K^+, HCO_3^-, Cl^-, PO_4^{2-}, Ca^{2+}, and Mg^{2+}. Essentially all filtered glucose, amino acids and varying amounts of some small organic acids (e.g., lactate, citrate, α-ketoglutarate, urate) are reabsorbed. The proximal tubule also reabsorbs those peptides and proteins that are filtered at the glomerulus. Toxicant-induced interruptions in the production of energy for Na^+ transport or the function of critical membrane-bound enzymes or transporters, for example, can profoundly affect proximal tubular function and thereby whole-kidney function. As an example, potassium dichromate produces dysfunction and necrosis of proximal tubular cells with the anticipated consequences. The ability of the proximal tubule to reabsorb glucose and filtered protein is reduced, and concomitant glucosuria and proteinuria are observed (Figure 11–5). Similarly, proximal tubular H_2O

reabsorption is decreased and urinary output increases more than four-fold in the 24 hours immediately following poisoning (Figure 11–5). Theoretically, the functional disturbances produced by toxicants can vary if one of the proximal tubule segments is damaged selectively.

MECHANISMS OF CELL DEATH

Reactive Oxygen Species (ROS) Generation

Toxic products derived from oxygen have been implicated as mediators of renal injury due to immunoinflammatory processes, ischemia, and a number of toxicants (Baud and Ardaillou, 1986; Weinberg, 1988; Shah, 1989). The reduction of oxygen by cells requires four electrons and results in conversion of O_2 directly to water. Incomplete reduction of O_2 leads to the generation of partially reduced and potentially toxic ROSs. Superoxide anion free radical is produced when oxygen accepts a single electron, whereas H_2O_2 is produced by a two-electron reduction of O_2. H_2O_2 formation can occur either directly or through the dismutation of superoxide anion. A second free radical species, hydroxyl radical, is formed from H_2O_2 and the superoxide anion free radical via the Haber-Weiss reaction. This reaction is slow and in biological systems is usually catalyzed by transition metal ions, a process termed the Fenton reaction. Ferrous iron (Fe^{2+}) appears to be the major intracellular mediator of the Fenton reaction; the precise source and form (e.g., organically bound) of the iron is unknown. Superoxide anion acts as a reductant for Fe^{3+}. The Fe^{2+} generated then reduces the hydrogen peroxide to hydroxyl radical (Baud and Ardaillou, 1986; Weinberg, 1988; Shah, 1989).

Superoxide anion is formed during natural oxidation reactions. These include the action of endoplasmic reticulum mixed-function oxidases, other NADPH oxidases such as those in the polymorphonuclear leukocytes (PMN), peroxisome-based oxidases, the mitochondrial electron transport system, and xanthine oxidase. Oxidation of arachidonic acid via cyclooxygenase and lipoxygenase may yield hydroxyl radical. A number of toxicants also produce ROS by redox cycling or other metabolic reactions (Kappus, 1987). Superoxide anion is far more reactive in nonaqueous environments such as biological membranes than in aqueous solutions; the toxicity of superoxide anion may arise from its direct reactivity within membranes. However, when generated in aqueous solutions, the toxicity of superoxide anion actually may be due to other ROS such as the hydroxyl radical. The hydroxyl radical is a highly reactive species and reacts rapidly with adjacent molecules; it does not

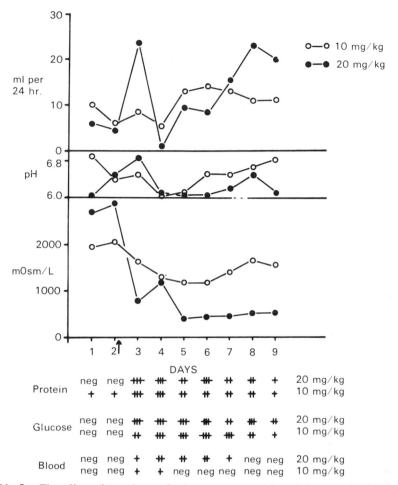

Figure 11–5. The effect of two doses of subcutaneous potassium dichromate (at the *arrow*) in rats. The rapidity of response and the quick return of function are illustrated. (From Berndt, W. O.: The effect of potassium dichromate on renal tubular transport processes. *Toxicol. Appl. Pharmacol.,* **32**:40–52, 1975.)

appear to cross biologic membranes. Superoxide anion and H_2O_2 are less reactive species and may diffuse from the initial site of formation to produce injury at a remote site within the cell. Although H_2O_2 readily crosses cell membranes, superoxide anion does not (Baud and Ardaillou, 1986; Weinberg, 1988; Shah, 1989).

ROS react with a variety of cellular constituents to induce toxicity. For example, ROSs are capable of: (1) inducing lipid peroxidation; (2) inactivating cellular enzymes by directly oxidizing critical -SH or -NH$_2$ groups; (3) depolymerizing polysaccharides; and (4) inducing DNA strand scission and chromosome breakage. Lipid peroxidation is a major deleterious effect of intracellular ROS generation. Peroxidation of membrane lipids usually involves the reaction of free radicals and the polyunsaturated fatty acid side chains of membrane phospholipids to form a

free radical and relatively stable lipid hydroperoxides. Decomposition of lipid hydroperoxides can be catalyzed by transition metals and results in the formation of alkoxy and peroxy free radicals that propagate the reaction. In addition, production of toxic lipid breakdown products such as hydroxylated fatty acids, alkanals, alk-2-enals, and 4-hydroxyalkenals occurs and contributes to organelle and cellular dysfunction. Thus, oxidative degradation of membrane lipids can result in altered membrane fluidity with concomitant alteration in membrane enzyme activity, altered membrane permeability and transport characteristics, as well as peroxidation-induced damage and dysfunction of nearby membrane proteins. ROSs can produce dramatic alterations in enzymatic activity and membrane structure/ function that contribute to the disruption of normal homeostatic mechanisms and eventually lead to cell death (Baud and Ardaillou, 1986; Weinberg, 1988; Shah, 1989).

A role for ROS production has been suggested in the renal dysfunction produced by reperfusion of the ischemic kidney (Baud and Ardaillou, 1986; Bonventre, 1988; Weinberg, 1988) and in several models (e.g., anti-GBM antibody disease, passive Heymann nephritis) of glomerular injury and dysfunction (Shah, 1989). Diamond et al. (1986) suggested that generation of ROS may be involved in the glomerular toxicity produced by PAN. PAN metabolism produces hypoxanthine, which can serve as a substrate for superoxide anion production via xanthine oxidase. Superoxide dismutase and allopurinol partially ameliorate the glomerular epithelial cell changes and proteinuria produced by PAN. Inhibition of superoxide anion formation (allopurinol) or scavenging of this ROS (superoxide dismutase) suggests that superoxide anion may mediate, in part, the glomerulotoxicity of PAN.

Other ROSs also may be produced in renal and/or extrarenal cells such as polymorphonuclear leukocytes (PMN; neutrophil). For example, singlet oxygen, an excited form of oxygen, may be produced. Similarly, H_2O_2 and chloride ion can be converted by PMN myeloperoxidase to hypochlorous acid, which is considered an ROS (Baud and Ardaillou, 1986; Weinberg, 1988; Shah, 1989).

Infiltration of PMNs is characteristic of a number of forms of glomerulonephritis. PMNs are capable of generating ROSs following a stimulus such as that provided by phorbol myristate acetate (PMA). Injection of PMA into the renal artery resulted in significant albuminuria with smaller amounts of other proteins being excreted into the urine; morphologic evidence of PMN infiltration and glomerular epithelial cell injury was present (Rehan et al., 1985). Depletion of neutrophils or treatment with catalase provided almost complete protection against PMA-induced proteinuria; superoxide dismutase (SOD), however, had no effect. This suggests that the glomerular injury was neutrophil dependent and involved H_2O_2, but not superoxide anion, production (Rehan et al., 1985). More recently, Yoshioka and Ichikawa (1989) reported that PMA stimulation of PMN reduced SNGFR by producing a profound reduction in K_f; R_E and P_{GC} were increased. Catalase pretreatment or PMN depletion prevented the changes in K_f, SNGFR, GFR, and R_E and P_{GC}. Thus, the glomerular injury produced by PMA administration appears to be due to infiltration of activated neutrophils into the glomerulus followed by a neutrophil-dependent ROS production. The mechanism(s) by which ROS decreased K_f is unclear but may involve secondary generation of vasoconstrictive leukotrienes or thromboxanes (Yoshioka and Ichikawa, 1989). A direct attack of ROS on the glomerular capillary wall also may be involved since ROS can increase the susceptibility of the GBM to degradation by proteolytic enzymes (Shah, 1989). Thus, while generation of ROS appears to be involved in a variety of forms of glomerular injury, the exact role of these toxic species likely involves a complex interaction with other mediators of glomerular injury (Shah, 1989).

Altered Calcium Homeostasis

The intracellular distribution of calcium exerts a profound influence on cell metabolism, motility, and division. Thus, intracellular calcium homeostasis is of importance to cell viability. The distribution of Ca^{2+} within renal cells is complex and involves binding to anionic sites on cell macromolecules (e.g., glycoproteins, proteins, phospholipids) and compartmentation within subcellular organelles. The critically important cellular calcium pool for regulation of intracellular calcium is the free Ca^{2+} present in the cytosol. The concentration of this pool is approximately $0.1~\mu M$ and is maintained at this level, although a large ($\sim 10,000:1$) extracellular/intracellular concentration gradient exists for Ca^{2+}. In addition, the proximal tubular cells (S_1 and S_2) reabsorb approximately 50 to 60 percent of the filtered load of calcium; the extent of S_3 Ca^{2+} reabsorption is unknown. Thus, there is a large transcellular flux of calcium from the lumen of the proximal tubule to the peritubular capillary blood; this Ca^{2+} flux also must be buffered to maintain the cytosolic free Ca^{2+} concentration ($[Ca^{2+}]_{fc}$) at $\sim 0.1~\mu M$. $[Ca^{2+}]_{fc}$ is regulated by energy-requiring transport systems located in the plasma membrane, endoplasmic reticulum, and mitochondrion.

Elevated cytosolic free Ca^{2+} concentrations may exert a number of detrimental effects on the cell. For example, an increase in $[Ca^{2+}]_{fc}$ can activate Ca^{2+}-dependent phospholipases, thereby initiating degradation of subcellular organelle and plasma membrane phospholipids with consequent alterations in membrane enzyme activity, permeability, and integrity. The lysophospholipids and nonesterified fatty acids produced by these reactions also can exert detrimental effects on cellular function. Ca^{2+} also may directly interact with membranes to alter permeability and transport characteristics. Uncoupling of mitochondrial phosphorylation has been observed with elevated calcium concentrations. In addition, elevated $[Ca^{2+}]_{fc}$ produces aberrations in the structure and function of cytoskeletal and contractile elements; blebbing of the cell surface results. Thus, alterations in intracellular calcium homeostasis can initiate several processes that could eventually lead to cell death (Cheung et al., 1986; Humes, 1986; Trump et al., 1989).

Altered intracellular Ca^{2+} homeostasis and/or uncompensated influx of Ca^{2+} has been implicated in initiation of proximal tubular cell death following ischemia/reperfusion. Depression of ATP concentration secondary to ischemia may diminish ATPase-dependent extrusion of Ca^{2+} from cells and inhibit the buffering of cytosolic Ca^{2+} concentration by decreasing sequestration within endoplasmic reticulum and mitochondria; efflux of Ca^{2+} from mitochondrial stores also would contribute to the increase in $[Ca^{2+}]_{fc}$. Reperfusion of the ischemic kidney presents a Ca^{2+} load to the tubule cell at a time when the mechanisms for maintenance of $[Ca^{2+}]_{fc}$ are not functioning at optimal rates. The resulting increase in $[Ca^{2+}]_{fc}$ may initiate processes leading to proximal tubular cell death subsequent to an ischemic insult (Cheung et al., 1986; Humes, 1986; Trump et al., 1989). In addition, alterations in $[Ca^{2+}]_{fc}$ also may play a role in the proximal tubular injury produced by $HgCl_2$ and gentamicin (see below).

SPECIFIC NEPHROTOXICANTS

As indicated above, not all compounds that influence renal function affect the kidney directly. Renal function may be altered secondarily to changes in blood pressure, blood volume, or neural or hormonal influences and to a variety of destructive systemic effects. The focus in this section will be on compounds that produce specific effects on the kidney. Many of these agents affect the kidney directly. In other cases, the ultimate toxicant might be a metabolic product formed within the kidney or produced in an extrarenal organ and transported to the kidney where it acts directly or requires further metabolism to a nephrotoxic product.

Heavy Metals

Most heavy metals are potent nephrotoxicants. Relatively low dosages of a variety of metals produce a similar set of signs and symptoms characterized by glucosuria, aminoaciduria, and polyuria (Figure 11–5). If the dosage of the metal is increased, renal necrosis, anuria, increased BUN, and death will follow. Most metals probably produce their nephrotoxicity by a similar mechanism. Following a toxic metal insult, the histologic picture is one of necrotic proximal tubules with lumens filled with proteinaceous material. It has been suggested that tissue destruction could lead to sloughing of proximal tubular cells into the lumen, resulting in tubular occlusion. Occlusion could be of sufficient magnitude to increase intratubular pressure, resulting in decreased glomerular filtration rate. However, this is probably an oversimplistic explanation. Oken (1976) has observed that when tubules are occluded after several nephrotoxicants, intraluminal pressure is reduced, not elevated. The apparently low glomerular filtration rate may be partially explained by increased permeability of the tubule to glomerular markers such as inulin, suggesting that the filtered inulin may leak back across the tubule membrane into the peritubular blood, thereby reducing inulin excretion and inulin clearance, producing an apparent decrease in glomerular filtration rate. Oken (1976), however, suggested that little leakage of inulin occurs. Rather, the fall in glomerular filtration rate was due to decreased glomerular permeability or reduced glomerular blood flow.

Indeed, there appears to be a significant vascular component of the nephrotoxicity of heavy metals. The severity of the renal damage produced by several heavy metals is reduced by feeding animals a high-salt diet prior to challenge with the poison. Since the high salt would decrease renin release by the kidney, a renin-angiotensin mechanism has been proposed to explain vasoconstriction. This interpretation has not, however, been universally accepted. Several investigators have recently suggested an involvement of renal prostaglandins in this vasoconstriction. However, even in the absence of vasoconstriction, changes in renal function, particularly in the proximal tubule, occur following heavy metals. Probably the frank nephrotoxicity that occurs in response to heavy metals is due to a combination of ischemia secondary to vasoconstriction and direct cellular toxicity of these materials. The direct cellular toxicity of metals is supported by in vitro studies demonstrating metal-induced damage to the proximal tubule.

Mercury. The toxicity of mercury has been recognized since antiquity. Elemental mercury undergoes biotransformation in the environment to various inorganic and organic salts; methylmercury, for example, is formed by microbial metabolism of both elemental and mercuric mercury. These mercurials can readily enter living organisms and thereby enter the food chain. In addition, organomercurial compounds have been used as fungicides and may enter the environment as industrial wastes. Organomercurials were once a mainstay of diuretic therapy. Thus, mercury may be introduced into the body as elemental mercury, as inorganic mercury, or as organic mercury.

Nephrotoxic potential varies widely between

the various forms of mercury (Berlin, 1986). The kidney and gastrointestinal system are the primary target organs of toxicity following accidental or suicidal ingestion of mercuric salts (Berlin, 1986). Necrosis of the proximal tubule occurs rapidly and can progress to renal failure within 24 to 48 hours of ingestion of a large dosage (acute lethal dose = 1 to 4 g) of a mercuric salt (Berlin, 1986). As with acute ingestion, the kidney is a primary target of chronic poisoning with mercuric salts, with both proximal tubular and glomerular damage being observed; glomerular damage may result from a mercury-induced autoimmune reaction (Berlin, 1986). In addition, nephrotoxicity has resulted from acute and chronic exposure to a variety of aryl and alkoxyalkyl mercury compounds. For example, phenylmercuric salts produce renal damage in mice and rats qualitatively similar to that observed with mercuric chloride. The metabolic breakdown of several aryl and alkoxyalkyl mercury compounds to inorganic mercury likely explains the similarity in nephrotoxic effects between these organomercurials and mercuric chloride. Although methylmercuric chloride has produced renal damage in humans and animals, the central nervous system (CNS) is the critical target of this and related alkyl mercury compounds (Berlin, 1986).

Extensive data have accumulated on the nephrotoxicity of mercury because it has been used frequently as a model compound to produce acute renal failure in animals. Mercuric chloride ($HgCl_2$) nephrotoxicity is characterized by an initial reduction in renal blood flow (RBF) coupled with an early and progressive decline in GFR; RBF may return to normal within 24 to 48 hours without restoration of GFR (Eknoyan et al., 1982; Lameire et al., 1982). For example, Eknoyan et al. (1982) found that GFR was reduced 35 percent within 6 hours of $HgCl_2$ (2 mg/kg) administration to rats and continued to decline when determined 12 (68 percent reduction) and 24 hours (84 percent reduction) after poisoning; elevations in the urea nitrogen and creatinine concentrations of serum were observed at 12 and 24 hours. The reduction in GFR results, in part, from the vasoconstriction produced by mercury but also may reflect reduction in K_f (Lameire et al., 1982). In addition to reducing GFR, $HgCl_2$ produces substantial tubular dysfunction. Fractional excretion of Na^+ is markedly increased, as is renal glucose excretion; proximal tubular organic anion secretion is diminished. Urinary volume often is increased early in $HgCl_2$-induced nephrotoxicity but declines as the extent of injury progresses (Kacew and Hirsch, 1981; Eknoyan et al., 1982). The major site of structural damage following a low

dosage of $HgCl_2$ (2 mg/kg) is the S_3 segment of the proximal tubule. Damage is most severe in those proximal tubule segments located in the medullary rays and outer stripe of the medulla (Eknoyan et al., 1982; Dobyan and Bulger, 1984). As the dosage of mercury is increased, toxicity occurs throughout the proximal nephron, and morphologic injury has been observed in the S_1 and S_2 segments of the proximal tubule following $HgCl_2$ dosages of 5 to 15 mg/kg (Weinberg et al., 1982; Knauss et al., 1983).

The sequence of events and their relative contributions to $HgCl_2$-induced proximal tubular cell necrosis are unclear. One of the earliest ultrastructural alterations induced by $HgCl_2$ is loss of the proximal tubule brush border. As early as eight hours after administering a small dosage of $HgCl_2$ (1 mg/kg) to rats, Ganote et al. (1974) were able to identify a variety of morphologic changes in the proximal tubule, including loss of brush border, dispersion of ribosomes, and formation of clumps of smooth membranes in the cytoplasm. These changes were followed by the appearance of vacuoles and other changes, including rupture of the plasma membrane and mitochondrial changes characteristic of cell necrosis. Subsequently, loss of brush border enzyme activity was shown to occur within 15 minutes of $HgCl_2$ administration (Zalme et al., 1976), and Weinberg et al. (1982) have observed ultrastructural evidence (e.g., focal brush border loss, increased numbers of vacuoles) of $HgCl_2$ proximal tubular injury three hours following treatment with 5 mg/kg of this toxicant. Thus, the brush border membrane may be the initial site of $HgCl_2$ injury.

Mercury combines with sulfhydryl groups and inhibits a great number of enzyme systems. Mitochondrial enzyme systems seem to be particularly sensitive to mercury, and the pathophysiologic effects often seen suggest inhibition of oxidative pathways. Sequential studies of adenine nucleotide concentrations following $HgCl_2$ administration found that [ATP] fell within one hour and continued to decline over a 48-hour period (Trifillis et al., 1981). In some studies, $HgCl_2$ produces aberrant mitochondrial function within one hour of administration. For example, mitochondria isolated from the renal cortex of rats two or three hours following treatment with a large $HgCl_2$ dosage (5 mg/kg) exhibited decreased adenine nucleotide translocase activity and respiratory rates (state 3); mitochondrial ADP uptake was reduced as early as one hour following $HgCl_2$ administration (Weinberg et al., 1982). Renal cortical slice oxygen consumption, ammonia production, and gluconeogenesis have been shown to be inhibited one to three hours following $HgCl_2$ administration (Preuss *et al.*, 1975). These data thus implicate mitochondria as an early intracellular site of Hg^{2+} action during the development of $HgCl_2$-induced proximal tubular necrosis. In the studies conducted by Ganote *et al.* (1974), however, oxygen consumption of tissue slices was not reduced until 24 hours after the $HgCl_2$ treatment, when the cells were frankly necrotic. Thus, these data suggest that mitochondrial injury does not play a primary role in the pathogenesis of mercury toxicity; rather, the data suggest that the mitochondrial damage occurred only at about the same time as general disruption of the plasma membrane.

Altered calcium homeostasis also has been implicated in $HgCl_2$-induced proximal tubular cell death. Chlorpromazine has been shown to ameliorate the renal functional and morphologic injury produced by $HgCl_2$ in rats (Dobyan and Bulger, 1984). Several phenothiazines act as calmodulin antagonists and may inhibit the entry of Ca^{2+} into injured cells and/or inhibit the deleterious effects associated with elevated concentrations of free Ca^{2+} in the cytosol (Dobyan and Bulger, 1984). Thus, Dobyan and Bulger suggested that alterations in cellular calcium homeostasis produced by $HgCl_2$ may elevate $[Ca^{2+}]_{fc}$ and contribute to the nephrotoxic properties of this metal.

Derangements in membrane phospholipid composition also may contribute to $HgCl_2$-induced nephrotoxicity. Phospholipids are major structural components of the plasma and subcellular organelle membranes and play a critical role in regulating cellular permeability characteristics, membrane enzyme activity, the activity of various transport systems, and membrane potential. Derangement of membrane phospholipid composition can have profound deleterious effects on membrane function and, consequently, cellular viability. Such derangements can be produced by inappropriate activation of soluble or membrane-bound phospholipases, inhibition of normal phospholipid synthesis, or direct toxicant binding to or modification of membrane phospholipids (Weinberg, 1988). However, owing to the wide variety of experimental protocols used to evaluate effects of mercury on phospholipids, definition of specific mechanisms remains unresolved.

The variety of experimental designs and paradoxical data make it impossible to define the specific etiology of $HgCl_2$-induced proximal tubular necrosis at this time. It is tempting to speculate that the alterations in mitochondrial bioenergetics produced by $HgCl_2$ result in an increase in $[Ca^{2+}]_{fc}$ with subsequent activation of Ca^{2+}-dependent phospholipases located within mitochondrial and plasma membranes. The derangements of membrane phospholipid composition then could contribute to the progressive decline in membrane function, aberrations in cellular function, and ultimately the proximal tubular cell necrosis induced by $HgCl_2$. However, yet to be eliminated are the possibilities that: (1) direct Hg^{2+} alteration in intracellular Ca^{2+} homeostasis is the initial event in $HgCl_2$ nephrotoxicity; or (2) Hg^{2+}-induced alterations in brush border membrane (BBM) phospholipid composition increase the permeability of this membrane to Ca^{2+}, thereby increasing $[Ca^{2+}]_{fc}$; or (3) several events initiated by $HgCl_2$ proceed in parallel to produce $HgCl_2$ renal dysfunction.

Cadmium. Cadmium is an interesting metal in that following administration of the metal there is enhanced synthesis in the liver of the metal-binding protein metallothionein. This compound seems to have a paradoxical effect on the systemic toxicity of cadmium. Metallothionein appears to bind cadmium and in this way protect certain organs such as the testes from cadmium toxicity. Yet, at the same time, metallothionein may enhance cadmium nephrotoxicity, possibly because the cadmium-metallothionein complex is taken up by the kidney more readily than is the free ion (Nordberg *el al.*, 1975; Nordberg, 1982). Injury produced by administration of the cadmium-metallothionein complex is localized to the first and second segments of the proximal tubule and is manifested by proteinuria, aminoaciduria, glucosuria, and decreased tubular reabsorption of phosphate (Goyer, 1982). The proteinuria is predominantly tubular in nature as indicated by an increased excretion of low-molecular-weight proteins (e.g., β_2-microglobulin); high-molecular-weight proteins have also been observed in the urine, suggesting a glomerular effect of cadmium as well (Goyer, 1982).

Other Metals. In sublethal doses, chromium produces proximal tubular necrosis similar to mercury except for its localization. Low doses of chromium produce relatively specific necrosis of the proximal convoluted tubule. Functionally, this leads to pronounced glucosuria (Figure 11–5). After low doses of chromium, the surface of the kidney shows marked signs of ischemia and tissue damage. As with mercury, when the dose of chromium is increased, toxicity is seen throughout the proximal tubule. Renal damage has also been observed following the administration of arsenic, gold, lead, iron, antimony, uranium, and thallium (Maher, 1976).

Halogenated Hydrocarbons

Chloroform. The renal lesions induced by acute administration of nephrotoxic doses of

CHCl$_3$ include increased kidney weight, swelling of tubular epithelium, fatty degeneration, tubular casts, and/or marked necrosis of proximal tubular epithelium. There is no primary glomerular damage and little involvement of the distal tubules. Functional changes include proteinuria, glucosuria, decreased secretion of organic anions, and increased BUN (Rush *et al.*, 1984a).

CHCl$_3$-induced nephrotoxicity depends, at least in part, on bioactivation to a toxic, reactive intermediate. There are dramatic species differences in susceptibility to CHCl$_3$ nephrotoxicity; certain strains of mice appear to be particularly susceptible to CHCl$_3$-induced renal injury (Hill *et al.*, 1975; Clemens *et al.*, 1979; Kluwe, 1981; Ahmadizadeh *et al.*, 1984). In addition, only male mice exhibit a nephrotoxic response to CHCl$_3$, whereas the hepatotoxic response is similar in both sexes (Smith *et al.*, 1983). This sex difference also appears to be related to differences in cytochrome P-450 content in the kidneys of male and female mice. The concentration of cytochrome P-450 is approximately fivefold greater in the kidneys of male as compared with female mice (Smith *et al.*, 1984). Castration of male mice reduced renal cytochrome P-450 content and reduced the susceptibility of the mice to CHCl$_3$-induced nephrotoxicity. Similarly, testosterone pretreatment of female mice substantially increased renal cytochrome P-450 content and rendered female mice as susceptible to the nephrotoxic effects of CHCl$_3$ as male mice (Smith *et al.*, 1984). Smith and Hook (1983) demonstrated that preincubation of renal cortical slices from male, but not female, mice with CHCl$_3$ resulted in a subsequent decrease of the ability of the slices to accumulate organic ions. Deuterated CHCl$_3$ was less effective than CHCl$_3$ in decreasing accumulation of organic ions by renal cortical slices from naive male mice. Similarly, carbon monoxide reduced CHCl$_3$ depression of slice organic ion accumulation, whereas the *in vitro* nephrotoxic effects of CHCl$_3$ were enhanced in glutathione (GSH)-depleted mice. These results suggested that the male, murine kidney may bioactivate CHCl$_3$ *in situ* to a nephrotoxic metabolite (Smith and Hook, 1983). Subsequently, Smith and Hook (1984) demonstrated that renal cortical microsomes prepared from male mice were capable of metabolizing CHCl$_3$ to CO$_2$ and a reactive metabolite that bound irreversibly to protein; however, little or no metabolism of CHCl$_3$ was observed in microsomes prepared from female mice. Addition of GSH to the microsomal mixture decreased the irreversible binding of the CHCl$_3$ metabolite to protein while increasing the formation of an

aqueous metabolite of CHCl$_3$. Branchflower *et al.*(1984) extended these observations by demonstrating that susceptibility of various mouse strains to CHCl$_3$ nephrotoxicity correlated with the capacity of the mouse kidney to metabolize CHCl$_3$ to phosgene. For example, homogenates of kidneys from male DBA/2J mice (susceptible strain) metabolized CHCl$_3$ to phosgene approximately twice as rapidly as renal homogenates from C57B1/6J mice (resistant strain). Thus, CHCl$_3$ appears to produce proximal tubular damage in the male mouse via a mechanism similar to that delineated in the liver (Kluwe, 1981; Branchflower *et al.*, 1984; Smith and Hook, 1984).

Bailie *et al.* (1984) have extended these experiments to rabbits. Pretreatment of rabbits with phenobarbital, a known inducer of rabbit renal cytochrome P-450, enhanced the *in vitro* toxic response of renal cortical slices to CHCl$_3$. Phenobarbital pretreatment also potentiated *in vitro* ^{14}CHCl$_3$ metabolism to CO$_2$ and increased covalently bound radioactivity in rabbit renal cortical slices and microsomes. Addition of L-cysteine reduced covalent binding in renal microsomes from both control and phenobarbital-pretreated rabbits. The reduction in covalent binding was associated with the formation of a radioactive phosgene-cysteine conjugate, 2-oxothiazolidine-4-carboxylic acid (OTZ). Formation of OTZ was enhanced in microsomes from phenobarbital-pretreated rabbits. These results also support the hypothesis that renal metabolism of CHCl$_3$ to a toxic, reactive intermediate (phosgene) occurs via cytochrome P-450.

Though the data above argue strongly for the formation of phosgene as the nephrotoxic metabolite of CHCl$_3$ in mouse and rabbit kidney, extrapolation of this mechanism to nephrotoxicity in other species should be made with caution. For other species, particularly humans and rats, the primary target of chloroform is the liver, and nephrotoxicity has been seen in human females as well as in female rats and dogs (Kluwe, 1981), suggesting possible alternate mechanisms of toxicity in these species. In addition, the chronic renal damage and tumor formation that may occur in humans and laboratory species following long-term exposure to low concentrations of chloroform and other halogenated hydrocarbons may be produced by mechanisms entirely distinct from those described above.

Other halogenated hydrocarbons have also been shown to be toxic to the kidney, producing effects similar to those of CHCl$_3$ (Kluwe, 1981). Interestingly, the nephrotoxicity of several of the halogenated hydrocarbons may be related to renal activation of a conjugate formed in the liver.

Hexachlorobutadiene. Hexachloro-1,3-butadiene (HCBD) is a by-product in the manufacture of solvents such as trichloroethylene and perchloroethylene and is a relatively potent nephrotoxicant in rats, mice, and other mammalian species. The kidneys appear to be the primary target of HCBD toxicity (Lock, 1988). In rats, HCBD produces a well-defined lesion in the pars recta of the proximal tubule, characterized by loss of brush border and accompanied by decreased urinary concentrating ability, glucosuria, proteinuria, and reduction of the renal clearances of inulin, *p*-aminohippuric acid (PAH), and tetraethylammonium (TEA) (Lock, 1988).

HCBD administration to rats depletes hepatic, but not renal, nonprotein sulfhydryl (GSH) content (Lock, 1988). However, inducers and/or inhibitors of hepatic and/or renal cytochrome P-450 have little or no effect on HCBD nephrotoxicity, suggesting that HCBD-induced hepatic GSH depletion and nephrotoxicity are not dependent on P-450 bioactivation (Lock and Ishmael, 1981, 1982; Hook *et al.*, 1982). Indeed, *in vitro* studies have indicated that rat hepatic microsomal and cytosolic fractions catalyze the formation of a GSH conjugate of HCBD, *S*-(1,2,3,4,4-pentachloro-1,3-butadienyl) glutathione (HCBD-GSH), independent of cytochrome P-450 activity (Wolf *et al.*, 1984). Furthermore, disposition and metabolism studies in rats suggest that the primary route of elimination of HCBD is the bile; the principal metabolite is HCBD-GSH (Nash *et al.*, 1984).

The involvement of biliary metabolites in HCBD nephrotoxicity has been suggested by the observations that: (1) administration of lyophilized bile, collected from HCBD-treated rats, to naive rats produces necrosis of the pars recta, a lesion that is similar to that observed following treatment with HCBD, and (2) interruption of the enterohepatic circulation, by cannulation and exteriorization of the bile duct, prevents HCBD nephrotoxicity (Nash *et al.*, 1984). Furthermore, administration of chemically synthesized HCBD-GSH or its degradative products, the cysteine conjugate (HCBD-CYS) or mercapturate (HCBD-NAC), also results in necrotic lesions of the pars recta that are indistinguishable from those produced by HCBD (Ishmael and Lock, 1986). Taken collectively, these data suggest that HCBD undergoes GSH conjugation in the liver and elimination in the bile. HCBD-GSH may be metabolized further by hepatic γ-glutamyltranspeptidase, followed by hydrolysis to HCBD-CYS within the intestine. Following enterohepatic circulation, HCBD-CYS may be delivered to the kidney without further extrarenal metabolism or may be *N*-acetylated (HCBD-NAC) within the liver prior to renal uptake. Alternatively, metabolism of HCBD-GSH to HCBD-CYS may occur in the brush border of proximal tubular cells via γ-glutamyltranspeptidase and cysteinyl glycine dipeptidase, prior to renal tubular uptake.

The susceptibility of the proximal tubule to HCBD conjugates appears to be related in part to its ability to transport and accumulate these molecules. Renal accumulation of radiolabeled HCBD is localized in the outer stripe of the outer medulla, coinciding with the site of renal necrosis in rats. Organic anion transport appears to play an important role in the renal cortical accumulation and nephrotoxicity of HCBD conjugates, since both accumulation and nephrotoxicity of HCBD or HCBD-NAC can be completely prevented by the organic anion transport inhibitor probenecid (Lock and Ishmael, 1985). Once accumulated within the cell, HCBD-NAC may be deacetylated to HCBD-CYS and covalent binding may result, suggesting further metabolism and bioactivation of HCBD-CYS in proximal tubular cells. Indeed, the cysteine conjugate of HCBD and trichloroethylene (dichlorovinyl-1-cysteine [DCVC]) are excellent substrates for cysteine conjugate β-lyase, resulting in formation of pyruvate, ammonia, chloride, and a reactive mercaptan moiety; the latter is believed to be the ultimate nephrotoxicant, reacting with intracellular proteins, nucleic acids, and/or thiols to produce cytotoxicity (Anders *et al.*, 1988). The role of renal cytosolic and/or mitochondrial β-lyase in HCBD and DCVC nephrotoxicity has been suggested by the observation that treatment with an inhibitor of this enzyme—for example, aminooxyacetate—prevents nephrotoxicity (Anders *et al.*, 1988). Cysteine conjugates rapidly impair succinate-dependent state 3 respiration, mitochondrial calcium sequestration, membrane potential, and metabolism *in vitro*, indicating that mitochondria are important cellular targets in cysteine conjugate cytotoxicity (Anders *et al.*, 1988).

Bromobenzene. Bromobenzene is nephrotoxic as well as hepatotoxic. *In vitro* studies on the metabolism and covalent binding of ^{14}C-bromobenzene suggest that renal necrosis is caused by a metabolite formed in extrarenal tissues and transported to the kidney. The metabolism of bromobenzene, however, is quite complex, and the exact metabolite(s) mediating bromobenzene toxicity is (are) not clear. Bromobenzene is metabolized to both ortho- and para-bromophenol, both of which are nephrotoxic *in vivo* and *in vitro* (Rush *et al.*, 1984a). 2-Bromohydroquinone, the major hepatic microsomal metabolite of both bromobenzene and ortho-bromophenol in rats, also produces proximal tubular necrosis (Lau *et al.*, 1984; Lau and Monks, 1988), suggesting that 2-bromohydroquinone or a metabolite thereof may mediate bromobenzene nephrotoxicity. Incubation of rat liver microsomes with 2-bromohydroquinone and ^{35}S-GSH results in the formation of GSH conjugates that, when incubated with rat kidney cytosol, result in covalent binding (Monks *et al.*, 1985; Lock, 1988). The involvement of 2-bromohydroquinone glutathione conjugate(s) in bromobenzene nephrotoxicity is suggested further by the observation that administration of a chemically synthesized diglutathione conjugate of bromobenzene, 2-bromo-(diglutathion-*S*-yl) hydroquinone [2-Br-(diGSyl)HQ], produces proximal tubular necrosis indistinguishable from that observed following administration of bromobenzene or 2-bromohydroquinone (Monks *et al.*, 1985). However, the relative involvement of 2-Br-(diGSyl)HQ and/or other identified or putative (e.g., 6-bromo-2,5-dihydroxy-thiophenol) metabolites in bromobenzene nephrotoxicity has not been clearly defined. It is likely, for example, that 2-Br-(diGSyl)HQ requires further metabolism to produce its toxic effects since its metabolism via γ-glutamyltranspeptidase and subsequent transport appear to be critical in the onset and development of nephrotoxicity (Monks *et al.*, 1988). However, in contrast to HCBD, nephrotoxicity of 2-Br-(diGSyl)HQ is not blocked by probenecid (Monks *et al.*, 1988). Similarly, aminooxyacetate, (inhibitor of β-lyase) offers only slight protection against 2-Br-(diGSyl)HQ nephrotoxicity (Monks *et al.*, 1988). Thus, mechanisms mediating the transport and intracellular bioactivation of 2-Br-(diGSyl)HQ appear to be somewhat different than those reported for other GSH conjugates such as DCVC or HCBD.

Petroleum Hydrocarbons. Acute exposure to unleaded gasoline vapors produces nephropathy in male rats characterized by increased protein (hyaline) droplet formation, degenerative intracellular changes, and subsequent regeneration in proximal tubular epithelium (Swenberg *et al.*, 1989). This nephropathy has been demonstrated following exposure of male, but not female, rats to other petroleum-derived hydrocarbons and mixtures including decalin, jet fuel, isophorone, 1,4-dichlorobenzene, and *d*-limonene (Swenberg *et al.*, 1989). Chronic exposure of male rats to unleaded gasoline ultimately leads to induction of renal adenomas and carcinomas, a phenomenon that appears to be mediated by epigenetic mechanisms since unleaded gasoline is not genotoxic.

Studies investigating the pathogenesis of hydrocarbon nephropathy have suggested that association of these hydrocarbons with α_{2u}-globulin plays an important role. α_{2u}-Globulin is a low-molecular-weight protein (18,700 daltons) synthesized by the liver of adult rats and is freely filtered by the glomerulus. Urinary excretion of α_{2u}-globulin by females is believed to be less than 1 percent of that excreted by male rats. Tubular reabsorption of α_{2u}-globulin, similar to that of other low-molecular-weight proteins, is mediated by an endocytotic mechanism, followed by fusion with, and sequestration by, phagolysosomes. It has been suggested that hydrocarbons and/or their metabolites reversibly bind to α_{2u}-globulin and are taken up by the proximal tubule cell (primarily S_2 segment) via endocytosis. These complexes appear to be resistant to, or impair, lysosomal catabolism, leading to their accumulation in the form of polyangular droplets. Lysosomal overload and individual cell necrosis result, followed by regeneration of the injured cell (Swenberg *et al.*, 1989). It is believed that a sustained increase in renal cell proliferation can promote initiated cells to form preneoplastic foci and renal neoplasia. Thus, it has been proposed that a pivotal step in the onset and development of hydrocarbon nephropathy is binding of these hydrocarbons and/or metabolites to α_{2u}-globulin. A corollary to this hypothesis is that the absence of such a protein, or the absence of a similar binding site to a related low-molecular-weight protein, precludes development of hydrocarbon nephropathy and, hence, renal carcinoma. Indeed, female rats or male and female mice, who excrete α_{2u}-globulin in negligible amounts, are not susceptible to the acute or chronic renal effects of these hydrocarbons. Similarly, humans do not synthesize α_{2u}-globulin and, by inference, may not be at risk. It is not known, however, whether these hydrocarbons can associate with binding sites of other low-molecular-weight proteins and, if so, whether the same biochemical sequelae observed with α_{2u}-globulin complexes will occur.

Therapeutic Agents

Some examples of nephrotoxic therapeutic agents are shown in Table 11–1.

Analgesics. Chronic ingestion of excessive amounts of nonnarcotic analgesics can lead to analgesic nephropathy in humans. Substantial morbidity is associated with this drug-induced nephrotoxicity. The functional aberrations associated with analgesic nephropathy include reduced GFR, salt wastage, hyperkalemia, meta-

Table 11–1. **EXAMPLES OF NEPHROTOXIC THERAPEUTIC AGENTS***

TOXICANT	REFERENCE

Antibiotics/Antivirals
  Aminoglycosides
  β-Lactams
  Vancomycin
  Sulfonamides
  Demeclocycline
  Amphotericin B
  Polymyxin B, E
	Humes and Weinberg, 1986;
	Bailie and Neal, 1988;
	Coggins and Fang, 1988;
	Humes and O'Connor, 1988

Antineoplastics
  Cisplatin
  Nitrosureas
  Mitomycin C
  Methotrexate
	Litterst and Weiss, 1987

Analgesics/Antiinflammatory
  Acetaminophen
  NSAIDs†
	Black, 1986;
	Sabatini, 1988

CNS/Anesthetics
  Enflurane
  Methoxyflurane
  Lithium
	Mazze, 1981;
	Humes and Weinberg, 1986;
	Porter and Bennett, 1989

Diuretics Organic mercurials	Kacew and Hirsch, 1981

Immunosuppressants
  Cyclosporine A
  d-Penicillamine
	Humes and Weinberg, 1986;
	Remuzzi and Bertani, 1989

Radiocontrast Agents
  Diatrizoates
  Iodohippurates
  Iodothalamates
	Golman et al., 1987;
	Cronin, 1988

* Only agents that have a direct effect on the nephron are cited. Examples represent some, not all, commonly cited nephrotoxicants.

† NSAIDs, = Nonsteroidal antiinflammatory drugs.

bolic acidosis, and a vasopressin-resistant concentrating defect (Sabatini, 1988). Severe analgesic nephropathy can lead to papillary necrosis with sloughing of the papilla (Sabatini, 1988). Although renal function may stabilize if ingestion of the offending analgesic is discontinued, complete anuria often results in the presence of continued abuse.

Most patients who develop analgesic nephropathy consume analgesics daily and may ingest between 2 and 5 mg for periods up to three years (Buckalew and Schey, 1986; Sabatini, 1988). Appreciable geographic variability exists in the incidence of analgesic abuse and analgesic nephropathy in habitual consumers. In the United States, for example, Buckalew and Schey (1986) estimated that 10 percent of patients with end-stage renal disease (ESRD) in one North Carolina city were heavy consumers of analgesics, whereas this was true only for 2.8 percent and 1.7 percent of ESRD patients in Washington, D.C., and Philadelphia, respectively. The prevalence of analgesic nephropathy in ESRD patients can be considerably higher in individual countries. The prevalence of analgesic nephropathy in ESRD patients in Switzerland was 18.1 percent (Wing et al., 1989), and earlier data (1967–74) suggested a prevalence as large as 30 percent in Australia (Sabatini, 1988).

Analgesic nephropathy can be produced in experimental animals; however, large quantities of analgesics must be given for long periods of time (i.e., weeks to months) to induce papillary necrosis similar to that produced by human analgesic abuse (Kincaid-Smith, 1978; Bach and Gregg, 1988). Molland (1978) fed rats relatively moderate doses of analgesics for extended times and observed that aspirin had a greater nephrotoxic effect than either phenacetin or acetaminophen, although aspirin toxicity was less alone than in combination with one of the nonsalicylates. Following aspirin alone, the earliest changes occurred in the medullary interstitial cells. Interestingly, the cortical lesions induced by this aspirin regimen did not depend on the presence of medullary necrosis, suggesting that the papillary and cortical damage might be separate events. This is consistent with the observation that medullary damage is a chronic event, whereas cortical damage alone is seen following acute ingestion of these nephrotoxicants.

Considerable controversy has arisen concerning the specific agent(s) in the mixture responsible for the nephrotoxicity and the mechanism(s) by which it might act. It was suggested that the early papillary changes produced by aspirin might be due to vasospasm in the vasa recta and thus represent an ischemic injury. Such an effect is consistent with the ability of aspirin to inhibit prostaglandin synthesis. Theoretically, inhibition of renal medullary prostaglandin synthesis might remove an endogenous vasodilator prostaglandin, leading to localized vasoconstriction. Significantly, other inhibitors of prostaglandin synthesis will produce renal medullary lesions in rats (Nanra, 1974). Phenacetin or one of its metabolites, primarily N-acetyl-para-amino-phenol (APAP, acetaminophen, paracetamol), has been implicated as a major contributor to the toxicity in man; however, removal of phenacetin from analgesic mixtures has not eliminated the problem (Kincaid-Smith, 1978). APAP, however, remains a frequently used analgesic and is capable of producing analgesic nephropathy in animals (Molland, 1978). Although neither aspirin nor phenacetin achieves increased concentrations in the medulla, APAP and its conjugates appear to concentrate in the renal medulla (Duggin and Mudge, 1976). Dehydration of animals leads to maximal concentrations of these materials in the medulla, a fact consistent with the enhanced toxicity that occurs during dehydration. Thus, trapping of APAP (or its metabolites) in the medulla by the countercurrent mechanism may play a role in the medullary toxicity produced by APAP.

APAP is metabolized to an arylating metabolite in vitro by an arachidonic acid–dependent pathway (Moldeus and Rahimtula, 1980; Mohandas et al., 1981; Boyd and Eling, 1981). In vitro, arachidonic acid–dependent covalent binding of APAP was greatest in the papilla and

least in the cortex, whereas NADPH-dependent binding was greatest in the cortex and undetectable in the papilla. Prostaglandin endoperoxide synthetase (PES)–dependent covalent binding of APAP to rabbit renal medullary microsomes was reduced by inhibitors of prostaglandin synthetase and antioxidants (Moldeus and Rahimtula, 1980; Mohandas et al., 1981; Moldeus et al., 1982). GSH also reduced the PES-dependent covalent binding of APAP; some of this was due to the generation of a GSH conjugate, but most could be accounted for by the oxidation of GSH to GSSG (Moldeus et al., 1982). The hydroperoxidase component of PES appeared to be responsible for the metabolic activation of APAP, and the inhibitory effect of antioxidants as well as the rapid oxidation of GSH support the hypothesis that a radical intermediate of APAP is formed in the renal papilla and may be responsible for initiating toxicity.

BEA (2-bromoethylamine) is proving to be a useful model of the morphologic and functional aberrations associated with papillary injury. This halogenated hydrocarbon produces complete papillary necrosis in virtually 100 percent of rats (Bach and Gregg, 1988; Sabatini, 1988). Histologic abnormalities are observed in the thin limbs and collecting ducts of the papilla in 24 hours, with complete necrosis of the thin limbs and more extensive collecting duct injury observable in 48 hours. The percentage of filtering juxtamedullary nephrons is markedly reduced by BEA, and the juxtamedullary glomeruli become sclerotic. BEA produces marked polyuria associated with a urine concentrating defect resistant to antidiuretic hormone. Renal wastage of Na^+ and Cl^- occurs and can result in extracellular fluid (ECF) volume contraction and metabolic alkalosis. Patients with analgesic nephropathy frequently become hyperkalemic, and potassium homeostasis is abnormal in BEA-treated rats. Phosphate, but not magnesium, wastage occurs in BEA-treated rats; however, papillary necrosis did not impair the adaptation to phosphate or magnesium deprivation. In contrast, urinary acidification remained normal in BEA-treated rats, suggesting that the hyperchloremic metabolic acidosis observed in some patients with papillary necrosis may not be related to a selective defect in acid excretion as a result of damage to the collecting duct. Thus, BEA-induced papillary necrosis in rats mimics several of the clinical features associated with analgesic nephropathy in humans. This feature, coupled with the rapid production and reproducibility of the papillary injury, suggests that BEA will become a major tool for examination of factors capable of ameliorating papillary necrosis as well as mechanisms important to the pathogenesis of this desease (Bach and Gregg, 1988; Sabatini, 1988).

Anesthetics. Several of the halogenated hydrocarbon anesthetics have been suggested to produce nephrotoxicity, but only one agent, methoxyflurane, has been documented to produce reproducible renal failure. In both animals and man, methoxyflurane produced a high-output renal failure, negative fluid balance, and increases in serum sodium, osmolality, and BUN. Patients or animals were unable to concentrate urine despite fluid deprivation and vasopressin administration, pointing to a defect in the renal concentrating mechanism. This toxicity had not originally been seen in animal studies. When Mazze (1981) and his collaborators studied a series of five rat strains, however, they found that the Fisher-344 and the Buffalo strains metabolized methoxyflurane to a greater extent than the other strains studied. The Fisher-344, with the greatest degree of metabolism, was the only strain that evidenced nephrotoxicity. Methoxyflurane appears to be metabolized primarily to inorganic fluoride and oxalate. Enhanced metabolism and nephrotoxicity were seen following phenobarbital treatment, whereas enzyme inhibition decreased metabolism and reduced nephrotoxicity. Subsequent studies indicated that it was the generation of the fluoride ion (acting in the ascending limb of the loop of Henle or in the collecting duct) that rendered the medulla antidiuretic hormone (ADH) resistant.

Antibiotics/Antivirals. *Aminoglycosides.* The incidence of acute renal failure in humans due to nephrotoxicants is approximately 15 percent. Antibiotics are the most frequently cited etiology of toxicant-induced acute renal failure. Within the antibiotic category, aminoglycosides are the leaders in producing renal injury, with about 10 percent of all cases of acute renal failure being attributed to the use of aminoglycoside antibiotics (Humes *et al.*, 1982; Bennett, 1983).

The severity of aminoglycoside nephrotoxicity runs the gamut from clinically trivial effects on tubular function to life-threatening acute tubular necrosis; severe nephrotoxicity seems to be rare if aminoglycosides are administered rationally (Leitman and Smith, 1983). Aminoglycoside nephrotoxicity is characterized primarily by a variety of renal functional alterations including: (1) enzymuria (brush border membrane and lysosomal); (2) tubular proteinuria (β_2-microglobulinuria); (3) transport defects (glycosuria, aminoaciduria, Mg^{2+} and K^+ wasting); (4) nephrogenic diabetes insipidus; and (5) diminished glomerular filtration rate (Humes *et al.*, 1982; Humes and O'Connor, 1988). The initial manifestation of aminoglycoside nephrotoxicity is enzymuria, which can occur as early as 24 hours after a single therapeutic dose. Most clinical descriptions of aminoglycoside-induced acute renal failure stress the nonoliguric character of the injury. Polyuria and nephrogenic diabetes insipidus develop early, prior to a fall in creatinine clearance. Aminoglycoside nephrotoxicity usually is reversible upon cessation of treatment.

The primary target of aminoglycoside toxicity is the proximal tubular cell. Movement across the apical membrane of the proximal tubular cell appears to be the dominant route by which aminoglycosides gain access into the cell. Aminoglycosides are reabsorbed by an endocytotic mechanism responsible for reabsorption of low-molecular-weight proteins. After filtration, a small fraction of the cationic antibiotic binds to anionic phospholipids, such as the polyphosphoinositides, in the brush border of the proximal tubule. The bound aminoglycoside is engulfed by adsorptive endocytosis and stored in secondary lysosomes. Aminoglycosides also have been shown to be localized in the cytoplasm prior to lysosomal uptake, and these antibiotics are capable of binding to membranes of other subcellular organelles, with potential for redistribution among them. Basolateral membrane binding and uptake occur, but this represents a minor contribution to cellular aminoglycoside concentration (Humes *et al.*, 1982; Kaloyanides, 1984; Humes and O'Connor, 1988; Weinberg, 1988). Once taken up by proximal tubular cells, the aminoglycosides reside in a poorly exchangeable pool. Renal cortical tissue half-lives of aminoglycosides may exceed those in serum by over 100-fold.

A variety of aminoglycoside-induced biochemical aberrations likely contribute to the proximal tubular cell injury produced by these antibiotics. Aminoglycosides inhibit several lysosomal phospholipases (Tulkens *et al.*, 1979; Hostetler and Hall, 1982) as well as phosphatidylinositol-specific phospholipase C activity in both renal cortical cytosol (Lipsky and Leitman, 1982) and proximal tubular cell brush border membrane (Schwetz *et al.*, 1984). Inhibition of these phospholipases would be expected to alter the amount and relative phospholipid composition of plasma and subcellular membranes within the proximal tubule.

The alterations in renal cortical phospholipid content and composition precede the appearance of appreciable renal dysfunction, suggesting that these alterations may alter organelle membrane permeability and transport as well as phospholipid-dependent enzyme activities. Gentamicin does inhibit the activity of two basolateral membrane phospholipid-dependent enzymes, Na^+-K^+-ATPase and adenylate cyclase. However, gentamicin treatment did not change the bulk fluidity of the basolateral membrane (Williams et al., 1984) and did not increase the phospholinositol (PI) content of this membrane (Knauss et al., 1983). Although a causal relationship between aminoglycoside-induced alterations in membrane phospholipid content/composition and proximal tubular cell injury has not been demonstrated, the nephrotoxic potential of an aminoglycoside, the potency of phospholipase inhibition, and the severity of phospholipidosis are closely related (Humes and O'Connor, 1988).

Alterations in membrane phospholipid composition, however, are not likely the sole mechanism by which aminoglycosides produce proximal tubular dysfunction. Mitochrondrial respiration is depressed by these antibiotics. Renal cortical mitochondria from gentamicin-treated rats exhibited depressed state 3 and DNP (2,4-dinitro-phenol)-uncoupled respiration; renal ATP content also was depressed, indicating that the mitochondrial dysfunction was sufficiently severe to impair cellular energetics (Humes and O'Connor, 1988). Gentamicin inhibits mitochondrial Ca^{2+} uptake (Sastrasinh et al., 1982) and displaces Ca^{2+} at binding sites on biological membranes (Williams et al.,1981; Humes et al., 1984; Ishikawa et al., 1985). Thus, gentamicin could elevate cytosolic free $[Ca^{2+}]$ first by displacing Ca^{2+} from membrane binding sites and second by preventing mitochondria from buffering the increased cytosolic free $[Ca^{2+}]$ (Inui et al., 1988). In addition, sequestration of aminoglycoside in lysosomes leads to myeloid body formation by impairment of phospholipid degradation. Lysosomal membrane integrity is reduced, and release of lysosomal enzymes into the cytosol with subsequent digestion of cytoplasmic components and organelles may occur. At present, the relative contribution of these events to initiation of proximal tubular cell injury is unclear (Humes and O'Connor, 1988).

Cephalosporins. Members of the cephalosporin class of antibiotics also are capable of producing acute proximal tubular injury. Cephaloridine is a broad-spectrum cephalosporin antibiotic that produces nephrotoxicity in both laboratory rats and humans when administered in large dosages. Like the aminoglycosides, cephaloridine has a relatively short plasma half-life. Cephaloridine accumulates in the kidney to a much greater extent than in other organs, most of it within the cortex (Wold, 1981; Tune, 1982). Several studies have indicated that the incidence and severity of cephaloridine nephrotoxicity are directly correlated with renal cortical accumulation of drug. The mechanisms mediating the renal cortical accumulation of cephaloridine involve an active transport process. Similar to PAH, cephaloridine is actively transported from the peritubular capillary into the proximal tubular cell via an organic anion transporter. However, in contrast to PAH, transport of cephaloridine across the luminal membrane is restricted. Consequently, high intracellular concentrations of cephaloridine are attained in the proximal tubular cell, potentially leading to cell damage. The role of an organic anion transporter in renal cortical accumulation and nephrotoxicity of cephaloridine is suggested by studies indicating that probenecid, an inhibitor of organic anion transport, markedly reduces cortical concentrations and nephrotoxicity of cephaloridine.

Although the role of tubular transport and accumulation in cephaloridine nephrotoxicity has been well defined, the exact biochemical mechanisms by which cephaloridine induces cytotoxicity are not well defined. However, several lines of evidence suggest that lipid peroxidation may play a role: (1) *In vivo* and *in vitro* exposure to cephaloridine increase renal cortical concentrations of peroxidative products, (2) cephaloridine nephrotoxicity is potentiated in rats fed antioxidant-deficient diets, (3) *in vitro* lipid peroxidation precedes the onset of cytotoxicity, and (4) antioxidant treatment protects against cephaloridine toxicity *in vitro* (Goldstein et al., 1988a). It has been postulated that cephaloridine may undergo redox cycling, resulting in reduction of molecular oxygen to superoxide anion, which may contribute to oxidative stress and lipid peroxidation (Kuo et al., 1983) (Figure 11–6). This hypothesis is supported by evidence indicating that cephaloridine undergoes anaerobic reduction by isolated renal cortical microsomes with subsequent production of superoxide anion radicals and hydrogen peroxide (Cojocel et al., 1985).

Another mechanism mediating cephaloridine nephrotoxicity may involve mitochondrial dysfunction. Mitochondrial function is impaired shortly following cephaloridine administration to rabbits and is characterized by marked depression in succinate-supported respiration (Tune et al., 1979). Furthermore, other nephrotoxic cephalosporins (i.e., cephaloglycin) produce similar patterns of respiratory depression, whereas nonnephrotoxic cephalosporins (i.e., cephalexin) do not affect mitochondrial function (Tune and Fravert, 1980). It has been proposed that nephrotoxic cephalosporins competitively inhibit the uptake of metabolic anionic substrates by the mitochondria; nontoxic cephalosporins do

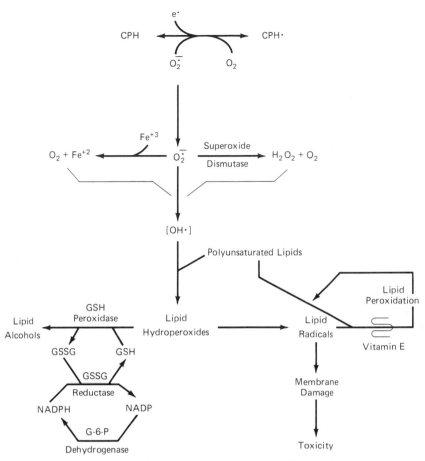

Figure 11–6. Postulated mechanism of toxicity of cephaloridine. Redox cycling leading to generation of ROSs; GSH depletion by oxidation and subsequent tissue damage.

not accumulate significantly within the proximal tubule and/or do not inhibit substrate transport as effectively (Tune *et al.*, 1989).

Other beta-lactam antibiotics also may be nephrotoxic. For example, imipenem, a beta-lactam antibiotic containing a carbapenem nucleus, produces proximal tubular necrosis in monkeys and rabbits. Similar to cephaloridine, rats are not very susceptible to imipenem nephrotoxicity (Birnbaum *et al.*, 1985). Coadministration of cilastatin, a dehydropeptidase inhibitor, markedly reduces renal cortical concentrations and nephrotoxicity of imipenem as well as cephaloridine (Birnbuam *et al.*, 1985), suggesting that renal cortical transport and accumulation of imipenem may be mediated by the same mechanism as that described for cephaloridine, and like cephaloridine, this mechanism plays an important role in the nephrotoxicity of imipenem.

Other Antibiotics. Tetracyclines, particularly demeclocycline, have on occasion produced renal medullary toxicity. Outdated tetracyclines may produce proximal tubular damage with polyuria, glucosuria, and aminoaciduria. In humans, penicillins and sulfonamides have been implicated in an inflammatory interstitial nephritis that is not dose related, apparently due to an immunologic-type mechanism (Appel and Neu, 1977a, 1977b).

Amphotericin B. Clinical utility of the antifungal agent amphotericin B is limited by its dose-related nephrotoxicity. Amphotericin B nephrotoxicity is unusual in that it impairs the functional integrity of all segments of the nephron including the glomerular capillary tuft and the proximal and distal portions of the tubule. Renal dysfunction has been reported to occur in 75 to 85 percent of amphotericin B–treated patients and is manifested as azotemia associated with decreased RPF and GFR, vasopressin-resistant polyuria, and renal tubular acidosis accompanied by potassium wasting and hypokalemia (Douglas and Healy, 1969; Burgess and Birchall, 1972). In addition, histological evidence of nephrocalcinosis, affecting both proximal and distal tubules, has been reported in amphotericin B–treated animals (Weldon and Schultz, 1974).

Two distinct mechanisms appear to be involved in amphotericin nephrotoxicity: (1) renal arteriolar vasoconstriction and (2) increased permeability of both proximal and distal tubules (Cheng et al., 1982; Capasso et al., 1986; Tolins and Raij, 1988a, 1988b). The renal hemodynamic effects of amphotericin are characterized by increased renal vascular resistance and decreased RPF (Cheng et al., 1982; Tolins and Raij, 1988a, 1988b). The exact mechanisms mediating amphotericin-induced renal vasoconstriction are not known; however, a role for activation of the tubuloglomerular feedback has been suggested (Tolins and Raij, 1988b). More recently, verapamil has been shown to block amphotericin-induced renal vasoconstriction completely, suggesting the possibility that vasoconstriction may be mediated by increased entry of calcium into vascular smooth muscle (Tolins and Raij, 1988a). Interestingly, verapamil did not completely block the fall in GFR, suggesting that decreased GFR is not exclusively due to vasoconstriction. It is unlikely that tubular toxicity associated with amphotericin can be attributed solely to ischemic effects associated with renal vasoconstriction (Tolins and Raij, 1988b). Rather, tubular toxicity most likely reflects the direct interaction of this polyene antibiotic with membrane-bound cholesterol to form aqueous channels, resulting in increased permeability to small solutes, particularly ions. This effect of amphotericin on membrane permeability could mediate the effects of this drug on concentrating ability and maintenance of acid-base balance. Indeed, formulation of amphotericin B as an emulsion markedly ameliorates amphotericin-induced polyuria without a concomitant loss of efficacy against fungal infections (Kirsh et al., 1988).

Antineoplastic Agents. *Cisplatin.* Nephrotoxicity is frequently a complication of cancer chemotherapy with the platinum coordination complex cisplatin. Although the primary target of cisplatin nephrotoxicity in laboratory rats is the pars recta of the proximal tubule, renal damage appears to be more widespread in cisplatin-treated humans, affecting the pars convoluta, distal tubule, and collecting duct (Tanaka et al., 1986). Kidney damage may persist in treated patients, lasting more than 12 months following cisplatin treatment, suggesting that cisplatin could exert continuing and irreversible damage to the kidneys (Fillastre and Raguenez-Viotte, 1989). In humans, renal dysfunction following cisplatin treatment is manifested by decreased RPF and GFR (and hence, increased BUN and serum creatinine concentrations), enzymuria, β_2-microglobulinuria, and inappropriate urinary losses of magnesium, resulting in hypomagnesemia (Fillastre and Raguenez-Viotte, 1989). In rats, cisplatin also induces polyuric renal failure, an effect that appears to be due to dissipation of the corticopapillary solute gradient (Safirstein et al., 1987).

The principal route of excretion of cisplatin is via the kidneys; consequently, the kidneys may be exposed to high concentrations of the drug. In laboratory rats, platinum is localized in the corticomedullary region, coinciding with the site of tubular necrosis in this species. Renal clearance of unbound platinum is comparable with or slightly greater than inulin clearance. Thus, cisplatin appears to be excreted predominantly by filtration and perhaps to a small extent by secretion; to date, there is no evidence for tubular reabsorption. Renal cortical accumulation and toxicity of cisplatin appear to be dependent on organic cation transport; *in vitro* uptake and *in vivo* nephrotoxicity of cisplatin are blocked by specific inhibitors of the organic cation transport system (Bird et al., 1984; Safirstein et al., 1984). Furthermore, cisplatin nephrotoxicity occurs in the nonfiltering isolated perfused rat kidney, suggesting that basolateral transport of cisplatin, presumably via organic cation transport, is critical to the onset and progression of cisplatin nephrotoxicity (Miura et al., 1987).

The exact biochemical mechanisms mediating cisplatin nephrotoxicity are not known. Cisplatin exists as a neutral complex in extracellular fluid. However, owing to the low intracellular concentrations of chloride, the chloride groups of the cisplatin complex are displaced by water, resulting in the intracellular formation of a positively charged hydrated or hydroxylated species. It has been hypothesized that these molecules may react with essential macromolecules of the tubular cell, resulting in nephrotoxicity (Goldstein and Mayor, 1983). Indeed, an early event in cisplatin nephrotoxicity in rats is inhibition of renal cortical DNA replication, an effect that precedes necrosis (Safirstein et al., 1987). Other mechanisms mediating cisplatin nephrotoxicity have been postulated, including binding to sulfhydryl groups of critical macromolecules, inhibition of renal ATPase, and mitochondrial dysfunction (Gordon and Gattone, 1986; Litterst and Weiss, 1987; Safirstein et al., 1987; Fillastre and Raguenez-Viotte, 1989).

Although heavy metals such as platinum are nephrotoxic, moieties other than, or in addition to, the platinum atom mediate cisplatin nephrotoxicity since the *trans* isomer of this platinum complex does not produce renal damage (Goldstein and Mayor, 1983). Moreover, structural modifications of the ligands of the cisplatin complex can alter the incidence and severity of nephrotoxicity. Promising analogues of cisplatin include carboplatin and iproplatin; both analogues appear to be less nephrotoxic than cisplatin, although hematologic effects persist (Litterst and Weiss, 1987).

Immunosuppressants. *Cyclosporine.* Cyclosporine A, a fungal cyclic polypeptide, is currently the immunosuppressant of choice for management of graft rejection in organ transplantation. However, nephrotoxicity of this agent limits its clinical utility; nearly all patients receiving therapeutic dosages of cyclosporine develop some form of renal dysfunction (Racusen and Solez, 1988). Clinically, cyclosporine nephrotoxicity may manifest as: (1) acute reversible renal dysfunction, (2) acute vasculopathy (thrombotic microangiopathy), and/or (3) chronic nephropathy with interstitial fibrosis (Racusen and Solez, 1988).

Acute renal dysfunction is manifested clinically as dose-related decreases in RPF and GFR and reflected by increased BUN and serum creatinine concentrations; these effects are reversible on reduction of dosage or cessation of cyclosporine therapy. Acute renal insufficiency in patients is probably related to drug-induced renal vasoconstriction. In humans and in laboratory rats, cyclosporine increases renal vascular resistance (Racusen and Solez, 1988). Furthermore, cyclosporine has been shown to decrease the ultrafiltration coefficient in rats, a factor that also may contribute to alterations in GFR (Racusen and Solez, 1988). Unfortunately, the site of cyclosporine-induced renal vasoconstriction (i.e., afferent versus efferent arterioles) is not known with certainty. Although the exact sites/mechanisms of cyclosporine-induced renal vasoconstriction are not known, stimulation of the renin-angiotensin system, an imbalance in vasoactive prostanoids (exaggerated intrarenal formation of potent vasoconstrictors; i.e., thromboxanes, coupled with inhibition of vasodilatory prostaglandins), and/or activation of the sympathetic nervous system have been suggested to play a role (Racusen and Solez, 1988; Remuzzi and Bertani, 1989). Clinical studies investigating the effects of drugs that interfere with the sympathetic nervous system, the renin-angiotensin system, and/or thromboxane and prostaglandin formation/activity may help unravel the mechanism of cyclosporine-induced renal vasoconstriction in humans.

Another form of cyclosporine nephrotoxicity, acute thrombotic microangiopathy, is a rather unusual nephrotoxic lesion. Cyclosporine microangiopathy is characterized by circular, nodular protein deposits (consisting of immunoglobulin M, complement, and/or fibrinogen) permeating the arteriolar wall, thrombosis of glomerular capillaries, and endothelial cell desquamation, effects that may narrow or even occlude the vascular lumen (Mihatsch *et al.*, 1989). The pathogenesis of these lesions is poorly understood, and the lesion itself has not been reproduced successfully in standard, normotensive laboratory rats. Clinically, this syndrome represents hemolytic uremic syndrome/thrombotic thryombocytopenia purpura (HUS/TTP), has a poor prognosis, and possibly results from a direct toxic effect of cyclosporine on vascular endothelium. Cyclosporine-induced arteriolopathy appears to be quite similar to reported cases of thrombotic microangiopathy in transplant rejection, independent of cyclosporine treatment. Thus, differentiation of drug-induced lesions from those related to organ rejection may be difficult, although the vessels primarily affected appear to be different with cyclosporine (arterioles) versus transplant rejection (arteries) (Mihatsch *et al.*, 1989).

A more chronic form of cyclosporine nephrotoxicity has been described in patients receiving the drug for 12 or more months. Although reductions in GFR are only modest, histopathological changes are quite profound, characterized by arteriolopathy, global and segmental glomerular sclerosis, striped interstitial fibrosis, and tubular atrophy (Remuzzi and Bertani, 1989). These lesions may not be reversible, are potentially progressive, and may result in end-stage renal failure. The irregular striped patterns of interstitial fibrosis induced by cyclosporine treatment are associated with atrophic tubules in the renal cortex; tubules in other areas may appear essentially normal (Mihatsch *et al.*, 1989). The pathogenesis of acute and chronic cyclosporine nephrotoxicity remains poorly understood, and the relationship between the acute and chronic lesions is not known.

Environmental Contaminants

A variety of pesticides and herbicides have reached sufficient concentrations in the environment to constitute potential hazards to man and animals (*see* Table 11–2). 2,4,5-Trichlorophenoxyacetic acid (2,4,5-T) has been a widely used herbicide. This compound has not been shown to be directly nephrotoxic, but it may influence renal function. The compound appears to be actively transported by the organic anion secretory system and is capable of inhibiting organic anion transport. Furthermore, in

Table 11–2. EXAMPLES OF OCCUPATIONAL/ENVIRONMENTAL AND EXPERIMENTAL NEPHROTOXICANTS*

TOXICANT	REFERENCE
Mycotoxins/Botanicals	Berndt, 1987
Aflatoxin B	
Citrinin	
Ochratoxin A	
Monocrotaline	
Pyrrolizidine alkaloids	
Rubratoxin B	
Halogenated Aliphatic Hydrocarbons	Lock, 1988; Kluwe, 1990
Bromobenzene	
Bromodichloromethane	
Carbon tetrachloride	
Chloroform	
Chlorotrifluoroethylene	
Dibromochloropropane	
Dibromoethane	
Dichloroethane	
Hexachlorobutadiene	
Pentachloroethane	
Trichloroethylene	
Tetrachloroethylene	
Tetrafluoroethylene	
Tris (2,3-dibromopropyl)-phosphate	
Volatile Hydrocarbons	Alden et al., 1984;
Petroleum fuels	Swenberg et al., 1989
Metals	Fowler et al., 1987;
Cadmium	Wedeen, 1988
Gold	
Lead	
Mercury	
Nickel	
Chromium	
Uranium	
Herbicides/Fungicides	Ecker et al., 1975;
Paraquat	Berndt, 1982a;
Diquat	Rankin et al., 1989
Succinimides	
2,4,5-Trichlorophenoxyacetate	
Organic Solvents	Gosselin et al., 1984
Ethylene glycol	
Diethylene glycol	
Toluene	
Experimental Tools/Miscellaneous	
p-Aminophenol	Newton et al., 1982
Adriamycin	Elema et al., 1988
Benzidine	Zenser and Davis, in press
Bromoethanamine hydrobromide	Sabatini, 1988
d-Serine	Carone and Ganote, 1975
d-Lysine	Racusen et al., 1985
Limonene	Lehman-McKeeman et al., 1989
Maleic acid	Berliner et al., 1950
Phenylanthranillic acid	Bach and Gregg, 1988
Puromycin aminonucleoside	Elema et al., 1988

* Only agents that have a direct effect on the nephron are cited. Examples represent some, not all, commonly cited nephrotoxicants.

high concentrations the compound appears to inhibit cation transport as well (Berndt, 1982a). The herbicide paraquat produces profound pulmonary damage following acute intoxication. In sublethal doses, paraquat appears to be actively secreted by the organic cation transport system of the kidney and is fairly rapidly removed from the body. Following high dosages, however, paraquat produces direct renal damage, thereby reducing its own elimination. This leads to prolonged high plasma concentrations of this agent, which enhance the lung damage (Ecker et al., 1975).

A number of industrial and agricultural chemicals may influence kidney function. Several of these compounds have a profound metabolic effect on the liver, and it is these abnormalities that have received most attention. However, it is not unlikely that in the future heretofore unrecognized abnormalities in renal function could be attributed to one or more of these agents. Polychlorinated biphenyls (PCBs) are a mixture of chemicals used in a wide variety of manufacturing processes, notably in the plastics industry, and as insulators. These compounds are ubiquitous contaminants of the environment and have been shown to have marked stimulating effects on drug metabolism in the liver and to increase liver size and liver weight. PCBs also have been shown to enhance drug-metabolizing enzyme activity in the kidney (Rush et al., 1984b). The polybrominated biphenyls (PBBs), although not so widespread, are also significant environmental contaminants. The PBBs similarly induce drug-metabolizing enzyme activity in the liver and kidney and thereby present a potential hazard (McCormack et al., 1978). Tetrachlorodibenzo-p-dioxin (TCDD) is an extremely toxic agent that has been known to produce a wide variety of toxic symptoms in animals and man. Like the polyhalogenated biphenyls, TCDD has not been shown to have a profound direct toxic effect on the adult kidney but does alter drug metabolism in this organ and could pose a potential hazard (Fowler et al., 1977). The presence of such potential stimulators of drug metabolism in the environment could lead to difficulty in interpreting experimental data. For instance, following accidental exposure to one of these stimulators, a relatively innocuous substance could be metabolically altered within the kidney and produce nephrotoxicity.

Mycotoxins are secondary fungal metabolites that can damage various organ systems upon ingestion of contaminated foodstuffs or feeds. Several mycotoxins have been reported to be nephrotoxicants (Hayes, 1980; Berndt, 1982b). For example, rubratoxin B, aflatoxin B_1, and sterigmatocystin induce renal lesions (Hayes, 1980). In rats, ochratoxin A and citrinin produced proteinuria, glucosuria, and reduction in urine osmolality. Proximal tubular transport of organic ions was also reduced by these mycotoxins. Interestingly, these mycotoxins may produce proximal tubular injury via different mechanisms. A single large dose of citrinin produced proximal tubular dysfunction and necrosis in rats. In contrast, repeated administration of small doses of ochratoxin A were required to elicit renal damage; a single large dose of this mycotoxin resulted in severe diarrhea and death without obvious effects on the kidney. Citrinin decreased rat renal cortical GSH concentration and appeared to bind covalently to renal constituents. Thus, citrinin (or a hepatic metabolite) may be activated to a toxic reactive metabolite within the kidney. Ochratoxin A and citrinin have been implicated in the production of porcine nephropathy. In addition, one or both of these mycotoxins may be involved in endemic Balkan nephropathy (EBN), a disease that is endemic to isolated rural populations of Bulgaria, Romania, and Yugoslavia (Hall, 1982). The renal pathology of EBN is characterized by extensive interstitial fibrosis and proximal tubular degeneration. This disease is comparable in many ways to porcine nephropathy, and ochratoxin A has been isolated from serum of patients with EBN (Hall, 1982).

EFFECT OF AGE ON RENAL SUSCEPTIBILITY TO TOXICANTS

Theoretically, both the young and old might be expected to be less susceptible to chemically induced nephrotoxicity based on renal functional considerations alone. Specifically, renal functions that normally render the adult kidney vulnerable to chemical toxicity may be less well developed in the young or may be impaired in the aged. For example, the immature and senescent kidneys are often characterized by decreased GFR, RPF, tubular transport, and concentrating ability, all of which are critical to the delivery, uptake, and concentration of toxicants in the renal epithelium. Organic anion transport, for instance, is incompletely developed at birth; thus, low intracellular concentrations of nephrotoxicants that are dependent on organic anion transport for renal uptake would be expected in newborns. Indeed, neonatal rabbits are not susceptible to cephaloridine nephrotoxicity (Wold et al., 1977). Furthermore, stimulation of the renal organic anion transport system with penicillin or PAH pretreatment enhances cephaloridine nephrotoxicity in neonatal rabbits, suggesting that cephaloridine nephrotoxicity is dependent on a mature organic anion transport system for proximal tubular transport and subsequent accumulation of drug (Wold *et al.*, 1977). An age-related decrease in susceptibility to gentamicin nephrotoxicity in the young also has been reported and attributed to decreased renal exposure and accumulation of gentamicin, an effect that may be due to decreased GFR in immature nephrons and, hence, decreased delivery of gentamicin to brush border membranes of proximal tubules (Goldstein and Hook, in press).

Similar to the young, kidneys of senescent rats (33 to 34 months) are characterized by decreased capacity for organic anion transport and, hence, decreased capacity to transport and accumulate cephaloridine, resulting in a blunted nephrotoxic response (Goldstein, 1990). However, in the absence of an age-related decline in organic anion transport, middle-aged (9 to 12 months) or old rats (27 to 29 months) are more susceptible to cephaloridine nephrotoxicity, a phenomenon that appears to be due to age-dependent effects on the pharmacokinetics and, hence, renal cortical accumulation of this agent (Goldstein *et al.*, 1986). Middle-aged rats also are more susceptible to acetaminophen nephrotoxicity, an effect that may be due in part to age-related changes in the pharmacokinetics and renal cortical accumulation of this drug (Tarloff *et al.*, 1989). However, factors other than age-dependent acetaminophen pharmacokinetics mediate the enhanced nephrotoxic response in middle-aged rats since at equivalent blood concentrations of acetaminophen age-dependent nephrotoxicity is still observed (Tarloff *et al.*, 1989). Indeed, factors other than drug metabolism and pharmacokinetics appear to play an important role in age-dependent nephrotoxicity since renal tubular injury is more severe in older rats following a biochemical insult that is independent of pharmacokinetics and disposition, that is, ischemia or anoxia (Goldstein *et al.*, 1988b). Thus, kidneys of old rats are intrinsically more susceptible to a toxic insult.

REFERENCES

Ahmadizadeh, M.; Echt, R.; Kuo, C. H.; and Hook, J. B.: Sex strain differences in mouse kidney: Bowman's capsule morphology and susceptibility to chloroform. *Toxicol. Lett.*, **20**:161–172, 1984.

Alden, C. L.; Kanerva, R. L.; Ridder, G.; and Stone, L. C.: The pathogenesis of the nephrotoxicity of volatile hydrocarbons in the male rat. In Mehlman, M. A. (ed.): *Renal Effects of Petroleum Hydrocarbons.* Princeton Scientific Publishers, Princeton, 1984, pp. 107–120.

Anders, M. W.; Lash, L.; Dekant, W.; Elfarra, A. A.; and Dohn, D. R.: Biosynthesis and biotransformation of glutathione *S*-conjugates to toxic metabolites. *CRC Crit. Rev. Toxicol.*, **18**:311–341, 1988.

Appel, G. B., and Neu, H. C.: The nephrotoxicity of antimicrobial agents (part 1). *N. Engl. J. Med.*, **296**:663–670, 1977a.

——: The nephrotoxicity of antimicrobial agents (part 2). *N. Engl. J. Med.*, **296**:722–728, 1977b.

Arendshorst, W. J., and Gottschalk, C. W.: Glomerular ultrafiltration dynamics: historical perspective. *Am. J. Physiol.*, **248**:F163–F174, 1985.

Bach, P. H., and Gregg, N. J.: Experimentally induced renal papillary necrosis and upper urothelial carcinoma. *Int. Rev. Exper. Pathol.*, **30**:1–54, 1988.

Bailie, G. R., and Neal, D.: Vancomycin ototoxicity and nephrotoxicity. *Med. Toxicol.*, **3**:376–386, 1988.

Bailie, M. B.; Smith, J. H.; Newton, J. F.; and Hook, J. B.: Mechanism of chloroform nephrotoxicity. IV: Phenobarbital potentiation of *in vitro* chloroform metabolism and toxicity in rabbit kidneys. *Toxicol. Appl. Pharmacol.*, **74**:285–292, 1984.

Baud, L., and Ardaillou, R.: Reactive oxygen species: production and role in the kidney. *Am. J. Physiol.*, **251**:F765–F776, 1986.

Bennett, W. M.: Aminoglycoside nephrotoxicity. *Nephron*, **35**:73–77, 1983.

Berlin, M.: Mercury. In Friberg, L.; Norberg, G. F.; and Vouk, V. (eds.): *Handbook on the Toxicology of Metals*, 2nd ed. Elsevier Science Publishers B.V., Amsterdam, 1986, pp. 387–445.

Berliner, R. W.; Kennedy, T. J.; and Hilton, J. G.: Effect of maleic acid on renal function. *Proc. Soc. Exp. Biol. Med.*, **75**:791–794, 1950.

Berndt, W. O.: The effect of potassium dichromate on renal tubular transport processes. *Toxicol. Appl. Pharmacol.*, **32**:40–52, 1975.

——: Renal methods in toxicology. In Hayes, A. W. (ed.): *Principles and Methods of Toxicology.* Raven Press, New York, 1982a, pp. 447–474.

——: Nephrotoxicity of natural products. Mycotoxin-induced nephropathy. In Porter, G. A. (Ed.): *Nephrotoxic Mechanisms of Drugs and Environmental Toxins.* Plenum Publishing Corp., New York, 1982b, pp. 241–254.

——: Naturally occurring environmental contaminants. In Bach, P. E., and Lock, E. A. (eds.): *Nephrotoxicity in the Experimental and Clinical Situation.* Martinus Nijhoff Publishers, Lancaster, England, 1987, pp. 683–700.

Bertolatus, J. A.; Foster, S. J.; and Hunsicker, L. G.: Stainable glomerular basement membrane polyanions and renal hemodynamics during hexadimethrine-induced proteinuria. *J. Lab. Clin. Med.*, **103**:632–642, 1984.

Bertolatus, J. A., and Hunsicker, L. G.: Glomerular sieving of anionic and neutral bovine albumins in proteinuric rats. *Kidney Int.*, **28**:467–476, 1985.

Bird, J. E.; Walser, M. M.; and Quebbemann, A. J.: Protective effect of organic cation transport inhibitors on *cis*-diamminiedichloroplatinum-induced nephrotoxicity. *J. Pharmacol. Exp. Ther.*, **231**:752–758, 1984.

Birnbaum, J.; Kahan, F. M.; Kropp, H.; and MacDonald, J. S.: Carbapenems, a new class of beta-lactam antibiotics. *Am. J. Med.*, **78**(Suppl. 6A):3–21, 1985.

Black, H. E.: Renal toxicity of non-steroidal anti-inflammatory drugs. *Toxicol. Pathol.*, **14**:83–90, 1986.

Bonventre, J. V.: Mediators of ischemic renal injury. *Annu. Rev. Med.*, **39**:531–544, 1988.

Boyd, J. A., and Eling, T. E.: Prostaglandin endoperoxide synthetase–dependent cooxidation of acetaminophen to intermediates which covalently bind *in vitro* to rabbit renal medullary microsomes. *J. Pharmacol. Exp. Ther.*, **219**:659–664, 1981.

Branchflower, R. V.; Nunn, D. S.; Highet, R. J.; Smith, J. H.; Hook, J. B.; and Pohl, L. R.: Nephrotoxicity of chloroform: metabolism to phosgene by the mouse kidney. *Toxicol. Appl. Pharmacol.*, **72**:159–168, 1984.

Brenner, B. M.; Bohrer, M. P.; Baylis, C.; and Deen, W. M.: Determinants of glomerular permselectivity: insights derived from observations *in vivo. Kidney Int.*, **12**:229–237, 1977.

Brenner, B. M.; Zatz, R.; and Ichikawa, I.: The renal circulations. In Brenner, B. M., and Rector, F. C., Jr. (eds.): *The Kidney*, Vol. 1, 3rd ed. W. B. Saunders Co., Philadelphia, 1986, pp. 93–123.

Buckalew, V. M., and Schey, H. M.: Analgesic nephropathy: a significant cause of morbidity in the United States. *Am. J. Kidney Dis.*, **7**:164–168, 1986.

Burg, M. B.: Renal handling of sodium, chloride, water, amino acids, and glucose. In Brenner, B. M., and Rector, F. C., Jr. (eds.): *The Kidney*, Vol. 1, 3rd ed. W. B. Saunders Co., Philadelphia, 1986, pp. 145–175.

Burgess, J. L., and Birchall, R.: Nephrotoxicity of amphotericin B, with emphasis on changes in tubular function. *Am. J. Med.*, **53**:77–84, 1972.

Capasso, G.; Schuetz, H.; Vickermann, B.; and Kinne, R.: Amphotericin B and amphotericin B methylester: effect on brush border membrane permeability. *Kidney Int.*, **30**:311–317, 1986.

Carone, F. A., and Ganote, C. E.: *d*-Serine nephrotoxicity. The nature of proteinuria, glucosuria, and aminoaciduria in acute tubular necrosis. *Arch. Pathol.*, **99**(12):658–662, 1975.

Cheng, J-T.; Witty, R. T.; Robinson, R. R.; and Yarger, W. E.: Amphotericin B nephrotoxicity: increased renal resistance and tubule permeability. *Kidney Int.*, **22**:727–733, 1982.

Cheung, J. Y.; Bonventre, J. V.; Malis, C. D.; and Leaf, A.: Calcium and ischemic injury. *N. Engl. J. Med.*, **314**:1670–1676, 1986.

Clemens, T. L.; Hill, R. N.; Bullock, L. P.; Johnson, W. D.; Sultatos, L. G.; and Vesell, E. S.: Chloroform toxicity in the mouse: Role of genetic factors and steroids. *Toxicol. Appl. Pharmacol.* **48**:117–130, 1979.

Coggins, C. H., and Fang, L. S-T.: Acute renal failure associated with antibiotics, anesthetic agents and radiographic contrast agents. In Brenner, B. M., and Lazarus, J. M. (eds.): *Acute Renal Failure*. Churchill Livingstone, New York, 1988, pp. 295–352.

Cojocel, C.; Hannemann, J.; and Baumann, K.: Cephaloridine-induced lipid peroxidation initiated by reactive oxygen species as a possible mechanism of cephaloridine nephrotoxicity. *Biochim. Biophys. Acta*, **834**, 402–410, 1985.

Cronin, R. E.: Radiocontrast media–induced acute renal failure. In *Nephrotoxin-Induced Diseases of Kidney*. 1988.

Diamond, J. R.; Bonventre, J. V.; and Karnovsky, M. J.: A role of oxygen free radicals in aminonucleoside nephrosis. *Kidney Int.*, **29**:478–483, 1986.

Dobyan, D. C., and Bulger, R. E.: Partial protection by chlorpromazine in mercuric chloride–induced acute renal failure in rats. *Lab. Invest.*, **50**:578–586, 1984.

Douglas, J. B., and Healy, J. K.: Nephrotoxic effects of amphotericin B, including renal tubular acidosis. *Am. J. Med.*, **46**:154–162, 1969.

Dousa, T. P.: Glomerular metabolism. In Seldin, D. W., and Giebisch, G. (eds.): *The Kidney: Physiology and Pathophysiology*, Vol. 1. Raven Press, New York, 1985, pp. 645–667.

Duggin, G. D., and Mudge, G. H.: Analgesic nephropathy: renal distribution of acetaminophen and its conjugates. *J. Pharmacol. Exp. Ther.*, **199**:1–9, 1976.

Dworkin, L. D., and Brenner, B. M.: Biophysical basis of glomerular filtration. In Seldin, D. W., and Giebisch, G. (eds.): *The Kidney: Physiology and Pathophysiology*, Vol. 1. Raven Press, New York, 1985, pp. 397–426.

Ecker, J. L.; Hook, J. B.; and Gibson, J. E.: Nephrotoxicity of paraquat in mice. *Toxicol. Appl. Pharmacol.*, **34**:178–186, 1975.

Eknoyan, G.; Bulger, R. E.; and Dobyan, D. C.: Mercuric chloride–induced acute renal failure in the rat. I. Correlation of functional and morphologic changes and their modification by clonidine. *Lab. Invest.*, **46**:613–620, 1982.

Elema, J. D.; Weening, J. J.; and Grond, J.: Focal glomerular hyalinosis and sclerosis in aminonucleoside and adriamycin nephrosis: pathogenetic and therapeutic considerations. *Contrib. Nephrol.*, **60**:73–82, 1988.

Fillastre, J. P., and Raguenez-Viotte, G.: Cisplatin nephrotoxicity. *Toxicol. Lett.*, **46**:163–175, 1989.

Fowler, B. A.; Hook, G. E. R.; and Lucier, G. W.: Tetrachlorodibenzo-*p*-dioxin induction of renal microsomal enzyme systems: ultrastructural effects of pars recta (S3) proximal tubule cells of the rat kidney. *J. Pharmacol. Exp. Ter.*, **203**:712–721, 1977.

Fowler, B. A.; Mistry, P.; and Goering, P. L.: Mechanisms of metal-induced nephrotoxicity. In Bach, P. E., and Lock, E. A. (eds.): *Nephrotoxicity in the Experimental and Clinical Situation*. Martinus Nijhoff Publishers, Lancaster, England, 1987, pp. 659–682.

Ganote, C. E.; Reimer, K. A.; and Jennings, R. B.: Acute mercuric chloride nephrotoxicity: an electron microscopic and metabolic study. *Lab. Invest.*, **31**:633–647, 1974.

Goldstein, R. S.: Drug-induced nephrotoxicity in middle-aged and senescent rats. In Volans, G. N., Sims, J., Sullivan, F. M., and Turner, P. (eds.): *Proceedings of the V International Congress of Toxicology: Basic Science in Toxicology*. Taylor and Francis, London, 1990, pp. 412–421.

Goldstein, R. S., and Hook, J. B.: Biochemical mechanisms of nephrotoxicity in the neonate and child. In Edelmann, C. M.; Bernstein, J.; Meadow, S.; Travis, L.; and Spitzer, A. (eds.): *Pediatric Kidney Disease*, 2nd ed. Little, Brown and Co., Boston, in press.

Goldstein, R. S., and Mayor, G. H.: The nephrotoxicity of cisplatin. *Life Sci.*, **32**:685–690, 1983.

Goldstein, R. S.; Pasino, D. A.; and Hook, J. B.: Cephalordine nephrotoxicity in aging male Fischer-344 rats. *Toxicology*, **38**:43–53, 1986.

Goldstein, R. S.; Smith, P. F.; Tarloff, J. B.; Contardi, L.; Rush, G. F.; and Hook, J. B.: Minireview: biochemical mechanisms of cephaloridine nephrotoxicity. *Life Sci.*, **42**:1809–1816, 1988a.

Goldstein, R. S.; Tarloff, J. B.; and Hook, J. B.: Age-related nephropathy in laboratory rats. *FASEB J.*, **2**:2241–2251, 1988b.

Golman, K.; Holtz, E.; and Almen, T.: Radiographic contrast media. In Bach, P. E., and Lock, E. A. (eds.): *Nephrotoxicity in the Experimental and Clinical Situation*. Martinus Nijhoff Publishers, Lancaster, England, 1987, pp. 701–726.

Gordon, J. A., and Gattone, V. H.: Mitochondrial alterations in cisplatin-induced acute renal failure. *Am. J. Physiol.*, **250**:F991–F998, 1986.

Gosselin, R. E.; Smith, R. P.; and Hodhe, H. C. (eds.): *Clinical Toxicology of Commercial Products*. Williams and Wilkins, Baltimore, 1984, pp. III172–III179.

Gottschalk, C. W.: Osmotic concentration and dilution of the urine. *Am. J. Med.*, **36**, 670–685, 1964.

Goyer, R. A.: Cadmium nephropathy. In Porter, G. A. (ed.): *Nephrotoxic Mechanism of Drugs and Environmental Toxins*. Plenum Publishing Corp., New York, 1982.

Grond, J.; Weening, J. J.; van Goor, H.; and Elema, J. D.: Application of puromycin aminonucleoside and adriamycin to induce chronic renal failure in the rat. *Contrib. Nephrol.*, **60**:83–93, 1988.

Hall III, P. W.: Endemic Balkan nephropathy. In Porter, G. A. (ed.): *Nephrotoxic Mechanisms of Drugs and Environmental Toxins.* Plenum Publishing Corp., New York, 1982, pp. 227–240.

Hayes, A. W.: Mycotoxins: a review of biological effects and their role in human diseases. *Clin. Toxicol.*, **17**:45–83, 1980.

Hill, R. N.; Clemens, T. L.; Liu, D. K.; Vesell, E. S.; and Johnson, W. D.: Genetic control of chloroform toxicity in mice. *Science*, **190**:159–160, 1975.

Hook, J. B.; Rose, M. S.; and Lock, E. A.: The nephrotoxicity of hexachloro-1:3-butadiene in the rat: studies of organic anion and cation transport in renal slices and the effect of monooxygenase inducers. *Toxicol. Appl. Pharmacol.*, **65**:373–382, 1982.

Hostetler, K. Y., and Hall, L. B.: Inhibition of kidney phospholipases A and C by aminoglycoside antibiotics: possible mechanism of aminoglycoside nephrotoxicity. *Proc. Natl. Acad. Sci. USA*, **79**:1663–1667, 1982.

Humes, H. D.: Role of calcium in pathogenesis of acute renal failure. *Am. J. Physiol.*, **250**:F579–F589, 1986.

Humes, H. D., and O'Connor, R. P.: Aminoglycoside nephrotoxicity. In Schrier, R. W., and Gottschalk, C. W. (eds.): *Diseases of the Kidney*, Vol. 2, 4th ed. Little, Brown, Boston, 1988, pp. 1229–1273.

Humes, H. D.; Sastrasinh, M.; and Weinberg, J. M.: Calcium is a competitive inhibitor of gentamicin-renal membrane binding interactions and dietary calcium supplementation protects against gentamicin nephrotoxicity. *J. Clin. Invest.*, **73**:134–147, 1984.

Humes, H. D., and Weinberg, J. M.: Toxic nephropathies. In Brenner, B. M., and Rector, F. C. (eds.): *The Kidney.* W. B. Saunders Co., Philadelphia, 1986, pp. 1491–1532.

Humes, H. D.; Weinberg, J. M.; and Knauss, T. C.: Clinical and pathophysiologic aspects of aminoglycoside nephrotoxicity. *Am. J. Kidney Dis.*, **11**:5–29, 1982.

Hunsicker, L. G.; Shearer, T. P.; and Shaffer, S. J.: Acute reversible proteinuria induced by infusion of the polycation hexadimethrine. *Kidney Int.*, **20**:7–17, 1981.

Inui, K-I.; Saito, H.; Iwata, T.; and Hori, R.: Aminoglycoside-induced alterations in apical membranes of kidney epithelial cell line (LLC-PK1). *Am. J. Physiol.*, **254**:C251–C257, 1988.

Ishikawa, Y.; Inui, K.; and Hori, R.: Gentamicin binding to brush border and basolateral membranes isolated from rat kidney cortex. *J. Pharmacobio-Dyyn.*, **8**:931–941, 1985.

Ishmael, J., and Lock, E. A.: Nephrotoxicity of hexachlorobutadiene and its glutathione-derived conjugates. *Toxicol. Pathol.*, **14**:258–262, 1986.

Kacew, S., and Hirsch, G. H.: Evaluation of nephrotoxicity of various compounds by means of *in vitro* techniques and comparison to *in vivo* methods. In Hook, J. B. (ed.): *Toxicology of the Kidney.* Raven Press, New York, 1981, pp. 77–98.

Kaloyanides, G. J.: Aminoglycoside-induced functional and biochemical defects in the renal cortex. *Fund. Appl. Toxicol.*, **4**:930–943, 1984.

Kanwar, Y. S.: Biophysiology of glomerular filtration and proteinuria. *Lab. Invest.*, **51**:7–21, 1984.

Kappus, H.: Oxidative stress in chemical toxicity. *Arch. Toxicol.*, **60**:144–149, 1987.

Kincaid-Smith, P.: Analgesic nephropathy. *Kidney Int.*, **13**:1–4, 1978.

Kirsh, R.; Goldstein, R.; Tarloff, J.; Parris, D.; Hook, J.; Hanna, N.; Bugelski, P.; and Poste, G.: An emulsion-based formulation of amphotericin B: improved

therapeutic index in treatment of systemic murine candidiasis. *J. Infect. Dis.*, **158**:1065–1070, 1988.

Klahr, S.; Schreiner, G.; and Ichikawa, I.: The progression of renal disease. *N. Engl. J. Med.*, **318**:1657–1666, 1988.

Kluwe, W. M.: The nephrotoxicity of low molecular weight halogenated alkane solvents, pesticides, and chemical intermediates. In Hook, J. B. (ed.): *Toxicology of the Kidney.* Raven Press, New York, 1981.

———: Chronic chemical injury to the kidney. In Goldstein, R. S.; Hewitt, W. R.; and Hook, J. B. (eds.): *Toxic Interactions.* Academic Press, New York, 1990, pp. 367–406.

Knauss, T. C.; Weinberg, J. M.; and Humes, D. H.: Alterations in renal cortical phospholipid content induced by gentamicin: time course, specificity, and subcellular localization. *Am. J. Physiol.*, **224**:F535–F546, 1983.

Kriz, W., and Kaissling, B.: Structural organization of the mammalian kidney. In Seldin, D. W., and Giebisch, G. (eds.): *The Kidney: Physiology and Pathophysiology*, Vol. 1. Raven Press, New York, 1985, pp. 265–306.

Kuo, C. H.; Maita, K.; Sleight, S. D.; and Hook, J. B.: Lipid peroxidation: a possible mechanism of cephaloridine-induced nephrotoxicity. *Toxicol. Appl. Pharmacol.*, **67**:78–88, 1983.

Lameire, N.; Vanholder, R.; Vakaet, L.; Pattyn, P.; Ringoir, S.; and Qautacker, J.: Renal hemodynamics in nephrotoxic acute renal failure. In Porter, G. A. (ed.): *Nephrotoxic Mechanisms of Drugs and Environmental Toxins.* Plenum Publishing Corp., New York, 1982, pp. 37–56.

Lau, S. S.; Monks, T. J.; and Gillette, J. R.: Identification of 2-bromohydroquinone as a metabolite of bromobenzene and *o*-bromophenol: implications for bromobenzene-induced nephrotoxicity. *J. Pharmacol. Exp. Ther.*, **230**:360–366, 1984.

Lau, S. S., and Monks, T. J.: Minireview: the contribution of bromobenzene to our current understanding of chemically-induced toxicities. *Life Sci.*, **42**:1259–1269, 1988.

Lehman-McKeeman, L. D.; Rodriguez, P. A.; Takigiku, R.; Caudill, D.; and Fey, M. L.: D-Limonene–induced male rat–specific nephrotoxicity: evaluation of the association between D-limonene and α_{2u}-globulin. *Toxicol. Appl. Pharmacol.*, **99**:250–259, 1989.

Leitman, P. S., and Smith, C. R.: Aminoglycoside nephrotoxicity in humans. *Rev. Infect. Dis.*, 5(Suppl. 2):S284–S293, 1983.

Lipsky, J. J., and Leitman, P. S.: Aminoglycoside inhibition of a renal phosphatidylinositol phospholipase C. *J. Pharmacol. Exp. Ther.*, **220**:287–292, 1982.

Litterst, C. L., and Weiss, R. B.: Clinical and experimental nephrotoxicity of chemotherapeutic agents. In Bach, P. H., and Lock, E. A. (eds.): *Nephrotoxicity in the Experimental and Clinical Situation.* Martinus Nijhoff Publishers, London, 1987, pp. 771–816.

Lock, E. A.: Studies on the mechanism of nephrotoxicity and nephrocarcinogenicity of halogenated alkenes. *CRC Crit. Rev. Toxicol.*, **19**:23–42, 1988.

Lock, E. A., and Ishmael, J.: Hepatic and renal nonprotein sulfhydryl concentration following toxic doses of hexachloro-1,3-butadiene in the rat: the effect of Aroclor 1254, phenobarbitone, or SKF 525A treatment. *Toxicol. Appl. Pharmacol.*, **57**:79–87, 1981.

———: The hepatotoxicity and nephrotoxicity of hexachlorobutadiene. In Yoshida, H.; Hagihara, Y.; and Ebashi, S. (eds.): *Advances in Pharmacology and Therapeutics II*, Vol. 5, *Toxicology and Experimental Models.* Pergamon Press, New York, 1982, pp. 87–96.

————: Effect of the organic acid transport inhibitor probenecid on renal cortical uptake and proximal tubular toxicity of hexachloro-1,3-butadiene and its conjugates. *Toxicol. Appl. Pharmacol.*, **81**:32–42, 1985.

Maher, J. F.: Toxic nephropathy. In Brenner, B. M., and Rector, F. C., Jr. (eds.): *The Kidney*. W. B. Saunders, Philadelphia, 1976.

Mazze, R. I.: Methoxyflurane nephropathy. In Hook, J. B. (ed.): *Toxicology of the Kidney*. Raven Press, New York, 1981, pp. 135–149.

McCormack, K. M.; Kluwe, W. M.; Rickert, D. E.; Sanger, U. L.; and Hook, J. B.: Renal and hepatic microsomal enzyme stimulation and renal function following three months of dietary exposure to polybrominated biphenyls. *Toxicol. Appl. Pharmacol.*, **44**: 539–553, 1978.

Mihatsch, M. J.; Thiel, G.; and Ryffel, B.: Cyclosporine A: action and side-effects. *Toxicol. Lett.*, **46**:125–139, 1989.

Miura, K.; Goldstein, R. S.; Pasino, D. A.; and Hook, J. B.: Cisplatin nephrotoxicity: role of filtration and tubular transport of cisplatin in isolated perfused kidneys. *Toxicology*, **44**:147–158, 1987.

Mohandas, J.; Duggin, G. G.; Horvath, J. S.; and Tiller, D. J.: Metabolic oxidation of acetaminophen (paracetamol) mediated by cytochrome P-450 mixed function oxidase and prostaglandin endoperoxidase synthetase in rabbit kidney. *Toxicol. Appl. Pharmacol.*, **61**:252–259, 1981.

Moldeus, P.; Andersson, B.; Rahimtula, A.; and Berggren, M.: Prostaglandin synthetase catalyzed activation of paracetamol. *Biochem. Pharmacol.*, **31**: 1363–1368, 1982.

Moldeus, P., and Rahimtula, A.: Metabolism of paracetamol to a glutathione conjugate catalyzed by prostaglandin synthetase. *Biochem. Biophys. Res. Commun.*, **96**:469–475, 1980.

Molland, E. A.: Experimental renal papillary necrosis. *Kidney Int.*, **13**:5–14, 1978.

Monks, T. J.; Highet, R. J.; and Lau, S. S.: 2-Bromo-(diglutathion-S-yl) hydroquinone nephrotoxicity: physiological, biochemical and electrochemical determinants. *Mol. Pharmacol.*, **34**:492–500, 1988.

Monks, T. J.; Lau, S. S.; Highet, R. J.; and Gillette, J. R.: Glutathione conjugates of 2-bromohydroquinone are nephrotoxic. *Drug Metab. Dispos.*, **13**:553–559, 1985.

Nanra, R. S.: Pathology, aetiology and pathogenesis of analgesic nephropathy. *Aust. N.Z. J. Med.*, **4**:602–603, 1974.

Nash, J. A.; King, L. J.; Lock, E. A.; and Green, T.: The metabolism and disposition of hexachloro-1:3-butadiene in the rat and its relevance to nephrotoxicity. *Toxicol. Appl. Pharmacol.*, **73**:124–137, 1984.

Newton, J. F.; Kuo, C.-H.; Gemborys, M. W.; Mudge, G. H.; and Hook, J. B.: Nephrotoxicity of *p*-aminophenol, a metabolite of acetaminophen in the Fischer 344 rat. *Toxicol. Appl. Pharmacol.*, **65**:336–344, 1982.

Nordberg, G. F.: Metabolism of cadmium. In Porter, G. A. (ed.): *Nephrotoxic Mechanisms of Drugs and Environmental Toxins*. Plenum Publishing Corp., New York, 1982.

Nordberg, G. F.; Goyer, R.; and Nordberg, M.: Comparative toxicity of cadmium-metallothionein and cadmium chloride on mouse kidney. *Arch. Pathol.*, **99**:192–197, 1975.

Oken, D. E.: Acute renal failure caused by nephrotoxins. *Environ. Health Perspect.*, **15**:101–109, 1976.

Porter, G. A., and Bennett, W. M.: Drug induced renal effects of cyclosporine, aminoglycoside antibiotics and lithium: extrapolation of animal data to man. In Bach, P. H., and Lock, E. A. (eds): *Nephrotoxicity: In Vitro to In Vivo Animals to Man*. Plenum Press, New York, 1989, pp. 147–170.

Preuss, H. G.; Tourkantonis, A.; Hsu, C. H.; Shim, P. C.; Barzyk, P.; Tio, F.; and Schreiner, G. E.: Early events in various forms of experimental acute tubular necrosis in rats. *Lab. Invest.*, **32**:286–294, 1975.

Racusen, L. C.; Finn, W. F.; Whelton, A.; and Solez, K.: Mechanisms of lysine-induced acute renal failure in rats. *Kidney Int.*, **27**:517–522, 1985.

Racusen, L. C., and Solez, K.: Cyclosporine nephrotoxicity. *Int. Rev. Exp. Pathol.*, **30**:107–157, 1988.

Rankin, G. O.; Yang, D. J.; Teets, V. J.; Shin, H. C.; and Brown, P. I.: Role of biotransformation in acute *N*-(3,5-dichlorophenyl)-succinimide–induced nephrotoxicity. In Bach, P. H., and Lock, E. A. (eds.): *Nephrotoxicity: In Vitro to In Vivo Animals to Man*. Plenum Press, New York, 1989, pp. 601–606.

Rehan, A.; Johnson, K. J.; Kunkel, R. G.; and Wiggins, R. C.: Role of oxygen radicals in phorbol myristate acetate–induced glomerular injury. *Kidney Int.*, **27**: 503–511, 1985.

Remuzzi, G., and Bertani, T.: Renal vascular and thrombotic effects of cyclosporine. *Am. J. Kidney Dis.*, **13**:261–272, 1989.

Rush, G. F.; Kuo, C.-H.; and Hook, J. B.: Nephrotoxicity of bromobenzene in mice. *Toxicol. Lett.*, **20**:23–32, 1984a.

Rush, G. F.; Smith, J. H.; Newton, J. F.; and Hook, J. B.: Chemically induced nephrotoxicity: role of metabolic activation. *CRC Crit. Rev. Toxicol.*, **13**:99–160, 1984b.

Sabatini, S.: Analgesic-induced papillary necrosis. *Semin. Nephrol.*, **8**:41–54, 1988.

Safirstein, R.; Miller, P.; and Guttenplan, J. B.: Uptake and metabolism of cisplatin by rat kidney. *Kidney Int.*, **25**:753–758, 1984.

Safirstein, R.; Winston, J.; Moel, D.; Dikman, S.; and Guttenplan, J.: Cisplatin nephrotoxicity: insights into mechanisms. *Int. J. Andrology*, **10**:325–346, 1987.

Sastrasinh, M.; Weinberg, J. M.; and Humes, H. D.: The effect of gentamicin on calcium uptake by renal mitochondria. *Life Sci.*, **30**:2309–2315, 1982.

Schnaper, H. W., and Robsen, A. M.: Nephrotic syndrome: minimal change disease, focal glomerulosclerosis, and related disorders. In Schrier, R. W., and Gottschalk, C. W. (eds.): *Diseases of the Kidney*, Vol. 2. Little, Brown and Co., Boston, 1988, pp. 1945–2004.

Schwertz, D. W.; Kreisberg, J. I.; and Venkatachalam, M. A.: Effects of aminoglycosides on proximal tubular brush border membrane phosphatidylinositol–specific phospholipase C. *J. Pharmacol. Exp. Ther.*, **231**:48–55, 1984.

Shah, S. V.: Role of reactive oxygen metabolites in experimental glomerular disease. *Kidney Int.*, **35**: 1093–1106, 1989.

Skorecki, K. L.; Nadler, S. P.; Badr, K. F.; and Brenner, B. M.: Renal and systemic manifestations of glomerular disease. In Brenner, B. M., and Rector, F. C., Jr. (eds.): *The Kidney*, Vol. 1, 3rd ed. W. B. Saunders Co., Philadelphia, 1986, pp. 891–928.

Smith, J. H., and Hook, J. B.: Mechanism of chloroform nephrotoxicity. II. *In vitro* evidence for renal metabolism of chloroform in mice. *Toxicol. Appl. Pharmacol.*, **70**:480–485, 1983.

————: Mechanism of chloroform nephrotoxicity. III. Renal and hepatic microsomal metabolism of chloroform in mice. *Toxicol. Appl. Pharmacol.*, **73**:511–524, 1984.

Smith, J. H.; Maita, K.; Sleight, S. D.; and Hook, J. B.: Mechanism of chloroform nephrotoxicity. I. Time course of chloroform toxicity in male and female mice. *Toxicol. Appl. Pharmacol.*, **70**:467–479, 1983.

————: Effect of sex hormone status on chloroform nephrotoxicity and renal mixed function oxidases in mice. *Toxicology, 30*:305–316, 1984.

Swenberg, J. A.; Short, B.; Borghoff, S.; Strasser, J.; and Charbonneau, M.: The comparative pathobiology of α_{2u}-globulin nephropathy. *Toxicol. Appl. Pharmacol., 97*:35–47, 1989.

Tanaka, H.; Ishikawa, E.; Teshima, S.; and Shimizu, E.: Histopathological study of human cisplatin nephrotoxicity. *Toxicol. Pathol., 14*:247–257, 1986.

Tarloff, J. B.; Goldstein, R. S.; Mico, B. A.; and Hook, J. B.: Role of pharmacokinetics and metabolism in the enhanced susceptibility of middle aged male Sprague-Dawley rats to acetaminophen nephrotoxicity. *Drug Metab. Dispos., 17*:139–146, 1989.

Tisher, C. C., and Madsen, K. M.: Anatomy of the kidney. In Brenner, B. M., and Rector, F. C., Jr. (eds.): *The Kidney,* Vol. 1, 3rd ed. W. B. Saunders Co., Philadelphia, 1986, pp. 3–60.

Tolins, J. P., and Raij, L.: Adverse effect of amphotericin B administration on renal hemodynamics in the rat. Neurohumoral mechanisms and influence of calcium channel blockade. *J. Pharmacol. Exp. Ther., 245*: 594–599, 1988a.

————: Chronic amphotericin B nephrotoxicity in the rat, protective effect of prophylactic salt loading. *Am. J. Kidney Dis., 11*:313–317, 1988b.

Trifillis, A. L.; Kahng, M. W.; and Trump, B. F.: Metabolic studies of $HgCl_2$-induced acute renal failure in the rat. *Exp. Mol. Pathol., 35*:14–24, 1981.

Trump, B. F.; Berezesky, I. K.; Smith, M. W.; Phelps, P. C.; and Elliget, K. A.: The relationship between cellular ion deregulation and acute and chronic toxicity. *Toxicol. Appl. Pharmacol., 97*:6–22, 1989.

Tulkens, G. A.; Van Hoof, F.; and Tulkens, P.: Gentamicin-induced lysosomal phospholipidosis in cultured rat fibroblasts. Quantitative ultrastructural and biochemical study. *Lab. Invest., 40*:481–491, 1979.

Tune, B. M.: Nephrotoxicity of cephalosporin antibiotics. Mechanisms and modifying factors. In Porter, G. A. (ed.): *Nephrotoxic Mechanisms of Drugs and Environmental Toxins.* Plenum Publishing Corp., New York, 1982, pp. 151–164.

Tune, B. M., and Fravert, D.: Cephalosporin nephrotoxicity. Transport, cytotoxicity and mitochondrial toxicity of cephaloglycin. *J. Pharmacol. Exp. Ther., 215*:186–190, 1980.

Tune, B. M.; Fravert, D.; and Hsu, C.-Y.: Oxidative and mitochondrial toxic effects of cephalosporin antibiotics in the kidney. *Biochem. Pharmacol., 38*:795–802, 1989.

Tune, B. M.; Wu, K. W.; Fravert, D.; and Holtzman, D.: Effect of cephaloridine on respiration by renal cortical mitochondria. *J. Pharmacol. Exp. Ther., 210*:98–100, 1979.

Wedeen, R. P.: Heavy metals. In Schrier, R. W., and Gottschalk, C. W. (eds.): *Diseases of the Kidney,* Vol.

2, 4th ed. Little, Brown and Co., Boston, 1988, pp. 1359–1376.

Weinberg, J. M.: The cellular basis of nephrotoxicity. In Schrier, R. W., and Gottschalk, C. W. (eds.): *Diseases of the Kidney,* Vol. 2, 4th ed. Little, Brown and Co., Boston, 1988, pp. 1137–1195.

Weinberg, J. M.; Harding, P. G.; and Humes, H. D.: Mitochondrial bioenergetics during the initiation of mercuric-chloride-induced renal injury. II. Functional alterations of renal cortical mitochondria isolated after mercuric chloride treatment. *J. Biol. Chem., 257*:68–74, 1982.

Weldon, M. W., and Schultz, M. E.: Renal ultrastructure after amphotericin B. *Pathology, 6*:191–200, 1974.

Williams, P. D.; Holohan, P. D.; and Ross, C. R.: Gentamicin nephrotoxicity. II. Plasma membrane changes. *Toxicol. Appl. Pharmacol., 61*:243–251, 1981.

Williams, P. D.; Trimble, M. E.; Crespo, L.; Holohan, P. D.; Freedman, J. C.; and Ross, C. R.: Inhibition of renal Na^+, K^+-adenosine triphosphatase by gentamicin. *J. Pharmacol. Exp. Ther., 231*:248–253, 1984.

Wing, A. J.; Brunner, F. P.; Geerlings, W.; Broyer, M.; Brynger, H.; Fassbinder, W.; Rissoni, G.; Selwood, N. H.; and Tufveson, G.: Contribution of toxic nephropathies to end-stage renal failure in Europe: a report from the EDTA-ERA registry. *Toxicol. Lett., 46*:281–292, 1989.

Wold, J. S.: Cephalosporin nephrotoxicity. In Hook, J. B. (ed.): *Toxicology of the Kidney.* Raven Press, New York, 1981, pp. 251–266.

Wold, J. S.; Joost, R. R.; and Owen, N. Y.: Nephrotoxicity of cephaloridine in newborn rabbits: role of the renal organic anionic transport system. *J. Pharmacol. Exp. Ther., 201*:778–785, 1977.

Wolf, C. R.; Berry, P. N.; Nash, J. A.; Green, T.; and Lock, E. A.: Role of microsomal and cytosolic glutathione *S*-transferases in the conjugation of hexachloro-1:3-butadiene and its possible relevance to toxicity. *J. Pharmacol. Exp. Ther., 228*:202–208, 1984.

Yoshioka, T., and Ichikawa, I.: Glomerular dysfunction induced by polymorphonuclear leukocyte–derived reactive oxygen species. *Am. J. Physiol., 257*:F53–F59, 1989.

Zalme, R. C.; McDowell, E. M.; Nagle, R. B.; McNeil, J. S.; Flamenbaum, N.; and Trump, B. F.: Studies on the pathophysiology of acute renal failure. II. A histochemical study of the proximal tubule of the rat following administration of mercuric chloride. *Virchows Arch. [Zellpathol.], 22*:197–216, 1976.

Zenser, T. V., and Davis, B. B.: Oxidation of xenobiotics by prostaglandin H synthase. In Goldstein, R. S.; Hewitt, W. R.; and Hook, J. B. (eds.): *Toxic Interactions.* Academic Press, New York, 1990. pp. 61–86.

Chapter 12

RESPONSES OF THE RESPIRATORY SYSTEM TO TOXIC AGENTS

Terry Gordon and *Mary O. Amdur*

INTRODUCTION

Inhalation is a very important route of exposure to toxic chemicals, especially in the workplace. By reason of its structure and function, the lung is efficient in absorbing many types of inhaled materials. In some cases, the distribution of inhaled toxicants to other organs can be very rapid because the lung receives all of the cardiac output. Thus, for many agents the lung is merely the route of systemic absorption whereas for other agents the lung is the primary target organ. It is thus appropriate to distinguish between "inhalation toxicology" which simply defines the route of exposure and "pulmonary toxicology" which assesses the response of the lung to toxic agents. For example, some materials such as the herbicide paraquat cause pulmonary damage when entering the body by ingestion or other routes of exposure.

Pulmonary toxicologists have rapidly progressed in their ability to assess subtle damage to the lung in terms of functional, biochemical, and morphologic alterations. The use of more sensitive methodologies has allowed examination of the responses of experimental animals and human subjects to concentrations at or approaching those that occur in industrial settings or atmospheric pollution. Epidemiologists now use a variety of pulmonary function tests to assess decrements in lung function in workers and in populations exposed to various air pollutants. These pulmonary function tests have been adapted for use in animals and are currently used by many investigators to examine the mechanisms responsible for the pulmonary effects observed in human subjects exposed to air pollutants. When similar data can be obtained in both experimental animals and human subjects (for example, effects on mucociliary clearance of particles or on increased responsiveness to bronchoconstrictive agents), such direct comparisons assist in the problems of extrapolation from animal to man. Progress has been made in understanding some of the mechanisms underlying the response of the lung to toxic agents. In response to toxic insult pulmonary cells are known to release a variety of potent chemical mediators that may critically affect lung function. Biochemical data are also useful in assessing the toxic potential of many agents and are available from the study of cells taken from exposed animals as well as from *in vitro* exposure of cells in culture. Bronchoalveolar lavage is now widely used in both experimental animals and human subjects to examine these factors following exposure. This chapter will discuss how the pulmonary toxicologist uses these methods to study the biochemical, structural, and functional changes produced by inhalation of pollutant gases and particles.

STRUCTURE OF THE RESPIRATORY TRACT

The structure of the mammalian respiratory tract is very complex and several interspecies differences have been described. For a comprehensive discussion of the structure of the respiratory tract and how this relates to the function of the lung, the reader is referred to *The Pathway for Oxygen: Structure and Function in the Mammalian Respiratory System* (Weibel, 1984) and *The Normal Lung* (Murray, 1986). This section is intended only as a brief orientation.

Major Divisions

The nasopharyngeal region extends from the anterior nares to the level of the larynx and is lined with vascularized mucous epithelium. Inhaled air is warmed and humidified during its passage through the nasopharynx. Large inhaled particles are filtered out and gases with very high water solubility are absorbed. Thus, the nasopharyngeal region serves to protect the lung. The significance of this protective function is amply demonstrated when a greater lung response is observed when a soluble gas such as formaldehyde or hydrogen chloride is administered via a tracheal cannula that bypasses this region. Historically, other than the perforated nasal septum observed in workers exposed to chromium compounds, little attention has been given to the nasopharynx as a site of toxic action. Currently, a greater interest is focusing on the nasal area, for example, the production of nasal cancer in rats following exposure to formaldehyde.

The tracheobronchial region consists of the trachea, bronchi, and bronchioles which serve as conducting airways between the nasopharynx and the peripheral lung where gas exchange occurs. In the human lung, these conducting airways are typically dichotomous, symmetric tubes that decrease in diameter with each division or generation. The human lung has about 23 generations. Overall, the rodent lung is similar, but it has fewer generations and slightly different branching patterns. In the rodent, the branching pattern is usually monopodal with a bifurcation resulting in major and minor daughter branches. These branching patterns and the physical dimensions of the airways are critical in determining the deposition of particles and the absorption of gases by the respiratory tract. Extrapolation of toxicity data between rodents and man, therefore, must take into account these differences in branching patterns.

Although the tracheobronchial system may serve merely as conducting tubes for the passage of gases to the exchange surfaces of the lung, these airways are comprised of many reactive elements such as smooth muscle, epithelium, nerves, and secretory cells. Each of these reactive elements may be affected by acute or chronic exposure to toxic agents that compromise the function of these conducting airways. The tracheobronchial region is lined with at least eight types of epithelial cells and is coated with a thin layer of mucus produced by a variety of secretory cells along the conducting airways. The beating of cilia moves this "mucus blanket" upwards. This mucociliary escalator serves as an important clearance mechanism for deposited particles that are carried to the oral cavity where they are swallowed and excreted. Some materials such as sulfuric acid or cigarette smoke are known to impair these clearance mechanisms and can prolong airway exposure to toxic particles or bacteria.

The pulmonary region is the area of the lung where gas exchange takes place. The acinus is the basic functional unit of the mammalian lung. It includes the respiratory bronchioles; alveolar ducts and sacs; and hundreds of alveoli and their associated capillaries, lymphatic tissues, and supportive tissues. The adult human lung contains about 200,000 acini. Alveoli are thin-walled polyhedral-shaped pouches with one side open to a respiratory bronchiole, an alveolar duct, or an alveolar sac. Gas exchange, the primary function of the pulmonary system, occurs between the lumen of these thin-walled alveoli and a dense pulmonary capillary network that covers about 85 to 95 percent of the alveolar surface. The air-blood barrier thus consists of a surfactant lining fluid, the alveolar epithelium and its basement membrane, interstitial space elements, and the vascular endothelium and its basement membrane. The total thickness of this barrier is only 0.4 to 2.5 μm. Moreover, the total alveolar surface area in an adult human is 140 to 150 m^2 which provides a total surface area for exposure to toxic agents that is approximately 70 times that for the skin. Therefore, by necessity, the mammalian lung has developed an elaborate defense system to preserve the alveolar-capillary barrier and its function (see below).

Lung Cell Types

Well over 40 cell types are required to perform the diverse functions of the respiratory tract. These include 17 types of epithelium, nine types of unspecified connective tissue, two types of bone and cartilage, seven types of cells related to blood vessels, two distinctive types of muscle cells, and five types associated with the pleural or nervous tissue elements. The cells of greatest interest are those that are unique to the respiratory tract, such as ciliated epithelium, nonciliated bronchiolar epithelium (Clara cells), type I (squamous alveolar) pneumocytes, type II (great alveolar) pneumocytes, and alveolar macrophages. Also of special interest are vascular endothelial cells and interstitial cells (fibroblasts and fibrocytes) which constitute the greatest percentage of total cells present, totaling over 60 percent of the number of cells in the adult human lung. Weibel (1985) presents an excellent discussion of lung cell biology.

The conducting airways, from the trachea to the respiratory bronchioles, are lined by epithelial cells that differ in type and function at the various levels. Ciliated epithelial cells are the predominant cells in the trachea, bronchi, and bronchioles of airways > 1 mm in diameter, where they outnumber mucus or serous-secreting cells five to one. As the terminal bronchiole diminishes in diameter and terminates in the respiratory bronchiole, the cilia-bearing cells gradually disappear. The mucus blanket, which is propelled upward by concerted beating of the cilia, is produced by several different cell types. The presence of these secretory cells and their contribution to the mucus blanket varies from the larger to the smaller airways and among species (Warheit, 1989): they include mucus (goblet) and serous epithelial cells as well as gland cells of both the mucus and serous types. Nonciliated bronchiolar cells (Clara cells) are typically present only in small bronchioles. The function of the Clara cell is not known, although ultrastructural and cytochemical evidence indicates that they are metabolically active and probably secretory. Clara cells are major sites of lung injury from xenobiotic compounds which are metabolized to reactive intermediates by a lung cytochrome P-450 system.

Airway smooth muscle has an important role in lending rigidity to the luminal walls and in regulating regional airflows and ventilation by changing airway caliber. The majority of airway smooth muscle is located in the conducting airways and lies anatomically beneath the epithelial lining cells. Bundles of smooth muscle have also been identified in the walls of respiratory bronchioles and at alveolar duct openings. The relaxation and contraction of airway smooth muscle is controlled by both neurogenic stimulation and by cellular mediators released locally. Cholinergic innervation produces contraction of airway smooth muscle, whereas both adrenergic and nonadrenergic inhibitory pathways lead to relaxation. Local mediators such as eicosanoids may participate in the regulation of airway smooth muscle tone in both the homeostatic state and during inflammation, whereas mediators such as histamine, tachykinins, and platelet activating factor contribute to the contractile state of airway smooth muscle during inflammation.

The alveolar surface on the luminal side of the basement membrane is lined by squamous alveolar type I pneumocytes and by great alveolar type II pneumocytes. The intracellular structure of type I and type II cells is a reflection of their function. The type I cell is believed to function predominantly as a barrier and thus has few organelles whereas the cytoplasm of the metabolically active type II cell has an endoplasmic reticulum, Golgi apparatus, and other cytosomes (Figure 12–1). The type I cells are very thin (0.1 to 0.3 μm) with a large surface area covering 93 percent of the alveolar surface area. Thus, type I cells, though fewer in number than the type II cells, make up most of the barrier of the blood-gas pathway. Type II cells are more numerous but due to their cuboidal shape make up only 7 percent of the surface area. Type II cells synthesize and release the surfactant material (lipids and proteins), which is vital in regulating surface tension for parenchymal support. Type II cells are now known to be the progenitor cells of type I cells both during lung development and after pulmonary injury from materials such as beryllium or oxidants.

Alveolar macrophages are resident phagocytic cells that are found free in the alveoli. They ingest inhaled particulate material and are the main clearance mechanism for the pulmonary region. Infectious particles are usually killed by the macrophages except in some chronic infectious diseases such as tuberculosis and in some viral diseases. Following oxidant injury to the alveolar epithelium, macrophages can release factors that promote growth of type II cells and thus play a role in the repair process. The effect of inhaled materials on macrophage function may be assessed by examination of cells obtained by bronchoalveolar lavage.

PULMONARY PHYSIOLOGY/FUNCTION

The primary purpose of the mammalian pulmonary system is the exchange of gases between the lumen of the air spaces and the pulmonary capillaries. Impairment of this process can affect the function of the entire body to a degree dependent on the severity of gas exchange dysfunction. The impairment of gas exchange in the lung can result from (1) a decrease in the delivery and removal of air to the alveoli which may occur during airway obstruction produced by an irritant gas such as sulfur dioxide or (2) the inefficient transfer of gases between the lumen of the airspaces and the blood which may result from pulmonary edema or a mismatch in the ventilation/vascular perfusion ratio.

Several physiologic techniques have been developed to monitor the function of the pulmonary system in man as well as in experimental animals. These tests allow the researcher or occupational health physician to detect the presence of impairment, the type of impairment, and the severity. Changes in lung function should reflect alterations in structure because lung function is tightly coupled to lung structure. Measurement of pulmonary function under normal conditions or in normal individuals allows the toxicologist to compare values obtained under experimental conditions or during actual workplace exposures. The presence of small yearly decrements in pulmonary function (greater than that which can be attributed to aging) may alert the occupational health physician to the early stages of occupationally induced pulmonary disease. In many cases, pulmonary function tests can be very sensitive and decrements in lung function can be detected prior to biochemical or histologic alterations. Detailed descriptions of the pulmonary physiology fundamentals that are the basis of pulmonary function tests may be obtained in texts by West (1985) and Grodins and Yamashiro (1978). Details for the performance and interpretation of pulmonary function tests may be found in Cotes (1979) and Clausen

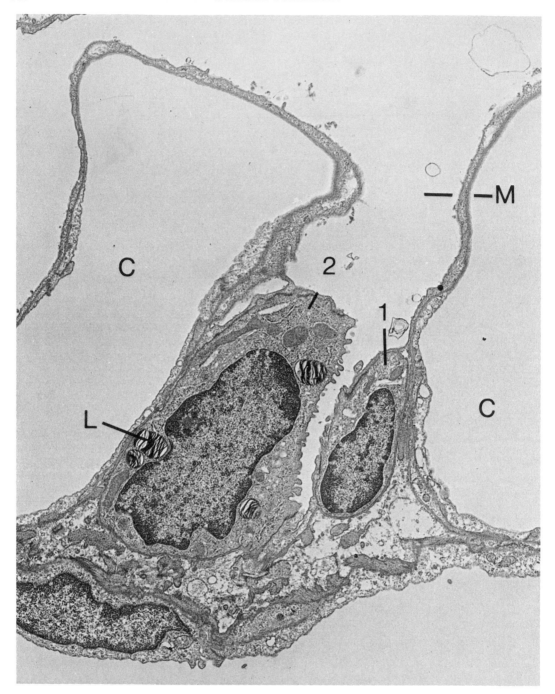

Figure 12–1. Electron micrograph of a rat lung. The alveolus is separated from the blood capillary *(C)* by a thin margin of the type I cell *(1)*. Note the closeness of approach of these two compartments at *M*. A type II cell *(2)* can be seen containing lamelli bodies *(L)* presumed to be storage sites for the lung surfactant.

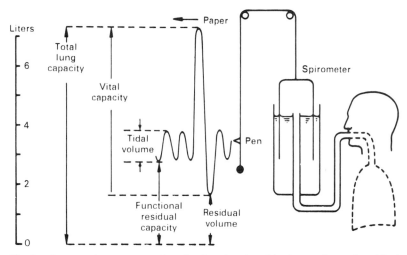

Figure 12–2. Lung volumes. Note that the functional residual capacity and residual volume cannot be measured with the spirometer. (From West, J. B.: *Respiratory Physiology—The Essentials.* © 1974 The Williams & Wilkins Co., Baltimore.)

(1984) for human testing and in Takezawa *et al.* (1980) and Mauderly (1989) for animal testing.

The three most common types of pulmonary function tests performed in human subjects and animals are measurement of (1) lung volumes, (2) the mechanical behavior of the lung, and (3) gas exchange proficiency. The first and simplest noninvasive pulmonary function examination entails the measurement of the gas volume in the lung at different points of respiration. These measurements require voluntary cooperation and forced expiratory maneuvers by the subject. Therefore, studies in animals are performed using anesthesia and artificial ventilation of the lungs. Although anesthesia can complicate the interpretation of experimental results, careful handling of the animals and the use of proper control groups has permitted the use of pulmonary function testing in numerous pulmonary toxicology studies in animals. With the use of minimal anesthesia and soft endotracheal tubes, pulmonary function tests have even been performed serially on the same animals throughout the course of long-term exposures to pollutants (Gross and White, 1986). Moreover, noninvasive measurements of pulmonary function in unanesthetized animals have been developed.

Figure 12–2 is a simplified diagram of the classification of the volumes within the adult human lung. The lung volumes are typically recorded as the subject breathes normally or maximally into a spirometer. *Tidal volume* is the relatively small volume of air exchanged during restful breathing. A tidal volume of 500 ml inhaled at a *frequency* of 15 breaths/minute provides a *minute volume* of 7500 ml/minute. Maximal inspiration and expiration can also be

recorded and the total volume represents the *vital capacity*. The approximately 1500 ml of gas remaining in the lung following maximal expiration is known as the *residual volume*. Addition of the residual volume to the vital capacity yields the *total lung capacity*. Significant changes in these lung volumes or in the dynamic flow of gas in the lung are used to interpret functional changes in the pulmonary system and detect the presence of pulmonary disease.

The impairment of the flow of gases to the gas exchange regions can be classified as either an obstructive or restrictive airway disease or pattern. As seen in Figure 12–3, analysis of lung volumes and comparison to normal values can differentiate between obstructive and restictive pulmonary disease. Typically, restrictive diseases are characterized by a decrease in lung volumes such as vital and total lung capacities. Restrictive defects may occur when the elastic properties of lung tissue are decreased and the lung becomes stiff in fibrotic diseases such as asbestosis, silicosis, and pneumonia. As observed in workers with occupational asthma due to agents such as western red cedar dust or toluene diisocyanate, obstructive injury is characterized by an obstruction to airflow. This increase in the resistance to airflow is characterized chiefly by a decrease in expiratory flow rates such as the forced expiratory volume in 1 second (FEV_1) and gas trapping (Figure 12–3). These obstructive changes may be reversible with medication if the obstruction is due to acute constriction of smooth muscle ringing the airways. Chronic obstructive airway disease may occur when airway caliber is decreased by an irreversible increase in airway smooth muscle

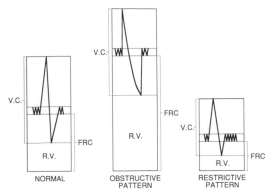

Figure 12–3. Typical lung volume measurements from individuals with normal lung function, obstructive airway disease, or restrictive lung disease. Note that there is (1) a slowing of forced expiration in addition to gas trapping (an increase in residual volume) in obstructive disease and (2) a general decrease in lung volumes in restrictive disease. Note that the measurements read from left to right.

tone, increased mucus thickness, or local airway restriction due to a neoplastic growth.

The mechanical behavior of the lung is affected by airway caliber, elastic properties of lung tissue, and the surfactant properties of the alveoli as well as the mechanical properties of the chest wall. The mechanical properties are determined quantitatively in terms of dynamic and static measurements of lung function. In both animals and human subjects, these measurements are typically performed by spirometry or with the use of a plethysmograph (or body box). Irritant air pollutants (such as sulfur dioxide) or bronchoconstrictive agents (such as histamine) that affect mainly the upper airways produce an increase in airway resistance. Physiologically, an increase in resistance to airflow usually indicates a decrease in airway caliber (resistance to airflow through a tube such as an airway is inversely proportional to tube radius to the fourth power). Irritants that have their actions mainly in the peripheral portions of the lung can produce a decrease in lung compliance. Compliance is an index of the functional stiffness of the lung tissues and is measured as the ratio of the change in volume produced by a change in the transpulmonary driving pressure to inflate and deflate the lung. Decreases in dynamic lung compliance suggest that the peripheral portions of the lung have lost their elasticity. Because dynamic lung compliance is not completely independent of a decrease in airway caliber in the peripheral airways, static lung compliance measurements are sometimes necessary

for interpretation of the structural basis of these mechanical changes. Whereas dynamic compliance is calculated at end expiration and inhalation (flow is zero) and is dependent on lung volume history, frequency, and airway caliber, static compliance is typically calculated at the nearly linear portion of the pressure-volume curve during deflation. Properly interpreted, measurement of pulmonary mechanics is a useful tool for pulmonary toxicologists. Kessler *et al.* (1973) demonstrated in dogs exposed to *Ascaris* antigen that measurement of pulmonary mechanics to indicate the site of action correlated well with localization of airway constriction demonstrated by tantalum bronchography. Responses to other specific irritant air pollutants are discussed in Chapter 25. Drazen (1984) presents an excellent discussion on the analysis of pulmonary mechanics changes in the determination of the site of toxic response.

Ultimately, the chief function of the lung is the exchange of oxygen and carbon dioxide across the alveolar-capillary barrier. The exchange of these gases depends not only on the ventilation of the airspaces with fresh air, the perfusion of the capillary bed, and the proper matching of these two processes, but also on the tissue barrier between these two compartments. Measurement of the diffusing capacity (or transfer factor) of the lung is an excellent research and diagnostic tool and in practice it is quantified by measuring the transfer rate of carbon monoxide from the lung into the pulmonary capillary bed. Decreases in diffusing capacity suggest that either the ventilation/perfusion ratio or the tissue barrier has been altered and that the effective diffusion distance for oxygen and carbon dioxide has been increased.

PHYSICAL CLASSIFICATION OF INHALED TOXIC MATERIAL

In common usage, the term *gas* is usually applied to a substance that is in the gaseous state at room temperature and pressure. The term *vapor* is applied to the gaseous phase of a material that is ordinarily a solid or liquid at room temperature and pressure. The vapor pressure of a solid or liquid is thus of importance in evaluating its potential hazard. For example, the vapor pressure of a very toxic material may be so low that the vapor would not reach a sufficient concentration to pose a hazard.

The general term *aerosol* is used for a relatively stable suspension of solid particles or liquid droplets in air. *Dusts* are solid particles formed by grinding, milling, or blasting. *Fumes* are formed by combustion, sublimation, or condensation of vaporized material. In general the size of fume tends to be < 0.1 μm though the

Table 12–1. HYGIENIC CLASSIFICATION OF GASES AND VAPORS

CLASSIFICATION	EXAMPLES
Irritants	Ammonia, sulfur dioxide, ozone, phosgene, halogens, acrolein
Asphyxiants	
Simple	Nitrogen, hydrogen, methane, helium
Chemical	Carbon monoxide, hydrogen, cyanide, nitriles, hydrogen sulfide
Central nervous system depressants	Aliphatic hydrocarbons, chloronated hydrocarbons, acetone, ethyl ether, benzene
Neurotoxic agents	Carbon disulfide, mercury, acrylamide, n-hexane, methyl n-butyl ketone
Hepatotoxic agents	Carbon tetrachloride, chloroform, allyl alcohol, bromobenzene
Nephrotoxic agents	Carbon tetrachloride, chloroform, trichlorethylene
Agents damaging blood	Nitrobenzene, arsine, naphthylene
Agents damaging bone marrow	Benzene, trinitrotoluene
Carcinogens	Vinyl chloride, 2-naphthylamine, bis(chloromethyl)ether

size can increase somewhat by flocculation (aggregation) as the fume ages. The syndrome known as "metal fume fever" is produced by freshly formed metal oxides such as zinc oxide. *Smoke* is produced by the combustion of organic material. *Mists* and *fogs* are aerosols of liquid droplets formed by condensation of liquid on particulate nuclei in the air or by the uptake of liquid by hygroscopic particles. *Smog* is currently used to describe the complex mixture of particles and gases formed in the atmosphere by irradiation of automobile exhaust. In the environment or the workplace, each of these aerosol types occurs as a complex mixture that depends on the generation process as well as secondary processes that may occur as a result of gas-particle interactions in the air. The physical and chemical interactions between gases and particles are extremely complex and depend on solubility and reactivity factors as well as the presence of water vapor. Gases and vapors may be adsorbed onto the surface of aerosols or dissolved in droplets. For example, polynuclear aromatic hydrocarbons frequently occur on the surface of atmospheric aerosols. During coal combustion, a variety of trace metals (Zn, As, Sb) as well as sulfuric acid are concentrated on the surface of the ultrafine fraction of the aerosol. These particles are of particular toxicologic importance because they are difficult to remove from the effluent and, when inhaled, penetrate to the sensitive pulmonary region of the lung.

Gases and Vapors

The absorption and distribution of gases and vapors depends on (1) the concentration in the inhaled air, (2) the duration of exposure, (3) solubility, and (4) the level of physical activity of the exposed individual. Active physical work or exercise increases the depth and frequency of breathing and therefore the total amount of toxic gas to which the lung is exposed. In addition, an increased heart rate increases blood flow which can lead to greater systemic absorption of inhaled gases. The factors governing systemic absorption and distribution in body tissues are extensively discussed in Chapter 3.

Gases and vapors may be classified according to the nature of their toxic action. Such a classification is often more appropiate than one based on chemical properties *per se*. Gases as chemically diverse as nitrogen and methane have similar toxic actions. Table 12–1 presents a classification of gases and vapors based on their toxic action. Examples are given of common industrial chemicals in each category. The classes of gases and vapors with toxic action in the lung are discussed below, whereas those that affect other organs are presented in other chapters.

Irritants produce inflammation in the mucus membranes with which they come in contact. They are sometimes subdivided into primary and secondary irritants. A primary irritant, for all practical purposes, exerts little systemic toxic action because either the product formed in the tissues of the respiratory tract is nontoxic or the respiratory irritant action is far in excess of any systemic toxic action. Secondary irritants do produce irritant action on respiratory mucus membranes, but this effect is overshadowed by systemic effects resulting from absorption.

Asphyxiants are materials that deprive the body of oxygen. Simple asphyxiants are physiologically inert gases that are present in the atmosphere in sufficient quantity to exclude an adequate supply of oxygen. Chemical asphyxiants are materials that render the body incapable of utilizing an adequate supply of oxygen. They are thus toxic in concentrations far below the level needed for damage from simple asphyxiants. Two classic examples of chemical asphyxiants are carbon monoxide and cyanide. Carbon monoxide interferes with the transport of oxygen to the tissues by its affinity for hemoglobin. Cyanide does not interfere with the transfer of oxygen to the tissues, but does alter cellular use of oxygen in energy production.

Aerosol Characterization and Behavior

The site of deposition of an aerosol in the respiratory tract, as well as its chemical makeup, is obviously of profound importance to its potential toxicity. Particle size is usually the critical factor that determines the region of the respiratory tract in which an aerosol deposits. Deposition of particles on the surface of the lung and airways is brought about by a combination of lung morphometry and the patterns of airflow in the respiratory system together with the physical factors that lead to the removal of particles from the air. This section presents a very brief summary of some of the terminology used to define particle size and outlines the physical factors that lead to particle deposition. Hinds (1982) provides a detailed discussion of these areas for the reader in need of further information.

Particle Size. Except under controlled experimental conditions, inhaled aerosols are heterogeneous in size. It is thus necessary to define the size distribution, which for most aerosols approximates a log-normal distribution. By assuming a log-normal function, the size distribution of particles may be described by the *median* or *geometric mean* and the *geometric standard deviation.* A plot of frequency of a given size against the log of the size produces a bell-shaped probability curve. Particle data are frequently handled by plotting the cumulative percentage of particles less than a stated size increment against the log of the stated size on log probability paper. This results in a straight line that may be fitted by eye or mathematically. In actual practice it is not unusual to have some deviation from a straight line at the largest or smallest particle sizes measured. The geometric mean is the 50 percent size as the mean bisects the curve. The geometric standard deviation (σg) is calculated as:

$$\sigma g = \frac{84.1\% \text{ size}}{50\% \text{ size}}$$

The σg of the particle size distribution is a measure of the heterogeneity of the aerosol. In the laboratory, values for σg of 1.8 to 3.0 are frequently encountered. In the field, values for σg may range from 2.0 to 4.5. For some laboratory studies it is desirable to have aerosols that are uniform or nearly so in size (a monodisperse aerosol). For practical purposes, an aerosol with a $\sigma g < 1.2$ may be considered as monodisperse.

The median diameter determined may reflect the number of particles as the count median diameter (CMD) or reflect mass as the mass median diameter (MMD). The latter is of particular significance in toxicology. The larger the mass of particles capable of penetrating the lung, the greater the probability of a toxic effect. Although the MMD is the most commonly used particle size parameter in toxicology, in some instances, smaller particles may be present in large numbers but contribute proportionately less to mass measurements than larger particles. In these cases, it is advantageous to use the CMD to describe the particle size distribution which relates to particle number. The size distribution in relation to other factors, such as area, may also be of interest. Surface area becomes of special importance when toxic materials are adsorbed on the surface of particles and thus carried to the lung.

Particles that are nonspheric in shape are frequently characterized in terms of equivalent spheres on the basis of equal mass, volume, or aerodynamic drag. The *aerodynamic diameter* takes into account both the density of the particle and aerodynamic drag. It represents the diameter of a unit density sphere having the same terminal settling velocity as the particle, whatever its size, shape, and density. Aerodynamic diameter is the proper measurement to consider for particles that are deposited by impaction and sedimentation. For very small particles, which are deposited primarily by diffusion, the critical factor is particle size, not density or shape.

Another factor that must be kept in mind is that the size of the particle may increase in the respiratory tract. Materials that are hygroscopic, such as sodium chloride, sulfuric acid, or glycerol, take on water and grow in size in the warm, saturated atmosphere of the respiratory tract.

Deposition Mechanisms. Deposition of particles may occur by interception, impaction, sedimentation, and diffusion (Brownian movement). In the lung, the last three mechanisms are the most important. Interception occurs only when the trajectory of a particle brings it near enough to a surface so that an edge of the particle contacts the surface. Interception is mainly important only for the deposition of fibers such as asbestos. Whereas fiber diameter determines the probability of deposition by impaction and sedimentation, interception is dependent on fiber length. Thus, a fiber with a diameter of 1 μm and a length of 200 μm would be deposited in the bronchial tree primarily by interception rather than by impaction.

Particles suspended in air, owing to inertia, tend to continue to travel along their original path. In a bending airstream, such as at an airway bifurcation, a particle may be impacted on the surface. At symmetric bifurcations, which typically occur in the human lung, the deposition rate is likely to be higher for particles moving in the center of the airway.

Sedimentation brings about deposition in the smaller bronchi, the bronchioles, and the alveolar spaces where the airways are small and the velocity of the airflow is low. As a particle moves downward through air, buoyancy and the resistance of air act on the particle in an upward direction while gravitational force acts on the particle in a downward direction. Eventually, the gravitational force equilibrates with the sum of the buoyancy and the air resistance, and the particle continues to settle with a constant velocity known as the terminal settling velocity. Sedimentation is no longer a significant route of particle deposition when the aerodynamic diameter is below 0.5 μm.

Diffusion is an important factor in the deposition of submicron particles. A random motion is imparted to the particles by the impact of gas molecules. This Brownian motion increases with decreasing particle size so that diffusion is an important deposition mechanism in small airways and alveoli for particles below about 0.5 μm.

Respiratory Tract Deposition

As indicated above, the site of deposition of particles in the respiratory tract is determined by a combination of the physical forces that govern particle behavior in an airstream and the anatomy of the respiratory tract. The measurement critical to assessment of toxicity is the regional deposition, rather than simply the total amount of material deposited in the whole lung. The site of deposition affects (1) the severity of the consequences of tissue damage to the respiratory tract, (2) the degree of absorption of systemic toxicants, and (3) the clearance mechanisms available for the ultimate removal of the particles.

Factors Influencing Regional Deposition. Figure 12–4 illustrates schematically the nature of the interaction of physical and biologic factors leading to regional deposition. The size relationships shown for the various compartments are not quantitative. They are intended merely to indicate the progressive increase in both size and surface area that occur in the respiratory tract. The directional changes imposed on the airflow during breathing become less abrupt and the velocity decreases as particles progress down the respiratory tract.

Particles having an aerodynamic diameter of 5 to 30 μm are largely deposited in the nasopharyngeal region by impaction. Because of their size, impaction is an important mechanism for their removal from an airstream. The high air

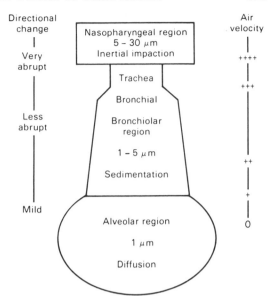

Figure 12–4. Parameters influencing particle deposition. [From Casarett, L. J.: The vital sacs: Alveolar clearance mechanisms in inhalation toxicology. In Blood, F. R. (ed.): *Essays in Toxicology*, Vol. 3. Academic Press, New York, 1972.]

velocity and the tortuous nature of the nasopharyngeal air passages force many sharp changes in airflow direction and provide an ideal environment for impaction. The majority of particles having an aerodynamic diameter of 1 to 5 μm pass through this region and are deposited in the tracheobronchial regions by sedimentation. This mechanism of deposition is favored by the slower airflows, which allow time for deposition by gravitational forces. As the alveolar regions are approached, the velocity of the airflow decreases markedly, allowing even more time for sedimentation. Generally, particles < 0.5 μm which have penetrated to the alveoli are deposited primarily by diffusion.

Additional physiologic or pathologic factors may act to affect particle deposition. One important factor is the pattern of breathing. During quiet breathing, in which the tidal volume is only two to three times the volume of the anatomic dead space, a large proportion of the inhaled particles may be exhaled. During exercise, where larger volumes are inhaled at higher velocities, impaction in the large airways and sedimentation and diffusion in the smaller airways and alveoli will increase. Breath holding also increases deposition from sedimentation and diffusion. This fact is often utilized in aerosol therapy by having the patient take a deep breath and hold it.

Table 12–2. RESPIRATORY TRACT DEFENSE MECHANISMS

Nonspecific defense
    Clearance—nasal, tracheobronchial, and alveolar
    Secretions—mucus, surfactant
    Cellular defenses
        Nonphagocytic—epithelium
        Phagocytic—macrophages and neutrophils
    Biochemical defenses—antiproteolytic enzymes and antioxidants

Specific (immunologic) defense
    Antibody-mediated (B-lymphocyte dependent)
        Serum immunoglobulins
        Secretory immunoglobulins
    Cell-mediated (T-lymphocyte)
        Lymphokine-mediated
        Direct cellular cytotoxicity

Factors that modify the diameter of the conducting airways can modify particle deposition. In patients with chronic bronchitis, the mucous layer is greatly thickened and may partially block the airways in some areas. Jets formed by the air flowing through such partially occluded airways have the potential to increase deposition of particles by impaction and turbulent diffusion in the small airways. Irritant materials that produce bronchoconstriction would tend to increase tracheobronchial deposition of particles. Cigarette smoking has been shown experimentally to produce such an effect (Lippmann *et al.*, 1971).

RESPONSE OF THE LUNG TO TOXIC MATERIAL

The lung is in direct constant contact with the external environment and is exposed to many infectious organisms as well as an increasing number of potentially hazardous particles and gases. The lung has developed extraordinary specific and nonspecific defense mechanisms that under most circumstances successfully prevent the development of pulmonary disease. The following sections will discuss: (1) the inherent defense mechanisms of the lung, (2) the types of pulmonary injury that can occur when these elaborate mechanisms are overcome, and (3) the underlying cellular and biochemical mechanisms leading to pulmonary disease from inhaled toxic material.

Lung Defense

When challenged by the absorption of toxic gases or the deposition of particles, the mammalian pulmonary system can respond by various mechanisms to neutralize or remove the harmful substance. The type of response mounted by the lung depends, of course, on the physical and chemical properties of the agent. Some agents may elicit nonspecific defense responses where-as others may elicit specific cell- or antibody-mediated immunologic mechanisms (Table 12–2).

Nonspecific Defense Mechanisms

Clearance of Particles. The clearance of particles deposited on the surface of the respiratory tract is an important aspect of lung defense against inhaled toxic particles. The speed and efficiency of clearance of deposited particles are critical in determining their toxic potential. Rapid removal lessens the time available to cause damage to the pulmonary tissues or to permit systemic absorption. Impairment of these clearance mechanisms is an important response of the lung to certain toxic agents. The specific mechanism available for the removal of particles from the respiratory tract varies with the site of deposition. Schlesinger (1990) reviews mechanistic aspects of clearance as well as discussing agents that can interfere with proper functioning of these mechanisms.

Tracheobronchial Clearance. The mucus layer covering this region is moved upward by the beating of the underlying cilia. This movement provides a mucociliary escalator that transports deposited particles and particle-laden macrophages upward to the mouth where they are swallowed and eliminated through the gastrointestinal tract. The rate of mucociliary clearance has been measured in both human subjects and experimental animals by using radiolabel-tagged particles. The rate of clearance may then be measured by external monitoring of the radioactivity. Mucociliary clearance is relatively rapid and is completed within 24 to 48 hours.

Pulmonary Clearance. There are three primary avenues by which particulate material is removed from the pulmonary region once it has been deposited: (1) particles may be phagocytized and cleared up the tracheobronchial tree via the mucociliary escalator, (2) particles may be phagocytized and removed via the lymphatic drainage, or (3) material may dissolve from the surfaces of particles and be removed via the bloodstream or lymphatics. Other particles, and perhaps some dissolved material, may be sequestered in the lung. The interaction of particles with lung tissue is very dynamic, with competition among each of the processes for removal, and perhaps with certain elements of lung tissue for retention of particles and complexed material. Within minutes after particles are inhaled, they may be found within alveolar macrophages, and essentially all particles are ultimately engulfed within a matter of hours. Many of the alveolar macrophages are ultimately transported to the mucociliary escalator. How they reach the ciliated surfaces from the alveoli is not clear. One of the most accepted theories is that the alveolar macrophages move via ameboid motion to the level of the respiratory bronchiole. It is also possible that the macrophages are carried to the bronchioles with alveolar fluid that contributes to the serous fluid layer in the airways.

Phagocytosis of inhaled particles is also performed by neutrophils, although neutrophils are not present in significant numbers in the normal lung nor do they phagocytize as rapidly or as many particles as do macrophages. Macrophages and neutrophils, as well as eosinophils, can release a large number of chemical mediators which can kill or neutralize inhaled microorganisms or inert particles. These mediators include toxic oxygen species (such as superoxide anion, hydrogen peroxide, hydroxyl radical, and hypochlorous acid), proteases, and lysozymes. The lung has developed a fine counterbalance system to keep these mediators in check: pulmonary cells are known to contain or release antioxidants and antiproteases. After exposure to inhaled gases and particles, an imbalance in these lung defense systems can occur and the stimulation of oxygen-derived free radicals, for instance, may result in lung tissue damage (see below).

The epithelial cells lining the conducting airways and the gas exchange areas provide several lines of defense for maintaining lung integrity during toxic insults. Adjacent epithelial cells are joined by tight junctions which are relatively resistant to the passage of fluid and macromolecules (compared to the junctions present between vascular endothelial cells) and protect underlying nerve receptors from irritant gases and particles. In addition to this barrier function, epithelial cells also produce protective secretions such as (1) the serous and mucous fluids which comprise the "mucus blanket" in the conducting airways and (2) the surfactant lining fluid in the alveoli. Airway epithelial cells also produce a variety of inflammatory mediators and proteins (see below) whose roles in defense of lung integrity are unclear at this time.

Specific Defense Mechanisms

Nonspecific defense mechanisms, such as clearance and phagocytosis, are present in the lung from birth and provide a considerable degree of protection against injury from a wide variety of inhaled agents. In contrast, specific defense mechanisms are acquired over time and are stimulated by the constant exposure to numerous species of airborne microorganisms as well as a variety of low- and high-molecular-weight antigenic material (Fine and Balmes, 1988). The immune system can mount either cellular or humorally mediated responses to these inhaled antigens which can add to the nonspecific mechanisms of lung defense. The immune response to foreign antigenic material is exceptional in its flexibility and the memory of its humoral and cell-mediated pathways. Pulmonary toxicologists are concerned with both direct and indirect immunologic effects resulting from exposure to inhaled material.

Direct immunologic effects occur when inhaled foreign material sensitizes the respiratory system to further exposure to the same material. Once sensitized to a particular antigen, the immune system can produce an amplified response to extremely small concentrations of that antigen. The mammalian lung has a well developed immune system. Lymphocytes reside in the hilar or mediastinal lymph nodes, lymphoid aggregates, and lymphoepithelial nodules, as well as in aggregates or as single cells throughout the airways. The response of the pulmonary immune system to inhaled antigens is very complex and not completely understood. Bronchoconstriction and chronic pulmonary disease can result from inhalation of materials that appear to act wholly or partly through an allergic response. The underlying mechanism is demonstrated by the presence of circulating or fixed antibodies to specific components of the inhaled material. In some instances these reactions are caused by spores of molds or by bacterial contaminants. Frequently, chemical components of the sensitizing dusts or gases are responsible for the allergic response. Small-molecular-weight compounds can act as haptens that combine with native proteins to form a new compound that is recognized as foreign by the immune system. Further exposure to the sensitizing compound can result in an allergic reaction that is characterized by the release of a variety of inflammatory mediators that produce an early and/or late bronchoconstrictor response. Such a response is observed in sensitized workers exposed to toluene diisocyanate (TDI), a chemical widely used in the manufacture of polyurethane plastics (Brooks, 1983).

The exact role of the immune system in occupationally induced asthma is unclear at present. For example, approximately 5 to 10 percent of exposed workers become sensitized to TDI. Sensitized workers develop bronchoconstriction after exposure to extremely low levels of TDI. However, circulating antibodies to TDI and nonspecific airway hyperresponsiveness (a central feature of asthma) are not found in all workers with occupationally induced asthma from TDI.

Indirect immune effects occur when exposure to air pollutants either suppresses or enhances the immune response to other material. Both sulfur dioxide and ozone can boost the response of the respiratory system to inhaled foreign material. Riedel *et al.* (1988) have demonstrated that ovalbumin-sensitized guinea pigs exposed to as little as 0.16 to 4.3 ppm sulfur dioxide for eight hours per day for five days develop significantly greater bronchoconstriction after a subsequent challenge with ovalbumin than control animals exposed to air. This increased responsiveness after sulfur dioxide exposure was associated with an increase in IgG levels in serum and lavage fluid. In a similar manner, repeated exposure to ozone can heighten the response to inhaled albumin in guinea pigs. Gershwin *et al.* (1981) have observed an increase in IgE antibody containing cells in the epithelial lining of the airways of animals exposed to ozone, suggesting that the potentiation of this immune response may be due to an increase in circulating or secretory antibodies to the sensitizing antigen. Although the majority of data suggest that ozone and sulfur dioxide can potentiate the immune response of the mammalian lung to inhaled foreign antigens, this effect has not been demonstrated in humans and may be species or exposure (concentration × time) dependent (Kleeberger *et al.*, 1989).

Acute Pulmonary Injury

The mammalian pulmonary system is exposed to a wide variety of toxic gases and particles and has evolved specialized mechanisms to defend itself against injury. Unlike most organs, the lung can respond to a toxic insult or agent by first trying to remove or neutralize it and then repairing the damage. The resulting inflammatory process involves the recruitment and activation of cells, typically from the vascular system, to the site of injury. The respiratory system also has a wide variety of resident inflammatory cells that can become activated under a barrage of foreign particles and gases. These cells include alveolar macrophages, which can engulf inhaled particles, and mast cells, which can amplify the re-

sponse to foreign antigens. The purpose of this inflammatory process is the resolution and repair of pulmonary injury and the return to normal lung function. Unfortunately, the repair process itself can often result in harm to the lung. The defense mechanisms that evolved to protect mammalian lungs from foreign matter and antigens often can result in more harm than good when activated by inhalation of toxic chemicals. The following paragraphs will describe the major classifications of pulmonary injury that can be produced by inhaled material and the inflammatory cells and mediators involved in the production of this injury. Because pulmonary injury can range from acute reversible bronchoconstriction in the conducting airways to mesothelioma cancer in the pleural space, the following discussions will be divided into conducting airway and peripheral lung effects and will examine the acute and chronic inflammatory processes that may result in the impairment of gas exchange, the primary function of the lung.

Conducting Airway Effects

The conducting airways can respond in a number of ways to the irritating gases and particles that are not removed by the nasopharyngeal passages. These include bronchoconstriction, airway edema, airway hyperresponsiveness, and impairment of defense mechanisms such as clearance. The type of effect depends not only on the chemical activity (reactivity and solubility) of the toxic agent, but also on the dose of the agent delivered to the target tissue. For example, at least two different mechanisms can be responsible for the bronchoconstriction produced by inhaled gases or particles. Acute exposure to sulfur dioxide for as little as three minutes can produce bronchoconstriction in the absence of airway cell injury or inflammation. Asthmatic individuals are especially sensitive to sulfur dioxide and undergo significant airway narrowing and wheezing at concentrations as low as 0.4 ppm. This response to sulfur dioxide is believed to be due to activation of irritant nerve receptors and a vagal reflex because the response can be inhibited by anticholinergic agents. Additional mechanisms are possible because treatment with chromoglycate, which blocks the release of inflammatory mediators from mast cells, inhibits the bronchoconstriction produced by sulfur dioxide.

Airway inflammation is another mechanism that can result in the production of bronchoconstriction. Damage to the epithelial lining of the airways can initiate a series of events that can alter airway caliber. Only recently have investigators determined that airway epithelial cells do not function merely as protective barrier cells and as a participant in the mucociliary escalator, but that they also play a critical role in the initiation of an inflammatory cascade that occurs after airway injury. Epithelial cells can produce many inflammatory mediators such as arachidonic acid metabolites which can alter vascular permeability and act as chemotactic factors. Injury to epithelial lining cells can also interfere with their homeostatic role in regulating airway smooth muscle tone. Epithelial cells produce prostaglandin E_2 and an unidentified relaxant factor that can control the degree of airway smooth muscle contraction. Airway epithelial cells also contain neutral endopeptidase, an enzyme that metabolizes tachykinins, such as substance P, after their release from afferent nerve endings in the airways. Release of tachykinins from afferent nerve endings occurs after inhalation of a variety of irritants, including cigarette smoke, formaldehyde, and ether. Disruption of the airway epithelium could thus remove important down-regulatory mechanisms of smooth muscle contraction.

Increased resistance to airflow due to airway narrowing can result from mechanisms other than contraction of airway smooth muscle. Acute airway injury can result in the release of several vasoactive mediators. These mediators can alter local vascular permeability and lead to the release of fluid and plasma proteins from the vasculature. The resulting interstitial edema could decrease airway caliber and thus increase airway resistance. Likewise, hypersecretion of mucus and serous fluids into the lumen of the airways could decrease airway caliber and produce airway obstruction. Although (1) airway inflammation has been described after exposure to high concentrations of many inhaled substances, (2) mucus plugging of airways occurs in severe asthma, and (3) hypersecretion follows inhalation of cigarette smoke or repeated exposure to high concentrations of sulfur dioxide, it is not clear whether these mechanisms play a significant role in airway obstruction after exposure to realistic concentrations of air pollutants.

Exposure to air pollutants can alter the response of airway smooth muscle to various endogenous bronchoconstrictors. Changes in the airway responsiveness to specific antigen challenges after pollutant exposures were discussed above. In a number of mammalian species, including man, inhalation of environmental and workplace chemicals such as ozone, nitrogen dioxide, and TDI causes an acute airway injury which is associated with an increase in the nonspecific responsiveness of airway smooth muscle (Boushey et al., 1980). Airway hyperresponsiveness is defined as the increased, yet reversible, airway constriction that occurs in response to agents such as histamine and methacholine. An increase in the nonspecific responsiveness of airway smooth muscle is an important consideration in the study of the adverse health effects of occupational and environmental air pollutants (Sheppard, 1986). First, airway hyperresponsiveness is a central feature of asthma and can be induced by acute exposure to inhaled agents that cause airway injury. In addition, the likelihood of environmental agents causing bronchoconstriction or exacerbations of preexisting asthma in patients may be predicted on the basis of the individual's degree of airway responsiveness. Moreover, studying the underlying mechanisms of chemically induced airway hyperresponsiveness may provide clues to the heightened airway responsiveness of asthmatics. There has been convincing evidence that inflammation is associated with the development of acute airway hyperresponsiveness after chemical inhalation (see review of Boushey et al., 1980). Each substance that has been shown to produce airway hyperresponsiveness in animals or man also causes airway inflammation. Various inflammatory cells and mediators have been implicated in this alteration of airway smooth muscle function, although the involvement of specific pathways of the inflammatory cascade appears to be dependent on the stimuli and species studied. Airway epithelial injury, altered vagal nerve sensitivity, polymorphonuclear leukocytes, and inflammatory mediators such as arachidonic acid metabolites and tachykinins appear to contribute to the airway hyperresponsiveness observed in animal and human studies. Thus, it is unlikely that a single unifying mechanism for acquired airway hyperresponsiveness is responsible for occupationally induced asthma. Regardless of the mechanism of induction, individuals with heightened responsiveness to bronchoprovocation, such as asthmatics (approximately 5 percent of the U.S. population), may be at increased risk during exposure to various pollutants. For example, exercising asthmatics are more sensitive to sulfur dioxide and acid particles than normal individuals.

Impairment of clearance mechanisms by inhaled pollutants can significantly affect the retention time of deposited material. Pollutants such as ozone, cigarette smoke, and sulfuric acid do alter particle clearance but the direction of this change depends on several factors. The alteration in clearance of particles or bacteria from the lung depends not only on the site of deposition in the respiratory tract, but also on the site of injury caused by the toxic pollutant. For instance, mucociliary clearance of 5-μm parti-

Table 12–3. MUCOCILIARY CLEARANCE AFTER CIGARETTE EXPOSURE—DONKEY AND MAN

Donkeys	2 cigarettes	Increase
	15 cigarettes	Decrease
Man	2 cigarettes	Increase
Donkeys	30 cigarettes	
	3 × week, 6 month	Large decrease
Man	Heavy smokers	Large decrease

cles deposited in the large conducting airways may be affected minimally by a relatively insoluble gas such as ozone that may cause pulmonary injury in the lung periphery. Impairment of mucociliary clearance, however, is a toxic action of many inhaled agents. This can occur when the beating of the cilia is impaired by injury to the cilia, depletion of its energy sources, or by an alteration in the chemical properties and viscosity of the gel/sol makeup of the mucus blanket. The latter alteration can significantly change the milieu in which the cilia beat. The present theory of ciliary beating suggests that cilia beat in the less viscous sol layer and movement in this layer may propel the thicker gel layer above. A change in the viscosity of either layer can significantly affect forward propulsion and may occur either (1) acutely after the stimulated release of mucus or serous material from epithelial cells or (2) chronically after a change in mucus or serous cell number or size.

A change in tracheobronchial clearance is one of the many toxic actions of cigarette smoke. Table 12–3 shows the effects of cigarette smoke on clearance in donkeys and human subjects. In donkeys, the smoking of two cigarettes speeded clearance and the smoking of 15 cigarettes slowed clearance. In human subjects, the smoking of two cigarettes produced a speeding of clearance as it had in the donkeys. In chronic studies, the donkeys showed a major slowing of mucociliary clearance similar to that observed in heavy smokers. These studies provide one example of the value of parallel data obtained in experimental animals and human subjects for meaningful prediction of response. The acute response of donkeys (and also of rabbits) to short-term exposures to sulfuric acid is similar to that for cigarette smoke. Thus, the data on the effect of cigarette smoke strengthen the prediction that the mucociliary response of human subjects to chronic exposure to sulfuric acid (which would be both impossible and unethical to do) would be similar to the response of the animals.

Peripheral Lung Effects

The gas exchange surfaces of the lung are lined with type I and type II epithelial cells. Because the type I cell covers the majority of the surface area of the lung, it is particularly susceptible to injury from inhaled substances. Changes in the distribution of type I and type II cells commonly occur after peripheral injury. For example, ultrastructural damage to type I epithelial cells occurs in rats shortly after exposure to ozone or nitrogen dioxide and repair of the lesion begins within 24 hours. Type I cell injury and loss is repaired by proliferation of type II cells as seen by histology and by incorporation of tritiated thymidine. Whereas the role of type II cell proliferation in the adaptation to oxidant injury has been demonstrated by many investigators, the source and type of mediator(s) that trigger this mitotic response in type II cells are not known.

Host defenses against particles that deposit in the peripheral regions of the lung were briefly described above. Pulmonary clearance of inert particles or microorganisms is mediated primarily by phagocytosis and removal by alveolar macrophages. Because macrophages reside primarily on the luminal surface of the alveoli, they are readily exposed to and injured by air pollutants that reach the peripheral lung. Functional changes in macrophage mobility or phagocytic properties have been observed after *in vivo* exposure to ozone, nitrogen dioxide, metals, and diesel exhaust. For example, ozone causes a decrease in the phagocytic activity of alveolar macrophages for latex beads and bacteria (Coffin *et al.*, 1968; Driscoll *et al.*, 1987). Several aspects of macrophage phagocytic function may be affected by oxidant injury: (1) recognition of particles as foreign material, (2) attachment of particles to the membrane, (3) membrane fluidity, and (4) internalization of particles. Thus, injury to alveolar macrophages can alter the normal clearance of particles from the lung and increase the exposure of pulmonary cells to toxic material or microorganisms.

Decrements in host lung defenses against microorganisms may be partially responsible for the increase in respiratory illnesses observed in susceptible populations after pollutant exposures. This increase has been observed after oxidant air pollution episodes and in children residing in homes with gas-burning stoves. Experimental work in animals has demonstrated increased infectivity with bacteria after exposure to ozone, nitrogen dioxide, or phosgene. In these experiments, the respiratory tracts of animals are infected with bacteria after exposure to the toxic agent. Exposure to the toxic agent is associated with an increase in mortality compared to control animals. As little as 0.1 ppm ozone can affect antibacterial defense mechanisms in the lung. Although macrophages play an important part in clearing bacteria from the lung, it is not clear if decreased macrophage phagocytosis has a role in the observed increases in infection (Gardner, 1984). Exposure to phosgene at concentrations greater than those that cause increased infectivity does not significantly alter phagocytic activity by macrophages. Moreover, ozone does not appear to have a significant effect on antiviral defenses in the lung (Selgrade *et al.*, 1988). This latter point is important in assessing the potential of air pollutants for adverse effects on host lung defense, because 90 percent of the respiratory infections in individuals under the age of 50 are viral rather than bacterial in origin.

Inflammation in the peripheral lung of exposed individuals or experimental animals often results in changes in mechanical properties that correlate with structural changes. However, changes in standard measures of pulmonary function are frequently not sensitive indices for pulmonary injury, especially low-level chronic effects which may progress to debilitating lung diseases only after years of exposure. Therefore, researchers and occupational health physicians have developed other techniques for studying the production of lung injury. One of the most powerful of these techniques is bronchoalveolar lavage. The procedures, rationale, and scientific validity of bronchoalveolar lavage in both man and experimental animals have been thoroughly reviewed by Reynolds (1988) and Henderson (1989), respectively. Lavage has been used successfully to diagnose pulmonary disease in man and to study the underlying mechanisms in the production of lung inflammation and injury in animal models. In addition, bronchoalveolar lavage is used as a tool to assay airborne agents for toxic potential and is now an established procedure for studying biomarkers of pulmonary injury from inhaled material.

To perform the lavage procedure, access to the airways must be established and the lung or lung segment filled with sterile, isotonic fluid which is then withdrawn by suction. The cells and mediators present in the recovered lavage fluid can be studied both quantitatively and qualitatively. Changes in the number and type of recovered cells are used to detect and differentiate inflammatory changes in the lung. A simple increase in the total number of recovered cells is often a sensitive indicator of pulmonary injury. Differential cell counts provide useful information on the stage, progression, and resolution of the inflammatory injury. Similar information is obtained by analysis of chemical mediators in bronchoalveolar lavage after exposure to the toxic agent. In evaluating mechanisms of pulmonary injury, data obtained from bronchoalveolar lavage must be interpreted with care and preferably in conjunction with either structural or functional observations. Acute inflammatory injury in the lung is characterized by the general release of many mediators and by the influx and activation of several cell types. The complexity of the role of inflammatory cells and mediators in acute airway injury can be seen in the study of the airway hyperresponsiveness observed in humans and animals after viral infection or exposure to ozone, nitrogen dioxide, TDI, or acrolein. Mediators released from nerves, neutrophils, eosinophils, airway epithelial cells, and platelets have all been demonstrated by various investigators to play the major role in the production of airway hyperresponsiveness and include tachykinins, leukotriene B_4, thromboxane, platelet activating factor, and major basic protein. Thus, the designation of specific cells or mediators to key roles in acute inflammatory injury is difficult.

Inflammatory Cells and Mediators in Acute Pulmonary Injury

The initial step in the inflammatory response in the pulmonary system involves the stimulation or injury of resident cells lining or in the lumen of the airspaces and the release of mediators that (1) increase the permeability of the vascular system locally and (2) attract blood-borne inflammatory cells to the site of injury. The type of inflammatory mediators released by resident cells of the pulmonary system is extensive (Table 12–4) and includes eicosanoids, kinins, cytokines, histamine, complement components, proteases, toxic oxygen species, and platelet activating factor.

The increase in permeability leads to the extravasation of plasma proteins and fluid resulting in localized interstitial edema. Alone, this edema can often lead to an acute impairment of lung function. Edema in the walls of the conducting airways can result in a decrease in airway caliber and thus an increase in resistance to airflow during breathing. In the peripheral lung, interstitial edema can increase the distance gases must diffuse during their exchange between the lumen of the alveoli and the pulmonary capillary bed. Several inflammatory mediators have chemotactic properties and can attract inflammatory cells

Table 12–4. CELLULAR EFFECTS AND SOURCES OF INFLAMMATORY MEDIATORS IN THE LUNG

MEDIATOR	MAJOR SOURCE	INFLAMMATORY EFFECT
Histamine	Mast cell	Vascular permeability, smooth muscle contraction
Complement factors	Macrophage	Regulate vascular permeability, smooth muscle contraction, chemotactic factors
Eicosanoids	Most cell types	Regulate vascular permeability, smooth muscle contraction, chemotactic factors
TNF	Macrophage/monocyte	Alter PMN-endothelial cell adherence, vascular permeability, fever
Interleukin-1	Macrophage, endothelium	Intercellular signaling, fever, vascular permeability
Proteases	Macrophage, PMN, eosinophil, mast cell	Digest proteins
PAF	Macrophage	Vascular permeability, smooth muscle contraction
Toxic oxygen species	Macrophage, PMN, eosinophil	Injure microorganisms and cells
Tachykinins	Afferent nerve endings	Smooth muscle contraction, vascular permeability

to the site of injury. For example, the arachidonic acid metabolite leukotriene B$_4$ is a potent chemotactic factor released by airway epithelial cells and may be responsible for the influx of polymorphonuclear leukocytes (neutrophils) to both the conducting airways and lung periphery after exposure to ozone.

The neutrophil is often the first cell to reach the site of injury and its presence, histologically, is often a sign of acute inflammation. The neutrophil is a pluripotent inflammatory cell that can phagocytize inhaled particles as well as release proteases and oxygen-derived free radicals to kill invading organisms such as bacteria. Morphologically, the neutrophil is unique in its multilobed nucleus and the presence of specific and azurophilic granules. Neutrophil activation can lead to degranulation and the release of proteases such as lysozyme, collagenase, and elastase. In addition, the neutrophil can undergo a respiratory burst with the release of superoxide anion, hydrogen peroxide, and hypochlorous acid. The release of these proteases and toxic oxygen species likely evolved to defend the mammalian lung against inhaled organisms such as bacteria and molds. When neutrophils are recruited and activated in response to an inhaled toxic gas or inert particle, the somewhat inadvertent release

of these factors can result in pulmonary injury. In addition, the neutrophil itself is capable of releasing chemotactic factors that can attract other inflammatory cells that could amplify the injury.

Like the neutrophil, the pulmonary macrophage is a multifaceted cell that can phagocytize inhaled particles as well as release a wide variety of inflammatory mediators and growth factors on activation. Although airway and pulmonary vascular macrophages have recently been described, the alveolar macrophage is the most numerous resident inflammatory cell type in the pulmonary system. Thus, the alveolar macrophage is often described as the first line of defense against particles that deposit in the lung. The alveolar macrophage has a huge capacity for phagocytizing inhaled particles and has been known to attempt phagocytosis of asbestos particles several times its size in length and to continue the ingestion of particles to the seeming exclusion of visible cytoplasm. After the initial phagocytosis, the macrophage can remove the ingested particles from the lung by either chemical attack and dissolution of the particle (if soluble), transporting the particle up the mucociliary escalator, or migrating from the lumen of the airspaces through the interstitium into the lymph system. The macrophage is also capable of the release of a wide variety of inflammatory mediators that can attract and activate other cells. The stimulated alveolar macrophage, like the neutrophil, undergoes a respiratory burst with the extracellular release of toxic oxygen species. Many other inflammatory mediators, including arachidonic acid metabolites, complement factors, and platelet activating factor are released upon macrophage activation. Macrophages are also capable of *de novo* synthesis of cytokines, such as tumor necrosis factor and interleukin-1, and growth factors. These cytokines can amplify the inflammatory process by altering vascular endothelial cell permeability, promoting the adhesion of circulating neutrophils to the vascular walls near the site of injury, and by acting as intercellular signals with lymphocytes. Macrophages also release growth factors that can stimulate fibroblast proliferation and collagen synthesis. Chronic activation of macrophages by mineral dusts such as silica and asbestos appears to play a central role in fibrotic occupational lung diseases (see below).

Numerous other cells play a role in the inflammatory response of the pulmonary system. Mast cells are specialized resident inflammatory cells which are usually associated with allergic responses to antigenic stimuli. When membrane-bound antibodies are activated by foreign antigen, mast cells release inflammatory mediators such as histamine and the proteases, chymase, and tryptase. Eosinophils are also potent inflammatory cells that release the cytotoxic granular component major basic protein as well as eicosanoids.

Chronic Pulmonary Injury

Despite the specific and nonspecific defenses of the lung, chronic injury to the lung from inhaled agents occurs all too often. Chronic pulmonary injury occurs when defenses and repair processes simply cannot resolve damage resulting from acute exposure to high concentrations of a toxic material or repeated exposure to low levels of material. The outcome of the struggle between repair and injury can produce a wide range of pulmonary diseases including cancer, chronic obstructive pulmonary diseases, and fibrotic restrictive diseases (Table 12–5). Although the etiology of these chronic diseases is generally unclear, a significant portion results from the exposure to occupational and environmental pollutants. Moreover, the contribution of occupational and environmental agents is overshadowed by that attributed to cigarette smoke. Understanding the involvement of these factors in the pathogenesis of chronic lung diseases is a major focus of pulmonary toxicology research

and is important in the design of effective epidemiologic studies.

Chronic Obstructive Airway Diseases

The incidence of chronic obstructive airway diseases has been increasing rapidly. One major obstructive disease in which inhaled pollutants appear to play a role is *emphysema*. Emphysema is a common disease and although it is estimated to be responsible for only 1 to 5 percent of deaths in the United States, the frequency of emphysematous lesions at autopsy is reported to be as high as 50 percent (Thurlbeck, 1976). Emphysema is characterized by the destruction of the walls of the air spaces distal to the terminal bronchioles resulting in the abnormal permanent enlargement of the airspaces. The development of these structural changes over a lifetime are associated with the steady progression of functional disability including dyspnea, wheezing, cough, a decrease in diffusing capacity, and a slowing of forced expiration. Emphysema is clearly associated with heavy cigarette smoking and occurs late in life and frequently in combination with chronic bronchitis. Although the exact components of cigarette smoke that are responsible for the development of emphysema are unidentified, the inflammatory changes involved in the destruction of the walls of the airspaces have been described. Neutrophils and macrophages are stimulated by cigarette particles and this activation has been hypothesized and shown to cause an imbalance in the levels of proteases and antiproteases in the lung. An increase in the release of proteases such as elastase from neutrophils and macrophages or a decrease in the level of the antiproteases α_1-antiprotease or α-macroglobulin would allow the destruction of structural elastin in the walls of the airspaces. Both of these events do occur in the lungs of cigarette smokers: increased elastolytic activity and decreased antiprotease activity. Toxic oxygen species released by phagocytes contribute to the tissue injury on their own or indirectly by inhibition of α_1-antiprotease activity.

Chronic bronchitis is characterized by excessive mucus secretion in the bronchial tree and a chronic or recurrent productive cough. Chronic irritation by inhaled agents and microbiologic infection are both important in the etiology of chronic bronchitis. There appears to be little question of a relationship between chronic bronchitis and both cigarette smoking and air pollution. Smoking is by far the greater of the two as a contributing factor to bronchitis. Therefore, careful data collection on smoking history is necessary to assess the contribution of air pollution toward chronic bronchitis. The following

Table 12–5. INDUSTRIAL TOXICANTS PRODUCING LUNG DISEASE

TOXICANT	COMMON NAME OF DISEASE	OCCUPATIONAL SOURCE	ACUTE EFFECT	CHRONIC EFFECT
Asbestos	Asbestosis	Mining, construction, shipbuilding, manufacture of asbestos-containing material		Fibrosis, pleural calcification, lung cancer, pleural mesothelioma
Aluminum dust	Aluminosis	Manufacture of aluminum products, fireworks, ceramics, paints, electrical goods, abrasives	Cough, shortness of breath	Interstitial fibrosis
Aluminum abrasives	Shaver's disease, corundum smelter's lung, bauxite lung	Manufacture of abrasives, smelting	Alveolar edema	Interstitial fibrosis, emphysema
Ammonia		Ammonia production, manufacture of fertilizers, chemical production, explosives	Upper and lower respiratory tract irritation, edema	Chronic bronchitis
Arsenic		Manufacture of pesticides, pigments, glass, alloys	Bronchitis	Lung cancer, bronchitis, laryngitis
Beryllium	Berylliosis	Ore extraction, manufacture of alloys, ceramics	Severe pulmonary edema, pneumonia	Fibrosis, progressive dyspnea, interstitial granulomatosis, cor pulmonale
Cadmium oxide		Welding, manufacture of electrical equipment, alloys, pigments, smelting	Cough, pneumonia	Emphysema, cor pulmonale
Carbides of tungsten, titanium, tantalum	Hard metal disease	Manufacture of cutting edges on tools	Hyperplasia and metaplasia of bronchial epithelium	Peribronchial and perivascular fibrosis
Chlorine		Manufacture of pulp and paper, plastics, chlorinated chemicals	Cough, hemoptysis, dyspnea, tracheobronchitis, bronchopneumonia	
Chromium (VI)		Production of Cr compounds, paint pigments, reduction of chromite ore	Nasal irritation, bronchitis	Lung cancer, fibrosis

Substance	Disease	Occupation/Source	Symptoms	Effects
Coal dust	Pneumoconiosis	Coal mining		Fibrosis
Cotton dust	Byssinosis	Manufacture of textiles	Chest tightness, wheezing, dyspnea	Reduced pulmonary function, chronic bronchitis
Hydrogen fluoride		Manufacture of chemicals, photographic film, solvents, plastics	Respiratory irritation, hemorrhagic pulmonary edema	
Iron oxides	Siderotic lung disease; silver finisher's lung, hematite miner's lung, arc welder's lung	Welding, foundry work, steel manufacture, hematite mining, jewelry making	Cough	Silver finisher's: subpleural and perivascular aggregations of macrophages; hematite miner's: diffuse fibrosis-like pneumoconiosis; arc welder's: bronchitis
Isocyanates		Manufacture of plastics, chemical industry	Airway irritation, cough, dyspnea	Asthma, reduced pulmonary function
Kaolin	Kaolinosis	Pottery making		Fibrosis
Manganese	Manganese pneumonia	Chemical and metal industries	Acute pneumonia, often fatal	Recurrent pneumonia
Nickel		Nickel ore extraction, smelting, electronic electroplating, fossil fuels	Pulmonary edema, delayed by 2 days (NiCO)	Squamous cell carcinoma of nasal cavity and lung
Oxides of nitrogen		Welding, silo filling, explosive manufacture	Pulmonary congestion and edema	
Ozone		Welding, bleaching flour, deodorizing	Pulmonary edema	Emphysema
Phosgene		Production of plastics, pesticides, chemicals	Edema	Bronchitis
Perchloroethylene		Dry cleaning, metal degreasing, grain fumigating	Edema	
Silica	Silicosis, pneumoconiosis	Mining, stone cutting, construction, farming, quarrying		Fibrosis
Sulfur dioxide		Manufacture of chemicals, refrigeration, bleaching, fumigation	Bronchoconstriction, cough, chest tightness	
Talc	Talcosis	Rubber industry, cosmetics		Fibrosis
Tin	Stanosis	Mining, processing of tin		Widespread mottling of X-ray without clinical signs
Vanadium		Steel manufacture	Airway irritation and mucus production	Chronic bronchitis

indices of air pollution have been shown to correlate with the aggravation of symptoms or the mortality associated with chronic bronchitis: population size of the community, amounts of fuel burned in large cities, airborne dust and smoke, decreased visibility, and levels of sulfur dioxide.

Bronchial *asthma* is a conducting airway disease characterized by the increased responsiveness of airway smooth muscle to a variety of stimuli. Although the role of ambient levels of environmental pollutants such as acid aerosols and ozone in the development of asthma is controversial, occupational agents are clearly associated with asthma (Sheppard, 1986). Occupational asthma is produced by a wide range of particles and gases including western red cedar dust, TDI, and platinum and chromium salts and a common underlying mechanism for all these agents is unlikely. For most of these agents, sensitive individuals develop wheezing after exposure to extremely low concentrations, suggesting that immunologic mechanisms are involved. Research efforts have not confirmed immunologic involvement in many types of occupational asthma and other theories are being examined such as altered adrenergic receptor sensitivity, increased accessibility to irritant nerve receptors, or the release of inflammatory mediators such as eicosanoids, platelet activating factor, tachykinins, and major basic protein.

Lung Cancer

Although the topic of cancer is thoroughly covered in Chapter 5, it is necessary to discuss environmental and occupational agents as causative factors in the development of lung cancer. In industrialized nations, lung cancer is the leading cause of mortality among cancer deaths in both men and women. The majority of lung cancer deaths occurs in individuals between the ages of 40 and 70 years. This apparent latency in the production of benign or malignant lung cancers makes the relationship between the incidence of cancer and environmental pollutant exposure difficult to establish. There is considerable controversy whether there is an increased risk of lung cancer in urban environments after the data are corrected for cigarette smoking. Smoking is the number one risk factor in lung cancer and 80 percent of lung cancers occur in smokers. Average smokers have a 10-fold and heavy smokers have a 20-fold greater risk of developing lung cancer than nonsmokers. Thus, it is difficult to dissect an increased lung cancer risk due to exposure to environmental air pollutants from the risk attributable to smoking. Occupational exposure to certain industrial chemicals, however, is clearly associated with the development of lung

cancer. Increases in the incidence of lung cancer have occurred in workers exposed to asbestos; bischloromethyl ether; and metals such as nickel, chromium, and beryllium. Although asbestos is no longer used for insulation purposes in the United States, it is still a special concern for health researchers because of the long latency period to the onset of its effects and the potential hazard from the deterioration of previously insulated buildings.

Fibrotic Lung Diseases

Numerous occupational agents induce an inflammatory process that involves all of the components of the alveolar wall: epithelial cells, interstitial cells such as fibroblasts, vascular endothelial cells, collagen, and elastin. Although there is no clear evidence that chronic exposure to environmental pollutants at ambient concentrations causes fibrotic changes in man, chronic inhalation of mineral dusts such as silica and asbestos produces a group of interstitial lung diseases termed pneumoconioses. The underlying inflammatory process may resolve or it may develop into fibrosis after a period of many years. Animal research and more recently human clinical studies have demonstrated that the fibrogenesis that characterizes several occupational lung diseases cannot be attributed to a single inflammatory cell. Activated cells may release a number of mediators and growth factors that act to promote or prevent cell proliferation and to stimulate or inhibit connective tissue production. Occupationally induced interstitial lung diseases have been characterized as a process of the initiation of injury, amplification, and repair or resolution (Davis and Calhoun, 1988). In most workplace settings, the initiating agent has been clearly identified. However, the participation of cells and mediators in the ensuing development of lung disease is not completely understood. These amplification and repair processes are critical to the understanding of fibrotic lung disease, because the primary inflammatory process appears to be the same regardless of the inhaled material. The important research questions to be answered are why pulmonary injury leads to fibrosis in only some cases and what cells and mediators prevent the restoration of normal lung function and structure.

While the neutrophil appears to play a key role in acute inflammatory injury, the alveolar macrophage is the central character in chronic lung injury and fibrosis. Activated macrophages produce inflammatory mediators such as toxic oxygen species, complement factors, eicosanoids, cytokines, and proteases. An early hypothesis regarding the role of macrophages in fibrotic lung injury was based on the observation that

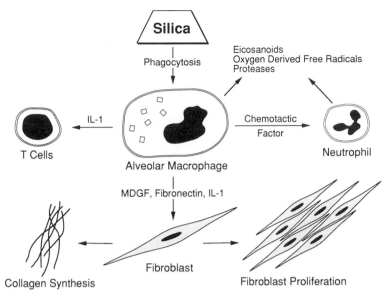

Figure 12–5. Inflammatory cells and mediators involved in the production of fibrosis by inhaled silica. (Adapted from Davis, G. S. and Calhoun, W. J.: Occupational and environmental causes of interstitial lung disease. In Schwarz, M. I., and King, R. E.: *Interstitial Lung Disease*. B. C. Decker, Toronto, 1988, pp. 63–109.)

repeated exposure to mineral dusts is cytotoxic to macrophages. The destruction of alveolar macrophages would thus cause the release of toxic oxygen species and enzymes that injure pulmonary tissue. It is now clear that the alveolar macrophage can undergo various levels of activation and that cell death is not necessary for the release of these and other inflammatory mediators. Chronic lung injury can result from the continued activation of macrophages by inert dust inhalation. Phagocytosis and destruction of inhaled particles by macrophages (and neutrophils) possibly evolved as a nonspecific lung defense in response to inhaled bacteria and other microorganisms. Phagocytosis of inert mineral dusts such as silica and asbestos likely results in the generation and unfortunate release of both toxic oxygen species and proteases into the local environment.

Silicon makes up approximately 25 percent of the earth's surface and exposure to crystalline silica is common in several different mining operations. Quartz is the most stable and common crystalline type of silica and exposure to the α-quartz form is responsible for the majority of clinically diagnosed silicosis. Silicosis is a fibronodular lung disease that occurs after occupational exposure to crystalline silica for 5 years or longer. The so-called silicotic nodule is the typical pulmonary lesion that positively identifies silicosis. These are firm nodules of concentrically arranged bundles of collagen fibers, usually 1 to 10 mm in diameter. They are composed of collagen and reticulin surrounded by macrophages, lymphocytes, and fibroblasts. The pathologic localization about the respiratory bronchiole appears to be related to the site of particle deposition. Brody *et al.* (1982) have established that the deposition of silica particles is focused at the alveolar duct bifurcations. Silica particles can be seen at the center of the nodule as well as in macrophages. Despite the fact that the incidence of silicosis dates from antiquity, current research still leaves many gaps in our knowledge relating to the precise manner in which the lesion develops, the relationship of the crystalline structure and size of the silica dust to the production of silicosis, and the correlation between retained dust load and the degree of pulmonary tissue reaction. The chronic pulmonary inflammation seen in silicosis appears to revolve around the macrophage (Figure 12–5). Besides the inflammatory mediators mentioned above, the macrophage releases several factors that modulate the development of fibrosis. These include factors that promote fibroblast proliferation and collagen synthesis: alveolar macrophage-derived growth factor, fibronectin, interleukin-1, and tumor necrosis factor. Mediators released from macrophages or other activated cells also appear to affect the type as well as the amount of collagen synthesized by fibroblasts. Changes in the ratio of type I to type III collagen have been observed in experimental models of silicosis and other fibrotic diseases. In addition, abnormal cross-linking of collagen helices can yield molecules more resistant to normal collagen metabolism and thus contribute to the development of interstitial fibrosis.

EXPOSURE SYSTEMS

To the toxicologist, inhalation exposure poses a variety of specialized problems that are not encountered when other routes of exposure are used. Exposure systems vary in complexity from those required to expose one or two rodents for an hour or less to those used for continuous exposure of dogs or primates for periods of months or years. Chambers have also been designed for exposure of human subjects who may be exercising on a bicycle during portions of an exposure period of several hours. A historical review by MacFarland (1983) discusses the design and operation of exposure chambers.

The most commonly used exposure chambers are so-called dynamic systems, which means that air flows continuously through the chamber and the toxic material being studied is continually metered into this airstream. The main airstream is purified of extraneous contaminants and maintained at constant temperature and humidity. Except for the control chamber, chambers are usually operated at a slight negative pressure. This is a safety precaution to ensure that any leaks will allow room air to enter the chamber rather than letting toxic material leak out to expose laboratory personnel. The control chamber is often kept at a slight positive pressure to ensure that unwanted airborne material from the room will not enter the control chamber.

The concentration of the toxic material in the chamber atmosphere is varied by altering the rate of addition of the substance to the main airstream and/or the rate of airflow through the chamber. From the respective flow rates it is possible to calculate the nominal concentration. It is, however, necessary to measure the concentration by techniques of collection and analysis appropriate to the material being studied. Material losses may occur in duct work, on chamber walls, and on the fur of animals if it is a whole-body exposure. The actual concentration is thus always slightly lower than the calculated nominal concentration. The concentration of importance, of course, is that in the breathing zone of the exposed animals. Samples should therefore be taken that are representative of that concentration. It is also necessary to take samples from various locations in the chamber to ensure that uniform mixing has been achieved. Animals should be randomly assigned to positions within the chamber during exposures and rotated at intervals to guard against accidental bias of dose. Individual cages should be used within the expo-

sure chamber to prevent animals from crowding together in one spot and reducing individual exposure. Groups of control animals are exposed for the same time periods to purified air in chambers of the same design and operated under the same conditions as those used for the exposure groups.

The method of generation of the material being tested varies with the nature of the material. Generation of gases or vapors is less complicated than generation of aerosols. The method chosen must be capable of generating a reproducible concentration of the material entering the airstream of the chambers over the time period of exposure. A most useful book by Willeke (1980) and an article by Rampe (1981) discuss the principles of generating experimental atmospheres for various types of materials.

Animals may be exposed with only the nose or head projecting into the chambers. Phalen (1984) gives a table summarizing the advantages, disadvantages, and special problems of these various modes of exposure. In whole-body exposure the animals are unrestrained, which has advantages and disadvantages for long-term experiments. The toxic material, especially if it is an aerosol, may be deposited on the animals' fur which can lead to oral ingestion via grooming. If the material is highly toxic or radioactive, such contamination can lead to exposure of personnel handling the animals. These problems are reduced or eliminated in nose or head-only systems. Restraint obviously adds some stress, but this can be minimized by appropriate design of the animal holders. The holder may double as a body plethysmograph, which makes possible measurement of pulmonary function during exposure.

Much useful information has been safely obtained by short-term exposure of human subjects, especially when the exposures are combined with toxicokinetic, physiologic, and biochemical measurements. Such data have been of particular value in assessing the response to low concentrations of air pollutants such as sulfur oxides, ozone, or nitrogen oxides. These exposures may be done in carefully designed chambers in which the subjects may freely move about or perform controlled exercise. They are more frequently done with the individual breathing through a mouthpiece or face mask connected to the contaminated atmosphere.

Tracheal instillation is frequently used to assess the toxic potential of particulate matter. The advantages to instillation are that the total dose to the lung is more easily quantified than that occurring during inhalation exposure and the procedure requires no specialized exposure systems or generation techniques for exposing animals. In addition, it is often difficult to correlate the initial events and injury responsible for the effects observed in chronic inhalation studies. The participating cells and mediators can easily be studied within hours to weeks after a single instillation of the particulate matter. The main disadvantage of tracheal instillation is the uncertaintity of the dose delivered to the specific target site observed to be affected in inhalation studies. Thus, the usefulness of tracheal instillation is limited to mechanistic studies in which the ease of delivery to the lung is very important.

In Vitro Studies

The study of mechanisms underlying the pulmonary injury produced by inhaled gases and particles is complicated by the wide variety of cells that comprise the respiratory tract. To focus on specific cells and the cellular injury that may be involved in the inflammatory response, several investigators have studied the effects of in vitro exposure of isolated cells to pollutants. The first step in conducting these experiments is the isolation and purification of sufficient numbers of viable cells of interest. Isolation of pulmonary macrophages is relatively simple and involves the repeated lavage of the entire lung via a tracheal cannula in anesthetized animals or specific lobes via a bronchoscope in human volunteers. The recovered cells are predominantly macrophages ($>$ 75 percent in nearly every specie examined) and can be subsequently purified by enrichment techniques such as adherence to plastic surfaces or the use of density gradients. The isolation of other pulmonary cells in sufficient quantities to perform in vitro exposures is significantly more difficult. In animal studies, the lung is removed and typically filled with a proteolytic enzyme solution (elastase, trypsin, or bacterial protease) and incubated at 37°C to release epithelial lining cells from their basement membranes. The lungs are then minced and filtered and the mixture of recovered cells separated by a number of methods including centrifugal elutriation, density gradient centrifugation, differential adherence, and flow cytometry. Similar cell separation techniques can be applied to human tissues recovered from autopsy specimens or resected lung sections. Once the desired cell type is isolated in sufficient numbers and viability, the cells are exposed in vitro as soon as possible to ensure that as little as possible of normal cell function is lost. Because the separation procedures themselves can harm the purified cell population, several investigators prefer to develop primary cell cultures of the isolated cells or transform the cells into immortal cell lines. These latter two techniques allow the researcher to perform many experiments on pro-

liferating cells from a single source and serve to reduce variability in experimental results.

After isolation of the cell of interest, the research toxicologist can expose the cells to toxic agents by a variety of methods. The simplest exposure technique is the addition of the toxic agent to the culture flask. The results obtained using this technique are difficult to interpret because of the undefined chemical interactions of the pollutant with the culture media. During in vivo exposure, epithelial lining cells or alveolar macrophages are exposed to airborne pollutants with a minimal layer of fluid protection such as the surfactant lining fluid or the mucus blanket. Therefore, exposure systems that are more relevant to the in vivo exposure of pulmonary cells to airborne pollutants are more commonly in use. Cells are grown on suitable substrates in vessels that facilitate the exposure of minimally covered cells to the pollutant. If the particular cell function being studied is not affected by drying, the culture media may simply be removed during short exposures to the pollutant gas in an exposure chamber. Usually, attempts are made to keep the exposure atmosphere saturated with water vapor. Because this is not always possible and several cell types are disturbed by drying, more elaborate exposure systems have been developed. These systems basically involve the cyclic mechanical manipulation of the media on the cells so that the cells are freely exposed to the pollutant gas at intervals in which little or no media covers them. This is accomplished by slow rocking of the cells or rotation of the cells on tilted platters (Valentine, 1985). A more recent exposure technique involves the culture of cells on collagen-coated membrane substrates which allows the feeding of nutrients from below the cells and no interference of media between the cell and the exposure gas. Using this method, Cohen et al. (1990) have demonstrated that as little as 0.05 ppm ozone produces cytotoxicity in cultured alveolar macrophages, whereas few if any effects have been observed in cells exposed to higher concentrations of ozone using the more conventional mechanical techniques. These results suggest that the interaction of pollutant gas and the target cells depends on the amount of culture media overlying the cells and the exposure methodology. Therefore, in vitro exposures are chiefly useful in examining the mechanisms responsible for toxicity observed in vivo and are not particularly useful for dose/response extrapolation. In addition, because cell-to-cell interactions occur in vivo and the toxic action of a particular agent may involve the participation of more than one cell type, results from single cell type exposures in vitro must be interpreted with caution. To overcome these difficulties, investigators have developed *in vitro* culture methodologies for examining biochemical changes in lung slices (Freeman and O'Neill, 1984) or isolated perfused lungs (Rhoades, 1984).

REFERENCES

Boushey, H. A.; Holtzman, M. J.; Sheller, J. R.; and Nadel, J. A.: Bronchial hyperreactivity: state of the art. *Am. Rev. Respir. Dis.,* **121**:389–413, 1980.

Brody, A. R.; Roe, M. W.; Evans, J. N.; and Davis, G. S.: Deposition and translocation of inhaled silica in rats. *Lab. Invest.,* **47**:533–542, 1982.

Brooks, S. M.: Bronchial asthma of occupational origin. In Rom, W. N. (ed.): *Environmental and Occupational Medicine.* Little, Brown and Company, Boston, 1983, pp. 233–250.

Clausen, J. L. (ed.): *Pulmonary Function Testing Guidelines and Controversies.* Grune & Stratton, Orlando, Florida, 1984.

Coffin, D. L.; Gardner, D. E.; Holzman, R. S.; and Wolock, F. J.: Influence of ozone on pulmonary cells. *Arch. Environ. Health,* **16**:633, 1968.

Cohen, D. S.; Welch, W. J.; and Sheppard, D.: Ambient concentrations of ozone cause cytotoxicity and suppression of protein synthesis in cultured alveolar macrophages and epithelial cells without inducing stress protein synthesis. *Am. Rev. Respir. Dis.,* **141**:A101, 1990.

Cotes, J. E.: *Lung Function.* Blackwell, Oxford, England, 1979.

Davis, G. S., and Calhoun, W. J.: Occupational and environmental causes of interstitial lung disease. In Schwarz, M. I., and King, R. E.: *Interstitial Lung Disease,* B. C. Decker, Toronto, 1988, pp. 63–109.

Drazen, J. M.: Physiologic basis and interpretation of indices of pulmonary mechanics. *Environ. Health Perspect.,* **56**:3–9, 1984.

Driscoll, K. E.; Vollmuth, T. A.; and Schlesinger, R. B.: Acute and subchronic ozone inhalation in the rabbit: response of alveolar macrophages. *J. Toxicol. Environ. Health,* **21**:27, 1987.

Fine, J. F., and Balmes J.: Airway inflammation and occupational asthma. In Fick, R. (ed.): *Airway Inflammation. Clin. Chest Med.* **4**:577–590, 1988.

Freeman, B. A., and O'Neill, J. J.: Tissue slices in the study of lung metabolism and toxicology. *Environ. Health Perspect.,* **56**:51–60, 1984.

Gardner, D. E.: Alterations in macrophage functions by environmental chemicals. *Environ. Health Perspect.,* **55**:343–358, 1984.

Gershwin, L. J.; Osebold, J. W.; and Zee, Y. C.: Immunoglobulin E-containing cells in mouse lung following allergen inhalation and ozone exposure. *Int. Arch. Allergy Appl. Immunology,* **65**:266–277, 1981.

Grodins, F. S., and Yamashiro, S. M.: *Respiratory Function of the Lung and Its Control.* Macmillan, New York, 1978.

Gross, D. B., and White, H. J.: Pulmonary functional and morphological changes induced by a 4-week exposure to 0.7 ppm ozone followed by a 9-week recovery period. *J. Toxicol. Environ. Health,* **17**:143–157, 1986.

Henderson, R. F.: Bronchoalveolar lavage: a tool for assessing the health status of the lung. In McClellan, R. O., and Henderson, R. F. (eds.): *Concepts in Inhalation Toxicology.* Hemisphere, New York, 1989, pp. 415–444.

Hinds, W. C.: *Aerosol Technology.* John Wiley & Sons, 1982.

Kessler, G.-F.; Austin, J. H. M.; Graf, P. D.; Gamsu, G.; and Gold, W. M.: Airway constriction in ex-

perimental asthma in dogs: tantalum bronchographic studies. *J. Appl. Physiol.,* **35**:703–708, 1973.

Kleeberger, S. R.; Kolbe, J.; Turner, C.; and Spannhake, E. W.: Exposure to 1 ppm ozone attenuates the immediate antigenic response of canine peripheral airways. *J.Toxicol. Environ. Health,* **28**:349–362, 1989.

Lippmann, M.; Albert, R. E.; and Peterson, H. T.: Regional deposition of inhaled aerosols in man. In Walton, W. H. (ed.): *Inhaled Particles and Vapours.* Unwin, Old Woking, Surrey, England, 1971, pp. 105–120.

MacFarland, H. N.: Design and operational characteristics of inhalation exposure equipment—a review. *Fund. Appl. Toxicol.,* **3**:603–613, 1983.

Mauderly, J. L.: Effect of inhaled toxicants on pulmonary function. In McClellan, R. O., and Henderson, R. F. (eds.): *Concepts in Inhalation Toxicology.* Hemisphere, New York, 1989, pp. 347–401.

Murray, J. F.: *The Normal Lung.* W. B. Saunders, Philadelphia, 1986.

Phalen, R. F.; Mannix, R. C.; and Drew, R. T.: Inhalation exposure methodology. *Environ. Health Perspect.,* **56**:23–34, 1984.

Rampe, L. W.: Generating and controlling atmospheres in inhalation chambers. In Gralla, E. J. (ed.): *Scientific Considerations in Monitoring and Evaluating Toxicological Research.* Hemisphere, Washington, D.C., 1981, pp. 57–69.

Reynolds, H. Y.: Bronchoalveolar lavage. In Murray J. F., and Nadel J. A. (eds.): *Textbook of Respiratory Medicine.* W. B. Saunders, Philadelphia, 1988, pp. 597–610.

Rhoades, R. A.: Isolated perfused lung preparation for studying altered gaseous environments. *Environ. Health Perspect.,* **56**:43–50, 1984.

Riedel, F.; Kramer, M.; Scheibenbogen, C.; and Rieger, C. H. L.: Effects of SO$_2$ exposure on allergic sensitization in the guinea pig. *J. Allergy Clin. Immunol.,* **82**:527–534, 1988.

Schlesinger, R. B.: The interaction of inhaled toxicants with respiratory tract clearance mechanisms. *Crit. Rev. Toxicol.,* **20**:257–286, 1990.

Selgrade, M. K.; Illing, J. W.; Starnes, D. M.; Steak, A. G.; Menache, M. G.; and Stevens, M. A.: Evaluation of effects of ozone exposure on influenza infection in mice using several indicators of susceptibility. *Fund. Appl. Toxicol.,* **11**:169–180, 1988.

Sheppard, D.: Significance of airway hyperresponsiveness to occupational and environmental lung disorders. *Semin. Respir. Med.* **7**:241–248, 1986.

Takezawa, J.; Miller, F. J.; and O'Neil, J. J.: Single breath diffusing capacity and lung volumes in small laboratory mammals. *J. Appl. Physiol.,* **48**:1052–1059, 1980.

Thurlbeck, W. M.: *Chronic Airflow Obstruction in Lung Disease.* W. B. Saunders, Philadelphia, 1976.

Valentine, R.: An *in vitro* system for exposure of lung cells to gases: effects of ozone on rat macrophages. *J. Toxicol. Environ. Health,* **16**:115–126, 1985.

Warheit, D. B.: Interspecies comparisons of lung responses to inhaled particles and gases. *Crit. Rev. Toxicol.,* **20**:1–29, 1989.

Weibel, E. R.: *The Pathway for Oxygen. Structure and Function in the Mammalian Respiratory System.* Harvard University Press, Cambridge, 1984.

Weibel, E. R.: Lung cell biology. In Fishman, A. P. (ed.): *Handbook of Physiology. Section 3: The Respiratory System.* American Physiology Society, Bethesda, 1985, pp. 47–91.

West, J. B.: *Respiratory Physiology—The Essentials.* Williams & Wilkins, Baltimore, 1985.

Willeke, D.: *Generation of Aerosols and Facilities for Exposure Experiments.* Ann Arbor Science, Ann Arbor, 1980.

Chapter 13

TOXIC RESPONSES OF THE NERVOUS SYSTEM

Douglas C. Anthony and *Doyle G. Graham*

INTRODUCTION

Neurotoxicology is an exciting area of science not only because of the importance of toxic injury to the nervous system in human disease, but also because specific toxicants and toxins have been invaluable tools for the advancement of neurobiology. In fact, much of our understanding of the organization and function of the nervous system is based on observations derived from the action of neurotoxicants. The binding of exogenous compounds to membranes has been the basis for the definition of specific receptors within the brain; an understanding of the roles of different cell types in the function of the nervous system has stemmed from the selectivity of certain toxicants in injuring only certain cell types; and important differences in basic metabolic requirements of different subpopulations of neurons have been inferred from the effects of toxicants.

At the same time that industrial progress has aided in the understanding of the nervous system has come the age in which neurotoxic exposures of humans are a major environmental concern. Human exposures have occurred throughout the world in epidemics in which thousands of individuals have been exposed to neurotoxicants; and perhaps of even greater concern, large numbers of people develop neurologic disorders and are exposed to environments containing known neurotoxicants and many more compounds whose effects on the nervous system are unknown. How many of these people are suffering from the neurotoxic effects of unidentified agents? This issue remains unclear, but it is a concern to all neurotoxicologists. The cause of Parkinson's disease is unknown, but epidemiologic data suggest that the incidence is related to components of the environment (Snyder and D'Amato, 1985), and while toxic exposure is a recognized cause of peripheral neuropathies, the cause of a particular neuropathy is never determined in many people with this neurologic condition. Although we do not know whether or how many of these people are suffering from the effects of toxic exposure, one thing is clear: there is reason to be concerned.

To understand neurotoxicologic diseases, one must appreciate something of the anatomy, physiology, development, and healing capacity of the nervous system. These complexities of the nervous system, however, can be reduced to a number of generalities that allow a basic understanding of the actions of toxicants. Some of these general principles are: (1) a privileged status of the nervous system that maintains a barrier between itself and the blood, (2) the importance of the energy requirements of the brain, (3) the extensions of the nervous system over space and the requirements of cells with such a complex geometry, (4) the maintenance of an environment rich in lipids, and (5) the transmission of information across extracellular space. Each of these features of the nervous system carries with it specialized metabolic requirements and unique vulnerabilities to toxic compounds.

BLOOD-BRAIN BARRIER

The nervous system is protected from entry of many potential toxicants through an anatomically defined barrier. In 1885, Ehrlich, while studying the distribution of dyes in the body, noticed that although other tissues become stained, the brain and spinal cord did not develop the color of the dyes (Ehrlich, 1885). One can only imagine the excitement on the realization that this observation pointed to the existence of an interface between the blood and the brain, or a blood-brain barrier. Most of the brain, spinal cord, retina, and peripheral nerve demonstrate this restricted entry of molecules, a barrier that is similar in its selectivity to the barrier between cells and extracellular space (Davson, 1989). The brain, spinal cord, and peripheral nerves are completely covered with a continuous lining of specialized cells that limits the entry of molecules from adjacent tissue. In the brain and spinal cord, this is the meningeal surface, and in peripheral nerves each fascicle of nerve is sur-rounded by perineurial cells.

The nervous system maintains a similar in-terface with the bloodstream. It appears that the principal basis of the blood-brain barrier is the tight junction that exists between endothelial cells only in the nervous system (Reese and Kar-novsky, 1967). To gain entry to the nervous system, molecules must pass through the cell membranes of the endothelial cell of the brain, rather than between endothelial cells as they do in other tissues. Thus, aside from molecules that are actively transported into the brain, the penetration of toxicants or their metabolites into the nervous system is largely related to their lipid solubility, and their ability to pass through the plasma membranes of the cells forming the bar-rier (Brightman, 1989), rather than between cells. There are two important exceptions to this general rule. First are those substances such as amino acids, which are actively transported into the nervous system. Second, ganglia, both spinal and autonomic, as well as a small number of other sites within the brain, contain capillaries with 4-nm gaps between endothelial cells as seen in tissues outside the nervous system, and thus are not protected by blood-tissue barriers. The discontinuity of the barrier allows the entry of the anti-cancer drug doxorubicin into the sensory ganglia, and leads to a selectivity of the neuro-toxicity of this compound for ganglionic neurons (Cho, 1977).

It should be noted that the blood-brain barrier is incompletely developed at birth, and even less so in premature infants. This predisposes the premature infant to brain injury by toxicants such as unconjugated bilirubin, which later in life would be excluded. Thus, unconjugated bilirubin enters the nervous system of premature infants (Lucey et al., 1964) where its toxic ac-tion leads to a permanent brain disability.

ENERGY REQUIREMENTS OF THE BRAIN

Neurons and cardiac myocytes are exquisitely sensitive to the deprivation of oxygen. This vul-nerability is a reflection of the high dependence of these cells on aerobic metabolism. These cells share the property of conduction of electrical impulses, and their dependence on aerobic respiration emphasizes the high metabolic de-mand associated with the maintenance and re-petitive reinstitution of ion gradients. The fact that these membrane depolarizations and re-polarizations occur so rapidly necessitates that the cell have the requisite energy to reestablish ion gradients through active ion transport. This process occurs with a frequency that requires that the cell be able to produce large quantities of high-energy phosphates even in a resting state. That the energy requirements of the brain are related to membrane depolarizations is supported by the fact that hyperactivity, as in epileptic foci, increases the energy requirements by as much as five times (Plum and Posner, 1985). The depen-dence on a continual source of energy, in the absence of energy reserves, places the neuron in a vulnerable position. To meet these high energy requirements, the brain utilizes aerobic glycoly-sis, and therefore, is extremely sensitive to even brief interruptions of the supply of oxygen or glucose.

For these reasons, prolonged hypoxia, regard-less of its cause, often results in injury to the brain. Drowning, or near-drowning, deprives an individual of oxygen, and can be viewed as re-latively pure hypoxia. If the patient is revived, the period of hypoxia and body temperature dur-ing the hypoxia will determine the severity of the damage. As temperature is lowered, the need for oxygen is lessened. Thus, the severity of neurologic damage is often less in individuals who suffer near-drowning episodes in ice-cold water than is the injury that occurs in warm water (Orlowski, 1987). Deprivation of oxygen for more than a few minutes initiates a lethal injury of neurons. Almost immediately, the cells can-not conduct impulses appropriately, and the brain fails to function, with a loss of conscious-ness (Ernsting, 1963). Within a few minutes, the damage is irreversible; the neurons have died and, if the individual survives, the neurons will be lost in the cortex, basal ganglia, and Purkinje cell layer of the cerebellum. In the most severe circumstance, glia as well as neurons die, result-ing in cerebral cortical "laminar necrosis."

Toxicants that inhibit aerobic respiration have a similar effect. Cyanide (Vogel and Sultan, 1981) and hydrogen sulfide (Beauchamp et al., 1984), for example, bind cytochrome oxidase irreversibly and prevent mitochondria from utilizing oxygen as an electron acceptor. Sim-ilarly, when carbon monoxide complexes with hemoglobin, the oxygen carrying capacity of hemoglobin is obliterated; high concentrations of carbon monoxide can render an organism ex-tremely hypoxic and result in widespread dam-age to the nervous system. Indeed, individuals who are injured sublethally by carbon monoxide sometimes show loss of cortical neurons in a laminar necrosis pattern, or severe degeneration of the globus pallidus (Brierley and Graham, 1984). The oligodendrocyte is not completely impervious to the deprivation of oxygen, and following exposure to carbon monoxide, the oli-godendrocyte may lose its ability to maintain myelin. This loss of myelin results in an entirely separate process known as demyelination. Each of these separate pathologic processes, cortical necrosis, basal ganglia infarction, and delayed demyelination, may occur in carbon monoxide poisoning either separately or in combination, and emphasize the vulnerable position of the nervous system to the deprivation of oxygen (Shepard, 1983).

THE OBSTACLE OF SPACE

Although simple multicellular organisms are able to survive without specialized means of intercellular communication, more complex invertebrates, and all vertebrates, have specialized systems to overcome the problem of the separation of cells in space. A vascular system allows for the transport of materials from one region of the organism to another. Some forms of intercellular communication can also be conducted through the vascular system, and these hormones transmit information to remote sites through the blood.

Some information, however, is too vital to be conducted in such a diffuse and slow manner, and the nervous system can be envisioned as the remedy to the obstacle of space in intercelluar communication. Impulses are conducted over great distances at rapid speed and provide information about the environment to the organism in a coordinated manner that allows an organized response to be carried out at a specific site. But the intricate organization of such a communication network places an unusual and unparalleled demand on the cells of the nervous system. Single cells, rather than being spherical and a few micrometers in diameter, are elongate and may extend over a meter in length!

The anatomy of such a complex intercellular network introduces variations in metabolism and cellular geometry that are peculiar to the nervous system. The two immediate demands placed on the neuron are the maintenance of a much larger cellular volume, and the transport of intracellular materials over great distances. Although the length of neurons may exceed 200,000 times the dimensions of most other cells, the cellular volume has not undergone a similar increase due to the unique attribute of very fine cylindrical extensions of the cell to span the long distances. By reducing the diameter of the cellular extension, the neuron is able to span the required distances but maintain less cytoplasmic volume.

Even so, the volume of the axon may be much greater than the volume of the cell body. If one considers the lower motor neuron in humans, the cell body is located in the spinal cord and the axon extends to the site of innervation of a muscle at a distant location. In spite of the smaller diameter of the axon, the tremendous distances traversed by the axon translate to an axonal volume that may be hundreds of times greater than that of the cell body itself (Cavanagh, 1984).

This places a great burden on the neuron to provide protein synthetic machinery for such a cytoplasmic volume. The machinery is readily visible in large neurons through the light microscope as the Nissl substance, which is formed by clusters of ribosomal complexes for the synthesis of proteins (Carpenter and Sutin, 1983). That this is a reflection of an unusual protein synthetic burden may be surmised from the fact that neurons are the only cell type with such a Nissl substance.

In addition to the increased burden of protein synthesis, the neuron is dependent on the ability to distribute materials over the distances encompassed by its processes. While analogous systems exist in all cell types and are referred to as cytoplasmic streaming, in the nervous system this process occurs over much greater distances and is referred to as axonal transport. Protein synthesis occurs in the cell body, and the protein products are then transported through the process of axonal transport to the appropriate site. Through studies of the movement of radiolabeled amino acid precursors, several major components of axonal transport are known (Baitinger et al., 1982).

The first component is referred to as fast axonal transport and carries a large number of proteins from their site of synthesis in the cell body into the axon. Many of these proteins are associated with vesicles (Grafstein and Forman, 1980) and migrate through the axon at a rate of 400 mm/day (Figure 13–1). An understanding of the molecular basis of this fast axonal transport is now evolving. The process has been known to be dependent on ATP for quite some time, but it was not until the description of a microtubule-associated ATPase activity that there rapidly emerged the concept of microtubule-associated motors. These proteins, kinesin and dynein being the prototypes of what may be a class of microtubule-associated motors, provide both the mechanochemical force in the form of a microtubule-associated ATP-ase and the interface between microtubules as the track, and vesicles as the cargo (Schnapp et al., 1985). Vesicles are transported rapidly in an anterograde direction by kinesin, and transported in a retrograde direction by dynein (Vale et al., 1985; Johnson, 1985; Schnapp and Reese, 1989). While this mechanism of cytoplasmic transport toward the cell periphery and back toward the nucleus appears to be a general feature of cells, the process is amplified within the nervous system by the distances encompassed by the axonal extensions of neurons.

The transport of some organelles, including mitochondria, comprises an intermediate component of axonal transport, moving at 50 mm/

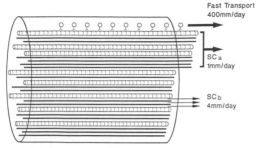

Figure 13–1. Schematic diagram of an axon. Fast axonal transport is depicted as spherical vesicles moving along microtubules with an intervening microtubule-associated motor. The slow component A (SCa) represents the movement of the cytoskeleton composed of neurofilaments and microtubules. Slow component B (SCb) moves at a faster rate than SCa, and includes soluble proteins which are apparently moving between the more slowly moving cytoskeleton.

day (Lorenz and Willard, 1978). As with the fast component, the function is apparently the continuous replacement of organelles within the axon. The slowest component of axonal transport represents the movement of the cytoskeleton itself, rather than the movement of enzymes or organelles through the cytosol (Figure 13–1). The cytoskeleton is composed of structural elements, including microtubules formed by the associaton of tubulin subunits, and neurofilaments formed by the association of three neurofilament protein subunits. Each of these structural elements of the cytoskeleton moves along the length of the axon at a specific rate. Initially described by Hoffman and Lasek as slow component A (SCa), to distinguish the movement from another slow component of axonal transport, slow component B (SCb) (Hoffman and Lasek, 1975), these same two components have also been termed components IV (SCb) and V (SCa) relative to the faster components (I-III) (Baitinger et al., 1982).

Neurofilaments and microtubules move at an approximate rate of 1 mm/day and comprise the majority of SCa. Moving at only a slightly more rapid rate of 2 to 4 mm/day is slow component B, which is composed of more than 200 proteins (Brady and Lasek, 1982). Included in SCb are several structural proteins, such as the component of microfilaments (actin) and several microfilament-associated proteins (M2 protein and fodrin), as well as clathrin and many soluble proteins.

This continual transport of proteins from the cell body through the various components of forward-directed, or anterograde, axonal transport is the mechanism through which the cell body provides the distal axon with its comple-ment of functional and structural proteins. Some vesicles are also moving in a retrograde direction and undoubtedly provide the cell body with information concerning the status of the distal axon. The evidence for such a dynamic interchange of materials and information stems not only from the biochemical detection of these components of axonal transport, but also from the observations of the effects of terminating this interchange by severing the axon from its cell body. The result of such an interruption of cell-axon exchange is that the axon is destined to degenerate, deprived of its only source of protein synthesis. The cell body responds to the transection of the axon as well, and undergoes a process termed chromatolysis, indicating that the cell body is "aware" of the status of its distal axon.

These dynamic relationships between the neuronal cell body and its axon are critical to understanding the basic pathologic responses to axonal and neuronal injuries caused by neurotoxicants. When the neuronal cell body has been lethally injured, it degenerates along with all of its cellular processes. In toxicology, as well as in all of neurobiology, this process is a "neuronopathy" and is characterized by the loss of the entire cell, body and processes, with no potential for regeneration. However, when the injury is at the level of the axon, the axon may degenerate while the neuronal cell body continues to survive, a condition known as an "axonopathy" (Figure 13–2). In this setting, there is a potential for regeneration and recovery from the toxic injury as the axonal stump sprouts and regenerates. It should come as little surprise that the axonal transport systems have become of major interest in attempts to understand the toxic degeneration of axons, or what has been viewed as chemical transection of the axon.

MAINTENANCE OF A LIPID-RICH ENVIRONMENT

Myelin is formed in the central nervous system (CNS) by oligodendrocytes, and in the peripheral nervous system (PNS) by Schwann cells. Both of these cell types form concentric layers of lipid-rich myelin by the progressive wrapping of their cytoplasmic processes around the axon in successive loops. Ultimately, these cells exclude water and ions from the cytoplasmic surface of their membranes to form the major dense line of myelin (Braun, 1977). In a similar process, the extracellular space is eliminated from the extracellular surface of the bilayers and the lipid membranes stack together separated only by a proteinaceous intraperiod line existing between successive layers.

The formation and maintenance of myelin requires metabolic machinery and structural proteins that are unique to the nervous system.

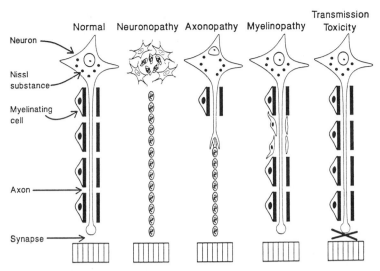

Figure 13–2. Patterns of neurotoxic injury. A neuronopathy results from the death of the entire neuron. Astrocytes often proliferate in response to the neuronal loss, creating the pathologic impression of neuronal loss and gliosis. When the axon is the primary site of injury, the axon may degenerate while the surviving neuron shows only chromatolysis with margination of its Nissl substance and nucleus to the cell periphery. This condition is termed an axonopathy. Myelinopathies result from disruption of myelin or from a selective injury to the myelinating cells. Adjacent cells divide and cover the denuded axon rapidly; however, the process of remyelination is much less effective in the CNS than in the PNS. Some compounds do not lead to cell death, but exert their toxic effects by interrupting the process of neurotransmission, either through blocking excitation, or by excessive stimulation.

Myelin basic protein, a basic protein of CNS myelin, is closely associated with the intracellular space (major dense line of myelin) (Braun *et al.,* 1980), and an analogous protein, P1 protein, is located in the peripheral nervous system. On the extracellular surface of the lipid bilayers is the CNS protein, proteolipid protein. The absence of this protein in several species, including humans, results in an hereditary disorder in which myelin of the CNS does not form normally (Nave *et al.,* 1986; Duncan *et al.,* 1987).

There are, in fact, a variety of hereditary disorders in which myelin is either poorly formed from the outset, or is not maintained after its formation. In addition to the absence of proteolipid protein, there are a variety of inherited abnormalities of lipid catabolism, including the abnormalities in the catabolism of certain ceramides, ceramide sulfates, and gangliosides. These genetic defects have provided some insight into the special processes required to maintain the lipid-rich environment of myelin. It is now known that the maintenance of myelin is dependent on a large number of membrane-associated proteins and complex lipid metabolism. In the context of toxic exposures, it is easy to imagine how some toxic compounds interfere with this complex process of the maintenance of myelin and result in the toxic "myelinopathies" (Figure 13–2).

TRANSMISSION OF INFORMATION ACROSS EXTRACELLULAR SPACE

Intercellular communication is established in the nervous system through the synapse. Neurotransmitters released from one axon act as the first messenger. Binding of the transmitter to the postsynaptic receptor is followed by the activation of a second messenger system leading to changes in the responding cell. In the case of neuromuscular transmission, acetylcholine crosses the synaptic cleft to bind the cholinergic receptor of the myocyte and leads to muscular contraction.

The process of neurotransmission is a target of a variety of therapeutic drugs and is a major component of the science of neuropharmacology. In addition, there are a variety of toxic compounds that interact directly with the process of neurotransmission, and hence form the basis of neurotransmitter-associated toxicity. Thus, the same process that is the target of many clinical neuropharmacologic strategies and drug designs, is also the target of certain neurotoxic compounds.

DEVELOPMENT OF THE NERVOUS SYSTEM

One feature important to understanding neuro-toxicity is the dynamic process of development of the nervous system. Both neuronal and glial precursors replicate in the germinal mantle, a collection of cells near the ventricular system. Successive layers of cerebral cortex, as well as other neurons, supportive astrocytes, and myelinating oligodendrocytes, migrate from the germinal mantle in a precisely ordered sequence both *in utero* and in early postnatal life.

Development of the brain continues during childhood and provides a certain resilience toward injuries. Much of this is due to the fact that the younger brain has greater plasticity, that ability of one portion of the nervous system to assume the function of a destroyed area. The brain of a child may compensate partially for an injury that would result in much greater disability in an adult (Goldberger and Murray, 1985). This plasticity of the immature nervous system appears to derive from the ability of dendrites to arborize and form new synapses. It is both curious and tragic that this capacity is progressively lost with age.

On the other hand, the developing nervous system is particularly vulnerable to certain agents. Ethanol exposure during pregnancy can result in abnormalities in the fetus, including abnormal neuronal migration, abnormal facial development leading to a characteristic appearance, and diffuse abnormalities in the development of neuronal processes, especially the dendritic spines (Stoltenburg-Didinger and Spohre, 1983; Abel *et al.*, 1983). The exposure may be of no consequence to the mother, while the fetus is devastated by it, with a resultant mental retardation. Although there remains a great deal of uncertainty concerning the molecular basis of this developmental aberration, it occurs in a variety of experimental animals, and it appears that acetaldehyde, a product of ethanol catabolism, can produce migration defects in developing animals similar to those which occur in the fetal alcohol syndrome (O'Shea and Kaufman, 1979).

FUNCTIONAL MANIFESTATIONS OF NEUROTOXICITY

Most of us are aware of the neurobehavioral effects of alcohol on the adult organism. Indeed, alterations in neurological or psychological health have frequently been the first clues that a given chemical is neurotoxic. What follows is a presentation of neurotoxicology from a molecular and cellular perspective. This chapter does not include effects on higher integrative func-

tions, such as cognition, or changes in an individual's emotional state. Neither does it detail the important neurobehavioral and physiological observations which can be made in the living animal; a cellular/molecular basis for each of these changes certainly exists but has not yet been identified in many cases. For an excellent discussion of these subjects, the reader is referred to the chapter by Dr. Stata Norton in the third edition of this book.

NEURONOPATHIES

Certain toxicants are specific for neurons, or sometimes a particular group of neurons, resulting in their injury, or when intoxication is severe enough, in their death. The loss of a neuron is irreversible and includes degeneration of all of its cytoplasmic extensions, dendrites and axons, and of the myelin ensheathing the axon (Figure 13–2). Although the neuron, as a cell, is similar to other cell types in many respects, some features of the neuron are unique, placing the neuron at risk for the action of cellular toxicants. Because many neurotoxic compounds act at the site of the cell body, when massive loss of axons and myelin are discovered in the peripheral or central nervous systems, the first question is whether the neuronal cell bodies themselves have been destroyed.

Although a large number of compounds are known to result in toxic neuronopathies (Table 13–1), all of these toxicants share certain features. Each of these toxic conditions is the result of a cellular toxicant that has a predilection for neurons, most likely due to one of the neuron's peculiar vulnerabilities. An initial injury of neurons is followed by necrosis, leading to their permanent loss. These agents tend to be diffuse

Table 13–1. COMPOUNDS ASSOCIATED WITH NEURONAL INJURY

Aluminum	Kanamycin
6-Aminonicotinamide	Lead
Azide	Manganese
Bismuth	Methanol
Carbon monoxide	Methylazoxymethanol
Carbon tetrachloride	acetate
Chloramphenicol	Methylbromide
Cyanide	Methylmercury
Dichlorodiphenylchlore-	1-Methyl-4-phenyl-
thane	1,2,3,6-tetrahydropyri-
Diphenylhydantoin	dine (MPTP)
Doxorubicin	Quinidone
Ethambutol	Quinine
Hydrogen sulfide	Streptomycin
Kainate	Thallium
	Thiophene
	Trimethyltin

in their action, although they may show some selectivity in the degree of injury of different neuronal subpopulations, or at times may show an exquisite selectivity for such a subpopulation. The expression of these cellular events is often a diffuse encephalopathy, with global dysfunctions; however, the symptomatology reflects the injury to the brain so that neurotoxicants that are selective in their action may lead to interruption of only a particular functionality.

Doxorubicin

Although it is the cardiac toxicity that limits the quantity of doxorubicin (Ariamycin®) that can be given to cancer patients, doxorubicin also injures neurons in the PNS, specifically those of the dorsal root ganglia and autonomic ganglia (Cho, 1977; Cho et al., 1980). Doxorubicin is an anthracycline antibiotic derivative whose antineoplastic properties derive from its ability to intercalate in double-stranded DNA, interfering with transcription. Because all neurons are dependent on the ability to transcribe DNA, it is quite interesting that the neurotoxicity of doxorubicin is so limited in its extent. The particular vulnerability of sensory and autonomic neurons appears to reflect the lack of protection of these neurons by a blood-tissue barrier within ganglia. If the blood-brain barrier is temporarily opened by the use of mannitol, the toxicity of doxorubicin is expressed in a much more diffuse manner, with injury of neurons in the cortex and subcortical nuclei of the brain (Kondo et al., 1987). Thus, in the presence of a competent blood-brain barrier doxorubicin gains a limited access to the nervous system, and it is at this site of restricted entry where it exerts its more general mechanism of toxicity.

Methylmercury

The neuronal toxicity of organomercurial compounds, such as methylmercury, was tragically manifested in large numbers of poisonings in Japan and Iraq. The residents of Minamata Bay in Japan whose diet was largely composed of fish from the bay were exposed to massive amounts of methylmercury when mercury-laden industrial effluent was rerouted into the bay (Kurland et al., 1960; Takeuchi et al., 1962). Methylmercury injured even more people in Iraq, with more than 400 deaths and 6000 people hospitalized. In this epidemic, as well as in several other smaller epidemics, the effects occurred after consuming grain that had been dusted with methylmercury as an inexpensive pesticide (Bakir et al., 1973).

The mechanism of methylmercury toxicity has been the subject of intense investigation. However, it is still unclear whether the ultimate toxicant is the methylmercury or liberated mercuric ion. While Hg^{2+} is known to bind strongly to sulfhydryl groups, it is not entirely clear that MeHg results in cell death through sulfhydryl binding. A variety of aberrations in cellular metabolism have been noted, including impaired glycolysis (Paterson and Usher, 1971), nucleic acid biosynthesis (Frenkel and Harrington, 1979), aerobic respiration (Fowler and Woods, 1977), and protein synthesis (Cheung and Verity, 1985). It seems likely that MeHg toxicity is mediated by numerous reactions and that no single critical target will be identified. As these cellular toxic events occur, the injured neurons eventually die and are lost. Exposure to methylmercury leads to a diffuse distribution of neuronal injury, and subsequently to a diffuse encephalopathy. Although the distribution of injury is diffuse, there is still some selectivity of the toxicant for some groups of neurons over others. The distribution of neuronal injury appears not to be related to the tissue distribution of either methylmercury or ionic mercury, but rather to particular vulnerabilities of some neurons.

The clinical picture varies both with the severity of exposure and the age of the individual at the time of exposure. In adults, the most dramatic sites of injury are the neurons of the visual cortex, and the small internal granular cell neurons of the cerebellar cortex, whose massive degeneration results in marked ataxia (Shiraki, 1979). In children, particularly those exposed to methylmercury in utero, the neuronal loss is widespread and, in settings of greatest exposure, produces profound mental retardation and paralysis (Reuhl and Chang, 1979).

Trimethyltin

Organotins are used industrially as plasticizers, antifungal agents, or other pesticides. Trimethyltin gains access to the nervous system where, by an undefined mechanism, it leads to a diffuse neuronal injury. Many neurons of the nervous system begin to accumulate cytoplasmic bodies composed of Golgi-like structures, followed by cellular swelling and necrosis (Bouldin et al., 1981). The hippocampus is particularly vulnerable to the process, and following acute intoxication, the cells of the fascia dentata degenerate while, with a chronic exposure, the cells of the corpus ammonis degenerate. Because the neurons of the corpus ammonis are the most vulnerable to hypoxia, interference with energy production is one possible mechanism of toxicity.

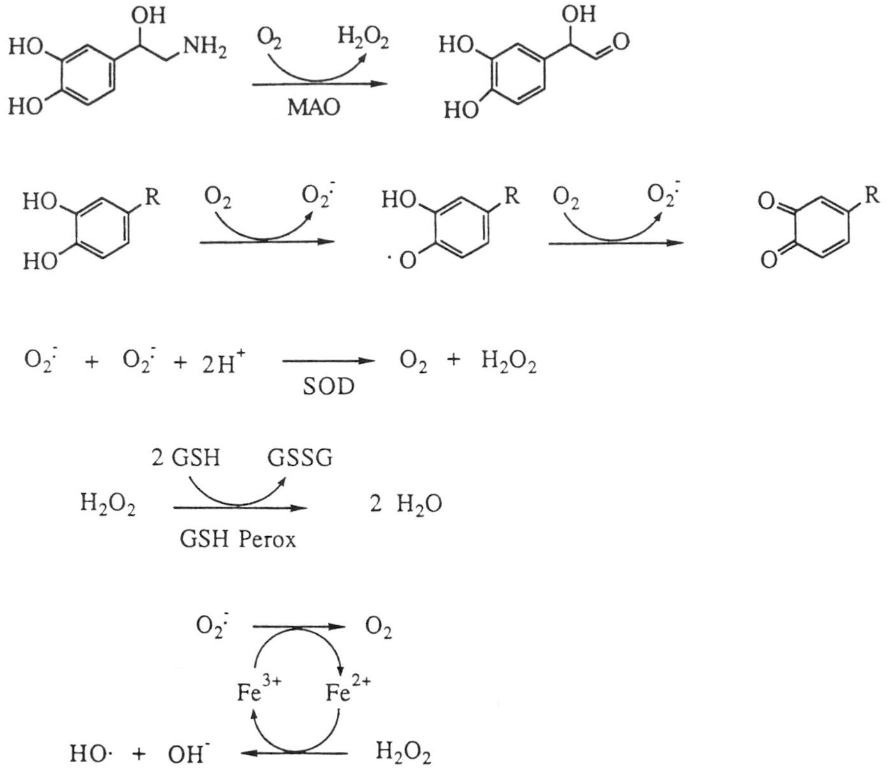

Figure 13–3. Catecholamine oxidation and activated oxygen species. Both the enzyme-catalyzed oxidation of catecholamines, here illustrating the action of monoamine oxidase (MAO) on norepinephrine, and the nonenzymatic oxidation of catecholamines generate activated oxygen species, hydrogen peroxide and superoxide. There are intracellular enzymes that together handle the flux of superoxide (superoxide dismutase, SOD) and hydrogen peroxide (glutathione peroxidase, GSH Perox). The hydroxyl radical (HO·) is a highly reactive molecule that may react with lipids, proteins, and nucleic acids. Although originally thought to arise through the direct reaction of peroxide and superoxide, it appears that the only likely source of the hydroxyl radical is through the metal-catalyzed Fenton reaction. In addition, the autoxidation of catecholamines generates the semiquinone and the catechomaine-derived quinone, which is a strong electrophile and reacts with available sulfhydryls.

Hydroxydopamine and Catecholamine Toxicity

The progressive loss of catecholaminergic neurons that occurs with age has been postulated to derive from the toxicity of the oxidation products of catecholamines as well as from the products of the partial reduction of oxygen. The oxidation of catecholamines by monoamine oxidase (MAO) yields H_2O_2, a known cytotoxic metabolite. The autoxidation of catecholamines, especially dopamine, results in the production of catecholamine-derived quinones as well as superoxide anion ($O_2^{-·}$), H_2O_2 from $O_2^{-·}$ dismutation, and OH⁻ from the Fenton reaction (Figure 13–3) (Cohen and Heikkila, 1977). The cell's content of glutathione affords protection from the flux of quinones, glutathione peroxidase from H_2O_2, and superoxide dismutase from

$O_2^{-·}$. Among the naturally occurring catecholamines, dopamine is the most cytotoxic, because of both its greater ease of autoxidation and the greater reactivity of its orthoquinone oxidation product (Graham *et al.*, 1978).

The analog of dopamine, 6-hydroxydopamine, is extremely potent in leading to a chemical sympathectomy. This compound fails to cross the blood-brain barrier, so its site of action is limited to the periphery. In addition, it does not cross into peripheral nerve and, in fact, gains access to nerves only at their terminals. Here, where 6-hydroxydopamine has access to many nerve terminals, it is actively transported into those neurons that have an uptake mechanism for the structurally similar catecholamines. These are, of course, the sympathetic terminals. The uptake of 6-hydroxydopamine results in an injury to sympathetic neurons due to an oxidative process of this catecholamine analog similar to that of dopamine (Figure 13–3). The result is a selective destruction of sympathetic innervation (Malmfors, 1971). The sympathetic fibers degenerate, resulting in an uncompensated parasympathetic tone, with a slowing of the heart rate and hypermotility of the gastrointestinal system. It is noteworthy that neurobiologists employ 6-hydroxydopamine to destroy specific groups of catecholaminergic neurons. Using stereotaxic injections, 6-hydroxydopamine is delivered to a particular anatomic site. If injected into the caudate nucleus, which is rich in dopaminergic synapses, neurite degeneration follows, but if injected into the *substantia nigra*, then the cell bodies of the dopamine neurons are destroyed (Marshall *et al.*, 1983).

MPTP

The illicit drug trade has injured thousands of individuals, perhaps among the most dramatic of those injuries were to those people who thought they were injecting themselves with a meperidine derivative, or "synthetic heroin." However, because of a chemist's error, they also received a contaminant, 1-methyl-4-phenyl-1,2,3,6-tetrahydropyridine (MPTP). Over hours to days, dozens of these patients developed the signs and symptoms of irreversible Parkinson's disease (Langston and Irwin, 1986), some becoming almost immobile with rigidity.

It is not only surprising that a compound like MPTP is neurotoxic, but it is equally surprising

that MPTP is a substrate for the B isozyme of monoamine oxidase (MAO-B). It appears that MPTP, an uncharged species at physiological pH, easily crosses the blood-brain barrier and diffuses into cells, including astrocytes. The MAO-B of astrocytes catalyzes the two electron oxidation to yield the corresponding dihydropyridinium ion, $MPDP^+$ (Trevor *et al.*, 1987). A further two-electron oxidation yields the pyridinium ion, MPP^+ (Figure 13–4). MPP^+ enters dopaminergic neurons of the *substantia nigra* via the dopamine uptake system resulting in injury or death of the neuron. Noradrenergic neurons of the *locus ceruleus* are also vulnerable to repeated exposures of MPTP (Langston and Irwin, 1986), although they are less affected by single exposures than the dopaminergic neurons. Once within the dopaminergic neuron, MPP^+ exerts its direct toxic effect as a general cellular poison, a process that may be related to the inhibition of oxidative phosphorylation (Singer *et al.*, 1988). In fact, the general toxicity of MPP^+ itself is great when administered to animals, although systemic exposure to MPP^+ does not result in neurotoxicity because it does not cross the blood-brain barrier.

The symptomatology reflects the unusual selectivity of this neurotoxicant for the neurons of the *substantia nigra*. Experimental animals and humans show the effects of the selective loss of neurons in the *substantia nigra*, the condition of Parkinsonism (Kopin, 1988). Masked facies,

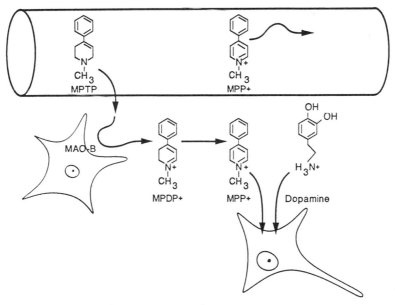

Figure 13–4. Diagram of MPTP toxicity. MPP^+, either formed elsewhere in the body following exposure to MPTP or injected directly, is unable to cross the blood-brain barrier. In contrast, MPTP gains access and is oxidized *in situ* to $MPDP^+$ and MPP^+. The same transport system that carries dopamine into the dopaminergic neurons also transports the cytotoxic MPP^+.

difficulties in initiating and terminating movements, resting "pill-rolling" tremors, rigidity, and bradykinesias are all features of Parkinson's disease, and of MPTP neurotoxicity.

Several issues remain to be resolved, including the exact molecular mechanism of MPP^+ toxicity, and why mice and especially rats are so much less sensitive than monkeys or humans. In addition, it has been observed recently that individuals who were exposed to insufficient MPTP to result in immediate Parkinsonism, are, years later, developing early signs of the disease (Calne *et al.*, 1985). This observation presents a frightening specter that the onset of a neurotoxicologic disease may follow toxic exposure by many years. It does not seem likely that an early sublethal injury to dopaminergic neurons later becomes lethal. Rather, smaller exposures to MPTP may cause a decrement in the population of neurons within the *substantia nigra*. Such a loss would most likely be silent because the symptoms of Parkinson's disease do not develop until approximately 80 percent of the *substantia nigra* neurons are lost. Then, in these prediposed individuals, the neurologic picture of Parkinson's disease develops at an earlier age as a further loss of catecholaminergic neurons occurs during the process of aging.

AXONOPATHIES

The neurotoxic disorders termed "axonopathies" are those in which the primary site of toxicity is the axon itself. The axon degenerates, and with it, the myelin surrounding that axon; however, the neuron cell body remains intact (Figure 13–2). John Cavanagh coined the term "dying back neuropathy" as a synonym for axonopathy (Cavanagh, 1964). The concept of "dying back" postulated that the focus of toxicity was the neuronal cell body itself and that the distal axon degenerated progressively from the synapse, back toward the cell body with increasing injury. It now appears that, in the best studied axonopathies, a different pathogenetic sequence occurs; the toxicant results in a "chemical transection" of the axon at some point along its length, and the axon distal to the transection, biologically separated from its cell body, degenerates.

Because longer axons have more targets for toxic damage than shorter axons, one would predict that longer axons would be more affected in toxic axonopathies. Indeed, such is the case. The involvement of long axons of the CNS, such as ascending sensory axons in the posterior columns or descending motor axons, along with long sensory and motor axons of the PNS, prompted Spencer and Schaumburg (1976) to suggest that the toxic axonopathies in which the distal axon was most vulnerable be called "central peripheral distal axonopathies," which, though cumbersome, accurately depicts the pathologic sequence.

A critical difference exists in the significance of axonal degeneration in the CNS compared to that in the PNS: peripheral axons can regenerate, whereas central axons cannot. Thus, partial recovery, complete in mild cases, can occur after axonal degeneration in the PNS, whereas the same event in the CNS is irreversible.

Axonopathies, then, can be considered to result from a chemical transection of the axon. The number of axonal toxicants is staggering (Table 13–2); however, they may be viewed as a group, all of which result in the pathologic loss of axons with the survival of the cell body. Because the axonopathies pathologically resemble the actual physical transection of the axon, axonal transport appears to be a likely target in many of the toxic axonopathies. Furthermore, as these axons degenerate, the result is most often the clinical condition of peripheral neuropathy in which sensations and motor strength are first impaired in the most distal extent of the axonal processes, the feet and hands. With time and with continued injury, the deficit progresses to involve more proximal areas of the body and the long axons of the spinal cord. The potential for regeneration is great when the insult is limited to peripheral nerves and may be complete in axonopathies in which the initiating event can be determined and removed.

Table 13–2. COMPOUNDS ASSOCIATED WITH AXONAL INJURY

Acrylamide	3,3'-Iminodipropionitrile
Amiodarone	Isoniazid
Amytriptiline	Lead
p-Bromophenylacetylurea	Leptophos
Carbon disulfide	Lithium
Chlordecane	Methyl n-butyl ketone
Colchicine	Metronidazole
Dapsone	Misonidazole
Dichlorophenoxyacetate	Nitrofurantoin
Dimethylaminopropionitrile	Perhexilene
	Platinum
Disulfiram	Polybrominated biphenyls
EPN (O-ethyl-O-4-nitrophenyl phenylphosphonothioate)	Polychlorinated biphenyls
	Pyridinethione
	Taxol
Ethylene oxide	Trichloroethylene
Glutethimide	Tri-ortho-cresyl phosphate (TOCP)
Gold	Vincristine
Hexane	
Hydralazine	

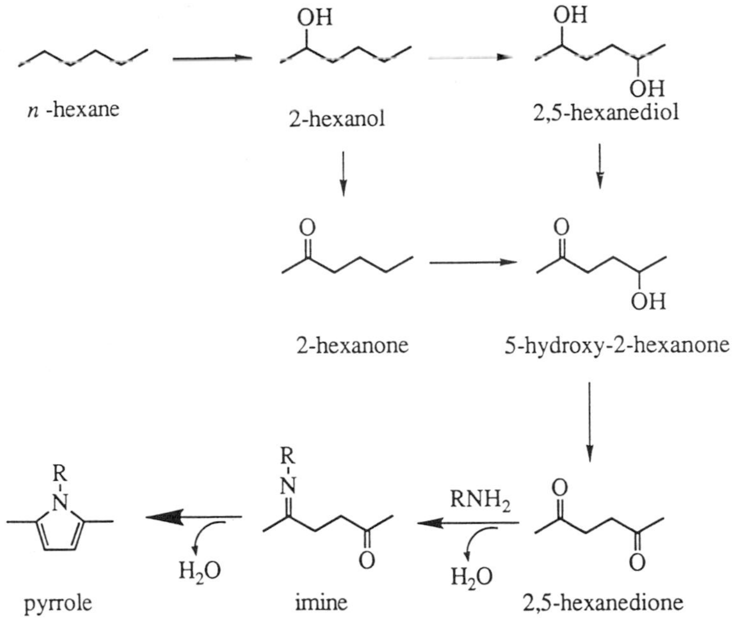

Figure 13–5. Metabolism of hexane. Both *n*-hexane and 2-hexanone (methyl *n*-butyl ketone) are neurotoxic, and both are activated through ω-1 oxidation to the ultimate toxic metabolite, 2,5-hexanedione. The toxicity of γ-diketones derives from the ability of these diketones to react with protein amino groups (RNH$_2$) to form an imine in an initial reversible step, and then to cyclize irreversibly to form a pyrrole.

γ-Diketones

Since the late 1960s and early 1970s, it has been appreciated that humans develop a progressive sensorimotor distal axonopathy when they are exposed to high concentrations of the simple alkane, *n*-hexane, day after day in work settings (Yamamura, 1969), or after repeated intentional inhalation of hexane-containing glues. This axonopathy can be reproduced in its entirety in rats and larger species after weeks to months of exposure to *n*-hexane or its oxidative metabolites (Spencer *et al.*, 1980).

The observation in a fabric printing plant in Ohio (Allen *et al.*, 1980) that methyl *n*-butyl ketone (2-hexanone) resulted in an identical neuropathy to that caused by *n*-hexane prompted elucidation of the metabolism of these two six-carbon compounds (Figure 13–5). The ω-1 oxidation of the carbon chain results ultimately in the γ-diketone, 2,5-hexanedione (HD). That HD is the ultimate toxic metabolite of both *n*-hexane and methyl *n*-butyl ketone is shown by the fact that other γ-diketones or γ-diketone precursors are similarly neurotoxic, while α- and β-diketones are not (Krasavage *et al.*, 1980).

The elucidation of the pathogenetic mechanism of γ-diketone neuropathy has come from an understanding of the biology of the axon and the chemistry of γ-diketone reactivity. The γ-diketones react with amino groups in all tissues to form pyrroles. That pyrrole formation is an actual step in the pathogenesis of this axonopathy has been established by two observations. First, 3,3-dimethyl-2,5-hexanedione, which cannot form a pyrrole, is not neurotoxic (Sayre *et al.*, 1986). Second, the *d,l*-diastereomer of 3,4-dimethyl-2,5-hexanedione (DMHD) both forms pyrroles faster than *meso*-DMHD, and is more neurotoxic than *meso*-DMHD (Genter *et al.*, 1987).

While proteins everywhere, including hemoglobin, are derivatized by γ-diketones, the cytoskeleton of the axon, and especially the neurofilament, are very stable proteins, making it the toxicologically significant target in γ-diketone intoxication. The cellular changes are identical in rats and humans: the development of neurofilament aggregates in the distal, subterminal axon, which, as they grow larger, form massive swellings of the axon, often just proximal to nodes of Ranvier. The neurofilament-filled axonal swellings result in marked distortions of nodal anatomy, including the retraction of paranodal myelin. Following labeling of neurofilament proteins with radioactive amino precursors, the neurofilament transport appears to be abnormal in the γ-diketone model, although results have shown both an acceleration and a slowing of transport depending on the particular diketone (Griffin *et al.*, 1984; Monaco *et al.*, 1989). With continued intoxication, swellings are seen more proximally, and there is degeneration of the distal axon along with its myelin. Long axons in the CNS also develop neurofilament-filled swellings distally, but axonal degeneration is seen much less often.

There are two unusual attributes of the neurofilament that may lead to its vulnerability to the γ-diketones. The three subunits, having molecular weights of 70, 160, and 200 kDa, are assembled in the perikaryon, into a filament which appears to be stable. Second, the neurofilament is the slowest moving component of axoplasm, transported at 1 mm/day (Baitinger *et al.*, 1982). Thus, with chronic γ-diketone intoxication, there is likely to be progressive pyrrole derivatization down the length of the axon. If this reaction results in covalent cross-linking of neurofilaments, as discussed below, this may present obstructions to the proximo-distal transport of growing masses of neuro-filaments.

Hexane neuropathy is one of the best understood of the toxic neuropathies, and much of this understanding has stemmed from controversy over whether pyrrole formation alone is the injury (an arylation reaction), or whether subsequent oxidation of pyrroles leading to covalent protein cross-linking is a necessary step (Graham *et al.*, 1982; DeCaprio *et al.*, 1983; Sayre *et al.*, 1985). The question was recently addressed again in experiments with a novel γ-

diketone, 3-acetyl-2,5-hexanedione (AcHD) (St. Clair *et al.*, 1988). AcHD results in very rapid pyrrole formation both *in vitro* and *in vivo*. However, the electron-withdrawing acetyl group renders the resulting pyrrole essentially inert, so that it does not undergo oxidation. Despite massive pyrrole derivatization, AcHD results in neither clinical nor morphologic evidence of neurotoxicity. Thus, pyrrole derivatization is not sufficient to produce the neurofilamentous swellings; pyrrole oxidation, followed by nucleophilic attack and neurofilament cross-linking seem to be necessary for the neurotoxicity.

The pathologic processes of neurofilament accumulation and degeneration of the axon are followed by the emergence of a clinical peripheral neuropathy. Experimental animals become progressively weak, beginning in the hindlimbs. With continued exposure, the axonopathy may progress, leading to successive weakness in more proximal muscle groups. This is precisely the sequence of events in humans as well, and the initial stocking-and-glove distribution of sensory loss progresses to involve more proximal sensory and motor axons.

IDPN

β,β'-Iminodipropionitrile (IDPN) is a bifunctional nitrile that, in addition to a bizarre "waltzing syndrome" that has defied explanation, results in massive neurofilament-filled swellings (Griffin and Price, 1980) of the proximal, instead of the distal, axon (Figure 13–6). Whether

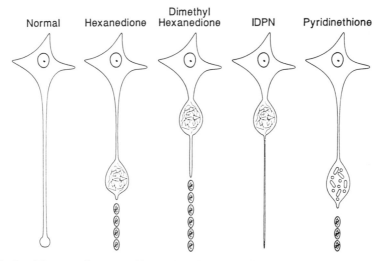

Figure 13–6. Diagram of axonopathies. While 2,5-hexanedione results in the accumulation of neurofilaments in the distal regions of the axon, 3,4-dimethyl-2,5-hexanedione results in identical accumulation within more proximal segments. These proximal neurofilamentous swellings are quite similar to those that occur in the toxicity of β,β'-iminodipropionitrile (IDPN), although the distal axon does not degenerate in IDPN axonopathy, but becomes atrophic. Pyridinethione results in axonal swellings that are distended with tubulovesicular material, followed by distal axonal degeneration.

these bifunctional groups undergo bioactivation to generate a bifunctional cross-linking reagent is unknown, but the similarity to the neurofilamentous neurotoxicity of the γ-diketones is a striking feature of this model neurotoxicant.

Understanding of the similarities of the γ-diketones and IDPN was extended when the potency of the γ-diketones was increased through molecular modeling. DMHD (3,4-dimethyl-2,5-hexanedione) is an analog of 2,5-hexanedione that accelerates the rates of both pyrrole formation and oxidation of the pyrrole. DMHD is 20 to 30 times more potent as a neurotoxicant, and, in addition, the neurofilament-filled swellings occur in the proximal axon (Anthony et al., 1983a), as in IDPN intoxication. In these models of proximal neurofilamentous axonopathies, there is a block of neurofilament transport down the axon; thus, in this situation, the accumulation of neurofilaments results from block of the slow component A of axonal transport (Griffin et al., 1978, 1984). Decreasing the rate of intoxication with DMHD changes the location of the swellings to more distal locations, suggesting that the neurofilamentous axonopathies have a common mechanism and that the position of the neurofilamentous swellings along the axon reflects the rate at which this process occurs (Anthony et al., 1983b).

An important difference is seen between the two proximal neurofilamentous axonopathies caused by IDPN and DMHD, however. After DMHD intoxication, animals become progressively paralyzed in all four limbs, corresponding with marked degeneration of the axon distal to the swellings. By contrast, the axon distal to IDPN-induced swellings undergoes atrophy, not degeneration, and the animal does not experience the same muscle weakness or paralysis. This observation suggests not only that axonal degeneration is required before muscle weakness develops, but also that the presence of neurofilamentous aggregates in the proximal axon is not incompatible with the survival of the distal axon.

Carbon Disulfide

The most significant exposures of humans to CS$_2$ have occurred in the vulcan rubber and viscose rayon industries. Manic psychoses were observed in the former setting and were correlated with very high levels of exposure (Seppäläinen and Haltia, 1980). In recent decades, interest in the human health effects has been focused on the nervous system and the cardiovascular system, where injury has been documented in workers exposed to much higher levels than those that are allowed today.

What is clearly established is the capacity of CS$_2$ to cause a distal axonopathy that is identical pathologically to that caused by 2,5-hexanedione. Indeed, at a molecular level, the sequence of events begins with the initial derivatization of lysyl residues to form a dithiocarbamate (Lam and DeStefano, 1986). The subsequent molecular events have not been fully resolved, but recent evidence suggests that CS$_2$ may also be a protein cross-linking agent (Amarnath et al., 1991).

The clinical effects of exposure to CS$_2$ in the chronic setting are quite similar to those of hexane exposure, with the development of sensory and motor symptoms occurring initially in a stocking-and-glove distribution. In addition to this chronic axonopathy, CS$_2$ can also lead to aberrations in mood and signs of diffuse encephalopathic disease. Some of these occur transiently at first and subsequently become more long lasting, a feature that is common in vascular insufficiency in the nervous system. This fact, in combination with the knowledge that CS$_2$ may accelerate the process of atherosclerosis, suggests that some of the effects of CS$_2$ on the CNS are vascular in origin.

Organophosphorus Esters

Many toxicologists and most physicians who practice in rural areas are aware of the acute cholinergic poisoning induced by certain organophosphorus esters. These compounds, which are used as pesticides and as additives in plastics and petroleum products, inhibit acetylcholinesterase and create a cholinergic excess. However, as tens of thousands of humans could attest, tri-ortho-cresyl phosphate (TOCP) may also cause a severe central peripheral distal axonopathy without inducing cholinergic poisoning. An epidemic of massive proportion occurred during Prohibition in the United States, when a popular drink (Ginger Jake) was contaminated with TOCP (Kidd and Langworthy, 1933). Another outbreak occurred in Morocco when olive oil was adulterated with TOCP. Humans cases of paralysis have also occurred after exposure to the herbicides and cotton defoliants, EPN (O-ethyl O-4-nitrophenyl phenylphosphonothioate) and leptophos [O-(4-bromo-2,5-dichlorophenyl) O-methyl phenylphosphonothioate] (Abou-Donia and Lapadula, 1990).

The hydrophobic organophosphorus compounds readily enter the nervous system, where they alkylate or phosphorylate macromolecules and lead to neurotoxicity which is delayed in its onset. There are probably multiple targets for attack by organophosphorus esters, but which is critically related to axonal degeneration is not clear. Not all of the organophosphorus esters that inhibit acetylcholinesterase lead to a delayed neurotoxicity. While these "nontoxic" organophosphorus esters inhibit most of the esterase activity of the nervous system, there is another esterase activity, or "neurotoxic esterase," that is inhibited by the neurotoxic organophosphorus esters. Furthermore, there is a good correlation between the potency of a given organophosphorus ester as an axonal toxicant and its potency as an inhibitor of this "neurotoxic esterase." Neither the normal function for this enzyme activity nor its relation to axonal degeneration is understood (Davis and Richardson, 1980; Johnson, 1982).

The degeneration of axons does not commence immediately after acute organophosphorus ester exposure, but is delayed for seven to ten days between the acute high-dose exposure and the clinical signs of axonopathy. The axonal lesion in the PNS appears to be readily repaired, and the peripheral nerve becomes refractory to degeneration after repeated doses (Abou-Donia and Graham, 1978). By contrast, axonal degeneration in the long tracks of the spinal cord is progressive, resulting in a clinical picture that may resemble multiple sclerosis.

Pyridinethione

Zinc pyridinethione has antibacterial and antifungal properties and is a component of shampoos that are effective in the treatment of seborrhea and dandruff. Because the compound is directly applied to the human scalp, it caused some concern when it was discovered that zinc pyridinethione is neurotoxic in rodents. Rats, rabbits, and guinea pigs all develop a distal axonopathy when zinc pyridinethione is a contaminant of their food (Sahenk and Mendell, 1979). Fortunately, however, zinc pyridinethione does not penetrate skin well, and it has not resulted in human injury to date.

Although the zinc ion is an important element of the therapeutic action of the compound, only the pyridinethione moiety is absorbed following ingestion, with the majority of zinc eliminated in the feces. In addition, sodium pyridinethione is also neurotoxic, establishing that it is the pyridinethione that is responsible for the neurotoxicity (Collum and Winek, 1967). Pyridinethione chelates metal ions, and, once oxidized to the disulfide, may lead to the formation of mixed disulfides with proteins. However, which of these properties, if either, is the molecular mechanism of its neurotoxicity remains unknown.

Although these molecular issues remain to be resolved, pyridinethione appears to interfere with the fast axonal transport systems. While the fast anterograde system is less affected, pyridinethione impairs the turnaround of rapidly transported vesicles, and slows the retrograde transport of vesicles (Sahenk and Mendell, 1980). This aberration of the fast axonal transport systems is the most likely physiologic basis of the accumulation of tubular and vesicular structures in the distal axon (Figure 13–6). As these materials accumulate in one region of the axon, they distend the axonal diameter, resulting in axonal swellings filled with tubulovesicular profiles. As in many other distal axonopathies, the axon degenerates in its more distal regions beyond the accumulated structures. Ultimately, the functional consequence of the axonal degeneration in this exposure is similar to that of other axonopathies—a peripheral neuropathy.

Microtubule-Associated Neurotoxicity

The role of microtubules in axonal transport and in the maintenance of axonal viability is still being elucidated; however, the biochemistry and toxicity of several alkaloids isolated from plants have greatly aided the understanding of these processes. The first of these historically are the vinca alkaloids and colchicine which bind to tubulin and inhibit the association of this protein subunit to form microtubules. Vincristine, one of the vinca alkaloids, has found clinical use in the treatment of leukemia due to the antimitotic activity of its microtubule-directed action. Colchicine, on the other hand, is used primarily in the treatment of gout. Both of these microtubule inhibitors have also been the cause of peripheral neuropathies in patients (Casey et al., 1973).

Much more recently, another plant alkaloid, taxol, has been described that has quite a different interaction with microtubules. Taxol binds to tubules when they are assembled, and stabilizes the polymerized form of tubules so that they remain assembled even in the cold or in the presence of calcium, conditions under which microtubules normally dissociate into tubulin subunits (Schiff and Horwitz, 1981). Taxol has also found its way into clinical usage as a treatment of certain cancers and has resulted in an axonopathy in patients receiving large doses of this compound (Lipton et al., 1989).

It is fascinating that both the depolymerization of tubules by colchicine and the vinca alkaloids and the stabilization of tubules by taxol lead to an axonopathy. It has been known for some time that microtubules are in a state of dynamic equilibrium in vitro, with tubules existing in equilibrium with dissociated subunits. This process almost certainly occurs in vivo as well, even as tubulin migrates down the axon. Thus, the tubules are constantly associating and dissociating. It is within this dynamic equilibrium that taxol and the vinca alkaloids exert their toxic

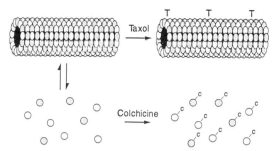

Figure 13–7. Neurotoxicants directed toward microtubules. Colchicine leads to the depolymerization of microtubules by binding to the tubulin monomers and preventing their association into tubules. Taxol stabilizes the microtubules, preventing their dissociation into subunits under conditions in which they would normally dissociate. Both compounds interfere with the normal dynamic equilibrium that exists between tubulin and microtubules, and both are neurotoxic.

effects, preventing the interchange of the two pools of tubulin (Figure 13–7).

The morphology of the axon is, of course, quite different in the two situations. In the case of colchicine, the axon appears to undergo atrophy, and there are fewer microtubules within the axons. In contrast, following exposure to taxol, microtubules are present in great numbers and are aggregated to create interesting arrays of microtubules (Roytta et al., 1984; Roytta and Raine, 1986). Both, however, probably interfere with the process of fast axonal transport, although this has not yet been demonstrated definitively with taxol. In both situations, the resultant clinical condition is a peripheral neuropathy.

MYELINOPATHIES

Myelin provides the electrical insulation of neuronal processes, and its absence leads to a slowing of conduction and aberrant conduction of impulses between adjacent processes, socalled "ephaptic transmission" (Rasminsky, 1980; Delio, et al., 1987). Toxicants exist that result in the separation of the myelin lamellae, termed intramyelinic edema, and in the selective loss of myelin, termed demyelination (Figure 13–2). Early in its evolution, intramyelinic edema is reversible, but this process may progress to segmental demyelination. Segmental demyelination may also result from direct toxicity to the myelinating cell. After segmental demyelination, remyelination of naked internodes by Schwann cells is often seen in the PNS, whereas remyelination in the CNS occurs to only a limited extent. Interestingly, remyelination after segmental demyelination in peripheral nerve

Table 13–3.   COMPOUNDS ASSOCIATED WITH INJURY OF MYELIN

Acetylethyltetramethyltetralin(AETT)	Hexachlorophene
	Isoniazid
Cuprizone	Lysolethicin
Cyanate	Tellurium
Dichloroacetate	Triethyltin
Ethidium bromide	

involves multiple Schwann cells and results, therefore, in internodal lengths (the distances between nodes of Ranvier) that are much shorter than normal and a permanent record of the demyelinating event.

The compounds in Table 13–3 each lead to a myelinopathy. Some of these compounds have created problems in humans, and many have been used as tools to explore the process of myelination of the nervous system and the process of remyelination following toxic disruption of myelin. In general terms, the functional consequences of demyelination depend on the extent of the demyelination and whether it is localized within the CNS, the PNS, or is more diffuse in its effects. Those toxic myelinopathies in which the disruption of myelin is diffuse generate a global neurologic deficit, whereas those that are limited to the PNS produce the symptoms of peripheral neuropathy.

Hexachlorophene

Hexachlorophene, or methylene 2,2'-methylenebis(3,4,6-trichlorophenol), resulted in human neurotoxicity when newborn infants, particularly premature infants, were bathed with the compound to avoid staphylococcal infections (Mullick, 1973). Following skin absorption of this hydrophobic compound, hexachlorophene enters the nervous system and results in intramyelinic edema, splitting the intraperiod line of myelin in both the CNS and the PNS. Experimental studies with erythrocyte membranes show that hexachlorophene binds tightly to cell membranes, resulting in the loss of ion gradients across the membrane (Flores and Buhler, 1974). It may be that hexachlorophene results in loss of the ability to exclude ions from between the layers of myelin, and that with ion entry comes water as well. Another, perhaps related, effect is the uncoupling of mitochondrial oxidative phosphorylation by hexachlorophene (Cammer and Moore, 1974) since this process is dependent on a proton gradient.

Early on, the intramyelinic edema is reversible, but with increasing exposure, hexachlorophene causes segmental demyelination, and the addition of water and ions to the myelin adds to the volume of the brain. The swelling of the brain causes increased intracranial pressure which may be fatal in and of itself. With high-dose exposure, axonal degeneration is seen, along with degeneration of photoreceptors in the retina. It has been postulated that the pressure from severe intramyelinic edema may also injure the axon leading to axonal degeneration, and endoneurial pressure measurements support this idea (Myers *et al.*, 1982). The toxicity of hexachlorophene expresses itself functionally in diffuse terms that reflect the diffuse process of myelin injury. Humans exposed acutely to hexachlorophene may have generalized weakness, confusion, and seizures. Progression may occur to include coma and death.

Tellurium

Although human cases have not been reported, neurotoxicity of tellurium has been demonstrated in animals. Young rats exposed to tellurium in their diet develop a severe peripheral neuropathy. Within the first two days of beginning a diet containing tellurium, the synthesis of myelin lipids in Schwann cells displays some striking changes (Harry *et al.*, 1989). There is a decreased synthesis of cholesterol and the cerebrosides, lipids richly represented in myelin, whereas the synthesis of phosphatidylcholine, a more ubiquitous membrane lipid, is unaffected. The synthesis of free fatty acids and cholesterol esters increases to some degree, and there is a marked elevation of squalene, a precursor of cholesterol. These biochemical findings demonstrate that there are a variety of lipid abnormalities, and the simultaneous increase in squalene and decrease in cholesterol suggest that tellurium or one of its derivatives may interfere with the normal conversion of squalene to cholesterol.

At the same time as these biochemical changes are occurring, lipids are accumulating in Schwann cells within intracytoplasmic vacuoles, and shortly afterwards, these Schwann cells lose their ability to maintain myelin. Axons and the myelin of the CNS are impervious to the effects of tellurium. However, individual Schwann cells in the PNS disassemble their concentric layers of myelin membranes, depriving the adjacent intact axon of its electrically insulated status. Not all Schwann cells are equally affected by the process, but rather those Schwann cells that encompass the greatest distances appear to be the most affected. These cells are associated with the largest diameter axons, and encompass the longest intervals of myelination and provide the thickest layers of myelin. Thus, it appears that these vulnerable cells are those with the largest volume of myelin to support (Bouldin *et al.*, 1988).

As the process of remyelination begins, several cells cooperate to reproduce the myelin layers that were previously formed by a single Schwann cell. Perhaps this diminished demand placed upon an individual cell is the reason that remyelination occurs even in the presence of continued exposure to tellurium (Bouldin *et al.*, 1988). As the cellular and biochemical events are limited, so the expression of the impairment is of short duration. The animals initially develop severe weakness in the hindlimbs, but then recover their strength after two weeks on the tellurium-laden diet.

Lead

Lead exposure in animals results in a peripheral neuropathy with prominent segmental demyelination, a process that bears a strong resemblance to tellurium toxicity (Dyck *et al.*, 1977). However, the neurotoxicity of lead is much more variable in humans than in rats and is asssociated with a variety of manifestations of toxicity in other organ systems.

That lead is toxic to the nervous system has been appreciated for centuries. In current times, adults are exposed to lead in occupational settings through lead smelting processes and soldering, and in domestic settings through lead pipes or through the consumption of "moonshine" contaminated with lead. In addition, even in the absence of definable exposures, some areas contain higher levels of environmental lead resulting in higher blood levels in the inhabitants. Children, especially those younger than five, have higher blood levels of lead than adults in the same environments, due to mouthing objects and the consumption of substances other than food. The most common acute exposure in children, however, is through the consumption of paint chips containing lead pigments (Perlstein and Attala, 1966).

In young children, acute massive exposures result in severe cerebral edema, perhaps from damage to endothelial cells. Children seem to be more susceptible to this lead encephalopathy than adults; however, adults may also develop an acute encephalopathy in the setting of massive lead exposure.

Chronic lead intoxication in adults results in peripheral neuropathy that is often accompanied by manifestations outside the nervous system, such as gastritis, colicky abdominal pain, anemia, and the deposition of lead in particular regions creating lead lines in the gums and in the epiphyses of long bones in children. The effects of lead in the peripheral nerve of humans is not entirely understood. Electrophysiological studies have demonstrated a slowing of nerve conduction (Buchthal and Behse, 1979). While this observation is consistent with the segmental demyelination that develops in experimental animals, pathologic studies in humans with lead neuropathy typically have demonstrated an axonopathy (Buchthal and Behse, 1979). Another curious finding in humans is the predominant involvement of motor axons, creating one of the few clinical situations in which patients present with a predominantly motor neuropathy.

Although the manifestations of acute and chronic exposures to lead have been long established, it is only in recent years that the concept has emerged that extremely low levels of exposure to lead in "asymptomatic" children may have an effect on their intellectual functions. Initial reports noted a relationship beween mild elevations of blood lead in children and school performance, and more recently the relationship between elevated lead levels in decidual teeth and performance on tests of verbal abilities, attention, and behavior (nonadaptive) (Needleman and Gatsonis, 1990). Although there is a clear association between lead level and intellectual performance, there has been some controversy as to whether lead is causal. The children with higher blood levels tend to share certain other environmental factors, such as socioeconomic status and parental educational level. The complex human situations have made it difficult to be completely certain about the role of lead in intellectual abilities in children, but the association between lead exposure and brain dysfunction is certainly of concern, and has received some support in animal models (Gilbert and Rice, 1987).

NEUROTRANSMISSION-ASSOCIATED TOXICITY

Many neurotoxicants destroy cellular structures within the nervous system providing anatomic footprints of their toxicity. In some instances, however, dysfunction of the nervous system may occur without overt evidence of altered cellular structures: rather, the neurotoxicity expresses itself in terms of altered behavior or impaired performance on neurologic tests. In fact, many of the neurotoxic agents that lead to anatomic evidence of cellular injury were first demonstrated to be neurotoxic through the detection of neurologic dysfunction.

Molecular mechanisms are not understood for many of these agents; however, there is a group of such compounds in which the chemical basis of their action is clear. These are the toxicants that impair the process of neurotransmission. A wide variety of naturally occurring toxins, as well as synthetic drugs, interact with specific mechanisms of intercellular communication. At times, interruption of neurotransmission is beneficial to an individual, and the subject becomes one of neuropharmacology. Yet, excessive exposure, or inappropriate exposure may be viewed as one of the patterns of neurotoxicology.

This group of compounds may interrupt the transmission of impulses, block or accentuate transsynaptic communication, or interfere with second-messenger systems. In general, the acute effects of these compounds are directly related to the immediate concentration of the compound at the active site, which bears a direct relationship to the level of the drug in the blood. The structural similarity of many compounds with similar actions has led to the recognition of specific categories of drugs and toxins. For example, some mimic the process of neurotransmission of the sympathetic nervous system, and are termed the sympathomimetic compounds. As the targets of these drugs are located throughout the body, the responses are not localized; however, the responses are stereotyped in that each member of a class tends to have similar biologic effects. In terms of toxicity, most of the side effects of these drugs may be viewed as short-term interactions that are easily reversible with time, or that may be counteracted by the use of appropriate antagonists. However, some of the toxicity associated with long-term use may be irreversible and is of considerable concern. For example, phenothiazines, which have been used to treat chronic schizophrenia for long periods to time, may lead to the condition of tardive dyskinesia in which the patient is left with a permanent disability of prominent facial grimaces (DeVeaugh-Geiss, 1982). Both reversible acute high dose toxicity and sustained effects following chronic exposure are common features of the agents which interact with the process of neurotransmission.

Nicotine

Widely available in tobacco products and in certain pesticides, nicotine has diverse pharmacologic actions and may be the source of considerable toxicity. These toxic effects range from acute poisoning to much more chronic effects. Nicotine exerts its effects by binding to a subset of cholinergic receptors, the nicotinic receptors. These receptors are located in ganglia, at the neuromuscular junction, and also within the central nervous system where the psychoactive and addictive properties most likely reside. Smoking and "pharmacologic" doses of nicotine accelerate heart rate, elevate blood pressure, and constrict blood vessels within the skin. Because the majority of these effects may be prevented by the administration of α- and β-adrenergic blockade, these consequences may be viewed as the result of stimulation of the ganglionic sympathetic nervous system (Benowitz, 1986). At the same time, nicotine leads to a sensation of "relaxation", and is associated with alterations of electroencephalographic (EEG) recordings in humans. These effects are probably related to the binding of nicotine with nicotinic receptors within the CNS, and the EEG changes may be blocked with an antagonist, mecamylamine.

Acute overdose of nicotine has occurred in children who accidentally ingest tobacco products, in tobacco workers exposed to wet tobacco leaves (Gehlbach *et al.,* 1974), or workers exposed to nicotine-containing pesticides. In each of these settings, the rapid rise in circulating levels of nicotine leads to excessive stimulation of nicotinic receptors, a process that is folowed rapidly by ganglionic paralysis. Initial nausea, rapid heart rate, and perspiration are followed shortly by marked slowing of heart rate with a fall in blood pressure. Somnolence and confusion may occur, followed by coma; death, when it occurs, is often the result of paralysis of the muscles of respiration.

Such acute poisoning with nicotine is, fortunately, uncommon. Exposure to lower levels for longer duration, in contrast, is quite common and the health effects of this exposure are of considerable epidemiologic concern. In humans, however, it has been impossible so far to separate the effects of nicotine from those of other components of cigarette smoke. The complications of smoking include cardiovascular disease, cancers (especially malignancies of the lung), chronic pulmonary disease, and attention deficit disorders in children of women who smoke during pregnancy. Nicotine may be a factor in some of these problems. For example, an increased propensity for platelets to aggregate is seen in smokers and this platelet abnormality correlates with the level of nicotine. Furthermore, nicotine places an increased burden on the heart through its acceleration of heart rate and blood pressure, suggesting that nicotine may play a role in the onset of myocardial ischemia (Benowitz, 1986).

It seems more clear that chronic exposure to nicotine has effects on the developing fetus. Along with decreased birth weights, attention deficit disorders are more common in children whose mothers smoke cigarettes during pregnancy, and nicotine has been shown to lead to analogous neurobehavioral abnormalities in animals exposed prenatally to nicotine (Lichensteiger *et al.,* 1988). Nicotinic receptors are expressed early in the development of the nervous system, beginning in the developing brainstem and later expressed in the diencephalon. The role of these nicotinic receptors during development is unclear; however, it is quite possible that the interaction of nicotine with its receptors in the CNS during the prenatal period is the basis of subsequent attention disorders in young animals and children.

Cocaine

Cocaine differs from nicotine in the eyes of the law, a feature of the compound that affects the willingness of users to discuss their patterns of use. Nonetheless, it has been possible to obtain estimates of the number of users. In 1972, approximately 9 million college-age adults were using the drug; in 1982, approximately 33 million (Fishburne *et al.,* 1983), a staggering number even prior to the epidemic use of smokable cocaine, or "crack."

Cocaine blocks the reuptake of catecholamines at nerve terminals, and its entry into the CNS across the blood-brain barrier allows a central effect that accounts for the euphoric sensation and the addictive properties. Acute toxicity due to excesive intake, or overdose, may result in unanticipated deaths. While these tragic accounts in celebrities may attract media attention, it is the chronic "recreational" consumption of cocaine that is of greatest epidemiologic concern. Perhaps the most alarming of these, considering the young populations who use cocaine, is the potential for cocaine-induced effects on the fetus.

Although cocaine increases maternal blood pressure during acute exposure, in pregnant animals, the blood flow to the uterus actually diminishes. Depending on the level of the drug in the mother, the fetus may develop marked hypoxia as a result of the diminished uterine blood flow (Woods *et al.,* 1987). In a study of women who used cocaine during pregnancy, there were more miscarriages and placental hemorrhages (abruptions) than in drug-free women (Chasnoff *et al.,* 1985). In addition, the newborn infants of cocaine users were less interactive than normal newborns and exhibited a poor response to stimuli in the environment (Chasnoff *et al.,* 1985). Although it is possible that this represents an expression of intoxication in the newborn, a more alarming possibility is that these observations reflect the consequences of cocaine-induced fetal hypoxia *in utero.* The answers to these questions may emerge in the future as the full impact of the "crack" epidemic is felt.

Excitatory Amino Acids

Glutamate and certain other acidic amino acids are excitatory neurotransmitters within the CNS. The discovery that these excitatory amino acids are neurotoxic at concentrations that are low relative to their concentrations in the brain has generated a great amount of interest in these "excitotoxins." *In vitro* systems have established that the toxicity of glutamate can be blocked by certain glutamate antagonists (Rothman and Olney, 1986), and the concept is rapidly emerging that the toxicity of excitatory amino acids may be related to such divergent conditions as hypoxia, epilepsy, and neurodegenerative diseases (Meldrum, 1987; Choi, 1988).

Glutamate neurotransmission is mediated by at least three subtypes of receptors that may be recognized by their specificity for kainate, quisqualate, and N-methyl-D-aspartate (NMDA). The entry of glutamate into the CNS is regulated at the blood-brain barrier, and following an injection of a large dose of glutamate in infant rodents, glutamate exerts its effects in the area of the brain in which the blood-brain barrier is least developed, the circumventricular organ. Within this site of limited access, glutamate injures neurons, apparently by opening glutamate-dependent ion channels, ultimately leading to neuronal swelling and neuronal cell death (Olney, 1978; Coyle, 1987). The toxicity affects the dendrites and neuronal cell bodies, but seems to spare axons. The only known related human condition is the "Chinese restaurant syndrome," in which consumption of large amounts of monosodium glutamate as a seasoning may lead to a burning sensation in the face, neck, and chest.

The cyclic glutamate analog kainate was initially isolated from a seaweed in Japan as the active component of this herbal treatment of ascariasis. Kainate is extremely potent as an excitotoxin, being 100-fold more toxic than glutamate and is selective at a molecular level for the kainate receptor (Coyle, 1987). Like glutamate, kainate selectively injures dendrites and neurons, and shows no substantial effect on glia or axons. As a result, this compound has found great use in neurobiology as a tool (McGeer et al., 1978). Injected into a region of the brain, kainate can destory the neurons of that area without disrupting all of the fibers that pass through the same region (Coyle, 1987). Neurobiologists, as a result of this neurotoxic tool, are able to study the role of neurons in a particular area independent of the axonal injuries that occur when similar lesioning experiments are performed by mechanical cutting.

Recently there has been renewed interest in the possibility that another excitotoxin, α-amino-β-methylaminopropionic acid (or β-N-methyl-amino-L-alanine, BMAA), present in the seeds of *Cycas circinalis,* is responsible for the neuronal degenerative disease amyotrophic lateral sclerosis-parkinsonism-dementia (ALS/PD) complex, which developed in the 1940s and 1950s in the Chamorro population of Guam. Kurland proposed that Guamanian ALS/PD was due to a component of the diet, and evulations of the diet at that time suggested the disorder may be related to the cycad (Kurland, 1963). However, acute exposures of rats to the cycad failed to reveal a neurodegenerative disorder, and the topic was not studied further until recently.

With the intervening years, however, several epidemiologic facts provide support that ALS/PD of Guam may be due to an environmental agent. First, the incidence of ALS/PD has decreased substantially, a finding compatible with an environmental factor. Second, ALS/PD of Guam has occurred in immigrants to Guam who adopted the lifestyle of the Chamorros (Garruto et al., 1981). Initial attempts to identify an environmental agent focused on heavy metals, and attention was drawn to concentrations of aluminum in Guam and in the brains of patients dying of ALS/PD (Rodgers-Johnson et al., 1986). However, if aluminum plays a role in this disease, it is not likely to be the only factor because the manifestations and pathologic features are quite different than "dialysis dementia" which appears to have a clear relationship to excessive exposure to aluminum in dialysis fluid (Elliott et al., 1978).

On the other hand, a toxicity associated with the cycad, or specifically with BMAA as an excitatory amino acid peculiar to the cycad, is attractive in explaining the regional and temporal distributions of ALS/PD on Guam. During World War II, the cycad was used as a source of food by the Chamorros, and it has long been suspected that this disease may be a delayed-onset of cycad-related toxicity. BMAA has been isolated from the cycad, and is excitotoxic producing seizures in animals. The toxicity of BMAA is similar to that of glutamate *in vitro,* and can be blocked by certain glutamate antagonists (Nunn et al., 1987). Studies *in vivo,* however, have not yet demonstrated a clear etiologic relationship between BMAA and ALS/PD. To date, the only evidence in whole animals that BMAA may be related to the disorder is the finding of motor symptoms in macaques exposed to BMAA in their diet (Spencer et al., 1987; Hugon et al., 1988). It therefore remains to be resolved what role BMAA and cycad consumption play in developing Guamanian ALS/PD; however, it seems quite likely that the disorder is due to an environmental agent and may be considered a form of neurotoxicity.

The growing field of the excitotoxic amino acids embodies many of the same attributes that characterize the more general discipline of neurotoxicology. Neurotoxicology is generally viewed as the study of compounds that are deleterious to the nervous system, and from this mold emerges the effects of glutamate and kainate. Exposure to these excitotoxic amino acids leads to neuronal injury, and when of sufficient degree, may kill neurons. However, the implications of these findings, as with the entire field of neurotoxicology, extend beyond the direct toxicity of the compounds in exposed populations. With kainate, as with many other neurotoxic compounds, has come a tool for the neurobiologist who seeks to explore the anatomy and function of the nervous system. Kainate, through its selective action on neuronal cell bodies, has provided a greater understanding of the functions of cells within a specific region of the brain while previous lesioning techniques addressed only regional functionalities. Finally, the questions surrounding BMAA, the cycad, aluminum, and Guamanian ALS/PD serve to remind the student of neurotoxicology that the causes of many neurologic diseases remain unknown. This void in understanding, and the implication that some neurodegenerative diseases may have toxic etiologies, provide a heightened desire to appreciate more fully the effects of elements of our environment on the nervous system.

REFERENCES

Abel, E. L.; Jacobsen, S.; and Sherwin, B. J.: *In utero* ethanol exposure: functional and structural brain damage. *Neurobehav. Toxicol. Teratol.*, **5**:139–146, 1983.

Abou-Donia, M. B., and Graham, D. G.: Delayed neurotoxicity of *O*-ethyl *O*-4-nitrophenyl phenylphosphonothioate: subchronic (90 days) oral administration in hens. *Toxicol. Appl. Pharmacol.*, **45**:685–700, 1978.

Abou-Donia, M. B., and Lapadula, D. M.: Mechanisms of organophosphorus ester-induced delayed neurotoxicity: Type I and Type II. *Annu. Rev. Pharmacol. Toxicol.*, **30**:405–440, 1990.

Allen, N.; Mendell, J. R.; Billmaier, J.; Fontaine, R. E.; and O'Neill, J.: Toxic polyneuropathy due to methyl *n*-butyl ketone: an industrial outlook. *Arch. Neurol.*, **32**:209–222, 1980.

Amarnath, V.; Anthony, D. C.; Valentine, W. M.; and Graham, D. G.: The mechanism of the carbon disulfide mediated crosslinking of proteins. *Chem. Res. Toxicol.*, in press.

Anthony, D. C.; Boekelheide, K.; Anderson, C. W.; and Graham, D. G.: The effect of 3,4-dimethyl substitution on the neurotoxicity of 2,5-hexanedione. II. Dimethyl substitution accelerates pyrrole formation and protein crosslinking. *Toxicol. Appl. Pharmacol.*, **71**:372–382, 1983a.

Anthony, D. C.; Boekelheide, K.; and Graham, D. G.: The effect of 3,4-dimethyl substitution on the neurotoxicity of 2,5-hexanedione. I. Accelerated clinical neuropathy is accompanied by more proximal swellings. *Toxicol. Appl. Pharmacol.*, **71**:362–371, 1983b.

Baitinger, C.; Levine, J.; Lorenz, T.; Simon, C.; Skene, P.; and Willard, M.: Characteristics of axonally transported proteins. In Weiss, D. G. (ed.): *Axoplasmic Transport*. Springer-Verlag, Berlin, 1982, pp. 110–120.

Bakir, F.; Damluji, S. F.; Amin-Zaki, L.; Murtadha, M.; Khalidi, A.; Al-Rawi, N. Y.; Tikriti, S.; Dhahir, H. I.; Clarkson, T. W.; Smith, J. C.; and Doherty, R. A.: Methylmercury poisoning in Iraq. *Science*, **181**:230–241, 1973.

Beauchamp, R. O., Jr.; Bus, J. S.; Boreiko, C. J.; and Andjelkovich, D. A.: A critical review of the literature on hydrogen sulfide toxicity. *CRC Crit. Rev. Toxicol.*, **13**:25–97, 1984.

Benowitz, N. L.: Clinical pharmacology of nicotine. *Annu. Rev. Med.*, **37**:21–32, 1986.

Bouldin, T. W.; Gaines, N. D.; Bagnell, C. R.; and Krigman, M. R.: Pathogenesis of trimethyltin neuronal toxicity. *Am. J. Pathol.*, **104**:237–249, 1981.

Bouldin, T. W.; Samsa, G.; Earnhardt, T. S.; and Krigman, M. R.: Schwann cell vulnerability to demyelination is associated with internodal length in tellurium neuropathy. *J. Neuropathol. Exp. Neurol.*, **47**:41–47, 1988.

Brady, S. T., and Lasek, R. J.: The slow components of axonal transport: movements, compositions and organization. In Weiss, D. G. (ed.): *Axoplasmic Transport*. Springer-Verlag, Berlin, 1982, pp. 206–217.

Braun, P. E.: Molecular architecture of myelin. In Morell, P. (ed.): *Myelin*. Plenum Press, New York, 1977, pp. 91–115.

Braun, P. E.; Pereyra, P. M.; and Greenfield, S.: Myelin organization and development: a biochemical perspective. In Hashim, G. A. (ed.): *Myelin: Chemistry and Biology*. Alan R. Liss, New York, 1980, pp. 1–17.

Brierley, J. B., and Graham, D. I.: Hypoxia and vascular disorders of the central nervous system. In Adams, J. H.; Corsellis, J. A. N.; and Duchen, L. W. (eds.): *Greenfield's Neuropathology*, 4th ed. John Wiley & Sons, New York, 1984, pp. 125–156.

Brightman, M. W.: The anatomic basis of the blood-brain barrier. In Neuwelt, E. A. (ed.): *Implications of the Blood-Brain Barrier and Its Manipulation*, Vol. 1. Plenum Press, New York, 1989, pp. 53–83.

Buchthal, F., and Behse, F.: Electrophysiology and nerve biopsy in men exposed to lead. *Br. J. Ind. Med.*, **36**:135–147, 1979.

Calne, D. B.; Langston, J. W.; Martin, W. R. W.; Stoeessl, A. J.; Adam, M. J.; Pate, B. D.; and Schulzer, M: Positron emission tomography after MPTP: observations relating to the cause of Parkinson's disease. *Nature*, **317**:246–248, 1985.

Cammer, W., and Moore, C. L.: The effect of hexachlorophene on the respiration of brain and liver mitochondria. *Biochem. Biophys. Res. Commun.*, **46**:1887–1894, 1974.

Carpenter, M. B., and Sutin, J: *Human Neuroanatomy*, 8th ed. Williams & Wilkins, Baltimore, 1983, pp. 85–133.

Casey, E. B.; Jeliffe, A. M.; LeQuesne, P. M.; and Millett, Y. L.: Vincristine neuropathy: clinical and electrophysiological observations. *Brain*, **96**:69–86, 1973.

Cavanagh, J. B.: The significance of the "dying-back" process in experimental and human neurological disease. *Int. Nat. Rev. Exp. Pathol.*, **7**:219–267, 1964.

Cavanagh, J. B.: Towards the molecular basis of toxic neuropathies. In Galli, C. L.; Manzo, L.; and Spencer, P. S. (eds.): *Recent Advances in Nervous System Toxicology*. Plenum Press, New York, pp. 23–42, 1984.

Chasnoff, I. J.; Burns, W. J.; Schnoll, S. H.; and Burns, K. A.: Cocaine use in pregnancy. *N. Engl. J. Med.*, **313**:666–669, 1985.

Cheung, M. K., and Verity, M. A.: Experimental

methyl mercury neurotoxicity: locus of mercurial inhibition of brain protein synthesis *in vivo* and *in vitro*. *J. Neurochem.*, **44**:1799–1808, 1985.

Cho, E. S.: Toxic effects of adriamycin on the ganglia of the peripheral nervous system: a neuropathological study. *J. Neuropathol. Exp. Neurol.*, **36**:907–915, 1977.

Cho, E. S.; Spencer, P. S.; Jortner, B. S.; and Schaumberg, H. H.: A single intravenous injection of doxorubicin (adriamycin) induces sensory neuropathy in rats. *Neurotoxicology*, **1**:583–590, 1980.

Choi, D. W.: Glutumate neurotoxicity and diseases of the nervous system. *Neuron*, **1**:623–634, 1988.

Cohen, G., and Heikkila, R. E.: *In vivo* scavenging of superoxide radicals by catecholamines. In Michelson, A. M., McCord, J. M.; and Fridovich, I. (eds.): *Superoxide and Superoxide Dismutases*. Academic Press, London, 1977, pp. 351–365.

Collum, W. D., and Winek, C. L.: Percutaneous toxicity of pyridinethiones in a dimethylsulfoxide vehicle. *J. Pharm. Sci.*, **56**:1673–1675, 1967.

Coyle, J. T.: Kainic acid: insights into excitatory mechanisms causing selective neuronal degeneration. In Bock, G., and O'Connor, M. (eds.): *Selective Neuronal Death*. John Wiley, New York, 1987, pp. 186–203.

Davis, C. S., and Richardson, R. J.: Organophosphorus compounds. In Spencer, P. S., and Schaumburg, H. H. (eds.): *Experimental and Clinical Neurotoxicology*. Williams & Wilkins, Baltimore, 1980, pp. 527–544.

Davson, H.: History of the blood-brain barrier concept. In Neuwelt, E. A. (ed.): *Implications of the Blood-Brain Barrier and Its Manipulation*, Vol. 1. Plenum Press, New York, 1989, pp. 27–52.

DeCaprio, A. P.; Strominger, N. L.; and Weber, P.: Neurotoxicity and protein binding of 2,5-hexanedione in the hen. *Toxicol. Appl. Pharmacol.* **68**:297–307, 1983.

Delio, D. A.; Gold, B. G.; and Lowndes, H. E.: Crosstalk between intraspinal elements during progression of IDPN neuropathy. *Toxicol. Appl. Pharmacol.*, **90**:253–260, 1987.

DeVeaugh-Geiss, J.: Tardive dyskinesia: phenomenology, pathophysiology, and pharmacology. In *Tardive Dyskinesia and Related Involuntary Movement Disorders*. John Wright PSG, Boston, 1982, pp. 1–18.

Duncan, I. D.; Hammang, J. P.; and Trapp, B. D.: Abnormal compact myelin in the myelin deficient rat: absence of proteolipid protein correlates with a defect in the intraperiod line. *Proc. Natl. Acad. Sci. USA*, **84**:6287–6291, 1987.

Dyck, P. J.; O'Brien, P. C.; and Ohnisi, A.: Lead neuropathy. 2. Random distribution of segmental demyelination among "old internodes" of myelinated fibers. *J. Neuropathol. Exp. Neurol.*, **36**:570–575, 1977.

Ehrlich, P.: *Das Sauerstoff-Bedurfnis des Organismus. Eine Farbenanalytische Studie*, Berlin, 1885, pp. 69–72.

Elliott, H. L.; Dryburgh, F.; Fell, G. S.; Sabet, S.; and MacDougall, A. I.: Aluminum toxicity during regular haemodialysis. *Br. Med. J.*, **1**:1101–1103, 1978.

Ernsting, J.: Some effects of brief profound anoxia upon the central nervous system. In Schadé, J. P., and McMenemey, W. M. (eds.): *Selective Vulnerability of the Brain in Hypoxemia*. Blackwell Scientific, Oxford, 1963, pp. 41–45.

Fishburne, P. M.; Abelson, H. I.; and Cisin, I.: *National Household Survey on Drug Abuse: National Institute of Drug and Alcohol Abuse Capsules, 1982*. Dept. of Health and Human Services, 1983.

Flores, G., and Buhler, D. R.: Hemolytic properties of hexachlorophene and related chlorinated biphenols. *Biochem. Pharmacol.*, **23**:1835–1843, 1974.

Fowler, B. A., and Woods, J. S.: The transplacental toxicity of methylmercury to fetal rat liver mitochondria. *Lab. Invest.*, **36**:122–130, 1977.

Frenkel, G. D., and Harrington, L.: Inhibition of mitochondrial nucleic acid synthesis by methylmercury. *Biochem. Pharmacol.*, **28**:651–655, 1979.

Garruto, R. M.; Gajdusek, D. C.; and Chen, K.-M.: Amyotrophic lateral sclerosis and parkinsonism-dementia among Filipino migrants to Guam. *Ann. Neurol.*, **10**:341–350, 1981.

Gehlbach, S. H.; Williams, W. A.; Perry, L. D.; and Woodall, J. S.: Green-tobacco sickness: an illness of tobacco harvesters. *JAMA*, **229**:1880–1883, 1974.

Genter, M. B.; Szákal-Quin, Gy.; Anderson, C. W.; Anthony, D. C.; and Graham, D. G.: Evidence that pyrrole formation is a pathogenetic step in γ-diketone neuropathy. *Toxicol. Appl. Pharmacol.*, **87**:351–362, 1987.

Gilbert, S. G., and Rice, D. C.: Low-level lifetime lead exposure produces behavioral toxicity (spatial discrimination reversal) in adult monkeys. *Toxicol. Appl. Pharmacol.*, **91**:484–490, 1987.

Goldberger, M. E., and Murray, M.: Recovery of function and anatomical plasticity after damage to the adult and neonatal spinal cord. In Cotman, C. W. (ed.): *Synaptic Plasticity*. Guilford Press, New York, 1985, pp. 77–110.

Grafstein, B., and Forman, D.: Intracellular transport in neurons. *Physiol. Rev.*, **60**:1167–1218, 1980.

Graham, D. G.; Tiffany, S. M.; Bell, W. R., Jr.; and Gutknecht, W. F.: Autoxidation versus covalent binding of quinones as the mechanism of toxicity of dopamine, 6-hydroxydopamine and related compounds for C1300 neuroblastoma cells *in vitro*. *Mol. Pharmacol.*, **14**:644–653, 1978.

Graham, D. G.; Anthony, D. C.; Boekelheide, K.; Maschmann, N. A.; Richards, R. G.; Wolfram, J. W.; and Shaw, B. R.: Studies of the molecular pathogenesis of hexane neuropathy. II. Evidence that pyrrole derivatization of lysyl residues leads to protein crosslinking. *Toxicol. Appl. Pharmacol.*, **64**:415–422, 1982.

Griffin, J. W., and Price, D. L.: Proximal axonopathies induced by toxic chemicals. In Spencer, P. S., and Schaumburg, H. H. (eds.): *Experimental and Clinical Neurotoxicology*. Williams & Wilkins, Baltimore, 1980, pp. 161–178.

Griffin, J. W.; Hoffman, P. N.; Clark, A. W.; Carroll, P. T.; and Price, D. L.: Slow axonal transport of neurofilament proteins: impairment by β,β'-iminodipropionitrile administration. *Science*, **202**:633–635, 1978.

Griffin, J. W.; Anthony, D. C.; Fahnestock, K. E.; Hoffman, P. N.; and Graham, D. G.: 3,4-Dimethyl-2,5-hexanedione impairs the axonal transport of neurofilament proteins. *J. Neurosci.*, **4**:1516–1526, 1984.

Harry, G. J.; Goodrum, J. F.; Bouldin, T. W.; Wagner-Recio, M.; Toews, A. D.; and Morell, P.: Tellurium-induced neuropathy: metabolic alterations associated with demyelination and remyelination in rat sciatic nerve. *J. Neurochem.*, **52**:938–945, 1989.

Hoffman, P. N., and Lasek, R. J.: The slow component of axonal transport: identification of major structural polypeptides of the axon and their generality among mammalian neurons. *J. Cell Biol.*, **66**:351–366, 1975.

Hugon, J.; Ludolph, A.; Roy, D. N.; Schaumburg, H. H.; and Spencer, P. S.: Studies on the etiology and pathogenesis of motor neuron diseasës. II. Clinical and electrophysiologic features of pyramidal dysfunction in macaques fed *Lathyrus sativus* and IDPN. *Neurology*, **38**:435–442, 1988.

Johnson, K. A.: Pathway of the microtubule-dynein ATPase and the structure of dynein: a comparison with actomyosin. *Annu. Rev. Biophys. Biophys. Chem.,* **14**:161–188, 1985.

Johnson, M. K.: The target for initiation of delayed neurotoxicity by organophosphorus esters: biochemical studies and toxicological applications. In Hodgson, E.; Bend, J. R.; and Philpot, R. M. (eds.): *Reviews in Biochemical Toxicology,* Vol. 4. Elsevier, New York, 1982, pp. 141–212.

Kidd, J. G., and Langworthy, O. R.: Paralysis following the ingestion of Jamaica ginger extract adulterated with tri-*ortho*-cresyl phosphate. *Johns Hopkins Med. J.,* **52**:39–60, 1933.

Kondo, A.; Inoue, T.; Nagara, H.; Tateishi, J.; and Fukui, M.: Neurotoxicity of adriamycin passed through the transiently disrupted blood-brain barrier by mannitol in the rat brain. *Brain Res.,* **412**:73–83, 1987.

Kopin, I. J.: MPTP effects on dopamine neurons. *Ann. NY Acad. Sci.,* **537**:451–461, 1988.

Krasavage, W. J.; O'Donoghue, J. L.; DiVincenzo, G. D.; and Terhaar, C. J.: The relative neurotoxicity of MnBK, *n*-hexane, and their metabolites. *Toxicol. Appl. Pharmacol.,* **52**:433–441, 1980.

Kurland, L. T.: Epidemiological investigations of neurological disorders in the Mariana islands. In Pemberton, J. (ed.): *Epidemiology Reports on Research and Teaching.* Oxford University Press, Oxford and New York, 1963, pp. 219–223.

Kurland, L. T.; Faro, S. N.; and Siedler, J.: Minamata disease. *World Neurol.,* **1**:370–395, 1960.

Lam, G.-W., and DiStefano, V.: Characterization of carbon disulfide binding in blood and to other biological substances. *Toxicol. Appl. Pharmacol.,* **86**:235–242, 1986.

Langston, J. W., and Irwin, I.: MPTP: current concepts and controversies. *Clin. Neuropharmacol.,* **9**:485–507, 1986.

Lichensteiger, W.; Ribary, U.; Schlumpf, M.; Odermatt, B.; and Widmer, R.: Prenatal adverse effects of nicotine on the developing brain. In Boer, G. J.; Feenstra, M. G. P.; Mirmiran, M.; Swaab, D. F.; and Van Haaren, F. (eds.): *Progress in Brain Research,* Vol. 73. Elsevier, Amsterdam, 1988, pp. 137–157.

Lipton, R. B.; Apfel, S. C.; Dutcher, J. P.; Rosenberg, R.; Kaplan, J.; Berger, A.; Einzig, A. I.; Wiernik, P.; and Schaumburg, H. H.: Taxol produces a predominantly sensory neuropathy. *Neurology,* **39**:368–373, 1989.

Lorenz, T., and Willard, M.: Subcellular fractionation of intra-axonally transported polypeptides in the rabbit visual system. *Proc. Natl. Acad. Sci. USA,* **75**:505–509, 1978.

Lucey, J. F.; Hibbard, E.; Behrman, R. E.; Esquivel, F. O.; and Windle, W. F.: Kernicterus in asphyxiated newborn Rhesus monkeys. *Exp. Neurol.,* **9**:43–58, 1964.

Malmfors, T.: The effects of 6-hydroxydopamine on the adrenergic nerves as revealed by fluorescence histochemical method. In Malmfors, T., and Thoenen, H. (eds.): *6-Hydroxydopamine and Catecholaminergic Neurons.* North-Holland, Amsterdam, 1971, pp. 47–58.

Marshall, J. F.; Drew, M. C.; and Neve, K. A.: Recovery of function after mesotelencephalic dopaminergic injury in senescence. *Brain Res.,* **259**:249–260, 1983.

McGeer, E. G., Olney, J. W., and McGeer, P. L. (eds.): *Kainic Acid as a Tool in Neurobiology.* Raven Press, New York, 1978.

Meldrum, B.: Excitatory amino acid antagonists as potential therapeutic agents. In Jenner, P. (ed.): *Neurotoxins and Their Pharmacological Implications.* Raven Press, New York, 1987, pp. 33–53.

Monaco, S.; Jacob, J.; Jenich, H.; Patton, A.; Autilio-

Gambetti, L.; and Gambetti, P.: Axonal transport of neurofilament is accelerated in peripheral nerve during 2,5-hexanedione intoxication. *Brain Res.,* **491**:328–334, 1989.

Mullick, F. G.: Hexachlorophene toxicity: human experience at the AFIP. *Pediatrics,* **51**:395–399, 1973.

Myers, R. R.; Mizisin, A. P.; Powell, H. C.; and Lampert, P. W.: Reduced nerve blood flow in hexachlorophene neuropathy: relationship to elevated endoneurial pressure. *J. Neuropathol. Exp. Neurol.,* **41**:391–399, 1982.

Nave, K.-A.; Lai, C.; Bloom, F. E.; and Milner, R. J.: Jimpy mouse: a 74-base deletion in the mRNA for myelin proteolipid protein and evidence for a primary defect in RNA splicing. *Proc. Natl. Acad. Sci. USA,* **83**:9264–9268, 1986.

Needleman, H. L., and Gatsonis, C. A.: Low-level lead exposure and the IQ of children. A meta-analysis of modern studies. *JAMA,* **263**:673–678, 1990.

Nunn, P. B.; Seelig, M.; Zagoren, J. C.; and Spencer, P. S.: Stereospecific acute neurotoxicity of "uncommon" plant amino acids linked to human motor-system diseases. *Brain Res.,* **410**:375–379, 1987.

Olney, J. W.: Neurotoxicity of excitatory amino acids. In McGeer, E. G.; Olney, J. W.; and McGeer, P. L. (eds.): *Kainic Acid as a Tool in Neurobiology.* Raven Press, New York, 1978, pp. 95–122.

Orlowski, J. P.: Drowning, near-drowning, and ice-water submersions. *Pediatr. Clin. North Am.,* **34**:75–92, 1987.

O'Shea, K. S., and Kaufman, M. H.: The teratogenic effect of acetaldehyde: implications for the study of fetal alcohol syndrome. *J. Anat.,* **128**:65–76, 1979.

Paterson, R. A., and Usher, D. R.: Acute toxicity of methylmercury on glycolytic intermediates and adenine nucleotides in rat brain. *Life Sci.,* **10**:121–128, 1971.

Perlstein, M. A., and Attala, R.: Neurologic sequelae of plumbism in children. *Clin. Pediatr.,* **5**:292–298, 1966.

Plum, F., and Posner, J. B.: Neurobiologic essentials. In Smith, L. H., Jr., and Thier, S. O. (eds.): *Pathophysiology: The Biological Principles of Disease.* W. B. Saunders, Philadelphia, 1985, pp. 1009–1036.

Rasminsky, M.: Ephaptic transmission between single nerve fibers in the spinal nerve roots of dystrophic mice. *J. Physiol. (Lond.),* **305**:151–169, 1980.

Reese, T. S., and Karnovsky, M. J.: Fine structural localization of a blood-brain barrier to exogenous peroxidase. *J. Cell. Biol.,* **34**:207–217, 1967.

Reuhl, K. R., and Chang, L. W.: Effects of methylmercury on the development of the nervous system: a review. *Neurotoxicology,* **1**:21–55, 1979.

Rodgers-Johnson, P.; Garruto, R. M.; Yanagihara, R.; Chen, K.-M.; Gajdusek, D. C.; and Gibbs, C. J.: Amytrophic lateral sclerosis and parkinsonism-dementia on Guam: a 30-year evaluation of clinical and neuropathological trends. *Neurology.* **36**:7–13, 1986.

Rothman, S. M., and Olney, J. M.: Glutamate and the pathophysiology of hypoxic-ischemic brain damage. *Ann. Neurol.,* **19**:105–111, 1986.

Roytta, M., and Raine, C. S.: Taxol-induced neuropathy: chronic effects of local injection. *J. Neurocytol.,* **15**:483–496, 1986.

Roytta, M.; Horwitz, S. B.; and Raine, C. S.: Taxol-induced neuropathy: short-term effects of local injection. *J. Neurocytol.,* **13**:685–701, 1984.

Sahenk, Z., and Mendell, J. R.: Ultrastructural study of zinc pyridinethione-induced peripheral neuropathy. *J. Neuropathol. Exp. Neurol.,* **38**:532–550, 1979.

Sahenk, Z., and Mendell, J. R.: Axoplasmic transport

in zinc pyridinethione neuropathy: evidence for an abnormality in distal turn-around. *Brain Res.*, **186**:343–353, 1980.

Sayre, L. M.; Autilio-Gambetti, L.; and Gambetti, P.: Pathogenesis of experimental giant neurofilamentous axonopathies: a unified hypothesis based on chemical modification of neurofilaments. *Brain Res. Rev.*, **10**:69–83, 1985.

Sayre, L. M.; Shearson, C. M.; Wongmongkolrit, T.; Medori, R.; and Gambetti, P.: Structural basis of γ-diketone neurotoxicity: non-neurotoxicity of 3,3-dimethyl-2,5-hexanedione, a γ-diketone incapable of pyrrole formation. *Toxicol. Appl. Pharmacol.*, **84**:36–44, 1986.

Schiff, P. B., and Horwitz, S. B.: Taxol assembles tubulin in the absence of exogenous guanosine 5'-triphosphate or microtubule-associated proteins. *Biochemistry*, **20**:3242–3252, 1981.

Schnapp, B. J., and Reese, T. S.: Dynein is the motor for retrograde axonal transport of organelles. *Proc. Natl. Acad. Sci. USA*, **86**:1548–1552, 1989.

Schnapp, B. J.; Vale, R. D.; Sheetz, M. P.; and Reese, T. S.: Single microtubules from squid axoplasm support bidirectional movement of organelles. *Cell*, **40**:455–462, 1985.

Seppäläinen, A. M., and Haltia, M.: Carbon disulfide. In Spencer, P. S., and Schaumburg, H. H. (eds.): *Experimental and Clinical Neurotoxicology.* Williams & Wilkins, Baltimore, 1980, pp. 356–373.

Shephard, R. J.: *Carbon Monoxide: The Silent Killer.* Charles C Thomas, Springfield, Illinois, 1983, pp. 68–109.

Shiraki, H.: Neuropathological aspects of organic mercury intoxication, including Minimata disease. In Vinken, P. J., and Bruyn, G. W. (eds.): *Handbook of Clinical Neurology,* Vol. 36. North-Holland, Amsterdam, 1979, pp. 83–145.

Singer, T. P.; Ramsay, R. R.; McKeown, K.; Trevor, A; and Castagnoli, N. E., Jr.: Mechanism of the neurotoxicity of 1-methyl-4-phenylpyridinium (MPP^+), the toxic bioactivation product of 1-methyl-4-phenyl-1,2,-3,6-tetrahydropyridine (MPTP). *Toxicology*, **49**:17–23, 1988.

Snyder, S. H., and D'Amato, R. J.: Predicting Parkinson's disease. *Nature*, **317**:198–199, 1985.

Spencer, P. S., and Schaumburg, H. H.: Central-peripheral distal axonopathy: the pathology of dying-back polyneuropathies. In Zimmerman, H. (ed.): *Progress in Neuropathology,* Vol. 3. Grune & Stratton, New York, 1976, pp. 253–295.

Spencer, P. S.; Schaumburg, H. H.; Sabri, M. I.; and Veronesi, B.: The enlarging view of hexacarbon neurotoxicity. *CRC Crit. Rev. Toxicol.*, **7**:279–356, 1980.

Spencer, P. S.; Nunn, P. B.; Hugon, J.; Ludolph, A. C.; Ross, S. M.; Roy, D. N.; and Robertson, R. C.: Guam amyotrophic lateral sclerosis-parkinsonism-dementia linked to a plant excitant neurotoxin. *Science*, **237**:517–522, 1987.

St. Clair, M. B. G.; Amarnath, V.; Moody, M. A.; Anthony, D. C.; Anderson, C. W.; and Graham, D. G.: Pyrrole oxidation and protein crosslinking are necessary steps in the development of γ-diketone neuropathy. *Chem. Res. Toxicol.*, **1**:179–185, 1988.

Stoltenburg-Didinger, G., and Spohre, H. L.: Fetal alcohol syndrome and mental retardation: spine distribution of pyramidal cells in prenatal alcohol exposed rat cerebral cortex. *Dev. Brain Res.*, **11**:119–123, 1983.

Takeuchi, T.; Morikawa, H.; Matusmoto, H.; Kambara, T.; and Shiraishi, Y.: A pathological study of Minamata disease in Japan. *Acta Neuropathol.*, **2**:40–57, 1962.

Trevor, A. J.; Singer, T. P.; Ramsay, R. R.; and Castagnoli, N. E., Jr.: Processing of MPTP by monoamine oxidases: implications for molecular toxicology. *J. Neural. Transm. (Suppl.)*, **23**:73–89, 1987.

Vale, R. D.; Reese, T. S.; and Sheetz, M. P.: Identification of a novel force-generating protein, kinesin, involved in microtuble-based motility. *Cell*, **42**:39–50, 1985.

Vogel, S. N., and Sultan, T. R.: Cyanide poisoning. *Clin. Toxicol.*, **18**:367–383, 1981.

Woods, J. R.; Plessinger, M. A., and Clark, K. E.: Effect of cocaine on uterine blood flow and fetal oxygenation. *JAMA*, **257**:957–961, 1987.

Yamamura, Y.: *n*-Hexane polyneuropathy. *Folia Psychiatr. Neurol.*, **23**:45–57, 1969.

Chapter 14

TOXIC RESPONSES OF THE HEART AND VASCULAR SYSTEMS

Joseph P. Hanig and Eugene H. Herman

INTRODUCTION

Chemicals can selectively affect the heart or the vasculature. The effect can be solely functional, lasting only during the exposure period, and its magnitude is usually dose related. The risk of irreversibility of the effect increases with the dose or duration of exposure. Generally, after a functional change in the heart, the risk of lethality is greater than that which occurs after changes in other parenchymatous organs. Sudden death due to arrhythmia contributes to a major portion of the mortality caused by a drug overdose. Chemicals can also produce structural—that is, degenerative and inflammatory—changes in the heart or blood vessels, and these in turn may lead to persistent functional changes. A structural change can develop even after a single exposure to drugs, for example, the myocardial necrosis induced by a large dose of β-adrenergic agonist drugs.

Cardiovascular functional effects develop after administration of a lethal dose of most chemicals and are usually secondary to the changes in other organ systems. Primary cardiovascular toxicity is the most common consequence of an exaggerated pharmacologic effect after an overdose of cardiovascular drugs. Similarly, other organotropic drugs, for example, those affecting the central nervous system (CNS) or the autonomic nervous system, may also affect the cardiovascular system; their toxicity can be unrelated to the therapeutic action and thus is a side effect.

Although cardiovascular diseases (hypertension, atherosclerosis, etc.) are the most prevalent chronic diseases of humans in industrialized societies today, the role of low-level chronic exposure to chemicals in the etiology of these conditions is unknown. A few chemicals such as lead, cadmium, and oral contraceptive steroids have been associated with the development of chronic cardiovascular disease in humans.

The mechanisms of selective, direct cardiovascular toxicity involve perturbations in membrane functions, particularly in ion transport and in the contractile or energy-supplying systems. Because of the great sensitivity of the heart to hypoxia and changes in acid-base balance and electrolytes, alterations via an effect of the chemical on other organs can indirectly lead to cardiovascular effects. It is conceivable that some of these conditions might play a role in the pathogenesis of insidiously developing cardiovascular diseases. For example, carbon monoxide reduces the amount of oxygen available to the heart, and tachycardia and electrocardiographic (ECG) changes suggestive of hypoxia can be the first sign of acute poisoning. Repeated long-term exposure to carbon monoxide can lead to structural damage of the blood vessels, which promotes the development of atherosclerosis. In addition to these toxicologic mechanisms, the immune system is involved in some of the cardiovascular reactions when the chemical acts as a hapten or directly affects the function of the immune system.

OVERVIEW OF CARDIOVASCULAR PATHOPHYSIOLOGIC AND PATHOLOGIC EFFECTS OF CHEMICALS

Cardiac Functions and Disorders

The most important manifestations of cardiac effects arise from alteration of electrical or contractile properties of the heart. Chemicals influence these properties by their actions on heart rate (chronotropic), conductivity (dromotropic), excitability (bathmotropic), or contractility (inotropic).

Arrhythmia. An arrhythmia can be caused by an alteration in the cardiac impulse rate, in

This chapter is dedicated to our colleague Tibor Balazs, D.V.M., in recognition of his outstanding scientific contributions to the discipline of toxicology and his many significant activities as a teacher and mentor.

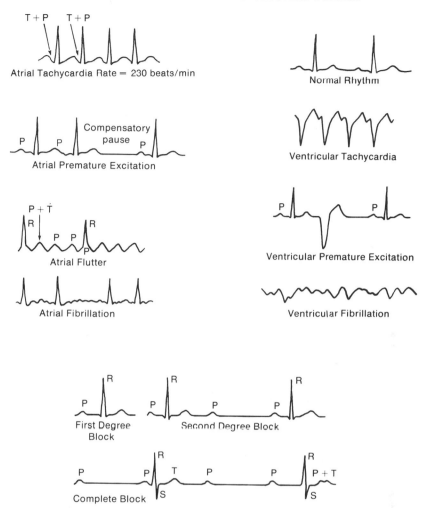

Figure 14–1. Electrocardiographic changes in various arrhythmias. (From Harvey, A. M. *et al.*, (eds.): *The Principles and Practice of Medicine,* 20th ed. Appleton-Century-Crofts, East Norwalk, Conn., 1980.)

the site of origin of the cardiac impulse, or in the velocity of cardiac impulse conduction. Arrhythmias are usually classified on the basis of ECG criteria (Figure 14–1). Some, such as sinus tachycardia or atrioventricular block, clearly result from disturbances of impulse formation or conduction, respectively. Others, such as ectopic beats arising in various parts of the heart, stem from excessive automaticity, from reentry excitation, or from impaired conduction, for example, escape beats.

Disturbances of Impulse Formation. Under normal conditions, impulses originate in the heart by the spontaneous depolarization of specialized cells in the sinoatrial node (SA node). The rate of the depolarization can be altered by changes in autonomic nervous system activity. Increased vagal activity can slow or stop sinus

nodal pacemakers, and increased sympathetic activity causes sinus tachycardia. Augmented automaticity in the His-Purkinje fibers of the cardiac conducting system is a common cause of arrhythmias.

In contrast to normal mechanisms of automaticity, impulses arising from abnormal automatic mechanisms in the diseased or chemically altered heart can originate from atrial or ventricular working muscle cells as well as from the specialized conduction tissue. Normally, the diastolic transmembrane potential of Purkinje fibers and ventricular cardiac cells is close to -90 mV and is largely the result of a potassium ion current in the resting cell. The action potential is initiated primarily by a rapid movement of sodium into the cell (fast current). However, when the diastolic transmembrane potential is

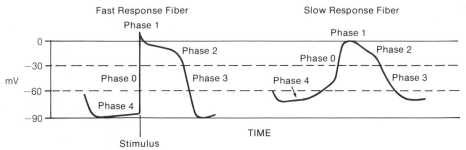

Figure 14–2. Action potential of cells of the cardiac conducting system. After depolarization during phase 0, the cell slowly recovers and is fully repolarized by the end of phase 3. A fast-response fiber is illustrated on the *left,* and a slow-response fiber on the *right.* Although the fast-response fiber may have some spontaneous diastolic depolarization during phase 4, most fibers are stimulated by an outside impulse, usually by propagation of an action potential from an adjacent cell in the conducting system. The slow-response fiber, on the *right,* has a less negative maximum diastolic potential, a slower rate of rise of phase 0, and has distinctly separated phases 1, 2, and 3. Working muscle cells and cells in the conducting system outside the SA and AV nodes have action potentials more similar to the fast-response fibers, with even less spontaneous diastolic depolarization. (From Harvey, A. M. *et al.* (eds.): *The Principles and Practice of Medicine,* 20th ed. Appleton-Century-Crofts, East Norwalk, Conn., 1980.)

reduced (shifted in the direction toward zero), depolarization can be mediated by the transport of other ions, particularly of calcium (slow current). Conditions predisposing to slow responses, such as regional acidosis or hyperkalemia accompanying ischemia, may result in an arrhythmia due to increased automaticity.

Chemicals can directly influence the initiation or propagation of the cardiac electrical impulse by altering the ionic gradients and fluxes that form the basis of these processes. For example, strontium and barium ions carry current through the slow channels in place of calcium ions, an action that initially stimulates the heart. However, they subsequently precipitate arrhythmias (ventricular extrasystoles and tachycardia leading to ventricular fibrillation) followed by cardiac standstill. These effects are thought to be due to impairment of the efflux of potassium ions from cardiac muscle cells.

If the action potential of a cardiac cell fails to return to the resting level along its normal time course so that repolarization is interrupted or delayed, a second action potential may arise (early afterdepolarization). Impulses can also arise by delayed afterdepolarization: in this instance, voltage swings to the resting diastolic level at the end of repolarization. However, rather than the voltage merely returning to the resting level, a secondary depolarization may occur in diastole. Delayed afterdepolarizations can cause either coupled extrasystoles or runs of tachyarrhythmias and can be triggered by premature systoles; by increases in spontaneous rate, calcium concentration, or sympathetic ac-

tivity; and by agents such as the digitalis glycosides (Koch-Weser, 1979; Bigger and Hoffman, 1980).

Disturbances of Impulse Conduction. The two types of electrical activity (fast and slow responses) that have been detected either in anatomically different cardiac tissue or in chemically altered cardiac cells are recognized for their important role in the genesis of arrhythmias (Figure 14–2).

The action potential of fast-response cells is characterized by a large resting potential (-90 mV), a threshold potential of about -70 mV, a rapid influx of Na^+ (phase 0 of the action potential), and a large amplitude, all of which result in rapid conduction. Fast-response cells are located in the working atria and ventricles and in most portions of the conducting system except the SA and AV nodes. The fast-response fibers also possess a second slow inward current, carried by Ca^{2+} ions through separate, specific membrane channels. The slow response develops only when the fast Na^+ depolarizing current has decreased the transmembrane potential to about -55 mV. Sustained depolarization of the membrane to about -60 mV, by abnormal conditions such as increased extracellular K^+ or hypoxia, inactivates the fast Na^+ channel while leaving the slow calcium component functional. The ability of the slow-response action potential to propagate can be enhanced by catecholamines or phosphodiesterase inhibitors. The initiation and conduction of the slow-response action potentials in fibers that are partially depolarized by damage or hypoxia may initiate abnormalities of cardiac rhythm. Quinidine and other antiarrhythmic agents, parodoxically, may provoke rhythm disturbances as a result of an inhibiting effect on the fast inward Na^+ channel, thereby allowing development of slow responses.

In general, the most common site of conduction disturbance is the AV node, but similar disturbances may occur in branches of the bundle of His or in the more peripheral Purkinje network. Agents that cause heart block do so by delaying propagation of electrical impulses in specialized myocardial conducting tissue. The digitalis glycosides increase the refractory period in the AV node and thus decrease impulse conduction velocity.

In certain situations, conduction delay and block paradoxically lead to tachyarrhythmias by the mechanism of reentry. Reentry consists of reexcitation caused by continuous propagation of the same impulse for one or more cycles. If the cardiac impulse enters a potentially reentrant pathway and conducts slowly through depolarized ischemic tissue in a circuitous pathway, it may reach normal myocardium, which has recovered its excitability. The SA and AV nodes are regions in which conduction is normally very slow, and further slowing by premature activation, disease, or certain agents leads to conditions that permit reentry. These factors also can create conditions that permit reentry in cells, such as the Purkinje fibers, that usually conduct cardiac impulses at very rapid rates. In most instances, marked slowing of conduction (the decrease of fast response or development of slow response) is the alteration that permits reentry.

Sensitization to Arrhythmias. The discovery that chloroform appeared to sensitize the heart to the effects of sympathomimetic amines was followed by the observation that a number of compounds, many of which are halogenated hydrocarbons, have the same property (Zakhari and Aviado, 1982; Reynolds, 1983). There are several actions by which the halogenated hydrocarbon chemicals can modify sensitivity of the cardiac pacemaking and conduction system to other agents. These include a marked suppression of SA nodal fibers with pacemaker migration to the AV junctional region and an enhanced propagation of premature beats due to a profound reduction of the refractory period of the Purkinje fibers. Some slowing of ventricular conduction may also contribute to enhanced arrhythmogenic activity by favoring reentry. Cardiac stimulation by catecholamines will result in a predictable sequence of events, regardless of the state of the organism. As the dose is increased, a sinus tachycardia followed by ventricular bigeminy, multifocal premature ventricular contractions, ventricular tachycardia, and finally ventricular

fibrillation is a typical sequence. These effects will occur at lower doses when the heart has been exposed to halogenated hydrocarbon substances.

The increased myocardial sensitivity to the arrhythmogenic action of cardiac glycosides after potassium depletion by agents acting on the kidney is also well known. Digitalis glycosides produce a variety of cardiac arrhythmias by causing alterations in impulse formation, impulse conduction, or both. The cardiac arrhythmias that occur as part of digitalis toxicity appear to be due to an extension of the alteration of membrane Na^+-K^+-ATPase activity. Digitalis glycosides and extracellular K^+ have competitive affinities for Na^+-K^+-ATPase. K^+ may simultaneously stimulate enzyme activity and decrease the binding of glycosides to the ATPase. Cardiac glycosides will inhibit the exchange mechanism, resulting in a loss of intracellular K^+ and an increase in intracellular Na^+ concentration. A decrease in extracellular K^+ would enhance the inhibitory effect of the glycosides on the (Na^+-K^+-ATPase) system, allowing additional Na^+ to enter the cell. Under these conditions, the magnitude of the membrane potential would approach the threshold for initiation of diastolic depolarization. This type of interaction can lead to severe arrhythmias, for example, ventricular fibrillation (Deglin *et al.*, 1977; Bigger and Hoffman, 1980; Bowman and Rand, 1980).

Cardiac Contraction. Cardiac contraction is initiated by depolarization of the cardiac cell membrane, the sarcolemma (Figure 14–3). Immediately after the sudden surge of sodium into the cell, an equally rapid decrease in Na^+ membrane permeability toward the resting level occurs. In many mammals (e.g., humans, monkeys, dogs) the membrane remains depolarized at a relatively stable plateau before repolarization proceeds. The prolonged plateau phase of the action potential is due to a combination of a decrease in K^+ conductance and the activation of slow inward Ca^{2+} and Na^+ currents. Termination of the plateau phase and repolarization of the membrane follows as the conductance increases. As a consequence of these and other intracellular ionic events, there is an increase in the intracellular free Ca^{2+} concentration obtained both from extracellular sources and by release of calcium stores loosely bound to sarcolemmal cisterns. The free calcium combines with one of the modulating myocardial proteins, troponin C, to alter the conformation of the troponin complex, releasing its inhibition on the myosin-ATPase contractile mechanism and thereby resulting in contraction. Relaxation follows as a result of active calcium uptake by the sarcoplasmic reticulum and possibly the

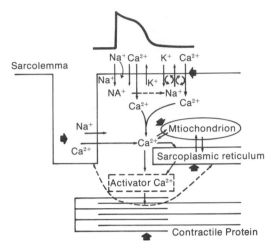

Figure 14-3. Schematic representation of organelles and molecular events of excitation-contraction coupling in the cardiac cell. *Large shaded arrows* indicate sites within the cardiac cell (sarcolemma, sarcoplasmic recticulum, mitochondria, and contractile proteins), where various agents, discussed in the text, may act to alter cardiac function and induce toxicity. (Reprinted with permission from Brody, T. M., and Chubb, J. M. In Balazs, T.(ed.): *Cardiac Toxicology,* Vol. 1. Copyright 1981. CRC Press, Inc., Boca Raton, Fla.)

sarcolemma and mitochondria (Bowman and Rand, 1980; Braunwald *et al.,* 1980a).

Effects of Chemicals on the Force of Contraction. Myocardial contraction is enhanced by an increase in availability of Ca^{2+} ions inside the cell. Catecholamines act through receptors located on the myocardial cell membrane that activate the adenyl cyclase system. The resulting increase in cyclic AMP ultimately affects membrane systems within the cells that deliver Ca^{2+} ions to the contractile proteins. Contraction is also increased to some degree by corticosteroids, angiotensin, serotonin, and glucagon. Myocardial contraction is decreased by hypoxia, by acidosis, and by many chemicals.

A decrease in force of contraction leading to acute heart failure may develop after an acute myocardial infarction or exposure to cardiodepressant substances. Certain conditions or substances (e.g., ethanol, haloalkanes, and cobalt) can also cause myocardial function to deteriorate slowly over many months or years. In this instance, cardiac output gradually becomes inadequate, and the overt signs of congestive heart failure develop.

Impaired cardiac contraction can result from interference with the autonomic nervous system control of the heart, from a decrease in cardiac energetics (availability of substrates for fuel, oxygen extraction, metabolic processes for energy production and/or utilization of energy), or from an alteration in the process of excitation contraction coupling.

Autonomic nervous system impulses reaching the heart result in the release of the neurochemical transmitters norepinephrine or acetylcholine. Sympathetic stimulation gives rise to an increased force of contraction. In contrast, interference with the release of norepinephrine attenuates sympathetic drive on the heart and decreases myocardial contractility.

Parasympathetic stimulation leads to a decrease in heart rate and force of contraction in the atria. Despite limited vagal innervation and muscarinic receptors in the ventricular muscle, vagal impulses or acetylcholine can also produce a negative inotropic effect in the ventricles of the intact heart.

Agents that interfere with the process of energy liberation and/or storage depress myocardial contractility (Merin, 1978; Van Stee, 1982). The energy contained in carbon-carbon and carbon-hydrogen bonds of substrates transported to the myocardial cells by blood in the coronary vascular bed is fundamental to the metabolic process. Cardiac muscle has the highest rate of oxygen consumption and the largest fractional extraction of arterial oxygen of any tissue. Oxygen availability becomes limited when coronary flow is reduced. When the coronary blood flow or oxygen extraction does not keep up with the demand, myocardial metabolism and function are disrupted.

Heart muscle can utilize energy from numerous fuel sources (Figure 14–4). Free fatty acids, ketone bodies, triglycerides, lactate, pyruvate, and glucose can all be extracted from the blood by the heart if the arterial concentrations are great enough. The energy available during oxidation of these substrates is conserved during oxidative phosphorylation and generation of adenosine triphosphate (ATP). Heart muscle obtains energy for contraction through hydrolysis of ATP. The heart stores this energy as both ATP and creatine phosphate (CP). CP is converted to ATP by reaction with adenosine diphosphate (ADP) under the influence of the enzyme creatine phosphokinase (CPK). Likely sites for chemical interference with energy metabolism would be the rate-limiting steps in the tricarboxylic acid cycle, electron transport systems, oxidative phosphorylation, and intracellular energy transport.

Energy utilization involves the conversion of chemical energy into mechanical energy and into the energy necessary to drive ion pumps. Calcium ions provide a vital link in energy utilization. Catecholamines, by increasing cyclic AMP

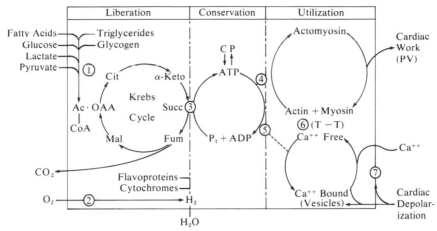

Figure 14–4.   Schema of energetics in cardiac muscle. (From Olson, R. E.; Dhalla, N. S.; and Sun, C. N.: Changes in energy stores in the hypoxic heart. *Cardiology,* **56**:114–124, 1971/72. Reprinted with permission of S. Karger AG, Basel.)

levels, regulate intracellular Ca^{2+} movements such as the entrance of Ca^{2+} during the cardiac action potential, the uptake of calcium into the sarcoplasmic reticulum, and phosphorylation of tropin. β-Adrenergic receptor blocking agents inhibit these actions and exert a negative inotropic effect. Interference with Ca^{2+} ion kinetics has been implicated as a locus of action of a number of substances that depress contractility (Braunwald, 1980; Braunwald *et al.,* 1980a, 1980b).

Chemicals can alter cardiac function by affecting any of the steps involved in the excitation-contraction coupling process (Brody and Chubb, 1981; Schlant and Sonnenblick, 1982).

Disturbances in the permeability of the cell membrane to ions or alterations in the activity of membrane-bound enzyme can change the shape and/or duration of the action potential and may influence myocardial contractile strength. Tetraethylammonium significantly alters the shape of the action potential and decreases the force of contraction by altering membrane potassium conductance. Inhibition of the cell membrane transport of calcium is yet another means by which drugs and chemicals can alter cardiac contractility and potentially cause cardiac toxicity. Verapamil blocks the slow inward calcium current, an action that decreases the concentration of intracellular calcium, and thus less calcium is available to interact with the contractile proteins and, as a result, contractile activity decreases. Alterations in membrane-bound enzyme activity can also affect cardiac function. For example, the ATP-dependent sodium pump (Na^+-K^+-ATPase), which maintains the normal transcellular gradient of Na^+ and K^+, is extremely sensitive to the cardiac glycosides, which inhibit its activity.

The smooth sarcoplasmic reticulum (SR) is involved in modulating calcium flux within the cell. The enzyme Ca^{2+}-Mg^{2+}-ATPase is embedded within the SR membrane. Experimental evidence indicates that this enzyme (the "calcium pump") causes accumulation of intracellular free Ca^{2+} to an extent sufficient to effect complete relaxation of the myocardial muscles. The SR is also thought to release bound Ca^{2+} upon excitation of the muscle to effect contraction. Quinidine is known to have a depressant effect on cardiac contractility. *In vitro* studies, in which calcium uptake by partially purified SR vesicles was determined, indicated that quinidine exerted a dose-dependent inhibitory effect on this process. Thus, the mechanism by which quinidine inhibits calcium uptake may be mediated by a direct inhibitory effect on the SR "calcium pump."

Mitochondria have also been implicated as regulators of the cytosolic Ca^{2+} concentration. Drugs and chemicals that decrease the rate or extent of Ca^{2+} accumulation by the mitochondria may disrupt heart function. Lead concentrations at one-tenth of that required to inhibit heart mitochondrial oxidative phosphorylation significantly decreased the rate and extent of Ca^{2+} accumulation by mitochondria. If a significant impairment in mitochondrial Ca^{2+} accumulation occurs and if other organelles involved in the modulation of intracellular Ca^{2+} cannot remove the excess Ca^{2+}, cardiac structural alterations result.

The force that the muscle develops and the shortening that occurs are the result of the interaction of several protein molecules that make up the myofibrils of the myocardial cells. Myofibrils are divided into sarcomeres, which are composed of the proteins actin and myosin. Contraction occurs as a result of crossbridge formation between the actin and myosin molecules and subsequent lateral movement of the two proteins relative to each other. In order for crossbridges of the contractile proteins to form and lead to shortening or to force development, chemical energy must be supplied to the system in the form of ATP. ATPase activity is associated with the myosin protein, and the activity of this ATPase correlates with the ability of myosin to bind actin. Agents that alter the activity of myosin ATPase could conceivably affect cardiac performance. For example, the general anesthetic halothane depresses contractility, and this effect is mediated in part by the inhibition of myosin ATPase activity.

Circulatory Regulation and Disorders

For proper functioning of the cardiovascular system, at least two important parameters must be carefully regulated: mean arterial blood pressure and cardiac output. Mean arterial blood pressure (MABP) is controlled within fairly narrow limits, whereas the cardiac output is regulated to match the work output or oxygen consumption of the organism and thus can vary over a wider range.

The short-term control of MABP is achieved through the arterial baroreceptors in the aortic arch and the carotid sinuses in conjunction with centers in the medulla, which have efferent connections to the heart, and to vascular smooth muscle in the arterioles and venules. The baroreceptors or pressoreceptors are maximally sensitive to arterial pressure changes near the normal range. Elevated arterial pressure increases the firing rate of the baroreceptor nerves and results in decreased output from the sympathetic regions and increased output from the parasympathetic regions of the brain. Decreased sympathetic discharge to the periphery decreases the heart rate and contractility in the heart, decreases arteriolar resistance, and increases venous capacitance. These effects combine to decrease peripheral resistance. A fall in MABP has the opposite effects.

The long-term regulation of MABP is primarily achieved by blood volume regulation and thus requires the integrity of kidney function along with the renin-angiotensin system, antidiuretic hormone, and aldosterone level. Maintenance of the MABP is important, since it is the driving force for blood flow through peripheral organs.

The cardiac output can vary over a five- to sixfold range. This variation is tightly linked to whole-body oxygen consumption. Of equal importance to the absolute level of the cardiac output is the distribution of the cardiac output to the vital organs. Important mechanisms that are responsible for the distribution of the cardiac output include neural control and local regulation. Neural control consists primarily of increasing or decreasing the level of sympathetic discharge to vascular smooth muscle in arterioles. The effects elicited by sympathetic stimulation are specific in each tissue and are largely dependent on the density and proportion of α- and β-adrenergic receptors. Stimulation of α receptors generally elicits vasoconstriction, and stimulation of β receptors usually causes vasodilation. α-Adrenergic agonists increase Ca^{2+} influx via the slow inward current. Cytoplasmic-bound Ca^{2+} activates an enzyme that phosphorylates myosin to interact with actin, leading to contraction of the vascular smooth muscle. β-Adrenergic agonists increase cyclic AMP, which, by activation of protein kinase, enhances the efflux of Ca^{2+} and results in relaxation of the vessel wall. Similarly, manganese, cobalt, and Ca^{2+} antagonists cause relaxation of the vascular smooth muscle.

In contrast to neural control is the local control of blood flow to certain tissues. The heart, brain, and skeletal muscles are very adept at regulating their own flow locally to match the metabolic needs of that particular tissue. The local control of blood flow, called autoregulation, is mediated by products of metabolism, so that increased work is accompanied by increased tissue metabolism along with an increased blood flow. Other organs of the body, such as the gastrointestinal (GI) tract and the skin, are more dependent on neural regulation of their flow and will exhibit an increase in blood flow with decreases in sympathetic discharge. This mechanism subserves GI function during digestion and also the important role of the skin in heat dissipation for temperature regulation.

The changes in cardiac output are the result of altered venous return from the periphery, along with changes in myocardial contractility and rate of contraction. The distribution of blood flow is primarily determined by neural mechanisms from the CNS as modified by local autoregulation in certain tissues. Thus, the cardiac output is generally distributed to organ systems in proportion to their activity, both mechanical and metabolic.

Hypotension, Shock. When cardiac output or the MABP falls to critically low levels, the perfusion of vital organs is reduced. Hypotension, a sustained reduction of systemic arterial pressure, is common in acute poisoning, for example, with CNS depressants, in anaphylactic reactions, or with an overdose of certain antihypertensive agents (orthostatic hypotension). Circulatory insufficiency may not develop, since increased sympathoadrenal activity results in compensatory circulatory changes. However, in poisoning with cytotoxic chemicals, e.g., heavy metals, when a large amount of plasma is lost in the areas of inflammation and hemorrhage or when endotoxins from the gut flora enter the circulation, a state of circulatory insufficiency (shock) may develop. Inadequate blood volume in the absence of hemorrhage follows increased loss of body fluids brought about by persistent vomiting or diarrhea due to gastroenteritis, as occurs in poisoning with a variety of chemicals. Decreased intravascular volume leads to a decreased cardiac output. Other causes of shock include inadequate myocardial contraction resulting from severe arrhythmia, from cardiomyopathies, or inadequate peripheral circulation brought about by an altered vasomotor tone due to the effects of chemical mediators, e.g., histamine, leukotriene, and kinins. In shock, all physiologic parameters concerned with the perfusion of tissues are disturbed. The most critical effect involves the small blood vessels, the microcirculation, which is ultimately responsible for the exchange between blood and tissue. When compromised, signs of tissue death due to hypoxia and acidosis appear.

Hypertension. Chemicals can increase systemic arterial (systolic and/or diastolic) blood pressure as an acute event or can contribute to the development of its sustained increase by a variety of mechanisms.

Arterial hypertension may occur in the course of an overdose with sympathomimetic and anticholinergic drugs. Sudden drug-induced hypertension can cause cerebrovascular accidents when diseased blood vessels cannot adapt to high perfusion pressures. The sympathomimetic amines (norepinephrine, epinephrine, phenylephrine, etc.) elevate blood pressure by stimulating vascular α receptors with or without increasing cardiac output. The administration of 10 percent phenylephrine, even as an eyedrop, may be followed by hypertension, especially in the neonate.

Mineralocorticoids, especially when administered with sodium chloride, cause sodium retention and elevate blood pressure via an increase in circulatory volume. Licorice, which contains glycyrrhizin, an aldosteronelike substance that exerts mineralocorticoid activity, can cause sustained hypertension. Agents that cause hyperreninemia, e.g., cadmium—raise blood pressure by the generation of angiotensinogen II, which acts directly on the vascular smooth muscle. Depletion of renomedullary vasodilator substances has been implicated in the hypertension associated with analgesic drug-induced nephropathy. Increased synthesis of angiotensinogen has been considered to be a factor in the hypertension produced by high dosages of estrogen-containing oral contraceptives.

Sustained hypertension is the most important risk factor predisposing to coronary and cerebral atherosclerosis. The mechanisms by which hypertension produces vascular degenerative lesions involve increased vascular permeability with entry of blood constituents into the vessel wall, activation of phospholipase, and release of free arachidonate. The role of oxygen-centered free radicals generated in the arachidonate-prostaglandin pathways has been implicated in the development of destructive lesions of endothelium and vascular smooth muscle (Kontos and Hess, 1983).

Hemorrhage. Although chemicals can affect the structure of large vessels, leading to hemorrhage, e.g., aneurysms produced by lathyrogens, the capillaries are more frequently affected, often by nonspecific mechanisms, e.g., anoxia. Capillaries are common targets of cytotoxic chemicals, and therefore petechial hemorrhages are common in several organs after acute poisonings. A chemically induced defect in the blood-clotting mechanism increases the probability that hemorrhage may occur after a trivial trauma. Several chemicals can decrease platelet count by either a toxic mechanism (certain antitumor drugs) or an immune system-mediated mechanism (antiplatelet antibodies). Chemicals can also inhibit the synthesis of clotting factors; for example, coumarin inhibits the synthesis of prothrombin.

Thrombosis, Embolism. Thrombosis, the formation of a semisolid mass from blood constituents in the circulation, can occur both in arteries and in veins. Chemically induced predisposition to thrombosis most frequently occurs by induction of platelet aggregation, by an increase of their adhesiveness, or by creation of a state of hypercoagulability via an increase or activation of clotting factors. Large doses of epinephrine can affect each of these events. Effects on the platelets play a role in the thrombogenic action of the azo dye Congo red; when injected intravenously, the effect on coagulation is responsible for the thrombogenic effect of intravenously injected free fatty acids. Other sites of action of chemicals in predisposing to thrombosis include effects on antithrombin III (by oral contraceptive steroids) and inhibition of fibrinolysis (by corticosteroids, mercurials). Sudden changes in blood flow brought about by vasoconstriction (e.g., by ergotamine) or a decrease in peripheral resistance (e.g., by an autonomic blocking drug) can trigger arterial thrombosis. Venous stasis contributes to the development of venous thrombosis (Zbinden, 1976). Table 14–1 presents a list of thrombogenic agents and conditions.

Injury to the vessel wall by intravenous infusion of an irritating drug produces phlebitis, or

Table 14–1.   COMPOUNDS PRODUCING THROMBOSIS*

AGENT	SITE OF ACTION AND/OR MECHANISM
Endothelial Damage	
Homocysteine	Deendothelialization
Endotoxin	Deendothelialization
Polyanethol sulfate	Deendothelialization
Sodium acetriozate (radiocontrast agent)	Disseminated thrombosis in capillaries and veins; formation of insoluble fibrinogen derivative due to extraction of glycoproteins
Pathophysiologic Circulatory Dynamics	
Ergotamine	Profound vasoconstriction in peripheral arteries
Pitressin	Profound vasoconstriction in coronary and mesenteric arteries
Oral contraceptives	Venous stasis in lower extremities
ACh and autonomic blockers	Hypovolemic hypotension and stasis
Sympathomimetic agents	Elevated blood pressure and turbulence at bifurcations; distensions of vessels to produce endothelial damage
Effects on Platelets	
Serotonin	Increase in platelet count (above $10^6/mm^3$) symptomatic thrombocythemia
Progesterone	
Testosterone	
Somatotropic hormone	
Vinblastine	
Vincristine	
Congo red	Increase in platelet aggregation
Ristocetin (antibiotic)	
Serotonin	
Thrombin	
Epinephrine	
Adenosine diphosphate	Increase in platelet adhesiveness
Epinephrine	
Thrombin	
Evans blue	
Effects on Clotting Factors	
Epinephrine	Increase in factors VIII and IX
Guanethidine	Secondary effects due to release of epinephrine
Debrisoquin	
Tyramine	
Lactic acid (iv infusion)	Activation of Hageman factor
Long-chain fatty acids (iv infusion)	Activation of Contact factors
Catecholamines	Elevation in circulating levels of fatty acids
ACTH	
Thymoleptics	
Nicotine	
Oral contraceptives	Decrease in antithrombin III levels
Mercuric chloride	Inhibition of fibrinolysis
Prednisolone (corticosteroids)	
ε-Aminocaproic acid	Plasminogen antiactivator
Tranexamic acid	
Aprotinine	Proteinase inhibitors
Iniprol	

* Data from Zbinden, G.: Evaluation of thrombogenic effects. In Elliott, H. W.; George, R.; and Okun, R. (eds.): *Annual Review of Pharmacology and Toxicology,* Vol. 16. Annual Review Inc., Palo Alto, Calif., 1976, pp. 177–188.

by generalized endothelial damage (*e.g.*, that caused by polyanethol sulfonate) produces thromboses at the sites of lesions. Portions of thrombi may break and travel in the vascular system until arrested—an embolus—in a vessel of smaller caliber than that of its origin. The consequence depends on the site of arrest. The most important drugs that produce thromboembolisms are the contraceptive steroids.

Chemically Induced Structural Changes in the Heart

Chemically induced structural effects in the heart usually are manifested in the myocardium as focal or diffuse degenerative changes. A predilectional site is the left ventricular subendocardium because of its great sensitivity to hypoxia due to the low perfusion pressure of this area. Histologically, the muscle cells show increased eosinophilia, loss of striations, and granularity of the cytoplasm. Acute inflammatory signs, such as vascular dilation, tissue edema, and leukocytic infiltration, accompany the lesion (Figure 14–5). Lymphocytes, monocytes, macrophages, and fibroblasts are present in the subacute lesion and are gradually replaced by collagen. By electron microscopic examination the earliest change, observed two minutes after injection of a necrosis-inducing intraperitoneal dose of isoproterenol HC1 to rats, consisted of hypercontraction of myofibrils in muscle cells in the apical subendocardium. Over the next few minutes, "contraction bands" developed. This event was attributable to an excessive calcium influx. In two hours, the bands disappeared, perhaps through the action of calcium-activated proteases. Doughnut-shaped granules then appeared in the mitochondria; they were identical to those observed when the mitochondria were calcium-loaded and are regarded as evidence of irreversible damage. Inflammatory cells appeared by eight hours. The lesion progressed to myocytolysis (Balazs and Bloom, 1982).

An increased Ca^{2+} contributes to ATP depletion by stimulating its hydrolysis and inhibiting mitochondrial ATP synthesis. As a result of ATP catabolism, hypoxanthine accumulates. Ca^{2+} activates neutral proteases, which convert xanthine dehydrogenase to xanthine oxidase, an enzyme that generates a superoxide radical from O_2 during hypoxia. The superoxide will react with itself and yields peroxide, which reacts with superoxide to yield oxygen, water, and the most ractive free OH radical (Titus, 1983).

In hypersensitivity myocarditis, focal or diffuse interstitial infiltrations with eosinophils, lymphocytes, and plasma cells are characteristic. Necrotic changes are usually absent. Vasculitis may be associated with this reaction, which

heals without a scar after withdrawal of the chemical. Penicillin-, sulfonamide-, and methyldopa–induced myocarditis fit into this category (Billingham, 1980).

Slowly developing cardiomyopathies occur in chronic alcoholics and in patients treated with the antineoplastic anthracyclines. In these patients, the heart fails progressively, and the clinical syndrome of congestive heart failure develops. Ventricular dilatation, diffuse myocardial cellular degeneration, and/or interstitial fibrosis are the main morphologic findings. Alcoholics have an accumulation of lipid droplets in the cardiac muscle cells. Anthracyclines produce myofibrillar loss and cytoplasmic vacuolization (Ferrans, 1982).

Prolonged administration of certain chemicals can lead to cardiac hypertrophy, an increase in the mass of the muscle due to the increase in size of the cells. In these cells, the nuclei, mitochondria, and Golgi complexes are enlarged and the ribosomes are increased. Prolonged treatment with very high doses of sympathomimetics, such as isoproterenol or thyroid hormones, produces hypertrophy.

Inflammation of the serous membranes of the heart is most commonly a part of hypersensitivity reactions, for example, a lupus erythematosus-like reaction induced by hydralazine or procainamide. Endocardial and valvular fibrosis has occurred in patients taking methysergide, a congener of LSD.

A few chemicals have produced tumors in the heart in rodents; for example, 1,3-butadiene and nitrosamines caused sarcomas (Billingham, 1980).

Teratogenic Effects

Cardiovascular teratologic changes have been produced by a variety of chemicals. In humans, the critical period for the cardiovascular teratogenesis is from the fifth to the eighth week after conception. Failures to form, to persist, or to involute a specific structure result in malformations. Ventricular or atrial septal defects, patent ductus arteriosus, and tetralogy of Fallot are the most common cardiovascular abnormalities that have been induced by chemicals. Trypan blue and bis(dichloroacetyl) diamine can produce a high incidence of these changes (Jackson, 1981). Cardiovascular functional disturbances, for example, systemic hypertension, can develop in the progeny after treatment with certain drugs (salicylate, indomethacin) during pregnancy (Balazs, 1982).

TOXICOLOGIC CLASSIFICATIONS OF CARDIOVASCULAR REACTIONS

Three mechanisms can be distinguished in the development of cardiovascular toxicity. The first

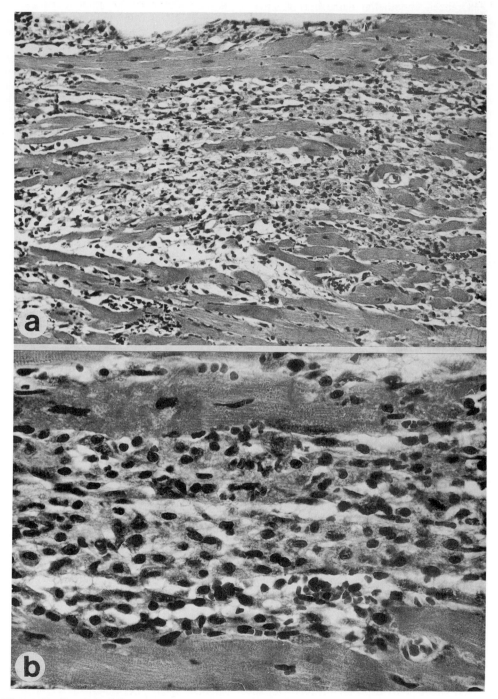

Figure 14–5. Hydralazine-induced lesions in a rat: *(a)* subendocardial region of left ventricular free wall, showing areas of necrosis and infiltrate of mononuclear cells; *(b)* high-power view shows fresh necrosis in some muscle cells at *top,* as evidenced by the loss of cross striations, presence of contraction bands, and apparent presence of mononuclear cells within the fibers. H&E ×130 and ×400. (From Balazs, T,; Ferrans, V. J.; El-Hage, A.; Ehrreich, S. J.; Johnson, G. L.; Herman, E. H.; Atkinson, J. C.; and West, W. L.: Study of the mechanism of hydralazine-induced myocardial necrosis in the rat. *Toxicol. Appl. Pharmacol.,* **59**:524–534. 1981.)

is related to an exaggerated pharmacologic effect of a compound, e.g., to overdoses of cardiovascular drugs. Drugs increase or decrease the intensity of organ function; an effect beyond the physiologic limits represents a dysfunction. The cardiotoxicity of β-adrenergic agonists, e.g., isoproterenol, is an example of such a mechanism. This drug affects both the cardiac β_1 and vascular and bronchial β_2 receptors and produces tachycardia and hypotension in low multiples of the bronchodilator doses. Tachycardia increases the myocardial oxygen demand, which may not be met, and ECG signs of myocardial hypoxia, ST segment depression and arrhythmia develop. The hypoxia is most marked in the least perfused left ventricular subendocardium, as evidenced by the greatest degree of ATP, phosphocreatine, and glycogen depletion and lactate accumulation. This is also the area where necrosis develops in experimental animals given a grossly very high dose of isoproterenol. β-Adrenergic-receptor blocking agents decrease both the pharmacologic and cardiotoxic effects of isoproterenol, indicating the role of the pharmacologic mechanism in the pathogenesis of the lesion (Balazs and Bloom, 1982).

Digitalis-, quinidine-, and procainamide-induced arrhythmias and antihypertensive-induced orthostatic hypotension are other examples of cardiovascular toxicities induced by exaggerated pharmacologic effects.

A second mechanism of cardiotoxicity involves an irreversible interaction of a chemical or its metabolite with a functional or structural molecule of vital significance. The binding is not a specific one, like that of a ligand to a receptor, but is nonspecific and covalent, like that of a free radical to a nucleophile. The development of the lesion depends on the rate of reactive metabolite formation and the concentration of protective substances in the cell. The protective mechanism against free radicals in the heart is at a lower level than that which exists in other parenchymatous organs, and therefore the heart is especially susceptible to the effects of these chemicals. A free radical mechanism plays a role in the chronic cardiotoxicity of antineoplastic anthracyclines. These drugs are activated to a free radical at multiple sites in the myocardial cell (Doroshow, 1988). Iron must be present for doxorubicin free radical formation to result in significant damage (Myers, 1988). Doxorubicin is an extremely active iron chelator. When formed, an iron-doxorubicin complex can readily catalyze the formation of a variety of free radical reactions capable of causing cellular damage. This process leads to the development of a cardiomyopathy. The first agent that was found to exert significant cardioprotective activity both experimentally and clinically is the EDTA derivative ICRF-187, an effective iron chelator (Herman et al., 1988; Speyer et al., 1988).

Another example of in situ formation of a reactive cardiotoxic metabolite is represented by acrolein, which is generated from allylamine by oxidative deamination. Oral administration of this compound to rats for a few weeks produces myocardial and vascular fibroses. Inhibition of the enzymatic transformation of allylamine to acrolein protects against the lesion (Boor, 1983). Acrolein conjugates with reduced glutathione and is excreted as mercapturic acid in the urine. Depletion of glutathione would be expected to enhance the toxicity.

A third mechanism of cardiovascular toxicity is represented by the immune system–mediated effects. In these "hypersensitivity" reactions, either the compound acts as a hapten that binds to an endogenous macromolecule, e.g., protein or nucleic acid, or the compound may act directly on the immune system, e.g., on helper or suppressor T cells. The cardiovascular system is affected in systemic anaphylaxis, where the protein-bound hapten binds to IgE on mast cells and basophils and elicits the release of histamine, serotonin, and leukotriene, the mediators of vascular effects. The haptenic antigen may bind to the cell membrane and, combining with the antibody produced or via lymphocytes, triggers a cytotoxic reaction. Antigen-antibody complexes deposited in the tissue can initiate—via complement fixation—inflammatory reactions, often in the blood vessels. Although a large number of commonly used drugs, e.g., aspirin, sulfonamides, and penicillin, can produce a cardiovascular hypersensitivity reaction, the incidence is very low. It is likely, as with other hypersensitivity reactions, that immunogenetic determinants, coded by the genes of the major histocompatibility complex, predispose to their development. The gene products are extremely polymorphic. The presence of a set of specific alleles (haplotypes) is required to produce the determinant on which the susceptibility to the antigen and the development of the reaction depends (Balazs, 1983).

Cardiotoxic Chemicals

Aliphatic Alcohols, Aldehydes, and Glycols. Ethanol decreases the force of cardiac contraction at a blood concentration of 75 mg/100 ml in humans. Although a negative dromotropic effect and a decreased threshold for ventricular fibrillation have been shown to occur in dogs after a single intravenous administration of ethanol, arrhythmias are prominent only after long-term treatment. These effects also occur in chronic alcoholics and may result in ventricular fibrillation and sudden death. Chronic alcohol consumption (alcoholism) decreases myocardial capacity on increased demand, resulting in dyspnea due to pulmonary congestion. Cardiomegaly or dilation of the chambers with mural thrombi are the postmortem findings. Interstitial fibrosis and increased lipid in the muscle cells are seen histologically (Billingham, 1980).

Although the acute cardiotoxicity of methanol is comparable to that of ethanol, those of the longer-chain alcohols are greater on a molar basis (Rubin and Rubin, 1982).

Acetaldehyde, the hepatic metabolic product of ethanol oxidation, has negative inotropic effects at blood concentrations that occur after a moderate ethanol intake. At higher concentrations, acetaldehyde releases catecholamines; hence it produces sympathomimetic effects. Such an effect gradually decreases with aldehydes of increasing chain length.

Dihydroxyalcohols, e.g., propylene glycol and polyethylene glycol-500, have cardiac effects in some instances when they are used as a vehicle for drugs. The former enhances the arrhythmogenic effect of digitalis and the latter the pressor effect of epinephrine in experimental animals (Van Stee, 1982).

The mechanism of the acute cardiodepressant effects of alcohols and aldehydes is related to an inhibition of intracellular calcium transport. The mechanism of chronic cardiotoxicity of ethanol involves several metabolic changes, such as increased triglyceride and proteoglycan formations.

Halogenated Alkanes. The cardiotoxicity of low-molecular-weight halogenated hydrocarbons is greater than that of unsubstituted hydrocarbons. They depress the heart rate, contractility, and conduction. The number of halogen atoms and unsaturated bonds influences the relative potency; e.g., negative inotropism of the substituted ethanes increases with up to four chlorines, and trichloroethylene is more potent than trichloroethanol. Some of these agents sensitize the heart to the arrhythmogenic effect of endogenous epinephrine or to β-adrenergic agonist drugs. Chloroform was one of the first agents to be recognized as having this sensitizing effect, and recently the low-pressure fluorocarbons, the Freons, have been reported to be sensitizing agents. Trichlorofluoromethane, one of the most toxic fluorocarbons, sensitized dogs to epinephrine at a concentration of 0.3 percent, and such an effect has also occurred in humans (Zakhari and Aviado, 1982).

Halogenated hydrocarbon anesthetics generally have effects similar to those described above. Halothane, methoxyflurane, and enflurane have negative chronotropic, inotropic, and dromotropic effects at the concentration used for anesthesia. Hence, they can produce myocardial depression and, although rarely, even cardiac arrest. Nevertheless, the stimulation of the sympathetic nervous system by respiratory acidosis, tracheal intubation, or surgical manipulation during an inadequate depth of anesthesia results in cardiac stimulation or even arrhythmia. The older and now obsolete anesthetics, e.g., cyclopropane and diethylether, were more potent sensitizers of the heart to epinephrine than are the modern anesthetics (Merin, 1981; Steffey, 1982).

The effects of the halogenated hydrocarbons are reversible, at least in patients without pre-existing cardiovascular disease. Chronic exposure to certain haloalkanes has been surmised to produce degenerative cardiac changes in humans. In investigations of the cardiodepressant mechanisms of these agents, interference with energy production and utilization and in the transfer of intracellular calcium between subcellular compartments has been postulated.

Heavy Metals. Among heavy metals causally associated with cardiovascular disease, cadmium, lead, and cobalt have selective cardiotoxic effects. They are negative inotropics and dromotropics and can also produce structural changes in the heart. A single dose of cadmium at 3 mg/kg intraperitoneally or six months of oral treatment (130 mg/liter in drinking water) in rats prolonged the P-R interval in the ECG. Chronic treatment also caused cardiac hypertrophy and vacuolation in the Purkinje cells. Lead given to rats for six weeks (100 mg/liter) produced degenerative changes in the heart. Such changes have also been detected in humans, in "moonshine" drinkers, and in children exposed to high doses of lead. A delayed effect of prenatal exposure of rats to lead manifested itself as a sensitization to the arrhythmogenic effect of norepinephrine postnatally. Similar phenomena were observed in adult rats receiving lead as neonates. Arrhythmias also occur in children exposed to lead and disappear after chelation therapy.

Cobalt, given orally to rats for eight weeks at doses of 26 mg/kg after an initial 100 mg/kg dose, produced cardiomyopathy. Rats kept on a low-protein diet developed vacuolar hydropic lesions after two weeks of treatment with cobalt at 4 to 12.5 mg/kg. The lesions were similar to those observed in heavy beer drinkers consuming a specific brand of beer that contained cobalt as a foam stabilizer; these individuals developed heart failure within a few months. The cardiotoxic effects of these heavy metals is attributed to their antagonistic action toward Ca^{2+}

as well as to their ability to form complexes with intracellular macromolecules.

Several other metals affect sarcolemmal ion channels. Manganese, nickel, and lanthanum block Ca^{2+} channels at a concentration similar to that of cobalt (1 mM). Barium is a potent arrhythmogen. $BaCl_2$ given intravenously at 5 mg/kg to rabbits produced ventricular tachycardia. This compound has been used as a model for screening antiarrhythmic agents. Traces of heavy metals are found in drinking water; however, calcium and magnesium in the water decrease their absorption (Revis, 1982).

Digitalis and Other Positive Inotropic Agents. Glycosides of digitalis, strophanthin, and oleandrin inhibit the sarcolemmal sodium pump. Na^+-K^+-ATPase, resulting in an increased intracellular Na^+ concentration, which in turn causes an elevation of intracellular Ca^{2+} concentration via Na^+/Ca^{2+} exchange. Consequently, cardiac contractility increases. However, the increased calcium enhances automaticity, which, along with other effects of digitalis, e.g., the increased vagal activity, and slowed AV conduction, leads to arrhythmias. Premature ventricular contractions may lead to ventricular fibrillation. The slowed AV conduction may progress to complete heart block.

Humans, dogs, and cats are the most sensitive species to digitalis, whereas rats are the least sensitive. Decreased concentration of potassium, brought about by certain diuretics, predisposes to the toxic effects. Decreased glomerular filtration rate prevalent in the elderly also predisposes to the toxicity of those glycosides that are eliminated by the kidney, e.g., digoxin. A moderately increased serum drug concentration (above the therapeutic level) can cause cardiotoxicity, and, indeed, the incidence of these reactions has been as high as 20 percent in hospitalized patients (Cliff *et al.*, 1975; Akera and Brown, 1982).

Several structurally unrelated chemicals increase the resting Na^+ permeability or slow the inactivation of the Na^+ channel; hence they have digitalislike cardiotoxic effects. Aconitine and *Veratrum* alkaloids and venoms secreted by lower animals (e.g., anemone toxins from coelenterata, palytoxin from corals, or batrachotoxin from the Columbian frog) produce arrhythmias and death by this mechanism. The extreme toxicity of palytoxin is shown by its intravenous LD50 value, which is 25 and 90 ng/kg in the rabbit and rat, respectively.

Other Cardiovascular Drugs and Biotoxins. Epinephrine and synthetic analogues, particularly the β-adrenergic-receptor agonists (e.g., isoproterenol) have positive chronotropic and inotropic effects, and the adverse reactions are related to these pharmacologic effects. In addition to tachycardia, ventricular arrhythmia can occur even at therapeutic doses on rare occasions. An overdose of these drugs can produce ECG signs of myocardial hypoxia (ST segment deviation and ectopic beats) and subendocardial necrosis. This lesion has been observed in several experimental animal species and has also been reported to occur in a few instances in humans. Myocardial hypoxia brought about by the increased oxygen demand that is not met and the consequent cellular calcium overloads has been a proposed mechanism for the observed toxicity (Balazs and Bloom, 1982).

Vasodilating antihypertensive drugs such as hydralazine can produce cardiotoxic effects similar to those mentioned above. These effects are elicited by a reflex tachycardia during hypotension.

The β-adrenergic-receptor blockers alone in overdose, as well as other antihypertensive drugs that inhibit adrenergic function (reserpine or guanethidine), decrease cardiac contractility and can cause AV block and possibly precipitate heart failure. Adverse cardiac effects (e.g., angina and even myocardial infarction) can occur after sudden withdrawal of β blockers, due to receptor supersensitivity brought about by an increased number of the β-adrenergic receptors, which is an adaptive event during treatment.

Antiarrhythmic drugs decrease the conductivity and irritability of the myocardium, which is the basis of their therapeutic use. They block the sodium channel during its conducting state. Quinidine and procainamide prolong the QRS and Q-T intervals in low multiples of the therapeutic doses. This condition predisposes to arrhythmia, e.g., by the reentry mechanism. Lidocaine and phenytoin in overdoses produce sinus bradycardia and cardiac arrest. Local anesthetics of the amide type, after inadvertent intravenous injection, cause ventricular fibrillation and cardiac arrest.

A variety of venoms from marine species, (e.g., saxitoxin or tetrodotoxin) decrease conduction in the sodium channel. Since the neurons are the most sensitive in poisoning, the nervous system symptoms are prominent.

Central Nervous System – Acting Drugs. Tricyclic antidepressants like imipramine and amitriptyline have quinidinelike effects on the heart. An overdose results in prolongation of the P-R, QRS, and Q-T intervals, in bundle branch block, and in supraventricular as well as ventricular arrhythmias.

Monoamine oxidase (MAO) inhibitor antidepressant drugs cause severe cardiovascular reactions (hypertensive crisis) when ingested with tyramine-containing foods or when used in combination with tricyclic antidepressants or sympathomimetic drugs. Tyramine is a sympathomimetic amine that is without effect when ingested in food because of its rapid biotransformation by MAO in the gut and liver. This reaction does not occur when MAO is inhibited.

Neuroleptic agents such as the phenothiazine and butyrophenone derivatives can produce dose-related tachyarrhythmias and other changes similar to those seen with the tricyclics, but the incidence is lower. In rare instances, sudden cardiac death preceded by ventricular fibrillation has been attributed to an overdose of these drugs. Aged patients with preexisting heart disease are at the greatest risk. Long-term or uncontrolled therapy with the antipsychotic drug lithium can produce ventricular arrhythmias and, rarely, myocardial lesions. Nonmedical use of psychoactive drugs (e.g., amphetamine, cocaine, and marijuana) can produce cardiovascular emergencies. These drugs increase the work load of the heart by increasing the heart rate and blood pressure and are particularly dangerous in individuals with angina, hypertension, coronary atherosclerosis, or cerebrovascular disease (Stimmel, 1979).

Chemotherapeutic Drugs. Among the antimicrobial antibiotics, the calcium antagonistic aminoglycosides, some of the macrolides, and chloramphenicol have weak negative inotropic effects. An overdose can cause adverse effects in patients with preexisting heart disease. Certain antibiotics from *Streptomyces* that are used in veterinary medicine or as feed additives (e.g., monensin and lasalocid) increase sarcolemmal cationic transport and may cause cardiac effects (Akera and Brown, 1982). Emetine, an obsolete antiparasitic drug, causes arrhythmias and myocardial necrosis of dose-related severity.

Antineoplastic antibiotics such as the anthracyclines (daunorubicin and doxorubicin) are potent cardiotoxic agents. The first therapeutic doses can produce arrhythmia, possibly due to histamine release. Chronic treatment leads to congestive cardiomyopathy; its development is delayed for months after treatment and is related to the cumulative dose. Cardiac dilatation, atrophy, and degeneration of the myocytes, as well as interstitial edema and fibrosis, are the postmortem findings in humans and also in experimental animals. Generation of reactive oxygen, peroxidation of membrane lipids, and consequent changes in permeability and in cellular homeostasis have been considered in the pathogenesis of this injury (Balazs and Ferrans, 1978). Table 14–2 presents general cardiotoxic effects of selected classes of agents and resulting structural alterations.

5-Fluorouracil, another antineoplastic drug, can produce signs of myocardial ischemia even during the early period of treatment and can ultimately precipitate cardiac arrest. Cyclophosphamide in large therapeutic doses can produce myocardial capillary microthrombosis, pericarditis, and cardiac failure. Radiation therapy combined with antineoplastic drugs produces capillary and pericardial lesions; e.g., anthracycline induces synergistic cardiotoxicity.

Table 14–3 presents the effects of selected chemicals on the heart.

Chemically Induced Structural Changes in Vasculature

Chemicals can produce degenerative and/or inflammatory changes in the blood vessels as a consequence of an excessive pharmacologic effect or by an interaction with a vascular structural or functional macromolecule. As a result of sustained arterial vasoconstriction, peripheral arterial lesions consisting of intimal proliferation and medial degenerative changes leading

Table 14–2. CARDIOTOXIC EFFECTS*

	CHRONO-TROPIC	DROMO-TROPIC	BATHMO-TROPIC	INO-TROPIC	ARRHYTH-MOGENIC	STRUCTURAL
Ethanol		–	+	–	+	Chronic cardiomyopathy
Haloalkanes	–	–	+	–	+	Chronic degenerative changes
Heavy metals		–		–	+	Chronic degenerative changes
Digitalis	–	–	+	+	+	
Catecholamines	+	+	+	+	+	Acute focal necrosis cardiac hypertrophy
Antiarrhythmics	–	–		–	+	
Tricyclic antidepressants	+	–	+			
Neuroleptics		–		–	+	
Antineoplastic anthracyclines				+		Chronic cardiomyopathy

* Negative = decreased. Positive = increased.

Table 14–3. SELECTED CARDIOTOXIC AGENTS*

AGENTS (CHEMICAL CLASS OR USE CATEGORY)	CARDIAC EFFECT AND/OR PRIMARY SITE	ASSOCIATED DISEASE STATE AND/OR MECHANISM
Substituted Aliphatic Hydrocarbons		
A. Haloalkanes	Negative chronotropic, inotropic, and dromotropic effects that depress heart rate, contractility, and conduction	Cardiotoxicity exceeds that of similar chain length unsubstituted hydrocarbons; maximum toxicity at 4 Cl atoms
1. Chloroform	Arrhythmias	Sensitizes the heart to endogenous catecholamines
2. Cyclopropane and di-ethylether[a,b]	Arrhythmias	Sensitize the heart to catecholamines
3. Freons (fluorocarbons)[c]	Reduces cardiac output and coronary flow	Reflex increases in sympathetic and parasympathetic impulses to heart via respiratory tract mucosa irritation
4. Haloanesthetics (halothane, methoxyflurane and enflurane)	Negative chronotropic, inotropic, and dromotropic effects; possible cardiac arrest	Myocardial depression
5. Substituted ethanes	Negative inotropism	
B. Alcohols and aldehydes		
1. Acetaldehyde	Negative inotropic effects (after moderate ethanol intake)	Release of catecholamines and resulting sympathetic effects (at higher doses); toxicity diminishes with increasing aldehyde chain length
2. Ethanol	Decreases cardiac contraction; causes arrhythmias and ventricular fibrillation with sudden death (after chronic exposure); cardiomegaly (found upon autopsy)	Pulmonary congestion; congestive heart failure; leakage of myocardial cells; depression of oxidative phosphorylation in heart mitochondria; interstitial fibrosis and increased lipid in muscle cells[d]
3. PEG 500[e]	Enhancement of the pressor effects of epinephrine	
4. Propylene glycol[e]	Enhancement of arrhythmogenic effects of digitalis	
Heavy Metals[f-g]		
1. Barium	Potent arrhythmogen; production of ventricular tachycardia	Greatly prolongs action potentials
2. Cadmium		
Acute	Prolongation of PR interval; heart failure in diastole	Antagonism of Ca^{2+} ion; shortens action potential
Chronic	Cardiac hypertrophy and vacuolation in the Purkinje cells	
3. Cobalt	Cardiac lesions, heart failure	Antagonism of endogenous Ca^{2+}, complexes of cobalt with macromolecules
4. Lanthanum	Effects upon sarcolemmal ion channels	Blocks Ca^{2+} channels
5. Lead		
Prenatal[h]	Postnatal sensitization to the arrhythmogenic effects of norepinephrine	
Adult[i]	Negative inotropism; ECG abnormalities and rhythm changes; deformation of T wave; prolongation of PR interval	Displacement of Ca^{2+}; interference with Ca availability; interference with energy metabolism and ATP synthesis in heart

445

Table 14–3. (*Continued*)

AGENTS (CHEMICAL CLASS OR USE CATEGORY)	CARDIAC EFFECT AND/OR PRIMARY SITE	ASSOCIATED DISEASE STATE AND/OR MECHANISM
6. Manganese	Effects upon sarcolemmal ion channels	Blocks Ca^{2+} channels
7. Nickel	Effects upon sarcolemmal ion channels	Blocks Ca^{2+} channels
8. Vanadium	Both positive and negative inotropic effects *in vitro* depending upon species; decrease of left ventricular contraction and negative chronotropic effects in intact animal	Inotropic changes related to alteration in available surface Ca^{2+}; effects upon phosphorylation reactions; inhibition of Na^+K^+ ATPase
Gases		
1. Carbon disulfide	Angina pectoris	Formation of thiocarbamates; inhibition of dopamine hydroxylase; disruption of lipid and thyroxine metabolism; development of coronary heart disease
2. Carbon monoxide (acute)	Tachycardia, bradycardia, extrasystoles; increased demand for oxygen by the heart; production of angina pectoris; myocardial infarction	Interference with myocardial energy metabolism
Drugs A. Cardioactive drugs 1. Antiarrhythmics		
a. Quinidine and procainamide	Decreased conductivity and automaticity of the myocardium Prolongation of QRS and QT intervals; ventricular fibrillation after i.v. injection; extrasystoles, low doses accelerate while large doses prolong AV conduction; cardiac arrest	
b. Lidocaine	Sinus bradycardia; depressed automaticity of Purkinje fibers and myocardial cells; depressed myocardial contractility	Shortened action potentials of Purkinje fibers and myocardial cells
c. Phenytoin	Suppression of automaticity; cardiac arrest	
2. Adrenergic agonists a. Epinephrine and[j] isoproterenol	Positive inotropic and chronotropic effects; ST segment deviation, ectopic beats, and subendocardial necrosis	Myocardial hypoxia; cellullar Ca^{2+} overload
b. Isoproterenol[j] (only)	Hypercontraction of myofibrils in apical subendocardium; appearance of donut-shaped granules in mitochondria, myocytolysis	Excessive Ca^{2+} influx
3. Adrenergic antagonists as well as reserpine and guanethidine	Deceased cardiac contractility; production of AV block; heart failure (effects of overdose); angina and possible myocardial infarction (effects of withdrawal)	Receptor supersensitivity; excess numbers of receptors
4. Glycosides of digitalis,[k,l] strophanthin, and oleandrin	Increase in cardiac contractility, irritability, and arrhythmias Premature ventricular contractions Prolonged PR interval	Inhibit the sarcolemmal Na^+ pump (Na^+K^+ ATPase) with elevation of intracellular Ca^{2+} via Na^+/Ca^{2+} exchange Ventricular fibrillation Complete heart block

Drug	Effect	Mechanism
5. Nicotine	Arrhythmias	Suppresses K^+ conductance
6. Vasodilators and antihypertensives (hydralazine, diazoxide, minoxidil)[g]	Similar effects to epinephrine, via reflex tachycardia during hypotension	
B. Ca^{2+} antagonists[g]		
1. Bepridil	Negative chronotropic and ionotropic effects	Blocks slow Ca^{2+} channels; depressed Ca^{2+} release from the SR
2. Papaverine	Negative chronotropic and ionotropic effects	Blocks slow channels; inhibits phosphodiesterase and elevates cAMP
3. Verapamil and nifedipine	Negative chronotropic and ionotropic effects	Excitation contraction uncoupling; block both slow Ca^{2+} and Na^+ channels; depress or block Ca^{2+} influx into myocardial cells
C. CNS active drugs[m]		
1. Amphetamine and cocaine[m]	Increased heart rate; blood pressure increase causing great risk when there is preexisting angina, hypertension, and atherosclerosis	Increased work load on the heart
2. Imipramine and amitryptyline	Low doses enhance cardiac contractility, whereas high doses depress it as well as coronary flow and heart rate; quinidinelike effects on the heart; prolongation of the PR, QRS, and QT interval; bundle branch block; supraventricular and ventricular arrhythmias	Cardiac arrest; catecholamine reuptake inhibition; anticholinergic effects
3. Lithium (long-term) (toxic dose)	Ventricular arrhythmias and in rare instances, myocardial lesions	
4. MAO inhibitors	Palpitation	Exaggerated sympathomimetic effects
5. Marijuana	Positive inotropic and chronotropic effects; premature ventricular contractions; enhanced ventricular automaticity	Facilitation of SA and AV nodal conduction; increased work load on heart
6. Methyldopa[d]	Focal or diffuse interstitial infiltration with eosinophils, lymphocytes, and plasma cells	Hypersensitivity myocarditis
7. Methysergide	Endomyocardial fibrosis; valvular defects	
8. Neuroleptics[a] (phenothiazines and butyrophenones)	Tachyarrhythmias, hypotension, ventricular tachycardia, and fibrillation (rare), conduction defects; prolongation of QT interval; abnormalities in T wave sinus tachycardia, widening of QRS complex	Quinidine-type toxicity; peripheral α receptor blockade; central and peripheral anticholinergic actions
9. Barbiturates	Depression of myocardial contractility	Inserts in lipid bilayer of membrane; stabilizes membranes
D. Chemotherapeutic agents		
1. Antimicrobial antibiotics a. Antimicrobial antibiotics b. Some macrolides and chloramphenicol	Weak negative inotropic effects	Depressed Ca^{2+} uptake
2. Antineoplastic antibiotics a. Anthracyclines[o,p] (doxorubicin and daunorubicin)	Arrhythmias (acute); Congestive cardiomyopathy (after chronic use); cardiac dilation, atrophy and degeneration of the myocytes, and interstitial edema and fibrosis (seen at autopsy)	Possibly due to histamine release; generation of reactive oxygen; peroxidation of membrane lipids and consequent changes in permeability and in cellular homeostasis

Table 14–3. (Continued)

AGENTS (CHEMICAL CLASS OR USE CATEGORY)	CARDIAC EFFECT AND/OR PRIMARY SITE	ASSOCIATED DISEASE STATE AND/OR MECHANISM
b. 5-Fluorouracil	Myocardial ischemia: cardiac arrest	Cardiac failure
c. Cyclophosphamide (large doses)	Myocardial capillary microthrombosis: pericarditis	
3. Emetine	Sinus tachycardia dose-related arrhythmias and myocardial necrosis, ventricular fibrillation	Conduction disturbances; effects upon K^+ ion movements
4. Monensin and lasalocid[l]	Positive inotropic effect; increased cardiac output; occasional increase in heart rate and automaticity; increased coronary blood flow	Increased excitation-contraction coupling; enhanced metabolism of cardiac cells; increased sarcolemmal cationic trap for Na^+, and lasalocid a cationic trap for K^+
5. Penicillin and sulfonamide[d]	Focal or diffuse interstitial infiltration with eosinophils, lymphocytes and plasma cells	Hypersensitivity myocarditis
E. Carcinogenic agents[d]		
1,3-Butadiene and nitrosamines	Sarcoma formation within heart	Induction of chemical carcinogenesis
F. Agents and drugs producing cardiovascular teratogenesis[q]		
1. Bis(dichloroacetyl) diamine	Ventricular septal defects; dextrocardia; ectopia; tetralogy of Fallot; pulmonic stenosis	
2. Caffeine	Ventricular septal defects	
3. Cortisone	Ventricular and atrial septal defects	
4. Dextroamphetamine	Ventricular septal defects	
5. Ethanol	Ventricular septal defects	
6. Phenobarbital		
7. Salicylate and indomethacin		Systemic hypertension
Toxins[g]		
1. Batrochotoxin	Ventricular arrhythmia, fibrillation, positive inotropic effects	Increase in resting Na^+ permeability; actions upon protein constituents of Na^+ channel
2. Cobra venom cardiotoxin	Systolic arrest; disruption of myocardial cell membranes and myofibrils	Depression of Ca^{2+} accumulation in SR; inhibition of Ca-ATPase; SR membranes become more leaky; depression of Ca^{2+} accumulation in mitochondria; ultimate Ca^{2+} overload
3. Endotoxin	Reduced coronary perfusion; depression of contractility; negative inotropic and chronotropic responses to NE and histamine	Depression of Ca-ATPase activity, depression of Ca^{2+} uptake, reduced Ca^{2+} release by action potentials
4. Grayanotoxins	Positive inotropic action	Increases Na^+ permeability; opens voltage-dependent Na^+ channels
5. Sea anemone toxins (ATX-II and CTX)	Conduction defects: negative chronotropic effect; positive inotropic effects	Greatly slows inactivation of Na^+ channels

6. Scorpion neurotoxin	Positive chronotropic effects; induction of fibrillation	Slows closing of Na^+ channel and opening of K^+ channel; causes neurotransmitter release
		Blocks fast Na^+ channels
7. Tetrodotoxin and saxitoxin	Conduction defects	Increased resting Na^+ permeability; slowed inactivation of Na^+ channel with prolonged action potentials
8. Veratridine, aconidine	Induction of cardiac arrhythmias; increase or enhancement of automaticity; positive inotropic effect (veratridine)	
9. Volvatoxin A	Cardiac arrest in systole; increase in diastole resting tension of cardiac muscle	Makes SR membrane leaky to Ca^{2+} alteration of ultrastructure of mitochondria, thereby inhibiting ability to accumulate Ca^{2+}

[a] **Merin, R. G.,** Cardiac toxicology of inhalation anesthetics, in *Cardiac Toxicology,* Vol. 2, Balazs, T., Ed., CRC Press, Boca Raton, Fla., 1981, 1.

[b] **Steffey, E. P.,** Cardiovascular effects of inhalation anesthetics, in *Cardiovascular Toxicology,* Van Stee, E. W., Ed., Raven Press, New York, 1982.

[c] **Zakhari, S. and Aviado, D. M.,** Cardiovascular toxicology and aerosol propellants, refrigerants and related solvents, in *Cardiovascular Toxicology,* Van Stee, E. W., Ed., Raven Press, New York, 1982, 281.

[d] **Billingham, M. F.,** Morphologic changes in drug-induced heart disease, in *Drug-Induced Heart Disease,* Bristow, M. R., Ed., Elsevier/North-Holland, Amsterdam, 1980, 128.

[e] **Van Stee, E. W.,** Cardiovascular toxicology: foundation and scope, in *Cardiovascular Toxicology,* Van Stee, E. W., Ed., Raven Press, New York, 1982.

[f] **Revis, N. W.,** Relationship of vanadium, cadmium, lead, nickel, cobalt and soft water to myocardial and vascular toxicity and cardiovascular disease, in *Cardiovascular Toxicology,* Van Stee, E. W., Ed., Raven Press, New York, 1982, 365.

[g] **Speralakis, N.,** Effects of cardiotoxic agents on the electrical properties of myocardial cells, in *Cardiac Toxicology,* Vol. 1, Balazs, T., Ed., CRC Press, Boca Raton, Fla., 1981, 39.

[h] **Magos, L.,** The effects of industrial chemicals on the heart, in *Cardiac Toxicology,* Vol. 2, Balazs, T., Ed., CRC Press, Boca Raton, Fla., 1981, 203.

[i] **Williams, J., Hejtmancik, M. R., Jr., and Abreu, M.,** Cardiac effects of lead, *Fed. Proc. Fed. Am. Soc. Exp. Biol.,* 42, 2989, 1983.

[j] **Balazs, T. and Bloom, S.,** Cardiotoxicity of adrenergic bronchodilator and vasodilating antihypertensive drugs, in *Cardiovascular Toxicology,* Van Stee, E. W., Ed., Raven Press, New York, 1982, 353.

[k] **Cliff, I. E., Caranasos, G. J., and Stewart, R. B.,** Clinical problems with drugs, in *Major Problems in Internal Medicine,* Smith, L. H., Ed., W. B. Saunders, Philadelphia, 1975, 115.

[l] **Akers, T. and Brown, B. S.,** Cardiovascular toxicology of cardiotonic drugs and chemicals, in *Cardiovascular Toxicology,* Van Stee, E. W., Ed., Raven Press, New York, 1982, 353.

[m] **Stimmel, B.,** *Cardiovascular Effects of Mood Altering Drugs,* Raven Press, New York, 1979.

[n] **Weiss, L. W.,** The cardiotoxicity of neuroleptic and tricyclic antidepressant drugs, in *Cardiac Toxicology,* Vol. 2, Balazs, T., Ed., CRC Press, Boca Raton, Fla., 1981, 125.

[o] **Balazs, T. and Ferrans, V. J.,** Cardiac lesions induced by chemicals, *Environ. Health Perspect.,* 26, 181, 1978.

[p] **Ferrans, V. J.,** Overview of morphological reactions of the heart to toxic injury, in *Cardiac Toxicology,* Vol. 3, Balazs, T., Ed., CRC Press, Boca Raton, Fla., 1981, 83.

[q] **Jackson, R.,** Developmental cardiotoxic effects of chemicals, in *Cardiac Toxicology,* Vol. 3, Balazs, T., Ed., CRC Press, Boca Raton, Fla., 1981, 163.

* Reprinted with permission from Cohen, G. M. (ed.): *Target Organ Toxicity,* Vol. 2, 1986, pp. 32—37. Copyright CRC Press, Inc., Boca Raton, Fla.

to gangrene develop with ergotamine intoxication. An example of a direct toxic mechanism is that produced by allylamine; when the compound was given orally to rats for a few weeks, it produced vascular smooth muscle hyperplasia that resulted in coronary artery and aortic lesions mimicking the atherosclerotic process. The active metabolite is acrolein, which denatures protein and disrupts nucleic acid synthesis. Deposition of fibrinlike material in the ground substance of collagen leads to fibrinoid necrosis. It is an early consequence of hypertension due to the entry of fibrinogen into the wall of small arteries.

Changes in the collagen of the large arteries leading to localized dilatations (aneurysms) occur in lathyrism or are produced by β-aminopropionitrile in young rats and various avian species.

Atherosclerosis is a degenerative process occurring within arteries; plaques containing lipids, complex carbohydrates, blood products, and calcium accumulate in the intima and inner portion of the media. This lesion generally occurs in major blood vessels such as the aorta and coronary, carotid, and femoral arteries. Early experiments have shown that diets high in saturated fats and cholesterol produce atheromas; however, recently the low-density β-lipoproteins have been implicated along with stress and hypertension as predisposing factors. The principal consequence of atheroma is narrowing of an artery. If the narrowing occurs in a renal artery, renal hypertension may develop. When this process occurs in the cerebral vessels, there is a potential for stroke; when it occurs in the coronary artery, myocardial ischemia can occur and may culminate in a myocardial infarction.

Chemicals can produce or enhance atheroma formation by several mechanisms. Carbon monoxide, which increases capillary permeability, accelerates plaque formation in animals on atherogenic, high-cholesterol diets. The effect of CO may actually be due, however, to a lack of oxygen, since atheroma formation is also enhanced in animals subjected to hypoxia. Another agent is carbon disulfide (CS_2), which has produced a two- to threefold increase in coronary heart disease in exposed industrial workers. In cholesterol-fed rabbits. CS_2 greatly accelerated the formation of atheroma. The mechanism for CS_2-atheroma production is thought to consist of direct injury to the endothelium coupled with changes in lipid metabolism associated with hypothyroidism, since thiocarbamate (thiourea), a potent antithyroid substance, is a principal urinary metabolite of CS_2. Homocysteine has

direct effects on the arterial and venous walls. The process involves platelet adhesion, proliferation of smooth muscle cells, accumulation of lipid into these cells with their subsequent transformation into foam cells, and finally loss of the endothelial layer at the site of the atherogenic defect (Van Stee, 1982).

Hypersensitivity, immune system–mediated vasculitis, generally occurs in small vessels (arterioles, venules, capillaries), although the coronary arteries can be involved. The presence of eosinophils and mononuclear cells is characteristic. The pathogenesis is associated with the deposition of soluble immune complexes in the vessel wall and with the activation of the complement system. Gold salts, methyldopa, penicillin, sulfonamides, and several other drugs can produce this reaction in humans (Ferrans, 1982). Some of these drugs have also been suspected to exacerbate preexisting polyarteritis (a necrotizing vasculitis) or cause a syndrome like periarteritis nodosa, a vascular disease of unknown origin (Billingham, 1980). Vascular alterations by agents are presented in Table 14–4.

Vascular Effects in Vital Organs

Brain. The integrity of the vascular components of the blood-brain barrier (BBB) relies on the metabolic status of the endothelial cells and the effectiveness of tight junctions between them.

Anoxia and ischemia of the brain will cause endothelial cells to swell and the junctions to widen, but it takes several hours for the barriers to break down, resulting in vascular disruption. In addition, hypercapnia (very high CO_2 concentrations) opens the BBB by abolishing autoregulation and producing brain edema. Cerebral blood flow is greatly increased, and hemorrhages may occur. Another process that increases cerebrovascular permeability is pinocytosis, and this is increased by agents such as divalent cations, high concentrations of norepinephrine and serotonin, and chemically induced convulsions (e.g., those caused by metrazol).

Lead is deleterious to sulfhydryl proteins that form structural units as well as biochemical enzyme systems. It produces encephalopathy with brain edema, and toxic effects on endothelial cells occur before those on the neurons and glia. Newborn rats exposed to lead showed separation at tight junctions, increase of permeability, and loss of a major portion of the BBB (Rapoport, 1976).

A variety of cytolytic agents break down the BBB by disruptive effects on cell membranes and capillaries. These agents include alcohols,

Table 14–4. VASCULAR ALTERATIONS*

ALTERATION	CAUSATIVE AGENTS
Atherosclerosis	Goiteragenic substances, carbon disulfide, benzpyrene, dimethyl-benzanthracene, homocysteine, CO, fluorocarbons, oral contraceptives (mainly progestins), hydrochlorthiazide + propranolol, Ca, lead, and soft water
Medial proliferation	Ergot alkaloids, pyrrolizidine alkaloids (due to prolonged constriction)
Intimal proliferation	Oral contraceptives, chronic ergotamine or methysergide maleate, talc or Mg silicate (in i.v. drug abusers), allylamine or phosphodiesterse inhibitors (in animals)
Calcification	Calcinogenic plants (*Cestrum diurnum, Trisetum flavescens, Solarum malacoxylon* and *Solanum tordum*), and vitamin D_3 toxicosis
Aneurysms	*Lathyrus* sp., β-aminoproprionitrile, penicillamine, and aminoacetonitrile (these all involve inhibition of lysyl oxidase, a copper-containing enzyme necessary for normal strength of vascular walls via crosslinking of collagen and elastin
Medial hemorrhagic necrosis	Fenoldopam mesylate (a dopaminergic vasodilator in rats), minoxidil, hydralazine, nicorandil, theobromine, diazoxide, digoxin, norepinephrine, other compounds that produce inotropy and vasodilatation
Fibrinoid necrosis	Organic mercury, lead toxicosis, phenylbutazone
Microangiopathy endothelial damage	Cadmium (testicular capillary damage), cyclophosphamide
Vasculitis (nonnecrotizing)	Drug-related hypersensitivity reactions from penicillin, ampicillin, chlortetracycline, chlorthalidone, cromolyn Na, diphenylhydantoin, isoniazid, procainamide, quinidine
Toxic necrotizing vasculitis	Arsenic, bismuth, gold, methamphetamine, sulfonamides

* Data from Van Fleet, J. F.; Ferrans, V. J.; and Herman, E.: Cardiovascular and skeletal muscle systems. In Haschek-Hock, W. M., and Rousseaux, C. G. (eds.): *Fundamentals of Toxicologic Pathology*. Academic Press, San Diego, in press.

other lipid solvents, cobra venom, surfactants, and high concentrations of sulfhydryl inhibitors (Bakay, 1956). Hypertonic solutions of NaC1, urea, and mannitol, cause reversible opening of the BBB due to shrinking of vascular endothelium and separation of tight junctions.

Lungs. Alveolar capillary fragility and permeability changes result in pulmonary edema and a serious decrease in oxygen exchange. This occurs often following inhalation of irritant gases. Excessive intravenous infusion of fluid is the most frequent cause of iatrogenic pulmonary edema, especially following replacement of blood loss by electrolyte solutions. Opiates (heroin, methadone) can produce delayed pulmonary edema after intravenous self-administration; neurogenic alterations of central origin of capillary permeability are implicated. Drug addicts who self-administer dissolved tablets intravenously develop pulmonary embolism and thrombosis because of the talc vehicle. Pulmonary thromboembolism has been associated with the use of high doses of oral contraceptive estrogens in women who are predisposed to thrombosis.

The pyrrolizidine alkaloid microcrotaline, at a single dose of 50 mg/kg in rats, produced pulmonary hypertension four weeks later. Ultra-structural changes consisted of evagination of vascular smooth muscle cells with loss of myofilament cells during the onset of hypertension (Smith and Heath, 1976). Pulmonary arterial hypertension often developed in obese patients taking large doses of an anorexic drug, aminorex fumarate. Histologically, intimal and medial thickening were detected. These changes could not be reproduced in animal experiments.

Carbamylhydrazine HC1 induced tumors in blood vessels of the lung after oral administration to mice (Toth *et al.*, 1975).

Liver. Hepatotoxins that produce hemorrhagic necrosis (e.g., dimethylnitrosamine) ultimately produce occlusion of veins. Pyrrolizidine alkaloids produce identical effects resulting in hepatic venoocclusive disease, which is not uncommon in children in South Asia. The initial lesion consists of a proliferation of the endothelium in the small efferent veins, followed by a proliferation of the vascular connective tissue, leading to an occusion of these veins. This can result in early death.

Oral contraceptives have produced thrombosis in the portal circulation, involving proliferation and thickening of the intima. A rare condition, peliosis, is induced by estrogenic and androgenic steroids. This lesion consists of islands of dilated portal sinusoids, and fatal bleeding may occur from their rupture. Endotoxins produce swelling of Kupffer and endothelial cells, as well as adhesion of platelets to sinusoid walls, all of which affect the microcirculation.

Chronic hepatitis induced by oxyphenisatin or nitrofurantoin and cirrhosis induced by ethanol, arsenicals, or methotrexate, lead to the development of portal hypertension. Tumors of the hepatic vasculature have been induced by thorium dioxide and vinyl chloride; hemangioendotheliomas and hemangiosarcomas, respectively, have been reported.

Kidney. Several nephrotoxins affect the renal blood vessels and can cause marked constriction of renal arteries. Preglomerular vasoconstriction and/or relaxation of the postglomerular vessels greatly depresses the glomerular filtration rate. A tubuloglomerular feedback control mediated by the vasoconstrictor effect of adenosine shuts down glomerular vessels following necrosis of the tubular epithelium. Nephropathies induced by cadmium, lead, and certain analgesics produce systemic arterial hypertension by affecting one or more components of the renal blood pressure regulatory systems. Structural changes of the renal vessels, consisting of diffuse fibrosis of the capillaries, have been reported after chronic exposure to cadmium in experimental animals.

Immune complex deposits on the basement membranes of glomerular capillaries are characteristic of hypersensitivity reactions induced by a large number of chemicals, e.g., gold salts, d-penicillamine in humans, and $HgCl_2$ in experimental animals.

Heart. A large number of endogenous substances (e.g., epinephrine, angiotensin, histamine, thromboxane, and leukotrienes) can cause marked constriction of the coronary arteries. Ergonovine and vasopressin are the most consistent provokers of coronary spasm in the clinical setting and also in experimental animals. Coronary constriction results in myocardial hypoxia with ECG signs such as ST segment deviation. It can precipitate death in patients with preexisting heart disease.

Withdrawal of coronary vasodilators such as nitroglycerin or nitroglycol caused sudden death in industrial workers who were exposed all week on the job and then abstained from the chemical on weekends. They were adapted and dependent on the continuous presence of these compounds to maintain a minimum level of coronary flow. A second mechanism for coronary artery toxicity due to nitrites and nitrates relates to the so-called aging of the coronary arteries due to repeated vasodilation and the metabolic sequelae of heme

redox reactions. This toxicity is nonspecific, since it is also seen after prolonged exposure to CS_2 (Magos, 1981).

Structural changes consisting of intimal proliferation and vascular occlusion or atherosclerotic lesions have been produced by methysergide and cigarette smoke, respectively, in chronic animal experiments.

Vasculotoxic Chemicals

Heavy Metals. In general, heavy metals produce their toxicity by destroying sulfhydryl proteins that comprise important structural components of vasculature.

Inorganic lead causes changes in arterial elasticity by specific effects upon the ground substance, and it has been shown to cause sclerosis of renal vessels. Severe lead intoxication has been linked with hypertension in humans, but lesser degrees of lead ingestion have not been implicated. Whereas pigeons have been shown to develop hypertension after exposure to 0.8 ppm Pb^{2+} for six months, a similar exposure in rats was without effect. Analysis of Pb^{2+} concentrations showed that the highest levels occurred in the aorta (Revis, 1982).

Cadmium is an insidiously acting compound on the vasculature, and it appears to play a role in the etiology of hypertension. Increased salt and water retention and hyperreninemia have been implicated in the mechanism. When Cd^{2+} is administered to rats in drinking water, hypertension results at exposure levels of 5 ppm, whereas hypotension occurs at levels of 50 ppm (Revis, 1982). Similarly, *in vitro,* low levels of Cd^{2+} (8.4 μg/liter) stimulate vascular contraction, whereas high doses (840 μg/liter) cause relaxation. In both rats and pigeons, the formation of atherosclerotic plaques has been enhanced by Cd^{2+} with a concomitant fall in serum high-density lipoproteins and cholesterol. In rats, chronic administration of Cd^{2+} caused renal arteriolar thickening as well as diffuse fibrosis of capillaries. Similar vascular changes are also responsibile for development of testicular damage and atrophy. In the uterus, Cd^{2+} produces lesions in the endothelial clefts as well as having deleterious effects on the microcirculation. Destruction of the placenta in rats has also been reported. Many of the vascular effects may be reversed by either a Cd^{2+} chelator or zinc. There appears to be biologic antagonism between Cd^{2+} and Zn^{2+}, and in many instances, humans dying of hypertension have a higher ratio of Cd/Zn than normal, as well as a higher absolute level of Cd^{2+} (Schroeder, 1971).

Inorganic mercury produces vasoconstriction of the preglomerular vessels. In addition, the integrity of the blood-brain barrier may be disrupted by mercury. The opening of the BBB results in extravasation of plasma proteins across vascular walls into adjoining brain tissues.

Arsenic, in the form of the hydride arsine, affects the vasculature of the lungs, leading to pulmonary edema. It has been proposed that the very high levels of As in soil and water of Taiwan is responsible for blackfoot disease, a severe form of arteriosclerosis. Arsenic has been reported to cause noncirrhotic portal hypertension in humans in India as a result of contamination of the water supply (Datta, 1976).

Chromium appears to play an important role in the maintenance of vascular integrity. A deficiency of this metal in animals results in elevated serum cholesterol levels and increased atherosclerotic aortic plaques. Autopsies of humans have revealed virtually no chromium in the aortas of individuals dying of atherosclerotic heart disease, in comparison with normal individuals dying of other causes (Schroeder, 1971).

Gases. Carbon monoxide exposure in rabbits, at 180 ppm exposure for four hours, results in focal intimal damage and edema. This is in the range of CO exposure that humans might experience from cigarette smoke (Thomsen and Kjeldsen, 1975). Atherogenesis may also be accelerated in rabbits exposed to CO while consuming an atherogenic diet. This phenomenon also occurred, however, during hypoxia in the absence of CO, so that the vascular wall deprived of oxygen, rather than being exposed to CO *per se,* may really be responsible for this effect. The conversion of more than 20 percent of the hemoglobin to carboxyhemoglobin increases the permeability of vascular walls to macromolecules, an incipient change in the pathogenesis of atherosclerosis.

Oxygen exposure causes toxicity primarily in the vasculature of the eye and the lungs. Administration of oxygen to the premature newborn can cause irreversible vasoconstriction and ultimate obliteration of retinal vasculature with resulting permanent blindness (Beehler, 1964). In the adult, high oxygen tension causes vascular effects that result in the shrinking of the visual field; however, these effects are reversible after cessation of exposure. In squirrel monkeys, exposure to 100 percent oxygen for 50 to 117 hours caused increases in vascular permeability with leakage and edema of the retina, as evidenced by fluorescein angiography. These effects are largely functional and reversible (Kinney *et al.,* 1977). In experimental studies in rats, exposure for two days to 60 percent O_2 did not produce tolerance but in fact lowered survival time after 100 percent O_2 exposure. In the pulmonary capillary bed, the volume and thickness of capillary endothelium decreased, and perivascular edema was present (Hayatdavoudi *et al.,* 1981). Exposure to a high oxygen pressure of 1 to 4 atmospheres for two to four hours produced partial or total occlusion of capillaries and electron microscopic evidence of damaged endothelial cells in several species (Nasseri *et al.,* 1976). Ozone affects the pulmonary vasculature. The injuries usually take the form of pulmonary arterial lesions that lead to thickening of the artery walls, which is associated with increased levels of serum trypsin protein esterase. Ultrastructural alterations in the alveolar capillaries have also been demonstrated.

The complex gas mixture of automobile exhausts has been shown to cause structural changes in the myocardium and aorta of guinea pigs, as well as exaggeration of hemorrhage and infarct in the hemispheres and basal ganglia in spontaneously hypertensive rats (Roggendorf *et al.,* 1981). In addition, composition and deposition of lipids in the wall of the aorta of rats were affected, presumably owing to the known atherogenic effect of CO present in the gas mixture. Exposure of animals to cigarette smoke, which is known to contain CO, tars, nicotine, and so on, has resulted in coronary artery disease.

Drugs and Other Medicinal Agents. Aspirin, the most widely consumed of all drugs, can produce endothelial damage as part of a pattern of gastric erosion. Studies in rats, utilizing transmission electron microscopy, have shown that there are very early changes in the basement membrane of the endothelial cell of the capillaries and postcapillary venules. This is the first step that may lead to obliteration of small vessels and ischemic infarcts in the gut (Robins, 1980).

The sympathomimetic amines cause damage to arterial vasculature. Amphetamine abuse caused damage to cerebral arteries in an experimental animal model. Large doses of norepinephrine produced toxic effects on the endothelium of rabbit thoracic aorta (Christensen, 1974). Animal studies have demonstrated that nicotine is, upon chronic exposure, toxic to the aortic endothelium. Degenerative changes in the aortic arch have taken the form of increased numbers of microvilli and many focal areas of unusual endothelial cytoarchitecture (Booyse *et al.,* 1981). Degenerative changes of myocardial arterioles have been produced experimentally in dogs forced to smoke. Similar changes have also been detected in humans who were heavy smokers and died of noncardiac causes (Wald and Howard, 1975; Auerbach and Carter, 1980).

Anticoagulants can cause toxic vascular effects. Warfarin has been shown to cause subdural hematoma of the posterior fossa as well as spontaneous epidural spinal hematoma. Studies of warfarin in rats have revealed changes in capillary ultrastructure as well as evidence of cases of vasculitis in humans (Howitt *et al.*, 1982).

Oral contraceptive steroids can produce thromboembolic disorders. An increased incidence of deep-vein phlebitis, pulmonary embolism, and myocardial infarction has been associated with their use in young women (Stolley, 1980). They have been shown to cause intracranial venous thrombosis, which greatly increases the risk of stroke (Fairburn, 1981). Administration of 0.1 percent cholesterol or 0.05 percent dietary estrogen in the form of estradiol to experimental animals produced vascular lesions involving lipid vacuoles in the smooth muscle cells of the aorta. A combination of these two compounds produced severe degenerative atherosclerotic effects on coronary arteries as well as lipid deposition along the ascending aorta. A combination of testosterone and estradiol caused increased vascular smooth muscle cell mitosis and degeneration (Toda *et al.*, 1981).

Antineoplastic drugs cause a variety of effects on different vascular beds. For example, cyclophosphamide causes cerebrovascular and viscerovascular lesions, resulting in hemorrhages (Levine and Sowinski, 1974). In studies with 5-fluoro-2-deoxyuridine in dogs, chronic infusions into the hepatic artery resulted in GI hemorrhage and portal vein thrombosis.

Another category of agents that has been reported to produce vasculotoxic effects are the iodinated radio contrast dyes used for visualization of blood vessels in angiography. In addition to anaphylactic reactions, they can cause thrombophlebitis. The cyanoacrylate adhesives that have found use in repairing blood vessels and other tissues have produced degenerative changes in the arteries of dogs. Certain rapidly polymerizing polyurethane preparations used for transcatheter-embolization techniques in surgery have produced dissolution of arterial walls (Doppman *et al.*, 1978). Dermal microvascular lesions have been reported after plastic film wound dressings were applied in various animal species.

Toxins. Bacterial endotoxins produce a variety of toxic effects in many vascular beds. In the liver, they cause swelling of endothelial cells and adhesion of platelets to sinusoid walls, which affects the microcirculation (McCuskey *et al.*, 1982). In the lung, endotoxins produce increased vascular permeability and pulmonary hypertension. Infusion of endotoxin into experimental animals produces thickening of endothelial cells and formation of fibrin thrombi in small veins. These thrombi were soon lysed, and this process was followed by extravasation of erythrocytes. The excessive hydration of endothelial cells may play a role in these processes (Baris *et al.*, 1980). In piglets, severe coronary artery damage was demonstrated. These changes included disappearance of microvilli from endothelial cells (exfoliation), followed by necrosis of medial smooth muscle cells. All these changes ultimately lead to stenosis of coronary arteries. The terminal phase of endotoxin effects on the systemic vasculature results in a marked hypotension (Personen *et al.*, 1981).

Staphylococcal α toxin in isolated mesenteric arteries caused delayed vasconstriction and, when administered intravenously, caused hypertension in several experimental animal species. Lethal doses, however, caused hypotension and circulatory collapse.

Vascular toxicities of selected chemicals are presented in Table 14–5.

METHODOLOGY FOR EVALUATING VASCULAR TOXICOLOGY

There are a variety of *in vivo* techniques that may be utilized for the evaluation of vascular toxicity. Electromagnetic flowmeters (Kolin, 1960) and ultrasonic Doppler flowmeters (Hartley and Cole, 1974) may be used to measure blood flow directly. These techniques are noninvasive in that they measure blood flow through the wall of vessels without penetrating them. Another approach that is quite useful to measure target organ blood flow relies on arteriovenous differences in the concentrations of dye, various chemical compounds, or gases via dilution that involves the Fick principle (Wood, 1962). The basic assumption in this procedure is that the organ in question removes material from blood flowing through it. Blood flow may also be measured directly using the semiisolated dog biceps or cat hindlimb preparations. Vascular reactivity after administration of toxic chemicals may be assessed in a perfused rat hindlimb preparation (Bekemeier and Hirschelmann, 1989). Angiography, utilizing injections of radiocontrast substances, may be utilized to visualize various vessels (Diamantopoulos *et al.*, 1975), although it is not always possible to separate the direct effects of some of the contrast media on vasculature from preexisting conditions that this procedure is used to diagnose. Finally, direct observations of microvasculature beds may be conducted using a microscope and transilluminating the thin membranes of the hamster cheek pouch, rat or mouse ear, or mesenteric beds.

In vitro preparations utilizing isolated vascular

Table 14-5. VASCULOTOXIC AGENTS*

AGENT (CHEMICAL CLASS OR USE CATEGORY)	VASCULAR EFFECT AND/OR PRIMARY SITE	ASSOCIATED DISEASE STATE AND/OR MECHANISM
A. Heavy Metals		
Arsenic (arsine)	Arteriosclerosis Pulmonary vascular lesions	Peripheral vascular disease Noncirrhotic portal hypertension Pulmonary edema
Beryllium	Decreased hepatic flow: hemorrhage	Occlusion of hepatic venous flow
Cadmium	Aortic damage to endothelium allowing lipid deposition; lesions in uterine endothelial cleft; renal arteriolar thickening; effect on microcirculation	Atherosclerosis Hypertension
Chromium (deficiency)	Atherosclerotic aortic plaques	Atherosclerosis; elevated serum cholesterol
Copper (chronic)	Acceleration of atherosclerosis	
(acute)	Hypotension	
Copper (deficiency)	Aortic aneurysms	
Germanium	Hemorrhage, edema in lungs and GI tract	
Indium	Hemorrhage and thrombosis in the kidney and liver	
Lead	Damage to endothelial cell with changes in blood-brain barrier permeability; changes in arterial elasticity; effects on ground substance; sclerosis of vessels in the kidney	Encephalopathy Hypertension
Mercury	Preglomerular vasoconstriction: glomerular immune complex deposits; lesions of the aorta; opening of blood-brain barrier	Glomerulonephritis; inhibition of amino acid uptake
Selenium	Atherosclerotic plaques	Atherosclerosis
Thallium	Perivascular cellular infiltration in the brain (cuffing)	
B. Industrial and Environmental Agents		
Allylamine	Renal artery lesion; intimal smooth muscle proliferation in coronary arteries	Endogenous formation of acrolein with destruction of vascular protein and nucleic acid components
β-Aminopropionitrile	Aortic lesions and atheroma formation	Damage to vascular connective tissue matrix; aneurysm
Boron	Hemorrhage; edema; increase in microvascular permeability in the lung Tumors of pulmonary blood vessels	Pulmonary edema
Carbamylhydrazine HCl		Cancer
Carbon disulfide	Microvascular effect on ocular fundus and retina; direct injury to endothelial wall; promoter of atheroma formation	Coronary vascular disease Atherosclerosis

Table 14–5. (*Continued*)

AGENT (CHEMICAL CLASS OR USE CATEGORY)	VASCULAR EFFECT AND/OR PRIMARY SITE	ASSOCIATED DISEASE STATE AND/OR MECHANISM
Chlorophenoxy herbicides		
Dimethylnitrosamine	Decreased hepatic flow; hemorrhage; necrosis	Hypertension
4-Fluoro-10-methyl-12-benzyanthracene	Pulmonary artery lesions; coronary vessel lesion	Occlusion of veins
Glycerol	Strong renal vasoconstriction	Acute renal failure
Hydrochloric acid (aspiration of stomach contents)	Increased microvascular permeability	Pulmonary edema
Hydrogen fluoride	Hemorrhage; edema in the lung	Pulmonary edema
Paraquat	Vascular damage in lungs and brain	Cerebral purpura
Pyrrolizidine alkaloids	Pulmonary vasculitis; damage to vascular smooth muscle cells; proliferation of endothelium and vascular connective tissue in the liver	Pulmonary hypertension Hepatic venoocclusive disease
Organophosphate pesticides		Cerebral arteriosclerosis
Vinyl chloride	Portal hypertension; tumors of hepatic blood vessels	Cancer
C. Gases		
Auto exhaust	Hemorrhage and infarct in cerebral hemispheres; atheroma formation in aorta	Atherosclerosis due to CO content
Carbon monoxide	Damage to intimal layer; edema; atheroma formation	Atherosclerosis
Nitric oxide	Vacuolation of arteriolar endothelial cells; edema, thickening of alveolar-capillary membranes	Pulmonary edema
Oxygen	Vasoconstriction-retinal damage; increased retinal vascular permeability-edema; increased pulmonary vascular permeability-edema	Blindness in neonate; shrinking of visual field in adults; pulmonary edema
Ozone	Arterial lesions in the lung	Pulmonary edema
D. Drugs and Related Compounds		
Antibiotic-Antimitotics		
Cyclophosphamide	Lesions of pulmonary endothelial cells	
5-Fluorodeoxyuridine	GI tract hemorrhage; portal vein thrombosis	
Gentamicin	Long-lasting renal vasoconstriction	Renal failure

Vasoactive Agents

Agent	Effect
Amphetamine	Cerebrovascular lesions secondary to drug abuse
	Disseminated arterial lesions similar to periarteritis nodosa
Dihydroergotamine	Spasm of retinal vessels
Ergonovine	Coronary artery spasm
Ergotamine	Vasospastic phenomena with and without thrombosis; medial atrophy
	Angina
	Gangrene of peripheral tissues
Epinephrine	Peripheral arterial thrombi in hyperlipemic rats
Histamine	Coronary spasm; damage to endothelial cells in hepatic portal vein
	Participates in thrombogenesis
Methysergide	Intimal proliferation; vascular occlusion of coronary arteries
	Coronary artery disease
Nicotine	Alteration of cytoarchitecture of aortic endothelium; increase in microvilli
	"Aging" of coronary arteries
Nitrites and nitrates	Spasm of coronary artery; endothelial damage
Norepinephrine	Repeated vasodilation

Metabolic Affectors

Agent	Effect
Alloxan	Microvascular retinopathy
	Diabetes; blindness
Chloroquine	Retinopathy
Fructose	Microvascular lesions in retina
	Diabeteslike condition
Iodoacetates	Vascular changes in retina

Anticoagulants

Agent	Effect
Sodium warfarin; warfarin	Spinal hematoma; subdural hematoma; vasculitis
	Uncontrolled bleeding; hemorrhage

Radiocontrast Dyes

Agent	Effect
Metrizamide; metrizoate	Coagulation; necrosis in celiac and renal vasculature

Cyanoacrylate Adhesives

Agent	Effect
2-Cyano-acrylate-n-butyl	Granulation of arteries with fibrous masses
Ethyl-2-cyanoacrylate	Degeneration of vascular wall with thrombosis
Methyl-2-cyanoacrylate	Vascular necrosis

Miscellaneous Drugs and Compounds

Agent	Effect
Aminorex fumarate	Intimal and medial thickening of pulmonary arteries
	Pulmonary arterial hypertension
Aspirin	Endothelial damage; gastric erosion obliteration of small vessels; ischemic infarcts
	Changes in the basement membrane of endothelial cells

Table 14-5. (*Continued*)

AGENT (CHEMICAL CLASS OR USE CATEGORY)	VASCULAR EFFECT AND/OR PRIMARY SITE	ASSOCIATED DISEASE STATE AND/OR MECHANISM
Cholesterol; oxygenated derivatives of cholesterol: noncholesterol steroids	Atheroma formation; arterial damage	Atherosclerosis
Homocysteine	Increase of vascular fragility; loss of endothelium; proliferation of smooth muscle cells promotion of atheroma formation	Atherosclerosis; effects on protein synthesis
Oral contraceptives	Thrombosis in cerebral and peripheral vasculature	Thromboembolic disorders
Penicillamine	Vascular lesion in connective tissue matrix of arterial wall; glomerular immune complex deposits	Glomerulonephritis; inhibits synthesis of vascular connective tissue
Talc and other silicates	Pulmonary arteriolar thrombosis; emboli	
Tetradecylsulfate Na	Sclerosis of veins (used as a sclerosing agent)	Cytotoxicity
Thromboxane A$_2$	Extreme cerebral vasoconstriction	Cerebrovascular ischemia

* Based on information gathered from sources listed in references.

strips or rings in muscle baths allow for perfusion of smooth muscle with agents in question (Trendelenburg, 1974). These preparations may include or omit the endothelial cells in order to determine the role of this vascular layer on responses (Furchgott and Zawadzki, 1980; Luscher and Vanhoutte, 1988). Electrophysiological procedures that utilize intracellular microelectrodes allow for recording and manipulation of resting membrane potentials, action potentials, and cell membrane resistance. Toxic materials that alter these parameters may be thus evaluated (Johansson and Somlyo, 1980). The use of *in vitro* techniques that involve tissue culture growth of smooth muscle cells from 10- to 20-day-old chick embryos or rat aorta may be used to determine direct effects of assorted vasculotoxic agents on noninnervated vascular smooth muscle cells (Sperelakis, 1982).

Finally, there are a variety of animal models for vascular disease found in humans. These include the use of various avian species, nonprimate mammals, and nonhuman primates to model atherosclerosis involving dietary manipulations or certain vasculotoxic agents. Different types of hypertension may be modeled using variations of the Goldblatt renal artery ligation procedure (Goldblatt *et al.*, 1934) as well as the genetic hypertensive SH rat (Okamoto, 1969), the Dahl salt-sensitive rat (Dahl *et al.*, 1962), or the DOCA-salt–induced water retention model.

DETECTION OF CARDIOVASCULAR TOXIC EFFECTS IN EXPERIMENTAL ANIMALS

The detectability of cardiovascular toxicities in animal experiments is a function of their mechanism. Although exaggerated pharmacologic effects are generally recognized, there are examples of species differences, as has already been mentioned for digitalis. Serotonin consistently increases the pulmonary blood pressure in dogs and cats but rarely in humans; L-dopa increases the systemic blood pressure in rats and cats but produces postural hypotension, at least with chronic administration, in humans; prostaglandin $F_2\alpha$ decreases the blood pressure in cats but increases it in humans (Brunner and Gross, 1979). Great differences in sensitivity of the contractile response to various agonists have been detected in the coronary arteries *in vitro* from the dog, pig, and cow (Ginsburg *et al.*, 1980). Some of these variations are most likely related to the differences in the distribution of subtypes of receptors that mediate different effects in the various species.

Since preclinical or premarketing toxicity studies of chemicals are done in healthy, well-nourished young adult animals, facultative toxicities, which require a predisposing condition, may be overlooked.

A preexisting cardiovascular disease can sensitize the cardiovascular system to toxicity. Patients with coronary artery disease have decreased exercise tolerance after the ingestion of 2 oz of ethanol; they may not tolerate the cardiovascular effects of inhalation anesthetics and may succumb with postsurgical myocardial infarction. Patients with valvular heart disease and congestive heart failure are at risk with respect to the slight negative inotropic effects of certain drugs (e.g., aminoglycoside antibiotics).

Obesity, poor nutritional status, or old age can contribute to cardiovascular toxicity. An example of the sensitizing role of overweight has been shown in animal experiments (e.g., with isoproterenol in rats). The subcutaneous LD50 is greatly reduced, and death is due to ventricular fibrillation (Balazs *et al.*, 1983). Poor nutritional status or deficiency of a specific vitamin (*e.g.*, thiamine) predisposes to the cardiotoxicity of cobalt and of arsenic compounds. The adaptability of the cardiovascular system is reduced with age; this reduction and the large use of drugs in the elderly are responsible for the majority of adverse drug effects, especially those of the antidepressants, on this organ system.

Drug interactions play a major role in the development of severe acute cardiovascular toxicity. Diuretics that cause excess loss of K^+ and Mg^{2+} sensitize to the effects of digitalis and also to those of other cardiotoxic agents. Concurrent administration of cardiovascular drugs having similar effects, but which act by a different mechanism, results in potentiation of specific adverse effects; e.g., propranolol a β-receptor blocker, with verapamil, a Ca^{2+} channel blocker, causes AV block and profound hypotension.

The detection of a toxic effect is uncertain when the mechanism is not related to a pharmacologic effect, that is, when a reactive metabolite produces the injury. The biotransformation of the chemical as well as the rate of reactive metabolite formation varies between species. The most difficult is the detection of the hypersensitivity reactions, particularly the antibody- or lymphocyte-mediated cytotoxicity, and the immune complex-induced injuries. They are not likely to be detected, even in early clinical trials in humans, because of genetically controlled individual differences in susceptibility to the antigen.

Detection of cardiovascular toxicity requires a complete physical examination in both experimental animals and humans. The ECG is a generally applicable indicator of cardiac function, whereas the blood pressure is the circulatory indicator, for diagnostic purposes. A comprehensive monograph deals with *in vivo* techniques as applied to toxicology in animal experiments (Brunner and Gross, 1979). Careful morphologic examinations should be conducted postmortem to detect and characterize the structural changes. In addition to *in vivo* pharmacologic measurements, *in vitro* electrophysiologic and biochemical methods are used to investigate the mechanism of action for various cardiovascular toxicities. These should be evaluated in relation to the desired pharmacologic effect in each tested species. Data obtained in experimental animals need to be studied further in humans; clinical pharmacologic and/or epidemiologic investigations should be performed to substantiate findings from animal experiments.

REFERENCES

Akera, T., and Brown, B. S.: Cardiovascular toxicology of cardiotonic drugs and chemicals. In Van Stee, F. W. (ed.): *Cardiovascular Toxicology*. Raven Press, New York. 1982. pp. 109–135.

Auerbach, O., and Carter, H. W.: Smoking and the heart. In Bristow, M. R. (ed.): *Drug-Induced Heart Disease*. Elsevier North-Holland Press, Amsterdam, 1980, pp. 359–376.

Bakay, L.: *The Blood Brain Barrier*. Charles C Thomas, Springfield, Ill., 1956, pp. 88–91.

Balazs, T.: An overview on delayed toxic effects of pre- and perinatal drug exposure. In Yoshida, H.; Hagrihara, Y.; and Ebashi, S. (eds.): *Advances in Pharmacology and Therapeutics II*. Pergamon Press, Ltd., Oxford, 1982, pp. 163–176.

———: Detection of rare adverse reactions induced by chemicals. In Homburger. R. (ed): *Safety Evaluation and Regulation of Chemicals*. S. Karger, Basel, 1983, pp. 243–250.

Balazs, T., and Bloom, S.: Cardiotoxicity of adrenergic bronchodilator and vasodilating antihypertensive drugs. In Van Stee, E. W. (ed.): *Cardiovascular Toxicology*. Raven Press, New York, 1982, pp. 199–221.

Balazs, T., and Ferrans, V. J.: Cardiac lesions induced by chemicals. *Environ. Health Perspect.*, **26**:181–191, 1978.

Balazs, T.; Ferrans, V. J.; El-Hage, A.; Ehrreich, S. J.; Johnson, G. L.; Herman, E. H.; Atkinson, J. C.; and West, W. L.: Study of the mechanism of hydralazine-induced myocardial necrosis in the rat. *Toxicol. Appl. Pharmacol.*, **59**:524–534, 1981.

Balazs, T.; Johnson, G.; Joseph, X.; Ehrreich, S.; and Bloom, S.: Sensitivity and resistance of the myocardium to the toxicity of isoproterenol in rats. In Spitzer, J. (ed.): *Myocardial Injury*. Plenum Publishing Corp., New York. 1983, pp. 563–577.

Baris, C.; Guest, M. M.; and Frazer, M. E.: Direct effects of endotoxin on the microcirculation. *Adv. Shock Res.*, **4**:153–160, 1980.

Beehler, C. C.: Oxygen and the eye. *Surv. Ophthalmol.*, **9**:549–560, 1964.

Bekemeier, H., and Hirschelmann, L.: Reactivity of resistance blood vessels *ex vivo* after administration of toxic chemicals to laboratory animals: arteriolotoxicity. *Toxicol. Lett.*, **49**:49–54, 1989.

Bigger, J. T., and Hoffman, B. F.: Antiarrhythmic drugs. In Gilman, A. G.; Goodman, L. S.; and Gilman. A. (eds.): *Goodman and Gilman's The Phar-*macological Basis of Therapeutics, 6th ed. Macmillan Publishing Co., New York, 1980, pp. 761–792.

Billingham, M. F.: Morphologic changes in drug-induced heart disease. In Bristow, M. R. (ed.): *Drug-Induced Heart Disease*. Elsevier/North-Holland Press, Amsterdam, 1980, pp. 128–149.

Boor, P. J.: Allylamine cardiotoxicity; metabolism and mechanism. In Spitzer, J. (ed.): *Myocardial Injury*. Plenum Publishing Corp., New York, 1983, pp. 533–543.

Booyse, F. M.: Osikowicz, G.; and Quarfoot, A. J.: Effects of chronic oral consumption of nicotine on the rabbit aortic endothelium. *Am. J. Pathol.*, **102**:229–238, 1981.

Bowman, W. C., and Rand, M. J.: The heart and drugs affecting cardiac function. In Bowman, W. C., and Rand, M. J. (eds.): *Textbook of Pharmacology*. Blackwell Scientific Publications, Oxford; C. V. Mosby Co., St. Louis, 1980, pp. 22.10–22.75.

Braunwald, E.: Pathophysiology of heart failure. In Braunwald, E. (ed.): *Heart Disease: A Texbook of Cardiovascular Medicine*. W. B. Saunders Co., Philadelphia, 1980, pp. 453–471.

Braunwald, E.; Ross, J., Jr.; and Sonnerblick, E. H.: Disorders of myocardinal function. In Isselbacher, K. J.; Adams, R. D.; Braunwald, E.; Petersdorf, R. G.; and Wilson, J. D. (eds.): *Harrison's Principles of Internal Medicine*, 9th ed. McGraw-Hill Book Co., New York, 1980a.

Braunwald, E.; Sonnerblick, E. H.; and Ross, J., Jr.: Contraction of the normal heart. In Braunwald, E. (ed.): *Heart Disease: A Textbook of Cardiovascular Medicine*. W. B. Saunders Co., Philadelphia, 1980b, pp. 413–452.

Brody, T. M., and Chubb, J. M.: Biochemical and ionic mechanisms of cardiotoxic agents. In Balazs, T. (ed.): *Cardiac Toxicology*, Vol. 1. CRC Press, Boca Raton, Fla., 1981, pp. 2–13.

Brunner, H., and Gross, F.: Cardiovascular pharmacology. In Zbinden, G., and Gross, F. (eds.): *Pharmacological Methods in Toxicology*. Pergamon Press, Ltd., Oxford, 1979, pp. 63–99.

Christensen, B. C.: Repair in arterial tissue. *Virchows Arch. Pathol. Anat.*, **363**:33–46, 1974.

Cliff, L. E.; Caranasos, G. J.; and Stewart, R. B.: Clinical problems with drugs. In Smith, L. H. (ed.): *Major Problems in Internal Medicine*. W. B. Saunders Co., Philadelphia, 1975, pp. 115–126.

Dahl, L. K.; Heine M.; and Tassinari, L.: Effect of chronic excess salt. Evidence that factors play an important role in susceptibility to experimental hypertension. *J. Exp. Med.*, **115**:1173–1190, 1962.

Datta, D. J.: Letter; arsenic and non-cirrhotic portal hypertension. *Lancet*, **21**:7956, 1976.

Deglin, S. M.; Deglin, J. M.; and Chung, E. K.: Drug-induced cardiovascular disease. *Drugs*, **14**:29–40, 1977.

Diamantopoulos, G.; Matthes, D.; and Goerttler, A.: Coronary angiographic demonstration of the dilation effect of dipyridamole on coronary arteries and its inhibition by caffeine. *Arzheim-Forsch.*, **25**:1396–1400, 1975.

Dontos, H. A., and Hess, M. L.: Oxygen radicals and vascular damage. In Spitzer, J. (ed.): *Myocardial Injury*. Plenum Publishing Corp., New York, 1983, pp. 365–377.

Doppman, J. L.; Aven, W.; Bowman, R. L.; Wood, L. L.; and Girton, M.: A rapidly polymerizing polyurethane for transcathetal embolization. *Cardiovasc. Radio.*, **1**:109–116, 1978.

Doroshow, J. H.: Role of reactive oxygen production in doxorubicin cardiac toxicity. In Hacker, M. P.; Lazo, J. S.; and Tritton, T. R. (eds.): *Organ Directed Toxicities of Anticancer Drugs*. Martinus Nijhoff, Boston, 1988, pp. 31–40.

Fairburn, B.: Intracranial venous thrombosis complicating oral contraceptive: treatment by anticoagulant drugs. *Br. Med. J.*, **2**:647, 1981.

Ferrans, V. J.: Overview of morphological reactions of the heart to toxic injury. In Balazs, T. (ed.): *Cardiac Toxicology III*. CRC Press Inc., Boca Raton, Fla., 1982, pp. 83–109.

Furchgott, R. F., and Zawadzki, J. V.: The obligatory role of endothelial cells in the relaxation of arterial smooth muscle by acetylcholine. *Nature*, **288**:373–376, 1980.

Ginsburg, R.; Bristow, M. R.; Schroeder, J. S.; Harrison, D. C.; and Stinson, E. B.: Potential pharmacological mechanisms involved in coronary artery spasm. In Bristow, M. R. (ed.): *Drug-Induced Heart Disease*. Elsevier North-Holland Press, Amsterdam, 1980, pp. 457–465.

Goldblatt, H.; Lynch, J.; Hanzel, R. F.; and Summerville, W. W.: Studies in experimental hypertension. 1. The production of resistent elevation of systolic blood pressure by means of renal ischemia. *J. Exp. Med.*, **59**:347–379, 1934.

Hartley, C. J., and Cole, J. S.: An ultrasonic pulsed doppler system for measuring blood flow in small vessels. *J. Appl. Physiol.*, **37**:626–629, 1974.

Harvey, A. M. (ed.): The *Principles and Practice of Medicine*, 20th ed. Appleton-Century-Crofts, East Norwalk, Conn., 1980.

Hayatdavoudi, G.; O'Neal, J. J.; Barry, B. E.; Freeman, B. A.; and Crapo, J. D.: Pulmonary injury in rats following continuous exposure to 60% O_2 for 7 days. *J. Appl. Physiol.*, **51**:1220–1231, 1981.

Herman, E. H., Ferrans, V. J.; Young, R. S. K.; and Hamlin, R. L.: Effect of pretreatment with ICRF-187 on the total cumulative dose of doxorubicin tolerated by beagle dogs. *Cancer Res.*, **48**:6918–6925, 1988.

Howitt, A. J.; Williams, A. J.; and Skinner, C.: Warfarin induced vasculitis: a dose-related phenomena in susceptible individuals. *Postgrad. Med. J.*, **58**:233–234, 1982.

Jackson, B.: Developmental cardiotoxic effects of chemicals. In Balazs, T. (ed.): *Cardiac Toxicology III*. CRC Press, Inc., Boca Raton, Fla., 1981, pp. 163–177.

Johansson, R., and Somlyo, A. P.: Electrophysiology and excitation-contraction coupling. In Bohr, D. F.; Somlyo, A. P.; and Sparks, H. V., Jr. (eds.): *Handbook of Physiology, Section 2, The Cardiovascular System*. Amer. Physiol. Soc., Bethesda, Md, 1980, pp. 301–323.

Kinney, J. A.; McKay, C. L.; and Gordon, R. A.: The use of fluoroscein angiography to study oxygen toxicity. *Ann. Ophthalmol.*, **9**:895–898, 1977.

Koch-Weser, J.: Drug-induced arrhythmias in man. *Pharmacol. Ther.*, **5**:125–131, 1979.

Kolin, A.: Circulatory system methods; blood flow determination by electromagnetic method. In Glasser, O. (ed.): *Medical Physics*, Vol. 3. Year Book Publishers, Chicago, 1960, pp. 141–154.

Kontos, H. A., and Hess, M. L.: Oxygen radicals and vascular damage. *Adv. Exp. Med. Biol.* **161**:363–375, 1983.

Levine, S., and Sowinski, R.: Cyclophosphamide induced cerebral and visceral lesions in rats. Enhancement by endotoxins. *Arch. Pathol.*, **98**:177–182, 1974.

Luscher, T. F., and Vanhoutte, P. M.: Endothelium-dependent responses in human blood vessels. *Trends Pharmacol. Sci.*, **9**:181–184, 1988.

Magos, L.: The effects of industrial chemicals on the heart. In Balazs, T. (ed.): *Cardiac Toxicology II*. CRC Press, Inc., Boca Raton, Fla., 1981, pp. 203–209.

McCuskey, R. S.; Urbaschek, R.; McCuskey, P. A.; and Urbaschek, B.: *In vivo* microscopic studies of responses of the liver to endotoxin. *Klin. Wochenschr.*, **60**:749–751, 1982.

Merin, R. G.: Myocardial metabolism for the toxicologist. *Environ. Health Perspect.*, **26**:169–174, 1978.

———: Cardiac toxicology of inhalation anesthetics. In Balazs, T. (ed.): *Cardiac Toxicology II*. CRC Press, Inc., Boca Raton, Fla., 1981, pp. 1–15.

Myers, C. E.: Role of iron in anthracycline action. In Hacker, M. P.; Lazo, J. S.; and Tritton, T. R. (eds.): *Organ Directed Toxicities of Anticancer Drugs*. Martinus Nijhoff, Boston, 1988, pp. 17–30.

Nasseri, M.; Eisele, R.; Kotter, D.; Kirstaedter, H.; and Wolf, J.: Comparative studies on the effect of oxygen high pressure (OHP) on different species with special reference to organ preservation. *Respiration*, **33**:70–83, 1976.

Olson, R. E.; Dhalla, N. S.; and Sun, C. N.: Changes in energy stores in the hypoxic heart. *Cardiology*, **56**:114–124, 1971–72.

Okamoto, K.: Spontaneous hypertension in rats. *Int. Rev. Exp. Pathol.* **7**:227–270, 1969.

Personen, E.; Kaprio, E.; Rapola, J.; Soveri, T.; and Okansen, H.: Endothelial cell damage in piglet coronary artery after i.v. adminstration of *E. coli* endotoxin. *Atherosclerosis*, **40**:65–73. 1981.

Rapoport, S.: *Blood-Brain Barrier in Physiology and Medicine*. Raven Press, New York. 1976. pp. 129–152.

Revis, N. W.: Relationship of vanadium, cadmium, lead, nickel, cobalt and soft water to myocardial and vascular toxicity and cardiovascular disease. In Van Stee, E. W. (ed.): *Cardiovascular Toxicology*. Raven Press, New York, 1982. pp. 365–377.

Reynolds, A. C.: Cardiac arrhythmias in sensitized hearts. *Res. Commun. Chem. Pathol. Pharmacol.*, **40**:3–14, 1983.

Robins, P. G.: Ultrastructural observations on the pathogenesis of aspirin-induced gastric erosions. *Br. J. Exp. Pathol.*, **61**:497–504, 1980.

Roggendorf, W.; Thron, N. L.; Ast, D.; and Kholer, P. R.: Effects of chronic exposure to auto exhaust gas on the CNS of normotensive and hypertensive rats. *Acta Neuropathol. (Suppl.) (Berl.)* **7**:17–19, 1981.

Rubin, J. T., and Rubin, E.: Myocardial toxicity of alcohols, aldehydes and glycols, including alcoholic cardiomyopathy. In Van Stee, E. W. (ed.): *Cardiovascular Toxicology*. Raven Press, New York, 1982, pp. 353–363.

Schlant, R. C., and Sonnenblick, E. H.: Pathophysiology of heart failure. In Hurst, J. W. (ed.): *The Heart*. McGraw-Hill Book Co., New York, 1982, pp. 382–407.

Schroeder, H. A.: Trace elements in degenerative cardiovascular disease. In Conn, H. L., Jr., and Horwitz, O. (eds.): *Cardiac and Vascular Disease*, Vol. II, Lea & Febiger, Philadelphia, 1971, pp. 973–977.

Smith, P., and Health, D.: Evagination of vascular smooth muscle during early stages of crotalaria pulmonary hypertension. *J. Pathol.*, **124**:177–183, 1976.

Sperelakis, N.: Cultured heart cell reaggregate model for studying problems in cardiac toxicology. In Van Stee, E. W. (ed.): *Cardiovascular Toxicology*. Raven Press, New York, 1982, pp. 57–108.

Speyer, J. L.; Green, M. D.; Sanger, J.; Ward, C.; Kramer, A.; Rey, M.; Wernz, J. C.; Blum, R. H.; Meyers, M.; Muggia, F.; Ferrans, V. J.; Stecy, P.; Felt, F.; Dubin, N.; Jacquotte, A.; Taubes, S.; and London, C.: A trial of ICRF-187 to selectively protect against chronic adriamycin cardiac toxicity: rational and preliminary results of a clinical trial. In Hacker, M. P.; Lazo, J. S.; and Tritton, T. R. (eds.): *Organ Directed Toxicities of Anticancer Drugs*. Martinus Nijhoff, Boston, 1988, pp. 64–73.

Steffey, E. P.: Cardiovascular effects of inhalation anesthetics. In Van Stee, E. W. (ed.): *Cardiovascular Toxicology*. Raven Press, New York, 1982, pp. 259–281.

Stimmel, B.: *Cardiovascular Effects of Mood Altering Drugs*. Raven Press, New York, 1979.

Stolley, P. D.: Drug, thromboembolism and myocardial infarction. In Bristow, M. R. (ed.): *Drug-Induced Heart Disease*. Elsevier/North-Holland Press, Amsterdam, 1980, pp. 313–321.

Thomsen, H. K., and Kjeldsen, K.: Aortic intimal injury in rabbit. An evaluation of a threshold limit. *Arch. Environ. Health,* **30**:604–607, 1975.

Titus, E. O.: A molecular biologic approach to cardiac toxicology. In Spitzer, J. (ed.): *Myocardial Injury*. Plenum Publishing Corp., New York, 1983, pp. 509–519.

Toda, J.; Leszozynski, D.; and Kummerow, F.: Vasculotoxic effects of dietary testosterone, estradiol and cholesterol on chick artery. *J. Pathol.,* **134**:219–231. 1981.

Toth, B.; Shimizeu, H.; and Erickson, J.: Carbamylhydrazine hydrochloride as a lung and blood vessel tumor inducer in Swiss mice. *Eur. J. Cancer,* **11**:17–22. 1975.

Trendelenburg, U.: The relaxation of rabbit aortic strips after a preceding exposure to sympathomimetic amines. *Naunyn-Schmiedeberg's Arch. Pharmacol.,* **281**:13–46, 1974.

Van Fleet, J. F.; Ferrans, V. J.; and Herman, E.: Cardiovascular and skeletal muscle systems. In Haschek-Hock, W. M., and Rousseaux, C. G. (eds.): *Fundamentals of Toxicologic Pathology*. Academic Press, San Diego, in press.

Van Stee, E. W.: Cardiovascular toxicology: foundation and scope. In Van Stee, E. W. (ed.): *Cardiovascular Toxicology*. Raven Press, New York, 1982, pp. 1–35.

Wald, N., and Howard, S.: Smoking, carbon monoxide and disease. *Ann. Occup. Hyg.,* **18**:1–14, 1975.

Wood, E. H. (ed.): *Symposium on the Use of Indicator-Dilution Techniques in the Study of the Circulation*. American Heart Association Monograph, No. 4, 1962.

Zakhari, S., and Aviado, D. M.: Cardiovascular toxicology and aerosol propellants, refrigerants and related solvents. In Van Stee, E. W. (ed.): *Cardiovascular Toxicology*. Raven Press, New York, 1982, pp. 281–327.

Zbinden, G.: Evaluation of thrombogenic effects. In Elliott, H. W.; George, R.; and Okun, R. (eds.): *Annual Review of Pharmacology and Toxicology*, Vol. 16. Annual Review Inc., Palo Alto, Calif., 1976, pp. 177–188.

Chapter 15

TOXIC RESPONSES OF THE SKIN

Edward A. Emmett

INTRODUCTION

In this chapter, a survey of toxicologic principles related to the skin will be given. No attempt will be made to be exhaustive. There is a large amount of information available, especially with regard to the effects of specific toxic agents for which more comprehensive works must be consulted. Several excellent sources are available (e.g., Foussereau *et al.,* 1982; Adams, 1983; Marzulli and Maibach, 1983). The discussion will generally be confined to the effects of chemical agents or to the combined effects of physical and chemical agents such as are responsible for photosensitization. The skin is, of course, vulnerable to the effects of physical agents; for example, both ionizing and nonionizing radiation have important and complex effects; and it is profoundly affected by heat, repeated trauma, cold, and humidity. However, these are not dealt with in this chapter.

The skin has great importance as an organ that interfaces with the external environment and constitutes a barrier and transition zone between the internal and external milieux. A major function of skin is to preserve the constituents and composition of the body contents—witness the massive and potentially lethal fluid losses in extensive burns.

The skin, and particularly the dead outer stratum corneum layer, is also an excellent barrier against certain external chemical agents, although others may penetrate readily. Indeed, there are many agents for which, under normal circumstances of exposure, the skin represents the major portal of entry. The subject of percutaneous absorption is thus of great importance both for general toxicology and for effects on the skin, since toxic reactions in the skin generally depend on interactions of toxicants with the less superficial, living layers of the skin. However, it remains very difficult to predict accurately penetration through the skin from theory or animal models (Grandjean *et al.,* 1988; Stoughton, 1989).

The skin displays a limited, but fairly large, variety of toxic responses reflecting the major patterns of possible structural and functional changes. Because the surface of the skin is so readily visible, toxic reactions have been described mainly on the basis of morphologic rather than functional changes. In the case of the skin, the biochemical sequence of toxic events is often less well understood than for certain other organs. It is important to recognize that similar morphologic changes could result from widely differing toxicologic mechanisms. Although some efforts have been made, rigid standardization of morphologic criteria is not yet widely practiced.

In actual practice, chemical injury to the skin is influenced by a large number of environmental factors that alter the interface. These include variations in heat and humidity, friction, pressure, trauma, abrasion, wind, vibration, ultraviolet and visible radiations, electrical current, and coincident effects of infestations or infection. There are morphologic, physiologic, and biochemical protective and homeostatic mechanisms in the skin; these include the epidermal barrier, eccrine sweating, phagocytic cells and processes, metabolic detoxication, specific immunologic processes, and protective mechanisms, such as melanin pigmentation, which protect against ultraviolet radiation. These may vary on a genetic or phenotypic basis and may be influenced by systemic or local disease or by the effects of other toxic substances. For example, individuals with atopy (characterized in part by infantile and adolescent eczema, hayfever, and asthma) seem particularly prone to develop irritant dermatitis. The actual expression or degree of expression of a toxic effect may thus be the end result of a markedly complex set of local and general factors. In experimental studies, these factors are also of crucial importance and may help to explain the rather poor concordance that has been reported between laboratories for assessment of effects such as irritation (Weil and Scala, 1971). Comparability of technique is of paramount importance in this field.

Although the actual burden of chemically induced human skin disease cannot be reliably computed from information currently available, it is clear that it is of significant proportions. Figures from the United States Department of Labor indicate that occupational skin disease, the vast majority of which is due to effects of toxic chemicals, is the most frequently reported occupational disease (Report to OSHA, 1979). In California, which has the most comprehensive occupational disease-reporting system, skin diseases accounted for 40 percent of reported diseases; eye conditions, 29 percent; and chemical burns, 9.7 percent. Thus, conditions primarily due to external contact constituted 79 percent of these diseases. By contrast, other conditions due to toxic materials accounted for 12.6 percent, namely, respiratory including pneumoconioses, 5.5 percent; digestive and other symptoms, 4.2 percent; and systemic effects, 3 percent (Baginsky, 1982). Irritant and allergic contact dermatitis account for the great majority of occupational skin disorders. In addition to occupational exposures from handling chemicals, there is a large variety of opportunities for potentially hazardous materials to contact the skin during the course of daily life, including contact with clothing, cosmetics, cleansing agents, contaminated surfaces, incompletely cured resins, plants, foods, jewelry, and a vast array of consumer products. Good epidemiologic data on the incidence of toxic cutaneous responses in nonoccupational settings are, however, sparse or nonexistent. The toxicity of agents contacting the skin is clearly of widespread interest and is vital to those interested in the safety of cosmetics, toiletries, and household products. A standard nomenclature and list of cosmetic ingredients have been established to assist in this task (CTFA, 1982).

The information available supports the conclusion that, other factors being equal, toxic effects on the skin are characterized by definable dose-response relationships, in which concentration, duration, extent of application, and the total dosage applied are important. However, in contrast to inhalation exposures to airborne substances, other than in experimental circumstances, our ability to assess accurately cutaneous exposures is poorly developed. In order to estimate exposure, levels on contaminated surfaces have been measured, absorbent pads applied to the skin, skin surface wipings taken, and for selected agents, quantitation of fluorescence or of indicator materials performed, but none of these is universally satisfactory. In the estimation of total dosage to the organism, biologic monitoring will satisfactorily measure total absorption by all routes including the percutaneous route. This is one of the reasons that it generally offers a better estimate of risk than ambient environmental monitoring (Lauwerys, 1983).

STRUCTURE AND FUNCTION

A diagrammatic representation of the structure of the skin is shown in Figure 15–1. The skin contains three main layers: an outer layer of epithelial tissue, the *epidermis;* a loose connective tissue layer, the *dermis;* and an inner layer of variable thickness containing adipose tissue and connective tissue, the *hypodermis* or *panniculus adiposus* (Montagna and Parakkal, 1974). The epidermis contains a number of cell types including keratinocytes, melanocytes, Langerhans cells, and Merkel cells. Most numerous are the keratinocytes, which serve to produce keratin in the process of keratinization or cornification.

The epidermis is divided into several layers based on the behavior of the keratinocytes. The *basal layer* consists of germinative cells, which are extremely active metabolically, divide rapidly, and display many mitotic figures and label with thymidine. Above this layer are two differentiated layers of viable cells, the *spinous* or *prickle cell layer* and the *granular cell layer.* The outer layer, the *stratum corneum,* consists of a multicellular membrane of dried, flattened keratinocytes, which have no metabolic activity and represent the nonviable end product of the synthetic activity of the lower layers. This layer is the main barrier site in the skin for water, electrolytes, most other chemicals, microorganisms, and electrical resistance. The epidermis also provides some mechanical resistance to stretching.

Keratinization begins with the synthesis of fibrous prekeratins in the basal layer; aggregated filaments run the length of the cell by the time it reaches the spinous layer. In the granular layer, protein granules are formed that contribute to the process. In the stratum corneum, the cells are cornified and filled with a filamentous network of keratins embedded in a matrix containing mucus and lipids surrounded by a highly chemically resistant thickened cell envelope. Between the cornified cells is an intercellular material that contains ceramides that appear to contribute to the permeability barrier. These structural components are closely related, and the complex multicomponent system results in the effectiveness of the barrier (Scheuplein and Blank, 1971; Matolsky, 1987). Retinoids have been shown to profoundly alter the differentiation pattern of human epidermal keratinocytes, but the underlying

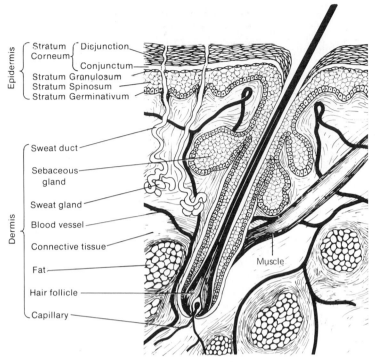

Epidermis
- Stratum Corneum
  - Disjunction
  - Conjunctum
- Stratum Granulosum
- Stratum Spinosum
- Stratum Germinativum

Dermis
- Sweat duct
- Sebaceous gland
- Sweat gland
- Blood vessel
- Connective tissue
- Fat
- Hair follicle
- Capillary

Muscle

Figure 15–1. Diagram of a cross section of human skin.

biochemical basis for this change is unknown (Eckert and Rorke, 1989). The water content of stratum corneum varies from around 10 percent to 70 percent, depending particularly on external environmental conditions. The chemical composition and structure are significantly different in certain skin diseases such as psoriasis.

The epidermis contains a constantly renewing cell population. In the human, the transit time from mitosis within the viable epidermis is on the order of 12 to 14 days and within the stratum corneum about 15 days, for a total of about 28 days. In psoriasis, however, it may be as short as four days. These times are shorter for certain experimental species, most of which have a much thinner epidermis than humans.

Roughly 5 to 10 percent of the epidermal cells are Langerhans cells. These are mesenchyme-derived dendritic cells that form a network in the viable dermis. They are responsible for antigen recognition and processing.

Melanocytes are dendritic cells derived from the neural crest that are responsible for the synthesis of melanin in a specialized organelle called the *melanosome*. These organelles are transferred to keratinocytes, where they are aggregated and destroyed by phagolysosomes in Caucasians but not in Negroids or Australoids. A number of morphologic differences exist between the races both in the production and lysis

of melanosomes and in the degree and type of melanization. The role, if any, that pigmentation plays in modifying chemical damage in the skin is still contentious, although melanin has a major role in protection against ultraviolet radiation. Melanin is both an oxygen scavenger and a sunscreen. It may also function to remove the mutagenic and carcinogenic toxic oxygens from the surrounding keratinocytes and Langerhans cells (Nordland *et al.*, 1989).

The epidermis is separated from and attached to the dermis by a basal lamina. The epidermal-dermal junction has a characteristically ridged shape. The underlying dermis consists of loose connective tissue, which envelopes the body in a strong, flexible envelope. The dermis contains collagen, reticulin and elastin fibers, glycosaminoglycan ground substance, and a variety of scattered cells including the predominant fibroblast, as well as macrophages, mast cells, and lymphocytes. The dermis actively determines wound repair. The ground substance provides a slow diffusion medium for constituent fluids.

The dermis has substantial vascular plexuses, unlike the epidermis, which is avascular. Thus, if bleeding is produced, the dermis must have been penetrated. The dermal blood supply is substantially greater than required for its metabolic activity; thus, dermal vessels can play an important role in thermoregulation by controlling the dissipation of heat to the surface. The dermis has a plexus of lymphatics, which drain to the regional lymph nodes and the thoracic duct. The dermis has abundant sensory and sensorimotor nerves.

There are a number of epithelial structures known collectively as the *epidermal appendages,* which are extensions of modified epidermal cells into the dermis. These include the eccrine sweat glands, apocrine sweat glands, hair follicles, and sebaceous glands. The eccrine sweat glands have a secretory portion located in the hypodermis immediately below the dermis and have a coiled duct leading to the epidermal surface. They are located over the entire body surface and produce sweat, a dilute aqueous solution whose function is evaporative cooling in thermoregulation. Eccrine sweating is produced by thermal, emotional, and gustatory stimuli, and the glands are under autonomic control. Apocrine glands, which have no known function, are confined to the axillary areas, genitalia, and nipples. Their secretion is emptied into the pilary (hair) canal. Initially odorless, it acquires odor through bacterial decomposition.

Hair follicles are located over the entire body surface. Each follicle appears to have the potential to be either a terminal hair, as in the scalp or the pubic region after puberty; a soft vellus hair; or fetal (lanugo) hair. The deepest portion of the hair follicle is the germinal matrix, one of the most metabolically active tissues in the body, which is surrounded by a highly vascularized connective tissue. The uppermost cells from the proliferating germinal follicle are pushed up into the external root sheath of the hair follicle, differentiate, become keratinized, and form the hair that protrudes from the canal. The keratin of hair and of nail, though similar, is immunologically distinct from that of the stratum corneum, has a higher cystine content, and may have an additional matrix protein with a high sulfur content that serves to cross-link filament bundles.

Sebaceous glands are associated with hair follicles except for the palms, soles, and dorsal of the foot. Sebaceous gland cells accumulate lipids, and as they break down, they discharge a holocrine secretion, sebum, into the pilary canal. These glands are under hormonal control. Sebum is expelled partly by the contraction of the small arrectores pili muscles. Lipids on the surface of the skin vary in quantity, depending on both the amount of sebum and the numbers of desquamating epidermal cells, which also contribute lipids. In areas where sebaceous glands are active and abundant, such as the scalp, forehead, and upper back, up to 90 percent of the surface lipids may originate from sebum.

There are substantial differences in the skin from one region of the body to another. The thickness of the epidermis varies greatly; whereas it is about 0.06 mm over much of the body, on the palms and soles the epidermis may be several millimeters thick. The distribution and activity of the appendages, the vascular and nerve supply, and other characteristics also vary markedly. These structural differences are matched by functional differences—for example, marked variations in percutaneous absorption, as discussed in the following section.

The skin is one of the body's largest organs and represents about 10 percent of body weight. It is an important contributor to the function, metabolism, and integrity of the whole organism.

PERCUTANEOUS ABSORPTION

Percutaneous absorption is both a critical determinant of the local effects of agents applied to the skin and a determinant of systemic toxicity. In general, the range of rates of percutaneous absorption is quite high. A number of materials, especially lipophilic substances, such as organophosphate insecticides and polychlorinated biphenyls, penetrate quite readily; for other substances, particularly those that are hydrophilic, penetration may be very slow.

The major barrier for almost all substances and particularly hydrophilic substances is the stratum corneum, across which penetration occurs by passive absorption (Schaefer *et al.,* 1982). It is felt that the major route for penetration is across the epidermis itself and that diffusion through the epidermal appendages plays relatively little role. This is based partly on stoichiometric considerations, as the appendages such as hair follicles and sebaceous glands constitute only about 0.1 percent of the cross-sectional surface area presented to a potential penetrant. The appendages may be responsible for more rapid transient diffusion, particularly of lipophilic materials, before a steady state is established.

There appear to be different molecular pathways for the passage of polar and nonpolar materials. Polar substances may diffuse through the outer surface of protein filaments of the hydrated stratum corneum, whereas nonpolar molecules diffuse through nonaqueous lipid matrix (Blank and Scheuplein, 1969). It can be deduced from such observations that variations in the water content of the stratum corneum will have a profound effect on penetration, particularly of polar substances. Once through the epidermal barrier, substances must diffuse through the living layers of the epidermis and the dermis to reach the vessels of the systemic blood circulation and lymphatics, to reach targets in the underlying tissues of the skin, or to be biotransformed. Relatively little barrier to penetration is presented at these levels. The circulation is the limiting factor only for a few substances that either penetrate the stratum corneum very rapidly, such as helium (Scheuplein and Blank, 1971), or that severely damage the stratum corneum.

Information about percutaneous absorption comes from two major lines of investigation, the use of *in vitro* techniques and the use of *in vivo* techniques. Although the two approaches have to date produced somewhat different types of information, there appears to be fairly good agreement between results obtained from equivalent techniques when special care is given to duplicating experimental conditions (Franz, 1975; Bronaugh et al., 1982).

In Vitro *Studies*

In vitro techniques generally use diffusion cells in which excised skin is used as the membrane. The compound whose absorption is to be assessed is placed on one side in a suitable vehicle; this side may be open or closed. The compound is assayed in the fluid on the other side of the membrane, which is sampled regularly. This fluid is usually physiologic saline, and the experiment takes place at physiologic temperature. For these experiments, human or animal skin can be used, either epidermis separated by heat or chemically (using cantharadin) or surgical slices produced by a dermatome. Full-thickness skin from humans or animals with a thick dermis is technically unsatisfactory (Bronaugh and Maibach, 1983).

Studies with homologous groups of molecules and particularly with aliphatic alcohols (Scheuplein and Blank, 1971; Schaefer and Jamoulle, 1988) have indicated that percutaneous absorption follows Fick's diffusion law, which can be expressed in integrated form as:

$$J_s \frac{K_m D C_s}{\gamma} = K_p C_s$$

and

$$K_p = \frac{K_m D}{\gamma}$$

where J_s is the steady-state flux of solute (moles · cm^{-2} · hr^{-1}), K_m is the solute sorbed per milliliter of tissue or solute, D is the average membrane diffusion coefficient for solute (cm^2 · sec^{-1}), C_s is the concentration difference of solute across membrane (moles · cm^{-3}), γ is the membrane thickness (cm), and K_p is the permeability constant for solute (cm · hr^{-1}).

Thus the flux (J_s) is related particularly to the solvent-membrane distribution coefficient (K_m). K_m, in turn, is a major factor in determining the permeability constant (K_p). The solvent-membrane partition coefficient (K_m) can be readily determined for stratum corneum by mixing the substance and solvent in a cell with a small piece of accurately weighed dry stratum corneum, followed by appropriate chemical analysis of the substance in the two phases.

Fick's law seems to hold fairly well for gases, ions, or nonelectrolytes; apparent exceptions occur when the applied substance damages tissue. Flux may be proportional to concentration for very dilute solutions of some substances such as butanol but may increase at higher concentrations, apparently owing to the absorption of nonpolar molecules into the skin. Highly lipid-soluble materials may be even more effective in this regard and when absorbed into the stratum corneum may increase the diffusivity of other test substances (Scheuplein and Ross, 1970; Scheuplein and Blank, 1971).

In Vivo *Studies*

In vivo studies of percutaneous absorption involve topical application of substances to the intact skin of whole animals for a defined time period. Radiolabeled tracers are generally used, especially as the levels of absorbed substances in blood or plasma are often very low, making chemical analysis difficult. The radiolabeled material may be measured in excreta so that the percentage absorbed is calculated. Alternatively, tracers can be given both topically and either intraperitoneally or intravenously. Radioactivity in excreta or elsewhere can be measured and percutaneous absorption measured by the ratio of the areas under the concentration versus time curves (AUC) for the two methods of administration (*see* Chapter 3). Such methods measure the percutaneous absorption of the substance to be assessed but, unless speciation of the radiolabeled material is performed, do not indicate the nature of the material absorbed. Methods comparing different routes of administration are invalid if biotransformation of the chemical by skin was extensive and differed from that in other organs (Wester and Maibach, 1976).

Other approaches to *in vivo* measurement of absorption have been used. These include the use of a biologic response, such as cutaneous vasoconstriction, which has been used to detect absorption of topical corticosteroids, and remainder analysis, where the loss of radioactivity or substance from the skin surface is measured; however, the latter is less satisfactory both as the skin may act as a reservoir for unabsorbed material and as full recovery of radioactivity is never assured.

The rhesus monkey appears to produce results reasonably similar to those from humans (Wester and Maibach, 1976). Rodents appear to have higher permeability than man, with guinea pig, rat, and rabbit, in that order, showing increasingly greater penetrability (Tregear, 1966).

Factors Affecting Percutaneous Absorption

A considerable number of factors have been shown to affect percutaneous absorption. For convenience, these may be loosely classified as those associated with the skin, vehicle, or type of penetrant.

Skin. The amount absorbed is obviously dependent on the applied dose, the time before contact is terminated as by washing or removal, the concentration, and the surface area of application. The efficiency of absorption may change and can fall as the actual concentration increases, although the total amount absorbed into the body seems always to increase (Wester and Maibach, 1976). The physical integrity of the stratum corneum is vital; partial or complete removal or changes in the composition and structure such as occur in certain diseases affect absorption. Important species differences exist, as previously indicated.

As with other cutaneous functions, there is a profound regional variation, as illustrated in Table 15–1, which shows relative permeability data for human skin regions (Feldmann and Maibach, 1969).

The penetration of polar substances is increased by hydration of the stratum corneum. There is also a linear increase in the penetration of polar substances with temperature up to 50°C. With lipids, temperature dependence may be nonlinear, perhaps reflecting changes in viscosity. Both hydration and local skin temperature

Table 15–1. RELATIVE REGIONAL PERMEABILITY OF HUMAN SKIN TO TOPICAL[14]C HYDROCORTISONE*

Plantar foot arch	1
Lateral ankle	3
Palm	6
Ventral forearm	7
Dorsal forearm	8
Back	12
Scalp	25
Axilla	26
Forehead	43
Jaw angle	93
Scrotum	300

* Data from Feldmann R. J., and Maibach, H. I.: Absorption of some organic compounds through the skin in man. *J. Invest. Dermatol.*, **54**:339–404, 1969.

are increased by occlusion of the site of application using an impervious material such as a sheet of polyethylene. This has been taken advantage of in dermatologic therapy, particularly to increase the penetration of topically applied corticosteroids.

Sweat can dissolve or leach substances from solid objects, after which they may cause skin damage. The allergen nickel is notably dissolved from metallic alloys by sweat (Hemingway and Molokhia, 1987). Plasma is even more effective than sweat in producing dissolution of nickel, which probably accounts for the high prevalence of nickel sensitization produced by ear piercing (Emmett *et al.*, 1988).

Vehicle. The vehicle or solvent has a profound effect on percutaneous absorption. The nature of the vehicle governs the vehicle/stratum corneum partition coefficient, which determines absorption. The vehicle may influence absorption in other ways. It may contain a damaging solvent or determine pH, thus altering the ionization of electrolytes. The presence of anionic and cationic surfactants such as soaps and detergents, even in dilute concentration, will increase the permeability for water and for other polar substances by damaging the stratum corneum, although the precise mechanisms are incompletely understood. Nonionic surfactants are less active in this regard. Marked variations in biologic potency, determined by differences in vehicles, are seen among topical glucocorticosteroids used therapeutically (Stoughton, 1989).

Substance. Although data are quite incomplete for many classes of compounds, some general principles can be derived (Scheuplein and Blank, 1971). The permeability of skin to water has been well studied. The stratum corneum is one of the most water impermeable of all biological membranes. Simple polar nonelectrolytes appear to penetrate the stratum corneum at approximately the same rate as water. Water-miscible alcohols have similar permeability constants; adding additional polar groups drastically reduces the rate. Introducing methylene groups into a simple polar nonelectrolyte increases the membrane solubility, resulting in a higher permeability. Electrolytes applied from aqueous solution penetrate poorly, and the ionization of a weak electrolyte radically reduces its permeability.

Organic liquids can be divided into those that are nondamaging to the membrane, such as alcohols higher than C_2, and those that damage, such as acetone, hexane, and other common solvents. Lipid solubility is an important determinant for nondamaging solvents; high permeability is guaranteed where the vehicle is polar. Damaging solvents delipidize the skin, producing functional interstices in skin that serve as low-energy diffusion pathways. The result is a fairly porous nonselective membrane.

In general, true gases, as opposed to vapor phase concentrations of volatile liquids and solvents, penetrate the skin relatively well, although the diffusion coefficients are very small compared with those typical of gaseous diffusion.

Biotransformation

The skin, and particularly the epidermis, is an actively metabolizing organ that is capable of significant biotransformation of xenobiotics (Pannatier *et al.*, 1978). A number of studies have addressed the presence of arylhydrocarbon hydroxylase (AHH) activity in the skin; benzo-[a]pyrene metabolites including epoxides may be formed in the skin. This activity is inducible (Bickers, 1988). Most of the enzymes are present in the lower epidermis rather than the dermis. The total AHH activity of skin toward benzo[a]pyrene is about 2 percent of that of liver.

Metabolic transformation may affect topically applied drugs. For example, it has been estimated that from 16 to 21 percent of a dose of glyceryl trinitrate applied to monkeys is biotransformed by the skin (Wester *et al.*, 1981).

In addition to metabolic transformation, substances in the superficial layers of the skin are subject to photochemical reactions if they absorb ultraviolet (UV) or visible radiation.

Biotransformation in other organs may also be important in the production of toxic effects in the skin. An example of how a number of processes may be involved is porphyria cutanea tarda, which is characterized by blistering and fragility of the skin, photosensitivity, pigmentary changes, and excessive hirsutism. An epidemic of this disease occurred among several thousand people in southeastern Turkey in the late 1950s when, during a famine, wheat treated with hexachlorobenzene was eaten rather than planted (Schmid, 1960).

Hexachlorobenzene produces excessive accumulation of uroporphyrins and coproporphyrins in liver as a result of interference with porphyrin metabolism (J. A. Goldstein *et al.*, 1977). Consequently, porphyrins accumulate in various tissues including the skin. These substances render the skin photosensitive as a result of intense absorption of porphyrins in the 400-nm, SORET band, with subsequent photoactivation and damage to cell membranes and/or cell constituents (B. D. Goldstein and Harber, 1972).

Excretion from the Skin

Integumentary loss of body constituents including xenobiotics may occur with loss of des-

quamated cells, hair, or nails; in the eccrine or apocrine sweat; or in secretions such as tears and milk.

The average human adult scalp contains about 100,000 hairs with a growth rate of about 0.37 mm/day. Human hair grows in a cyclic manner, with a resting (telogen) phase lasting about three months and a growth phase (anagen) lasting for two to six years. There is also a brief involutional phase (catagen). Normally, about 70 scalp hairs are lost daily. Certain metals are incorporated into the matrix of the growing hairs and remain in the hair tissue until it is eventually lost (Brown and Crounse, 1980). Measurement of the hair content of As, Cd, and Pb (after suitable washing to remove material externally deposited on hair) has been shown to reflect exposures reliably; however, this is not true for Zn and Cu (Hammer *et al.*, 1971).

There has been relatively little study of excretion in the eccrine sweat. Sweat volume varies from 250 ml to many liters per day. Sweat rates of greater than 1 liter per hour are seen in hot conditions or heavy work rates. Thus, the total amount of sweat loss is variable. Furthermore, acclimatization to heat is characterized both by decreased sweating and by decreased solute concentrations. Sodium and chloride are the main solutes in sweat, but many other substances are present. Substantial amounts of many metals are excreted in the sweat, including Cu, Zn, and Fe; concentrations of Pb, Cd, and Ni in sweat are equal to or higher than those in urine (Cohn and Emmett, 1978). Thus, the potential exists, depending on sweat rates and acclimatization, for substantial losses of these metals in sweat. A number of water-soluble drugs are excreted in sweat. The excretion of aminopyrine, antipyrene, sulfaguanidine, and sulfadiazine has been studied (Johnson and Maibach, 1971). These show a high sweat-to-plasma concentration, and their excretion behavior is consistent with partitioning between plasma of pH 7.4 and a fluid of pH near 5.

Animal models for eccrine sweating are sparse since apocrine glands predominate in other species.

Sweat can be obtained from collection in occlusive plastic bags applied to the skin, but use of this technique may alter sweat composition. The alternate approach of total-body washdown to collect human sweat is more accurate but tedious and cumbersome.

TOXIC SKIN REACTIONS

Irritant Responses

By the term *cutaneous irritant*, we generally refer to an agent that produces a local cutaneous inflammatory response (dermatitis) by direct action on skin without the involvement of an immunologic mechanism. In this sense, *irritation* is not used to describe noninflammatory reactions such as subjective sensations (itch, burning, etc.) or more subtle biochemical or histologic changes such as epidermal thickening, although these could represent variations of the same effect. Irritation of the skin is important, and it is commonly thought to account for about 60 to 80 percent of the burden of clinically recognized human contact dermatitis, although this figure no doubt varies from location to location. Most of the remaining contact dermatitis represents allergic contact dermatitis. Contact dermatitis is manifest by signs of erythema (redness) and edema in experimental test animals. In humans, more varied responses are seen, and erythema and edema frequently progress to vesiculation, scaling, and thickening of the epidermis. Histologically, the hallmark is spongiosis or intracellular edema of the epidermis (Soter and Fitzpatrick, 1987).

It is useful to distinguish two reasonably distinct types of cutaneous irritation and two related conditions (NAS, 1977; McCreesh and Steinberg, 1983):

Acute irritation. A local, reversible inflammatory response of normal living skin to direct injury caused by a single application of a toxic substance, without the involvement of an immunologic mechanism

Cumulative irritation. Reversible irritation resulting from repeated or continued exposures to materials that do not in themselves cause acute irritation

Corrosion. Direct chemical action on normal living skin that results in its disintegration and irreversible alteration at the site of contact; corrosion is manifested by ulceration and necrosis with subsequent scar formation

Phototoxicity (photoirritation). Irritation resulting from light-induced molecular changes in the structure of chemicals applied to the skin; phototoxicity is dealt with elsewhere in this chapter

Acute irritation is produced by a relatively large number of substances of varying chemical types, many of which are highly chemically active such as relatively strong solvents, acids, and bases. However, no demonstrably reliable method for assessing irritancy based on chemical structure has been advanced.

In practice, a significant amount of irritant dermatitis appears to result from cumulative irritation, resulting in so-called cumulative insult dermatitis. Substances that produce this type of reaction are termed *marginal irritants*. This type of dermatitis is often multifactorial, with both physical factors and multiple chemical exposures playing a role.

Figure 15–2 shows the results of the application of an aliquot of a concentrated synthetic laundry waste water to the same position on the backs of 20 human subjects under an occlusive patch for 21 consecutive days in a cumulative insult patch test. A response scored as +1 indicates erythema with a definable margin; +2, erythema with induration; and +3, vesiculation or pustulation. Once a +3 reaction was observed, the treatment was suspended. It is

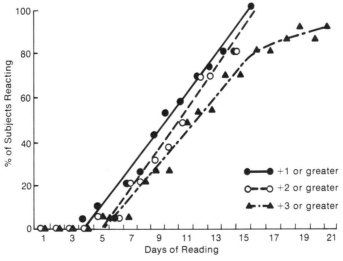

Figure 15–2. Cumulative percentage of subjects with grade 1, grade 2, or grade 3 reaction to repeated application of synthetic laundry waste water in cumulative insult patch test.

seen that no reactions were observed in any individual for the first several days; however, from day 4 to day 16, all subjects developed erythema, which progressed rapidly in virtually all individuals within a few days of its onset. It should be added that the rate of progression of cumulative irritation changes shows significant variation for different applied substances.

The biochemical mechanisms involved in irritation are not well characterized. Substances that are keratin solvents, dehydrating agents, oxidizing agents, reducing agents, and others may be irritants. To date, there has not been a good correlation between measured biochemical changes in the skin and development of irritation.

A large number of tests for predicting irritation have been proposed over recent years. Those in more widespread use fall into the general categories of single-application tests or cumulative-insult tests. The most widely used test is based on that described by Draize and colleagues in 1944.

Substances are applied to abraded and intact skin of the albino rabbit, clipped free of hair. A minimum of six rabbits are used in abraded and intact skin tests. The substance is inserted under a square patch such as surgical gauze measuring 2.5 cm by 2.5 cm (1 inch by 1 inch) and two single layers thick, using 0.5 ml (in the case of liquids) or 0.5 g (in the case of solids and semisolids) of the test substance. Solids are dissolved in an appropriate solvent, and the solution applied as for liquids. The animals are immobilized with patches secured in place by adhesive tape. The entire trunk of the animal is then wrapped with an impervious material such as rubberized cloth for the 24-hour period of exposure. This material aids in maintaining the test patches in position and retards the evaporation of volatile substances. After 24 hours of exposure, the patches are removed and the resulting reactions are evaluated on the basis of certain designated values. Readings are made again at the end of 72 hours (CFR, 1980).

A number of modifications have been made in this test over the years by different authors. Although there is considerable dispute about a number of experimental details and its predictive competency, it is frequently a legal requirement (McCreesh and Steinberg, 1983). Different testing methods have been recommended, depending on product usage, for example, shorter four-hour testing for certain household substances (NAS, 1977). Considerable variation in results obtained has been noted, particularly between laboratories (Weil and Scala, 1971). Nevertheless, the test is widely considered to be a relatively satisfactory method of identifying strong irritants.

For mild to moderate irritants, cumulative irritancy tests appear to give better predictive results (Phillips et al., 1972). There is reasonable concordance between the results of such testing in albino rabbits and humans (Steinberg et al., 1975). All such test procedures are sensitive to methodologic variations, including such factors as site of application, hair pattern, depilation technique, strain, species, occlusive technique, vehicle, size of application area, lighting, procedure for reading reactions, and others. In humans, there are marked variations in the responses of different individuals to the same substance and of one individual to different substances, so that one is unable in any subject to predict the intensity of reaction to one irritant on the basis of the reaction to another.

Chemical Burns. Corrosive substances can cause severe ulceration in humans. Although terminology is not standardized, more severe corrosive changes are often designated as *chemical burns*.

Characteristics of these lesions vary depending on the nature of the toxic material. Severe burns from acids usually cause a dry crust from coagulation necrosis, the color varying with the anion. Alkalies produce softer burns, which may be extremely painful. Phenolics can result in local anesthesia so that pain will be absent after a short time. Some materials, such as nitrogen mustard and certain organotins, produce characteristically delayed reactions. The action of some corrosives differs from thermal burns in that toxic effects may continue indefinitely. In the case of alkyl mercury, it has been shown that evacuation of blister fluid containing the toxin helps prevent extension of the lesion.

A vital step in limiting tissue damage is rapid removal of the causal material. In practice, this is almost always best done with copious soap and water. Among the few exceptions are quicklime (CaO), whose reaction with water is extremely exothermic, the solution of 1 g generating over 18,000 calories, and titanium tetrachloride and tin tetrachloride, which rapidly hydrolyze to form hydrochloric acid.

Specific therapeutic approaches are necessary with some substances including white phosphorus and hydrogen fluoride (Curreri et al., 1970; Emmett, 1980). White phosphorus, which burns in air, can produce severe thermal and chemical injury. It may reignite as it dries. After washing, debridement is performed under water. Initial luminescence in the dark may help in particle identification. Treatment with 1 percent copper sulfate, sufficiently brief to avoid systemic absorption and copper poisoning, converts the phosphorus to copper phosphide, which is then removed. Hydrogen fluoride may produce extensive painful necrosis locally, which may progress over a few days. Hypocalcemia from the precipitation of calcium contributes to the local injury and may result in profound systemic hypocalcemia. Treatment with calcium gluconate locally and monitoring of serum calcium levels with calcium administration, as required, are necessary.

The effects of systemic absorption of toxic materials must always be considered.

Allergic Contact Responses

Allergic contact dermatitis occurs as a result of cell-mediated or type IV immune reactions (see Baer and Bickers, 1981; Dahl, 1981; Bergstresser, 1989). Allergic contact dermatitis is important because of both the specificity of the response and the quite low amounts of allergen that may elicit an inflammatory reaction.

Immunobiologic Process. A number of phases may be distinguished in the development of contact allergy. For a varying period of time, which may be a lifetime or only a few days, there is a *refractory period* during which sensitization does not take place. Sensitization develops in an *induction period,* which generally takes from 10 to 21 days. After the induction of sensitization is complete, reexposure to the antigen will result in *elicitation* of the reaction after a characteristic delay of usually 12 to 48 hours (hence the name *delayed hypersensitivity).* Once induced, the allergic sensitivity will persist for a varying period, possibly for a lifetime.

Why some exposures and not others initiate sensitization is not entirely clear but appears to depend on the nature of the chemical, concentration, type of exposure, genetic susceptibility, and nongenetic idiosyncrasies. It is clear that some allergens (e.g., poison ivy extract) are very potent sensitizers, whereas others rarely sensitize despite extensive exposure.

Cutaneous antigens (haptens) are generally of low molecular weight. The first step in the allergic process appears to be absorption of the hapten into the skin and covalent binding to a carrier protein. The antigen is bound to cell surfaces especially of the epidermal Langerhans cell (Baer and Berman, 1981) or macrophages. These cells *process* the antigen by altering the configurational arrangement and *present* the antigen by holding it to the cell surface for subsequent interaction with histocompatible T lymphocytes. The T lymphocyte–macrophage interaction can occur in skin and does not appear to require cooperation of cells in the regional lymph node. Either Langerhans cells or T lymphocytes migrate from the skin to the regional lymph node. The antigen-bearing lymphocyte

settles in the paracortical area of the lymph nodes. Following clonal proliferation to form immunoblasts in the paracortical areas, two populations of sensitized lymphocytes are formed, *effector* T lymphocytes, which travel to the skin surface in the peripheral blood, and long-lived *memory cells,* which will proliferate to form new populations of sensitized lymphocytes on recontact with the antigen.

The elicitation phase can take place once the sensitization phase has been completed and may occur as a result of reintroduction or persistence of the antigen. Effector T lymphocytes in the skin become activated as they recognize the hapten-protein complex, enlarge, and resemble lymphoblasts (blast transformation). The activated lymphocytes, and other cells, synthesize a variety of substances called *cytokines,* which mediate the response. More than 30 cytokines have been described, although it is not clear that they are all distinct substances. These include chemotactic, macrophage migration inhibition, macrophage-activating, leukocyte-inhibiting, and lymph node permeability factors; lymphotoxins; transfer factors; and others. In addition to sensitized lymphocytes, other lymphocytes not specifically sensitized to the antigen as well as monocytes and macrophages may be recruited to the reaction to contribute to the inflammatory response and to manufacture lymphokines. A variety of other cells including B lymphocytes and possibly cutaneous basophils may play a role in these responses.

Although it is considered prudent to assume that allergic contact sensitization persists indefinitely, it has been shown that the prevalence of positive patch tests to poison ivy extract declines with age, suggesting that some individuals may lose their sensitization. As memory cells appear to have a finite life, it is theoretically possible that sensitization could be lost.

Causes of Contact Allergy. Contact allergy may occur from a very large number of antigens; it seems possible that most substances may at least very rarely be antigens. A list of selected important allergens is seen in Table 15–2. However, there is a great range in antigenic potency, and a relatively small number of strong sensitizers have been identified experimentally or in humans. Strong allergens are often aromatic substances with molecular weights less than 500; they tend to be highly lipid soluble and quite reactive with protein, although exceptions occur.

Two groups of dermatologists, the North American Contact Dermatitis Group (NACDG) and the International Contact Dermatitis Research Group (ICDRG), use a limited standard

Table 15–2. SELECTED IMPORTANT ALLERGIC CONTACT SENSITIZERS

Metals
  Nickel and nickel salts
  Chromium salts
  Cobalt salts
  Organomercurials
Plant sensitizers
  Toxicodendron genus: pentadecylcatechols
    and other catechols
  Primula obconica: α-methylene-γ-butyrolactone
  Compositae family: sesquiterpene lactones
Rubber additives
  Mercaptobenzthiazole
  Thiuram sulfides
  p-Phenylenediamine and derivatives
  Diphenylguanidine
  Resorcinol monobenzoate
Epoxy oligomer (M.W. 340)
Methyl methacrylate and other acrylic monomers
Pentaerythritol triacrylate and other multifunctional
  acrylates
Hexamethylenediisocyanate
p-Tertiary butyl phenol
Ethylenediamine, hexamethylenetetramine, and
  other aliphatic amines
Formaldehyde
Neomycin
Benzocaine
Captan

set of antigens for patch testing and centrally report and periodically publish results. The reported prevalence of contact allergic sensitivity on diagnostic patch testing in patients of both groups is shown in Table 15–3, taken from Rudner (1973). It is seen that reactions to nickel were most frequent in each group. These statistics are an interesting guide to some of the more frequent antigens; they have important limitations, however, as they are not population based and do not necessarily contain all important antigens; for example, in the United States, because of ease of diagnosis, poison ivy reactions are not included. The reported prevalence of sensitization in human populations is clearly a function of relative antigenic potency, extent of hazardous exposure, and the diagnostic test used. Figure 15–3 shows the structural formulas of a number of important contact allergens.

There are a wide number of situations in which sensitized subjects can contact antigens in a manner that will lead to development of contact dermatitis (Fregert, 1981; Foussereau *et al.,* 1982; Adams, 1983). Common sources include, but are certainly not limited to, contact with metals (nickel); metal compounds (nickel, chromium, cobalt salts, and organomercurials); perfumes; preservatives; hair dyes; colorants in cosmetics and toiletries; resins and dyes in cloth-

Table 15–3. REPORTED PREVALENCE OF SELECTED ALLERGIC SENSITIVITY REACTIONS ON DIAGNOSTIC PATCH TESTING WITH STANDARD SET OF ANTIGENS*

COMPOUND, TEST CONCENTRATION, AND VEHICLE		NORTH AMERICA (n = 1200), PERCENT POSITIVE REACTIONS	EUROPE[†] (n = 4824), PERCENT POSITIVE REACTONS
Nickel sulfate	2.5% petrolatum	11	6.7
Potassium dichromate	0.5% petrolatum	8	
Thiomerosal	0.1% petrolatum	8	
p-Phenylenediamine	1% petrolatum	8	4.7
Ethylenediamine	1% petrolatum	7	
Neomycin sulfate	20% petrolatum	6	3.7
Benzocaine	5% petrolatum	5	4
Mercaptobenzothiazole	2% petrolatum	4	2
Formalin	2% aqueous	4	3.5
Tetramethylthiuram disulfide	2% petrolatum	4	2

* Modified from Rudner, E. F.: Epidemiology of contact dermatitis in North America. *Arch. Dermatol.,* **108**:537–540, 1973.
† Data for Europe and North America are both given only where test concentration and vehicle were similar.

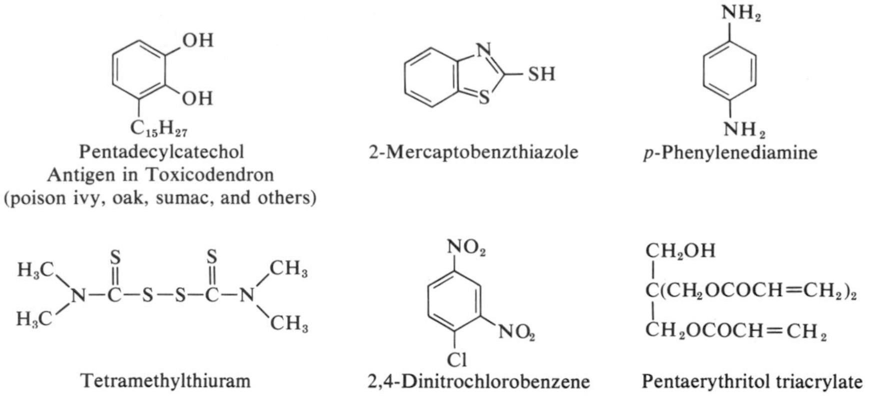

Figure 15-3. Structural formulas of some potent contact sensitizers.

ing, additives, and adhesives in rubber and leather products; typical medicaments; many plants and plant products; pesticides; monomers used in plastics such as acrylates, polyurethanes, and epoxys; additives in coolants and cutting oils; photographic chemicals; and a wide variety of industrial chemicals. Fully cured plastics are usually not antigenic unless they release formaldehyde or contain leachable additives.

Either flareups of cutaneous reactions or possibly systemic symptoms may occur on ingestion of antigens to which contact allergic sensitization has been previously induced, although the frequency of such reactions is debated (Menne, 1983).

A number of terms are used in connection with allergic contact sensitivity. These include:

> *Sensitizing potential.* The relative capacity of a given agent to induce sensitization in a group of humans or animals
> *Index of sensitivity.* The prevalence of sensitivity to a substance in a given population at a given time
> *Allergen replacement.* The removal of antigens from products, replacing them with substances of a lower sensitizing potential

Cross-Sensitization and Multiple Sensitization.

Cross-sensitization may occur when two or more potential antigens share similar groups. This may depend on a particular chemical group, e.g., a primary para amine (R-NH$_2$) attached directly to an aromatic ring, or on structural similarity (*e.g.*, some quinolines). The structural formulas for several substances with para-amino groups that frequently appear to cross-react are shown in Figure 15-4. Cross-sensitization might be explained by the formation of similar reaction products *in vivo*, by the formation of common metabolites, or by the induction of similar changes in carrier proteins. Satisfactory explanations do not yet exist for all purported examples of cross-sensitization.

Terms used in connection with *multiple sensitization* include:

> *Cross-sensitization.* A is the primary allergen (antigen). Induction of sensitization to it is combined with the acquisition of sensitization to a chemically related molecule such as B, which is called a *secondary allergen* (antigen).
> *Concomitant sensitization.* This occurs when different substances A and B are present in the same product and sensitization to both takes place on the same occasion.
> *Simultaneous sensitization.* Simultaneous sensitization occurs when an individual is sensitized to different substances in different products.
> *False cross-sensitivity.* This occurs when the same antigen is present in different products (e.g., eugenol in perfumes, soft drinks, and underarm deodorants).

Diagnostic Patch Testing.

The existence of allergic contact dermatitis is confirmed by diagnostic patch testing. The principle is simple: A concentration of the test substance that is known to be nonirritating and does not induce sensitization is applied to the skin in a suitable vehicle, commonly white petrolatum. It is also necessary that the application concentration be sufficient to elicit an allergic reaction in those sensitized. Nonirritancy is established by testing on a suitably large control population. In practice, suitable test concentrations have generally been established through trial and error, and the test is properly standardized and validated for only a limited number of substances. The material to be tested is applied to normal skin, usually on the back, and suitably occluded for 48 hours. Readings are generally made from 24 to 96 hours after removal of the patch. Adherence to exacting

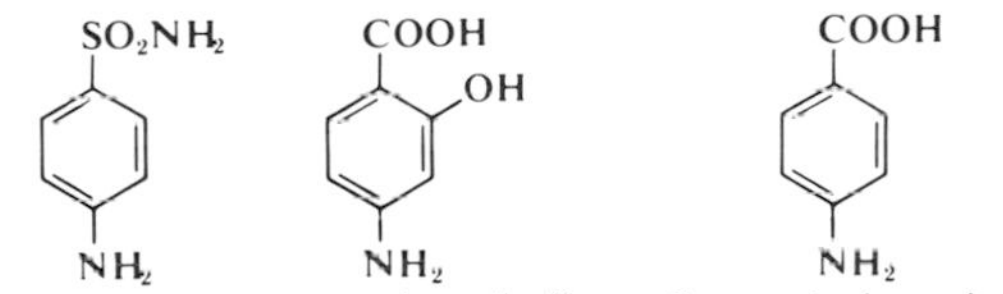

SO$_2$NH$_2$ COOH   COOH
                OH

NH$_2$ NH$_2$ NH$_2$
Sulfamide   Para-aminosalicylic   Para-aminobenzoic
              acid   acid

Figure 15–4. Structural formulas of selected para-amino compounds that show cross-reactions in allergic contact sensitization.

techniques in application and reading is very important (Cronin, 1980). In order to determine the relevance of positive patch test reactions to product exposure, usage testing with a product may be performed by daily application to skin such as at the elbow flexure. It has been possible to use *in vitro* tests such as lymphocyte transformation tests and macrophage migration inhibition tests to demonstrate type IV hypersensitivity in selected instances of allergic contact sensitization, but no *in vitro* test is yet sufficiently reliable for routine diagnostic use (Nordquist and Rosenthal, 1978).

A number of predictive tests have been developed to identify potential allergic contact sensitizers. To date, no satisfactory *in vitro* tests are available; all tests require the use of intact mammals with functioning immunologic systems. Humans or guinea pigs of Hartly or Pinbright strains are generally used. In guinea pigs, the induction phase consists of a number of epicutaneous applications, intradermal injections, or both. Epicutaneous applications are generally considered most realistic and relevant to human exposure. Complete Freund's adjuvant may be administered to increase immunologic reactivity. After a rest period, a challenge test is performed by closed or open epicutaneous testing. An increase in reactivity compared with presensitization or control animals is considered to indicate sensitization. Compounds that induce a high incidence of contact sensitivity tend to be fairly well identified in currently available predictive tests; weak sensitizers less well. This creates a difficulty as the identification of relatively weak sensitizers may be very important for materials such as toiletries that will be used by millions of people. A number of different test variations are in current use (Klecak, 1983), and comparative studies are relatively limited. These tests are sensitive to variations in technique, and many experimental variables affecting the induction of sensitization in the guinea pig have been described (Magnusson and Kligman, 1970).

Test procedures in human volunteers generally follow a similar pattern, with exposures to multiple occlusive patches followed by a rest period and challenge testing and nonirritant concentrations. Procedures to increase the yield of sensitization may be used; these include the use of local sodium lauryl sulfate applications and the use of high induction concentrations. Significant differences in results are seen from different techniques (Marzulli and Maibach, 1980). In these tests, it is necessary to use a sufficiently large experimental sample to allow a reasonable extrapolation of results to exposed populations.

Photosensitization

A number of physiologic and pathologic changes occur in the skin as a result of exposure to the UV component of sunlight. These include erythema (sunburn); thickening of the epidermis; darkening of existing pigment (immediate pigment darkening); new pigment formation (delayed tanning); actinic elastosis (premature skin ageing); proliferative and other changes in epidermal cells; selective defects in immunologic function (Krutmann and Elmets, 1988); actinic keratosis, a precancerous condition; and the development of squamous cell cancers, basal cell cancers, and probably some malignant melanomas (Parrish *et al.,* 1979; Kripke, 1980). These changes appear to occur as a result of the photochemical interaction of UV with normal components of the skin.

Foreign substances, either absorbed locally into the skin or reaching the skin through the systemic circulation, may be the subject of photochemical reactions within the skin, leading to either chemically induced photosensitivity reactions or altering the "normal" pathologic effects of light described above. Such reactions may augment pathologic changes like photocarcinogenesis or ameliorate them by absorbing potentially hazardous radiation or by scavenging potentially damaging excited molecular states. In recent times, advantage has been taken of light as a therapeutic agent, for example, in the phototherapy of neonatal hyperbilirubinemia; the use of ultraviolet radiation and photosensitizers such as psoralens to treat psoriasis; and visible light and hematoporphyrin derivatives to treat malignancy (photodynamic therapy).

Photobiologic Principles. Photochemical changes in the skin are important because humans have opportunities for extensive exposure both to sunlight and to a wide variety of artificial sources. That part of the solar spectrum of major toxicologic interest is from 290 to 700 nm. Shorter wavelengths are absorbed by the atmosphere, mostly by the ozone layer of the stratosphere, whereas longer wavelengths may cause tissue heating but generally lack the energy to cause photochemical changes.

Electromagnetic radiation may be regarded as consisting of waves (characterized by their frequency or wavelength in a particular medium) or photons (characterized by their energy). For photobiologic purposes, it is convenient to define particular wavebands that have certain physical or toxicologic characteristics. Currently accepted divisions of the spectrum are UV-C (germicidal UV), 220 to 280 nm; UV-B, 280 to 320 nm; UV-A, 320 to 400 nm; and visible, 400 to 760 nm. Progressively shorter than the UV-C are the vacuum UV and soft X rays; longer than the visible is the infrared. UV-C is not present in sunlight received at the earth's surface; it is, however, capable of profound photochemical damage to DNA and proteins. UV-B is the main region of sunlight responsible for "normal" pathologic changes in skin, although increasingly the UV-A is felt to play an important role (Parrish *et al.*, 1978). UV-A is responsible for most photosensitivity reactions. Visible radiations lack the energy to produce photochemical reactions in most proteins and in DNA but are well absorbed by certain highly specialized molecules such as rhodopsin or chlorophyll and by colored substances in general.

The radiation actually delivered to any target in the skin will be dependent on the skin optics (Anderson and Parrish, 1981). Skin is an optically inhomogeneous medium; reflection, refraction, scattering, and absorption all modify the radiation that reaches deeper structures. Important UV absorbers within the epidermis include melanin, which varies greatly in content and location between individuals and races; urocanic acid, a deamination product of histidine found in sweat; and for shorter wavelengths, proteins containing tryptophan and tyrosine. The net optical effect is that shorter wavelengths are selectively absorbed in the superficial layers, although a biologically significant amount of UV-B reaches the dermis. In addition, variations in epidermal thickness, water content of the skin, and the application of oils or sunscreens alter optical properties of skin.

The First Law of Photochemistry states that to produce an effect radiation must be absorbed. Absorption of specific wavelengths of radiation by a chromophore results in electronically excited molecules. An excited singlet state has a lifetime of 10^{-8} seconds or less before either returning to the ground state or undergoing the process of intersystem crossing to a metastable triplet state with a lifetime in the range of 10^{-4} to 10^{-1} seconds. Triplet excited states may relax to the ground state by transfer of energy to another molecule, and both singlet and triplet excited states may return to the ground state by emission of light (fluorescence or phosphorescence); by emission of heat; or by undergoing photochemistry such as *cis-trans* isomerization, ionization, rearrangement, fragmentation, and

intermolecular reactions. Through what is no doubt a complex series of events, initial, almost instantaneous photochemical events lead to longer-term biologic effects. The entire sequence is not yet well understood for any particular effect.

A most important concept in photobiology is that of *action spectrum,* the relative response of a system to different wavelengths. In theory, the action spectrum should reflect the absorption spectrum of the responsible chromophore. In practice, the relationship appears less exact for one or more of several reasons. The *in vivo* absorption spectrum may differ from that determined in a solvent system *in vitro* (Cripps and Enta, 1970), and the wavelength distribution of radiation actually reaching the target molecules in tissue will be modified as a result of the optical properties of overlying layers.

Mechanisms of Chemically Induced Photosensitization. *Photosensitization* designates an abnormal adverse reaction to ultraviolet and/or visible radiation. Xenobiotics may produce such reactions in a number of ways (Emmett, 1979), as indicated in Table 15–4. Of these reactions, the most important are phototoxicity and photoallergy. Phototoxicity designates a chemically induced increased reactivity of a target tissue to UV and/or visible radiation on a nonimmunologic basis. Each response is governed by a dose-response relationship between the intensity of the reaction and both the concentration of the inciting chemical in the target tissue and the amount of radiation of appropriate wavelengths (weighted for the action spectrum) to which that target tissue is exposed, provided that the time of administration is sufficiently short that photorecovery is not a factor.

Photoallergy designates an increased reactivity of the skin to UV and/or visible radiation produced by a chemical agent on an immunolog-

Table 15–4. SELECTED MECHANISMS OF CHEMICALLY INDUCED PHOTOSENSITIZATION

Phototoxicity
  e.g., 8-methoxypsoralen
Photoallergy
  e.g., tribromosalicyclanilide
Depigmentation, with subsequent alteration in cutaneous optical properties
  e.g., *p*-tertiary-butylphenol
Induction of endogenous photosensitizer
  e.g., hexachlorobenzene-induced porphyria cutanea tarda
Induction of disease characterized by photosensitivity
  Lupus erythematosus   e.g., procainamide
  Pellagra   e.g., INH
Undetermined mechanisms
  e.g., quinidine

ic basis. This type of response can be elicited only in individuals who have been previously allergically sensitized by exposure to the chemical agent and appropriate radiation. Photoallergy is distinctly less common than phototoxicity, although a few agents such as tetrachlorosalicylanilide are very potent photoallergens.

Phototoxicity. Phototoxic reactions have been described after contact, ingestion, or injection of causal agents. In addition to reactions in humans, they are responsible for certain economically important diseases of domestic animals. The skin and eyes are the major organs affected. The actual skin changes vary with the agent and circumstances of exposure. Swelling and redness frequently occur, and blistering may be seen. Hyperpigmentation, associated with long-standing morphologic changes in melanosomes, may follow a reaction. Possible eye changes may include keratoconjunctivitis or corneal and lens opacities (Bernstein *et al.*, 1970; Emmett *et al.*, 1977).

Phototoxic reactions are broadly divided into those that are oxygen dependent (photodynamic action) and a lesser number that do not require oxygen. In photodynamic mechanisms, either the excited triplet state is reduced, leading to the generation of highly reactive free radicals, which subsequently attach biological substrates (type I reaction), or the chromophore transfers its energy to O_2, generating singlet oxygen ($^1O_2$), an active oxidizing agent (type II reaction).

Nonphotodynamic compounds may in their excited state react directly with a target molecule. An example is the reaction of furocoumarins such as 8-methoxypsoralen with specific sites on DNA to form covalent bonds between the pyrimidine base and the furocoumarin (2 + 2 cycloaddition). Upon absorption of another photon, a second 2 + 2 cycloaddition reaction can take place, resulting in cross-linked DNA (Dall'Acqua, 1977). It is believed that these lesions are responsible for the major photosensitization effects of psoralens including photocarcinogenesis. Other substances such as chlorpromazine and protriptyline form stable toxic photoproducts after irradiation (Kochevar, 1981). Important subcellular targets for phototoxic reactions include nuclei, cytoplasmic organelles, and cell membranes.

A list of selected phototoxic agents is shown in Table 15–5.

Forbes *et al.* (1976) have nicely demonstrated that the phototoxic agent 8-methoxypsoralen is capable of markedly enhancing experimental UV carcinogenesis. Enhanced skin cancer formation has been described in humans treated with psoralens and UV-A for psoriasis (Stern *et al.*, 1979).

Table 15–5. SELECTED PHOTOTOXIC CHEMICALS

Furocoumarins
  8-Methoxypsoralen
  5-Methoxypsoralen (bergapten)
  trimethoxypsoralen
Polycyclic aromatic hydrocarbons
  Anthracene
  Fluoranthene
  Acridine
  Phenanthrene
Tetracyclines
  Demethylchlortetracycline
Sulfonamides
Chlorpromazine
Nalidixic acid
Nonsteroidal antiinflammatory drugs
  Benoxaprofen
Amyl *o*-dimethylaminobenzoic acid
Dyes
  Eosin
  Acridine orange
Porphyrin derivatives
  Hematoporphyrin

A number of assay systems for phototoxic substances exist. They include the use of biochemical tests, anuclear cells, nucleated cells in suspension or culture, small organisms, nonhuman mammalian skin, and human skin (Emmett, 1979). This seems to be an area in which the use of alternative methods to whole-animal predictive testing may enjoy early success. There are currently no regulatory guidelines on whole-animal methods of testing for phototoxic potential, so it is not surprising that no standardized method is available. Because so many variables are involved—species, light source, light dose, route of administration, interval between chemical treatment and irradiation, and so on—it is very difficult to compare the different published methods (Maurer, 1987).

Photoallergy. Photoallergy reactions (Emmett, 1978; Harber and Bickers, 1981) result from type IV, cell-mediated immune reactions similar to allergic contact dermatitis. In selected instances, the immunologic nature of the reactions has been demonstrated by a variety of techniques: experimental induction of sensitization in guinea pigs and humans, passive transfer of sensitization, *in vitro* lymphocyte transformation, and macrophage migration inhibition tests. The vast majority of these reactions appear to be elicited by UV-A and to result from topical exposure. A number of reports have described apparent photoallergy resulting from systemically administered agents, but documentation is generally incomplete. Clinical photoallergy is usually manifest as dermatitis on exposed areas, which may eventually spread to areas covered by clothes; lichenification (thickening with increased skin markings) and chronic pigmentary changes may also develop.

The main role of light in photoallergy appears to be in the conversion of the hapten to a complete allergen, although other roles are possible. The mechanisms may be complex and may differ depending on the allergen, but two types of reactions are thought to play a role. Radiation absorbed by the photosensitizer may result in its conversion to a photoproduct that is a more potent allergic sensitizer than the parent compound. Alternatively, the short-lived, highly reactive, excited state species formed on irradiation of a number of photoallergens may combine with proteins, forming light-induced hapten-protein complexes that could act as the complete allergens.

Table 15–6 lists some photoallergens. All are substances that absorb UV. They generally have a resonating structure and are at least weakly phototoxic in an appropriate experimental system. Photoallergy can be induced experimentally in the guinea pig, and human and predictive screening tests have been described, though their universality is open to question (Kochevar *et al.*, 1979; Harber *et al.*, 1982).

An important complication of photoallergy from some agents, such as halogenated salicylanilides and phenothiazines, is the development of *persistent light reaction*. In this condition, marked sensitivity to light persists despite the apparent removal of further exposure to the photoallergen, and the action spectrum broadens to include the UV-B as well as the UV-A. This condition may be very long-lived and troublesome.

Photoimmunology and Toxic Responses.
In the 1970s, it was observed that UV-B exposure produced selective defects in immunologic function and that these defects played a major role in facilitating the growth of UV-induced skin cancers. Subsequently, it was shown that UV-B also modulates the immune response to contact allergens, as well as to microorganisms such as herpes simplex types I and II.

There are direct effects on immunocompetent cells, particularly damage to the antigen-presenting Langerhans cells at the site of irradiation, produced by relatively low doses of UV-B. Additionally, indirect effects to suppress contact hypersensitivity occur from high doses of UV, which appear to be caused by the release of soluble mediators that may include prostaglandins, interleukin-1, and *cis*-urocanic acid. Urocanic acid is a natural component of the stratum corneum that undergoes a *trans-cis* isomerization when irradiated by UV-B.

Like UV-B, photosensitization with psoralens and porphyrins can also down-regulate the contact hypersensitivity response, although there may be subtle differences in the mechanisms of suppression (Krutmann and Elmets, 1988).

Chemical Acne, Including Chloracne

A number of agents produce acneiform lesions similar to those seen in acne vulgaris. These include greases and oils, coal tar pitch, creosote, and a number of cosmetic preparations (acne cosmetica). These forms of acne typically start with comedones and inflammatory folliculitis on areas of the body contacted by the causal agent, which stimulates proliferation of the follicular epithelium of the sebaceous gland. The duct cells, which are usually lipid filled, keratinize, leading to the formation of keratin cysts and a sac filled with retained sebaceous lipid and keratin lamellae. A perifollicular inflammatory response may be seen. Some systemically administered drugs, including iodides, bromides, and isoniazid, can also cause acne.

Chloracne is a somewhat more specific type of acneiform eruption due to poisoning by halogenated aromatic compounds with a specific molecular shape (Poland and Glover, 1977). A list of certain well-defined causal agents is given in Table 15–7. Structural formulas for TCDD, TCDF, and TCAB are shown in Figure 15–5. A number of these substances, including PCDDs, PCDFs, TCAB, and TCAOB, are formed as contaminants during the manufacture or use of other polychlorinated substances.

The primary response to TCDD appears to be

Table 15–6. SELECTED REPORTED PHOTOALLERGENS

Halogenated salicylanilides and related agents
  3,3',4',5-Tetrachlorosalicylanilide
  Bithional
  3,4',5-Tribomosalicylanilide
  4',5-Dibromosalicylanilide
  4-Chloro-2-hydroxybenzoic acid *n*-butylamide
    (Jadit)
Sulfonamides
Phenothiazides
  Promethazine hydrochloride
4,6-Dichlorophenylphenol
Quinoxaline 1,4-di-*N*-oxide
Coumarin derivatives
  6-Methylcoumarin
  4-Methyl-7-ethoxycoumarin
  7-Methylcoumarin
Musk ambrette
Sunscreen components
  Glyceryl *p*-aminobenzoic acid
Plants
  Compositae (ragweed, Australian bush dermatitis)

Table 15-7. CAUSES OF CHLORACNE

Polyhalogenated dibenzofurans
  Polychlorodibenzofurans (PCDF), especially tri-,
    tetra- (TCDFs), penta- (PCDFs), and
    hexachlorodibenzofuran
  Polybromodibenzofurans (PBDFs), especially
    tetrabomodibenzofuran (TBDF)
Polychlorinated dibenzodioxins (PCDDs)
  2,3,7,8-Tetrachlorodibenzo-*p*-dioxin (TCDD)
  Hexachlorodibenzo-*p*-dioxin
Polychloronaphthalenes (PCNs)
Polyhalogenated biphenyls
  Polychlorobiphenyls (PCBs)
  Polybromobiphenyls (PBBs)
3,4,3',4'-Tetrachloroazoxybenzene (TCAOB)
3,3',4,4'-Tetrachloroazobenzene (TCAB)

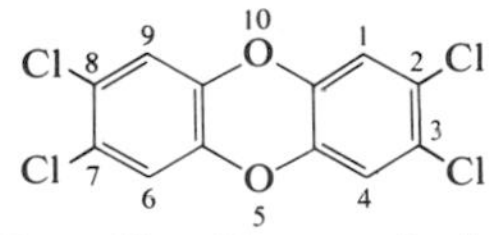

2,3,7,8-Tetrachlorodibenzo-*p*-dioxin (TCDD)

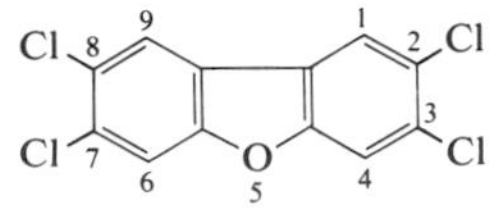

2,3,7,8-Tetrachlorodibenzofuran (TCDF)

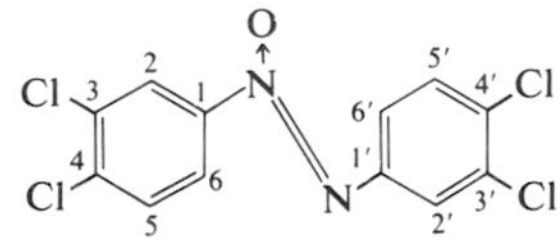

3,3'4,4'-Tetrachloroazoxybenzene (TCAB)

Figure 15-5. Structural formulas of certain potent chloracnegens.

hyperplasia and/or altered differentiation, and nearly all affected cells are epithelial. The effect is one of altered cellular regulation without a mutational effect on DNA. TCDD is a potent inducer of cytochrome P-450 and certain associated enzymatic activity, in particular microsomal-monooxygenase arylhydrocarbon hydroxide (AHH). The interaction of TCDD and related compounds with the Ah (arylhydrocarbon) receptor mediates the coordinate expression of a number of enzymes in addition to AHH. This induction is determined by a regulatory gene or genes known as the *Ah* locus. There is a good relationship between the binding of various halogenated dioxins and related compounds to the Ah receptor and the induction. The Ah receptor has not yet been purified and sequenced, but it is known to undergo a temperature-dependent biochemical and/or conformational change following binding of TCDD (Silbergeld and Gasiewicz, 1989).

A model has been proposed by Gillner *et al.* (1985) for receptor fit that provides a basis for explaining the similar enzyme-inducing properties and structure-activity relationships of TCDD, 3,3'4,4'-tetrachlorobiphenyl, and other compounds including certain naturally occurring indoles and photoxidized tryptophan derivatives that bind to the Ah receptor.

Chloracne is characterized by small, straw-colored cysts and comedones (Taylor, 1979). Inflammatory pustules and abscesses may occur but are not prominent features except in severe cases where large cysts may be seen as well as follicular hyperkeratosis. The most sensitive areas of skin, which may be the only ones involved, are below and to the outer side of the eye (the malar crescent) and behind the ear. The eruption typically involves exposed areas but may also involve covered areas, particularly the scrotum. Chloracne may continue to appear after

exposure to the chloracnegen has ceased, possibly as a result of its release from body stores. The clinical picture is distinctive but may not always be pathognomonic. Histologic changes commence with keratinization of the epithelium of the sebaceous gland ducts and outer root sheath of the hair. The sebaceous gland becomes replaced by a keratinous cyst, which is always attached to the epidermis (Crow, 1983).

Chloracne is a symptom complex whose other features vary depending on the actual chloracnegen and the circumstances of exposure.

TCDD is the most potent chloracnegen. Over 20 serious accidents with TCDD overexposure have occurred worldwide. Acute effects of exposure may include nausea, vomiting, headache, mucosal irritation, and chemical burns of the skin, sometimes with blistering; the latter occur particularly from handling contaminated objects or, as at Seveso, Italy, from being caught in the toxic cloud containing reactor contents following a reactor explosion. Chloracne is the first and most constant finding in the chronic stage. Other more variable findings have included: elevated porphyrin excretion, hyperpigmentation, hypertichosis, central and peripheral nervous system effects, and hepatic effects. Experimental effects of TCDD include teratogenicity, immunosuppression, and tumor induction.

The effects of PCBs may depend largely on the contaminants and on the route of absorption. In industrially exposed populations where percutaneous absorption may be the main route of uptake, chloracne is uncommon (Kimbrough, 1987). In these situations, the serum levels of PCBs may be correlated with the levels of hepatic enzymes and serum lipids, particularly triglycerides, but other toxic effects are less prominent. In contrast are epidemics in both Japanese and

Taiwanese populations who ingested rice oil contaminated with PCBs and developed Yusho show chloracne, a variety of other mucocutaneous symptoms including pigmentation, and meibomian gland metaplasia, as well as a number of systemic changes including increased porphyrin excretion and immunologic changes (Chang *et al.*, 1982). This rather different clinical syndrome may be related to the high concentrations of TCDF, chlorinated terphenyls, and other contaminants present in the oil rather than to PCBs.

Chloracne may be produced experimentally in the rhesus monkey, which develops facial lesions similar to those in humans, and on the inner surface of the rabbit ear but not elsewhere on rabbit skin.

Other Cutaneous Reaction Patterns

In addition to the conditions discussed to this point, a wide variety of other types of toxic reaction patterns are known. Because of the visibility of skin changes, these are best grouped according to the observed morphology. No exhaustive description is possible here.

Physical Dermatitis—Fiberglass. Fiberglass produces an intense pruritus (itching) of the skin in the presence or absence of pinpoint-sized papules, which are often excoriated and petechial. Urticaria and linear erosions are seen, generally secondary to scratching. The condition appears to be due to the physical properties of fiberglass. The likelihood of developing the condition appears directly related to the fiber diameter (which must be greater than 4.5 μm) and inversely to fiber length (Possick *et al.*, 1970; Konzen, 1982).

Urticarial Reactions. Urticarial (wheal-and-flare) reactions may be produced after cutaneous exposure to a relatively large number of agents, usually within 30 to 60 minutes of contact (Odum and Maibach, 1976; vonKrogh and Maibach, 1983). Causal agents may directly release histamine and other vasoactive substances (Zweiman, 1988). Biogenic polymers released from plants (nettles), animals (caterpillars, jellyfish), and a number of other substances fall into this category. Alternatively, some reactions depend on immediate immunologic reactions, whereas for a number of substances the mechanism is uncertain. Severe reactions may involve other organs including angioedema, bronchial asthma, anaphylactoid reactions, rhinoconjunctivitis, and gastrointestinal dysfunction. Urticaria is a frequent component of immediate hypersensitivity reactions to ingested or parenterally administered agents.

Cutaneous Granulomas. Cutaneous granulomas are usually seen as slightly erythematous, more or less flesh-colored papules, which may be grouped and may be associated with inflammatory changes. They are generally localized to sites of contact and result from a dermal response of mononuclear cells to poorly soluble substances (Epstein, 1980). Granulomas may represent a purely foreign body reaction as to talc and silica, or an immunologic response as in the case of beryllium, zirconium, and more rarely, chromium salts in tattoos. In the latter cases, appropriate immunologic testing may confirm sensitization.

Hair Damage and Loss. Hair is susceptible to damage both from agents contacting the hair externally and from those reaching the hair matrix through the dermis. Two major types of damage must be differentiated, keratolytic damage and matrix cell damage; the latter includes effluvium (hair loss) in the anagen or telogen phases.

Alkali, thioglycolates, and oxidizing agents such as peroxides and perborates produce keratolysis (dissolution of hair keratin) on local contact with the hair. Softening, matting, and increased fragility of hair ensues, which, depending on the extent of exposure, may involve local patches or the entire scalp. Regrowth of hair generally occurs, as the dermal hair matrix cells are not damaged.

Agents that damage the hair matrix (Reeves and Maibach, 1983) may directly poison active cells in the anagen phase. This leads either to cessation of growth and the loss of the entire hair or to the later loss of excessively brittle hair at the site of a weak constricted area in the shaft. Hair loss (anagen effluvium) may occur within one to two weeks of exposure to the agent. Causes of anagen effluvium include antimitotic agents such as alkylating agents, antimetabolites, and colchicine.

A number of substances precipitate telogen effluvium by precipitating hairs into the telogen phase. Hair shedding in the telogen phase occurs two to four months after exposure. Causes include oral contraceptives, a number of anticoagulants, propranolol, and triparanol. Some agents such as thallium, phenyl glycidyl, and dixyrazine cause hair loss of a mixed type. Hair loss in anagen and telogen phases can be distinguished by examination of shed hairs or hairs plucked from the scalp. Other causes of hair loss must be distinguished from chemical hair loss.

Hair may be discolored by chemical exposure—for example, green hair from copper, blue from indigo or cobalt, yellow from picric acid.

Hypopigmentation. A number of substances produce localized pigmentary loss, particularly phenols and catechols including hydroquinone, monobenzyl ether of hydroquinone,

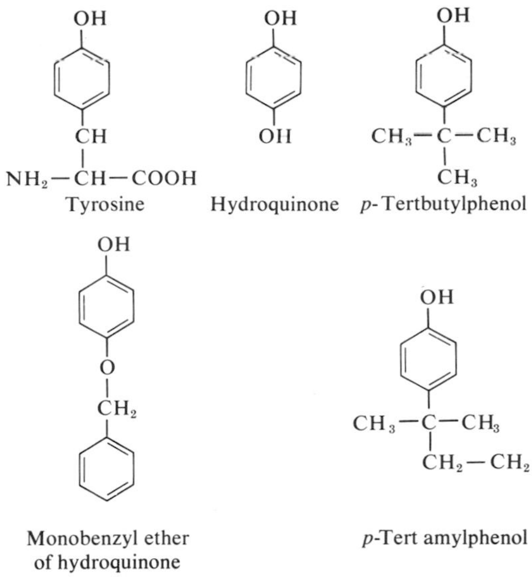

OH

CH

NH$_2$—CH—COOH
Tyrosine

OH

OH

Hydroquinone

OH

CH$_3$—C—CH$_3$

CH$_3$

p-Tertbutylphenol

OH

O

CH$_2$

OH

CH$_3$—C—CH$_3$

CH$_2$—CH$_2$

Monobenzyl ether
of hydroquinone

p-Tert amylphenol

Figure 15–6. Chemical structure of tyrosine and of selected depigmenting agents.

monomethyl ether of hydroquinone (*p*-hydroxyanisole), *p*-tertiary butyl phenol, *p*-tertiary amyl phenol, and 4-tertiary butyl catechol. These agents appear to have selective melanotoxicity. As shown in Figure 15–6, they bear structural similarity to tyrosine, the major building block of melanin (Gellin *et al.*, 1979).

The cosmetic disfiguration produced by these agents may be substantial, particularly in heavily pigmented individuals. Other agents such as arsenic can produce mixed pigmentary changes including circumscribed areas of pigment loss together with generalized increase in pigmentation.

As predictive skin testing is usually performed on albino animals in order that erythema may be better detected, these tests are generally not sensitive to effects on the pigment system, so that a false sense of security may ensue.

Hyperpigmentation. A number of chemical agents have been described that produce localized or diffuse increases in pigmentation. Localized changes occur secondary to phototoxic responses, especially with coal tar pitch and psoralens. Certain drugs including phenolphthalein and barbiturates produce a recurrent localized erythematous or dermatitic lesion that leaves a localized pigmented area, the so-called fixed drug eruption. These reactions recur at the same site on readministration of the agent; their pathogenesis is obscure. Large amounts of melanin-containing macrophages are found in the upper dermis in fixed drug eruptions.

Other causes of diffuse or local hyperpigmentation include heavy metals such as silver (argyria), bismuth, arsenic, and mercury; various

acridines and 4-aminoquinolines used as antimalarials; phenothiazines; tetracyclines; busulfan; and other alkylating agents (Granstein and Sober, 1983). Color changes in the skin may occur from the accumulation of exogenous or endogenous pigments, for example, the yellow-orange color of carotenaemia from carotenoids.

Cancer of the Skin. Carcinogenesis is dealt with elsewhere in this book. Important causes of skin cancer in humans in addition to UV and ionizing radiation are polycyclic aromatic hydrocarbons, arsenic, and combined exposures to psoralens and UV radiation. It is clear that a number of chemical agents influence the carcinogenic effects of UV radiation (Emmett, 1973; Forbes *et al.*, 1976).

REFERENCES

Adams, R. M.: *Occupational Skin Disease.* Grune & Stratton, Inc., New York, 1983.

Anderson, R. R., and Parrish, J. A.: The optics of skin. *J. Invest. Dermatol.,* **77**:13–19, 1981.

Baer, R. L., and Berman, B.: Role of Langerhans cells in cutaneous immunological reactions. In Safai, B., and Good, R. A. (eds.): *Immunodermatology.* Plenum Publishing Corp., New York, 1981.

Baer, R. L., and Bickers, D. R.: Allergic contact dermatitis, photoallergic contact dermatitis and phototoxic dermatitis. In Safai, B., and Good, R. A. (eds.): *Immunodermatology.* Plenum Publishing Corp., New York, 1981.

Baginsky, E.: *Occupational Skin Disease in California.* Division of Labor Statistics and Research, California Department of Industrial Relations, San Francisco, 1982.

Bergstresser, P. R.: Contact allergic dermatitis—old problems and new techniques. *Arch. Dermatol.,* **125**:276–279, 1989.

Bernstein, H. N.; Curtis, J.; Earl, F. L; and Kuwzbara, T.: Phototoxic corneal and lens opacities in dogs receiving a fungicide: 2,6-dichloro-4-nitroaniline. *Arch. Ophthalmol.,* **83**:336–348, 1970.

Bickers, D. R.: Metabolic activation of carcinogens by keratinocytes. *Ann. N.Y. Acad. Sci.,* **548**:102–107, 1988.

Blank, I. H., and Scheuplein, R. J.: Transport into and within the skin. *Br. J. Dermatol.,* **81**(Suppl. 4):4–10, 1969.

Bronaugh, R. L., and Maibach, H. I.: *In vitro* percutaneous absorption. In Marzulli, F. N., and Maibach, H. I. (eds.): *Dermatotoxicology,* 2nd ed. Hemisphere Publishing Co., Washington, D.C., 1983.

Bronaugh, R. L.; Steart, R. F.; Congdon, E. R.; and Giles, A. L.: Methods for *in vitro* percutaneous absorption studies. I. Comparison with *in vivo* results. *Toxicol. Appl. Pharmacol.,* **62**:474–480, 1982.

Brown, A. C., and Crounse, R. G.: *Hair, Trace Elements and Human Illness.* Praeger, New York, 1980.

CFR: United States, Code of Federal Regulations, Title 16, part 1500.41, 1980.

Chang, K. J.; Hsieh, K. H.; Lee, T. P.; and Tung, T. C.: Immunologic evaluation of patients with polychlorinated biphenyl poisoning: determination of phagocyte Fc and complement receptors. *Environ. Res.* **28**:329–334, 1982.

Cohn, J. R., and Emmett, E. A.: The excretion of trace metals in human sweat. *Ann. Clin. Lab. Sci.,* **8**:270–275, 1978.

Cripps, D. J., and Enta, T.: Absorption and action

spectra studies on bithional and halogenated salicylanilide photosensitivity. *Br. J. Dermatol.*, **82**:230–242, 1970.

Cronin, E.: *Contact Dermatitis*. Churchill-Livingstone, Edinburgh, 1980.

Crow, K. D.: Chloracne (halogen acne). In Marzulli, F. N., and Maibach, H. I. (eds.): *Dermatotoxicity*, 2nd ed. Hemisphere Publishing Co., Washington, D.C., 1983.

CTFA: *Cosmetic Ingredient Dictionary*. Cosmetic, Toiletry, and Fragrance Association, Washington, D.C., 1982.

Curreri, W. P.; Asch, M. J.; and Pruitt, B. A.: The treatment of chemical burns: specialized diagnostic and prognostic considerations. *J. Trauma*, **10**:634–642, 1970.

Dahl, M. V.: *Clinical Immunodermatology*. Year Book Medical Publishers, Chicago, 1981, chap. 9.

Dall'Acqua, F.: New chemical aspects of the photoreaction between psoralen and DNA. In Castellani, A. (ed.): *Research in Photobiology*. Plenum Publishing Corp., New York, 1977, pp. 245–255.

Eckert, R. L., and Rorke, E. A.: Molecular biology of keratinocyte differentiation. *Environ. Health Perspect.*, **80**:109–116, 1989.

Emmett, E. A.: Ultraviolet radiation as a cause of skin tumors. *Crit. Rev. Toxicol.*, **2**:211–255, 1973.

———: Drug photoallergy. *Int. J. Dermatol.*, **17**:370–379, 1978.

———: Phototoxicity from endogenous agents. *Photochem. Photobiol.*, **40**:429–436, 1979.

———: Topical agents. In Hanenson, I. B. (ed.): *Quick Reference to Clinical Toxicology*. J. B. Lippincott Co., Philadelphia, 1980.

Emmett, E. A.; Risby, T. H.; Jiang, L.; Ng, S. K.; Feinman, S.: Allergic contact dermatitis to nickel: bioavailability from consumer products and provocation threshold. *J. Am. Acad. Dermatol.*, **19**(2):314–322, 1988.

Emmett, E. A.; Stetzer, L.; and Taphorn, B.: Phototoxic keratoconjunctivitis from coal tar pitch volatiles. *Science*, **198**:841–842, 1977.

Epstein, W. L.: Foreign body granulomas. In Boros, D., and Yoshida, H. (eds.): *Basic and Clinical Aspects of Granulomatous Diseases*. Elselvier/North Holland, Amsterdam, 1980.

Feldmann, R. J., and Maibach, H. I.: Absorption of some organic compounds through the skin in man. *J. Invest. Dermatol.*, **54**:339–404, 1969.

Forbes, P. D.; Davies, R. E.; and Urbach, F.: Phototoxicity and photocarcinogenesis. Comparative effects of anthracene and 8-methoxypsoralen in the skin of mice. *Food Cosmet. Toxicol.*, **14**:303–306, 1976.

Foussereau, J.; Benezra, C.; and Maibach, H. I.: *Occupational Contact Dermatitis: Clinical and Chemical Aspects*. Munksgaard, Copenhagen, 1982.

Franz, T. J.: Percutaneous absorption. On the relevance of *in vitro* data. *J. Invest. Dermatol.*, **64**:190–195, 1975.

Fregert, S.: *Manual of Contact Dermatitis*, 2nd ed. Munksgaard, Copenhagen, 1981.

Gellin, G. A.; Maibach, H. I.; Misiaszek, M. H.; and Ring, M.: Detection of environmentally depigmenting substances. *Contact Dermatitis*, **5**:201–213, 1979.

Gillner, M.; Bergman, J.; Cambillau, C.; Fernstrom, B.; and Gunstafsson, J. A.: Interactions of indoles with specific binding sites for 2,3,7,8-tetrachlorodibenzo-*p*-dioxin in rat liver. *Mol. Pharmacol.*, **28**:357–363, 1985.

Goldstein, B. D., and Harber, L. C.: Erythropoetic protoporphyria: lipid peroxidation and red cell membrane damage associated with photohemolysis. *J. Clin. Invest.*, **51**:892–902, 1972.

Goldstein, J. A.; Friesen, M.; Linder, R. E.; Hickman, P.; Hass, J. R.; and Bergman, H.: Effects of pentachlorphenol on hepatic drug-metabolizing enzymes and porphyria related to contamination with chlorinated dibenzo-*p*-dioxins and dibenzofurans. *Biochem. Pharmacol.*, **26**:1549–1557, 1977.

Grandjean, P.; Berlin, A.; Gilbert, M.; and Penning, W.: Preventing percutaneous absorption of industrial chemicals: the "skin" notation. *Am. J. Indust. Med.*, **14**:97–107, 1988.

Granstein, R. D., and Sober, A. J.: Drug and heavy metal induced hyperpigmentation. In Marzulli, F. N., and Maibach, H. I. (eds.): *Dermatotoxicity*, 2nd ed. Hemisphere Publishing Co., Washington, D.C., 1983.

Hammer, D. I.; Finklea, J. F.; Hendricks, R. H.; Shy, C. M.; and Horton, R. J. M.: Hair, trace metals and environmental exposure. *Am. J. Epidemiol.*, **69**:84, 1971.

Harber, L. C.; Armstrong, R. B.; Walther, R. R.; and Ichikawa, H.: Current status of predictive animals for drug photoallergy and the correlation with humans. In Kligman, A., and Leyden, J. (eds.): *Assessment of Safety and Efficacy of Topical Drugs and Cosmetics*. Grune & Stratton, New York, 1982.

Harber, L. C., and Bickers, D. R.: *Photosensitivity: Principles of Diagnosis and Treatment*. W. B. Saunders Co., Philadelphia, 1981.

Hemingway, J. D., and Molokhia, M. M.: The dissolution of metallic nickel in artificial sweat. *Contact Dermatitis*, **16**:99–105, 1987.

Johnson, H. C., and Maibach, H. I.: Drug excretion in human eccrine sweat. *J. Invest. Dermatol.*, **56**:182–188, 1971.

Kimbrough, R. D.: Human health effects of polychlorinated biphenyls (PCBs) and polybrominated biphenyls (PBBs). *Annu. Rev. Pharmacol. Toxicol.*, **27**:87–111, 1987.

Klecak, G.: Identification of contact allergens. In Marzulli, F. N., and Maibach, H. I. (eds.): *Dermatotoxicology*, 2nd ed. Hemisphere Publishing Co., Washington, D.C., 1983.

Kochevar, I.: Phototoxicity mechanisms: chlorpromazine photosensitized damage to DNA and cell membranes. *J. Invest. Dermatol.*, **77**:59–64, 1981.

Kochevar, I. E.; Kaler, G. L.; Embinder, J.; and Harber, L. C.: Assay of contact photosensitivity to musk ambrette in guinea pigs. *J. Invest. Dermatol.*, **73**:144–146, 1979.

Konzen, J. K.: Fiberglass and the skin. In Maibach, H. I., and Gellin, G. A. (eds.): *Occupational and Industrial Dermatology*. Year Book Medical Publishers, Chicago, 1982.

Kripke, M. L.: Immunologic effects of UV radiation and their role in photocarcinogenesis. *Photochem. Photobiol. Rev.*, **5**:257–292, 1980.

Krutmann, J., and Elmets, C. A.: Recent studies on mechanisms in photoimmunology. *Photochem. Photobiol.*, **48**:787–798, 1988.

Lauwerys, R. R.: *Industrial Chemical Exposure: Guidelines for Biological Monitoring*. Biomedical Publications, Davis, Calif., 1983.

Magnusson, B., and Kligman, A. M.: *Allergic Contact Dermatitis in the Guinea Pig. Identification of Contact Allergens*. Charles C. Thomas, Springfield, Ill., 1970.

Marzulli, F. N., and Maibach, H. I.: Contact allergy: predictive testing of fragrance ingredients in humans by Draize and maximization methods. *J. Environ. Pathol. Toxicol.*, **3**:235–245, 1980.

———(eds.): *Dermatotoxicology*, 2nd ed. Hemisphere Publishing Co., Washington, D.C., 1983.

Matolsky, A. G.: Concluding remarks and future directions in the molecular and developmental biology of keratins. *Curr. Top. Dev. Biol.* **22**:255–264, 1987.

Maurer, T.: Phototoxicity testing—*in vivo* and *in vitro*. *Fund. Chem. Toxicol.*, **25**:407–414, 1987.

McCreesh, A. H., and Steinberg, M.: Skin irritation testing in animals. In Marzulli, F. N., and Maibach, H. I. (eds.): *Dermatotoxicology*, 2nd ed. Hemisphere Publishing Co., Washington, D.C., 1983.

Menne, T.: Reactions to systemic exposure to contact allergies. In Marzulli, F. N., and Maibach, H. I. (eds.): *Dermatotoxicology*, 2nd ed. Hemisphere Publishing Co., Washington, D.C., 1983.

Montagna, W., and Parakkal, P. F.: *The Structure and Function of Skin*. Academic Press, Inc., New York, 1974.

NAS: *Principles and Procedures for Evaluating the Toxicity of Household Substances*. National Academy of Sciences, Washington, D.C., 1977.

Nordlund, J. J.; Abdel-Malek, Z. A.; Boussy, R. E.; and Rheinis, L. A.: Pigment cell biology: an historical review. *J. Invest. Dermatol.*, **92**(4 Supp.):53–60, 1989.

Nordquist, B., and Rosenthal, S. A.: Studies on DNCB contact sensitivity in guinea pigs by the macrophage migration test. *Int. Arch. Allergy Appl. Immunol.*, **56**:73–78, 1978.

Odum, R. B., and Maibach, H. I.: Contact urticaria: a different contact dermatitis. *Cutis*, **18**:672–676, 1976.

Pannatier, A.; Jenner, P.; Testa, B.; and Etter, J. C.: The skin as a drug-metabolizing organ. *Drug Metab. Rev.*, **8**:319–343, 1978.

Parrish, J. A.; Anderson, R. R.; Urbach, F.; *et al.: UV-A Biologic Effects of Ultraviolet Radiation with Emphasis on Human Responses to Longwave Ultraviolet*. Plenum Press, New York, 1978.

Parrish, J. A.; White, H. A. D.; and Pathak, M. A.: Photomedicine. In Fitzpatrick, T. B.; (eds.): *Dermatology in General Medicine*, 2nd ed. McGraw-Hill Book Co., New York, 1979.

Phillips, L.; Steinberg, M.; Maibach, H.I.; and Akers, W. A.: A comparison of rabbit and human skin responses to certain irritants. *Toxicol. Appl. Pharmacol.*, **21**:369–382, 1972.

Poland, A., and Glover, E.: Chlorinated biphenyl induction of amyl hydrocarbon hydroxylase activity: a study of the structure activity relationships. *Mol. Pharmacol.*, **13**:924–938, 1977.

Poland, A., and Knutson, J. C.: 2,3,7,8-Tetrachlorodibenzo-*p*-dioxin and related halogenated aromatic hydrocarbons: examination of the mechanism of toxicity. *Annu. Rev. Pharmacol. Toxicol.*, **22**:517–554, 1982.

Possick, P. A.; Gellin, G. A.; and Key, M. D.: Fibrous glass dermatitis. *Am. Ind. Hyg. Assoc. J.*, **31**:12–15, 1970.

Reeves, J. R. T., and Maibach, H. I.: Drug and chemical-induced hair loss. In Marzulli, F. N., and Maibach, H. I. (eds.): *Dermatotoxicology*, 2nd ed.

Hemisphere Publishing Co., Washington, D.C., 1983.

Report of the OSHA Advisory Committee on Cutaneous Hazards. Office of Consumer Affairs, U.S. Department of Labor, Washington, D.C., 1979.

Rudner, E. J.: Epidemiology of contact dermatitis in North America. *Arch. Dermatol.*, **108**:537–540, 1973.

Schaefer, H., and Jamoulle, J. C.: Skin pharmacokinetics. *Int. J. Dermatol.*, **27**:351–359, 1988.

Schaefer, H.; Zesch, A.; Stuttgen, G.: Skin permeability. Springer-Verlag, Berlin, 1982.

Scheuplein, R. J., and Blank, I. H.: Permeability of the skin. *Physiol. Rev.*, **51**:702–747, 1971.

Scheuplein, R. J., and Ross, L.: Effects of surfactants and solvents on the permeability of epidermis. *J. Soc. Cosmetic Chemists*, **21**:853–873, 1970.

Schmid, R.: Cutaneous porphyria in Turkey. *N. Engl. J. Med.*, **263**:397–398, 1960.

Silbergeld, E. K., and Gasiewicz, T. A.: Dioxins and the Ah receptor. *Am. J. Ind. Med.*, **16**:455–474, 1989.

Soter, N. A., and Fitzpatrick, T. B.: Introduction and classification. In Fitzpatrick, T. B. (ed.): *Dermatology in General Medicine*, 3rd ed. McGraw-Hill Book Co., New York, 1987.

Steinberg, M.; Akers, W. A.; Weeks, M.: McCreesh, A. H.; and Maibach, H. I.: A comparison of test techniques. In Maibach, H. I. (ed.): *Animal Models in Dermatology*. Churchill Livingstone, New York, 1975.

Stern, R. S.; Thibodeu, L. A.; Kleinerman, R. A.; Parrish, J. A.; Fitzpatrick, T. B.; and 22 Participating Investigators: Risk of cutaneous carcinoma in patients treated with oral methoxsalen photochemotherapy for psoriasis. *N. Engl. J. Med.*, **300**:809–813, 1979.

Stoughton, R. B.: Percutaneous absorption of drugs. *Annu. Rev. Pharmacol. Toxicol.*, **29**:55–69, 1989.

Taylor, J. S.: Environmental chloracne: update and overview. *Ann. N.Y. Acad. Sci.*, **320**:295–307, 1979.

Tregear, R. T.: *Physical Functions of the Skin*. Academic Press, Inc., New York, 1966.

vonKrogh, G., and Maibach, H. I.: The contact urticaria syndrome. *J. Am. Acad. Dermatol.*, **5**(3):328–342, 1981.

Weil, C. S., and Scala, R. A.: Study of intra- and interlaboratory variability in the results of rabbit eye and skin irritation tests. *Toxicol. Appl. Pharmacol.*, **19**:276–360, 1971.

Wester, R. C., and Maibach, H. I.: Relationship of topical dose and percutaneous absorption in rhesus monkey and man. *J. Invest. Dermatol.*, **67**:518–520, 1976.

Wester, R. C.; Noonan, P. K.; Smeach, S.; and Kosobud, L.: Estimate of nitroglycerin percutaneous first pass metabolism. *Pharmacologist*, **23**:203, 1981.

Zweiman, B.: Mediators of allergic inflammation in the skin. *Clin. Allergy*, **18**:419–433, 1988.

Chapter 16

TOXIC RESPONSES OF THE REPRODUCTIVE SYSTEM

John A. Thomas

INTRODUCTION

The endocrine function of the gonads is primarily concerned with perpetuation of the species. The survival of any species depends on the integrity of its reproductive system. Sexual reproduction involves a very complex process for the gonads. Genes located in the chromosomes of the germ cells transmit genetic information and modulate cell differentiation and organogenesis. Germ cells ensure the maintenance of structure and functions in the organism in its own lifetime and from generation to generation.

The twentieth century has undergone an industrial renaissance, and through scientific and technical advances there has been a significant extension in life expectancy and generally an enhanced quality of life. Concomitantly with this industrial renaissance has come an estimated 50,000 to 60,000 chemicals into common use. Approximately 600 or more new chemicals enter commerce each year. The impact of new chemicals (or drugs) on the reproductive system was tragically accentuated by the thalidomide incidence in the 1960s (cf. Fabrio, 1985). This episode led to an increased awareness on a worldwide basis and brought forth laws and guidelines pertaining to reproductive system safety and testing protocols. This new awareness of reproductive hazards in the workplace has led to corporate policies and legal considerations (Bond, 1986; McElveen, 1986). In 1985, an AMA Council on Scientific Affairs charged an Advisory Panel on Reproductive Hazards in the Work Place to consider over 100 chemicals with the intent to estimate their imminent hazards (AMA Council on Scientific Affairs, 1985).

Concern for reproductive hazards is not a new concern but dates back to the Roman empire. Lead, found in high concentration in pottery and water vessels, probably played a role in the increased incidence of stillbirths. Lead is now known to be an abortifacient as well as capable of producing teratospermias. In the United

States, male factory workers occupationally exposed to 1,2-dibromo-3-chloropropane (DBCP) became sterile, as evidenced by oligospermia, azoospermia, and germinal aplasia. Factory workers in battery plants in Bulgaria, lead mine workers in the state of Missouri, and workers in Sweden who handle organic solvents (toluene, benzene, and xylene) suffer from low sperm counts, abnormal sperm, and varying degrees of infertility. Diethylstilbestrol (DES), lead, chlordecone methylmercury, and many cancer chemotherapeutic agents have been shown to be toxic to the male and female reproductive system and possibly capable of inflicting genetic damage to germ cells (*cf.* Barlow and Sullivan, 1982; Office of Technology Assessment Report, 1985).

The potential hazard of chemicals to reproduction and the risks to humans from chemical exposure are difficult to assess because of the complexity of the reproductive process, the unreliability of laboratory tests, and the quality of human data. In the human, it is estimated that one in five couples are involuntarily sterile; over one-third of early embryos die, and about 15 percent of recognized pregnancies abort spontaneously. Among the surviving fetuses at birth, approximately 3 percent have developmental defects (not always anatomic), and with increasing age, over twice that many become detectable. It should be obvious that even under normal physiological conditions the reproductive system does not function in a very optimal state. Not surprisingly, the imposition of chemicals (or drugs) on this system can further interfere with a number of biological processes or events.

GENERAL REPRODUCTIVE BIOLOGY

The developing gonad is very sensitive to chemical insult, with some cellular populations being more vulnerable than others to an agent's toxic actions. Further, the developing embryo is uniquely sensitive to changes in its environment whether such changes are caused by exposure to foreign chemicals or certain viruses. The toxicologist must be mindful of the teratogenic potential of a chemical as well as be aware of its potential deleterious actions on maternal biochemical processes. The development of normal reproductive capacity may offer particularly susceptible targets for toxins. Environmental factors might alter the genetic determinants of gonadal sex, the hormonal determinants of phenotypic sex, fetal gametogenesis, and reproductive tract differentiation, as well as postnatal integration of endocrine functions and other processes essential for the propagation of the species. The effects of environmental agents on sexual differentiation and development of reproductive capacity are largely unknown. Of the chemicals that have been studied, it is noteworthy that they possess a wide diversity in molecular structure and that they may affect specific cell populations within the reproductive system.

SEXUAL DIFFERENTIATION

An understanding of reproductive physiology requires consideration of the process of sexual differentiation or that pattern of development of the gonads, genital ducts, and external genitalia (cf. Simpson, 1980; De La Chapelle, 1987; Goldberg, 1988).

Gonadal Sex

A testes-determining gene on the Y chromosome is responsible for determining gonadal sex (cf. De La Chapelle, 1987). It converts an undifferentiated gonad into a testes. The organization of the gonadal anlage into the seminiferous or spermatogenic tubules of the male may be mediated by testes-determining genes. The H-Y antigen is a surface glycoprotein present in all male cells (cf. Goldberg, 1988). The testes produces two separate hormones: the Müllerian inhibiting factor (MIF) and testosterone. Testosterone-induced masculine differentiation is modulated by androgen receptors regulated by genes on the X chromosome. Alterations of the sex chromosomes may be transmitted by either one of the parents (gonadal dysgenesis) or may occur in the embryo itself. Failure of the sex chromosomes of either of the parents to separate during gametogenesis is called *nondisjunction* and can result in gonadal agenesis. Klinefelter's syndrome is characterized by testicular dysgenesis with male morphology and an XXY karyotype; Turner's syndrome includes ovarian agenesis with female morphology, an XO karyotype, and a single X chromosome.

Hermaphroditism (true and pseudo) may occur secondary to nondisjunction of sex chromosomes during the initial cleavage mitosis of the egg. Such a condition results in sex mosaics of XY/XX or XY/XO. Pseudohermaphrodites are characterized by secondary sex characteristics that differ from those predicted by genotype.

Chemically induced nondisjunction is a common genetic abnormality. Nondisjunction of Y chromosomes may be detected by the presence or absence of fluorescent bodies on the chromatin of sperm (YFF spermatozoa). YFF sperm are increased in patients treated with certain antineoplastic agents as well as with x-radiation.

Genotypic Sex

The normal female chromosome complement is 44 autosomes and 2 sex chromosomes, XX. The two X chromosomes contained in the germ cells are necessary for the development of a normal ovary. Apparently, autosomes also are involved in ovarian development, differentiation of the genital ducts, and external genitalia characteristic of a normal female. This requires that only a single X chromosome be involved in genetic events within the cell. Generally speaking, the second X chromosome of a normal XX female is genetically inactive in nongonadal cells, although it has been shown that the tip of the short arm of the chromosome is genetically active.

The Y chromosome is consistent with the male determinant. The normal male has a chromosome complement of 44 autosomes and 2 sex chromosomes, X and Y. An additional X chromosome does not change the fundamental maleness caused by the Y chromosome, but the gonads are often dysfunctional (Klinefelter's syndrome). Genetic coding on the X chromosome may be involved in transforming the gonad into a testis.

The presence of chromatin material on the short (p) arm of the (Y_p) chromosome directs the development of the testes. Chromatin material (Y_q) on the long (q) arm directs the development of spermatogenesis.

Phenotypic (Genital) Sex

In the early stages of fetal development, sexual differentiation does not require any known hormonal products. The differentiation of the genital ducts and the external genitalia, however, requires hormones. The onset of testosterone synthesis by the male gonad is necessary for the initiation of male differentiation. Although the testes are required in male differentiation, the embryonic ovaries are not needed to attain the female phenotype. Female characteristics develop in the absence of androgen secretion.

Two principal types of hormones are secreted by the fetal testes, an androgenic steroid responsible for male reproductive tract development and a nonsteroid factor that causes regression of the Müllerian ducts. Sertoli cells are the likely source of Müllerian inhibiting factor (MIF) or anti-Müllerian hormone (AMH). Leydig cell differentiation and regression correspond well with the onset and subsequent decline in testosterone synthesis by the fetal testis. Thus, the embryonic testis suppresses the development of the Müllerian ducts, allows the development of the Wolffian duct and its derivatives, and thereby imposes the male phenotype on the embryo.

Three periods for testosterone production have been described with regard to sexual differentiation. The first period occurs on days 14 to 17 of gestation in the rat and weeks 4 to 6 in the human. The second period occurs about day 17 of gestation to about 2 weeks postnatal age in the rat and from month 4 of pregnancy to 1 to 3 months of postnatal age in man. The third period follows a long period of testicular inactivity in both species when testosterone production is reinitiated between 40 and 60 days of age in the rat and 12 to 14 years of age in man.

The dynamics of testosterone and dihydrotestosterone production and cellular interactions are an important prerequisite to knowing which chemicals might affect sexual differentiation. Factors that reduce the ability of testosterone to be synthesized, activated, enter the cell, and/or affect the cell nucleus's ability to regulate the synthesis of androgen-dependent proteins would have a potential to alter sexual differentiation. Some of these are summarized in Table 16–1. Chemicals are capable of exerting a testosterone-depriving action on the developing systems. These include effects on the feedback regulation of gonadotropin secretion, gonadotropin effectiveness, testosterone and dihydrotestosterone synthesis, plasma binding, as well as cytoplasmic receptor and nuclear chromatin binding.

Insufficient amounts of androgens can feminize the male fetus with otherwise normal testes and an XY karyotype. Slight deficiencies affect only the later stages of differentiation of the external genital organs and result in microphallus, hypospadia (urethra opens on under surface of penis), and valviform appearance of the scrotum with masculine general morphology. However, a severe androgen deficiency (or resistance) allows the Müllerian system to persist and results in external genital organs of a female type (vagina and uterus) that coexist with ectopic testes and normal male efferent ducts. A lack of androgen receptors can also lead to a testicular feminization–type syndrome, even when normal levels of testosterone are present. Finally, sexual behavior also appears to be "imprinted" in the central nervous system by androgens from the testis and could be affected by endogenous and exogenous chemicals.

Estrogens exert an important developmental effect. Nearly 20 years have elapsed since the association between maternal diethylstilbestrol administration and vaginal adenocarcinoma in female offspring was reported. Diethylstilbestrol, or DES, a synthetic estrogen, has been used extensively both in human medicine and formerly in the feed of livestock. Other nonsteroidal

Table 16–1. FACTORS AFFECTING ANDROGEN EFFECTIVENESS*

TARGET	EFFECT	EXAMPLE
Hypothalamic-pituitary interaction	Feedback control of LHRH-mediated gonadotropin secretion	Estrogens, progestins
Gonadotropin action	Disrupt reproductive control processes involving gonadotropins	LH-FSH antibodies
Androgen synthesis	Inhibit key enzymes, e.g., cholesterol desmolase, 17α-hydroxylase, 3β-hydroxy-steroid oxidoreductase, C17-20 lyase, 17-keto reductase, 5α-reductase	Steroid analogues, diphenylmethylanes (amphenone B,DDD), pyridine derivatives (SU series), disubstituted glutartic acid imides (glutethimides), triazines, hydrazines, thiosemicarbazones
DHT synthesis	Inhibit 5α-reductase in target tissue	Androstene-17-carboxylic acid, progesterone
Plasma binding	Alter ratio of bound and free androgen in systemic circulation	Estrogens
Cytoplasmic receptors	Alter effect on target tissue by affecting binding to cytoplasmic receptors	Cyproterone acetate, 17α-methyl-β-testosterone, flutamide
DHT cellular binding	Block DHT effect on target tissue	Cyproterone acetate, spironolactone, dihydroprogesterone, RU-22930

* From Dixon, R. L.: Potential of environmental factors to affect development of reproductive system. *Fund. Appl. Toxicol.*, **2:**5–12, 1982.

estrogens—namely, the insecticides kepone and DDT (and its metabolites)—exhibit uterotropic actions in experimental animals (cf. Thomas, 1975). Similarly, polychlorinated biphenyls (PCBs) are uterotropic. Zearalenones, a plant mycotoxin, also exhibits female sex hormone properties.

GONADAL FUNCTION

Regardless of sex, the gonads possess a dual function: an endocrine function—that is, the secretion of sex hormones—and a nonendocrine function—that is, the production of germ cells (gametogenesis). The testes secrete male sex steroids, including testosterone and dihydrotestosterone. The testes also secrete small amounts of estrogens. The ovaries, depending on the phase of the menstrual cycle, secrete various amounts of estrogens and progesterone. Estradiol is the principal steroid estrogen secreted by the ovary in most mammalian species. The ovary is the chief source of progesterone secretion. The corpus luteum and the placenta are also primary sites of secretion of progesterone.

The gametogenic and the secretory functions of either the ovary or testes are dependent on the secretion of adenohypophyseal gonadotropins, follicle stimulating hormone (FSH), and luteinizing hormone (LH). LH, in the male, is also referred to as ICSH (interstitial cell stimulating hormone). FSH in the female stimulates follicular development and maturation in the ovary. FSH in the male stimulates the process of spermatogenesis. The secretion of pituitary FSH and LH are modulated by gonadal hormones. Sex steroids secreted by the testes or ovaries regulate the secretion of pituitary gonadotropins. The Sertoli cell of the testes secretes small amounts of estrogen and a proteinaceous hormone called inhibin. Inhibin aids in the modulation of spermatogenesis. ICSH(LH) provokes the process of steroidogenesis in the testes.

The onset of puberty results in the cyclic secretion of pituitary gonadotropins in the female. The cyclic secretion establishes the normal menstrual cycle. In males, puberty is evidenced by the continuous and noncyclic secretion of gonadotropins.

TESTICULAR FUNCTION

Spermatogenesis

The production of sperm, termed *spermatogenesis,* is a unique process in which the timing and stages of differentiation are known with a considerable degree of certainty. In producing spermatozoa by the process of spermatogenesis,

the germinal epithelium plays a dual function: It must produce millions of spermatozoa each day and also continuously replace the population of cells that give rise to the process, the spermatogonia (cf. Amann, 1989).

The sperm is among the smallest cells in man. In humans, its length is about 50 μm or only about one-half the diameter of the ovum, the largest cell of the female organism. The relative volume of a sperm is about 1/100,000 that of the egg. The sperm has a head, middle piece, and tail, which correspond, respectively, to the following functions: activation and genetics, metabolism, and motility.

Whereas only a few hundred human ova are released as cells ready for fertilization in a lifetime, millions of motile sperm are formed in the spermatogenic tubules each day. Several physiological factors affect the regulation of sperm motility (e.g., spermine, spermidine, "quiescence" factor, cAMP, motility stimulating factor, etc.) (Lindemann and Kanous, 1989). Oogenesis and spermatogenesis are compared in Figure 16–1.

Spermatogenesis starts at puberty and continues almost throughout life. The primitive male germ cells are spermatogonia, which are situated next to the basement membrane of the seminiferous tubules. Following birth, spermatogonia are dormant until puberty, when proliferative activity begins again. The onset of spermatogenesis accompanies functional maturation of the testes. Two major types of spermatogonia are present—type A, which generates other spermatogonia, and type B, which becomes a mature sperm. The latter type develops into primary spermatocytes, which undergo meiotic divisions to become secondary spermatocytes. The process of meiosis results in the reduction of the normal complement of chromosomes (diploid) to half this number (haploid) (Figure 16–2). Meiosis ensures the biologic necessity of evolution through the introduction of controlled variability. Each gamete must receive one of each pair of chromosomes. Whether it receives the maternal or paternal chromosome is a matter of chance. In the male, meiosis is completed within several days. In the female, meiotic division begins during fetal life but then is suspended until puberty. Meiosis may be the most susceptible stage for chemical insult.

Secondary spermatocytes give rise to spermatids. Spermatids complete their development into sperm by undergoing a period of transformation (spermiogenesis) that involves extensive nuclear and cytoplasmic reorganization. The nucleus condenses and becomes the sperm head; the two centrioles give rise to the flagellum or axial filament. Part of the Golgi apparatus be-

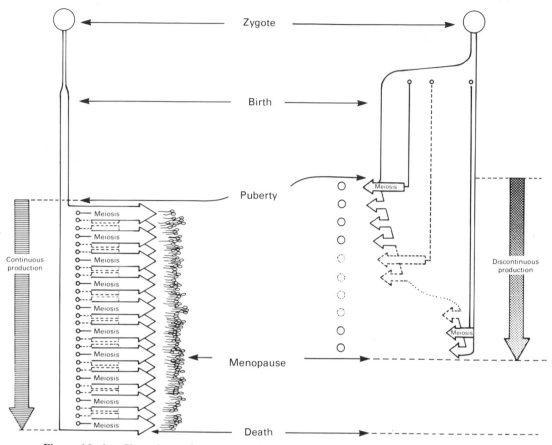

Figure 16–1. Chronology of gametogenesis. (Modified from Tuchmann-Duplessis, H.; David, G.; and Haegel, P.: *Illustrated Human Embryology: Embryogenesis*, Vol. I. Springer-Verlag, New York, 1972.)

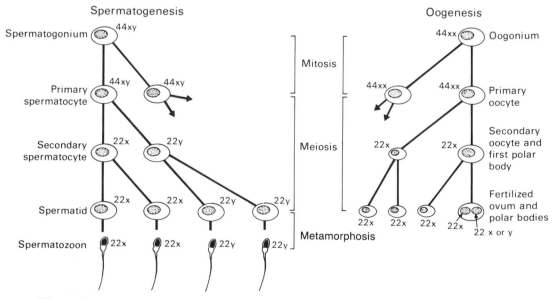

Figure 16–2. Cellular replication (mitosis) and cellular reductive divisions (meiosis) involved in spermatogenesis, oogenesis, and fertilization.

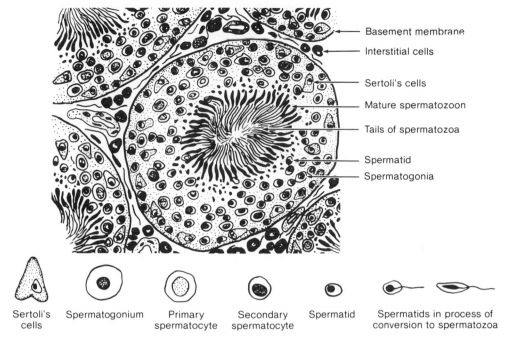

Basement membrane

Interstitial cells

Sertoli's cells

Mature spermatozoon

Tails of spermatozoa

Spermatid

Spermatogonia

Sertoli's cells | Spermatogonium | Primary spermatocyte | Secondary spermatocyte | Spermatid | Spermatids in process of conversion to spermatozoa

Figure 16–3.   Schematic cross section of seminiferous tubules of testes. Morphology of the Sertoli cell along with the cellular events involved in spermatogenesis (spermatogonium through spermatid).

comes the acrosome, and the mitochondria concentrate into a sheath located between two centrioles.

Seminiferous tubules contain germ cells at different stages of differentiation and Sertoli cells. In a cyclical fashion, spermatogonia A of certain areas of a tubule become committed to divide synchronously, and the cohorts of the resulting cells differentiate in unison. Thus, a synchronous population of developing germ cells occupies a defined area within a seminiferous tubule. Cells within each cohort are connected by intercellular bridges.

The anatomical relationships of the mammalian testes reveal that the process of spermatogenesis occurs within the seminiferous tubules (Figure 16–3). The germ cells, along with the Sertoli cells, are contained within the membranous boundaries of the seminiferous tubules. Conversely, the Leydig cells are situated in the interstitium or outside the seminiferous tubules. It may be seen that in several different species the seminiferous tubules contain single cellular associations. In humans, however, such cellular associations differ and are intermingled in a mosaiclike pattern. Varying among species, several cellular associations may be detected. Each cellular association contains four or five types of germ cells organized in a specific, layered pattern. Each layer represents one cellular generation. Fourteen cellular associations are observed in the seminiferous epithelium in the

rat (LeBlond and Clermont, 1952; Heller and Clermont, 1964).

Presuming a fixed point within the seminiferous tubule could be viewed in the developing germ cell, there would be a sequential appearance of each of these cellular associations that would be characteristic of the particular specie. This progression through the series of cellular associations would continue to repeat itself in a predictable fashion. The interval required for one complete series of cellular associations to appear at one point within a tubule is termed the *duration of the cycle of the seminiferous epithelium*. The duration of one cycle of the seminiferous epithelium depends on, and is thus equal to, the cell turnover rate of spermatogonia. Thus, the duration of the cycle of seminiferous epithelium varies among mammals, being a low of about 9 days in the mouse to a high of about 16 days in man (Table 16–2) (Galbraith *et al.*, 1982). Spermatids, emanating from spermatogonia committed to differentiate approximately 4.5 cycles earlier, are continuously released from the germinal epithelium.

Maturation changes occur in the sperm as they traverse along the tubules of the testes and the epididymides. During this passage, sperm acquire the capacity for fertility and become more motile. There is a progressive dehydration of the cytoplasm, decreased resistance to cold shock, changes in metabolism, and variations in membrane permeability. Each ejaculate contains a

Table 16–2. CRITERIA FOR SPERMATOGENESIS IN LABORATORY ANIMALS AND MAN*

	MOUSE	RAT	RABBIT (NEW ZEALAND WHITE)	DOG (BEAGLE)	MONKEY (RHESUS)	MAN
Duration of cycle of seminiferous epithelium (days)	8.6	12.9	10.7	13.6	9.5	16.0
Life span of						
B-type spermatogonia (days)	1.5	2.0	1.3	4.0	2.9	6.3
L + Z[†] spermatocytes (days)	4.7	7.8	7.3	5.2	6.0	9.2
P + D[†] spermatocytes (days)	8.3	12.2	10.7	13.5	9.5	15.6
Golgi spermatids (days)	1.7	2.9	2.1	6.9	1.8	7.9
Cap spermatids (days)	3.5	5.0	5.2	3.0	3.7	1.6
Fraction of a life span as						
B-type spermatogonia	0.11	0.10	0.08	0.19	0.19	0.25
Primary spermatocyte	1.00	1.00	1.00	1.00	1.00	1.00
Round spermatid	0.41	0.40	0.43	0.48	0.35	0.38
Testes wt (g)	0.2	3.7	6.4	12.0	49	34
Daily sperm production						
Per gram testis (10^6/g)	28	24	25	20	23	4.4
Per male (10^6)	5	86	160	300	1100	125
Sperm reserves in caudia (at sexual rest: 10^6)	49	440	1600	?[‡]	5700	420
Transit time (days) through (at sexual rest)						
Caput + corpus epididymides	3.1	3.0	3.0	?	4.9	1.8
Cauda epididymides	5.6	5.1	9.7	?	5.6	3.7

* From Galbraith, W. M.; Voytek, P.; and Ryon, M. G.: *Assessment of Risks to Human Reproduction and to Development of the Human Conceptus from Exposure to Environmental Substances.* Oak Ridge National Laboratory, U.S. Environmental Protection Agency, 1982. Available as order number DE82007897 from the National Technical Information Service, Springfield, VA.

[†] L = leptotene, Z = zygotene, P = pachytene, D = diplotene.
[‡] A question mark indicates unclear or inadequate data.

spectrum of normal sperm as well as those that are either abnormal or immature.

Normalcy of spermatogenesis can be evaluated from two standpoints: the number of spermatozoa produced per day and the quality of spermatozoa produced. The number of spermatozoa produced per day is defined as daily sperm production (Amann, 1981). The efficiency of sperm production is the number of sperm produced per day per gram of testicular parenchyma. The efficiency of sperm production in humans is only about 20 to 40 percent of that in other mammals (Amann, 1986). Sperm production in a young man is about 7 million sperm per day per gram, and by the fifth to ninth decade of life it drops to approximately one-half or about 3.5 million per day per gram, (cf. Johnson, 1986).

Blazak *et al.* (1985) have provided an assessment of the effects of chemicals on the male reproductive system using several parameters including sperm production, sperm number, sperm transit time, and sperm motility. These authors concluded that testes weights and epididymal sperm numbers were unreliable indicators of sperm production rates.

Sertoli Cells

In early fetal life, the Sertoli cells secrete anti-Müllerian hormone (AMH). The exact physiological role is not understood, but after puberty, they begin to secrete the hormone inhibin, which may aid in modulating pituitary FSH.

The Sertoli cell junctions form the blood-testis barrier that partitions the seminiferous epithelium into a basal compartment containing spermatogonia and early spermatocytes and an adluminal compartment containing more fully developed spermatogenic cells. An ionic gradient is maintained between the two tubular compartments. Nutrients, hormones, and other chemicals must pass either between or through Sertoli cells in order to diffuse from one compartment to another. Germinal cells are found either between adjacent pairs of Sertoli cells or inside their luminal margin.

Sertoli cells secrete a number of hormones and/or proteins. These secretory products can be used to measure Sertoli function in the presence of chemical insult. The Sertoli cells secrete tissue plasminogen activator, androgen-binding protein (ABP), inhibin, AMH, transferrin, and other proteases. ABP is a protein similar to plasma sex steroid–binding globulin (SSBG). In rodents, ABP acts as a carrier for testosterone and dihydrotestosterone. Sertoli cells probably synthesize estradiol and estrone in response to FSH stimulation.

Normal spermatogenesis requires Sertoli cells. Many chemicals affecting spermatogenesis act indirectly through their effect on the Sertoli cell (e.g., dibromochloropropane[DBCP], monoethylhexyl phthalate[MEHP]) rather than directly on the germ cells. Tetrahydrocannabinol (THC) acts at several sites in the reproductive system, including the Sertoli cell where it acts by inhibiting FSH-stimulated cAMP accumulation (Heindel and Keith, 1989).

Interstitium

The Leydig cells or interstitial cells are the primary site of testosterone synthesis (Figure 16–3). These cells are closely associated with the testicular blood vessels and the lymphatic space. The spermatic arteries to the testes are tortuous, and their blood flows parallel to, but in the opposite direction of, blood in the pampiniform plexus of the spermatic veins (Figure 16–8). This anatomic arrangement seems to facilitate a countercurrent exchange of heat, androgens, and other chemicals.

LH stimulates testicular steroidogenesis. Androgens are essential to spermatogenesis, epididymal sperm maturation, the growth and secretory activity of accessory sex organs, somatic masculinization, male behavior, and various metabolic processes.

POSTTESTICULAR PROCESSES

The end product of testicular gametogenesis is immature sperm. Posttesticular processes involve ducts that move maturing sperm from the testis to storage sites where they await ejaculation. A number of secretory processes exist that control fluid production and ion composition; secretory organs contribute to the chemical composition (including specific proteins) of the semen.

Efferent Ducts

The fluid produced in the seminiferous tubules moves into a system of spaces called the rete testis. The chemical composition of the rete testis fluid is unique and has a total protein concentration much lower than that of the blood plasma. The efferent ducts open into the caput epididymis.

Although the rete testis fluid normally contains inhibin, ABP, transferrin, myoinositol, steroid hormones, amino acids, and various enzymes, only ABP and inhibin appear to be specific products and useful indicators of the functional integrity of the seminiferous epithelium or Sertoli cells (Mann and Lutwak-Mann, 1981). However, relative concentrations of other constituents may indicate alterations in membrane barriers or active transport processes. The concentration of chemicals in the rete testis fluid relative to unbound plasma concentration has been used to estimate the permeability of the blood-testis barrier for selected chemicals (Okumura et al., 1975).

Epididymides

The epididymis is a single, highly coiled duct measuring approximately 5 meters in humans. It is arranged anatomically into three parts called the caput, the corpus, and the cauda epididymides (cf. Cooper, 1986; Amann, 1987).

From the rete testis, testicular fluid first enters efferent ducts and then the epididymides. Here the sperm are subjected to a changing chemical environment as they move through the organ.

The first two sections together (the caput plus the corpus) are regarded as making up that part of the epididymis involved with sperm maturation, whereas the terminal (the cauda) segment is regarded as the site of sperm storage. There are, however, differences in the position and extent of the segments in various species of mammals.

From 1.8 to 4.9 days are required for sperm to move through the caput to the corpus epididymis where maturation takes place. In contrast, the transit time for sperm through the cauda epididymis in sexually rested males differs greatly among species and ranges from 3.7 to 9.7 days. Average sperm transit time for a 21- to 30-year-old man is six days. The number of sperm in the caput and corpus epididymis is similar in sexually rested males and in males ejaculating daily. The number of sperm in the cauda epididymis is more variable, being lower in sexually active males.

Active transport processes affect the amount of fluid flowing through the epididymis. Because much of the fluid produced by the testis is apparently absorbed in the epididymis, the relative concentration of sperm is increased.

Hence, important functions of the epididymis are reabsorption of rete testis fluid, metabolism, epithelial cell secretions, sperm maturation, and sperm storage. The chemical composition of the epididymal plasma plays an important role in both sperm maturation and sperm storage. Environmental chemicals perturb these processes and can produce adverse effects.

Accessory Sex Organs

The anatomical relationship of accessory sex organs in the male rodent is depicted on Figure

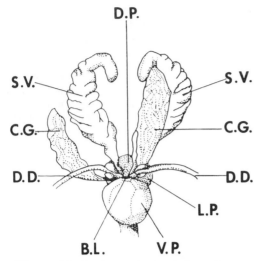

Figure 16–4. Anatomical relation of components of rodent sex accessory glands. *D.D.*, ductus deferens; *B.L.*, bladder; *V.P.*, ventral prostate; *L.P.*, lateral prostate; *C.G.*, coagulating gland (also called anterior prostate); *S.V.*, seminal vesicle; *D.P.*, dorsal prostate. (From Hayes, A. W.: *Principles and Methods of Toxicology*. Raven Press, New York, 1982.)

16–4. Most mammals possess seminal vesicles (exceptions—cats and dogs) and most have prostate glands. However, the physiological and anatomical characteristics of the prostate gland may vary considerably among mammals.

The seminal plasma functions as a vehicle for conveying the ejaculated sperm from the male to the female reproductive tract. The seminal plasma is produced by the secretory organs of the male reproductive system, which, along with the epididymides, include the prostate, seminal vesicles, bulbourethral (Cowper's) glands, and urethral (Littre's) glands. Any abnormal function of these organs can be reflected in altered seminal plasma characteristics. Seminal plasma is normally an isotonic, neutral medium, which, in many species, contains sources of energy such as fructose and sorbitol that are directly available to sperm. Functions of the other constituents such as citric acid and inositol are not known. In general, the secretions from the prostate and seminal vesicles contribute little to fertility (Mann and Lutwak-Mann, 1981).

The accessory sex organs are androgen dependent. They serve as indicators of the Leydig cell function and/or androgen action. The weights of the accessory sex glands are an indirect measure of circulating testosterone levels. The ventral prostate of rats has been used to study the actions of testosterone and to investigate the molecular basis of androgen-regulated gene function.

Human semen emission initially involves the urethral and Cowper's glands, with the prostatic secretion and sperm coming next and the seminal vesicle secretion delivered last. There is a considerable overlap between the presperm, sperm-rich, and postsperm fractions. Therefore, even if an ejaculate is collected in as many as six (split-ejaculate) fractions, it is rarely possible to obtain a sperm-free fraction consisting exclusively of prostatic or vesicular secretions.

Acid phosphatase and citric acid are markers for prostatic secretion; fructose is an indicator for seminal vesicle secretion. It is estimated that about one-third of the entire human ejaculate is contributed by the prostate and about two-thirds by the seminal vesicles. Both the vas deferens and the seminal vesicles apparently synthesize prostaglandins. Semen varies both in volume and composition between species. Human, bovine, and canine species have a relatively small semen volume (1 to 10 ml); semen of stallions and boars is ejaculated in much larger quantities. Sperm move from the distal portion of the epididymis through the vas deferens (ductus deferens) to the urethra. Vasectomy is the surgical removal of the vas deferens or a portion of it. The semen of some animals, including rodents and man, tends to coagulate on ejaculation. The clotting mechanism (e.g., "copulatory plug") involves enzymes and substrates from different accessory organs.

Although all mammals have a prostate, the organ differs anatomically, physiologically, and chemically among species, and lobe differences in the same species may be pronounced. The rat prostate is noted for its complex structure and its prompt response to castration and androgen stimulation. The human prostate is a tubuloalveolar gland made up of two prominent lateral lobes that contribute about a third of the ejaculate.

Prostate secretion in men and many other mammal species contains acid phosphatase, zinc, and citric acid. The prostatic secretion is the main source of acid phosphatase in human semen; its concentration provides a convenient method for assessing the functional state of the prostate. The human prostate also produces spermine. Certain proteins and enzymes (acid phosphatase, γ-glutamyl transpeptidase, glutamic-oxaloacetic transaminase), cholesterol, inositol, zinc, and magnesium have also been proposed as indicators of prostatic secretory function. Radioactive zinc (^{65}Zn) uptake by rodent prostate glands has been used as an index for androgenic potency (Gunn and Gould, 1956). An ionic antagonism exists between zinc and cadmium. Cadmium can induce metallothionein in the prostate glands of experimental animals (Waalkes *et al.*, 1982).

The anatomical structure of the seminal vesicle varies among animals. The seminal vesicle is a compact glandular tissue arranged in the form of multiple lobes that surround secretory ducts. Like the prostate, the seminal vesicle is responsive to androgens and is a useful indicator of Leydig cell function. The vesicular glands can be used as a gravimetric indicator for androgens.

In man, the seminal vesicle contributes about 60 percent of the seminal fluid. The seminal vesicles also produce more than half of the seminal plasma in laboratory and domestic animals such as the rat, guinea pig, and bull. In man, bull, ram, and boar (but not rat), most of the seminal fructose is secreted by the seminal vesicles, and consequently, in these species the chemical assay of fructose in semen is a useful indicator of the relative contribution of the seminal vesicles toward whole semen. Seminal vesicle secretion is also characterized by the presence of proteins and enzymes, phosphorylcholine, and prostaglandins.

Erection and Ejaculation

The physiologic processes are controlled by the central nervous system (CNS) but are modulated by the autonomic nervous system.

Parasympathetic nerve stimulation results in dilatation of the arterioles of the penis, which initiates an erection. Erectile tissue of the penis fills with blood, veins are compressed to block outflow, and the turgor of the organ increases. In man, afferent impulses from the genitalia and descending tracts, which mediate erections in response to erotic psychic stimuli, reach the integrating centers in the lumbar segments of the spinal cord. The efferent fibers are located in the pelvic splanchnic nerves.

Ejaculation is a two-stage spinal reflex involving emission and ejaculation. Emission is the movement of the semen into the urethra; ejaculation is the propulsion of the semen out of the urethra at the time of orgasm. Afferent pathways involve fibers from receptors in the glans penis that reach the spinal cord through the internal pudendal nerves. Emission is a sympathetic response effected by contraction of the smooth muscle of the vas deferens and seminal vesicles. Semen is ejaculated out of the urethra by contraction of the bulbocavernosus muscle. The spinal reflex centers for this portion of the reflex are in the upper sacral and lowest lumbar segments of the spinal cord; the motor pathways traverse the first to third sacral roots of the internal pudendal nerves.

Little is known concerning the effects of chemicals on erection or ejaculation (Woods, 1984). Pesticides, particularly the organophosphates, are known to affect neuroendocrine processes involved in erection and ejaculation. Many drugs act on the autonomic nervous system and affect potency (Table 16–3) (*see also* Papadopoulas, 1980; Buchanan and Davis, 1984; Stevenson and Umstead, 1984). Impotence, the failure to obtain or sustain an erection, is rarely of endocrine origin; more often, the cause is psychologic. The occurrence of nocturnal or early-morning erections implies that the neurologic and circulatory pathways involved in attaining an erection are intact and suggests the possibility of a psychologic cause.

OVARIAN FUNCTION

Oogenesis

Ovarian germ cells with their follicles have a dual origin; the theca or stromal cells arise from fetal connective tissues of the ovarian medulla, the granulosa cells from the cortical mesenchyme (Figure 16–5).

Between 300,000 and 400,000 follicles are present at birth in each human ovary. After birth, many undergo atresia, and those that survive are

Table 16–3.   DRUG-INDUCED IMPOTENCE*

	AGENT	CNS	ANS	ENDO.
Narcotics	Morphine	+	+	?
	Ethanol	+		
Psychotropic	Chlorpromazine		+	
	Diazepam	+		
	Tricyclic antidepressants		+	?
	MAO inhibitors		+	
Hypotensives	Methyldopa	+	+	+
	Clonidine	+	+	
	Reserpine	+	+	
	Guanethidine		+ +	
Hormones/antagonists	Estrogens			+
	Cyproterone			+

* From Millar, J. G. B.: Drug-induced impotence. *Practitioner*, **223**:634–639, 1979.

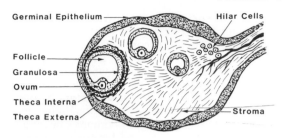

Figure 16–5. Schematic representation of ovarian morphology. (From Thomas, J. A., and Keenan, E. J.: *Principles of Endocrine Pharmacology*. Plenum Press, New York, 1986.)

continuously reduced in number. Any agent that damages the oocytes will accelerate the depletion of the pool and can lead to reduced fertility in females. About one-half of the number of oocytes present at birth remain at puberty; the number is reduced to about 25,000 by 30 years of age. About 400 primary follicles will yield mature ova during a woman's reproductive life span (Figure 16–1). During the 30 years or more that constitute the reproductive period, follicles in various stages of growth can always be found. After menopause, follicles are no longer present in the ovary.

Follicles remain in a primary follicle stage following birth until puberty, when a number of follicles start to grow during each ovarian cycle. However, most fail to achieve maturity. For the follicles that continue to grow, the first event is an increase in size of the primary oocytes. During this stage, fluid-filled spaces appear among the cells of the follicle, which unite to form a cavity or antrum. This is the graafian follicle.

Primary oocytes undergo two specialized nuclear divisions, which result in the formation of four cells containing one-half the number of chromosomes (Figure 16–2). The first meiotic division occurs within the ovary just before ovulation, and the second occurs just after the sperm fuses with the egg. In the first stage of meiosis, the primary oocyte is actively synthesizing DNA and protein in preparation for entering prophase. The DNA content doubles as the prophase chromosomes each produce their mirror image. Each doubled chromosome is attracted to its homologous mate to form tetrads. The members of the tetrads synapse or come to lie side by side. Before separation, the homologous pairs of chromosomes exchange genetic material by a process known as crossing over. Thus, qualitative differences occur between the resulting gametes. Subsequent meiotic stages distribute the members of the tetrads to the daughter cells in such a way that each cell receives the haploid number of chromosomes. At telophase, one secondary oocyte and a polar body have been formed, which are no longer genetically identical.

The secondary oocyte enters the next cycle of division very rapidly; each chromosome splits longitudinally; the ovum and the three polar bodies now contain the haploid number of chromosomes and half the amount of genetic material. Although the nuclei of all four eggs are equivalent, the cytoplasm is divided unequally. The end products are one large ovum and three rudimentary ova known as polar bodies, which subsequently degenerate. The ovum is released from the ovary at the secondary oocyte stage; the second stage of meiotic division is triggered in the oviduct by the entry of the sperm.

Ovarian Cycle

The cyclic release of pituitary gonadotropins involving the secretion of ovarian progesterone and estrogen is depicted in Figure 16–6. These female sex steroids determine ovulation and prepare the female accessory sex organs to receive the male sperm. Sperm, ejaculated into the vagi-

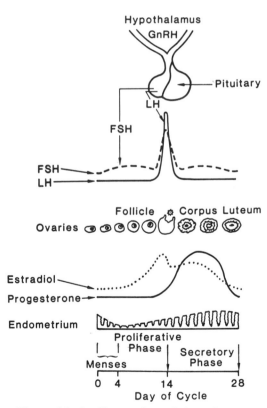

Figure 16–6. Hormonal regulation of menstrual function. *FSH*, follicle stimulating hormone; *GnRH*, gonadotropin releasing hormone; *LH*, luteinizing hormone. (From Thomas, J. A., and Keenan, E. J.: *Principles of Endocrine Pharmacology*. Plenum Press, New York, 1986.)

na, must make their way through the cervix into the uterus where they are capacitated. Sperm then move into the oviducts where fertilization takes place. The conceptus then returns from the oviducts to the uterus and implants into the endometrium.

POSTOVARIAN PROCESSES

Female accessory sex organs function to bring together the ovulated ovum and the ejaculated sperm. Chemical composition and viscosity of reproductive tract fluids, as well as the epithelial morphology of these organs, are controlled by ovarian (and trophoblastic) hormones.

Oviducts

The oviducts provide the taxis of the fimbria, which is under muscular control. The involvement of the autonomic nervous system in this process, as well as in oviductal transport of both the male and female gametes, raises the possibility that pharmacologic agents known to alter the autonomic nervous system may alter function and, therefore, fertility.

Uterus

Uterine endometrium reflects the cyclicity of the ovary as it is prepared to receive the conceptus. The myometrium's major role is contractile. In primates, at the end of menstruation, all but the deep layers of the endometrium are sloughed. Under the influence of estrogens from the developing follicle, the endometrium increases rapidly in thickness. The uterine glands increase in length but do not secrete to any degree. These endometrial changes are called proliferative. After ovulation, the endometrium becomes slightly edematous, and the actively secreting glands become tightly coiled and folded under the influence of estrogen and progesterone from the corpus luteum. These are secretory (progestational) changes (Figure 16–6).

When fertilization fails to occur, the endometrium is shed, and a new cycle begins. Only primates menstruate. Other mammals have a sexual or estrus cycle. Female animals come into "heat" (estrus) at the time of ovulation. This is generally the only time during which the female is receptive to the male. In spontaneously ovulating species (e.g., rodents), the endocrine events are comparable with those in the menstrual cycle. In the rabbit, ovulation is a reflex produced by copulation.

Cervix

The mucosa of the uterine cervix does not undergo cyclic desquamation, but there are regular changes in the cervical mucus. Estrogen, which makes the mucus thinner and more alkaline, promotes the survival and transport of sperm. Progesterone makes the mucus thick, tenacious, and cellular. The mucus is thinnest at the time of ovulation and dries in an arborizing, fernlike pattern on a slide. After ovulation and during pregnancy, it becomes thick and fails to form the fern pattern. Disruptions of the cervix may be expressed as disorders of differentiation (including neoplasia), disturbed secretion, and incompetence. Exfoliative cytologic (Papanicolaou's stain) and histologic techniques are currently used to assess disorders of differentiation. Various synthetic steroids (e.g., oral contraceptives) can affect the extent and pattern of cervical mucus.

Vagina

Estrogen produces a growth and proliferation of vaginal epithelium. The layers of cells become cornified and can be readily identified in vaginal smears. Vaginal cornification has been used as an index for estrogens. Progesterone stimulation produces a thick mucus; the epithelium proliferates, becoming infiltrated with leukocytes. The cyclic changes in the vaginal smear in rats are easily recognized. The changes in humans and other species are similar but less apparent. Analysis of vaginal fluid or cytologic studies of desquamated vaginal cells (quantitative cytochemistry) reflects ovarian function. Vaginal sampling of cells and fluid might offer a reliable and easily available external monitor of internal function and dysfunction. Alteration in vaginal flora can be a toxicologic condition associated with the use of vaginal tampons (*viz.* toxic shock syndrome [TSS]).

FERTILIZATION

During fertilization, the ovum contributes the maternal complement of genes to the nucleus of the fertilized egg and provides food reserves for the early embryo. The innermost of the egg is the vitelline membrane. Outside the ovum proper lies a thick, tough, and highly refractile capsule termed the zona pellucida, which increases the total diameter of the human ovum to about 0.15 mm. Beyond the zona pellucida is the corona radiata derived from the follicle; it surrounds the ovum during its passage in the oviduct.

Formation, maturation, and union of a male and female germ cell are all preliminary events leading to a combined cell or zygote. Penetration of ovum by sperm and the coming together and pooling of their respective nuclei constitute the process of fertilization.

Only minutes are required for the sperm to penetrate the zona pellucida after passing through the cumulus oophorus *in vitro* and probably sooner *in vivo*. The sperm traverse along a curved oblique path. Entering the perivitelline space, the sperm head immediately lies flat on the vitellus; its plasma membrane fuses with that of the vitellus and then embeds into the ovum. The cortical granules of the egg disappear, the vitellus shrinks, and the second maturation division is reinitiated, which results in extrusion of the second polar body. A specific factor in the ovum appears to trigger the development of the male pronucleus; the chromatin of the ovum forms a female pronucleus.

As syngamy approaches, the two pronuclei become intimately opposed but do not fuse. The nuclear envelopes of the pronuclei break up; nucleoli disappear and chromosomes condense and promptly aggregate. The chromosomes mingle to form the prometaphase of the first spindle, and the egg divides into two blastomeres. From sperm penetration to first cleavage usually requires about 12 hours in laboratory animals.

From a single fertilized cell (the zygote), cells proliferate and differentiate until more than a trillion cells of about 100 different types are present in the adult organism.

IMPLANTATION

The developing embryo migrates through the oviduct into the uterus. Upon contact with the endometrium, the blastocyst becomes surrounded by an outer layer or syncytiotrophoblast, a multinucleated mass of cells with no discernible boundaries, and an inner layer of individual cells, the cytotrophoblast. The syncytiotrophoblast erodes the endometrium, and the blastocyst implants. Placental circulation is then established and trophoblastic function continues. The blastocysts of most mammalian species implant about day 6 or 7 following fertilization. At this stage, the differentiation of the embryonic and extraembryonic (trophoblastic) tissues is apparent.

Trophoblastic tissue differentiates into cytotrophoblast and syncytiotrophoblast cells. The syncytiotrophoblast cells produce chorionic gonadotropin, chorionic growth hormones, placental lactogen, estrogen, and progesterone, which are needed to achieve independence from the ovary in maintaining the pregnancy. Rapid proliferation of the cytotrophoblast serves to anchor the growing placenta to the maternal tissue.

The developing placenta consists of proliferating trophoblasts, which expand rapidly and infiltrate the maternal vascular channels. Shortly after implantation, the syncytiotrophoblast is bathed by maternal venous blood, which supplies nutrients and permits an exchange of gases. Histotrophic nutrition involves yolk sac circulation; hemotrophic nutrition involves the placenta. Placental circulation is established quite early in women and primates and, relatively, much later in rodents and rabbits. Interestingly, placental dysfunction due to vascular compromise caused by cocaine leads to increased fetal risk, causing growth retardation and prematurity. Fetal loss due to abruptio placentae may occur (cf. Doering *et al.,* 1989).

Placentation varies considerably among various domestic animals, experimental animals, and primates. Man and monkey possess a hemochorial placenta. Pigs, horses, and donkeys have an epitheliochorial type of placenta, whereas sheep, goats, and cows have a syndesmochorial type of placenta. In laboratory animals (e.g., rat, rabbit, and guinea pig), the placenta is termed a hemoendothelial type. Among the various species, the number of maternal and fetal cell layers ranges from six layers (e.g., pig, horse) to a single layer (e.g., rat, rabbit). Primates, including man, have three layers of cells in the placenta that a substance must pass across. Thus, the placentas of some species are "thicker" than others.

Generally, the placenta is quite impermeable to chemicals/drugs with molecular weights of 1000 daltons or more. Most medications have molecular weights of 500 daltons or less. Hence, molecular size is rarely a factor in denying a drug's entrance across the placenta and into the embryo/fetus.

INTEGRATIVE PROCESSES

Hypothalamo-Pituitary-Gonadal Axis

FSH and LH are glycoproteins synthesized and released from a subpopulation of the basophilic gonadotropic cells of the pituitary gland. Hypothalamic neuroendocrine neurons secrete specific releasing or release-inhibiting factors into the hypophyseal portal system, which carries them to the adenohypophysis where they act to stimulate or inhibit the release of anterior pituitary hormones (Table 16–4). Luteinizing hormone–releasing hormone (LHRH) acts on gonadotropic cells, thereby stimulating the release of FSH and LH. LHRH and follicle stimulating hormone–releasing hormone (FSHRH) appear to be the same substance. Native and synthetic forms of LHRH stimulate the release of both gonadotrophic hormones; thus, it has been proposed to call this compound gonadotropin-releasing hormone (GnRH).

The neuroendocrine neurons have nerve terminals containing monoamines (norepinephrine,

Table 16–4.   HYPOTHALAMIC HORMONES OR FACTORS CONTROLLING THE RELEASE OF ANTERIOR PITUITARY HORMONES*

NOMENCLATURE	ABBREVIATION
Corticotropin (ACTH)-releasing hormone	CRH
Thyrotropin-releasing hormone	TRH
Luteinizing hormone (LH)–releasing hormone/follicle stimulating hormone (FSH)–releasing hormone	LHRH/FSHRH (GnRH)
Growth hormone (GH)–inhibitory factor, somatostatin	GHIF, SRIF
Growth hormone (GH)–releasing factor	GHRF
Prolactin-inhibitory factor	PIF
Prolactin-releasing factor	PRF
Melanocyte-stimulating hormone (MSH)–inhibitory factor	MIF
Melanocyte-stimulating hormone (MSH)–releasing factor	MRF

* From Thomas, J. A. and Keenan, E. J.: *Principles of Endocrine Pharmacology.* Plenum, New York, 1986, p. 18.

dopamine, serotonin) that impinge on them. Reserpine, chlorpromazine, and monoamine oxidase (MAO) inhibitors modify the content or actions of brain monoamines that affect gonadotropins.

FSH probably acts primarily on the Sertoli cells, but it also appears to stimulate the mitotic activity of spermatogonia. LH stimulates steroidogenesis. A defect in the function of the testis (in the production of spermatozoa or testosterone) will tend to be reflected in increased levels of FSH and LH in serum because of the lack of the "negative feedback" effect of testicular hormones (Figure 16–7).

The hypothalamo-pituitary-gonadal feedback system is a very delicate modulated hormonal process. Several sites in the endocrine process can be perturbed by drugs (e.g., oral contraceptives) and by different chemicals (Figure 16–7). Gonadotoxic agents may act on neuroendocrine processes in the brain or they may act directly on the target organ (e.g., gonad). Toxicants that adversely or otherwise alter the hepatic and/or renal biotransformation of endogenous sex steroid might be expected to interfere with the pituitary feedback system.

Puberty

From the early newborn period to the onset of puberty, the testes remain hormonally dormant. After birth, the androgen-secreting Leydig cells in the mammalian fetal testes become quiescent, and a period follows in which the gonads of both sexes await final maturation of the reproductive system.

The onset of puberty begins with secretion of increasing levels of gonadotropins. The physiological trigger for puberty is poorly understood, but somehow a hypothalamic gonadostat changes the rate of secretion of LHRH, resulting in increases in LH. As puberty approaches, a pulsatile pattern of LH and FSH secretion is observed.

The gonad itself is not required for activating FSH or LH at the onset of puberty. It is a CNS phenomenon. Female puberty is affected by a wide range of influences including climate, race, heredity, athletic activity, and degree of adiposity.

SEXUAL BEHAVIOR AND LIBIDO

Physiologic processes that account for sexual behavior are poorly understood. The external environment greatly affects sexual behavior, and libido components of reproductive activity de-

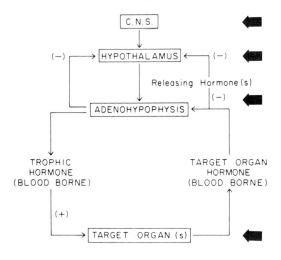

Figure 16–7. Relation between adenohypophyseal-hypothalamic axis and hormone target organs. (From Thomas, J. A. *et al.* Hormone assays and endocrine function, in Hayes, A. W.: *Principles and Methods of Toxicology.* Raven Press, New York, 1982.)

pend on a close interplay between neural and endocrine events. For example, a correlation of behavior and receptivity for insemination is attained by complex neuroendocrine mechanisms involving the brain, the pituitary, and sex steroid hormones. This complexity varies even among higher vertebrates. Thus, in reproductive studies involving rodents, the investigator must determine whether the animals actually mate. In the rat, this can be determined by inspecting females each day for vaginal plugs. The number of mountings, thrusts, and ejaculations each can be quantified as indicators of reproductive behavior. It is also important to determine whether the male animal mounts females or other males. If the male copulates and is still sterile, indicators of male fertility such as testicular function should be considered. Failure to copulate suggests either a neuromuscular and/or behavioral defect in the experimental animal.

GENERAL TOXICOLOGIC/ PHARMACOLOGIC PRINCIPLES

Many of the principles that govern absorption, distribution, metabolism, and excretion of a chemical or drug also apply to the reproductive system. There are, however, some rather unique barriers that affect a chemical's action on the mammalian reproductive system. The maternal-fetal interface occurring at the placenta represents a barrier to chemicals coming in contact with the developing embryo. Unfortunately, the placenta is not so restrictive as to deny most chemicals from crossing the placenta. Most chemicals are not denied entrance into a number of compartments or secretions of the reproductive tract. Indeed, xenobiotic and certain drugs can be readily detected in uterine secretions, in milk of the lactating mother, and in seminal fluid (Mann and Lutwak-Mann, 1981). No specialized barriers appear to prevent chemicals or drugs from acting on the ovary. Several drugs are known to interfere with ovarian function (Table 16-5). Unlike the female gonad, a somewhat

Table 16–5. CHEMOTHERAPEUTIC AGENTS AND OVARIAN DYSFUNCTION*

Prednisone	Busulfan
Vincristine	Methotrexate
Vinblastine	Cytosine arabinoside
6-Mercaptopurine	L-Asparginase
Nitrogen mustard	5-Fluorouracil
Cyclophosphamide	Adriamycin
Chlorambucil	

* Haney, A. F.: Effects of toxic agents on ovarian function. In Thomas, J. A.; Korach, K. S.; and McLachlan, J. A. (eds.): *Endocrine Toxicology*. Raven Press, New York, 1985.

specialized barrier is present in the male gonad. This specialized biologic barrier is referred to as the blood-testis barrier.

BLOOD-TESTIS BARRIER

There are a number of specialized anatomical barriers in the body. Tissue permeability barriers include the blood-brain barrier, the blood-thymus barrier, and the blood-bile barrier. Important barriers within the endocrine system are the placental barrier and the blood-testis barrier. The blood-testis barrier is situated somewhere between the lumen of an interstitial capillary and the lumen of a seminiferous tubule (Neaves, 1977). Several anatomically related features intervene between the two luminal spaces, including the capillary endothelium, capillary basal lamina, lymphatic endothelium, myoid cells, basal lamina of the seminiferous tubule, and Sertoli cells. The barrier that impedes or denies the free exchange of chemicals/drugs between the blood and the fluid inside the seminiferous tubules is located in one or more of these structures. The apparent positioning of distances relative to transepithelial permeability can affect the passage (or blockage) of a substance through the blood-testis barrier. These epithelial cell anatomical relationships can affect the tightness of fit between cells and the extent to which a chemical's passsage can occur. Such junctions or cell unions are often leaky and may allow for a substance's passage. These so-called gap junctions may even be less developed in the immature or young mammalian testes, hence affording greater opportunities for foreign chemicals to permeate the seminiferous tubule. Setchell and coworkers (1969) first demonstrated that immunoglobulins and iodinated albumin, inulin, and a number of small molecules were excluded from the seminiferous tubules by the blood-testis barrier. Dym and Fawcett (1970) suggested that the primary permeability barrier for the seminiferous tubules was composed of the surrounding layers of myoid cells while specialized Sertoli cell–to–Sertoli cell junctions within the seminiferous epithelium constituted a secondary cellular barrier. Okumura and coworkers (1975) quantified permeability rates for nonelectrolytes and certain chemicals/drugs. Small-molecular weight molecules (e.g., water, urea) can readily cross the blood-testis barrier; larger-sized substances (e.g., inulin) are impeded. The degree of lipid solubility and ionization are important determinants as to whether a substance can permeate the blood-testis barrier. A number of factors are known to affect the permeability of the blood-testis barrier, including ligation of the efferent ductules, autoimmune orchiditis, and vasectomy.

BIOTRANSFORMATION OF EXOGENOUS CHEMICALS

The mammalian gonad is capable of metabolizing a host of foreign chemicals that have traversed the blood-testis barrier. While mixed-function oxidases and epoxide-degrading enzymes may not be as active as hepatic systems, they are nevertheless present. Cytochrome P-450 is present in the testes. Cytochrome P-450, in general, is quite sensitive to the effects of a number of chemicals. Gonadal cytochrome P-450 is no exception. Arylhydrocarbon hydroxylase (AHH) is present in testicular microsomes (I. P. Lee *et al.*, 1981). Consequently, the pathways for steroidogenesis contain a number of enzymes that are affected by chemicals or drugs (Table 16–6). Like the process of steroidogenesis in the gonads, the adrenal cortex is also vulnerable to chemical insult (cf. Colby, 1988). Both parent compound and its metabolite(s) can adversely affect the gonad (Table 16–7). Whether biotransformation occurs gonadally or extragonadally, the end result can be interference of spermatogenesis and/or steroidogenesis. Their mechanism(s) of toxicity varies considerably. The microsomal oxidation of *n*-hexane yields 2,5-hexanedione (2,5-HD). *n*-Hexane, an environmental toxicant, causes peripheral poly-

neuropathy and testicular atrophy (Boekelheide, 1987, 1988). 2,5-HD produces gonadal toxicity by altering testicular tubulin. From these findings, Boekelheide suggested that damage to the microtubules of the Sertoli cell results in germ cell loss in 2,5-HD–treated rats. Ethylene glycol monoethyl ether, along with its metabolites, is a gonadal toxin (Nagano *et al.*, 1979). 2-Methoxyacetaldehyde (MALD) produces specific cellular toxicity to pachytene spermatocytes (Foster *et al.*, 1986). Diethylhexyl phthalate (DEHP) and its metabolite(s) monoethylhexyl phthalate (MEHP) are both gonadal toxicants whose mechanism(s), in part, is due to depletion of testicular zinc. DEHP, and other plasticizers, can adversely affect spermatogenesis (cf. Thomas and Thomas, 1984). Gray and Beamand (1984) have proposed that the mechanism of DEHP-induced testicular atrophy involves a membrane alteration leading to separation of the germ cells (spermatocytes and spermatids) from the underlying Sertoli cells. The separation of spermatocytes and spermatids would interfere with the transfer of nutrients from the Sertoli cells, leading to death and disintegration of the germ cells. MEHP, and not DEHP, is most likely the principal gonadal toxicant (Albro *et al.*, 1989). A summary of the effects of various phthalates on parameters in the reproductive tract may be seen in Table 16–8. While dietary zinc deficiency in humans causes an inhibition of spermatogenesis, there are no reports of

Table 16–6.   INHIBITORS OF STEROIDOGENIC ENZYMES*

ENZYME	INHIBITOR
Cholesterol side chain cleavage	Aminoglutethimide, 3-methoxybenzidine, cyanoketone, estrogens, azastene, danazol
Aromatase	4-Acetoxy-androstene-3,17-dione, 4-hydroxy-androstene-3,17-dione, 1,4,6-androstatriene-3,17-dione, 6-bromoandrostene-3,17-dione, 7α(4'amino)phenylthioandrostenedione, δ'-testolactone, fenarimol[†]
11-Hydroxylase	Danazol, metyrapone
21-Hydroxylase	Danazol, spironolactone
17-Hydroxylase	Danazol, spironolactone
17,20-Desmolase	Danazol, spironolactone
17-Hydroxysteroid dehydrogenase	Danazol
3-Hydroxysteroid dehydrogenase	Danazol
c-17-L-20-lyase	Ketoconozole[‡]

* Modified from Haney, A. F.: Effects of toxic agents on ovarian function. In Thomas, J. A.; Korach, K. S.; and McLachlan, J. A. (eds.): *Endocrine Toxicology.* Raven Press, New York, 1985.
[†] *See* Hirsch *et al., 1987.*
[‡] *See* Effendy and Krause, 1989.

Table 16–7. REPRESENTATIVE DRUGS, CHEMICALS AND THEIR METABOLITES AND THEIR ABILITY TO EXERT TOXIC ACTIONS UPON THE MALE GONAD*

PARENT COMPOUND	METABOLITE	REFERENCE
Amiodarone (antiarrhythmic drug)	Desethylamiodarone	Holt *et al.*, 1984
Cephalosporin analogues (antimicrobial drug)	*N*-Methyltetrazolethiol[†]	Comereski *et al.*, 1987
Valproic acid (antiepileptic drug)	Isomers of 2-ethyl hexanol (?)[‡]	Ritter *et al.*, 1987
Diethylhexyl phthalate (DEHP; plasticizer)	Mono-ethylhexyl phthalate and 2-ethyl hexanol (?)[‡]	Thomas *et al.*, 1982
Dibromochloropropane[§] (DBCP; fungicide)	Dichloropropene(s) derivatives (?)[‡]	Torkelson *et al.*, 1961
Ethylene glycol monoethyl ether (industrial solvent)	2-Methoxyacetaldehyde	Foster *et al.*, 1986
n-Hexane (environmental toxicant)	2,5-Hexanedione	Boekelheide, 1987
Acrylamide (industrial use)	*N*-Methylacrylamide, *N*-isopropylacrylamide	Sakamoto and Hashimoto, 1986

* Modified from Thomas, J. A., and Ballantyne, B.: *J. Occup. Med.*, **32**:547–553, 1990.
† Only substituent is a testicular toxin, not cephalosporin.
‡ Questionable testicular toxin but probably teratogenic.
§ Radiometabolities of (^{3}H)-DBCP are not preferentially labeled in the testes (*see* Shemi *et al.*, 1987).

phthalate-induced zinc deficiency causing infertility in human males. Epichlorohydrin, a highly reactive electrophile used in the manufacture of glycerol and epoxy resins, produces spermatozoal metabolic lesions (cf. Toth *et al.*, 1989). Tri-*o*-cresyl phosphate (TOCP), an industrial chemical used as a plasticizer in lacquers and varnishes, decreases epididymal sperm motility and density. TOCP interferes with spermatogenic processes and sperm motility directly and not via an androgenic mechanism or decreased vitamin E (Somkuti *et al.*, 1987).

2-Methoxylethanol (2-ME), an industrial solvent, is toxic to both the male and female reproductive system (Mebus *et al.*, 1989). 2-ME must be metabolized to 2-methoxyacetic acid (2-MAA) by alcohol and aldehyde dehydrogenases in order to attain its testicular toxicity. All stages of spermatocyte development and some stages of spermatid development are affected by 2-ME. 2-ME is also embryotoxic and teratogenic in

Table 16–8. EFFECTS OF PHTHALATE ACID ESTERS ON THE MALE REPRODUCTIVE SYSTEM*

SPECIES	PAE	EFFECT
Rat	DEHP	Testicular degeneration
Rat	DOP	Decreased testes weight
Rat	DEHP	Semisterility
Ferret	DEHP	Testicular degeneration
Rat	DEHP	Testis histological damage
Rat	DEHP	↓ Testes weight, ↓ zinc
Rat	DEHP	Testicular atrophy
Mouse	DEHP	↓ Testosterone, ↑ testes weight, ↓ zinc
Mouse	MEHP	↔ Testes
Rat	DEHP	↓ Testes weight, ↓ zinc
Rat	DMP	↓ Testes weight, ↑ zinc excretion
Rat	MEHP	Testicular atrophy, ↓ zinc
Rat	DEHP	Testicular atrophy, ↓ zinc
Rat	DEHP, DA79P	↓ Testicular weight

* Thomas, J. A.; Curto, K. A.; and Thomas, M. J.: MEHP/DEHP gonadal toxicity and effects on rodent accessory sex organs. *Environ. Health Perspect.*, **45**:85–92, 1982.

several species (Hanly *et al.*, 1984). 2-ME (also known as methyl cellosolve) when applied dermally can produce a decline in epididymal sperm and testicular spermatid counts in rats (Feuston *et al.*, 1989). Ethanol also causes delayed testicular development and may affect the Sertoli cell and/or the Leydig cell (Anderson *et al.*, 1989). Trifluoroethanol and trifluoroacetaldehyde produce specific damage to pachytene and dividing spermatocytes and round spermatids in rats (Lloyd *et al.*, 1988).

Metabolites of cephalosporin reportedly cause testicular toxicity in rats (Comereski *et al.*, 1987). Testicular degeneration from analogues of cephalosporin is most likely to occur with cefbuperazone, cefamandole, and cefoperazone. Cyclosporin can also inhibit testosterone biosynthesis in the rat testes (Rajfer *et al.*, 1987). Amiodarone and its desethyl metabolite can be detected in high concentrations in the testes and semen, but their action(s) on spermatogenesis or sperm motility is (are) not known (Holt *et al.*, 1984).

Like the testes, the ovary possesses the metabolic capability to biotransform certain exogenous substrates. Furthermore, the process of ovarian steroidogenesis, like the testes and the adrenal cortex (*cf.* Colby, 1988), is susceptible to different agents that interfere with the biosynthesis of estrogens (*see* Table 16–6). Less is known about how chemicals or drugs interfere with ovarian metabolism. The ovary has not been studied as extensively because of its more difficult and complex hormonal relationships. Nevertheless, several chemotherapeutic agents can inhibit ovarian function (Table 16–5). Recently, Faustman *et al.* (1989) have studied the toxicity of direct-acting alkylating agents on rodent embryos. Their findings failed to reveal any specific structure activity pattens among various alkylating agents. Like the testes, mixed-function oxidases and various cytochrome systems are found in the ovary. Primordial oocyte toxicity as well as other sites of action can be affected by certain chemicals or drugs (Haney, 1985).

DNA REPAIR

Depending on the specie, there are varying degrees of capacity for spermatogenic cells to repair DNA damage due to environmental toxicants (J. P. Lee, 1983). It is well known that UV and X rays can damage DNA molecules; lethal mutation (i.e., cell deaths) and mutation resulting from transformed cells can also occur. Spermatogenic cells can be used to study unscheduled DNA synthesis (Dixon and Lee,

1980). Unscheduled DNA repair in spermatogenic cells is dose and time dependent. Spermiogenic cells are less able to repair DNA damage resulting from alkylating agents. This DNA repair system provides a protective mechanism from certain toxicants; it is also a sensitive index of chromosome damage.

Drug-induced unscheduled DNA synthesis in mammalian oocytes reveals that female gametes possess an excision repair capacity (R. A. Pedersen and Brandriff, 1980). Unlike mature sperm, the mature oocyte maintains a DNA repair ability. However, this ability decreases at the time of meiotic maturation.

Different occupations can result in varying degrees of chromosomal aberrations (Table 16–9). In particular, lead toxicity can induce a variety of chromatid and chromosome breaks. Lead is one of the earliest substances associated with causing deleterious effects on the reproductive system (Thomas and Brogan, 1983). Lead poisoning has been associated with reduced fertility, miscarriages, and stillbirth since antiquity (Lancranjan *et al.*, 1975). Lead salts are among the oldest known spermicidal agents; lead has long been known to be an abortifacient (*cf.* Hildebrand *et al.*, 1973).

TARGETS FOR CHEMICAL TOXICITY

There are several sites of interference by chemicals upon the mammalian reproductive system (Figure 16–7). Drugs and chemicals can act directly on the CNS, particularly the hypothalamus and the adenohypophysis. A number of drugs (e.g., tranquilizers, sedatives, etc.) can modify the CNS leading to alterations in the secretion of hypothalamic-releasing hormones and/or gonadotropins (Table 16–4). Synthetic steroids (viz., 19-nortestosterones) are very effective in suppressing gonadotropin secretion and hence block ovulation.

The gonads are also targets for a host of drugs and chemicals (Table 16–10) (Chapman, 1983; Thomas and Keenan, 1986). The majority of these agents are representatives from major chemical classes of cancer chemotherapeutic agents, particularly the alkylating agents. Procarbazine, an antineoplastic drug, causes severe damage to the acrosomal plasma membrane and the nucleus of the sperm head in hamsters (Singh *et al.*, 1989). Alkylating agents are effective against rapidly dividing cells. Not surprisingly, cellular division of germ cells is also affected, leading to arrest of spermatogenesis.

Different cell populations of the mammalian testis exhibit somewhat different thresholds of sensitivity to different toxicants (Figure 16–8). Thus, the germ cells are most sensitive to chemi-

Table 16–9. OCCUPATIONAL EXPOSURE TO LEAD AND ITS RELATIONSHIP TO CHROMOSOMAL ABERRATIONS*

EXPOSED SUBJECTS	TYPE OF ABERRATION
Positive Findings	
Lead oxide factory workers	Chromatid and chromosome breaks
Chemical factory workers	Chromatid gaps, breaks
Zinc plant workers	Gaps, fragments, rings, exchanges, dicentrics
Blast-furnace workers, metal grinders, scrap metal workers	Gaps, breaks, hyperploidy, structural abnormalities
Battery plant workers and lead foundry workers	Gaps, breaks, fragments
Lead oxide factory workers	Chromatid and chromosome aberrations
Battery melters, tin workers	Dicentrics, rings, fragments
Ceramic, lead, and battery workers	Breaks, fragments
Smelter workers	Gaps, chromatid and chromosome aberrations
Battery plant workers	Chromatid and chromosome aberrations
Negative Findings	
Policemen	
Lead workers	
Shipyard workers	
Smelter workers	
Volunteers (ingested lead)	
Children (near a smelter)	

* From Thomas, J. A., and Brogan, W. C.: Some actions of lead on the sperm and on the male reproductive system. *Am. J. Ind. Med.*, **4**:127–134, 1983.

cal insult (i.e., spermatogenesis). The Sertoli cells possess a somewhat intermediate sensitivity to chemical inhibition; Leydig cells are quite resistant to environmental toxicants. Dibromochloropropane (DBCP), a fungicide, causes infertility in a number of species, including man. DBCP causes sterility, but it may do so by acting through the Sertoli cell. DBCP may also inhibit sperm carbohydrate metabolism at the NADH dehydrogenase step in the mitochondrial electron transport chain (Greenwell *et al.*, 1987). Despite DBCP propensity to cause degeneration of the seminiferous tubules, toxicokinetic studies fail to reveal any preferential uptake by the testes (Shemi *et al.*, 1987). DBCP gonadotoxicity appears to be sex specific since only testicular injury has been reported; it does not cause comparable adverse effects in the female rat (Shaked *et al.*, 1988). Analogues of DBCP cause testicular necrosis as well as DNA damage in the rat (Soderlund *et al.*, 1988).

The production of lactate and pyruvate are indicators of Sertoli cell function (Williams and Foster, 1988). Either dinitrobenzene (DNB) or mono-(2-ethylhexyl)phthalate (MEHP) can affect lactate (and pyruvate) production by rat Sertoli cell cultures. The Sertoli cell appears to be a prime target for the toxic actions of DNB (Blackburn *et al.*, 1988). R. E. Chapin *et al.* (1988) have also indicated that MEHP adversely

affects the mitochondria of the Sertoli cell *in vitro*. Likewise, dinitrotoluene (DNT) has a locus of toxic action that is the Sertoli cell (Bloch *et al.*, 1988).

Anti-LH peptides can affect Leydig cell steroidogenesis. LHRH analogues (e.g., buserelin) can reduce testicular and uterine weights in rats (Donaubauer *et al.*, 1987).

In some species, the pampiniform plexus, which functions as an effective heat exchange system to ensure that the blood profusing the testes is at a temperature compatible with sper-

Table 16–10. DRUGS THAT ARE GONADOTOXIC IN HUMANS*

MALES	FEMALES
Busulfan	Busulfan
Chlorambucil	Chlorambucil
Cyclophosphamide	Cyclophosphamide
Nitrogen mustard	Nitrogen mustard
Adriamycin	
Corticosteroids	
Cytosine-arabinoside	
Methotrexate	
Procarbazine	
Vincristine	
Vinblastine	Vinblastine

* From Chapman, R. M.: Gonadal injury resulting from chemotherapy. *Am. J. Ind. Med.*, **4**:149–161, 1983.

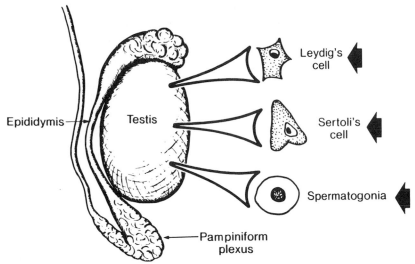

Figure 16–8. Some possible sites of action of selected gonadotoxins. (From Thomas, J. A. *et al.* Hormone assays and endocrine function, in Hayes, A. W.: *Principles and Methods of Toxicology.* Raven Press, New York, 1982.)

matogenesis, is destroyed by cadmium, leading to necrosis of the blood vessels supplying the testes. Another anatomical structure of the testes, namely, the epididymis, is less vulnerable to chemical insult, although halogenated hexoses and substituted glycerol moieties can alter electrolyte passage and sugar transport.

The liver and the kidney contain enzyme systems that affect the biological half-life of steroids and other hormones. Hence, xenobiotics that interfere with excretory processes might be expected to alter the endocrine system. For example, a number of hepatic steroid hydroxylases can be induced by either organophosphates or organochlorine pesticides. Such hydroxylation reactions can be expected to render the endogenous steroid more polar and hence more readily excreted by the kidney.

EVALUATING REPRODUCTIVE FUNCTION

The endocrine system of the female is more complex and dynamic than that of the male. Hence, evaluating reproductive function in the female is more difficult. Immediate distinctions must also be made between the pregnant and the nonpregnant female. Regardless of sex, both behavioral and physiologic factors must be considered in evaluating reproductive toxicity. Further, the physiologic events involved in reproduction have inherent time factors that are species specific. Oftentimes, evaluating a chemical's or drug's potential to affect the reproductive system is costly and time-consuming. Furthermore, many of the end points used to evaluate the reproduc-

tive system are not always reliable and have limitations (Table 16–11).

The fact that such a wide variety of chemicals or drugs can perturb the reproductive system adds another dimension of difficulty in attempting to evaluate reproductive toxicity. Not only is there considerable diversity in chemical configuration of the toxicant, but sites of action and mechanisms of action can be very different (Table 16–12).

Several classes of therapeutic agents can affect the male reproductive system (Table 16–13) as well as the female reproductive system (Table 16–14). Some of these agents act on the neural component of the endocrine system, whereas others act directly on the gonad.

TESTING MALE REPRODUCTIVE CAPACITY

A host of tests have been used or proposed for evaluating the male reproductive system (Table 16–15). Several cellular sites or processes are vulnerable to chemical and/or drug insult. Perturbing many of the endocrine or biochemical events associated with the male reproductive system seldom occurs after a single exposure to a toxicant(s). Rather, multiple exposure extended over some duration of time are most likely required to detect male reproductive toxicity. Most of the tests are invasive and hence limited to animals and not generally acceptable for use in humans. Indeed, in humans, the noninvasive approaches involve sperm counts, blood gonadotrophin levels, and a nonbarren marriage. Testicular biopsy can be used in selected circum-

Table 16–11. ADVANTAGES AND LIMITATIONS OF STANDARD REPRODUCTIVE PROCEDURES*

END POINT	LIMITATIONS	VALUE
Fertility	Insensitive	Integrates all reproductive functions
Testicular histology	Subjective; not quantitative	Information on target cell
Testis weights	Less sensitive than sperm counts; affected by edema	Rapid; quantitative

* From Meistrich, M. L.: Evaluation of reproductive toxicity by testicular sperm head counts. *J. Am. Coll. Toxicol.,* **8:**551–567, 1989.

stances to evaluate spermatogenesis (i.e., infertility/sterility), but this procedure is obviously invasive. Azoospermia can be caused by agents, genetic disorders (e.g., Klinefelter's syndrome), infections (e.g., mumps), irradiation, and hormonal defects. Dietary deficiencies are well known to cause spermatogenic arrest (Table 16–16). Similarly, lead can produce infertility, sterility, and varying abnormalities in sperm function and morphology (Table 16–17). Pogach *et al.* (1989) have reported that *cis*-platinum causes Sertoli cell dysfunction in rodents. These changes in Sertoli cell function appear to be responsible for *cis*-platinum–induced impairment in spermatogenesis. Other heavy metals such as cobalt, iron, cadmium, mercury, molybdenum, and silver can adversely affect spermatogenesis and accessory sex organ function. Dietary zinc deficiency can produce sterility (Prasad *et al.*, 1967). Likewise, chemically induced zinc depletion (e.g., phthalates) can produce testicular damage as evidenced by sterile seminiferous tubules (Thomas *et al.*, 1982). In experimental animals, zinc prevents cadmium carcinogenicity in the rat testes (Koizumi and Waalkes, 1989). The major preventive effect of zinc against cadmium-induced testicular tumors may be due to its ability to reduce the cytotoxicity of cadmium in interstitial cells.

Sensitivity of the various parameters used to evaluate the male reproductive system varies considerably. There are advantages as well as limitations to a number of standard reproductive procedures. Testicular weights are a rapid quantitative index, but this measurement is less sensitive than sperm counts and is affected by water imbibition (edema). In normal males, the number of sperm produced per day per testis is largely determined by testicular size. In many mammals, testis size is correlated to daily sperm production. Fertility as an index is quite insensitive, although it does incorporate all reproductive functions. Fertility profiles using serial mating studies to assess the biologic status of sperm cells have constituted a useful test for both dominant lethal mutations (Epstein *et al.*, 1972) and male reproductive capacity (I. P. Lee and

Dixon, 1972). Testicular histology provides information on target cell morphology, although it too is subjective and not particularly quantitative. Histologic evaluation of the seminiferous tubules can establish the cellular integrity and provide information about the process of spermatogenesis (Figure 16–9). It is more difficult to detect morphologic changes in Leydig cells and to some extent Sertoli cells. Leydig cell function is better determined by evaluating androgen levels (or gonadotropins) or, in the case of Sertoli cells, the measurement of androgen-binding protein (ABP).

Flow cystometric analyses of the testes can be used to evaluate specific cell populations (Selden *et al.*, 1989). This technique has the advantage of being able to assess simultaneously multiple characteristics on a cell-to-cell basis with the results being rapidly correlated for each cell type or property. Cell size, cell shape, cytoplasmic granularity and pigmentation, along with measurements of surface antigens, lectin binding, DNA/RNA, and chromatin structure, are among some of the intrinsic and extrinsic parameters that can be evaluated. The toxicity of

Table 16–12. POSSIBLE SITES OF ACTION OF AGENTS AFFECTING THE REPRODUCTIVE SYSTEM

ANATOMICAL SITE	ENDOCRINE EFFECT(S)
Central Nervous System	
Cerebral cortex	Altered secretion of FSH/LH
Median eminence	Altered releasing hormone secretion
Adenohypopysis	Changes in gonadotrophin secretion
Peripheral Target Organs	
Ovary	Altered secretion of estrogens
Testes	Altered secretion of androgens
Liver	Increased catabolism of steroids
Kidney	Increased excretion of steroids

Table 16-13. AGENTS REPORTED TO AFFECT MALE REPRODUCTIVE CAPACITY*

Steroids
Natural and synthetic androgens (antiandrogens), estrogens (antiestrogens), and progestins

Antineoplastic Agents
Alkaloids—vinca alkaloids (vinblastine, vincristine)
Alkylating agents—esters of methanesulfonic acid (MMS, EMS, busulfan); ethylenimines (TEM, TEPA); hydrazines (procarbazine); nitrogen mustards (chlorambucil, cyclophosphamide); nitrosoureas (CCNU, BCNU, MNU)
Antimetabolites—azauridine, 5-bromodeoxyuridine, cytosine arabinoside, 5-fluorouracil, 6-mercaptopurine)
Antitumor antibiotics—actinomycin D, adriamycin, bleomycin, daunomycin, mitomycin C

Drugs That Modify the Nervous System
Alcohols
Anesthetic gases and vapors—enflurane, halothane, methoxyflurane, nitrous oxide
Antiparkinsonism drugs—levodopa
Appetite suppressants
Narcotic and nonnarcotic analgesics—opioids
Neuroleptics—phenothiazines, imipramine, and amitriptyline
Tranquilizers—phenothiazines, reserpine, monoamine oxidase inhibitors
Antiadrenergic drugs—clonidine, methyldopa, guanethidine, bretylium, reserpine

Other Therapeutic Agents
Alcoholism—tetraethylthiuram disulfide (antabuse)
Analgesics and antipyretics—phenacetin
Anticonvulsants—diphenylhydantoin (phenytoin)
Antiinfective agents—amphotericin B, hexachlorophene, hycanthone, nitrofurans
Antischistosomal agents—niridazole, hycanthone
Antiparasitic drugs—quinine, quinacrine, chloroquine
Diuretics—aldactone, thiazides
Gout suppressants—colchicine
Histamines and histamine antagonists—chlorcyclizine, cimetidine
Oral hypoglycemic agents—chlorpropamide
Xanthines—caffeine, theobromine

Metals and Trace Elements
Al, boranes, boron, Cd, Co, Pb, Hg, methylmercury, Mo, Ni, Ag, U

Insecticides
Benzene hexachlorides—lindane
Carbamates—carbaryl
Chlorobenzene derivatives—chlorophenothane (DDT), methoxychlor
Indane derivatives—aldrin, chlordane, dieldrin
Phosphate esters (cholinesterase inhibitors)—dichlorvos(DDVP), hexamethylphosphoramide
Miscellaneous—chlordecone (kepone)

Herbicides
Chlorinated phenoxyacetic acids—(2,4-D), (2,4,5-T)
Quaternary ammonium compounds—diquat, paraquat

Rodenticides
Metabolic inhibitors—fluoroacetate (fluoroacetamide)

Fungicides, Fumigants, and Sterilants
Apholate, captan, carbon disulfide, dibromochloropropane (DBCP), ethylene dibromide, ethylene oxide, thiocarbamates (cineb, maneb), triphenyltin, carbendazim

Food Additives and Contaminants
Aflatoxins, cyclamate, diethylstilbestrol (DES), dimethylnitrosamine, gossypol, metanil yellow, monosodium glutamate, nitrofuran derivatives

Industrial Chemicals
Chlorinated hydrocarbons—hexafluoroacetone, PBBs, PCBs, dioxin (TCDD)
Hydrazines—dithiocarbamoylhydrazine
Monomers—vinyl chloride, chloroprene
Polycyclic aromatic hydrocarbons (PAHs)—dimethylbenzanthracene (DMBA), benzo[a]pyrene
Solvents—benzene, carbon disulfide, glycolethers, hexane, thiophene, toluene, xylene

Miscellaneous
Personal habits—alcohol consumption, tobacco smoking
Agents of abuse—marijuana, heroin, cocaine, anabolic steroids, etc.
Physical factors—heat, light, hypoxia
Radiation—α, β and γ radiation: x-rays
Stable isotopes—deuterium oxide

---

* Modified from Dixon, R. L.: Toxic responses of the reproductive system. In Klaassen, C. D.; Amdur, M. O.; and Doull, J. (eds.): *Casarett and Doull's Toxicology: The Basic Science of Poisons,* 3rd ed. Macmillan Publishing Co., New York, 1986.

Table 16–14. AGENTS REPORTED TO AFFECT FEMALE REPRODUCTIVE CAPACITY*

Steroids
Natural and synthetic androgens (antiandrogens), estrogens (antiestrogens), and progestins

Antineoplastic Agents
Alkylating agents—cyclophosphamide, busulfan
Antimetabolites—folic acid antagonists (methotrexate)

Other Therapeutic Agents
Anesthetic gases and vapors—halothane, enflurane, methoxyflurane
Antiparkinsonism drugs—levodopa
Antiparasitic drugs—quinacrine
Appetite suppressants
Narcotic and nonnarcotic analgesics—opioids
Neuroleptics, phenothiazines, imipramine, and amitriptyline
Serotonin
Sympathomimetic amines—epinephrine, norepinephrine, amphetamines
Tranquilizers—phenothiazines, reserpine, monoamine oxidase inhibitors

Metals and Trace Elements
Arsenic, lead, lithium, mercury and methylmercury, molybdenum, nickel, selenium, thallium

Insecticides
Benzene hexachlorides—lindane
Carbamates—carbaryl
Chlorobenzene derivatives—chlorophenothane (DDT), methoxychlor
Indane derivatives—aldrin, chlordane, dieldrin
Phosphate esters (cholinesterase inhibitors)—parathion
Miscellaneous—chlordecone (kepone), mirex, hexachlorobenzene, ethylene oxide

Herbicides
Chlorinated phenoxyacetic acids—2,4-D, 2,4,5-T

Food Additives and Contaminants
Cyclohexylamine, diethylstilbestrol (DES), dimethylnitrosamines, monosodium glutamate, nitrofuran
(AF$_2$), nitrosamines, sodium nitrite

Industrial Chemicals and Processes
Building materials—formaldehyde
Chlorinated hydrocarbons—polychlorinated biphenyls (PCBs), chloroform, trichloroethylene
Paints and dyes—aniline
Plastic monomers—caprolactam, styrene, vinyl chloride
Polycyclic aromatic hydrocarbons (PAHs)—benzo[a]pyrene
Rubber manufacturing—chloroprene
Solvents—benzene, carbon disulfide, chloroform, ethanol, glycol ethers, hexane, toluene, trichloroethylene, xylene
Miscellaneous—cyanoketone, hydrazines

Consumer Products
Flame retardants—TRIS, polybrominated biphenyls (PBBs)
Plasticizers—phthalic acid ester (DEHP)

Miscellaneous
Ethanol, nicotine, marijuana, cocaine, heroin

* Modified from Dixon, R. L.: Toxic responses of the reproductive system. In Klaassen, C. D.; Amdur, M. O.; and Doull, J. (eds.): *Casarett and Doull's Toxicology: The Basic Science of Poisons,* 3rd ed. Macmillan Publishing Co., New York, 1986.

thiotepa on mouse spermatogenesis has been determined using dual-parameter flow cytometry. The dual parameters of DNA stainability versus RNA content provide excellent resolution of testicular cell types (Evenson *et al.,* 1986). Flow cytometry has also been used to study the effects of methyl-benzimidazol-2-yl-carbamate (MBC) on mouse germ cells. MBC exposure results in an altered ratio of testicular cell types, abnormal sperm head morphology, and altered sperm chromatin structure (Evenson *et al.,* 1987).

Oxidative damage to spermatogenic cells has also been associated with reproductive dysfunction in laboratory animals, and this too can provide an index for assessing risk. Angioli *et al.* (1987) have proposed an *in vitro* spermatogenic cell model for assessing reproductive toxicity that involves the ability of bleomycin to reduce oxidative changes in male germ cell populations.

Penetration of zona-free hamster eggs by human sperm has also been suggested as a useful chemical test to assess male fertility. Recently,

**Table 16–15. POTENTIALLY USEFUL TESTS OF MALE
REPRODUCTIVE TOXICITY FOR LABORATORY
ANIMALS AND/OR MAN***[†]

Testis
  Size *in situ*
  Weight
  Spermatid reserves
  Gross and histologic evaluation
  Nonfunctional tubules (%)
  Tubules with lumen sperm (%)
  Tubule diameter
  Counts of leptotene spermatocytes

Epididymis
  Weight and histology
  Number of sperm in distal half
  Motility of sperm, distal end (%)
  Gross sperm morphology, distal
    end (%)
  Detailed sperm morphology, distal
    end (%)
  Biochemical assays

Accessory Sex Glands
  Histology
  Gravimetric

Semen
  Total volume
  Gel-free volume
  Sperm concentration
  Total sperm/ejaculate
  Total sperm/day of abstinence
  Sperm motility, visual (%)
  Sperm motility, videotape (%
    and velocity)
  Gross sperm morphology
  Detailed sperm morphology

Endocrine
  Luteinizing hormone
  Follicle stimulating hormone
  Testosterone
  Gonadotropin-releasing
    hormone

Fertility
  Ratio exposed: pregnant females
  Number embryos or young per
    pregnant female
  Ratio viable embryos:corpora lutea
  Number 2–8 cell eggs
  Number unfertilized eggs; abnormal
    eggs
  Sperm per ovum

In Vitro
  Incubation of sperm in agent
  Hamster egg penetration test

Other Tests Considered
  Tonometric measurement of testicular
    consistency
  Qualitative testicular histology
  Stage of cycle at which spermiation
    occurs
  Quantitative testicular histology

Sperm Motility
  Time-exposure photography
  Multiple-exposure photography
  Cinemicrography
  Videomicrography
  Sperm membrane characteristics
  Evaluation of sperm metabolism
  Fluorescent Y bodies in spermatozoa
  Flow cytometry of spermatozoa
  Karyotyping human sperm pronuclei
  Cervical mucus penetration test

* *See* Galbraith *et al.* (1982) for complete table and discussion of the relative usefulness of these tests.
[†] Modified from Dixon, R. L.: Toxic responses of the reproductive system. In Klaassen, C. D.; Amdur, M. O.; and Doull, J. (eds.): *Casarett and Doull's Toxicology: The Basic Science of Poisons,* 3rd ed. Macmillan Publishing Co., New York, 1986.

this assay has also been recommended as a prognostic indicator in *in vitro* fertilization programs (Nahhas and Blumenfeld, 1989).

The epididymis and the sex accessory organs can also be used to evaluate the status of male reproductive processes. While the epididymis has an important physiologic role in the male reproductive tract, it is less useful as a parameter for assessing gonadotoxins. Its histologic integrity may be examined, but the most meaningful determinations are the number of sperm stored within the cauda epididymis and a measure of

sperm motility and morphology. Epididymal sperm may be extruded onto a glass slide and viewed under the microscope for motility and abnormalities. Epididymal sperm may also be extruded, diluted with saline in a hemocytometer, and counted. Sperm morphology may be evaluated using either wet preparations or properly prepared, stained smears but requires an appropriate classification scheme (Wyrobek, 1983; Wyrobek *et al.*, 1983). Chromosomal analysis is used in the laboratory and clinic to diagnose genetic diseases. Sex accessory organs,

Table 16–16. DIETARY DEFICIENCY(S) AND SPERMATOGENIC ARREST*

DEFICIENCY(S)	SPECIE
Manganese	Rats and rabbits
Vitamin A	Mice, rats, and guinea pigs
Vitamin B(pyridoxine)	Rats
Vitamin E	Rats, hamsters, and guinea pigs
Zinc	Mice, rats, dogs, and sheep

* From Mann, T., and Lutwak-Mann, C.: *Male Reproductive Function and Semen: Themes and Trends in Physiology, Biochemistry and Investigative Andrology.* Springer-Verlag, New York, 1981.

usually the prostate (e.g., ventral lobes in the rodent) and the seminal vesicles (empty), are a rapid and quantitative measure of the male reproductive processes that are androgen dependent. Chemical indicators in sex accessory glands such as fructose and citric acid have also been used to evaluate male sex hormone function (cf. Mann and Lutwak-Mann, 1981).

Semen analysis can be used as an index of testicular and posttesticular organ function. Semen can be collected from a number of experimental and domestic animals using an artificial vagina. Electroejaculatory techniques and chemically induced ejaculations have also been employed to produce semen samples, particularly in animal husbandry.

Both quantitative and qualitative characteristics of more than one ejaculate must be evaluated to ensure that conclusions concerning testicular function are valid. Since semen represents contributions from accessory sex glands as well as the testes and epididymides, only the total number of sperm in an ejaculate is a reliable estimate of sperm production. The number of sperm introduced into the pelvic urethra during emission and the volume of fluid from the accessory sex glands are independent. The potential sources of error in measuring ejaculate volume, concentration, and the seminal characteristics necessary to calculate total sperm per ejaculate must be considered (Amann, 1981).

Several factors affect the number of sperm in an ejaculate including age, testicular size, frequency, degree of sexual arousal, and season (particularly domestic animals). Although ejaculation frequency or the interval since the last ejaculation alters the total number of sperm per ejaculate, ejaculation frequency does not influence daily sperm production. However, because of epididymal storage, frequent ejaculation is necessary if the number of sperm counted in ejaculated semen is to reflect sperm production accurately. If only one or two ejaculates are collected weekly, a 50 percent reduction in sperm production probably would remain undetected. Ejaculates should be collected daily (or every other day) over a period of time. The analysis of isolated ejaculate or even several ejaculates collected at irregular intervals cannot estimate daily sperm production or output. The first several ejaculates in each series contain more sperm than subsequent ejaculates because the number of sperm available for ejaculation is being reduced.

There have been recent advances in the automation of semen analysis (Boyers *et al.,* 1989). Semiautomated measures of sperm motility may be categorized as indirect or direct methods. Indirect methods of sperm analysis estimate mean swimming speed of cells by measuring properties of the whole sperm suspension. Spectrometry or turbidimetric methods record changes in optical density. Direct methods involve visual assessment of individual sperm cells and stem from early efforts to quantitate sperm swimming speed. Such direct measurements may include photographic methods like time-exposure photography, multiple-exposure photography, and cinematography. Computer-aided sperm motion analysis (CASMA) may be applied to morphology, physiology, motility, or flagellar analysis. CASMA allows visualization of both digitized static and dynamic sperm images.

Androgen receptors for testosterone and dihydrotestosterone (DHT) have also been used to evaluate the effects of various gonadotoxins. A number of divalent metal ions (Zn, Hg, Cu, Cd, etc.) can inhibit androgen-receptor binding in rodent prostate glands (Donovan *et al.,* 1980). Likewise, TCDD, a reproductive toxin in

Table 16–17. SOME ACTIONS OF LEAD ON THE MALE REPRODUCTIVE SYSTEM*

SPECIES	EFFECT
Rat	Infertility
Rat	Germinal epithelial damage
Rat	Oligospermia and testicular degeneration
Rat	Decreased sperm motility and prostate hyperplasia
Mouse	Infertility
Mouse	Abnormal sperm
Human	Teratospermia, hypospermia, and asthenospermia

* From Bell, J. U., and Thomas, J. A.: Effects of lead on the reproductive system. In Singhal, R. L., and Thomas, J. A. (eds.): *Basic and Clinical Toxicity of Lead.* Urban and Schwarzenberg, Medical Publishers, Baltimore, 1980, pp. 169–189.

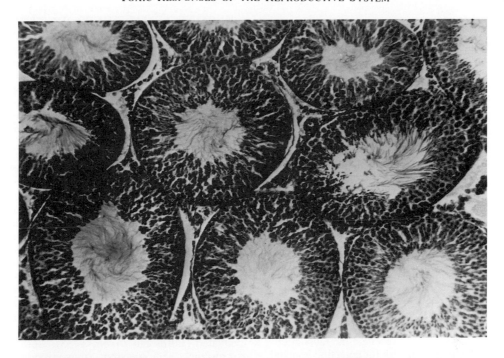

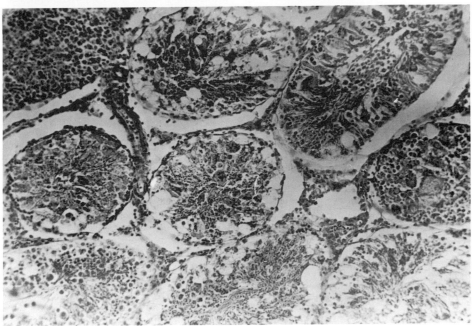

Figure 16–9.   Histology section of rat testes. *Above:* Normal H&E section revealing morphologic integrity of seminiferous tubules. *Below:* Chemical-induced testicular damage resulting in vacuolation of seminiferous tubules. Note partially sterile tubules. (From Thomas J. A. *et al.* Hormone assays and endocrine function, in Hayes, A. W.: *Principles and Methods of Toxicology.* Raven Press, New York, 1982.)

females, has an avidity for the estrogen receptor (cf. Hruska and Olson, 1989). Such receptor studies have been used primarily to gain insight into aspects of molecular mechanisms of toxicity and not for routine evaluation procedures.

Efforts have been made to identify so-called testicular marker enzymes as indicators of normal or abnormal cellular differentiation in the gonad (Hodgen, 1977; Shen and Lee, 1977; Chapin *et al.*, 1982). At least eight enzymes— namely, hyaluronidase (H); lactate dehydrogenase isoenzyme-X (LDH-X); and the dehydrogenases of sorbitol (SDH), α-glycerophosphate (GPDH), glucose-6-phosphate (G6PDH), malate (MDH), glyceraldehyde-3-phosphate (G3PDH), and isocitrate (ICDH)—have been studied with regard to their usefulness as predictors of gonadal toxicity.

A number of secretory products of the Sertoli cell hold some potential for evaluating male reproductive function. Of the several secretory products of the Sertoli cell (e.g., transferrin, ceruloplasmin, tissue plasminogen activator, sulfated glycoproteins), androgen-binding protein (ABP) has perhaps received the most attention as a potential indicator for detecting gonadal injury. Sertoli cell ABP and testicular transferrin may be affected by similar regulatory agents (e.g., FSH, insulin) (Skinner *et al.*, 1989). Leydig cell cultures can also be considered as a potential indicator to evaluate endocrine function of the gonad. Leydig cells, like the Sertoli cell, secrete a number of proteins, peptides, and other substances (e.g., β-endorphin, corticotropin-releasing factor [CRF]) (Eskeland *et al.*, 1989). Other than the inhibitory actions of DBCP on Sertoli cell ABP secretions, neither this cell and its secretions nor the Leydig cell has been used in reproductive toxicology evaluation.

TESTING FEMALE REPRODUCTIVE CAPACITY

Evaluating female mammalian reproductive processes is far more complex than in the male. Female reproductive processes involve oogenesis, ovulation, the development of sexual receptivity, coitus, gamete and zygote transport, fertilization, and implantation of the concepters. All these processes or events are potential sites of chemical or drug interference.

Evaluation of the female reproductive tract for toxicologic perturbations not surprisingly may overlap with testing methods for assessing teratogenicity and mutagenicity. Indeed, reproductive end points that indicate dysfunction in the female (Table 16–18), including perinatal parameters, often overlap with developmental toxicity end points (Table 16–19). The neonate is particularly sensitive to a variety of drugs and chemicals (Thomas, 1989).

Gross pathology (*e.g.*, gravimetric responses—ovary, uteri, *etc.*) and histopathology are important to reproductivity and should be evaluated (Ettlin and Dixon, 1985). Both light microscopy and electron (transmission and scanning) may be useful in assessing ovarian and pituitary ultrastructure. As in the male (Table 16–15), there are a number of useful tests to evaluate the female reproductive system (Table 16–20). These tests can be performed on a wide variety of end points, at different anatomical sites, and can include both biochemical, hormonal, or morphologic parameters.

Methods to assess directly the effects of test compounds on oogenesis and/or folliculogenesis include histologic determination of oocytes and/ or follicle number (Dobson *et al.*, 1978). Chemical effects on oogenesis can be measured in-

---

Table 16–18. REPRODUCTIVE END POINTS TO INDICATE REPRODUCTIVE DYSFUNCTION

Decreased libido; impotence
Sperm abnormalities: decreased number/motility; morphology
Subfecundity: abnormal gonads/ducts of external genitalia; abnormal pubertal development; infertility of male/female; amenorrhea; anovulatory cycles; delay in conception
Illness during pregnancy/parturition: toxemia; hemorrhage
Early fetal loss (to 28 weeks)
Late fetal loss (after 28 weeks)/stillbirth
Intrapartum death
Death in first week
Decreased birth weight
Gestational age at delivery: prematurity; postmaturity
Altered sex ratio; chromosome abnormalities
Multiple births; birth defects
Infant death
Childhood morbidity; childhood malignancies

Table 16-19.   DEVELOPMENTAL TOXICITY END POINTS*

Type I Changes
(Outcomes Permanent, Life-Threatening, and Frequently Associated with Gross
   Malformations)
Reduction of number of live births (litter size)
Increased number of stillbirths
Reduced number of live fetuses (litter size)
Increased number of resorptions
Increased number of fetuses with malformations

Type II Changes
(Outcomes Nonpermanent, Non–Life-Threatening, and Not Associated with Mal-
   formations)
Reduced birth weights
Reduced postnatal survival
Decreased postnatal growth, reproductive capacity
Increased number of fetuses with retarded development

* From Frankos, V. H.: FDA perspectives on the use of teratology data for human risk.
Fund. Appl. Toxicol., **5**:615–625, 1985.

directly by determining fertility of the offspring
(McLachlan *et al.,* 1981). Other indirect measures of ovarian toxicity in animals include
assessment of age at vaginal opening, onset of
reproductive senescence, and total reproductive
capacity (Gellert, 1978).

Morphologic tests can quantify and assess primordial germ cell number, stem cell migration,
oogonial proliferation, and urogenital ridge development. *In vitro* techniques can be used to
evaluate primordial germ cell proliferation,
migration, ovarian differentiation, and folliculogenesis (Ways *et al.,* 1980; Thompson, 1981).

Serial oocyte counts can monitor oocyte and/
or follicle destruction in experimental animals
(I. Pedersen and Peters, 1968). This approach is
a reliable means of quantifying the effects of
chemicals on oocytes and follicles.

Follicular growth may be assayed in experimental animals using (^{3}H)-thymidine uptake, ovarian response to gonadotropins, and follicular kinetics (Hillier *et al.,* 1980). These
approaches identify both direct and indirect
effects on follicular growth and identify drugs
and other environmental chemicals that are
ovotoxic (Mattison and Nightingale, 1980).

Serum levels of estrogen or estrogenic effects
on target tissues are indicators of normal follicular function. Tissue and organ responses include
time of vaginal opening in immature rats, uterine
weight, endometrial morphology, and/or serum
levels of FSH and LH. Granulosa cell culture
techniques provide direct screens of the ability of
chemicals to inhibit cell proliferation and/or estrogen production (Zeleznik *et al.,* 1979). The
biosynthesis of estradiol and its metabolism to
estrone and estriol by the ovary constitutes another indicator of the reproductive process. The

peripheral catabolism of these steroids is principally a function of the liver.

Nuclear and cytoplasmic estrogen/progester-
one may provide important toxicologic applications. Estradiol and progesterone receptors are
especially important since chemicals (e.g., DDT
and other organochlorine pesticides) compete for
these receptors and perhaps alter their molecular
conformation (Thomas, 1975).

The process of ovulation differs among various mammalian species. Some animals ovulate
spontaneously upon copulation (e.g., rabbit),
whereas other species (e.g., humans and subhuman primates) have a hormonally dependent cycle. Several steroidal and nonsteroidal agents
can interfere with this neuroendocrine process of
ovulation. In the estrus cycle of rodents, ovulation occurs at intervals from four to five days.
Ovulation occurs during estrus and can be readily detected by cornification of vaginal epithelium. The rat's estrus cycle can be divided into
four stages and can be recognized by changes in
vaginal cytology: proestrus, estrus, metestrus,
and diestrus.

The processes of fertilization and implantation
can be affected by both chemicals and drugs.
The formation, maturation, and union of germ
cells compose a complex physiologic event that
is sensitive to foreign substances. Fertilization
can also be achieved *in vitro* with sperm and ova
extradited from a variety of different mammalian
species including humans.

Reproductive performance is best assessed by
pregnancy, and this represents a successful index
for evaluating endocrine toxicity (or lack thereof). Mating studies using rats is a fundamental
procedure that determines total reproductive
capacity.

Table 16–20. POTENTIALLY USEFUL TESTS OF FEMALE REPRODUCTIVE TOXICITY*

Body Weight

Ovary
  Organ weight
  Histology
  Number of oocytes
  Rate of follicular atresia
  Follicular steroidogenesis
  Follicular maturation
  Oocyte maturation
  Ovulation
  Luteal function

Hypothalamus
  Histology
  Altered synthesis and release of neurotransmitters,
    neuromodulators, and neurohormones

Pituitary
  Histology
  Altered synthesis and release of trophic hormones

Endocrine
  Gonadotropin
  Chorionic gonadotropin levels
  Estrogen and progesterone

Oviduct
  Histology
  Gamete transport
  Fertilization
  Transport of early embryo

Uterus
  Cytology and histology
  Luminal fluid analysis (xenobiotics, proteins)
  Decidual response
  Dysfunctional bleeding

Cervix/Vulva/Vagina
  Cytology
  Histology
  Mucus production
  Mucus quality (sperm penetration test)

Fertility
  Ratio exposed: pregnant females
  Number of embryos or young per pregnant female
  Ratio viable embryos: corpora lutea
  Ratio implantation: corpora lutea
  Number 2–8 cell eggs
  Number of unfertilized eggs; abnormal eggs
  Number of corpora lutea

In Vitro
  In vitro fertilization of superovulated eggs, either ex-
    posed to chemical in culture or from treated females

* Modified from Dixon, R. L.: Toxic responses of the reproductive system. In Klaassen, C. D.; Amdur, M. O.; and Doull, J. (eds.): *Casarett and Doull's Toxicology: The Basic Science of Poisons,* 3rd ed. Macmillan Publishing Co., New York, 1986.

REPRODUCTIVE TESTS AND REGULATORY REQUIREMENTS

Some regulatory agencies have adopted standard toxicologic testing programs for drugs, food additives, and pesticides (*see* Table 16–21) (*see also* Lamb, 1985; Lamb *et al.,* 1986). Both the U.S. Food and Drug Administration (FDA) and the U.S. Environmental Protection Agency (EPA) have established study designs to assess the reproductive risks of chemicals and drugs. The FDA imposes guidelines for drugs that include three different protocols on development, fertility, and general reproductive performance. Segment I includes fertility and reproductive function in males and in females. Segment II involves studies pertaining to developmental toxicology and teratology, whereas segment III encompasses perinatal and postnatal studies. Segment I studies are initial studies usually requiring additional protocols leading to conventional teratology experiments that emphasize detecting any morphological defects in the offspring of laboratory animals. By using pregnant animals (segment III) that are treated for the last third of their period of gestation, including lactation and weaning, assessment can be made about the effects of chemicals/drug exposure on late fetal development, particularly lactation and offspring survival.

The U.S. FDA uses multigeneration studies for food additives to evaluate chemical effects on fertility, gestation, parturition, lactation, and offspring development and reproduction. Such assessments of reproductive toxicity provide important information on chemical safety, but they require at least a year to complete. Such tests can therefore be very expensive.

Table 16–21. SUMMARY OF REPRODUCTIVE TOXICITY TESTING USED BY U.S. REGULATORY AGENCIES AND BY THE NATIONAL TOXICOLOGY PROGRAM*

AGENCY	TEST(S)
FDA	Segment I: fertility and reproductive function in male and female
FDA	Segment II: development toxicology and teratology
FDA	Segment III: perinatal and postnatal toxicity
FDA	Multigeneration (three-generation) (e.g., drugs)
EPA	Two-generation (e.g., pesticides)
NTP	Fertility Assessment by Continuous Breeding (FACB)

* Modified from Lamb, J. C.: Reproductive toxicity testing: evaluating and developing new testing systems. *J. Am. Coll. Toxicol.,* **4**:163–178, 1985.

The EPA has adopted a set of test guidelines for assessing reproductive toxicity, particularly as they apply to pesticides. In general, EPA tests are less costly and of shorter duration than those required by the FDA, in particular, the FDA's requirement for multigeneration testing. The EPA guidelines necessitate that the highest dose level reveals some toxicologic manifestations but not mortality. Such a procedure gives a degree of assurance that a chemical is not a reproductive toxicant where toxicity is present, but the reproductive system is unaffected.

The National Toxicology Program (NTP) adopted the Fertility Assessment by Continuous Breeding (FACB) protocol in the early 1980s. The FACB protocol was introduced by McLachlan *et al.* (1981) and was designed to reduce the time for reproductive toxicity testing yet still provide data comparable with other testing systems. FACB tests take no longer than the improved and shortened EPA test designs. The FACB protocol uses more animals per group and, in general, increases the statistical power of the assay. Recently, Morrissey *et al.* (1988) have evaluated the effectiveness of continuous breeding reproduction studies. This subtle modification of increasing the statistical power of the assay is important, since fertility is an especially important indicator of reproductive toxicity, and is one of the least sensitive indicators in the assessment of the reproductive system (Schwetz *et al.*, 1980).

Reproductive toxicity studies extending over multiple generations are scientifically and logistically difficult to manage, interpret, and finance (Johnson, 1986). While the FDA segment tests are collectively very meaningful in assessing reproductive toxicity (or safety), none of these batteries of tests can replace the other, and the multigeneration evaluation has considerable scientific merit for justifying their expense. However, current multigeneration protocols could be revised in order to improve on the toxicologic information collected.

FDA reproductive testing guidelines requiring preclinical animal testing for each new drug depends on how women might be exposed to the drug itself. The FDA further categorizes drugs on five different levels, depending on potential risk (e.g., category A—no evidence of human development toxicity—to category D or X—demonstrated birth defects) (cf. Frankos, 1985). Present FDA Bureau of Foods testing guidelines recommend a two-generation reproductive study, including a teratology phase, to be undertaken for food additives and color additives.

The classic three-generation reproduction study requires continuous exposure of the parental generation (F_0) and the offspring of each succeeding generation to the test chemical (Collins, 1978). Mating indices can be calculated:

Mating index
$$= \frac{\text{Number of copulations}}{\text{Number of estrus cycles required}} \times 100$$

Fecundity index
$$= \frac{\text{Number of pregnancies}}{\text{Number of copulations}} \times 100$$

Male fertility index
$$= \frac{\begin{array}{c}\text{Number of males}\\\text{impregnating females}\end{array}}{\begin{array}{c}\text{Number of males exposed to}\\\text{fertile nonpregnant females}\end{array}} \times 100$$

Female fertility index
$$= \frac{\text{Number of females conceiving}}{\begin{array}{c}\text{Number of females exposed to}\\\text{fertile males}\end{array}} \times 100$$

Incidence of parturition
$$= \frac{\text{Number of parturitions}}{\text{Number of pregnancies}} \times 100$$

Pups are examined for physical abnormalities at birth. The numbers of viable, stillborn, and cannibalized members of each litter are recorded. Observations for clinical signs are made daily. The number of survivors on days 1, 4, 12, and 21 postparturition is recorded. The following survival indices can be calculated:

Live birth index
$$= \frac{\text{Number of viable pups born}}{\text{Total number of pups born}} \times 100$$

24-hour survival index
$$= \frac{\begin{array}{c}\text{Number of pups viable}\\\text{at lactation day 1}\end{array}}{\text{Number of viable pups born}} \times 100$$

4-day survival index
$$= \frac{\begin{array}{c}\text{Number of pups viable}\\\text{at lactation day 4}\end{array}}{\text{Number of viable pups born}} \times 100$$

12-day survival index
$$= \frac{\begin{array}{c}\text{Number of pups viable}\\\text{at lactation day 12}\end{array}}{\begin{array}{c}\text{Number of pups viable}\\\text{at lactation day 4}\end{array}} \times 100$$

21-day survival index
$$= \frac{\begin{array}{c}\text{Number of pups viable}\\\text{at lactation day 21}\end{array}}{\begin{array}{c}\text{Number of pups retained}\\\text{at lactation day 4}\end{array}} \times 100$$

Recently, the International Life Sciences Institute—Nutrition Foundation convened to discuss criteria for listing substances that might be developmental toxicants under the provisions of California's Safe Drinking Water and Toxic Enforcement Act of 1986 ("Proposition 65"). Such criteria are very difficult to establish, but they should emphasize human relevancy and biological plausibility (Mattison et al., 1989).

It is evident that a number of test systems are available to assess the degree of changes on the reproductive system. Some such tests employ many animals and follow their reproductive histories for more than one generation, whereas still other tests employ cell systems that are perhaps representative of a molecular approach to determining mechanism(s) of toxicologic action(s).

HUMAN RISK FACTORS AFFECTING FERTILITY

Most humans are exposed to a vast number of chemicals that may be hazardous to their reproductive capacity. Many chemicals have been identified as reproductive hazards in laboratory studies (Clegg et al., 1986; Zenick and Clegg, 1986; Working, 1988). Although the extrapolation of data from laboratory animals to humans is inexact, a number of these chemicals have also been shown to exert detrimental effects on human reproductive performance. The list includes drugs, especially steroid hormones and chemotherapeutic agents; metals and trace elements; pesticides; food additives and contaminants; industrial chemicals; and consumer products.

Fertility in humans, like that in experimental animals, is susceptible to environmental and/or industrial chemicals. Infertility is a problem of increasing concern among several industrialized countries. Levine (1983) has suggested methods for detecting occupational causes of male infertility. The decrease in sperm density purportedly having occurred over the past 30 years has been associated with the increased use of recreational drugs and the use of certain medications that can secondarily affect the reproductive system. Furthermore, a comparison of the production of spermatozoa from the testes of different species reveals that the output of human sperm is approximately four times less than other mammals in terms of the number of sperm produced per gram of tissue (Amann and Howard, 1980).

It has also been suggested that the human male is more vulnerable to environmental and occupational toxins than other mammals (Overstreet, 1984; Overstreet et al., 1988). The somewhat fragile nature of the male reproductive system to occupational exposure to the fungicide DBCP

was reinforced when Whorton et al. (1977) described its injurious actions upon the testes. Fortunately, recovery from severe oligospermia after DBCP exposure has been reported by Lantz et al. (1981). Levine et al. (1983), however, have indicated that reproductive histories are superior to sperm counts in assessing male infertility caused by DBCP.

It has been extremely difficult to correlate directly human exposure to occupational chemicals with alterations in the reproductive system. A particularly complicating factor(s) in this lack of correlation is that the normal reproductive processes seldom operate at a physiologic optimum. For example, as many as 15 percent of all married couples in the United States are defined as being clinically infertile (MacLeod, 1971), whereas another 25 percent of the women exhibit impaired fecundity (Mosher, 1981). At least 30 percent of early human conceptions and up to 15 percent of recognized pregnancies are terminated by spontaneous abortions (cf. Haney, 1985). Of the 15 percent spontaneous abortions terminating as recognized pregnancies, about 25 percent have abnormalities that are related to genetic etiologies and another 7 percent are caused by so-called environmental agents. By far, most of these abortions are due to unknown factors, and this constitutes about 7 percent of the cases of spontaneous abortions.

Many other factors can affect the normalcy of the female reproductive system as evidenced by variations in the menstrual process. Hence, physiological, sociological, and psychological factors have been linked with menstrual disorders. Factors that are known to affect menstruation yet are for the most part completely unrelated to occupational settings include age, body weight extremes, liver disease, thyroid dysfunction, IUDs, stress, exercise, and marital status. It is, therefore, obvious that a number of factors can affect menstruation and that these factors do not even include such things as therapeutic drugs (Selevan et al., 1985), so-called recreational drugs, or potentially toxic substances present in occupational environments. Even the choice of control populations in studies involving the adverse effects on the reproductive system can affect the risk estimates. Environmental chemical exposure can produce reproductive dysfunction in males (Table 16–22) as well as in females (Table 16–23).

Extrapolation of Animal Data to Humans

The exclusive use of animal experimental results to predict outcomes in humans still represents an uncertainty. This uncertainty can be somewhat relieved if findings from multiple species are known, particularly subhuman pri-

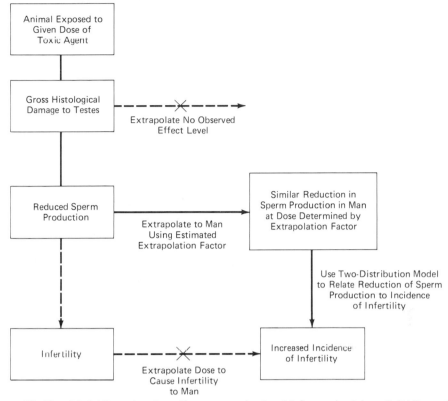

Figure 16–10. Model for estimation of human reproductive risk from animal data. *Solid lines with arrows* indicate useful approaches. *Dashed lines* indicate approaches that are not useful, and a *cross* on the line indicates that extrapolation in this manner is not useful. (From Meistrich, M. L.: Evaluation of reproductive toxicity by testicular sperm head counts. *J. Am. Coll. Toxicol.*, **8**:551–567, 1989.)

mates, and there are epidemiologic studies that help substantiate laboratory experiments. While there are many general similarities among mammals with respect to their response to drugs and/or chemicals, there are nevertheless some notable differences. Many of these species differences can be attributed to toxicokinetics, especially biotransformation. Greater predictability can be seen in results from well-validated animal models. A model for estimating human reproductive risk from animal data may be seen in Figure 16–10. Zenick and Clegg (1989), Buiatti *et al.* (1984), and Paul (1988) have reviewed several factors that are important in assessing risk to the male reproductive system. It is considerably easier to extrapolate controlled drug studies in animals to exact therapeutic regimens in humans than it is to simulate a chemical's exposure in an animal to a presumed environmental exposure in humans. Occupational exposures are inexact, and environmental levels are even more difficult to document (cf. Lemast-

Table 16–22. ENVIRONMENTAL CHEMICAL EXPOSURE ASSOCIATED WITH PRODUCTIVE DYSFUNCTION IN MEN[*][†]

Carbon disulfide
Chlordecone (Kepone)
Chloroprene
Dibromochloropropane (DBCP)
Ethylene dibromide
Ethylene oxide
Ethanol consumption
Glycol ethers
Hexane
Inorganic lead and other smelter emissions
Organic lead
Pesticides (occupational exposure)
Vinyl chloride

[*] Effects of nontherapeutic agents were selected from *Chemical Hazards to Human Reproduction* (Nisbet and Karch, 1983), *Reproductive Hazards of Industrial Chemicals* (Barlow and Sullivan, 1982), and *Occupational Exposure Associated with Male Reproductive Dysfunction* (Schrag and Dixon, 1985). As modified by Dixon, 1986.
[†] *See also* Thomas, 1981, 1986.

Table 16–23. ENVIRONMENTAL CHEMICAL EXPOSURE ASSOCIATED WITH REPRODUCTIVE DYSFUNCTION IN WOMEN*†

Anesthetic gases (operating room personnel)
Aniline
Benzene
Carbon disulfide
Chloroprene
Ethanol consumption
Ethylene oxide
Glycol ethers
Formaldehyde
Inorganic lead and other smelter emissions
Organic lead
Methylmercury
Pesticides (occupational exposure)
Phthalic acid esters (PAEs)
Polychlorinated biphenyls (PCBs)
Styrene
Tobacco smoking
Toluene
Vinyl chloride

* Effects of nontherapeutic agents were selected from *Chemical Hazards to Human Reproduction* (Nisbet and Karch, 1983) and *Reproductive Hazards of Industrial Chemicals* (Barlow and Sullivan, 1982). As modified from Dixon, 1986.
† See also Thomas, 1981, 1986.

ers and Selevan, 1984). Exposures usually involve mixtures of chemicals, and individuals may not be aware of all the chemicals with which they come into contact. Thus, the effect of individual chemicals is difficult to assess, and cause-and-effect relationships are nearly impossible to establish.

Epidemiologic Studies

Epidemiology is increasingly important in establishing cause-and-effect relationships. Epidemiology and risk assessment are inextricably related. Reproductive surveillance programs are important underpinnings for monitoring endocrine processes. By closely monitoring worker exposures to industrial/environmental toxicants, safer conditions will be established.

If exposure to a chemical has occurred in a human population, or if concern surrounds the use of a certain chemical, epidemiologic studies may be used to identify effects on reproduction. Sheikh (1987) has pointed out factors that are important in selecting control populations for studying adverse reproductive effects on occupational environments. The design of epidemiologic studies may involve either retrospective or prospective gathering of data. Statistical aspects to be considered in epidemiologic studies include power, sample size, significance level, and magnitude of the effect.

REFERENCES

Albro, P. W.; Chapin, R. E.; Corbett, J. T.; Schroeder, J.; and Phelps, J. L.: Mono-2-ethylhexyl phthalate, a metabolite of di-(2-ethylhexyl) phthalate, causally linked to testicular atrophy in rats. *Toxicol. Appl. Pharmacol.,* **100**:193–200, 1989.

AMA Council on Scientific Affairs: Effects of toxic chemicals on the reproductive system. *JAMA,* **253**:3431–3437, 1985.

Amann, R. P.: A critical review of methods for evaluation of spermatogenesis from seminal characteristics. *J. Androl.,* **2**:37–58, 1981.

————: Detection of alterations in testicular and epididymal function in laboratory animals. *Environ. Health Perspect,* **70**:149–158, 1986.

————: Function of the epididymis in bulls and rams. *J. Reprod. Fertil.,* (Suppl.):115–131, 1987.

————: Structure and function of the normal testis and epididymis. *J. Am. Coll. Toxicol.,* **8**:457–471, 1989.

Amann, R. P., and Howard, S. S.: Daily spermatozoal production and epididymal spermatozoal reserves of the human male. *J. Urol.,* **124**:211–219, 1980.

Anderson, R. A., Jr.; Berryman, S. H.; Phillips, J. F.; Feathergill, K. A.; Zaneveld, L. J. D.; and Russell, L. D.: Biochemical and structural evidence for ethanol-induced impairment of testicular development: apparent lack of Leydig cell involvement. *Toxicol. Appl. Pharmacol.,* **100**:62–85, 1989.

Angioli, M. P.; Ramos, K.; and Rosenblum, I. Y.: Interactions of bleomycin with reduced and oxidized ion in rat spermatogenic cells. *In Vitro Toxicol.,* **1**:45–54, 1987.

Barlow, S. M., and Sullivan, F. M.: *Reproductive Hazards of Industrial Chemicals.* Academic Press, London, 1982.

Bell, J. U., and Thomas, J. A.: Effects of lead on the reproductive system. In Singhal, R. L., and Thomas, J. A. (eds.): *Basic and Clinical Toxicity of Lead.* Urban and Schwarzenberg Medical Publishers, Baltimore, 1980, pp. 169–189.

Blackburn, D. M.; Gray, A. J.; Lloyd, S. C.; Sheard, C. M.; and Foster, P. M. D.: A comparison of the effects of the three isomers of dinitrobenzene on the testis in the rat. *Toxicol. Appl. Pharmacol.,* **92**:54–64, 1988.

Blazak, W. F.; Ernest, T. L.; and Stewart, B. E.: Potential indicators of reproductive toxicity: testicular sperm production and epididymal sperm number, transit time, and motility in Fischer 344 rats. *Fund. Appl. Toxicol.* **5**:1097–1103, 1985.

Bloch, E.; Gondos, B.; Gatz, M.; Varma, S. K.; and Thyson, B.: Reproductive toxicity of 2,4-dinitrobenzene in the rat. *Toxicol. Appl. Pharmacol.,* **94**:466–472, 1988.

Boekelheide, K.: 2,5-Hexanedione alters microtubule assembly. I. Testicular atrophy, not nervous system toxicity, correlates with enhanced tubulin polymerization. *Toxicol. Appl. Pharmacol.,* **88**:370–382, 1987.

————: Rat testis during 2,5-hexanedione intoxication and recovery. II. Dynamic of pyrrole reactivity, tubulin content, and microtubule assembly. *Toxicol. Appl. Pharmacol.,* **92**:28–33, 1988.

Bond, M. B.: Role of corporate policy on reproductive hazards of the workplace. *J.O.M.* **28**:193–199, 1986.

Boyers, J. N.; Davis, L. U.; and Katz, D. F.: Automated semen analysis. *Curr. Probl. Obstet. Gynecol. Fertil.,* Sept./Oct., pp. 169–195, 1989.

Buchanan, J. F., and Davis, L. J.: Drug-induced infertility. *Drug Intellig. Clin. Pharm.* **18**:122–132, 1984.

Buiatti, E.; Barchielli, A.; Geddes, M.; Nastasi, L.; and Kriebel, D.: Risk factors in male infertility: a case-control study. *Arch. Environ. Health*, **39**:266–270, 1984.

Chapin, R. E.; Gray, T. J. B.; Phelps, J. L.; and Dutton, S. L.: The effects of mono-(2-ethylhexyl)-phthalate on rat Sertoli cell-enriched primary cultures. *Toxicol. Appl. Pharmacol.*, **92**:467–479, 1988.

Chapin, R. E.; Norton, R. M.; Popp, J. A.; and Bus, J. S.: The effects of 2,5-hexanedione on reproductive hormones and testicular enzyme activities in the F-344 rat. *Toxicol. Appl. Pharmacol.*, **62**:262–272, 1982.

Chapman, R. M.: Gonadal injury resulting from chemotherapy. *Am. J. Ind. Med.*, **4**:149–161, 1983.

Clegg, E. D.; Sakai, C. S.; and Voytek, P. E.: Assessment of reproductive risks. *Biol. Reprod.*, **34**:5–16, 1986.

Colby, H.: Adrenal gland toxicity: chemically-induced dysfunction. *J. Am. Coll. Toxicol.*, **7**:45–69, 1988.

Collins, T. F. X.: Reproduction and teratology guidelines: review of deliberations by the National Toxicology Advisory Committee's reproduction panel. *J. Environ. Pathol. Toxicol.*, **2**:141–147, 1978.

Comereski, C. R.; Bergman, C. L.; and Buroker, R. A.: Testicular toxicity of *N*-methyltetrazolethiol cephalosporin analogues in the juvenile rat. *Fund. Appl. Toxicol.*, **8**:280–289, 1987.

Cooper, T. G.: *The Epididymis, Sperm Maturation and Fertilization*. Springer-Verlag, Berlin, 1986.

De La Chapelle, A.: The Y-chromosomal and autosomal testis-determining genes. In Goodfellow, P. N.; Craig, I. W.; Smith, J. C.; and Wolfe, J. (eds.): *The Sex-Determining Factor. Development 101* (Suppl.), 1987, pp. 33–38.

Dixon, R. L.: Potential of environmental factors to affect development of reproductive system. *Fund. Appl. Toxicol.*, **2**:5–12, 1982.

———: Toxic responses of the reproductive system. In Klaassen, C. D.; Amdur, M. O.; and Doull, J. (eds.): *Casarett and Doull's Toxicology: The Basic Science of Poisons*, 3rd ed. Macmillian Publishing Co., New York, 1986.

Dixon, R. L., and Lee, I. P.: Pharmacokinetic and adaptation factors in testicular toxicity. *Fed. Proc.*, **39**:66–72, 1980.

Dobson, R. L.; Koehler, C. G.; Felton, J. S.; Kwan, T. C.; Wuebbles, B. J.; and Jones, D. C. L.: Vulnerability of female germ cells in developing mice and monkeys to tritium, gamma rays, and polycyclic aromatic hydrocarbons. In Mahlum, D. D.; Sikor, M. R.; Hackett, P. L.; and Andrew, F. D. (eds.): *Developmental Toxicology of Energy-Related Pollutants.* Conference 771017, U.S. Department of Energy Technical Information Center, Washington, D.C., 1978.

Doering, P. L.; Davidson, C. L.; LaFauce, L.; and Williams, C. A.: Effects of cocaine on the human fetus: a review of clinical studies. *Drug Intellig. Clin. Pharm.*, **23**:639–645, 1989.

Donaubauer, A. H.; Kramer, M.; Krein, K.; Mayer, D.; Von Rechenberg, W.; Sandow, J.; and Schutz, E.: Investigations of the carcinogenicity of the LH-RH analog buserelin (HOE 766) in rats using the subcutaneous route of administration. *Fund. Appl. Toxicol.*, **9**:738–752, 1987.

Donovan, M. P.; Schein, L. G.; and Thomas, J. A.: Inhibition of androgen-receptor interaction in mouse prostate gland cytosol by divalent metal ions. *Mol. Pharmacol.*, **17**:156–162, 1980.

Dym, M., and Fawcett, D. W.: The blood-testis barrier in the rat and the physiological compartmentation of the seminiferous epithelium. *Biol. Reprod.*, **3**:300–326, 1970.

Eckols, K.; Williams, J.; and Uphouse, L.: Effects of chlordecone on progesterone receptors in immature and adult rats. *Toxicol. Appl. Pharmacol.*, **100**:506–516, 1989.

Effendy, I., and Krause, W.: *In vivo* effects of terbinafine and ketoconazole on testosterone plasma levels in healthy males. *Dermatologica*, **178**:103–106, 1989.

Epstein, S. S.; Arnold, E.; Andrea, J.; Bass, W.; and Bishop, Y.: Detection of chemical mutagens by the dominant lethal assay in mice. *Toxicol. Appl. Pharmacol.*, **23**:288–325, 1972.

Eskeland, N. L.; Lugo, D. I.; Pintar, J. E.; and Schachter, B. S.: Stimulation of beta-endorphin secretion by corticotropin-releasing factor in primary rat Leydig cell cultures. *Endocrinology*, **124**:2914–2919, 1989.

Ettlin, R. A., and Dixon, R. L.: Reproductive toxicology. In Mottet, N. K. (ed.): *Environmental Pathology, Chemicals*. Oxford University Press, New York, 1985.

Evenson, D. P.; Baer, R. K.; Jost, L. K.; and Gesch, R. W.: Toxicity of thiotepa on mouse spermatogenesis as determined by dual-parameter flow cytometry. *Toxicol. Appl. Pharmacol.*, **82**:151–163, 1986.

Evenson, D. P.; Janca, F. C.; and Jost, L. K.: Effects of the fungicide methyl-benzimidazol-2-yl carbamate (MBC) on mouse germ cells as determined by flow cytometry. *J. Toxicol. Environ. Health*, **20**:387–399, 1987.

Fabrio, S.: On predicting environmentally-induced human reproductive hazards: an overview and historical perspective. *Fund. Appl. Toxicol.*, **5**:609–614, 1985.

Faustman, E. M.; Kirby, Z.; Gage, D.; and Varnum, M.: *In vitro* developmental toxicity of five direct acting alkylating agents in rodent embryos: structure-activity patterns. *Teratology*, **40**:199–210, 1989.

Gilfillan, S. C.: Lead poisoning and the fall of Rome. *J.O.M.*, **7**:53–60, 1965.

Feuston, M. H.; Bodnar, K. R.; Kerstetter, S. L.; Grink, C. P.; Belcak, M. J.; and Singer, E. J.: Reproductive toxicity of 2-methoxyethanol applied dermally to occluded and nonoccluded sites in male rats. *Toxicol. Appl. Pharmacol.*, **100**:145–161, 1989.

Foster, P. M. D.; Blackburn, D. M.; Moore, R. B.; and Lloyd, S. C.: Testicular toxicity of 2-methoxyacetaldehyde, a possible metabolite of ethylene glycol monomethyl ether, in the rat. *Toxicol. Lett.*, **32**:73–80, 1986.

Frankos, V. H.: FDA perspectives on the use of teratology data for human risk. *Fund. Appl. Toxicol.*, **5**:615–625, 1985.

Galbraith, W. M.; Voytek, P.; and Ryon, M. G.: *Assessment of Risks to Human Reproduction and to Development of the Human Conceptus from Exposure to Environmental Substances*. Oak Ridge National Laboratory, U.S. Environmental Protection Agency, National Technical Information Service, Springfield, Va., 1982.

Gellert, R. J.: Uterotrophic activity of polychlorinated biphenyls (PCB) and induction of precocious reproductive aging in neonatally treated female rats. *Environ. Res.*, **16**:123–130, 1978.

Goldberg, E. H.: H-Y antigen and sex determination. *Philos. Trans. R. Soc. Lond.* [*Biol.*], **322**:73–81, 1988.

Gray, T. J. B., and Beamand, J. A.: Effect of some phthalate esters and other testicular toxins on primary cultures of testicular cells. *Food Cosmet. Toxicol.*, **22**:123–131, 1984.

Greenwell, A.; Tomaszewski, K. E.; and Melnick, R. L.: A biochemical basis for 1,2-dibromo-3-chloropropane-induced male infertility: inhibition of sperm mitochondrial electron transport activity. *Toxicol. Appl. Pharmacol.*, **91**:274–280, 1987.

Gunn, S. A., and Gould, T. C.: Difference between

dorsal and lateral components of dorsolateral prostate in Zn^{65} uptake. *Proc. Soc. Exp. Biol. Med.,* **92**:17–20, 1956.

Haney, A. F.: Effects of toxic agents on ovarian function. In Thomas, J. A.; Korach, K. S.; and McLachlan, J. A. (eds.): *Endocrine Toxicology.* Raven Press, New York, 1985.

Hanly, J. R., Jr.; Yano, B. L.; Nitschke, K. D.; and John, J. A.: Comparison of the teratogenic potential of inhaled ethylene glycol monomethyl ether in rats, mice and rabbits. *Toxicol. Appl. Pharmacol.,* **75**:409–422, 1984.

Hayes, A. W.: *Principles and Methods of Toxicology.* Raven Press, New York, 1982.

Heindel, J. J., and Keith, W. B.: Specific inhibition of FSH-stimulated cAMP accumulation by delta-9 tetrahydro-cannabinol in cultures of rat Sertoli cells. *Toxicol. Appl. Pharmacol.,* **101**:124–134, 1989.

Heller, C. G., and Clermont, Y.: Kinetics of the germinal epithelium in man. *Recent Prog. Horm. Res.,* **20**:545–575, 1964.

Hildebrand, D. C.; Der, R.; Griffin, W. T.; and Fahim, M. S.: Effect of lead acetate on reproduction. *Am. J. Obstet. Gynecol.,* **115**:1058–1065, 1973.

Hillier, S. G.; Zeleznik, A. J.; Knazek, R. A.; and Ross, G. T.: Hormonal regulation of preovulatory follicle maturation in the rat. *J. Reprod. Fertil.,* **60**:219–229, 1980.

Hirsch, K. S.; Weaver, D. E.; Black, L. J.; Falcone, J. F.; and MacLusky, N. J.: Inhibition of central nervous system aromatase activity: a mechanism for fenarinol-induced infertility in the male rat. *Toxicol. Appl. Pharmacol.,* **91**:235–245, 1987.

Hodgen, G. D.: Enzyme markers of testicular function. In Johnson, A. D., and Gomes, W. R. (eds.): *The Testis,* Vol. 4. *Advances in Physiology, Biochemistry, and Function.* Academic Press, Inc., New York, 1977.

Holt, D. W.; Adams, P. C.; Campbell, R. W. J.; Morley, A. R.; and Storey, G. C. A.: Amiodarone and its desethyl metabolite: tissue distribution and ultrastructural changes in amiodarone-treated patients. *Br. J. Clin. Pharmacol.,* **17**:195–196, 1984.

Hruska, R. E., and Olson, J. R.: Species differences in estrogen receptors and in response to 2,3,7,8-tetrachlorodibenzo-*p*-dioxin exposure. *Toxicol. Lett.,* **48**:289–299, 1989.

Johnson, E. M.: The scientific basis for multigeneration safety evaluations. *J. Am. Coll. Toxicol.,* **5**:197–201, 1986.

Koizumi, T., and Waalkes, M. P.: Effects of zinc on the distribution and toxicity of cadmium in isolated interstitial cells of the rat testis. *Toxicology,* **56**:137–146, 1989.

Lamb, J. C.: Reproductive toxicity testing: evaluating and developing new testing systems. *J. Am. Coll. Toxicol.,* **4**:163–178, 1985.

Lamb, J. C.; Ross, M. D.; and Chapin, R. E.: Experimental methods for studying male reproductive function in standard toxicology studies. *J. Am. Coll. Toxicol.,* **5**:225–234, 1986.

Lancranjan, I.; Papescu, H. I.; Gavanescu, O.; Klepsch, I.; and Serbanescu, M.: Reproductive ability of workmen occupationally exposed to lead. *Arch. Environ. Health,* **30**:396–401, 1975.

Lantz, G. D.; Cunningham, G. R.; Huckins, C.; and Lipshultz, L.I.: Recovery from severe oligospermia after exposure to dibromochloropropane. *Fertil. Steril.,* **35**:46–53, 1981.

LeBlond, C. P., and Clermont, Y.: Definition of the stages of the cycle of the seminiferous epitehlium of the rat. *Ann. N.Y. Acad. Sci.,* **55**:548–571, 1952.

Lee, I. P., and Dixon, R. L.: Effects of procarbazine on

spermatogenesis studied by velocity sedimentation cell separation and serial mating. *J. Pharmacol. Exp. Ther.,* **181**:219–226, 1972.

Lee, I. P.; Suzuki, K., and Nagayama, J.: Metabolism of benzo(a)pyrene in rat prostate glands following 2,3,7,8-tetrachlorodibenzo-*p*-dioxin exposure. *Carcinogenesis,* **2**:823–831, 1981.

Lee, J. P.: Adaptive biochemical repair response toward germ cell DNA damage. *Am. J. Ind. Med.,* **4**:135–147, 1983.

Lemasters, G. K., and Selevan, S. G.: Use of exposure data in occupational reproductive studies. *Scand. J. Work Environ. Health,* **10**:1–6, 1984.

Levine, R. J.: Methods for detecting occupational causes of male infertility. *Scand. J. Work Environ. Health,* **9**:371–376, 1983.

Levine, R. J.; Blunden, P. B.; DalCorso, R. D.; Starr, T. B.; and Ross, C. E.: Superiority of reproductive histories to sperm counts in detecting infertility at a DBCP manufacturing plant. *J. O. M.,* **25**:591–597, 1983.

Lindemann, C. B., and Kanous, K. S.: Regulation of mammalian sperm motility. *Arch. Andrology,* **23**:1–22, 1989.

Lloyd, S. C.; Blackburn, D. M.; and Foster, P. M. D.: Trifluoroethanol and its oxidative metabolites: comparison of *in vivo* and *in vitro* effects in rat testis. *Toxicol. Appl. Pharmacol.,* **92**:390–401, 1988.

MacLeod, J.: Human male infertility. *Obstet. Gynecol. Surv.,* **26**:335–351, 1971.

Mann, T., and Lutwak-Mann, C.: *Male Reproductive Function and Semen: Themes and Trends in Physiology, Biochemistry and Investigative Andrology.* Springer-Verlag, New York, 1981.

Mattison, D. R.; Hanson, J. W.; Kochhar, D. M.; and Rao, K. S.: Criteria for identifying and listing substances known to cause developmental toxicity under California's Proposition 65. *Reprod. Toxicol.,* **3**:3–12, 1989.

Mattison, D. R., and Nightingale, M. S.: The biochemical and genetic characteristics of murine ovarian aryl hydrocarbon (benzo[a]pyrene)hydroxylase activity and its relationship to primordial oocyte destruction by polycyclic aromatic hydrocarbons. *Toxicol. Appl. Pharmacol.,* **56**:399–408, 1980.

McElveen, J. C., Jr.: Reproduction hazards in the workplace: some legal considerations. *J. Occup. Med.,* **28**:103–110, 1986.

McLachlan, J. A.; Newbold, R. R.; Korach, K. S.; Lamb, J. C.; and Suzuki, Y.: Transplacental toxicology: prenatal factors influencing postnatal fertility. In Kimmel, C. A. and Buelke-Sam, J. (eds.): *Developmental Toxicology.* Raven Press, New York, 1981.

Mebus, C. A.; Welsch, F.; and Working, P. K.: Attenuation of 2-methoxyethanol–induced testicular toxicity in the rat by simple physiological compounds. *Toxicol. Appl. Pharmacol.,* **99**:110–121, 1989.

Meistrich, M. L.: Evaluation of reproductive toxicity by testicular sperm head counts. *J. Am. Coll. Toxicol.,* **8**:551–567, 1989.

Millar, J. G. B.: Drug-induced impotence. *Practitioner,* **223**:634–639, 1979.

Morrissey, R. E.; Lamb IV, J. C.; Schwetz, B. A.; Teague, J. L.; and Morris, R. W.: Association of sperm, vaginal cytology, and reproductive organ weight data with results of continuous breeding reproduction studies in Swiss (CD-1) mice. *Fund. Appl. Toxicol.,* **11**:359–371, 1988.

Mosher, W. D.: Contraceptive utilization: United States. *Vital Health Stat.,* **23**:1–58, 1981.

Nagano, K.; Nakayama, E.; Koyano, M.; Dobayaski, H.;

Adachi, H.; and Yamada, T.: Testicular atrophy of mice induced by ethylene glycol monoakyl ethers. *Jpn. J. Ind. Health,* **21**.29–35, 1979.

Nahhas, F., and Blumenfeld, F.: Zona-free hamster egg penetration assay and prognostic indicator in an IVF program. *Arch. Andrology,* **23**:33–37, 1989.

Neaves, W. B.: The blood-testis barrier. In Johnson, A. D., and Gomes, W. R. (eds.): *The Testis,* Vol. 6. Academic Press, New York, 1977, pp. 125–153.

Nisbet, I. C., and Karch, N. J.: *Chemical Hazards to Human Reproduction.* Noyes Data, Park Ridge, N.J., 1983.

Office of Technology Assessment Report. *Reproductive Health Hazards in the Workplace.* U.S. Government Printing Office, Washington, D.C., 1985.

Okumura, K.; Lee, I. P.; and Dixon, R. L.: Permeability of selected drugs and chemicals across the blood-testis barrier of the rat. *J. Pharmacol. Exp. Ther.,* **194**:89–95, 1975.

Overstreet, J. W.: Reproductive risk assessment. *Terat. Carcin. Mut.,* **4**:67–75, 1984.

Overstreet, J. W.; Samuels, S. J.; Day, P.; Hendrickx, A. G.; Prahalada, S.; Mast, T.; Katz, D. F.; and Sakai, C.: Early indicators of male reproductive toxicity. *Risk Analysis,* **8**:21–26, 1988.

Papadopoulas, C.: Cardiovascular drugs and sexuality. *Arch. Intern. Med.,* **140**:1341–1345, 1980.

Paul, M. E.: Reproductive fitness and risk. *Occup. Med: State Art Rev.,* **3**:323–340, 1988.

Pedersen, I., and Peters, H.: Proposal for a classification of oocytes and follicles in the mouse ovary. *J. Reprod. Fertil.,* **17**:555–557, 1968.

Pedersen, R. A., and Brandriff, B.: Radiation- and drug-induced DNA repair in mammalian oocytes and embryos. In Generoso, W. M.; Shelby, M. D.; and DeSerres, F. J. (eds.): *DNA Repair and Mutagenesis in Eukaryotes.* Plenum Publishing Corp., New York, 1980.

Pogach, L. M.; Lee, Y.; Gould, S.; Giglio, W.; Meyenhofer, M.; and Huang, H. F. S.: Characterization of *cis*-platinum-induced Sertoli cell dysfunction in rodents. *Toxicol. Appl. Pharmacol.,* **98**:350–361, 1989.

Prasad, A. S.; Obeleas, D.; Wolf, P.; and Horowitz, J. P.: Studies on zinc deficiency: changes in trace element and enzyme activities in tissues of zinc-deficient rats. *J. Clin. Invest.,* **46**:549–557, 1967.

Rajfer, J.; Sikka, S. C.; Lemmi, C.; and Koyle, M. A.: Cyclosporine inhibits testosterone biosynthesis in the rat testis. *Endocrinology,* **121**:586–589, 1987.

Ritter, E. J.; Scott, W. J., Jr.; Randall, J. L.; and Ritter, J. M.: Teratogenicity of di(ethylhexyl) phthalate, 2-ethylhexanol, 2-ethylhexanoic acid, and valproic acid, and potentiation by caffeine. *Teratology,* **35**:41–46, 1987.

Sakamoto, J., and Hashimoto, K.: Reproductive toxicity of acrylamide and related compounds in mice—effects on fertility and sperm morphology. *Arch. Toxicol.,* **59**:201–205, 1986.

Schrag, S. D., and Dixon, R. L.: Occupational exposure associated with male reproductive dysfunction. *Annu. Rev. Pharmacol. Toxicol.,* **25**:567–592, 1985.

Schwetz, B. A., Roa, K. S.; and Park, C. N.: Insensitivity of tests for reproductive problems. *J. Environ. Pathol. Toxicol.,* **3**:81–98, 1980.

Selden, J. R.; Robertson, R. T.; Miller, J. E.; Vetter, C.; Minsker, D. H.; Huber, A. C.; and Nichols, W. W.: The rapid and sensitive detection of perturbations in spermatogenesis: assessment by quantitative dual parameter (DNA/RNA) flow cytometry. *J. Am. Coll. Toxicol.,* **8**:507–523, 1989.

Selevan, S. G.; Lindhohm, M. L.; Hornung, R. W.; and Hemminki, K.: A study of occupational exposure to antineoplastic drugs and fetal loss in nurses. *New Engl. J. Med.,* **313**:1173–1178, 1985.

Setchell, B. P.; Vogimayr, J. K.; and Waites, G. M. H.: A blood-testis barrier restricting passage from blood lymph into rete testis fluid but not into lymph. *J. Physiol.,* **200**:73–85, 1969.

Shaked, I.; Sod-Moriah, U. A.; Kaplanski, J.; and Potashnik, G.: Reproductive performance of dibromochloropropane-treated female rats. *Int. J. Fertil.,* **33**:129–133, 1988.

Sheikh, K.: Choice of control population in studies of adverse reproductive effects of occupational exposures and its effect on risk estimates. *Br. J. Ind. Med.,* **44**:244–249, 1987.

Shemi, D.; Sod-Moriah, U. A.; Kaplanski, J.; Potashnik, G.; Bitan, A. P.; and Buchman, O.: Gonadotoxicity and kinetics of dibromochloropropane in male rats. *Toxicol. Lett.,* **36**:209–212, 1987.

Shen, R. S., and Lee, I. P.: Developmental patterns of enzymes in mouse testis. *J. Reprod. Fertil.,* **48**:301–305, 1977.

Simpson, J. L.: Genes, chromosomes, and reproductive failure. *Fertil. Steril.* **33**:107–116, 1980.

Singh, H.; Kozel, T.; and Jackson, S.: Effect of procarbazine on sperm morphology in Syrian hamsters. *J. Toxicol. Environ. Health,* **27**:107–121, 1989.

Skinner, M. K.; Schlitz, S. M.; and Anthony, C. A.: Regulation of Sertoli cell differentiated function: testicular transferrin and androgen-binding protein expression. *Endocrinology,* **124**:3015–3024, 1989.

Soderlund, E. J.; Brunborg, G.; Omichinski, J. G.; Holme, J. A.; Dahl, J. E.; Nelson, S. D.; and Dybing, E.: Testicular necrosis and DNA damage caused by deuterated and methylated analogues of 1,2-dibromo-3-chloropropane in the rat. *Toxicol. Appl. Pharmacol.,* **94**:437–447, 1988.

Somkuti, S. G.; Lapadula, D. M.; Chapin, R. E.; Lamb IV, J. C.; and Abou-Donia, M. B.: Reproductive tract lesions resulting from subchronic administration (63 days) of tri-*o*-cresyl phosphate in male rats. *Toxicol. Appl. Pharmacol.,* **89**:49–63, 1987.

Stevenson, J. G., and Umstead, G. S.: Sexual dysfunction due to antihypertensive agents. *Drug Intellig. Clin. Pharm.,* **18**:113–121, 1984.

Thomas, J. A.: Effects of pesticides on reproduction. In Thomas, J. A., and Singhal, R. L. (eds.): *Molecular Mechanisms of Gonadal Hormone Action.* University Park Press, Baltimore, 1975, pp. 205–223.

———: Reproductive hazards and environmental chemicals: a review. *Toxic Substances J.,* **2**:318–348, 1981.

———: Survey of reproductive hazards. *J. Am. Coll. Toxicol.,* **5**:203–207, 1986.

———: Pharmacologic and toxicologic responses in the neonate. *J. Am. Coll. Toxicol.* **5**:957–962, 1989.

Thomas, J. A., and Brogan, W. C.: Some actions of lead on the sperm and on the male reproductive system. *Am. J. Ind. Med.,* **4**:127–134, 1983.

Thomas, J. A.; Curto, K. A.; and Thomas, M. J.: MEHP/DEHP gonadal toxicity and effects on rodent accessory sex organs. *Environ. Health Perspect.,* **45**:85–92, 1982.

Thomas, J. A., and Keenan, E. J.: *Principles of Endocrine Pharmacology.* Plenum Press, New York, 1986.

Thomas, J. A., and Thomas, M. J.: Biological effects of di-(2-ethylhexyl) phthalate and other phthalic acid esters. *Crit. Rev. Toxicol.,* **13**:283–317, 1984.

Thompson, E. A., Jr.: The effects of estradiol upon the thymus of the sexually immature female mouse. *J. Steroid Biochem.,* **14**:167–174, 1981.

Torkelson, R. R.; Sadek, S. E.; and Rowe, V. K.: Toxicologic investigations of 1,2-dibromo-3-chlorpropane. *Toxicol. Appl. Pharmacol.*, **3**:545–557, 1961.

Toth, G. P.; Zenick, H.; and Smith, M. K.: Effects of epichlorohydrin on male and female reproduction in Long-Evan rats. *Fund. Appl. Pharmacol.*, **13**:16–25, 1989.

Tuchmann-Duplessis, H.; David, G.; and Haegel, P.: *Illustrated Human Embryology*, Vol. I. Springer-Verlag, New York, 1972.

Waalkes, M. P.; Donovan, M. P.; and Thomas, J. A.: Cadmium-induced prostate metallothionein in the rabbit. *Prostate*, **3**:23–25, 1982.

Ways, S. C.; Blair, P. B.; Bern, H. A.; and Staskawicz, M. D.: Immune responsiveness of adult mice exposed neonatally to diethylstilbestrol, steroid hormones, or vitamin A. *J. Environ. Pathol.*, **3**:207–227, 1980.

Whorton, D. M.; Kraus, R. M.; Marshall, S.; and Milby, T. H.: Infertility in male pesticide workers. *Lancet*, **2**:1259–1267, 1977.

Williams, J., and Foster, P. M. D.: The production of lactate and pyruvate as sensitive indices of altered rat Sertoli cell function *in vitro* following the addition of various testicular toxicants. *Toxicol. Appl. Pharmacol.*, **94**:160–170, 1988.

Woods, J. S.: Drug effects on human sexual behavior. In Woods, N. F. (ed.): *Human Sexuality in Health and Illness*, 3rd ed. C. V. Mosby Co., St. Louis, 1984.

Working, P. K.: Male reproductive toxicology: comparison of the human to animal models. *Environ. Health Perspect.*, **77**:37–44, 1988.

Wyrobek, A. J.: Methods for evaluating the effects of environmental chemicals on human sperm production. *Environ. Health Perspect.*, **48**:53–59, 1983.

Wyrobek, A. J.; Gordon, L. A.; Burkhart, J. G.; Francis, M. C.; Kapp, R. W., Jr.; Letz, G.; Malling, H. V.; Topham, J. C.; and Whorton, M. D.: An evaluation of the mouse sperm morphology test and other sperm tests in nonhuman mammals. A report of the U.S. Environmental Protection Agency Gene-Tox Program. *Mutat. Res.*, **115**:1–72, 1983.

Zeleznik, A. J.; Hillier, S. G.; Knazek, R. A.; Ross, G. T.; and Coon, H. G.: Production of long-term steroid producing granulosa cell cultures by cell hybridization. *Endocrinology*, **105**:156–162, 1979.

Zenick, H., and Clegg, E. D.: Tissues in risk assessment in male reproduction toxicology. *J. Am. Coll. Toxicol.*, **5**:249–261, 1986.

———: Assessment of male reproductive toxicity: a risk assessment approach. In Hayes, A. W. (ed.): *Principles and Methods of Toxicology*, 2nd ed. Raven Press, New York, 1989, pp. 275–309.

Chapter 17

TOXIC RESPONSES OF THE EYE

Albert M. Potts

INTRODUCTION

As in previous editions, space limitations require similar restriction of subject matter here. It is proposed to treat damage by chemical agents only. Structures dealt with are the globe and its contents, the adnexae, and CNS portions of the visual system only to the end of the retinal ganglion cell neuron in the lateral geniculate body. Major emphasis is on substances demonstrated to be harmful to humans. No distinction will be made between substances that have known therapeutic value and those that have none. It is axiomatic that a substance with pharmacologic activity can be toxic in high doses or when acting on a susceptible subject. Exceptions to these stipulations will be for good cause.

Treatment will emphasize varieties of toxic phenomena and mechanisms where known. Exhaustive treatment of ophthalmic toxicology requires volumes of text. Such texts exist and should be consulted for details on specific substances (see Galezowski, 1878; Uhthoff, 1911; Lewin and Guillery, 1913; Duke-Elder and Mac-Faul, 1972; Grant, 1986; Fraunfelder, 1989). References are also given on ocular anatomy and physiology (Duke-Elder and Wybar, 1961; Davson, 1972; *Handbook,* 1972–1977).

The eye, despite its small mass, contains derivatives of surface ectoderm (corneal epithelium and conjunctiva) and of mesoderm (choroid, iris, and ciliary body stroma). It contains true neural tissue (the inner retinal layer and optic nerve) and a highly specific light-sensitive modification of neural tissue (the photoreceptors). It contains two relatively large avascular areas (the lens and cornea), which are bounded by unique active transport systems responsible for maintaining a steady state of hydration and hence transparency. It contains a small private cerebrospinal fluid system (the aqueous system) where ciliary body processes are analogous to choroid plexus, where the barrier to circulating blood is as specific as that of the brain, and where the outflow system is so critical that loss of sight is the price

of dysfunction. Unique chemical substances in significant concentration are the organ-specific lens proteins; the (at least) four photosensitive pigments; and the avid electron acceptor, melanin, present in ocular tissues at higher levels than anywhere else in the human body. These unique features in a small physical compass make for a multiplicity of types of reactions to injury and a potentially high sensitivity to toxic substances.

Since the appearance of the third edition of this book, there has been above-average concentration of new publication in two subject areas. One area is the study of the effect of various substances on intraocular structures when the substances are introduced into the vitreous cavity. The search for adjuvants to the procedure of vitrectomy seems to be the dynamic for this activity.

The second area that has stimulated attention is that of the Draize test for corneal damage. Each of the above subjects will be treated in its pertinent anatomical category.

CORNEA, CONJUNCTIVA, AND NEIGHBORING TISSUES

Special Considerations

The cornea (Figure 17–1) and its neighboring partial analogue, the conjunctiva, are the portions of the eye directly exposed to external insults. The cornea must maintain its transparency to remain functional. A scar, the normal body reparative process, with or without vascularization, is tolerated by other body structures with no adverse effects. In the case of the cornea, a scar or vascularization can destroy function completely. Hence, a very small amount of corrosive substance—an amount of no consequence elsewhere on the body—can be the cause of blindness if it reaches the cornea.

There is convincing evidence that corneal transparency is maintained by the boundary layers of epithelium and endothelium, which have

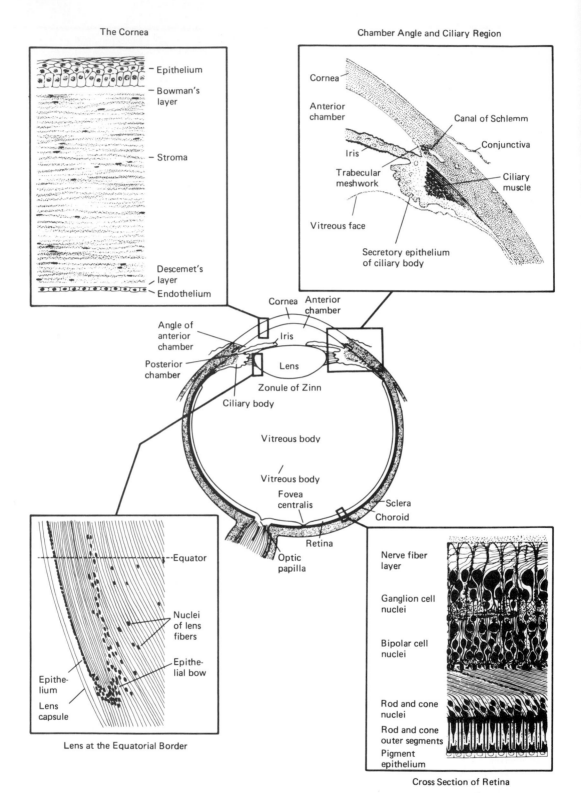

The Cornea

- Epithelium
- Bowman's layer
- Stroma
- Descemet's layer
- Endothelium

Chamber Angle and Ciliary Region

Cornea

Anterior chamber

Iris

Trabecular meshwork

Vitreous face

Canal of Schlemm

Conjunctiva

Ciliary muscle

Secretory epithelium of ciliary body

Cornea Anterior chamber

Angle of anterior chamber

Iris

Posterior chamber

Lens

Zonule of Zinn

Ciliary body

Vitreous body

Vitreous body

Fovea centralis

Sclera

Choroid

Retina

Optic papilla

Lens at the Equatorial Border

Equator

Nuclei of lens fibers

Epithelial bow

Epithelium

Lens capsule

Cross Section of Retina

Nerve fiber layer

Ganglion cell nuclei

Bipolar cell nuclei

Rod and cone nuclei

Rod and cone outer segments

Pigment epithelium

Figure 17–1. Digrammatic horizontal cross section of the eye, with medium-power enlargement of details in cornea, chamber angle, lens, and retina. (The enlarged retina diagram *[lower right]* is taken from Polyak, S.: *The Retina.* University of Chicago Press, Chicago, 1941. By permission of Mrs. Stephen Polyak.)

small mass and relatively high metabolic activity (Maurice, 1969). Thus, death of these boundary layers—20 to 25 mg of tissue in the adult eye—is responsible for imbibition of water and loss of transparency. The stoichiometric implications of these minute quantities are impressive.

External Contact Agents

Acids. A splash of acid in the eye is a medical emergency and offers a poor setting for gathering scientific data. We must rely on adequately controlled experimental studies for much of our knowledge of corneal burns. An excellent set of studies was performed during World War II under the auspices of the Office of Scientific Research and Development and was reported by Friedenwald and coworkers (Friedenwald et al., 1944, 1946). These authors established standard techniques for applying acids (and bases) to the eye and set standards by which damage could be evaluated. Their results bore out the clinical impression that damage by acid was a dual function of pH and of the capacity of the anion in question to combine with protein. Acid burns vary in severity from those that heal completely to those that cause complete opacity or even perforation of the globe.

It has been assumed in the past that the degree of damage seen shortly after an acid burn is an accurate indicator of the eventual result to be expected. In view of some of the new developments in the treatment of alkali burns (see below), it may be that we will be able to abort the late sequellae of acid burns more effectively than in the past.

Special aspects of some acids complicate the picture. The dehydrating effect of concentrated sulfuric acid as well as the high heat of hydration adds to its acid properties in determining the severity of the burn. The affinity of the anion for the corneal tissue also plays a role in the severity of damage. Friedenwald and coworkers (1946) showed that buffered solutions of picric, tungstic, and tannic acids produced lesions of significant severity in the rabbit eye and with no great differences in severity from pH 1.5 to pH 9.

This effect was in sharp contrast to that of hydrochloric acid, which caused severe damage at pH 1, with virtually no effect at pH 3 and above. As the pH of buffered solutions applied to the human eye is decreased from 7.4, the onset of discomfort begins at about pH 4.5. Between pH 4.5. and 3.5, one creates punctate breaks in the corneal epithelium that are stainable with fluorescein but heal in a few hours' time.

Another special instance is that of compressed sulfur dioxide. When many industrial refrigeration plants used SO_2 as the refrigerant, eye damage caused by a high-pressure jet of sulfur dioxide was not uncommon. The anhydrous liquid hitting the cornea under pressure not only combines with corneal water to form H_2SO_3, but because of its relative fat solubility, it penetrates the cornea into the aqueous and hydrolyzes there, causing deep keratitis and iritis. Studies on the mechanism of SO_2 injury were done by Grant (1947). In view of the new ban on halogenated hydrocarbons as refrigerants, because of their contribution to depletion of the ozone layer, it is possible that some SO_2 cooling systems may reappear.

It is universally agreed that the one best treatment for acid burns is rapid irrigation with large volumes of water. The reduction of concentration, including hydrogen ion concentration, by dilution is most important. Mechanical removal from the site of injury by the stream of water is accomplished simultaneously. Attempts to obtain some special buffered solution or mildly alkaline wash only delay the start of treatment. Washing should begin as close in time and place to the site of the accident as possible. All industrial safety personnel should know this fact and be prepared to begin treatment by washing. Even in the case of concentrated sulfuric acid burns, where it is expected that the addition of water will generate heat, the water wash is best, using a large enough volume and a fast enough rate to dissipate heat as well as wash out acid.

Strong Alkalies—Ammonia, Collagenase. In addition to considerations of pH, there are several factors specific to alkali burns. First, alkalies in concentrations that can cause serious eye burns exist in many homes. Household ammonia and sodium hydroxide–containing drain cleaners are the chief offenders. The second problem specific to alkalies is the serious late effects of alkali burns. Even burns that at the time of injury appear to be mild can go on to opacification, vascularization, ulceration, or perforation (Hughes, 1946a, 1946b). The photographs presented in Hughes's experimental paper (Hughes, 1946b) are eloquent on this subject. It should be noted that in experimental animals Hughes produced burns of all degrees of severity by exposure of the cornea to isotonic $N/20$ sodium hydroxide. Exposure for 30 seconds followed by washing caused signs that lasted for several weeks only and usually cleared with no residues. Exposure to the same agent for three minutes followed by washing caused severe early opacification, marked vascularization at three months, and residues of opacity, pigment, and vessels after ten months. Irrigation with $N/20$ NaOH for more than three minutes could cause catastrophic changes in the cornea and surrounding tissues, leading to complete opacification and purulent infiltration within a week or ten days with ulceration and perforation.

One of the exceptions to the uniform behavior

of alkali cations is that of ammonia. Of all the alkali cations measured, ammonium ion as ammonium hydroxide penetrates epithelium, stroma, and anterior chamber more rapidly than any other. Grant speculates on whether this is due to the fat solubility of nonionized NH_3, to rapid diffusion, or to the ability of NH_4OH to injure corneal epithelium (Grant, 1986). However this may be, it has been shown that ammonia is detectable in the anterior chamber 15 seconds after exposure of the cornea to concentrated NH_4OH (Siegrist, 1920). Uveitis may be an early manifestation in ammonia burns.

The Special Case of Lime Burns. The second exception to the generalizations about cations is the case of calcium oxide, known popularly as unslaked lime. This substance, a component of Portland cement and of most commercial wall plasters, absorbs water to form calcium hydroxide with the liberation of heat. Calcium hydroxide is sparingly soluble in water but in solution (saturated solution, 0.15 percent, pH = 12.4) causes the usual alkali burn. In addition to the generation of heat, the special problem in lime burns is that lime, plaster, or cement on reaching the eye tends to react with the moisture and protein found there and form clumps of moist compound, very difficult to remove by the usual irrigation. Such clumps tend to lodge deep in the cul-de-sacs inferiorly and superiorly and act as reservoirs for the liberation of $Ca(OH)_2$ over long periods of time. This is why physicians have been especially concerned about lime burns in the past and why special care must be taken in treatment of this condition. This treatment consists of (Grant, 1986) (1) rapid irrigation, to remove as much material as can be quickly washed away; (2) debridement, to remove physically whatever gross particles of lime can be seen on the cornea and in the cul-de-sacs; and (3) use of a complexing agent, preferably ethylenediaminetetraacetic acid disodium salt (EDTA), to remove the remainder of the $Ca(OH)_2$-generating material that cannot be handled grossly. With observation of these extra requirements, lime burns can be made to follow the pattern of other alkali burns.

The Late Effects. The fact that early appearance of an alkali burn is not an adequate guide to prognosis and the possible appearance of infiltration, ulceration and perforation about a week after the injury have caused much speculation about the mechanism of these late serious sequelae.

More recent reviews dealing with alkali burns are those of Pfister and Koski (1982) and Reim and Schmidt-Martens (1982). The first reviewers emphasize: (1) delayed epithelial repair after severe stromal burns; (2) rapid and prolonged rise of intraocular pressure secondary to prostaglandin release (Pfister and Burstein, 1976); (3) the release of lytic enzymes, particularly collagenase, from polymorphonuclear leukocytes presumably attracted to the site by the prostaglandins. This chain of events clarifies the finding by Slansky and coworkers (1968), confirmed by Brown *et al.* (1969), that significant amounts of collagenase are present in alkaliburned cornea. The amount is greater than that present in normal corneal epithelium and was correctly attributed by the Brown group to exogenous neutrophils (1970). The use of locally applied collagenase inhibitors improved the treatment of alkali burns measurably (Brown *et al.*, 1972). (4) The observation that ascorbic acid in the aqueous humor falls to 30 percent of its normal value (normal = 15 to 20 times plasma) in alkali burns (Levinson *et al.*, 1976) has led the Pfister group to postulate that the lower ascorbate causes localized scurvy of the cornea with inhibition of formation of repair collagen (Pfister and Paterson, 1977; Pfister *et al.*, 1978). The two papers cited show significant reduction of corneal ulceration and perforation in alkaliburned rabbits when ascorbate is given subcutaneously or topically.

A more recent report from the Pfister group on alkali burns in the rabbit suggests that for established corneal ulcers 10 percent citrate is demonstrably therapeutic; ascorbate is not (Pfister *et al.*, 1988).

Aspects of the Reim and Schmidt-Martens review are: (1) an extended discussion of the appropriateness of antiinflammatory steroids as therapy in alkali burns and the conclusion—based on Reim's work, and contrary to generally held opinion in the United States—that the use of steroids is indicated; (2) consideration not only of collagenase inhibitors but also of inhibitors of prostaglandin synthesis as therapeutic agents. This introduces the whole category of nonsteroidal antiinflammatory agents, but of these only topical indomethacin is mentioned as having clinical trial. J. A. Anderson and coworkers (1982) advocate such a trial for 2-(2-fluoro-4-biphenylyl) propionic acid, flurbiprofen, on the basis of animal experiments.

An item of additional interest is the report of Nirankari *et al.* (1981) suggesting that the mechanism of action of ascorbate is as a superoxide radical scavenger and that both superoxide dismutase and ascorbate are effective in preventing ulceration after standard alkali burns.

Adding to the catalog of enzyme activities liberated from neutrophils in the alkali-burned cornea is the report of Chayakul and Reim (1982) on beta-N-acetylglucosaminidase.

Thus, renewed interest in the subject has revealed new mechanisms of injury, which, in turn, point to new therapeutic approaches.

Organic Solvents. Neutral organic solvents such as ethanol, acetone, ethyl ether, ethyl acetate, hexane, benzol, and toluene may contact the eye in industrial or laboratory accidents. These substances have in common their ability to dissolve fats. As a result, they cause pain on contacting the eye, and examination after a generous splash of solvent shows dulling of the cornea. The epithelium will show punctate staining with fluorescein. The damage appears to be scattered loss of epithelial cells due to solution of some of the fats that occur in these cells. The sensation is due to trauma of some of the populous and sensitive corneal nerve endings. Damage is never extensive or long-lasting if the splash is at room temperature. Hot solvents of low volatility add the problem of thermal burn to that of solvent action, and the end result is potentially more serious and less predictable.

One must note an industrial hazard introduced by the needs of high technology. Trichlorosilane ($SiHCl_3$) is used to clean the surface of silicon wafers in the manufacture of microcircuit chips. The solvent has a low flash point; the mixture of its vapors with air is highly explosive; it decomposes violently in contact with water, giving off voluminous HCl-containing vapors with eye burn capability. The report of Hübner and coworkers (1979) deals with a thermal burn plus chemical burn but serves to underline the existence of the hazard.

Detergents. An increasing number of substances are used in technology as detergents, emulsifying agents, wetting agents, antifoaming agents, and solubilizers. They have the common property of lowering the surface tension of aqueous solutions, and they possess discrete nonpolar and polar portions in the same molecule. The nonpolar portion is frequently a long aliphatic chain. The polar portion can be cationic, anionic, or nonionic.

Curiously, there appears to be no relation between surface tension–lowering ability and the amount of damage caused by any given detergent, and the mechanism of damage is not at all clear.

In general, cationic detergents are more damaging than anionic agents and both of these more than nonionics. For a rabbit eye test that has become the FDA standard and for a table of the maximum tolerated concentrations of 23 surface-active agents, see Draize and Kelley (1952). It is remarkable that such tolerated concentrations vary from 0.5 percent for the cationic lauryl dimethyl benzyl ammonium chloride through 20 percent for sodium lauryl sulfate to 100 percent for the nonionic sorbitan mono-laurate or mono-oleate. Note that one-third of the animals in the rabbit test have no washing of the eye after instillation of 0.1 ml of test substance, one-third have the eye washed after two seconds, and one-third have the eye washed after four seconds. A "tolerated concentration" is one in which there is no residual irritation after seven days.

An unprecedented departure affecting the field of ophthalmic toxicology in particular and animal experimentation in general is attributable to the "animal rights activists." These are not the "animal welfare" groups with whom we share the sincere desire for the humane treatment of animals under all circumstances, not least in the laboratory. The "activists" wish to outlaw all animal experimentation. To support their contention, they have committed violent acts that include destruction of laboratory installations and destruction of research records.

A more subtle consequence is the undertaking by some well-meaning workers to devise substitutes for animal experiments in a host of *in vitro* procedures. For a survey, see the proceedings of an international workshop held in April 1984 (Reinhardt *et al.*, 1985). For a reasoned approach whose logical conclusions are soft pedaled by its authors, see A. M. Goldberg and Frazier (1989).

Much of the anger of the activists has been directed against the Draize test. Inadequate education prevents such people from realizing how many functional systems are being tested with a single application of a corrosive substance to an organ as complex as the eye. Temporary disability, permanent scarring, an ulcer that goes on to perforation, uveitis and its consequences, and glaucoma and its consequences are some of the things the Draize test rules in or out. Valid *in vitro* tests for the function of organ subsystems are probably decades away and will come as the result of general development in biological science—not from external pressures.

Suggestions for alternatives made since 1983 include (1) quantitative fluorescence microscopy of the posterior segment (Baurman *et al.*, 1983); (2) tests on cell cultures or cornea held in an ussing cell (Andermann and Erhart, 1983); (3) inhibition of spontaneous contractions of mouse and rabbit isolated ileum (Muir *et al.*, 1983); (4) Papanicolou cytology of exfoliated corneal cells washed out of the cul-de-sac (Walberg, 1983); (5) cultures of the ciliated protozoan *Tetrahymena thermophylia* reacted with the test substance; (6) cultures of mouse LS cells as test object (Kemp *et al.*, 1983); (7) uptake of tritiated uridine in Balb/c 3T3 cells as test (Shopsis and Sathe, 1984); (8) localized application to chick chorioallantoic membrane (Leighton *et al.*, 1985; Parish, 1985).

All of the above represent presumably valid and well-executed experiments. However, if the experimenter does not understand the question to be asked, he or she cannot possibly come up with the correct answer. Ostensibly simple systems like the above (which have their own complexities) cannot simulate the interrelations of the complex set of systems that constitute the eye.

An excellent evaluation is that of Frederick K. Goodwin (Goodwin, 1989), who points out that the objective of the extremists is to stop all research without regard to the cost in human life or health and that time devoted to the presently impossible search for an *in vitro* alternative plays into their hands.

One piece of beneficial fallout from all this disturbance is the reexamination of the statistical basis of the Draize test as originally proposed and as engraved in stone by the FDA. The report of DeSousa *et al.* (1984) compared the use of two, three, four, five, and six rabbit samples for each of 67 petrochemicals. It showed that even two rabbit samples were 88 percent accurate. The suggestion is that although evolving an alternative test will take many man-centuries of work, one could instantly reduce the number of animals used with only a small and known decrease in accuracy.

Some of the surface-active agents, especially the cationic substances, in higher concentrations can cause severe burns with permanent opacity and vascularization. In human accidents, the immediate severe pain leads to rapid washing out of the eye, and only in the most extreme circumstances will permanent damage result. One exceptional circumstance with hazard potential is that some nonionic detergents actually cause topical anesthesia of the cornea (Martin *et al.*, 1962). It is conceivable that if a formulation contains such a surfactant in combination with an anionic or a cationic detergent, the anesthetic surfactant might eliminate the pain warning and allow severe damage to occur.

Vesicant War Gases. A group of chemical substances have in common the property of causing severe skin burns on contact in very low concentrations. They have been used or their use has been considered as chemical warfare agents—thus, the rubric for this section. All these agents cause severe eye burns on contact with the liquid or vapor. The biochemistry of the "mustard" vesicants was reviewed by Gilman and Philips (1946) and need not be repeated here. Lawley and Brookes (1965) presented evidence that these alkylating agents reacted selectively with the DNA synthesis mechanism.

Without reference to chemical warfare, a ni-trogen mustard is an intermediate in the manufacture of meperidine (Pethidine®, Demerol®), and eye irritation has been reported among plant personnel (Minton, 1949). Furthermore, numerous variants on nitrogen mustards are now standard therapeutic agents for a number of neoplastic diseases, especially lymphomas and blood dyscrasias. The manufacture and utilization of these drugs will continue to present a finite eye hazard.

Lacrimators and Smog. A number of chemically reactive substances in very high dilution are able to stimulate corneal sensory endings and cause reflex tearing. These contrast sharply with the mustards, which show a long latent period for subjective symptoms and then cause severe damage. The lacrimators in threshold concentrations cause instant sensation and no tissue damage. However, in higher concentrations, lacrimators can cause chemical burns with loss of corneal epithelium.

Typical lacrimators are as follows:

α-Chloroacetophenone   α-Brombenzyl cyanide

$$C_2H_5-O\overset{O}{\overset{\|}{C}}-CH_2I$$

Ethyl iodoacetate

See M. B. Jacobs (1942).

Lacrimator eye damage is complicated by the method of delivery. The two most common forms of delivery are the pencil-like tear-gas gun, purchasable by individuals in many states, and the aerosol can, used by law enforcement agencies under the trade name Mace®. The pencil gun has a charge of powdered α-chloroacetophenone propelled by the equivalent of a 22-caliber blank cartridge. When the gun is discharged near the eye, the force of the propellant can drive the powdered lacrimator deep into the cornea. The cartridge wadding can also strike the eye with force, causing mechanical injury (Levine and Stahl, 1968). The chemical alone causes mechanical damage, and its concentration in the eye exceeds the lacrimatory threshold by many, many times. This type of injury may lead to permanent corneal opacity. A similar but less severe injury can result if an aerosol can containing dissolved chloroacetophenone is discharged close to the eye instead of at a distance of several feet or more as recommended by the manufacturer (Thatcher *et al.*, 1971).

The mechanism of action of the lacrimators was investigated during World War II, notably by Dixon (1948) and Mackworth (1948). Their investigations showed that whatever the chemical nature of the lacrimator, they all shared the property of inhibiting sulfhydryl enzymes. They had no effect on enzymes not dependent on SH groups for their activity.

There are a few incongruities not well explained by this theory. Iodoacetate is a sulfhydryl reagent but is not a lacrimator. Lewisite is a good sulfhydryl reagent; even under the conditions of the Dixon experiments, it combines with 65 percent of the available SH groups; but it is not a lacrimator. The mustards react with SH groups. Whereas this reaction is a slow one and happens in minutes rather than seconds, the latent period for eye symptoms from the mustards is a matter of hours. Dixon himself pointed to another incongruity in the simple sulfhydryl reaction theory. The instant lacrimation on exposure to above-threshold concentration, the rapid cessation of effect on stopping exposure, and the resumption of irritation on restoring the lacrimator all speak against an irreversible combination of agent with critical tissue constituent. Dixon's suggestion that the nerve might respond to a *change* in −SH seems improbable. Recent publications on lacrimators have made no contribution to mechanism of action (Bleckmann and Sommer, 1981; Pfannkuch and Bleckmann, 1982). The whole subject of lacrimators is past due for reinvestigation.

The likely stimulus for such an investigation is the upsurge of an environmental lacrimator that must be dealt with expeditiously. This is photochemical smog. Not to be confused with industrial smog, this entity results from the interaction of automobile exhaust emissions and ultraviolet radiation from sunlight. It was first noticed in the Los Angeles area in the 1940s about the time when the last definitive work on chemical warfare lacrimators reached print.

It is now a major blight in every metropolitan area of the United States. We appear to be dealing with substances formed by ultraviolet-activated oxygen, with oxides of nitrogen, and the olefins, aromatics, and perhaps aliphatic hydrocarbons of automobile exhaust. Of the products, the major identified component is the class of peroxyacyl nitrates, which have distinct lacrimator action. This is not the whole story, however, for artificially generated smog used in laboratory studies is several times more active a lacrimator than peroxyacetyl nitrate. For a competent review of this subject, see Jaffe (1967).

Despite tightened emission control standards for new cars, and despite the avoidance of urban respiratory disasters with their help, the harder problems of chronic respiratory disease and chronic eye irritation have not been tackled. Still more remote, the esthetic problem of visibly clean air stands little chance of near-term solution when the short-term costs to large commercial interests are significant. Thus, half measures and extended studies are likely to be the order of the day. As a result, our knowledge of the eye effects of photochemical smog will be expanded, and it may be that we will be able to restudy the general problem of lacrimators with new understanding as a result.

Miscellaneous Substances.

Metallic Salts. Heavy metal ions combine with protein functional groups. In high enough concentration, metal salts cause tissue destruction. Thus, workers with such materials have the hazard of corneal opacity and ulceration, should a splash hit the eye. Adequate protection is indicated.

The more subtle deposition of metal components in the tissues of cornea, conjunctiva, and lids secondary to chronic overuse for therapeutic purposes is a phenomenon of the recent preantibiotic past when heavy-metal salts were the only available antibacterial agents. The tissue discoloration is a striking cosmetic defect. The chief offenders in the United States have been mild silver proteinate and yellow oxide of mercury (Wheeler, 1947; Wilkes, 1953). Outside of the United States there have been reports of argyrosis secondary to a silver-containing eyelash dye (Velhagen, 1953).

Hydroquinone. In many industries, a fine dust of particles can be generated, and in the absence of adequate exhaust velocity, these particles can reach the eye. This set of events can occur in the manufacture of any noxious solid substance. A particularly striking report was that of B. Anderson (1947) on workers engaged in the manufacture of hydroquinone for many years. The colorless hydroquinone dust on reaching the eye (with a distribution corresponding to the palpebral fissure) oxidizes to brown benzoquinone. This material is stored in large granules in or near the basal layer of the corneal epithelium and in smaller granules in the more superficial epithelium. It is visible as a brown band keratopathy.

Dichloroethane. A remarkable note on species specificity is provided by the reaction of the dog cornea to the systemic administration of 1,2-dichloroethane. Milky-white opacity results after exposure to 1000 ppm for seven hours. This appears not to be related to direct contact of the eye with the agent but is due to secondary action of the drug or a metabolic product on the corneal endothelium. Of many species of vertebrates tested, only the dog and the fox show the effect. For a report on a number of experiments, see the review by Heppel and coworkers (1944).

Lash Lure. In the past when there were few restrictions on the composition of cosmetics in this country, hair dyes and eyelash dyes were sold whose principal ingredient was *p*-phenylenediamine. It was the severe reaction to such a preparation sold under the proprietary name Lash Lure® that encouraged more stringent federal regulation. It appears that *p*-phenylenediamine and its analogues can easily sensitize the lid skin and external ocular structures. Continued application of the haptene can cause severe damage to the contacted tissues. Corneal ulceration with loss of vision and even a fatality have been reported. A concentration of papers appeared in the *Journal of the American Medical Association* in 1933 and 1934. For a review, see Linksz (1942).

Corneal Involvement by Internally Administered Substances

Uncommonly, a systemic drug may affect the cornea selectively.

Quinacrine. The antimalarial quinacrine (Atabrine®) is such a substance, and the effect is corneal edema. A typical report is that of Chamberlain and Boles (1946). This edema was a relatively rare occurrence in the Pacific theater during World War II where some 25 cases were recognized among many thousands of men taking the usual daily 100-mg prophylactic dose. The precise mechanism of action is unclear, though it is tempting to postulate a specific effect on the corneal endothelium.

Chloroquine. A second antimalarial substance affecting the cornea after oral administration is chloroquine. However, just as with the retinal lesions (*see* below), chloroquine keratopathy is seen chiefly in patients receiving 250 to 500 mg/day for rheumatoid arthritis or systemic lupus. The subjective symptoms are intolerance to glare and halos around lights. At ordinary levels of illumination, vision is not impaired. Slit lamp examination shows grayish turbidity in the deep layers of the epithelium. Biopsy has shown that these particles fluoresce; so they are presumably chloroquine or a metabolic product. The involvement disappears on cessation of drug administration. For a good early report, see Calkins (1958). For retinal effects of chloroquine. see below.

Chlorpromazine. The eye effects of chlorpromazine are minimal, but in patients who have received daily doses of 500 mg or more for at least three years granular deposits have been noted on the corneal endothelium and the lens capsule. These findings were first reported by Greiner and Berry (1964) in 12 of 70 patients. DeLong and coworkers (1965) described an additional series of 49 involved patients in a series of 131. In this latter series, only patients who received a cumulative dose of 1000 g or more of the drug showed corneal changes.

It is reasonable to assume that these chlorpromazine effects are due to the compound coming out of solution in the aqueous humor and depositing on surfaces bathed in the aqueous. A second type of deposition exists where the compound appears to come out of tear solution and deposit on corneal epithelium. This appears to be the case with tamoxifen and amiodarone (*see* the end of the retina section).

Lids and Lacrimal Apparatus

As mentioned in a previous section, the lids are usually involved in heavy-metal pigmentation. Another function that may be disturbed by lid damage is the drainage of tears through the lacrimal puncta at the inner nasal margins of the upper and lower lids. The normal tear flow enters the lacrimal canaliculi in the lid margins via the puncta and continues on through common canaliculus, lacrimal sac, and nasolacrimal duct into the nasopharynx. Action of any of the corrosives discussed above can cause scarring shut of the puncta or canaliculi or both with obstruction of tear flow and annoying epiphora—tears running down the cheek. Indeed, the scar need not even obstruct the drainage system. If it distorts lid position enough so that the lacrimal punctum is everted and no longer in contact with the tear film, this is enough to cause epiphora. Because the drainage system of the upper lid is often inefficient, sometimes involvement of the lower lid alone is enough to cause epiphora. Other effects of scarring can be turning in of the lids (entropion) with abrasion of the cornea by eyelashes. Turning out of the lids (ectropion) can cause desiccation of the cornea if it is exposed. The surgical correction of these scarring effects is difficult and not uniformly successful.

One medication that has the property of lowering intraocular pressure was found after ten years of general use to block the lacrimal drainage system. The structure of the drug, furfuryl trimethyl ammonium iodide (Furmethide®), is as follows:

$$\text{O} \diagdown \text{CH}_2\text{N}^+(\text{CH}_3)_3\text{I}^-$$

It was introduced to ophthalmic practice by Meyerson and Thau (1940) and was used in 10 percent solution for cases of intractable glaucoma until the report of Shaffer and Ridgway in 1951 described numerous cases of lacrimal obstruction in patients who used the drug continuously for three months or more. The obstruction was caused by nonspecific inflammatory tissue. Biopsy showed such inflammation in conjunctiva and at multiple points in the lacrimal drainage system.

The toxicology of the sclera is peculiar in that for practical purposes it does not exist. Externally applied corrosives reach the cornea before the sclera. Since loss of transparency of the cornea is accomplished by relatively low concentrations of corrosives and since cornea and sclera are equally susceptible to extreme burns that might cause perforation, selective scleral damage by corrosives just does not happen. Similarly, when collagen synthesis is inhibited as in lathyrism, the greater exposure of the cornea makes it more susceptible to perforation, other things being equal.

The very real threat of cicatricial lid disease posed by the beta-adrenergic blocker Practolol® has turned out to be a property of that drug and not of the group as a whole. In the United States, propranolol has been used without reliably reported adverse ocular effects. Timolol (Timoptic®), a topically applied beta blocker, has proved an effective antiglaucoma medication with minimal ocular side effects.

In a limited number of patients, practolol causes an "oculocutaneous syndrome" with atrophy of the lacrimal gland, corneal ulceration, and even corneal perforation. Because of its appearance and immunologic behavior, the syndrome has been called ocular cicatricial pemphigoid (Van Joost et al., 1976).

Elevated antinuclear antibodies caused by practolol have been demonstrated by Garner and Rahi (1976) and by Jachuck et al. (1977). Considering the structure of practolol versus that

of innocuous propranolol, it would appear that the β-blocking property is conferred by N-isopropyl propanolamine side chains, ether-linked to an aromatic nucleus. This suggests that the disease-producing property of practolol resides in the dissimilar portion of the molecule. The p-acetamidophenol of practolol suggests similarity to the sulfonamide moiety, which can cause the oculocutaneous syndrome Stevens-Johnson disease.

Apparently unrelated to hypersensitivity is the cicatricial ectropion reported to occur secondary to prolonged systemic 5-fluorouracil therapy (Straus et al., 1977). The condition is reversible on stopping the drug.

THE IRIS, AN INDICATOR OF AUTONOMIC ACTIVITY

Peripheral Effects

The special aspect of the iris (Figure 17–1) for pharmacology is its double innervation (sympathetic for dilator and parasympathetic for sphincter) and its being behind a transparent window, the cornea. Thus, as one would expect, sympathomimetic and parasympatholytic substances dilate the pupil, and parasympathomimetic and sympatholytic substances constrict the pupil—events easily observed in the intact subject. Allowing for the poor ocular penetration of very polar substances and for the coexistence of centrally initiated impulses, the pupil is an excellent indicator of autonomic activity of topically or systemically administered drugs and poisons.

The eye effects of extracts of mandragora and hyoscyamus were known to Galen in the second century A.D. These effects in sixteenth century Venice gave rise to the plant name belladonna (Matthiolus, 1598). The early experiments of Thomas Fraser on physostigma (Fraser, 1863) and those of T. R. Elliott on epinephrine (Elliott, 1905) utilized observations of the iris in intact animals.

The greatest potential, happily unrealized, for observation of these types of effects in human toxicology is from the effects of so-called "nerve gases" in combat. All these substances are so-called "irreversible" cholinesterase inhibitors. Diisopropyl fluorophosphate is an early synthesized example of such compounds. The acetylcholine constantly manufactured at cholinergic nerve endings and unhydrolyzed by normally present cholinesterase causes pupillary constriction in poisoning by these substances.

Since World War II, such cholinesterase inhibitors have been synthesized as insecticides. An occasional accidental toxic episode has been reported—usually concerning a worker standing

Practolol

Propranolol

Timolol

in a field being dusted with insecticide from an airplane. Further, the pilot of such a plane may experience visual symptoms from the same cause (Upholt *et al.*, 1956).

A somewhat odd iris effect has been labeled "cornpicker's pupil." It is mydriasis caused by operating farm machinery in a cornfield containing jimson weed, *Datura stramonium*. Enough hyoscyamine and related parasympatholytic substances from the plant reach the eye to dilate the pupil over a period of days (Goldey *et al.*, 1966).

It is understood that accidental poisoning by any of the agents in the autonomic group will, if severe enough, cause pupillary signs that may be helpful in establishing a diagnosis.

Central Effects

Not all pupillary changes due to toxic substances are demonstrably direct effects on the iris. The markedly constricted pupil characteristic of morphine poisoning appears to be due to central reinforcement of the physiologic light reflex. Constriction of the pupil caused by morphine is abolished by section of the optic nerve. The consensual reflex caused in the optic nerve-sectioned eye by light stimulation of the intact eye is enhanced by systemic administration of morphine. There is a small residual pupillary constriction caused by morphine in the absence of light. This may be direct action on the pupillary constrictor center or on the muscle itself, but this effect is small in comparison to light reflex enhancement (McCrea *et al.*, 1942).

Similarly, any drug effects observed in the alert animal are algebraically additive with centrally originating reflexes such as sympathetic dilation in the startle reflex, or pupillary constriction that accompanies concentration on a near object. These tend to be transient and are able to be sorted out from toxic drug effects. Similarly, the effects of general anesthetics in first constricting, then dilating, the pupil are superimposed on other pharmacologic and toxicologic effects.

Inflammatory Iris Reactions

The highly vascular iris is quite sensitive to physical and chemical trauma. Its response to all types of insults is nonspecific and consists primarily of increase in vascular permeability. The result of this is, first, liberation of protein into the normally low-protein aqueous humor. Both serum proteins and fibrin can enter the anterior chamber, and fibrin coagulum can eventually cause blockage of outflow of the aqueous humor (see below). The second reaction to insult is entry of leukocytes from inflamed iris vessels into the aqueous humor. Subsequent fibroblast metaplasia is again a threat to the aqueous outflow system.

Any of the corrosive substances discussed earlier can cause iritis if they reach the cornea in sufficient concentration to penetrate the anterior chamber or if they rapidly destroy the corneal epithelial barrier and then penetrate. In a special category are the relatively fat-soluble bases like ammonia and pyridine and acids or acid anhydrides such as sulfur dioxide, acetic acid, and acetic anhydride. These penetrate intact corneal epithelium rapidly and reach the iris in concentrations high enough to cause iritis.

The ciliary body (see below) is a pigmented vascular structure, protected by the iris from initial assault by harmful substances penetrating the cornea, but susceptible to leakage of protein and leukocytes if sufficient concentrations of noxious agent reach it. The vessels of iris plus ciliary body constitute the "blood-aqueous barrier." Evidence is adequate to implicate prostaglandins in the disruption of this barrier by corrosive substances or, more gently, by rapid lowering of the intraocular pressure. The latter experimental situation was used by van Haeringen *et al.* (1982) to test the effectiveness of nonsteroidal antiinflammatory agents, presumably in their role as inhibitors of prostaglandin synthesis.

Some insults to the iris are severe enough to cause loss of cellular integrity. This is most easily observable as liberation of melanin granules from the highly pigmented posterior iris epithelium into the aqueous humor. These granules may contribute to blockage of the aqueous outflow channels with consequent secondary glaucoma. The deposits on corneal endothelium and anterior lens capsule caused by high doses of phenothiazines resemble very tiny pigment granules. It seemed on personal observation that the white granules reported by others were diffraction halos around the tiny pigment particles as seen in the slit lamp. The remarkable storage of phenothiazines in the pigmented structures of the eye has already been reported (Potts, 1962b). It seems highly probable, in view of this storage and in view of the fact that the chlorpromazine opacities are confined to surfaces bathed by the aqueous humor, that (1) the drug is responsible for very chronic and very low-grade loss of posterior pigment epithelial cells of the iris and (2) the pigment granules liberated from these cells accumulate on corneal endothelium and lens capsule and even may be eventually incorporated into these structures, giving rise to the clinical effects of chlorpromazine on the anterior segment.

THE AQUEOUS OUTFLOW SYSTEM

General Considerations

As was mentioned at the beginning of this chapter, the eye, a small segregated portion of the central nervous system, has its own equivalent of the cerebrospinal fluid system. Disturbances of this system are as disastrous to the eye as disturbances of the cerebrospinal fluid system are to the brain. The ocular equivalent of cerebrospinal fluid is the aqueous humor, which is actively secreted into the posterior chamber by the double epithelial layer covering the ciliary processes (Figure 17–1). The aqueous humor flows between the posterior surface of the iris and the anterior lens surface, enters the anterior chamber through the pupillary aperture, and leaves the eye at the anterior chamber angle via the trabecular meshwork, the canal of Schlemm, and the aqueous veins (Figure 17–1). Although pathways have not yet been worked out completely, there appears to be a homeostatic mechanism that maintains normal intraocular pressure within the physiologic limits of approximately 10 to 22 mm Hg. However, the mechanism does not have the capacity for 100 percent modulation, for when the aqueous outflow system becomes severely incompetent due to disease, aqueous secretion is not shut off and intraocular pressure rises. When this pressure exceeds 28 to 30 mm Hg, ischemic damage occurs to the optic nerve fibers just before they pierce the lamina cribrosa to exit from the eye. This damage due to increased intraocular pressure is glaucoma and may lead to complete blindness unless treated.

There are two major mechanisms by which glaucoma may originate. The first involves gradual diminution of the ability of the trabecular meshwork—canal of Schlemm—system to pass fluid as with the inflammatory changes discussed in the previous section. This type of disease is characterized by insidious rise in pressure into the 30 to 40-mm-Hg range, absence of pain, and slow loss of peripheral visual field, usually unnoticed by the patient. This type of disease is known as "chronic simple glaucoma" or "chronic open-angle glaucoma." When it follows an identifiable inflammatory episode such as a chemical burn, it may be called "secondary," but it is still in the open-angle glaucoma category. The second mechanism is operative only in certain susceptible individuals who because of an inherited narrow chamber angle, or an angle narrowed by a swelling cataractous lens, can experience sudden and complete occlusion of the chamber angle filtration system by the most peripheral portion of the iris on iris dilation (cf. Figure 17–1). This type of disease is charac-terized by rapid rise in intraocular pressure to 60, 70, or even 100 mm Hg, severe pain, conjunctival and deep scleral injection, and rapid loss of vision. This type of disease is known as "acute congestive" or "angle-closure" glaucoma.

Open-Angle Glaucoma

Glaucoma of the first type, open-angle glaucoma, can occur secondary to any toxic inflammation. Burns by acid, alkali, and vesicant gases have been documented as initiators of open-angle disease (Duke-Elder, 1969). A more unusual cause of open-angle glaucoma is "epidemic dropsy" reported from India. Individuals show edema of the extremities, gastrointestinal disturbances, and cardiac hypertrophy as well as glaucoma (Maynard, 1909). The occurence has been attributed to contamination of cooking oil by oil from the seeds of *Argemone mexicana,* and the offending agent has been said to be the alkaloid sanguinarine from the argemone oil (S. L. Sarkar, 1926; S. N. Sarkar, 1948). Claims have been made in the past that the disease could be reproduced in experimental animals by argemone oil and by sanguinarine administration (Hakim, 1954). A recent reevaluation of the problem suggests that administration of sanguinarine orally, intravenously, or by cardiac puncture to rabbits, cats, and chickens does not reproduce the effects of epidemic dropsy; however, administration of argemone oil to chickens does cause edema of wattles (Dobbie and Langham, 1961). There seems little question that the disease is attributable to contaminated cooking oil. One of the problems is that since the first reports of epidemic dropsy the term "sanguinarine" has changed its meaning from an impure mixture of substances obtained from *Sanguinaria canadensis,* the Canadian bloodroot (Dana, 1828), to a pure chemical substance—a naphthaphenanthridine alkaloid (Manske, 1954). It is by no means impossible that in this process the actual toxic agent of argemone oil has been lost and that we have been defeated by a change in semantics. Thus, although sanguinarine is probably not the toxic agent, some component of argemone oil is. This does not make the problem less real or less deserving of reinvestigation.

Another type of open-angle glaucoma that has been recognized is that caused by long-term topical administration of antiinflammatory corticosteroids for eye disease (François, 1961; Goldman, 1962; Armaly, 1963). Armaly showed further that eyes already glaucomatous had greater rises in intraocular tension after corticoids than did normal eyes. Not only can steroid glaucoma be caused by topical application to the eye, but it may be caused by systemic administration as well (see Bernstein *et al.*, 1963a, for early literature references). The additional hazard with systemic administration is that therapy for allergic, rheumatic, and other disease will not be conducted by an ophthalmologist, and the idea of checking intraocular pressure or visual field may not occur to the physician until severe damage has occurred.

Angle-Closure Glaucoma

The second type of glaucoma, angle-closure glaucoma, can be induced in an individual who is susceptible because of a genetically narrow anterior chamber angle or who has an angle narrowed by intraocular changes. This disease is frequently iatrogenic, and the precipitating event is often mydriasis for eye examination or for the treatment of iritis. The most commonly offending drug is atropine because of the effectiveness of its action and its difficult reversibility. However, any mydriatic can be the precipitating cause, and all have been implicated at one time or another. For a partial list, see Duke-Elder (1969).

THE CILIARY BODY

The ciliary body, which lies just posterior to the root of the iris (Figure 17–1), is a structure with dual function. By means of the collagenous zonular fibers that stretch from lens to ciliary processes, the ciliary body acts as the structure physically supporting the lens. Increase in tension of the radially directed and parasympathetically innervated ciliary muscle allows the tension on the zonular fibers to relax. This in turn allows the natural elasticity of the lens capsule to make the lens more spheric and to change the focus of the retinal image from distant to near objects. This is the mechanism of accommodation that is stimulated by parasympathomimetic agents and paralyzed by parasympatholytic agents. Thus, in poisoning by cholinesterase inhibitors the small pupil caused by action of acetylcholine on the iris sphincter is accompanied by spasm of accommodation due to action on the ciliary muscle. This causes blurring of distant objects that were previously in focus. The converse is true in atropine poisoning. The pupil is wide and accommodation is paralyzed, making it difficult to see near objects. When atropine or other parasympatholytics are used as medication in gastrointestinal disease, it is rare that the dose is high enough to cause measurable pupillary effects. However, it is not uncommon, particularly in a patient whose accommodation is already limited by presbyopia, that the medication will cause discomfort in near vision.

There are numerous medications said to cause blurring of vision where the mechanism of action is less understandable. One such instance is the blurring experienced from large doses of phenothiazines. It appears to be possible, at least, that the blurring described is due to ciliary muscle weakness secondary to very high concentrations of the drug in the ciliary body due to storage of the polycyclic phenothiazine on melanin pigment in the ciliary body.

The second function of the ciliary body depends on its vascularity and on the two specialized layers of epithelium that cover it. The epithelium secretes aqueous humor at the rate of approximately 1 μl/min. Although it is problematic whether any substance can increase aqueous secretion, there is evidence that both epinephrine and carbonic anhydrase inhibitors such as acetazolamide can decrease aqueous humor formation. Diuretics based on the property of carbonic anhydrase inhibition can lower intraocular pressure as a side effect, but there is no record of any of them causing serious difficulty such as phthisis bulbi.

THE LENS

Description

Normal Function and Composition. The lens (Figure 17–1) is an avascular, transparent tissue surrounded by an elastic, acellular, collagenous capsule. It has the property of acting with the transparent cornea as an essential element in the image-forming system of the eye.

The lens is composed of only a single cell type and continually grows throughout life without losing a single cell; growth rate is inversely related to age. The lens can be arbitrarily divided into its anterior and posterior parts, with an equatorial region separating the two. On the anterior or corneal side, lying just beneath the capsule, is a layer of cuboidal epithelial cells: the only area where the cells possess the organelles typically found in all cells. The epithelial cells undergo mitosis and migrate toward the equatorial region where they elongate into fibers, become layered over older fibers, and continue migrating toward the anterior and posterior poles. Consequently, the major portion of the lens is composed of long, thin fibers that have a hexagonal cross section and form closely packed, onionlike layers. The oldest fibers occupy the center of the lens or nucleus, whereas younger fibers surrounding the nucleus occupy the area known as the cortex. The most superficial cortical cells possess some cytoplasmic organelles, but as the cells continue to differentiate, these organelles gradually disappear, giving way to a low-density fibrillar material, which in turn allows greater transparency. The tips of the fibers differentiating from either side of the anterior pole eventually join and form a special arrangement called suture-lines.

Water and protein are the primary chemical constituents of the lens (Paterson, 1972). The fibers are mostly composed of the soluble proteins α-, β-, and γ-crystallins and the insoluble protein albuminoid. These proteins are unique in being organ specific, not species specific, immunologically. With such a great proportion of protein, it is not surprising that the lens actively synthesizes proteins; in fact, lenticular growth and development depend on a continuous and abundant supply of biosynthetic proteins (Waley, 1969). Protein synthesis may also be the prime consumer of energy generated in the lens, which is necessary in the synthetic mechanics itself and in actively transporting amino acids against a concentration gradient from the aqueous humor into the epithelium (Kuck, 1970b).

Maintenance of an ionic equilibrium with a high intracellular K^+/Na^+ ratio through active transport of K^+ across the epithelium into the lens and Na^+ out of the lens expends a large quantity of energy. The flow of these ions through the lens has been attributed to the existence of a "pump-leak" mechanism (van Heyningen, 1969; Kuck, 1970b; Paterson, 1972). The high level of K^+ in the lenticular epithelium as a result of active transport from the aqueous humor favors diffusion of K^+ along a concentration gradient across the posterior capsule and into the vitreous. On the other hand, high vitreal content of Na^+ favors diffusion of Na^+ in the opposite direction, proceeding toward the epithelial cell layer where it is actively transported out of the lens and into the aqueous humor. The enzyme presumed to be associated with active transport, Na^+- and K^+-activated adenosine triphosphatase, is almost exclusively located in the epithelium. The energy necessary to drive active transport and other endergonic reactions is derived from the metabolism of glucose and primarily from anerobic glycolysis (van Heyningen, 1969; Kuck, 1970b). However, glucose degradation via the Krebs cycle with subsequent synthesis of ATP by the mitochondrial respiratory chain located solely in the anterior epithelium and superficial cortical fibers may possibly contribute as much as 30 percent to the total lenticular energy output (van Heyningen, 1969; Trayhurn and van Heyningen, 1971a, 1971b).

Other biochemical reactions important to lenticular metabolism include nucleic acid synthesis in areas undergoing mitosis, pentose shunt pathway supplying reduced nicotinamide adenine dinucleotide phosphate, sorbitol pathway, and the α-glycerophosphate cycle. Other cellular constituents include small amounts of lipids and glycoproteins, ophthalmic acid, and a relatively large quantity of reduced glutathione, whose role in lenticular metabolism has not been fully evaluated. Small amounts of Ca^{2+} are also necessary to maintain membrane integrity.

Cataract

Normal lenses are transparent, permitting light to pass through and allowing it to be focused on the retina. Transparency is dependent not only on the highly ordered cellular arrangement but also on fiber size, uniformity of dimension and shape, molecular structure, and regularity of packing (Kuck, 1970a, 1970c). In fact, the primary function of lenticular metabolism appears to be directed toward maintaining this organized structure and resulting transparency. Interference with normal lens metabolism, interference with active transport across the cell boundaries, breakage of the lens capsule, and many other types of insult cause alteration in optical properties. Such alterations take various morphologic appearances. Layers of cells in anterior or posterior cortex can change refractive index, the axial lens nucleus can change refractive index, or the anterior or posterior subcapsular layers can change refractive index. Although in medical jargon these changes are termed "opacities," they merely represent the change from perfect transparency to translucency. The result is that image quality in the optical system of the eye deteriorates and visual acuity falls. All such changes, whatever the cause, are lumped under the common term "cataract." Cataracts can be caused by a variety of unrelated circumstances (van Heyningen, 1969), for example, senile cataract due to age, congenital cataracts possibly related to immunologic or pathologic infections, inborn errors of metabolism such as in galactosemia, endocrine cataracts as in diabetes, and drug-induced cataracts. It is this latter category that will be described here, although similarities in mechanism may exist in all the above classes.

2,4-Dinitrophenol. In addition to a variety of toxic effects, systemic administration of 2,4-dinitrophenol (DNP) causes cataracts in some individuals. The classic instances of human dinitrophenol poisoning occurred during 1935 to 1937 when the substance was introduced as an antiobesity agent and was sold without prescription. Several hundred human cataracts resulted. For a review of these events, see Horner (1942). Lenticular opacity first develops in the anterior capsule and eventually spreads to include the cortex and the nucleus. Although cataracts may not develop until after months of treatment or until after drug withdrawal, the subcapsular and the posterior poles of the lens are the more severely affected. Vision is not immediately hindered but rapidly deteriorates as the cataract develops.

Experimental animals are insensitive to the cataractogenic activity of DNP, with the exception of young fowl and rabbits. A reversible cataract can be induced in chicks within one hour after systemic treatment. Analysis of aqueous humor, vitreous humor, and lens after a dose of DNP indicated a higher DNP concentration present in the young animal than in the adult, suggesting a possible explanation for both species and age sensitivity for DNP cataractogenic activity (Gehring and Buerge, 1969b). Within four to six hours after feeding a diet containing 0.25 percent DNP, vacuolization of the anterior lens can be induced in ducklings and chicks. *In vitro* incubation of lens with DNP forms cataracts (Gehring and Buerge, 1969a), with an increase in sodium influx and potassium efflux and swelling prior to cortical opacification (Ikemoto, 1971).

The cataractogenic activity of DNP may be related to its ability to uncouple oxidative phosphorylation, that is, inhibiting ATP synthesis without influencing electron transfer along the mitochondrial respiratory chain. Although experimental studies with other species indicate that lens metabolism is essentially anerobic, with ATP synthesis depending on glycolysis and therefore insensitive to DNP, mitochondrial oxidative phosphorylation in the epithelial cells may play a greater role in ATP synthesis in fowl and human lenses (Kuck, 1970b). As with any cell, removal of sodium ions from the lenticular cells may be the major energy utilizing reaction, in order to maintain proper ionic balances (Trayhurn and van Heyningen, 1971a). Other inhibitors of mitochondrial respiration, such as cyanide and amytal, also lead to increases in lenticular sodium content, which would be followed by decreases in ATP concentration, swelling, and opacification of the fibers.

Steroids. The first controlled study on the cataractogenic activity of corticosteroids was reported in 1960 (Black *et al.*, 1960). Thirty-nine percent of patients receiving prolonged therapy with either cortisone, prednisone, or dexamethasone for rheumatoid arthritis developed posterior subcapsular cataracts. A good correlation existed between cataract formation and dose and duration of therapy. No cataracts were observed in patients receiving low doses for a year or longer and medium or high doses for less than a year. In this study, there was no serious impairment of vision. Further investigation revealed that corticosteroid-induced cataracts could be distinguished by clinical morphology from cataracts caused by diabetes, 2,4-dinitrophenol, and trauma but could not be distinguished from cataracts caused by intraocular disease and ionizing radiation (Oglesby *et al.*, 1961a). Later reports confirmed the etiology and morphology, and a correlation was clearly established between the incidence of posterior subcapsular opacities and having received 15 mg of prednisone per day or equivalent for a year or longer (Oglesby *et al.*, 1961a; Crews, 1963; Williamson *et al.*, 1969; Williamson, 1970). In contrast, four children developed posterior subcapsular cataracts after receiving 1 to 3 mg of prednisolone or equivalent dose of paramethazone for only three to ten months, suggesting either a genetic or an age-dependent sensitivity (Loredo *et al.*, 1972). The clinical progression of the posterior subcapsular opacity has been graded I to IV by Williamson and coworkers (1969). Once vacuoles have formed, they are not reversible even if the drug is withdrawn during the early phases of opacification, although further progression to advanced stages will not occur (Lieberman, 1968). Grade III has been established as the point where visual difficulties become evident and vacuole extension into the cortex will progress in spite of drug withdrawal (Williamson, 1970). Similar findings have been reported after topical administration of corticosteroids (Becker, 1964). A useful review is that of Lubkin (1977).

Experimentally, steroidal cataracts were first observed in two out of four rabbits receiving 2 mg of betamethasone subconjunctivally for 41 weeks (Tarkkanen *et al.*, 1966). Long-term topical administration of several steroids also caused lenticular changes that were confined to the anterior subcapsular and cortical areas (D. C. Wood *et al.*, 1967) and therefore different from human cataracts. In contrast, short- or long-term systemic administration of prednisone or prednisolone did not result in cataracts when administered alone, although it did potentiate the cataractogenic activity of 2,4-dinitrophenol (Bettman *et al.*, 1964) and galactose (Bettman *et al.*, 1968) but not xylose, triparanol, or radiation. Betamethasome, applied topically, did enhance the formation of galactose cataracts (Cotlier and Becker, 1965).

The mechanism of steroid-induced cataracts has not been sufficiently investigated. *In vitro* studies (Ono *et al.*, 1971, 1972b) indicated that the lens can not only accumulate cortisol but also can biotransform it to its sulfate and glucuronide conjugates. Cortisol also binds to the soluble proteins β-crystallin and α-crystallin (Ono *et al.*, 1972b). Alterations in Na^+ and K^+ ion transport have been reported resulting in increased hydration of the lens (Harris and Gruber, 1962). Inhibition of synthesis of lenticular proteins has been suggested as a possible mechanism of steroidal cataracts (Ono et al., 1972a). It has been known since the work of Axelsson and Holmberg (1966) that long-acting cholinesterase inhibitors cause anterior and posterior subcapsular cataracts. This has been amply confirmed in humans and in monkeys (Shaffer and Hetherington, 1966; Kaufman et al., 1977a). The mechanism of cataractogenesis is unknown. A curious finding is that topical application of atropine prevents the experimental cataract in monkeys (Kaufman et al., 1977b).

Chlorpromazine. It was noted in the cornea section above that pigment granules appear on the anterior lens surface as well as the corneal endothelium in individuals who have received large doses of chlorpromazine over long periods of time. Although these granules are almost certainly exogenous to the lens in origin, they become incorporated into lens substance and cause loss of transparency. By these criteria, this phenomenon is cataract and should be mentioned here.

Thallium. The soluble salts of thallium acetate and thallium sulfate have been used as insecticides, as rodenticides, and at one time, as a systemic or topical depilatory agent. Thallous ion (Tl^+) is readily absorbed through the skin or gastrointestinal epithelium. Ingestion or application causes a variety of toxic symptoms, such as disturbances of the gastrointestinal tract, hair loss, polyneuritis of feet and legs, weakness or paralysis of the legs, psychic disturbances, neuritis of the optic nerve (described below), and in rare instances, cataracts (Duke-Elder, 1969; Grant, 1986). Thallium acetate induces cataracts in rats within six weeks after initiating a daily dose of 0.1 mg, appearing first as radial striations in the anterior cortex between the sutures and the equator. While the early phases will remain stationary if thallium administration ceases, development of subcapsular opacities will occur if administration continues. Microscopic examination reveals areas of proliferation or deletion of subcapsular epithelium and accumulation of a homogeneous or granular material axially to the fibers (Duke-Elder, 1969). The nuclear region is spared.

Thallous ion rapidly accumulates in the lens both in vivo (Potts and Au, 1971) and in vitro (Kinsey et al., 1971), possibly by an active transport mechanism dependent on the action of Na^+-K^+-ATPase. Thallium especially accumulates in those tissues with high K^+ levels, suggesting a competition for the same cellular transport mechanisms. In fact, thallium sub-stitutes for potassium in many enzymes requiring K^+ for activity but is effective at a concentration ten times lower than is needed for K^+. Examples of some enzymes studied are the following: (1) brain K^+-activated phosphatases (Inturrisi, 1969a), (2) brain microsomal Na^+-K^+-ATPase (Inturrisi, 1969b), (3) muscle pyruvate kinase (Kayne, 1971), and (4) skin Na^+-K^+-ATPase (Maslova et al., 1971). Whether any of the above reactions are affected in the lens has not been reported, but substitution for K^+ in the frog skin Na^+-K^+-ATPase results in inhibition of the Na^+ pump. Electron microscopic examination of the kidney, liver, and intestine from rats chronically receiving subacute doses (10 to 15 mg Tl^+ per kilogram) of thallium acetate reveals a possible primary lesion of the mitochondria, exhibiting swelling, loss of cristae, deposition of granular material, and aggregation of mitochondrial granules (Herman and Bensch, 1967). Additional morphologic changes include disruption of the endoplasmic reticulum and formation of autophagic vacuoles.

Busulfan. Busulfan (Myleran®) is a 1,4-bis(methanesulphonyloxy)-butane alkyating agent used in treating chronic myeloid leukemia.

$$CH_3 \cdot \overset{\overset{O}{\uparrow}}{\underset{\underset{O}{\downarrow}}{S}} \cdot (CH_2)_4 \cdot O \cdot \overset{\overset{O}{\uparrow}}{\underset{\underset{O}{\downarrow}}{S}} \cdot CH_3$$

Busulfan (Myleran®)

Posterior subcapsular opacities or irregularities may result following chronic busulfan therapy (Podos and Canellos, 1969; Ravindranathan et al., 1972; Grant, 1986; Hamming et al., 1976), although the incidence or conditions surrounding these cataracts have not been fully investigated.

Experimentally induced cataracts can be obtained by feeding rats a diet containing 7.5 to 20.0 mg/kg of busulfan. An irreversible cataract is completely developed in five to seven weeks (Solomon et al., 1955; von Sallmann, 1957). The earliest observation includes an increased mitotic activity of the epithelium primarily in the equatorial region, which eventually returns to and drops below normal levels. White dots or small vacuoles appear in the posterior and anterior lens, rapidly followed by opacification progressing from the equator to the posterior and anterior subcapsular zones. Similarities have been drawn between busulfan and ionizing radiation cataracts, suggesting that those species with the slowest lens mitotic activity will develop cataracts more slowly (von Sallmann, 1957). The underlying mechanism may involve altered epithelial cell division. Injection of a single 12.5 mg/kg dose intraperitoneally reveals that busulfan acts during the relatively long G phase (Grimes *et al.,* 1964) of the cell cycle (Harding *et al.,* 1971), permitting normal synthesis of DNA but preventing subsequent mitosis. Consequently, the affected epithelial cells accumulate in preprophase, containing bizarre clumps of nuclear chromatin and twice the normal DNA content. Some of these cells undergo nuclear fragmentation and disintegration, while the remainder return to interphase with a tetraploid level of DNA. A similar mechanism occurs after chronic administration of busulfan (Grimes and von Sallmann, 1966). Following each cycle of DNA synthesis, mitosis is inhibited; and since the cells in the equatorial zone have the shortest intermitotic time (19 days), these are affected first. The cells in the equatorial zone normally migrate through the meridional rows and differentiate into lens fibers. However, death of these cells occurs after three days of busulfan treatment, leading to a decrease in cell density and disorganization of the meridional rows and finally opacification. Continuous administration of this drug results in a depletion in the number of epithelial cells and complete disruption of the equatorial zone.

Triparanol. Triparanol (MER-29) was developed in the late 1950s as a blood cholesterol–lowering agent. Subsequent experiments in rats revealed decreased serum and tissue cholesterol levels and concomitant elevation in desmosterol levels. Triparanol inhibits cholesterol synthesis by inhibiting the $C_{24,25}$ double-bond reduction in desmosterol (Avigan *et al.,* 1960; Steinberg and Avigan, 1960). Two reports published prior to the removal of triparanol from the market due to other toxicities confirmed the development of posterior and anterior subcapsular opacities following a dose of at least 250 mg per day for 15 to 18 months (Kirby *et al.,* 1962; Laughlin and Carey, 1962).

Triparanol can induce cataracts in rats fed a diet containing 0.1 percent of the drug (von Sallmann *et al.,* 1963). Small sudanophilic vesicles form on the fibers and eventually aggregate into large clusters. Prior to central and peripheral opacification, triparanol causes a tenfold increase in lens sodium content, causing hydration and swelling (Harris and Gruber, 1969, 1972). Upon returning to a normal diet, the cataracts are reversed as new fibers are laid down in the periphery, excess Na^+ and water are pumped out, and K^+ levels return to normal. Morphologic alterations have been observed under the electron microscope with other tissues sensitive to triparanol toxicity. Abnormalities consist of crystalloid and membranous intracytoplasmic inclusion bodies in neurons (Schutta and Neville, 1968), mitochondrial swelling, and rupture and fragmentation of the endoplasmic reticulum in the liver (Otto, 1971). Since cholesterol is an essential component of cellular membranes, inhibition of its synthesis could result in an overall inhibition of membrane synthesis (Rawlins and Uzman, 1970), involving all subcellular membranous structures, including mitochondria. Changes in mitochondrial oxidative metabolism (Otto, 1971) could conceivably result in deficiencies of the Na^+-pump mechanism in extruding intracellular Na^+ from the lens and consequently lead to Na^+ accumulation in the lens. Further experimental evidence concerning the mechanism of triparanol cataracts is lacking.

Naphthalene. In addition to its retinotoxic action, systemic absorption of naphthalene vapor may result in cataracts (Grant, 1986). Oral administration of 1 g/kg/day to rabbits leads to lenticular changes, initially observed as a swelling in the peripheral portion of the lens. Vacuoles form between the epithelium cells within six hours after the first dose, spread toward the nucleus, and within two weeks the whole lens is affected with a mature cataract. Mitosis of the epithelial cells is inhibited after two or three doses, and the cells break down later. After one week, swelling and striations extend into the cortex and mitotic arrest is observed. Finally, after two weeks of naphthalene treatment, the epithelium shows areas of cell duplication, nuclear degeneration, and normal and abnormal mitosis. Since abnormal mitotic areas become partly denuded of cells, cells are irregularly arranged in the periphery (Pirie, 1968). The stages of naphthalene-induced cataract are similar to those that occur in the development of human senile cataract.

The biochemical basis for naphthalene cataract has been investigated (van Heyningen and Pirie, 1967) and shown to be related to the liver metabolite of naphthalene, 1,2-dihydro-1,2-dihydroxynaphthalene. Lenticular catechol reductase biotransforms 1,2-dihydro-1,2-dihydroxynaphthalene to 1,2-dihydroxynaphthalene, which in turn is autooxidized in air at neutral pH to 1,2-naphthoquinone and hydrogen peroxide. Ascorbic acid reverses the latter reaction and forms dehydroascorbic acid, which can be reduced by glutathione. Since ascorbic acid diffuses out of the lens very slowly, it accumulates in the lens of the naphthalene-fed rabbit and in the lens incubated *in vitro* with 1,2-dihydro-1,2-dihydroxynaphthalene (van Heyningen, 1970a). The sequence of reactions involves reduction of ascorbic acid by 1,2-naphthoquinone in the aqueous humor to dehydroascorbic acid, which rapidly penetrates the lens and is reduced by glutathione. Oxidized glutathione and 1,2-naphthoquinone may compete for the enzyme glutathione reductase, which normally maintains high lenticular levels of reduced glutathione. A reduction in the concentration of these coupled with the removal of oxygen from the aqueous humor due to the autooxidation of 1,2-dihydroxynaphthalene may make the lens sensitive to naphthoquinone toxicity. Other diols that do not form quinones in similar *in vitro* experiments do not result in lenticular opacities or increased ascorbic acid levels (van Heyningen, 1970b).

In addition to the reduction of glutathione levels and aqueous humor oxygen content, 1,2-naphthoquinone is a very active compound and reacts with lenticular glutathione, amino acids, and proteins (Rees and Pirie, 1967). Interaction with the structural proteins results in the brown color of the lens characteristic of naphthalene cataracts and insoluble complexes of β- and γ-crystallins. However, combination with these proteins does not inhibit naphthoquinone oxidation of ascorbic acid. Reactions between coenzymes and enzymes and 1,2-naphthoquinone can cause changes in the oxidation/reduction potential of the lens and abnormal metabolic reactions, which either alone or in combination would lead to cellular disruption and, finally, cataracts.

Galactose. An unusual experimental cataract results from feeding animals a diet containing high levels of galactose. The morphologic changes in the lens during galactose feeding were photographed and described by Sippel (1966a). Within two days after initiating a diet containing 50 percent galactose, rats show water clefts situated between lenticular fibers in the anterior equatorial region. After ten days the cortex is almost completely liquefied and more transparent to light as a result of vacuole aggregation. Total lenticular opalescence is complete after 28 days of galactose feeding. Accompanying these changes is an increase in DNA synthesis (Weller and Green, 1969) and mitosis of the epithelial cells (Kuwabara et al., 1969; van Heyningen, 1969) after three days of feeding. Eventually mitosis returns to and drops below normal activity as the cataract progresses.

The mechanism of galactose- and other sugar-related cataracts has been explained by excessive hydration of the lens observed as early as 12 hours after initiating a galactose-enriched diet. Galactose and other sugars are transported across the capsule and epithelial cell membrane by facilitated transport and diffusion (Elbrink and Bihler, 1972), and on entering the lens, galactose is either slowly phosphorylated to galactose-6-phosphate or reduced by the NADPH-dependent aldose reductase to dulcitol. While other sugar alcohols formed by aldose reductase are converted by polyol-NADP oxidoreductase to readily diffusible products, dulcitol is not further biotransformed. Since it diffuses out of the lens only very slowly, dulcitol accumulates to high levels and consequently exerts a strong osmotic force, drawing water into the lens in order to maintain osmotic equilibrium. Therefore, increases in dulcitol levels are accompanied by a parallel increase in water content (Kinoshita, 1965; van Heyningen, 1971). If dulcitol synthesis is depressed by inhibiting aldose reductase with 3,3-tetramethyleneglutaric acid, water uptake and fiber vacuolization are prevented (van Heyningen, 1971). Furthermore, feeding young Carworth Farms Webster (CFW) mice a galactose-enriched diet does not produce cataracts, since lenses of this strain fail to biotransform galactose to dulcitol (Kuck, 1970c). Therefore, lenticular hydration resulting from the osmotic force due to dulcitol accumulation and retention explains fiber vacuolization and the initial structural alterations in galactose cataracts. Further investigations verified the lack of or very low activity of other lenticular enzymes that could biotransform dulcitol, e.g., galactokinase or 1-gulonate NADP oxidoreductase (van Heyningen, 1971).

Additional biochemical changes consist of a very early loss in amino acids due to a deficiency in the amino acid–concentrating mechanism and a marked drop in glutathione content (Kinoshita, 1965; Sippel, 1966a; Kinoshita et al., 1969; van Heyningen, 1969, 1971). Both decreases are probably related to increased membrane permeability following swelling. Glycolysis and respiration decrease to 60 percent of normal after two days of galactose feeding but remain at this level of activity as the cataract progresses (Sippel, 1966b). Adenosine triphosphate levels decrease slightly during the early stages, but progressive vacuolization and opacification are accompanied by a 75 percent loss in ATP content. (Sippel, 1966b; Kuck, 1970c). Decreased aldolase activity correlates with progressive vacuolization of the cortex and glutathione loss during the first week of galactose diet; however, decreases in glucose-6-phosphate dehydrogenase, lactic acid dehydrogenase, and α-glycerophosphate dehydrogenase activity correlate with protein diminution occurring during the development of nuclear cataract (Sippel, 1967; Kuck, 1970c). Alterations in electrolyte balance do not occur until the late vacuolar stage. Surprisingly, the increased water uptake observed during the initial stages of cataract development is not accompanied by an increased Na^+ uptake and a loss of K^+ ions from the lens. In fact, Na^+ ion is pumped out of the lens during the initial development as effectively as from a normal lens, with only a slight loss in K^+. Only in the late vacuolar stage, with the development of nuclear opacification, does the lens fail to extrude Na^+, suggesting a second dramatic increase in membrane permeability to water during the terminal stages (Kinoshita, 1965). This is in the face of a still very much active cation pump mechanism. Decreases are observed in Mg^{2+}-dependent adenosine triphosphatase activity after six days of feeding a galactose-enriched diet, whereas Na^+-K^+-activated adenosine triphosphatase activity is markedly depressed after 15 days (Fournier and Patterson, 1971).

The lenticular opacities that develop on galactose feeding can be reversed if the sugar is withdrawn from the diet prior to nuclear involvement. After 10 to 12 days on the galactose diet, membrane permeability alters so that dulcitol leaks out as fast as it is formed. At this time, little, if any, protein is lost, but there is an increasing concentration of lens amino acids derived from protein, either from proteolysis or from inhibition of protein synthesis (Barber, 1972). As the cataract develops further, amino acids are suddenly reduced. Parallel accumulation of dulcitol and water in the lenticular fibers definitely causes the initial stages of cortical vacuolization and opacification. However, only failure of the lens to synthesize proteins or alterations in enzymic activity essential in maintaining lens integrity could explain the irreversible nature of the mature nuclear cataract. The entire biochemistry of the lens would be deleteriously affected by the removal of reduced pyridine dinucleotide phosphate (NADPH) consumed during the reduction of galactose to dulcitol catalyzed by aldose reductase. Consequently, the reduced NADPH/NADP ratio alters the oxidation-reduction potential of the lens (Kuck, 1970b).

Experimentally induced galactose cataract has its counterpart in human physiology. Galactosemia is an autosomal recessive genetic deficiency in galactose metabolism. Affected infants on a milk diet show high blood and urine galactose levels, hepatomegaly, splenomegaly, eventual mental retardation, and cataracts. The genetic defect is deficiency in the enzymes galactose-1-phosphate-uridyl transferase or galactokinase (Kinoshita, 1965; Monteleone et al., 1971; Nordmann, 1971; Levy et al., 1972). These enzymes are necessary in transforming unusuable galactose into usable glucose-1-phosphate. Galactose or galactose-1-phosphate reaches excessive levels in the blood and aqueous humor, triggering dulcitol synthesis in the lens and subsequent fibril vacuolization (van Heyningen. 1969). Removal of galactose from the diet can reverse the symptoms.

The multiple causes of cataract suggest multiple mechanisms rather than a final common pathway. This, in turn, suggests that we are not close to the multiple required solutions even though the sugar cataract problem appears to be solved brilliantly. Thus, new experimental test situations are to be welcomed. Merriam and Kinsey (1950) demonstrated that rabbit lenses could be maintained in organ culture for at least a week without loss of transparency, and this system has been exploited at various times. Mikuni et al. (1981) showed that microtubules disappear in cultured rat lenses in parallel with cataract formation. The size and orientability of microtubules suggest that they may well play a role in maintenance of lens transparency, and that this may be a profitable lead. Giblin et al. (1982), using cultured rabbit lenses, showed that glutathione and the hexose monophosphate shunt are vital in the detoxication of hydrogen peroxide in the culture medium. Since an early drop in glutathione level is characteristic in a number of cataracts including human ones, this lead, too, has promise. Sodium selenite injected into the intact rat causes large nuclear cataracts within 72 hours. Bunce and Hess (1981) showed that this event was also accompanied by a decrease in glutathione in lens. One is entitled to speculate whether this is a manifestation of selenium being an imperfect substitute for sulfur or whether it has a more basic significance for chemical cataractogenesis.

THE VITREOUS CAVITY

A major innovation in ophthalmic surgical practice during the last decade has been the "pars plana vitrectomy," which seems to be executable without inevitable disaster. A natural consequence of the procedure (accomplished by simultaneous aspiration of vitreous contents and replacement with fluid) is the investigation of how the composition of the replacement fluid will affect the structures that line the vitreous cavity, particularly the retina.

There are two major motivations behind the experimental use of a wide variety of substances placed in the vitreous cavity. The first is the possibility that endophthalnitis, difficult to combat, might be treated more effectively by vitrectomy plus an appropriate chemotherapeutic agent. The second motivation is the desire to find a magic inhibitor of proliferative vitreoretinopathy—the chief cause of blindness in diabetics.

Results are expressed as tolerated doses and tolerated concentrations because this is the way results are expressed by the authors. The reader may be assured that in each case cited doubling the intravitreal dose or doubling the concentration will cause retinal damage.

Considering the second category first, antineoplastic fluorouracil was examined for toxicity when placed in the vitreous space. Stern et al. (1983) found that 0.5 mg fluorouracil in the vitreous cavity of rabbits was tolerated every 24 hours for seven days with no signs of damage. On the same schedule, 1.25 mg. caused marked damage. According to Barrada et al. (1984), fluorouracil was tolerated by primate eyes in a single dose of 750 μg. Figures were also presented by these authors on combinations with etopside and with vincristine. Apparently, 0.5 μg/ml of vincristine in the vitreous perfusion fluid of primates was well tolerated. The later report of Orr et al. (1986) dealt with recovery of ^{14}C-labeled fluorouracil from the rabbit eye. Recovery was greatest if both vitrectomy and lensectomy had been done. The presence of silicone oil reduced the recovery.

Thinking along similar lines, Kirmani et al. (1983) devised a test object for proliferative vitreoretinopathy by injecting cultured rabbit dermal fibroblasts in the rabbit vitreous. Six cytotoxic drugs were tested using this test object. Daunomycin at 10 nanomoles per eye stopped cellular proliferation and prevented subsequent traction detachment. Equivalent doses of actinomycin C, colchicine, cytosine arabinoside, 5-fluorodeoxyuridine, and vinblastine sulfate showed no such effect. Therapeutic use was recommended against by these authors, just as the use of doxorubicin was recommended against by Sunalp et al. (1985).

Let us now return to the antiinfectious agents. Moxalactam, a third-generation, semisynthetic, cephalosporinlike antibiotic, enters the eye when given parenterally, but vitreous concentrations are disappointing (Fett et al., 1984). The rabbit retina tolerates 1.25 mg injected into the vitreous, but higher doses damage the retina. A related compound, cefoperazone, is harmless when a single dose of 8 mg is injected into the vitreous of Dutch Belted rabbits. Doses of 16 mg and higher cause retinal damage (O'Hara et al., 1986). In the same series ceftriaxone was tolerated in a maximum intravitreal dose of 20 mg (Shockley et al., 1984). Still in the same series, ceftazidine showed transient decrease of the b wave of the electroretinogram (ERG). The injection of 2 mg into the vitreous of a phakic rabbit gave what are judged to be bactericidal levels for at least 72 hours (Jay et al., 1987).

The aminoglycoside antibiotics were tested for toxicity on intravitreal injection by D'Amico et al. (1985). Their injections began at the level of 100 μg per eye. They found gentamycin the most toxic, followed by netlimycin and tobramycin

(about equal), followed by amikacin and kanamycin (also about equal).

The semisynthetic beta lactam antibiotic imipinem was found by Derick et al. (1987) to be tolerated in vitrectomy infusion fluid at concentrations of up to 16 μg/ml in rabbits.

Pflugfelder et al. (1987) found that otherwise resistant strains of gram-positive organisms isolated from endophthalmitis eyes were sensitive to vancomycin. Vitrectomized rabbit eyes appeared to tolerate up to 2 mg of the drug without damage. Further, the effect of vancomycin plus gentamycin appeared to be additive.

A newer glycopeptide antibiotic with activity similar to that of vancomycin was tolerated in intravitreal infusion solution for the rabbit eye at a concentration of 8 μg/ml.

Note should be taken of the use by Alghadyan et al. (1988) of liposome-bound cyclosporine with a view toward reducing toxicity; 500 μg injected into the vitreous cavity were tolerated with no damage to rabbit retina.

A number of publications have dealt with intravitreal tolerance to antiviral agents. Pulido et al. (1984) recommended using up to 30 μg vidarbine intraocularly or 8 to 16 μg/ml in infusion fluid. For acyclovir, the recommendation was 80 μg intraocularly or 40 μg/ml in infusion fluid.

Hydroxyacyclovir was evaluated in the same laboratory a year later (Pulido et al., 1985). These workers found no changes from intravitreal doses as high as 400 μg. The effectiveness of this drug against cytomegalovirus was pointed out as a special application.

Yoshizumi et al. (1986) applied vidarbine intravitreally dissolved in DMSO. Tolerated was 100 μg/ml in the infusion fluid. The drug has in vitro effectiveness against herpes simplex virus. The innocuousness of two separate foreign substances must be proved.

In the same order of magnitude of toxicity is trifluorothymidine. It is tolerated at a single dose of 200 μg and at a level of 60 μg/ml on perfusion (Pang et al., 1986). The same laboratory reports that gancyclovir, active against cytomegalovirus, is tolerated in infusion fluid at levels of 30 μg/ml or less (Kao et al., 1987). Further, it appears that in combinations of antiviral drugs toxicity is not additive. Useful combinations must be defined (Small et al., 1987).

Publications on antifungal agents have been fewer in number. However, the upper therapeutic level of 5-fluorocytosine has been found to be 100 μg on intravitreal injection (Yoshizumi and Silverman, 1985). A comparable single dose of fluconazole (anticandida) is tolerated in similar conditions (Schulman et al., 1987).

The unique immunosuppressive cyclosporin is

tolerated at 100 μg intravitreally; 200 μg causes histological damage (Grisolano and Peyman, 1986).

THE RETINA AND CHOROID

The retina is the very compact and highly complex neural structure responsible for transducing the ocular light image and doing considerable preprocessing of the neural impulses before sending them toward the brain (Figure 17–1). The layer of rods and cones—modified neural structures containing photosensitive pigments—is the receptor of the light image. The receptor cells synapse with bipolar cells, which in turn synapse with ganglion cells. In addition, lateral synapses occur with horizontal cells and feedback synapses occur with amacrine cells. The Müller cells, the glia equivalent in retina, have nuclei near the center of the retinal thickness and long processes that extend through the whole retinal thickness. Finally, the single layer of retinal pigmented epithelium underlies the receptors and sends processes that envelop the receptor outer segments. It should be evident from these relationships—all of which exist in the 100- to 500-μm retinal thickness—that studies on the overall biochemistry and physiology of such a structure are likely to be confusing and misleading. To dispel any lingering hope that the retinal layers are uniform metabolically if not morphologically, one need only read below how specific toxic substances affect specific retinal layers. After one has recognized with Warburg (1926) that the retina as a whole is the most actively metabolizing structure in the normal body, one must view metabolic studies on whole retina with healthy skepticism. The extremely compact structure of the retina creates a real dilemma when one wishes to study a single cell type. One solution is that worked out by Lowry and coworkers (1956, 1961), who microdissected freeze-dried retina and picked out nuclei of each cell type for metabolic studies. Other approaches utilize histochemical techniques on retinas with individual cell layers destroyed by toxic substances. This subject is still very much open for definitive study, and its incomplete state will hinder us greatly in reaching satisfying conclusions on the mechanism of action of retinotoxic substances.

The choroid is a vascular layer whose chief constituents in addition to the blood vessels are collagenous connective tissue and cells containing large numbers of melanin granules. The latter are important because of the affinity of melanin for polycyclic aromatic compounds. In primates, which have a well-established retinal blood supply, the choroid is responsible for nutrition of the receptor cell layer only. In lower vertebrates the choroidal vasculature supplies all of the retina.

Because of this dependence and because of physical proximity, many diseases primary in the choroid cause retinal damage and some diseases primary in retina cause choroidal damage. Thus, *chorioretinitis* is a commonly encountered term. It is based on clinical observation and does not imply which structure is primary for the disease process.

Chloroquine

The 4-aminoquinoline chloroquine is effective as (1) an antimalarial, requiring doses of 500 mg

Chloroquine

per week for three to four weeks, with maintenance on 250 mg per week, and (2) an antiinflammatory agent, requiring doses of at least 250 mg per day to be effective. The low-dose therapy used for malaria is essentially free from any toxic side effects; however, the chronic, high-dose therapy used for rheumatoid arthritis and discoid and systemic lupus erythematosus frequently causes a number of side effects, the most serious of which involves an irreversible loss of retinal functions. In 1959, the first cases of chloroquine-induced retinopathy were reported (Hobbs *et al.*, 1959), but since then numerous reports have confirmed the etiology of similar observations as resulting from chloroquine therapy (see reviews by Nylander, 1967; Duke-Elder and MacFaul, 1972). Hydroxychloroquine has also been reported to cause a similar

Hydroxychloroquine

retinopathy (Crews, 1967; Shearer and Dubois, 1967), although the incidence of toxicity may be less (Shearer and Dubois, 1967; Sassaman *et al.*, 1970).

The clinical findings accompanying chloroquine retinopathy may generally be thought of in terms of early and late phenomena. Among the early findings are (1) a "bull's-eye retina," visualized as a dark, central pigmented area involving the macula, surrounded by a pale ring of depigmentation, which in turn is surrounded by another ring of pigmentation; (2) diminished electrooculogram; (3) possible granular pigmentation of the peripheral retina; and (4) subjective visual disturbances, observed as blurred vision and difficulty in reading, with words or letters missing in long sentences or long words. Late findings are (1) progressive scotoma, (2) constriction of the peripheral fields commencing in the upper temporal quadrant, (3) narrowing of the retinal artery, (4) color and night blindness, (5) absence of a typical pigment pattern, and (6) abnormal electrooculograms and electroretinograms; these symptoms are irreversible. Indeed, there have been reports of irreversible chloroquine retinopathy where the entire development of the disease has occurred after cessation of the drug (R. P. Burns, 1966). It is generally recognized that the incidence of these chloroquine-induced toxic effects increases as the daily dose, total dose, and duration of therapy increase. The absence of permanent damage has been reported in patients receiving not more than 250 mg of chloroquine or 200 mg of hydroxychloroquine per day (Scherbel et al., 1965). Nevertheless, utilization of sensitive testing methods such as "macular dazzling" and retinal threshold tests has indicated some degree of retinal malfunction in all patients receiving even small doses of these drugs (Carr, 1968). Thus, there is a qualitative difference between the depression of visual function observed in all patients and the specific damage seen in relatively few individuals. Approximately 20 to 30 percent of the patients receiving higher doses of chloroquine will exhibit some type of retinal abnormality, while 5 to 10 percent show severe changes in retinal function (Butler, 1965; Crews, 1967; Nylander, 1967). One interesting paradox is worth noting. Despite severe retinopathy and "extinguished" ERG, normal or nearly normal dark adaptation performance is characteristic of chloroquine toxicity. This is in marked contrast to phenothiazine retinopathy (see below) (Krill et al., 1971).

Experimentally induced chloroquine retinopathy was first produced in the cat after long-term, oral administration of subtoxic doses, 1.5 to 6.0 mg daily (Meier-Ruge, 1965b). A light pigmentation appeared in the cat's fundus four to seven weeks after the daily dosage schedule, and the retinopathy was fully developed after eight weeks. Histologic and histochemical analysis revealed a thickening of the pigment epithelial cell layer, increases in the mucopolysaccharide and sulfhydryl group content, decreases in enzymatic activity of the pigment epithelium, migration of pigment into the outer nuclear layer, and finally total atrophy of the photoreceptors (Meier Ruge, 1968). Similar findings were observed in rabbits (Dale et al., 1965; Meier-Ruge, 1965a; François and Maudgal, 1967) and humans (Bernstein and Ginsberg, 1964; Wetterholm and Winter, 1964).

A report on miniature pigs fed chloroquine at 1000 times the human therapeutic level describes massive storage of gangliosides in the CNS and in retinal ganglion cells (Klinghardt et al., 1981). Early in the 200-day feeding program, epileptic and myoclonic fits were observed. Later "visual impairment" was observed. One wonders whether this finding is more related to the "myeloid bodies" seen in the retinal ganglion cells of experimental animals within a week of beginning chloroquine (e.g., Kolb et al., 1972) than it is to the retinotoxicity of humans.

Because of its high affinity for melanin, the mechanism of chloroquine-induced retinopathy has been related to the extremely high concentrations that are attained in the pigmented eye and that remain at these high levels (Bernstein et al., 1963b; Potts, 1964a, 1964b) long after other tissue levels have been depleted. Both hydroxychloroquine and desethylchloroquine, the major metabolite of chloroquine, behave similarly (McChesney et al., 1965, 1967). Accumulation of chloroquine in the pigmented structures of the human choroid and pigmented epithelium has been reported, and the amount depends on dosage and duration of drug therapy (Lawwill et al., 1968). In addition, small amounts of chloroquine and its metabolites are excreted in the urine years after cessation of drug treatment (Bernstein, 1967). The prolonged exposure of the retinal cell layers to chloroquine probably explains the irreversible nature of human retinopathy, which may not only progress (Okun et al., 1963) but also develop after chloroquine has been withdrawn (R. P. Burns, 1966).

Investigations concerning the primary retinotoxic lesion caused by chloroquine have led to two schools of thought. Based on the histologic and histochemical findings and the melanin-binding property of chloroquine described above, one theory indicates a primary biochemical lesion in the pigmented epithelium cell layer of the retina. It is clear that storage in pigment in itself is not a sufficient cause for toxicity. It is simply that a toxic substance such as chloroquine like any other poison increases its effect as the concentration in tissue multiplied by time of exposure ($C \times T$) increases. Storage on melanin causes enormous increases in this $C \times T$

factor for the melanin-containing tissue—in this case, the retinal pigment epithelium.

Many biochemical reactions can be inhibited by chloroquine (reviewed by Bernstein, 1967; Mackenzie, 1970). Inhibition of protein metabolism of the pigment epithelium has been proposed as the primary cause for the retinotoxic effects of chloroquine (Meier-Ruge, 1968). *In vitro* experiments utilizing only whole-pigment epithelial cells have indicated that chloroquine and hydroxychloroquine markedly inhibit amino acid incorporation in protein (Gonasun and Potts, 1972).

Phenothiazines

The potency of phenothiazines as tranquilizers is related to the chemical constituent attached to the N-atom of the three-ring base: Group I compounds processing an aminopropyl side chain are least potent; group II compounds with a piperidine group in the side chain are more potent; and group III drugs composed of a piperazine group in the side chain are the most potent antipsychotic drugs (Boet, 1970). Successful remission of psychotic states requires persistent drug therapy at relatively high doses. Therefore, it is not surprising that many side effects are associated with long-term high-dose phenothiazine therapy. Ocular complications may involve the cornea and the lens, described above, and the retina, described in this section.

Chlorpromazine
(aminopropyl side chain)

Thioridazine
(piperidyl group in the side chain)

Prochlorperazine
(piperazinyl group in the side chain)

The first phenothiazine derivative reported to alter retinal function belonged to group II: piperidylchlorophenothiazine (Sandoz NP-207). During clinical trials, the initial symptoms of visual disturbances were observed as impairment to adaptation in dim light. Further disturbances involved reduced visual acuity, constricted visual fields, and abnormal pigmentation of the retina, appearing in the periphery or macula as fine salt-and-pepper clumps of pigment (Kinross-Wright, 1956). Abnormalities in dark adaptation, color vision, and the ERG coupled with severe pigment clumping during the advanced stages indicated toxic effects in both rod and cone receptors. Disturbances of retinal function usually developed within two to three months after receiving 400 to 800 mg of the drug per day and a total of 20 to 30 g. Higher dosages required only 30 days to develop toxic symptoms. On withdrawal of the drug, some symptoms may be reversed, although pigment clumping remains visible in the fundus. However, total reversal is not possible, and in some cases, severe visual loss and blindness result. The strong evidence that NP-207 was the causative agent in these visual disturbances resulted in its removal from clinical study (Boet, 1970).

Replacement of the 2-chlorine of NP-207 with a methylmercapto group yields thioridazine, a phenothiazine derivative effective in treating schizophrenia and nonpsychotic severe anxiety without possessing some of the side effects common to the aminopropyl phenothiazines. Thioridazine also causes pigmentary and visual disturbances similar to those caused by NP-207, but dosages of over 1200 mg per day for 30 days are required to affect retinal function (Weekley *et al.*, 1960). Initially, a loss of visual acuity is observed, followed by night blindness, difficulty in adapting to average light conditions after being exposed to bright sunlight, and finally retinal pigmentary changes. In severe toxicity, excessive pigment deposition and an extinguished ERG are found. Usually, cessation of the medication is accompanied by complete or partial restoration of retinal function, although the pigmentary disturbances remain (Potts, 1968). Additional reports of thioridazine-induced retinopathy have been summarized (Siddall, 1966; Boet, 1970; Cameron et al., 1972). The dosages required to produce these retinopathies are usually in excess of the recommended therapeutic levels. Normal dosages do not cause disturbances in retinal function even after years of treatment.

The group I phenothiazine chlorpromazine is generally free from retinotoxic effects. Rare cases have been reported (Siddall, 1965, 1966, 1968) of a reversible, fine granular pigmentation in the retinal background after 2.4 g of chlorpromazine per day for two years following 1 to 2 g per day for 6 to 28 months. Only one patient recorded heavy pigmentation.

The piperazine derivatives (group III) have not been reported to affect retinal function (Duke-Elder and MacFaul, 1972). Since these drugs are the most potent phenothiazine derivatives, less drug is needed to control the psychotic individual, resulting in a lessening of side effects.

Experimentally induced phenothiazine retinopathy was accomplished by orally administering NP-207 to cats; the initial dose of 10 mg/kg/day was slowly increased to 120 mg/kg/day (Meier-Ruge and Cerletti, 1966; Cerletti and Meier-Ruge, 1967). The first retinal changes appeared as fine grayish-blackish spots on the fundus after four to five weeks of treatment. These fine granules gradually coalesced and formed irregular patches of pigment as the retinopathy became fully developed after six to seven weeks of treatment. A partial explanation for the retinal changes was made by the finding that phenothiazine derivatives accumulate in very high concentrations in the uveal tract (Potts, 1962a, 1962b). Experiments utilizing labeled chlorpromazine, prochlorperazine, and NP-207 have indicated binding of these drugs to the melanin-containing tissues of the eye, allowing high concentrations to accumulate and remain in the eye for extended periods of time (Potts, 1962a, 1962b; Green and Ellison, 1966; Cerletti and Meier-Ruge, 1967). In vitro studies employing isolated choroidal melanin granules or synthetic melanin (Potts, 1964a, 1964b) have indicated that several phenothiazine derivatives bind to melanin, therefore verifying the result obtained in vivo that tissue melanin content is the essential component responsible for concentrating these N-substituted phenothiazines. As stated above for chloroquine, concentration on pigmented structures merely gets the phenothiazine to the tissue in high concentration. Both toxic and nontoxic phenothiazines participate in this effect. After storage the specific toxic activity (possibly one of the effects detailed below) must cause tissue damage.

Histologic examination of retinas from NP-207–treated cats has shown initial posterior vacuolization of outer segments one to two weeks after retinal pigmentation, followed by disorganization of the entire lamellar structure of the disk, and finally atrophy and disintegration of the rods and cones. Other cellular layers appear normal with the exception of a proliferative pigment epithelium (Cerletti and Meier-Ruge, 1967). Histochemical enzymic analysis of the same tissues revealed an increase in lactic acid dehydrogenase activity of the Müller cells, followed shortly by a decrease of this enzyme's activity in the rod and cone ellipsoids, both changes occurring prior to retinal pigmentation and structural changes. Similar but less marked alterations were noted for glutamic dehydrogenase, glucose-6-phosphate dehydrogenase, and 6-phosphogluconate dehydrogenase activities. Loss in enzymic activities of adenosine triphosphatase, succinic acid dehydrogenase, and DPN diaphorase paralleled the loss of rods and cones (Cerletti and Meier-Ruge, 1967). An increased amount of lipid-staining material in the pigment epithelium, due to the disintegration of outer segments, an increase of glycogen in the Müller cells, and a decreased amount of phospholipid-staining material were observed shortly before major morphologic changes.

Despite the plethora of metabolic activities attributable to phenothiazines (e.g., Guth and Spirtes, 1964), none have been identified that are restricted to the retinotoxic substances and are not shown by the innocuous ones. Thus, a pathophysiologic mechanism for the toxic effect is not in hand.

Indomethacin

Administration of the antiinflammatory drug indomethacin in dosages of 50 to 200 mg per day for one to two years may result in decrease of visual acuity, visual field changes, and abnormalities in dark adaptation, ERG, and the EOG (C. A. Burns, 1966, 1968; Henkes and van Lith, 1972; Hekes et al., 1972). In one study of 34 patients (C. A. Burns, 1968), all exhibited a decreased retinal sensitivity, manifested as a lowered ERG or an altered threshold for dark adaptation. Ten of these patients had macular area disturbances, evidenced by paramacular depigmentation varying from mottled depigmentation to areas of pigment atrophy. Greater decreases in the scotopic component of the ERG than in the phototopic component have been re-

Indomethacin

ported (Palimeris *et al.,* 1972). However, except for the pigmentary disturbances, visual function improves upon cessation of drug treatment accompanied by a return to normal amplitudes in the a and b waves of the ERG.

Coupled to its antiinflammatory properties, indomethacin prevents the release of lysosomal enzymes and stabilizes liver lysosomes when exposed to labilizing conditions (Ignarro, 1972). Inhibition of Ca^{2+} accumulation in injured tissue (Northover, 1972) and Ca^{2+} influx into stimulated smooth muscle by indomethacin (Northover, 1971) have been reported. However, the role of the metabolic reactions on indomethacin-induced retinopathy is unclear, since no experimental studies have been carried out involving indomethacin and the retina.

Oxygen

The therapeutic use of oxygen in concentrations greater than in ambient air has increased during the past several years. Healthy adults can usually tolerate breathing pure oxygen for up to three hours without exhibiting any uncomfortable symptoms; however, further inhalation at atmospheric pressure or short-term inhalation of high concentrations of oxygen at 2 to 3 atmospheres results in bilateral progressive constriction of the peripheral fields, impaired central vision, mydriasis, and constriction of the retinal vasculature (Grant, 1986; Nichols and Lambertsen, 1969; Mailer, 1970). All the symptoms are reversible upon inhalation of air. Although severe retinal damage in adults is rare during hyperoxia, one case was reported concerning an individual suffering from myasthenia gravis who developed irreversible retinal atrophy after breathing 80 percent oxygen for 150 days (Kobayashi and Murakami, 1972). The retinal vasculature was markedly constricted with no blood flowing through both eyes. The vascular disorder was limited only to retinal circulation.

Although there is a dose-dependent vasocon-

striction of the retinal vessels and decrease in blood flow during hyperoxia, there is actually an increase in the oxygenation of the retina (Dollery *et al.,* 1969). Since the choriocapillaris can now supply the inner retinal layers with oxygen in addition to the supply from the retinal vessels, toxic levels of oxygen may accumulate and inhibit certain metabolic reactions essential for vision. More important, a decrease in the supply of nutrients, and especially glucose, to the visual cells results from the secondary decrease in blood flow, and only when the endogeneous supply of nutrients is metabolized and exhausted will deficiencies in vision be noticed (Nichols and Lambertsen, 1969).

A selective effect of hyperoxia on mature visual cells is exemplified by exposing adult rabbits to 100 percent oxygen for 48 hours. The result is loss of the ERG and visual cell death (Noell, 1955). Further experimentation with rabbits indicated that the centrally located rods, characterized by a low glycogen content and rich choroidal blood supply and therefore analogous to the human macula, are the most sensitive cells to oxygen toxicity (Bresnick, 1970). Peripheral rods and cones are less sensitive and spared from the toxic effects, whereas other retinal layers—the inner nuclear layer, the ganglion cell layer, and the pigmented epithelial layer—appear normal. Rods containing a single synaptic ribbon appear to be more sensitive than rods with multisynaptic ribbons. The earliest morphologic changes in the outer nuclear layer include the formation of membrane-bound vesicles in the inner segment, swelling of the endoplasmic reticulum and Golgi apparatus followed by nuclear pyknosis, mitochondrial abnormalities, degeneration of the synaptic bodies, and vesiculation of the outer segment (Bresnick, 1970).

Although adults are not seriously affected by breathing high concentrations of oxygen, this is not true for premature infants. Frequently, premature infants are placed in incubators and breathe oxygen in concentrations greater than in air. On removal from hyperoxia, they develop an irreversible bilateral ocular disease known as retrolental fibroplasia. Critical in the development of this oxygen-induced disease is the embryologic nature of the human retinal vasculature. Beginning with the fourth month of gestation, the retinal vascular system develops from the hyaloid vascular stalk in the optic nerve, and by the eighth month, the retina is vascularized only in its nasal periphery. Development into the peripheral retina is not complete until after birth of a full-term infant (Patz, 1969–70). Only the incompletely developed retinal circulation is susceptible to toxic levels of oxygen, whereas a mature retinal vascular system and other incompletely formed circulations are not sensitive to oxygen toxicity. Within six hours after an infant is placed in a high-oxygen-containing atmosphere, vasoconstriction of the immature vessels occurs, which is reversible if the child is immediately returned to air but is irreversible if hyperoxia therapy is continued (Beehler, 1964). Obliteration of the capillary lumen takes place as the vessel walls adhere to each other. This is followed by degeneration of the capillary endothelial cells and depression of the normal anterior forward growth of the retinal vessels. Immediately after returning to a normal oxygen atmosphere, vessels adjacent to the damaged area rapidly proliferate, invade the retina, penetrate the internal limiting membrane, and enter the vitreous. During the advanced stages, retinal fibrosis may cause retinal detachment. The opaque retrolental mass causes leukocoria (Beehler, 1964; Patz, 1969–70).

Experimental investigations with kittens have indicated a similar and selective degeneration and proliferation of the developing retinal capillary endothelium. The vasoconstriction and lumen obliteration are directly related to the degree of immaturity of the retinal vascular system and to the concentration and duration of exposure to oxygen (Ashton and Pedler, 1962; Ashton, 1966, 1970; Patz, 1969–70; Flower and Patz, 1971). While hyperoxia is selectively toxic to the immature retinal vascular system, no toxic effects are evident on the retina itself. Glycolytic and respiratory rates are unchanged (Graymore, 1970). These results contrast with the oxygen-induced photoreceptor atrophy observed in adult animals.

High concentrations of oxygen inhibit a number of enzymatic paths (Davies and Davies, 1965). Inhibition of respiration, electron transport, ATP synthesis, glycolysis, and a number of enzyme and coenzyme functions requiring free sulfhydryl groups for activity has been reported (reviewed by Haugaard, 1965, 1968; Menzel, 1970). The toxicity induced during maturation of the retinal vascular system, causing retrolental fibroplasia, may be explained by any of the above deficiencies, although no specific mechanism has been proposed. However, the toxicity on the mature photoreceptor cells may be explained by inhibition of glycolysis, which is essential for retinal function.

Epinephrine

In eyes that are aphakic, postcataract extraction cystoid macular edema has been described after the use of epinephrine (Kolker and Becker, 1968; Obstbaum et al., 1976). Recovery is expected but not invariable on cessation of use of the drug.

Iodate

In the preantibiotic era of the 1920s, attempts were made to combat systemic septic disease, such as septicemia, by intravenous injection of inorganic antiseptics. It was found after the use of one of these—concentrated Pregl solution, known under the trade name of Septojod®—that a number of individuals became blind (Riehm, 1927). It was demonstrated by Riehm (1929) that the primary retinal involvement was of the pigment epithelium and that this disease could be induced experimentally by injecting Septojod® into pigmented rabbits. Vito (1935) was able to demonstrate that the actual toxic agent involved was sodium iodate. However, the exact way in which iodate causes degeneration and the reason for the particular susceptibility of the pigment epithelium have not been adequately worked out. Although iodate is known to be a relatively stable oxidizing agent, and though the probability of this mechanism of action is reinforced by the fact that the iodate effect can be completely neutralized by the reducing agent, cysteine (Sorsby and Harding, 1960), the effect has not been reproduced by other oxidizing agents, such as manganese dioxide, perborate, and persulfate (Sorsby, 1941). It is true, however, that none of these agents has the relative stability of iodate, and a dose comparable with that of iodate could not be given intravenously without killing the experimental animals.

Various experiments verified a primary effect of iodate on the pigment epithelium cell layer, followed by a secondary lesion and degeneration of the rod outer segments. Within hours after the administration of iodate, the thickness of the pigment epithelium layer is reduced, accompanied by loss of cellular limits, loss of definition, and formation of a granular cytoplasm (Garymore, 1970). Since the pigment epithelium cell layer lies between the choroidal vasculature and photoreceptors, it is responsible for exchange of nutrients and metabolites from the blood to the visual cells. Iodate-induced interruption in this flow of nutrients by possibly affecting the energy supply of the pigment epithelium or the rhodopsin cycle in the pigment epithelium would subsequently lead to photoreceptor degeneration.

Sparsomycin

The antibiotic sparsomycin, prepared from *Streptomyces sparsogenes*, is useful as an anticancer drug. One report (McFarlane et al., 1966) described two patients who received sparsomycin intravenously and developed pigmentary disturbances corresponding to bilateral ring scotomas. The total dose was 12 and 7.5 mg over a period of 13 to 15 days, respectively. Postmortem histologic examination of the eyes disclosed primary degeneration of the pigment epithelium and a closely associated secondary degeneration of the rods and cones, with a decrease in the acid mucopolysaccharide content of the damaged areas. As an inhibitor of protein synthesis, sparsomycin exerts its action by inhibiting peptide bond formation in both bacterial, mammalian (Trakatellis, 1968; I. H. Goldberg and Friedman, 1971), and human test systems (Neth and Winkler, 1972); but whether a similar effect occurs in the pigment epithelium as part of the sparsomycin-induced visual disturbances is not known.

Retinoids

Derivatives of the naturally occurring retinol, retinal, retinoic acid family appear to be useful in dermatological disease but not without some ocular side effects. Isoretinoin, which is 13-cis retinoic acid, is effective against cystic acne, but a small percentage of patients develop poor night vision and glare sensitivity (Weleber et al., 1986). Although various tests of retinal function show abnormalities, there is no correlation between the medication and a single test. Etretinate is an aromatic retinoid, effective against acne. However, a few patients show decreased rod sensitivity, reduced amplitudes of the scotopic ERG, and a deutan color vision abnormality (Weber et al., 1988). The hypothesis that the drug substitutes for the retinoids of the normal photoreceptors has yet to be substantiated.

Tamoxifen

This drug, which is a triphenyl ethylene derivative, has marked antiestrogen properties and appears to be effective in certain circumstances against carcinoma of the breast. Kaiser-Kupfer and Lippman (1978) reported perimacular deposits and macular edema in four patients who had received high doses of tamoxifen for more than a year. Vinding and Nielsen (1983) reported similar lesions in 2 of 17 patients who received tamoxifen at a total dose some 10 percent of that reported previously. The nature of these lesions in uncertain.

In addition, both sets of authors describe subepithelial corneal deposits of granules in a whorl configuration. This corneal phenomenon is most reminiscent of the findings in patients receiving the antiarrythmic drug amiodarone (Wilson et al., 1980; Hirst et al., 1982; Kaplan and Cappaert, 1982). The present reviewer has observed several such cases and is convinced that the whorls originate because the drug is relatively insoluble in tears and that the whorls are created by the successive positions of the lid margins as the tear film evaporates.

Experimental Retinopathy

Iodoacetate. An important technique used in examining metabolic interrelationships between the different cell layers in the retina and also in determining which cells contribute to the components of the electroretinogram is to destroy selectively individual cell layers in experimental animals. A most potent tool for such studies is iodoacetate, which in carefully controlled doses rapidly and thoroughly obliterates receptor cells in rabbits (Schubert and Bornschein, 1951; Noell, 1952).

Graymore and Tansley (1959) were able to reproduce the effect in rats with the help of sodium maleate in addition to the iodoacetate. Examination of the fundus of rabbits, cats, or monkeys indicates the development of a grayish retinal opacity after the first day of treatment, which persists for about a week. Retinal pigmentation, superficially similar to human retinitis pigmentosa, appears about a week following the initial dose. Electron microscopic examination of rabbit retinas indicates lesions in the rod and cone outer segments within three hours after treatment with iodoacetate in albino rabbits and within 12 hours after iodoacetate treatment in pigmented rabbits with marked disintegration of outer segments in albinos observed after 12 hours (Lasansky and de Robertis, 1959). Disorganization of the outer segment through vesiculation and lysis of the membrane structure is accompanied by swelling and vacuolization of the endoplasmic reticulum and Golgi apparatus in the inner segment, by disintegration of mitochondria in the ellipsoid, by pyknosis of the nuclei, and by lysis of the synaptic vessicles. Widespread capillary closure rapidly follows destruction of the photoreceptor cell layer (Dantzker and Gerstein, 1969). Iodoacetate causes an irreversible decrease in the amplitudes of the a, b, and c waves of the electroretinogram (Noell, 1959; François et al., 1969a). All the evidence indicates a selective retinotoxic effect of iodoacetate on the photoreceptor cells since even one week after a small dose both the pigment epithelium and inner nuclear cell layers are intact (Dantzker and Gerstein, 1969).

The mechanism of iodoacetate-induced retinopathy may be twofold. Iodoacetate inhibits glyceraldehyde-3-phosphate dehydrogenase and therefore prevents the conversion of 1,3-diphosphoglyceraldehyde into 1,3-glyceric acid, a necessary reaction in pyruvate and lactate production during the glycolytic catabolism of glucose (Noell, 1959). Glycolysis provides the major source of energy to the photoreceptor cells, and inhibition of this reaction would necessarily lead to cell destruction. Moreover, anerobic glycolysis was inhibited 75 percent after ten minutes of treatment with iodoacetate in a dose that yielded visual cell damage (Graymore, 1970). However, this theory is inconsistent with other experimental observations. The ERG is diminished within minutes after infusion of iodoacetate (Noell, 1959), and decreases in enzyme activity do not always appear prior to morphologic and structural changes of these cells. Alteration in the free sulfhydryl group content of the visual cells has been reported (Reading and Sorsby, 1966), suggesting that damage to the membrane structure of the photoreceptor cells and outer segments may be the primary retinotoxic effect of iodoacetate. An additional effect on glycolysis may contribute to the irreversible nature of iodoacetate toxicity.

Dithizone. Administration of the diabetogenic (Kadota, 1950; Okamoto, 1955) chemical dithizone intravenously to rabbits in doses be-

Dithizone (diphenylthiocarbazone)

tween 17.5 and 40 mg/kg causes retinal lesions (Grignolo et al., 1952; Weitzel et al., 1954; Sorsby and Harding, 1960). Ophthalmoscopic and histologic examination reveal severe retinal edema developing within 24 to 48 hours, followed by the appearance of red islets indicating recovery from edema and pigmentary disturbances in the fundus. When the edema finally disappears, usually in six to eight days, the irregular pigmentation has spread throughout the retina (Sorsby and Harding, 1962). While the rabbit receptors appear to be the cell layer most sensitive to dithizone toxicity, there is swelling of the nerve fiber layer. The diffuseness of the lesion is reflected in the decreased amplitudes of the ERG and the EOG (Babel and Ziv, 1957, 1959; François et al., 1969a), initially observed as a suppression of the c-wave (Wirth et al., 1957) and b-wave amplitudes (Babel and Ziv, 1957). Eventually, the entire ERG is completely obliterated. Finally, as the retina becomes disorganized, optic atrophy (François et al., 1969b) and proliferation of the pigment epithelium (Karli, 1963) are observed. Pretreatment of rabbits with cysteine does not protect against the retinotoxic action of dithizone as it does against iodate and iodoacetate poisoning (Sorsby and Harding,

1960). This suggests a difference in mechanisms between the three retinotoxic agents.

Dithizone-induced retinopathy appears to be species-specific, developing in those species possessing a tapetum, for example, dogs and rabbits, but not developing in those species lacking a tapetum, for example, rats, monkeys (Budinger, 1961; Delahunt et al., 1962), and man. A possible relationship, at least in the dog, has been suggested (Weitzel et al., 1954; Budinger, 1961; Delahunt et al., 1962) between the Zn^{2+}-chelating properties of dithizone and retinal degeneration. Dithizone depletes the canine tapetum of its rich supply of Zn^{2+}, leading to severe tapetal necrosis, retinal edema, and finally loss of retinal structure and function. On the other hand, in the rabbit, an early decrease of ERG amplitude and swelling of the neuroepithelium followed rapidly by complete retinal disorganization suggest that additional factors are involved in dithizone retinopathy. Experiments with ethambutol, another zinc chelator, show that tapetal zinc in dogs is lowered by an amount comparable with the lowering caused by dithizone. The green color of the tapetum is lost, but no retinopathy results (Figueroa et al., 1971). Possible interference in the active transport of ions from the choriocapillaris through the pigment epithelium (François et al., 1969b) and alterations in the total and free sulfhydryl group content resulting from protein denaturation (Reading and Sorsby, 1966) have been reported. A similar compound, sodium diethyldithiocarbamate, not only causes tapetal necrosis in dogs but also inhibits oxygen consumption, pyruvate utilization, and citrate synthesis (DuBois et al., 1961) in liver and kidney. Perhaps dithizone exerts a similar inhibitory effect on retinal metabolism.

Diaminodiphenoxyalkanes. A set of toxic substances that appear to be specific for pigment epithelium is the family of the diaminodiphenoxyalkanes.

The series, in which $n = 5$, 6, and 7 are the most active, was originally synthesized for schistosomacidal properties. No human use was ever reported, but in susceptible animals—monkey, dog, and cat—a single oral or intravenous dose causes eventual pigmented retinopathy (Edge et al., 1956; Sorsby and Nakajima, 1958) and complete loss of the electroretinogram within a few days (Nakajima, 1958). There is selective action on the pigmented epithelium, but when these cells are destroyed, the overlying receptor cells also degenerate (Ashton, 1957). This is like the iodate situation above.

An approach to the mechanism of toxic action was begun when Glocklin and Potts (1962) showed that uptake of ^{32}P into acid-soluble phosphorus fractions was inhibited by diaminodiphenoxyheptane in pigment epithelium *in vitro* but not in neuroretina.

THE GANGLION CELL LAYER AND OPTIC NERVE

General Considerations

The attribute that separates the ganglion cell (Figure 17–1) from the remainder of the retina is that it is the cell body of a neuron that extends into the depth of the central nervous system. The axons from the ganglion cell layer form the nerve fiber layer of the retina and exit from the eye at the optic papilla. Most of the fibers, carrying visual information, travel some 120 mm from the globe via optic nerve, optic chiasm, and optic tract to the point where they synapse in the lateral geniculate body of the midbrain. Like any other central nervous system neuron, the optic nerve fiber degenerates in both directions from a cut. Thus, the ganglion cell of the retina may be damaged by direct action upon it, the cell body, or it may degenerate secondary to toxic destruction of the optic nerve. Instances of both types of damage will be cited below.

A second unique property of the ganglion cell-optic nerve is its behavior as a physiologically dual structure. The central 5 percent of the field of vision is the sole portion that possesses high visual acuity. This corresponds to an area of retinal receptors of 1.5-mm diameter centered on the fovea centralis. Although there is considerable preprocessing of visual information in the retina, there is still correspondence between receptor location and ganglion cell type or ganglion cell location or both. The result of this is that the information from that central-most acute 5 percent of visual field runs in an identifiable bundle of fibers—the so-called papillomacular bundle—whose position can be identified by myelin degeneration stains at each position in the optic nerve and optic tract after damage to the central retina (Brouwer and Zeeman, 1926). Moreover, this fiber bundle acts as a separate entity in its behavior toward a number of toxic substances as well as toward some diseases.

It is not clear why this should be the case. We do know that papillomacular fibers are predominantly small fibers (Potts *et al.*, 1972). It is possible that these fibers with the greatest ratio of surface area to volume have the highest metabolic demand of all optic nerve fibers.

However, in the case of some toxic substances the papillomacular bundle is spared and the peripheral fibers are hit. Thus, it appears that specific chemical affinities may play a role. The opposite effect, the loss of the peripheral visual field to the action of a toxic substance, may not represent a case of selective affinity at all. If the substance has its primary action on the ganglion cell, and if there is uniform loss of absolute number of cells across the entire retinal area, the peripheral retina will be wiped out. The macular area will survive with at most a decrease in acuity, because there are so many more cells in the macular area. However this may be, some toxic substances affect the ganglion cell body; others affect the fibers of the papillomacular bundle; others affect peripheral fibers only. In each case, death of a portion of the neuron means death of the entire neuron and loss of that specific information transmission channel. To take cognizance of this attribute where damage to a retinal cell body can cause loss of function through an entire tract, we will designate this section as dealing with the ganglion cell neuron (GCN).

One other special consideration deals with a clinical entity, pallor of the disk. When any considerable number of optic nerve fibers die, their lack of demand for nutrition is somehow conveyed to the surrounding capillaries. These disappear over a period of months. In the one place where optic nerve capillaries may be inspected with ease, the optic papilla, the nerve head becomes abnormally pale on ophthalmoscopic inspection, owing to loss of capillary supply. There is a very good correlation between the pallor observed after the loss of a large number of fibers and optic atrophy. This has reached the point where many clinicians report "optic atrophy" on ophthalmoscopic examination when they mean "pale disk." Such an examination in marginal cases or done by a poor observer could lead to erroneous results. It is important for the reader of a report on toxicology to know whether the description of optic atrophy is a clinical or a histologic one.

Specific Substances

Methanol. A well-publicized and uniquely American poison affecting the GCN is methanol. The first practical distillation process that created a preparation potable by the unwary and the clinical report of the first 275 cases of methanol poisoning appeared in the United States (Wood and Buller, 1904). Whenever access to ethanol has been restricted, as in prohibition or in wartime, the incidence of methanol poisoning has risen, and epidemics centering on some local source of supply are reported in significant number. The characteristic results of an epidemic are that a third of those exposed to methanol recover with no residues, a third have severe visual loss or blindness, and a third die. Thus, in sufficiently high doses methanol has profound systemic effects. Studies in the 1950s showed that methanol poisoning was a primate disease (Gilger and Potts, 1955) and that it was a palimpsest of three different diseases (Potts et al., 1955). Those diseases are (1) organic solvent poisoning (which is the only disease the subprimates show), (2) systemic acidosis, and (3) central nervous system effects, including changes in the eye and the basal ganglia. It was shown that the LD90 for primates gave only transient solvent toxicity signs and that a lucid interval set in, followed by systemic acidosis. Acidosis was enough to kill the animal unless it was combatted with base. If the acidosis was treated, the animal died later of the CNS disease. In many monkeys at the peak of the CNS signs, retinal edema was a common finding. In its most severe form, it covered the entire retina and produced the rhesus equivalent of the cherry-red spot.

Because methanol poisoning in humans is a medical emergency and it is usually impossible to determine the dose ingested, this kind of unified picture is difficult to come by. However, all the phases seen in the rhesus disease are seen in human disease, even to the basal ganglion lesion (Orthner, 1950).

The specific eye effects are definite as far as they go. Everyone agrees that nerve-head pallor is a constant finding in human cases who recover from methanol poisoning with permanent visual impairment. In monkeys, marked demyelination of temporal retina has been demonstrated, along with marginal loss of ganglion cells (Potts et al., 1955). Thus, optic atrophy is a definite finding in methanol poisoning, but there is some question of whether the disease is primary in the ganglion cell layer. Arguments in favor are the observed retinal edema in the acute phase and the finding of loss of ganglion cells. Arguments against are lack of ganglion cell loss reported by McGregor (1943) and Orthner (1950).

The proximal toxic agent is generally accepted to be the methanol oxidation product formaldehyde (Potts, 1952; Cooper and Kini, 1962). It has now been established after some controversy that the mechanism of oxidation of methanol differs in primates and subprimates. In primates the principal metabolic pathway is via alcohol dehydrogenase (Kini and Cooper, 1961). In subprimates the favored pathway is via the catalase system (Tephly et al., 1963). It is tempting to attribute the primate nature of methanol poisoning to some difference in availability of formal-

dehyde from alcohol dehydrogenase oxidation. This does not seem to be the case. In unpublished results from our laboratory, equal amounts of ^{14}C label from $^{14}CH_3OH$ are bound to eye and brain in rabbits and monkeys.

The report of Martin-Amat et al. (1978) that optic disk edema may be produced by infusions of formate in the monkey reopens the question of the proximal toxic agent in methanol poisoning. Since their experimental conditions require constant infusions of formate, it is difficult to design an experiment of long-enough duration to determine whether the other criteria observed in human methanol poisoning can be met—that is, death with destruction of the basal ganglia. Clearly, more work on the one-carbon metabolism of the primate is called for.

The treatment of methanol poisoning involves both combatting acidosis and preventing methanol oxidation. With the general availability of hemodialysis in the United States, prompt hemodialysis appears to be the method of choice in preventing methanol oxidation by removing it from the body. For a review of the literature on human cases treated by hemodialysis, see Gonda et al. (1978). Comparison of small groups of patients by Keyvan-Larijarni and Tannenberg (1974) appears to demonstrate that peritoneal dialysis is measurably less effective than hemodialysis.

Where dialysis is not available or is delayed, prevention of methanol oxidation may be achieved by administration of ethanol, which competes successfully for alcohol dehydrogenase. This allows time for methanol to be excreted unoxidized in urine and breath. The value of ethanol administration during dialysis is marginal because it is removed from blood at about the same rate as methanol. However, since dialysis requires a finite time for completion, there may be some benefit in attempting to maintain a blood ethanol level.

It was suggested by Gilger and coworkers (1956) that treatment for a 70-kg man be 4.5 oz of 50 percent ethanol initially, followed by 3.0 oz every four hours for 48 hours or until blood methanol reached negligible levels. In a number of sporadic cases, this has appeared to be effective therapy.

A curious addendum to the methanol literature in the 1980s was caused by the rediscovery of the typical lesions of the basal ganglia. These had been described by Orthner in humans (Orthner, 1950) and in monkeys by this author (Potts et al., 1955) some 30 years earlier. The new factor was the availability of the computerized tomography (CT) scan. With it there was no prerequisite for a fatal outcome plus autopsy. Neurologists examining survivors of severe methanol poisoning became aware for the first time of diminished density in the region of the putamen. They correlated this finding with the observation of extrapyramidal symptoms and with typical hemorrhagic necrosis in the basal ganglia of those patients who did come to autopsy (Bourrat *et al.*, 1986; Henze *et al.*, 1986; Wagner, 1986; Friedman *et al.*, 1987; Guillaume *et al.*, 1987; Rosenberg, 1987; Betta and Forno, 1988; Koopmans *et al.*, 1988; Phang *et al.*, 1988).

It may be that at long last the information conveyed by rhesus experiments will be appreciated. Methanol poisoning can only be understood as the composite of three separate diseases.

Ethambutol. This substance was found by *in vivo* screening to be most effective against

$$CH_2OH \diagdown \qquad\qquad\qquad C_2H_5$$
$$\qquad HC-HN-(CH_2)_2-NH-CH \diagup \quad \cdot 2HCl$$
$$C_2H_5 \diagup \qquad\qquad\qquad CH_2OH$$
d-2-2'-(Ethylenediimino)-di-1-butanol dihydrochloride

tuberculosis in mice (J. P. Thomas *et al.*, 1961). The drug, because of its relatively good tolerance and its efficacy against isoniazid-resistant tuberculosis, has become an established member of the antituberculosis armamentarium. In some 10 percent of patients receiving 25 to 50 mg/kg/day, loss of vision appears one to seven months after start of dosage (Carr and Henkind, 1962; Place and Thomas, 1963). (For a thorough review of human and animal toxicity, see Leibold, 1966; Place *et al.*, 1966; Schmidt, 1966.)

The typical toxic phenomenon is "retrobulbar neuritis" in the sense that there is visual field involvement without obvious swelling of the nerve head. However, in addition to central scotoma, which is thought of as the typical finding in retrobulbar neuritis, a smaller proportion of patients show loss of peripheral field with preservation of central vision (Leibold, 1966). All visual symptoms are dose-related. Figures collected from various sources in the literature by Citron (1969) suggest:

DOSAGE (mg/kg/day)	CASES	INCIDENCE OF COMPLICATIONS
50	60	15%
>35	59	18%
<30	59	5%
25	130	3%
15	—	Negligible

Visual disturbances appear to regress completely on cessation of drug administration.

The mechanism of therapeutic action and the mechanism of toxicity are far from clear. Etham-

butol is a chelating agent that will remove zinc from the tapetum lucidum of dogs. However, it does not cause the pigmentary retinopathy that a chelating agent such as dithizone causes (Figueroa *et al.*, 1971). When *Mycobacterium smegmatis* is used as a model for *M. tuberculosis*, ethambutol-inhibited cells become deficient in RNA. As a consequence, protein synthesis is inhibited (Forbes *et al.*, 1965). A recent recommendation of substituting biweekly high-dose therapy for daily intermediate-dose therapy is said to eliminate visual system toxicity (Trumbull *et al.*, 1977).

Carbon Disulfide. This inflammable and volatile liquid (BP = 46.3°C) was important in the past as a solvent for sulfur in the rubber industry and as a solvent for alkali-treated cellulose in the viscose process for rayon and cellophane. Improved ventilation and substitution of other solvents have made classical carbon disulfide poisoning a thing of the past. The impressive complex of central scotoma, drop in visual acuity, widespread peripheral neuritis, personality changes, vascular encephalopathy, and generalized arteriosclerosis with cardiovascular and renal sequelae is not seen. However, there are recent disquieting reports from Japan and from Finland of subtle eye effects, seen at solvent levels that do not produce the classic symptoms, and that until now were thought to be safe (Raitta and Tolonen, 1980; Sugimoto and Goto, 1980).

Curiously, the retinopathy seen in Japan, which consists of microaneurysms and small hemorrhages, was not observed in Finnish workers to exceed the incidence in controls. In Finland the positive findings were delayed peripapillary filling on fluorescein angiography, widening of retinal arterioles, and lower peak to the ocular pulse wave. Clearly, carbon disulfide in industry needs another look.

A curious aspect of CS_2 poisoning is the lack of correspondence between anatomic and physiologic findings (Birch-Hirschfeld, 1900; Ide, 1958). One possible reason for this is restriction of the experimental situation to rodents, which do not appear to have a dual optic nerve. Much experimentation will be required to exploit the little we now know of carbon disulfide poisoning.

Thallium. Considerable clinical experience in thallium poisoning has arisen from use of thallous acetate in the 1920s as an epilating agent by dermatologists and its use as a rat poison (Celio Paste®) with consequent accidental and intentional poisonings. For a short time in the early 1930s, a cosmetic depilatory cream (Koremlu®) caused additional chronic cases. (For reviews of this material, *see* Heyroth, 1947;

Prick *et al.*, 1955). Systemic symptoms in thallium poisoning include gastroenteritis, polyneuritis, and allopecia. Ocular involvement is cataract, especially in rats, and optic neuritis in humans.

The unifying concept that made the behavior of lens and optic nerve understandable was developed in the 1960s when it became apparent that thallous ion is in many ways a stand-in for potassium ion. For a review of this, see Gehring and Hammond (1967). The University of Chicago laboratory was able to show that lens and optic nerve, two high-potassium tissues, were also able to store Tl^+ (Potts and Au, 1971). The ionic similarities are great enough that Tl^+ can activate (Na^+-K^+)-activated ATPase (Britten and Blank, 1968). Kinsey and coworkers (1971) demonstrated that thallous ion accumulation in lens was by active transport and by the alkali metal–transporting system. An additional and unexpected finding was high storage of Tl^+ in melanin-containing eye structures (Potts and Au, 1971). Although Tl^+ can act for K^+ in many systems, it is clear that it cannot do so in every case. It seems logical that accumulation of thallium where potassium should normally be, without its being able to substitute for potassium in every enzyme system, is the basis for thallium toxicity. It is not clear which parts of the GCN are most affected.

Needless to say, prophylaxis is the only practical therapy in thallium poisoning.

Pentavalent Arsenic. Pentavalent arsenicals have been found in the past to be effective against trypanosomiasis (H. W. Thomas, 1905).

$$NaO-\overset{\overset{\displaystyle OH}{|}}{\underset{\underset{\displaystyle O}{\|}}{As}}-\bigcirc-NH_2$$

Sodium arsanilate (Atoxyl®)

$$NaO-\overset{\overset{\displaystyle OH}{|}}{\underset{\underset{\displaystyle O}{\|}}{As}}-\bigcirc-NH-CH_2-C\overset{\displaystyle O}{\underset{\displaystyle NH_2}{}}$$

Sodium *N*-(carbamoylmethyl)-arsanilate (Tryparsamide®)

The same ability to pass the blood-brain barrier that allowed effectiveness against trypanosomes also made possible treatment of neurosyphilis. Numerous derivatives of sodium arsanilate were synthesized by Ehrlich in his early investigations of trypanocidal and spirochetocidal activity. Tryparsamide®, a substance of relatively low toxicity, was synthesized

at the Rockefeller Institute (W. A. Jacobs and Heidelberger, 1919) and introduced into tropical medicine shortly thereafter (Pearce, 1921). Tryparsamide® was then found effective against neurosyphilis (Henrichsen, 1939).

Eye effects were a constant accompaniment of the use of pentavalent arsenicals and were a prime reason for their eventual abandonment. The clinical figures of Neujean and coworkers (1948) suggest that 3 to 4 percent of trypanosomiasis cases treated with Tryparsamide® show visual effects, and a third of these—for example, 1 percent of all cases—show peripheral contraction of visual fields. There are anatomic findings to accompany the clinical symptoms, and here the peripheral area of the ganglion cell layer is most severely involved (Birch-Hirschfeld and Köster, 1910). There is considerable evidence that at the cellular level all the arsenicals reach the same oxidation state, whatever their form at introduction (P. Ehrlich, 1909).

Interest has been maintained in organic arsenicals in recent years by the finding that when they are included in the feed of poultry and swine at an optimal level, the animals thrive and gain weight. Errors on the farm can expose the animals and the growers to a toxic hazard. Studies like the thesis of Ledet (1979) should be extended.

Quinine. Although the massive use of quinine decreased abruptly with the advent of new synthetic antimalarials in the 1940s, plasmodia resistant to these new compounds appeared rapidly. Quinine is the drug of choice in these situations (Nieuwveld *et al.*, 1982). Thus, quinine has an established place in today's pharmacopoeia. An additional therapeutic effect is said to be relief of nocturnal recumbancy leg cramps. The availability of the drug allows ingestion in excessive doses for intended abortion and intended suicide as in the past. Hence, quinine poisoning is still with us, as are the poorly understood eye effects.

It is now clear that there are two dosage levels at which quinine (and its congeners) may be toxic. The first is a very low level caused by a single dose of as little as 12 mg (Belkin, 1967). The symptoms are those of thrombocytopenic purpura. The cause is an immune reaction in which the drug acts as a haptene. This phenomenon was treated exhaustively by Shulman (1958) where the offender was quinidine. The visual system is affected as much or as little as it would be in purpura caused by any other haptene. Its blood vessels are subject to hemorrhage secondary to thrombocytopenia as any set of vessels would be, but there is no specific selectivity for the eye.

The usual therapeutic regime for malaria is 1.3

g/day in four divided doses for seven days. Experiments on human volunteers have shown that eye effects of blurring, decrease of visual acuity, and loss of peripheral field occur with single doses of 2.5 to 4.0 g (Duke-Elder and MacFaul, 1972). A single dose of 8.0 can be fatal. It is doses of 2.5 g and above that have specific eye effects. The eye effects have been attributed by some to arteriolar constriction, by others to direct action on the ganglion cell body, and by still others to effects on the whole retina. See the reports of François et al. (1967), Cibis et al. (1973), Brinton et al. (1980), and Gangitano and Keltner (1980) for the various arguments adduced and additional literature reviews. In cats given a sublethal dose of quinine sulfate, early electroretinographic changes that show whole-retina involvement are transient. Early peripapillary and retinal edema, which suggests ganglion cell involvement, is also transient. The earliest anatomic changes that become permanent are pyknosis and then generalized loss of retinal ganglion cells. This is almost certainly the locus of high-dose specific eye effects.

Hemodialysis has been recommended as the treatment of choice, but some reservations are expressed by Dickinson et al. (1981).

Glutamate. An experimental entity involving the ganglion cell neuron is glutamate poisoning. Lucas and Newhouse (1957) reported that administration of high doses of sodium 1-glutamate to suckling mice caused degeneration of the retinal ganglion cell layer and failure of formation of the inner nuclear layer. Freedman and Potts (1962) were able to reproduce this phenomenon in newborn albino rats. They showed that glutaminase I was repressed in the retinas of these animals and postulated this as the mechanism of glutamate toxicity.

Later work has revealed an extensive series of compounds related to glutamate that have neuroexcitatory or neurotoxic properties or both. The term "excitotoxin," which implies that there is a relation between the two properties, has been coined. At all events, the entire subject area is in flux; some feel for this may be obtained from the review of Olney (1982).

Perhaps most important is the fact that whereas glutamate affects the developing retina only, some of the newer compounds cause selective cell loss when injected intravitreally in mature animals. This represents no human hazard but promises to be a powerful experimental tool. DL-2-Aminoadipic acid, the next higher homolog of glutamic, destroys Müller cells and in high doses causes swelling of astrocytes and oligodendrocytes (Pedersen and Karlsen, 1979; Ishikawa and Mine, 1983). Kainic acid, a sterically hindered analogue of glutamic acid, destroys the "displaced amacrine cells" of the chicken retina (D. Ehrlich and Morgan, 1980).

In research performed during World War II on the vesicant methyl nitrosocarbamate (see section on vesicant gases, nitrosamines), it was found that there was selective chromatolysis and destruction of the retinal ganglion cell layer. The experiments were done in cats allowed to inhale

$$Cl-CH_2-CH_2-N-\overset{\displaystyle O}{\overset{\|}{C}}-OCH_3$$
$$\underset{N=O}{|}$$

Methyl N-β-chlorethyl-N-nitrosocarbamate

the vapor at a concentration of 50 μg/liter for ten minutes (Gates and Renshaw, 1946). The compound is an alkylating agent like the nitrogen mustards, and it alkylates functional groups of proteins and nucleic acids in a more or less random manner. Unlike the amino acid series described above, this compound represents a hazard to its user during synthesis and during exposure of the test animal.

SMON. Special mention should be made of the optic nerve damage (accompanying widespread demyelination in the CNS) caused by 7-iodo-5-chloro-8-hydroxyquinoline, iodochlorhydroxyquin known as Clioquinol®. Entero-Vioform®, and Vioform®.

The drug is an effective amebicide and is useful in the treatment of amebiasis when given at the level of 500 to 750 mg three times a day for ten days. An eight-day interval must be observed before a second ten-day course is given.

However, this drug has been available over the counter outside the United States principally to combat "traveler's diarrhea" where a specific diagnosis has not been made and where physician control of dosage is lacking. Particularly in Japan, an entity has been recognized and labeled "subacute myeloopticoneuropathy" (SMON) attributable to use of this substance. It is said that from 1955 to 1970, 10,000 cases of SMON were diagnosed in Japan. A national commission was formed by the Japanese government, and in 1970 the sale of the drug was prohibited. For a bibliography of the Japanese literature, see Shigematsu (1975).

The entity is characterized clinically by paresthesias and numbness of the extremities, ataxia, and weakness in the legs. Twenty-seven percent of SMON patients have visual disturbances attributed to demyelination of the optic nerve (Sobue and Ando, 1971).

The extremely high incidence in Japan has not been explained satisfactorily. High dosage levels, additive effects of environmental pollutants, and as-yet-unidentified factors have all been invoked. A representative of the manufacturer claims that since 1935 only 50 cases of SMON with a history of iodochlorhydroxyquin consumption have been identified in the rest of the world (Burley, 1977).

The disease can be reproduced in experimental animals by feeding the drug, and optic nerve demyelination is demonstrable in dogs and cats (Tateishi and Otsuki, 1975).

ORGANOMERCURIALS

Metallic mercury has been recognized to present a relatively low-level hazard to the individual and the eye. The eye does not appear to be involved in poisoning by inorganic salts of mercury. This is treated well by Grant (1986). The marked toxicity of organic compounds of mercury and their effect on vision have been known since the report of Edwards (1865), but this remained a laboratory caution until the multiple epidemics of the last decades. The presently accepted site of damage to the visual system puts the subject beyond the avowed scope of this chapter, but its importance requires that it be treated here.

Epidemics of organomercurial poisoning have originated in two major and diverse manners. The earliest cases of both series were found in 1956. The subtler, hence the more difficult, of the two to identify occurred in Japan, and in retrospect cases seen in 1951 were part of the epidemic. To summarize years of active research sponsored by the Japanese government, the hazard originated when metallic mercury, used as a catalyst in the acetaldehyde plant near Minamata Bay, was discharged into the bay as waste sludge. The aquatic plant life in the bay was able to convert elemental mercury to organomercurials, especially to methyl mercury. The fish and shellfish of the bay acquired methyl mercury from the plants and the contaminated water. The local inhabitants, many of whom were fishermen, were poisoned by the contaminated seafood and began to present with neurologic complaints at the local hospitals. In February 1963, the disease was identified as organomercurial poisoning. From 1965 to 1974, a series of 520 patients was seen in Nigata prefecture who were identified as having organomercurial poisoning. The source of the epidemic was a similar factory. The excellent account of the findings edited by Tsubaki and Irukayama (1977), entitled *Minamata Disease,* is a model of reporting.

The second type of epidemic arose in multiple sites and always with the same causation. Seed grain treated with an organomercurial antifungal agent was used by peasant farmers to make bread. Iraq had epidemics in 1956, 1960, and 1971–72 (Bakir *et al.,* 1973). The last caused 6530 cases admitted to hospitals, of whom 459 died. Similar but lesser outbreaks are recorded for Guatemala in 1963 to 1965, for Pakistan in 1961 and 1969, and Ghana in 1967.

The textbook description of organomercurial poisoning is that of Hunter, Bomford, and Russell (1940); the disease complex is often designated "Hunter-Russell syndrome." The components are: (1) ataxia, (2) impairment of speech, and (3) constriction of visual field. The Minamata cases also showed a high incidence of hearing loss and somatosensory change.

Histopathology was done on monkeys by Hunter *et al.* and by Shaw *et al.* (1975) and by Takeuchi and Ito (1977) (in Tsubaki and Irukayama, 1977) on the Minamata deaths. All of them agree that eye findings are negligible and that the major and consistent finding is necrosis of neurons in the cerebral cortex, particularly in the depth of the sulci, and most particularly in the calcarine fissure of the visual cortex.

Clinically, there is some description of disk hyperemia, and later disk pallor in Iraqi patients (Sabelaish and Hilmi, 1976). A curious and disturbing finding is the remarkable bilateral symmetry of the reported visual field defects, presumably caused by two parallel but separate pathologic events in the right and left calcarine cortex. One might expect some asymmetry and some difference in projection of the two hemifields to the right and left eye. This has not been reported.

REFERENCES

Alghadyan, A. A.; Peyman, G. A.; Khoobehi, B.; and Lin, K. R: Liposome-bound cyclosporine: retinal toxicity after intravitreal injection. *Int. Ophthalmol.,* **12**:105–107, 1988.

Andermann, G., and Erhart, M.: Are local tolerance tests in animals always necessary? *Methods Find. Exp. Clin. Pharmacol.,* **5**:321–333, 1983.

Anderson, B.: Corneal and conjunctival pigmentation among workers engaged in the manufacture of hydroquinone. *Arch. Ophthalmol.,* **38**:812–826, 1947.

Anderson, J. A.: Chen, C. C.; Vita, J. B.; and Shackleton, M.: Disposition of topical flurbiprofen in normal and aphakic rabbit eyes. *Arch. Ophthalmol.,* **100**:642–645, 1982.

Armaly, M.: Effect of corticosteroids on intraocular pressure and fluid dynamics. *Arch. Ophthalmol.,* **70**:482–491, 492–499, 1963.

Ashton, N.: Degeneration of the retina due to 1 : 5-di(*p*-aminophenoxy) pentane dihydrochloride. *J. Pathol. Bacteriol.,* **74**:103–112, 1961.

———: Oxygen and the growth and development of retinal vessels: *in vivo* and *in vitro* studies. *Am. J. Ophthalmol.,* **62**:412–435, 1966.

———: Some aspects of the comparative pathology of oxygen toxicity in the retina. *Ophthalmologica.,* **160**:54–71, 1970.

Ashton, N., and Pedler, C.: Studies on developing retinal vessels. IX. Reaction of endothelial cells to oxygen. *Br. J. Ophthalmol.,* **46**:257–276, 1962.

Avigan, J.; Steinberg, D.; Vroman, H. E.; Thompson,

M. J.; and Mosettig, E.: Studies on cholesterol biosynthesis. I. The identification of desmosterol in serum and tissues of animals and man treated with MER-29. *J. Biol. Chem.*, **235**:3123–3126, 1960.

Axelsson, U., and Holmberg, A.: The frequency of cataract after miotic therapy. *Acta Ophthalmol.*, **44**:421–429, 1966.

Babel, J., and Ziv, B.: L'action du dithizone sur la rétine du lapin étude electrophysiolôgique. *Experientia*, **13**:122–123, 1957.

———: L'action du métabolisme des hydrates de carbone sur l'électrorétinogramme du lapin. *Ophthalmologica*, **137**:270–281, 1959.

Bakir, F.; Damluji, S. F.; Amin-Zaki, L.; Murtadha, M.; Khalidi, A.; Al-Rawi, N. Y.; Tikriti, S.; Dhahir, H. I.; Ciarkson, T. W.; Smith, J. C.; and Doherty, R. A.: Methylmercury poisoning in Iraq. *Science*, **181**:230–241, 1973.

Barber, G. W.: Physiological chemistry of the eye. *Arch. Ophthalmol.*, **87**:72–106, 1972.

Burrada, A.; Peyman, G. A.; Case, J.; Fishman, G.; Thomas, A.; and Fiscella, R.: Evaluation of intravitreal 5-fluorouacil, vincristine, VP-16, doxorubicin and thiotepa in primate eyes. *Ophthalmic Surg.*, **15**:767–769, 1984.

Baurmann, H.; Chioralia, G.; and Seifert, H.: Fluorescence microscopy study of fluorescein in the posterior segment of the eye following local application of drugs. *Klin. Monatsbl. Augenheilkd.*, **183**:32–36, 1983.

Becker, B.: Cataracts and topical corticosteroids. *Am. J. Ophthalmol.*, **58**:872–873, 1964.

Beehler, C. C.: Oxygen and the eye. *Surv. Ophthalmol.*, **9**:549–560, 1964.

Belkin, G. A.: Cocktail purpura: an unusual case of quinine sensitivity. *Ann. Intern. Med.*, **66**:583–585, 1967.

Bernstein, H. N.: Chloroquine ocular toxicity. *Surv. Ophthalmol.*, **12**:415–477, 1967.

Bernstein, H. N., and Ginsberg, J.: The pathology of chloroquine retinopathy. *Arch. Ophthalmol.*, **71**:238–245, 1964.

Bernstein, H. N.; Mills, D. W.; and Becker, B.: Steroid-induced elevation of intraocular pressure. *Arch. Ophthalmol.*, **70**:15–18, 1963a.

Bernstein, H. N.; Zvaifler, N.; Rubin, M.; and Mansour, Sister A. M.: The ocular deposition of chloroquine. *Invest. Ophthalmol.*, **2**:384–392, 1963b.

Betta, P. G., and Forno, G.: Necrosi emorragica del putamen da intossicazione acuta da alcool metilico. *Patologica*, **80**:215–218, 1988.

Bettman, J. W.; Fung, W. E.; Webster, R. G.; Noyes, P. P.; and Vincent, N. J.: Cataractogenic effect of corticosteroids on animals. *Am. J. Ophthalmol.*, **65**:581–586, 1968.

Bettman, J. W.; Noyes, P.; and DeBoskey, R.: The potentiating action of steroids in cataractogenesis. *Invest. Ophthalmol.*, **3**:459, 1964.

Birch-Hirschfeld, A.: Beitrag zur Kenntnis der Netzhautganglienzellen unter physiologischen und pathologischen Verhältnissen. *Albrecht von Graefes Arch. Ophthalmol.*, **50**:166–246, 1900.

Birch-Hirschfeld, A., and Köster, G.: Die Schädigung des Auges durch Atoxyl. *Albrecht von Graefes Arch. Ophthalmol.*, **76**:403–463, 1910.

Black, R. L.; Oglesby, R. B.; von Sallmann, L.; and Bunim, J. L.: Posterior subcapsular cataracts induced by corticosteroids in patients with rheumatoid arthritis. *J.A.M.A.* **174**:166–171, 1960.

Bleckmann, H., and Sommer, C.: Hornhauttrubungen durch chloracetophenon. *Graefes Arch. Klin. Exp. Ophthalmol.*, **216**:61–67, 1981.

Boet, D. J.: Toxic effects of phenothiazines on the eye. *Doc. Ophthalmol.*, **28**:1–69, 1970.

Bourrat, C.; Ribouliard, L.; Flocard, F.; Chalumeau, A.; and Guillaume, C.: Intoxication volontaire par le methanol. *Rev. Neurol. (Paris)*, **142**:530–534, 1986.

Bresnick, G. H.: Oxygen-induced visual cell degeneration in the rabbit. *Invest. Ophthalmol.*, **9**:372–387, 1970.

Brinton, G. S.; Norton, E. W. D.; Zahn, J. R.; and Knighton, R. W.: Ocular quinine toxicity. *Am. J. Ophthalmol.*, **90**:403–410, 1980.

Britten, J. S., and Blank, W.: Thallium activation of the (Na^+-K^+) activated ATPase of rabbit kidney. *Biochim. Biophys. Acta*, **159**:160–166, 1968.

Brouwer, B., and Zeeman, W. P. C.: The protection of the retina in the primary optic neuron in monkeys. *Brain*, **49**:1–35, 1926.

Brown, S. I.; Tragakis, M. P.; and Pearce, D. B.: Treatment of the alkali-burned cornea. *Am. J. Ophthalmol.*, **74**:316–320, 1972.

Brown, S. I.; Weller, C. A.; and Akiya, S.: Pathogenesis of ulcers of the alkali-burned cornea. *Arch. Ophthalmol.*, **83**:205–208, 1970.

Brown, S. I.; Weller, C. A.; and Wassermann, H. E.: Collagenolytic activity of alkali-burned corneas. *Arch. Ophthalmol.*, **81**:370–373, 1969.

Budinger, J. M.: Diphenylthiocarbazone blindness in dogs. *Arch. Pathol.*, **71**:304–310, 1961.

Bunce, G. E., and Hess, J. L.: Biochemical changes associated with selenite-induced cataract in the rat. *Exp. Eye Res.*, **33**:505–514, 1981.

Burley, D.: Clioquinol: time to act. *Lancet*, **1**:1256, 1977.

Burns, C. A.: Ocular effects of indomethacin. Slit lamp and electroretinographic (ERG) study. *Invest. Ophthalmol.*, **5**:325, 1966.

———: Indomethacin, reduced retinal sensitivity and corneal deposits. *Am. J. Ophthalmol.*, **66**:825–835, 1968.

Burns, R. P.: Delayed onset of chloroquine retinopathy. *N. Engl. J. Med.*, **275**:693–696, 1966.

Butler, I.: Retinopathy following the use of chloroquine and allied substances. *Ophthalmologica*, **149**:204–208, 1965.

Calkins, L. L.: Corneal epithelial changes occurring during chloroquine (Aralen) therapy. *Arch. Ophthalmol.*, **60**:981–988, 1958.

Cameron, M. E.; Lawrence, J. M.; and Obrich, J. G.: Thioridazine (Mellaril) retinopathy. *Br. J. Ophthalmol.*, **56**:131–134, 1972.

Carney, M.; Kao, G.; Peyman, G. A.; Fiscella, R.; and Staneck, J.: The intraocular penetration and retinal toxicity of teicoplanin. *Ophthalmic Surg.*, **19**:119–123, 1988.

Car, R. E.: Chloroquine and organic changes in the eye. *Dis. Nerv. Syst.*, **29** (Suppl.):36–39, 1968.

Carr, R. E., and Henkind, P.: Ocular manifestations of ethambutol. Toxic amblyopia after administration of an antituberculous drug. *Arch. Ophthalmol.*, **67**:566–571, 1962.

Cerletti, A., and Meier-Ruge, W.: Toxicological studies on phenothiazine induced retinopathy. In *Toxicity and Side Effects of Psychotropic Drugs. Proc. Eur. Soc. Drug Toxic.*, **9**:170–188, 1967.

Chamberlain, W. P., Jr., and Boles, D. J.: Edema of cornea precipitated by quinacrine (Atebrine). *Arch. Ophthalmol.*, **35**:120–134, 1946.

Chayakul, V., and Reim, M.: Enzymatic activity of beta-N-acetylglucosaminidase in the alkali-burned rabbit cornea. *Graefes Arch. Klin. Exp. Ophthalmol.*, **218**:149–152, 1982.

Cibis, G. W.; Burian, H. M., and Blodi, F. C.:

Electroretinogram changes in acute quinine poisoning. *Arch. Ophthalmol.*, **90**:307–309, 1973.

Citron, K. M.: Ethambutol: a review with special reference to ocular toxicity. *Tubercle*, **50** (Suppl.):32–36, 1969.

Cooper, J. R., and Kini, M. M.: Biochemical aspects of methanol poisoning. *Biochem. Pharmacol.*, **11**:405–416, 1962.

Cotlier, E., and Becker, R.: Topical steroids and galactose cataracts. *Invest. Ophthalmol.*, **4**:806–814, 1965.

Crews, S. J.: Posterior subcapsular lens opacities in patients on long-term corticosteroid therapy. *Br. Med. J.*, **1**:1644–1646, 1963.

————: The prevention of drug induced retinopathies. *Trans. Ophthalmol. Soc. U.K.*, **86**:63–76. 1967.

Dale, A. J.; Parkhill, E. M.; and Layton, D. D.: Studies on chloroquine retinopathy in rabbits. *J.A.M.A.* **193**:241–243, 1965.

D'Amico, D. J.; Caspers-Velu, L.; Libert, J.; Shanks, E.; Schrooyen, M.; Hanninen, L. A.; and Kenyon, K. R.: Comparative toxicity of intravitreal aminoglycoside antibiotics. *Am. J. Ophthalmol.*, **100**:264–275, 1985.

Dana: Sanguinarin, ein neues organisches Alkali in Sanguinaria. *Mag. Pharm.*, **23**:124, 1828.

Dantzker, D. R., and Gerstein, D. D.: Retinal vascular changes following toxic effects on visual cells and pigment epithelium. *Arch. Ophthalmol.*, **81**:106–114, 1969.

Davies, H. C., and Davies, R. E.: Biochemical aspects of oxygen poisoning. In Fenn, W. D., and Rahn, H. (eds.); *Handbook of Physiology*, Vol. 2, Sect. 3. American Physiological Society, Washington, D.C., 1965.

Davson, H.: *The Physiology of Eye*, 3rd ed. Academic Press, Inc., New York and London, 1972.

Delahunt, C. S.; Stebbins, R. B.; Anderson, J.; and Bailey, J.: The cause of blindness in dogs given hydroxypyridinethione. *Toxicol. Appl. Pharmacol.*, **4**:286–291, 1962.

DeLong, S. L.; Poley, B. J.; and McFarlane, J. R., Jr.: Ocular changes associated with long-term chloropromazine therapy. *Arch. Ophthalmol.*, **73**:611–617, 1965.

Derick, R. J.; Paylor, R.; and Peyman, G. A.: Toxicity of imipenen in vitreous replacement fluid. *Ann. Ophthalmol.*, **19**:338–339, 1987.

DeSousa, D. J.; Rouse, A. A.; and Smolon, W. J.: Statistical consequences of reducing the number of rabbits utilized in eye irritation testing: data on 67 petrochemicals. *Toxicol. Appl. Phramocol.*, **76**:234–242, 1984.

Dickinson, P.; Sabto, J.; and West, R. H.: Management of quinine toxicity. *Trans. Ophthamol. Soc. N.Z.*, 3356–3358, 1981.

Dixon, M.: Reactions of lachrymators with enzymes and proteins. *Biochem. Soc. Symp.*, **2**:39–49, 1948.

Dobbie, G. C., and Langham, M. E.: Reaction of animal eyes to sanguinarine argemone oil. *Br. J. Ophthalmol.*, **45**:81–95, 1961.

Dollery, C. T.; Bulpitt, D. J.; and Kohner, E. M.: Oxygen supply to the retina from the retinal and choroidal circulations at normal and increased arterial oxygen tensions. *Invest. Ophthalmol.*, **8**:588–594, 1969.

Draize, J. H., and Kelley, E. A.: Toxicity to eye mucosa of certain cosmetic preparations containing surface active agents. *Proc. Sci. Sect. Toilet Goods Assoc.*, **17**:1–4, 1952.

DuBois, K. P.; Raymund, A. B.; and Hietbrink, B. E.: Inhibitory action of dithiocarbamates on enzymes of animal tissues. *Toxicol. Appl. Pharmacol.*, **3**:236–255, 1961.

Duke-Elder, Sir S.: Cataract. In Duke-Elder, Sir S. (ed.): *System of Ophthalmology*, Vol. XI. *Diseases of the Lens and Vitreous: Glaucoma and Hypotony*. Henry Kimpton, London, 1969.

Duke-Elder, Sir S., and Jay, B.: Disease of the lens and vitreous: glaucoma and hypotony. In Duke-Elder, Sir S. (ed.): *System of Ophthalmology*, Vol. XI. Henry Kimpton, London, 1969.

Duke-Elder, Sir S., and MacFaul, P. A.: Injuries. In Duke-Elder, Sir S. (ed.): *System of Ophthalmology*, Vol. XIV, Part II. C. V. Mosby, St. Louis, 1982, pp. 1011–1356.

Duke-Elder, Sir S., and Wybar, K. C.: The anatomy of the visual systems. In Duke-Elder, Sir S. (ed.): *System of Ophthalmology*, Vol. II. C. V. Mosby, St. Louis, 1961.

Edge, N. D.; Mason, D. F. J.; Wein, R.; and Ashton, N.: Pharmacological effects of certain diaminodiphenoxy alkanes. *Nature (Lond.)*, **178**:806–807, 1956.

Edwards, G. N.: *St. Barth. Hosp. Rep.*, **i**:141, 1865; **ii**:211, 1866.

Ehrlich, D., and Morgan, I. G.: Kainic acid destroys displaced amacrine cells in post-hatch chicken retina. *Neurosci. Lett.*, **17**:43–48, 1980.

Ehrlich, P.: Uber den jetzigen stand der Chemotherapie. *Ber. Dtsch. Chem. Ges.*, **42**:17–47, 1909.

Elbrink, J., and Bihler, I.: Membrane transport of sugars in the rat lens. *Can. J. Ophthalmol.*, **7**:96–101, 1972.

Elliott, T. R.: The action of adrenalin. *J. Physiol.*, **32**:401–467, 1905.

Fett, D. R.; Silverman, C. A.; and Yoshizumi, M. O.: Moxolactan retinal toxicity. *Arch. Ophthalmol.*, **102**:435–438, 1984.

Figueroa, R.; Weiss, H.; Smith, J. C., Jr.; Hackley, B. M.; McBean, L. D.; Swassing, C. R.; and Halstead, J. A.: Effect of ethambutol on the ocular zinc concentration of dogs. *Am. Rev. Respir. Dis.*, **104**:592–594, 1971.

Flower, R. W., and Patz, A.: Oxygen studies in retrolental fibroplasia. IV. The effects of elevated oxygen tension in retinal vascular dynamics in the kitten. *Arch. Ophthalmol.*, **85**:197–203, 1971.

Forbes, M.; Kuck, N. A.; and Peets, E. A.: Effect of ethambutol on nucleic acid metabolism in mycobacterium smeginatis and its reversal by polyamines and divalent cations. *J. Bacteriol.*, **89**:1299–1305, 1965.

Fournier, D. J., and Patterson, J. W.: Variations in ATPase activity in the development of experimental cataracts. *Proc. Soc. Exp. Biol. Med.*, **137**:826–832, 1971.

François, J.: Glaucome apparement simple, secondaire à la cortisonothérapie locale, *Ophthalmologica* (Suppl.), **142**:517–523, 1961.

François, J.; Jönsas, C.; and de Rouck, A.: Étude expérimentale sur l'effect de l'iodo-acétate de soude sur l'électro-rétinogramme et l'électro-oculogramme du lapin. *Ann. Ocul. (Paris)*, **202**:637–642, 1969a.

————: Experimental studies on the effect of dithizone on the electro-retinogram and the electro-oculogram in rabbits. *Ophthalmologica*, **159**:472–477, 1969b.

François, J., and Maudgal, M. C.: Experimentally induced chloroquine retinopathy in rabbits. *Am. J. Ophthalmol.*, **64**:886–893, 1967.

François, J,; Verriest, G.; and DeRouck, A.: Etude des fonctions visuelles dans deux cas d'intoxication par la quine. *Ophthalmologica*, **153**:324–335, 1967.

Fraser, T. R.: On the characters, actions and therapeutical uses of the ordeal bean of Calabar. *Edinburgh Med. J.*, **9**:36–56, 123–132, 235–248, 1863.

Fraunfelder, F. T.: *Drug Induced Ocular Side Effects*

and Drug Interactions, 3rd ed. Lea & Febiger, Philadelphia, 1989.

Freedman, J. K., and Potts, A. M.: Repression of glutaminase I in the rat retina by administration of sodium-1-glutamate. *Invest. Ophthalmol.,* **1**:118–121, 1962.

Friedenwald, J. S.; Hughes, W. F.; and Herrmann, H.: Acid-base tolerance of the cornea. *Arch. Ophthalmol.,* **31**:279–283, 1944.

———: Acid burns of the eye. *Arch. Ophthalmol.,* **35**:98–108, 1946.

Friedman, L.; O'Keefe, D.; Patel, M.; and Tchang, S.: Computed tomography findings in methanol intoxication. *S. Afr. Med. J.,* **71**:800, 1987.

Galen: De Methodo Medendi. In Kuhn, C. G. (ed.): *Opera Omnia,* (Lib. III. Cap. 2) Vol. 10. Knobloch, Leipzig, 1825, p. 171.

Galezowski, X.: *Des Amlyopies et des Amauroses Toxiques.* P. Assaebin, Paris, 1878.

Gangitano, J. L., and Keltner, J. L.: Abnormalities of the pupil and visual-evoked potential in quinine amblyopia, *Am. J. Ophthalmol.,* **89**:425–430, 1980.

Garner, A., and Rahi, A. H. S.: Practolol and ocular toxicity. *Br. J. Ophthalmol.,* **60**:684–686, 1976.

Gates, M., and Renshaw, B.: Chemical warfare agents and related chemical problems. *Sum. Tech. Rep. Div. 9.* NDRC, Washington, D.C., 1946.

Gehring, P. J., and Buerge, J. F.: The cataractogenic activity of 2,4-dinitrophenol in ducks and rabbits. *Toxicol. Appl. Pharmacol.,* **14**:475–486, 1969a.

———: The distribution of 2,4-dinitrophenol relative to its cataractogenic activity in ducklings and rabbits. *Toxicol. Appl. Pharmacol.,* **15**:574–592, 1969b.

Gehring, P. J., and Hammond, P. B.: The interrelationship between thallium and potassium in animals. *J. Pharmacol. Exp. Ther.,* **155**:187–201, 1967.

Giblin, F. J.; McCready, J. P.; and Reddy, V. N.: The role of glutathione metabolism in the detoxification of H_2O_2 in rabbit lens. *Invest. Ophthalmol. Vis. Sci.,* **22**:330–335. 1982.

Gilger, A. P., and Potts, A. M.: Studies on the visual toxicity of methanol. V. The role of acidosis in experimental methanol poisoning. *Am. J. Ophthalmol.,* **39**:63–86. 1955.

Gilger, A. P.; Potts, A. M.; and Farkas, I.: Studies on the visual toxicty of methanol. IX. The effect of ethanol on methanol poisoning in the rhesus monkey. *Am. J. Ophthalmol.,* **42**:244–252, 1956.

Gilman, A., and Philips, F. S.: The biological actions and therapeutic applications of the β-chlorethyl amines and sulfides. *Science,* **103**:409–415, 1946.

Glocklin, V. C., and Potts, A. M.: The metabolism of retinal pigment cell epithelium. I. The *in vitro* incorporation of P-32 and the effect of diaminodiphenoxyalkane. *Invest. Ophthalmol.,* **1**:111–117, 1962.

Goldberg, A. M., and Frazier, J. M.: Alternatives to animals in toxicity testing. *Sci. Am.,* **261**:24–30, 1989.

Goldberg, I. H., and Friedman, P. A.: Specificity in the mechanism of action of antibiotic inhibitors of protein and nucleic acid synthesis. *Pure Appl. Chem.,* **28**:499–524, 1971.

Goldey, J. A.; Dick, D. A.; and Porter, W. L.: Cornpicker's pupil: a clinical note regarding mydriasis from Jimson weed dust (Stramonium). *Ohio State Med. J.,* **62**:921, 1966.

Goldmann, H.: Cortisone glaucoma. *Arch. Ophthalmol.,* **68**:621–626, 1962.

Gonsaun, L. M., and Potts, A. M.: Possible mechanism of chloroquine induced retinopathy. Presented at the Fifth International Congress on Pharmacology, San Francisco, California, July 23–28, 1972.

———: *In vitro* inhibition of protein synthesis in the retinal pigment epithelium by chloroquine. *Invest. Ophthalmol. Vis. Sci.,* **13**:107–115, 1974.

Gonda, A.; Gault, H.; Churchill, D.; and Hollomby, D.: Hemodialysis for methanol intoxication. *Am. J. Med.,* **64**:749–758, 1978.

Goodwin, F. K.: Animal research versus humane use: the struggle to sustain our research advances. *FASEB J.,* **3**:2455–2456, 2463–2464, 1989.

Grant, W. M.: Ocular injury due to sulfur dioxide. *Arch. Ophthalmol.,* **38**:755–761, 762–774, 1947.

———: A new treatment for calcific corneal opacities. *Arch. Ophthalmol.,* **48**:681–685, 1952.

———: *Toxicology of the Eye,* 3rd ed. Charles C Thomas Pub., Springfield, Ill., 1986.

Graymore, C. N.: Biochemistry of the retina. In Graymore, C. N. (ed.): *Biochemistry of the Eye.* Academic Press, Inc., New York, 1970.

Graymore, C. N., and Tansley, K.: Iodoacetate poisoning of the rat retina. I. Production of retinal degeneration. *Br. J. Ophthalmol.,* **43**:177–185, 1959.

Green, J., and Ellison, T.: Uptake and distribution of chlorpromazine in animal eyes. *Exp. Eye Res.,* **5**:191–197, 1966.

Greiner, A. C., and Berry, K.: Skin pigmentation and corneal and lens opacities with prolonged chlorpromazine therapy. *Can. Med. Assoc., J.,* **90**:663–665, 1964.

Grignolo, A.; Butturini, U.; and Baronchelli, A.: Ricerchi preliminari sul diabete sperimentale da ditizone. III. Manifestazioni oculari. *Boll. Soc. Ital. Biol. Sper.,* **28**:1416–1418, 1952.

Grimes, P., and von Sallmann, L.: Interference with cell proliferation and induction of polyploidy in rat lens epithelium during prolonged myleran treatment. *Exp. Cell Res.,* **42**:265–273, 1966.

Grimes, P.; von Sallmann, L.; Frichette, A.: Influence of myleran on cell proliferation in the lens epithelium. *Invest. Ophthalmol.,* **3**:566–576, 1964.

Grisolano, J., Jr. and Peynan, G. A.: Retinal toxicity study of intravitreal cyclosporia. *Ophthalmic Surg.,* **17**:155–156, 1986.

Guillaume, C.; Perrot, D.; Bouffard, Y.; Delafosse, B.; and Motin, J.: L'intoxication methanolique. *Ann. Fr. Anesth. Reanim.* **6**:17–21, 1987.

Guth, P. S., and Spirtes, M.A.: The phenothiazine tranquilizers: biochemical and biophysical actions. *Int. Rev. Neurobiol.,* **7**:231–278, 1964.

Hakim, S. A. E.: Argemone oil, sanguinarine, and epidemic-dropsy glaucoma. *Br. J. Ophthalmol.,* **38**:193–216, 1954.

Hamming, N. A.; Apple, D. J.; and Goldberg, M. F.: Histopathology and ultrastructure of busulfan-induced cataract. *Albrecht von Graefes Arch. Ophthalmol.,* **200**:139–147, 1976.

Handbook of Sensory Physiology, Vol. VII. Autrum, H.; Jung, R.; Loweenstein, W. R.; MacKay, D. M., and Teubner, H. L. (eds.). Springer-Verlag, Berlin, Heidelberg, New York, 1972–77.

Harding, C. V.; Reddan, J. R.; Unakar, N. J.; and Bagchi, M.: The control of cell division in the ocular lens. *Int. Rev. Cytol.,* **31**:215–300, 1971.

Harris, J. E., and Gruber, L.: The electrolyte and water balance of the lens. *Exp. Eye Res.,* **1**:372–384, 1962.

———: The reversal of triparanol induced cataracts in the rat. *Doc. Ophthalmol.,* **26**:324–333, 1969.

———: Reversal of triparanol-induced cataracts in the rat. II. Exchange of ^{22}Na, ^{42}K, ^{86}Rb in cataractous and clearing lenses. *Invest. Ophthalmol.,* **11**:608–616, 1972.

Haugaard, N.: Poisoning of cellular reactions by oxygen. *Ann. N.Y. Acad. Sci.,* **117**, Art. **2**:736–744, 1965.

————: Cellular mechanisms of oxygen toxicity. *Physiol. Rev.*, **48**:311–372, 1968.

Henkes, H. E., and van Lith, G. H. M.: Retinopathy due to indomethacin. *Ophthalmologica*, **164**:385–386, 1972.

Henkes, H. E.; van Lith, G. H. M.; and Canta, L. R.: Indomethacin retinopathy. *Am. J. Ophthalmol.*, **73**:846–856, 1972.

Henrichsen, J.: Tryparsamide in the treatment of syphilis—a review of the literature. *Venereal Dis. Inform.*, **20**:293–322, 1939.

Henze, T.; Scheidt, P.; and Prange, H. W.: Die Methanol-Intoxikation. *Nervenartzt*, **57**:658–661, 1986.

Heppel, L. A.; Neal, P. A.; Endicott, K. M.; and Porterfield, V. T.: Toxicology of dichloroethane. I. Effect on the cornea. *Arch. Ophthalmol.*, **32**:391–394. 1944.

Herman, M. M., and Bensch, K. G.: Light and electron microscopic studies of acute and chronic thallium intoxication in rats. *Toxicol. Appl. Pharmacol.*, **10**:199–222, 1967.

Heyroth, F. F.: Thallium, a review and summary of medical literature. *Public Health Service Reports* (Suppl.). U.S. Government Printing Office, Washington, D.C., 1947.

Hirst, L. W.; Sanborn, G.; Green, W. R.; Miller, N. R.; and Heath, W. D.: Amodiaquine ocular changes. *Arch. Ophthalmol.*, **100**:1300–1304, 1982.

Hobbs, H. E.; Sorsby, A.; and Friedman, A.: Retinopathy following chloroquine therapy. *Lancet.* **2**:478–480. 1959.

Horner, W. D.: Dinitrophenol and its relation to formation of cataract. *Arch. Ophthalmol.*, **27**:1097–1121, 1942.

Hüber, U.; Emmerlich, P.; and Heidenbluth, I.: Kandidose bei Explosionsverbrennung und Verätzung durch Trichlorsilan. *Dermatol. Monatsschr.*, **165**:795–798, 1979.

Hughes, W. F.: Alkali burns of the eye. I. Review of the literature and summary of present knowledge. *Arch. Ophthalmol.*, **35**:423–449, 1946a.

————: Alkali burns of the eye. II. Clinical and pathological course. *Arch. Ophthalmol.*, **36**:189–214, 1946b.

Hunter, D.; Bomford, R. R.; and Russell, D. S.: Poisoning by methyl mercury compounds. *Q. J. Med. N.S.*, **9**:192–219, 1940.

Ide, T.: Histopathological studies on retina, optic nerve and arachnoidal membrane of mouse exposed to carbon disulfide poisoning. *Acta Soc. Ophthalmol. Jap.*, **62A**:85–108, 1958.

Ignarro, L. J.: Lysosome membrane stabilization *in vivo*. Effects of steroidal and nonsteroidal antiinflammatory drugs on the integrity of rat liver lysosomes. *J. Pharmacol. Exp. Ther.*, **182**:179–188, 1972.

Ikemoto, K.: Effects of cataractogenic compounds, fatty acids and related compounds on cation transport of incubated lens. *Osaka City Med. J.*, **71**:1–18, 1971.

Inturrisi, C. E.: Thallium activation of K^+-activated phosphatases from beef brain. *Biochem. Biophys. Acta.* **173**:567–569, 1969a.

————: Thallium-induced dephosphorylation of a phosphorylated intermediate of the (sodium and thallium-activated) ATPase. *Biochim. Biophys. Acta*, **178**:630–633, 1969b.

Ishikawa, Y., and Mine, S.: Aminoadipic acid toxic effects on retinal glial cells. *Jpn. J. Ophthalmol.*, **27**:107–118, 1983.

Jachuck, S. J.; Stephenson, J.; Bird, T.; Jackson, F. S.; and Clark, F.: Practolol induced autoantibodies and their relation to oculocutaneous complications. *Postgrad. Med. J.*, **53**:75–77, 1977.

Jacobs, M. B.: *War Gases*. Interscience, New York, 1942.

Jacobs, W. A., and Heidelberger, M.: Aromatic arsenic compounds. II. The amides and alkyl amides of N-arylglycine arsonic acids. *J. Am. Chem. Soc.*, **44**:1587–1600, 1919.

Jaffe, L. S.: Photochemical air pollutants and their effect on men and animals. I. General characteristics and community concentrations. *Arch. Environ. Health*, **15**:782–791, 1967.

Jay, W. M.; Fishman, P.; Aziz, M.; and Shockey, R. K.: Intravitreal ceftazidine in a rabbit model: dose- and time-dependent toxicity and pharmacokinetic analysis. *J. Ocul. Pharmacol.*, **3**:257–262, 1987.

Kadota, I.: Studies on experimental diabetes mellitus, as produced by organic reagents. Oxine diabetes and dithizone diabetes. *J. Lab. Clin. Med.*, **35**:568–591, 1950.

Kaiser-Kupfer, M. I., and Lippman, M. E.: Tamoxifen retinopathy. *Cancer Treat. Res.*, **62**:315–320, 1978.

Kao, G. W.; Peyman, G. A.; Fiscella, R.; and House, B.: Retinal toxicity of gancyclovir in vitrectomy infusion solution. *Retina*, **7**:80–83, 1987.

Kaplan, L. J., and Cappaert, W. E.: Amiodarone keratopathy: correlation to dosage and duration. *Arch. Ophthalmol.*, **100**:601–602, 1982.

Karli, P.: Les dégénérescences rétiniennes spontanées et expérimentales chez l'animal. *Progr. Ophthalmol.*, **14**:51–89, 1963.

Kaufman, P. L.; Axelsson, U.; and Bárány, E. H.: Induction of subcapsular cataracts in cynomolgus monkeys by echothiophate. *Arch. Ophthalmol.*, **95**:499–504. 1977a.

————: Atropine inhibition of echothiophate cataractogenesis in monkeys. *Arch. Ophthalmol.*, **95**:1262–1268, 1977b.

Kayne, F. J.: Thallium (I) activation of pyruvate kinase. *Arch. Biochem. Biophys.*, **143**:232–239, 1971.

Kemp, R. B.; Meredith, R. W.; Gamble, S.; and Frost, M.: A rapid cell culture technique for assessing the toxicity of detergent-based products *in vitro* as a possible screen for eye irritancy *in vivo*. *Cytobios*, **36**:153–159, 1983.

Keyvan-Larijarni, H., and Tannenberg, A. M.: Methanol intoxication, comparison of peritoneal dialysis and hemodialysis treatment. *Arch. Intern. Med.*, **134**:293–296. 1974.

Kini, M. M., and Cooper, J. R.: Biochemistry of methanol poisoning. III. The enzymatic pathway for the conversion of methanol to formaldehyde. *Biochem. Pharmacol.*, **8**:207–217, 1961.

Kinoshita, J. H.: Cataracts in galactosemia. *Invest. Ophthalmol.*, **4**:786–799, 1965.

Kinoshita, J. H.; Barber, G. W.; Merola, L. O.; and Fung, B.: Changes in the levels of free amino acids and myoinositol in the galactose-exposed lens. *Invest. Ophthalmol.*, **8**:625–632, 1969.

Kinross-Wright, V.: Clinical trial of a new phenothiazine compound NP-207. *Psychiatr. Res. Rep. Am. Psychiatr. Assoc.*, **4**:89–94, 1956.

Kinsey, V. E.; McLean, I. W.; and Parker, J.: Studies on the crystalline lens. XVIII. Kinetics of thallium (Tl^+) transport in relation to that of the alkali metal cations. *Invest. Ophthalmol.*, **10**:932–942, 1971.

Kirby, T. J.; Achor, R. W. P.; Perry, H. O.; and Winkelmann, R. K.: Cataract formation after triparanol therapy. *Arch. Ophthalmol.*, **68**:486–489. 1962.

Kirmani, M.; Santana, M., Sorgente, N.; Wiedemann, P.; and Ryan, S. J.: Antiproliferative drugs in the treatment of experimental proliferative retinopathy. *Retina*, **3**:269–272, 1983.

Klinghardt, G. W.; Fredman, P.; and Svennerholm,

L.: Chloroquine intoxication induces ganglioside storage in nervous tissue: a chemical and histopathological study of brain, spinal cord, dorsal root ganglia, and retina in the miniature pig. *J. Neurochem.*, **37**:897–908. 1981.

Kobayashi, T., and Murakami, S.: Blindness of an adult caused by oxygen. *J.A.M.A.* **219**:741–742, 1972.

Kolb, H.; Rosenthal, A. R.; Juxsoll, D.; and Bergsma, D.: Preliminary results on chloroquine induced damage to retina of rhesus monkey. Presented at Association for Research in Vision and Ophthalmology, Sarasota, Fla., Spring 1972.

Kolker, A. E., and Becker, B.: Epinephrine maculopathy, *Arch. Ophthalmol.*, **79**:552–562. 1968.

Koopmans, R. A.; Li, D. K.; and Paty, D. W.: *J. Comput. Assist. Tomogr.*, **12**:168–169, 1988.

Krill, A. E.; Potts, A. M.; and Johanson, C. E.: Chloroquine retinopathy. Investigation of discrepancy between dark adaptation and electroretinographic findings in advanced stages. *Am. J. Ophthalmol.*, **71**:530–543. 1971.

Kuck, J. F. R., Jr.: Chemical constituents of the lens. In Graymore, C. N. (ed.): *Biochemistry of the Eye.* Academic Press, Inc., New York, 1970a.

———: Metabolism of the lens. In Graymore, C. N. (ed.): *Biochemistry of the Eye.* Academic Press, Inc., New York, 1970b.

———: Cataract formation. In Graymore, C. N. (ed.): *Biochemistry of the Eye.* Academic Press, Inc., New York, 1970c.

———. Response of the mouse lens to high concentrations of glucose and galactose. *Ophthalmic Res.*, 1:166–174, 1970d.

Kuwabara, T.; Kinoshita, J. H.; and Cogan, D. G.: Electron microscopic study of galactose-induced cataract. *Invest. Ophthalmol.*, **8**:133–149, 1969.

Lasansky, A., and de Robertis, E.: Submicroscopic changes in visual cells of the rabbit induced by iodoacetate. *J. Biophys. Biochem. Cytol.*, **5**:245–250, 1959.

Laughlin, R. C., and Carey, T. F.: Cataracts in patients treated with triparanol, *J.A.M.A.* **181**:339–340, 1962.

Lawley, P. D., and Brookes, P.: Molecular mechanism of the cytotoxic action of difunctional alkylating agents and of resistance to this action. *Nature*, **206**:480–483, 1965.

Lawwill, T.; Appleton, B.; and Altstatt, L.: Chloroquine accumulation in human eyes. *Am. J. Ophthalmol.*, **65**:530–532, 1968.

Ledet, A. E.: Clinical, toxicological and pathological aspects of arsanilic acid poisoning in swine. Ph.D. thesis, Iowa State University, Ames, Iowa, 1970; University Microfilms, Ann Arbor, Mich., 1979.

Leibold, J. E.: The ocular toxicity of ethambutol and its relation to dose. *Ann. N.Y. Acad. Sci.*, **135**:904–909. 1977.

Leighton, J.; Nassauer, J.; and Tchao, R.: The chick embryo in toxicology: an alternative to the rabbit eye. *Food. Chem. Toxicol.*, **23**:293–298, 1985.

Levine, R. A., and Stahl, C. J.: Eye injury caused by tear-gas weapons. *Am. J. Ophthalmol.*, **65**:497–508. 1968.

Levinson, R. A.; Paterson, C. A.; and Pfister, R. R.: Ascorbic acid prevents corneal ulceration and perforation following experimental alkali burns. *Invest. Ophthalmol. Visual Sci.*, **15**:986–993, 1976.

Levy, N. S.; Krill, A. E.; and Beutler, E.: Galactokinase deficiency and cataracts. *Am. J. Ophthalmol.*, **74**:41–48, 1972.

Lewin, L., and Guillery, H.: *Die Wirkung von Arzneimitteln und Giften auf das Auge*, Vols. 1 and 2. A. Hirshwald, Berlin, 1913.

Lieberman, T. W.: Prolonged pharmacology and the eye. Ocular effects of prolonged systemic drug administration. *Dis. Nerv. Syst.*, **29** (Suppl.):44–50, 1968.

Linksz, A.: Applied pharmacology of the skin in the ophthalmologists everyday practice. *Arch. Ophthalmol.*, **28**:959–982, 1942.

Loredo, A.; Rodriguez, R. S.; and Murillo, L.: Cataracts after short-term corticosteroid treatment. *N. Engl. J. Med.*, **286**:160, 1972.

Lowry, O. H.; Roberts, N. R.; and Lewis, C.: The quantitative histochemistry of the retina. *J. Biol. Chem.*, **220**:879–892, 1956.

Lowry, O. H.; Roberts, N. R.; Schulz, D. W.; Clow, J. E.; and Clark, J. R.: Quantitative histochemistry of retina. II. Enzymes of glucose metabolism. *J. Biol. Chem.*, **236**:2813–2820, 1961.

Lubkin, V. L.: Steroid cataract—a review and a conclusion, *J. Asthma Res.*, **14**:55–59, 1977.

Lucas, D. R., and Newhouse, J. P.: The toxic effect of sodium 1-glutamate on the inner layers of the retina. *Arch. Ophthalmol.*, **58**:193–201, 1957.

Mackenzie, A. H.: An appraisal of chloroquine. *Arthritis Rheum.*, **13**:280–291, 1970.

Mackworth, J. F.: The inhibition of thiol enzymes by lachrymators. *Biochem. J.*, **42**:82–90, 1948.

Mailer, C. M.: Paradoxical differences in retinal vessel diameters and the effect of inspired oxygen. *Can. J. Ophthalmol.*, **5**:163–168, 1970.

Manske, R. H. F.: α-Napthaphenanthredine alkaloids. In Manske, R. H. F., and Holmes, H. L. (ed.): *The Alkaloids, Chemistry and Physiology*, Vol. IV. Academic Press, Inc., New York, 1954, pp. 253–263.

Martin, G.; Draize, J. H.; and Kelley, E. A.: Local anesthesia in eye mucosa produced by surfactants in cosmetic formulations. *Proc. Sci. Sect. Toilet Goods Assoc.*, **37**:2–3. 1962.

Martin-Amat, G.; McMartin, K. E.; Hayreh, S. S.; Hayreh, M. S.; and Tephly, T. R.: Methanol poisoning: ocular toxicity produced by formate. *Toxicol. Appl. Pharmacol.*, **45**:201–208, 1978.

Maslova, M. N.; Natochin, Y. V.; and Skulsky, I. A.: Inhibition of active sodium transport and activation of Na^+-K^+-ATPase by ions Tl^+ in frog skin. *Biokhimiia*, **36**:867–869, 1971.

Matthiolus, P. A.: *Commentarius in sex libros super Dioscorides.* N. Baseus, 1598.

Maurice, D. M.: The cornea and the sclera. In Davson, H. (ed.): *The Eye*, Vol, I, 2nd ed. Academic Press, Inc., New York, 1969.

Maynard, F. P.: Preliminary note on increased intraocular tension met within cases of epidemic dropsy. *Indian Med. Gaz.*, **44**:373–374, 1909.

McChesney, E. W.; Banks, W. F., Jr.; and Fabian, R. J.: Tissue distribution of chloroquine, hydroxychloroquine and desethylchloroquine in the rat. *Toxicol. Appl. Pharmacol.*, **10**:501–513, 1967.

McChesney, E. W.; Banks, W. F., Jr.; and Sullivan, D. J.: Metabolism of chloroquine and hydroxychloroquine in albino and pigmented rats. *Toxicol. Appl. Pharmacol.*, **7**:627–636, 1965.

McCrea, F. D.; Eadie, G. S.; and Morgan, J. E.: The mechanism of morphine miosis. *J. Pharmacol. Exp. Ther.*, **74**:239–246, 1942.

McFarlane, J. R.; Yanoff, M.; and Scheie, H. G.: Toxic retinopathy following sparsomycin therapy. *Arch. Ophthalmol.*, **76**:532–540, 1966.

McGregor, I. S.: Study of histopathologic changes in retina and late changes in the visual field in acute methanol poisoning. *Br. J. Ophthalmol.*, **27**:523–543, 1943.

Meier-Ruge, W.: Die Morphologie der experimentellen

Chlorochinretinopathie des Kaninchens. *Ophthalmologica*, **150**:127–137, 1965a.

————: The pathophysiological morphology of the pigment epithelium and its importance for retinal structure and function. *Med. Probl. Ophthalmol.*, **8**:32–48, 1968.

————: Experimental investigation of the morphogenesis of chloroquine retinopathy. *Arch. Ophthalmol.*, **73**:540–544. 1965b.

Meier-Ruge, W., and Cerletti, A.: Zur experimentellen Pathologie der Phenothiazin-Retinopathie. *Ophthalmologica*, **151**:512–533, 1966.

Menzel, D. B.: Toxicity of ozone, oxygen, and radiation. *Annu. Rev. Pharmacol.*, **10**:379–394, 1970.

Merriam, F. C., and Kinsey, V. E.: Studies on the crystalline lens. I. Technique for *in vitro* culture of crystalline lenses and observations on the metabolism of the lens. *Arch. Ophthalmol.*, **43**:979–988, 1950.

Meyerson, A., and Thau, W.: Ocular pharmacology of furfuryl trimethyl ammonium iodide with special reference to intraocular tension. *Arch. Ophthalmol.*, **24**:758–760, 1940.

Mikuni, I.; Fujiwara, T.; and Obazawa, H.: Microtubules in experimental cataracts: disappearance of microtubules of epithelial cells and lens fibers in colchicine-induced cataracts. *Tokai J. Exp. Clin. Med.*, **6**:297–303, 1981.

Minton, J.: *Occupational Eye Diseases and Injuries*. Grune & Stratton, Inc., New York, 1949, p. 46.

Monteleone, J. A.; Beutler, E.; Monteleone, P. L.; Utz, C. L.; and Casey, E. C.: Cataracts, galactosuria and hypergalactosemia due to galactokinase deficiency in a child. *Am. J. Med.*, **50**:403–407, 1971.

Muir, C. K.; Flower, C; and VanAbbe, N. J.: A novel approach to the search for *in vitro* alternatives to *in vivo* eye irritancy testing. *Toxicol. Lett.*, **18**:1–5, 1983.

Nakajima, A.: The effect of amino-phenoxy-alkanes on rabbit ERG. *Ophthalmologica*, **136**:332–344, 1958.

Neth, R., and Winkler, K.: Proteinsynthese in menschlichen Leukocyten. II. Wirkung einiger Antibiotica auf die Proteinsyntheseleistung von Zellsuspensionen und auf die Peptidyltransferase-Aktivität in zellfreien Systemen. *Klin. Wochenschr.*, **50**:523–524, 1972.

Neujean, G.; Weyts, E.; Bacq, Z. M.: Action du B.A.L. sur les accidents ophthalmologiques de la thérapeutique à la tryparsamide. *Bull. Acad. R. Med. Belg.*, **13**:341–350, 1948.

Nichols, C. W., and Lambertsen, C. J.: Effects of high oxygen pressures on the eye. *N. Engl. J. Med.*, **281**:25–30, 1969.

Nieuwveld, R. W.; Halkett, J. A.; and Spracklen, F. H. N.: Drug resistant malaria in Africa: a case report and review of the problem and treatment. *South Afr. Med. J.*, **62**:173–175, 1982.

Nirankari, V. S.; Varma, S. D.; Lakhanpal, V.; and Richards, R. D.: Superoxide radical scavenging agents in treatment of alkali burns. *Arch. Ophthalmol.*, **99**:886–887, 1981.

Noell, W. K.: The impairment of visual cell structure by iodoacetate. *J. Cell Comp. Physiol.*, **40**:25–45, 1952.

————: Metabolic injuries of the visual cell. *Am. J. Ophthalmol.*, **40**:60–70, 1955.

————: The visual cell: electric and metabolic manifestations of its life processes. *Am. J. Ophthalmol.*, **48**:347–370, 1959.

Nordmann, J.: L'oculiste et la detection preventive systematique de la galactosemie. *Ophthalmologica*, **163**:129–135, 1971.

Northover, B. J.: Mechanism of the inhibitory action of indomethacin on smooth muscle. *Br. J. Pharmacol.*, **41**:540–551, 1971.

————: The effects of indomethacin in calcium,

sodium, potassium and magnesium fluxes in various tissues of the guinea pig. *Br. J. Pharmacol.*, **45**:651–659, 1972.

Nylander, U.: Ocular damage in chloroquine therapy. *Acta Ophthalmol.*, **92** (Suppl.):1–71, 1967.

Obstbaum, S. A.; Galin, M. A.; and Poole, T. A.: Topical epinephrine and cystoid macular edema. *Ann. Ophthalmol.*, **8**:455–458, 1976.

Oglesby, R. B.; Black, R. L.; von Sallmann, L.; and Bunim, J. J.: Cataracts in patients with rheumatic diseases treated with corticosteroids. *Arch. Ophthalmol.*, **66**:625–630, 1961a.

————: Cataracts in rheumatoid arthritis patients treated with corticosteroids. *Arch. Ophthalmol.*, **66**: 519–523, 1961b.

O'Hara, M. A.; Bode, D. D.; Kincaid, M. C.; and Perkins, M. C.: Retinal toxicity of intravitreal cefoperazone. *J. Ocul. Pharmacol.*, **2**:177–184, 1986.

Okamoto, K.: Experimental pathology of diabetes melitus. (Report II) I. Experimental studies on production and progress of diabetes mellitus by zinc reagents. *Tohoku J. Exp. Med.*, **61** (Suppl. III):1–35, 1955.

Okun, E.; Gouras, P.; Bernstein, H.; and von Sallmann, L.: Chloroquine retinopathy. *Arch Ophthalmol.*, **69**:59–71, 1963.

Olney, J. W.: The toxic effects of glutamate and related compounds in the retina and the brain. *Retina*, **2**:341–359, 1982.

Ono, S.; Hirano, H.; and Obara, K. O.: Absorption of cortisol-4-^{14}C into rat lens. *Jpn. J. Exp. Med.*, **41**:485–487, 1971.

————: Presence of cortisol-binding protein in the lens. *Ophthalmic Res.*, **3**:233–240, 1972a.

————: Study on the conjugation of cortisol in the lens. *Ophthalmic Res.*, **3**:307–310, 1972b.

Orr, E.; Tervaert, D. C.; Lean, J. S.: Aqueous concentrations of fluorouracil after intravitreal injection. Normal, vitrectomized, and silicone-filled eyes. *Arch. Ophthalmol.*, **104**:431–434, 1986.

Orthner, H.: *Methanol Poisoning*. Springer, Berlin, 1950.

Otto, H. F.: Tierexperimentelle Untersuchungen zur Hepato-Toxizität von Triparanol. *Beitr. Pathol.*, **142**:177–193, 1971.

Palimeris, G.; Koliopoulos, J.; and Velissaropoulos, P.: Ocular side effects of indomethacin. *Ophthalmologica*, **164**:339–353, 1972.

Pang, M. P.; Peyman, G. A.; Nikoleit, J.; Fiscella, R.; and Kao, G.: Intravitreal trifluorothymidine and retinal toxicity. *Retina*, **6**:260–263, 1986.

Parish, W. E.: Ability of *in vitro* (corneal injury-eye organ-and chorioallantoic membrane) tests to represent histopathological features of acute eye inflammation. *Food Chem. Toxicol.*, **23**:215–227, 1985.

Paterson, C. A.: Distribution and movement of ions in the ocular lens. *Doc. Ophthalmol.*, **31**:1–28, 1972.

Patz, A.: Retrolental fibroplasia. *Surv. Ophthalmol.*, **14**:1–29, 1969–70.

Pearce, L.: Studies on the treatment of human tyrpanosomiasis with tryparsamide (the sodium salt of *N*-phenylglycineamide-*p*-arsonic acid). *J. Exp. Med.*, **34** (Suppl. 1):1–104, 1921.

Pedersen, O. O., and Karlsen, R. L.: Destruction of Müller cells in the adult rat by intravitreal injection of D.L-alpha-aminoadipic acid. An electron microscopic study. *Exp. Eye Res.*, **28**:569–575, 1979.

Pfannkuch, F., and Bleckmann, H.: Morphologische Befunde an der Kaninchencornea nach Tränengasverätzung. *Graefes Arch. Klin. Exp. Ophthalmol.*, **218**:177–184, 1982.

Pfister, R. R., and Burstein, N.: The alkali burned cornea. I. Epithelial and stromal repair. *Exp. Eye Res.*, **23**:519–535, 1976.

Pfister, R. R.; Haddox, J. L.; and Lank, K. M.: Citrate or ascorbate/citrate treatment of established corneal ulcers in the alkali-injured rabbit eye. *Invest. Ophthalmol. Visual Sci.,* **29**:1110–1115, 1988.

Pfister, R. R., and Koski, J.: Alkali burns of the eye: pathophysiology and treatment. *South. Med. J.,* **75**:417–422, 1982.

Pfister, R. R., and Paterson, C. A.: Ascorbic acid in the treatment of alkali burns of the eye. *Invest. Ophthalmol. Visual Sci.,* **16**:1050–1057, 1977.

Pfister, R. R.; Paterson, C. A.; and Hayes, S. A.: Topical ascorbate decreases the incidence of corneal ulceration after experimental alkali burns. *Invest. Ophthalmol. Visual Sci.,* **17**:1019–1024, 1978.

Pflugfelder, S. C.; Hernandez, E.; Fliesler, S. J.; Alvarez, J.; and Pflugfelder, M. E.: Intravitreal vancomycin. Retinal toxicity, clearance, and interaction with gentamycin. *Arch. Ophthalmol.,* **105**:831–837, 1987.

Phang, P. T.; Passerini, L.; Mielke, B; Berendt, R.; and King, E. G.: Brain hemorrhage associated with methanol poisoning. *Crit. Care Med.,* **16**:137–140, 1988.

Pirie, A.: Pathology in the eye of the naphthalene-fed rabbit. *Exp. Eye Res.,* **7**:354–357, 1968.

Place, V. A.; Peets, E. A.; Buyske, D. A.; and Little, R. R.: Metabolic and special studies of ethambutol in normal volunteers and tuberculous patients. *Ann. N.Y. Acad. Sci.,* **135**:775–795, 1966.

Place, V. A., and Thomas, J. P.: Clinical pharmacology of ethambutol. *Am. Rev. Respir. Dis.,* **87**:901–904, 1963.

Podos, S. M., and Canellos, G. P.: Lens changes in chronic granulocytic leukemia. *Am. J. Ophthalmol.,* **68**:500–504, 1969.

Polyak, S.: *The Retina.* University of Chicago Press, Chicago, 1941.

Potts, A. M.: Methyl aclohol poisoning. *ONR Resp. Rev.,* pp. 4–9, Nov. 1952.

———: The concentration of phenothiazines in the eyes of experimental animals. *Invest. Ophthalmol.,* **1**:522–530, 1962a.

———: Uveal pigment and phenothiazine compounds. *Trans. Am. Ophthalmol. Soc.,* **60**:517–552, 1962b.

———: Further studies concerning the accumulation of polycyclic compounds on uveal melanin. *Invest. Ophthalmol.,* **3**:399–404, 1964a.

———: The reaction of uveal pigment *in vitro* with polycyclic compounds. *Invest Ophthalmol.,* **3**:405–416, 1964b.

———: Agents which cause pigmentary retinopathy. *Dis. Nerv. Syst.,* **29** (Suppl.):16–18, 1968.

Potts, A. M., and Au, P. C.: Thallous ion and the eye. *Invest. Ophthalmol.,* **10**:925–931, 1971.

Potts, A. M.; Hodges, D.; Shelman, C. B.; Fritz, K. J.; Levy, N. S.; and Mangnall, Y.: Morphology of the primate optic nerve. III. Fiber characteristics of the foveal outflow. *Invest. Ophthalmol.,* **11**:1004–1016, 1972.

Potts, A. M.; Praglin, J.; Farkas, I.; Orbison, L.; and Chickering, D.: Studies on the visual toxicity of methanol. VIII. Additional observations on methanol poisoning in the primate test object. *Am. J. Ophthalmol.,* **40**:76–82, 1955.

Prick, J. J. G.; Sillevis-Smitt, W. G.; and Muller, L.: *Thallium Poisoning.* Elsevier Publishing Co., New York. 1955.

Pulido, J. S.; Palacio, W.; Peyman, G. A.; Fiscella, R.; Greenberg, D.; and Stelmack, T.: Toxicity of intravitreal antiviral drugs. *Ophthalmic. Surg.,* **15**:666–669, 1984.

Pulido, J.; Peyman, G. A.; Lesar, T.; and Vernot, J.: Intravitreal toxicity of hydroxyacyclovir (BW-B7590), a new antiviral agent. *Arch. Ophthalmol.,* **103**:840–841, 1985.

Raitta, C., and Tolonen, M.: Microcirculation of the eye in workers exposed to carbon disulfide. In Merrigan, W. H., and Weiss, B. (eds.): *Neurotoxicity of the Visual System.* Raven Press, New York, 1980.

Ravindranathan, M. P.; Paul, V. J.; and Kuriakose, E. T.: Cataract after busulphan treatment. *Br. Med. J.,* **1**:218–219, 1972.

Rawlins, F. A., and Uzmana, B. G.: Retardation of peripheral nerve myelination in mice treated with inhibitors of cholesterol biosynthesis. A quantitative electron microscopic study. *J. Cell Biol.,* **216**:505–517, 1970.

Reading, H. W., and Sorsby, A.: Retinal toxicity and tissue—SH levels. *Biochem. Pharmacol.,* **15**:1389–1393, 1966.

Rees, J. R., and Pirie, A.: Possible reactions of 1,2-naphthaquinone in the eye. *Biochem. J.,* **102**:853–863, 1967.

Reim, M., and Schmidt-Martens, F. W.: Behandlung von Veratzungen. *Klin. Monatsbl. Augenheilkd.,* **181**:1–9, 1982.

Reinhardt, C. A.; Bosshard, E.; and Schlatter, C. (eds.): Proceedings of an international workshop on irritation testing of skin and mucus membranes, 3–5 April 1984, Kartause Ittingen near Frauenfeld, Switzerland. *Food Chem. Toxicol.,* **23**:247–252, 1985.

Riehm, W.: Ueber Presojod-Schädigung des Auges. *Klin. Monatsbl. Augenheilkd.,* **78**:87, 1927.

———: Akute Pigmentdegeneration der Netzhaut nach Intoxikation mit Septojod. *Arch. Augenheilkd.,* **100**:872–882, 1929.

Roe, O.: The ganglion cells of the retina in cases of methanol poisoning in human beings and experimental animals. *Acta Ophthalmol. Scand.,* **26**:169–182, 1948.

Rosenberg, N. L.: Methyl malonic acid, methanol, metabolic acidosis, and lesions of the basal ganglia. *Ann. Neurol.,* **22**:96–97, 1987.

Rösner, H.: Untersuchungen zur Wirkung von Chlorpromazin im ZNS von Teleosteern. I. Einfluss auf das Normalverhalten sowie den Einbau von ^{3}H-Uridin und ^{3}H-Histidin. *Psychopharmacologia,* **23**:125–135, 1972.

Sebelaish, S., and Hilmi, G.: Ocular manifestations of mercury poisoning. *W.H.O. Reports,* **53** (Suppl.):83–86, 1976.

Sarkar, S. L.: Katakar oil poisoning. *Indian Med. Gaz.,* **61**:62–63, 1926.

Sarkar, S. N.: Isolation from argemone oil of dihydrosanguinarine and sanguinarine: toxicity of sanguinarine. *Nature (Lond.),* **162**:265–266, 1948.

Sassaman, F. W.; Cassidy, J. J.; Alpern, M.; and Maaseidvaag, F.: Electroretinography in patients with connective tissue diseases treated with hydroxychloroquine. *Am. J. Ophthalmol.,* **70**:515–523, 1970.

Scherbel, A. L.; Mackenzie, A. H.; Nousek, J. E.; and Atdjian, M.: Ocular lesions in rheumatoid arthritis and related disorders with particular reference to retinopathy. A study of 741 patients treated with and without chloroquinine drugs. *N. Engl. J. Med.,* **273**:360–366, 1965.

Schmidt, I. G.: Central nervous system effects of ethambutol in monkeys. *Ann. N.Y. Acad. Sci.,* **135**:759–774, 1966.

Schubert, G., and Bornschein, H.: Spezifische Schädigung von Netzhautelementen durch Jodazetat. *Experientia,* **7**:461–462, 1951.

Schulman, J. A.; Peyman, G. A.; Fiscella, R.; Small, G.; Coats, M.; Wajaszczak, C. P.; and Steahly, L.: Toxicity of intravitreal injection of fluconazole in the rabbit. *Can. J. Ophthalmol.,* **22**:304–306, 1987.

Schutta, H. S., and Neville, H. E.: Effects of cholesterol synthesis inhibitors on the nervous system. A light and electron microscopic study. *Lab Invest.*, **19**:487–493, 1968.

Shaffer, R. N., and Hetherington, J.: Anticholinesterase drugs and cataracts. *Am. J. Ophthalmol.*, **62**:613–628, 1966.

Shaffer, R. N., and Ridgway, W. L.: Furmethide iodide in the production of dacryostenosis. *Am. J. Ophthalmol.*, **34**:718–720, 1951.

Shaw, C.-M.; Mottet, N. K.; Body, R. L.; and Luschei, E. S.: Variability of neuropathologic lesions in experimental methylmercurial encephalopathy in primates. *Am. J. Pathol.*, **80**:451–470, 1975.

Shearer, R. V., and Dubois, E. L.: Ocular changes induced by long-term hydroxychloroquine (Plaquenil®) therapy. *Am. J. Ophthalmol.*, **64**:245–252, 1967.

Shigematsu, I.: Subacute myelo-optico-neuropathy (SMON) and clioquinol. *Jpn. J. Med. Sci. Biol.*, **28** (Suppl.):35–55, 1975.

Shockley, R. K.; Jay, W. M.; Friberg, T. R.; Aziz, A. M.; Rissing, J. F.; Aziz, M. Z.: Intravitreal ceftriaxone in a rabbit model. Dose- and time-dependent toxic effects and pharmacokinetic analysis. *Arch. Ophthalmol.*, **102**:1236–1238, 1984.

Shopsis, C., and Sathe, S.: Uridine uptake inhibition as a cytotoxicity test: correlations with the Draize test. *Toxicology*, **33**:195–206, 1984.

Shulman, N. R.: Immunoreactions involving platelets. *J. Exp. Med.*, **107**:665–729, 1958.

Siddall, J. R.: The ocular toxic findings with prolonged and high dosage chlorpromazine intake. *Arch. Ophthalmol.*, **74**:460–464, 1965.

———: Ocular toxic changes associated with chlorpromazine and thioridazine. *Can. J. Ophthalmol.*, **1**:190–198, 1966.

———: Ocular complications related to phenothiazines. *Dis. Nerv. Syst.*, **29** (Suppl.):10–13, 1968.

Siegrist, A.: Konzentrierte Alkali-und Säurewirkung auf das Auge. *Z. Augenheilkd.*, **43**:176–194, 1920.

Silverman, J.: Preliminary findings on the use of protozoa *(Tetrahymena thermophyla)* as models for ocular irritation testing in rabbits. *Lab. Anim. Sci.*, **33**:56–59, 1983.

Sippel, T. O.: Changes in water, protein, and glutathione contents of the lens in the course of galactose cataract development in rats. *Invest. Ophthalmol.*, **5**:568–575, 1966a.

———: Energy metabolism in the lens during development of galactose cataract in rats. *Invest. Ophthalmol.*, **5**:576–587, 1966b.

———: Enzymes of carbohydrate metabolism in developing galactose cataracts of rats. *Invest. Ophthalmol.*, **6**:59–63, 1967.

Slansky, H. H.; Freeman, M. I.; and Itoi, M.: Collagenolytic activity in bovine corneal epithelium. *Arch. Ophthalmol.*, **80**:496–498, 1968.

Small, G. H.; Peyman, G. A.; Srinivasan, A.; Smith, R. T.; and Fiscella, R.: Retinal toxicity of combination antiviral drugs in an animal model. *Can. J. Ophthalmol.*, **22**:300–303, 1987.

Sobue, I., and Ando, K.: Myeloneuropathy with abdominal symptoms—5 clinical features and diagnostic criteria. *Clin. Neurol.*, **11**:244–248, 1971.

Solomon, C.; Light, A. E.; and De Beer, E. J.: Cataracts produced in rats by 1,4-dimethanesulfonoxybutane (myleran). *Arch. Ophthalmol.*, **54**:850–852, 1955.

Sorsby, A.: The nature of experimental degeneration of the retina. *Br. J. Ophthalmol.*, **25**:62–65, 1941.

Sorsby, A., and Harding, R.: Protective effect of cysteine against retinal degeneration induced by iodate and iodoacetate. *Nature (Lond.)*, **187**:608–609, 1960.

Sorsby, A., and Nakajima, A.: Experimental degeneration of the retina. IV. Diaminodiphenoxyalkanes as inducing agents. *Br. J. Ophthalmol.*, **42**:563–571, 1958.

Steinberg, D., and Avigan, J.: Studies on cholesterol biosynthesis. II. The role of desmosterol in the biosynthesis of cholesterol. *J. Biol. Chem.*, **235**:3127–3129, 1960.

Stern, W. N.; Guerin, C. J.; Lewis, G. P.; Anderson, D. H.; and Fisher, S. K.: Ocular toxicity of fluorouracil after vitrectomy. *Am. J. Ophthalmol.*, **96**:43–51, 1983.

Straus, D. J.; Mausolf, F. A.; Ellerby, R. A.; and McCracken, J. D.: Cicatricial ectropion secondary to 5-fluorouracil therapy. *Med. Pediat. Oncol.*, **3**:15–19, 1977.

Sugimoto, K., and Goto, S.: Retinopathy in chronic carbon disulfide exposure. In Merrigan, W. H., and Weiss, B. (eds.): *Neurotoxicity of the Visual System.* Raven Press, New York, 1980.

Sunalp, M. A.; Wiedemann, P.; Sorgente, N.; and Ryan, S. J.: Effect of adriamycin on experimental proliferative retinopathy in the rabbit. *Exp. Eye Res.*, **41**:105–115, 1985.

Tarkkanen, A.; Esila, R.; and Liesmaa, M.: Experimental cataracts following long-term administration of corticosteroids. *Acta Ophthalmol.*, **44**:665–668, 1966.

Tateishi, J., and Otsuki, S.: Experimental reproduction of SMON in animals by prolonged administration of clioquinol: clinico-pathological findings. *Jpn. J. Med. Sci. Biol.*, **28** (Suppl.):165–186, 1975.

Tephly, T. R.; Parks, R. E., Jr.; and Mannering, G. J.: Methanol metabolism in the rat. *J. Pharmacol. Exp. Ther.*, **143**:292–300, 1963.

Thatcher, D. B.; Blaug, S. M.; Hyndiuk, R. A.; and Watzke, R. C.: Ocular effects of chemical Mace in the rabbit. *Clin. Med.*, **78**:11–13, 1971.

Thomas, H. W.: Some experiments in the treatment of trypanosomiasis. *Br. Med. J.*, **1**:1140–1143, 1905.

Thomas, J. P.; Baughn, C. O.; Wilkinson, R. G.; and Shepard, R. G.: A new synthetic compound with antituberculous activity in mice: ethambutol dextro 2,2' ethylenediimino di-1-butanol. *Am. Rev. Respir. Dis.*, **83**:891–893, 1961.

Trakatellis, A. C.: Effect of sparsomycin on protein synthesis in the mouse liver. *Proc. Natl. Acad. Sci. USA*, **59**:854–860, 1968.

Trayhurn, P., and van Heyningen, R.: Aerobic metabolism in the bovine lens. *Exp. Eye Res.*, **12**:315–327, 1971a.

———: The metabolism of glutamate, aspartate and alanine in the bovine lens. *Biochem. J.*, **124**:72P–73P, 1971b.

Trumbull, G. C.; Sbarbaro, J. A.; and Iseman, M.: (Correspondence) High dose ethambutol. *Am. Rev. Respir. Dis.*, **115**:889–890, 1977.

Tsubaki, T., and Irukayama, K. (eds.): *Minamata Disease.* Kodansha Ltd., Tokyo; Elsevier Scientific Pub. Co., Amsterdam, 1977.

Uhthoff, W.: Die Augenstörungen bei Vergiftungen. In Graefe-saemisch *Handbuch der Gesamten Augenheilkunde*, **11**:1–180, Engelmann, Leipzig, 1911.

Upholt, W. M.; Quinby, G. E.; Batchelor, G. S.; and Thompson, J. P.: Visual effects accompanying TEPP-induced miosis. *Arch. Ophthalmol.*, **56**:128–134, 1956.

van Haeringen, N. J.; Oosterhuis, J. A.; and van Delft, J. L.: A comparison of the effects of non-steroidal compounds on the disruption of the blood-aqueous barrier. *Exp. Eye Res.*, **35**:271–277, 1982.

van Heyningen, R.: The lens: metabolism and cataract. In Davson, H. (ed.): *The Eye, Vegetative Physiology and Biochemistry*, Vol. 1, 2nd ed. Academic Press, Inc., New York, 1969.

————: Ascorbic acid in the lens of the naphthalene-fed rabbit. *Exp. Eye Res.*, **9**:38–48, 1970a.

————: Effect of some cyclic hydroxy compounds on the accumulation of ascorbic acid by the rabbit lens *in vitro*. *Exp. Eye Res.*, **9**:49–56, 1970b.

————: Galactose cataract: a review. *Exp. Eye Res.*, **11**:415–428, 1971.

van Heyningen, R., and Pirie, A.: The metabolism of naphthalene and its toxic effect on the eye. *Biochem. J.*, **102**:842–852, 1967.

Van Joost, T. H.; Crone, R. A.; and Overdijk, A. D.: Ocular cicatricial pemphigoid associated with practolol therapy. *Br. J. Dermatol.*, **94**:447–50, 1976.

Velhagen, K.: Zur Hornhautargyrose. *Klin. Monatsbl. Augenheilkd.*, **122**:36–42, 1953.

Vinding, T., and Nielsen, N. V.: Retinopathy caused by treatment with tamoxifen in low dosage. *Acta Ophthalmol.*, **61**:45–50, 1983.

Vito, P.: Contributo allo studio della degenerazione pigmentaria della retina indotta dalla soluzione iodica di Pregl. *Boll. Ocul.*, **14**:945–957, 1935.

von Sallmann, L.: The lens epithelium in the pathogenesis of cataract. *Am. J. Ophthalmol.*, **44**:159–170, 1957.

von Sallmann, L.; Grimes, P.; and Collins, E.: Triparanol induced cataract in rats. *Arch. Ophthalmol.*, **70**:522–530, 1963.

Wagner, A.: CT-forandringer i cerebrum ved akut metanolforgiftning. *Ugeskr. Laeger*, **148**:178–179, 1986.

Walberg, J.: Exfoliative cytology as a refinement of the Draize eye irritancy test, *Toxicol. Lett.*, **18**:49–55, 1983.

Waley, S. G.: The lens: function and macromolecular composition. In Davson, H. (ed.): *The Eye*, Vol. 1, 2nd ed. Academic Press, Inc., New York, 1969.

Warburg, O.: *Über den Stoffwechsel der Tumoren.* Springer, Berlin, 1926, p. 138.

Weber, U.; Goerz, G.; Michaelis, L.; and Melnik, B.: Disorders of retinal function in long-term therapy with retinoid etretinate. *Klin. Monatsbl. Augenheilkd.*, **192**:706–711, 1988.

Weekley, R. D.; Potts, A. M.; Reboton, J.; and May, R. H.: Pigmentary retinopathy in patients receiving high doses of a new phenothiazine. *Arch. Ophthalmol.*, **64**:65–74, 1960.

Weitzel, G.; Strecker, F. J.; Roester, U.; Buddecke, E.;

and Fretzdorff, A. M.: Zinc im tapetum lucidum. *Hoppe Seylers Z. Physiol. Chem.*, **296**:19–30, 1954.

Weleber, R. G.; Denman, S. T.; Hanifin, J. M.; and Cunningham, W. J.: Abnormal retinal function associated with isoretinoin therapy for acne. *Arch. Ophthalmol.*, **104**:831–837, 1986.

Weller, C. A., and Green, M.: Methionyl-tRNA synthetase detected by [^{76}Se]-selenomethionine in lenses from normal and galactose-fed rats. *Exp. Eye Res.*, **8**:84–90, 1969.

Wetterholm, D. H., and Winter, F. C.: Histopathology of chloroquine retinal toxicity. *Arch. Ophthalmol.*, **71**:82–87, 1964.

Wheeler, M. C.: Discoloration of the eyelids from prolonged use of ointments containing mercury. *Trans. Am. Ophthalmol. Soc.*, **45**:74–80, 1947.

Wilkes, J. W.: Argyrosis of cornea and conjunctiva. *J. Tenn. Med. Assoc.*, **46**:11–13, 1953.

Williamson, J.: A new look at the ocular side-effects of long-term systemic corticosteroid and adenocorticotrophic therapy. *Proc. R. Soc. Med.*, **63**:791–792, 1970.

Williamson, J.; Paterson, R. W. W.; McGavin, D. D. N.; Jasani, M. K.; Boyle, J. A.; and Doig, W. M.: Posterior subcapsular cataracts and glaucoma associated with long-term oral corticosteroid therapy. In patients with rheumatoid arthritis and related conditions. *Br. J. Ophthalmol.*, **53**:361–372, 1969.

Wilson, F. M., II; Schmitt, T. E.; and Grayson, M.: Amiodarone-induced cornea verticillata. *Ann. Ophthalmol.*, June 1980, pp. 657–660.

Wirth, A.; Quaranta, C. A.; and Chistoni, G.: The effect of dithizone on the electroretinogram of the rabbit. *Bibl. Ophthalmol.*, **48**:66–73, 1957.

Woods, C. A., and Buller, F.: Poisoning by wood alcohol. Cases of death and blindness from Columbian spirits and other methylated preparations. *J.A.M.A.*, **43**:972–977; 1058–1062; 1117–1123; 1213–1221; 1289–1296, 1904.

Wood, D. C.; Contaxis, I.; Sweet, D.; Smith, J. C., II; and Van Dolah, J.: Response of rabbits to corticosteroids. I. Influence on growth, intraocular pressure and lens transparency. *Am. J. Ophthalmol.*, **63**:841–849, 1967.

Yoshizumi, M. O.; Niizawa, J. M.; and Meyers-elliott, R.: Ocular toxicity of intravitreal vidarbine solubilized in dimethylsulfoxide. *Arch. Ophthalmol.*, **104**:426–430, 1986.

Yoshizumi, M. O., and Silverman, C.: Experimental intravitreal 5-fluorocytosine. *Ann. Ophthalmol.*, **58**–61, 1985.

UNIT III

TOXIC AGENTS

Chapter 18

TOXIC EFFECTS OF PESTICIDES

Donald J. Ecobichon

INTRODUCTION

The United States Environmental Protection Agency (U.S. EPA) definition of *pesticide* is any substance or mixture of substances intended for preventing, destroying, repelling, or mitigating any pest. Pesticides may also be described as any physical, chemical, or biologic agent that will kill an undesirable plant or animal pest. The term *pest* includes harmful, destructive, or troublesome animals, plants, or microorganisms. The term *pesticide* is a generic name for a variety of agents that are usually more specifically classified on the basis of the pattern of use and organism killed. In addition to the major agricultural classes that encompass insecticides, herbicides, and fungicides, one finds pest control agents grouped as acaricides, larvacides, miticides, molluscides, pediculicides, rodenticides, scabicides, plus attractants (pheromones), defoliants, desiccants, plant growth regulators, and repellants.

Over the centuries, man has developed many ingenious methods in his attempts to control the invertebrates, vertebrates, and microorganisms that constantly threatened his supply of food and fiber and his health. The historical literature is replete with descriptions of plant diseases and insect plagues and measures taken to control them. Sulfur was used as a fumigant by the Chinese before 1000 B.C. Because of its fungicidal properties, elemental sulfur was used in the 1800s in Europe against powdery mildew on fruit and is still the major pesticide used in California today. In Japan in the sixteenth century, poor quality rendered whale oil was mixed with vinegar and sprayed on paddies and fields, this mixture preventing the development of insect larvae by weakening the cuticle. The Chinese were applying moderate amounts of arsenic-containing compounds as insecticides in the sixteenth century. As early as 1690, water extracts of tobacco leaves *(Nicotiana tabacum)* were sprayed as insecticides and nux vomica, the seed of *Strychnos nux-vomica* (strychnine), was in-

troduced to kill rodents. In the mid-1800s, the pulverized root of *Derris eliptica,* containing rotenone, was used as an insecticide as was pyrethrum extracted from the flowers of chrysanthemums *(Chrysanthemum cinerariaefolium).* In the late 1800s, arsenic trioxide was used as a weed killer, particularly for dandelions. Bordeaux mixture {copper sulfate, lime [Ca(OH)$_2$, water]} was introduced in 1882 to combat vine downy mildew *(Plasmopara viticola),* a disease introduced into France from the United States when phylloxera-resistant vine rootstocks were imported. Sulfuric acid, at a concentration of 10 percent v/v, was used in the early 1900s to destroy dicotyledonous weeds that would absorb the acid, whereas cereal grains, and so forth, having a smooth and waxy monocotyledon, were protected. Paris Green (copper arsenite) was introduced for the control of Colorado beetle in the late 1800s and was used extensively by the 1900s. Calcium arsenate replaced Paris Green and lead arsenate was a major cornerstone in the agriculturalist's armamentarium against insect pests in the early 1900s. By the 1920s, the widespread use of arsenical pesticides caused considerable public concern because some treated fruits and vegetables were found to have toxic residues. It can be appreciated that, although some of these early pesticides caused minimal harm to humans exposed to them, other agents were exceedingly toxic and the medical literature of the era is sprinkled with anecdotal reports of poisonings. Looking back over the early years of pesticide development before the 1930s, it is somewhat surprising to realize just how few pesticides were available (Cremlyn, 1978).

The 1930s ushered in the era of modern synthetic chemistry including the development of a variety of agents such as alkyl thiocyanate insecticides, dithiocarbamate fungicides, ethylene dibromide, methyl bromide, ethylene oxide, and carbon disulfide as fumigants (Cremlyn, 1978). By the beginning of World War II, there were a number of pesticides including dichlorodi-

Table 18–1. TYPE OF OCCUPATIONAL DISEASE REPORTED CAUSED BY PESTICIDES AND OTHER AGRICULTURAL CHEMICALS IN CALIFORNIA IN 1969*

	TYPE OF DISEASE				
TYPE OF CHEMICAL	*Systemic Poisoning*	*Respiratory Condition*	*Skin Condition*	*Other and Unspecified*	*Total All Types*
Organic phosphate pesticides	140	4	12	75	231
Halogenated hydrocarbon pesticides	9	7	19	22	57
Herbicides	3	9	50	14	76
Fertilizers	—	8	28	7	43
Fungicides	2	3	21	1	27
Phenolic compounds	2	1	10	2	15
Sulfur	1	2	25	3	31
Organomercury compounds	1	—	—	1	2
Lead or arsenic	2	—	2	5	9
Miscell.—specified	5	1	15	7	28
Unspecified	9	12	162	21	204
Total	175	47	345	160	727

* From California Department of Public Health: *Occupational Diseases in California Attributed to Pesticides and Other Agricultural Chemicals, 1969*. Bureau of Occupational Health and Environment Epidemiology, Sacramento, 1969.

phenyltrichloroethane (DDT), dinitrocresol, 4-chloro-2-methyloxyacetic acid (MCPA), and 2,4-dichlorophenoxyacetic acid (2,4-D) under experimental investigation, much of this activity being kept under wraps of secrecy during the war (Kirby, 1980). In the postwar era, there was rapid development in the agrochemical field, with a plethora of insecticides, fungicides, herbicides, and so forth being introduced. In no field of synthetic organic chemistry has there been such a diversity of structures arising from the application of principles of chemistry to the mechanism(s) of action in pests to develop selectivity and specificity in agents toward certain species while reducing toxicity to other forms of life.

It is important to appreciate that, despite the modern day development of second- and third-generation derivatives of the early chemical pesticides, all pesticides possess an inherent degree of toxicity to some living organism; otherwise they would be of no practical use. Unfortunately, the target species selectivity of pesticides is not as well developed as might be hoped for, nontarget species frequently being affected because they possess physiologic and/or biochemical systems similar to those of the target organisms. There is no such thing as a "completely safe" pesticide. There are, however, pesticides that can be used safely and/or present a low level of risk to human health when applied with proper attention to the labeling instructions. Despite the current conflagration over pesticide use and the presence of low levels of residues in food, groundwater, and air, these agents comprise integral components of our crop and health protection programs. As long as they continue to be used, accidental and/or intentional poisoning of wildlife, domestic stock, and humans can be anticipated and will require treatment.

On a worldwide basis, intoxications attributed to pesticides have been estimated to be as high as 500,000 illnesses annually, with as many as 20,000 deaths (Copplestone, 1977). These estimates have been criticized as inflated. In many countries, the documentation of pesticide poisonings is very inadequate. With good reporting systems in place, the above values may not be too far off the mark. Poisonings reported under the requirements of the California State Workmen's Compensation Law revealed that, in 1969, there were 727 occupational disease reports attributed to agricultural chemicals (Table 18–1). Thirty-two percent of these cases involved organophosphorus ester insecticides, 10 percent herbicides, 8 percent halogenated hydrocarbon insecticides, 6 percent fertilizers, and 44 percent miscellaneous or unidentified chemicals. As is indicated in the table, the majority of the poisonings were found among agricultural workers. Hayes and Vaughn (1977) reported that, in the United States in 1974, there were only 52 fatal accidental poisonings with pesticides compared to 152 in 1956. More recent results from California, a state that uses a vast amount of chemical pesticides, revealed that 1087 occupationally related exposures occurred in 1978. A breakdown of these poisonings by job category, as is shown in Figure 18–1, revealed that ground applicators were at greatest risk whereas aerial applicators and workers involved in mosquito abatement programs had the least pesticide-related illness (Kilgore, 1988). Such data are not representative of the rest of the agricultural

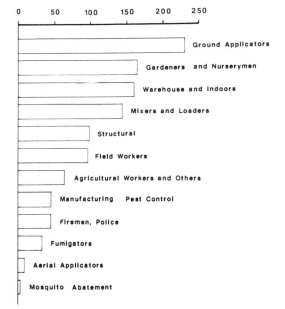

Figure 18–1. Frequency of pesticide poisoning related to occupational and potential for exposure. Data compiled from the records of the California Department of Public Health (Kilgore, 1988).

world. It is important to appreciate that the incidence of poisoning is 13 times higher in developing countries than in highly industrialized nations which "consume" 85 percent of the world pesticide production (Forget, 1989). In 1983, the Labor Compensation Fund of Thailand reported only 117 pesticide poisoning cases per 100,000 agricultural workers with 0.8 deaths per 100,000 workers (Boon-Long *et al.*, 1986). However, a survey of hospital admissions/deaths due to pesticides conducted by the Ministry of Public Health of Thailand in the same year estimated a total of 8268 pesticide poisonings within an agricultural community of 100,000 workers. The differences between these two national estimates of pesticide-related toxicity

can be explained by the fact that only companies having more than 20 employees must submit claims, whereas a large number of pesticide applicators would be individual farmers, members of cooperatives, or those working for small companies. These totals, of course, do not include individuals who were affected but not seriously enough to seek medical attention. In Sri Lanka, the national average for incidence of pesticide poisonings was 79 per 100,000 population in 1979 with a range of 17 to 367, depending on the reporting region and fatalities being approximately 8 or 9 percent (Jeyaratnam *et al.*, 1982). In a survey of patients hospitalized in the years 1975–80, it was found that 79,961 patients were admitted because of pesticide poisoning and 6083 of these died. Some 73 percent of pesticidal poisonings were attributed to suicide attempts, 17 percent to occupational exposures, and 8 percent to accidental exposure. In contrast to such figures, results from Dade County, Florida, for 1956–67 revealed a total of 122 fatalities with 57 percent being suicide-related, 29 percent accidental, 10 percent homicidal, and 2.5 percent occupational (Reich *et al.*, 1968).

No one can doubt the efficacy of pesticides to protect crops in the field, thereby providing us with abundant, inexpensive, wholesome, and attractive fruits and vegetables. It has been estimated that, in 1830, it took 58 man-hours to tend and harvest an acre of grain, whereas today it takes approximately two man-hours (Kirby, 1980). Over this time period, the price of cereal grain has not risen proportionally to the costs of the labor to produce it. Along with improved strains of crops, insecticides, fungicides, and herbicides have played important roles in crop improvements and yields. Even with such advances, it is estimated that up to 50 percent of harvested crops can be damaged by post-harvest infestation by insects, fungi, rodents, and so forth (Table 18–2).

The medical miracles accomplished by pesticides have been documented: the suppression of

Table 18–2. WORLDWIDE HARVEST LOSSES IN FIVE IMPORTANT CROPS*

| CROP | POTENTIAL HARVEST (1000t) | HARVEST 1978 (1000t) | LOSSES THROUGH | | |
			Weeds (%)	*Diseases* (%)	*Insects* (%)
Rice	715,800	378,645	10.6	9.0	27.5
Maize	563,016	362,582	13.0	9.6	13.0
Wheat	578,400	437,236	9.8	9.5	5.1
Sugarcane	1,603,200	737,483	15.1	19.4	19.5
Cotton	63,172	41,757	5.8	12.1	16.0

* From *GIFAP Bulletin*, Vol. 12, March/April, 1986. GIFAP, International Group of National Associations of Agrochemical Manufacturers, Brussels, Belgium.

a typhus epidemic in Naples, Italy, by DDT in the winter of 1943–1944 (Brooks, 1974); the control of "river blindness" (onchocerciasis) in West Africa by killing the insect vector (blackfly) carrying the filaria for this disease with temephos (Abate®) (Walsh, 1986); and the control of malaria in Africa, the Middle East, and Asia by eliminating the plasmodia-bearing mosquito populations with a variety of insecticides (Matsumura, 1985). There is still a great need for advancement in disease vector control by pesticides: 600 million people are at risk from schistosomiasis in the Middle East and Asia; 200 million suffer from filariasis in tropical Africa, Asia, Indonesia, and the Caribbean region; 20 million people in tropical Africa, Arabia, Mexico, and Guatemala are infected by the filarium causing onchocerciasis; and 1000 million worldwide harbor pathologic intestinal worm infestations (Albert, 1987). Although the benefits of pesticides are recognized by those who require them, certain parts of the world are experiencing an environmentalist- and media-evoked backlash toward all pesticide use because of the carelessness, misuse, and/or abuse of some agents by a relatively few individuals in a limited number of well-publicized incidents. With no direct involvement in health care or food or fiber production, some environmental and consumer advocacy groups propose a total ban on pesticide use. Between the two extremes of overwhelming use and total ban lies a position of careful and rational use of these beneficial chemicals.

The widespread use and misuse of the early, toxic pesticides created an awareness of the potential hazard to the health of agriculturalists and others, and a concern regarding the protection of the consumer from residues in foods. Although some legislation was introduced by individual states during the late 1800s, it was not until 1906 that the Wiley or Sherman Act was passed, creating the first Federal Food and Drugs Act. This was replaced by the Federal Food Drug and Cosmetic Act (FDCA) in 1938. Specific pesticide amendments were passed in 1954 and 1958 requiring that pesticide tolerances be established for all agricultural commodities. The 1958 amendment contained the famous Delaney Clause (Section 409) which states that "no additive shall be deemed safe if it is found to induce cancer when ingested by man or animal or, if it is found, after tests which are appropriate for the evaluation of the safety of food additives, to induce cancer in man or animals" (National Academy of Sciences, 1987). It should be noted that the Delaney Clause does not require proof of carcinogenicity in humans. Pesticides fall under this "additive" legislation.

Dealing specifically with pesticides, the Federal Insecticide, Fungicide, and Rodenticide Act (FIFRA) was originally passed by Congress in 1947 as a labeling statute that would group all pest control products, initially only insecticides, fungicides, rodenticides, and herbicides, under one law to be administered by the U.S. Department of Agriculture (USDA). Amendments in 1959 and 1961 added nematicides, plant growth regulators, defoliants, and desiccants to FIFRA jurisdiction plus the authorization to deny, suspend, or cancel registrations of products although assuring the registrant's right to appeal. In 1972, FIFRA was reorganized and the administrative authority was turned over to the newly formed Environmental Protection Agency (EPA). The new Act, along with subsequent amendments in 1975, 1978, 1980, and 1984, defines the registration requirements and appropriate chemical, toxicologic, and environmental impact studies, label specifications, use restrictions, the establishment of tolerances for pesticide residues on raw agricultural products, and the responsibility to monitor pesticide residue levels in foods. However, FIFRA is not all-encompassing because the Food and Drug Administration retains the basic responsibility for both monitoring residue levels and seizure of foods not in compliance with the regulations and the USDA continues to be the responsible authority for the monitoring of meat and poultry for pesticides as well as for other chemicals.

FIFRA regulations set out the requirements essential before an EPA (Office of Pesticide Programs) review of any pesticide and formulated product for registration can occur. This information base includes product and residue chemistry, environmental fate, toxicology, biotransformation/degradation, occupational exposure and reentry protection, spray drift, environmental impact on nontarget species, and product performance and efficacy. Depending on the proposed use pattern of the pesticide, results from different "groups" of toxicologic studies are required to support the registration. The typical spectrum of basic pesticide toxicity data required under FIFRA regulations is summarized in Table 18–3. Extensive ancillary studies of environmental impact (birds, mammals, aquatic organisms, plants, and so forth), environmental persistence and bioaccumulation, and so forth are also required. A schematic diagram showing the "information package" required in support of a registration and the appropriate time span required to develop this data base from the point of patenting the newly synthesized chemical until its registration, production, marketing, and user acceptability is shown in Figure 18–2. One can only visualize the enormous costs involved in "guiding" a new pesticidal chemical through to a finished, efficacious, and marketable product.

Table 18–3. BASIC REQUIREMENTS REGARDING TOXICITY DATA FOR NEW PESTICIDE REGISTRATIONS

Acute	Oral (rat)
	Dermal (rabbit)
	Inhalation (usually rat)
	Irritation studies
	Eye (rabbit)
	Skin (rabbit, guinea pig)
	Dermal sensitization (guinea pig)
	Delayed neurotoxicity (hen)
Subchronic	90-Day feeding study
	Rodent (rat, mouse)
	Nonrodent (dog)
	Dermal Dependent upon use pat-
	Inhalation tern and potential for
	Neurotoxicity occupational exposure
Chronic	One- or two-year oral study
	Rodent (usually rat)
	Nonrodent (dog)
	Oncogenicity study (rat or mouse)
Reproductive	*In vitro* mutagenicity (microorganisms, etc.)
	Fertility/reproduction (rat, mouse, rabbit)
	Teratogenicity (rat, mouse, rabbit)

Although the ultimate uses of the particular chemical will govern the extent of the information base required prior to registration, estimates of average development costs of the order of $30 to $50 million are not unrealistic.

Other nations including Canada, the United Kingdom, Japan and, more recently, the European Economic Community (EEC) have promulgated legislation similar to that of the United States as safeguards in human exposure to pesticides in food commodities. Many developing nations, with a lack of trained manpower to develop their own legislation, have adopted the regulatory framework of one or another of the industrialized nations, permitting the sale and use of pesticides registered under the legislation of that country but prohibiting the use of agents unable to meet the stringent requirements.

Exposure

Despite the fact that organic chemists are well on their way in the synthesis of third- and fourth-generation derivatives of those earlier toxic agents and the fact that extensive preregistration toxicity testing is required for each new chemical, a glance at the media and the scientific literature in any one week will reveal that we are still experiencing many problems with pesticides. In addition to severe, life-threatening, accidental exposures and suicide attempts that no amount of legislation or study can prevent, occu-

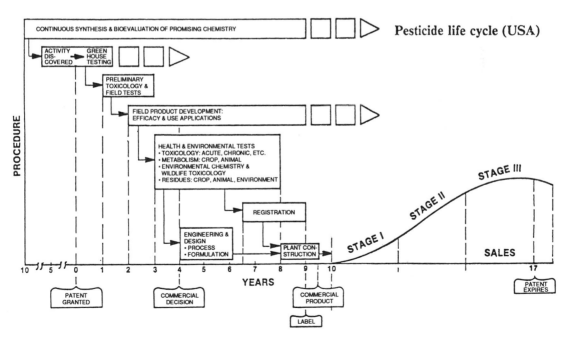

Figure 18–2. A schematic diagram depicting the generation of an appropriate toxicity data base, the time frame for data acquisition, and the significant milestones in the life cycle of a pesticide in the United States. (GIFAP Bulletin, Sept. 1983, with permission.)

pational exposure to pesticide concentrates occurs at the point of mixing and loading, whereas exposure to end-use (diluted) formulation occurs during routine application throughout the growing season. The exposure of pickers, handlers, and packagers to deposited residues on harvested fruits and vegetables continues to be a concern to both management and union organizations. Bystander exposure to off-target drift and deposition of pesticides has become a significant concern. At the extreme end of the exposure spectrum lies the ultimate consumer of the food item containing residues of a pesticide that (1) is used illegally as in the recent case of aldicarb on melons and cucumbers (Jackson *et al.*, 1986); (2) is misused in terms of the application rate; (3) is present at higher than anticipated levels as a consequence of picking and shipping the sprayed product before a suitable time period of residue degradation has occurred; or (4) is present at concentrations above the tolerance levels established by government agencies. The media is replete with documented incidents of environmental contamination by pesticides: (1) of surface and/or groundwater essential as sources of potable drinking water; (2) of commercial fish stocks as well as sportfish; (3) of other wildlife upon which native peoples, parti-

cularly those living in the Arctic, depend as a major source of dietary protein; and (4) of long distance aerial transport of undeposited and/or revolatilized pesticide.

An evaluation of the hazards of pesticides to human health frequently begins with the development of a dose-effect relationship based on documented and anecdotal information on human exposure. As is shown in Figure 18–3, several populations of individuals may be identified as having possible exposure to a range of concentrations of a particular agent, including accidental and/or suicidal poisonings, pesticide workers (manufacturing, mixer/loader, applicators, harvesting, handling, and so forth), bystanders inadvertently sprayed or exposed to off-target drift from spraying operations, and the general public. The shape of the dose-effect curve is dependent on detailed knowledge of the amount of exposure received by each of these groups. Within each group, variability will be considerable. Frequently, exposure evaluations begin at the top of the relationship where exposure is greatest, more easily estimated, and, in most cases, the acute biologic effects are clearly observed and may be associated with a specific agent or a class of chemicals over a relatively narrow dosage range. It has been stated that, if

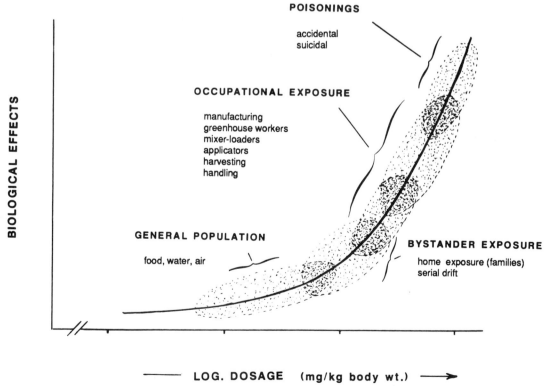

Figure 18–3. A theoretical dose-effect relationship for acute toxicity comparing the potential for exposure in terms of occupation, level of exposure, and possible biologic effects.

Table 18–4. ESTIMATED SURFACE AREA OF EXPOSED PORTIONS OF A BODY OF A CASUALLY DRESSED INDIVIDUAL*

UNCLOTHED SURFACE	SURFACE AREA (sq ft)	PERCENT OF TOTAL
Face	0.70	22.0
Hands	0.87	27.6
Forearms	1.30	41.3
Back of neck	0.12	3.8
Front of neck and "v" of chest	0.16	5.1

* Data from Batchelor, G. S., and Walker, K. C.: *AMA Arch. Ind. Hyg. Occup. Med.*, **10**:522–529, 1954.

Table 18–5. PERCENT OF TOTAL BODY SURFACE AREA REPRESENTED BY BODY REGIONS*

BODY REGION	SURFACE AREA (% OF TOTAL)
Head	5.60
Neck	1.20
Upper arms	9.70
Forearms	6.70
Hands	6.90
Chest, back, shoulders	22.80
Hips	9.10
Thighs	18.00
Calves	13.50
Feet	6.40

* Estimated proportions from the "50 percentile man" having a surface area of 1.92 m², height of 175 cm, and body weight of 78 kg. Data by Spear, R. C. et al.: *J. Occup. Med.*, **19**,406–410, 1977.

no discernible adverse health effect(s) are seen at high levels of exposure, it is unlikely that anything will be observed at lower levels of exposure. Although this hypothesis may be true for acute systemic effects, it is not applicable to chronic effects (changes in organ function, mutagenicity, teratogenicity, carcinogenicity) that may develop at some latent period of time after either a single high level exposure, repeated moderate or high level exposures, or annual exposure to low levels of the agents for decades.

As has been documented by Hayes (1982), there is sufficiently detailed documentation on many pesticidal poisonings so that a possible level of exposure can be identified. In some 48 suicide attempts by ingestion of the herbicide glyphosate, the average volume of product (concentrate containing active ingredient and a surfactant) ingested was 120 ml [range of 104 ml (nonfatal) to 206 ml (fatal)] (Sawada et al., 1988). An estimate of what constitutes a toxic dose can be readily obtained. In other cases, such as one involving the insecticide fenitrothion, where the individual was exposed by dermal contact to a 7.5 percent solution of the agent in corn oil wiped up with facial tissues by a bare hand, exposure was more difficult to assess (Ecobichon et al., 1977). It is imperative that forensic and clinical toxicologists and emergency service personnel attempt to ascertain how much of the material was involved in the poisoning.

Worker exposure can be estimated within reason by considering the various job functions performed (i.e., diluting concentrated formulations, loading diluted end-use formulations into tanks, spray application, harvesting sprayed crops, post-harvest handling of sprayed crops, and so forth). The potential level(s) of pesticide encountered in each job category and the route(s) of exposure can be estimated. The majority of occupational illnesses arising from pesticides involve dermal exposure enhanced, however, in certain job categories by acquisition of a portion of the dosage by the inhalation of aerosolized spray. Many exposures appear to be entirely dermal in character. The surface area of the unclothed parts of the body of a casually dressed, unprotected worker is shown in Table 18–4, the values having been determined by Batchelor and Walker (1954) using the method of Berkow (1931). More recent data for the entire surface area of a "50 percentile man," as determined by Spear et al. (1977), are shown in Table 18–5. With surface patch (gauze, fabric) testing on various parts of the body, accurate estimates of dermal exposure can be obtained. The reader is referred to the following studies for details: Wolfe et al. (1967, 1972), Wojeck et al. (1981), and Franklin et al. (1981). Where inhalation can be considered to contribute significantly to the total exposure, as in greenhouse and other structural spraying operations in enclosed environments, drivers in tractor cabs, operators of rotary fan mist sprayers, and so forth, measurements of aerial concentrations in the working environment can be made and related to respiratory rates and length of time spent in that environment. A more direct means of assessing the contribution of the inhalation component of an exposure can be obtained with personal air sampling monitors worn during the day (Turnbull et al., 1985; Grover et al., 1986). More direct estimates of total exposure can be made by measuring excretory products (parent chemical, degradation products) in urine and feces over a suitable post-exposure time interval (Durham et al., 1972; Kolmodin-Hedman et al., 1983; Frank et al., 1985; Grover et al., 1986).

It is important to appreciate that minimal protection of certain parts of the body can markedly reduce exposure to an agent. Depending on the task of the worker, protection of the hands (5.6 percent of body surface) by appropriate chemical-resistant gloves may reduce contamination by 33 percent (forest spraying with knapsack sprayer having single nozzle lance), by 66 percent (weed control using tractor-mounted booms equipped with hydraulic nozzles), or by 86 percent (filling tanks on tractor-powered sprayers) (Bonsall, 1985). Studies monitoring the absorption of pesticides applied to the skin of different areas of the human body have revealed marked regional variations in percutaneous absorption, greatest uptake being in the scrotal region, followed by the axilla, forehead, face, scalp, the dorsal aspect of the hand, the palm of the hand, and the forearm in decreasing order (Feldman and Maiback, 1974).

The exposure of a bystander, an individual accidentally but directly sprayed or exposed to aerial off-target drifting aerosol, is considerably more difficult to assess. The levels encountered may be several-fold lower than those in the occupational setting, making the analysis of residue and the detection of meaningful biologic changes more difficult. Greater variation in exposure estimates and biologic effects can be anticipated. The adverse health effects may be subtle in appearance and rather nonspecific, reflecting a slow deterioration of physiologic function clouded by the individual's adjustment or adaptation to the changes, taking many years to develop to the point of detection. In a similar fashion, the identification of pesticide-related adverse health effects in the general population, who inadvertently acquire low levels of pesticides daily via food and water, is extremely difficult. Frequently, the residue levels in these media are orders of magnitude lower than those encountered in occupational or bystander exposure and are at or near the limits of analytical detection by sophisticated techniques. Any biologic effects resulting from such low level exposure are unlikely to be distinctive and any causal association with a particular chemical or class of agents is likely to be tenuous and confounded by many other factors of lifestyle, and so forth.

It must be emphasized that many of the public concerns about pesticides are related to "older" chemicals, many of them having entered the market in the 1950s and 1960s without the benefit of the extensive toxicity and environmental impact studies demanded prior to distribution of new chemicals today. It must also be pointed out that many of these older pesticides have received little reassessment using the more definitive techniques and protocols required today. Although government agencies and industry have been slow in their reevaluation of a vast array of pesticides in use "out there," it frequently appears that reassessment comes in the wake of or concomitant with some recently exposed, adverse environmental or health effect.

Given the previously mentioned costs of conducting a full battery of studies, the time frame required, and the limited market for some of these chemicals in North America or even worldwide, the registration of many of these pesticides will be withdrawn voluntarily by industry, and the answers to the public concerns will never be obtained. Hazardous chemicals will be removed from use but, unfortunately, it is possible that some very beneficial and essential pesticides will be lost. Given the situation of today, created by the last generation and inherited by the present one, the problems still must be dealt with. It is imperative that one has a thorough understanding of the toxicity associated with pesticides and, wherever possible, an in-depth knowledge of the basic mechanisms of action of these chemicals.

INSECTICIDES

The literature pertaining to the chemistry and development of the various classes of insecticides over the past 45 years is extensive and the reader is referred to the monographs of O'Brien (1960, 1967), Melnikov (1971), Fest and Schmidt (1973), Brooks (1974a,b), Eto (1974), Hayes (1975, 1982), Kuhr and Dorough (1976), Ecobichon and Joy (1982), and Leahey (1985), and previous editions of this text for detailed discussions of the chemistry, nomenclature (chemical, common, and trade names), biotransformation and degradation, environmental effects, as well as target and nontarget species toxicity. Compilations of LD_{50} values in the laboratory rat may be found in Gaines (1969), Frear (1969), and Worthing (1987). Acute toxicity data for laboratory animals, fish, and wildlife are recorded in a number of reports (Pickering et al., 1962; Tucker and Crabtree, 1970; Worthing, 1987). Only selected examples of the classes of insecticides will be discussed in this chapter, with emphasis being placed on their toxicity to the human.

All of the chemical insecticides in use today are neurotoxicants and act by poisoning the nervous systems of the target organisms. The central nervous system (CNS) of insects is highly developed and not unlike that of the mammal (O'Brien, 1960). Although the peripheral nervous system (PNS) of insects is not as complex as that of the mammal, there are striking similarities (O'Brien, 1960). The development of insecticides has been based on specific structure-activity relationships requiring the manipulation of a basic chemical structure to obtain an optimal shape and configuration for specificity toward a unique biochemical or physiologic feature of the

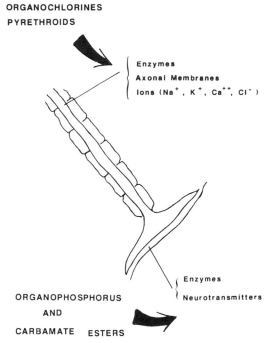

ORGANOCHLORINES
PYRETHROIDS

{ Enzymes
  Axonal Membranes
  Ions (Na$^+$, K$^+$, Ca^{++}, Cl$^-$) }

ORGANOPHOSPHORUS
AND
CARBAMATE ESTERS

{ Enzymes
  Neurotransmitters }

Figure 18–4. Potential sites of action of classes of insecticides on the axon and the terminal portions of the nerve.

nervous system of the target organism. Given the fact that insecticides are not selective and affect nontarget species as readily as target organisms, it is not surprising that a chemical that acts on the insect nervous system will elicit similar effects in higher forms of life. The target sites and/or mechanism(s) of action may be similar in all species; only the dosage (level of exposure and duration) will dictate the intensity of biologic effects. It is sufficient at this stage to indicate the potential sites of action of the insecticide classes (Figure 18–4) and their interference with the membrane transport of sodium, potassium, calcium, or chloride ions; inhibition of selective enzymatic activities; or contribution to the release and/or the persistence of chemical transmitters at nerve endings.

Organochlorine Insecticides

Although DDT (dichlorodiphenyltrichloroethane) was first synthesized by Zeidler in 1874, it remained for Paul Müller, a Swiss chemist working for J. R. Geigy AG, to rediscover DDT in 1939 while searching for a contact poison against clothes moths and carpet beetles. The effectiveness of DDT against a variety of household and crop insect pests was quickly demonstrated, earning Müller a Nobel Price in 1948 for

his research. Before the end of World War II, DDT was available to the Allies and saw its first medical use in the suppression of a typhus epidemic in Naples, Italy, during the winter of 1943–44 when it was applied directly to humans to control lice (Brooks, 1972a). The discovery of the insecticidal properties of other organochlorine compounds including aldrin, dieldrin, endrin, chlordane, and benzene hexachloride before 1945 had immediate consequences and introduced the era of the synthetic chemical insecticides and their remarkable impact on food production and human health (Metcalf, 1972; Brooks, 1974a,b).

The organochlorine (chlorinated hydrocarbon) insecticides are a diverse group of agents belonging to three distinct chemical classes including the dichlorodiphenylethane-, the chlorinated cyclodiene-, and the chlorinated benzene- and cyclohexane-related structures (Table 18–6). From the mid-1940s to the mid-1960s, the organochlorine insecticides were used extensively in all aspects of agriculture and forestry, in building and structural protection, and in human situations to control a wide variety of insect pests. The properties (low volatility, chemical stability, lipid solubility, slow rate of biotransformation and degradation) that made these chemicals such effective insecticides also brought about their demise because of persistence in the environment, bioconcentration, and biomagnification within various food chains and the acquisition of biologically active body burdens in many wildlife species that, if not lethal, certainly interfered with the reproductive success of the species. The publication of Rachel Carson's book, *Silent Spring,* did much to draw attention to the plight of wildlife, particularly avian species such as grebes, pelicans, falcons, and eagles that occupied the top trophic level of their respective food chains (Carson, 1962). Definitive studies both in wildlife and laboratory species have demonstrated the potent estrogenic and enzyme-inducing properties of the organochlorine insecticides, particularly the dichlorodiphenylethane-type, which interfered directly or indirectly with fertility and reproduction (Stickel, 1968; McFarland and Lacy, 1969; Longcore *et al.,* 1971; McBlain *et al.,* 1977). In avian species, such interference is related to steroid metabolism and the inability of the bird to mobilize sufficient calcium to produce a strong enough eggshell to withstand the rigors of being buffeted around in a nest, the resultant cracking allowing the entry of bacteria and death of the developing embryo (Carson, 1962; Peakall, 1970). The reproduction in fish is adversely affected by the bioconcentration of these agents in the yolk sac

Table 18–6. STRUCTURAL CLASSIFICATION OF ORGANOCHLORINE INSECTICIDES

DICHLORODIPHENYLETHANES		DDT, DDD Dicofol Perthane Methoxychlor Methlochlor
CYCLODIENES		Aldrin, Dieldrin Heptachlor Chlordane Endosulfan
CHLORINATED BENZENES CYCLOHEXANES		HCB, HCH Lindane (α-BHC)

of the fry. Many studies have demonstrated the gradual accumulation of residues of these chemicals and their metabolites in body tissues as well as the slow elimination from the system (Laben *et al.,* 1965; Dustman and Stickel, 1969). Despite the fact that the widespread use of organochlorine insecticides has been banned in North America and Europe, these chemicals are used extensively in third-world, developing nations because they are inexpensive to manufacture, they are highly effective and relatively safe, there are few substitutes available, and the risk benefit ratio is highly weighted in favor of their continued use for the control of insects causing devastation to crops and human health. Thus, these insecticides are still important toxicologically.

Signs and Symptoms of Poisoning. Given the diversity of chemical structure, it is not surprising that the signs and symptoms of toxicity and the mechanism(s) of action are somewhat different (Table 18–7).

Exposure of humans and animals to high oral doses of DDT results in paresthesia of the tongue, lips, and face; apprehension, hypersusceptibility to external (light, touch, sound) stimuli; irritability; dizziness, vertigo; tremor; and tonic and clonic convulsions. Motor unrest and fine tremors associated with voluntary movements progress to coarse tremors without interruption in moderate to severe poisonings. Symptoms generally appear several hours (6 to 24 hours) after exposure to large doses. Little toxicity is seen following the dermal exposure to DDT, presumably because the agent is poorly absorbed through the skin, a physiologic phenomenon that has contributed to the rather good safety record of DDT, despite careless handling

by applicators and formulators (Hayes, 1971). It has been estimated that a dose of 10 mg/kg will cause signs of poisoning in humans. Chronic exposure to moderate concentrations of DDT causes somewhat milder signs of toxicity as listed in Table 18–7.

Although the functional injury of DDT poisoning can be associated with effects on the CNS, few pathologic changes can be demonstrated in that tissue in animals. However, following exposure to moderate or high nonfatal doses or subsequent to subacute or chronic feeding, major pathologic changes are observed in the liver and reproductive organs. Morphologic changes in mammalian liver include hypertrophy of hepatocytes and subcellular organelles such as mitochondria, proliferation of smooth endoplasmic reticulum and the formation of inclusion bodies, centrolobular necrosis following exposure to high concentrations, and an increase in the incidence of hepatic tumors (Hayes, 1959; Hansell and Ecobichon, 1974; IARC, 1974). However, there has been no epidemiologic evidence linking DDT to carcinogenicity in humans (Hayes, 1975, 1982). When technical DDT (20 percent *o,p'*-DDT plus 80 percent *p,p'*-DDT) was administered to male cockerels or rats, reduced testicular size was observed and, in female rats, the estrogenic effects of the *o,p'*-isomer were observed in the edematous, blood-engorged uteri (Hayes, 1959; Ecobichon and MacKenzie, 1974). The *o,p'*-isomer has been shown to compete with estradiol for binding the estrogen receptors in rat uterine cytosol (Kupfer and Bulger, 1976).

Unlike the situation with DDT where there have been few recorded fatalities following poisoning, there have been a number of fatalities

Table 18–7.   SIGNS AND SYMPTOMS OF ACUTE AND CHRONIC TOXICITY FOLLOWING EXPOSURE TO ORGANOCHLORINE INSECTICIDES

INSECTICIDE CLASS	ACUTE SIGNS	CHRONIC SIGNS
Dichlorodiphenylethanes		
DDT	Parathesia (oral ingestion)	Loss of weight, anorexia
DDD (Rothane)	Ataxia, abnormal stepping	Mild anemia
DMC (Dimite)	Dizziness, confusion, headache	Tremors
Dicofol (Kelthane)	Nausea, vomiting	Muscular weakness
Methoxychlor	Fatigue, lethargy	EEG pattern changes
Methiochlor	Tremor (peripheral)	Hyperexcitability, anxiety
Chlorbenzylate		Nervous tension
Hexachlorocyclohexanes		
Lindane (γ-isomer)		
Benzene hexachloride (mixed isomers)		
Cyclodienes		
Endrin	Dizziness, headache	Headache, dizziness, hyperexcitability
Telodrin	Nausea, vomiting	
Isodrin	Motor hyperexcitability	Intermittent muscle twitching and myoclonic jerking
Endosulfan	Hyperreflexia	
Heptachlor	Myoclonic jerking	Psychological disorders including insomnia, anxiety, irritability
Aldrin	General malaise	
Dieldrin	Convulsive seizures	
Chlordane	Generalized convulsions	EEG pattern changes
Toxaphene		Loss of consciousness
		Epileptiform convulsions
Chlordecone (Kepone)		
Mirex		Chest pains, arthralgia
		Skin rashes
		Ataxia, incoordination, slurred speech, opsoclonus
		Visual difficulty, inability to focus and fixate
		Nervousness, irritability, depression
		Loss of recent memory
		Muscle weakness, tremors of hands
		Severe impairment of spermatogenesis

following poisoning by the cyclodiene and hexachlorocyclohexane type insecticides. The chlorinated cyclodiene insecticides are among the most toxic and environmentally persistent pesticides known (Hayes, 1982). Even at low doses, these chemicals tend to induce convulsions before less serious signs of illness occur. Although the sequence of signs generally follows the appearance of headaches, nausea, vertigo and mild clonic jerking, motor hyperexcitability, and hyperreflexia, some patients have convulsions without warning symptoms (Hayes, 1971). An important difference between DDT and the chlorinated cyclodienes is that the latter are efficiently absorbed through the skin and, therefore, pose an appreciable hazard to occupationally exposed individuals. Chronic exposure to low or moderate concentrations of these agents elicits a spectrum of signs and symptoms, including both sensory and motor components of the CNS (Table 18–7). In addition to the recognized neurotoxicity, aldrin and dieldrin interfere with reproduction, increased pup losses (vitality, viability) being reported in studies in rats and dogs (Kitselman, 1953; Treon and Cleveland, 1955). Treatment with dieldrin during pregnancy caused a reduction in fertility and increased pup mortality (Treon and Cleveland, 1955). The treatment of pregnant mice with dieldrin resulted in teratologic (delayed ossification, increases in supernumerary ribs) effects (Chernoff *et al.*, 1975).

Exposure to lindane (the γ-isomer of hexachlorocyclohexane, HCH) produces signs of poisoning that resemble those caused by DDT (i.e., tremors, ataxia, convulsions, stimulated respiration, and prostration). In severe cases of acute poisoning, violent tonic and clonic convulsions occur and degenerative changes in the liver and in renal tubules have been noted. Technical grade HCH used in insecticidal preparations contains a mixture of isomers: the γ- and α-isomers are convulsant poisons; the β- and δ-isomers are CNS depressants. The mechanisms of action remain unknown. Lifetime feeding studies in mice have revealed that technical HCH and some of the isomers caused an increase in hepatocellular tumors (IARC, 1974). Only the γ-isomer (lindane) sees any medicinal use today, being a component of a pediculicide shampoo for head lice. One undocumented case, known to the author, resulted in mild tremors in a child on whose head the shampoo was used vigorously and repeatedly for more than a week. The symptoms disappeared rapidly when the treatment was terminated.

Industrial carelessness during the manufacture of an organochlorine compound chlordecone (Kepone) brought this agent and the closely related insecticide, mirex, to the attention of toxicologists in 1975 when 76 of 148 workers in a factory in Hopewell, Virginia, developed a severe neurologic syndrome (Cannon *et al.*, 1978; Taylor *et al.*, 1978; Guzelian, 1982). This condition, known as the "Kepone shakes," was characterized by tremors, altered gait, behavioral changes, ocular flutter (opsoclonus), arthralgia, headache, chest pains, weight loss, hepatomegaly, splenomegaly, and impotence, the onset of symptoms generally occurring with a latency of approximately 30 days from the initiation of exposure and persisting for many months after the termination of exposure (Joy, 1982). Laboratory tests showed a reduced sperm count and reduced sperm motility. Routine neurologic studies revealed nothing untoward, but microscopic examination of biopsies of the sural nerve revealed relative decreases in the populations of small myelinated and unmyelinated axons. With electron microscopy, a number of abnormalities were visible and the significant findings included damage to Schwann cells (membranous inclusions, cytoplasmic folds), prominent endoneural collagen pockets, vacuolization of unmyelinated fibers, focal degeneration of axons with condensation of neurofilaments and neurotubules, focal interlamellar splitting of myelin sheaths, and the formation of myelin "bodies" and a complex infolding of inner mesaxonal membranes into axoplasm (Martinez *et al.*, 1978). The involvement of unmyelinated fibers and small myelinated fibers may partially explain the clinical picture. It has been suggested that chlordecone may interfere with metabolic

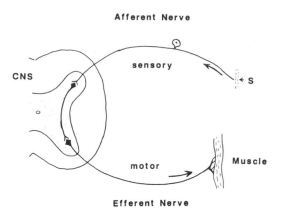

Figure 18–5. A simple, intact reflex arc involving a peripheral, afferent (sensory) neuron, interneurons in the CNS, and a peripheral, efferent (motor) neuron that innervates a muscle.

processes in Schwann cells. However, it should be noted that all of these degenerative changes are nonspecific in nature and are commonly seen in other toxic polyneuropathies. Many of the toxic manifestations of chlordecone poisoning in these workers have been confirmed in animal studies, the major target organs being the CNS, the liver, the adrenals, and the testes (Huber *et al.*, 1965; Eroschenko and Wilson, 1975; Egle *et al.*, 1978; Larson *et al.*, 1979; Baggett *et al.*, 1980). As with other organochlorine insecticides, chlordecone is an excellent inducer of hepatic microsomal monooxygenase enzymes and, in rats and mice, has been associated with the formation of hepatomas and malignant tumors in organs other than the liver, female animals being more susceptible than male (Guzelian, 1982). In many ways, mirex behaves like chlordecone and there is evidence for the oxidative biotransformation of mirex to chlordecone *in vivo*. Mirex causes hepatomegaly and a dose-dependent increase in neoplastic nodules and hepatocellular carcinomas, particularly in male animals (Innes *et al.*, 1969; Waters *et al.*, 1977).

Site and Mechanism of Toxic Actions. Essential to the action of organochlorine insecticides is an intact reflex arc consisting of afferent (sensory) peripheral neurons impinging on interneurons in the spinal cord, with accompanying ramifications and interconnections up and down the CNS and interactions with efferent, motor neurons as shown schematically in Figure 18–5. Examining the mechanism of action of the DDT-type insecticides, the most striking observation in a poisoned insect or mammal is the display of periodic sequences of persistent tremoring and/or convulsive seizures suggestive of repetitive discharges in neurons. These characteristic episodes of hyperactivity

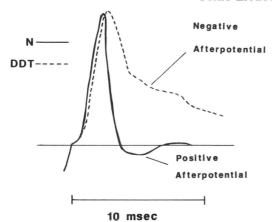

Figure 18–6. A schematic diagram of an oscilloscope recording of the depolarization and repolarization of a normal neuron (——) and one from a DDT-treated animal (- - - - -), showing the prolongation of the negative afterpotential (NAP).

interspersed with normal function were recognized as early as 1946. The second most striking observation is that these repetitive tremors, seizures, and electrical activity can be initiated by tactile and auditory stimuli, suggesting that the sensory nervous system appears to be much more responsive to stimuli. An examination of the sequence of electrical events in normal and DDT-poisoned nerves reveals that, in the latter, a characteristic prolongation of the falling phase of the action potential (the negative afterpotential) occurs (Figure 18–6). The nerve membrane remains in a partially depolarized and partially repolarized state and is extremely sensitive to complete depolarization again by very small stimuli (Joy, 1982). Thus, following exposure to DDT, the repetitive stimulation of the peripheral sensory nerves by touch or sound is magnified in the CNS, causing generalized tremoring throughout the body.

How does DDT elicit this effect? There are at least four mechanisms, possibly all functioning simultaneously (Matsumura, 1985). At the level of the neuronal membrane, DDT affects the permeability to potassium ions, reducing potassium transport across the membrane. DDT alters the porous channels through which sodium ions pass—these channels activate (open) normally but, once open, are inactivated (closed) slowly, thereby interfering with the active transport of sodium out of the nerve axon during repolarization. DDT inhibits neuronal adenosine triphosphatase (ATPase), particularly the Na^+, K^+-ATPase and Ca^{2+}-ATPase that play vital roles in neuronal repolarization. DDT also inhibits the ability of calmodulin, a calcium mediator in nerves, to transport calcium ions essential for the

intraneuronal release of neurotransmitters. All of these inhibited functions reduce the rate at which repolarization occurs and increase the sensitivity of the neurons to small stimuli that would not elicit a response in a fully repolarized neuron.

The chlorinated cyclodiene, benzene, and cyclohexane type insecticides are different from DDT in many respects, both in the appearance of the intoxicated individual and possibly also in the mechanism(s) which appear to be localized more in the CNS than in the sensory division of the PNS. The overall appearance of the intoxicated individual is one of CNS stimulation. As is shown in Figure 18–7, the cyclodiene compounds mimic the action of the chemical picrotoxin, a nerve excitant and antagonist of the neurotransmitter γ-aminobutyric acid (GABA) found in the CNS (Eldefrawi *et al.*, 1985; Matsumura, 1985). GABA induces the uptake of chloride ions by neurons. The blockage of this activity by picrotoxin, picrotoxinin, or cyclodiene insecticides results in only partial repolarization of the neuron and a state of uncontrolled excitation. The cyclodiene insecticides are also potent inhibitors of Na^+, K^+-ATPase and, more importantly, the enzyme Ca^{2+}, Mg^{2+}-ATPase that is essential for the transport (uptake and release)

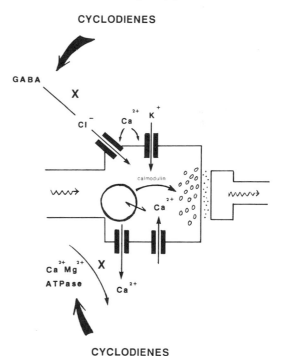

Figure 18–7. Proposed sites of action of cyclodiene-type organochlorine insecticides on chloride ion transport by antagonizing GABA receptors in the chloride channel as well as inhibition of Ca^{2+}, Mg^{2+}-ATPase.

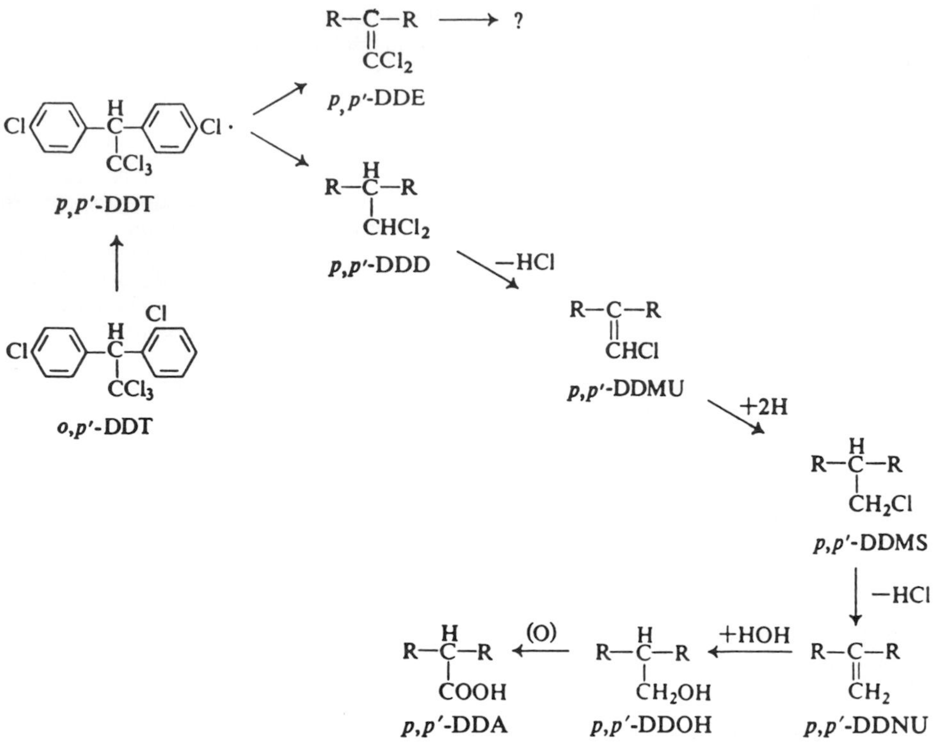

Figure 18–8. Degradation of DDT by mammalian and avian tissues. *Abbreviations:* DDD, 1,1-dichloro-2,2-bis(*p*-chlorophenyl)ethane; DDE, 1,1-dichloro-2,2-bis(*p*-chlorophenyl)ethylene; DDMU, 1-chloro-2,2-bis(*p*-chlorophenyl)ethylene; DDMS, 1-chloro-2,2-(*p*-chlorophenyl)ethane; *DDNU,* unsym-bis(*p*-chlorophenyl)ethylene; DDOH, 2,2-bis(*p*-chlorophenyl)ethanol; DDA, bis(*p*-chlorophenyl)acetic acid. (From Ecobichon and Saschenbrecker, 1968.)

of calcium across membranes (Matsumura, 1985; Wafford *et al.,* 1989). The inhibition of Ca^{2+}, Mg^{2+}-ATPase, located in the terminal ends of neurons in synaptic membranes, results in an accumulation of intracellular free calcium ions with the promotion of calcium-induced release of neurotransmitters from storage vesicles and the subsequent depolarization of adjacent neurons and the propagation of stimuli throughout the CNS.

Biotransformation, Distribution, and Storage. The phenomenon of bioconcentration and biomagnification of the organochlorine insecticides in food chains has already been mentioned. Once the chemical is acquired by the organism, its biotransformation, proceeds at an exceptionally slow rate due, in part, to the complex aromatic ring structures and to the extent of chlorination, these ring substituents being exceedingly difficult to remove by the enzymatic processes available in body tissues. DDT undergoes slow but extensive biotransformation in mammals, one major metabolite, DDE, being formed nonenzymatically as well as by enzymatic dechlorination (Figure 18–8) (Ecobichon and

Saschenbrecker, 1967, 1968). Other degradation products such as DDD and DDA are formed by a series of reductive dechlorination and oxidative reactions, only the latter agent being sufficiently water soluble to be readily excreted (Ecobichon and Saschenbrecker, 1968). Not surprisingly, analysis of body tissues yields a mixture of DDT and various metabolites, all of which possess a relatively high degree of lipid solubility. The results of such analyses are frequently presented in terms of total DDT-derived material. In contrast, the biotransformation of the cyclodiene-type insecticides is extremely slow, aldrin and heptachlor being converted by oxidative reactions to dieldrin and heptachlor epoxide, respectively, without altering significantly either the lipid solubility characteristics or their toxicologic properties (Keane and Zavon 1969, Matthews and Matsumura, 1969). Although the α-, β-, and γ-isomers of hexachlorocyclohexane are biotransformed at significantly different rates *in vivo* by dehydrochlorination, glutathione conjugation, and aromatic ring hydroxylation to produce a variety of excretable phenolic products, the β-isomer is much more slowly metabolized and is found as the predominant tissue residue (Egan *et al.,* 1965; O'Brien, 1967; Abbott *et al.,* 1968). Toxophene, a complex mixture of chlorinated camphenes (chlorobornanes) possessing widely varying biologic activities, is extensively biotransformed by both oxidative and reductive cytochrome P-450 monooxygenases (Saleh *et al.,* 1977; Turner *et al.,* 1977). Considering the complex cage-structured chlordecone and mirex, there is little evidence of any biotransformation of these chemicals *in vivo* other than the oxidative conversion of mirex into the ketone, chlordecone, prior to either slow excretion in the feces or storage in body fat.

The highly lipid-soluble nature of the organochlorine insecticides, characterized by large fat:water partition coefficients, guarantees that these chemicals will be sequestered in body tissues (liver, kidneys, nervous system, adipose tissue) having a high lipid content where the residues either elicit some biologic effect or, as in the case of adipose tissue, remain stored and undisturbed. Studies in both humans and laboratory animals have demonstrated that there was a log-log relationship between the daily intake of DDT and adipose residues, with a state of equilibrium being attained between intake and elimination from the body and plateau residue concentrations being related to the amount of agent acquired daily. Following the termination of exposure, the organochlorine insecticides are slowly eliminated from the storage sites *in vivo.* The elimination of DDT from the body occurs at a rate of approximately 1.0 percent of the stored quantity per day (Hayes, 1971). The elimination rates from animals are exceedingly slow, biologic half-lives of DDT in exposed cattle being of the order of 335 days (Laben *et al.,* 1965). The elimination rate and depletion of body storage sites may be enhanced by fasting which results in the mobilization of adipose tissue and the insecticide contained therein (Ecobichon and Saschenbrecker, 1969). However, with a high body burden of toxicant, there is the possibility of enhanced toxicity from circulating agent being redistributed to target organs as was seen in a study in cockerels (Ecobichon and Saschenbrecker, 1969). In animals with a body burden of DDT, treatment with phenobarbital has resulted in an enhanced elimination of the agent and metabolites as measured by residue levels in biologic fluids and tissues (Alary *et al.,* 1971; Lambert and Brodeur, 1976).

Given the physicochemical properties of the organochlorine insecticides, it is not surprising that humans acquired body burdens of these chemicals during the 1950s and 1960s when they were used on almost all food crops. Depending on the region of the world, the intensity of use, the extent of occupational and accidental exposure, and dietary habits, the bioconcentration and bioaccumulation of DDT in human adipose tissue resulted in levels of the order of 5 ppm DDT and approximately 15 ppm of total DDT-derived material (Fiserova-Bergerova *et al.,* 1967; Abbott *et al.,* 1968; Morgan and Roan, 1970). The levels of other organochlorine insecticides sequestered in body fat were never as high as that of DDT. With declining use and the eventual ban of this class of insecticides from the North American market, body burdens of these insecticides declined slowly. By the late 1960s adipose levels of 2 ppm DDT (9 ppm of total DDT-derived material) were detectable. Whereas the daily intake of DDT in the United States was approximately 0.2 mg/day in 1958, this had decreased to about 0.04 mg/day by 1970 (Hayes, 1971). Today, only trace levels of DDT, of the order of 2.0 ppm of total DDT-derived material, are detectable in human adipose tissue (Mes *et al.,* 1982). Currently, major concerns are centered on the Inuit living in Arctic regions where the sources of dietary protein (fish, seals, walruses, whales, and so forth) have proven to be major depositories of organochlorine insecticides and other chlorinated hydrocarbons (PCBs, PCDDs, PCDFs). As the "ripple effect" of global pollution spreads to these distant regions, the resident animal species, possessing significant adipose tissue depots, have acquired body burdens of these chemicals and the human occupies the top position in these food chains.

Treatment of Poisoning. The life-threatening situation in organochlorine insecticide poisoning is associated with the tremors, the motor seizures, and the interference with respiratory function (hypoxemia and resulting acidosis) arising from repetitive stimulation of the CNS. In addition to the general decontamination and supportive treatment, diazepam (0.3 mg/kg i.v.; maximum dose of 10 mg) or phenobarbital (15 mg/kg i.v.; maximum dose of 1.0 g) may be administered by slow injection to control the convulsions. It many be necessary to repeat the treatment.

Although such treatment was not available when the organochlorine insecticides were at their peak use, recent experience with chlordecone intoxications introduced a regimen of therapy to enhance the rate of excretion of stored chlordecone from the body. The oral administration of the anion-exchange resin, cholestyramine, to intoxicated patients resulted in a 3- to 18-fold enhanced fecal excretion of chlordecone, significantly reduced the biologic half-life of stored chlordecone, and enhanced the rate of recovery from toxic manifestations (Cohn *et al.,* 1978). The rationale for the use of cholestyr-

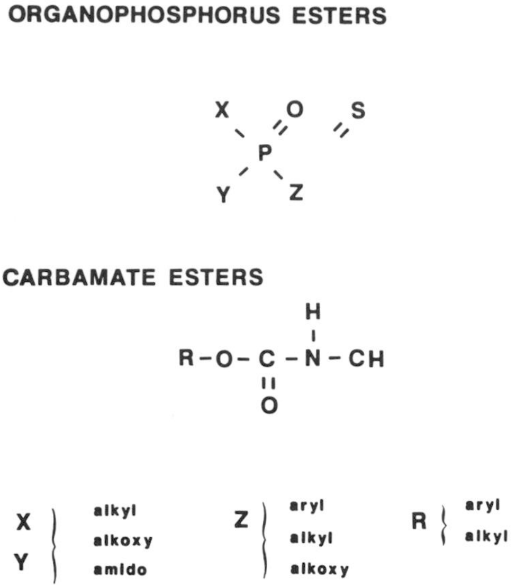

ORGANOPHOSPHORUS ESTERS

CARBAMATE ESTERS

Figure 18–9. The basic "backbone" structures of the two types of anticholinesterase class insecticides, the organophosphorus and the carbamate esters. With the organophosphorus compounds the esters may be of phosphoric acid (P = O) or of phosphorothioic (P = S) acids. The substituents X, Y, Z, and R denote the variety of groups attached directly to or through an oxygen to the phosphorus.

amine rests on the biliary-enterohepatic circulation of chlordecone, the anion-exchange resin binding the secreted insecticide, reducing reabsorption and retaining the bound agent in the lumen of the intestinal tract for fecal excretion. Indirectly, cholestyramine may reduce chlordecone reabsorption by binding bile salts and thereby reducing the formation of emulsions and the uptake of this lipid-soluble agent. Whether or not such therapy would be suitable for other organochlorine insecticides would be dependent on the extent of biliary secretion of the agents and/or their metabolites. It is possible that cholestyramine might prove efficacious in treating organochlorine insecticide intoxications.

Anticholinesterase Insecticides

The agents comprising this type of insecticide have a common mechanism of action but arise from two distinctly different chemical classes, the esters of phosphoric or phosphorothioic acid and those of carbamic acid (Figure 18–9). The anticholinesterase insecticides are represented by a vast array of structures that have demonstrated the ultimate in structure-activity relationships in attempts to produce potent and selective insect toxicity while minimizing the toxicity toward nontarget species. Today, there are some 200 different organophosphorus ester

and approximately 25 carbamic acid ester insecticides in the marketplace, formulated into literally thousands of products. For detailed discussions on nomenclature, chemistry, and development of these insecticides, the reader is referred to the books of O'Brien (1960), Heath (1961), Melnikov (1971), Fest and Schmidt (1973), Eto (1974), Kuhr and Dorough (1976), Ecobichon and Joy (1982), Matsumura (1985), and a review by Holmstedt (1959).

The organophosphorus ester insecticides were first synthesized in 1937 by a group of German chemists led by Gerhard Schrader at Farbenfabriken Bayer AG (Schrader and Kukenthal, 1937). Many of their trial compounds proved to be exceedingly toxic and, unfortunately, under the management of the Nazis in World War II, some were developed as potential chemical warfare agents. Although it is true that all of the organophosphorus esters were derived from "nerve gases" (chemicals such as soman, sarin, and tabun), a fact that the media continually emphasizes, the insecticides used today are at least three "generations" of development away from those highly toxic chemicals. The first organophosphorus ester insecticide to be used commercially was tetraethylpyrophosphate (TEPP) and, although effective, it was extremely toxic to all forms of life and chemical stability was a major problem in that TEPP hydrolyzed readily in the presence of moisture. Further development was directed toward the synthesis of more stable chemicals having moderate environmental persistence, giving rise to parathion (*O,O*-diethyl-*O-p*-nitrophenyl phosphorothioate, E-605) in 1944 and the oxygen analog, paraoxon (*O,O*-diethyl-*O-p*-nitrophenyl phosphate) at a later date. Although these two chemicals had the properties desired in an insecticide (low volatility, chemical stability in sunlight and in the presence of water, environmental persistence for efficacy), they both exhibited a marked mammalian toxicity and were unselective with respect to target and nontarget species. The replacement of DDT with parathion in the 1950s resulted in a series of fatal poisonings and bizarre accidents arising from the fact that workers did not appreciate that this agent was far different from the relatively innocuous organochlorine insecticides with which they were familiar (Ecobichon, 1982a). The number of severe poisonings attributed to parathion provided the stimulus for a search for analogs that would be more selective in their toxicity to target species and less toxic to nontarget organisms, including wildlife, domestic stock, and humans.

The first pesticidal carbamic acid esters were synthesized in the 1930s and were marketed as fungicides. These aliphatic esters possessed poor insecticidal activity and interest in this chemical class lay dormant until the mid-1950s when renewed interest in insecticides having anticholinesterase activity but reduced mammalian toxicity led to the synthesis of several potent aryl esters of methylcarbamic acid. The insecticidal carbamates were synthesized on purely chemical grounds as analogs of the drug physostigmine, a toxic anticholinesterase alkaloid extracted from the seeds of the plant *Physostigma venenosum,* the Calabar bean.

Signs and Symptoms of Poisoning. Although the structures are diverse in nature, the mechanism by which the organophosphorus and carbamate ester insecticides elicit their toxicity is identical and is associated with the inhibition of the nervous tissue acetylcholinesterase (AChE), the enzyme responsible for the destruction and termination of the biologic activity of the neurotransmitter acetylcholine (ACh). With the accumulation of free, unbound ACh at the nerve endings of all cholinergic nerves, there is continual stimulation of electrical activity. The signs of toxicity include those resulting from stimulation of the muscarinic receptors of the parasympathetic autonomic nervous system (increased secretions, bronchoconstriction, miosis, gastrointestinal cramps, diarrhea, urination, bradycardia); those resulting from the stimulation and subsequent blockade of nicotinic receptors, including the ganglia of the sympathetic and parasympathetic divisions of the autonomic nervous system as well as the junctions between nerves and muscles (causing tachycardia, hypertension, muscle fasciculations, tremors, muscle weakness, and/or flaccid paralysis); and those resulting from effects on the CNS (restlessness, emotional lability, ataxia, lethargy, mental confusion, loss of memory, generalized weakness, convulsion, cyanosis, coma) (Table 18–8).

The classic picture of anticholinesterase insecticide intoxication which was first described by DuBois (DuBois, 1948; DuBois *et al.,* 1949) has become more complicated in recent years by the recognition of additional and persistent signs of neurotoxicity not previously associated with these chemicals. First, and frequently associated with exposure to high concentrations of the insecticides (suicide attempts, drenching with dilute or concentrated chemicals) are effects that may persist for several months following exposure and involve neurobehavioral, cognitive, and neuromuscular functions (Ecobichon, 1982a). The first evidence of this type of syndrome, delayed psychopathologic-neurologic lesions, was reported by Spiegelberg (1963), who had been studying workers involved in the production and handling of the highly toxic nerve

gases in Germany during World War II. The characteristic symptomatology subdivided these patients into two distinct groups. The first and largest group was characterized by persistently lowered vitality and ambition; defective autonomic regulation leading to cephalagia, gastrointestinal and cardiovascular symptoms; premature decline in potency and libido; intolerance to alcohol, nicotine, and various medicines; and an impression of premature aging. The second group, in addition to the above symptoms, showed one or more of the following: depressive or subdepressive disorders of vital function; cerebral vegetative (syncopal) attacks; slight or moderate amnestic or demential effects; and slight organoneurologic defects. These symptoms developed and persisted for some five to ten years following exposure to these most toxic organophosphorus esters during the war years. The controversial paper of Gershon and Shaw (1961), a study of 16 cases of pesticide applicators exposed primarily to organophosphorus ester insecticides for 10 to 15 years, reported a wide range of persistent signs of toxicity, including tinnitus, nystagmus, pyrexia, ataxia, tremor, paresthesia, polyneuritis, paralysis, speech difficulty (slurring), loss of memory, insomnia, somnambulism, excessive dreaming, drowsiness, lassitude, generalized weakness, emotional lability, mental confusion, difficulty in concentration, restlessness, anxiety, depression, dissociation, and schizophrenic reactions. Although the results of other studies have been equivocal in their support of such an array of long-term signs and symptoms, there is a persistent recurrence of the symptomatology in a number of anecdotal and documented reports (Ecobichon, 1982a). The literature on potential, suspected, and established sequelae of organophosphorus ester insecticide intoxications does not confirm the frequently seen statement that clinical recovery from nonfatal poisoning is always complete in a few days. Continuous and close observation of the acutely intoxicated patients for some weeks following their recovery from the initial toxicity and treatment thereof would be necessary to identify the subtle changes indicated above. The emergency service physician rarely sees the patient following stabilization and initial "recovery." Definitive examples where such observation has been possible are few but one such fortuitous case illustrates what can be achieved if there is close follow-up (Ecobichon *et al.,* 1977).

A 33-year-old female technician was exposed dermally to an unknown amount of a 7.5 percent v/v solution of fenitrithion [*O,O*-dimethyl-*O*-(4-nitro-*m*-tolyl) phosphorothioate] prepared in corn oil, having wiped up the spilled material with facial tissues and

Table 18–8. SIGNS AND SYMPTOMS OF ANTICHOLINESTERASE INSECTICIDE POISONING*

NERVOUS TISSUE AND RECEPTORS AFFECTED	SITE AFFECTED	MANIFESTATIONS
Parasympathetic autonomic (muscarinic receptors) postganglionic nerve fibers	Exocrine glands	Increased salivation, lacrimation, perspiration
	Eyes	Miosis (pinpoint and nonreactive), ptosis, blurring of vision, conjunctival injection, "bloody tears"
	Gastrointestinal tract	Nausea, vomiting, abdominal tightness, swelling and cramps, diarrhea, tenesmus, fecal incontinence.
	Respiratory tract	Excessive bronchial secretions, rhinorrhea, wheezing, edema, tightness in chest, bronchospasms, bronchoconstriction, cough, bradypnea, dyspnea
	Cardiovascular system	Bradycardia, decrease in blood pressure
	Bladder	Urinary frequency and incontinence
Parasympathetic and sympathetic autonomic fibers (nicotinic receptors)	Cardiovascular system	Tachycardia, pallor, increase in blood pressure
Somatic motor nerve fibers (nicotinic receptors)	Skeletal muscles	Muscle fasciculations (eyelids, fine facial muscles), cramps, diminished tendon reflexes, generalized muscle weakness in peripheral and respiratory muscles, paralysis, flaccid or rigid tone
		Restlessness, generalized motor activity, reaction to acoustic stimuli, tremulousness, emotional lability, ataxia
Brain (acetylcholine receptors)	Central nervous system	Drowsiness, lethargy, fatigue, mental confusion, inability to concentrate, headache, pressure in head, generalized weakness
		Coma with absence of reflexes, tremors, Cheyne–Stokes respiration, dyspnea, convulsions, depression of respiratory centers, cyanosis

* From Ecobichon, D. J., and Joy, R. M. *Pesticides and Neurological Diseases.* CRC Press, Boca Raton, Florida, 1982.

bare hands. Distinctive symptoms (memory loss, tremors, fatigue) were observed two days after exposure accompanied by a 45 percent reduction in plasma cholinesterase activity but only minimal change in erythrocyte AChE activity. She was hospitalized for treatment and the signs and symptoms became more intense, being characteristic of those associated with intoxication by organophosphorus esters (see Table 18–8). The patient responded to repeated antidotal (pralidoxime) treatment (see Treatment). Although the plasma cholinesterase activity returned to normal levels some 15 to 20 days after exposure, moderate neuromuscular (fasciculations, generalized muscle weakness) and psychiatric (emotional lability, decreased ability to concentrate on tasks, memory impairment, lethargy) sequelae persisted for upwards of four months after exposure, although recovery was complete within nine months of the incident.

A second distinct manifestation of exposure to organophosphorus ester insecticides has recently been described by clinicians in Sri Lanka involved in the treatment of suicide attempts (Senanayake and Karalliedde, 1987). This paralytic condition, called the "intermediate syndrome," consisted of a sequence of neurologic signs that appeared some 24 to 96 hours after the acute cholinergic crisis but before the expected onset of delayed neuropathy, the major effect being muscle weakness, primarily affecting muscles innervated by the cranial nerves (neck flexors, muscles of respiration) as well as those of the limbs. Cranial nerve palsies were common. There was a distinct risk of death during this time interval because of respiratory depression and distress which required urgent ventilatory support and was responsive to atropine. The chemicals involved in these distinctive intoxications included fenthion, dimethoate, monocrotophos, and methamidophos. There were no obvious clinical differences during the acute intoxication phase between those patients who developed the intermediate syndrome and others who did not, all patients being treated in the same manner.

A third syndrome, that of organophosphate-induced delayed neurotoxicity (OPIDN), is caused by some phosphate, phosphonate, and phosphoramidate esters, only a few of which

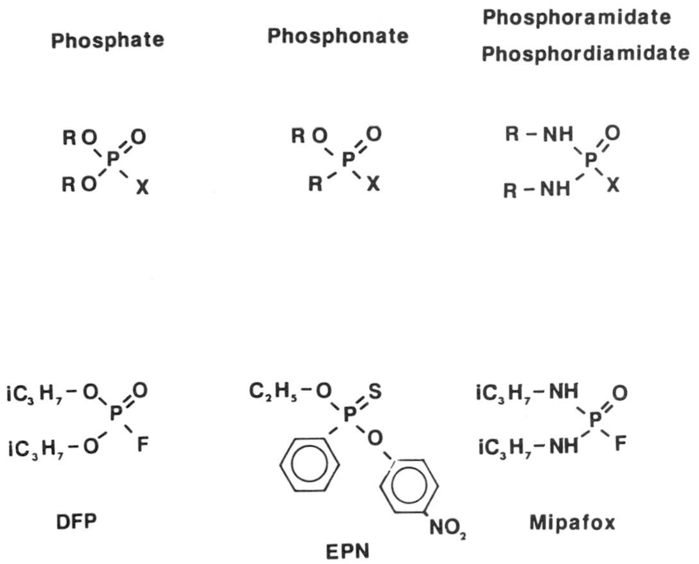

Figure 18–10. The basic structures and nomenclature of organophosphorus esters, with examples, capable of causing organophosphate-induced delayed neurotoxicity (OPIDN).

have ever been used as insecticides (Figure 18–10). Historically, this syndrome has been known for almost 100 years, being associated with the chemical tri-*o*-tolyl phosphate (TOTP) (Ecobichon, 1982a). The first major epidemic of OPIDN occurred during the prohibition years in the United States, resulting from the consumption of a particular brand of alcoholic extract of Jamaican ginger contaminated or adulterated with mixed tolyl phosphate esters. The syndrome, affecting some 20,000 individuals to varying degrees, was known as "ginger jake paralysis" or "jake leg" and was studied in detail by Maurice Smith of the U.S. Public Health Service. He not only confirmed that the condition could be reproduced in animals (rabbits, dogs, monkeys, calves) but also demonstrated that only one of the three isomers found in commercial tri-tolyl phosphate, the *ortho*-isomer, was responsible for the toxicity (Smith *et al.,* 1931). The initial flaccidity, muscle weakness in the arms and legs giving rise to a clumsy, shuffling gait, were replaced by a spasticity, hypertonicity, hyperreflexia, clonus, and abnormal reflexes, indicative of damage to the pyramidal tracts and a permanent upper motor neuron syndrome (Ecobichon, 1982a). In many patients, recovery was limited to the arms and hands, damage to the lower extremities (foot drop, spasticity, and hyperactive reflexes) being permanent and suggesting damage to the spinal cord (Morgan and Penovich, 1978). A similar neuropathy occurred with an experimental organophosphorus ester insecticide, mipafox, following an accident in a manufacturing pilot plant. Details

of the effects on two of the workers were described by Bidstrup *et al.* (1953) and Ecobichon (1982a). The poisoning of water buffalo in the early 1970s in Egypt by an insecticide, leptophos, revealed a neurologic syndrome similar to that observed following exposure to TOTP (Abou-Donia, 1981). There was also evidence of leptophos-induced neuropathies among workers in a manufacturing plant in the United States, but the controversial observations were obscured by concomitant exposure of the workers to *n*-hexane, another neurotoxic chemical (Xintaris *et al.,* 1978).

Concern that many of the over 200 organophosphorus ester insecticides in use might cause this unique neuropathy has resulted in an intensive study of the syndrome, the identification of the most susceptible species (the hen and the cat), the development of standard protocols to test all insecticides, and at least a partial elucidation of the mechanisms by which agents elicit this condition. Histologic examination of the nervous systems of hens treated with a suitable agent (TOTP, DFP, mipafox, leptophos) has revealed a Wallerian, "dying-back" degeneration of large diameter axons and their myelinic sheaths in distal parts of the peripheral nerves and of long spinal cord tracts, i.e., the rostral ends of ascending tracts and the distal ends of descending tracts (Cavanagh, 1954; Sprague and Bickford, 1981). Biochemical studies have demonstrated that the above-mentioned agents inhibit a neuronal, nonspecific carboxylesterase, neuropathic target esterase (NTE), which appears to have some, as yet unknown, role in lipid metabolism in neurons (Johnson, 1982). If acute exposure to an appropriate organophosphorus ester results in >70 percent inhibition of NTE, the characteristic OPIDN usually follows, with ataxia being observed some 7 to 14 days following treatment and progression to moderate to severe muscular weakness and paralysis with concomitant changes in neuronal morphology (Johnson, 1982; Slott and Ecobichon, 1984). It is the considered opinion of many investigators that many of the commonly used phosphate and phosphorothioate ester insecticides might be capable of causing this syndrome if only sufficient concentrations of the agents could be obtained *in vivo*. However, taking paraoxon as an example of such a phosphate ester, the animal(s) would either die as a consequence of other acute toxic effects or would rapidly detoxify the agent, thereby preventing the acquisition of sufficient paraoxon to inhibit NTE. There also appear to be subtle structure-activity relationships between organophosphorus esters and the active site on the NTE protein because many phosphate esters are not good inhibitors of NTE (Ohkawa *et al.*, 1980; Abou-Donia, 1981). It should be emphasized that, although NTE inhibition remains a useful function for monitoring the potential of organophosphorus esters to induce OPIDN, the role of this enzyme in the initiation of the syndrome remains unknown and histopathologic evidence is a requirement of the U.S. EPA protocol.

The signs and symptoms of acute intoxication by carbamate insecticides are quite similar to those described above for organophosphorus compounds, differing only in the duration and intensity of the toxicity. The most apparent reasons for the relatively short duration of action and the mild to moderate severity of signs are that (1) carbamate insecticides are reversible inhibitors of nervous tissue AChE, unlike most of the organophosphorus esters (see following section) and (2) they are rapidly biotransformed *in vivo*. Despite the extensive toxicologic research demonstrating that the pesticidal carbamate esters are "relatively safe" chemicals producing only transient, short-term toxicity following acute administration, carbamate insecticide toxicity has been reported in humans and fatalities have occurred (Ecobichon, 1982b; Hayes, 1982). Invariably, these serious poisonings have involved carbaryl and have occurred as a consequence of accidental or purposeful (suicidal) exposure to high concentrations (Hayes, 1982; Cranmer, 1986). Information on the incidences of human intoxication by carbaryl can be found in the Carbaryl Decision Document (EPA, 1980). For the period 1966–80, 195 human

intoxication cases were reported (3 fatalities, 16 hospitalizations, and 176 cases receiving medical attention). A single oral dose of 250 mg of carbaryl (2.8 mg/kg body weight) is sufficient to elicit moderately severe poisoning in an adult man (Cranmer, 1986). Moderate but transient toxicity has also been observed following exposure to a few of the more potent carbamate ester insecticides such as methomyl (Lannate®) and propoxur (Baygon®) (Vandekar *et al.*, 1968, 1971; Liddle *et al.*, 1979). More recently, the illegal use of aldicarb (Temik®), a very acutely toxic carbamate ester, on watermelons in California and on English cucumbers in British Columbia, Canada, resulted in moderate to severe toxicity in consumers of these products, the signs and symptoms including nausea, vomiting, gastrointestinal cramps, and diarrhea (Jackson *et al.*, 1986).

There is little evidence of prolonged neurotoxicity following the exposure of humans to carbamate ester insecticides. However, this statement should be made cautiously. One case of a farmer who handsprayed a vegetable garden with a water-wettable formulation of carbaryl, drenching himself in the process, resulted in a chronic polyneuropathy which included such signs as persistent photophobia, mild and persistent paresthesia, memory loss, muscular weakness, fatigue, and lassitude (Ecobichon, 1982b). Although no other references have been seen in the literature describing long-term, persistent effects of any of the carbamic ester insecticides in humans, there is evidence in animal studies, albeit at near toxic doses, of a Wallerian-type degeneration of spinal cord tracts in rabbits and hens following treatment with sodium diethyldithiocarbamate (Edington and Howell, 1969). Carbaryl, when fed to hogs (150 mg/kg per day for 72 or 83 days), caused a rear leg paralysis that was minimal while resting but, when the animals were forced to move, resulted in marked incoordination, ataxia, tremors, clonic muscle contractions, and prostration (Smalley *et al.*, 1969). There was histologic evidence of lesions in the CNS and in skeletal muscle. Carbamate ester insecticides do not inhibit NTE or elicit OPIDN-type neurotoxicity. Behavioral changes have been noted in a number of animal studies following the subchronic or chronic administration of different carbamate insecticides (Santalucito and Morrison, 1971; Desi *et al.*, 1974). There is sufficient evidence to indicate that carbamate insecticides can initiate neurologic and behavioral changes at dosages causing no apparent clinical signs (Ecobichon, 1982b; Hayes, 1982). However, the signal danger from pesticidal carbamates and neurologic problems appears to involve acute single exposures to

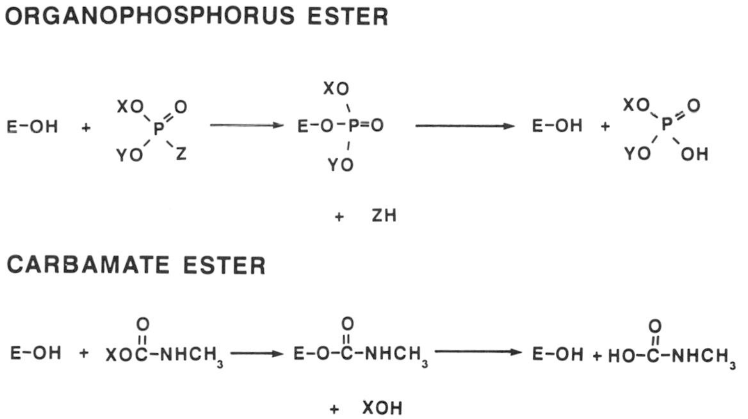

ORGANOPHOSPHORUS ESTER

$$E-OH \; + \; \begin{array}{c} XO \\ \diagdown \\ YO \end{array}\hspace{-0.3em}\begin{array}{c} O \\ \diagup\hspace{-0.3em}\diagup \\ P \\ \diagdown \end{array}\hspace{-0.3em}Z \longrightarrow \begin{array}{c} XO \\ \diagdown \\ E-O-P=O \\ \diagup \\ YO \end{array} \longrightarrow E-OH \; + \; \begin{array}{c} XO \\ \diagdown \\ YO \end{array}\hspace{-0.3em}\begin{array}{c} O \\ \diagup\hspace{-0.3em}\diagup \\ P \\ \diagdown \end{array}\hspace{-0.3em}OH$$

$$+ \quad ZH$$

CARBAMATE ESTER

$$E-OH \; + \; XO\overset{O}{\overset{\|}{C}}-NHCH_3 \longrightarrow E-O-\overset{O}{\overset{\|}{C}}-NHCH_3 \longrightarrow E-OH + HO-\overset{O}{\overset{\|}{C}}-NHCH_3$$

$$+ \quad XOH$$

Figure 18–11. The interaction between an organophosphorus or carbamate ester with the serine hydroxyl group in the active site of the enzyme acetylcholinesterase (E–OH). The intermediate, unstable complexes formed before the release of the "leaving" groups (ZH and XOH) are not shown. The dephosphorylation or decarbamoylation of the inhibited enzyme is the rate-limiting step to forming free enzyme.

massive doses of the agents or at least repeated exposure to large doses.

Site and Mechanism of Toxic Action. Although the anticholinesterase-type insecticides have a common mode of action, there are significant differences between organophosphorus and carbamate esters. The reaction between an organophosphorus ester and the active site in the AChE protein (a serine hydroxyl group) results in the formation of a transient intermediate complex that partially hydrolyzes with the loss of the "Z" substituent group, leaving a stable, phosphorylated, and largely unreactive, inhibited enzyme that, under normal circumstances, can be reactivated only at a very slow rate (Figure 18–11). With many organophosphorus ester insecticides, an irreversibly inhibited enzyme is formed, and the signs and symptoms of intoxication are prolonged and persistent, requiring vigorous medical intervention and including the reactivation of the enzyme with specific chemical antidotes (see Treatment). Without intervention, the toxicity will persist until sufficient quantities of "new" AChE are synthesized in 20 to 30 days to destroy efficiently the excess neurotransmitter. The nature of the substituent groups at "X," "Y," and "Z" plays an important role in the specificity for the enzyme, the tenacity of binding to the active site, and the rate at which the phosphorylated enzyme dissociates to produce free enzyme. Many of the more recently introduced organophosphorus esters (acephate, temephos, dichlorvos, trichlorfon) are less tenacious inhibitors of nervous tissue AChE, the phosphorylated enzyme being more readily and spontaneously dissociated.

In contrast, carbamic acid esters, attaching to the reactive site of the AChE, undergo hydrolysis in two stages: the first stage is the removal of the "X" substituent (an aryl or alkyl group) with the formation of a carbamylated enzyme; the second stage is the decarbamylation of the inhibited enzyme with the generation of free, active enzyme (Figure 18–11). Carbamic acid esters are nothing more than poor substrates for the cholinesterase-type enzymes.

Presenting the concept of the interaction between organophosphorus and carbamic esters with AChE in another manner (Table 18–9), one can see that the only distinctive difference between the two anticholinesterase-type insecticides lies in the rate at which the dephosphorylation or decarbamoylation takes place. The rate is exceedingly slow for organophosphorus esters, so much so that the enzyme is frequently considered to be irreversibly inhibited. The rate of decarbamoylation is sufficiently rapid that these esters are often considered to be reversible inhibitors or poor substrates with low turnover rates. The characteristics of the various rate constants for the natural substrate (ACh), organophosphorus and carbamate esters are shown in Table 18–9. It is important to appreciate that the rate at which step 3 proceeds is thousands of times slower with carbamate esters than with ACh whereas with organophosphorus esters, it is several orders of magnitude slower (Ecobichon, 1979). This subject has been extensively reviewed by Aldridge and Reiner (1972).

A number of organophosphorus (phosphate, phosphonate, and phosphoramidate) esters (Figure 18–10), the chemical warfare agents sarin, soman, and tabun and a few other compounds

Table 18–9. KINETICS OF ESTER HYDROLYSIS*

$$EH + AB \rightleftarrows EHAB \rightarrow BH + EA \rightarrow EH + AOH$$

ESTERS	COMPLEX FORMATION $(K_A = k_{-1}/k_{+1})$	ACYLATION (k_2)	DEACYLATION (k_3)
Substrates	Small	Extremely fast	Extremely fast
Organophosphorus esters	Small	Moderately fast	Slow or extremely slow
Carbamate esters	Small	Slow	Slow

* From Ecobichon, D. J. In Geissbuhler, H. (ed.): *Advances in Pesticide Science, Part 3, Biochemistry of Pests and Mode of Action of Pesticides, Pesticide Degradation, Pesticide Residues and Formulation Chemistry.* Pergamon Press, New York, 1979, pp. 516–524.

such as DFP, mipafox, and leptophos, have the ability to bind tenaciously to the active site of AChE and of NTE to produce an irreversibly inhibited enzyme by a mechanism known as "aging." The aging process is dependent on the size and configuration of the alkyl (R) substituent, the potency of the ester increasing in the order diethyl, dipropyl, and dibutyl for such analogs as DFP and mipafox (Aldridge and Johnson, 1971). The aging process is generally accepted as being due to the dealkylation of the intermediate dialkylphosphorylated enzymes by one of two possible mechanisms (Figure 18–12). The first involves the hydrolysis of a P–O bond following a nucleophile (base) attack on the phosphorus atom. The second mechanism

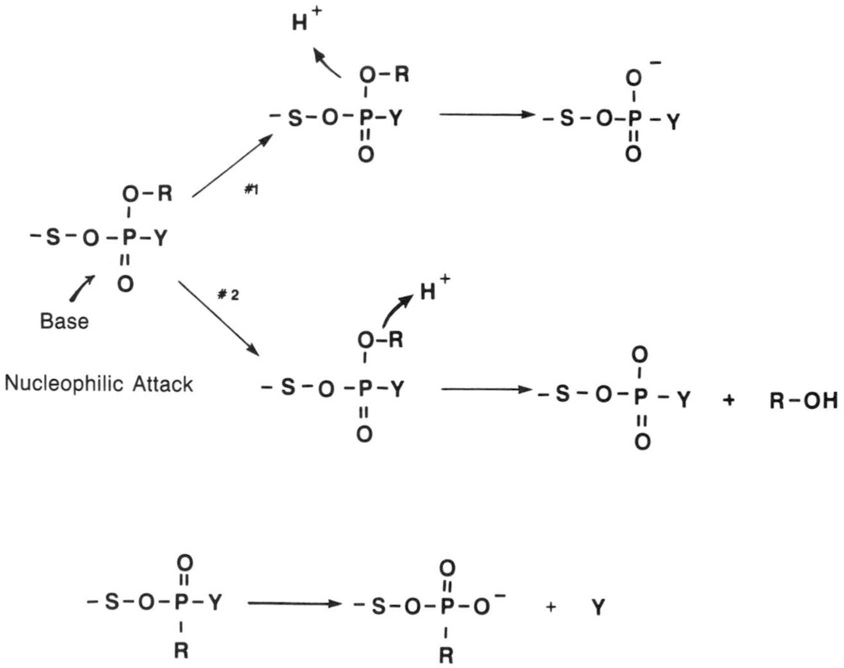

If one or two R-P bonds are P-O-C (phosphate, phosphonate), aging results.
If R-P bonds are P-C (phosphinate), no aging occurs.

Figure 18–12. A schematic diagram illustrating two mechanisms by which the "aging" of organophosphorus ester inhibited acetylcholinesterase may occur. See text for details.

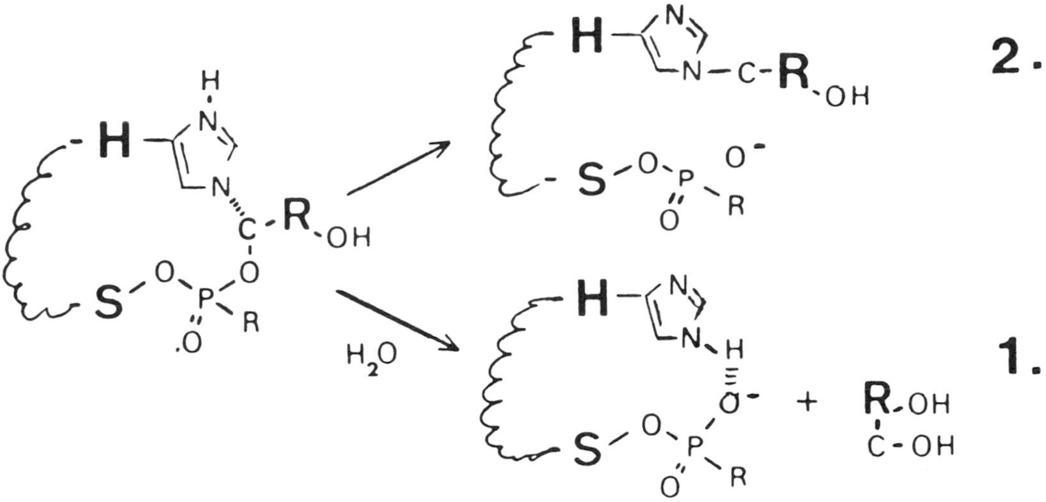

Figure 18–13. The phosphorylation, aging, and possible alkylation reactions of saligenin cyclic phosphorus esters with α-chymotrypsin to yield two possible stabilized forms of the aged enzyme, both utilizing an imidazole group of a neighboring histidine in close proximity to the active center of the enzyme. (Toia and Casida, 1979)

involves the hydrolysis of an O–C bond by an acid catalysis, resulting in the formation of a carbonium ion as the leaving group (O'Brien, 1960; Eto, 1974; Johnson, 1982). The aging process is believed to fix an extra charge to the protein, causing some perturbation to the active site, thereby preventing dephosphorylation. While the exact nature of this reaction has not been demonstrated for AChE and NTE, evidence from experiments with saligenin cyclic phosphorus esters (derivatives of TOTP) and α-chymotrypsin points to the possibility of two stabilized forms of "aged" enzyme (Toia and Casida, 1979). As is shown in Figure 18–13, both of the reactions utilize the imidazole group of a neighboring histidine. In one reaction, the hydroxylated substituent is released and the phosphorylated enzyme is stabilized by a hydrogen on the imidazole group. In the other reaction, the leaving substituent becomes attached to the imidazole, yielding a N–C-hydroxylated derivative of the phosphorylated enzyme. Johnson (1982) proposed that, in the case of NTE, if one or two of the P–R bonds were P–O–C (as in phosphates and phosphonates), aging would occur rapidly whereas if the P–R bonds were P–C (as in phosphinates), aging would not be possible.

Biotransformation, Distribution, and Storage. Both the organophosphorus and carbamate ester insecticides undergo extensive biotransformation in all forms of life, both the route(s) and the rate(s) of metabolism

being highly species specific and dependent on the substituent chemical groups attached to the basic "backbone" structure of these esters (Figure 18–9). Tissue enzymes of both Phase I (oxidative, reductive, hydrolytic) and Phase II (transfer or conjugative reactions with glutathione, glucuronic acid, glycine, and so forth) types are found widespread in plant, invertebrate, and vertebrate species and, indeed, are responsible for some aspects of the species sensitivity and/or both natural and acquired resistance to many of these insecticides. The biotransformation of anticholinesterase type insecticides has been extensively reviewed in the literature and the reader is referred to such sources as O'Brien (1967), Menzie (1969), Eto (1974), Kulkarni and Hodgson (1984), Ecobichon and Joy (1982), and Matsumura (1985) for details on the various mechanisms involved.

Exogenous (xenobiotic or foreign) compounds undergo metabolic transformation *in vivo* to less toxic and more polar metabolites that can be eliminated from the organism more readily. The Phase I detoxification processes usually form reactive metabolites whereas Phase II processes conjugate the polar Phase I metabolites with some natural body substituent to form a product with enhanced water solubility and excretability. (See Chapter 4.)

As is shown in Figure 18–14, organophosphorus esters may undergo simultaneous, enzymatic attack at a number of different points in the molecule. Only one reaction, that of the oxida-

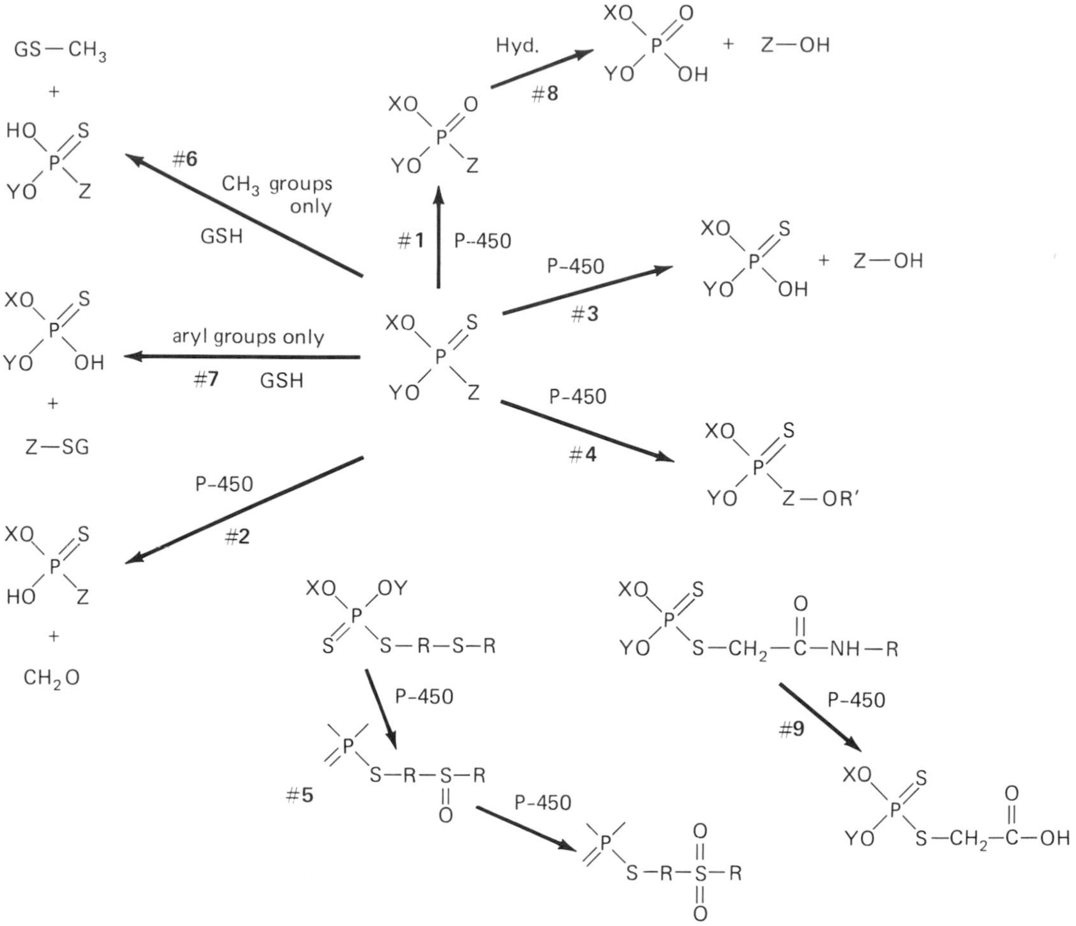
GS—CH3
+
HO S P YO Z
#6
CH3 groups only
GSH
XO O P YO Z
Hyd.
#8
XO O P YO OH
+ Z—OH
#1
P-450
P-450
#3
XO S P YO OH
+ Z—OH
XO S P YO OH
aryl groups only
#7 GSH
+
Z—SG
XO S P YO Z
P-450
#4
XO S P YO Z—OR′
P-450
#2
XO S P HO Z
+
CH2O
XO OY P S S—R—S—R
P-450
#5
S—R—S—R
O
P-450
S—R—S—R
O
O
XO S P YO S—CH2—C—NH—R
O
P-450
#9
XO S P YO S—CH2—C—OH
O

Figure 18–14. A schematic diagram depicting the various Phase I and Phase II biotransformation pathways of an organophosphorus ester and the nature of the products formed as a consequence of oxidative, hydrolytic, GSH-mediated transfer and conjugation of intermediate metabolites in mammals. See text for details.

tive desulfuration of phosphorothioate esters (Mechanism 1), results in a significant increase in the toxicity of the biotransformation product, an oxygen analog. Many of the organophosphorus esters in use today are phosphorothioate (parathion, methyl parathion, fenitrothion, and so forth) or phosphorodithioate (azinophos-methyl, malathion) esters. The presence of this thiono-group reduces the AChE-inhibiting properties of the ester, and confers greater chemical stability (nonenzymatic hydrolysis) on the molecule but also confers species selectivity. Although oxidative desulfuration in insects and mammals results in the formation of a more toxic oxygen analog of the parent insecticide, this intermediate can be readily hydrolyzed by aryl and aliphatic hydrolases found in mammalian tissues, whereas insect species are frequently deficient in these enzymes, making insects more susceptible to such agents (Mechanism 8).

Oxidative dealkylation and dearylation reactions (Mechanisms 2 and 3) involve enzymes that utilize the coenzyme reduced nicotinamide adenine dinucleotide phosphate (NADPH), the ubiquitously distributed cytochrome P-450 system and an NADPH-regenerating system to provide the necessary oxygen, and electrons to produce polar metabolites. Demethylation, with the formation of an aldehyde, occurs quite readily, whereas the reaction becomes significantly reduced when the alkyl group becomes longer (i.e., ethyl, propyl, and so forth) (Mechanism 2). Dearylation occurs in a similar fashion with the formation of a phenol and a dialkylphosphoro- or dialkylphosphorothioic acid (Mechanism 3). The monooxygenase system can also catalyze a number of reactions involving substitutents on side groups resulting in (1) aromatic ring hydroxylation (Mechanism 4); (2) thioether oxidation (Mechanism 5); (3) deamination; (4) alkyl and *N*-hydroxylation; (5) *N*-oxide formation; and (6) *N*-dealkylation. A number of transferases use glutathione (γ-glutamyl-L-cysteinyl glycine, GSH) as a cofactor and acceptor for *O*-alkyl and *O*-aryl groups (Mechanisms 6 and 7) to yield monodesmethyl products plus *S*-methylglutathione or dialkylphosphoro- or dialkylphosphorothioic acids plus aryl-glutathione derivatives, respectively.

Hydrolysis of phosphoro- and phosphorothioic acid esters occurs via a number of different tissue hydrolases (nonspecific carboxylesterases, arylesterases, phosphorylphosphatases, phosphotriesterases, carboxyamidases) scattered ubiquitously throughout the plant and animal kingdoms, with activity being highly dependent on the nature of the substituents (Ecobichon, 1979). Slight structural modifications to substituents on the insecticide molecule can dramatically alter the specificity of these enzymes toward an agent and affect species selectivity. The arylesterases [aromatic or A-esterases (ArE), EC 3.1.1.2] preferentially hydrolyze aryl (phenol, naphthol, indole, and so forth) esters of short-chain aliphatic or phosphorus acids, particularly if there is a double bond present in the alcohol moiety in position α with respect to the ester bond (Mechanism 8). Carboxylesterases [carboxylic acid ester hydrolases (CE), EC 3.1.1.1] are capable of hydrolyzing a variety of aliphatic and aryl esters of short-chain fatty acids. The most important example of this reaction involving organophosphorus ester insecticides is with malathion [*O*,*O*-dimethyl-*S*-(1,2-dicarbethoxyethyl) phosphorodithioate] where one of the two available ethylated carboxylic ester groups is hydrolyzed to yield malathion (or malaoxon) α-monoacids that are biologically inactive (Dauterman and Main, 1966). This CE-catalyzed reaction is an important feature of resistance to this insecticide in insects and to tolerance in mammals. Potentiation of anticholinergic effects can be produced by the combined administration of certain pairs of organophosphate ester insecticides such as EPN (*O*-ethyl-*O*-*p*-nitrophenylbenzenethiophosphonate) and malathion (Frawley *et al.*, 1957). The mechanism for this effect involves the inhibition of carboxyesterases by EPN (Murphy, 1969, 1972, 1980). Carboxyamidases (acylamide amidohydrolase, EC 3.5.1.4), found extensively in plant, insect, and vertebrate tissues, are of limited current interest in the degradation of insecticides, dimethoate [*O*,*O*-dimethyl-*S*-(*N*-methylcarbamoylmethyl) phosphorodithioate] having been the only organophosphorus ester insecticide shown to be hydrolyzed by mammalian tissue amidases (Mechanism 9). Phosphorylphosphatases and phosphotriesterases have limited involvement in the biotransformation of organophosphorus ester insecticides but play a role in the detoxification of some of the chemical warfare agents.

Phase II conjugative reactions are of limited necessity in the biotransformation of organophosphorus ester insecticides, usually being relegated to the task of glucuronidating or sulfating the aromatic phenols, cresols, and so forth, hydrolyzed from the ester (Yang, 1976). However, one must be wary of these enzyme systems because metabolism studies of chlorfenvinphos [2-chloro-1-(2', 4'-dichlorophenyl)vinyl diethylphosphate] revealed the presence of glucuronide and glycine conjugates of several products whereas studies with trichlorfon (*O*,*O*-dimethyl-1-hydroxy-2,2,2-trichloroethyl phosphonate) revealed direct glucuronidation of the insecticide without prior biotransformation (Hutson *et al.*, 1967; Bull, 1972).

In a similar fashion, carbamate ester insecticides can undergo simultaneous attack at several points in the molecule depending on the nature of the substituents attached to the basic structure (Figure 18–15). In addition to the hydrolysis of the carbamate ester group by tissue CE and the release of a substituted phenol, carbon dioxide, and methylamine (Mechanism 1), several oxidative and reductive reactions involving cytochrome P-450 related monooxygenases can proceed, the ultimate products being considerably more polar than the parent insecticide. The extent of hydrolysis of carbamate ester insecticides varies greatly between species, ranging from 30 to 95 percent hydrolysis. The type of oxidative reactions observed with carbamate esters can be simplified into two main groups: (1) direct ring hydroxylation (Mechanism 2) and (2) oxidation of appropriate side chains as is shown for this "mythical" methylcarbamate, resulting in the hydroxylation of *N*-methyl groups or methyl groups to form hydroxymethyl groups (Mechanism 3), *N*-demethylation of secondary and tertiary amines (Mechanism 4), *O*-dealkylation of alkoxy side chains (Mechanism 5), thioether oxidation (Mechanism 6), and so forth. Phase II conjugative reactions can occur at any free, reactive grouping with glucuronide and sulfate derivatives (Mechanism 7), as well as GSH conjugates (mercapturates) being formed (Mechanism 8). For a comprehensive understanding of the various mechanisms involved, the reader is referred to those reviews mentioned above, as well as to pertinent articles by Ryan (1971), Fukuto (1972), and Kuhr and Dorough (1976).

Treatment of Poisoning. Despite the qualitative and quantitative differences between organophosphorus and carbamate insecticide in-

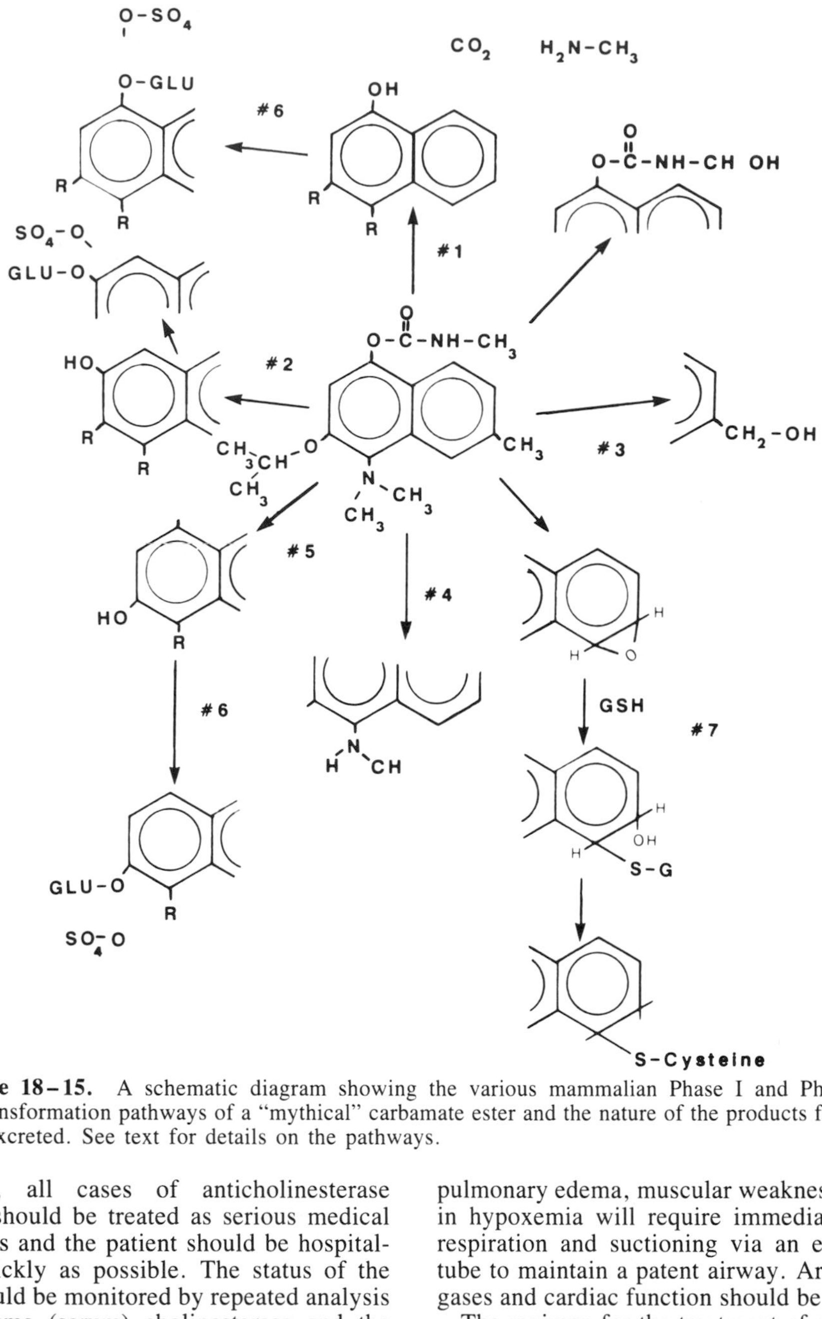

Figure 18–15. A schematic diagram showing the various mammalian Phase I and Phase II biotransformation pathways of a "mythical" carbamate ester and the nature of the products formed and excreted. See text for details on the pathways.

toxications, all cases of anticholinesterase poisoning should be treated as serious medical emergencies and the patient should be hospitalized as quickly as possible. The status of the patient should be monitored by repeated analysis of the plasma (serum) cholinesterase and the erythrocyte AChE, the inhibition of the activities of these two enzymes being good indicators of the severity of organophosphorus ester poisoning while only the erythrocytic AChE is inhibited by carbamate esters (except at excessively high levels of exposure). As a consequence of the extensive involvement of the entire nervous system, the life-threatening signs (respiratory depression, bronchospasm, bronchial secretions,

pulmonary edema, muscular weakness) resulting in hypoxemia will require immediate artificial respiration and suctioning via an endotracheal tube to maintain a patent airway. Arterial blood gases and cardiac function should be monitored.

The regimen for the treatment of organophosphorus ester insecticide intoxication, based on the analysis of serum pseudocholinesterase, is described in Table 18–10 (Namba et al., 1971; Ecobichon et al., 1977). Atropine is used to counteract the initial muscarinic effects of the accumulating neurotransmitter. However, atropine is a highly toxic antidote and great care must be taken. Frequent small doses of atropine (subcutaneously or intravenously) are indicated

Table 18–10. CLASSIFICATION AND TREATMENT OF ORGANOPHOSPHORUS INSECTICIDE POISONING BASED ON PLASMA PSEUDOCHOLINESTERASE ACTIVITY MEASUREMENTS*

| CLASSIFICATION OF POISONING | ENZYME ACTIVITY (% OF NORMAL) | TREATMENT | |
		Atropine	*Pralidoxime*
Mild	20–50	1.0 mg s.c.	
Moderate	10–20	1.0 mg i.v. every 20 to 30 minutes until sweating and salivation disappear and slight flush and mydriasis appear	1.0 g i.v. over 20 to 30 minutes
Severe	10	5.0 mg i.v. every 20 to 30 minutes until sweating and salivation disappear and slight flush and mydriasis appear	1.0 g i.v. as above. If no improvement, administer another 1.0 g i.v. If no improvement, start i.v. infusion at 0.5 g/hour

* From Ecobichon, D. J., Ozere, R. L., Reid, E., and Crocker, J. F. S.: *Can. Med. Assoc. J.,* **116**:377–379, 1977.

for mild signs and symptoms following a brief, intense exposure. Relatively large, cumulative doses of atropine, up to 50 mg daily, may be essential to control severe muscarinic symptoms. The status of the patient must be monitored continuously by examining for the disappearance of secretions (dry mouth and nose) and sweating, facial flushing, and mydriasis (dilatation of pupils).

Supplementary treatment to offset moderate to severe nicotinic and CNS signs and symptoms usually takes the form of one of the specific antidotal chemicals, the oximes (pralidoxime or 2-PAM, toxogonin), administered intravenously to reactivate the inhibited nervous tissue AChE. The use of this agent may not be necessary for cases of mild intoxication and it should be reserved for moderate to severe poisonings. Treatment, by slow intravenous infusion of doses of 1.0 g, should be initiated as soon as possible, because the longer the interval between exposure and treatment, the less effective the oxime will be. In many poisonings, a single treatment with pralidoxime will be sufficient to elicit a reversal of the signs and symptoms and reduces the amount of atropine needed. If absorption, distribution, and/or metabolism of the organophosphorus ester is delayed in the body, it may be essential to administer pralidoxime repeatedly over several days after initial treatment. Care should be taken with repeated dosing because pralidoxime effectively binds calcium ions and causes muscle spasms not unlike those elicited by the organophosphorus esters. Severe muscle cramping, particularly in the extremities, may be alleviated by oral or intravenous calcium solutions (Ecobichon et al., 1977).

The therapeutic action of the oxime com-

pounds resides in their capacity to reactivate AChE without contributing markedly toxic actions of their own. Those organophosphorus esters possessing good "leaving groups," i.e., the "X" moiety, phosphorylate the nervous tissue AChE by a mechanism similar to that of acetylation by the substrate ACh. These esters are frequently called irreversible inhibitors because the hydrolysis of the phosphorylated enzyme by water is exceedingly slow (Table 18–9). However, various nucleophilic agents containing a substituted ammonium group will dephosphorylate the phosphorylated enzyme at a much more rapid rate than water. The basic requirements for a reactivating molecule consisted of a rigid structure containing a quaternary ammonium group and an acidic nucleophile that would be complementary with the phosphorylated enzyme in such a way that the nucleophilic oxygen would be positioned close to the electrophilic phosphorus atom. These structure-activity requirements led to the development of the pralidoxime compounds, the syn-isomer of 2-PAM (2-formyl-N-methylpyridinium chloride oxime) being particularly active (Childs et al., 1955; Askew, 1956; Kewitz and Wilson, 1956; Namba and Hiraki, 1958). The reaction of 2-PAM with the phosphorylated enzyme proceeds as shown in Figure 18–16.

The reactivation is an equilibrium reaction, the oxime reacting either with the phosphorylated enzyme or free, unbound organophosphorus ester, the product being a phosphorylated oxime which, in itself, can be a potent cholinesterase inhibitor if it is stable in an aqueous medium (Schoene, 1972). In general, the phosphorylated oxime degrades quickly in water.

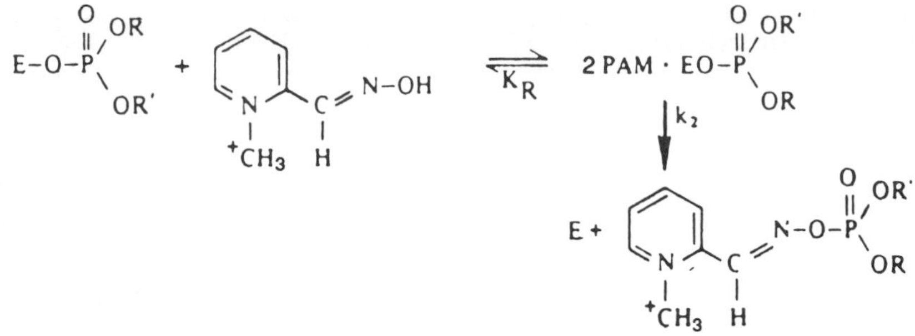

Figure 18–16. The pralidoxime-catalyzed reactivation of an organophosphate-inhibited molecule of AChE, showing the release of active enzyme and the formation of an oxime-phosphate complex.

A practical limitation on the usefulness of oxime reactivators lies in the inability of these agents to reactivate "aged" AChE, that enzyme in which the phosphorylated enzyme has been further dealkylated and the phosphoryl group becomes tightly bound to the reactive site (*see* Figure 18–12). Success with the pyridinium analogs led to an intensive search for more effective oximes and the discovery of the bispyridinium compounds, toxogonin or obidoxime [bis(4-formyl-*N*-methylpyridinium oxime) ether dichloride], TMB-4 [*N,N*-trimethylene bis(pyridine-4-aldoxime) bromide], and, more recently, the H-series compounds. However, these agents are not without toxicity and only pralidoxime has seen antidotal use (Engelhard and Erdmann, 1964; Steinberg *et al.*, 1977). Toxogonin is less toxic than TMB-4 and is capable of reactivating AChE inhibited by a variety of organophosphorus esters.

The clinical treatment of carbamate toxicity is similar to that for organophosphorus ester insecticide intoxication with the exception that the use of oximes is contraindicated. Early reports, in which pralidoxime or toxogonin was used in treating carbaryl intoxications, revealed that the oxime enhanced the carbaryl-induced toxicity (Sterri *et al.*, 1979; Ecobichon and Joy, 1982). With other carbamate esters, pralidoxime had no obvious beneficial effect. Pralidoxime is not an effective antidote in carbamate intoxication because it does not interact with the carbamylated AChE in the same manner as with phosphorylated AChE.

Diazepam (10 mg s.c. or i.v.) may be included in the treatment regimen of all but the mildest cases of organophosphorus and/or carbamate intoxications. In addition to relieving any mental anxiety associated with the exposure, diazepam counteracts some aspects of the CNS and neuromuscular signs that are not affected by atropine. Doses of 10 mg (s.c. or i.v.) are appropriate and may be repeated. Other centrally acting drugs that may depress respiration are not recommended in the absence of artificial respiration.

It is important to appreciate that vigorous treatment of anticholinesterase type insecticide intoxications does not offer protection against the possibility of delayed onset neurotoxicity or the persistent sensory, cognitive, and motor defects discussed earlier. These deficits, albeit reversible over a long time interval, appear consistently in intoxications and are caused by mechanisms as yet unknown. Certain evidence points to severe damage to the neuromuscular junctions in skeletal muscle resulting in a persistent, peripheral muscular weakness (Wecker *et al.*, 1978).

Pyrethroid Insecticides

The newest major class of insecticides is the synthetic pyrethroids, a group of chemicals just entering the marketplace in 1980 but, by 1982, accounting for approximately 30 percent of the worldwide insecticide usage (Anon, 1977; Vijverberg and van den Bercken, 1982). However, these synthetics arise from a much older class of botanical insecticides, pyrethrum, a mixture of six insecticidal esters (pyrethrins, cinerins, and jasmolins) extracted from dried pyrethrum or chrysanthemum flowers (*Chrysanthemum cinerariaefolium, C. coccineum*) (Hartley and West, 1969). Although it is believed that the natural pyrethroids were discovered by the Chinese in the first century A.D., the first written accounts of these agents are found in the seventeenth century literature and commercial preparations made their appearance in the mid-1800s (Neumann and Peter, 1987). Japanese woodblock prints from the early 1800s exist in which one can see smouldering insecticide coils of pressed pyrethrum powder not unlike those manufactured and used today. The chrysanthemum varieties grown in Kenya yield the highest proportions of active ingredients, but the plants are grown commercially in many regions of the world. In 1965, the world output of pyrethrum was approximately 20,000 tons with Kenya alone producing some 10,000 tons (Cremlyn, 1978). The steady increase in use of this prepara-

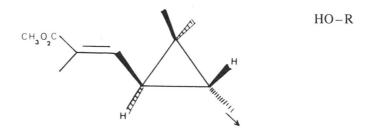

Chrysanthemic Acid

HO–R

Pyrethric Acid

Figure 18–17. The basic structures of the pyrethroid ester insecticides, showing the two characteristic acidic portions, chrysanthemic and pyrethric acids. Variations in the alcoholic (HO-R) moieties include alkyl- and aryl-ether chains of complex structure.

tion despite the extensive introduction of other synthetic insecticides lies in the fact that it has a rapid knockdown or paralytic action on flying insects, appearing to be very potent although having a very low toxicity in both insects and mammals due to efficient enzymatic degradation. The demand for this product has far exceeded the limited world production, leading chemists to focus attention on the synthesis of new analogs, hopefully with better stability in light and air, persistence, more selectivity in target species, and a further reduction in mammalian toxicity. In addition to extensive agricultural use, the synthetic pyrethroids are components of household sprays, flea preparations for pets, plant sprays for home and greenhouse use, and so forth. For an in-depth discussion of the development of the pyrethroid ester insecticides, their chemistry and biologic activity, the reader is referred to Elliott (1976), Cremlyn (1978), Casida *et al.* (1983), Leahey (1985), Matsumura (1985), and Narahashi *et al.* (1985).

The major active principles in pyrethrum are pyrethrin I, esters of chrysanthemic acid (pyrethrin I, cinerin I, and jasmolin I), and pyrethrin II which are esters of pyrethric acid (pyrethrin II, cinerin II, and jasmolin II) (Figure 18–17). Pyrethrin I is the most active ingredient for

lethality whereas pyrethrin II possesses remarkable knockdown properties for a wide range of household, veterinary, and post-harvest storage insects. The natural pyrethrins and early synthetic chrysanthemic acid derivatives are more active as contact than as stomach poisons, whereas the more recent synthetic agents show particular potency when ingested and are less susceptible to biotransformation by insects and mammals. Several of the pyrethroid esters exist in isomeric forms which have distinctively different toxicities and potencies (Casida *et al.*, 1983). Distinct molecular structures convey selectivity toward certain insect species and, in certain cases, to toxicity in mammals.

Signs and Symptoms of Poisoning. Based on the symptoms produced in animals receiving acute toxic doses, the pyrethroids fall into two distinct classes of chemicals (Table 18–11). The Type I poisoning syndrome or "T syndrome" is produced by esters lacking the α-cyano substituent and is characterized by restlessness, incoordination, prostration, and paralysis in the cockroach, whereas in the rat such signs as sparring and aggressive behavior, enhanced startle response, whole body tremor, and prostration are seen. The Type II syndrome, also known as the "CS syndrome," is produced by those esters containing the α-cyano substituent and elicits

Table 18–11.   CLASSIFICATION OF PYRETHROID ESTER INSECTICIDES ON THE BASIS OF CHEMICAL STRUCTURE AND OBSERVED BIOLOGICAL ACTIVITY

	STRUCTURE	SIGNS AND SYMPTOMS		
		Cockroach	*Rat*	*Chemicals*
Type I syndrome ("T" syndrome)	$R{-}C({=}O){-}O{-}R$	Restlessness Incoordination Prostration Paralysis	Hyperexcitation Sparring Aggressiveness Enhanced startle response Whole body tremor Prostration	Pyrethrin I Allethrin Tetramethrin Kadethrin Resmethrin Phenothrin Permethrin
Type II syndrome ("CS" syndrome)	$R{-}C({=}O){-}O{-}C(CN){-}R$	Hyperactivity Incoordination Convulsions	Burrowing Dermal tingling Clonic seizures Sinuous writhing Profuse salivation	Cypermethrin Fenpropanthrin Deltamethrin Cyphenothrin Fenvalerate Fluvalinate

intense hyperactivity, incoordination, and convulsions in cockroaches, whereas rats display burrowing behavior, coarse tremors, clonic seizures, sinuous writhing (choreoathetosis), and profuse salivation without lacrimation; hence the term CS (choreoathetosis/salivation) syndrome. A few of these agents, fenpropanthrin, for example, cause a mixture of Type I and II effects, depending on the species (rat or mouse) treated and possibly on the route of administration (Verschoyle and Aldridge, 1980; Gammon *et al.*, 1981; Lawrence and Casida, 1982). The bulk of evidence points to the fact that the Type II syndrome involves primarily an action in the mammalian CNS, whereas with the Type I syndrome, peripheral nerves are also involved. This hypothesis was based initially on the observed symptomatology, but more recent evidence has revealed a correlation between the severity of Type II responses and brain concentrations of deltamethrin in mice, regardless of the route of administration (Barnes and Verschoyle, 1974; Ruzo *et al.*, 1979). Agents eliciting the Type II syndrome have greater potency when injected intracerebrally, relative to intraperitoneal injection, than those causing Type I syndrome effects (Lawrence and Casida, 1982). There is no indication of a fundamental difference between the mode of action of pyrethroids on neurons of target and nontarget species, and the neurotoxicologic responses depend on a combination of physicochemical properties of the particular pyrethroid ester, the dose applied, the time interval after treatment, and the physiologic properties of the particular model used (Leake *et al.*, 1985).

Although these insecticides cannot be considered to be highly toxic to mammals, their use indoors in enclosed and poorly ventilated spaces

has resulted in some interesting signs and symptoms of toxicity to humans. Exposure to pyrethrum is known to cause contact dermatitis, the descriptions of the effects ranging from localized erythema to a severe vesicular eruption (McCord *et al.*, 1921). The allergenic nature of this natural product is not surprising, with asthma-like attacks and anaphylactic reactions with peripheral vascular collapse being observed. Human toxicity associated with the natural pyrethrins stems from the allergenic properties rather than direct neurotoxicity. There has been little evidence of the allergic-type reactions in humans exposed to synthetic pyrethroid esters.

One notable form of toxicity associated with synthetic pyrethroids has been a cutaneous paresthesia observed in workers spraying esters containing α-cyano substituent (deltamethrin, cypermethrin, fenvalerate). The paresthesia developed several hours following exposure, being described as a stinging or burning sensation on the skin which, in some cases, progressed to a tingling and numbness, the effects lasting some 12 to 18 hours (LeQuesne *et al.*, 1980; Tucker and Flannigan, 1983).

Recent reports have appeared in the literature from the People's Republic of China, where synthetic pyrethroids have been used on a large scale on cotton crops since 1982 (Stuart-Harle, 1988; He *et al.*, 1988, 1989). Associated with the sloppy handling of deltamethrin and fenvalerate, both Type II compounds, some 573 cases of acute poisoning have occurred with some 229 cases of occupational exposure. Some 45 cases of intoxication involved cypermethrin. Occupational exposure resulted in some dizziness plus a burning, itching, or tingling sensation of the exposed skin which was exacerbated by sweating and washing with warm water. The signs and symptoms disappeared by 24 hours after exposure. Spilling these agents on the head, face, and eyes resulted in pain, lacrimation, photophobia, congestion, and edema of the conjunctiva and eyelids. Ingestion of pyrethroid esters caused epigastric pain, nausea and vomiting, headache, dizziness, anorexia, fatigue, tightness in chest, blurred vision, paresthesia, palpitations, coarse muscular fasciculations in large muscles in extremities, and disturbances of consciousness. In severe poisonings, convulsive attacks persisting from 30 to 120 seconds were accompanied by flexion of upper limbs and extension of lower limbs with opisthotonos and loss of consciousness. The frequency of these seizures was of the order of 10 to 30 times a day in the first week after exposure, gradually decreasing in incidence, with recovery within two to three weeks (He *et al.*, 1989). The signs and symptoms of acute intoxication appear to be reversible and no chronic toxicity has been reported to date.

Site and Mechanism of Toxicity.   Most of the research to investigate the mechanism(s) by which the pyrethroid esters elicit their effects has been conducted *in vitro* using cockroach, crayfish, or squid giant axon preparations (Narahashi, 1971, 1976; Casida *et al.*, 1983). In contrast, as a consequence of the complexity of the mammalian nervous system, studies on intact animals have not yielded conclusive, fundamental information concerning the mechanism of action of these agents. Type I pyrethroid esters affect sodium channels in nerve membranes, causing repetitive neuronal discharge and a prolonged negative after-potential, the effects being quite similar to those produced by DDT. There appears to be a prolongation of sodium influx with a delay in the closing of the sodium activation "gate," resulting in an increased and prolonged sodium tail current. Although the repetitive discharges could occur in any region of the nervous system, those at presynaptic nerve terminals would have the most dramatic effect on synaptic transmission, i.e., the CNS and peripheral ganglia, giving rise to the signs documented in Table 18–11. These changes are not accompanied by a large membrane depolarization so that no blockage of impulse conduction occurs (Narahashi, 1985). Type II pyrethroid esters produce an even longer delay in sodium channel inactivation, leading to a persistent depolarization of the nerve membrane without repetitive discharge, a reduction in the amplitude of the action potential, and an eventual failure of axonal conduction and a blockade of impulses (Narahashi, 1985). The depolarizing action would have a dramatic effect on the sensory nervous system because such neurons tend to discharge

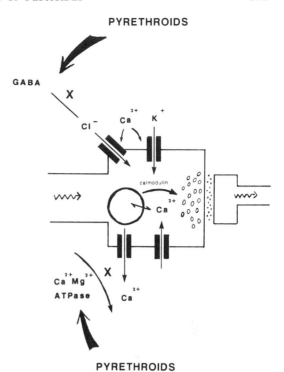

Figure 18–18.   Proposed cellular mechanisms by which pyrethroid esters interfere with neuronal function: (1) by inhibition of Ca^{2+}, Mg^{2+}-ATPase, thereby interfering with calcium removal from the ending; (2) binding to GABA receptors in the chloride channel; (3) inhibition of calmodulin which binds calcium ions, thereby increasing the levels of free calcium in the nerve ending to act on neurotransmitter release.

when depolarized even slightly, resulting in an increase in the number of discharges (van den Bercken and Vijverberg, 1983). This alone could account for the tingling and/or burning sensation felt on exposed skin. In addition, a slight depolarization at presynaptic nerve terminals would result in increased release of neurotransmitter, serious disturbance of synaptic transmission, and the generation of the symptomatology associated with Type II esters.

Other sites of action have been noted for pyrethroid esters (Figure 18–18). Several agents (permethrin, cypermethrin, deltamethrin) inhibit Ca^{2+}, Mg^{2+}-ATPase, the effect of which would result in increased intracellular calcium levels accompanied by increased neurotransmitter release and postsynaptic depolarization (Clark and Matsumura, 1982). The protein calmodulin, responsible for the intracellular binding of calcium ions to reduce spontaneous neurotransmitter release, can be inhibited by both permethrin and cypermethrin *in vitro* (Rashatwar and Matsumura, 1985). There is strong evidence that Type II esters bind to the GABA-receptor chloride channel complex, impeding chloride ion transport (Eldefrawi *et al.*, 1985). It is important to emphasize the similarities between the actions of the pyrethroid esters and the organochlorine insecticides at the membrane and macromolecular level.

Biotransformation, Distribution, and Storage. Evidence to date suggests that pyrethroid esters elicit little chronic toxicity either in animals or the human. Chronic animal feeding studies yield high "no-effect" levels, suggesting that there is little storage or accumulation of a body burden of these agents and, perhaps, an efficient detoxification of the chemicals.

Examination of the chemical structure of the pyrethroid esters reveals the presence of two ester linkages, a terminal methyl ester (pyrethrin II) and one more centrally located adjacent to the cyclopropane moiety (allethrin, tetramethrin, phenothrin, deltamethrin) and/or the α-cyano substituent (deltamethrin, cypermethrin, fenvalerate, cyphenothrin). Pyrethroid esters should be susceptible to degradation by hydrolytic enzymes, possibly by nonspecific carboxylesterases found associated with the microsomal fraction of tissue homogenates in various species (Ecobichon, 1979, Casida *et al.*, 1983). Hydrolysis of the methoxycarbonyl group in pyrethrin II by an esterase in rat liver has been reported but the major site of hydrolytic activity would appear to be at the central ester linkage (Elliott *et al.*, 1972; Shono *et al.*, 1979; Glickman and Casida, 1982). The importance of ester hydrolysis as a route of detoxification is verified by the fact that many organophosphorus esters, capable of inhibiting tissue esterases, potentiate pyrethroid ester toxicity in many species (Casida *et al.*, 1983). Species susceptibility to pyrethroid ester toxicity would appear to be highly dependent on the nature of the tissue esterase, the level of activity detected, the substrate specificity, and rate of hydrolysis encountered in target and nontarget species.

The microsomal monooxygenase system, found in the tissues of almost all species, is extensively involved in the detoxification of every pyrethroid ester in mammals and of some of these agents in insect and fish species. Much of the research in this field has been summarized by Shono *et al.* (1979), Kulkarni and Hodgson (1980), and Casida *et al.* (1983). The importance of the oxidative mechanisms in detoxification is demonstrated by the inclusion of the synergist, piperonyl butoxide, a classic monooxygenase inhibitor, in preparation for houseflies and other insects to enhance the potency of pyrethroid esters in the 10- to 300-fold range (Casida *et al.*, 1983; Matsumura, 1985).

Treatment of Poisoning. Limited experience with intoxications by pyrethroid esters has restricted the development of any protocols for treating such poisonings. No specific treatment has been reported other than symptomatic and supportive therapies (He *et al.*, 1989).

Botanical Insecticides

In the early days of insecticide usage, a number of naturally occurring agents of plant origin were employed to control insect pests. These chemicals ranged from highly toxic (to both target and nontarget species) agents such as nicotine to relatively innocuous substances such as derris root. Interestingly, despite the overwhelming number of synthetic insecticide formulations on the market, the above two agents can still be purchased and are still considered as effective insecticides.

Nicotine. Nicotine, first used as an insecticide in 1763, has been used as a contact insecticide, stomach poison, and fumigant in the form of nicotine alkaloid, the sulfate salt, or other derivatives. Commercially, it is extracted from the leaves of *Nicotiana tabacum* and *Nicotiana rustica* by alkali treatment and steam distillation or by extraction with benzene, trichloroethylene, or diethyl ether. Nicotine comprises some 97 percent of the alkaloid content of commercial tobacco. It is marketed under the trade name of Black Leaf 40®, an aqueous solution of the sulfate salt of nicotine, containing 40 percent nicotine.

Nicotine is extremely toxic, the acute oral LD50 in rats being of the order of 50 to 60 mg/kg. It is readily absorbed through the skin, and any contact with nicotine solutions should be washed off immediately. Anecdotal accounts of experiences by people who sprayed this chemical as an agricultural insecticide make an interesting collection of stories, all pointing to the fact that nicotine mimics the action of acetylcholine at all ganglionic synapses and at neuromuscular junctions, causing muscular fasciculations, convulsions, and death from paralysis of the respiratory muscles via blockade of the neuromuscular junctions (see Table 18–8). It functions as an insecticide in much the same manner, causing a blockade of synapses associated with motor nerves in insects.

Rotenoids. Six rotenoid esters occur naturally and are isolated from the plant *Derris eliptica* found in Southeast Asia or from the plant *Lonchocarpus utilis* or *L. urucu* native to South America. Rotenone, one of the alkaloids, is the most potent and can be purified by solvent extraction and recrystallization. It can be used either as a contact or a stomach poison. However, it is unstable in light and heat and almost all toxicity can be lost after two to three days during the summer.

Rotenone is very toxic to fish, one of its main uses by native people over the centuries being to paralyze fish for capture and consumption. The mammalian toxicity varies greatly with the species exposed, the method of administration, and the type of formulation. Crystalline rotenone has an acute oral LD50 of 60, 132, and 3000 mg/kg for guinea pigs, rats, and rabbits, respectively (Matsumura, 1985). Because the toxicity of derris powders exceeds that of the equivalent content of rotenone, it is obvious that the other esters in crude preparations have significant biologic activity. Acute poisoning in animals is characterized by an initial respiratory stimulation followed by respiratory depression, ataxia, convulsions, and death by respiratory arrest (Shimkin and Anderson, 1936). The anesthetic-like action on nerves appears to be related to the ability of rotenone to block electron transport in mitochondria by inhibiting oxidation linked to $NADH_2$, this resulting in nerve conduction blockade (O'Brien, 1967; Corbett, 1974). Although toxicity in laboratory and domestic animals has been reported with acute LD50 values of 10 to 30 mg/kg being reported, human intoxications are rare. The estimated fatal oral dose for a 70-kg man is of the order of 10 to 100 g. Rotenone has been used topically for treatment of head lice, scabies, and other ectoparasites, but the dust is highly irritating to the eyes (conjunctivitis), the skin (dermatitis), and to the upper respiratory tract (rhinitis) and throat (pharyngitis).

HERBICIDES

An herbicide, in the broadest definition, is any compound that is capable of either killing or severely injuring plants and may be used for the elimination of plant growth or the killing off of plant parts (Jager, 1983). For more than a century, chemicals have been used to control unwanted vegetation, but many of the early chemicals such as sulfuric acid, sodium chlorate, arsenic trioxide, sodium arsenite, petroleum oils, iron and copper sulfate, or sodium borate were frequently hard to handle and/or were very toxic, were relatively nonspecific, or were phytotoxic to the crop as well as the unwanted plant life if not applied at exactly the proper time. In the late 1930s, many studies were initiated to find agents that would selectively destroy certain plant species. Many of these early chemicals were more effective but still possessed mammalian toxicity. However, a few compounds served as prototype chemicals for further development. Summaries of the early days of herbicide development are presented by Cremlyn (1978) and by Kirby (1980).

In the past two decades, the herbicides have represented the most rapidly growing section of the agrochemical pesticide business due in part to (1) movement into monocultural practices where the risk of weed infestation has increased because fallowing and crop rotation which would change weed species are no longer in vogue; and (2) mechanization of agricultural practices (planting, tending, harvesting) because of increased labor costs. The annual rate of growth of herbicide production on a worldwide basis between 1980 and 1985 was 1.9 percent per year, more than double the rate of growth for insecticides during the same period (Marquis, 1986). The result of this extensive development has been a plethora of chemically diverse structures rivalling the innovative chemistry of the insecticides, the aim being to protect desirable crops and to obtain high yields by selectively eliminating unwanted plant species, thereby reducing the competition for nutrients. For a more complete discussion of the development of herbicides, the reader is referred to Cremlyn (1978), McEwen and Stephenson (1979), and Jager (1983).

Herbicides may be classified in a number of ways. The first classification is by chemical structure although this is not very enlightening, because there is tremendous overlapping of biologic effects for a variety of chemical structures. The second method of classification pertains to how and when the agents are applied. *Preplanting* herbicides are applied to the soil before a crop is seeded. *Preemergent* herbicides are applied to the soil before the usual time of appearance of the unwanted vegetation. *Postemergent* herbicides are applied to the soil or foliage after the germination of the crop and/or weeds. Plant biochemists classify herbicides according to their mechanism of toxicity in plants, i.e., *selective* (toxic to some species), *contact* (act when impinging on the plant foliage), or *translocated* (being absorbed via the soil or through the foliage into the plant xylem and phloem.) In this chapter, herbicides will be classified by their ability to interfere with specific biochemical processes essential for normal growth and development, such interaction(s) resulting in severe injury to and the eventual death of the plant. In Table 18–12, the various mechanisms by which herbicides exert their biologic effects are shown along with the generic and chemical names of the classes of herbicides and some examples of each class. The claim has been made that, because the mode(s) of action

Table 18–12.   MECHANISMS OF ACTION OF HERBICIDES

MECHANISM(S)	CHEMICAL CLASSES
Inhibition of photosynthesis by disruption of light reactions and blockade of electron transport	Ureas, 1,3,5-triazines, 1,4-triazines, uracils, pyridazones, 4-hydroxybenzonitriles, N-arylcarbamates, acylanilides (some)
Inhibition of respiration by blockade of electron transfer from NADH or blocking the coupling of electron transfer to ADP to form ATP.	Dinitrophenols Halophenols
Growth stimulants, "auxins"	Aryloxyalkylcarboxylic acids Benzoic acids
Inhibitors of cell and nucleus division	Alkyl N-arylcarbamates Dinitroanilines
Inhibition of protein synthesis	Chloracetamide
Inhibition of carotenoid synthesis, protective pigments in chloroplasts to prevent chlorophyll from being destroyed by oxidative reactions	O-substituted diphenyl ethers Hydrazines
Inhibition of lipid synthesis	S-alkyl dialkylcarbamodithioates Aliphatic chlorocarboxylic acids
Unknown mechanisms, nonselective chemicals	Inorganic agents (copper sulfate, sulfuric acid, sodium chlorate, sodium borate) Organic agents (dichlobenil, chlorthiamid, bentazone, diphenamid, benzoylpropethyl)

From Jager, G.: In Büchel, K. H. (ed.): *Chemistry of Pesticides*. John Wiley & Sons, New York, 1983.

involve biochemical phytoprocesses having no counterparts in mammalian systems, there is no risk of mammalian toxicity associated with these chemicals. With the exception of a few chemicals, the herbicides have demonstrated low toxicity in mammals. However, the current controversy around these chemicals centers on demonstrated or suspected mutagenicity, teratogenicity, and/or carcinogenicity associated either with the agent(s) or with contaminants and by-products of manufacture found in trace amounts in technical grade material. The presence of some of these contaminants has been largely ignored without realizing that the toxicities associated with them are both different from those observed with the herbicidal chemical and occur frequently at far lower dosages.

In terms of general toxicity, because the major route of exposure to herbicides is dermal, and because these agents tend to be strong acids, amines, esters, and phenols, they are dermal irritants, causing skin rashes and contact dermatitis even when exposure involves diluted formulations. There appear to be subpopulations of individuals who are hypersensitive to dermal contact with solutions or aerosolized mists of certain types of herbicides, moderate to severe urticaria being observed that may persist for 5 to 10 days following exposure. Certain individuals, particularly those prone to allergic reactions, may experience severe contact dermatitis, asthmalike attacks, and even anaphylactic reactions, following dermal or inhalation contact with formulated herbicides. Whether these effects are chemical-specific for the herbicide or for emulsifiers, cosolvents, and so-called "inerts" found in formulations has not been established. Although skin patch testing of herbicidal chemicals has usually proven to be negative, it is possible that the patients' responses may be associated with a generalized, nonspecific irritant effect of the formulation. Many of these dermal and pulmonary reactions respond satisfactorily to treatment with antihistaminic agents.

In contrast, there are other herbicides that can elicit a range of acute and chronic effects following exposure, and it is on these chemicals that attention will be focused.

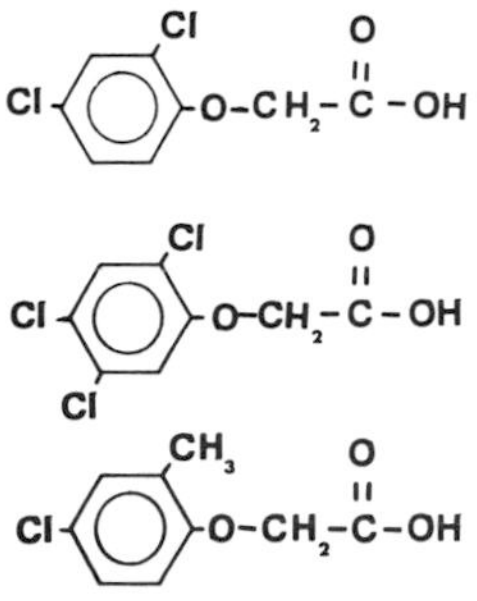

Figure 18–19. The molecular structure of the three most common chlorophenoxyacetic acid herbicides: 2,4-D, 2,4-dichlorophenoxyacetic acid; 2,4,5-T, 2,4,5-trichlorophenoxyacetic acid; and MCPA, 4-chloro-*o*-toloxyacetic acid. In addition to the salts of the acids, ester and amine derivatives are also marketed.

Chlorophenoxy Compounds

During World War II, considerable effort was directed toward the development of effective, broad-spectrum herbicides in both the United States and the United Kingdom with a view to both increasing food production and to finding potential chemical warfare agents (Kirby, 1980). The chlorophenoxy compounds (Figure 18–19), including the acids, salts, amines, and esters, were the first commercially available products evolving from this research in 1946. This class of herbicides has seen continuous, extensive, and uninterrupted use since 1947 in agriculture for broad-leafed weeds and in the control of woody plants along roadside, railway, and utilities rights of way and in forest management programs, particularly in reforestation. In plants, these chemicals mimic the action of auxins, hormones chemically related to indoleacetic acid that stimulate growth. No hormonal activity is observed in mammals and other species, and beyond target organ toxicity that can be associated with the pharmacokinetics, biotransformation, and/or elimination of these chemicals, their mechanism(s) of toxic action are poorly understood.

A tremendous volume of mammalian toxicity data has been collected over the past 42 years from both animal studies and incidents of human exposure (Hayes, 1975, 1982). It is of interest to note that, in a recent toxicologic reevaluation of 2,4-D for the purposes of providing the U.S. EPA with a new toxicity data base for the chemical, an industry task force discovered nothing of toxicologic significance that was not already known about the chemical, with one exception (Mullison, 1986). The exceptional finding was the appearance of astrocytomas in the brains of male Fischer 344 strain rats exposed to the highest (45 mg/kg per day) dosage. A subsequent review of the findings suggested that this tumor incidence was not treatment related (Koestner, 1986; Solleveld *et al.*, 1986). The acute toxicity elicited by chlorophenoxy herbicides has been described by Hayes (1982). The oral LD50 values ranged from 300 to >1000 mg/kg in different animal species, only the dog appearing to be particularly sensitive, possibly on the basis that it has considerable difficulty in the renal elimination of such organic acids (Gehring *et al.*, 1976). Animals will tolerate repeated oral exposure to doses of chlorophenoxy herbicides marginally below the single, toxic oral dose without showing significant signs of toxicity, an observation suggesting that there is little cumulative effect on target organs. At dosages causing toxicity, few specific signs other than muscular and neuromuscular involvement were observed in animals although tenseness, stiffness in extremities, muscular weakness, ataxia, and paralysis have been reported. Hepatic and renal injury in addition to irritation of the gastrointestinal mucosa have been observed in acute lethality studies in animals.

The case of accidental and/or occupational intoxications by chlorophenoxy herbicides have been reviewed by Hayes (1982). Most patients complained of headache, dizziness, nausea, vomiting, abdominal pains, diarrhea, respiratory complications, aching and tender muscles, myotonia, weakness, and fatigue. Clinically, there is some evidence of renal dysfunction, transient albuminuria being observed in some cases. There is little documented evidence of neurotoxicity associated with chlorophenoxy herbicides with the exception of one study where decreased peripheral nerve conduction velocities were observed in workers employed in manufacturing 2,4-D and 2,4,5-T (Singer *et al.*, 1982). A wide range of human lethal dosages of 2,4-D has been reported in the literature, the average lethal dose being in excess of 300 mg/kg. The oral dose required to elicit symptoms is of the order of 50 to 60 mg/kg. In one poisoning, death occurred in a 75-kg male following the intentional ingestion of 6 g (80 mg/kg), although the actual dose may have been much higher because the individual had vomited (Nielsen *et al.*, 1965). In another case, the daily ingestion of 500 mg of 2,4-D over a three-week period elicited no symptoms (Berwick, 1970). The clinical course of one patient who intentionally ingested a "large" volume of a mixture of the butyl esters of 2,4-D and 2,4,5-T was characterized by increased body temperature, increased pulse and respiratory rates, decreased blood pressure, respiratory alkalosis, profuse sweating, oliguria, hemoconcentration, increased blood urea nitrogen, and a deepening coma. At autopsy, focal submucosal hemorrhage, moderate congestion, and edema of the intestine were seen along with congestion in the lungs. Necrosis of the intestinal mucosa as well as necrosis and fatty infiltration of the liver were observed. Pneumonitis and inflammation of terminal bronchioles was observed and renal damage included degeneration of the convoluted tubules, fatty infiltration, and the presence of proteinaceous material in the glomerular spaces (Hayes, 1982). Earlier literature reported significant peripheral neuropathies in three people acquiring toxic concentrations via percutaneous absorption while spraying 2,4-D ester for weeds (Goldstein *et al.*, 1959). In each case, the signs and symptoms began several hours after exposure and progressed until pain, paresthesia, and paralysis were severe. The diagnosis of peripheral neuropathy was supported by electromyographic analysis and recovery was incomplete even after a lapse of some years. In a more recent report of a suicidal ingestion of a 2,4-D concentrate, the morphologic examination of nervous tissue revealed extensive plaques of acute demyelination in all parts of the brain that resembled those observed in acute multiple sclerosis (Dudley and Thapar, 1972). In an unusual "experiment," 2,4-D was administered either by intramuscular or by intravenous injection to two moribund patients with disseminated coccidioidomycosis (Seabury, 1963). The patient treated intramuscularly (40 mg of 2,4-D, sodium salt) showed no symptoms. The patient receiving daily intravenous injections of 120 to 960 mg of 2,4-D sodium salt/day for 16 days showed few adverse effects but, on receiving 3600 mg two days after the administration of a 2000 mg dose, showed toxicity in the form of fibrillary twitching in the facial, hand, and forearm muscles that persisted for several hours; stupor; hyporeflexia (knees, ankles, biceps tendons) that persisted for 24 hours; lethargy; and marked muscular weakness. Within 48 hours the patient had returned to his prereaction status.

Immediately following the industrial accident that occurred at the Monsanto plant in Nitro, West Virginia, on March 8, 1949 where 2,4,5-T was being synthesized, acute symptoms of exposure to the reaction products included skin, eye, and respiratory tract irritation; headache; dizziness; nausea; acneiform eruptions; severe pain in the muscles of the thorax, shoulders, and extremities; fatigue; nervousness; irritability; dyspnea; complaint of decreased libido; and intolerance to cold (Ashe and Suskind, 1953). In a 1984 epidemiologic study of active and retired employees from this plant, clinical evidence of chloracne persisted in some 55.7 percent of those exposed (113 out of 204) and an association was found between the persistence of chlor-

acne and the presence and severity of actinic elastosis of the skin (Suskind and Hertzberg, 1984). Although there was some evidence of exposure and a history of gastrointestinal tract ulcers, there was no evidence of increased risk for cardiovascular, hepatic, or renal disease or of central or peripheral nervous tissue damage.

Serious reservations have been raised about the toxic properties of the chlorophenoxy herbicides because such neuropathies have not been observed in recent years with occupational and/or accidental exposure to high concentrations of these agents. In earlier times, before the method of synthesis was altered, workers involved in the manufacture of this class of herbicides, particularly 2,4,5-T, experienced a severe type of contact dermatitis called "chemical worker chloracne" (Schultz, 1968; Poland *et al.*, 1971). Herbicide sprayers of a few decades ago developed a persistent condition known as "weed bumps" following daily and seasonal exposure to chlorophenoxy herbicides. Chloracne, however, is not a unique condition associated only with chlorophenoxy herbicides and can be caused by a number of chlorinated aromatic compounds including polychlorinated biphenyls, dibenzo-*p*-dioxins, dibenzofurans, and chlorinated naphthalenes (Schultz, 1968). The true culprit was unmasked when teratologic studies revealed that commercial 2,4,5-T caused cleft palate and renal malformations in mice and renal anomalies in rats (Courtney *et al.*, 1970). Today, the evidence is quite conclusive that many of these biologic effects were not related to the herbicide but to a contaminant, 2,3,7,8-tetrachloro-dibenzo-*p*-dioxin (TCDD or the news media's dioxin), a by-product formed during synthesis if the temperature is not rigidly controlled (Courtney and Moore, 1971). Levels of TCDD of the order of 30 to 50 μg/g have been estimated to have occurred in commercial 2,4,5-T. The sample of 2,4,5-T used in the teratological studies was found to contain 30 μg TCDD/g (Courtney and Moore, 1971). More recent teratologic studies, conducted with "clean" (i.e., <0.5 ppm) TCDD have demonstrated that dosages of the order of 15 to 100 mg/kg per day during organogenesis were required to elicit birth defects (cleft palate, cystic kidney) and fetotoxic effects in mice and hamsters, whereas rats and monkeys appeared to be resistant to 2,4,5,-T-induced teratogenicity (Hayes, 1982). The carcinogenicity of 2,4-D and 2,4,5-T in laboratory rodents has not been conclusively demonstrated, but TCDD has caused an increased incidence of tumors at multiple sites when fed in the diet at low (ng or pg/g) concentrations (Van Miller *et al.*, 1977; Kociba *et al.*, 1978). Currently, levels of TCDD detectable in commercial 2,4,5-T are of the order of 0.005

to 0.010 μg/g, thereby presenting one possible explanation for the absence of present-day toxicity observed with this chemical (Ecobichon, unpublished results). The above studies focussed the direction of research toward two classes of contaminants, the chlorinated dibenzo-p-dioxins and the dibenzofurans, and two important endpoints of toxicity identified from animal studies, birth defects and carcinogenesis.

Tetrachlorodibenzo-p-dioxin has been shown to be extremely toxic to a number of animal species, the acute oral LD50 values ranging from 0.0006 to 0.283 mg/kg, the guinea pig being the most susceptible species (Schwetz et al., 1973; Moore et al., 1979). However, it should be emphasized that mortality does not occur immediately, the animals undergoing a slow but progressive decline into a moribund state associated with an increased incidence of infections and the eventual death some 14 to 28 days after treatment. It appears that the animals' "environment" suddenly becomes toxic to them, leading investigators to examine the immune response and the discovery that TCDD and related compounds caused a marked atrophy of the thymus gland, the source of the T-cell components of the immune response (Vos et al., 1983). Although a complete discussion of the toxicity of chlorinated dioxins and furans is beyond the scope of this chapter, the TCDD story emphasizes the toxicologic importance of minor contaminants found in pesticides, the necessity for testing these chemicals independently from the pesticide, and, furthermore, the need for cautious interpretation of results from animal experiments in relation to effects in the human. This statement should not minimize the fact that serious toxicologic problems in both animals and humans can arise as a consequence of exposure to high concentrations of polychlorinated dibenzo-p-dioxins and dibenzofurans, as was encountered in the Missouri incident (Kimbrough et al., 1977; Hoffman et al., 1986). Rather than stress the reader with the voluminous literature on the subject of associations of dioxins, 2,4-D, and 2,4,5-T with adverse health effects (neuropathies, birth defects, cancer, and so forth), a perusal of cogent and responsible reviews such as those of Hay (1982), Tucker et al. (1983), Whelan (1985), Gough (1986), and Tschirley (1986) is recommended for an overview of the dioxin literature.

The extensive use of Agent Orange, a 50:50 mixture of the n-butyl esters of 2,4-D and 2,4,5-T, as a defoliant during the Vietnam conflict raised the spectre of possible adverse health effects among service personnel handling and spraying the material (Operation Ranchhand) as well as among soldiers during field operations who might acquire body burdens by dermal exposure or ingestion of contaminated drinking water. The facts that: (1) some 11.5 million gallons of Agent Orange were used up to 1971; (2) contamination by TCDD occurred to a maximum of 47 μg/g; and (3) birth defects and cancers were produced in animals did nothing to reduce the concerns of both those potentially exposed individuals and government departments. Unfortunately, despite many claims of adverse health effects of diverse nature among veterans of this war, various epidemiologic studies conducted in Australia, New Zealand, and the United States have provided inconclusive evidence that exposure was high enough to have elicited such effects (Buckingham, 1982; Hay, 1982; Walsh, 1983; Greenwald et al., 1984; Gough, 1986; CDC, 1988; Gochfeld, 1988; Stellman et al., 1988).

The most conclusive evidence of toxicologic effects of TCDD in the human comes from a dozen or more separate industrial accidents where upward of a total of 1500 workers have been exposed to high but unknown levels of TCDD and related material. The best description of these incidents can be found in Hay (1982). As was mentioned above for the Nitro, West Virginia accident, the only consistent effects observed have been persistent chloracne. Other effects observed included porphyria, reversible liver damage expressed as elevated blood serum transaminases [serum glutamic-oxaloacetic transaminase (SGOT), serum glutamic-pyruvic transaminase (SGPT)], some disturbance of lipid metabolism, polyneuropathies, and possible psychiatric disturbances. In contrast, TCDD-induced effects in animals have included liver damage, porphyria, changes in lipid metabolism, hepatic microsomal enzyme induction, reproductive problems including fetotoxicity and teratogenicity, tissue wasting, suppression of the immune response, and increased tumor incidence (IARC, 1977).

The inability to demonstrate conclusively adverse health effects in military and civilian personnel exposed to TCDD-contaminated Agent Orange in Vietnam led investigators to examine larger populations of individuals potentially exposed to chlorophenoxy herbicides, including workers in agriculture and forestry and herbicide manufacturing and formulating who have used 2,4,5-T and/or 2,4-D extensively and, in some cases, almost exclusively since the introduction of these chemicals in 1947. However, the results of a number of studies that focussed on the incidence of carcinogenicity have not resolved the issue. Early studies in Sweden suggested that exposure to chlorophenoxy herbicides and chlorophenols produced a sixfold increase in soft tissue sarcomas, Hodgkin's disease, and non-Hodgkin's lymphoma whether or not the chemicals were contaminated by polychlorinated dibenzodioxins and dibenzofurans (Hardell and Sandstrom, 1979; Eriksson et al., 1981; Hardell et al., 1981). Some studies confirmed the Swedish results but, due to small sample sizes, incidence rates, and so forth, lacked significant statistical power (Axelson et al., 1980; Cantor, 1982; Thiess et al., 1982). Other studies have failed to confirm these results (Ott et al., 1980; Lynge, 1985; Pearce et al., 1986; Wiklund et al., 1988; Bond et al., 1988). A study conducted in Kansas demonstrated an association between farm herbicidal use and non-Hodgkin's lymphoma, the incidence of which appeared to increase with the number of days exposure per year (Hoar et al., 1986). In the opinion of some, this study went one step too far in associating the blame to 2,4-D even though this chemical was the dominant herbicide used on corn. It is, however, obvious that, within the agricultural workforce, there is a higher incidence of certain types of cancer (Cantor, 1982; Woods et al., 1986; Council on Scientific Affairs, 1988; Wiklund et al., 1988). A recent but still incomplete study of prairie wheat farmers in Saskatchewan, Canada, has revealed no increase in non-Hodgkin's lymphoma above the incidence observed in the nonfarming population (Wigle et al., 1990). In relation to the general population of this province in which 2,4-D has seen highest and most consistent use since 1947 (60 percent of national total), farmers had lower overall mortality and cancer rates than expected. Lacking the ideal "definitive" and "clean" cancer study, it is certain that this controversy will continue in the scientific literature (Barinaga, 1989).

Bipyridyl Derivatives

One chemical class of herbicides deserving of particular attention is the bipyridyl group, specifically paraquat (1,1'-dimethyl-4-,4'-bipyridylium dichloride, methyl viologen) and diquat (1,1'-ethylene-2,2'-bipyridylium dibromide) (Figure 18–20). Paraquat was first synthesized in 1882, but its pesticidal properties were not discovered until 1959 (Haley, 1979). This agent, a nonselective contact herbicide, is one of the most exquisite pulmonary toxicants known and has been the subject of intensive investigation because of the startling toxicity observed in humans. Many countries have banned or severely restricted the use of paraquat because of the debilitating or life-threatening hazards from occupational exposure and the large number of reported accidental and suicidal

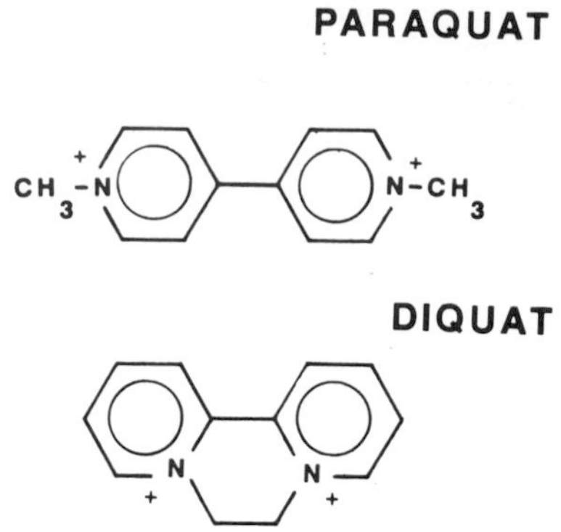

Figure 18–20. The chemical structures of paraquat and diquat, marketed as the dichloride and dibromide salts respectively.

fatalities (Campbell, 1968; Davies et al., 1977; Haley, 1979). By 1977, the number of fatalities had reached 564 (Hayes, 1982). The analog, diquat, is considerably less potent than paraquat, but nonetheless can cause severe acute and chronic poisoning.

In animals, paraquat shows moderate acute toxicity, the oral LD50 values for the rat ranging from 40 to 200 mg/kg. Intoxication involves a combination of signs and symptoms that include lethargy, hypoxia, dyspnea, tachycardia, hyperapnea, adipsia, diarrhea, ataxia, hyperexcitability, and convulsions, depending on the dosage and the species being studied (Smith and Heath, 1976; Haley, 1979). Necropsy reveals hemorrhagic and edematous lungs, intraalveolar hemorrhage, congestion and pulmonary fibrosis, centrilobular hepatic necrosis, and renal tubular necrosis. Lung weights of intoxicated animals increase significantly despite marked losses in body weight. From a catalogue of all the signs and symptoms, it is obvious that the lung is the most susceptible target organ, the same histopathologic picture of pulmonary lesions being observed in mice, rats, dogs, and humans (Clarke et al., 1966). Regardless of the route (ingestion, injection, inhalation) of exposure to moderate doses, immediate effects are usually not seen in animals but, within 10 to 14 days, respiration becomes impaired, rapid, and shallow and the morphologic changes seen include degeneration and vacuolization of pneumocytes, damage to type I and type II alveolar epithelial cells, destruction of the epithelial membranes, and the proliferation of fibrotic cells.

Paraquat, being a highly polar compound, is poorly absorbed from the gastrointestinal tract, experiments in rats demonstrating that 52 percent of the administered dose was still localized in the intestinal tract some 32 hours after administration (Murray and Gibson, 1974). Approximately 5 to 10 percent of an ingested dose is absorbed (Haley, 1979). In human intoxications by formulation concentrates, it has been suggested that the presence of emulsifiers and/or cosolvents may well enhance absorption. It is the consensus of opinion that paraquat is not extensively metabolized *in vivo* although intestinal microflora may be responsible for some 30 percent of the excreted, unidentifiable metabolites in animal studies (Daniel and Gage, 1966). The high levels of paraquat found in renal tissue of intoxicated animals point to the role of this organ in excreting the unchanged herbicide (Rose *et al.*, 1976). Measurable amounts of paraquat were found in urine for up to 21 days posttreatment in rats and monkeys, even though some 45 percent of the dose administered had been excreted in the urine and feces within 48 hours of treatment (Murray and Gibson, 1974).

Lung tissue acquires much higher concentrations of paraquat than do most tissues of the body with the exception of the kidney and, over a 30-hour posttreatment period, pulmonary concentrations increase disproportionately to those levels found in other tissues (Sharp *et al.*, 1972; Rose *et al.*, 1976). The same phenomenon is observed with the *in vitro* uptake of paraquat by tissue slices, the lung acquiring relatively high concentrations of unbound (free) paraquat whereas tissue slices from other organs were unable to accumulate paraquat (Rose *et al.*, 1976). Biochemical studies have revealed that paraquat is actively acquired by alveolar cells by a diamine/polyamine transport system where it undergoes NADPH-dependent, one-electron reduction to form a free radical capable of reacting with molecular oxygen (in abundant supply) to reform the cation paraquat plus a reactive oxygen (superoxide anion, O_2^-) that is converted into hydrogen peroxide by the enzyme superoxide dismutase. The hydrogen peroxide and superoxide anion can attack polyunsaturated lipids present in cell membranes to produce lipid hydroperoxides which, in turn, can react with other unsaturated lipids to form more lipid-free radicals thereby perpetuating the system (Smith, 1987). The resulting cellular membrane damage reduces the functional integrity of the cell, affects efficient gas transport and exchange, and induces respiratory impairment. The severity of the cellular effects can be modulated by the availability of oxygen, animals kept in air with only 10 percent oxygen faring better than those kept in room air (Rhodes, 1974). In paraquat poisonings, even though the patients may suffer from hypoxia and respiratory insufficiency, hyperbaric oxygen is contraindicated because it appears to promote cellular toxicity.

Cases of paraquet poisonings, of both children and adults, have been described in detail in the literature (Almog and Tal, 1967; Davies *et al.*, 1977; Haley, 1979; Hayes, 1982). The ingestion of commercial paraquat formulations, concentrates containing up to 20 percent active ingredient, is invariably fatal and runs a time course of three to four weeks. The initial irritation and burning of the mouth and throat, the necrosis and sloughing of the oral mucosa, severe gastroenteritis with esophageal and gastric lesions, abdominal and substernal chest pains, and bloody stools gives way to the characteristic and dominant pulmonary symptoms, including dyspnea, anoxia, opacity in the lungs as seen by chest X-ray, coma, and death. Paraquat induces multiorgan toxicity with necrotic damage to the liver, kidneys, and myocardial muscle plus extensive hemorrhagic incidents throughout the body. Although most of the paraquat intoxications involve the ingestion of the compound, there are reports of toxicity following dermal exposure with blistering and erythema being observed. There is evidence of nonfatal chronic impairment of pulmonary function in sprayers who inhaled aerosolized paraquat from diluted (0.2 percent w/v) spray formulations over a number of years (Hayes, 1982).

Treatment of paraquat poisoning should be vigorous and initiated as quickly as possible. Gastric lavage should be followed by the administration of mineral adsorbents such as Fuller's earth (kaolin), bentonite clay, or activated charcoal to bind any unabsorbed paraquat remaining in the gastrointestinal tract. Purgatives may be given. Absorbed paraquat may be removed from the bloodstream by hemoperfusion through charcoal or by hemodialysis, although this is of limited value because blood levels of the herbicide are generally low. To avoid excessive pulmonary damage, supplemental oxygen should be reduced to a level just sufficient to maintain acceptable arterial oxygen tension (>40 to 50 mm Hg) (Haley, 1979; Hayes, 1982).

Diquat is a rapidly acting contact herbicide used as a desiccant, for the control of aquatic weeds and to destroy potato halums before harvesting. Diquat is slightly less toxic than paraquat, the oral LD50 values in animals being of the order of 100 to 200 mg/kg. Part of the reduced toxicity may be related to the fact that it is poorly absorbed from the gastrointestinal tract, only 6 percent of an ingested dose being excreted in the urine, whereas following subcutaneous administration, 90 to 98 percent of the dose is eliminated via the urine (Daniel and Gage, 1966). A latency period of 24 hours is seen prior to visible toxic effects.

Following acute, high-dose exposure or

Table 18–13. HERBICIDAL CHEMICALS: CLASSES, COMMON NAMES, AND ACUTE TOXICITY

CHEMICAL CLASS	GENERIC NAME	TRADE NAME	ORAL LD50 (mg/kg)
Acetanilides		Alachlor	1,200
		Metolachlor	2,780
Amides	3,4-Dichloropropionanilide	Propanil	
Arylaliphatic Acids	2-Methoxy-3,6-dichloroben-zoic acid	Dicamba	3,500
	3-Amino-2,5-dichlorobenzoic acid	Chloramben	5,000
Carbamates	Isopropyl carbanilate	Propham	5,000
	4-Chloro-2-butynyl-*m*-chlorocarbanilate	Barban	600
Dinitroanilines	*a,a,a*-Trifluoro-2,6-dinitro-*N,N*-dipropyl-*p*-toluidine	Trifluralin	10,000
Nitriles	2,6-Dichlorobenzonitrile	Dichlobenil	270
	4-Hydroxy-3,5-diiodobenzoni-trile	Ioxynil	110
Substituted ureas	3-(*p*-chlorophenyl)-1,1-di-methylurea	Monuron	3,000
	3-(3,4-Dichlorophenyl)1,1-dimethylurea	Diuron	
Triazines	2-Chloro-4-(ethylamino)-6-(isopropylamino)-*S*-triazine	Atrazine	1,000
	2-Chloro-4,6-bis (ethylamino)-*S*-triazine	Simazine	1,000

chronic exposure of animals to diquat, the major target organs were the gastrointestinal tract, the liver, and the kidneys (Hayes, 1982; Morgan, 1982). Chronic feeding studies resulted in an increased incidence of cataracts in both dogs and rats (Clark and Hurst, 1970). It is considered that diquat can form free radicals, the tissue necrosis being associated with the same mechanism(s) of superoxide-induced peroxidation as observed with paraquat. However, unlike paraquat, diquat shows no special affinity for the lung and does not appear to fit the mechanism that selectively concentrates paraquat in the lung (Rose and Smith, 1977).

Few diquat-related human intoxications have been reported to date (Schonborn *et al.*, 1971; Narita *et al.*, 1978; Hayes, 1982). In the few cases of suicidal intent described, ulceration of mucosal membranes, gastrointestinal symptoms, acute renal failure, hepatic damage, and respiratory difficulties were observed. Central nervous system effects were more severe. Interestingly, no fibrosis was evident in the lungs. One individual died of cardiac arrest.

A variety of herbicides representative of several chemical classifications and diverse structures have been introduced over the years into agricultural practices (Table 18–13). In general, these chemicals have relatively low acute toxicity, the oral LD50 values in rats being

of the order of 100 to 10,000 mg/kg. Large doses can be administered in subchronic and chronic toxicity studies without eliciting significant biologic effects. Poisonings in humans have usually been associated with occupational exposure to high concentrations during the manufacturing or mixing/loading phases of application or with a few, atypical but sometimes well publicized incidents (Hayes, 1982). However, as was encountered with the chlorophenoxy herbicides, many of these chemicals are old and were registered at a time when the protocols and quality of the toxicologic assessment were not as stringent as those required today by regulatory agencies. In reexamining these chemicals by state-of-the-art techniques in vogue today, the chemicals themselves or minor contaminant by-products of synthesis have elicited mutagenic, teratogenic, or carcinogenic potential not detected before. In addition, the application of sophisticated analytical techniques to residue analysis of groundwater, food, and air has revealed the presence of low concentrations of many of these agents in media to which the general public is exposed. This has necessitated closer scrutiny of the chemicals and testing procedures and changes in registration, and has heightened concerns among consumer groups to the point that they have lost faith in the system of registration. The task of retesting and reevaluating these

ALACHLOR

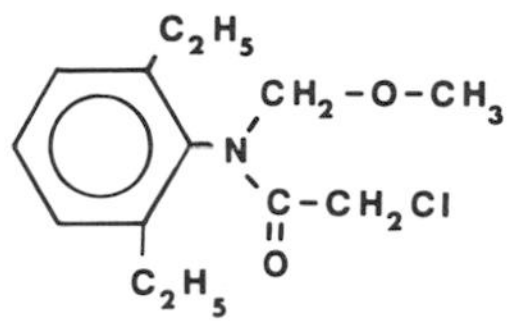

METOLACHLOR

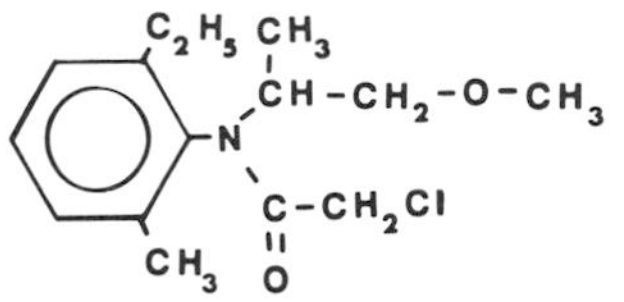

Figure 18–21. The chemical structures of alachlor (2-chloro-2',6'-diethyl-*N*-(methoxymethyl)acetanilide) and metolachlor (2-chloro-6'-ethyl-*N*-(2-methoxy-1-methylethyl)acet- *o*-toluidide.

chemicals is a tedious and costly endeavor. The dilemma faced by manufacturers and regulators alike is that such reevaluation must be done for all chemical pesticides because a number of untoward adverse biologic effects have been identified among chemicals presently undergoing reassessment.

One good example of the problems encountered is that observed with alachlor (Lasso®) and the closely related analog, metolachlor (Dual®, Primextra®) (Figure 18–21). Alachlor was registered in the mid-to-late 1960s, the application being supported by toxicity studies carried out on behalf of the manufacturer by the Industrial Biotest Laboratories (IBT). During the investigations carried out by the United States and Canadian committees on IBT practices, some alachlor studies were deemed to be invalid or inadequate, and the manufacturer was requested to provide replacement studies on long-term effects to support the continued registration of the product. A major controversy arose in Canada and the United States following the submission of the studies in the early 1980s, giving rise in Canada to an official review board (Alachlor Review Board, 1987). Concerns were raised about the incidence of adenocarcinomas in the stomachs and nasal turbinates of Long-Evans rats and in the lungs of CD-1 mice receiving the highest dosages of 126 mg/kg per day (rats) and 260 mg/kg per day (mice). The results were such that, using the IARC classification system, alachlor was considered to be a category 2B carcinogen, a probable human carcinogen. There were concerns about potentially hazardous expo-

sure of agricultural workers to the chemical during mixing and loading, with levels ranging from 0.00038 to 2.7 mg/kg per day, depending on the exposure model used and whether or not protective clothing was worn. In regions where alachlor was used, the analysis of selected wells revealed alachlor at 0.10 to 2.11 μg/liter with one sample showing 9.1 μg/liter. Identified carcinogenicity in two species plus the presence of alachlor in the environment in a medium from which the general populace could acquire residues set the stage for the cancellation of alachlor's registration in Canada in February, 1985.

Unfortunately, during the assessment of alachlor, a competitor's product, another chloroacetanilide that could substitute for alachlor, was dragged into the discussion, evidence pointing to the fact that metolachlor caused significant increases in hepatocellular carcinomas and adenocarcinomas in nasal turbinates of female and male Sprague-Dawley rats, respectively. A more detailed study of well water in a region where both herbicides were used revealed contamination by either one or the other compounds in a number of samples, the mean concentration of metolachlor being between one and two orders of magnitude higher than that observed for alachlor, even though most positive samples were below the IMAC values for alachlor (5.0 μg/liter) and metolachlor (105 μg/liter). Despite the fact that the Canadian federal regulatory agency was of the opinion that metolachlor was much "safer," the Review Board concluded that there was no difference between the safety of alachlor and metolachlor to humans, both analogs being animal carcinogens.

FUNGICIDES

Fungicidal chemicals are derived from a variety of structures ranging from simple inorganic compounds such as sulfur and copper sulfate, through the aryl- and alkyl-mercurial compounds and chlorinated phenols to metal-containing derivatives of thiocarbamic acid (Figure 18–22). The chemistry of fungicides and their properties have been discussed by Cremlyn (1978) and by Kramer (1983). Some 80 million pounds of fungicides are used annually in the United States, being applied as dusts or liquid sprays as protectant or surface fungicides. According to the site of the fungal infestation and application pattern, one or more of these chemicals may be used as a foliar, soil, or dressing fungicide and, in some cases, the same compound may be used in all three stages. *Foliar fungicides* are applied to the aerial green parts of plants, producing a protective barrier on the cuticular surface and being systemically toxic to the developing fungus. *Soil*

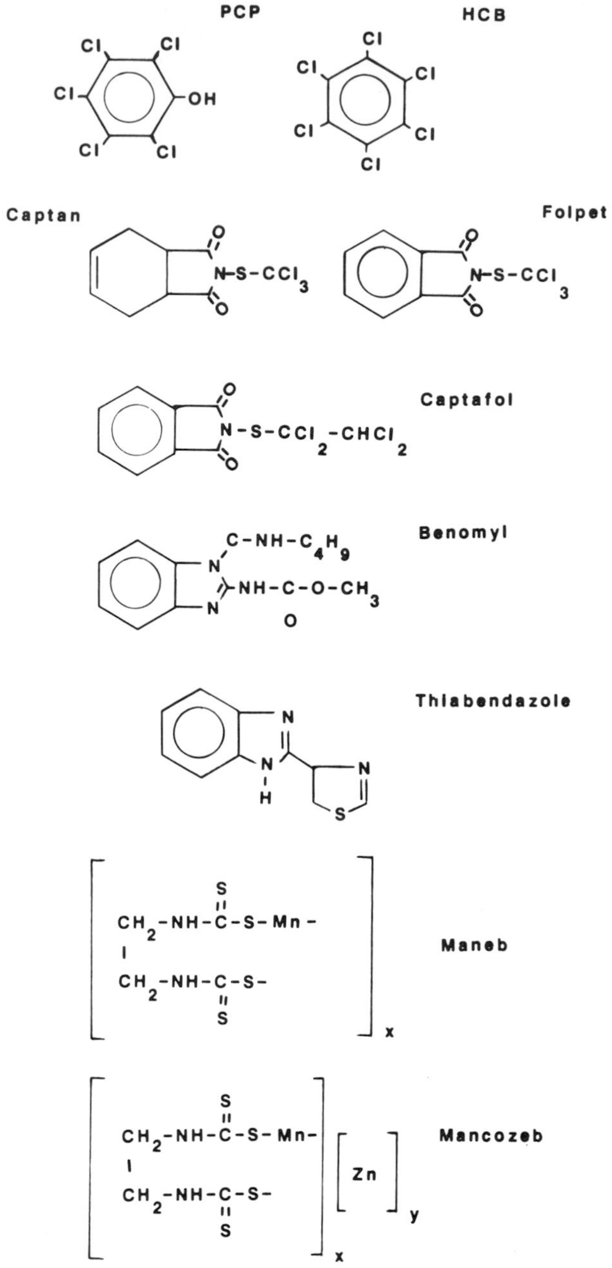

Figure 18–22. Chemical structures of fungicides representative of various chemical classifications.

fungicides are applied as liquids, dry powders, or granules, acting either through the vapor phase or by systemic properties. *Dressing fungicides* are applied to the post-harvest crop (cereal grains, tubers, corms, and so forth) as liquids or dry powders to prevent fungal infestation of the crop, particularly if it may be stored under less than optimum conditions of temperature and humidity. The post-harvest loss of food crops to disease is a serious worldwide problem (Table 18–2).

Fungicides may be described as protective, curative, or eradicative according to their mode of action. *Protective fungicides,* applied to the plant before the appearance of any phytopathic fungi, prevent infection by either sporicidal activity or by changing the physiologic environment on the leaf surface. *Curative fungicides* are used when an infestation has already begun to invade the plant, these chemicals penetrating the plant cuticle and destroying the young fungal mycelium (the hyphae) growing in the epidermis of the plant and preventing further development. *Eradicative fungicides* control fungal development following the appearance of symptoms, usually after sporulation, killing both the new spores and the mycelium by penetrating the cuticle of the plant to the subdermal level (Kramer, 1983).

To be an effective fungicide, a chemical must possess the following properties: (1) it must have very low toxicity to the plant but high toxicity to the particular fungus; (2) it must be active *per se* or be capable of conversion (by plant or fungal enzymes) into a toxic intermediate; (3) it must have the ability to penetrate fungal spores or the developing mycelium to reach a site of action; and (4) it must form a protective, tenacious deposit on the plant surface that will be resistant to weathering by sunlight, rain, and wind (Cremlyn, 1978). As might be expected, these properties are never met entirely by any single fungicide, all commercially available compounds showing some phytotoxicity, lack of persistence due to environmental degradation, and so forth. Thus, the timing of the application is quite critical in terms of the development of the plant as well as the fungus.

The topic of fungicidal toxicity has been extensively reviewed by Hayes (1975, 1982). With a few exceptions, most of these chemicals have a low order of toxicity to mammals, the oral LD50 values in the rat being of the order of 800 to 10,000 mg/kg. However, all fungicides are cytotoxic and most produce positive results in the usual *in vitro* microbial mutagenicity test systems. Such results are not surprising because the microorganisms (salmonella, coliforms, yeasts, and fungi) used in these test systems are not dissimilar from those cell systems for which fungicides were designed to kill either through a direct lethal effect or via lethal genetic mutations (Lukens, 1971). A "safe" fungicide (nonmutagenic in test cell systems) would be useless for the protection of food and health. Public concern has been focussed on the positive mutagenicity tests obtained with many fungicides and the predictive possibility of both teratogenic and carcinogenic potential. The fact that nearly 90 percent of all agricultural fungicides are carcinogenic in animal models has not reassured the public, especially when this is translated into the fact that some 75 million pounds of the fungicides used annually fall into this category (NAS, 1987). An evaluation of 11 fungicides concluded that, although the area treated with these chemicals represented only 10 percent of the acreage treated annually with pesticides, they could account for 60 percent of the total estimated dietary carcinogenic risk. Although tolerances have been set for such agents as captan, mancozeb, and benomyl on a few specific crops, no oncogenic fungicides other than benomyl have any section 409 (Delaney clause) tolerances, making regulation of carcinogenic risk a complex and delicate task. The EPA has used level-of-detection tolerances, but these have been set without the benefit of present-day sensitive analytical chemistry. In other words, the "zero" level of detection has been pushed backward, extremely low levels of these chemicals being detected today that could not be measured five or ten years ago.

The entire discipline of fungicidal chemistry and use is in a state of fluctuation. Many older agents, mentioned briefly below, have been deregistered because of overt toxicity encountered during their use. However, they are still being used in certain parts of the world. Other chemicals are being removed from the market because of perceived potential hazards to health. Still other fungicides are undergoing current reinvestigation and reevaluation because of suspicions of possible toxicity or incomplete toxicity data, particularly in the area of teratogenicity and carcinogenicity.

Hexachlorobenzene

The mammalian toxicity of hexachlorobenzene (HCB), not to be confused with the insecticide hexachlorocyclohexane (lindane, HCH), has been reviewed by Hayes (1975, 1982). From the late 1940s through the 1950s, HCB saw extensive use as fungicidal dressing, being applied to seed grain as a dry powder. Between 1955 and 1959, a spectacular epidemic of HCB poisoning, ultimately involving some 4000 patients, occurred in Turkey where people consumed treated grain during times of crop failure. The syndrome was called the "new disease" or "black sore" and was characterized by dermal blistering and epidemolysis, infection with pigmented scars on healing, and alopecia (Schmid, 1960; Wray *et al.*, 1962). The skin was photosensitive, pigmentation of exposed as well as covered parts of the body being seen. The initial diagnosis of the condition was congenital porphyria cutanea tarda. Because it appeared so suddenly, physicians looked for other causes and symptoms. More severe cases developed a suppurative arthritis, osteomyelitis, and osteoporosis of the bones of the hands (Cam and Nigogosyan, 1963). Hepatomegaly was observed in most hospitalized patients and some 30 percent of the cases showed enlarged thyroid glands, although functional changes were not observed. The disease was seen predominantly within families, in males (76 percent) and in children 4 to 14 years of age (81 percent). Young children were particularly at risk, nursing infants developing a lesion known as "pink sore" that was associated with a 95 percent mortality rate and was related to transplacental and milk acquisition of HCB from women who had consumed contaminated grain. The causative agent was identified in 1958 and the Turkish government stopped the practice of using HCB in 1959, with a gradual disappearance of new cases by 1963.

Like the organochlorine insecticides, HCB possesses all of the properties of chemical stability and environmental persistence, slow rate of degradation, slow metabolism, bioaccumulation in adipose tissue and other organs having high content of lipid membranes, and the ability to induce tissue microsomal monooxygenase enzymes. Chronic exposure of animals resulted in hepatomegaly and porphyria, focal alopecia with dermal itching and eruptions followed by pigmented scars, anorexia, and neurotoxicity expressed as increased irritability, ataxia, and tremors. Immunosuppression was observed in both mice and rats. A dose-dependent increase in hepatic and thyroid tumors was observed in hamsters during a chronic (70-week) study (Lambrecht et al., 1982). Although HCB was not mutagenic in microbial test systems and was negative in dominant lethal mutation tests, it did cause terata in mice (renal and palate malformations) and in rats (increased incidence of 14th rib). It would appear that there are considerable differences among laboratory rat strains in susceptibility to teratogenicity. Hexachlorobenzene was particularly toxic to developing perinatal animals, transplacental acquisition and, more importantly, acquisition via the milk causing enlarged kidneys, hydronephrosis, hepatomegaly, and possible effects on the immune system.

Organomercurials

In the past, alkyl-, alkoxyalkyl-, and aryl-mercurial compounds such as methyl- or methoxyethyl-mercuric chloride and dicyandiamide, phenylmercuric acetate, tolylmercuric acetate, ethylmercuric p-toluene sulfanilide, and so forth were used extensively as dressing fungicides for the prevention of seed-borne diseases of cereal grains, vegetables, cotton, soybeans, and sugar beets. Despite the recognized neurotoxicity of these chemicals, their use continued up until the early 1970s when individual tragic poisonings as well as a large-scale poisoning epidemic resulted in decisions to ban their use. Once again, the problem was generally associated with either the ingestion of fungicide-treated grain as in the Iraq epidemic or, as in the New Mexico incident, the consumption of meat from animals (hogs) to whom treated grain had been fed (Curley et al., 1971; Bakir et al., 1973).

The toxicology of the mercurial fungicides has been reviewed and the incidents of human poisoning have been described in detail (Ecobichon, 1982c; Hayes, 1982). Following acute intoxication, the signs and symptoms arise generally from the mercuric cation and the classic picture emerges of effects primarily in two organ systems, the gastrointestinal tract and the kidney (Koos and Longo, 1976). On the other hand, chronic poisoning is generally slow, insidious in onset and eventually will involve most organ systems. However, the major effects will be associated with the debilitation of the peripheral sensory and motor nerves and the CNS (Zepp et al., 1974). The perinatal individual is particularly vulnerable to organomercurial poisoning as will be recalled from the Minamata incident when seafood contaminated by methylmercury from an industrial process was consumed. Whereas the pregnant mothers were usually asymptomatic, the fetuses acquired most of the methylmercury with such disastrous effects on the developing CNS that postnatal brain development virtually ceased (Matsumoto et al., 1965; Chang et al., 1977; Tsubaki et al., 1978).

Fortunately for all, these chemicals no longer see commercial use although queries might be raised about continued use in developing countries.

Pentachlorophenol

Once used in tremendous volumes as an insecticide and fungicide in preserving wood products, this chemical is being phased out of use because of the discovery that many commercial products were contaminated by polychlorinated dibenzodioxins and dibenzofurans, predominantly by hexa-, hepta-, and octachlorinated congeners. These congeners are considerably less toxic than TCDD, but evidence from animal studies has pointed to the fact that the contaminants in commercial or technical pentachlorophenol (PCP) were responsible for the toxicity observed. Technical grade PCP fed to rats caused altered plasma enzymes, increased hepatic and renal weights, and hepatocellular degeneration, in addition to changes in blood biochemistry (decreased erythrocyte count, decreased hemoglobin, and serum albumin). The administration of purified PCP resulted only in increased liver and kidney weight. Prolonged treatment of female rats with technical PCP caused hepatic porphyria, increased microsomal monooxygenase activity, and increased liver weight, whereas purified PCP caused no changes over the dosage range studied (Goldstein *et al.*, 1977). Pentachlorophenol was not teratogenic in rats and is not considered to be carcinogenic in mice or rats (Innes *et al.*, 1969; Johnson *et al.*, 1973; Schwetz *et al.*, 1977). A number of environmental problems have been associated with PCP (Eisler, 1989).

Human poisoning by commercial PCP has occurred, usually associated with occupational exposure and instances of sloppy handling and neglect of hygienic principles. Some of the signs and symptoms may be due to the contaminants (polychlorinated dibenzodioxins and dibenzofurans) found in older technical grade product. The chemical is absorbed readily through the skin, the most usual route of acquisition, several products including PCP being detected in the urine. High level exposure can result in death preceded by an elevated body temperature (42°C or 108°F), profuse sweating and dehydration, marked loss of appetite, decrease in body weight, tightness in the chest, dyspnea following exercise, rapid pulse, nausea and vomiting, headache, incoordination, generalized weakness, and early coma (Hayes, 1982). Pentachlorophenol acts cellularly to uncouple oxidative phosphorylation, the target enzyme being Na^+, K^+-ATPase (Desaiah, 1977). Survivors frequently display dermal irritation and exfoliation, irritation of the upper respiratory tract, and possible impairment of autonomic function and circulation.

Phthalimides

Of the three chemicals belonging to this classification, only folpet and captofol are true phthalimides, the prototype chemical, captan, being structurally different with a cyclohexene ring (Figure 18–22). To study these agents, one must study captan because it is the oldest chemical, the most effective of the class, and has been embroiled in a prolonged controversy concerning teratogenicity and carcinogenicity.

As early as 1951, compounds containing an *N*-trichloromethylthio group were recognized as being potent surface fungicides. Captan was an effective, persistent foliar fungicide, particularly for Botrytis mold on soft fruit, apple, and pear scab; black spot on roses; and as a seed dressing (Cremlyn, 1978). Captafol and folpet were subsequently developed as foliar fungicides. All three chemicals have oral LD50 values of approximately 10,000 mg/kg in the rat. Unfortunately, these chemicals became embroiled in a testing laboratory controversy and, because the structures were similar to that of the drug

thalidomide, concerns were raised over potential teratogenicity. At daily doses of 500 mg/kg on days 7 and 8 of gestation in the hamster, teratogenicity was reported. Studies in other species either failed to confirm this effect or produced equivocal results open to speculative interpretation. Mutagenicity associated with these chemicals was confirmed and more recent long-term studies, conducted to support continued registration, revealed that captan caused duodenal tumors in the animal model (rat) being used (Anon., 1982). Studies were to be repeated to ascertain a no-observable-effect level because tumors were observed at all captan concentrations fed in the diet in the replacement studies. There, the matter rests.

Although the mechanism(s) by which captan and its analogs exert their cellular toxicity is not known, it has been demonstrated that captan reacts with cellular thiols to produce thiophosgene, a potent unstable chemical. Thiophosgene could poison cells by interacting with sulfhydryl-, amino-, or hydroxyl-containing enzymes, a hypothesis that is supported by the fact that the fungitoxicity of these three chemicals can be nullified by the addition of thiols (Cremlyn, 1978). Other investigators state that the entire molecule is required to react with thiol groups in fungal cells. It is possible that there are several mechanisms by which these chemicals can induce cellular toxicity. Experiments have shown that a volatile breakdown product of captan was responsible for the mutagenic activity, the volatile mutagen being short lived and formed at much higher levels at an alkaline pH, possibly related to hydrolysis of the molecule. There is also a diffusible mutagen causing biologic activity distinct from that produced by the volatile component (Bridges *et al.*, 1972). Interestingly, fungal resistance has never developed to captan, whereas fungi have become resistant to both folpet and captofol.

Dithiocarbamates

Dimethyl- and ethylene-bisdithiocarbamate (EBDC) compounds have been employed since the early 1950s as fungicides, the EBDC chemicals seeing widespread use on a large variety of small fruits and vegetables. The nomenclature of these agents arises from the metal cations with which they are associated: i.e., dimethyldithiocarbamic acid bound to iron or zinc are ferbam and ziram, respectively, whereas EBDC compounds associated with sodium, manganese, or zinc are nabam, maneb, and zineb, respectively. As is shown in Figure 18–22, these chemicals are polymeric structures possessing environmental stability and yielding good foliar protection as well as a low order of acute toxicity with

LD50 values in excess of 6000 mg/kg with the exception of nabam (395 mg/kg). Mancozeb is a polymeric mixture of a zinc salt and the chemical maneb.

Although toxicity is negligible in animal feeding trials even at high doses, acceptance of these agents has been marred by reported adverse health effects. Maneb, nabam, and zineb have been reported to be teratogenic (Petrova-Vergieva and Ivanova-Chemischanka, 1973). Mancozeb has not been demonstrated to be teratogenic in the rat, but maneb has been associated with adverse reproductive outcomes (embryotoxicity, number of offspring per litter, pregnancy rate, estrous cycle, fetal development) (Lu and Kennedy, 1986). Maneb caused pulmonary tumors in mice but studies in the rat have been equivocal (IARC, 1976). Environmental and mammalian degradation of the EBDC compounds into ethylene thiourea (ETU), a known mutagen, teratogen, and carcinogen, as well as an antithyroid compound, has raised suspicions about these agents and fostered requests for more in-depth studies (IARC, 1976). There is also evidence that ETU may be formed while processing and cooking EBDC-contaminated products. Few additional, definitive, and more recent studies have yielded any evidence of consequence concerning health hazards.

FUMIGANTS

Such agents are used to kill insects, nematodes, weed seeds, and fungi in soil, silo-stored cereal grains, fruit, and vegetables, clothes, and so forth, generally with the treatment being carried out in enclosed spaces because of the volatility of most of the products. Fumigants range from acrylonitrile and carbon disulfide to carbon tetrachloride, ethylene dibromide, chloropicrin, and ethylene oxide; their toxicologic properties are discussed under other headings because many have other uses. Attention in this section will be directed only to a very few agents although all of the chemicals mentioned have the potential for inhalation exposure and, for some of them, dermal and ingestion exposure.

Fumigants may be liquids (ethylene dibromide, dibromochloropropane, formaldehyde) that readily vaporize at ambient temperature, solids that can release a toxic gas on reacting with water (Zn_2P_3, AlP) or with acid [NaCN, $Ca(CN)_2$], or gases (methyl bromide, hydrogen cyanide, ethylene oxide). These chemicals are nonselective and extremely toxic at elevated concentrations. The physicochemical properties of these agents and hence their pattern(s) of use vary considerably (Cremlyn, 1978). In general, with proper attention to use and with appropriate safety precautions, there should be little other than occasional occupational exposure, the volatility of the agents being such that when the enclosed space is opened, the gas or vapor escapes readily. However, reports in the literature have indicated the presence of low residue levels of ethylene dibromide, methyl bromide, and so forth in various samples of foods treated with these chemicals. More extensive descriptions of fumigant toxicity can be found in Hayes (1982) and Morgan (1982).

Phosphine

Used extensively as a grain fumigant, phosphine is released from aluminum phosphide (AlP) by the natural moisture in the grain over a long period of time, giving continual protection during transhipment of the grain. One serious accident with this chemical has been reported, the author of this chapter playing a small role in identifying the causative agent, as the problem originated in the port of Montreal, Canada (Wilson et al., 1980). Grain leaving Canada for European destinations is fumigated by adding a certain number of sachets of AlP per ton of grain in the hold of the ship while loading. Phosphine (PH_3), being heavier than air, sinks slowly through the grain. The particular ship in question ran into a bad storm off Nova Scotia and began to leak, hastening the breakdown of the AlP to form PH_3. The toxicant penetrated the quarters of the crew and officers where 29 out of 31 crew members became acutely ill and two children, family of one of the officers, were seriously affected, one dying before reaching a hospital in Boston. Symptoms of PH_3 intoxication in the adults included shortness of breath, cough and pulmonary irritation, nausea, headache, jaundice, and fatigue. The highest concentrations of PH_3 (20 to 30 ppm) were measured in a void space on the main deck near the air intake for the ship's ventilation system. In some of the living quarters, PH_3 levels of 0.5 ppm were detected. Although this could be considered a bizarre situation, it does illustrate an apparent problem of the use of this type of agent in an atmosphere of excess moisture.

Ethylene Dibromide/Dibromochloropropane

When inhaled, at relatively high (>200 ppm) concentrations, ethylene dibromide can cause pulmonary edema and inflammation in the exposed animals. As one might expect, repeated exposures to lower concentrations produced hepatic and renal damage visualized as morphologic changes. Centrolobular hepatic necrosis and proximal tubular damage in the kidneys were observed in one fatal poisoning where the individual ingested 4.5 ml of ethylene dibromide. This chemical, along with 1,2-dibromo-3-chloropropane (DBCP), was found to elicit malignant gastric squamous cell carcinomas in mice and rats (IARC, 1977). DBCP was also found to cause sterility in male animals, concentrations as low as 5 ppm having an adverse effect on testicular morphology and spermatogenesis. However, these results in animals came to light only when a similar situation was detected in workers who manufactured the agent. Equivocal results have been reported for the mutagenicity of DBCP, the agent causing base pair-substitution but not a frame-shift mutation in salmonella strains. In animal studies of the dominant lethal assay, DBCP was positive (mutagenic) in rats but not in mice. DBCP was a reproductive toxicant in rabbits and rats but not in mice (IARC, 1977).

RODENTICIDES

Many vertebrates, including rats, mice, squirrels, bats, rabbits, skunks, monkeys, and even elephants, on occasion can be considered to be pests. Rodents, the most important of which are the black rat *(Rattus rattus)*, the brown or Norway rat *(Rattus norvegicus)*, and the house mouse *(Mus musculus)*, are particularly serious problems because they act as vectors for several human diseases. They can consume large quantities of post-harvest, stored food and/or foul or contaminate even greater amounts of foodstuffs with urine, feces, hair, and bacteria that cause diseases.

A rodenticide, to be effective yet safe, must satisfy the following criteria: (1) it must not be unpalatable to the target species and, therefore, must be quite potent; (2) it must not induce bait shyness so that the animal will continue to eat it; (3) death should occur in a manner that does not raise the suspicions of the survivors; (4) it should make the intoxicated animal go out into the open to die (otherwise the rotting corpses create health hazards); and (5) it should be species specific with considerably lower toxicity to other animals that might inadvertently consume the bait or eat the poisoned rodent (Cremlyn, 1978). The agents used constitute a diverse range of chemical structures having a variety of mechanisms of action in partially successful attempts to attain species selectivity (Figure 18–23). With some chemicals, advantage has been taken of the physiology and biochemistry unique to rodents. With other rodenticides, the site(s) of action are common to most mammals but advantage is taken of the habits of the pest animal and/or the dosage, thereby minimizing toxicity to nontarget species.

Although most rodenticides are formulated in

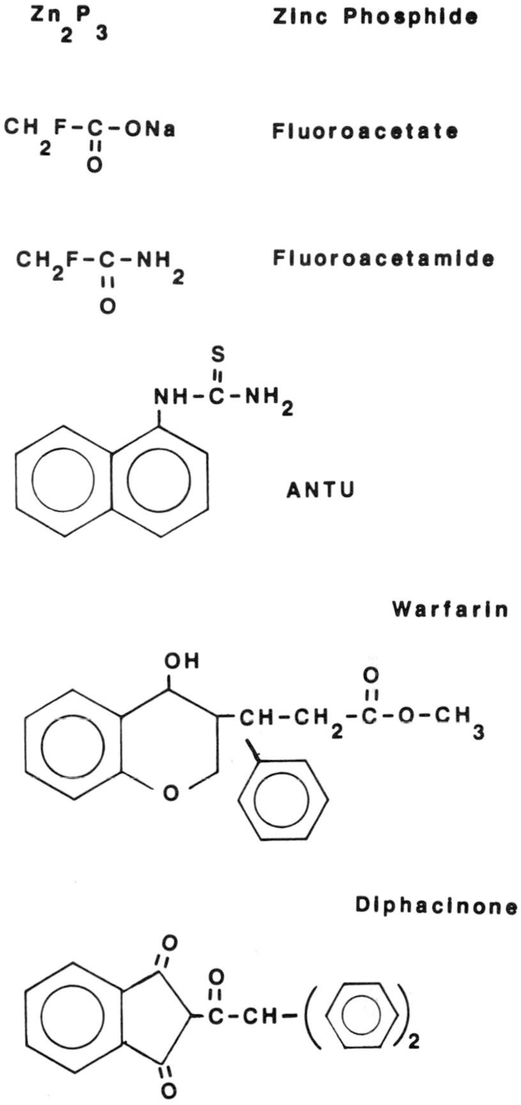

Figure 18–23. Representative structures of inorganic and organic rodenticides from various chemical classifications.

baits that are unpalatable to humans, thereby minimizing the potential hazard, there are surprising numbers of rodenticide intoxications each year. With only a few exceptions, the accidental or intentional ingestion of most rodenticides poses a serious, acute toxicologic problem because, invariably, the dosage ingested is high and the signs and symptoms of intoxication are generally well advanced and quite severe when the patient is seen by a physician. As with other household products, rodenticide poisoning is more frequently seen in children, the added hazard being the small body weight in relation to the dosage ingested. The toxicology of the various classes of rodenticides has been extensively reviewed and the reader is referred to Hayes (1982) and to Ellenhorn and Barceloux (1988) for in-depth coverage of the subject.

A number of inorganic compounds including thallium sulfate, arsenious oxide, other arsenic salts, barium carbonate, yellow phosphorus, aluminum phosphide, and zinc phosphide have been used as rodenticides. A mixture of sodium cyanide with magnesium carbonate and anhydrous magnesium sulfate has been used in rabbit and mole burrows, hydrogen cyanide gas being liberated slowly on contact with moisture. Natural or synthetic organic chemicals including strychnine, red squill (scillaren glycosides), and DDT have been used in the past. All of these agents are nonselective, highly toxic, and hazardous to other forms of life and, with the exception of zinc phosphide, have been abandoned in favor of target specific, selective chemicals.

Zinc Phosphide

This agent is used in developing nations because it is both a cheap and effective rodenticide. The toxicity of the chemical can be accounted for by the phosphine (PH_3) formed following a hydrolytic reaction with water in the stomach on ingestion. Phosphine causes widespread cellular toxicity with necrosis of the gastrointestinal tract and injury to other organs such as the liver and kidneys. Although moist zinc phosphide emits an unpleasant, rotten-fish odor, it is accepted in baits at concentrations of 0.5 or 1.0 percent by rodents.

Accidental poisonings are rare in adults but a definite problem in children. Hayes (1982) recounts a poisoning attributed to the inhalation of zinc phosphide dust from treated grain, the signs of intoxication including vomiting, diarrhea, cyanosis, tachycardia, rhales, restlessness, fever, and albuminuria several hours following exposure. It is a favorite chemical in suicides in Egypt (Amr, personal communication). The signs and symptoms include nausea, vomiting, headache, lightheadedness, dyspnea, hypertension, pulmonary edema, dysrrhythmias and convulsions. Doses of the order of 4000 to 5000 mg have been fatal, but other individuals have survived doses of 25,000 to 100,000 mg if early vomiting has occurred. The usual decontamination measures and supportive therapy are often successful if initiated early.

Fluoroacetic Acid and Derivatives

Sodium fluoroacetate (Compound 1080) and fluoroacetamide (Compound 1081) are white in color, odorless, and tasteless. The extreme toxicity of these two chemicals has restricted their use to prepared baits. Both agents are well absorbed from the gastrointestinal tract. Acute oral toxicity of fluoroacetate in the rat is of the order of 0.2 mg/kg whereas that of fluoroacetamide is 4 to 15 mg/kg. The mechanism of action involves the incorporation of the fluoroacetate into fluoroacetyl-coenzyme A which condenses with oxaloacetate to form fluorocitrate, this product inhibiting the enzyme aconitase and preventing the conversion of citrate to isocitrate in the tricarboxylic (Krebs) cycle. Inhibition of this system by fluorocitrate results in reduced glucose metabolism and cellular respiration and affects tissue energy stores. These chemicals are uniquely effective in mice and rats because of the high metabolic rate in tissues which are susceptible to inhibition.

Estimates of the lethal dose of fluoroacetate in humans lie in the range of 2 to 10 mg/kg. Gastrointestinal symptoms are seen initially at some 30 to 100 minutes following ingestion. Initial nausea, vomiting, and abdominal pain are replaced by sinus tachycardia, ventricular tachycardia or fibrillation, hypotension, renal failure, muscle spasms, and such CNS symptoms as agitation, stupor, seizures, and coma. Histopathologic examination of postmortem samples has revealed cerebellar degeneration and atrophy. There are no known antidotes to fluoroacetate intoxication, although glycerol monoacetate proved beneficial in the treatment of poisoned monkeys.

α-Naphthyl Thiourea (ANTU)

Following the discovery that phenylthiourea was lethal to rats but was not toxic to humans, ANTU was introduced as a relatively selective rodenticide (Richter, 1945, 1946). A wide range of acute oral LD50 values has been reported for different species, the rat being the most sensitive at 3 mg/kg, whereas the monkey was the least susceptible at 4 g/kg. The exact mechanism of action is not known, but it is suspected that ANTU must be biotransformed in vivo into a reactive intermediate. Young rats are resistant to the chemical whereas older rats become tolerant to it, evidence suggesting that perhaps microsomal monooxygenases in young rats metabolize the agent too rapidly into nontoxic products whereas, in older rats, either the lower levels of monooxygenases or the inhibition of these enzymes results in less activation and affords protection (Boyd and Neal, 1976). ANTU causes extensive pulmonary edema and pleural effusion as a consequence of action on the pulmonary capillaries. Studies with [35]S- and ^{14}C-labelled ANTU revealed that covalent binding to macromolecules in the lung and liver occurred following treatment (Boyd and Neal, 1976). Following exposure to ANTU, there are a number of biochemical effects such as alterations in carbohydrate metabolism, adrenal stimulation, and interaction of the chemical with sulfhydryl groups, but none of these appear to bear any relationship to the observed signs of toxicity.

Although it would appear that the human is quite resistant to ANTU intoxication, probably because insufficient quantities are ingested, poisonings have occurred, with tracheobronchial hypersecretion of a white, nonmucous froth containing little protein, pulmonary edema, and respiratory difficulty (Hayes, 1982).

Pyrinimil

Norway rats, roof rats, and mice are all highly susceptible to this more recently developed substituted urea compound, N-(3-pyridinylmethyl)-N'-(4-nitrophenyl) urea (PNU, Vacor®). The acute oral LD50 in the rat is of the order of 5 mg/kg, whereas the oral LD50 for most other species is in excess of 500 mg/kg (Peardon, 1974). Cats, however, are quite susceptible.

Pyrinimil interferes with nicotinamide metabolism and has a direct effect on glucose metabolism on the basis that it is diabetogenic, destroying the β islet cells of the pancreas. There are other effects, obviously caused by different mechanisms of action, most of these having been observed in cases of human intoxication. The clinical picture is similar to diabetic ketoacidosis. An initial hyperglycemia is followed by a persistent (48 hour) hypoglycemia with, subsequently, permanent glucose intolerance and ketoacidosis. Orthostatic hypotension and postural lightheadedness may be observed. Dysphagia, impotence, urinary retention, and constipation or diarrhea may occur as manifestations of an autonomic neuropathy (LeWitt, 1980). Symptoms also include nausea, vomiting, abdominal pain, diffuse myalgias, polyuria, polydypsia, dyspnea, malaise, and general weakness. The importance of the neurologic impairment has only recently been appreciated with both peripheral sensory and motor neuropathies with ataxia being reported (LeWitt, 1980; Ellenhorn and Barceloux, 1988). Neurologic disorders frequently appeared within hours of ingestion and various spurious symptoms persisted for weeks and months after exposure.

Anticoagulants

With the discovery that coumadin [3-(α-acetonylbenzyl)-4-hydroxycoumarin, warfarin), isolated from spoiled sweet clover, acted as an anticoagulant by antagonizing the actions of vitamin K in the synthesis of clotting factors (factors II, VII, IX, and X), it was introduced as a rodenticide. The onset of anticoagulation is delayed 8 to 12 hours after the ingestion of warfarin, this latent period of onset being dependent on the half-lives of the various clotting factors (Katona and Wason, 1986). The safety of warfarin as a rodenticide rests with the fact that multiple doses are required before toxicity develops, single doses having little effect. However, the development of resistance to warfarin in rats in the 1950s prompted reseach into newer compounds, the exploration of structure-activity relationships leading to the development of the superwarfarins (brodifacoum, bromadiolone, coumachlor, diphencoumarin) and a new class of anticoagulant compounds, the indanediones (diphacinone, chlorophacinone, pindone) which are more water soluble. All of these newer agents differ from one another in terms of acute toxicity, rapidity of action, and acceptance by the rodent. Resistance toward these chemicals has not developed to date.

Human poisonings by these agents are quite rare because they are dispensed in grain-based baits. However, there are sufficient numbers of suicide attempts, attempted murder, and a rather famous classic case of inadvertent consumption of warfarin-laden corn meal bait by an unsuspecting Korean family to provide adequate documentation of the signs and symptoms of poisoning (Lange and Terveer, 1954; Hayes, 1982; Jones, 1984; Lipton, 1984; Katona and Wason, 1986). Following consumption over a period of days, bleeding of the gingiva and nose occurs, with bruising and hematomas developing at the knee and elbow joints and on the buttocks, gastrointestinal bleeding with dark tarry stools, hematuria accompanied by abdominal or low back (flank) pain, epistaxis, and cerebrovascular accidents. The signs and symptoms will persist for many days after cessation of exposure, particularly so in the case of the superwarfarins which have prolonged biologic half-lives, i.e., brodifacoun with 156 hours compared to 37 hours for warfarin (Katona and Wason, 1986). In the Korean episode, consumption of warfarin was estimated to be of the order of 1 to 2 mg/kg per day for a period of 15 days, signs and symptoms appearing 7 to 10 days after initial exposure, 2 out of the 14 affected individuals dying as a consequence of not receiving any treatment (Lange and Terveer, 1954).

Norbormide

This chemical, with a particularly complex structure, was introduced in 1964. The chemical is lethal to rats at concentrations of 5 to 15 mg/kg but is nontoxic to other species, including the human. Although the mechanism of action remains unknown, the site of action is on the smooth muscle of peripheral blood vessels, caus-

Table 18–14. THE WHO RECOMMENDED CLASSIFICATION OF PESTICIDES BY HAZARD*

| | | LD50 FOR THE RAT (mg/kg BODY WEIGHT) | | | |
| | | Oral | | Dermal | |
CLASS		Solids	Liquids	Solids	Liquids
Ia	Extremely hazardous	≤5	≤20	≤10	≤40
Ib	Highly hazardous	5–50	20–200	10–100	40–400
II	Moderately hazardous	50–500	200–2000	100–1000	400–4000
III	Slightly hazardous	>500	>2000	>1000	>4000
III+	Unlikely to present hazard in normal use	>2000	>3000	—	—

* From Copplestone, J. F.: *Bull. WHO*, **66**:545–551, 1988.

ing irreversible vasoconstriction and initiating widespread tissue ischemia, necrosis, and subsequent death (Hayes, 1982). This effect is not observed in other animal species, making the rat unique in this respect. Toxicity was not observed in human volunteers subjected to intradermal injections (0.1 ml of a 0.1 percent solution) or to oral doses of 20 to 300 mg (Hayes, 1982).

CONCLUSIONS

With the advent of the chemical pesticides, their diverse nature, structures, and biologic activity, the problem of ranking the hazard that each one poses to health has arisen. Should a classification system be based on acute toxicity alone or should some numerical scoring system be used to evaluate other endpoints of toxicity? Should the classification scheme be based on the oral, dermal, or inhalation routes of exposure to the active ingredient or to a formulation concentrate? If one chooses acute toxicity and a definitive endpoint expressed as the LD50, one must be cognizant of the fact that the LD50 is an estimate, the range and confidence limits for any particular chemical possibly overlapping a class "boundary." To establish a classification system on the basis of other toxicologic endpoints would be impossible given the variability of biologic effects, the dosages required to attain them, and the significance of such results in terms of human exposure.

In 1972, the WHO Expert Committee on Insecticides recommended the preparation of a classification of pesticides that would serve as a guide for developing countries (WHO, 1973). The classification was to distinguish between the more and the less hazardous forms of each pesticide and should permit formulations to be classified according to the percentage of the active ingredient and its physical state. Only acute hazard to health was considered, i.e., that resulting from single or multiple exposures over a relatively short period of time from handling the product in accordance with the manufacturer's directions. In 1975, the categories of the classification were established and, with only one modification to Class III, are essentially as appear in Table 18–14. It is important to appreciate that the LD50 value quoted for any pesticide is not the median value but the lower confidence limit value for the most sensitive sex, thereby ensuring that a large safety factor has been built into the classification. A recent paper by Copplestone (1988) discusses the advantages and disadvantages of the system and the placement of problem chemicals such as rodenticides (highly toxic to rats but not presenting the same hazard to humans) and paraquat (having a low dermal toxicity but causing fatal effects if ingested).

From experience, the WHO is of the opinion that this classification scheme has worked well in practice, faithfully reflecting the toxicity of these chemicals for humans. Only a few changes in classification have been made for chemicals and/or their formulations since the introduction of the scheme, signifying that the system functions effectively. It would appear that acute toxicity is the most effective parameter by which to judge the hazard to human health. With the move away from animal experimentation to *in vitro* testing, this classification system can be modified to reflect other endpoints of toxicity if they can be quantitated, correlated, and validated to be equivalent to the LD50 results. As stated by Dr. Copplestone, "the classification has been a meeting point between science and administration and a useful tool in the armamentarium of preventive medicine" (Copplestone, 1988).

REFERENCES

Abbott, D. C.; Goulding, R.; and Tatton, J. O. 'G.: Organochlorine pesticide residues in human fat in Great Britain. *Br. Med. J.*, **3**:146–149, 1968.

Abou-Donia, M. B.: Organophosphorus ester-induced delayed neurotoxicity. *Annu. Rev. Pharmacol. Toxicol.*, **21**:511–548, 1981.

Alachlor Review Board: *Report of the Alachlor Review Board*. Agriculture Canada, Canadian Government Publishing Centre, Ottawa, Canada, 1987.

Alary, J. G.; Guay, P.; and Brodeur, J.: Effect of phenobarbital pretreatment on the metabolism of DDT in the rat and the bovine. *Toxicol. Appl. Pharmacol.*, **18**:457–468, 1971.

Albert, A.: *Xenobiosis, Food, Drugs and Poisons in the Human Body*. Chapman and Hall, London, 1987, pp. 113–116.

Aldridge, W. N., and Johnson, M. K.: Side effects of organophosphorus compounds: delayed neurotoxicity. *Bull. WHO*, **44**:259–263, 1971.

Aldridge, W. N., and Reiner, E.: *Enzyme Inhibitors as Substrates*. North-Holland/American Elsevier, Amsterdam and New York, 1972.

Almog, C., and Tal, E.: Death from paraquat after subcutaneous injection. *Br. Med. J.*, **3**:721, 1967.

Anon.: A look at world pesticide markets. *Farm Chem.*, **141**:38–42, 1977.

Anon.: Captan. *A Report by the Consultative Committee on Industrial Bio-Test Pesticides*. Agriculture Canada, 1982.

Ashe, W., and Suskind, R. R.: Chloracne cases of the Monsanto Chemical Company, Nitro, West Virginia. In *Reports of the Kettering Laboratory*, University of Cincinnati, October 1949, April 1950, July 1953.

Askew, B. M.: Oximes and hydroxamic acids as antidotes in anticholinesterase poisoning. *Br. J. Pharmacol. Chemother.* **11**:417–423, 1956.

Axelson, O.; Sundell, L.; Andersson, K.; Edling, C.; Hogstedt, C.; and Kling, H.: Herbicide exposure and tumor mortality. *Scand. J. Work Environ. Health*, **6**:73–79, 1980.

Baggett, J. McC.; Thureson-Klein, A.; and Klein, R. L.: Effects of chlordecone on the adrenal medulla of the rat. *Toxicol. Appl. Pharmacol.*, **52**:313–322, 1980.

Bakir, F.; Damluji, S. F.; Amin-Zaki, L.; Murtadha, M.; Khalidi, A.; Al-Rawi, N. Y.; Tikriti, S.; Dhahir, H. I.; Clarkson, T. W.; Smith, J. C.; and Doherty, R. A.: Methylmercury poisoning in Iraq. *Science*, **181**:230–241, 1973.

Barinaga, M.: Agent Orange: Congress impatient for answers. *Science*, **245**:249–250, 1989.

Barnes, J. M., and Verschoyle, R. D.: Toxicity of new pyrethroid insecticides. *Nature*, **248**:711, 1974.

Batchelor, G. S., and Walker, K. C.: Health hazards involved in use of parathion in fruit orchards of north central Washington. *AMA Arch. Ind. Hyg. Occup. Health*, **10**:522–529, 1954.

Berkow, S. G.: Value of surface-area proportions in the prognosis of cutaneous burns and scalds. *Am. J. Surg.*, **11**:315–320, 1931.

Berwick, P.: Dichlorophenoxyacetic acid poisoning in man. Some interesting clinical and laboratory findings. *JAMA*, **214**:1114–1117, 1970.

Bidstrup, P. L.; Bonner, J. A.; and Beckett, A. G.: Paralysis following poisoning by a new organic phosphorus insecticide (Mipafox). *Br. Med. J.*, **1**:1068–1072, 1953.

Bond, G. G.; Wetterstroem, N. H.; Roush, G. J.; McLaren, E. A.; Lipps, T. E.; and Cook, R. R.: Cause specific mortality among employees engaged in the manufacture, formulation or packaging of 2,4-dichlorophenoxyacetic acid and related salts. *Br. J. Indust. Med.*, **45**:98–105, 1988.

Bonsall, J. L.: Measurement of occupational exposure to pesticides. In Turnbull, G. S. (ed.): *Occupational Hazards of Pesticide Use*. Francis and Taylor, London, 1985, pp. 13–33.

Boon-Long, J.; Glinsukon, T.; Pothisiri, P.; Srianujata, S.; Suphakarn, V.; and Wongphanich, M.: Toxicological problems in Thailand. In Ruchirawat, M., and Shank, R. C. (eds.): *Environmental Toxicity and Carcinogenesis*. Text and Journal Corporation, Bangkok, Thailand.

Boyd, M. R., and Neal, R. A.: Studies on the mechanism of toxicity and of development of tolerance to the pulmonary toxic α-naphthylthiourea (ANTU). *Drug Metab. Dispos.*, **4**:314–322, 1976.

Bridges, B. A.; Mottershead, R. P.; Rothwell, M. A.; and Green, M. H. L.: Repair-deficient bacterial strains suitable for mutagenicity screening: tests with the fungicide captan. *Chem. Biol. Interact.*, **5**:77–84, 1972.

Brooks, G. T.: *Chlorinated Insecticides*. Vol. 1. *Technology and Application*. CRC Press, Cleveland, Ohio, 1974a.

———: *Chlorinated Insecticides*. Vol. II. *Biological and Environmental Aspects*. CRC Press, Cleveland, Ohio. 1974b.

Buchel, K. H. (ed.): *Chemistry of Pesticides*. John Wiley & Sons, New York, 1983.

Buckingham, W. A.: *Operation Ranch Hand: The Air Force and Herbicides in Southeast Asia, 1961–1971*. U.S. Air Force, Washington, D.C. 1982.

Bull, D. L.: Metabolism of organophosphorus insecticides in animals and plants. *Residue Rev.*, **43**:1–22, 1972.

Cam, C., and Nigogosyan, G.: Acquired toxic porphyria cutanea tarda due to hexachlorobenzene. *JAMA*, **183**:88–91, 1963.

Campbell, S.: Paraquat poisoning. *Clin. Toxicol.*, **1**:245–249, 1968.

Cannon, S. B.; Veasey, J. M. Jr.; Jackson, R. S.,; Burse, V. W., Hayes, C.; Straub, W. E.; Landrigan, P. J.; and Liddle, J. A.: Epidemic kepone poisoning in chemical workers. *Am. J. Epidemiol.*, **107**:529–537, 1978.

Cantor, K. P.: Farming and mortality from non-Hodgkin's lymphoma: a case-control study. *Int. J. Cancer*, **29**:239–247, 1982.

Carson, R.: *Silent Spring*. Houghton Mifflin, Boston, 1962.

Casida, J. E.; Gammon, D. W.; Glockman, A. H.; and Lawrence, L. J.: Mechanisms of selective action of pyrethroid insecticides. *Annu. Rev. Pharmacol. Toxicol.* **23**:413–438, 1983.

Cavanagh, J. B.: The toxic effects of tri-ortho-cresyl phosphate on the nervous system, an experimental study in hens. *J. Neurol. Neurosurg. Psychiatry*, **17**:163–172, 1954.

Centers for Disease Control Veterans Health Studies. Serum 2,3,7,8-tetrachlorodibenzo-*p*-dioxin levels in U.S. Army Vietnam-era veterans. *JAMA*, **260**:1249–1254, 1988.

Chang, L. W.; Reuhl, K. R.; and Lee, G. W.: Degenerative changes in the developing nervous system as a result of in utero exposure to methyl mercury. *Environ. Res.*, **14**:414–423, 1977.

Chernoff, N.; Kavlock, R. J.; Kathrein, J. R.; Dunn, J. M.; and Haseman, J. K.: Prenatal effects of dieldrin and photodieldrin in mice and rats. *Toxicol. Appl. Pharmacol.*, **31**:302–308, 1975.

Childs, A. F.; Davies, D. R.; Green, A. L.; and Rutland, J. P.: The reactivation by oximes and hydroxamic acids of cholinesterase inhibited by organophosphorus compounds. *Br. J. Pharmacol., Chemother.* **10**:462–465, 1955.

Clark, D. G., and Hurst, E. W.: The toxicity of diquat. *Br. J. Ind. Med.*, **27**:51–55, 1970.

Clark, D. G.; McElligott, T. F.; and Hurst, E. W.: The toxicity of paraquat. *Br. J. Ind. Med.*, **23**:126–132, 1966.

Clark, J. M., and Matsumura, F.: Two different types of inhibitory effects of pyrethroids on nerve Ca and Ca-Mg-ATPase activity in the squid, *Loligo pealei. Pestic. Biochem. Physiol.*, **18**:180–190, 1982.

Cohn, W. J.; Boylan, J. J.; Blanke, R. V.; Fariss, M. W.; Nowell, J. R.; and Guzelian, P. S.: Treatment of chlordecone (Kepone) toxicity with cholestyramine. *N. Engl. J. Med.*, **298**:243–248, 1978.

Committee on Scientific and Regulatory Issues Underlying Pesticide Use Patterns and Agricultural Innovation: *Regulating Pesticides in Food.* National Academy Press, Washington, D. C., 1987.

Copplestone, J. F.: In Watson, D. L., and Brown, A. W. A. (eds.): *Pesticide Management and Pesticide Resistance.* Academic Press, New York, 1977.

———: The development of the WHO Recommended Classification of Pesticides by Hazard. *Bull. WHO*, **66**:545–551, 1988.

Corbett, J. R.: *The Biochemical Mode of Action of Pesticides.* Academic Press, New York, 1974.

Council on Scientific Affairs.: Cancer risk of pesticides in agricultural workers. *JAMA*, **260**:959–966, 1988.

Courtney, K. D., and Moore, J. A.: Teratology studies with 2,4,5-trichlorophenoxyacetic acid and 2,3,7,8-tetra-chlorodibenzo-dioxin. *Toxicol. Appl. Pharmacol.*, **20**:396–403, 1971.

Courtney, K. D.; Gaylor, D. W.; Hogan, M. D.; Falk, H. L.; Bates, R. R.; and Mitchell, I.: Teratogenic evaluation of 2,4,5-T. *Science*, **168**:864–866, 1970.

Cranmer, M. F.: Carbaryl. A toxicological review and risk analysis. *Neurotoxicology*, **1**:247–332, 1986.

Cremlyn, R.: *Pesticides. Preparation and Mode of Action.* John Wiley & Sons, New York, 1978.

Curley, A.; Sedlak, V. A.; Girling, E. F.; Hawk, R. E.; Bartnel, W. F.; Pierce, P. E.; and Likosky, W. H.: Organic mercury identified as the cause of poisoning in humans and hogs. *Science*, **172**:65–67, 1971.

Dale, W. E., and Quinby, G. E.: Chlorinated insecticides in the body fat of people in the United States. *Science*, **142**:593–595, 1963.

Daniel, J. W., and Gage, J. C.: Absorption and excretion of diquat and paraquat in rats. *Br. J. Ind. Med.*, **23**:133–136, 1966.

Dauterman, W. C., and Main, A. R.: Relationship between acute toxicity and in vitro inhibition and hydrolysis of a series of homologs of malathion. *Toxicol. Appl. Pharmacol.*, **9**:408–418, 1966.

Davies, J. E.; Edmundson, W. F.; Schneider, N. J.; and Cassady, J. C.: Problems of prevalence of pesticide residues in humans. In Davies, J. E., and Edmundson, W. F. (eds.): *Epidemiology of DDT.* Futura, Mount Kisco, New York, 1972, pp. 27–37.

Davies, D. S.; Hawksworth, G. M.; and Bennett, P. N.: Paraquat poisoning. *Proc. Eur. Soc. Toxicol.*, **18**:21–26, 1977.

Desaiah, D.: Effects of pentachlorophenol on the ATPases in rat tissue. In Rao, K. R. (ed.): *Pentachlorophenol.* Plenum Press, New York, 1977, pp. 277–283.

Desi, I.; Gonczi, L.; Simon, G.; Farkas, I.; and Kneffel, Z.: Neurotoxicologic studies of two carbamate pesticides in subacute animal experiments. *Toxicol. Appl. Pharmacol.*, **27**:465–476, 1974.

DuBois, K. P.: New rodenticidal compounds, *J. Am. Pharm. Assoc.*, **37**:307–310, 1948.

DuBois, K. P.; Doull, J.; Salerno, P. R.; and Coon, J. M.: Studies on the toxicity and mechanisms of action of *p*-nitrophenyl-diethyl-thionophosphate (Parathion): *J. Pharmacol. Exp. Ther.*, **95**: 75–91, 1949.

Dudley, A. W., Jr., and Thapar, N. T.: Fatal human ingestion of 2,4-D, a common herbicide. *Arch. Pathol.*, **94**:270–275, 1972.

Durham, W. F.; Wolfe, H. R.; and Elliott, J. W.: Absorption and excretion of parathion by spraymen. *Arch. Environ. Health*, **24**: 381–387, 1972.

Dustman, E. H., and Stickel, L. F.: The occurrence and significance of pesticide residues in wild animals. *Ann. NY Acad. Sci.*, **160**:162–172, 1969.

Ecobichon, D. J.: Hydrolytic mechanisms of pesticide degradation. In Geissbuhler, H. (ed.): *Advances in Pesticide Science, Part 3, Biochemistry of Pests and Mode of Action of Pesticides, Pesticide Degradation, Pesticide Residues and Formulation Chemistry.* Pergamon Press, New York, 1979, pp. 516–524.

———: Organophosphorus ester insecticides. In Ecobichon, D. J., and Joy, R. M.: *Pesticides and Neurological Diseases.* CRC Press, Boca Raton, Florida, 1982a, pp. 151–203.

———: Carbamic acid ester insecticides. In Ecobichon, D. J., and Joy, R. M.: *Pesticides and Neurological Diseases.* CRC Press, Boca Raton, Florida, 1982b, pp. 205–233.

———: The mercurial fungicides. In Ecobichon, D. J., and Joy, R. M.: *Pesticides and Neurological Diseases.* CRC Press, Boca Raton, Florida, 1982c, pp. 235–261.

Ecobichon, D. J., and Joy, R. M.: *Pesticides and Neurological Diseases.* CRC Press, Boca Raton, Florida, 1982.

Ecobichon, D. J., and MacKenzie, D. O.: The uterotropic activity of commercial and isomerically pure chlorobiphenyls in the rat. *Res. Commun. Chem. Pathol. Pharmacol.*, **9**:85–95, 1974.

Ecobichon, D. J., and Saschenbrecker, P. W.: Pharmacodynamic study of DDT in cockerels. *Can. J. Physiol. Pharmacol.*, **46**:785–794, 1968.

———: The redistribution of stored DDT in cockerels under the influence of food deprivation. *Toxicol. Appl. Pharmacol.*, **5**:420–432, 1969.

Ecobichon, D. J.; Ozere, R. L.; Reid, E.; and Crocker, J. F. S.: Acute fenitrothion poisoning. *Can. Med. Assoc. J.*, **116**:377–379, 1977.

Edington, N., and Howell, J. M.: The neurotoxicity of sodium diethyl-diethio-carbamate in the rabbit. *Acta Neuropathol.*, **12**:339–346, 1969.

Egan, H.; Goulding, R.; Toburn, J. and Tatton, J. O'G: Organochlorine residues in human fat and human milk. *Brit. Med. J.*, **2**:66–69, 1965.

Egle, J. L., Jr.; Guzelain, P. S.; and Borzelleca, J. F.: Time course of the acute toxic effects of sublethal doses of chlordecone (Kepone). *Toxicol. Appl. Pharmacol.*, **48**:533–536, 1979.

Eisler, R.: *Pentachlorophenol Hazards to Fish, Wildlife and Invertebrates: A Synoptic Review.* U.S. Department of the Interior, Fish and Wildlife Service. Biological Report 85 (1.17), April, 1989.

Eldefrawi, M. E. S.; Sherby, S. M.; Abalis, I. M.; and Eldefrawi, A. T.: Interactions of pyrethroid and cyclodiene insecticides with nicotinic acetylcholine and GABA receptors. *Neurotoxicology* **6**:47–62, 1985.

Ellenhorn, M. J., and Barceloux, D. G.: Pesticides. In *Medical Toxicology. Diagnosis and Treatment of Human Poisoning.* Elsevier, New York, 1988, pp. 1081–1108.

Elliott, M.: Future use of natural and synthetic pyrethroids. In Metcalf, R. L., and McKelvey, J. J., Jr. (eds.): *The Future for Insecticides: Needs and Prospects.* John Wiley & Sons, New York, 1976, pp. 163–193.

Elliott, M.; Janes, N. F.; Kimmel, E. C.; and Casida, J. E.: Metabolic fate of pyrethrin I, pyrethrin II and allethrin administered orally to rats. *J. Agric. Food Chem.*, **20**:300–313, 1972.

Englehard, H., and Erdmann, W. D.: Beziehangen zwischen chemischer struktur und cholinesterase reaktivierendes wirksamkeit bei einen reihe neuer bisquartarer pyridin-4-aldoxime. *Arznem. Forsch.*, **14**:870 – 875, 1964.

EPA: *Carbaryl Decision Document.* U.S. Environmental Protection Agency. Government Printing Office, Washington, D.C., 1980.

Eriksson, M.; Hardell, L.; Berg, N. O.; Moller, T.; and Axelson, O.: Soft-tissue sarcomas and exposure to chemical substances: a case-referent study. *Br. J. Indust. Med.*, **38**:27 – 33, 1981.

Eroschenko, V. P., and Wilson, W. O.: Cellular changes in the gonads, livers and adrenal glands of Japanese quail as affected by the insecticide Kepone. *Toxicol. Appl. Pharmacol.*, **31**:491 – 504, 1975.

Eto, M.: *Organophosphorus Pesticides: Organic and Biological Chemistry.* CRC Press, Cleveland, Ohio. 1974.

FAO/WHO: *The Monographs on Fenitrothion. Evaluations of Some Pesticide Residues in Food.* WHO Pesticide Residue Series No. 14, 1975, pp. 335 – 381.

Feldman, R. J., and Maiback, H. I.: Percutaneous penetration of some pesticides and herbicides in man. *Toxicol. Appl. Pharmacol.*, **28**:126 – 132, 1974.

Fest, C., and Schmidt, K.-J.: *The Chemistry of Organophosphorus Pesticides.* Springer-Verlag, New York, 1973.

Fiserova-Bergerova, V.; Radomski, J. L.; Davies, J. E.; and Davis, J. H.: Levels of chlorinated hydrocarbon pesticides in human tissues. *Indust. Med. Surg.,* **36**:65 – 70, 1967.

Forgct, G.: Pesticides: necessary but dangerous poisons. *IDRC Rep.*, **18**:4 – 5, 1989.

Frank, R.; Campbell, R. A.; and Sirons, G. J.: Forestry workers involved in aerial application of 2,4-dichlorophenoxyacetic acid (2,4-D): exposure and urinary excretion. *Arch. Environ. Contam. Toxicol.,* **14**:427 – 435, 1985.

Franklin, C. A.; Fenske, R. A.; Greenhalgh, R.; Mathieu, L.; Denley, H. V.; Leffingwell, J. T.; and Spear, R. C.: Correlation of urinary pesticide metabolite excretion with estimated dermal contact in the course of occupational exposure to guthion. *J. Toxicol. Environ. Health,* **7**:715 – 731, 1981.

Frawley, J. P.; Fuyat, H. N.; Hagan, E. C.; Blake, J. R.; and Fitzhugh, O. G.: Marked potentiation in mammalian toxicity from simultaneous administration of two anticholinesterase compounds. *J. Pharmacol. Exp. Ther.,* **121**:96 – 106, 1967.

Frear, D. E. H.: *Pesticide Index,* 4th ed. College Science Publishers, State College, Pennsylvania, 1969.

Fukuto, T. R.: Metabolism of carbamate insecticides. *Drug Metab. Rev.,* **1**:117 – 147, 1972.

Gaines, T. B.: Acute toxicity of pesticides. *Toxicol. Appl. Pharmacol.,* **14**:515 – 534, 1969.

Gammon, D. W.; Brown, M. A.; and Casida, J. E.: Two classes of pyrethroid action in the cockroach. *Pestic. Biochem. Physiol.,* **15**:181 – 191, 1981.

Gehring, P. J.; Watanabe, P. G.; and Blau, G. E.: Pharmacokinetic studies in evaluation of the toxicological and environmental hazard of chemicals. In Mehlman, M. A.; Shapiro, R. E.; and Blumenthal, H. (eds.): *New Concepts in Safety Evaluation.* John Wiley & Sons, New York, 1976, pp. 195 – 270.

Gershon, S., and Shaw, F. H.: Psychiatric sequelae of chronic exposure to organophosphorus insecticides. *Lancet* **i**:1371 – 1374, 1961.

Glickman, A. H., and Casida, J. E.: Species and structural variations affecting pyrethroid neurotoxicity. *Neurobehav. Toxicol. Teratol.,* **4**:793 – 799, 1982.

Gochfeld, M.: New light on the health of Vietnam veterans. *Environ. Res.,* **47**:109 – 111, 1988.

Goldstein, N. P.; Jones, P. H.; and Brown, J. R.: Peripheral neuropathy after exposure to an ester of dichlorophenoxyacetic acid. *JAMA,* **171**:1306 – 1309, 1959.

Goldstein, J. A.; Fridsen, M.; Linder, R. E.; Hickman, P.; Hass, J. R.; and Bergman, H.: Effects of pentachlorophenol on hepatic drug-metabolizing enzymes and porphyria related to contamination with chlorinated dibenzo-*p*-dioxins and dibenzofurans. *Biochem. Pharmacol.,* **26**:1549 – 1557, 1977.

Gough, M.: *Dioxin, Agent Orange. The Facts.* Plenum Press, New York, 1986.

Greenwald, W.; Kovasznay, B.; Collins, D. N.; and Therriault, G.: Sarcomas of soft tissues after Vietnam service. *J. Natl. Cancer Inst.,* **73**:1107 – 1109, 1984.

Grover, R.; Cessna, A. J.; Muir, N. I.; Riedel, D.; Franklin, C. A.; and Yoshida, K.: Factors affecting the exposure of ground-rig applicators to 2,4-dimethylamine salt. *Arch. Environ. Contam. Toxicol.,* **15**:677 – 686, 1986.

Guzelian, P. S.: Comparative toxicology of chlordecone (kepone) in humans and experimental animals. *Annu. Rev. Pharmacol. Toxicol.,* **22**:89 – 113, 1982.

Haley, T. J.: Review of the toxicology of paraquat (1,1'-dimethyl-4,4'-bipyridinium chloride). *Clin. Toxicol.,* **14**:1 – 46, 1979.

Hansell, M. M., and Ecobichon, D. J.: Effects of chemically pure chlorobiphenyls on the morphology of rat liver. *Toxicol. Appl. Pharmacol.,* **28**:418 – 427, 1974.

Hardell, L., and Sandstrom, A.: Case-control study: soft-tissue sarcomas and exposure to phenoxyacetic acids or chlorophenols. *Br. J. Cancer,* **39**:711 – 717, 1979.

Hardell, L.; Eriksson, M.; Lenner, P.; and Lundgren, E.: Malignant lymphoma and exposure to chemicals, especially organic solvents, chlorophenols and phenoxy acids: a case-control study. *Br. J. Cancer,* **43**:169 – 176, 1981.

Hartley, G. S., and West, T. F.: *Chemicals for Pest Control.* Pergamon Press, Oxford, 1969, p. 26.

Hay, A.: *The Chemical Scythe. Lessons of 2,4,5,-T and Dioxin.* Plenum Press, New York, 1982.

Hayes, W. J., Jr.: The pharmacology and toxicology of DDT. In Muller, P. (ed.): *The Insecticide DDT and Its Importance.* Birkhauser Verlag, Basel, Switzerland, 1959.

———: Insecticides, rodenticides and other economic poisons. In DiPalma, J. R. (ed.): *Drill's Pharmacology in Medicine,* 4th ed. McGraw-Hill, New York, 1971, pp. 1256 – 1276.

———: *Toxicology of Pesticides.* Williams & Wilkins, Baltimore, 1975.

———: *Pesticides Studied in Man.* Williams & Wilkins, Baltimore, 1982.

Hayes, W. J., Jr.; Dale, W. E.; and Pirkle, C. I.: Evidence of the safety of long-term, high, oral doses of DDT for man. *Arch. Environ. Health,* **22**:19 – 35, 1971.

Hayes, W. J., Jr., and Vaughn, W. K.: Mortality from pesticides in the United States in 1973 and 1974. *Toxicol. Appl. Pharmacol.,* **42**:235 – 252, 1977.

He, F.; Sun, J.; Han, K.; Wu, Y.; Wang, S., and Liu, L.: Effects of pyrethroid insecticides on subjects engaged in packaging pyrethroids. *Br. J. Indust. Med.* **45**:548 – 551, 1988.

He, F.; Wang, S.; Liu, L.; Chen, S.; Zhang, Z.; and Sun, J.: Clinical manifestations and diagnosis of acute pyrethroid poisoning. *Arch. Toxicol.,* **63**:54 – 58, 1989.

Heath, D. F.: *Organophosphorus Poisons. Anticholinesterases and Related Compounds.* Pergamon Press, London, 1961.

Hoar, S. K.; Blair, A.; Holmes, F. F.; Boysen, C. D.; Robel, R. J.; Hoover, R.; and Fraumeni, J. F., Jr.:

Agricultural herbicide use and risk of lymphoma and soft-tissue sarcoma. *JAMA,* **256**:1141–1147, 1986.

Hoffman, R. E.; Stehr-Green, P. A.; Webb, K. B.; Evans, G.; Knutsen, A. P.; Schramm, W. F.; Staake, J. L.; Gibson, B. B.; and Steinberg, K. K.: Health effects of long-term exposure to 2,3,7,8-tetrachlorodibenzo-*p*-dioxin. *JAMA,* **255**:2031–2038, 1986.

Holmstedt, B.: Pharmacology of organophosphorus cholinesterase inhibitors. *Pharmacol. Rev.,* **11**:567–688, 1959.

Huber, J.: Some physiologic effects of the insecticide Kepone in the laboratory mouse. *Toxicol. Appl. Pharmacol.,* **7**:516–524, 1965.

Hutson, D. H.; Akintonwa, D. A. A.; and Hathway, D. E.: The metabolism of 2,chloro-1-(2', 4', dichlorophenyl) vinyl diethylphosphate (chlorfenvinphos) in the dog and rat. *Biochem. J.,* **102**:133–142, 1967.

IARC: *Monograph on the Evaluation of Carcinogenic Risk of Chemicals to Man.* Vol. 5. *Some Organochlorine Pesticides.* International Agency for Research on Cancer, Lyon, France, 1974.

———: *Monographs on the Evaluation of Carcinogenic Risk of Chemicals to Man.* Vol. 12. *Some Carbamates, Thiocarbamates and Carbazines.* International Agency for Research on Cancer, Lyon, France, 1976.

———: *Monographs on the Evaluation of Carcinogenic Risk of Chemicals to Man.* Vol. 15. *Some Fumigants, the Herbicides 2,4-D and 2,4,5-T, Chlorinated Dibenzodioxins and Miscellaneous Industrial Chemicals.* International Agency for Research on Cancer, Lyon, France, 1977.

Innes, J. R. M.; Ulland, B. M.; Valerio, M. G.; Petrucelli, L.; Fishbein, L.; Hart, E. R.; Pallotta, A. J.; Bates, R. R.; Falk, H. L.; Gart, J. J.; Klein, M.; Mitchell, I.; and Peters, J.: Bioassay of pesticides and industrial chemicals for tumorigenicity in mice: a preliminary note. *J. Natl. Cancer Inst.,* **42**:1101–1114, 1969.

Jackson, R. J.; Stratton, J. W.; Goldman, L. R.; Smith, D. F.; Pond, E. M.; Epstein, D.; Neutra, R. R.; Kelter, A.; and Kizer, K. W.: Aldicarb food poisoning from contaminated melons—California. *Mortal. Morbid. Wkly. Rep.* **35**:254–258, 1986.

Jager, G.: Herbicides. In Buchel, K. H. (ed.): *Chemistry of Pesticides.* John Wiley & Sons, New York, 1983, pp. 322–392.

Jeyaratnam, J.; DeAlwis Seneviratne, R. S.; and Copplestone, J. F.: Survey of pesticide poisoning in Sri Lanka. *Bull. WHO* **60**:615–619, 1982.

Johnson, M. K. The target for initiation of delayed neurotoxicity by organophosphorus esters: biochemical studies and toxicological applications. In Hodgson, E.; Bend, J. R.; and Philpot, R. M. (eds.): *Reviews of Biochemical Toxicology.* Vol. 4. Elsevier, New York, 1982, pp. 141–212.

Johnson, R. L.; Gehring, P. J.; Kociba, R. J.; and Schwetz, B. A.: Chlorinated dibenzodioxins and pentachlorophenol. *Environ. Health Perspect.,* **5**:171–175, 1973.

Jones, E. C.; Growe, G. H.; and Naiman, S. C.: Prolonged anticoagulation in rat poisoning. *JAMA,* **252**:3005–3007, 1984.

Joy, R. M.: Chlorinated hydrocarbon insecticides. In Ecobichon, D. J., and Joy, R. M.: *Pesticides and Neurological Diseases.* CRC Press, Boca Raton, Florida, 1982, pp. 91–150.

Katona, B., and Wason, S.: Anticoagulant rodenticides. *Clin. Toxicol. Rev.,* **8**:1–2, 1986.

Keane, W. T., and Zavon, M. R.: The total body burden of dieldrin. *Bull. Environ. Contam. Toxicol.,* **4**:1–16, 1969.

Kewitz, H., and Wilson, I. B.: A specific antidote against lethal alkylphosphate intoxication. *Arch. Biochem. Biophys.* **60**:261–263, 1956.

Kilgore, W.: Human exposure to pesticides. In Newberne, P. M.; Shank, R. C.; and Ruchirawat, M. (eds.): *International Toxicology Seminar: Environmental Toxicology.* Chulabhorn Research Institute and Mahidol University, 1988.

Kilgore, W. W., and Akesson, N. B.: Minimizing occupational exposure to pesticides; populations at exposure risk. *Residue Rev.,* **75**:21–31, 1980.

Kimbrough, R. D.; Carter, C. D.; Liddle, J. A.; Cline, R. E.; and Philips, P. E.: Epidemiology and pathology of a tetrachlorodibenzodioxin poisoning episode. *Arch. Environ. Health,* **32**:77–86, 1977.

Kirby, C.: *The Hormone Weedkillers.* BCPC Publications, Croydon, U.K., 1980.

Kitselman, C. H.: Long-term studies on dogs fed aldrin and dieldrin in sublethal dosages with reference to the histopathological findings and reproduction. *J. Am. Vet. Med. Assoc.,* **123**:28–36, 1953.

Kociba, R. I.; Keyes, D. G.; and Beyer, J. E.: Results of a two year chronic toxicity and oncogenicity study of 2,3,7,8-tetrachlorodibenzo-*p*-dioxin in rats. *Toxicol. Appl. Pharmacol.,* **46**:279–303, 1978.

Koestner, A.: The brain-tumor issue in long-term toxicity studies in rats. *Food Chem. Toxicol.,* **24**:139–143, 1986.

Kolmodin-Hedman, B.; Hoglund, S.; and Akerblom, M.: Studies on phenoxy acid herbicides. I. Field Study. Occupational exposure to phenoxy acid herbicides (MCPA, dichlorprop, mecoprop and 2,4-D) in agriculture. *Arch. Toxicol.,* **54**:257–275, 1983.

Koos, B. J., and Longo, L. D.: Mercury toxicity in the pregnant woman, fetus and newborn infant. *Am. J. Obstet. Gynecol.,* **126**:390–409, 1976.

Kramer, W.: Fungicides and bacteriocides. In Buchel, K. H. (ed.): *Chemistry of Pesticides.* John Wiley & Sons, New York, 1983, pp. 227–321.

Kuhr, R. J., and Dorough, H. W.: *Carbamate Insecticides: Chemistry, Biochemistry and Toxicology.* CRC Press, Boca Raton, Florida, 1976.

Kulkarni, A. P., and Hodgson, E.: The metabolism of insecticides: the role of monooxygenase enzymes. *Annu. Rev. Pharmacol.,* **24**:19–42, 1984.

Kupfer, D., and Bulger, W. H.: Studies on the mechanism of estrogenic actions of *o,p*-DDT: interactions with the estrogen receptor. *Pestic. Biochem. Physiol.,* **6**:461–470, 1976.

Laben, R. C.; Archer, T. E.; Crosby, D. G.; and Peoples, S. A.: Lactational output of DDT fed postpartum to dairy cattle. *J. Dairy Sci.,* **48**:701–708, 1965.

Lambert, G., and Brodeur, J.: Influence de certains inducteurs ou de certaines combinaisons d'inducteurs enzymatiques sur l'elimination des residus du DDT chez le rat. *Rev. Can. Biol.* **35**:33–39, 1976.

Lambrecht, R. W.; Erturk, E.; Grunden, E.; Headley, D. B.; Morris, C. R.; Peters, H. A.; and Bryan, G. T.: Hepatotoxicity and tumorigenicity of hexachlorobenzene (HCB) in Syrian golden hamsters after subchronic administration. *Fed. Proc.* **41**:329, 1982.

Lange, P. F., and Terveer, J.: Warfarin poisoning. *U.S. Armed Forces J.,* **5**:872–877, 1954.

Larson, P. S.; Egle, J. L., Jr.; Hennigar, G. R.; Lane, R. W.; and Borzelleca, J. F.: Acute, subacute and chronic toxicity of chlordecone. *Toxicol. Appl. Pharmacol.,* **48**:29–41, 1979.

Lawrence, L. J., and Casida, J. E.: Pyrethroid toxicology: mouse intracerebral structure-toxicity relationships. *Pestic. Biochem. Physiol.,* **18**:9–14, 1982.

Leahey, J. P.: *The Pyrethroid Insecticides.* Taylor and Francis, London, 1985.

Leake, L. D.; Buckley, D. S.; Ford, M. G.; and Salt, D.

W.: Comparative effects of pyrethroids on neurones of target and non-target organisms. *Neurotoxicology,* **6**:99–116, 1985.

LeQuesne, P. M.; Maxwell, I. C.; and Butterworth, S. T.: Transient facial sensory symptoms following exposure to synthetic pyrethroids: a clinical and electrophysiological assessment. *Neurotoxicology,* **2**:1–11, 1980.

LeWitt, P. A.: The neurotoxicity of the rat poison Vacor. A clinical study of 12 cases. *N. Engl. J. Med.,* **302**:73–77, 1980.

Liddle, J. A.; Kimbrough, R. D.; Needham, L. L.; Cline, R. E.; Smrek, A. L.; Yert, L. W.; Bayse, D. D.; Ellington, A. C.; and Dennis, P. A.: A fatal episode of accidental methomyl poisoning. *Clin. Toxicol.,* **15**:159–167, 1979.

Lipton, R. A., and Klass, E. M.: Human ingestion of a "superwarfarin" rodenticide resulting in prolonged anticoagulant effect. *JAMA,* **252**:3004–3005, 1984.

Longcore, J. R.; Samson, F. B.; and Whittendale, T. W., Jr.: DDE thins eggshells and lowers reproductive success of captive black ducks. *Bull. Environ. Contam. Toxicol.,* **6**:485–490, 1971.

Lu, M.-H., and Kennedy, G. L., Jr.: Teratogenic evaluation of mancozeb in the rat following inhalation exposure. *Toxicol. Appl. Pharmacol.,* **84**:355–368, 1986.

Lukens, R. J.: *Chemistry of Fungicidal Action.* Springer-Verlag, New York, 1971.

Lynge, E.: A follow-up study of cancer incidence among workers in manufacture of phenoxy herbicides in Denmark. *Br. J. Cancer,* **52**:259–270, 1985.

Marquis, J. K.: *Contemporary Issues in Pesticide Toxicology and Pharmacology.* S. Karger A. G., Basel, Switzerland, 1982, pp. 87–95.

Martinez, A. J.; Taylor, J. R.; Houff, S. A.; and Isaacs, E. R.: Kepone poisoning: cliniconeuropathological study. In Roizin, L., Shiraki, H., and Greevic, N. (eds.): *Neurotoxicology.* Raven Press, New York, 1977, pp. 443–456.

Matsumoto, H.; Koya, G.; and Takeuchi, T.: Fetal Minamata disease. A study of two cases of intrauterine intoxication by a methyl mercury compound. *J. Neuropathol. Exp. Neurol.,* **24**:563–574, 1965.

Matsumura, F.: *Toxicology of Insecticides.* Plenum Press, New York, 1985.

Matthews, H. B., and Matsumura, F.: Metabolic fate of dieldrin in the rat. *J. Agric. Food Chem.,* **17**:845–852, 1969.

McBlain, W. A.; Lewin, V.; and Wolfe, F. H.: Estrogenic effects of the enantiomers of *o,p'*-DDT in Japanese quail. *Can. J. Zool.,* **55**:562–568, 1977.

McCord, C. P.; Kilker, C. H.; and Minster, D. K.: Pyrethrum dermatitis: a record of the occurrence of occupational dermatoses among workers in the pyrethrum industry. *JAMA,* **77**:448–449, 1921.

McEwen, F. L., and Stephenson, G. R.: *The Use and Significance of Pesticides in the Environment.* John Wiley & Sons, New York, 1979, pp. 91–154.

McFarland, L. Z., and Lacy, P. B.: Physiologic and endocrinologic effects of the insecticide kepone in the Japanese quail. *Toxicol. Appl. Pharmacol.,* **15**:441–450, 1969.

Melnikov, N. N.: Chemistry of pesticides. *Residue Rev.* **36**:1–480, 1971.

Menzie, C. M.: *Metabolism of Pesticides.* Bureau of Sport Fisheries and Wildlife. Special Scientific Report. Wildlife No. 127, Washington, D.C., 1969.

Mes, J.; Davies, D. J.; and Turton, D.: Polychlorinated biphenyl and other chlorinated hydrocarbon residues in adipose tissue of Canadians. *Bull. Environ. Contam. Toxicol.,* **28**:97–104, 1982.

Metcalfe, R. L.: Development of selective and biodegradable pesticides. In *Pest Control Strategies for the Future.* Agriculture Board, Division of Biology and Agriculture, National Research Council, National Academy of Science, Washington, D.C., 1972, pp. 137–156.

———: A century of DDT. *J. Agric. Food Chem.,* **21**:511–519, 1973.

Moore, J. A.; McConnell, E. E.; Dalgard, D. W.; and Harris, M. W.: Comparative toxicity of three halogenated dibenzofurans in guinea pigs, mice and rhesus monkeys. *Ann. NY Acad. Sci.,* **320**:151–163, 1979.

Morgan, D. P.: *Recognition and Management of Pesticide Poisonings.* 3rd ed. Publication EPA-540/9-80-005, U.S. Environmental Protection Agency, 1982.

Morgan, D. P., and Roan, C. C.: Chlorinated hydrocarbon pesticide residue in human tissues. *Arch. Environ. Health,* **20**:452–457, 1970.

Morgan, J. P., and Penovich, P.: Jamaica ginger paralysis. Forty-seven year follow-up. *Arch. Neurol.,* **35**:530–532, 1978.

Mullison, W. R.: An Interim Report Summarizing 2,4-D Toxicological Research Sponsored by the Industry Task Force on 2,4-D Research Data and a Brief Review of 2,4-D Environmental Effects. Technical and Toxicology Committees of the Industry Task Force on 2,4-D Research Data, 1986.

Murphy, S. D.: Mechanisms of pesticide interactions in vertebrates. *Residue Rev.,* **25**:201–221, 1969.

———: The toxicity of pesticides and their metabolites. In *Degradation of Synthetic Organic Molecules in the Biosphere.* Proceedings of a Conference. National Academy of Sciences, Washington, D.C., 1972, pp. 313–335.

———: Toxic interactions with dermal exposure to organophosphate insecticides. In Holmstedt, B.; Lauwerys, R.; Mercier M.; and Roberfroid, M. (eds.): *Mechanisms of Toxicity and Hazard Evaluation.* Elsevier/North Holland Biomedical Press, Amsterdam, 1980, pp. 615–621.

Murray, R. E., and Gibson, J. E.: Paraquat disposition in rats, guinea pigs and monkeys. *Toxicol. Appl. Pharmacol.,* **27**:283–291, 1974.

Namba, T., and Hiraki, K.: PAM (pyridine-2-aldoxime methiodide therapy for alkylphosphate poisoning. *JAMA,* **166**:1834–1839, 1958.

Namba, T.; Nolte, C. T.; Jackrel, J.; and Grob, D.: Poisoning due to organophosphate insecticides. *Am. J. Med.,* **50**:475–492, 1971.

Narahashi, T.: Mode of action of pyrethroids. *Bull. WHO,* **44**:337–345, 1971.

———: Effect of insecticides on nervous conduction and synaptic transmission. In Wilkinson, C. F. (ed.): *Insecticide Biochemistry and Physiology.* Plenum Press, New York, 1976, pp. 327–352.

———: Nerve membrane ionic channels as the primary target of pyrethroids. *Neurotoxicology,* **2**:3–22, 1985.

Narahashi, T.; Cranmer, J. M.; and Wooley, D. E. (eds.): Pyrethroids and neuroactive pesticides. *Proceedings of the Third International Conference on Neurotoxicology of Selected Chemicals,* Sept. 9–12, 1984. *Neurotoxicology* **6**: 1985.

Narita, S.; Motojuku, H.; Sato, J.; and Mori, H.: Autopsy in acute suicidal poisoning with diquat dibromide. *Jpn. J. Rural Med.,* **27**: 454–455, 1978.

National Academy of Science: Regulating Pesticides in Food. *The Delaney Paradox. Report of Committee on Scientific and Regulatory Issues Underlying Pesticide Use Patterns and Agricultural Innovation.* National Academy Press, Washington, D. C., 1987.

Neuman, R., and Peter, H. N.: Insecticidal organophosphates: nature made them first. *Experientia* **43**:1235–1237, 1987.

Nielsen, K.; Kaempe, B.; and Jensen-Holm, J.: Fatal poisoning in man by 2,4-dichlorophenoxyacetic acid

(2,4-D). Determination of the agent in forensic materials. *Acta Pharmacol. Toxicol.* **22**:224–234, 1965.

O'Brien, R. D.: *Toxic Phosphorus Esters. Chemistry, Metabolism and Biological Effects.* Academic Press, New York, 1960.

———: *Insecticides, Action and Metabolism.* Academic Press, New York, 1967.

Ohkawa, N.; Oshita, H.; and Miyamoto, J.: Comparison of inhibitory activity of various organophosphorus compounds against acetylcholinesterase and neurotoxic esterase of hens with respect to delayed neurotoxicity. *Biochem. Pharmacol.,* **29**:2721–2727, 1980.

Ott, M. G.; Holder, B. B.; and Olson, R. D.: A mortality analysis of employees engaged in the manufacture of 2,4,5-trichlorophenoxyacetic acid. *J. Occup. Med.,* **22**:47–50, 1980.

Peakall, D. B.: Pesticides and the reproduction of birds. *Sci. Am.,* **222**:72–78, 1970.

Pearce, N. E.; Smith, A. H.; Howard, J. K.; Sheppard, R. A.; Giles, H. J.; and Teague, C. A.: Non-Hodgkin's lymphoma and exposure to phenoxyherbicides, chlorophenols, fencing work and meat works employment: a case-control study. *Br. J. Indust. Med.,* **43**:75–83, 1986.

Peardon, D. L.: RH-787, a new selective rodenticide. *Pest Control,* **42**:14–27, 1974.

Peters, H. A.; Johnson, S. A. M.; Cam, S.; Oral, S.; Muftu, Y.; and Ergene, T.: Hexachlorobenzene induced porphyria: effect of chelation on the disease, porphyrin and metal metabolism. *Am. J. Med. Sci.,* **251**:314–322, 1966.

Petrova-Vergieva, T., and Ivanova-Chemishanska, L.: Assessment of the teratogenic activity of dithiocarbamate fungicides. *Food Cosmet. Toxicol.,* **11**:239–244, 1973.

Pickering, Q. H.: Henderson, C.; and Lemke, A. E.: The toxicity of organic phosphorus insecticides to different species of warmwater fishes. *Trans. Am. Fish. Soc.,* **91**:175–184, 1962.

Poland, A. P.; Smith, D.; Metter, G.; and Possick, P.: A health survey of workers in a 2,4-D and 2,4,5-T plant with special attention to chloracne, porphyria cutanea tarda and psychologic parameters. *Arch. Environ. Health,* **22**:316–327, 1971.

Quinby, G. E.; Hayes, W. J., Jr.; Armstrong, J. F.; and Durham, W. F.: DDT storage in the U.S. population. *JAMA,* **191**:175–179, 1965.

Rashatwar, S. S., and Matsumura, F.: Interaction of DDT and pyrethroids with calmodulin and its significance in the expression of enzyme activities of phosphodiesterase. *Biochem. Pharmacol.,* **34**:1689–1694, 1985.

Reich, G. A.; Davis, J. H.; and Davies, J. E.: Pesticide poisoning in South Florida: an analysis of mortality and morbidity and a comparison of sources of incidence data. *Arch. Environ. Health,* **17**:768–775, 1968.

Rhodes, M. L.: Hypoxic protection in paraquat poisoning. A model for respiratory distress syndrome. *Chest,* **66**:341–342, 1974.

Richter, C. P.: Biological factors involved in poisoning rats with alpha-naphthylthiourea (ANTU). *Proc. Soc. Exp. Biol. Med.,* **63**:364–372, 1946.

Rose, M. S.; Lock, E. A.; Smith, L. L. and Wyatt, I.: Paraquat accumulation: tissue and species specificity. *Biochem. Pharmacol.* **25**:419–423, 1976.

Rose, M. S.; Lock, E. A.; Smith, L. L.; and Wyatt, I.: Paraquat accumulation: tissue and species specificity. *Biochem. Pharmacol.,* **25**:429–423, 1976.

Rose, M. S., and Smith, L. L.: Tissue uptake of paraquat and diquat. *Gen. Pharmacol.,* **8**:173–176, 1977.

Ruzo, L. O.; Engel, J. L.; and Casida, J. E.: Decamethrin metabolites from oxidative, hydrolytic and conjugative reactions in mice. *J. Agric. Food Chem.,* **27**:725–731, 1979.

Ryan, A. J.: The metabolism of pesticidal carbamates. *CRC Crit. Rev. Toxicol.,* **1**:33–54, 1974.

Saleh, M. A.; Turner, W. A.; and Casida, J. E.: Polychlorobornane components of toxaphene: structuretoxicity relations and metabolic reductive dechlorination. *Science,* **198**:1256–1258, 1977.

Santalucito, J. A., and Morrison, G.: EEG of Rhesus monkeys following prolonged low-level feeding of pesticides. *Toxicol. Appl. Pharmacol.,* **19**:147–154, 1971.

Sawada, V.; Nagai, Y.; Ueyama, M.; and Yamamoto, I.: Probable toxicity of surface-active agent in commercial herbicide containing glyphosate. *Lancet,* **i**:299, 1988.

Schmid, R.: Cutaneous porphyria in Turkey. *N. Engl. J. Med.,* **263**:397–398, 1960.

Schoene, K.: Reaktivierung von *O,O*-diethylphosphorylacetylcholinesterase. Reaktivierungs-re-phosphorylierungs gleichgewicht. *Biochem. Pharmacol.,* **21**: 163–170, 1972.

Schonborn, H.; Schuster, H. P.; and Koessling, F. K.: Klinik und morphologie der akuten peroralen diquatintoxikation (re-lone). *Arch. Toxicol.,* **27**:204–216, 1971.

Schrader, G., and Kukenthal, H.: Farbenfabriken Bayer AG: DBP 767153 and 767723, 1937.

Schulz, K. N.: Clinical picture and etiology of chloracne. *Arb. Med. Sozialmed. Areitshyg.,* **3**:25–29, 1968.

Schumacher, M. C.: Farming occupations and mortality from non-Hodgkin's lymphoma in Utah. *J. Occup. Med.,* **27**:580–584, 1985.

Schwetz, B. A.; Norris, J. M.; Sparschu, G. L.; Rowe, V. K.; Gehring, P. J.; Emerson, J. L.; and Gerbig, C. G.: Toxicology of chlorinated dioxins. *Adv. Chem.* **120**:55–69, 1973.

Schwetz, B. A.; Quast, J. F.; and Keeler, P. A.: Results of two-year toxicity and reproduction studies on pentachlorophenol in rats. In Rao, K. R. (ed.): *Pentachlorophenol.* Plenum Press, New York, 1977, pp. 301–315.

Seabury, J. H.: Toxicity of 2,4-dichlorophenoxyacetic acid for man and dog. *Arch. Environ. Health,* **7**:202–209, 1963.

Senanayake, N., and Karalliedde, L.: Neurotoxic effects of organophosphorus insecticides. *N. Engl. J. Med.* **316**:761–763, 1987.

Sharp, C. W. M.; Ottolenghi, A.; and Posner, H. S.: Correlation of paraquat toxicity with tissue concentrations and weight loss of the rat. *Toxicol. Appl. Pharmacol.,* **22**:241–251, 1972.

Shimkin, M. B., and Anderson, N. N.: Acute toxicities of rotenone and mixed pyrethrins in mammals. *Proc. Soc. Exp. Biol. Med.* **34**:135–138, 1936.

Shono, T.; Ohsawa, K.; and Casida, J. E.: Metabolism of *trans*- and *cis*-permethrin, *trans*- and *cis*-cypermethrin and decamethrin by microsomal enzymes. *J. Agric. Food Chem.,* **27**:316–325, 1979.

Singer, R.; Moses, M.; Valciukas, J.; Lilis, R.; and Selikoff, I. J.: Nerve conduction velocity studies of workers employed in the manufacture of phenoxy herbicides. *Environ. Res.,* **29**:297–311, 1982.

Slott, V., and Ecobichon, D. J.: An acute and subacute neurotoxicity assessment of trichlorfon. *Can. J. Physiol. Pharmacol.,* **62**:513–518, 1984.

Smalley, H. E.; O'Hara, P. J.; Bridges, C. H.; and Radeleff, R. D.: The effects of chronic carboryl administration on the neuromuscular system of swine. *Toxicol. Appl. Pharmacol.,* **14**:409–419, 1969.

Smith, L. L.: The mechanisms of paraquat toxicity in the lung. *Rev. Biochem. Toxicol.,* **8**:37–71, 1987.

Smith, M. I., and Lillie, R. D.: The histopathology of triorthocresyl phosphate poisoning. The etiology of so-called ginger paralysis (third report). *Arch. Neurol. Psychiatry,* **26**:976–992, 1931.

Smith, P., and Heath, D.: Paraquat. *Crit. Rev. Toxicol.* **4**:411–445, 1976.

Solleveld, H. A.; Haseman, J. K.; and McConnell, E. E.: Natural history of body weight gain, survival and neoplasia in the F344 rat. *J. Natl. Can. Inst.* **72**:929–940, 1984.

Spear, R. C.; Popendorf, W. J.; Leffingwell, J. T.; Milby, T. H.; Davies, J. E.; and Spencer, W. F.: Field workers' response to weathered residues of parathion. *J. Occup. Med.* **19**:406–410, 1977.

Spiegelberg, U.: Psychopathologisch-neurologische spat und dauerschaden nach gewerblicher intoxikation durch phosphorsaureester (alkylphosphate). In *Proc. 14th Int. Cong. Occup. Health. Excerpta Med. Found. Int. Congr. Ser. No. 62,* pp. 1778–1780, 1963.

Sprague, G. L., and Bickford, A. A.: Effect of multiple diisopropylfluorophosphate injections in hens: behavioral, biochemical and histological investigation. *J. Toxicol. Environ. Health,* **8**:973–988, 1981.

Steinberg, G. M.: Cranmer, J.; and Ash, A. B.: New reactivators of phosphonylated acetylcholinesterase. *Biochem. Pharmacol.,* **26**:439–441, 1977.

Stellman, S. D.; Stellman, J. M.; and Sommer, J. F.: Health and reproductive outcomes among American legionnaires in relation to combat and herbicide exposure in Vietnam. *Environ. Res.,* **47**:150–174, 1988.

Sterri, S. H.; Rognerud, B.; Fiskum, S. E.; and Lyngaas, S.: Effect of toxogonin and P2S on the toxicity of carbamates and organophosphorus compounds. *Acta Pharmacol. Toxicol.,* **45**:9–15, 1979.

Stickel, L. F.: Organochlorine Pesticides in the Environment. United States Department of the Interior, Fish and Wildlife Service. Special Scientific Report—Wildlife No. 119. Washington, D. C., 1968.

Stuart-Harle, M.: "Safe" pesticides found toxic. *Biotechnology,* **3**:16, 1988.

Suskind, R. R., and Hertzberg, V. S.: Human health effects of 2,4,5-T and its toxic contaminants. *JAMA,* **251**:2372–2380, 1984.

Taylor, J. R.; Selhorst, J. B.; Houff, S. A.; and Martinez, A. J.: Chlordecone intoxication in man. I. Clinical observations. *Neurology,* **28**:626–630, 1978.

Thiess, A. M.; Frentzel-Beyme, R.; and Link, R.: Mortality study of persons exposed to dioxin in a trichlorophenol process accident that occurred in the BASF AG on November 17, 1953. *Am. J. Indust. Med.,* **3**:179–189, 1982.

Toia, R. F., and Casida, J. E.: Phosphorylation, "aging" and possible alkylation reactions of saligenin cyclic phosphorus esters with α-chymotrypsin. *Biochem. Pharmacol.,* **28**:211–216, 1979.

Tschirley, F. H.: Dioxin. *Sci. Am.,* **254**:29–35, 1986.

Tsubaki, T.; Hirota, K.; Shirakawa, K.; Kondo, K.; and Sato, T.: Clinical, epidemiological and toxicological studies of methylmercury poisoning. In Plaa, G. L., and Duncan, W. A. M. (eds.): *Proceedings of the First International Congress of Toxicology. Toxicology as a Predictive Science.* Academic Press, New York, 1978, pp. 339–357.

Tucker, R. E.; Young, A. L.; and Gray, A. P. (eds.): *Human and Environmental Risks of Chlorinated Dioxins and Related Compounds.* Plenum Press, New York, 1983.

Tucker, R. K., and Crabtree, D. G.: *Handbook of Toxicity of Pesticides to Wildlife.* United States Department of Interior, Fish and Wildlife Service. Resource Publication No. 84. United States Printing Office, Washington, D.C., 1970.

Tucker, S. B., and Flannigan, S. A.: Cutaneous effects from occupational exposure to fenvalerate. *Arch. Toxicol.,* **54**:195–202, 1983.

Turnbull, G. J.; Sanderson, D. M.; and Crome, S. J.: Exposure to pesticides during application. In Turnbull, G. J. (ed.): *Occupational Hazards of Pesticide Use.* Taylor and Francis, London, 1985, pp. 35–49.

Turner, W. A.; Engel, J. L.; and Casida, J. E.: Toxaphene components and related compounds: Preparation and toxicity of some hepta-, octa- and nonachlorobornanes, hexa- and heptachlorobornenes and a hexachlorobornadiene. *J. Agric. Food Chem.,* **25**:1394–1401, 1977.

Treon, J. F., and Cleveland, F. P.: Toxicity of certain chlorinated hydrocarbon insecticides for laboratory animals with special reference to aldrin and dieldrin. *J. Agric. Food Chem.,* **3**:402–408, 1955.

Vandekar, M.; Heyadat, S.; Plestina, R.; and Ahmady, G.: A study of the safety of *o*-isopropoxyphenylmethylcarbamate in an operational field-trial in Iran. *Bull. WHO,* **38**:609–623, 1968.

Van den Bercken, J., and Vijverberg, H. P. M.: Interaction of pyrethroids and DDT-like compounds with the sodium channels in the nerve membrane. In Miyamoto, J., and Kearney, P. C. (eds.): *Pesticide Chemistry. Human Welfare and the Environment.* Vol. 3. *Mode of Action, Metabolism and Toxicology.* Pergamon Press, Oxford, 1983, pp. 115–121.

Van Miller, J. P.; Lalich, J. J.; and Allen, J. R.: Increased incidence of neoplasm in rats exposed to low levels of 2,3,7,8-tetrachlorodibenzo-*p*-dioxin. *Chemosphere,* **6**:537–544, 1977.

Verschloyle, R. D., and Aldridge, W. N.: Structure-activity relationships of some pyrethroids in rats. *Arch. Toxicol.,* **45**:325–329, 1980.

Vijverberg, H. P. M., and Van den Bercken, J.: Structure related effects of pyrethroid insecticides on the lateral line sense organ and on peripheral nerves of the clawed frog, *Xenopus laerus. Pestic. Biochem. Physiol.,* **18**:315–324, 1982.

Vos, J. G.; Krajnc, E. I.; Beekhof, P. K.; and van Looten, M. J.: Methods for testing immune effects of toxic chemicals: evaluation of the immunotoxicity of various pesticides in the rat. In Miyamoto, J., and Kearney, P. C. (eds.): *Pesticide Chemistry. Human Welfare and the Environment.* Vol. 3. *Mode of Action, Metabolism and Toxicology.* Pergamon Press, Oxford, 1983, pp. 497–504.

Wafford, K. A.: Sattelle, D. B.; Gant, D. B.; Eldefrawi, A. T.; and Eldefrawi, M. E.: Non competitive inhibition of GABA receptors in insect and vertebrate CNS by endrin and lindane. *Pestic. Biochem. Physiol.,* **33**:213–219, 1989.

Walsh, J.: River blindness: a gamble pays off. *Science,* **232**:922–925, 1986.

Walsh, R. J.: Chairman, Case-Control Study of Congenital Anomalies and Vietnam Service (Birth Defects Study). Report to the Minister for Veterans' Affairs. Jan. 1983. Australian Government Publishing Service, Canberra, 1983.

Waters, E. M.; Huff, J. E.; and Gerstner, H. B.: Mirex. An overview. *Environ. Res.,* **14**:212–222, 1977.

Wecker, L.; Kiauta, T.; and Dettbarn, W.-D.: Relationship between acetylcholinesterase inhibition and the development of a myopathy. *J. Pharmacol. Exp. Ther.,* **206**:97–104, 1978.

Whelan, E.: *Toxic Terror.* Jameson Books, Ottawa, Illinois, 1985.

Wigle, D. T.; *et al.*: Mortality study of Canadian male farm operators: non-Hodgkin's lymphoma mortality and agricultural practices in Saskatchewan. *J. Nat. Cancer Inst.* **82**:575–582. 1990.

Wiklund, K.; Lindefors, B.-M.; and Holm, L.-E.: Risk of malignant lymphoma in Swedish agricultural and forestry workers. *Br. J. Indust. Med.*, **45**:19–24, 1988.

Wilson, R.; Lovejoy, F. H.; Jaeger, R. J.; and Landrigan, P. L.: Acute phosphine poisoning aboard a grain freighter. *JAMA* **244**:148–150, 1980.

Wojeck, G. A.; Nigg, H. N.: Stamper, J. H.; and Bradway, D. E.: Worker exposure to ethion in Florida citrus. *Arch. Environ. Contam. Toxicol.*, **10**:725–735, 1981.

Wolfe, H. R.; Durham, W. F.; and Armstrong, J. F.: Exposure of workers to pesticides. *Arch. Environ. Health*, **14**:622–633, 1967.

Wolfe, H. R.; Armstrong, J. F.; Staiff, D. C.; and Comer, S. W.: Exposure of spraymen to pesticides. *Arch. Environ. Health*, **25**:29–31, 1972.

Woods, J.; Polissar, L.; Severson, R.; and Heuser, L.: Phenoxy herbicides and chlorophenols as risk factors for soft tissue sarcoma and non-Hodgkin's lymphoma. *Am. J. Epidemiol.*, **124**:529, 1980.

World Health Organization: *WHO Technical Report Series 513* (Safe use of pesticides: twentieth report of the WHO Expert Committee on Insecticides). WHO, Geneva, Switzerland, 1973, pp. 43–44.

Worthing, C. R. (ed.): *The Pesticide Manual. A World Compendium. British Crop Protection Council.* Lavenham Press, Lavenham, U.K., 1987.

Wray, J. E.; Muftu, Y.; and Dogramaci, I.: Hexachlorobenzene as a cause of porphyria turcica. *Turk. J. Pediatr.*, **4**:132–137, 1962.

Xintaris, C.; Burg, J. R.; Tanaka, S.; Lee, S. T.; Johnson, B. L.; Cottrill, C. A.; and Bender, J.: *Occupational Exposure to Leptophos and Other Chemicals.* DHEW (NIOSH) Publication No. 78-136. U.S. Government Printing Office, Washington, D.C., 1978.

Yang, R. S. H.: Enzymatic conjugation and insecticide metabolism. In Wilkinson, C. F. (ed.): *Insecticide Biochemistry and Physiology.* Plenum Press, New York, 1976, pp. 177–225.

Zepp, E. A.; Thomas, J. A.; and Knotts, G. R.: The toxic effects of mercury. A survey of the newer clinical insights. *Clin. Pediatr.*, **13**:783–787, 1974.

Chapter 19

TOXIC EFFECTS OF METALS

Robert A. Goyer

INTRODUCTION

Metals differ from other toxic substances in that they are neither created nor destroyed by humans. Nevertheless, utilization by humans influences the potential for health effects in at least two major ways: first, by environmental transport, that is, by human or anthropogenic contributions to air, water, soil, and food, and second, by altering the speciation or biochemical form of the element (Li, 1981; Beijer and Jernelöv, 1986).

Metals are redistributed naturally in the environment by both geologic and biologic cycles (Figure 19–1). Rainwater dissolves rocks and ores and physically transports material to streams and rivers, adding and deleting from adjacent soil, and eventually to the ocean to be precipitated as sediment or taken up in rainwater to be relocated elsewhere on earth. The biologic cycles include bioconcentration by plants and animals and incorporation into food cycles. These natural cycles may exceed the anthropogenic cycle, as is the case for mercury. Human industrial activity, however, may greatly shorten the residence time of metals in ore, form new compounds, and greatly enhance worldwide distribution. The role of human activity in redistribution of metal is demonstrated by the 200-fold increase in lead content of Greenland ice beginning with a "natural" low level (about 800 B.C.) and a gradual rise in lead content of ice through the evolution of the industrial age, followed by a nearly precipitous rise in lead corresponding to the period when lead was added to gasoline in the 1920s (Ng and Patterson, 1981). Metal contamination of the environment, therefore, reflects both natural sources and contribution from industrial activity.

Metals emitted into the environment from combustion of fossil fuels in the United States are shown in Table 19–1. These include many of the metals most abundant in particulates in ambient air. The only metals or metal-like elements that may be emitted in gaseous discharges

in measurable concentrations are mercury or selenium. Metals in raw surface water reflect erosion from natural sources, fallout from the atmosphere, and additions from industrial activities. Lowering pH as occurs with acid precipitation or the acid rain phenomenon may enhance solubilization and mobilization and perhaps change chemical species for many metals (Goyer, 1985). Metals in soil and water may enter the food chain. For persons in the general population, food sources probably represent the largest source of exposure to metals, with an additional contribution from air. Further potential sources of human exposure include consumer products and industrial wastes as well as the working environment.

Occupational exposure to metals is restricted to "safe" levels, defined as the threshold limit value for an eight-hour day, five-day workweek. These levels are intended to provide a margin of safety between maximum exposure and minimum levels that will produce illness. Permissible levels vary widely, and the differences reflect, in a sense, the toxicologic potency of the metal. As a general rule, the metals that are most abundant in the environment have lesser potential for toxicity as evidenced by the prevailing standard for permissible occupational exposure.

Metals are probably the oldest toxins known to humans. Lead usage may have begun prior to 2000 B.C. when abundant supplies were obtained from ores as a by-product of smelting silver. Hippocrates is credited in 370 B.C. with the first description of abdominal colic in a man who extracted metals. Arsenic and mercury are cited by Theophrastus of Erebus (387–372 B.C.) and Pliny the Elder (A.D. 23–79). Arsenic was obtained during the melting of copper and tin, and an early use was for decoration in Egyptian tombs. On the other hand, many of the metals of toxicologic concern today are only recently known to humans. Cadmium was first recognized in ores containing zinc carbonate in 1817. About 80 of the 105 elements in the periodic table are regarded as metals, but less than 30

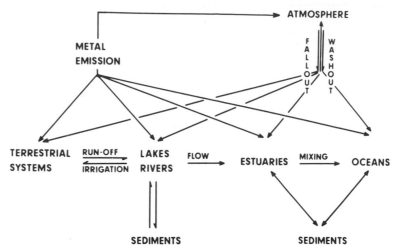

Figure 19–1. Routes for transport of trace elements in the environment. (From Beijer, K., and Jernelöv, A.: Sources, transport and transformation of metals in the environment. In Friberg, L.; Nordberg, G. F.; and Vouk, V. B. [eds.]: *Handbook on the Toxicology of Metals,* Vol. 1, 2nd ed., *General Aspects.* Elsevier Scientific Publ., Amsterdam, 1986, pp. 68–74.

Table 19–1. **TOXICOLOGICALLY IMPORTANT METALS MOBILIZED BY COMBUSTION OF FOSSIL FUEL IN THE UNITED STATES (COLUMN A), CONCENTRATIONS IN PARTICULATES IN AMBIENT AIR (COLUMN B) AND IN RAW SURFACE WATER (COLUMN C), AND BEST (WORLDWIDE) PREVAILING STANDARDS FOR THRESHOLD LIMIT VALUES (TLV) FOR EIGHT-HOUR OCCUPATIONAL EXPOSURE (COLUMN D)**

	A: FROM FOSSIL FUELS U.S.* (10^3 tons)	B: IN PARTICULATES IN AIR[†] TYPICAL (ng/m³)	C: IN WATER, μg/liter AND FREQUENCY OF DETECTION[‡] *maximum*			D: *TLV*[¶] (mg/m³)
			maximum	*mean*	%	
Al	6000	3080	2760	74	31	10
As	27	10	§			0.2
Ba	300	100	340	43	99	0.5
Be	15	0.2	1.22	0.19	5.4	0.002
Cd	1	1	120	10	2.5	0.05
Co	15	5	48	17	2.8	0.05
Cr	0	20	112	10	25	0.05 CrVI
Cu	9	500	280	15	75	0.2 fume
Fe	6002	4000	4600	52	76	3.5
Li	39	4				0.025
Mg	1200	2000				10.0
Mn	33	100	3230	60	58	5.0 dust
Mo	5	1	1500	68	38	10
Ni	11	20	30	19	16	0.1 sol.
Pb	126	2000	140	13	19	0.15
Sn		50				2.0 inorg.
Se	2	1				0.2
V	27	30	300	2	5	0.1 fume
Zn	30	500	2010	79.2	80	5.0

* From Vouk and Piver, 1983, data from 1977 fuel consumption.
† From Thompson, 1979, ten-day period, six U.S. cities.
‡ From NAS, 1977.
§ Arsenic in water is extremely variable, 10 to 1100 μg/liter 728 samples surface water 22 percent in the 10 to 20 μg range.
¶ ACGIH, 1985.

have compounds that have been reported to produce toxicity in humans. The importance of some of the rarer or lesser known metals such as indium or tantalum might increase with new applications in microelectronics or other new technologies.

The conceptual boundaries of what is regarded as toxicology of metals continues to broaden. Historically, metal toxicology largely concerned acute or overt effects, such as abdominal colic from lead toxicity or the bloody diarrhea and suppression of urine formation from ingestion of corrosive (mercury) sublimate. There must still be knowledge and understanding of such effects, but with present-day occupational and environmental standards, such effects are uncommon. Beyond this, however, is growing inquiry regarding subtle, chronic, or long-term effects where cause-and-effect relationships are not obvious or may be subclinical. This might include a level of effect that causes a change that resides within the generally regarded norm of human performance, for example, lower I.Q. and childhood lead exposure. Assigning responsibility for such toxicologic effects is extremely difficult and not always possible, particularly when the end point in question lacks specificity in that it may be caused by a number of agents or even combinations of substances. The challenges, therefore, for the toxicologist are multiple. The major ones include the need for quantitative information regarding dose and tissue levels, greater understanding of the metabolism of metals particularly at the tissue and cellular level where effects that have specificity may occur, and finally, recognition of factors that influence toxicity of a particular level of exposure such as dietary factors or protein-complex formation that enhance or protect from toxicity. Treatment, particularly the administration of chelating agents, remains an important topic especially for those metals that are cumulative and persistent, for example, Pb, Cd, and Ni. However, prevention of toxicity is the major objective of public health policies and occupational hygiene programs. There is increasing emphasis on the use of biologic indicators of toxicity such as heme enzymes in lead toxicity, renal tubular dysfunction in cadmium exposure, and neurologic effects in mercury toxicity to serve as guidelines for preventive or therapeutic intervention.

ESTIMATES OF DOSE-EFFECT RELATIONSHIPS

Estimates of the relationship of dose or level of exposure to a particular metal are, in many ways, a measure of dose-response relationships, discussed in greater detail in Chapter 2. The conceptual background for this topic is also considered elsewhere (Friberg *et al.*, 1986b). Dose or estimate of exposure to a metal may be a multidimensional concept and is a function of time as well as concentration of metal. The most precise definition of *dose* is the amount of metal within cells or organs manifesting a toxicologic effect. Results from single measurements may reflect recent exposure or longer-term or past exposure, depending on retention time in the particular tissue. Blood, urine, and hair are the most accessible tissues in which to measure dose and are sometimes referred to as *indicator tissues*. *In vivo*, quantitation of metals within organs is not yet possible, although techniques such as neutron activation and fluorescence spectroscopy may hold promise for the future. Indirect estimates of quantities in specific organs may be calculated from metabolic models derived from autopsy data.

At the cellular level, toxicity is related to availability, so that chemical form and ligand binding become critical factors. Alkyl compounds are lipid soluble and pass readily across biologic membranes unaltered by their surrounding medium. They are only slowly dealkylated or transformed to inorganic salts. Hence, their excretion tends to be slower than inorganic forms, and the pattern of organic toxicity differs. For example, alkyl mercury is primarily a neurotoxin versus the renal toxicity of mercuric chloride. Metals that have strong affinity for osseous tissue like lead and radium have a long retention time and tend to accumulate with age. Other metals are retained in soft tissues because of affinities for intracellular proteins, such as renal cadmium bound to metallothionein.

Blood and urine usually reflect recent exposure and correlate best with acute effects. An exception is urine cadmium where increased metal in urine may reflect renal damage related to accumulation of cadmium in the kidney. Partitioning of metal between cells and plasma and between filterable and nonfilterable components of plasma should provide more precise information regarding the presence of biologically active forms of a particular metal. Such partitioning is now standard laboratory practice for blood calcium; ionic calcium is by far the most active form of the metal. Speciation of toxic metals in urine may also provide diagnostic insights. For example, cadmium metallothionein in urine may be of greater toxicologic significance than cadmium chloride.

Hair can be useful in assessing variations in exposure to metals over the long term. Analysis may be performed on segments so that metal content of the newest growth can be compared with past exposures. Correlation between blood levels of metal and concentration in hair is not expected because blood levels reflect only current exposures. Caution must be taken in washing hair prior to analysis to ensure removal of metal deposits from external contamination.

FACTORS INFLUENCING TOXICITY OF METALS

There are only a few general principles available that contribute to understanding the pathophysiology of metal toxicity. Most metals affect multiple organ systems, and the targets for toxicity are specific biochemical processes (enzymes) and/or membranes of cells and organelles. The toxic effect of the metal usually involves an interaction between the free metal ion and the toxicologic target. There may be multiple reasons why a particular toxic effect occurs. For instance, the metabolism of the toxic metal may be similar to a metabolically related essential element. Such is the case for some of the effects of lead—for example, lead and calcium in the central nervous system; lead, iron, and zinc in heme metabolism. Cells that are involved in the transport of metals, such as gastrointestinal, liver, or renal tubular cells, are particularly susceptible to toxicity. However, for many metals, these cells have protective mechanisms involving protein complex formation that permits intracellular accumulation of potentially toxic metals without causing cell injury.

Metal–protein complexes involved in detoxication or protection from toxicity have now been described for a few metals (Goyer, 1984). Morphologically discernible cellular inclusion bodies are present with exposures to lead, bismuth, and a mercury-selenate mixture. Metallothioneins form complexes with cadmium, zinc, copper, and other metals, and ferritin and hemosiderin are intracellular iron-protein complexes. The protein complexes formed by lead, bismuth, mercury-selenate, and iron, at least for hemosiderin, have attracted interest because these complexes are insoluble in tissues and can be observed histologically. However, it is this lack of solubility that has made detailed biochemical study very difficult. On the other hand, for those metal–protein complexes that are stable and soluble in aqueous media, such as metallothionein and ferritin, there is considerable biochemical information. More is known about ferritin than perhaps any of these protein complexes since it is soluble and at the same time it has a unique ultrastructural appearance so that it can be readily identified in cells and organelles. None of these proteins or metal–protein complexes have any known enzymatic activity. From these considerations, it becomes clearer why

speciation—that is, how much metal in a tissue that is in a particular biochemical form and what it is bound to—may be the ultimate determinant of toxicity.

Numerous exogenous factors influence the occurrence of toxicity in any particular subject (Nordberg *et al.*, 1978). These include age, diet, and interactions and concurrent exposure with other toxic metals. Persons at either end of the life span, young children or elderly, are believed to be more susceptible to toxicity from exposure to a particular level of metal than adults. Rapid growth and cell division represent opportunities for genotoxic effects. Intrauterine toxicity to methyl mercury is well documented. There is no impediment to the transplacental transport of lead, so that fetal blood lead levels are similar to maternal levels.

The major pathway of exposure to many toxic metals in children is with food, and children consume more calories per body weight than adults. Moreover, children have higher gastrointestinal absorption of metals, particularly lead. Experimental studies have extended these observations to many metals, and milk diet, probably because of lipid content, seems to increase metal absorption.

Effects of some dietary factors on metal toxicity are at the level of absorption from the gastrointestinal tract. There is an inverse relationship between protein content of diet and cadmium and lead toxicity. Vitamin C reduces lead and cadmium absorption, probably because of increased absorption of ferrous ion. On the other hand, metabolically related essential metals may alter toxicity by interaction at the cellular level. Lead, calcium, and vitamin D have a complex relationship affecting mineralization of bone and more directly through impairment of 1-25-dihydroxy vitamin D synthesis in the kidney. Metal-metal interaction may have considerable influence on dose-effect relationships and is commented on in discussions of specific metals.

"Life-style" factors such as smoking or alcohol ingestion may have indirect influences on toxicity. Cigarette smoke in itself contains some toxic metals such as cadmium, and cigarette smoking may influence pulmonary effects. Alcohol ingestion may influence toxicity indirectly by altering diet and reducing essential mineral intake. For instance, a decrease in dietary calcium will influence toxicity of major toxic metals, including lead and cadmium.

Chemical form or speciation of the metal may be an important factor, not only for pulmonary and gastrointestinal absorption but in terms of body distribution and toxic effects. Dietary phosphate generally forms less soluble salts of metals than other anions. Alkyl compounds, such as tetraethyl lead and methyl mercury, are lipid soluble and more soluble in myelin than inorganic salts of these metals.

For metals that produce hypersensitivity reactions, the immune status of an individual becomes an additional toxicologic variable. Metals that provoke immune reactions include mercury, gold, platinum, beryllium, chromium, and nickel. Clinical effects are varied but usually involve any of four types of immune responses. In anaphylactic or immediate hypersensitivity reactions, the antibody IgE reacts with the antigen on the surface of mast cells, releasing vasoreactive amines. Clinical reactions include conjunctivitis, asthma, urticaria, or even systemic anaphylaxis. Cutaneous, mucosal, and bronchial reactions to platinum have been attributed to this type of hypersensitivity reaction. Cytotoxic hypersensitivity is the result of a complement-fixing reaction of IgG immunoglobulin with antigen or hapten bound to the cell surface. The thrombocytopenia sometimes occurring with exposure to organic gold salts may be brought about in this manner. Immune complex hypersensitivity occurs when soluble immune complex deposits (antigen, antibody, and complement) within tissues, producing an acute inflammatory reaction. Immune complexes are typically deposited on the epithelial (subepithelial) side of glomerular basement membrane, resulting in proteinuria, and occur following exposure to mercury vapor or gold therapy. Cell-mediated hypersensitivity, also known as the *delayed hypersensitivity reaction*, is mediated by thymus-dependent lymphocytes and usually occurs 24 to 48 hours after exposure. The histologic reaction consists of mononuclear cells and is the typical reaction seen in the contact dermatitis following exposure to chromium or nickel. The granuloma formation occurring with beryllium and zirconium exposure may be a form of cell-mediated immune response.

CARCINOGENESIS

Given the long history of human exposure to metals, knowledge of the potential carcinogenicity of metal compounds has evolved slowly, and most of this information has only been obtained in recent years (Friberg and Nelson, 1981; IARC, 1987).

Furthermore, predictive *in vitro* methods using nonmammalian systems, such as the Ames test, do not seem as responsive as for organic compounds (Costa, 1980). Evidence of carcinogenicity for metals relates more precisely with specific compounds of metals than with the metal itself. That is, some chemical forms of a metal

may have more potency for carcinogenesis than others; for example, nickel subsulfide (Ni_3S_2) is more carcinogenic than amorphous nickel monosulfide (NiS); but such differences may be explained on the basis of cell uptake rates or solubility. Similar debates concern various compounds of chromium. Nevertheless, if any form of a metal is carcinogenic, the metal itself must be regarded as a carcinogen.

Although only a few metals show any evidence of carcinogenicity, this is an exceedingly important topic because of the ubiquity of most metals, their wide industrial use, and their persistence in the environment. Identification of metal carcinogens in industry is made even more perplexing because seldom is exposure to a single metal—it is usually to mixtures. And there is the added question of the role of metals as promoters or cocarcinogens with organic carcinogens because of their persistence in tissues, as may be the case for lead.

The chronology of observation on the carcinogenicity of metals is shown in Figure 19–2. Specific details pertaining to the carcinogenicity of each metal are discussed later in the chapter, along with other toxicologic effects. However, the figure does provide an overview. Human case reports of skin cancer due to arsenic exposure were recognized in the nineteenth century, but epidemiologic support from case study observations did not occur until over 50 years later, and there has not yet been confirmation in experimental animals. On the other hand, lead is the only metal shown to be carcinogenic in animal models by oral administration. Yet evidence in humans is limited to a couple of recent case reports. How much of what kind of evidence, animal and/or human, is required to label a metal as a carcinogen must be decided for each metal. Animal studies that use routes of administration different from those by which humans may be exposed, such as by injection, have limitations for extrapolation to humans.

CHELATION

Chelation is the formation of a metal ion complex in which the metal ion is associated with a charged or uncharged electron donor referred to as a ligand. The ligand may be monodentate, bidentate, or multidentate; that is, it may attach or coordinate using one or two or more donor atoms. Bidentate ligands form ring structures that include the metal ion and the two ligand atoms attached to the metal (Williams and Halstead, 1982–83).

Chelating agents are generally nonspecific in regard to their affinity for metals. To varying degrees, they will mobilize and enhance the ex-

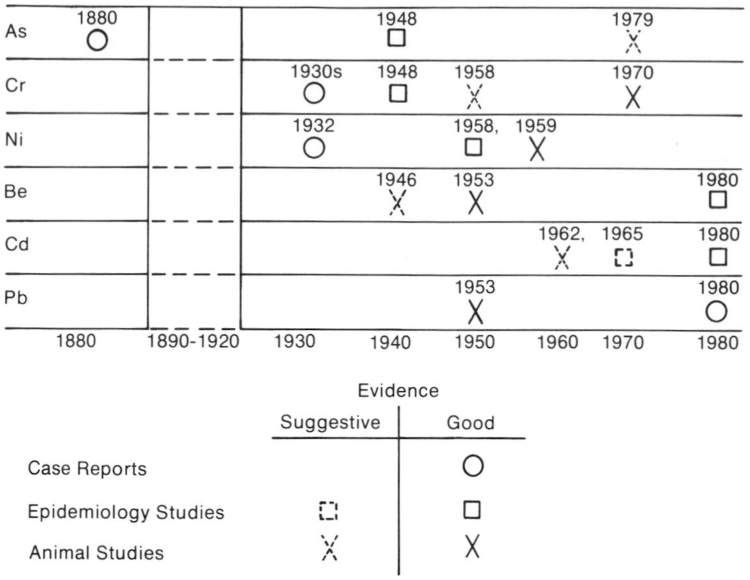

	1880			1948			1979	
As	O			□			X	

			1930s	1948	1958		1970	
Cr			O	□	X		X	

			1932		1958, 1959			
Ni			O		□ X			

				1946	1953			1980
Be				X	X			□

						1962, 1965		1980
Cd						X []		□

					1953			1980
Pb					X			O

1880   1890–1920   1930   1940   1950   1960   1970   1980

Evidence

	Suggestive	Good
Case Reports		O
Epidemiology Studies	[]	□
Animal Studies	X	X

Figure 19–2. Chronology of observations on the carcinogenicity of metals. (Modified from Friberg, L., and Nelson, N.: Introduction, general findings and general recommendations. Workshop/Conference on the Role of Metals in Carcinogenesis. *Environ. Health Perspect.*, **40**:5–10, 1981.)

cretion of a rather wide range of metals, including essential metals such as calcium and zinc (Table 19–2). Their efficacy depends not solely on their affinity for the metal of interest but also on their affinity for endogenous metals, mainly Ca, which compete in accordance with their own affinities for the chelator. Properties of a few of the commonly used chelators will be described.

BAL

BAL (British Anti Lewisite), or 2,3-dimercaptopropanol, was the first clinically useful chelating agent. It was developed during World War II as a specific antagonist to vesicant arsenical war gases based on the observation that arsenic has an affinity for sulfhydryl-containing substances. BAL, a dithiol compound with two sulfur atoms on adjacent carbon atoms, competes with the critical binding sites responsible for the toxic effects. These observations led to the prediction that the "biochemical lesion" of arsenic poisoning would prove to be a thiol with sulfhydryl groups separated by one or more intervening carbon atoms. This prediction was borne out a few years later with the discovery that arsenic interferes with the function of 6,8-dithiooctanoic acid in biologic oxidation (Gunsalus, 1953).

BAL has been found to form stable chelates *in vivo* with many toxic metals including inorganic mercury, antimony, bismuth, cadmium, chromium, cobalt, gold, and nickel. However, it is not necessarily the treatment of choice for toxicity to these metals. BAL has been used as an adjunct in the treatment of the acute encephalopathy of lead toxicity. It is a potentially toxic drug, and its use may be accompanied by multiple side affects. Although BAL will increase the excretion of cadmium, there is a concomitant increase in renal cadmium concentration, so that its use in cadmium toxicity is to be avoided. It does, however, remove inorganic mercury from kidneys but is not useful in treatment of alkyl or phenylmercury toxicity. BAL also enhances the toxicity of selenium and tellurium, so it is not to be used to remove these metals.

Table 19–2. LIGANDS (CHELATING AGENTS) PREFERRED FOR REMOVAL OF TOXIC METALS

LIGAND	METAL
BAL	Arsenic, lead (with Ca-EDTA), mercury, inorganic
DMPS	Methyl mercury, inorganic mercury, cadmium, copper, and nickel
Calcium EDTA	Lead
Penicillamine	Copper, lead
Calcium DPTA	Cadmium (with BAL)
Desferrioxamine	Iron
Dithiocarb	Nickel carbonyl

DMPS

DMPS (2,3-dimercapto-1-propanesulfonic acid) is a water-soluble derivative of BAL developed to reduce the toxicity and unpleasant side effects of BAL. DMPS has been shown to reduce blood lead levels in children (Chisolm and Thomas, 1985). It has the advantage over EDTA in that it is administered orally and does not appear to have toxic side effects. It has been widely used in the Soviet Union to treat many different metal intoxications and even atherosclerosis by the adherents of the notion that this degenerative disorder of blood vessels in due to metal-ion accumulations in the blood vessel wall, leading to inhibition of enzyme metabolism.

DMPS is effective in removal of both inorganic and methyl mercury, probably because it is not lipophilic like BAL and does not penetrate tissues but removes extracellular metal (Gabard, 1976). Experiments in rats suggest that DMPS can be used to estimate the renal burden of lead (Twarog and Cherian, 1984) and inorganic mercury (Cherian *et al.*, 1988). It may also be effective in removal of copper, nickel, and cadmium immediately after exposure but not from tissue stores.

EDTA

Calcium EDTA is the calcium disodium salt of ethylenediaminetetraacetic acid. The calcium salt must be used clinically because the sodium salt has greater affinity for calcium and will produce hypocalcemic tetany. However, the calcium salt will bind lead with displacement of calcium from the chelate. It is poorly absorbed from the gastrointestinal tract, so it must be given parenterally, and it becomes rapidly distributed in the body. It is the current method of choice for treatment of lead toxicity (Chisolm, 1974). The peak excretion is within the first 24 hours and represents excretion of lead from soft tissues. Removal from the skeletal system occurs more slowly with restoration of equilibrium with soft tissue compartments. Calcium EDTA does have the potential for nephrotoxicity, so it should be administered only when indicated clinically (Chisolm and O'Hara, 1982; EPA, 1986).

Penicillamine

Penicillamine (B,B^1-dimethylcystein), a hydrolytic product of penicillin, is the choice for therapy of Wilson's disease (copper toxicity) and is effective in removal of lead, mercury, and iron (Walshe, 1964). It is also important to note that penicillamine removes other physiologically essential metals including zinc, cobalt, and man-

ganese. It also has the risk of inducing a hypersensitivity reaction with a wide spectrum of undesired immunologic effects including skin rash, blood dyscrasias, and possibly proteinuria and the nephrotic syndrome. It has cross-sensitivity to penicillin, so it should be avoided by persons with penicillin hypersensitivity. Recent studies have shown the effectiveness of a new orally active chelating agent, triethylene tetramine 2HCl (Trien), in Wilson's disease, particularly in those persons who have developed sensitivity to pencillamine (Walshe, 1983).

DTPA

DTPA, or diethylenetriamine-pentaacetic acid, has chelating properties similar to those of EDTA. The calcium salt (CaNa$_2$ DPTA) must be used clinically because of its high affinity for calcium. It has been used for chelation of plutonium and other radioactive metals but with mixed success.

Desferrioxamine

Desferrioxamine is a hydroxylamine isolated as the iron chelate of *Streptomyces pilosus* and is used clinically in the metal-free form (Keberle, 1964). It has a remarkable affinity for ferric iron and a low affinity for calcium and competes effectively for iron in ferritin and hemosiderin but not transferrin, or the iron in hemoglobin or heme-containing enzymes. It is poorly absorbed from the gastrointestinal tract, so it must be given parenterally. Clinical usefulness is limited by a variety of toxic effects including hypotension, skin rashes, and possibly cataract formation. It seems to be more effective in hemosiderosis due to blood transfusion but is less effective in treatment of hemochromatosis.

Dithiocarb

Dithiocarb (diethyldithiocarbamate [DDC]) has been recommended as the drug of choice in the treatment of acute nickel carbonyl poisoning. The drug may be administered orally for mild toxicity but parenterally for acute or severe poisoning (Sunderman, 1979). It has also been used experimentally for removal of cadmium bound to metallothionein (Kojima *et al.*, 1989).

MAJOR TOXIC METALS WITH MULTIPLE EFFECTS

Arsenic

Arsenic is particularly difficult to characterize as a single element because its chemistry is so complex and there are many different compounds of arsenic. It may be trivalent or pentavalent and is widely distributed in nature. The most common inorganic trivalent arsenic compounds are arsenic trioxide, sodium arsenite, and arsenic trichloride. Pentavalent inorganic compounds are arsenic pentoxide, arsenic acid, and arsenates, such as lead arsenate and calcium arsenate. Organic compounds may also be trivalent or pentavalent, such as arsanilic acid, or even in methylated forms as a consequence of bimethylation by organisms in soil and fresh and seawaters. A summary of environmental sources of arsenic as well as potential health effects is contained in a World Health Organization (WHO) criteria document (WHO, 1981) and U.S. Environmental Protection Agency (EPA) documents on arsenic (EPA, 1984, 1987b).

Inorganic arsenic is released into the environment from a number of anthropogenic sources that include primary copper, zinc and lead smelters, glass manufacturers that add arsenic to raw materials, and chemical manufacturers. The National Air Sampling Network conducted by the U.S. EPA indicates that in areas not influenced by copper smelters, maximum 24-hour concentrations do not exceed 0.1 $\mu g/m^3$. Near point emissions (copper smelters), concentrations may exceed 1 $\mu g/m^3$. Drinking water usually contains a few micrograms per liter or less. More than 18,000 community water supplies in the United States have concentrations less than 0.01 mg/liter, but levels exceeding 0.05 mg/liter have been found in Nova Scotia, where arsenic content of bedrock is high. Even higher concentrations have been reported from various mineral springs—for example, Japan—1.7 mg As/liter; Cordoba, Argentina—3.4 mg/liter; Taiwan (artesian well water)—1.8 mg/liter. Most foods (meat and vegetables) contain some level of arsenic, but the daily diet in the United States contains below 0.04 mg but may contain 0.2 mg per day if the diet contains seafood. The total daily intake of arsenic by humans without industrial exposure, however, is usually less than 0.3 mg per day.

The major source of occupational exposure to arsenic in the United States is in the manufacture of pesticides, herbicides, and other agricultural products. High exposure to arsenic fumes and dust may occur in the smelting industries; the highest concentrations most likely occur among roaster workers.

Disposition. Airborne arsenic is largely trivalent arsenic oxide, but deposition in airways and absorption from lungs are dependent on particle size and chemical form.

Studies show that 6 to 9 percent of orally administered ^{74}As-labeled trivalent or pentavalent arsenic is eliminated in feces in mice, indicating almost complete absorption from the gastrointestinal tract. Limited data also suggest nearly complete absorption of soluble forms of trivalent and pentavalent arsenic (Tam et al., 1979). Excretion of absorbed arsenic is mainly via urine. The biologic half-life of ingested inorganic arsenic is about ten hours, and 50 to 80 percent is excreted in about three days. The biologic half-life of methylated arsenic was found to be 30 hours, in one study (Crecelius, 1977).

Arsenic has a predilection for skin and is excreted by desquamation of skin and in sweat, particularly during periods of profuse sweating. It also concentrates in nails and hair. Arsenic in nails produces Mee's lines (transverse white bands across fingernails) appearing about six weeks after onset of symptoms of toxicity. Time of exposure may be estimated from measuring the distance of the line from the base of the nail and the rate of nail growth, which is about 0.3 cm/month or 0.1 mm/day. Arsenic in hair may also reflect past exposure, but intrinsic or systematically absorbed arsenic in hair must be distinguished from arsenic that is deposited from external sources. Human milk contains about 3 μg/liter of arsenic.

Placental transfer of arsenic has been shown in hamsters injected intravenously with high doses (20 mg/kg body weight) of sodium arsenate (Ferm, 1977), and studies of tissue levels of arsenic in fetuses and newborn babies in Japan show that the total amount of arsenic in the fetus tends to increase during gestation, indicating placental transfer. A study of women in the United States found cord blood levels of arsenic to be similar to maternal blood levels (Kagey et al., 1977).

Biotransformation of Arsenic In Vivo. The metabolism and potential for toxicity of arsenic are further complicated by in vivo transformation of inorganic forms by methylation to monomethyl and dimethyl arsenic. Current knowledge of this process has been summarized by the EPA (1984). Dimethyl arsenic is the principal transformation product. This is presumed to be a process of detoxification of the more toxic inorganic forms, and dimethyl arsenic appears to be a terminal metabolite that is rapidly formed and rapidly excreted. However, exposure to inorganic arsenic may exceed rate of transformation, resulting in toxicity from the inorganic form so that consideration of toxic dose responses to inorganic arsenic must be assessed in the light of what is known about metabolic transformation.

Ingestion of arsenic-containing seafood does not result in increased excretion of inorganic arsenic and methyl- and dimethylarsinic acid but results in large increases of cacodylic acid (Buchet *et al.*, 1980).

Oxidation-Reduction Reactions of Inorganic Arsenic. There are a number of experiments in animals suggesting that reduction of pentavalent arsenic to arsenic trioxide occurs *in vivo*. The biochemical mechanism for *in vivo* methylation of inorganic arsenic is a reductive process, and it is presently presumed that reduction of arsenic *in vivo* is related to biomethylation (EPA, 1984). Lerman *et al.* (1983) found in the rat, using *in vitro* techniques, that isolated hepatocytes readily methylate trivalent arsenic, whereas there is virtually no methylation of pentavalent arsenic. These studies suggest that pentavalent arsenic must first be converted to arsenite prior to methylation. Trivalent inorganic arsenic undergoes extensive oxidation in aerated water. The pH of aqueous solutions appears to be a major factor in the relative stability of either valency form. Trivalent arsenic in alkaline solutions is more rapidly oxidized than at acidic pH. Pentavalent inorganic arsenic, on the other hand, is relatively stable at neutral or alkaline pH but undergoes reduction with decreasing pH.

Cellular Effects. It has been known for some years that trivalent compounds of arsenic are the principal toxic forms, and pentavalent arsenic compounds have little effect on enzyme activity. A number of sulfhydryl-containing proteins and enzyme systems have been found to be altered by exposure to arsenic. Some of these can be reversed by addition of an excess of a monothiol such as glutathione; those enzymes containing two thiol groups can be reversed by dithiols such as 2,3-dimercaptopropanol (BAL) but not by monothiols.

Arsenic affects mitochondrial enzymes and impairs tissue respiration (M. M. Brown *et al.*, 1976), which seems to be related to the cellular toxicity of arsenic. Mitochondria accumulate arsenic, and respiration mediated by NAD-linked substrates is particularly sensitive to arsenic and is thought to result from reaction between arsenite ion and dihydrolipoic acid cofactor, necessary for oxidation of the substrate (Fluharty and Sanadi, 1961). Arsenite also inhibits succinic dehydrogenase activity and uncouples oxidative phosphorylation, which results in stimulation of mitochondrial ATPase activity. Mitchell *et al.* (1971) proposed that arsenic inhibits energy-linked functions of mitochondria in two ways: competition with phosphate during oxidative phosphorylation and inhibition of energy-linked reduction of NAD.

Information from experimental studies with rats, chicks, minipigs, and goats have shown that arsenic in its inorganic form may be an essential nutrient, but the nutritional essentiality for humans has not been established (EPA, 1987b).

Toxicology. Ingestion of large doses (70 to 180 mg) may be acutely fatal. Symptoms consist of fever, anorexia, hepatomegaly, melanosis, and cardiac arrhythmia with electrocardiograph changes that may be the prodroma of eventual cardiovascular failure. Other features include upper respiratory tract symptoms, peripheral neuropathy, and gastrointestinal, cardiovascular, and hematopoietic effects. Acute ingestion may be suspected from damage to mucous membranes such as irritation, vesicle formation, and even sloughing. Sensory loss in the peripheral nervous system is the most common neurologic effect, appearing one or two weeks after large exposures and consisting of Wallerian degeneration of axons, but is reversible if exposure is stopped. Anemia and leukopenia, particularly granulocytopenia, occur in a few days and are reversible.

Chronic Toxicity. Chronic exposure to inorganic arsenic compounds may lead to neurotoxicity of both the peripheral and central nervous systems. Neurotoxicity usually begins with sensory changes, paresthesias, and muscle tenderness, followed by weakness, progressing from proximal to distal muscle groups.

Peripheral neuropathy may be progressive, involving both sensory and motor neurons, leading to demyelination of long axon nerve fibers, but effects are dose related. Acute exposure to a single high dose can produce onset of paresthesia and motor dysfunction, within 10 days. More chronic occupational exposures producing more gradual, insidious effects may be on the order of years, and it has been difficult to establish dose-response relationships.

Liver injury is characteristic of longer-term or chronic exposure, is initially reflected by jaundice, and may progress to cirrhosis and ascites. Toxicity to hepatic parenchymal cells results in elevations of liver enzymes in blood, and studies in experimental animals show granules and alterations in the ultrastructure of mitochondria, nonspecific manifestations of cell injury including loss of glycogen (EPA, 1984).

Peripheral vascular disease has been observed in persons with chronic exposure to arsenic in drinking water in Taiwan and Chile. It is manifested by acrocyanosis and Raynaud's phenomenon, and may progress to endarteritis obliterans and gangrene of the lower extremities (blackfoot disease). This specific effect seems to be related to the cumulative dose of arsenic, but prevalence is uncertain because of difficulties in separating arsenic-induced peripheral vascular disease from other causes of gangrene (Tseng, 1977).

Carcinogenicity. The potential carcinogenicity of arsenic has been extensively reviewed (WHO, 1981; EPA, 1987b).

In humans, chronic exposure to arsenic induces a series of characteristic changes in skin epithelium proceeding from hyperpigmentation to hyperkeratosis. The hyperkeratosis has been described histologically as showing hematin proliferation of a verrucous nature with derangement of the squamous portions of the epithelium or squamous cell carcinoma in some cases. There may actually be two cell types of arsenic-induced skin cancer, basal cell carcinomas and squamous cell carcinomas arising in keratotic areas. The basal cell cancers are usually only locally invasive, but squamous cell carcinomas may have distant metastases.

The skin cancers related to arsenic differ from the ultraviolet light–induced tumors in that they generally occur on areas of the body not exposed to sunlight, for example, palms and soles, and occur as multiple lesions.

Occupational exposure to airborne arsenic may also be associated with lung cancer, usually a poorly differentiated form of epidermoid bronchogenic carcinoma. The time period between initiation of exposure and occurrence of arsenic-associated lung cancer has been found to be on the order of 35 to 45 years. Enterline and Marsh (1980) report a latency period of 20 years in their study of copper smelter workers in Tacoma, Washington.

Other visceral tumors that have been associated with arsenic exposure include hemangiosarcoma of the liver (Popper *et al.*, 1978). Other cancers noted in arsenic-exposed subjects include lymphomas and leukemia, renal adenocarcinoma, and nasopharyngeal carcinoma.

The EPA (1987b) and the IARC (1987) classify arsenic as a carcinogen for which there is sufficient evidence from epidemiological studies to support a causal association between exposure to arsenic and skin cancer. However, in contrast to most other human carcinogens, it has been difficult to confirm in experimental animals. Intratracheal instillations of arsenic trioxide produced an increased incidence of pulmonary adenomas, papillomas, and adenomatoid lesions, suggesting that arsenic trioxide can induce lung carcinomas (Pershagan *et al.*, 1984), but other studies testing trivalent and pentavalent arsenic compounds by oral administration or skin application have not shown potential for either promotion or initiation of carcinogenicity. Similarly, experimental studies for carcinogenicity of organic arsenic compounds have been negative.

Studies on mutagenic effects of arsenic have been generally negative. Arsenic does not induce gene mutations in bacteria and was found to be inactive in inducing reverse mutation and mitotic gene conversion in yeast. Arsenate was found not to increase forward mutations at the thymidine kinase locus in mouse L51784 cells, whereas other known or suggested mutagenic metals (cadmium, nickel, and *trans*-platinum) were positive.

Several studies suggest that both trivalent and pentavalent arsenic compounds are capable of producing chromosome breaks and chromosome aberrations in human peripheral lymphocyte and human skin cultures. The majority of studies indicate, however, that people who have workplace or pharmaceutical exposure to arsenic have increased levels of chromosomal aberrations and sister chromosome exchanges in peripheral lymphocytes, although the scientific rigidity of some of these studies has been questioned (EPA, 1987b).

Reproductive Effects and Teratogenicity. High doses of inorganic arsenic compounds administered to pregnant experimental animals produce various malformations somewhat dependent on time and route of administration. However, no such effects have been noted in people with excessive occupational exposures to arsenic compounds.

Arsine. Arsine gas is formed by the reaction of hydrogen with arsenic and is generated as a by-product in the refining of nonferrous metals. Arsine is a potent hemolytic agent, producing acute symptoms of nausea, vomiting, shortness of breath, and headache accompanying the hemolytic reaction. Exposure may be fatal and may be accompanied by hemoglobinuria and renal failure, and even jaundice and anemia in nonfatal cases where exposure persists (Fowler and Weissberg, 1974).

Biologic Indicators. Biologic indicators of arsenic exposure are blood, urine, and hair (Table 19–3). Because of the short half-life of arsenic, blood levels are only useful within a few days of acute exposure but are not useful to assess chronic exposure. Urine arsenic is the best indicator of current or recent exposure and has been noted to be several hundred micrograms per liter with occupational exposure. However, some marine organisms may contain very high concentrations of organoarsenicals that do not have significant toxicity and are rapidly excreted in urine without transformation (Lauwerys, 1983). Workers should be advised not to ingest marine food for a day or two before testing. Hair or even fingernail concentration of arsenic may be helpful to evaluate past exposures, but interpretation is made difficult because of the problem of differentiating external contamination.

Table 19–3. BIOLOGIC INDICATORS OF ARSENIC EXPOSURE

	NORMAL	EXCESSIVE EXPOSURE
Whole blood	< 10 μg/liter	Up to 50 μg/liter
Urine*	< 50 μg/liter	> 100 μg/liter
Hair	< 1 μg/kg	

* Best indicator of current or recent exposure.

There are no specific biochemical parameters that reflect arsenic toxicity, but evaluation of clinical effects must be interpreted with knowledge of exposure history.

Treatment. BAL is used to treat acute dermatitis and pulmonary symptoms. BAL has also been used for the treatment of chronic arsenic poisoning, but there are no established biologic criteria or measures of effectiveness. BAL has been used most often in cases with dermatitis, but there is usually no change in the keratotic lesions or influence on progression to skin cancer.

Arsine toxicity is best treated symptomatically. BAL is not considered helpful (Fowler and Weissberg, 1974).

Beryllium

The major toxicologic effects of beryllium are on the lung. It may produce an acute chemical pneumonitis, hypersensitivity, and chronic granulomatous pulmonary disease (berylliosis). A variety of beryllium compounds and some of its alloys have induced malignant tumors of the lung in rats and monkeys and osteogenic sarcoma in rabbits. Human epidemiologic studies are strongly suggestive of a carcinogenic effect in humans (Kuschner, 1981). The EPA criteria document provides details regarding environmental sources of beryllium and reviews toxicological literature (EPA, 1987a).

Beryllium in the environment largely results from coal combustion. Illinois and Appalachian coal contains an average of about 2.5 ppm; oil contains about 0.08 ppm. The combustion of coal and oil contributes about 1250 or more tons of beryllium to the environment each year (mostly from coal), which is about five times the annual production for industrial use. The major industrial processes that release beryllium into the environment are beryllium extraction plants, ceramic plants, and beryllium alloy manufacturers. These industries also provide the greatest potential for occupational exposure. The major current use is as an alloy, but about 20 percent of world production is for applications utilizing the free metal in nuclear reactions, X-ray windows, and other special applications related to space optics, missile fuel, and space vehicles.

Knowledge of the disposition of beryllium has largely been obtained from experimental animals, particularly the rat. Clearance of inhaled beryllium is multiphasic; half is cleared in about two weeks; the remainder is removed slowly, and a residuum becomes fixed in the tissues, probably within fibrotic granulomata.

Gastrointestinal absorption of ingested beryllium probably only occurs in the acidic milieu of the stomach, where it is in the ionized form, but passes through the intestinal tract as precipitated phosphate. Removal of radiolabeled beryllium chloride from rat blood is rapid, having a half-life of about three hours. It is distributed to all tissues, but most goes to the skeleton. High doses go predominantly to liver, but it is gradually transferred to bone. The half-time in tissues is relatively short, except in the lung, and a variable fraction of an administered dose is excreted in the urine, where it has a long biological half-time. Normal beryllium excretion is on the order of a few nanograms per liter.

Skin Effects. Contact dermatitis is the commonest beryllium-related toxic effect. Exposure to soluble beryllium compounds may result in papulovesicular lesions on the skin. It is a delayed-type hypersensitivity reaction. The hypersensitivity is cell mediated, and passive transfer with lymphoid cells has been accomplished in guinea pigs. If contact is made with an insoluble beryllium compound, a chronic granulomatous lesion develops, which may be necrotizing or ulcerative. If insoluble beryllium-containing material becomes embedded under the skin, the lesion will not heal and may progress in severity. Use of a beryllium patch test to identify beryllium-sensitive individuals may in itself be sensitizing, and use of this procedure as a diagnostic test is discouraged.

Pulmonary Effects.

Acute Chemical Pneumonitis. Acute pulmonary disease from inhalation of beryllium is a fulminating inflammatory reaction of the entire respiratory tract, involving the nasal passages, pharynx, tracheobronchial airways, and the alveoli and in the most severe cases produces an acute fulminating pneumonitis. It occurs almost immediately following inhalation of aerosols of soluble beryllium compounds, particularly fluoride—an intermediate in the ore extraction process. Severity is dose related. Fatalities have occurred, although recovery is generally complete after a period of several weeks or even months.

Chronic Granulomatous Pulmonary Disease (Berylliosis). This syndrome was first described among fluorescent lamp workers exposed to insoluble beryllium compounds, particularly beryllium oxide. The major symptom is shortness of breath but in severe cases may be accompanied by cyanosis and clubbing of fingers (hypertrophic osteoarthropathy—a characteristic manifestation of chronic pulmonary disease). Chest X rays show miliary mottling. Histologically, the alveoli contain small interstitial granulomata, which resemble those seen in sarcoidosis. In the early stages, the lesions are composed of fluid, lymphocytes, and plasma cells. Multinucleated giant cells are common. Later, the granulomas become organized with proliferation of fibrosis tissue, eventually forming small, fibrous nodules. As the lesions progress, interstitial fibrosis increases with loss of functioning alveoli and effective air/capillary gas exchange and increasing respiratory dysfunction.

Beryllium is one metal in which evidence for carcinogenicity was observed in experimental studies, beginning in 1946, before the establishment of carcinogenicity in humans (Kuschner, 1981). Epidemiologic confirmation in humans has been evolving so that there is increasing acceptance that beryllium is, in fact, a human carcinogen. Studies of humans with occupational exposure to beryllium prior to 1970 were negative. However, reports of two worker populations and a registry of berylliosis cases studied earlier show a small excess of lung cancer, but the total number of cases is small. Both the IARC (1987) and the EPA (1987a) regard evidence for carcinogenicity to be sufficient from animals but limited in man.

In vitro studies of genotoxicity have shown that beryllium will induce morphologic transformation in mammalian cells (DiPaolo and Casto, 1979). Beryllium will also decrease fidelity of DNA synthesis but is negative when tested as a mutagen in bacterial systems.

Cadmium

Cadmium is a modern toxic metal. It was only discovered as an element in 1817, and industrial use was minor until about 50 years ago. But now it is a very important metal with many applications. Its main use is electroplating or galvanizing because of its noncorrosive properties. It is also used as a color pigment for paints and plastics and cathode material for nickel-cadmium batteries. Cadmium is a by-product of zinc and lead mining and smelting, which are important sources of environmental pollution. The toxicology of cadmium is extensively reviewed by Friberg *et al.* (1986a).

Airborne cadmium in the present-day workplace environment is generally 0.05 to 0.02 $\mu g/m^3$. Typical concentrations in ambient air in rural areas are 0.001 to 0.005 $\mu g/m^3$ and up to 0.050 or 0.060 $\mu g/m^3$ in urban areas (Kneip *et al.*, 1970).

Meat, fish, and fruit contain 1 to 50 $\mu g/kg$, grains contain 10 to 150 $\mu g/kg$, and the greatest concentrations are in liver and kidney of animals. Shellfish, such as mussels, scallops, and oysters, may be a major source of dietary cadmium and contain 100 to 1000 $\mu g/kg$. Shellfish accumulate cadmium from the water and then bind to cadmium-binding peptides. Total daily intake from food, water, and air in North America and Europe varies considerably but is estimated to be about 10 to 40 $\mu g/day$.

Cadmium is more readily taken up by plants than other metals such as lead (EPA, 1981). Factors contributing to soil content of cadmium are fallout from air, cadmium content of water irrigating fields, and cadmium added with fertilizers. Commercial phosphate fertilizers usually contain less than 20 mg/kg, but Anderson and Hahlin (1981) found an annual increase in soil and barley grain from continued use of phosphate fertilizer over a 15-year period. Another concern is use of commercial sludge to fertilize agricultural fields. Commercial sludge may contain up to 1500 mg of cadmium per kilogram of dry material.

Respiratory absorption of cadmium is about 15 to 30 percent. Workplace exposure to cadmium is particularly hazardous where there are cadmium fumes or airborne cadmium. Most airborne cadmium is respirable. A major nonoccupational source of respirable cadmium is cigarettes. One cigarette contains 1 to 2 μg cadmium, and 10 percent of the cadmium in a cigarette is inhaled (0.1 to 0.2 μg) (Elinder *et al.*, 1983). Smoking one or more packs of cigarettes a day may double the daily absorbed burden of cadmium.

Disposition. Gastrointestinal absorption is less than respiratory absorption and is about 5 to 8 percent. It is enhanced by dietary deficiencies of calcium and iron, and diets low in protein. Low dietary calcium stimulates synthesis of calcium-binding protein, which enhances cadmium absorption. Women with low serum ferritin levels have been shown to have twice the normal absorption of cadmium (Flanagan *et al.*, 1978). Zinc decreases cadmium absorption probably by stimulating production of metallothionein.

Cadmium is transported in blood bound to red blood cells and large-molecular-weight proteins in plasma, particularly albumin. A small fraction of blood cadmium may be transported by metallothionein. Blood cadmium levels in adults without excessive exposure are usually less than 1 $\mu g/dl$. Newborns have low body content of cadmium, usually less than 1 mg total body burden. The placenta synthesizes metallothionein and may serve as a barrier to maternal cadmium, but the fetus may be exposed with increased maternal exposure. Human breast milk and cow's milk are low in cadmium content, less than 1 $\mu g/kg$ of milk. About 50 to 75 percent of the body burden of cadmium is in liver and kidneys; half-life in the body is not exactly known but is many years and may be as long as 30 years. With continued retention, there is progressive accumulation in soft tissues, particularly kidney, through ages 50 to 60 years, when it begins to decline slowly. Because of the potential for accumulation in kidney, there is considerable concern for levels of dietary intake of cadmium by persons in the general population. Studies from Sweden have shown a slow but steady increase in cadmium content of vegetables over the years. Increase in body burden has been determined from a historic autopsy study (Friberg *et al.*, 1986a).

Toxicity. Acute toxicity may result from ingestion of relatively high concentrations of cadmium, as may occur in contaminated beverages or food. Nordberg (1972) relates an instance in which nausea, vomiting, and abdominal pain occurred from consumption of drinks containing approximately 16 mg/liter of cadmium. Recovery was rapid without apparent long-term effects. Inhalation of cadmium fumes or other heated cadmium-containing materials may produce an acute chemical pneumonitis and pulmonary edema.

The principal long-term effects of low-level exposure to cadmium are chronic obstructive pulmonary disease and emphysema and chronic renal tubular disease. There may also be effects on the cardiovascular and skeletal systems (Friberg *et al.*, 1986b).

Chronic Pulmonary Disease. Toxicity to the respiratory system is proportional to the time and level of exposure. Obstructive lung disease results from chronic bronchitis, progressive fibrosis of the lower airways, and accompanying alveolar damage leading to emphysema. The lung disease is manifested by dyspnea, reduced vital capacity, and increased residual volume. The pathogenesis of the lung lesion is turnover and necrosis of alveolar macrophages. Released enzymes produce irreversible damage to alveolar basement membranes including rupture of septa and interstitial fibrosis. It has been found that cadmium reduces α-1-antitrypsin activity, perhaps enhancing pulmonary toxicity. However, no difference in plasma α-1-antitrypsin activity could be found between cadmium-exposed workers with and without emphysema (Lauwerys *et al.*, 1979).

Kidney. The effects of cadmium on proximal renal tubular function are manifested by increased cadmium in the urine, proteinuria, aminoaciduria, glucosuria, and decreased renal tubular reabsorption of phosphate. Morphologic changes are nonspecific and consist of tubular cell degeneration in the initial stages, progressing to an interstitial inflammatory reaction and fibrosis. Analysis of kidney cadmium levels by *in vivo* neutron activation analysis and X-ray fluorescence has made it possible to study the relationship between renal cadmium levels and occurrence of effects (Roels *et al.*, 1983; Ellis *et al.*, 1984; Skerfving *et al.*, 1987). The critical concentration of cadmium in the renal cortex that produces tubular dysfunction in 10 percent of the population is about 200 $\mu g/g$ and 300 $\mu g/kg$ for 50 percent of the population. There is a pattern of liver and kidney cadmium levels increasing simultaneously until the average renal cortex cadmium concentration is about 300 $\mu g/g$ and the average liver level is about 60 $\mu g/g$. At higher liver levels, the renal cortex level is disproportionately low, as cadmium is lost from the kidney (Ellis *et al.*, 1985). Daily intakes in food of 140 to 260 μg cadmium per day for more than 50 years or workroom air exposures of 50 $\mu g/m^3$ for more than 10 years have produced renal dysfunction (Thun, 1989; WHO 1989). An epidemiological study on dose-response relationship of cadmium intake of rice from historical data using B_2-microglobulinuria as an index of renal tubular dysfunction found that the total cadmium intake over lifetime that produced an adverse health effect was 2000 mg for both men and women (Nogawa *et al.*, 1989).

The proteinuria is principally tubular, consisting of low-molecular-weight proteins whose tubular reabsorption has been impaired by cadmium injury to proximal tubular lining cells. The predominant protein is a B_2-microglobulin, but a number of other low-molecular-weight proteins have been identified in the urine of workers with excessive cadmium exposure, such as retinol-binding protein, lysozyme, ribonuclease, and immunoglobulin light chains (Lauwerys *et al.*, 1979). High-molecular-weight proteins in the urine, such as albumin and transferin, indicate that some workers may actually have a mixed proteinuria and suggest a glomerular effect as well. The pathogenesis of the glomerular lesion in cadmium nephropathy is not presently understood.

Role of Metallothionein in Cadmium Toxicity. Accumulation of cadmium in the kidney without apparent toxic effect is possible because of formation of cadmium-thionein or metal-lothionein, a metal–protein complex with a low molecular weight (about 6500 daltons) (Suzuki, 1982).

The amino acid composition of metallothionein is characterized by approximately 30 percent cysteine and the absence of aromatic amino acids. Specific optical absorption is due to location of metal thiolate complexes in the protein. Metallothionein contains 61 amino acids, and 20 are cysteine. Structural studies using nuclear magnetic resonance spectroscopy and electron spin resonance spectroscopy have identified two distinct metal clusters in mammalian metallothionein. The clusters seem to have significant differences in their affinity for different metal ions; one of the clusters has a high level of specificity for zinc. Metal binding is by trimercaptide bridges (Boulanger et al., 1983). Metallothionein is primarily a tissue protein and is ubiquitous in most ograns but is in highest concentration in liver, particularly following recent exposure, and in kidney where it accumulates with age in proportion to cadmium concentration.

Cadmium bound to metallothionein within tissues is thought to be nontoxic; however, when the levels of cadmium exceed the critical concentration, it becomes toxic. The factors that determine the level of cadmium or cadmium-metallothionein complex that is toxic are not clear, but several hypotheses have been proposed. A favored hypothesis attributes the nephrotoxicity of cadmium to that fraction of cadmium within cells that is not bound to metallothionein, that is, when the level of cadmium exceeds that of metallothionein available for binding (Nomiyama and Nomiyama, 1986; Goyer et al., 1989a). Another hypothesis is that extracellular cadmium bound to metallothionein is toxic (Cherian et al., 1976). Cadmium-metallothionein derived from cadmium-induced synthesis in reticulocytes (Tanaka et al., 1985) or released from liver cells is filtered by the renal glomeruli and reabsorbed by proximal tubular lining cells, where it is catabolized, releasing cadmium ions, which cause renal damage (Dudley et al., 1985). Support for this hypothesis is that parenterally administered cadmium-metallothionein is very toxic to renal tubular cells and that the plasma level of metallothionein increases with cadmium exposure (Lauwerys et al., 1980). Another proposal is that cadmium displaces essential metals from metallothionein, depriving important metalloenzymes of essential metal cofactors (Petering et al., 1984).

These hypotheses are not mutually exclusive, and the relative significance of each mechanism may differ under particular circumstances.

Reversibility of Renal Effects. Follow-up studies of persons with renal tubular dysfunction (β_2-microglobulinuria) from occupational exposure to cadmium have shown that the proteinuria is irreversible and that there is a significant increase of creatinine in serum with time, suggesting a progressive glomerulopathy (Roels et al.,

1989). Also, persons with renal tubular dysfunction from excess dietary ingestion of cadmium (cadmium-polluted rice) do not have reversal of defect as long as 10 years after reduced exposure in cases when the β_2-microglobulinuria exceeds 1000 μg/g creatinine (Kido et al., 1988). Ellis et al. (1985) have shown, however, that liver cadmium in workers no longer exposed to cadmium gradually declines. Persistence of renal tubular dysfunction after cessation of exposure may reflect the level of body burden and shifting of cadmium from liver to kidney.

Skeletal System. Cadmium toxicity affects calcium metabolism, and individuals with severe cadmium nephropathy may have renal calculi and excess excretion of calcium, probably related to increased urinary loss, but with chronic exposure, urine calcium may be less than normal. Associated skeletal changes are probably related to calcium loss and include bone pain, osteomalacia, and/or osteoporosis. Bone changes are part of a syndrome recognized in postmenopausal multiparous women living in the Fuchu area of Japan prior to and during World War II. The syndrome consisted of severe bony deformities and chronic renal disease. Excess cadmium exposure has been implicated in the pathogenesis of the syndrome, but vitamin D and perhaps other nutritional deficiencies are thought to be cofactors. "Itai-Itai" translates to "ouch-ouch", reflecting the accompanying bone pain (Nomiyama, 1980). Also, cadmium can affect calcium, phosphorus, and bone metabolism in both industrial workers and people exposed in the general environment. These effects may be secondary to the cadmium effects on the kidneys, but there has been little study of calcium metabolism in people with excess exposure to cadmium. The increased prevalence of renal stones reported from certain industries is probably one manifestation of the cadmium-induced kidney effects. It is not known if certain factors other than cadmium may play a role.

Osteomalacia has been reported in a few heavily exposed industrial workers and people with Itai-Itai disease. The industrial cases were mainly male, whereas Itai-Itai cases were almost exclusively female. However, the clinical features and biochemical findings are similar except Itai-Itai patients may have osteoporosis as well.

Nogawa et al. (1987) reported that serum $1\alpha,25(OH)_2$ vitamin D levels were lower in Itai-Itai disease patients and cadmium-exposed subjects with renal damage than in nonexposed subjects. Decrease in serum $1\alpha,25(OH)_2$ vitamin D levels was closely related to serum concentrations of parathyroid hormone, B_2-microglobulin, and percentage TRP, suggesting that cadmium-induced bone effects were mainly due to a disturbance in vitamin D and parathyroid hormone metabolism. Friberg *et al.* (1986a) suggest that cadmium in the proximal tubular cells depresses cellular functions, which may be followed by the depressed conversion of 25(OH) vitamin D to $1\alpha,25(OH)_2$ vitamin D. This is likely to lead to a decreased calcium absorption and a decreased mineralization of bone, which in turn may lead to osteomalacia.

Hypertension and Cardiovascular Disease. Epidemiology studies suggest that cadmium is an etiological agent for essential hypertension. A recent study found an increase in systolic and diastolic blood pressures in cadmium workers. Only systolic, but not diastolic, blood pressure was significantly associated with cadmium dose in multivariate analyses (Thun *et al.*, 1989). Studies from Japan have found a twice-as-high cerebrovascular disease mortality rate among people who had cadmium-induced renal tubular proteinuria as among people in cadmium-polluted areas without proteinuria (Nogawa *et al.*, 1979).

Rats exposed to cadmium in drinking water (Kopp *et al.*, 1983) developed electrocardiographic and biochemical changes in the myocardium and impairment of the functional status of the myocardium. These effects may be related to (1) decreased high-energy phosphate stored in the myocardium, (2) reduced myocardial contractility, and (3) diminished excitability of the cardiac conduction system. Jamall and Sprowls (1987) found that rats supplemented with copper, selenium, and cadmium in diets had marked reduction in heart cytosolic glutathione peroxidase, superoxide desmutase, and catalase. They suggest that heart mitochondria are the site of the cadmium-induced biochemical lesion in the myocardium.

Carcinogenicity. There have been a number of epidemiologic studies intended to determine a relationship between occupational (respiratory) exposure to cadmium and lung cancer and prostatic cancer. A follow-up study of cadmium-nickel battery workers in Britain (Sorahan and Waterhouse, 1983) and in Sweden (Kjellstrom *et al.*, 1979) found increased risks to lung and prostate cancer. Increase in respiratory cancers was also found in a restudy of a cohort in a U.S. cadmium-recovery plant (Thun *et al.*, 1985). These and other studies have been reviewed by the IARC (1987), with the conclusion that long-term occupational exposure to cadmium may contribute to lung cancer, but confounding exposures to arsenic, nickel, and possibly other respiratory carcinogens including cigarette smoking prevent a definitive conclusion. For prostatic cancer, the risk appears debatable.

The evidence for carcinogenicity of cadmium from experimental studies, however, is regarded by the IARC (1987) as sufficient. Cadmium chloride, oxide, sulfate, and sulfide produced local sarcomas in rats after their subcutaneous injection, and cadmium powder and cadmium sulfide produced local sarcomas in rats following their intramuscular administration. Cadmium chloride produced a dose-dependent increase in the incidence of lung carcinomas in rats after exposure by inhalation and a low incidence (5/100) of prostatic carcinomas after injection into the ventral prostate (Takenaka *et al.*, 1983).

Biologic Indicators. The most important measure of excessive cadmium exposure is increased cadmium excretion in urine. In persons in the general population, without excessive cadmium exposure, urine cadmium excretion is both small and constant. That is, it is usually on the order of only 1 or 2 μg/day, or less than 1 μg/g creatinine. With excessive exposure to cadmium as might occur in workers, increase in urine cadmium may not occur until all the available cadmium binding sites are saturated. However, when binding sites (metallothionein) are saturated, increased urine cadmium reflects recent exposure and body burden and renal cadmium concentration, so that urine cadmium measurement does provide a good index of excessive cadmium exposure. Nogawa *et al.* (1979) determined the urinary concentration of cadmium corresponding to a 1 percent prevalence rate of a number of abnormal urinary findings (Table 19–4). Tubular proteinuria, as indicated by measurable excretion of β_2-microglobulin, occurred at the 1 percent prevalence rate with a urinary cadmium concentration of 3.2 μg/g of creatinine. This was at a slightly lower urine cadmium level than other signs of renal tubular dysfunction. Retinol binding protein may be a more practical and reliable test of proximal tubular function than β_2-microglobulin because sensitive immunologic analytic methods are now available, and it is more stable in urine (Lauwerys *et al.*, 1984). Urinary excretion of N-acetyl-β-D-glucosaminidase activity may be an even more sensitive indicator of cadmium-induced renal tubular dysfunction than β_2-microglobulin (Kawada *et al.*, 1989). Changes in urinary excretion of low-molecular-weight proteins are mainly observed in workers excreting more than 10 μg cadmium per gram creatinine (Buchet *et al.*, 1980).

Most of the cadmium in urine is bound to metallothionein, and there is good correlation between metallothionein and cadmium in urine in cadmium workers with normal or abnormal renal function. Therefore, measurement of metallothionein in urine provides the same toxicologic information as measurement of cadmium

Table 19–4. URINARY CADMIUM CONCENTRATION CORRESPONDING TO 1 PERCENT PREVALENCE RATE FOR PARAMETERS OF RENAL DYSFUNCTION*

	URINARY CADMIUM μg/g CREATININE	
URINARY FINDING	*Male*	*Female*
Tubular proteinuria		
β_2-microglobulin	3.2	5.2
Retinal binding protein	4.4	7.4
Aminoaciduria (proline)	10.4	5.1
Proteinuria with glucosuria	7.4	7.4

* Data from Nogawa, K.; Kobayashi, E.; and Honda, R.: A study of the relationship between cadmium concentrations in urine and renal effects of cadmium. *Environ. Health Perspect.*, 28, 161–168, 1979.

and, in addition, does not have the problem of external contamination. Radioimmunoassay techniques for measurement of metallothionein are available (Chang *et al.*, 1980).

Treatment. Susceptibility to cadmium-induced toxicity is influenced by a number of factors, particularly ability of the body to provide binding sites on metallothionein. Protection is provided by dietary zinc, cobalt, or selenium. Treatment of the toxicity of cadmium on the kidney is to cease exposure to cadmium (Nordberg *et al.*, 1978).

The thiol-containing chelators such as BAL and penicillamine increase the biliary excretion of cadmium, whereas EDTA, DTPA, and related chelators increase urinary excretion if given shortly after cadmium exposure before new metallothionein is synthesized (Cherian and Rodgers, 1982). For chronic cadmium exposure, when cadmium is bound to metallothionein, the most promising compounds are derivatives of dithiocarbamates (Jones *et al.*, 1988). N-Benzyl-D-glucamin dithiocarbamate will reduce body burden of cadmium from chronically exposed rats and mice (Kojima *et al.*, 1989).

Chromium

Chromium is a generally abundant element in the earth's crust and occurs in oxidation states ranging from Cr^{2+} to Cr^{6+}, but only trivalent and hexavalent forms are of biologic significance. The trivalent is the more common form. However, hexavalent forms of chromate compounds are of greater industrial importance. Sodium chromate and dichromate are the principal substances for the production of all chromium chemicals. Sodium dichromate is produced industrially by the reaction of sulfuric acid

on sodium chromate. The major source of chromium is from chromite ore. Metallurgic-grade chromite is usually converted into one of several types of ferrochromium or other chromium alloys containing cobalt or nickel. Ferrochrome is used for the production of stainless steel. Chromates are produced by a smelting, roasting, and extraction process. The major uses of sodium dichromate are for the production of chrome pigments; for the production of chrome salts used for tanning leather, mordant dying, and wood preservatives; and as an anticorrosive in cooking systems, boilers, and oil drilling muds (Fishbein, 1981).

Chromium in ambient air originates from industrial sources, particularly ferrochrome production, ore refining, chemical and refractory processing, and combustion of fossil fuels. In rural areas, chromium in air is usually less than 0.1 ng/m^3 and from 0.01 to 0.03 μg/m^3 in industrial cities. Particulates from coal-fired power plants may contain from 2.3 to 31 ppm, but this is reduced to 0.19 to 6.6 ppm by fly-ash collection. Cement-producing plants are another important potential source of atmospheric chromium. Chromium precipitates and fallout are deposited on land and water; land fallout is eventually carried to water by runoff, where it is deposited in sediments. A controllable source of chromium is waste water from chrome-plating and metal-finishing industries, textile plants, and tanneries. Chromium in food is low, and estimates of daily intake by humans are under 100 μg, mostly from food, with trivial quantities from most water supplies and ambient air.

Disposition. Trivalent chromium is the most common form found in nature, and chromium in biologic materials is probably always trivalent. There is no evidence that trivalent chromium is converted to hexavalent forms in biologic systems. However, hexavalent chromium readily crosses cell membranes and is reduced intracellularly to trivalent chromium.

The known harmful effects of chromium in humans have been attributed to the hexavalent form, and it has been speculated that the biologic effects of hexavalent chromium may be related to the reduction to trivalent chromium and the formation of complexes with intracellular macromolecules. High concentrations of chromium are normally found in RNA, but its role is unknown. Chromium (III) is considered an essential trace nutrient serving as a component of the "glucose tolerance factor" (Mertz, 1969). It is a cofactor for insulin action and has a role in the peripheral activities of this hormone by forming a ternary complex with insulin receptors, facilitating the attachment of insulin to these sites. The most biologically active form of insulin appears to be a naturally occurring complex containing niacin as well as glycine, glutamic acid, and cysteine.

Human chromium deficiency may be occurring in infants suffering from protein-caloric malnutrition and elderly people with impaired glucose tolerance, but this is not well documented. Prolonged use of a synthetic diet without chromium supplementation may lead to chromium deficiency, impaired glucose metabolism, and possibly effects on growth and on lipid and protein metabolism. Half-time for elimination of chromium from rats is 0.5, 5.9, and 83.4 days, according to a three-compartment model (Mertz, 1969).

Human kinetic studies have identified an erythrocyte chromium compartment that corresponds to the survival time of the red blood cell and is almost exclusively excreted in urine.

Toxicology. Systemic toxicity to chromium compounds occurs largely from accidental exposures, occasional attempts to use chromium as a suicidal agent, and previous therapeutic uses. The major acute effect from ingested chromium is acute renal tubular necrosis.

Exposure to chromium, particularly in the chrome production and chrome pigment industries, is associated with cancer of the respiratory tract (Langard and Norseth, 1986). As early as 1936, German health authorities recognized cancer of the lung among workers exposed to chromium dust. In a review paper from 1950, Baetjer described 109 cases of cancer in the chromate-producing industry, 11 cases in the chrome pigment industry, and two cases in other industries. In a review of the histologic classification of 123 cases of lung cancer in chromate workers, Hueper (1966) found 46 squamous cell carcinomas, 66 anaplastic tumors, and 11 adenocarcinomas. The greatest risk of cancer is attributed to exposure to acid-soluble, water-insoluble hexavalent chromium as occurs in the roasting or refining processes. Other studies have supported the greater risk of cancer from exposure to slightly soluble, hexavalent compounds rather than trivalent chromium compounds. Hexavalent chromium is corrosive and causes chronic ulceration and perforation of the nasal septum. It also causes chronic ulceration of other skin surfaces, which is independent of hypersensitivity reactions on skin. Allergic chromium skin reactions readily occur with exposure and are independent of dose. Trivalent chromium compounds are considerably less toxic than the hexavalent compounds and are neither irritating nor corrosive. Nevertheless, nearly all workers in industries are exposed to both forms of chromium compounds, and at present, there is no information as to whether there is a gradient of risk from predominant exposure to hexavalent or insoluble forms of chromium to exposure to soluble trivalent forms.

Whether chromium compounds cause cancer at sites other than the respiratory tract is not clear. A slight increase in cancer of the gastrointestinal tract has been reported in other studies, but each involved only small groups of workers.

Animal studies support the notion that the most potent carcinogenic chromium compounds are the slightly soluble hexavalent compounds. Studies on *in vitro* bacterial systems, however, show no difference between soluble and slightly soluble compounds. Trivalent chromium salts have little or no mutagenic activity in bacterial systems. Since there is preferred uptake of the hexavalent form by cells and it is the trivalent form that is metabolically active and binds with nucleic acids within the cell, it has been suggested that the causative agent in chromium mutagenesis is trivalent chromium bound to genetic material after reduction of the hexavalent form.

Human Body Burden. Tissue concentrations of chromium in the general population have considerable geographic variation, as high as 7 μg/kg in lungs of persons in New York or Chicago with lower concentrations in liver and kidney. In persons without excess exposure, blood chromium concentration is between 20 and 30 μg/liter and is evenly distributed between erythrocytes and plasma. With occupational exposure, increase in blood chromium is related to increase in chromium in red blood cells. Urinary excretion is generally less than 10 μg/day in the absence of excess exposure.

Lead

If we were to judge of the interest excited by any medical subject by the number of writings to which it has given birth, we could not but regard the poisoning by lead as the most important to be known of all those that have been treated of, up to the present time.

ORFILA, 1817

Lead, the most ubiquitous toxic metal, is detectable in practically all phases of the inert environment and in all biologic systems. Because it is toxic to most living things at high exposures and there is no demonstrated biologic need, the major issue regarding lead is at what dose does it become toxic. Specific concerns vary with the age and circumstances of the host, and the major risk is toxicity to the nervous system. The most susceptible populations are children, particularly toddlers and infants in the neonatal period and the unborn fetus. Several reviews and multi-authored books on the toxicology of lead are available (NAS, 1972; Goyer and Rhyne, 1973; WHO, 1977b; Mahaffey, 1985; EPA, 1986, 1989a; Landrigan, 1989).

Sources. The principal route of exposure is food, but it is usually environmental and presumably controllable sources that produce excess exposure and toxic effects. These sources include lead-based indoor paint in old dwellings, lead in air from combustion of lead-containing auto exhausts or industrial emissions, lead-based paint, hand-to-mouth activities of young children living in polluted environments, and less commonly, lead dust brought home by industrial workers on their clothes and shoes, and lead-glazed earthenware.

Dietary intake of lead has been thought to decrease since the 1940s when estimates were 400 to 500 μg/day for U.S. populations to present levels of under 100 μg/day for adults (EPA, 1986).

Most municipal water supplies measured at the tap contain less than 0.05 μg/ml, so that daily intake from water is usually about 10 μg and unlikely to be more than 20 μg. Adults absorb 5 to 15 percent of ingested lead and usually retain less than 5 percent of what is absorbed. Children are known to have a greater absorption of lead than adults; one study found an average net absorption of 41.5 percent and 31.8 percent net retention in infants on regular diets.

Lead in the atmosphere exists either in solid forms, dust or particulates of lead dioxide, or in the form of vapors, particularly alkyl lead that has escaped by evaporation from automobile fuel systems.

Lead absorption by the lungs also depends on a number of factors in addition to concentration. These include volume of air respired per day, whether the lead is in particle or vapor form, and size distribution of lead-containing particles. Only a very minor fraction of particles over 0.5 μm in mean maximal external diameter is retained in the lung but is cleared from the respiratory track and swallowed. However, the percentage of particles less than 0.5 μm retained in the lung increases with reduction in particle size. About 90 percent of lead particles in ambient air that are deposited in the lungs are small enough to be retained. Absorption of retained lead through alveoli is relatively efficient and complete.

Concentrations of lead in air vary widely and may be lower than 1.0 μg/m^3 in certain urban environments. For the contemporary urbanite in the United States, air lead today is a minor component of total daily lead exposure.

More than 90 percent of lead in blood is in the red blood cells. There seem to be at least two major compartments for lead in the red blood

cell, one associated with the membrane and the other with hemoglobin. Small fractions may be related to other red blood cell components. Plasma ligands are not well defined, but it has been suggested that plasma and serum may contain diffusible fractions of lead in equilibrium with soft tissue or end-organ binding sites for lead. This fraction is difficult to measure accurately, but there is an equilibrium between red cell and plasma lead.

National estimates of the present extent and severity of recent human exposure to lead are based on blood lead level measurements from the second National Health and Nutrition Examination Survey of 1976–80. These data give estimates of the distribution of blood lead levels in the general United States population aged 6 months to 74 years. Lead in blood was found to vary with age and sex (Figure 19–3).

Preschool children aged 6 months to 5 years and adults of 25 to 54 years showed the highest blood lead levels, with a decreasing trend with increasing age from 6 months until late adolescence. Mean values declined from 16.3 μg/dl at 6 months to 2 years to 12.1 μg/dl at 15 to 17 years. Among adults ages 18 to 74 years, the mean blood lead levels increased significantly across successive age groups, reaching a maximum of 15.3 μg/dl at 45 to 54 years and then declining slightly in the older age groups. The trend with age in mean blood lead levels was generally similar among males and females. However, the mean levels were significantly lower in females than males (mean of 11.9 and 16.1 μg/dl, respectively).

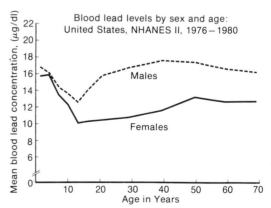

Figure 19–3. National estimates of blood lead levels in the United States. (From Mahaffey, K. R.; Annest, J. L.; Roberts, J. H.; and Murphy, R. S.: Estimates of blood lead levels: United States 1976–1980. Association with selected demographic and socioeconomic factors. *N. Engl. J. Med.*, **307**:573–579, 1982. Reprinted by permission of *The New England Journal of Medicine.*)

The total body burden of lead may be divided into at least two kinetic pools, which have different rates of turnover. The largest and kinetically slowest pool is the skeleton with a half-life of more than 20 years and a much more labile soft tissue pool. The total lifetime accumulation of lead may be about 200 mg and over 500 mg for an occupationally exposed worker. Kidney lead accumulates with age; lead in lung does not change. Lead in the central nervous system tends to concentrate in gray matter and certain nuclei. The highest concentrations are in the hippocampus, followed by cerebellum, cerebral cortex, and medulla. Cortical white matter seems to contain the least amount, but these comments are based on only a few reported human and animal studies.

Renal excretion of lead is usually with glomerular filtrate with some renal tubular resorption. With elevated blood lead levels, excretion may be augmented by transtubular transport.

Transplacental Transport of Lead. There is no impediment to the transplacental transport of lead (Goyer, in press). Cord blood generally correlates with maternal blood lead levels but is slightly lower. Maternal blood lead decreases slightly during pregnancy, suggesting that maternal lead is transferred to the fetus. Fetal tissues, including brain, maintain a steady concentration of lead regardless of increase in size.

Toxicity. The toxic effects of lead and the minimum blood lead level at which the effect is likely to be observed are shown in Table 19–5. The toxic effects from lead form a continuum from clinical or overt effects to subtle or biochemical effects. These effects involve several organ systems and biochemical activities. The critical effects or most sensitive effects in infants and children involve the nervous system (Rutter and Jones, 1983; ATSDR, 1989; EPA, 1989b; Needleman *et al.*, 1990). For adults with excess occupational exposure, or even accidental exposure, the concerns are peripheral neuropathy and/or chronic nephropathy. However, the critical effect or most sensitive effect for adults in the general population may be hypertension (EPA, 1989b). Effects on the heme system provide biochemical indicators of lead exposure in the absence of chemically detectable effects, but anemia due to lead exposure is uncommon without other detectable effects or other synergistic factors. Other target organs are the gastrointestinal and reproductive systems.

Nearly all environmental exposure to lead is to inorganic compounds, even lead in food. Organolead exposures, including tetraethyl lead, have unique toxicologic patterns (Grandjean and Grandjean, 1984).

Neurological, Neurobehavioral, and Developmental Effects in Children. Clinically overt lead encephalopathy may occur in children with high exposure to lead, probably at blood lead levels of 80 μg/dl or higher. Symptoms of lead encephalopathy begin with lethargy, vomiting, irritability, loss of appetite, and dizziness and progress to obvious ataxia and reduced level of consciousness, which may progress to coma and death. The pathological findings at autopsy are severe edema of the brain due to extravasation of fluid from capillaries in the brain. This is accompanied by loss of neuronal and increase in glial cells. Recovery is often accompanied by sequelae including epilepsy, mental retardation, and optic neuropathy and blindness in some cases (Perlstein and Attala, 1966).

Studies conducted during the 1970s indicate children with blood lead levels in 50- to 70-μg range, but without clinical symptoms of lead poisoning, may have decrements in expected cognitive abilities by as much as 5 or more I.Q points (Rutter and Jones, 1983).

In 1979, Needleman and coworkers reported that first- and second-grade children without symptoms of lead toxicity, but with elevated dentine lead levels, had deficits in psychometric intelligence, speech and language processing, attention, and classroom performance. At the fifth-grade level, those subjects with higher dentine levels had lower I.Q. scores and a greater need for special academic services (Bellinger *et al.*, 1986). In a ten-year follow-up of 122 of these children, neurobehavioral deficits were found to persist (Needleman *et al.*, 1990). These effects are termed "low-level lead toxicity," and they are now believed to be associated with blood lead levels of approximately 30 to 50 μg/dl or possibly even lower blood lead levels. These effects are also termed "subclinical lead toxicity" because they can only be detected by assessment of neuropsychologic behavior, such as hyperactivity or poor classroom behavior (decreased attention span).

For blood lead levels below 30 μg/dl, the evidence for I.Q. decrements are quite mixed, with some studies showing no deficit of I.Q. with blood lead levels below 30 if all variables are controlled (M. A. Smith *et al.*, 1983; McMichael *et al.*, 1988). The effects of low-level lead exposure (blood lead, 30 to 50 μg/dl) on CNS function is further supported by the finding of changes in EEG brain wave patterns and CNS-evoked potential responses in children displaying neuropsychologic deficits (Burchfiel *et al.*, 1980). A large-scale study conducted by M. A. Smith *et al.* (1983) of blood and tooth lead, behavior, intelligence, and a variety of other psychological skills in a population of

Table 19–5. LOWEST OBSERVED EFFECT LEVELS FOR INDUCED HEALTH EFFECTS,* BLOOD LEAD CONCENTRATION, μg/dl

EFFECT	CHILDREN	ADULTS
Heme Effects		
Anemia	80–100	80–100
U-ALA	40	40
B-EPP	15	15
ALA inhibition	10	<10
Py-5-N inhibition	<10	—
Neuro Effects		
Encephalopathy (overt)	80–100	100–120
Subclinical encephalopathy	—	50
I.Q. deficits	<30	—
In utero effects	<15	—
Peripheral neuropathy	40	40
Renal Effects		
Acute nephropathy (aminoaciduria)	80–100	?
Chronic nephropathy	—	60
Vit. D metabolism	<30	—
B.P. (males)	—	30 ?

* Modified from EPA: *Air Quality Criteria for Lead,* Vols. I–IV. EPA–600/8–83/02aF. U.S. Environmental Protection Agency, Washington, D.C., 1986.

4000 children aged six to seven years in three London boroughs found, on initial analysis, no statistically significant association between lead level and I.Q. or academic performance. However, further analysis of these data by Pocock *et al.* (1985) found that the I.Q. of the group of children with average blood lead levels of 12 to 15 μg/dl was 2 points below average for the control group. A prospective study of newborns in Boston not only supports concern for blood lead levels in the 10- to 15-μg/dl range but suggests that deficits in mental development may occur with umbilical cord blood lead levels of 6 to 7 μg/dl in lower socioeconomic strata children (Bellinger *et al.*, 1988). Since the studies involved concern effects associated with blood lead levels in pregnant women, umbilical cords, and infants up to two years of age, it is not clear whether this level applied to only fetuses or infants or preschool-age children. Therefore, a blood lead level of 10 to 15 μg/dl and possibly lower should be avoided in pregnant women, although they *per se* are not necessarily the population at risk. Other risk factors are emerging from these studies (EPA, 1989b).

SIGNIFICANCE OF 4-POINT REDUCTION IN I.Q. The biologic importance of a 4- to 7-point reduction in I.Q. may on first appearance seem unimportant, but further analyses suggest small changes to be of considerable significance when the actual cumulative frequency distributions of I.Q. between high- and low-lead subjects are

plotted and compared. There is a nearly fourfold increase in the number of children with a severe deficit, that is, I.Q. scores below 80. Also, the same shift truncates the upper end of the curve where there is a 5 percent reduction in children with superior function (I.Q. > 125). There is presently no estimate of the cost of this effect at the high end of the curve, but it may be of considerable importance to society (Needleman, 1989).

MECHANISMS OF NEUROTOXICITY. Experimental studies have shown that lead in the absence of morphologic changes does produce deficits in neurotransmission through inhibition of cholinergic function, possibly by reduction of extracellular calcium. Other noted changes in neurotransmitter function include impairment of dopamine uptake by synaptosomes and impairment of the function of the inhibitory neurotransmitter γ-aminobutyric acid (Rossouw *et al.*, 1987). Also, the fetal brain may have greater sensitivity to lead toxicity than the more mature brain. Studies of capillaries from children poisoned with lead and from experimental studies suggest that the immature endothelial cells forming the capillaries of the developing brain are less resistant to the effects of lead than capillaries from mature brains and permit fluid and cations including lead to reach newly formed components of the brain, particularly astrocytes and neurons. More recently, Markovac and Goldstein (1988) found lead may replace calcium in the activation of phospholipid-dependent protein kinase (protein kinase C) in brain microvessels.

Human data relating the effects of lead on heme metabolism and neurotoxicity are limited. The EPA criteria document for lead (1986) concludes that D-ALA may be neurotoxic by impairing γ-aminobutyric acid (GABA) functions by interaction with presynaptic receptors. Decreased levels of heme in the liver due to lead exposure may inhibit the activity of tryptophan pyrrolase, resulting in increased levels of tryptophan, serotonin, and 5-hydroxyindoleacetic acid in brain. Also, the fetal brain may have greater sensitivity to lead toxicity than the more mature brain because of immaturity in the blood-brain barrier.

PERIPHERAL NEUROPATHY. Peripheral neuropathy is a classic manifestation of lead toxicity, particularly the footdrop and wristdrop that characterized the house painter and other workers with excessive occupational exposure to lead more than a half-century ago. Segmental demyelination and possibly axonal degeneration follow lead-induced Schwann cell degeneration. Wallerian degeneration of posterior roots of sciatic and tibial nerves is possible, but sensory nerves are less sensitive to lead than motor nerve structure and function. Motor nerve dysfunction, assessed clinically by electrophysiologic measurement of nerve conduction velocities, has been shown to occur with blood lead levels as low as 40 μg/dl (EPA, 1986).

Hematologic Effects. Lead has multiple hematologic effects. In lead-induced anemia, the red blood cells are microcytic and hypochromic, as in iron deficiency, and usually there are increased numbers of reticulocytes with basophilic stippling, which results from inhibition of the enzyme pyrimidine-5-nucleotidase (Py-5-N)

(Paglia *et al.*, 1975). There is an inverse relationship between Py-5-N inhibition with blood lead concentration. A threshold for Py-5-N inhibition has been found to be 44 μg/dl or higher, but a study of 21 children two to five years of age found no threshold of effects of lead on activity of this enzyme or cell nucleotide contents even below 10 μg/dl. There was also a significant positive correlation of pyrimidine accumulation and the accumulation of zinc protoporphyrin (ZPP). Inhibition of Py-5-N activity and nucleotide accumulation with lead exposure affects erythrocyte membrane stability and survival by altering cell energy metabolism.

The anemia that occurs in lead poisoning results from two basic defects: shortened erythrocyte life span and impairment of heme synthesis. Shortened life span of the red blood cell is thought to be due to increased mechanical fragility of the cell membrane. The biochemical basis for this effect is not known but is accompanied by inhibition of sodium- and potassium-dependent ATPases (EPA, 1986).

A schematic presentation of effects of lead on heme synthesis is shown in Figure 19–4. Probably the sensitive effect is inhibition of δ-aminolevulinic acid dehydratase (ALA-D), resulting in a negative exponential relationship between ALA-D and blood lead. There is also depression of coproporphyrinogen oxidase, resulting in increased coproporphyrin activity. Lead also decreases ferrochelatase activity. This enzyme catalyzes the incorporation of the ferrous ion into the porphyrin ring structure. Bessis and Jensen (1965) have shown that iron in the form of apoferritin and ferruginous micelles may accumulate in mitochondria of bone marrow reticulocytes from lead-poisoned rats. Failure to insert iron into protoporphyrin results in depressed heme formation. The excess pro-

MITOCHONDRION

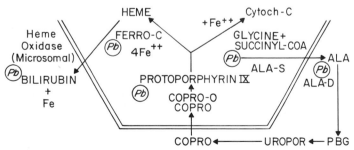

Figure 19–4. Scheme of heme synthesis showing sites where lead has an effect. *COA,* coenzyme A; *ALA-S,* aminolevulinic acid synthetase; *ALA,* d-aminolevulinic acid; *ALA-D,* aminolevulinic acid dehydratase; *PBG,* porphobilinogen; *UROPOR,* uroporphyrinogen; *COPRO,* coproporphyrinogen; *COPRO-O,* coproporphyrinogen oxidase; *FERRO-C,* ferrochelatase; *CYTOCH-C,* cytochrome c; Ⓟ, site for lead effect.

toporphyrin takes the place of heme in the hemoglobin molecule, and as the red blood cells containing protoporphyrin circulate, zinc is chelated at the center of the molecule at the site usually occupied by iron. Red blood cells containing zinc-protoporphyrin are intensely fluorescent and may be used to diagnose lead toxicity. Depressed heme synthesis is thought to be the stimulus for increasing the rate of activity of the first step in the heme synthetic pathway, δ-aminolevulinic acid synthetase, by virtue of negative feedback control. As a consequence, the increased production of δ-aminolevulinic acid and decreased activity of ALA-D result in a marked increase in circulating blood levels and urinary excretion of δ-ALA. Prefeeding of lead to experimental animals also raises heme oxygenase activity, resulting in some increase in bilirubin formation. The change in rates of activity of these enzymes by lead produces a dose-related alteration in activity of affected enzymes, but anemia only occurs in very marked lead toxicity. The changes in enzyme activities, particularly ALA-D in peripheral blood and excretion of ALA in urine, correlate very closely with actual blood lead levels and serve as early biochemical indices of lead exposure (EPA, 1986).

The sensitivity of specific individuals to lead effects on heme metabolism may be related to genetic polymorphisms of heme among people in the general population (EPA, 1986). The *ALA-D* gene has two common alleles, *ALA-D¹* and *ALA-D²*, which results in a polymorphic enzyme system with three distinct isozyme phenotypes, identified as ALA-D1-1, ALA-D1-2, ALA-D2-2. Frequencies of the isoenzyme phenotypes determined in an Italian population are 1-1, 81 percent; 2-1, 17 percent; and 2-2, 2 percent, whereas expression of *ALA-D²* was not observed in blacks in Liberia. At the biochemical level, no differences in reactivation of the isoenzymes have been reported. It has been suggested that individuals with 2-2 phenotype may develop increased lead accumulation and associated physiological effects (Ziemsen *et al.*, 1986). The *D²* allele may provide a basis for increased sensitivity to lead (Astrin *et al.*, 1987).

Renal Effects. Toxicologic effects of lead on the kidney divide into two major concerns: (1) reversible renal tubular dysfunction that occurs mostly in children with acute exposure to lead, usually associated with overt central nervous system effects, and (2) irreversible chronic interstitial nephropathy characterized by vascular sclerosis, tubular cell atrophy, interstitial fibrosis, and glomerular sclerosis (Goyer, 1971a). It is most often seen in workmen with years of exposure to lead. In the early stages of excess lead exposure, morphologic and functional

changes in the kidney are confined to the renal tubules and are most pronounced in proximal tubular cells. Mitochondria from kidney of lead-exposed rats have impaired oxidation and phosphorylation, which may be responsible for decrease in resorptive function of proximal tubular cells.

A pathognomonic feature of lead poisoning is the presence of characteristic nuclear inclusion bodies. By light microscopy the inclusions are dense, homogeneous eosinophilic bodies. They are acid-fast when stained with carbolfuchsin. Ultrastructurally, the bodies have a dense central core and outer fibrillary region, as shown in Figure 19–5. The bodies are composed of a lead-protein complex (Moore *et al.*, 1973). The protein is acidic and contains large amounts of aspartic and glutamic acids and little cystine. It is suggested that lead binds loosely to the carboxyl groups of the acidic amino acids. Most of the lead in the tubular cell is bound to the inclusion body. The sequestering of lead in these complexes may protect more susceptible organelles like mitochondria and endoplasmic reticulum (Goyer, 1971b). Experimental studies have shown that nuclear inclusion bodies are the earliest evidence of lead exposure and may be observed before any of the functional changes are detectable.

The pathogenesis of the inclusion bodies may be related to renal tubular cell transport and excretion of lead. Treatment of lead-exposed animals with chelating agents such as EDTA is accompanied by a sudden spike of urinary lead, which is maximum 12 to 24 hours after treatment (Goyer and Wilson, 1975). Also, no inclusion

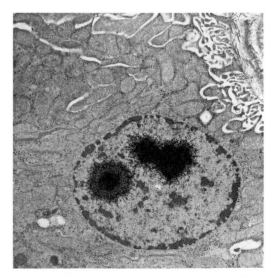

Figure 19–5. Lead-induced inclusion bodies in nucleus of renal tubular lining cell.

bodies can be found by morphologic study of renal tubular cells after EDTA therapy. The bodies may also be found intact in the urinary sediment of workmen with heavy exposure to lead (Schumann *et al.*, 1980). The bodies account for the major fraction of intracellular lead, and their loss in the urine may reflect a major pathway for lead excretion.

The origin of the protein-forming lead-induced inclusion bodies is uncertain. Egle and Shelton (1986) have shown that a nuclear matrix protein termed $p^{32}/6.3$ is the most abundant protein constituent of the inclusion bodies. This protein is normally present in neural tissue, but the metabolic mechanism responsible for its accumulation in the inclusion bodies induced by lead is not known. Lead has been shown to induce inclusion bodies in cytoplasm of kidney cells grown in culture. The bodies then tend to migrate into nuclei of the lead-exposed cells (McLaughlin *et al.*, 1980).

With continued exposure to lead, there is a gradual change in morphology beginning with the appearance of peritubular and periglomerular fibrosis, particularly in the deep cortex or juxtamedullary zone (Goyer, 1971a). This is accompanied by atrophy of some tubules and hyperplasia of others. There are also fewer inclusion bodies present in the advanced stages of lead-induced nephrosclerosis, and it may be impossible to find any inclusion bodies in lead-induced nephrosclerosis. Recognition of interstitial fibrosis induced by lead, therefore, from any other forms of interstitial fibrosis is not possible morphologically but must be made from history and knowledge of progression of the disease, if this is available.

The most important feature of the changes associated with acute lead nephropathy is that they are reversible, either by reduction of lead exposure or by chelation therapy, but the interstitial fibrosis of chronic lead nephropathy is not reversible. It is very important, therefore, to diagnose this disorder as early as possible so that exposure to lead can be discontinued and decrease in function halted. At the present time, there is no single definitive diagnostic test that will recognize lead-induced interstitial nephropathy except possibly renal biopsy, but this is not a practical measure. There have been several clinical studies in recent years of renal function in workmen with long-term occupational exposure to lead. If looked at together, the conclusion is reached that an early functional accompaniment of interstitial fibrosis is a reduction in glomerular filtration rate (Goyer, 1982).

Experimental studies in the rat suggest that there is a threshold for lead nephropathy with a blood lead level of about 45 μg/dl (Goyer

et al., 1989b), consistent with current occupational health standards and clinical observations.

The relationship between chronic lead exposure and gouty nephropathy, suggested more than a hundred years ago by the English physician Farrod, has received recent support from studies showing that gout patients with renal disease have a greater chelate-provoked lead excretion than do renal patients without gout. Lead reduces uric acid excretion. Elevated blood uric acid has been demonstrated in rats with chronic lead nephropathy (Goyer, 1971a).

Effect on Blood Pressure. Increase in blood pressure in probably the most sensitive adverse health effect from lead exposure occurring in the adult population. The addendum to the 1986 EPA *Air Quality Criteria for Lead* document (1989b) noted that a number of epidemiologic studies provided generally consistent evidence for the association between increased blood pressure and elevated body burden of lead in adults.

The largest study populations have been the second National Health and Nutrition Examination Survey (N-HANES II) for the U.S. population performed during the years 1976–80 and the British Regional Heart Study, an ongoing evaluation of men aged 40 to 59 from 24 British towns. The data collectively provide highly convincing evidence demonstrating small but statistically significant associations between blood lead levels and increased blood pressure in adult men; the strongest association was for males aged 40 to 59 and for systolic somewhat more so than for diastolic pressure. Virtually all the analyses demonstrate positive associations for the 40–59 age group, which remain or become significant (at $p < 0.05$) when adjustments are made for geographic site. Quantitatively, the relationship appears to hold across a wide range of blood lead values, extending down to as low as 7 μg/dl for middle-aged men. An estimated increase of about 1.5 to 3.0 mm Hg in systolic blood pressure occurs for every doubling of blood lead concentration in adult males but less than 1.0 to 2.0 mm Hg for adult females (Tyroler, 1988).

Lead may affect blood pressure by altering sensitivity of vascular smooth muscle to vasoactive stimuli or indirectly by altering neuroendocrine input to vascular smooth muscle. Lead-exposed persons may have higher plasma renin activity than normal during periods of modest exposure but normal or depressed plasma renin activity during more chronic severe exposures (Vander, 1988). Boscolo *et al.* (1981) found a slight but significant relationship between plasma renin and urinary kallikrein in men with occupational exposure to lead. Lead exposure may alter calcium-activated functions of vascular smooth muscle cells, including contractility, by decreasing Na^+/K^+-ATPase activity and stimulation of the Na/Ca exchange pump.

Carcinogenicity. Lead is classified as a 2B carcinogen by the IARC (1987). Evidence for carcinogenicity is adequate in animals but inadequate in humans.

A study of workmen in England many years ago with occupational exposure to lead did not show an increased incidence of cancer (Dingwall-Fordyce and Lane, 1963). Causes of mortality in 7000 lead workers in the United States showed a slight excess of deaths from cancer (Cooper and Gaffey, 1975), but the statistical significance of these findings has been debated (Cooper, 1980; Kang et al., 1980). The most common tumors found were of the respiratory and digestive systems, not the kidney. However, case reports of renal adenocarcinoma in workmen with prolonged occupational exposure to lead have appeared (Baker et al., 1980; Lilis, 1981).

Lead compounds stimulating proliferation of renal tubular epithelial cells (D. D. Choie and Richter, 1980) and similar effects have been noted in liver of rats (Columbano et al., 1983). Lead compounds induce cell transformation in Syrian hamster embryo cells (DiPaolo and Casto, 1979; Zelikoff et al., 1988).

Lead induction of renal adenocarcinoma in rats and mice is dose related and has not been reported at levels below that which produces nephrotoxicity (EPA, 1989a). The pathogenesis of lead-related renal tumors may be a related direct genetic effect on renal tubular cells but may also be a nonspecific response to epithelial hyperplasia, as has been noted in other experimental nephropathies and human diseases where renal tubular cysts and hyperplasia occur (Bernstein et al., 1987).

Other Effects. Severe lead toxicity has long been known to cause sterility, abortion, and neonatal mortality and morbidity. Studies have demonstrated gametotoxic effects in both male and female animals. However, the impact of levels of lead exposure occurring in today's society on reproductive effects is uncertain. The greatest concern is for intrauterine effects on the unborn fetus. Umbilical cord blood levels are the same as those of mother's blood, and because of the greater sensitivity of the fetus, pregnancy must be regarded as a period of increased susceptibility to lead (Goyer, in press).

A few clinical studies have found increased chromosomal defects in workers with blood lead levels above 60 μg/dl. Experimental studies suggest that lead alters the humoral immune system, and lead-induced immunosuppression

occurs at low dosages in experimental animals in which there is no apparent evidence of toxicity.

Lead lines (Burton's lines) or purple-blue discoloration of gingiva is a classical feature of severe lead toxicity in children with lead encephalopathy. However, this feature of lead toxicity and the presence of lead lines at the epiphyseal margins of long bones seen on X-rays of children with severe lead exposure are uncommon today.

Treatment. Chelation usually has a role in the treatment of the symptomatic worker or child. Institution of chelation therapy is probably warranted in workmen with blood lead levels over 60 μg/100 ml, but this determination must be made after assessment of exposure factors, including biologic estimates of clinical and biochemical parameters of toxicity.

For children, criteria have been established that may serve as guidelines to assist in evaluating the individual case (Chisholm and O'Hara, 1982). These include blood lead levels from 30 μg/dl up to 60 μg/dl, depending on free erythroprotoporphyrin (FEP) levels, and results of a lead mobilization test.

Also, cautionary measures for the safe use of chelating agents have been expressed particularly for Ca EDTA (Lilis and Fischbein, 1976). Serum blood urea nitrogen and creatinine are followed as indicators of renal function, and serum calcium is measured to monitor untoward effects of EDTA. In children with severe lead poisoning including encephalopathy, the mortality rate may be 25 to 38 percent when EDTA or BAL is used singly; combination therapy of EDTA and BAL has been shown to be effective in reducing mortality.

Mercury

No other metal better illustrates the diversity of effects caused by different chemical species than does mercury. On the basis of toxicologic characteristics, there are three forms of mercury; elemental, inorganic, and organic compounds. The major source of mercury is the natural degassing of the earth's crust, including land areas, rivers, and the ocean, and is estimated to be on the order of 25,000 to 150,000 tons per year (WHO, 1976; NRCC, 1979). Metallic mercury in the atmosphere represents the major pathway of global transport of mercury. Although anthropogenic sources of mercury have reached about 8,000 to 10,000 tons per year since 1973, nonanthropogenic sources are the predominating factors. Nevertheless, mining, smelting, and industrial discharge have been factors in environmental contamination in the past. For instance, it is estimated that loss in water effluent from chloralkali plants, one of the largest users of mercury, has been reduced 99 percent in recent years. Also, the use of mercury in the paper pulp industries has been reduced dramatically and has been banned in Sweden since 1966. Industrial activities not directly employing mercury or mercury products give rise to substantial quantities of this metal. Fossil fuel may contain as much as 1 ppm of mercury, and it is estimated that about 5000 tons of mercury per year may be emitted from burning coal, natural gas, and the refining of petroleum products. Calculations based on mercury content of the Greenland ice cap show an increase from the year 1900 to the present day and suggest that the increment is related to increase in background levels in rainwater and is related to man-made release. As much as one-third of atmospheric mercury may be due to industrial release of organic or inorganic forms. Regardless of source, both organic and inorganic forms of mercury may undergo environmental transformation. Metallic mercury may be oxidized to inorganic divalent mercury, particularly in the presence of organic material such as in the aquatic environment. Divalent inorganic mercury may, in turn, be reduced to metallic mercury when conditions are appropriate for reducing reactions to occur. This is an important conversion in terms of the global cycle of mercury and a potential source of mercury vapor that may be released to the earth's atmosphere. A second potential conversion of divalent mercury is methylation to dimethyl mercury by anaerobic bacteria. This may diffuse into the atmosphere and return to earth crust or bodies of water as methyl mercury in rainfall. If taken up by fish in the food chain, it may eventually cycle through humans.

Disposition. Toxicity of various forms or salts of mercury is related to cationic mercury *per se,* whereas solubility, biotransformation, and tissue distribution are influenced by valence state and anionic component (Berlin, 1986). Metallic or elemental mercury volatilizes to mercury vapor at ambient air temperatures, and most human exposure is by inhalation. Mercury vapor readily diffuses across the alveolar membrane and is lipid soluble, so that it has an affinity for red blood cells and the central nervous system. Metallic mercury, such as may be swallowed from a broken thermometer, is only slowly absorbed by the gastrointestinal tract (0.01 percent) at a rate related to the vaporization of the elemental mercury and is generally thought to be of no toxicologic consequence.

Inorganic mercury salts may be divalent (mercuric) or monovalent (mercurous). Gastrointestinal absorption of inorganic salts of mercury from food is less than 15 percent in mice and about 7 percent in a study of human volunteers, whereas absorption of methyl mercury is on the order of 90 to 95 percent. Distribution between red blood cells and plasma also differs. For inorganic mercury salts, cell-plasma ratio ranges from a high of two with high exposure to less than one, but for methyl mercury it is about ten. The distribution ratio of the two forms of mercury between hair and blood also differs; for organic mercury, it is about 250.

Kidneys contain the greatest concentrations of mercury following exposure to inorganic salts of mercury and mercury vapor, whereas organic mercury has a greater affinity for the brain, particularly the posterior cortex. However, mercury vapor has a greater predilection for the central nervous system than do inorganic mercury salts but less than organic forms of mercury.

Excretion of mercury from the body is by way of urine and feces, again differing with the form of mercury, size of dose, and time after exposure. Exposure to mercury vapor is followed by exhalation of a small fraction, but fecal excretion is the major route and is predominant initially after exposure to inorganic mercury. Renal excretion increases with time. About 90 percent of methyl mercury is excreted in feces after acute or chronic exposure and does not change with time (Miettenen, 1973).

All forms of mercury cross the placenta to the fetus, but most of what is known has been learned from experimental animals. Fetal uptake of elemental mercury in rats probably because of lipid solubility has been shown to be 10 to 40 times higher than uptake after exposure to inorganic salts. Concentrations of mercury in the fetus after exposure to alkylmercuric compounds are twice those found in maternal tissues, and methyl mercury levels in fetal red blood cells are 30 percent higher than in maternal red cells. The positive fetal-maternal gradient and increased concentration of mercury in fetal red blood cells enhance fetal toxicity to mercury, particularly following exposure to alkylmercury. Although maternal milk may contain only 5 percent of the mercury concentation of maternal blood, neonatal exposure to mercury may be greatly augmented by nursing.

Metabolic Transformation and Excretion. Elemental or metallic mercury is oxidized to divalent mercury after absorption to tissues in the body probably mediated by catalases. Inhaled mercury vapor absorbed into red blood cells is transformed to divalent mercury, but a portion is also transported as metallic mercury to more distal tissues, particularly the brain where biotransformation may occur. Methyl mercury undergoes biotransformation to divalent mercury compounds in tissues by cleavage of the carbon-mercury bond. There is no evidence of formation of any organic form of mercury in mammalian tissues. The aryl (phenyl) compounds are converted to inorganic mercury more rapidly than the shorter-chain alkyl (methyl) compounds. The relationship of these differences in rate of biotransformation versus rate of excretion and toxicity is not well understood. In those instances where the organomercurial is more rapidly excreted than inorganic mercury, increasing the rate of biotransformation will decrease the rate of excretion. Phenyl and methoxyethylmercury are excreted at about the same rate as inorganic mercury, whereas methyl mercury excretion is slower (Berlin, 1986).

Biologic half-times are available for a limited number of mercury compounds. Biologic half-time for methyl mercury is about 70 days and is virtually linear, whereas the half-time for retaining salts of inorganic mercury is about 40 days. There are few studies on biologic half-times for elemental mercury or mercury vapor, but it also appears to be linear with a range of values from 35 to 90 days.

Cellular Metabolism. Within cells, mercury may bind to a variety of enzyme systems including those of microsomes and mitochondria, producing nonspecific cell injury or cell death. It has a particular affinity for ligands containing sulfhydryl groups. In liver cells, methyl mercury forms soluble complexes with cysteine and glutathione, which are secreted in bile and reabsorbed from the gastrointestinal tract. Organomercurial diuretics are thought to be absorbed in the proximal tubule–binding specific receptor sites that inhibit sodium transport. In general, however, organomercury compounds undergo cleavage of the carbon-mercury bond, releasing ionic inorganic mercury.

Mercuric mercury, but not methyl mercury, induces synthesis of metallothionein probably only in kidney cells, but unlike cadmium-metallothionein it does not have a long biologic half-life. Mercury within renal cells becomes localized in lysosomes (Madsen and Christensen, 1978).

Toxicology. *Mercury Vapor.* Inhalation of mercury vapor may produce an acute, corrosive bronchitis and interstitial pneumonitis and, if not fatal, may be associated with symptoms of central nervous system effects such as tremor or increased excitability.

With chronic exposure to mercury vapor, the major effects are on the central nervous system. Early signs are nonspecific and have been termed the "asthenic-vegetative syndrome" or "micromercurialism." Identification of the syndrome requires neurasthenic symptoms and three or more of the following clinical findings: tremor, enlargement of the thyroid, increased uptake of radioiodine in the thyroid, labile pulse, tachycardia, dermographism, gingivitis, hematologic changes, or increased excretion of mercury in urine. With increasing exposure, the symptoms become more characteristic, beginning with intentional tremors of muscles that perform fine-motor functions (highly innervated), such as fingers, eyelids, and lips, and may progress to generalized trembling of the entire body and violent chronic spasms of the extremities. This is accompanied by changes in personality and behavior, with loss of memory, increased excitability (erethism), severe depression, and even delirium and hallucination. Another characteristic feature of mercury toxicity is severe salivation and gingivitis.

The triad of increased excitability, tremors, and gingivitis has been recognized historically as the major manifestation of mercury poisoning from inhalation of mercury vapor and exposure in the fur, felt, and hat industry to mercury nitrate (Goldwater, 1972).

Sporadic instances of proteinuria and even nephrotic syndrome may occur in persons with exposure to mercury vapor, particularly with chronic occupational exposure. The pathogenesis is probably immunologic similar to that which may occur following exposure to inorganic mercury.

In recent years, it has been claimed that mercury (vapor) released from dental amalgam may cause various health effects, but this topic is controversial. The uptake of mercury from amalgam is considerably less than has been associated with effects from occupational exposure to mercury (Fan, 1987). However, increase in mercury in urine and accumulation in several organs including the central nervous system and kidneys, from the release from amalgam, have been reported (Clarkson *et al.*, 1988; Langworth *et al.*, 1988).

Mercuric Mercury. Bichloride of mercury (corrosive sublimate) is the best-known inorganic salt of mercury, and the trivial name suggests its most apparent toxicologic effect when ingested in concentrations greater than 10 percent. A reference from the Middle Ages in Goldwater's book on mercury describes oral ingestion of mercury as causing severe abdominal cramps, bloody diarrhea, and suppression of urine (Goldwater, 1972). This is an accurate report of effects following accidental or suicidal ingestion of mercuric chloride or other mercuric salts. Corrosive ulceration, bleeding, and necrosis of the gastrointestinal tract are usually accompanied by shock and circulatory collapse. If the patient survives the gastrointestinal damage, renal failure occurs within 24 hours, owing to necrosis of the proximal tubular epithelium followed by oliguria, anuria, and uremia. If the patient can be maintained by dialysis, regeneration of tubular lining cells is possible. These may be followed by ultrastuctural changes consistent with irreversible cell injury including actual disruption of mitochondria, release of lysosomal enzymes, and rupture of cell membranes.

Injection of mercuric chloride produces necrosis of the epithelium of the pars recta kidney (Gritzka and Trump, 1968). Cellular changes include fragmentation and disruption of the plasma membrane and its appendages, vesiculation and disruption of the endoplasmic reticulum and other cytoplasmic membranes, dissociation of polysomes and loss of ribosomes, mitochondrial swelling with appearance of amorphous intramatrical deposits, and condensation of nuclear chromatin. These changes are common to renal cell necrosis due to various causes. Slight tubular cell injury may occur in workers with low-level exposure to metallic mercury vapor manifested by enxymuria and low-molecular-weight proteinuria (Roels et al., 1985).

Although exposure to a high dose of mercuric chloride is directly toxic to renal tubular lining cells, chronic low-dose exposure to mercuric salts or even elemental mercury vapor levels may induce an immunologic glomerular disease. This form of chronic mercury injury to the kidney is clinically the most common form of mercury-induced nephropathy. Exposed persons may develop a proteinuria that is reversible after workers are removed from exposure. It has been stated that chronic mercury-induced nephropathy seldom occurs without sufficient exposure to also produce detectable neuropathy.

Experimental studies have shown that the pathogenesis of chronic mercury nephropathy has two phases: an early phase characterized by an antibasement membrane glomerulonephritis followed by a superimposed immune complex glomerulonephritis with transiently raised concentrations of circulating immune complexes (Henry et al., 1988). The pathogenesis of the nephropathy in humans appears similar, although antigens have not been characterized. Also, the early glomerular nephritis may progress in humans to an interstitial immune complex nephritis (Tubbs et al., 1982).

Mercurous Compounds. Mercurous compounds of mercury are less corrosive and less toxic than mercuric salts, presumably because they are less soluble. Calomel, a powder containing mercurous chloride, has a long history of use in medicine. Perhaps the most notable modern usage has been as teething powder for children and is now known to be responsible for acrodynia or "pink disease." This is most likely a hypersensitivity response to the mercury salts in skin, producing vasodilation, hyperkeratosis, and hypersecretion of sweat glands. Children develop fever, a pink-colored rash, swelling of the spleen and lymph nodes, and hyperkeratosis and swelling of fingers. The effects are independent of dose and are thought to be a hypersensitivity reaction (Matheson et al., 1980).

Methyl Mercury. Methyl mercury is the most important form of mercury in terms of toxicity, and health effects from environmental exposures and many of the effects produced by short-term alkyls are unique in terms of mercury toxicity but are nonspecific in that they may be found in other disease states. Most of what is known about the clinical signs and symptoms and neuropathology of high-level or overt methyl mercury toxicity has been learned from studies of epidemics in Japan and Iraq (WHO, 1976; Berlin, 1986), from studies of populations eating mercury-contaminated fish (Skerfving, 1974), and from published reports of occupational exposures (Eyssen et al., 1983). Observations of changes in nonhuman primates studied experimentally are consistent with findings in humans and therefore provide additional information about time, dose, and tissue burden relationship, particularly for subclinical and subtle, low-level effects (Mottet et al., 1985).

The major human health effects are neurotoxic effects in adults (Bakir et al., 1973), and toxicity to the fetus of mothers exposed to methyl mercury during pregnancy (Cox et al., 1989). The brain is the critical organ. A genotoxic effect resulting in chromosomal aberrations has also been demonstrated in methyl mercury exposed populations.

Clinical manifestations of neurotoxic effects are (1) parathesia, a numbness and tingling sensation around the mouth, lips and extremities, particularly the fingers and toes; (2) ataxia, a clumsy stumbling gait, difficulty in swallowing and articulating words; (3) neuraesthenia, a generalized sensation of weakness, fatigue and inability to concentrate; (4) vision and hearing loss; (5) spacticity and tremor; and, finally, (6) coma and death.

Neuropathologic observations have shown the cortex of the cerebrum and cerebellum are selectively involved with focal necrosis of neurons, with lysis and phagocytosis and replacement by supporting gial cells. These changes are most prominent in the deeper fissures (sulci) such as in the visual cortex and insula. The overall acute effect is cerebral edema but with prolonged destruction of grey matter and subsequent gliosis. Cerebral atrophy results (Takeuchi, 1977).

MECHANISMS OF NEUROTOXICITY OF METHYL MERCURY. Experimental studies on mechanisms of methyl mercury toxicity provide some insight into the basis for the clinical observations as well as the greater sensitivity of the developing brain (Clarkson, 1983).

Exposure of the fetus *in utero* to high levels of mercury results in abnormal neuronal migration and deranged organization of brain nuclei (clusters of neurons) and layering of neurons in the cortex. Methyl mercury interacts with DNA and RNA and binds with sulfhydryl groups, resulting in changes of the secondary structure of DNA and RNA synthesis. Studies in mice have demonstrated an effect of methyl mercury on the microtubules of neurons. These observations may provide the cellular basis for the observed neuropathological changes in the migration pattern of neurons during development and is thought to be the basis for the developmental effects in the central nervous system. Male mice are more sensitive than females, consistent with the findings in humans (Sager *et al.*, 1984; B. H. Choie *et al.*, 1978).

DOSE-RESPONSE RELATIONSHIPS BETWEEN HEALTH AND RISK AND INTAKE OF METHYL MERCURY. The relationship between health risks and intake of methyl mercury has been developed from toxicological data obtained from studies of epidemics due to accidental poisoning in Minamata and Niigeta, Japan, in the 1950s and from studies of the episode in Iraq in 1972 (Berlin, 1986).

The critical or lowest observed adverse health effect in adults is paresthesia. By combining the two relationships—body burden versus intake and effect versus body burden—it was possible to calculate the average long-term daily intake associated with health effects in the most susceptible individual. This was estimated to be about 300 μg/day for an adult or 4300 ng Hg/day/kg body weight.

The critical effect from prenatal exposure to methyl mercury is psychomotor retardation. The infant may appear normal at birth, but there is a 12-month or more delay in learning to walk and talk and an increased incidence of seizures. The "threshold" or point where occurrence of critical effect exceeds background occurs at a lower dose for prenatal effect than that seen for adult exposure. Epidemiological studies relating dose to effects from prenatal exposures have now been conducted in Iraq, Canada, and New Zealand. From information obtained in these studies, C. Cox *et al.* (1989) have calculated that LOAEL (lowest observed adverse effect level) for psychomotor retardation occurs when maternal hair concentrations during pregnancy are between 10 and 20 ppm. Assuming that the relationship between intake and body burden of methyl mercury is the same in the pregnant and nonpregnant adult, this hair value would correspond to an intake of 800 to 1700 ng Hg/kg/day, and mother's red blood cell level of 40 to 80 μg/liter. In more severe cases from higher levels of exposure *in utero*, the child may develop ataxis motor disturbance and mental symptoms similar to those occurring in a child with cerebral palsy of unknown etiology. Postnatal poisoning may occur from transfer of methyl mercury via breast milk. Symptoms of this type of poisoning are similar to those of the adult.

The potential for recovery from the neurological effects may be better in cases of acute poisoning compared with prolonged exposure, but generally, neurotoxicity is irreversible.

Biologic Indicators. *Metallic Mercury.* The recommended standard (time-weight average [TWA]) for permissible exposure limits for inorganic mercury in air in the workplace is 0.05 mg Hg/m^3 (DHEW, 1977) and is equivalent to an ambient air level of 0.015 mg/m^3 for the general population (24-hour exposure).

Alkyl Mercury. The federal standard for alkyl mercury exposure in the workplace is 0.01 mg/m^3 as an eight-hour TWA with an acceptable ceiling of 0.04 mg/m^3. Although a precise correlation has not been found between exposure levels and mercury content of blood and urine, study of the Iraq epidemic has provided estimates of body burden of mercury and onset and frequency of occurrence of symptoms (Figure 19–6; Table 19–6).

The kinetics of methyl mercury excretion from the body correspond to a single biological half-time of about 70 days. Human adults attain a steady-state body burden where intake equals excretion after an exposure period of about one year (five biological half-times). From there, the body burden should be directly proportional to the average daily intake. Such dose-response calculations are subject to certain statistical error, as well as interindividual variation in critical body burden.

Treatment. Therapy of mercury poisoning should be directed to lowering the concentration of mercury at the critical organ or site of injury. For the most severe cases, particularly with acute renal failure, hemodialysis may be the first measure along with infusion of chelating agents for mercury such as cysteine or penicillamine. For less severe cases of inorganic mercury poisoning, chelation with BAL may be effective. However, chelation therapy is not very helpful for alkyl mercury exposure. Biliary excretion and reabsorption by the intestine and the enter-

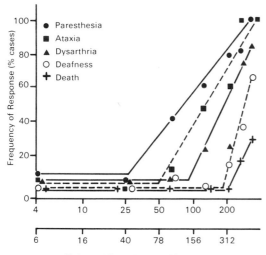

Figure 19–6. Dose-response relationships for methyl mercury. The upper scale of estimated body burden of mercury was based on the authors' actual estimate of intake. The lower scale is based on the body burden, which was calculated based on the concentration of mercury in the blood and its relationship to intake derived from radioisotopic studies of methyl mercury kinetics in human volunteers. (From Bakir, F.; et al.: Methyl mercury poisoning in Iraq. *Science,* **181:**230–241, 1973. Copyright 1973 by the American Association for the Advancement of Science.)

ohepatic cycling of mercury may be interrupted by surgically establishing gallbladder drainage or by the oral administration of a nonabsorbable thiol resin that binds mercury and enhances intestinal excretion (Berlin, 1986).

Nickel

Nickel is a respiratory tract carcinogen in workmen in the nickel-refining industry. Other serious consequences of long-term exposure to nickel are not apparent, but severe acute and sometimes fatal toxicity may follow nickel carbonyl exposure. Allergic contact dermatitis is common among persons in the general population. Deficiency of nickel alters glucose metabolism and decreases tolerance to glucose. From studies on rats, there is growing evidence that nickel may be an essential trace metal for mammals (Anke et al., 1983).

Disposition. Nickel is only sparsely absorbed from the gastrointestinal tract. It is transported in the plasma bound to serum albumin and multiple small organic ligands, amino acids, or polypeptides. Excretion in the urine is nearly complete in four or five days. Kinetics have been

described in rodents as a two-compartment model.

Dietary nickel intake by adults in the United States was estimated by Schroeder et al. (1962) to be in the range of 300 to 600 μg/day. In a study of nickel content of diets prepared in university or hospital kitchens in the United States, Myron et al. (1978) found nickel intake to average 165 (S.D. ± 11) μg/day or 75 ± 10 μg/1000 calories.

In one study, serum nickel was found to be 2.6 ± 0.9 μg/liter (range: 0.8 to 5.2) and mean excretion of nickel in urine of 2.6 ± 1.4 μg/day (range: 0.5 to 6.4) (McNeely et al., 1972). Serum nickel is influenced by environmental nickel or nickel concentration in the ambient air. Serum nickel measured in persons living in Sudbury, Ontario, which is in the vicinity of a large nickel mine, showed concentrations of 4.6 ± 1.4 μg/liter (range: 2.0 to 7.3), and urinary concentrations were 7.9 ± 3.7 μg/day (range: 2.3 to 15.7). Generally, fecal nickel is about 100 times urine nickel concentration.

Nickel administered parenterally to animals is rapidly distributed to kidney, pituitary, lung, skin, adrenal, and ovary and testis (Sunderman, 1981).

The intracellular distribution and binding of nickel are not well understood. Ultrafiltrable ligands seem to be of major importance in transport in serum and bile and urinary excretion as well as intracellular binding. The ligands are not well characterized, but Sunderman (1981) suggests that cysteine, histidine, and aspartic acid form nickel complexes either singly or as nickel-ligand species. *In vivo* binding with metallothionein has been demonstrated, but nickel at best

Table 19–6. THE TIME-WEIGHTED AVERAGE AIR CONCENTRATIONS ASSOCIATED WITH THE EARLIEST EFFECTS IN THE MOST SENSITIVE ADULTS FOLLOWING LONG-TERM EXPOSURE TO ELEMENTAL MERCURY VAPOR. THE TABLE ALSO LISTS THE EQUIVALENT BLOOD AND URINE CONCENTRATIONS[*†]

AIR (mg/m³)	BLOOD (μg/100 ml)	URINE (μg/liter)	EARLIEST EFFECTS
0.05	3.5	150	Nonspecific symptoms
0.1–0.2	7–14	300–600	Tremor

* Blood and urine values may be used only on a group basis owing to gross individual variations. Furthermore, these average values reflect exposure only after exposure for a year or more. After shorter periods of exposure, air concentrations would be associated with lower concentrations in blood and urine.
† From WHO: *Environmental Health Criteria 1. Mercury.* World Health Organization, Geneva, 1976.

induces metallothionein synthesis in liver or kidney only slightly.

A nickel-binding metalloprotein has also been identified in plasma with properties suggesting an α-1-glycoprotein with serum α-1-macroglobulin complex.

Evidence has accumulated over the past few years indicating that nickel is a nutritionally essential trace metal. Jackbean urease has been identified as a nickel metalloenzyme, and nickel is required for urea metabolism in cell cultures of soybean. However, a nickel-containing metalloenzyme has not yet been recovered from animal tissues. Nickel deficiency in rats is associated with retarded body growth and anemia, probably secondary to impaired absorption of iron from the gastrointestinal tract. In addition, there is significant reduction in serum glucose concentration. An interaction of nickel with copper and zinc is also suspected since anemia-induced nickel deficiency is only partially corrected with nickel supplementation in rats receiving low dietary copper and zinc (Spears et al., 1978).

Toxicology. *Carcinogenesis.* It has been known for 40 years that occupational exposure to nickel predisposes to lung and nasal cancer (Doll et al., 1977). Epidemiologic studies in 1958 showed that nickel refinery workers in Britain had a fivefold increase in risk to lung cancer and a 150-fold increase in risk to nasal cancers compared with people in the general population. More recently, increase in lung cancer among nickel workers has been reported from several different countries including suggestions of increased risks to laryngeal cancer in nickel refinery workers in Norway (Pedersen et al., 1978) and gastric carcinoma and soft tissue sarcomas from the Soviet Union. Six cases of renal cancer have been reported among Canadian and Norwegian workers employed in the electrolytic refining of nickel (Sunderman, Jr., 1981). McEwan (1978) has been able to detect early cytologic changes in sputum of exposed workers prior to chest X-ray or clinical indicators of respiratory tract cancer.

Because the refining of nickel in the plants that were studied involved the Mond process with the formation of nickel carbonyl, it was believed for some time that nickel carbonyl was the principal carcinogen. However, additional epidemiologic studies of workers in refineries that do not use the Mond process also showed increased risk of respiratory cancer, suggesting that the source of the increased risk is the mixture of nickel sulfides present in molten ore. Indeed, studies with experimental animals have shown that the nickel subsulfide (Ni_3S_2) produces local tumors at injection sites and by inhalation in rats, and in vitro mammalian cell tests demonstrate that Ni_3S_2 and $NiSO_4$ compounds give rise to mammalian cell transformation (Costa, 1980). Differences in the carcinogenic activities of nickel compounds may be attributable to variations in their capacities to provide nickel ion at critical sites within target cells, but this has not been established experimentally (Sunderman, Jr., 1989). However, the order of lung toxicity corresponds to water solubility of various compounds, with nickel sulfate being most toxic, followed by nickel subsulfide and nickel oxide (Dunick et al., 1989).

Nickel Carbonyl Poisoning. Metallic nickel combines with carbon monoxide to form nickel carbonyl ($Ni[CO]_4$), which decomposes to pure nickel and carbon monoxide on heating to 200°C (Mond process). This reaction provides a convenient and efficient method for the refinement of nickel. However, nickel carbonyl is extremely toxic, and many cases of acute toxicity have been reported. The illness begins with headache, nausea, vomiting, and epigastric or chest pain, followed by cough, hyperpnea, cyanosis, gastrointestinal symptoms, and weakness. The symptoms may be accompanied by fever and leukocytosis, and the more severe cases progress to pneumonia, respiratory failure, and eventually cerebral edema and death. Autopsy studies show the largest concentrations of nickel in lungs, with lesser amounts in kidneys, liver, and brain (Sunderman, Jr., 1981).

Dermatitis. Nickel dermatitis is one of the most common forms of allergic contact dermatitis: 4 to 9 percent of persons with contact dermatitis react positively to nickel patch tests. Sensitization might occur from any of the numerous metal products in common use, such as coins and jewelry. The notion that increased ingestion of nickel-containing food increases the probability of external sensitization to nickel is supported by finding increased urinary nickel excretion in association with episodes of acute nickel dermatitis (Menne and Thorboe, 1976).

Indicators of Nickel Toxicity. Blood nickel levels immediately following exposure to nickel carbonyl provide a guideline as to severity of exposure and indication for chelation therapy (Sunderman, Sr., 1979). Sodium diethyldithiocarbamate is the preferred drug, but other chelating agents, such as *d*-penicillamine and triethylenetetraamine, provide some degree of protection from clinical effects.

ESSENTIAL METALS WITH POTENTIAL FOR TOXICITY

This group includes seven metals generally accepted as essential: cobalt, copper, iron, manganese, molybdenum, selenium, and zinc. Each of the seven essential metals has three levels of biologic activity: trace levels required for optimium growth and development, homeostatic levels (storage levels), and toxic levels. For these metals, environmental accumulations are generally less important routes of excess exposure than accidents or occupation.

Although chromium and arsenic are regarded as essential to humans and animals, respectively, the toxicologic significance of chromium and arsenic warrants their being discussed as major toxic metals in the context of this chapter. Tin and vanadium are also essential to animals but are of less importance toxicologically and are included in the group of minor toxic metals.

Cobalt

Cobalt is essential as a component of vitamin B_{12} required for the production of red blood cells and prevention of pernicious anemia. There are 0.0434 μg of cobalt per microgram of vitamin B_{12}. If other requirements for cobalt exist, they are not well understood. Deficiency diseases of cattle and sheep, caused by insufficient natural levels of cobalt, are characterized by anemia and loss of weight or retarded growth. The occurrence, metabolism, and toxicity of cobalt are reviewed by I. C. Smith and Carson (1981), Elinder and Friberg (1986), and Angerer and Heinrich (1987).

Cobalt is a relatively rare metal produced primarily as a by-product of other metals, chiefly copper. It is used in high-temperature alloys and in permanent magnets. Its salts are useful in paint driers, as catalysts, and in the production of numerous pigments.

Cobalt salts are generally well absorbed after oral ingestion, probably in the jejunum. Despite this fact, increased levels tend not to cause significant accumulation. About 80 percent of the ingested cobalt is excreted in the urine. Of the remaining, about 15 percent is excreted in the feces by an enterohepatic pathway, whereas the milk and sweat are other secondary routes of excretion. The total body burden has been estimated as 1.1 mg.

The muscle contains the largest total fraction, but the fat has the highest concentration. The liver, heart, and hair have significantly higher concentrations than other organs, but the concentration in these organs is relatively low. The normal levels in human urine and blood are about 98 and 0.18 μg/liter, respectively. The blood level is largely in association with the red cells.

Significant species differences have been observed in the excretion of radiocobalt. In rats and cattle, 80 percent is eliminated in the feces.

Polycythemia is the characteristic response of most mammals, including humans, to ingestion of excessive amounts of cobalt. Toxicity resulting from overzealous therapeutic administration has been reported to produce vomiting, diarrhea, and a sensation of warmth. Intravenous administration leads to flushing of the face, increased blood pressure, slowed respiration, giddiness, tinnitus, and deafness due to nerve damage (Browning, 1969).

High levels of chronic oral administration may result in the production of goiter. Epidemiologic studies suggest that the incidence of goiter is higher in regions containing increased levels of cobalt in the water and soil. The goitrogenic effect has been elicited by the oral administration of 3 to 4 mg/kg to children in the course of sickle cell anemia therapy.

Cardiomyopathy has been caused by excessive intake of cobalt, particularly from the drinking of beer to which 1 ppm cobalt was added to enhance its foaming qualities. Why such a low concentration should produce this effect in the absence of any similar change when cobalt is used therapeutically is unknown. The signs and symptoms were those of congestive heart failure. Autopsy findings revealed a tenfold increase in the cardiac levels of cobalt. Alcohol may have served to potentiate the effect of the cobalt (Morin and Daniel, 1967).

Hyperglycemia due to β-cell pancreatic damage has been reported after injection into rats. Reduction of blood pressure has also been observed in rats after injection and has led to some experimental use in humans (Schroeder et al., 1967).

Occupational inhalation of cobalt-containing dust in the cemented tungsten carbide industry may cause respiratory irritation at air concentrations of 0.002 to 0.01 mg/m^3 and may be a cause of "hard-metal" pneumoconiosis. This may result in interstitial fibrosis. Allergic dermatitis of an erythematous papular type may also occur, and affected persons may have positive skin tests.

Single and repeated subcutaneous or intramuscular injection of cobalt powder and salts to rats may cause sarcomas at the site of injection, but there is no evidence of carcinogenicity from any other route of exposure (Gilman, 1962).

Copper

Copper is widely distributed in nature and is an essential element. Copper deficiency is characterized by hypochromic, microcytic anemia resulting from defective hemoglobin synthesis. Oxidative enzymes, such as catalase, peroxidase, cytochrome oxides, and others, also require copper. Medicinally, copper sulfate is used as an emetic. It has also been used for its astringent and caustic action and as an anthelmintic. Copper sulfate mixed with lime has been used as a fungicide. The potential health effects associated with copper are reviewed by the EPA (1987c).

Gastrointestinal absorption of copper is normally regulated by body stores (Sarkar *et al.*, 1983). It is transported in serum bound initially to albumin and later more firmly bound to α-ceruloplasmin, where it is exchanged in the cupric form. The normal serum level of copper is 120 to 145 μg/dl. The bile is the normal excretory pathway and plays a primary role in copper homeostasis. Most copper is stored in liver and bone marrow, where it may be bound to metallothionein. The amount of copper in milk is not enough to maintain adequate copper levels in the liver, lung, and spleen of the newborn. Tissue levels gradually decline up to about ten years of age, remaining relatively constant thereafter. Brain levels, on the other hand, tend almost to double from infancy to adulthood. The ratios of newborn to adult liver copper levels show considerable species difference: human, 15:4; rat, 6:4; and rabbit, 1:6. Since urinary copper levels may be increased by soft water, under these conditions, concentrations of approximately 60 μg/liter are not uncommon.

Copper is an essential part of several enzymes, including tyrosinase, involved in the formation of melanin pigments, cytochrome oxidase, superoxide dismutase, amine oxidases, and uricase. It is essential for the utilization of iron. Iron-deficiency anemia in infancy is sometimes accompanied by copper deficiency as well. Molybdenum also influences tissue levels of copper.

There are two genetically inherited inborn errors of copper metabolism that are in a sense a form of copper toxicity (Sarkar *et al.*, 1983). Wilson's disease is characterized by excessive accumulation of copper in liver, brain, kidneys, and cornea. Serum copper and ceruloplasmin are low, but serum copper, not bound to ceruloplasmin, is elevated. Urinary excretion of copper is high. The disorder is sometimes referred to as *hepatolenticular degeneration* in reference to the major symptoms. Clinical abnormalities of the nervous system, liver, kidneys, and cornea are related to copper accumulation. Although the etiology of this disorder is genetic, the basic defect at the biochemical level is not known. Increased binding of copper to an abnormal intracellular thionein or altered tissue excretion has been proposed. Cultured fibroblasts from persons with Wilson's disease have increased intracellular copper when cultured in Eagle's minimum essential medium with fetal bovine serum (Chan *et al.*, 1983). Clinical improvement can be achieved by chelation of copper with penicillamine (Walshe, 1964). Trien (triethylene tetramine [2HCl]) is also effective and has been used in patients with Wilson's disease who have toxic reactions to penicillamine (Walshe, 1983).

Menke's disease or Menke's "kinky-hair syndrome" is a sex-linked trait characterized by peculiar hair, failure to thrive, severe mental retardation, neurologic impairment, and death before three years of age. There is extensive degeneration of the cerebral cortex and of white matter. Again, the basic defect is not known. There are low levels of copper in liver and brain but high concentrations in other tissues. Even in cells with increased copper concentration, there is a relative deficiency in activities of some copper-dependent enzymes. Some laboratories have reported that larger-than-normal quantities of copper-thionein accumulated in fibroblasts, so that the basic defect may be in regulation of metallothionein synthesis. The finding of increased amounts of other metallothionein-binding metals (zinc, cadmium, mercury) in kidneys of patients with this disease supports this hypothesis (Riordan, 1983).

Acute poisoning resulting from ingestion of excessive amounts of oral copper salts, most frequently copper sulfate, may produce death. The symptoms are vomiting, sometimes with a blue-green color observed in the vomitus, hematemesis, hypotension, melena, coma, and jaundice. Autopsy findings have revealed centrilobular hepatic necrosis (Chuttani *et al.*, 1965). A few cases of copper intoxication as a result of burn treatment with copper compounds have resulted in hemolytic anemia. Copper poisoning producing hemolytic anemia has also been reported as the result of using copper-containing dialysis equipment (Manzer and Schreiner, 1970). Individuals with glucose-6-phosphate deficiency may be at increased risk to the hematologic effects of copper, but there is uncertainty as to the magnitude of the risk (Goldstein *et al.*, 1985).

Infants and children are susceptible to the effects of copper as evidenced by the incidence of childhood cirrhosis and the reports of copper intoxication in young children in India caused by drinking milk boiled and stored in brass vessels. There is some debate whether this specific disorder actually occurs outside of India. Nevertheless, it is thought that infants and children have increased susceptibility to copper toxicity because of the normally high hepatic copper levels in early life and homeostatic mechanisms are not fully developed at birth.

Indian childhood cirrhosis has not been noted in the United States, but there are case reports of severe liver disorders resulting from ingestion of 10 mg Cu per 10-kg child per day in contaminated milk.

Iron

The major interest in iron is as an essential metal, but toxicologic considerations are important in terms of accidental acute exposures and chronic iron overload due to idiopathic hemochromatosis or as a consequence of excess dietary iron or frequent blood transfusions. The complex metabolism of iron and mechanisms of toxicity are detailed by Jacobs and Worwood, (1981) and Spivey Fox and Rader (1988).

Disposition. The disposition of iron is regulated by a complex mechanism to maintain homeostasis. Generally, about 2 to 15 percent is absorbed from the gastrointestinal tract, whereas elimination of absorbed iron is only about 0.01 percent per day (percent body burden or amount absorbed). During periods of increased iron need (childhood, pregnancy, blood loss), absorption of iron is greatly increased. Absorption occurs in two steps: (1) absorption of ferrous ions from the intestinal lumen into the mucosal cells and (2) transfer from the mocusal cell to plasma where it is bound to transferrin for transfer to storage sites. Transferrin is a β_1-globulin with a molecular weight of 75,000 and is produced in the liver. As ferrous ion is released into plasma, it becomes oxidized by oxygen in the presence of ferroxidase I, which is identical to ceruloplasmin. There are 3 to 5 g of iron in the body. About two-thirds is bound to hemoglobin, 10 percent is bound to myoglobin and iron-containing enzymes, and the remainder is bound to the iron storage proteins ferritin and hemosiderin. Exposure to iron induces synthesis of apoferritin, which then binds ferrous ions. The ferrous ion becomes oxidized, probably by histidine and cysteine residues and carbonyl groups. Iron may be released from ferritin by reducing agents; ascorbic acid, cysteine, and reduced glutathione release iron slowly. Normally, excess ingested iron is excreted, and some is contained within shed intestinal cells and in bile and urine and in even smaller amounts in sweat, nails, and hair. Total iron excretion is usually on the order of 0.5 mg/day.

With excess exposure to iron or iron overload, there may be a further increase in ferritin synthesis in hepatic parenchymal cells. In fact, the ability of the liver to synthesize ferritin exceeds the rate at which lysosomes can process iron for excretion. Lysosomes convert the protein from ferritin to hemosiderin, which then remains in situ (Trump et al., 1973). The formation of hemosiderin from ferritin is not well understood but seems to involve denaturation of the apoferritin molecule. With increasing iron loading, ferritin concentration appears to reach a maximum, and a greater portion of iron is found in hemosiderin. Both ferritin and hemosiderin are, in fact, storage sites for intracellular metal and are protective in that they maintain intracellular iron in bound form.

A portion of the iron taken up by cells of the reticuloendothelial system enters a labile iron pool available for erythropoiesis, and part becomes stored as ferritin.

Toxicity. Acute iron toxicity is nearly always due to accidental ingestion of iron-containing medicines, and most often occurs in children. As of 1970, there were about 2000 cases in the United States each year, generally among children aged one to five years, who eat ferrous sulfate tablets with candylike coatings. Decrease of this occurrence should follow use of "child-proof" lids on prescription medicines. Severe toxicity occurs after ingestion of more than 0.5 g of iron or 2.5 g of ferrous sulfate. Toxicity becomes manifest with vomiting, one to six hours after ingestion. The vomitus may be bloody, owing to ulceration of the gastrointestinal tract. Stools may be black. This is followed by signs of shock and metabolic acidosis, liver damage, and coagulation defects within the next couple of days. Late effects may include renal failure and hepatic cirrhosis. The mechanism of the toxicity is thought to begin with acute mucosal cell damage, absorption of ferrous ions directly into the circulation, which cause capillary endothelial cell damage in liver.

Chronic iron toxicity or iron overload in adults is a more common problem. There are three basic ways in which excessive amounts of iron can accumulate in the body. The first circumstance is idiopathic hemochromotosis due to abnormal absorption of iron from the intestinal tract. The condition may be genetic. A second possible cause of iron overload is excess dietary iron. The African Bantu who prepares his daily food and brews fermented beverages in iron pots is the classic example of this form of iron overload. Sporadic other cases occur owing to excessive ingestion of iron-containing tonics or medicines. The third circumstance in which iron overload may occur is from the regular requirement for blood transfusion for some form of refractory anemias and is sometimes referred to as *transfusional siderosis* (Muller-Eberhard et al., 1977).

The pathologic consequences of iron overload are similar regardless of basic cause. The body iron content is increased to between 20 and 40 g. Most of the extra iron is hemosiderin. Greatest concentrations are in parenchymal cells of liver and pancreas, as well as endocrine organs and heart. Iron in reticuloendothelial cells (spleen) is greatest in transfusional siderosis and in the Bantu. Further clinical effects may include disturbances in liver function, diabetes mellitus, and even endocrine disturbances and cardiovascular effects. At the cell level, increased lipid peroxidation occurs with consequent membrane damage to mitochondria, microsomes, and other cellular organelles (Jacobs, 1977).

Treatment of acute iron poisoning is directed toward removal of the ingested iron from the gastrointestinal tract by inducing vomiting or gastric lavage and providing corrective therapy for systemic effects such as acidosis and shock. Deferrioxamine is the chelating agent of choice for treatment of iron absorbed from acute exposure as well as for removal of tissue iron in hemosiderosis. Repeated phlebotomy can remove as much as 20 g of iron per year. Ascorbic acid will also increase iron excretion as much as twofold normal (E. B. Brown, 1983).

Inhalation of iron oxide fumes or dust by workers in metal industries may result in deposition of iron particles in lungs, producing an X-ray appearance resembling silicosis. These effects are seen in hematite miners, iron and steel workers, and arc welders. Hematite is the most important iron ore (mainly Fe_2O_3). A report of autopsies of hematite miners noted an increase in lung cancer, as well as tuberculosis and interstitial fibrosis (Boyd *et al.*, 1970). The etiology of the lung cancer may be related to concomitant factors such as cigarettes or other workplace carcinogens. Hematite miners are also exposed to silica and other minerals, as well as radioactive materials; other iron workers have exposures to polycyclic hydrocarbons (A. I. G. McLaughlin, 1956). Dose levels of iron among iron workers developing pneumoconiosis have been reported to exceed 10 mg Fe/m^3.

Manganese

Manganese is an essential element and is a cofactor for a number of enzymatic reactions, particularly those involved in phosphorylation, cholesterol, and fatty acids synthesis. Manganese is present in all living organisms. While it is present in urban air and in most water supplies, the principal portion of the intake is derived from food. Vegetables, the germinal portions of grains, fruits, nuts, tea, and some spices are rich in manganese (NAS, 1973; Underwood, 1977; Keen and Leach, 1988).

Daily manganese intake ranges from 2 to 9 mg. Gastrointestinal absorption is less than 5 percent. It is transported in plasma bound to a β_1-globulin, thought to be transferrin, and is widely distributed in the body. Manganese concentrates in mitochondria, so that tissues rich in these organelles have the highest concentrations of manganese including pancreas, liver, kidney, and intestines. Biologic half-life in the body is 37 days. It readily crosses the blood-brain barrier, and half-time in the brain is longer than in the whole body.

Manganese is eliminated in the bile and is reabsorbed in the intestine, but the principal route of excretion is with feces. This system apparently involves the liver, auxiliary gastrointestinal mechanisms for excreting excess manganese, and perhaps the adrenal cortex. This regulating mechanism, plus the tendency for extremely large doses of manganese salts to cause gastrointestinal irritation, accounts for the lack of systemic toxicity following oral administration or dermal application.

Manganese and its compounds are used in making steel alloys, dry-cell batteries, electrical coils, ceramics, matches, glass, dyes; in fertilizers, welding rods; as oxidizing agents; and as animal food additives.

Industrial toxicity from inhalation exposure, generally to manganese dioxide in mining or manufacturing, is of two types: The first, manganese pneumonitis, is the result of acute exposure. Men working in plants with high concentrations of manganese dust show an incidence of respiratory disease 30 times greater than normal. Pathologic changes include epithelial necrosis followed by mononuclear proliferation.

The second and more serious type of disease resulting from chronic inhalation exposure to manganese dioxide, generally over a period of more than two years, involves the central nervous system. In iron-deficiency anemia, the oral absorption of manganese is increased, and it may be that variations in manganese transport related to iron deficiency account for individual susceptibility (Mena *et al.*, 1969). Those who develop chronic manganese poisoning (manganism) exhibit a psychiatric disorder characterized by irritability, difficulty in walking, speech disturbances, and compulsive behavior that may include running, fighting, and singing. If the condition persists, a masklike face, retropulsion or propulsion, and a Parkinson-like syndrome develop (Mena *et al.*, 1967). The outstanding feature of manganese encephalopathy has been classified as severe selective damage to the subthalamic nucleus and pallidum (Pentschew *et al.*, 1963). These symptoms and the pathologic lesions, degenerative changes in the basal ganglia, make the analogy to Parkinson's disease feasible. In addition to the central nervous

humoral factors including adrenocorticotropic hormone, parathyroid hormone, and endotoxin. In the liver, as well as other tissues, zinc is bound to metallothionein. The greatest concentration of zinc in the body is in the prostate, probably related to the rich content of zinc-containing enzyme acid phosphatase.

Deficiency. More than 70 metalloenzymes require zinc as a cofactor, and deficiency results in a wide spectrum of clinical effects depending on age, stage of development, and deficiencies of related metals.

Zinc deficiency in humans was first characterized by Prasad and coworkers (1963) in adolescent Egyptian boys with growth failure and delayed sexual maturation and is accompanied by protein-caloric malnutrition, pellagra, iron, and folate deficiency. Zinc deficiency in the newborn may be manifested by dermatitis, loss of hair, impaired healing, susceptibility to infections, and neuropsychologic abnormalities. Dietary inadequacies coupled with liver disease from chronic alcoholism may be associated with dermatitis, night blindness, testicular atrophy, impotence, and poor wound healing. Other chronic clinical disorders, such as ulcerative colitis and the malabsorption syndromes, chronic renal disease, and the hemolytic anemias, are also prone to zinc deficiency. Many drugs affect zinc homestasis, particularly metal-chelating agents and some antibiotics, such as penicillin and isoniazid. Less common zinc deficiency may occur with myocardial infarction, arthritis, and even hypertension.

Biologic Indicators of Abnormal Zinc Homeostasis. The range of normal plasma zinc level is from 85 to 110 μg/dl. Severe deficiency may decrease plasma zinc to 40 to 60 μg/dl, accompanied by increased serum β_2-globulin and decreased α-globulin. Urine zinc excretion may decrease from over 300 μg/day to less than 100 μg/day. Zinc deficiency may exacerbate impaired copper nutrition, and of course, zinc interactions with cadmium and lead may modify the toxicity of these metals (Sanstead, 1981).

Toxicity. Zinc toxicity from excessive ingestion is uncommon, but gastrointestinal distress and diarrhea have been reported following ingestion of beverages standing in galvanized cans or from use of galvanized utensils. However, evidence of hematologic, hepatic, or renal toxicity has not been observed in individuals ingesting as much as 12 g of elemental zinc over a two-day period.

With regard to industrial exposure, metal fume fever resulting from inhalation of freshly formed fumes of zinc presents the most significant effect. The disorder has been most commonly associated with inhalation of zinc oxide fume, but it may be seen after inhalation of fumes of other metals, particularly magnesium, iron, and copper. Attacks usually begin after four to eight hours of exposure—chills and fever, profuse sweating, and weakness. Attacks usually last only 24 to 48 hours and are most common on Mondays or after holidays. The pathogenesis is not known but is thought to be due to endogenous pyrogen released from cell lysis. Extracts prepared from tracheal mucosa and lungs of animals with experimentally induced metal fume fever produce similar symptoms when injected into other animals. Other aspects of zinc toxicity are not well established. Experimental animals have been given 100 times dietary requirements without discernible effects (Goyer *et al.*, 1979).

Exposure of guinea pigs three hours per day for six consecutive days to 5 mg/m^3 freshly formed ultrafine zinc oxide (the recommended TLV) produced decrements in lung volumes and carbon monoxide diffusing capacity that persisted 72 hours after exposure. These functional changes were correlated with microscopic evidence of interstitial thickening and cellular infiltrate in alveolar ducts and alveoli (Lam *et al.*, 1985).

Testicular tumors have been produced by direct intratesticular injection in rats and chickens. This effect is probably related to the concentration of zinc normally in the gonads and may be hormonally dependent. Zinc salts have not produced carcinogenic effects when administered to animals by other routes (Furst, 1981).

METALS WITH TOXICITY RELATED TO MEDICAL THERAPY

Metals considered in this group include aluminum, bismuth, gold, lithium, and platinum. Metals at one time were used to treat a number of human ills, particularly heavy metals like mercury and arsenic. Gold salts are still useful for the treatment of forms of rheumatism, and organic bismuth compounds are used to treat gastrointestinal disturbances. Lithium has become an important aid in the treatment of depression. The toxicologic hazards from aluminum are not from its use as an antacid but rather the accumulations that occur in bone and neurotoxicity in patients with chronic renal failure receiving hemodialysis therapy. A more recent concern regarding the potential neurotoxicity of aluminum involves its relationship to Alzheimer dementia and increase in bioavailability from change in soil and water pH from acid rain. Platinum is receiving attention as an antitumor agent. Barium and gallium are used as a radiopaque and radiotracer material, respectively, so they do have importance in medical therapy. Toxicologic effects are unlikely and seldom occur.

Aluminum

Aluminum is one of the most ubiquitous elements in the environment. It has, until recently, existed predominantly in forms not available to man and most other species. Acid rain, however, has increased dramatically the amount of aluminum appearing in biologic ecosystems, resulting in well-described destructive effects on fish and plant life species. Whether man is vulnerable to changes in aluminum bioavailability is a major scientific question.

Metabolism. Daily intake of aluminum for people in the general population has been reported to range from 9 mg/day to 36 mg/day, with an average of about 20 mg/day. The body attempts to maintain a balance between aluminum exposure and content of body tissues, so that little is absorbed. However, with intakes of greater than 1000 mg per day, retention does occur. Bone and lung have the largest concentrations of aluminum, suggesting bone may be a "sink" for aluminum. Aluminum does not normally accumulate in blood to any great extent (Ganrot, 1986).

Aluminum compounds can affect absorption of other elements in the gastrointestinal tract and alter intestinal function. Aluminum inhibits fluoride absorption and may decrease the absorption of calcium and iron compounds and possibly the absorption of cholesterol by forming an aluminum-pectin complex that binds fats to nondigestible vegetable fibers (Nagyvary and Bradbury, 1977). The binding of phosphorus in the intestinal tract can lead to phosphate depletion and osteomalacia. Aluminum may alter gastrointestinal tract motility by inhibition of acetylcholine-induced contractions and may be the explanation of why aluminum-containing antacids often produce constipation.

Experimental Toxicity Studies. Aluminum has marked differences in its effects on animals at different points in their life span and in different species. The normal concentration of aluminum in the mammalian brain is approximately 1 to 2 μg/g. In certain aluminum-sensitive species such as cats and rabbits, increasing aluminum by intrathecal infusion so that brain concentration is greater than 4 μg/g induces a characteristic clinical and pathological response. Initially, animals show subtle behavioral changes including learning and memory deficits and poor motor function. These changes progress to tremor, incoordination, weakness, and ataxia. This is followed by focal seizures and death within three or

four weeks of initial exposure. With lesser doses, there is longer survival but no recovery (DeBoni et al., 1976).

The most prominent early pathological change is an accumulation of neurofibrillary tangles (NFTs) in cell body, proximal axons, and dendrites of neurons of many brain regions. This is associated with loss of synapsis and atrophy of the dendritic tree. Not all species show this reaction to aluminum, however. The rat fails to develop NFTs or encephalopathy, and the monkey does so only after more than a year following aluminum infusion. NFTs are found primarily in large neurons such as Purkinje cells of the cerebellum and large neurons of the cerebral cortex. There is marked reduction in numbers of neurotubules and rate of cytoplasmic transport with impairment of intracellular transport. Aluminum also interacts with neuronal chromatin or DNA and is associated with a decreased rate of DNA synthesis. RNA polymerase activity is also reduced.

Aluminum competes with or alters calcium metabolism in several organ systems including the brain. Brain tissue calcium rises following aluminum exposure. Aluminum also binds to calmodulin and induces changes in its structure, leading to the suggestion that aluminum impairs the function of calmodulin as a calcium regulator. This would have profound effects on CNS function and disrupt neurotubular integrity and transport. While these studies in animals have provided some insights into mechanisms of neurotoxicity of aluminum in experimental models, the relationship to human disease is presently uncertain (Siegel and Haug, 1983; Bizzi and Gambetti, 1986; Birchall and Chappell, 1988).

Human Dementia Syndromes. *Dialysis Dementia.* A progressive fatal neurologic syndrome has also been reported in patients on long-term intermittent hemodialysis treatment for chronic renal failure (Alfrey et al., 1972). The first symptom in these patients is a speech disorder followed by dementia, convulsions, and myoclonus. The disorder, which typically arises after three to seven years of dialysis treatment, may be due to aluminum intoxication. Aluminum content of brain, muscle, and bone tissues increases in these patients.

Sources of the excess aluminum may be from oral aluminum hydroxide commonly given to these patients or from aluminum in dialysis fluid derived from tap water used to prepare the dialysate fluid. The high serum and aluminum concentrations may be related to increased parathyroid hormone due to low blood calcium and osteodystrophy common in patients with chronic renal disease. The syndrome may be prevented by avoidance of the use of aluminum-containing oral phosphate binders and monitoring of aluminum in the dialysate. Chelation of aluminum may be achieved with use of desferrioxamine, and progression of the dementia may be arrested or slowed (Wills and Savory, 1983).

Amyotrophic Lateral Sclerosis and Parkinsonism-Dementia Syndromes of Guam (Guam ALS-PD Complex). The Chammaro peoples of the Mariana Islands in the western Pacific Ocean, particularly Guam and Rota, have an unusually high incidence of neurodegenerative diseases associated with nerve cell loss and neurofibrillary degeneration of the Alzheimer type. Garruto *et al.* (1984) noted that the volcanic soils of the regions of Guam with high incidence of ALS-PD contained high concentrations of aluminum and manganese and were low in calcium and magnesium. They postulated that low intake of calcium and magnesium induced secondary hyperparathyroidism resulting in an increase in calcium, aluminum, and other toxic metals, resulting in neuronal injury and death. How and why aluminum enters the brain of these people are unclear. A recent study of mineral content of food did not indicate high exposure to aluminum or low dietary calcium (Crapper-McLachlan *et al.*, 1989). These authors suggest the diets of Guam may be the sources of the aluminum, particularly through the respiratory tract. Perl and Good (1987) have shown that aluminum may be taken up through nasal-olfactory pathways.

Alzheimer's Disease. Two observations have provided a suspected link between Alzheimer's disease and aluminum. First, increased amounts of aluminum have been found in brains of persons dying of Alzheimer's disease, although brain aluminum content has been found to vary greatly (from 0.4 to 107.9 μg/g). The overall mean aluminum content is approximately 5 to 10 μg/g, similar to levels related to encephalopathy in animal models. These levels of aluminum, however, are also found in dialysis patients, even those who are not demented (see "Dialysis Dementia").

The second major finding that relates aluminum encephalopathy to Alzheimer's disease is the finding of NFTs in both conditions (Klatzo *et al.*, 1965).

Perl and Brody (1980) developed a sensitive technique using the scanning electron microscope in conjunction with energy dispersive X-ray spectrometry for analysis of trace element constituents of the nervous system at the cellular level of resolution. With this technique, they were able to identify intraneuronal accumulations of aluminum in association with neurofibrillary tangle formation in the hippocampal neurons of brain tissues obtained from patients with Alzheimer's disease. However, it is now clear that the NFTs induced by the two conditions are different both structurally and chemically. Also, neurofibrillary tangles are present in a wide variety of neurologic disorders. Using X-ray spectrometry, Perl and Brody (1980) found aluminum in the nuclei of virtually all NFT-containing neurons and in virtually no non–NFT-containing neurons, so that aluminum may in some way be a secondary or interactive factor producing a different type of cellular dysfunction in Alzheimer's disease.

The question that has been raised about the increase in aluminum in brains of persons with Alzheimer's disease has not so much to do with exposure to aluminum as with how aluminum gets into the brain. The aluminum accumulations identified in brains of Alzheimer's disease patients reflect a defect in the functioning of various biologic barriers that normally serve to exclude aluminum from the central nervous system. The nature of the blood-brain barrier leak may be related to genetically inherent deficits or result from viral or immune-mediated damage. Another factor may be the chemical form of the aluminum presented to the individual. Relatively little is known about the role of speciation on the bioavailability of aluminum (Perl and Good, 1988).

Epidemiological Studies of Alzheimer's Disease and Aluminum Exposure. Studies of the prevalence of dementia have been reviewed by Henderson (1986) and Ineichen (1987). Prevalence rates varied from 2.5 percent in people over 65 years in London to 25 percent in people over 60 in the Soviet Union. Such variation most probably indicates differences in criteria for ascertainment but may also reflect differences in environment.

Epidemiological studies relating geographical variation in the rate of Alzheimer's disease and its relation to differences in the population exposure to aluminum are limited. A recent study in England found that where aluminum concentrations in the water supplies were high, daily intake of aluminum by people living in these areas was likely to be increased (Martyn *et al.*, 1989). A Norwegian study reported that mortality from dementia was higher in areas of the country where higher concentrations of aluminum in the water supply were found. In each of these studies, however, there are inconsistencies in the criteria for dementia and in information available from death certificates.

Bismuth

Bismuth has a long history of use in pharmaceuticals in Europe and North America. Both inorganic and organic salts have been used, depending on the specific application. There are three major categories of uses: antisyphilitic agents, topical creams, and antacids. Trivalent insoluble bismuth salts are used medicinally to control diarrhea and other types of gastrointestinal distress. Various bismuth salts have been used externally for their astringent and slight antiseptic property. Bismuth salts have also been used as radiocontrast agents. Further potential for exposure comes from the use of insoluble bismuth salts in cosmetics. Injections of soluble and insoluble salts, suspended in oil to maintain adequate blood levels, have been used to treat syphilis. Bismuth sodium thioglycollate, a water-soluble salt, was injected intramuscularly for malaria *(Plasmodium vivax)*. Bismuth glycolyarsanilate is one of the few pentavalent salts that have been used medicinally. This material was formerly used for treatment of amebiasis (Fowler and Vouk, 1986). Exposure to various bismuth salts for medicinal use has decreased with the advent of newer therapeutic agents. However, in the 1970s, reports appeared from France and Australia of unique encephalopathy occurring in colostomy and ileostomy patients using bismuth subgallate, bismuth subnitrate, and tripotassium-dicitrate-bismuthate for control of fecal odor and consistency. The symptoms included progressive mental confusion, irregular myoclonic jerks, a distinctive pattern of disordered gait, and a variable degree of dysarthria. The disorder was fatal to patients who continued use of the bismuth compounds, but full recovery was rapid in those in whom therapy was discontinued. The severity of the disorder seemed to be independent of dose and duration of therapy (Thomas *et al.*, 1977).

Most bismuth compounds are insoluble and poorly absorbed from the gastrointestinal tracts or when applied to the skin, even if the skin is abraded or burned. Symptomatic patients taking bismuth subgallate had an elevated median blood bismuth level of 14.6 μg Bi/dl, patients with clinical symptoms had a median blood level of 3 μg/dl, and colostomy patients not on bismuth therapy had a median bismuth blood level of 0.8 μg/dl. Health laboratory workers had a median bismuth blood level of 1.0 μg/dl. Binding in blood is thought to be largely to a plasma protein with a molecular weight greater than 50,000 daltons. A diffusible equilibrium between tissues, blood, and urine is established. Tissue distribution, omitting injection depots, reveals the kidney as the site of the highest concentration. The liver concentration is considerably lower at therapeutic levels, but with massive doses in experimental animals (dogs), the kidney/liver ratio is decreased. Passage of bismuth into the amniotic fluid and into the fetus has been demonstrated. The urine is the major route of excretion. Traces of bismuth can be found in milk and saliva. The total elimination of bismuth after injection is slow and dependent on mobilization from the injection site.

Acute renal failure can occur following oral administration of such compounds as bismuth sodium triglycocollamate or thioglycollate, particularly in children (Urizar and Vernier, 1966). The tubular epithelium is the primary site of toxicity, producing degeneration of renal tubular cells and nuclear inclusion bodies composed of a bismuth-protein complex analogous to those found in lead toxicity (Fowler and Goyer, 1975).

The symptoms of chronic toxicity in humans consist of decreased appetite, weakness, rheumatic pain, diarrhea, fever, metal line on the gums, foul breath, gingivitis, and dermatitis. Jaundice and conjunctival hemorrhage are rare but have been reported. Bismuth nephropathy with proteinuria may occur.

Chelation therapy using dimercaprol (BAL) is said to be helpful in removal of bismuth from children with acute toxicity (Arena, 1974).

Gallium

Gallium is of interest because of the use of radiogallium as a diagnostic tool for localization of bone lesions. It is obtained as a by-product of copper, zinc, lead, and aluminum refining and is used in high-temperature thermometers, as a substitute for mercury in arc lamps, as a component of metal alloys, and as a seal for vacuum equipment. It is only sparsely absorbed from the gastrointestinal tract, but concentrations of less than 1 ppm can be localized radiographically in bone lesions. Higher doses will visualize liver, spleen, and kidney as well (Hayes, 1988). Urine is the major route of excretion.

Administration of gallium arsenide results in arsenic intoxication (Webb *et al.*, 1984).

There are no reported adverse effects of gallium following industrial exposure. Therapeutic use of radiogallium produced some adverse effects, mild dermatitis, and gastrointestinal disturbances. Bone marrow depression has been reported and may be due largely to the radioactivity. In animals, gallium acts as a neuromuscular poison and causes renal damage. Photophobia, blindness, and paralysis have been reported in rats. Renal damage ranging from cloudy swelling to tubular cell necrosis has been reported. Large doses given to rats cause renal precipitates consisting of gallium, calcium, and phosphate (Newman *et al.*, 1979).

Gold

Gold is widely distributed in small quantities, but economically usable deposits occur as the free metal in quartz veins or alluvial gravel. Seawater contains 3 or 4 mg/ton, and small amounts, 0.03 to 1 mg percent, have been reported in many foods. Gold has a number of industrial uses because of its electrical and thermal conductivity.

While gold and its salts have been used for a wide variety of medicinal purposes, their present uses are limited to the treatment of rheumatoid arthritis and rare skin diseases such as discoid lupus. Gold salts are poorly absorbed from the gastrointestinal tract. Normal urine and fecal excretions of 0.1 and 1 mg/day, respectively, have been reported. After injection of most of the soluble salts, gold is excreted via the urine, whereas the feces account for the major portion of insoluble compounds. Gold seems to have a long biologic half-life, and detectable blood levels can be demonstrated for ten months after cessation of treatment.

Dermatitis is the most frequently reported toxic reaction to gold and is sometimes accompanied by stomatitis. Increase in serum IgE has been noted in patients with dermatological side effects.

Use of gold in the form of organic salts to treat rheumatoid arthritis may be complicated by development of proteinuria and the nephrotic syndrome, which morphologically consists of an immune complex glomerulonephritis with granular deposits along the glomerular basement membrane and in the mesangium. The pathogenesis of the immune complex disease is not certain, but gold may behave as a hapten and generate the production of antibodies with subsequent disposition of gold protein-antibody complexes in the glomerular subepithelium. Another hypothesis is that antibodies are formed against damaged tubular structures, particularly mitochondria, providing immune complexes for the glomerular deposits (Voil *et al.*, 1977).

Gold Salts. The pathogenesis of the renal lesions induced by gold therapy also has a direct toxicity to renal tubular cell components. From experimental studies, it appears that gold salts have an affinity for mitochondria of proximal tubular lining cells, which is followed by autophagocytosis and accumulation of gold in amorphous phagolysosomes (Stuve and Galle, 1970), and gold particles can be identified in degenerating mitochondria in tubular lining cells and in glomerular epithelial cells by X-ray microanalysis (Ainsworth *et al.*, 1981).

Lithium

Lithium carbonate is an important aid in the treatment of depression. There must be careful monitoring of usage to provide optimal therapeutic value and not to produce toxicity. Lithium is a common metal and is present in many plant and animal tissues. Daily intake is about 2 mg. It is readily absorbed from the gastrointestinal tract. Distribution in the human organs is almost uniform. The normal plasma level is about 17 μg/liter. The red cells contain less. Excretion is chiefly through the kidneys, but some is eliminated in the feces. The greater part of lithium is contained in the cells, perhaps at the expense of potassium. In general, the body distribution of lithium is quite similar to that of sodium, and it may be competing with sodium at certain sites, for example, in renal tubular reabsorption.

Lithium has some industrial uses, in alloys, as a catalytic agent, and as a lubricant. Lithium hydride produces hydrogen on contact with water and is used in manufacturing electronic tubes, in ceramics, and in chemical synthesis. From the industrial point of view, except for lithium hydride, none of the other salts or the metal itself is hazardous. Lithium hydride is intensely corrosive and may produce burns on the skin because of the formation of hydroxides (M. Cox and Singer, 1981). The therapeutic use of lithium carbonate may produce unusual toxic responses. These include neuromuscular changes (tremor, muscle hyperirritability, and ataxia), central nervous system changes (blackout spells, epileptic seizures, slurred speech, coma, psychosomatic retardation, and increased thirst), cardiovascular changes (cardiac arrhythmia, hypertension, and circulatory collapse), gastrointestinal changes (anorexia, nausea, and vomiting), and renal damage (albuminuria and glycosuria). The latter is believed to be due to temporary hypokalemic nephritis. These changes appear to be more frequent when the serum levels increase above 1.5 mEq/liter, suggesting that careful monitoring of this parameter is needed rather than reliance on the amount given.

Chronic lithium nephrotoxicity and interstitial nephritis can occur with long-term exposure, even when lithium levels remain within the therapeutic range (Singer, 1981). Animal studies have shown a similarity between lithium and sodium handling and that lithium may cause an ADH-resistant polyuria and secondary polydipsia. This abormality appears to be mediated by a central pituitary effect that reduces ADH release. Treatment with lithium salts has also been associated with nephrotic syndrome with minimal glomerular changes.

The cardiovascular and nervous system changes may be due to the competitive relationship between lithium and potassium and may thus produce a disturbance in intracellular metabolism. Thyrotoxic reactions, including goiter formation, have also been suggested

(Davis and Fann, 1971). While there has been some indication of adverse effects on fetuses following lithium treatment, none was observed in rats (4.05 mEq/kg), rabbits (1.08 mEq/kg), or primates (0.67 mEq/kg). This dose to rats was sufficient to produce maternal toxicity and effects on the pups of treated lactating dams (Gralla and McIlhenny, 1972).

Lithium overdosage and toxicity may be treated by administration of diuretics and lowering of blood levels. Acetazolamide, a carbonic anhydrase inhibitor, has been used clinically. Animal studies have shown that urinary excretion of lithium can be further enhanced by the combined administration of acetazolamide and furosemide. Treatment with diuretics must be accompanied by replacement of water and electrolytes (Steele, 1977).

Platinum

Platinum group metals include a relatively light triad of ruthenium, rhodium, and palladium and the heavy metals osmium, iridium, and platinum. They are found together in sparsely distributed mineral deposits or as a by-product of refining other metals, chiefly nickel and copper. Osmium and iridium are not important toxicologically. Osmium tetroxide, however, is a powerful eye irritant. The other metals are generally nontoxic in their metallic states but have been noted to have toxic effects in particular circumstances. Platinum is interesting because of its extensive industrial applications and use of certain complexes as antitumor agents.

Toxicological information for ruthenium is limited to references in the literature indicating that fumes may be injurious to eyes and lungs (Browning, 1969).

Rhodium trichloride produced death in rats and rabbits within 48 hours after intravenous administration at doses near the LD50 (approximately 200 mg/kg). It was suggested that death was attributable to central nervous system effects. In a single study, incorporation of rhodium (rhodium chloride) or palladium (palladous chloride) into the drinking water of mice at a concentration of 5 ppm over the lifetime of the animals produced a minimally significant increase in malignant tumors. Most of these tumors were classified as of the lymphoma-leukemia type (Schroeder and Mitchener, 1972).

Palladium chloride is not readily absorbed from subcutaneous injection, and no adverse effects have been reported from industrial exposure. Colloid palladium (Pd[OH]$_2$) is reported to increase body temperature, produce discoloration and necrosis at the site of injection, decrease body weight, and cause slight hemolysis.

Platinum metal itself is generally harmless, but an allergic dermatitis can be produced in susceptible individuals. Skin changes are most common between the fingers and in the antecubital fossae. Symptoms of respiratory distress, ranging from irritation to an "asthmatic syndrome" with coughing, wheezing, and shortness of breath, have been reported following exposure to platinum dust. The skin and respiratory changes are termed platinosis. They are mainly confined to persons with a history of industrial exposure to soluble compounds such as sodium chloroplatinate, although cases resulting from wearing platinum jewelry have been reported.

The complex salts of platinum may act as powerful allergens, particularly ammonium hexachloroplatinate and hexachloroplatinic acid. The allergenicity appears to be related to the number of chlorine atoms present in the molecule, but other soluble nonchlorinated platinum compounds may also be allergenic. Major considerations for this group of metals are the potential antitumor and carcinogenic effects of certain neutral complexes of platinum such as cis-dichlorodiamine, platinum (II) (or cis-platin), and various analogues (Kazantzis, 1981). They can inhibit cell division and have antibacterial properties as well. These compounds can react selectively with specific chemical sites in proteins such as disulfide bonds and terminal-NH$_2$ groups, with functional groups in amino acids, and in particular with receptor sites in nucleic acids. These compounds also exhibit neuromuscular toxicity and nephrotoxicity.

For antitumor activity, the complexes should be neutral and should have a pair of cis-leaving groups. Other metals in the group give complexes that are inactive or less active than the platinum analogue. At dosages that are therapeutically effective (antitumor), these complexes produce severe and persistent inhibition of DNA synthesis and little inhibition of RNA and protein synthesis. DNA polymerase activity and transport of DNA precursors through plasma membranes are not inhibited. The complexes are thought to react directly with DNA in regions that are rich in guanosine and cytosine.

Mutagenic and Carcinogenic Effects of Platinum Complexes. Cis-platin has been used clinically to treat some cancers of the head and neck, certain lymphomas, and testicular and ovarian tumors. Cis-platin is a strong mutagen in bacterial systems and has been shown to form both intra- and interstrand cross-links probably involving the whole molecule with human DNA in HeLa cell cultures. There is also a correlation between antitumor activity of cis-platin and its ability to bind DNA and induce phage from bacterial cells. It also causes chromosome aberration in cultured hamster cells and a dose-dependent increase in sister chromosome exchanges.

Although *cis*-platin has antitumorigenic activity in experimental animals, it also seems to increase the frequency of lung adenomas and give rise to skin papillomas and carcinomas in mice. These observations are consistent with the activity of other alkylating agents used in cancer chemotherapy. There are no reports of increased risk to cancer from occupational exposure to platinum compounds.

Nephrotoxicity. *Cis*-platin is a nephrotoxin. It produces compounds with antitumor activity and produces proximal and distal tubular cell injury mainly in the corticomedullary region, where the concentration of platinum is highest (Madias and Harrington, 1978). Although 90 percent of administered *cis*-platin becomes tightly bound to plasma proteins, only unbound platinum is rapidly filtered by the glomerulus and has a half-life of only 48 minutes. Within tissues, platinum is protein bound, with largest concentrations in kidney, liver, and spleen, and has a half-life of two or three days. Tubular cell toxicity seems to be directly related to dose, and prolonged weekly injection in rats causes atrophy of cortical portions of nephrons and cystic dilatation of inner cortical or medullary tubules and chronic renal failure due to tubulointerstitial nephritis (D. D. Choie *et al.*, 1981).

MINOR TOXIC METALS

Antimony

Antimony may have a tri- or pentavalence, and it belongs to the same periodic group as arsenic. Its disposition metabolism is thought to resemble that of arsenic. It is absorbed slowly from the gastrointestinal tract, and many antimony compounds are gastrointestinal irritants. Antimony tartar has been used as an emetic. The disposition of the tri and penta forms differs. Trivalent antimony is concentrated in red blood cells and liver, whereas the penta form is mostly in plasma. Both forms are excreted in feces and urine, but more trivalent antimony is excreted in urine, whereas there is greater gastrointestinal excretion of pentavalent antimony. Antimony is a common air pollutant from industrial emissions, but exposure for the general population is largely from food.

Antimony is included in alloys in the metals industry and is used for producing fireproofing chemicals, ceramics, glassware, and pigments. It has been used medicinally as an antiparasitic agent. Accidental poisonings can result in acute toxicity, which produces severe gastrointestinal symptoms including vomiting and diarrhea.

Most information about antimony toxicity has been obtained from industrial experiences. Occupational exposures are usually by inhalation of dust containing antimony compounds, antimony penta- and trichloride, trioxide, and trisulfide. Effects may be acute, particularly from the penta- and trichloride exposures, producing a rhinitis and even acute pulmonary edema. Chronic exposures by inhalation of other antimony compounds result in rhinitis, pharyngitis, tracheitis, and over the longer term, bronchitis and eventually pneumoconiosis with obstructive lung disease and emphysema. Antimony does accumulate in lung tissue (Elinder and Friberg, 1986).

Oral feeding of antimony to rats does not produce an excess of tumors. However, increased chromosome defects occur when human lymphocytes are incubated with a soluble antimony salt (Paton and Allison, 1972), and Syrian hamster embryo cells show and undergo neoplastic transformation when treated with antimony acetate (Casto *et al.*, 1979). Transient skin eruptions, "antimony spots," may occur in workers with chronic exposure.

Antimony may also form an odorless toxic gas, stibine (H_3Sb), which, like arsine, causes hemolysis.

Barium

Barium is used in various alloys; in paints, soap, paper, and rubber; and in the manufacture of ceramics and glass. Barium fluorosilicate and carbonate have been used as insecticides. Barium sulfate, an insoluble compound, is used as a radiopaque aid to X-ray diagnosis. Barium is relatively abundant in nature and is found in plants and animal tissue. Plants accumulate barium from the soil. Brazil nuts have very high concentrations (3000 to 4000 ppm). Some water contains barium from natural deposits.

The toxicity of barium compounds depends on their solubility. The soluble compounds of barium are absorbed, and small amounts are accumulated in the skeleton. The lung has an average concentration of 1 ppm (dry weight). The kidney, spleen, muscle, heart, brain, and liver concentrations are 0.10, 0.08, 0.05, and 0.03 ppm, respectively. Although some barium is excreted in urine, it is reabsorbed by the renal tubules. The major route of excretion is the feces. Occupational poisoning to barium is uncommon, but a benign pneumoconiosis (baritosis) may result from inhalation of barium sulfate (barite) dust and barium carbonate. It is not incapacitating and is usually reversible with cessation of exposure. Accidental poisoning from ingestion of soluble barium salts has resulted in gastroenteritis, muscular paralysis, decreased pulse rate, and ventricular fibrillation and extrasystoles. Potassium deficiency occurs in acute poisoning, and treatment with intravenous potassium appears beneficial. The digitalislike toxicity, muscle stimulation, and central nervous system effects have been confirmed by experimental investigation (Reeves, 1986).

Indium

Indium is a rare metal whose toxicologic importance was related to its use in alloys and solders and as a hardening agent for bearings. Use in the electronic industry for production of semiconductors and photovoltaic cells may greatly expand worker exposure. It is currently being used in medicine for scanning of organs and treatment of tumors. Indium is poorly absorbed from the gastrointestinal tract. It is excreted in the urine and feces. Its tissue distribution is relatively uniform. The kidney, liver, bone, and spleen have relatively high concentrations. Intratracheal injections produce similar concentrations, but the concentration in the tracheobronchial lymph nodes is increased.

There are no meaningful reports of human toxicity to indium. From animal experiments, it is apparent that toxicity is related to the chemical form. Indium chloride given intravenously to mice produces renal toxicity and liver necrosis. These effects are accompanied by induction of P-450–dependent microsomal enzyme activity and decreased activity of heme-synthesizing enzymes (Woods *et al.*, 1979). Hydrated indium oxide produces damage to phagocytic cells in liver and the reticuloendothelial system (Fowler, 1982).

Magnesium

Magnesium is used in lightweight alloys, as an electrical conductive material, and for incendiary devices such as flares. It is also an essential nutrient whose deficiency causes neuromuscular irritability, calcification, and cardiac and renal damage, which can be prevented by supplementation. The deficiency is called "grass staggers" in cattle and "magnesium tetany" in calves. Magnesium is a cofactor of many enzymes; it is apparently associated with phosphate in these functions.

Magnesium citrate, oxide, sulfate, hydroxide, and carbonate are widely taken as antacids or cathartics. The hydroxide, milk of magnesia, is one of the constituents of the universal antidote for poisoning. Topically, the sulfate is also used widely to relieve inflammation. Magnesium sulfate may be used as a parenterally administered central depressant. Its most frequent use for this purpose is in the treatment of seizures associated with eclampsia of pregnancy and acute nephritis.

Nuts, cereals, seafoods, and meats are high dietary sources of magnesium. The average city water contains about 6.5 ppm but varies considerably, increasing with the hardness of the water (Schroeder *et al.*, 1969).

Disposition. Magnesium salts are poorly absorbed from the intestine. In cases of overload, this may be due in part to their dehydrating action. Magnesium is absorbed mainly in the small intestine. The colon also absorbs some. Calcium and magnesium are competitive with respect to their absorptive sites, and excess calcium may partially inhibit the absorption of magnesium.

Magnesium is excreted into the digestive tract by the bile and pancreatic and intestinal juices. A small amount of radiomagnesium given intravenously appears in the gastrointestinal tract. The serum levels are remarkably constant. There is an apparent obligatory urinary loss of magnesium, which amounts to about 12 mg/day, and the urine is the major route of excretion under normal conditions. Magnesium found in the stool is probably not absorbed. Magnesium is filtered by the glomeruli and reabsorbed by the renal tubules. In the blood plasma, about 65 percent is in the ionic form, whereas the remainder is bound to protein. The former is that which appears in the glomerular filtrate. Mercurial diuretics cause excretion of magnesium as well as potassium, sodium, and calcium. Excretion also occurs in the sweat and milk. Endocrine activity, particularly of the adrenocortical hormones, aldosterone, and parathyroid hormone, has an effect on magnesium levels, although these effects may be related to the interaction of calcium and magnesium.

Tissue distribution studies indicate that of the 20-g body burden, the majority is intracellular in the bone and muscle. Bone concentration of magnesium decreases as calcium increases. Most of the remaining tissues have higher concentrations than blood, except for fat and omentum. With age, the aorta tends to accumulate magnesium along with calcium, perhaps as a function of atherosclerotic disease.

Toxicity. Freshly generated magnesium oxide can cause metal fume fever if inhaled in sufficient amounts analogous to the effect caused by zinc oxide. Both zinc and magnesium exposure of animals produced similar effects. It is reported that particles of magnesium in the subcutaneous tissue produce lesions that resist healing. In animals, magnesium subcutaneously or intramuscularly administered produces gas gangrene as a result of interaction with the body fluids and subsequent generation of hydrogen and magnesium hydroxide. The tissue lesion is reversible.

Conjunctivitis, nasal catarrh, and coughing up of discolored sputum result from industrial inhalation exposure. With industrial exposures, increases of serum magnesium up to twice the normal levels failed to produce ill effects but were accompanied by calcium increases. Intoxication occurring after oral administration of magnesium salts is rare but may be present in the face of renal impairment. The symptoms include a sharp drop in blood pressure and respiratory paralysis due to central nervous system depression (Browning, 1969).

Silver

The principal industrial use of silver is as silver halide in the manufacture of photographic plates. Other uses are for jewelry, coins, and eating utensils. Silver nitrate is used for making indelible inks and for medicinal purposes. The use of silver nitrate for prophylaxis of ophthalmia neonatorum is a legal requirement in some states. Other medicinal uses of silver salts are as a caustic, germicide, antiseptic, and astringent.

Silver does not occur regularly in animal or human tissue. The major effect of excessive absorption of silver is local or generalized impregnation of the tissues where it remains as silver sulfide, which forms an insoluble complex in elastic fibers, resulting in argyria. Silver can be absorbed from the lungs and gastrointestinal tract. Complexes with serum albumin accumulate in the liver, from which a fractional amount is excreted. Intravenous injection produces accumulation in the spleen, liver, bone marrow, lungs, muscle, and skin. The major route of excretion is via the gastrointestinal tract. Urinary excretion has not been reported to occur even after intravenous injection.

Industrial argyria, a chronic occupational disease, has two forms, local and generalized. The local form involves the formation of gray-blue patches on the skin or may manifest itself in the conjunctiva of the eye. In generalized argyria, the skin shows widespread pigmentation, often spreading from the face to most uncovered parts of the body. In some cases, the skin may become black, with a metallic luster. The eyes may be affected to such a point that the lens and vision are disturbed. The respiratory tract may also be affected in severe cases.

Large oral doses of silver nitrate cause severe gastrointestinal irritation owing to its caustic action. Lesions of the kidneys and lungs and the possibility of arteriosclerosis have been attributed to both industrial and medicinal exposures. Large doses of colloidal silver administered intravenously to experimental animals produced death due to pulmonary edema and congestion. Hemolysis and resulting bone marrow hyperpla-

sia have been reported. Chronic bronchitis has also been reported to result from medicinal use of colloidal silver (Browning, 1969; Luckey *et al.*, 1975).

Tellurium

Tellurium is found in various sulfide ores along with selenium and is produced as a by-product of metal refineries. Its industrial uses include applications in the refining of copper and in the manufacture of rubber. Tellurium vapor is used in "daylight" lamps. It is used in various alloys as a catalyst and as a semiconductor.

Condiments, dairy products, nuts, and fish have high concentrations of tellurium. Food packaging contains some tellurium; higher concentrations are found in aluminum cans than tin cans. Some plants, such as garlic, accumulate tellurium from the soil. Potassium tellurate has been used to reduce sweating.

The average body burden in humans is about 600 mg; the majority is in bone. The kidney is the highest in content among the soft tissues. Some data suggest that tellurium also accumulates in liver (Schroeder and Mitchener, 1972). Soluble tetravalent tellurites, absorbed into the body after oral administration, are reduced to tellurides, partly methylated, and then exhaled as dimethyl telluride. The latter is responsible for the garlic odor in persons exposed to tellurium compounds. Tellurium in the food is probably in the form of tellurates. The urine and bile are the principal routes of excretion. Sweat and milk are secondary routes of excretion.

Tellurates and tellurium are of low toxicity, but tellurites are generally more toxic. Acute inhalation exposure results in decreased sweating, nausea, a metallic taste, and sleeplessness. A typical garlic breath is a reasonable indicator of exposure to tellurium by the dermal inhalation, or oral route. Serious cases of tellurium intoxication from industrial exposure have not been reported. In rats, chronic exposure to high doses of tellurium dioxide has produced decreased growth and necrosis of the liver and kidney (Cerwenka and Cooper, 1961; Browning, 1969).

Sodium tellurite at 2 ppm in drinking water or potassium tellurate at 2 ppm of tellurium plus 0.16 μg/g in the diet of mice for their lifetime produced no effects in the tellurate group. The females of the tellurite (tetravalent) group did not live as long. In rats, 500 ppm in the diet of pregnant females induced hydrocephalus in the offspring. Abnormalities of and reduction in numbers of mitochondria were thought to be possible cellular causes of the transplacental effect.

One of the few serious recorded cases of tellurium toxicity resulted from accidental poisoning by injection of tellurium into the ureters during retrograde pyelography. Two of the three victims died. Stupor, cyanosis, vomiting, garlic breath, and loss of consciousness were observed in this unlikely incident.

Dimercaprol treatment for tellurium increases the renal damage. While ascorbic acid decreases the characteristic garlic odor, it may also adversely affect the kidneys in the presence of increased amounts of tellurium (Fishbein, 1977).

Thallium

Thallium is one of the more toxic metals and can cause neural, hepatic, and renal injury. It may also cause deafness and loss of vision. It is obtained as a by-product of the refining of iron, cadmium, and zinc. It is used as a catalyst, in certain alloys, optical lenses, jewelry, low-temperature thermometers, semiconductors, dyes and pigments, and scintillation counters. It has been used medicinally as a depilatory. Thallium compounds, chiefly thallous sulfate, have been used as rat poison and insecticides. This is one of the commonest sources of thallium poisoning.

Disposition.   Thallium is not a normal constituent of animal tissues. It is absorbed through the skin and gastrointestinal tract. After parenteral administration, a small amount can be identified in the urine within a few hours. The highest concentrations after poisoning are in the kidney and urine. The intestines, thyroids, testes, pancreas, skin, bone, and spleen have lesser amounts. The brain and liver concentrations are still lower. Following the initial exposure, large amounts are excreted in urine during the first 24 hours, but after that period, excretion is slow and the feces may be an important route of excretion.

Toxicology.   There are numerous clinical reports of acute thallium poisoning in humans characterized by gastrointestinal irritation, acute ascending paralysis, and psychic disturbances. Acute toxicity studies in rats have indicated that thallium is quite toxic. It has an oral LD50 of approximately 30 mg/kg. The estimated lethal dose in humans, however, is 8 to 12 mg/kg. Rat studies also indicate that thallium oxide, while relatively insoluble, is more toxic orally than by the intravenous or intraperitoneal route (Downs et al., 1960). The acute cardiovascular effects of thallium ions probably result from competition with potassium for membrane transport systems, inhibition of mitochondrial oxidative phosphorylation, and disruption of protein synthesis. It also alters heme metabolism.

The signs of subacute or chronic thallium poisoning in rats were hair loss, cataracts, and hindleg paralysis occurring with some delay af-ter the initiation of dosing. Renal lesions were observed at gross necropsy. Histologic changes revealed damage of the proximal and distal renal tubules. The central nervous system changes were most severe in the mesencephalon where necrosis was observed. Perivascular cuffing was also reported in several other brain areas. Electron microscope examination indicated that the mitochondria in the kidney may have been the first organelles affected. Liver mitochondria also revealed degenerative changes. The livers of newborn rats whose dams had been treated throughout pregnancy showed these changes. Similar mitochondrial changes were observed in the intestine, brain, seminal vesicle, and pancreas. It has been suggested that thallium may combine with the sulfhydryl groups in the mitochondria and thereby interfere with oxidative phosphorylation (Herman and Bensch, 1967). A teratogenic response to thallium salts characterized as achondroplasia (dwarfism) has been described in rats (Nogami and Terashima, 1973).

In humans, fatty infiltration and necrosis of the liver, nephritis, gastroenteritis, pulmonary edema, degenerative changes in the adrenals, degeneration of peripheral and central nervous system, alopecia, and in some cases, death have been reported as a result of long-term systemic thallium intake. These cases usually are caused by the contamination of food or the use of thallium as a depilatory. Industrial poisoning is a special risk in the manufacture of fused halides for the production of lenses and windows. Loss of vision plus the other signs of thallium poisoning have been related to industrial exposures (Browning, 1969; Fowler, 1982).

Tin

Tin is used in the manufacture of tinplate, in food packaging, and in solder, bronze, and brass. Stannous and stannic chlorides are used in dyeing textiles. Organic tin compounds have been used in fungicides, bactericides, and slimicides, as well as in plastics as stabilizers. The disposition and possible health effects of inorganic and organic tin compounds have been summarized in a WHO report (1980).

Disposition.   There is only limited absorption of even soluble tin salts such as sodium stannous tartrate after oral administration. Ninety percent of the tin administered in this manner is recovered in the feces. The small amounts absorbed are reflected by increases in the liver and kidneys. Injected tin is excreted by the kidneys, with smaller amounts in bile. A mean normal urine level of 16.6 μg/liter or 23.4 μg/day has been reported. The majority of inhaled tin or its salts remains in the lungs, most extracellularly, with some in the macrophages, in the form of SnO_2. The organic tins, particularly triethyltin, may be somewhat better absorbed. The tissue distribution of tin from this material shows highest concentrations in the blood and liver, with smaller amounts in the muscle, spleen, heart, or brain. Tetraethyltin is converted to triethyltin *in vivo.*

Chronic inhalation of tin in the form of dust or fumes leads to benign pneumoconiosis. Tin hydride (SnH_4) is more toxic to mice and guinea pigs than is arsine; however, its effects appear mainly in the central nervous system and no hemolysis is produced. Orally, tin or its inorganic compounds require relatively large doses (500 mg/kg for 14 months) to produce toxicity. The use of tin in food processing seems to demonstrate little hazard. The average U.S. daily intake, mostly from foods as a result of processing, is estimated at 17 mg. Inorganic tin salts given by injection produce diarrhea, muscle paralysis, and twitching.

Toxicology. Some organic tin compounds are highly toxic, particularly triethyltin. Trialkyl compounds including triethyltin cause an encephalopathy and cerebral edema. Toxicity declines as the number of carbon atoms in the chain increases. An outbreak of almost epidemic nature took place in France owing to the oral ingestion of a preparation (Stalinon®) containing diethyltin diodide for treatment of skin disorders.

Excessive industrial exposure to triethyltin has been reported to produce headaches, visual defects, and EEG changes that were very slowly reversed (Prull and Rompel, 1970). Experimentally, triethyltin produces depression and cerebral edema. The resulting hyperglycemia may be related to the centrally mediated depletion of catecholamines from the adrenals. Acute burns and subacute dermal irritation have been reported among workers as a result of tributyltin. Triphenyltin has been shown to be a potent immunosuppressant (Verschuuren *et al.,* 1970). Inhibition in the hydrolysis of adenosine triphosphate and uncoupling of oxidative phosphorylation taking place in the mitochondria have been suggested as the cellular mechanisms of tin toxicity (WHO, 1980).

Titanium

Most titanium compounds are in the oxidation state 4+ (titanic), but oxidation state 3+ (titanous) and oxidation state 2+ compounds as well as several organometallic compounds do occur. Titanium dioxide, the most widely used compound, is a white pigment used in paints and plastics; as a food additive to whiten flour, dairy products, and confections; and as a whitener in cosmetic products. Because of its resistance to corrosion and inertness, it has many metallurgical applications, particularly as a component of surgical implants and prostheses. It occurs widely in the environment; it is present in urban air, rivers, and drinking water and is detectable in many foods.

Disposition. Approximately 3 percent of an oral dose of titanium is absorbed. The majority of that absorbed is excreted in the urine. The normal urine concentration has been estimated at 10 µg/liter (Schroeder *et al.,* 1963; Kazantzis, 1981).

The estimated body burden of titanium is about 15 mg. Most of it is in the lungs, probably as a result of inhalation exposure. Inhaled titanium tends to remain in the lungs for long periods. It has been estimated that about one-third of the inhaled titanium is retained in the lungs. The geographic variation in lung burden is to some extent dependent on air concentration. For example, concentrations of 430, 1300, and 91 ppm is ashed lung tissue have been reported for the United States, Delhi, and Hong Kong, respectively. Mean concentrations of 8 and 6 ppm for the liver and kidney, respectively, were reported in the United States. Newborns have little titanium. Lung burdens tend to increase with age.

Toxicology. Occupational exposure to titanium may be heavy, and concentrations in air up to 50 mg/m^3 have been recorded. Titanium dioxide has been classified as a nuisance particulate with a TLV of 10 mg/m^3. Nevertheless, slight fibrosis of lung tissue has been reported following inhalation exposure to titanium dioxide pigment, but the injury was not disabling. Otherwise, titanium dioxide has been considered physiologically inert by all routes (ingestion, inhalation, dermal, and subcutaneous). The metal and other salts are also relatively nontoxic except for titanic acid, which, as might be expected, will produce irritation (Berlin and Nordman, 1986).

A titanium coordination complex, titanocene, suspended in trioctanoin, administered by intramuscular injection to rats and mice, produced fibrosarcomas at the site of injection and hepatomas and malignant lymphomas (Furst and Haro, 1969). A titanocene is a sandwich arrangement of titanium between two cyclopentadiene molecules. Titanium dioxide was found not to be carcinogenic in a bioassay study in rats and mice (NCI, 1979).

Uranium

The chief raw material of uranium is pitchblende or carnotite ore. This element is largely limited to use as a nuclear fuel.

The uranyl ion is rapidly absorbed from the gastrointestinal tract. About 60 percent is carried as a soluble bicarbonate complex, whereas the remainder is bound to plasma protein. Sixty percent is excreted in the urine within 24 hours. About 25 percent may be fixed in the bone (P. S. Chen *et al.*, 1961). Following inhalation of the insoluble salts, retention by the lungs is prolonged. Uranium tetrafluoride and uranyl fluoride can produce a typical toxicity because of hydrolysis to HF. Skin contact (burned skin) with uranyl nitrate has resulted in nephritis.

The soluble uranium compound (uranyl ion) and those that solubilize in the body by the formation of bicarbonate complex produce systemic toxicity in the form of acute renal damage and renal failure, which may be fatal. However, if exposure is not severe enough, the renal tubular epithelium is regenerated and recovery occurs. A study of uranium mill workers suggested that workers' long-term low-level exposure is associated with β_2-microglobulinuria and aminoaciduria (Thun *et al.*, 1985). Renal toxicity with the classic signs of impairment, including albuminuria, elevated blood urea nitrogen, and loss of weight, is brought about by filtration of the bicarbonate complex through the glomerulus, reabsorption by the proximal tubule, liberation of uranyl ion, and subsequent damage to the proximal tubular cells. Uranyl ion is most likely concentrated intracellularly in lysosomes (Ghadially *et al.*, 1982).

Inhalation of uranium dioxide dust by rats, dogs, and monkeys at a concentration of 5 mg U/m^3 for up to five years produced accumulation in the lungs and tracheobronchial lymph nodes that accounted for 90 percent of the body burden. No evidence of toxicity was observed despite the long duration of observation (Leach *et al.*, 1970).

Vanadium

Vanadium is a ubiquitous element. It is a by-product of petroleum refining, and vanadium pentoxide is used as a catalyst in various chemicals including sulfuric acid. It is used in the hardening of steel, in the manufacture of pigments, in photography, and in insecticides. It is common in many foods; significant amounts are found in milk, seafoods, cereals, and vegetables. Vanadium has a natural affinity for fats and oils; food oils have high concentrations. Municipal water supplies may contain on the average about 1 to 6 ppb. Urban air contains some vanadium, perhaps owing to the use of petroleum products or from refineries (Table 19–1), about 30 ng/m^3. The largest single compartment is fat. Bone and teeth stores contribute to the body burden. It has been postulated that some homeostatic mechanism maintains the normal levels of vanadium in the face of excessive intake, since the ele-

ment, in most forms, is moderately absorbed. The principal route of excretion of vanadium is the urine. The normal serum level is 35 to 48 μg/100 ml. When excess amounts of vanadium are in the diet, the concentration in the red cells tends to increase. Parenteral administration increases levels in the liver and kidney, but these increased amounts may only be transient. The lung tissue may contain some vanadium, depending on the exposure by that route, bur normally the other organs contain negligible amounts.

The toxic action of vanadium is largely confined to the respiratory tract. Bronchitis and bronchopneumonia are more frequent in workers exposed to vanadium compounds. In industrial exposures to vanadium pentoxide dust, a greenish-black discoloration of the tongue is characteristic. Irritant activity with respect to skin and eyes has also been ascribed to industrial exposure. Gastrointestinal distress, nausea, vomiting, abdominal pain, cardiac palpitation, tremor, nervous depression, and kidney damage, too, have been linked with industrial vanadium exposure.

Ingestion of vanadium compounds (V_2O_5) for medicinal purposes produced gastrointestinal disturbances, slight abnormalities of clinical chemistry related to renal function, and nervous system effects. Acute vanadium poisoning in animals is characterized by marked effects on the nervous system, hemorrhage, paralysis, convulsions, and respiratory depression. Short-term inhalation exposure of experimental animals tends to confirm the effects on the lungs as well as the effects on the kidney. In addition, experimental investigations have suggested that the liver, adrenals, and bone marrow may be adversely affected by subacute exposure at high levels (Waters, 1977; Wennig and Kirsch, 1988).

REFERENCES

Ainsworth, S. K.; Swain, R. P.; Watabe, N.; Brackett, N. C.; Pilia, P.; and Hennigar, G. R.: Gold nephropathy, ultrastructural fluorescent, and energy-dispersive x-ray microanalysis study. *Arch. Pathol. Lab. Med.*, **105**:373–378, 1981.

Alfrey, A. C.: Aluminum and tin. In Bonner, F., and Coburn, J. W. (eds.): *Disorders of Mineral Metabolism.* Academic Press, Inc., New York, 1981, pp. 353–369.

Alfrey, A. C.; Mishell, J. M.; Burks, J.; Contiguglia, S. R.; Rudolph, H.; Lewin, E.; and Holmes, J. H.: Syndrome of dyspraxia and multifocal seizures associated with chronic hemodialysis. *Trans. Am. Soc. Artif. Intern. Organs,* **18**:257–261, 1972.

American Conference of Governmental Industrial Hygienists (ACGIH): *Threshold Limit Values (TLV) and Biological Exposure Indices for 1985–1986.* ACGIH, Cincinnati, Ohio, 1985.

Anderson, A., and Hahlin, M.: Cadmium effects from phosphorus fertilization in field experiments. *Swed. J. Agric. Res.,* **11**:2, 1981.

Angerer, J., and Heinrich, R.: Cobalt. In Seiler, H. G., and Sigel, H. (eds.): *Handbook on Toxicity of Inorganic Compounds*. Marcel Dekker, New York, 1987, pp. 251–263.

Anke, M.; Grun, M.; Gropped, B.; and Kronemann, H.: Nutritional requirement of nickel. In Sarkar, B. (ed.): *Biologic Aspect of Metals and Metal-Related Diseases*. Raven Press, New York, 1983, pp. 88–105.

Araki, S., and Ushio, K.: Mechanism of increased osmotic resistance of red cells in workers exposed to lead. *Br. J. Ind. Med.*, **39**:157–160, 1982.

Arena, J. M.: *Poisoning*, 3rd ed. Charles C. Thomas, Publ., Springfield, Ill., 1974.

Astrin, K. H.; Bishop, D. F.; Wetmur, J. G.; Kaul, B.; Davidow, B.; and Desnick, R. J.: Delta-aminolevulinic acid dehydratase isozymes and lead toxicity. *Ann. N.Y. Acad. Sci.*, **514**:23–29, 1987.

ATSDR.: *The Nature and Extent of Lead Poisoning in Children in the United States: A Report to Congress*. Agency for Toxic Substances and Disease Registry, U.S. Department of Health and Human Services, Atlanta, Ga., 1989.

Baker, E. L.; Goyer, R. A.; Fowler, B. A.; Khettry, U.; Bernard, O. B.; Adler, S.; White, R.; Babayan, R.; and Feldman, R. G.: Occupational lead exposure, nephropathy and renal cancer. *Am. J. Ind. Med.*, **1**:139–148, 1980.

Bakir, R.; Damluji, S. F.; Amin-Zaki, L.; Murtadha, M.; Khalidi, A.; Al-Rawi, N. Y.; Tikriti, S.; Dhahir, H. I.; Clarkson, T. W.; Smith, J. C.; and Doherty, R. A.: Methyl mercury poisoning in Iraq. *Science*, **181**:230–241, 1973.

Beijer, K., and Jernelöv, A.: Sources, transport and transformation of metals in the environment. In Friberg, L.; Nordberg, G. F., and Vouk, V. B. (eds.): *Handbook on the Toxicology of Metals*, Vol. I, 2nd ed., *General Aspects*. Elsevier Scientific Publ., Amsterdam, 1986, pp. 68–74.

Bellinger, D.; Leviton, A.; Waternaux, C.; Needleman, H.; and Rabinowitz, M.: Low-level lead exposure, social class and infant development. *Neurotoxicol. Teratol.*, **10**:497–503, 1988.

Bellinger, D.; Needleman, H. L.; Bromfield, R.; and Mintz, M.: A follow-up study of the academic attainment and classroom behavior of children with elevated dentine lead levels. *Biol. Trace Elem. Res.*, **6**:207–223, 1986.

Berlin, M.: Mercury. In Friberg, L.; Nordberg, G. F.; and Vouk, V. B. (eds.): *Handbook on the Toxicology of Metals*, Vol. II, 2nd ed., *Specific Metals*. Elsevier Scientific Publ., Amsterdam, 1986, pp. 386–445.

Berlin, R., and Nordman, C.: Titanium. In Friberg, L.; Nordberg, G. F.; and Vouk, V. B. (eds.): *Handbook on the Toxicology of Metals*, Vol. II, 2nd ed., *Specific Metals*. Elsevier Scientific Publ., Amsterdam, 1986, pp. 594–609.

Bernstein, J.; Evan, A. P.; and Gardner, K. D.: Epithelial hyperplasia in human polycystic kidney disease. Its role in pathogenesis and risk of neoplasia. *Am. J. Pathol.*, **129**:92–101, 1987.

Bertholf, R. L.: Zinc. In Seiler, H. G., and Sigel, H. (eds.): *Handbook on Toxicity of Inorganic Compounds*. Marcel Dekker, New York, 1988, pp. 787–800.

Bessis, M. D., and Jensen, W. N.: Sideroblastic anemia, mitochondria and erythroblastic iron. *Br. J. Haematol.*, **11**:49–51, 1965.

Birchall, J., and Chappell, J.: The chemistry of aluminum and silicon in relation to Alzheimer's disease. *Clin. Chem.*, **34**:265–267, 1988.

Bizzi, A., and Gambetti, P.: Posphorylation of neurofilaments is altered in aluminum intoxication. *Acta Neuropathol.*, **71**:154–158, 1986.

Boscolo, P., and Carmignani, M.: Neurohumoral blood pressure regulation in lead exposure. *Environ. Health Perspect.*, **78**:101–106, 1988.

Boscolo, R.; Galli, G.; Iannaccone, A.; Martino, F.; and Porcelli, G.: Plasma renin activity and urinary kallirein excretion in lead-exposed workers as related to hypertension and neuropathy. *Life Sci.*, **28**:175–184, 1981.

Boulanger, Y.; Goodman, C. M.; Forte, C. P.; Fesik, S. W.; and Armitage, I. M.: Model for mammalian metallothionein structure. *Proc. Natl. Acad. Sci. USA*, **80**:1501–1505, 1983.

Boyd, J. T.; Doll, R.; Foulds, J. S.; and Leiper, J.: Cancer of the lung in iron ore (haematite) miners. *Br. J. Ind. Med.*, **27**:97–103, 1970.

Brown, E. B.: Therapy for disorders of iron excess. In Sarkar, B. (ed.): *Biological Aspects of Metal-Related Diseases*. Raven Press, New York, 1983, pp. 263–278.

Brown, M. M.; Rhyne, B. C.; Goyer, R. A.; and Fowler, B. A.: Intracellular effects of chronic arsenic administration on renal proximal tubule cells. *J. Toxicol. Environ. Health*, **1**:505–514, 1976.

Browning, E.: *Toxicity of Industrial Metals*, 2nd ed. Butterworths, London, 1969.

Buchet, J. -P.; Roels, H.; Bernard, A.; and Lauwerys, R.: Asssessment of renal function of workers exposed to inorganic lead, cadmium, or mercury vapor. *J.O.M.*, **22**:741–750, 1980.

Burchfiel, J.L.; Duffy, F. H.; Bartels, P. H.; and Needleman, H. L.: The combined discriminating power of quantitative electroencephalography and neuropsychologic measures in evaluating central nervous system effects of lead at low levels. In Needleman, H. D. (ed.): *Low Level Lead Exposures*. Raven Press, New York, 1980, pp. 75–90.

Burk, R. F.: Selenium in man. In Prasad, A. S., and Oberleas, D. (eds.): *Trace Elements in Human Health and Disease*, Vol. II. Academic Press, Inc., New York, 1976, pp. 105–134.

Casto, B. C.; Meyers, J.; and DiPaolo, J. A.: Enhancement of viral transformation for evaluation of the carcinogenic or mutagenic potential of inorganic metal salts. *Cancer Res.*, **39**:193–198, 1979.

CDC.: *Preventing Lead Poisoning in Young Children—A Statement by the Centers for Disease Control, Atlanta, Ga.* U.S. Department of Health and Human Services. No. 99–2230. Government Printing Office, Washington, D.C., 1985.

Cerwenka, E. A., and Cooper, W. C.: Toxicology of selenium and tellurium and their compounds. *Arch. Environ. Health*, **3**:189–200, 1961.

Chan, W. Y.; Tease, L. A.; Liu, H. C.; and Rennert, O. M.: Cell culture studies in Wilson's disease. In Sarkar, B. (ed.): *Biological Aspects of Metals and Metal-Related Diseases*. Raven Press, New York, 1983, pp. 147–158.

Chang, C. C.; Vander Mallie, R. J.; and Garvey, J. S.: A radioimmunoassay for human metallothionein. *Toxicol. Appl. Pharmacol.*, **55**:94–102, 1980.

Chen, P. S.; Terepka, R.; and Hodge, H. C.: The pharmacology and toxicology of the bone seekers. *Annu. Rev. Pharmacol.*, **1**:369–393, 1961.

Chen, X.; Yang, G.; Chen, J.; Chen, X.; Wen, Z.; and Ge, K.: Studies on the relationship of selenium and Keshan disease. *Biol. Trace Elem. Res.*, **2**:91–107, 1980.

Cherian, M. G.; Goyer, R. A.; and Delaquerriere-Richardson, L.: Cadmium-metallothionein induced nephropathy. *Toxicol. Appl. Pharmacol.*, **38**:399–408, 1976.

Cherian, M. G.; Miles, E. F.; Clarkson, T. W.; and Cox, C.: Estimation of mercury burdens in rats by chelation with dimercaptopropane sulfonate. *J. Pharmacol. Exp. Ther.*, **245**:479–484, 1988.

Cherian, M. G., and Rodgers, K.: Chelation of cadmium from metallothionein *in vivo* and its excretion in rats repeatedly injected with cadmium chloride. *J. Pharmacol. Exp. Ther.*, **222**:699–704, 1982.

Chisholm, J. J., Jr.: Chelation therapy in children with subclinical plumbism. *Pediatrics*, **53**:441–443, 1974.

Chisholm, J. J., Jr., and O'Hara, D. M. (eds.): *Lead Absorption in Children. Management, Clinical and Environmental Aspects.* Urban and Schwarzenberg, Baltimore, 1982.

Chisholm, J. J., Jr., and Thomas, D.: Use of 2,3-dimercaptopropane-1-sulfonate in treatment of lead poisoning in children. *J. Pharmacol. Exp. Ther.*, **235**:665–669, 1985.

Choie, B. H.; Lapham, L. W.; Amin-Zaki, L.; and Al-Saleem, T.: Abnormal neuronal migration, deranged cerebral cortical organization and diffuse white matter astrocytosis of human fetal brain. *J. Neuropathol. Exp. Neurol.*, **37**:719–733, 1978.

Choie, D. D.; Longenecker, D. S.; and Del Campo, A. A.: Acute and chronic cisplatin neophropathy in rats. *Lab. Invest.*, **44**:397–402, 1981.

Choie, D. D., and Richter, G. W.: Effect of lead on the kidney. In Singhal, R. O., and Thomas, J. A. (eds.): *Lead Toxicity.* Urban and Schwarzenberg, Baltimore, 1980.

Chuttani, H. K.; Gupti, P. S.; and Gultati, S.: Acute copper sulfate poisoning. *Am. J. Med.*, **39**:849–854, 1965.

Clarkson, T. W.: Methylmercury toxicity to the mature and developing nervous system: possible mechanisms. In Sarkar, B. (ed.): *Biological Aspects of Metals and Metal-Related Diseases.* Raven Press, New York, 1983, pp. 183–197.

Clarkson, T. W.; Friberg, L.; Hursh, J. B.; and Nylander, M.: The prediction of intake of mercury vapor from amalgams. In Clarkson, T. W.; Friberg, L.; Nordberg, G. F.; and Sager, P. (eds.): *Biological Monitoring of Metals.* Plenum Press, New York, 1988, pp. 247–264.

Columbano, A.; Ledda, G. M.; Siriqu, P.; Perra, T.; and Pani, P.: Liver cell proliferation induced by a single dose of lead nitrate. *Am. J. Pathol.*, **110**:83–88, 1983.

Cooper, W. C.: Occupational lead exposure. What are the risks? *Science*, **180**:129, 1980.

Cooper, W. C., and Gaffey, W. R.: Mortality of lead workers. J.O.M., **17**: 100–107, 1975.

Costa, M.: *Metal Carcinogenesis Testing, Principles and In Vitro Methods.* Humana Press, Clifton, N.J., 1980.

Cotzias, G. C.; Papavasiliou, P. S.; Ginos, J.; Stechk, A.; and Duby, S.: Metabolic modification of Parkinson's disease and of chronic manganese poisoning. *Annu. Rev. Med.*, **22**:305–336, 1971.

Cox, C.; Clarkson, T. W.; Marsh, D. O.; Amin-Zaki, L.; Tikriti, S.; and Myers, G. G.: Dose-response analysis of infants prenatally exposed to methyl mercury: an application of a single compartment model to single-strand hair analysis. *Environ. Res.*, **49**:318–332, 1989.

Cox, M., and Singer, I.: Lithium. In Bronner, F., and Coburn, J. W. (eds.): *Disorders of Mineral Metabolism.* Academic Press, Inc., New York, 1981, pp. 369–438.

Crapper, D. R.; McLachlan, C. D.; Krishnan, B.; Krishnan, S. S.; Dalton, A. J.; and Steele, J. C.: Aluminum and calcium in soil and food from Guam, Palau and Jamaica: implications for amyotropic lateral sclerosis and parkinsonism-dementia syndromes of Guam. *Environ. Geochem. Health*, **11**:47–53, 1989.

Crecelius, E. A.: Changes in the chemical speciation of arsenic following ingestion by man. *Environ. Health Perspect.*, **19**:147–150, 1977.

Curzon, M. E.; Adkins, B. L.; Bibby, B. G.; and Losee, F. L.: Combined effect of trace elements and fluorine on caries. *J. Dent. Res.*, **49**:526–528, 1970.

Davies, N. T.: Studies on the absorption of zinc by rat intestine. *Br. J. Nutr.*, **43**: 189–203, 1980.

Davis, J. W., and Fann, W. E.: Lithium. *Annu. Rev. Pharmacol.*, **11**:285–298, 1971.

DeBoni, U.; Otvos, A.; Scott, J. W.; and Crapper, D. R.: Neurofibrillary degeneration induced by system aluminum. *Acta Neuropathol.*, **35**:285–294, 1976.

DHEW.: *Occupational Diseases: A Guide to Their Recognition.* U.S. Department of Health, Education and Welfare, Publication No. 77–1811. Washington, D.C., 1977, p. 305.

Dingwall-Fordyce, I., and Lane, R. E.: A follow-up study of lead workers. *Br. J. Ind. Med.*, **20**:313–315, 1963.

DiPaolo, J. A., and Casto, B. C.: Quantitative studies of *in vitro* morphologic transformation of Syrian hamster cells by inorganic metal salts. *Cancer Res.*, **39**:1008–1019, 1979.

Diplock, A. T.: Metabolic aspects of selenium action and toxicity. *Crit. Rev. Toxicol.*, **4**:271–329, 1976.

Doll, R.; Mathews, J. D.; and Morgan, L. G.: Cancers of the lung and nasal sinuses in nickel workers: reassessment of the period of risk. *Br. J. Ind. Med.*, **34**:102–106, 1977.

Downs, W. L.; Scott, J. K.; Steadman, L. T.; and Maynard, E. A.: Acute and subacute toxicity studies of thallium compounds. *Am. Ind. Hyg. Assoc. J.*, **21**:399–406, 1960.

Dudley, R. E.; Gammal, L. M.; and Klaassen, C. D.: Cadmium-induced hepatic and renal injury in chronically exposed rats: likely role of hepatic cadmium-metallothionein in nephrotoxicity. *Toxicol. Appl. Pharmacol.*, **77**:414–426, 1985.

Dunick, J. K.; Elwell, M. R.; Benson, J. M.; Hobbs, C. H.; Hahn, F. F.; Haly, P. J.; Cheng, Y. S.; and Edison, A. F.: Lung toxicity after 13-week inhalation exposure to nickel oxide, nickel subsulfide or nickel sulfate hexahydrate in F344/N rats and B6C3F mice. *Fund. Appl. Toxicol.*, **12**:584–594, 1989.

Editorial. Selenium perspective. *Lancet*, **1**:685, 1983.

Egle, P. M., and Shelton, K. R.: Chronic lead intoxication causes a brain-specific nuclear protein to accumulate in the nuclei of cells lining kidney tubules. *J. Biol. Chem.*, **261**:2294–2298, 1986.

Elinder, C. -G., and Friberg, L.: Antimony. In Friberg, L.; Nordberg, G. F.; and Vouk, V. B. (eds.): *Handbook on the Toxicology of Metals*, Vol. II, 2nd ed., *Specific Metals.* Elsevier Scientific Publ., Amsterdam, 1977, pp. 56–85.

———: Cobalt. In Friberg, L.; Nordberg, G. F.; and Vouk, V. B. (eds.): *Handbook of the Toxicology of Metals.* Vol. II, 2nd ed., *Specific Metals.* Elsevier Scientific Publ., Amsterdam, 1986, pp. 211–232.

Elinder, C. -G.; Kjellstrom, T.; Lind, B.; Linnman, L.; Piscator, M.; and Sundstedt, K.: Cadmium exposure from smoking cigarettes. Variations with time and country where purchased. *Environ. Res.*, **32**:220–227, 1983.

Ellis, K. J.; Cohn, S. H.; and Smith, T.: Cadmium inhalation exposure estimates: their significance with respect to kidney and liver cadmium burden. *J. Toxicol. Environ. Health*, **15**:173–187, 1985.

Ellis, K. J.; Yuen, K.; Yasumura, S.; and Cohn, S. H.: Dose-response analysis of cadmium in man: body burden vs. kidney dysfunction. *Environ. Res.*, **33**:216–226, 1984.

Enterline, P. E., and Marsh, G. M.: Mortality studies

of smelter workers. *Am. J. Ind. Med.*, **1**:251–259, 1980.

EPA.: *Health Assessment Document for Cadmium.* EPA 60/8–81/023. U.S. Environmental Protection Agency, Washington, D.C., 1981.

———: *Health Assessment Document for Arsenic.* EPA 600/8–83–021F. U.S. Environmental Protection Agency, Washington, D.C., 1984.

———: *Air Quality Criteria for Lead,* Vols. I–IV. EPA–600/8–83/02aF. U.S. Environmental Protection Agency, Washington, D.C., 1986.

———: *Health Assessment Document for Beryllium.* EPA/600/8–84/026F. U.S. Environmental Protection Agency, Washington, D.C., 1987a.

———: *Special Report on Ingested Inorganic Arsenic: Skin Cancer and Nutritional Essentiality. Risk Assessment Form.* U.S. Environmental Protection Agency, Washington, D.C., 1987b.

———: *Summary Review of the Health Effects Associated with Copper. Health Issue Assessment.* EPA/600/8–87/001. U.S. Environmental Protection Agency, Washington, D.C., 1987c.

———: *Evaluation of the Potential Carcinogenicity of Lead and Lead Compounds.* EPA–600/8–89/045A. U.S. Environmental Protection Agency, Washington, D.C., 1989a.

———: *Supplement to the 1986 EPA Air Quality Criteria for Lead,* Vol. 1, *Addendum* EPA/600/8–89/049A. Office of Health and Environmental Assessment, U.S. Environmental Protection Agency, Washington, D.C., 1989b (pp. A1–A67).

Eyssen, G. E. M.; Reudy, J.; and Neims, A.: Methylmercury exposure in northern Quebec: II. Neurological finds in children. *Am. J. Epidemiol.*, **118**:470–478, 1983.

Fan, P. L.: Safety of amalgam. *CDA J.*, Sept.:**53**:34–36, 1987.

Ferm, V. H.: Arsenic as a teratogenic agent. *Environ. Health Perspect.*, **19**:215–217, 1977.

Fishbein, L.: Toxicology of selenium and tellurium. In Goyer, R. A., and Mehlman, M. A. (eds.): *Toxicology of Trace Metals.* John Wiley & Sons, New York, 1977, pp. 191–240.

———: Sources, transport and alteration of metal compounds: an overview. I. Arsenic, beryllium, cadmium, chromium, and nickel. *Environ. Health Perspect.*, **40**:43–64, 1981.

Flanagan, P. R.; McLellan, J.; Haist, J.; Cherian, M. G.; Chamberlain, M. J.; and Valberg, L. S.: Increased dietary cadmium absorption in mice and human subjects with iron deficiency. *Gastroenterology*, **74**:841–846, 1978.

Fluharty, A. L., and Sanadi, D. R.: On the mechanism of oxidative phosphorylation. II. Effect of arsenite alone and in combination with 2,3-dimercaptopropanol. *J. Biol. Chem.*, **236**:2772–2778, 1961.

Fowler, B. A.: Indium and thallium in health. In Rose, J. (ed.): *Trace Metals in Human Health.* Butterworth, London, 1982, pp. 74–82.

Fowler, B. A., and Goyer, R. A.: Bismuth localization within nuclear inclusions by x-ray microanalysis. *J. Histochem. Cytochem.*, **23**:722–726, 1975.

Fowler, B. A., and Vouk, V.: Bismuth. In Friberg, L.; Nordberg, G. F.; and Vouk, V. B. (eds.): *Handbook on the Toxicology of Metals,* Vol. II, 2nd ed., *Specific Metals.* Elsevier Scientific Publ., Amsterdam, 1986, pp. 117–129.

Fowler, B. A., and Weissberg, J. B.: Arsine poisoning. *N. Engl. J. Med.*, **291**:1171–1174, 1974.

Friberg, L.; Elinder, C. G.; Kjellstrom, T.; and Nordberg, G. (eds.): *Cadmium and Health. A Toxicological and Epidemiological Appraisal,* Vol. I, *General Aspects;* Vol. II, *Effects and Response.* CRC Press, Inc., Boca Raton, Fla., 1986a.

Friberg, L., and Lener, J.: Molybdenum. In Friberg, L.; Nordberg, G. F., and Vouk, V. B. (eds.): *Handbook on the Toxicology of Metals,* Vol. II, 2nd ed., *Specific Metals.* Elsevier Scientific Publ., Amsterdam, 1986.

Friberg, L., and Nelson, N.: Introduction, general findings and general recommendations. Workshop/Conference on the Role of Metals in Carcinogenesis. *Environ. Health Perspect.*, **40**:5–10, 1981.

Friberg, L.; Nordberg, G. F.; and Vouk, V. B. (eds.): *Handbook on the Toxicology of Metals,* Vol. 1, *General Aspects.* Elsevier Scientific Publ., Amsterdam, 1986b.

Furst, A.: Bioassay of metals for carcinogenesis: whole animals. *Environ. Health Perspect.*, **40**:83–91, 1981.

Furst, A., and Haro, R. T.: A survey of metal carcinogenesis. *Prog. Exp. Tumor Res.*, **12**:102–133, 1969.

Gabard, B.: Treatment of methyl mercury poisoning in the rat with sodium 2,3-dimercaptopropane-i-sulfonate: influence of dose and mode of administration. *Toxicol. Appl. Pharmacol.*, **38**:415–424, 1976.

Ganrot, P. O.: Metabolism and possible health effects of aluminum. *Environ. Health Perspect.*, **65**:363–441, 1986.

Garruto, R. M.; Fukatsu, R.; Yanaghara, R.; Gajdusek, D. C.; Hook, G.; and Fiori, C. E.: Imaging of calcium and aluminum in neurofibrillary tangle-bearing neurons in parkinsonism-dementia of Guam. *Proc. Natl. Acad. Sci. USA*, **81**:1875–1879, 1984.

Ghadially, F. N.; Lalonde, J. A.; and Yang-Steppuhn, S.: Uraniosomes produced in cultured rabbit kidney cells by uranyl acetate. *Virchows Arch. (Cell Pathol.)*, **39**:21–30, 1982.

Gilman, W.: Metal carcinogenesis. II. Study on the carcinogenicity of cobalt, copper, iron, and nickel compounds. *Cancer Res.*, **22**:158–170, 1962.

Goldstein, B. D.; Amoruso, M.; and Witz, G.: Erythrocyte glucose-6-phosphate dehydrogenase deficiency does not pose an increased risk for Black Americans exposed to oxidant gases in the workplace or general environment. *Toxicol. Ind. Health*, **1**:75–80, 1985.

Goldwater, L. J.: *Mercury: A History of Quicksilver.* York Press, Baltimore, 1972, pp. 270–277.

Goyer, R. A.: Lead and the kidney. *Curr. Top. Pathol.*, **55**:147–176, 1971a.

———: Lead toxicity: a problem in environmental pathology. *Am. J. Pathol.*, **64**:167–182, 1971b.

———: The nephrotoxic effects of lead. In Bach, P.; Bonner, F. W.; Bridges, J. W.; and Lock, E. A. (eds.): *Nephrotoxicity, Assessment and Pathogenesis.* John Wiley and Sons, Publ., Chichester, England, 1982, pp. 338–348.

———: Metal-protein complexes in detoxification process. In Brown, S. S. (ed.): *Clinical Chemistry and Clinical Toxicology,* Vol. 2. Academic Press, Inc., London, 1984, pp. 199–209.

———: Overview of conference on health effects of acid precipitation. *Environ. Health Perspect.*, **63**:3–4, 1985.

———: Transplacental transport of lead. *Environ. Health Perspect.*, in press.

Goyer, R. A.; Apgar, J.; and Piscator, M.: Toxicity of zinc. In Henkin, R. I., and Committee (eds.): *Zinc.* University Park Press, Baltimore, 1979, pp. 249–268.

Goyer, R. A.; Miller, C. R.; Zhu, S. -Y.; and Victery, W.: Non-metallothionein bound cadmium in the pathogenesis of cadmium nephropathy in the rat. *Toxicol. Appl. Pharmacol.*, **101**:232–244, 1989a.

Goyer, R. A., and Rhyne, B.: Pathological effects of lead. *Int. Rev. Exp. Pathol.*, **12**:1–77, 1973.

Goyer, R. A.; Weinberg, C. R.; Victery, W. M.; and Miller, C. R.: Lead induced nephrotoxicity: kidney calcium as an indicator of tubular injury. In Bach, P.

H., and Lock, E. A. (eds.): *Nephrotoxicity*. Plenum Publishing Co., 1989b, pp. 11–20.

Goyer, R. A., and Wilson, M. H.: Lead-induced inclusion bodies: results of EDTA treatment. *Lab. Invest.*, **32**:149–156, 1975.

Gralla, E. J., and McIlhenny, H. M.: Studies in pregnant rats, rabbits, and monkeys with lithium carbonate. *Toxicol. Appl. Pharmacol.*, **21**:428–433, 1972.

Grandjean, P., and Grandjean, E. (eds.): *Effects of Organolead Compounds*. CRC Press, Boca Raton, Fla., 1984.

Gritzka, T. L., and Trump, B. F.: Renal tubular lesions caused by mercuric chloride. *Am. J. Pathol.*, **52**:1225–1277, 1968.

Gunsalus, I. C.: The chemistry and function of the pyruvate oxidation factor (lipoic acid). *J. Cell. Comp. Physiol.*, **41** (Suppl. 1):113–136, 1953.

Hayes, R. L.: Gallium. In Seiler, H. G., and Sigel, N. (eds.): *Handbook on Toxicity of Inorganic Compounds*. Marcel Dekker, New York, 1988, pp. 297–300.

Henderson, A. S.: The epidemiology of Alzheimer's disease. *Br. Med. Bull.*, **42**:3–10, 1986.

Henry, G. A.; Jarnot, B. M.; Steinhoff, M. M.; and Bigazzi, P. E.: Mercury-induced autoimmunity in the MAXX rat. *Clin. Immunol. Immunopathol.*, **49**:187–203, 1988.

Herman, M. M., and Bensch, K. G.: Light and electron microscopic studies of acute and chronic thallium intoxication in rats. *Toxicol. Appl. Pharmacol.*, **10**:199–222, 1967.

Hogberg, J., and Alexander, J.: Selenium. In Friberg, L.; Nordberg, G. F.; and Vouk, V. B. (eds.): *Handbook on the Toxicology of Metals*, Vol. II, 2nd ed., *Specific Metals*. Elsevier Scientific Publ., Amsterdam, 1986, pp. 482–512.

Hueper, W. C.: *Occupational and Environmental Cancers of the Respiratory System*. Springer-Verlag, New York, 1966.

IARC: *Monograph on the Evaluations of Carcinogenicity: An Update of IARC Monographs*, Vols. 1–42, Suppl. 7. World Health Organization, International Agency for Research on Cancer, Lyon, France, 1987.

Ineichen, B.: Measuring the rising tide. How many dementia cases will there be by 2001? *Br. J. Psychol.*, **11**:26–35, 1987.

Jacobs, A.: Iron overload—clinical and pathological aspects. *Semin. Hematol.*, **14**:89–113, 1977.

Jacobs, A., and Worwood, M.: Iron. In Bronner, F., and Coburn, J. W. (eds.): *Disorders of Mineral Metabolism*, Vol. 1, *Trace Minerals*. Academic Press, Inc., New York, 1981, pp. 2–59.

Jamall, I. S., and Sprowls, J. T.: Effects of cadmium and dietary selenium on cytoplasmic and mitochondrial antioxidant defense systems in the heart of rats fed high dietary copper. *Toxicol. Appl. Pharmacol.*, **87**:102–110, 1987.

Johnson, J. L.; Jones, H. P.; and Rajagopalan, K. V.: *In vitro* reconstitution of demolybdosulfite oxidase by a molydenum cofactor from rat liver and other sources. *J. Biol. Chem.*, **252**:4994–5003, 1977.

Jones, S. G.; Singh, P. K.; and Jones, M. M.: Use of the Topliss scheme for the design of more effective chelating agents for cadmium decorporation. *Chem. Res. Toxicol.*, **1**:2234–2237, 1988.

Kagey, B. T.; Bumgarner, J. E.; and Creason, J. P.: Arsenic levels in maternal-fetal tissue sets. In Hemphill, O. D. (ed.): *Trace Substances in Environmental Health XI*. University of Missouri Press, Columbia, 1977, pp. 252–256.

Kang, H. K.; Infante, P. F.; and Carra, J. S.: Occupational lead exposure and cancer. *Science*, **207**:935–936, 1980.

Kawada, T.; Koyama, H.; and Suzuko, S.: Cadmium, NAG activity and β_2-microglobulin in the urine of cadmium pigment workers. *Br. J. Ind. Med.*, **46**:52–55, 1989.

Kazantzis, G.: Renal tubular dysfunction and abnormalities of calcium metabolism in cadmium workers. *Environ. Health Perspect.*, **28**:155–160, 1979.

———:Role of cobalt, iron, lead, manganese, mercury, platinum, selenium and titanium in carcinogenesis. *Environ. Health Perspect.*, **40**:143–161, 1981.

Keberle, H.: The biochemistry of desferrioxamine and its relation to iron metabolism. *Ann. N.Y. Acad. Sci.*, **119**:758–768, 1964.

Keen, C. L., and Leach, R. M.: Manganese. In Seiler, H. G., and Sigel, H. (eds.): *Handbook on Toxicity of Inorganic Compounds*. Marcel Dekker, New York, 1988, pp. 405–415.

Kido, T.; Honda, R.; Tsuritani, I.; Yamaya, H.; Ishizaki, M.; Yamada, Y.; and Nogawa, K.: Progress of renal dysfunction in inhabitants environmentally exposed to cadmium. *Arch. Environ. Health*, **43**:213–217, 1988.

Kjellstrom, T.; Friberg, L.; and Rahnster, B.: Mortality and cancer morbidity among cadmium-exposed workers. *Environ. Health Perspect.*, **28**:199–204, 1979.

Klatzo, I.; Wisniewski, H.; and Streicher, E.: Experimental production of neurofibrillary degenerations I. Light microscopic observations. *J. Neuropathol. Exp. Neurol.*, **24**:187–199, 1965.

Kneip, T. J.; Eisenbud, M.; Strehlow, C. D.; and Freudenthal, P. C.: Airborne particulates in New York City. *J. Air Pollut. Control Assoc.*, **20**:144–149, 1970.

Kojima, S.; Ono, H.; Kiyozumi, M.; Honda, T.; and Takadate, A.: Effect of *N*-benzyl-D-glucamine dithiocarbamate on the renal toxicity produced by subacute exposure to cadmium in the rat. *Toxicol. Appl. Pharmacol.*, **98**:39–48, 1989.

Kopp, S. J.; Perry, H. M.; Perry, E. F.; and Erlanger, M.: Cardiac physiologic and tissue metabolic changes following chronic low-level cadmium and cadmium plus lead ingestion in the rat. *Toxicol. Appl. Pharmacol.*, **69**:149–160, 1983.

Kuschner, M.: The carcinogenicity of beryllium. *Environ. Health Perspect.*, **40**:101–106, 1981.

Lam, H. F.; Conner, M. W.; Rogers, A. E.; Fitzgerald, S.; and Amdur, M. O.: Functional and morphological changes in the lungs of guinea pigs exposed to freshly generated ultrafine zinc oxide. *Toxicol. Appl. Pharmacol.*, **78**:29–38, 1985.

Landrigan, P. J.: (Editorial). Toxicity of lead at low dose. *Br. J. Ind. Med.*, **46**:593–596, 1989.

Langard, S., and Norseth, T.: Chromium. In Friberg, L.; Nordberg, G. F.; and Vouk, V. B. (eds.): *Handbook on Toxicology of Metals*, Vol. II, 2nd ed., *Specific Metals*. Elsevier Scientific, Amsterdam, 1986, pp. 185–210.

Langworth, S.; Elinder, C. G.; and Akesson, A.: Mercury exposure from dental fillings. *Swed. Dent. J.*, **12**:69–70, 1988.

Lauwerys, R. R.: *In vivo* tests to monitor body burdens of toxic metals in man. In Brown, S., and Savory, J. (eds.): *Clinical Toxicology and Clinical Chemistry of Metals*. Academic Press, Inc., New York, 1983, pp. 113–122.

Lauwerys, R. R.; Bernard, A.; Roels, H. A.; Buchet, J. -P.; and Viau, C.: Characterization of cadmium proteinuria in man and rat. *Environ. Health Perspect.*, **54**:147–152, 1984.

Lauwerys, R. R.; Roels, H. A.; Bernard, A.; and Buchet, J. -P.: Renal response to cadmium in a population living in a nonferrous smelter area in Belgium. *Int. Arch. Occup. Environ. Health*, **45**: 271–274, 1980.

Lauwerys, R. R.; Roels, H. A.; Buchet, J. -P.; Bernard,

A.; and Stanescu, D. D.: Investigations on the lung and kidney function in workers exposed to cadmium. *Environ. Health Perspect.*, **28**:137–146, 1979.

Leach, L. J.; Maynard, E. A.; Hodge, H. C.; Scott, J. K.; Yuile, C. L.; Sylvester, G. E.; and Wilson, H. B.: A five year inhalation study with uranium dioxide (UO^2) dust. I. Retention and biologic effect in the monkey, dog and rat. *Health Phys.*, **18**:599–612, 1970.

Lerman, S. A.; Clarkson, T. W.; and Gerson, R. J.: Arsenic uptake and metabolism by liver cells is dependent on arsenic oxidation state. *Chem. Biol. Interact.*, **45**:401–406, 1983.

Levander, O. A.: Considerations on the assessment of selenium status. *Fed. Proc.*, **44**:2579–2583, 1985.

Li, Y. -H.: Geochemical cycles of elements and human perturbation. *Geochim. Cosmochim. Acta*, **45**:2073–2084, 1981.

Lilis, R.: Long-term occupational lead exposure: chronic nephropathy and renal cancer: a case report. *Am. J. Ind. Med.*, **2**:293–297, 1981.

Lilis, R., and Fischbein, A.: Chelation therapy in workers exposed to lead—a critical review. *J.A.M.A.*, **235**:2823–2824, 1976.

Luckey, T. D.; Venugopal, B.; and Hutcheson, D.: *Heavy Metal Toxicity Safety and Hormonology.* Academic Press, Inc., New York, 1975.

Madias, N. E., and Harrington, J. T.: Platinum nephrotoxicity. *Am. J. Med.*, **65**:307–314, 1978.

Madsen, K. M., and Christensen, E. F.: Effects of mercury on lysosomal protein digestion in the kidney proximal tubule. *Lab. Invest.*, **38**:165–171, 1978.

Mahaffey, K. R. (ed.): *Dietary and Environmental Lead: Human Health Effects.* Elsevier Scientific, New York, 1985.

Mahaffey, K. R.; Annest, J. L.; Roberts, J. H.; and Murphy, R. S.: Estimates of blood lead levels: United States 1976–80. Association with selected demographic and socioeconomic factors. *N. Engl. J. Med.*, **307**:573–579, 1982.

Manzer, A. D., and Schreiner, A. W.: Copper-induced acute hemolytic anemia. A new complication of hemodialysis. *Ann. Intern. Med.*, **73**:409–412, 1970.

Markovac, J., and Goldstein, G. W.: Lead activates protein kinase C in immature rat brain microvessel. *Toxicol. Appl. Pharmacol.*, **96**:14–23, 1988.

Martyn, C. N.; Barber, D. J.; Osmond, C.; Harris, E. C.; Edwardson, J. A.; and Lacey, R. F.: Geographical relation between Alzheimer's disease and aluminum in drinking water. *Lancet*, **1**:59–62, 1989.

Matheson, D. S.; Clarkson, T. W.; and Gelfand, E. W.: Mercury toxicity (acrodynia) induced by long-term injection of gamma globulin. *J. Pediatr.*, **97**:153–155, 1980.

McConnell, K. P., and Hoffman, J. G.: Methionine selenomethionine parallels in *E. coli* polypeptide chain initiation and synthesis. *Proc. Soc. Exp. Biol. Med.*, **140**:638–641, 1972.

McEwan, J. C.: Five-year review of sputum cytology in workers at a nickel sinter plant. *Ann. Clin. Lab. Sci.*, **8**:503–509, 1978.

McLaughlin, A. I. G., and Harding, H. E.: Pneumoconiosis and other causes of death in iron and steel foundry workers. *Arch. Ind. Health*, **14**:350–362, 1956.

McLaughlin, J. R.; Goyer, R. A.; and Cherian, M. G.: Formation of lead-induced inclusion bodies in primary rat kidney epithelial cell cultures: effect of actinomycin D and cycloheximide. *Toxicol. Appl. Pharmacol.*, **56**:418–431, 1980.

McMichael, A. J.; Baghurst, P. A.; Wigg, N. R.; Vimpani, G. V.; Robertson, E. F.; and Roberts, R. J.: Port Pirie cohort study: environmental exposure to lead and children's abilities at the age of four years. *N. Engl. J. Med.*, **319**:468–475, 1988.

McNeely, M. D.; Nechay, M. W.; and Sunderman, F. W., Jr.: Measurements of nickel in serum and urine as indices of environmental exposure to nickel. *Clin. Chem.*, **18**:992–995, 1972.

Mena, I.; Kazuko, H.; Burke, K.; and Cotzias, G. C.: Chronic manganese poisoning. Individual susceptibility and absorption of iron. *Neurology*, **19**:1000–1006, 1969.

Mena, I.; Neurin, O.; Feunzobda, S.; and Cotzias, G. C.: Chronic manganese poisoning. Clinical picture and manganese turnover. *Neurology*, **17**:128–136, 1967.

Menne, T., and Thorboe, A.: Nickel dermatitis—nickel excretion. *Contact Dermatitis*, **2**:353–354, 1976.

Mertz, W.: Chromium occurrence and function in biological systems. *Physiol. Rev.*, **49**:163–239, 1969.

Miettenen, J. K.: Absorption and elimination of dietary mercury (Hg^{++}) and methyl mercury in man. In Miller, M. W., and Clarkson, T. W. (eds.): *Mercury Mercurials and Mercaptans.* Charles C. Thomas, Publ., Springfield, Ill., 1973, p. 233.

Mitchell, R. A.; Change, B. F.; Huang, C. H.; and DeMaster, E. G.: Inhibition of mitochondrial energy-linked functions by arsenate. *Biochemistry*, **10**:2049–2054, 1971.

Moore, J. F.; Goyer, R. A.; and Wilson, M. H.: Lead-induced inclusion bodies, solubility amino acid content and relationship to residual acidic nuclear proteins. *Lab. Invest.*, **29**:488–494, 1973.

Morin, Y., and Daniel, P.: Quebec beer-drinkers cardiomyopathy: etiological consideration. *J. Can. Med. Assoc.*, **97**:926–931, 1967.

Mottet, N. K.; Shaw, C. -M.; and Burbacher, T. M.: Health risks from increases in methylmercury exposure. *Environ. Health Perspect*, **63**:133–140, 1985.

Muller-Eberhard, U.; Miescher, P. A.; and Jaffe, E. R.: *Iron Excess. Aberrations of Iron and Porphyrin Metabolism.* Grune & Stratton, New York, 1977.

Myron, D. R.; Zimmerman, T. J.; Schuler, T. R.; Klevay, L. M.; Lee, D. E.; and Nielsen, F. H.: Intake of nickel and vanadium by humans. A survey of selected diet. *Am. J. Clin. Nutr.*, **31**:527–531, 1978.

Nagyvary, J., and Bradbury, E. L.: Hypocholesterolemic effects of Al^{3+} complexes. *Biochem. Res. Commun.*, **2**:592–598, 1977.

NAS: *Lead: Airborne Lead in Perspective.* National Academy of Sciences, Washington, D.C., 1972.

————: *Manganese.* National Academy of Sciences, Washington, D.C., 1973.

————: *Chromium.* Committee on Medical and Biological Effects of Atmospheric Pollutants, National Academy of Sciences, Washington, D.C., 1974.

————: *Selenium.* National Academy of Sciences, Washington, D.C., 1975.

————: *Drinking Water and Health.* National Acedemy of Sciences, Washington, D.C.,1977.

————: *Recommended Dietary Allowances.* 9th Rev. Natl. Res. Council (ed.). National Academy of Sciences, Food and Nutrition Board, Washington, D.C., 1980, pp. 162–164.

NCI: *Bioassay of Titanium Dioxide for Possible Carcinogenicity.* National Cancer Institute Carcinogenesis Technical Report Series No. 97, Department of Health, Education and Welfare Publication No. (NIH) 79–1347, Washington, D.C., 1979.

Needleman, H. L.: The persistent threat of lead: a singular opportunity. *Am. J. Public Health*, **79**:643–645, 1989.

Needleman, H. L.; Gunnoe, E. E.; Leviton, A.; Reed, R.; Peresie, H.; Maher, C.; and Barrett, P.: Deficits in psychologic and classroom performance of children with elevated blood lead levels. *N. Engl. J. Med.*, **300**:689–695, 1979.

Needleman, H. L.; Schell, A.; Bellinger, D.; Leviton, A.; and Allred, E.: Long-term effects of childhood exposure to lead at low dose; an eleven-year follow-up report. *New Engl. J. Med.*, **322**:83–88, 1990.

Newman, R. A.; Brody, A. R.; and Krakoff, I. H.: Gallium nitrate induced toxicity in the rat: a pharmacologic histopathologic and microanalytical investigation. *Cancer*, **44**:1728–1740, 1979.

Ng, A., and Patterson, C.: Natural concentrations of lead in ancient Arctic and Antarctic ice. *Geochim. Cosmochim. Acta*, **45**:2109–2121, 1981.

Nogami, H., and Terashima, Y.: Thallium-induced achondroplasia in the rat. *Teratology*, **8**:101–102, 1973.

Nogawa, K.; Honda, R.; Kido, T.; Tsuritani, I.; Yamada, Y.; Ishizaki, M.; and Yamaya, H.: A dose-response analysis of cadmium in the general environment with special reference to total cadmium intake limit. *Environ. Res.*, **48**:7–16, 1989.

Nogawa, K.; Kobayashi, E.; and Honda, R.: A study of the relationship between cadmium concentrations in urine and renal effects of cadmium. *Environ. Health Perspect.*, **28**:161–168, 1979.

Nogawa, K.; Tsuritani, I.; Kido, T.; Honda, R.; Yamada, Y.; and Ishizaki, M.: Mechanism for bone disease found in inhabitants environmentally exposed to cadmium: decreased 1,25-dihydroxy vitamin D level. *Int. Arch. Occup. Environ. Health*, **59**:21–30, 1987.

Nomiyama, K.: Recent progress and perspectives in cadmium health effects studies. *Sci. Total Environ.*, **14**:199–232, 1980.

Nomiyama, K., and Nomiyama, H.: Critical concentration of 'unbound' cadmium in the rabbit renal cortex. *Experientia*, **42**:149, 1986.

Nordberg, G. F.: Cadmium metabolism and toxicity. *Environ. Physiol. Biochem.*, **2**:7–36, 1972.

Nordberg, G. F.; Fowler, B. A.; Friberg, L.; Jernelov, A.; Nelson, N.; Piscator, M.; Sandstead, H. H.; Vostal, J.; and Vouk, V. B.: Factors influencing metabolism and toxicity of metals: a consensus report. *Environ. Health Perspect.*, **25**:3–42, 1978.

NRCC: *Effects of Mercury in the Canadian Environment*. National Research Council of Canada Publication No. 16739, Ottawa, Canada, 1979.

Orfilia, M. P.: *A General System of Toxicology*. M. Carey & Sons, Philadelphia, 1817.

Paglia, D. E.; Valentine, W. N.; and Dahlgren, J. G.: Effects of low level lead exposure on pyrimidine-5'-nucleotidase and other erythrocyte enzymes. *J. Clin. Invest.*, **56**:1164–1169, 1975.

Paton, F. R., and Allison, A. C.: Chromosome damage in human cell cultures induced by metal salts. *Mutat. Res.*, **16**:332–336, 1972.

Pedersen, E.; Anderson, A.; and Hogetveit, A.: A second study of the incidence and mortality of cancer of respiratory organs among workers at a nickel refinery. *Ann. Clin. Lab. Sci.*, **8**:503–510, 1978.

Pentschew, W.; Ebner, F. F.; and Kovatch, R. M.: Experimental manganese encephalopathy in monkeys. *J. Neuropathol. Exp. Neurol.*, **22**:488–499, 1963.

Perl, D. P., and Brody, A. R.: Detection of aluminum by SEM-X-ray spectrometry within neurofibrillary tangle-bearing neurons of Alzheimer's disease. *Neurotoxicology*, **1**:133–137, 1980.

Perl, D. P., and Good, P. F.: Uptake of aluminum in central nervous system along nasal-olfactory pathways. *Lancet*, **1**:1087, 1987.

———: Aluminum, environment and central nervous system disease. *Environ. Technol. Lett.*, **9**:901–906, 1988.

Perlstein, M. A., and Attala, R.: Neurologic sequelae of plumbism in children. *Clin. Pediatr.*, **5**:292–298, 1966.

Pershagan, G.; Nordberg, G.; and Bjorklund, N. -E.: Carcinoma of the respiratory tract in hamsters given arsenic trioxide and/or benzo[a]pyrene by the pulmonary route. *Environ. Res.*, **34**:227–241, 1984.

Petering, D. H.; Loftsgaarden, J.; Schneider, J.; and Fowler, B.: Metabolism of cadmium, zinc and copper in the rat kidney: the role of metallothionein and other binding sites. *Environ. Health Perspect.*, **54**:73–82, 1984.

Pocock, S. J.; Ashby, D.; and Smith, M. A.: Lead exposure and children's intellectual performance. *Inst. J. Epidemiol.*, **16**:57–67, 1985.

Popper, H.; Thomas, L. B.: Telles, N. C.; Falk, H.; and Selikoff, I. J.: Development of hepatic angiosarcoma in man induced by vinyl chloride thorotrast, and arsenic. *Am. J. Pathol.*, **92**:349–369, 1978.

Prasad, A. S.: Human zinc deficiency. In Sarkar, B. (ed.): *Biological Aspects of Metals and Metal-Related Diseases*. Raven Press, New York, 1983, pp. 107–119.

Prasad, A. S.; Miale, A., Jr.; Farid, Z.; Sandstead, H. H.; Schulert, A. R.; and Darby, W. J.: Biochemical studies on dwarfism, hypogonadism and anemia. *Arch. Intern. Med.*, **111**:407–428, 1963.

Prull, G., and Rompel, K.: EEG changes in acute poisoning with organic tin compounds. *Electroenceph. Clin. Neurophysiol.*, **29**:215–222, 1970.

Reeves A. L.: Barium. In Friberg, L.; Nordberg, G. F.; and Vouk, V. B. (eds): *Handbook on the Toxicology of Metals*, Vol. II, 2nd ed., *Specific Metals*. Elsevier Scientific Publ., Amsterdam, 1986, pp. 84–94.

Riordan, J. R.: Handling of heavy metals by cultured cells from patients with Menke's disease. In Sarkar, B. (ed.): *Biological Aspects of Metals and Metal-Related Diseases*. Raven Press, New York, 1983, pp. 159–170.

Roels, H.; Gennart, J. -P.; Lauwerys, R.; Buchet, J. -P.; Malchaire, J.; and Bernard, A.: Surveillance of workers exposed to mercury vapor: validation of a previously proposed biological threshold limit value for mercury concentration in urine. *Am. J. Ind. Med.*, **7**:45–71, 1985.

Roels, H. A.; Lauwerys, R. R.; Buchet, J. P.; Bernard, A. M.; Vos, A.; and Onersteyns, M.: Health significance of cadmium induced renal dysfunction: a five-year follow-up. *Br. J. Ind. Med.*, **46**:755–764, 1989.

Roels, H.; Lauwerys, R. R.; and Dardenne, A. N.: The critical level of cadmium in human renal cortex: a re-evaluation. *Toxicol. Lett.*, **15**:357–360, 1983.

Rossouw, J.; Offermeier, J.; and van Rooyen, J. M.: Apparent central neurotransmitter receptor changes induced by low-level lead exposure during different developmental phases in the rat. *Toxicol. Appl. Pharmacol.*, **91**:132–139, 1987.

Rutter, M., and Jones, R. R. (eds.): *Lead versus Health Sources and Effects of Low Level Lead Exposure*. John Wiley & Sons, New York, 1983.

Sager, P. R.; Aschner, M.; and Rodier, P. M.: Persistent differential alterations in developing cerebellar cortex of male and female mice after methylmercury exposure. *Dev. Brain Res.*, **12**:1–11, 1984.

Sanstead, H. H.: Zinc in human nutrition. In Bronner, F., and Coburn, J. W. (eds.): *Disorders of Mineral Metabolism*. Academic Press, Inc., New York, 1981, pp. 94–159.

Sarkar, B.; Laussac, J. -P.; and Lau, S.: Transport forms of copper in human serum. In Sarkar, B. (ed.): *Biological Aspects of Metals and Metal-Related Diseases*. Raven Press, New York, 1983, pp. 23–40.

Schroeder, H. A.; Balassa, J. J.; and Tipton, I. H.: Abnormal trace elements in man: nickel. *J. Chronic Dis.*, **15**:51–65, 1962.

——: Abnormal trace metals in man: titanium. *J. Chronic Dis.*, **16**:55–69, 1963.

Schroeder, H. A., and Mitchener, M.: Selenium and tellurium in mice. *Arch. Environ. Health*, **24**:66–71, 1972.

Schroeder, H. A.; Nason, A. P.; and Tipton, I. H.: Essential trace metals in man: cobalt. *J. Chronic Dis.*, **20**:869–890, 1967.

——: Essential trace metals in man: magnesium. *J. Chronic Dis.*, **21**:815–841, 1969.

Schumann, G. B.; Lerner, S. I.; Weiss, M. A.; Gawronski, L.; and Lohiya, G. K.: Inclusion bearing cells in industrial workers exposed to lead. *Am. J. Clin. Pathol.*, **74**:192–196, 1980.

Shamberger, R. J.: *Biochemistry of Selenium*. Plenum Press, New York, 1983, p. 243.

Siegel, N., and Haug, A.: Aluminum interaction with calmodulin. Evidence for altered structure and function from optical enzymatic studies. *Biochim. Biophys. Acta*, **14**:36–45, 1983.

Singer, I.: Lithium and the kidney. *Kidney Int.*, **19**:374–387, 1981.

Skerfving, S.: Methylmercury exposure, mercury levels in blood and hair, and health status in Swedes consuming contaminated fish. *Toxicology*, **2**:3–23, 1974.

Skerfving, S.; Christoffersson, J. -O.; Schutz, A.; Welinder, H.; Spang, G.; Ahlgren, L.; and Mattsoon, S.: Biological monitoring by *in vivo* XRF measurement of occupational exposure to lead cadmium and mercury. *Biol. Trace Ele. Res.*, **13**:241–251, 1987.

Smith, I. C., and Carson, L.: *Trace Metals in the Environment*. Ann Arbor Science, Ann Arbor, Mich., 1981.

Smith, M. A.; Delves, T.; Lansdown, R.; Clayton, B.; and Graham, P.: The effects of lead exposure on urban children: the Institute of Child Health/ Southampton study. *Dev. Med. Child Neurol.*, **25** (Suppl.):47, 1983.

Sorahan, T., and Waterhouse, J. A. J.: Mortality study of nickel cadmium battery workers by the method of regression models in life tables. *Br. J. Ind. Med.*, **40**:293–300, 1983.

Spears, J. W.; Hatfield, E. E.; Forbes, R. M.; and Koenig, S. E.: Studies on the role of nickel in the ruminant. *J. Nutr.*, **108**:313–320, 1978.

Spivey Fox, M. R., and Rader, J. I.: Iron. In Seiler, H. G., and Sigel, H. (eds.): *Handbook on Toxicity of Inorganic Compounds*. Marcel Dekker, New York, 1988, pp. 346–358.

Steele, T. N.: Treatment of lithium intoxication with diuretics. In Brown, S. S. (ed.): *Clinical Chemistry and Chemical Toxicology of Metals*. Elsevier Scientific Publ., Amsterdam, 1977, pp. 289–292.

Stuve, J., and Galle, P.: Role of mitochondria in the renal handling of gold by the kidney. *J. Cell Biol.*, **44**:667–676, 1970.

Sunderman, F. W., Jr.: Nickel. In Bronner, F., and Coburn, J. W. (eds.): *Disorders of Mineral Metabolism*, Vol. 1. Academic Press, Inc., New York, 1981, pp. 201–232.

——: Mechanisms of nickel carcinogenesis. *Scand. J. Work Environ. Health*, **15**:1–12, 1989.

Sunderman, F. W., Sr.: Efficacy of sodium diethyldithiocarbamate (dithiocarb) in acute nickel carbonyl poisoning. *Ann. Clin. Lab. Sci.*, **9**:1–10, 1979.

Suzuki, K. T.: Induction and degradation of metallothioneins and their relation to the toxicity of cadmium. In Foulkes, E. C. (ed.): *Biological Roles of Metallothionein*. Elsevier Scientific Publ., Amsterdam, 1982, pp. 215–235.

Takenaka, S.; Oldiges, H.; Konig, H.; Hochrainer, D.; and Oberdorster, G.: Carcinogenicity of cadmium chloride aerosols in W rats. *J. Natl. Cancer Inst.*, **70**:367–373, 1983.

Takeuchi, T.: Neuropathology of Minamata disease in Kumamoto: especially at the chronic stage. In Roizin, L.; Shiraki, H.; and Grcevic, N. (eds.): *Neurotoxicology*, Vol. 1. Raven Press, New York, 1977, pp. 235–246.

Tam, G. K. H.; Charbonneau, S. M.; Bryce, F.; Pomroy, C.; and Sandi, E.: Metabolism of inorganic arsenic in humans following oral ingestion. *Toxicol. Appl. Pharmacol.*, **50**:319–322, 1979.

Tanaka, K.; Min, K. -S.; Onasaka, S.; Fukuhara, C.; and Ueda, M.: The origin of metallothionein in red blood cells. *Toxicol. Appl. Pharmacol.*, **78**:63–66, 1985.

Thayer, J. S.: *Organometallic Compounds and Living Organisms*. Academic Press, New York, 1984.

Thomas, D. W.; Hartly, T. F.; and Sobecki, S.: Clinical and laboratory investigations of the metabolism of bismuth containing pharmaceuticals by man and dogs. In Brown, S. S. (ed.): *Clinical Chemistry and Clinical Toxicology of Metals*. Elsevier Scientific Publ., Amsterdam, 1977, pp. 293–296.

Thompson, R. J.: Collection and analysis of airborne metallic elements. In Risby, T. H. (ed.): *Ultratrace Metal Analysis in Biological Sciences and Environment*. American Chemical Society, Washington, D.C., 1979, pp. 54–72.

Thun, M. J.; Baker, D. B.; Steenland, K.; Smith, A. B.; Halperin, W.; and Berl, T.: Renal toxicity in uranium mill workers. *Scand. J. Work Environ. Health*, **11**:83–90, 1985.

Thun, M. J.; Osorio, A. M.; Schober, S.; Hannon, W. H.; Lewis, B.; and Halperin, W.: Nephropathy in cadmium workers: assessment of risk from airborne occupational exposure to cadmium. *Br. J. Ind. Med.*, **46**:689–697, 1989.

Thun, M. J.; Schnorr, T. M.; Smith, A. B.; Halperin, W. E.; and Lemen, R. A.: Mortality among a cohort of U.S. cadmium production workers—an update. *J. Natl. Cancer Inst.*, **74**:325–333, 1985.

Trump, B. F.; Valigersky, J. N.; Arstila, A. U.; Mergner, W. J.; and Kinney, T. D.: The relationship of intracellular pathways of iron metabolism to cellular iron overload and the iron storage diseases. *Am. J. Pathol.*, **72**:295–324, 1973.

Tseng, W. -P.: Effects and dose-response relationships of skin cancer and blackfoot disease with arsenic. *Environ. Health Perspect.*, **19**:109–119, 1977.

Tubbs, R. R.; Gephardt, G. N.; McMahon, J. T.; Phol, M. C.; Vidt, D. G.; Barenberg, S. A.; and Valenzuela, R.: Membranous glomerulonephritis associated with industrial mercury exposure. *Am. J. Clin. Pathol.*, **77**:409–413, 1982.

Twarog, T., and Cherian, M. G.: Chelation of lead by dimercaptopropane sulfonate and a possible diagnostic use. *Toxicol. Appl. Pharmacol.*, **72**:550–556, 1984.

Tyroler, H. A.: Epidemiology of hypertension as a public health problem: an overview as background for evaluation of blood lead–blood pressure relationship (symposium). *Environ. Health Perspect.*, **78**:3–8, 1988.

Underwood, E. J.: *Trace Elements in Human and Animal Nutrition*, 4th ed. Academic Press, Inc., New York, 1977.

Urizar, R., and Vernier, R. L.: Bismuth nephropathy. *J.A.M.A.*, **198**:187–189, 1966.

Vander, A. J.: Chronic effects of lead on renin-angiotensin system. *Environ. Health Perspect.*, **78**:77–83, 1988.

Verschuuren, H. G.; Ruitenberg, E. J.; Peetoom, F.;

Helleman, P. W.; and Van Esch, G. J.: Influence of triphenyltin acetate on lymphatic tissue and immune response in guinea pigs. *Toxicol. Appl. Pharmacol.,* **16**:400–410, 1970.

Voil, G. W.; Minielly, J. A.; and Bistricki, T.: Gold nephropathy tissue analysis by x-ray fluorescent spectroscopy. *Arch. Pathol. Lab. Med.,* **101**:635–640, 1977.

Vouk, V. B., and Piver, W. T.: Metallic elements in fossil fuel combustion and products: amounts and form of emissions and evaluation of carcinogenicity and mutagenicity. *Environ. Health Perspect.,* **47**:201–226, 1983.

Walshe, J. M.: Endogenous copper clearance in Wilson's disease: a study of the mode of action of penicillamine. *Clin. Sci.,* **26**:461–469, 1964.

———: Assessment of treatment of Wilson's disease with triethylene tetramine 2HC1 (trien 2HC1). In Sarkar, B. (ed.): *Biological Aspects of Metals and Metal-Related Diseases.* Raven Press, New York, 1983, pp. 243–261.

Waters, M. D.: Toxicology of vanadium. In Goyer, R. A., and Mehlman, M. A. (eds.): *Toxicology of Trace Metals.* John Wiley & Sons, New York, 1977, pp. 147–189.

Webb, D. R.; Sipes, I. G.; and Carter, D. E.: *In vitro* solubility and *in vivo* toxicity of gallium arsenide. *Toxicol. Appl. Pharmacol.,* **76**:96–104, 1984.

Wenning, R., and Kirsch, N.: Vanadium. In Seiler, H. G., and Sigel, H. (eds.): *Toxicity of Inorganic Compounds.* Marcel Dekker, New York, 1988, pp. 749–758.

WHO: *Environmental Health Criteria 1. Mercury.* World Health Organization, Geneva, 1976.

———: *Environmental Health Criteria for Cadmium. Ambio,* **6**:287–290, 1977a.

———: *Environmental Health Criteria 3. Lead.* World Health Organization, Geneva, 1977b.

———: *Environmental Health Criteria 15. Tin and Organotin Compounds: A Preliminary Review.* World Health Organization, Geneva, 1980.

———: *Environmental Health Criteria 19. Arsenic.* World Health Organization, Geneva, 1981.

———: *Environmental Health Criteria 58. Selenium.* World Health Organization, Geneva, 1986.

———: *Evaluation of Certain Food Additives and Contaminants.* World Health Organization Technical Report, Series 776. World Health Organization, Geneva, 1989.

Wilber, C. G.: *Selenium: A Potential Environmental Poison and a Necessary Food Constituent.* Charles C. Thomas, Publ., Springfield, Ill., 1983.

Williams, D. R., and Halstead, B. W.: Chelating agents in medicine. *Clin. Toxicol.,* **19**:1081–1115, 1982–83.

Wills, M. R., and Savory, J.: Aluminum poisoning: dialysis encephalopathy, osteomalacia and anemia. *Lancet,* **2**:29–33, 1983.

Winston, P. W.: Molybdenum. In Bonner, F., and Coburn, J. W. (eds.): *Disorders of Mineral Metabolism,* Vol. 1, *Trace Minerals.* Academic Press, Inc., New York, 1981, pp. 295–315.

Woods, J. S.; Carver, G. T.; and Fowler, B. A.: Altered regulation of hepatic heme metabolism by indium chloride. *Toxicol. Appl. Pharmacol.,* **49**:455–461, 1979.

Yang, G. Q.; Wang, S. Z.; Zhou, R. H.; and Sun, S. Z.: Endemic selenium intoxication of humans in China. *Am. J. Clin. Nutr.,* **37**:872–881, 1983.

Zelikoff, J. T.; Li, J. H.; Hartwig, A.; Wang, X. W.; Costa, M.; and Rossman, T. G.: Genetic toxicology of lead compounds. *Carcinogenesis,* **9**:1727–1732, 1988.

Ziemsen, B.; Angerer, J.; Lehnert, G.; Bernkmann, H. -G.; and Goedde, H. W.: Polymorphism of delta-aminolevulinic acid dehydratase in lead-exposed workers. *Int. Arch. Occup. Environ. Health,* **58**:245–247, 1986.

Chapter 20

TOXIC EFFECTS OF SOLVENTS AND VAPORS

Larry S. Andrews and *Robert Snyder*

INTRODUCTION

Nearly everyone is exposed to solvents. The utility of these fluids as solubilizers, dispersants, or diluents leads to the manufacture and use of billions of pounds each year. Occupational exposures can involve applications ranging from a secretary using correction fluid to a gas station attendant pumping gasoline. A refinery worker may be exposed to solvents on the job and upon returning home may paint a room, change the oil in the family car, or glue together an item in need of repair, thereby extending his exposure to solvents. Although the solvents, which are usually mixtures, have different trade names, they frequently contain similar chemicals. Clearly, exposure should not be equated with toxicity. The fundamental principle of toxicology, that is, the dose-response relationship, requires that there be (1) exposure and (2) a toxic effect. Nevertheless, the potential for toxicological interaction increases as exposure increases, and exposure to mixtures leads to the possibility of unpredictable additivity, synergism, or potentiation of effects. In the long run, we must learn to understand the interactive effects of solvents because exposure of human populations in the environment is not usually to a single chemical. Until we have developed that needed body of knowledge, we must make use of the data base available to us, which is the toxicology of individual solvents and the relationship between the structures of solvents and their toxicity within chemical classes.

PROPERTIES OF SOLVENTS

Exposure

Many solvents exhibit appreciable volatility under conditions of use, and consequently the worker is exposed to solvent vapors. The concentrations of gases and vapors in air are given in volume/volume (v/v) units, which include vol%, parts per million (ppm), and so on. In physiological fluids, such as blood and urine, we often express concentrations as weight/volume (w/v), e.g., μg/ml, mg/liter. Concentrations of gas mixtures given in w/v units depend on both temperature and pressure, since mass depends on the number of molecules present, but the volume occupied by that mass depends on temperature and pressure and is described by the ideal gas law (PV = nRT). For regulatory purposes, and in many experimental situations, vapor concentrations are expressed as parts of vapor per million parts of contaminated air (ppm) by volume at a specified temperature and pressure. Often ppm values are converted into mg solvent/m^3 air in order to estimate total exposure to a solvent over a period of time. Examples of methods for interconverting these values are shown in the Appendix to Chapter 20.

The volatility of solvents indicates that a major route of exposure will be by the respiratory system. Once vapors enter the lungs, they may readily diffuse across a large surface area of respiratory membranes and enter the bloodstream. The ability of solvent vapors to enter the bloodstream depends on their lipid solubility, since lipoprotein cell membranes must be traversed. Many solvents are quite lipid soluble and will enter the blood with ease. Since diffusion occurs from relatively high concentrations in lung air to low concentrations in blood and tissues, the driving force for the movement is the vapor concentration in inspired air.

Many factors including rate and depth of respiration will affect blood solvent concentrations (Astrand, 1975). The rate at which the solvent distributes to the body organs through the blood is controlled by the cardiac output. The rate at which it leaves the blood to enter the organs is a function of the partition (Ostwald) coefficient. Agents having a high blood/air partition coefficient, such as diethyl ether, leave the blood and enter the organs at a slow rate, whereas agents such as halothane have a low partition coefficient and thereby distribute more rapidly.

A second major potential route of exposure is

the skin. The ubiquity of solvents and the casual approach to their use almost ensure skin contact. Frequent contact with lipid-soluble solvents can lead to a defatting of skin or to skin irritation. Of more importance for systemic toxicity is that some solvents may penetrate skin barriers to absorption (from both liquid and vapor phases) and enter the bloodstream (Rihimaki and Pfaffli, 1978; Marzulli and Maibach, 1983). Susten *et al.* (1985) have estimated that dermal exposure to benzene in tire-building operations could account for 20 to 40 percent of the total dose. These observations have raised the possibility that toxic amounts of solvents may be absorbed through the skin as a result of occupational and consumer exposures. This question has not, as yet, been approached in a systematic fashion. However, it does not seem likely that the percutaneous route will be a major contributor to establishing a body burden of most solvents since (1) the lung provides a much more efficient transfer of vapors to the bloodstream than does skin and (2) the area of skin in contact with a liquid solvent must be large for there to be absorption of appreciable amounts. Clearly, abraded or burned skin will be less of a barrier to absorption of solvents, and the likelihood for production of systemic effects from dermal exposure will be increased.

Another aspect of exposure to solvents is the frequency of exposure. Consumers, by virtue of the fact that they use small amounts of products, are generally not exposed to large amounts of solvents over long periods of time. Exposure to low background levels with intermittent exposure to much higher levels is a likely exposure scenario in the consumer setting. For example, solvent from an opened can of paint stripper may evaporate into the garage over a period of time, but furniture refinishing is an infrequent activity. In the occupational setting, a similar situation exists, where there may be continuous exposure to low levels of solvent with brief exposure to high concentrations of solvents. It seems axiomatic that toxicity testing of solvents in experimental animals should incorporate these exposure realities into test protocols; however, little information is currently available on effects of intermittent exposure.

The American Conference of Governmental Industrial Hygienists (ACGIH, 1989) has recognized these aspects of solvent exposure in their program for establishing threshold limit values (TLVs). ACGIH defines TLVs as airborne concentrations of substances that represent conditions under which it is believed that nearly all workers may be exposed day after day without adverse effect. TLVs are based on the best available information from industrial experience, animal tests, and studies in human volunteers. This information is detailed in ACGIH's *Documentation of Threshold Limit Values* series. The ACGIH develops three categories of TLVs: (1) time-weighted average (TWA), a value for a normal 8-hour workday and 40-hour workweek; (2) short-term exposure limit (STEL), a value for a short period of time (usually 15 minutes); and (3) ceiling (TLV-C), a value that should not be exceeded even briefly. The ACGIH meets each year to consider new information and revises TLVs when warranted by new data.

The official U.S. government body assigned the task of establishing exposure levels in industry is the Occupational Safety and Health Administration (OSHA) of the Department of Labor. Standards are established based largely on information supplied by the National Institute of Occupational Safety and Health and other agencies concerned with the effects of chemicals on human health. Opinions are solicited from all interested parties, and decisions are made on the basis of weight of evidence and the intent to act conservatively with respect to the protection of the health of the worker. In many instances, OSHA has adopted standards established by ACGIH. In others, OSHA standards are more stringent than those of ACGIH. The availability of the expertise of both agencies is to the advantage of the worker and the health professional charged with ensuring the safety of the workplace.

Toxicity

The toxic effects of solvents are both general and specific. The effect observed in studies in experimental animals or in the occupational exposure setting will depend on many factors including: solvent structure, exposure level, frequency and coexposure, and subject sensitivity. General sources on the toxicology of specific solvents and on solvents contained in trade name products are the texts by Browning (1965) and by Gosselin *et al.* (1984).

General. Many organic solvents, including hydrocarbons, chlorinated hydrocarbons, alcohols, ethers, esters, and ketones, have the potential on acute high-level vapor exposure to cause narcosis and death. A typical exposure scenario is the worker who enters a reaction vessel or holding tank without appropriate respiratory equipment. In such a confined space, solvent vapor concentrations may reach many hundreds or thousands of parts per million, and the worker may be quickly overcome. Of course, the experimental animal analogy to this scenario is the acute inhalation toxicity study (LC50).

Workers exposed to solvents under these conditions will typically show signs of central nervous system disturbance. While there is some variation in signs and symptoms with solvent structure, results of high-level exposure are quite similar. The scenario of disorientation, euphoria, giddiness, confusion, progressing to unconsciousness, paralysis, convulsion, and death from respiratory or cardiovascular arrest is typically observed (Browning, 1965). The rapidity of the development of these symptoms almost ensures that the acute narcotic effects of solvents are due to the solvent itself and not metabolites. In the majority of subjects, recovery from central nervous system effects is rapid and complete following removal from exposure. Less certain are the effects of acute high-level exposure on the extent and reversibility of specific toxicity discussed below.

The similarity of the narcosis produced by solvents of diverse structure suggests that these effects result from a physical interaction of a solvent with cells of the central nervous system. If a purely physical interaction is assumed, then the narcotic effect of the solvent will be dependent only on the molar concentration of the solvent in the central nervous system cell. Equimolar concentrations of different solvents will result in narcotic effects of equal intensity. A more detailed discussion of solvent-induced narcosis is found in the discussion of ethanol in this chapter. Although an increased emphasis on worker protection has lessened the likelihood of acute high-level exposure to solvents, it is important to realize that solvent-induced narcosis remains an important aspect of solvent toxicity.

Other effects of solvents in workers that may be related to solvents in general and to relatively nonspecific actions on the central nervous system are those seen in behavioral toxicity tests. A list of such tests has been compiled from several recent reviews and is presented in Table 20–1 (Tilson and Cabe, 1978; Buelke-Sam and Kimmel, 1979; Feldman *et al.*, 1980). A brief examination of the tests and symptomatology leads to the conclusion that most tests are not applicable for experimental animals. Thus, results in human studies cannot usually be correlated and explored in an animal model because we do not yet know how animals "think" or "feel" or "react." Of course, the inability to establish a closely related animal model is not a reason in and of itself to discount results of behavioral tests in humans. However, the inability to establish an animal model does make more critical problems generic to testing in humans. For example: What was the subject's baseline behavioral function prior to exposure? What is the degree of exposure? Is there coexposure to other materials? How does one match an exposed population with a control population to minimize confounding effects on behavior? An additional question that needs to be addressed is: Do behavioral effects precede in time or dose, coexist with, or extend beyond demonstrable organic tissue damage? The study of a human population will make the answer to such a question very difficult to obtain.

Despite these obvious difficulties in study and interpretation, some recent studies on behavioral toxicity are of note. Behavioral toxicity studies on carbon disulfide (CS_2) are perhaps most conclusive of all solvents for which studies have been conducted.

Several researchers have shown that reaction time, psychomotor performance, and distractibility are sensitive indicators of CS_2 exposure in occupational settings (Tuttle, 1977; Hanninen *et al.*, 1978; Tolonen *et al.*, 1978). Behavioral effects precede the obvious neurological effects of CS_2 discussed below.

Acute and chronic occupational exposure to several other solvents and solvent mixtures have been reported to affect behavior adversely.

Table 20–1. SYMPTOMATOLOGY AND COMMONLY USED TESTS FOR BEHAVIORAL EFFECTS

SYMPTOMATOLOGY	TEST
Sensory—paresthesias, visual or auditory deficits	Neurologic, sight, and hearing examinations
Cognitive—memory (both short-term and long-term), confusion, disorientation	Wechsler memory scale Wechsler Adult Intelligence Scale (WAIS)
Affective—nervousness, irritability, depression, apathy, compulsive behavior	Eysenck Personality Inventory Rorschach Test Digit-Symbol Substitution Task Bourdon-Wiersma Vigilance Task
Motor—weakness in hands, incoordination, fatigue, tremor	Neurologic examination Santa Ana Dexterity Test Finger-tapping Test Simple or Choice Reaction Time

Among individual chemicals reported to affect behavior adversely are toluene, trichloroethylene, and styrene. Recent reviews include: Baker (1988) and Grasso (1988). A number of epidemiology studies on workers exposed to solvent mixtures have also recently been reported (Knave *et al.*, 1978; Elofsson *et al.*, 1980; Seppalainen *et al.*, 1980; Linz *et al.*, 1986). These studies involved painters, workers occupationally exposed to jet fuel, and workers with a diagnosis of "solvent poisoning."

Detection and interpretation of neurotoxic or neurobehavioral effects of solvents constitutes a controversial and rapidly expanding area in toxicology. Recent efforts by the U.S. Environmental Protection Agency (EPA) and other regulatory agencies to require screening of chemicals for neurobehavioral effects in acute and repeated-exposure animal studies appear to offer an increased potential to identify materials with unique effects on the CNS. It is important, however, that results obtained in these screening tests be further evaluated in definitive tests. Further, doses and end points of toxicity should be selected to have relevance to exposure and observed effects in the occupational setting (Zbinden, 1983).

Specific. Distinct from general acute central nervous system depressant actions of solvents are specific organ toxicities associated with them. Such effects include the hemopoietic toxicity of benzene, the CNS depressant effects of alkylbenzenes, hepatotoxicity of certain chlorinated hydrocarbons, the ocular toxicity of methanol, the hepatotoxicity and CNS depressant effects of ethanol, neurotoxicity of *n*-hexane and certain diketones, reproductive toxicity of ethylene glycol ethers, and the carcinogenicity of dioxane. Each of these effects will be described in more detail below, but first two important aspects of evaluating solvents for specific adverse effects are discussed.

Exposure

In contrast to general effects of solvents, specific toxicity usually results from repeated exposure to tolerable levels of solvents rather than to acute exposure to very high levels. A typical exposure scenario is a worker who is exposed day after day to a material. Solvent, a toxic metabolite of the solvent, or tissue damage from either may accumulate until a worker develops a clinically recognizable illness. Good estimates of dose or time required to develop an illness are generally not available for solvents for which specific human toxicities are recognized. Such exposure data are important to evaluate the sensitivity of animal models for these toxic effects.

Metabolism

Specific toxicities of solvents, as distinct from general effects discussed above, are directly related to the metabolism of the solvent. Thus, the hemopoietic toxicity of benzene, the neurotoxicity of *n*-hexane, and the reproductive toxicity of ethylene glycol ethers have all been attributed to toxic metabolites of these materials. This general phenomenon is termed *bioactivation* and is largely mediated by the family of enzymes termed *cytochrome P-450–dependent mixed-function oxidases* (*see* Chapter 4). Of course, not all metabolism of a given solvent need result in bioactivation. Typically, one or more cytochrome P-450 mixed-function oxidases may mediate the conversion of a large percentage of the dose of solvent to a harmless metabolite, a process termed *detoxication*.

Mixed-function oxidases are a family of enzymes, consisting primarily of the hemoprotein cytochrome P-450, and are located in the smooth endoplasmic reticulum of liver as well as most other tissues. These enzymes catalyse the oxidation or reduction of a wide variety of chemical structures. A postulated mechanism for mixed-function oxidative reactions is visualized in Chapter 4.

The chemical is reversibly bound by the oxidized form of cytochrome P-450. The resulting chemical complex is next reduced by an electron supplied by NADPH-cytochrome P-450 reductase. The reduced chemical P-450 complex binds a molecule of oxygen, and on addition of further reducing equivalents, one atom of oxygen is introduced into the chemical and the other is reduced to water. Upon release of the oxidized product, cytochrome P-450 returns to its oxidized state and is again capable of binding another drug molecule. As a result of this process, oxygen is introduced into any chemical that contains a favorably positioned C—H, N—H, S—H, or C—X (X = halogen) bond.

Several aspects of the cytochrome P-450 mixed-function oxidases are of importance for the conduct and interpretation of toxicity tests for solvents.

Interactions. Since mixed-function oxidases have a broad specificity, it is not surprising that one solvent can compete with another for available catalytic sites. Thus, toluene has been shown to be a competitive inhibitor of the metabolism of benzene (Andrews *et al.*, 1977; Sato and Nakajima, 1979). This competitive interaction alleviates the metabolite-mediated toxicity of benzene, as discussed below. Another example of metabolic interactions among solvents is presented in the chapter on the liver in this text. Prior exposure to a number of alcohols or ketones can potentiate the liver damage caused by chlorinated hydrocarbons.

Inducibility. The mixed-function oxidase system contains a group of isozymes termed *cytochromes P-450*. Treatment of animals, and presumably humans, with any of a great number of chemicals leads to increases in the metabolism of these and other chemicals because of elevations in the levels of the cytochromes P-450. The specificity of the induced enzymes varies. Some chemicals, such as benzene, are capable of increasing their own metabolism and that of a few other chemicals (R. Snyder *et al.*, 1967), whereas drugs like phenobarbital or environmental chemicals such as polychlorinated biphenyls can increase the metabolism of a wide variety of chemicals.

The toxicity of a chemical may be dramatically altered as a result of enzmye induction. If metabolic activation of a solvent to its toxic metabolite is limited by the constitutive concentration of the specific species of cytochrome P-450 through which it is metabolized, enzyme induction may lead to greater toxicity. Thus, bromobenzene given to rats at doses that do not produce serious toxicity in noninduced animals yields massive hepatic necrosis in animals pretreated with phenobarbital. Alternatively, toxicity of a given dose may be reduced by decreasing the fraction processed by the bioactivation pathway. Thus, treating rats with 3-methylcholanthrene prior to dosing with bromobenzene led to a reduction in expected hepatotoxicity. In this case, an alternative pathway leading to less toxic metabolites was induced, thereby reducing the fraction of the dose that passed through the bioactivation pathway.

Saturation. Implicit in the concept of enzyme-mediated detoxication or bioactivation is the phenomenon of enzymatic saturation. Exposure to massive amounts of a solvent may result in saturation of detoxication pathways, resulting in a spillover into bioactivation pathways. Metabolic saturation has been demonstrated for a number of solvents including *n*-hexane, vinylidene chloride, methyl chloroform, perchloroethylene, and ethylene dichloride (McKenna *et al.*, 1978; Baker and Rickert, 1981; Reitz *et al.*, 1982; Schumann *et al.*, 1982).

Occurrence of metabolic saturation may be of profound importance for the design and interpretation of safety evaluation studies employing maximum tolerated doses. Under these conditions, experimental animals may be exposed to doses that not only saturate detoxication pathways but are many times human exposure levels. Under conditions of high-level exposure (poisoning), saturation of metabolic pathways may prevail. When considering exposures at, or below, permissible standards, however, metabolic saturation may be less important in determining ultimate toxicity. Thus, Andersen *et al.* (1980) have found that at low vapor concentrations of several solvents respiration and hepatic perfusion indices were rate-limiting factors in metabolism and hence in the production of toxic metabolites.

Species, Genetics, and Age. Among many factors that can affect cytochrome P-450 mixed-function oxidase reactions are species, genetics, and age. Such confounding factors can greatly influence the metabolism and toxicity of solvents and are discussed elsewhere in this book.

AROMATIC HYDROCARBONS

Benzene

Benzene has had a long history of extensive use in industry, first as a volatile solvent and later as a starting material for the synthesis of other chemicals. Thus, in the late nineteenth century benzene facilitated the rapid development of the rubber industry because of its ability to dissolve rubber latex and then rapidly evaporate, leaving formed or coated rubber products. It played a similar role in high-speed printing processes because it is an excellent solvent for inks that must dry rapidly. Many other industries also use benzene as a solvent or as starting material for chemical syntheses. The manufacturers of paints and plastics have been among the heaviest users. Today, because of its antiknock properties, a mixture of benzene-rich aromatics is added to gasoline as a replacement for alkyl lead compounds.

Because benzene has an appreciable vapor pressure at ambient temperatures, hazardous occupational exposure usually occurs via inhalation. Acute exposure to high concentrations of benzene may kill by depressing the central nervous system, leading to unconsciousness and death, or by producing fatal cardiac arrhythmias (R. Snyder and Kocsis, 1975).

Hematopoietic, Leukemogenic, and Clastogenic Effects. The major toxic effect of benzene is hematopoietic toxicity, an effect unique to benzene among the simple aromatic hydrocarbons. Chronic exposure of humans to low levels of benzene in the workplace is associated with blood disorders including aplastic anemia and leukemia (Browning, 1965; R. Snyder and Kocsis, 1975; R. Snyder *et al.*, 1977). The bone marrow toxicity of benzene is characterized by a progressive decrease in each of the circulating formed elements of the blood, that is, erythrocytes, thrombocytes, and each of the various types of leukocytes. The extent to which each of the cell types is depleted varies with the individual and the degree of exposure to benzene. In both human and animal studies, it appears that benzene-induced bone marrow depression is a dose-dependent phenomenon. When all three cell types have been sufficiently depressed, the disease is called *pancytopenia* and results from benzene-induced damage resulting in necrosis and fatty replacement of bone marrow. Pancytopenia in the face of severely compromised bone marrow functionality is termed *aplastic anemia*.

In man, signs of chronic benzene toxicity have been observed since the turn of the century. Studies generally show that a decreased level of circulating erythrocytes or leukocytes is a relatively good indication of early benzene toxicity; among leukocytes, granulocyte levels are usually depressed more than lymphocyte levels. Although individual workers vary in their reactions to benzene, the toxicity appears to be a function of both exposure level and duration of exposure. The present OSHA standard for occupational exposure to benzene is 1 ppm as an eight-hour time-weighted average, with a ceiling value of 5 ppm for no more than 15 minutes (Federal Register, 1985). OSHA estimates that approximately 2 million workers are exposed to benzene.

In animals, benzene-induced bone marrow depression has been produced experimentally in a number of species. In each case, exposure to benzene caused significant leukopenia, and in contrast to humans, lymphocytes were decreased in number more than were granulocytes. The producion of anemia, first reported in 1897, has recently been studied using decreases in ^{59}Fe incorporation into red cell hemoglobin as a measure of benzene-induced depression of erythropoietic function (Lee et al., 1981; Bolcsak and Nerland, 1983).

Leukemia is a neoplastic type of blood dyscrasia associated with exposure to benzene. Leukemias are acute or chronic diseases that are further classified according to the cell type involved. The leukemia most commonly associated with benzene exposure is acute myelogenous leukemia. Acute myelogenous leukemia is characterized by an increased number of cells morphologically similar to the myeloblast. To date, benzene-induced leukemia has only been observed in humans; unlike bone marrow depression leading to aplastic anemia, no satisfactory animal model for benzene-induced leukemia exists that consistently reproduces the human diseases. It has, accordingly, been difficult to study the etiology and development of benzene-induced leukemia in animal systems. However, recent reports have stressed the production of

solid tumors in animals given benzene orally (Maltoni et al., 1983).

Evidence that benzene is a human leukemogen is primarily epidemiological but is strongly supported by a large number of case control studies (IARC, 1982). In 1964, Vigliani reported several cases of leukemia in workers exposed to benzene (Vigliani and Saita, 1964). Aksoy and coworkers (Aksoy et al., 1974, 1976; Aksoy and Erdem, 1978) reported on an increased incidence of leukemia in shoe workers occupationally exposed to benzene. McMichael et al. (1974, 1975) and Infante et al. (1977a, 1977b) reported cancers of the lymphatic and hemopoietic systems in workers in the U.S. rubber industry.

Exposure of experimental animals to benzene can result in cytogenetic aberrations in bone marrow and peripheral blood. These effects generally occur at high exposure levels and are largely limited to gaps and deletions. Abnormal forms are rare (Dean, 1978; Cortina et al., 1982). Workers exposed to benzene in levels sufficient to disturb hemopoiesis display a greater incidence of chromosome aberrations in peripheral blood and bone marrow than do unexposed controls. It has not been possible to estimate a minimum exposure level or exposure period needed to produce cytogenetic changes (Dabney, 1981).

Morimoto and coworkers (Morimoto et al., 1983) have shown that benzene metabolism is necessary for benzene-induced sister chromatid exchanges (SCEs). Working with whole blood cultures from human donors, they found that benzene could induce SCEs but only in the presence of microsomal enzymes. Addition of glutathione to blood cultures decreased benzene-induced SCEs. The benzene metabolites catechol and hydroquinone also induced SCEs. Significantly, addition of microsomal enzymes enhanced, and addition of glutathione inhibited, this response. Thus, the benzene metabolites catechol and hydroquinone and their metabolites are implicated in DNA damage induced by benzene. The ability of glutathione to inhibit SCE induction suggests the electrophilic nature of the toxic metabolites. Tice et al. (1982) have shown that production of SCEs is directly related to benzene biotransformation *in vivo* since toluene, a competitive inhibitor of benzene metabolism (Andrews et al., 1977), protected against the benzene effect.

Tunek and coworkers (Toft et al., 1982; Tunek et al., 1982) have related benzene's ability to induce micronuclei in bone marrow cells with benzene metabolism *in vivo*. Toft et al. (1982) exposed male mice to benzene vapors (1 to 200 ppm) for varying periods of time and reported that continuous exposure to 14 ppm benzene after one week resulted in a significant elevation in micronuclei. No effect was seen at the 1- to 10-ppm dose range, but at higher doses, the effect seemed to be related to a function of dose times time. Repeated subcutaneous injection of hydroquinone induced micronuclei formation at doses above 20 mg/kg. Doses of catechol up to 42 mg/kg/day for six consecutive days did not induce micronuclei formation. Simultaneous injection of toluene (876 mg/kg) decreased the benzene- or hydroquinone-induced micronuclei formation. In related experiments, benzene also produced micronuclei when administered parenterally.

Although human case reports and cytogenetic studies indicate a strong correlation between benzene exposure and leukemia, there are several reasons why a cause-and-effect relationship has not been universally accepted. Since all studies correlating exposure with effect are retrospective epidemiological studies, data regarding duration and level of benzene exposure are usually deficient or cannot be obtained. Furthermore, there are no animal models for benzene-induced leukemia, and although there is evidence that benzene has caused chromosome damage, it has not been demonstrated to be mutagenic using *in vitro* cell assays. As discussed above, benzene exposure in industry does not occur in total isolation from other solvents, and this is another complicating factor in trying to assign a cause-and-effect relationship between benzene exposure and leukemia. Nevertheless, on balance it must be accepted that benzene is a carcinogenic substance and is probably an important cause of acute myelogenous and perhaps other types of leukemia in humans.

Benzene Metabolism. In order to understand the mechanism of benzene toxicity, it is essential to study its disposition. Parke and Williams (1953) were among the first to suggest that one of its metabolites might be responsible for benzene toxicity. Several studies have demonstrated that modification of benzene metabolism leads to alterations in benzene toxicity. Longacre *et al.* (1981a, 1981b) demonstrated that benzene metabolites were found at higher levels in bone marrow of DBA/2 mice, which were sensitive to benzene, than in C57B1/6 mice, which were relatively resistant to benzene. On the other hand, Ikeda and Ohtsuki (1971) reported that stimulation of detoxication processes by phenobarbital protected rats against benzene-induced leukopenia. On the basis of these and other studies, it is well accepted that one, or more, of its metabolites is responsible for the production of the adverse hematological effects of benzene.

Although the major route of human exposure is by inhalation, many animal studies have been performed in which benzene was administered by a parenteral route. There is no evidence to suggest that variations in the route of administration can qualitatively alter the toxicity of ben-

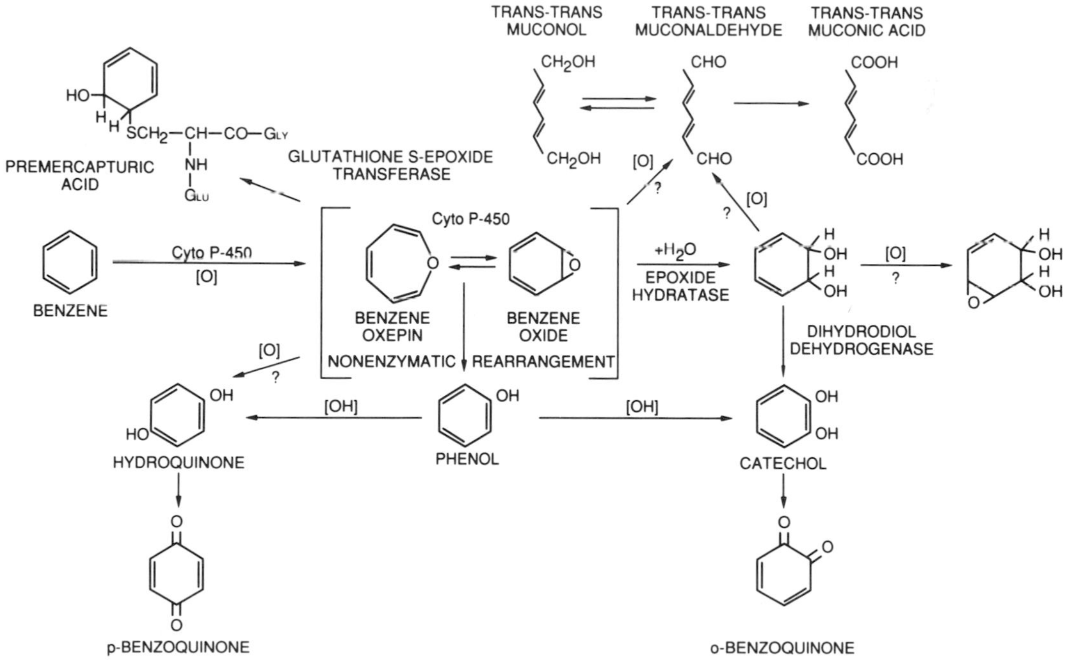

Figure 20–1. Biotransformation of benzene. Question marks refer to suggested but as yet unproven pathways.

zene. A significant portion of any dose of benzene is exhaled unchanged or stored in fat both in animals and humans. Rickert *et al.* (1979) reported that following inhalation of benzene in rats excretion via the lung followed a biphasic pattern indicative of a two-compartment model.

The bulk of the evidence suggests that benzene toxicity is produced by one or more metabolites of benzene rather than by benzene itself (R. Snyder *et al.*, 1981). The broad outlines of benzene metabolism were best established by Parke and Williams (1953) using ^{14}C-labeled benzene. Phenol, catechol, hydroquinone, and 1,2,4-trihydroxybenzene were recovered as ethereal sulfates and glucuronide conjugates in urine of treated animals. Other metabolites included 1-phenylmercapturic acid and *trans-trans*-muconic acid.

The metabolic pathway for benzene (R. Snyder *et al.*, 1981) may be pictured as a diagram of the fate of benzene oxide (Figure 20–1). Benzene is converted to benzene oxide (Figure 20–1) by the hepatic microsomal mixed-function oxidase. The oxide (Figure 20–2) may rearrange nonenzymatically to form phenol; react with glutathione to form a premercapturic acid, which is subsequently converted to *l*-phenyl-mercapturic acid; or it may react with epoxide hydrolase, which converts it to benzene dihydrodiol. The mixed-function oxidase and epoxide hydrolase are microsomal enzymes, but the dihydrodiol is oxidized to catechol by a cytosolic dehydrogenase. Catechol may also be formed by the hydroxylation of phenol. Hydroquinone is the primary product of further hydroxylation of phenol. Studies by Gilmour *et al.* (1986) suggested that it may be possible to form hydroquinone without the production of free phenol as an intermediate. Since this pathway has yet to be proven, it is shown with a question mark (Figure 20–1). Another question mark relates to the mechanism by which the ring is opened to yield muconaldehyde, another potential toxic metabolite, which may arise either at the epoxide stage or from the dihydrodiol (Latriano *et al.*, 1986). 1,2,4-Trihydroxybenzene is thought to arise from the hydroxylation of catechol.

Jerina and Daly (1974) suggest that the hydroxylation involves the intermediate formation of an epoxide, and much of the theory of carcinogenesis by bay region diol-epoxides is founded upon this concept. Although the epoxide of benzene has never been isolated and identified during the enzymatic oxidation of benzene, Tunek *et al.* (1982) reported that the addition of an excess of purified epoxide hydrolase to a rat liver microsomal system during benzene metabolism resulted in the production of the dihydrodiol. This could only have been the result of the intermediate formation of the epoxide. However, Ingelman-Sundberg and Hagbjork (1982) suggested that hydroxylation could occur via the insertion of a hydroxyl free radical (Figure 20–2). They postulate that the free radicals are generated by an iron-catalyzed cytochrome P-450–dependent Haber-Weiss reaction, and their data are supported by the demonstration that several compounds that prevent free radical formation or act as free radical scavengers can inhibit the hydroxylation of benzene by an isolated, reconstituted rabbit liver microsomal mixed-function oxidase. Gorsky and Coon (1985) proposed that a free radical mechanism occurs only at very low substrate concentrations when cytochrome P-450 could be uncoupled and yield hydrogen peroxide. Post and Snyder (1983) demonstrated that there are at least two different rat liver mixed-function oxidases active in benzene hydroxylation. The evidence suggests that these are cytochromes P-450 IIB1 in rat liver (R. Snyder, in press) and cytochrome P-450 IIE1 in rat (R. Snyder, 1990) and rabbit liver (Koop *et al.*, 1989).

The formation of the dihydroxylated metabolites, hydroquinone and catechol, seems to occur by different pathways. The dihydrodiol can be aromatized by a cytosolic dehydrogenase to yield catechol. Hydroquinone can be formed from phenol (Gilmour and Snyder, 1983a, 1983b) in a further hydroxylation step. Small amounts of catechol have also been observed arising from phenol (Sawahata and Neal, 1982; Gilmour and Snyder, 1983a, 1983b). The formation of these compounds and possibly the trihydroxy compound have been postulated by Tunek *et al.* (1980) and by Irons *et al.* (1982) to occur via the intermediate formation of quinones and/or semiquinones. In each case of hydroxylation, a free radical insertion may be postulated. The metabolism of phenol to hydroquinone appears to be such a reaction. It has been postulated that this reaction may be mediated by myeloperoxidase or a similar peroxidase in bone marrow (Eastmond *et al.*, 1987). Pirozzi *et al.* (1989) have suggested that this reaction may be mediated by the cyclooxygenase component of pros-

(a) Jerina and Daly (1974)

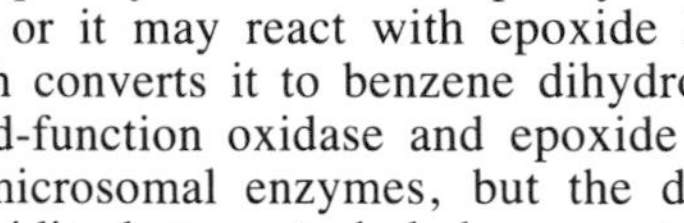

(b) Ingleman-Sundberg and Hagbjork (1982)

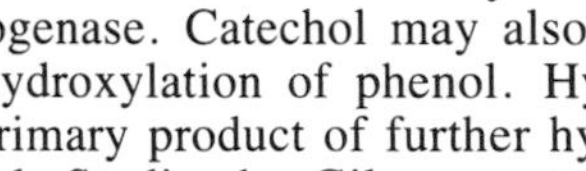

Figure 20–2. Mechanisms of benzene hydroxylation.

taglandin H synthetase. Thus, although the cytochrome P-450 system of the liver appears to be primarily concerned with benzene metabolism in the liver, other oxidative enzymes may play significant roles in further metabolism of benzene metabolites in the bone marrow.

Still another mechanism must be developed to explain the formation of muconic acid. Muconic acid was first identified as a metabolite of benzene produced by rabbits (Parke and Williams, 1953) and is also a known metabolite of catechol degradation by plant dioxygenases. Goldstein *et al.* (1982), however, have suggested that muconaldehyde might be the toxic metabolite that results from ring opening and is subsequently converted to muconic acid. Kirley *et al.* (1989) demonstrated the intermediate formation of a monoaldehydic, monocarboxylic intermediate, suggesting a two-step process leading from muconaldehyde to muconic acid.

Benzene metabolites that appear in the urine include etheral sulfates and glucuronides of the phenolic metabolites, muconic acid resulting from ring opening, and mercapturic acids resulting from glutathione conjugation. Medinsky *et al.* (1989), using data on the levels of these metabolites in urine, have published a model for the simulation of benzene metabolism by mice and rats. They assumed that benzene metabolism follows Michaelis-Menten kinetics, that all metabolism occurs via benzene oxide, and that conjugated phenolic metabolites, including mercapturic acids, as well as muconic acid in urine, account for the total metabolism. The results suggest that formation of toxic metabolites occurs via high-affinity, low-capacity pathways, whereas detoxication is accomplished via low-affinity, high-capacity pathways. These authors infer that at low substrate concentration a significant percentage of the metabolism follows pathways leading to the production of toxic metabolites. These simulations were supported by studies in animals that indicated that detoxication pathways predominated in rats, which are known to be less susceptible to benzene toxicity, but not in more susceptible mice where the production of toxic metabolites was more important. The model is deserving of further study and may well play a critical role in future deliberations on setting exposure standards for benzene.

Mechanism of Benzene Toxicity. An alternative fate for benzene metabolites is the covalent binding to cellular macromolecules, which many investigators believe is related to the mechanism of benzene toxicity and/or carcinogenicity. Radiolabeled benzene was used to detect covalent binding. C. A. Snyder *et al.* (1978) and Longacre *et al.* (1981a, 1981b) reported that benzene metabolites bind to proteins in mouse liver, bone marrow, kidney, spleen, blood, and muscle. Less covalent binding in bone marrow, blood, and spleen was observed in mice relatively resistant to benzene toxicity, that is, C56B1/6, than in more sensitive mice, that is, DBA/2. Irons *et al.* (1980) found covalent binding to protein in perfused bone marrow preparations. The observation of covalent binding demonstrates the chemical reactivity of one or more benzene metabolites. The ultimate significance of covalent binding to proteins will depend on the identification of the proteins, their function, and the degree to which it is modified by adduct formation.

Covalent binding of benzene metabolites to DNA offers a potential mechanism for inhibition of cell replication or for the initiation of leukemia. Lutz and Schlatter (1977) reported that in rats exposed to benzene vapor liver DNA contained labeled benzene residues. Bauer *et al.* (1989) reported on DNA adduct formation in both nuclei and mitochondria in the liver of rabbits treated with benzene and suggested the presence of several different adducts on the basis of the $[^{32}P]$post-labeling technique (Randerath *et al.*, 1981). Gill and Ahmed (1981) have suggested that the mitochondria represent an important site of covalent binding for benzene. Kalf *et al.* (1982) have demonstrated that the inhibition of RNA synthesis in mitochondria from both liver and bone marrow was correlated with covalent binding of benzene metabolites to DNA. It appears that phenol, hydroquinone, catechol, benzoquinone, and 1,2,4-trihydroxy benzene can lead to adduct formation in bone marrow mitochondria. The significance of inhibited RNA synthesis in mitochondria relates to inhibition of the synthesis of critical mitochondrial proteins and the resulting impairment of mitochondrial function. Furthermore, the demonstration by Post *et al.* (1984) that the benzene metabolites hydroquinone and benzoquinone inhibit nuclear mRNA synthesis adds further weight to the significance of the interactions of benzene metabolites and DNA.

The search for the ultimate mechanism of benzene-induced bone marrow depression or leukemia is complicated by the fact that neither the specific target cell nor the intracellular location of the target has been clearly identified. The data suggest that benzene metabolites may damage both the pluripotential stem cell and/or the early proliferating committed cell in either the erythroid or myeloid line. Thus, Lee *et al.* (1974) suggested that early proliferating cells and maturing cells in marrow, such as the pronormoblast and the normoblast in the erythroid line, were most sensitive to benzene. Uyeki *et al.* (1977), who reported on the inhibition of spleen colony formation by cells from benzene-exposed animals, were the first to report effects of benzene on stem cells. Boyd *et al.* (1982) have reported on effects of benzene and its metabolites on colony-forming units for granulocytes. There have been many other reports that support the concept that stem cells provide an important target for benzene.

The stem and progenitor cells cannot develop normally in marrow without the presence of a functional hematopoietic microenvironment. The stromal cells of the microenvironment form a supporting matrix for the development of cells in the bone marrow. Benzene has been demonstrated to impair mouse bone marrow stromal cells by Gaido and Wierda both *in vitro* (1984) and *in vivo* (1985). Among these cells are lymphocytes and macrophages. Post *et al.* (1985) reported that treatment with benzene or its metabolites hydroquinone or benzoquinone inhibited the production of interleukin-2 in T lymphocytes; MacEachern *et al.* (1989) and F. M. Robertson *et al.* (1989) reported that treatment of mice *in vivo* with benzene, or with a combination of the metabolites phenol and hydroquinone, resulting in release of elevated levels of hydrogen peroxide, interleukin-I, and tumor necrosis factor from stromal macrophages. These and other studies suggest that the hematopoietic microenvironment is another target for benzene.

In humans, the adverse effects of benzene are variants of either aplastic anemia or leukemia. It is likely that in each case metabolites of benzene initiate the disease process and also appear to be implicated in mutational events such as increases in sister chromatid exchange and micronucleus formation. These effects could be produced as a result of any of several actions of benzene metabolites in bone marrow cells. Multiple sites have been identified as potential targets for benzene metabolites. Irons *et al.* (1982) and Irons and Neptun (1980) have shown that microtubule assembly, a critical process for cell replication, is inhibited by benzene metabolites. The data cited above demonstrate that benzene metabolites can covalently bind to DNA, RNA, and protein. Benzene metabolites may also inhibit specific enzymes. In each case, an argument can be made that one of these events is responsible for the inhibition of cell replication. However, it may not be necessary to attempt to exclude any of these from consideration as a contributing event.

In addition to the possibility of multiple targets, we must consider the possibility that toxicity may result from the complementary action of more than one metabolite. To emphasize this point, an important publication by Eastmond *et al.* (1987) indicated that simultaneous administration of two benzene metabolites, phenol and hydroquinone, resulted in potentiation of their toxicities. While there are several possible explanations for this observation, it indicates that the interaction between benzene metabolites may be important for the eventual development of benzene-related disease. Thus, R. Snyder *et al.* (1989) found that there are a number of mixtures of benzene metabolites that result in either addition of the toxicities of the components or potentiation of their effects. The most effective and potent mixture observed was hydroquinone plus muconaldehyde, which rapidly produced serious bone marrow depression. Thus, a useful approach to further work in this area might be to consider that benzene toxicity is the result of (1) effects of benzene metabolites on more than one target and (2) effects of more than one metabolite.

Alkylbenzenes

The alkylbenzenes are single ring aromatic compounds containing one or more saturated aliphatic side chains. The major products of commerce and, therefore, those to which humans are most likely to be exposed include toluene (methylbenzene), ethylbenzene, cumene (isopropylbenzene), and the three xylenes (1,2-, 1,3-, and 1,4-dimethylbenzene). These compounds are primarily derived from petroleum distillation and coke oven effluents. The National Academy of Sciences (NAS/NRC, 1980) reported that in 1980 the production of the alkylbenzenes in the United States, expressed in millions of metric tons, was: toluene, 6.4; xylenes, 3.7; ethylbenzene, 3.9; and cumene, 1.8. It is clear that these compounds are major commodity chemicals and there is a high potential for many workers to be exposed. It should also be recognized that mixtures of these compounds may account for levels as high as 38 percent of unleaded gasoline (NAS/NRC, 1980). The potential for human exposure, albeit often at low levels, is accordingly expanded beyond industrial workers to gasoline station workers and the general public at large. It is, therefore, necessary to have a full understanding of the potential effects of these compounds.

The acute toxicity of inhaled alkylbenzenes is best described as CNS depression. In effect, these compounds appear to act as general anesthetics. Inhaled alkylbenzene vapors cause death in animal models at air levels that are relatively similar. Thus, the LC50 for toluene in mice is 5320 ppm/eight hours, for mixed xylenes in rats the value is 6700 ppm/four hours, for cumene in rats the value is 8000 ppm/four hours, and the lowest dose of ethylbenzene reported to kill rats—LC_{Lo} is 4000 ppm/four hours. It is likely that the mechanisms of action of the alkylbenzenes under conditions of acute exposure resemble those of the general anesthetics.

Less information is available regarding long-term exposure to alkylbenzenes. Cragg *et al.* (1989) reported effects of four-week exposures (six hours/day, five days/week) of mice, rats, and rabbits to ethylbenzene vapors. Rats and mice were exposed to 0, 99, 382, or 782 ppm ethylbenzene, whereas rabbits received 0, 382, 782, or 1610 ppm. Exposures did not increase mortality nor adversely affect clinical chemistries or gross/microscopic pathology. At the higher exposure levels, mice and rats exhibited increases in liver weights consistent with microsomal enzyme induction previously reported by Elovaara *et al.* (1985). The significance of this finding in the liver is uncertain. However, Bardodej and Cirek (1988) recently reported no adverse responses in hematological and liver function tests for workers exposed to ethylbenzene and monitored over 20 years.

Commercial xylenes from petroleum sources typically consist of 20 percent *o*-xylene, 44 percent *m*-xylene, 20 percent *p*-xylene, and up to 15 percent ethylbenzene. Carpenter *et al.* (1975) failed to identify target organs or any significant adverse effects in rats and dogs exposed to either 460 ppm or 810 ppm xylene vapors six hours/day, five days/week for a total of 66 days. Workers repeatedly exposed to xylene vapor concentrations in excess of 100 ppm frequently complain of gastrointestinal disturbances (Browning, 1965; Carpenter *et al.*, 1975). The toxicity of xylenes was recently reviewed by Low *et al.* (1989).

Epidemiological studies in workers (Matsushita *et al.*, 1975; Benignus, 1981) and in chronic solvent abusers (Morton, 1987) as well as animal studies (Sullivan *et al.*, 1989) have identified the central nervous system as a target organ for injury following repeated exposure to toluene. Workers exposed repeatedly to 200 to 300 ppm have been observed to have an impaired simple and choice reaction time and speed of perception. Very high levels of toluene encountered by "glue sniffers" will result in cerebellar damage as well as changes in CNS integrative functions.

Studies of genetic toxicity with toluene, xylene, and cumene have shown that they do not produce mutations in the various *Salmonella* strains used in the Ames test, with or without metabolic activation (NAS/NRC, 1980). Toluene and xylene are inactive as mutagens in the *Saccharomyces cerevisiae* D4 test for mitotic gene conversion and in the mouse lymphoma test. Toluene, but not ethylbenzene or xylene

isomers, was weakly active in the mouse micronucleus test (Mohtashamipur *et al.*, 1985). Although chromosome aberrations have been observed in rats exposed to toluene, they have not been seen in toluene-exposed humans. Weak or absent activity in genotoxicity tests suggests that alkylbenzenes are not carcinogenic, although they have not been systematically evaluated in animal tests.

Although it is important, with respect to the production of toxicity by most compounds, to ask why they are toxic, in the case of the alkylbenzenes, an important question may be why they are relatively nontoxic except during acute exposure to high concentrations. The toxicity of many chemicals requires metabolic activation to reactive species that then cause adverse effects. In the case of the alkylbenzenes, however, the major metabolic pathways appear to be toward metabolites that have a low order of toxicity and are readily excreted. Thus, toluene is oxidized at the methyl group, and a series of oxidations leads to benzoic acid, which is conjugated with glycine to form hippuric acid, which is then excreted. Hippuric acids are also metabolites of xylene and ethylbenzene. There is no evidence at present to indicate that these metabolic pathways can be saturated, leading to spillover into alternative metabolic pathways and the formation of toxic reactive intermediates and subsequent toxic or mutagenic effects.

CHLORINATED ALIPHATIC HYDROCARBONS

Dichloromethane

Dichloromethane (methylene chloride, CH_2Cl_2) is a widely used solvent that has been used for removing paint and degreasing, as a solvent for extracting foods (e.g., for the removal of caffeine from coffee), in the manufacture of plastics, and for other purposes. There has been concern about its potential carcinogenicity. Dichloromethane does not appear to pose a threat as a genotoxic agent. Neither rats (Serota *et al.*, 1986a) nor mice (Serota *et al.*, 1986b) displayed neoplastic lesions after administration of dichloromethane in drinking water at concentrations of 0, 0.15, 0.45, or 1.5 percent for two years, although hepatotoxicity was noted at higher doses. Nitschke *et al.* (1988) exposed male and female rats to dichloromethane vapors (0, 50, 200, or 500 ppm) for five days per week for two years. While the highest dose resulted in hepatocellular vacuolization in both sexes and the females developed benign breast tumors, there was no incidence of malignant neoplastic disease, and the no-observed-effect level

(NOEL) was set at 200 ppm. However, a separate inhalation study in mice and rats conducted by the National Toxicology Program in 1986 identified tumors in the livers and lungs of male and female mice and mammary tumors in female rats. Accordingly, dichloromethane was banned from use as a component of aerosol cosmetics (Federal Register, 1989).

The hepatotoxic or carcinogenic effects of the halocarbons are thought to require metabolic activation by mixed-function oxidases. The breakage of the C—H bond is usually the rate-limiting step (Ahmed *et al.*, 1980). Metabolism of the dihalomethanes leads to dehalogenation, and the end product is carbon monoxide. As a result, an elevation in carboxyhemoglobin levels may be observed (Nitschke *et al.*, 1988). The CO appears to arise from a formyl halide intermediate resulting from the loss of one halide atom from the halocarbon. This intermediate as an alternative to losing CO can covalently bind to cellular protein or lipid. The involvement of nonmicrosomal enzymes in dihalomethane metabolism leads to the production of formaldehyde and halide. A necessary step is the reaction of the dihalomethane with glutathione, which results in the loss of one halide. The resulting halomethylglutathione is postulated to undergo nonenzymatic hydrolytic dehalogenation, leaving hydroxymethylglutathione. The next step in the metabolic sequence results in the release of the hydroxymethyl group as formaldehyde. In the presence of formaldehyde dehydrogenase and NAD, formic acid can be formed.

Chloroform

The primary effect of high-level exposure to chloroform ($CHCl_3$) is its effect on the central nervous system. Owing to the early interest in developing chloroform as an anesthetic, there is extensive information on effects in humans. Concentrations up to about 400 ppm can be endured for 30 minutes without complaint; 1000 ppm exposure for seven minutes can cause dizziness and gastrointestinal upset; 14,000 ppm can cause narcosis.

Exposure to very high levels of $CHCl_3$ can cause liver and kidney damage as well as cardiac arrhythmias apparently due to sensitization of the myocardium to epinephrine. Orth (1965) has emphasized, however, that in human anesthesia the major effect on the heart is more likely to be cardiac arrest secondary to vagal stimulation. He suggests that ventricular fibrillation occurs only after the heart has stopped, anoxia develops, and carbon dioxide levels are elevated. These effects can be prevented by adequate anticholinergic therapy. Nevertheless, the use of chloroform in anesthesia in this country has been discouraged since 1912 (Pohl, 1979).

In humans who have developed liver failure following anesthesia, symptoms were observed within a few days following surgery. Nausea and vomiting were followed by jaundice and coma. Upon autopsy, evidence for centrilobular necrosis extending into periportal areas was seen. The intermeditate zones separating healthy and necrotic tissue contained ballooned and vacuolated cells laden with fat.

Repeated exposure to lower, subnarcotic levels of chloroform can also cause liver and kidney toxicity. However, these effects have typically not been seen in workers, despite the extensive and long history of use of $CHCl_3$. Challen *et al.* (1958) reported on workers exposed in an industrial setting to 21 to 237 ppm $CHCl_3$. Worker complaints were of depression and gastrointestinal distress. Liver function tests did not reveal any evidence of liver damage.

Chloroform-induced liver damage is also well recognized in experimental animal models. Torkelson *et al.* (1976) exposed rabbits, rats, guinea pigs, and dogs to 25, 50, or 85 ppm $CHCl_3$, seven hours/day, five days/week for six months. Histopathological evaluation of animals indicated centrilobular necrosis and cloudy swelling of kidneys. The effects of the 25-ppm dose were characterized as mild and reversible. Following oral administration of chloroform in a National Cancer Institute bioassay, it was concluded that male rats developed an excess of renal epithelial cell tumors and mice developed liver tumors (Pohl, 1979).

The mechanism by which chloroform produces liver toxicity has been reviewed by Pohl (1979). Chloroform is metabolized to reactive metabolites that covalently bind to hepatic proteins of the liver and deplete the liver of glutathione. The postulated toxic metabolite was phosgene. Protection against chloroform-induced nephrotoxicity is afforded by sulfhydryl compounds such as L-cysteine (Bailie *et al.*, 1984) and GSH (Kluwe and Hook, 1981). Alternatively, the inhibition of chloroform metabolism by piperonyl butoxide (Kluwe and Hook, 1981) or by methoxsalen (Letteron *et al.*, 1987) resulted in protection. Dietz *et al.* (1982) have suggested that although reactive metabolites are formed from chloroform, the carcinogenic effect is not related to formation of a DNA adduct but rather to recurrent cytotoxicity with chronic tissue regeneration.

J. H. Smith *et al.* (1983) proposed that hepatotoxic and nephrotoxic effects of chloroform occur independently and are related to differential metabolism of chloroform in the two organs. Whereas male mice display both hepatotoxicity and nephrotoxicity, only hepatotoxicity was observed in females. The underlying mechanism was postulated to be the conversion of chloroform to a reactive metabolite, probably phosgene, by male-specific cytochrome P-450, in male mouse kidney (J. H. Smith and Hook, 1984; J. H. Smith et al., 1984). A similar phenomenon is observed in male rabbits (Bailie et al., 1984). Chloroform is metabolized by cytochrome P-450 IIE1 (also called cytochrome P-450 j) (Brady et al., 1989). Hong et al. (1989) reported that in mouse kidney a specific form of cytochrome P-450 IIE1 was found in males and in testosterone-treated females. The corresponding enzyme in liver was not sex-specific. This enzyme is induced by secondary ketones in both liver and kidney, which suggests that the potentiation of both hepatotoxicity and nephrotoxicity by chloroform after treating animals with methyl-n-butyl ketone (Branchflower and Pohl, 1981) or acetone, 2-butanone, 2-pentanone, 2-hexanone, or 2-heptanone results from increased production of a reactive metabolite.

Carbon Tetrachloride

The mechanism of carbon tetrachloride–induced hepatic necrosis has been the subject of extensive research. Zimmerman (1978) has thoroughly reviewed the hepatotoxicity of CCl_4. In humans, monkeys, rats, mice, rabbits, guinea pigs, hamsters, cats, dogs, sheep, and cattle, CCl_4 causes centrilobular necrosis and fat accumulation. The extent of injury may be modified by factors such as species differences, age, and sex. Less sensitive models include birds, fish, amphibians, and some types of monkeys, female rats, and newborn rats and dogs. It is likely that the differences in sensitivity are more closely related to the relative ability of the various models to metabolically activate CCl_4 to toxic species than to differences in sensitivity of target sites. This concept is supported by the observation of Recknagel and Glende (1973) that administration of small doses of CCl_4 to rats one day before administration of a large dose results in protection against the toxicity otherwise produced by the large dose. The reason is that the small dose was sufficient to inactivate the mixed-function oxidase and thereby prevent metabolic activation to toxic metabolites.

The effects of nutritional alterations have been difficult to interpret but suggest that diets sufficiently low in protein to reduce mixed-function oxidase activity may be protective because of the reduced ability to yield metabolic activation of CCl_4. More prolonged protein deprivation, however, in the presence of residual mixed-function oxidase activity may lead to more severe liver damage because of the loss of protective sulfhydryl compounds such as glutathione.

The hepatic injury follows a well-studied course. After a single dose of CCl_4 given by gavage, or by most other routes, centrilobular necrosis begins to develop, with evidence of the lesion by 12 hours and full-blown necrosis by 24 hours. However, evidence for the beginning of recovery as indicated by the appearance of mitotic figures begins to appear within 24 hours, and the liver may be restored to normal within 14 days with removal of the residues of necrotic tissue (Smuckler, 1975). During the initial 48-hour period, liver enzymes, such as glutamic oxalacetic transaminase, glutamic pyruvic transaminase, and lactic dehydrogenase, appear and then recede from the serum and can be used as a measure of the extent of liver damage.

Lipid accumulation develops early, with the first drops of lipid seen under the electron microscope within the first hour; these become observable under the light microscope within three hours. Single cell necrosis is observable within five to six hours (Smuckler, 1975). Damage to mitochondria and the Golgi apparatus is evident. Other early signs of cell injury include disassociation of ribosomes from the rough endoplasmic reticulum to scattered sites in the cytoplasm and disarray of the smooth endoplasmic reticulum. This apparent membrane denaturing effect described by Reynolds (1972) is probably reflected in the loss of basophilia seen under the light microscope.

Although CCl_4-induced hepatotoxicity is dependent on its metabolism, there is much discussion concerning the precise nature of the reactive metabolite. Biochemically, damage to the endoplasmic reticulum leads to the accumulation of lipid and to depression of protein synthesis and of mixed-function oxidase activity. The mechanism of impaired mixed-function oxidase activity is thought to be the irreversible binding of a CCl_4 metabolite to cytochrome P-450, thereby rendering it inactive. Eventually, decreased mitochondrial function is also observed (Recknagel and Glende, 1973).

Recknagel and coworkers (1973, 1977) and Slater (1972) have argued that the mechanism of toxicity of CCl_4 involves the initial homolytic cleavage of a C—Cl bond by cytochrome P-450 to yield trichloromethyl and chlorine free radicals (Figure 20–3). The trichloromethyl free radical is then thought to attack enoic fatty acids in the membranes of the endoplasmic reticulum, leading to secondary free radicals within the fatty acids. These fatty acids are now subject to attack by oxygen, and the subsequent process, which is termed *lipid peroxidation*, produces damage to membranes and enzymes. Slater

(1) Rechnagel and Glende (1973)
$$CCl_4 \longrightarrow CCl_3\cdot + Cl\cdot$$

(2) Slater (1982)
$$CCl_3\cdot + O_2 \longrightarrow Cl_3COO\cdot$$

(3) Reiner and Uehleke (1971)
Mansby *et al.* (1974)
$$CCl_4 \longrightarrow Cl_3C:$$
$$\text{(carbene)}$$

Figure 20–3. Proposed reactive metabolites of CCl_4.

(1982) has suggested that the trichloromethyl free radical is less reactive than was once thought and that it is more likely that the reaction of O_2 with the trichloromethyl radical leads to a more reactive species, that is, $Cl_3COO\cdot$, the trichloromethylperoxy free radical. This free radical would readily interact with unsaturated membrane lipids to produce lipid peroxidation. The net effect of lipid peroxidation is to set in motion the series of inevitable cellular degradations described above that follow upon this initial insult.

An alternative hypothesis to free radical involvement is that covalent binding of CCl_4 metabolites to critical cellular macromolecules may lead to cell damage as in the case of acetaminophen and bromobenzene (Jollow and Smith, 1977). Mansuy *et al.* (1974) and Reiner and Uehleke (1971) have studied the splitting of carbon-halogen bonds under anaerobic conditions to yield highly reactive metabolites having the general structure $R_3C:$ and called carbenes. Uehleke (1977) reported on the covalent binding of CCl_4, $CHCl_3$, and halothane to macromolecules and suggests that under anaerobic conditions covalent binding is probably mediated by the carbene metabolites. Sipes and Gandolfi (1982) showed that halothane-induced liver damage produced under relatively anaerobic conditions is probably related to the formation of a carbene intermediate.

Thus, it appears that aerobic covalent binding and hepatotoxicity may be accounted for by the trichloromethyl free radical or the trichloromethyl peroxy free radical, whereas carbenes may play a more important role when oxygen tension is low (Uehleke, 1977; Sipes and Gandolfi, 1982; Slater, 1982).

LaCagnin *et al.* (1988) have identified another free radical metabolite of carbon tetrachloride, namely, the carbon dioxide anion radical, $\cdot CO_2^-$. They have demonstrated the appearance of this radical at the time of onset of LDH release from the liver, which is indicative of the onset of hepatotoxicity. Although the role played by the radical in hepatotoxicity is not yet defined, it appears to be an early marker of cell damage.

Other Haloalkanes and Haloalkenes

Many of the haloalkanes and haloalkenes are used as solvents and appear to have related mechanisms of toxic actions. Carbon tetrachloride is the prototype for these compounds, and its ability to cause both fatty infiltration and hepatic necrosis serves as the model for comparison. It should be stressed that although carbon tetrachloride, chloroform, and 1,1,2-trichloroethane also produce renal toxicity, there is no indication that this is a common property of other haloalkanes or haloalkenes (Plaa and Larson, 1965).

Zimmerman (1978) has collected the data on the hepatotoxicity of the haloalkanes and haloalkenes and has classified them according to the severity of the hepatic effects. Thus, methyl chloride, methyl bromide, methyl iodide, dichlorodifluoromethane, *trans*-1,2-dichloroethylene, ethyl chloride, ethyl bromide, ethyl iodide, and *n*-butylchloride produce no liver damage and only slight fat accumulation in liver. Chlorobromomethane, dichloromethane, *cis*-1,2-dichloroethylene, tetrachloroethylene, and 2-chloro-*n*-butane produce fatty liver without necrosis. Similarly, biochemical analyses, which attempted to relate both potential carcinogenicity and hepatotoxicity, showed that with respect to their ability to induce ornithine decarboxylase and serum alanine aminotransferase, on an equimolar basis, carbon tetrachloride > chloroform > dichloromethane (Kitchin and Brown, 1989). The following are characterized by the production of both fatty liver and necrosis:

Carbon tetrachloride	1,1,2,2,-Tetrachloroethane
Carbon tetraiodide	1,2-Dichloroethane
Carbon tetrabromide	1,2-Dibromoethane
Bromotrichloromethane	1,1,1-Trichloroethane
Chloroform	Pentamethylethane
Iodoform	1,1,2-Trichloroethylene
Bromoform	2-Chloro-*n*-propane
	1,2-Dichloro-*n*-propane

The hepatotoxicity of these agents has been associated with the ease with which a halogen can be removed to produce a reactive metabolite. The factors associated with increasing toxicity are increasing numbers of halogens in the molecule, increasing size (*i.e.* atomic number or weight of the halogens), and increasing ease of homolytic cleavage. By the same token, there is an inverse relationship between the severity of toxicity and the electronegativity of the halogens, or the chain length.

The metabolism of the haloforms (trihalomethanes) also involves the mixed-function oxidase. The initial step is the loss of a halide. Subsequent metabolism may lead to CO production. Covalent binding to macromolecules resulting from the metabolism of haloforms has been postulated to occur via the formation of phosgene, in the case of chloroform, and its analogue, dibromocarbonyl, in the case of bromoform.

The metabolism and the production of reactive intermediates from the haloethylenes appear to proceed by a different mechanism. The first step in the metabolism of vinyl chloride, trichloroethylene, perchloroethylene, vinyl bromide, vinyl fluoride, vinylidene chloride, and vinylidene fluoride has been proposed to involve microsomal oxidation leading to epoxide formation across the double bond (Figure 20–4) (Henschler and Hoos, 1982). These authors have suggested that the resulting oxiranes are highly reactive and therefore can covalently bind to nucleic acids with the eventual end result of mutations and cancer.

Bolt et al. (1982) collected the data on covalent binding to protein, both in vivo and in vitro, covalent binding to nucleic acids, mutagenicity in bacterial test systems, and carcinogenicity for these compounds. Although not all of these data points were available for each compound, some important comparisons result. Vinyl chloride and vinyl bromide exhibited positive responses in each category studied, whereas trichloroethylene, which displayed some degree of positive response in each of the other categories, was not carcinogenic. Vinylidene chloride, which covalently bound to protein and nucleic acids and was mutagenic, was an equivocal carcinogen. They postulated that based on carcinogenic potency the relative carcinogenicity of compounds that produced significant preneoplastic foci in livers of treated rats in this series was: vinyl chloride > vinyl fluoride > vinyl bromide. Furthermore, a comparison of the monohaloethylenes and the 1,1-dihaloethylenes indicated that monohalo compounds were more carcinogenic.

The chemical reactivity of chlorinated ethylene epoxides was studied by Politzer et al. (1981), who compared the ease with which the two C—O bonds could be broken as a function of halogenated substituents on the carbons using ethylene oxide as the standard of reference. They showed that in a comparison of ethylene oxide, vinyl chloride, and vinylidene chloride, with increasing chlorination of one carbon there is an increase in the bond strength of the chlorinated carbon to the oxygen and a decrease in the bond strength to the other (i.e., nonchlorinated) carbon. When both carbons are substituted with single chloride, the C—O bonds are equal. When there are two chlorines on one carbon and one on the other, there is again weakening of the less chlorinated carbon to oxygen bond. These authors suggest that the unsymmetrical chloroethylenes are more carcinogenic than the symmetrical because the ease of bond breakage potentiates covalent binding to DNA.

While reactivity appears to be a fundamental principle of covalent binding—i.e., the toxic or carcinogenic metabolite must indeed be a highly reactive compound—Bolt et al. (1982) suggest that there are limits to the effectiveness of highly reactive species. For example, they postulate that a major reason for the weak activity of vinylidene chloride as a carcinogen may be related to the instability of its putative metabolite, 1,1-dichlorooxirane. It is likely to be largely degraded before it reaches its site of action. Thus, these authors suggest that there is an optimum degree of stability that allows the intermediate to be formed by the mixed-function oxidase, reach the DNA, and form the covalent bond. If the reactivity is too low, covalent binding may be poor. If the reactivity is too high, it may never reach the target.

In addition to the well-described hepatotoxicity related to the haloalkanes and haloalkenes, several haloalkenes—e.g., tetrafluoroethylene, chlorotrifluoroethylene, 1,1-dichloro-2,2-difluoroethylene, hexafluoropropene, trichloroethylene, tetrachloroethylene, and hexachloro-1,3-butadiene—are nephrotoxic (Dekant et al., 1989). The early demonstration that trichloroethylene-extracted soybean meal yielded S-(dichlorovinyl)-L-cysteine, which in turn produced aplastic anemia in cattle, led to the observation that in rodents this compound caused nephrotoxicity. The mechanism appears to involve the cleavage of the cysteine derivative to 1,2-dichlorovinylthiol by renal cysteine conjugate beta-lyase. It has been suggested that those haloalkenes that induce nephrotoxicity act by first undergoing glutathione conjugation in the liver and are then transported to the kidney where they are metabolized to the cysteine conjugate. They are ultimately acted on by beta-lyase to yield highly reactive episulfonium ions that covalently bind to proteins and DNA. While

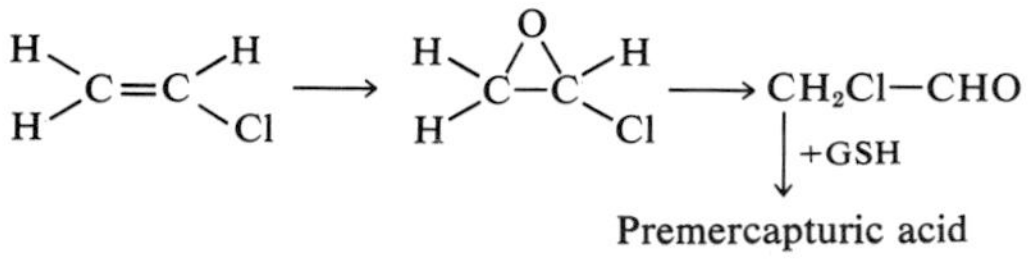

Figure 20–4. Biotransformation of vinyl chloride as an example of metabolism of haloalkenes.

the predominant effect is nephrotoxicity, in some cases the end result may be renal carcinogenesis.

Simple aliphatic halocarbons will continue to be an important area of research for some time to come. Some are found in drinking water as a result of chlorination procedures or because they enter groundwater from leachates at chemical dump sites. Although some have been shown to be carcinogenic in long-term bioassays, it will be essential for us to assess accurately the risk of human exposure to these chemicals at the levels at which they are found in the environment.

ALIPHATIC ALCOHOLS

Ethyl Alcohol (Ethanol, Alcohol)

There is probably greater exposure to ethanol than to any other solvent with the exception of water. Not only is it used as a solvent in industry, but it is heavily consumed by large numbers of people as a component of potentially intoxicating beverages. As a result of the petroleum shortage, plans call for diluting gasoline with ethanol to form a combustible product termed "gasohol." At that point, it is likely that we will experience universal exposure to ethanol. Nevertheless, historically, occupational exposure has been less important as a cause of injury than the fact that the worker may imbibe alcohol and thereby be rendered less likely to use safety precautions on the job. By the same token, the most important cause of death in auto accidents is drunken driving. Thus, most instances of death or injury related to ethanol come via abuse of ethanol as a beverage rather than to occupational exposure.

Blood Levels. Our information on the toxicity of ethanol comes from either clinical observations of human drinkers or controlled studies in animals and humans where ethanol has been administered either orally or parenterally. Although a TLV for ethanol at a level of 1000 ppm has been established (ACGIH, 1989), of greater concern has been the dose level likely to cause inebriation. As a practical matter, the legal definition of *intoxication* has been set on the basis of the blood alcohol level detected in alleged drunken drivers. Thus, in many states the demonstration that the driver has a blood alcohol level of 100 mg/100 ml of blood (100 mg%) is *prima facie* evidence of "driving under the influence of alcohol." In a 70-kg man, it would require approximately 3 ounces of pure alcohol to achieve a blood alcohol level in the range of 90 to 150 mg%. In terms of intake of alcoholic beverages, it would probably require that the individual would have to drink about 6

ounces of 100-proof whiskey, 12 ounces of fortified wine (i.e., sherry), or eight, 12-ounce bottles of beer to achieve that concentration. It is likely that most people would demonstrate inebriation under these conditions.

The blood alcohol level and the time necessary for it to be achieved are controlled largely by the quantity of food in the GI tract. Once absorbed, the alcohol equilibrates with body water, and when drinking is complete, the blood alcohol level begins to drop to some extent because of excretion of alcohol in the breath and urine but, more important, because it is metabolized in the liver. Ethanol is metabolized at a rate sufficient to reduce the blood alcohol level linearly by approximately 15 to 20 mg% per hour until low concentrations are reached, at which time the rate becomes asymptotic. Thus, if a blood alcohol concentration of 120 mg% were detected, it could be assumed that it would require approximately six to eight hours for ethanol to reach negligible levels in the blood.

CNS Effects. The pharmacological and toxicological effects of alcohol relate to the fact that alcohol acts as both a general anesthetic and a nutrient. As a general anesthetic, ethanol causes a dose-dependent central nervous system depression. Although many people appear to be animated under the influence, it is likely that this is a manifestation of the release of inhibitions and is a mild form of the stage II excitement and delirium observed during anesthesia with diethyl ether.

The overt display of inebriation occurs at different blood alcohol levels depending on the extent to which the subject has had previous experience with alcohol. In heavy drinkers, tolerance to the low-level effects of ethanol can be observed, and even social drinkers may not show obvious signs of intoxication at blood alcohol levels that would render novice drinkers clearly "under the influence." There are two reasons for these effects. Heavy drinkers may actually demonstrate a greater rate of ethanol metabolism. More important may be the fact that experienced drinkers have learned not to display their inebriation at the lower blood levels at which inexperienced drinkers clearly respond.

The literature on the biological and medical effects of alcohol is the largest single literature in medical science. Ethanol is distributed with body water, and its adverse effects to most organs have been reported. For the purposes of this discussion, some specific areas of the pharmacology and toxicology of ethanol will be discussed. These will include the effects of ethanol on the CNS, the fetal alcohol syndrome, the metabolism of ethanol, and the effects of ethanol on the liver. For additional detailed reports on current trends in alcohol research, the student is referred to compendia edited by Avogadro *et al.* (1979), Sherlock (1982), and Thurman and Hoffman (1983). Among the areas covered are interaction of ethanol with the endocrine system; interactions with xenobiotics; effects on renal, cardiovascular, and gastrointestinal systems; hematopoietic effects; enzymology; dependence and withdrawal; and other effects that indicate that alcoholism is a disease that encompasses the entire body.

The obvious behavioral effects of alcohol are well known. Loss of inhibitions have been eloquently described through several editions of a noted textbook of pharmacology: "Confidence abounds, the personality becomes expansive and vivacious, and speech may become eloquent and occasionally brilliant" (Ritchie, 1970). Although some reflexes may be enhanced at low blood ethanol concentrations because of release of higher center control, they soon deteriorate as the blood level increases. It can be demonstrated that contrary to what outer appearances may be, objective tests of manual dexterity and simple intellectual challenges demonstrate impairment at relatively low blood alcohol levels.

With increasing blood alcohol levels, there is gradual reduction of visual acuity, decreased sense of smell and taste, increased pain threshold, impaired muscular coordination, and possibly nystagmus. A staggering gait becomes apparent. Eventually, nausea and vomiting, diplopia, hypothermia, and loss of consciousness ensue. As an anesthetic, ethanol is thought to have a very low therapeutic index, and the subject is not far from death when anesthetic concentrations of ethanol are reached. While the level necessary to achieve loss of consciousness is not clearly defined, it is likely that at a blood alcohol level of 350 to 400 mg% most people would be asleep.

The mechanism by which ethanol causes these effects is not known. By the same token, it is not known how any of the general anesthetics function. Because the structure of general anesthetics is so varied, theories of anesthesia have developed that consider generalized interactions with the central nervous system rather than effects at specific receptors. A number of physicochemical theories have been proposed to explain the mechanism of action of general anesthetics. For example, the Meyer-Overton theory as described by Meyer (1937) suggested that the potency of a general anesthetic was directly related to its solubility in lipid membranes and was otherwise unrelated to its structure. Ferguson (1939) argued that the chemical potential or thermodynamic activity was more closely related to anesthetic activity, whereas Wulf and Feather-

stone (1957) argued that the critical property was the van der Waals constant. Pauling (1961) and S. L. Miller (1961) built their arguments around the effect of ethanol on water and suggested that clathrate formation in cells of the CNS created a structure for water that was conducive to anesthesia. The observation that elevation of ambient pressure caused experimental animals to awaken from anesthesia led K. W. Miller *et al.* (1973) to formulate a hypothesis that suggested that there was a linear relationship linking elevation of atmospheric pressure with decrease in anesthetic potency. It could then be suggested that the gas enters and distorts the membrane, taking up a given volume of space. According to the thermodynamic gas laws, the volume of the gas must decrease as the pressure increases, suggesting that the volume of the anesthetic in the membranes or the CNS decreases with increasing pressure, leading to reversal of anesthesia.

Singer and Nicolson (1972) have visualized the cell membrane as a two-dimensional solution of proteins and lipids. They visualize a bilayer composed largely of phospholipids in which the polar ends are in contact with water and the lipid ends meet in the membrane. The lipid bilayer is studded with proteins that are partially embedded in the lipid and partially extend into the aqueous medium. It has been suggested that ethanol interacts with the bilayer to distort and expand the membrane, thereby increasing its fluidity (Seeman, 1972; Rubin and Rottenberg, 1983). The result is displacement of critical membrane enzymes and alterations in membrane function. The outward signs of ethanol inebriation and anesthesia would then be a function of the significance of the role of the membranes of various CNS cells in controlling these physiological functions. It has been suggested that ethanol plays a role in depressing the activities of the reticular activating system in the CNS and thereby releases many functions from integrating control (Kalant, 1961). If that is true, the cell membranes of the reticular activating system may be especially sensitive to ethanol-induced changes in membrane fluidity, or their activity is so critical that small alterations in their function lead rapidly to readily observed changes in behavior.

Several recent observations *in vitro* may shed further light on the molecular mechanisms underlying the effects of ethanol. Ethanol has been shown to block the *N*-methyl-D-aspartate (NMDA) receptor in brain cells (Lovinger *et al.*, 1989) and to inhibit the related production of cyclic GMP (Hoffman *et al.*, 1989) at levels in the range that would be expected to produce mild intoxication. These events are associated with a decrease in calcium uptake into cerebellar cells, an event normally stimulated by NMDA. It has been suggested that these effects may help to explain short-term memory loss and impairment of motor function associated with drinking.

Fetal Alcohol Syndrome. One of the more serious consequences of ethanol consumption is the effect on the development of the embryo and fetus *in utero* (Pratt, 1982). The so-called fetal alcohol syndrome (FAS) is characterized by mental deficiency and microcephaly. The infants are generally small and demonstrate poor muscular coordination. These children also exhibit a characteristic facies recognizable to the specialist. The severity appears to be related to the extent of alcohol consumption by the mother during pregnancy. In addition to the suggestion that ethanol may interfere with membrane function during development, other factors may be related to the cause of FAS. These include the possibility that acetaldehyde may escape the damaged liver of the alcoholic mother and reach the developing fetal brain, changes in the patterns of amino acids in the maternal circulation available to the fetus, and alcohol-induced hypoglycemia. These effects individually or in concert could cause damage to the developing brain and lead to FAS.

Metabolism. It is recognized that the toxic effects of alcohol on the liver are directly related to its metabolism, and it is therefore important to understand the pathways of alcohol metabolism. In a large sense, these have been well worked out over a considerable period of time. In recent years, there has been considerable discussion over the relative toxicological significance of the various enzymes capable of mediating the first step in alcohol metabolism, namely, its oxidation to acetaldehyde. Alcohol dehydrogenase is a soluble enzyme found in high concentrations in the liver that appears to play the major role in alcohol metabolism. NAD is the coenzyme, and the products are acetaldehyde and NADH. The reverse of the reaction—that is, the conversion of acetaldehyde to ethanol—is favored, but during metabolism the products are rapidly removed, thereby preventing reversal of the reaction.

$$CH_3CH_2OH + NAD \xrightarrow{\text{Alcohol Dehydrogenase}} CH_3CHO + NADH$$

A second ezyme capable of converting ethanol to acetaldehyde is catalase, which by virtue of its peroxidative activity uses hydrogen peroxide to perform the oxidation. However, normally there is very little peroxide available to support the reaction in hepatocytes, and it is unlikely that catalase can account for more than 10 percent of ethanol metabolism. This situation could change if peroxide levels in hepatocytes were elevated. For example, clofibrate, which stimulates peroxisomal fatty acid oxidation, increases peroxide levels and thereby enhances ethanol oxidation by catalase. However, it would only be under such unusual circumstances that catalase would be expected to play a significant role in ethanol metabolism.

$$CH_3CH_2OH + H_2O_2 \xrightarrow{\text{Catalase}} CH_3CHO + H_2O$$

The third enzyme is located in the microsomes and has been termed by Lieber and DiCarli (1970) MEOS (microsomal ethanol oxidizing system) because it can be demonstrated that the addition of ethanol to isolated microsomes fortified with NADPH and oxygen results in the oxidation of ethanol to acetaldehyde.

$$CH_3CH_2OH + NADPH + O_2 \xrightarrow{\text{MEOS}} CH_3CHO + NADP + H_2O$$

Ohnishi and Lieber (1977) isolated a cytochrome P-450 that mediates this reaction. Coon and Koop (1987) suggested that although this nomenclature was useful in the early days of these investigations, it has several drawbacks including the fact that the enzyme is induced by many chemicals in addition to ethanol and that it metabolizes a wide range of substrates. They termed the enzyme *cytochrome P-450 3a* based on its electrophoretic characteristics. Its official nomenclature is *cytochrome P-450 IIE1*.

The contribution made by each of these enzymes to ethanol metabolism has been estimated by various authorities. Damgaard (1982) and Havre *et al.* (1977) have argued that non–alcohol dehydrogenase–mediated metabolism of ethanol accounts for no more than 10 percent of total ethanol metabolism. Vind and Grunnet (1983), on the other hand, estimate that non–alcohol dehydrogenase metabolism of ethanol may account for as much as 20 percent and may increase to 30 percent or higher when substrates such as xylitol, which are capable of generating exceedingly high levels of NADH, are added. The argument is that at these high NADH levels electron transfer into the mixed-function oxidase pathway via cytochrome b_5 is stimulated, and therefore, MEOS activity is enhanced. Nevertheless, regardless of which estimate more accurately reflects the percentage of non–alcohol dehydrogenase–mediated ethanol metabolism, it appears that the major enzyme involved in ethanol oxidation is alcohol dehydrogenase. It is unlikely that catalase plays a significant role in ethanol metabolism at concentrations of peroxide normally present in liver. The quantitative significance of the role of mixed-function oxidases in ethanol metabolism has yet to be established.

The further metabolism of ethanol relates to the metabolism of acetaldehyde. In the past, the fate of acetaldehyde has been linked to several enzymes located in various parts of the cell. In recent years, however, it has been postulated that acetaldehyde dehydrogenase, an NAD-requiring enzyme, plays the major role in its degradation, and this enzyme, although largely mitochondrial in rat liver, is a cytosolic enzyme in humans.

$$CH_3CHO + NAD \xrightarrow{\text{Acetaldehyde Dehydrogenase}} CH_3COO^- + NADH$$

The resulting acetate is released from the liver and oxidized peripherally, probably because during ethanol oxidation there is an increase in the NADH/NAD ratio that leads to decreased availability of oxaloacetate, decreased pyruvic dehydrogenase activity, and inhibition of citrate synthetase, which taken together inhibit the oxidation of acetate in the liver.

Liver Injury. The drinking of alcohol remains a leading cause of death due to liver cirrhosis. The diagnosis of early alcohol-induced liver disease involves recognition that the patient drinks alcohol to excess, that the patient may be experiencing social problems indicative of alcoholism, and that these are coupled with the finding of hepatomegaly, elevated serum transaminase, and possibly other clinical signs. At more advanced stages, patients may exhibit acute alcoholic hepatitis following heavy bouts of drinking. Signs include vomiting, diarrhea, jaundice, and psychiatric disturbances. The liver is enlarged and painful to palpation, whereas the spleen may be impalpable. The enlarged liver is due to fat accumulation as well as swelling of liver cells and accumulation of other components such as proteins, which would otherwise be secreted. A wide variety of changes in serum enzymes and proteins can be determined that reflect impairment of hepatic function. Eventually, with continued heavy drinking, frank hepatic cirrhosis, not unlike end-stage liver disease derived from other causes, will be observed and may be fatal.

The mechanism by which alcohol mediates liver damage has also generated much discussion. The underlying issue is whether alcoholic liver disease is the result of a direct toxic effect of ethanol on the liver or is the result of nutritional deficiencies that accompany excessive alcohol consumption. Alcohol provides 7.1 kcal/g. A pint of 100-proof whiskey would provide 1400 kcal, which is a significant portion of total caloric intake for most people. If alcoholics would maintain their normal diet plus large quantities of alcohol, they would gain weight at a rapid pace. Since obesity is not a usual corollary of alcoholism, it appears that alcohol replaces other sources of calories in the alcoholic's diet. Because alcohol contains no essential nutrients such as proteins, vitamins, or minerals and it replaces food that would contain these dietary components, it would be expected that alcoholics would develop nutritional deficiencies.

Clinical experience with alcoholics (Morgan, 1982) suggests that the stage of alcoholism in which the individual is viewed is critical to making nutritional judgments. Early clinical studies of patients with advanced alcohol-induced liver disease, especially involving patients from poor socioeconomic backgrounds, have reported that the patients exhibited weight loss and nutritional deficiencies. However, studies of alcoholics who did not display overt liver disease revealed normal nutrition. In another study in which a segment of the alcoholic study group displayed liver disease and a segment were clinically malnourished, there did not appear to be a relationship between nutritional status and the severity of the disease. Morgan (1982) suggests that although the intake of nutrients in the diet in a controlled experiment may be similar between control and alcoholic groups, the greater percent of calories derived from alcohol led to significantly different nutritional status. Among the nutritional problems caused by alcohol consumption are decreases in thiamine absorption, decreased enterohepatic circulation of folate, degradation of pyridoxal-5'-phosphate, and disturbances in the metabolism of both vitamins A and D (Mezey, 1985). Other factors that together can be considered as contributing to malabsorption and may contribute to the development of malnourishment despite adequate intake of essential nutrients include the effects of alcohol on gastric emptying time and changes in the physiology and morphology of the small intestine, secretion by the pancreas and biliary system, and splanchnic blood and lymph flow.

An alternative view offered by Lieber (1979) is that alcohol has a direct toxic effect on the liver that is not dependent on nutritional deficiency. The data come from studies in which humans given nutritional supplements while consuming excessive quantities of alcohol developed fatty livers. Furthermore, in a long-term study in which 15 baboons fed alcohol and given nutritional supplements all developed fatty liver, 5 developed hepatitis and 5 cirrhosis (Lieber *et al.*, 1975). These results were not confirmed, however, by Ainley *et al.* (1988), who performed a similar study in baboons with the aim of determining whether enrichment of the diet with Zn protected against hepatic fibrosis and cirrhosis.

Several questions remain to be answered before a conclusion can be reached on this issue. The central feature of the disease appears to be that the liver is unable to secrete lipid in the alcoholic, regardless of whether it is synthesized in the liver from ethanol or is taken in via the diet. Hence, liver lipid accumulates, alcoholic liver disease ensues, and cirrhosis may be the eventual outcome. The essence of the argument is that in humans, and perhaps in baboons, these events proceeded despite nutritionally adequate diets. The definition of the nutritionally adequate diet is stated in terms of a diet sufficient to prevent liver disease in a nondrinking individual. The diets were then supplemented to ensure adequacy. Nevertheless, there is no yardstick for the nutritional requirements of the alcoholic. An increase in lipotrope content several fold would represent excessive protection for the nondrinker but may not be adequate protection for the drinker. For example, Klatskin et al. (1954) reported on the increased choline requirement of the alcohol-fed rat, and Thompson and Reitz (1976) suggested that ethanol consumption led to an increase in choline oxidation in rats. Furthermore, alterations in the absorption and degradation of nutritional requirements under the influence of ethanol are well known, and therefore, adding the nutrients to the diet may be insufficient to ensure against nutritional derangements during alcohol intake.

The conclusions that can be drawn at this time are that given the severe derangement of hepatic metabolism produced by chronic alcohol feeding, the effects of ethanol on the GI tract, and the frequency of malnourishment among alcoholics, it is likely that nutritional factors play a major role in the development of alcoholic liver disease. However, the challenging suggestion that there may be a direct effect of ethanol on the liver provides a stimulus for further research to segregate out the proposed direct effect from the nutritional effects. The development of a readily available animal model in which the disease can be accurately reproduced would help to settle the question because it would permit the determination of the nutritional requirements of the alcoholic.

Interaction with Other Chemicals. The toxicological interaction of ethanol with other hepatotoxic agents is a well-recognized phenomenon (Zimmerman, 1978; Strubelt, 1980). The earliest reported indication of an interaction was between ethanol and CCl_4 used as a vermifuge in the treatment of hookworm in humans who drank alcoholic beverages. The observation that ethanol potentiates CCl_4 toxicity has also been made in several species of laboratory animals (Zimmerman, 1978; Strubelt, 1980; Shibayama, 1988). Reinke et al. (1988) reported that ethanol stimulated the production of trichloromethyl free radicals from carbon tetrachloride.

Pretreatment with ethanol also increases the hepatotoxicity of chloroform, trichloroethane, trichloroethylene, thioacetamide, dimethylnitrosamine, paracetamol, and aflatoxin B_1. Ethanol was less effective in increasing hepatotoxicity of allyl alcohol and galactosamine and did not alter the effects of bromobenzene, phalloidin, or praseodymium. The toxic effects of α-amantidine were reduced by ethanol.

Methanol, 2-propanol, 2-butanol, and 2-methyl-propanol mimicked the effects of ethanol and were more active in potentiating hepatotoxic effects of other agents. Whereas the ketone metabolites of the secondary alcohols—i.e., acetone and 2-butanone—increase the hepatotoxicity of CCl_4 and other halocarbons, acetaldehyde is lacking in this property, and inhibition of ethanol metabolism by pyrazole does not protect against the potentiating effect.

Although the mechanism of ethanol-enhanced hepatotoxicity is not fully understood, it may be a direct effect of ethanol rather than of a metabolite because of the lack of activity by acetaldehyde. Several possible mechanisms have been proposed to explain the effects of ethanol. These include attempts to demonstrate that ethanol acts by enhancing CCl_4 absorption, by inducing mixed-function oxidase, by depleting hepatic glutathione, by increasing lipid peroxidation, or by producing hypoxia. None of these proposed mechanisms has been entirely successful, and work in this field continues.

Ethanol as a Carcinogen. Because of the widespread use of alcoholic beverages, there has been understandable concern regarding the role of ethanol in carcinogenesis. The International Agency for Research on Cancer, an arm of the World Health Organization, convened an expert panel to review all the literature in this field (IARC, 1988). They concluded that whereas the evidence for the carcinogenicity of ethanol and alcoholic beverages in animals was inadequate, there is "sufficient evidence" for the carcinogenicity of alcoholic beverages in humans. The panel agreed that the evidence linked tumors of the oral cavity, pharynx, larynx, esophagus, and liver to the consumption of alcoholic beverages. Seitz and Simanowski (1986) suggested that ethanol did not act as an initiator but was more likely to be a cocarcinogen that interacts with other carcinogens to cause tumorigenic responses. Unlike most environmental carcinogens to which people are exposed either infrequently or at a low dose, the consumption of alcoholic beverages is common to millions of people on a relatively frequent basis at dietary dose levels. Further studies are required to define accurately the risk to the general population of users and to specific populations at risk.

Methanol

Methanol, or wood alcohol, is another potential neurotoxin that finds extensive use in industry as a solvent. The proposal to add methanol to gasoline or to design automobiles that use neat methanol as a fuel will necessarily widen consumer exposure to the material.

Blindness. The target of methanol toxicity is the retina, a fact that has been documented in many case reports of unfortunate individuals who ingested large amounts of the solvent. At high doses, methanol can cause reversible or permanent blindness and, in severe cases, death. Intoxication is characterized by initial mild inebriation followed by an asymptomatic period of 12 to 24 hours. At this time, a marked metabolic acidosis develops, which if not treated can be fatal. Visual problems include eye pain, blurred vision, constriction of visual fields, and other visual complaints. Permanent blindness can develop after as little time as 48 hours. The pathology of the visual lesion has been described in some detail. A marked optic disk edema and dilated pupils with greatly reduced reaction to light are observed. Intraaxonal swelling in the areas of the optic disk and anterior optic nerve are observed with light microscopy (Benton and Calhoun, 1952).

This syndrome has not been described in most common laboratory species. Indeed, while metabolic acidosis and ocular toxicity are observed in humans and monkeys, rodents, dogs, and cats display only mild central nervous system depression following dosing with comparable doses of methanol (Tephly, 1977). A description of the species differences in methanol metabolism has led to a better appreciation of the pathogenesis and treatment of methanol poisoning.

Metabolism. Methanol is rapidly and well absorbed by inhalation, oral, and topical exposure routes (Dutkiewicz *et al.*, 1980). Following absorption, the alcohol is rapidly distributed to organs according to the distribution of body water (Yant and Schrenk, 1937).

An abbreviated scheme for the metabolism of methanol is presented below:

$$CH_3OH \rightarrow HCHO \rightarrow$$
Methanol   Formaldehyde
$$HCOOH \rightarrow CO_2$$
Formic Acid   Carbon Dioxide

There are two pathways available in the mammalian organism for oxidation of methanol: a catalase peroxidative pathway and an alcohol dehydrogenase system. Studies by Mannering, Tephly, and their colleagues (Mannering and Parks, 1975; Makàr and Tephly, 1977) have shown that in the rat, guinea pig, and rabbit the major route of methanol oxidation is through a catalase-dependent pathway, whereas in the monkey and in man, an alcohol dehydrogenase system functions *in vivo*. Metabolism to formic acid is quite rapid. Indeed, in monkeys or humans poisoned with very large amounts of methanol, formaldehyde is not detected even in very low levels in tissues at autopsy. Formic acid is further oxidized to carbon dioxide by an enzymatic pathway dependent on the presence of the cofactor folic acid. The enzyme is active in both rodents and primates, but conversion of formic acid to CO_2 appears to be slower in primates than in rodents (Tephly *et al.*, 1979).

Tephly has shown that the monkey appears to be an appropriate animal model for studying methanol poisoning since the resulting syndrome closely resembles that seen in humans (McMartin *et al.*, 1975). Using the primate as a model, Tephly and coworkers have elucidated in detail the relationship between methanol metabolism and toxicity (McMartin *et al.*, 1977, 1979, 1980). In rodents, a species that is not susceptible to methanol-induced ocular toxicity, methanol is rapidly metabolized to CO_2. In contrast, in primates and humans, alcohol dehydrogenase— and folate-dependent pathways slowly metabolize methanol to CO_2. The kinetics of metabolism and elimination of large doses of methanol in primates are such that formic acid accumulates in tissues including the eye (McMartin *et al.*, 1975, 1977; Tephly *et al.*, 1979; Noker and Tephly, 1980). A metabolic acidosis and the characteristic ocular toxicity of methanol exposure result. The ocular toxicity appears to be due to the presence of elevated levels of formic acid in blood (McMartin *et al.*, 1975, 1977; Tephly *et al.*, 1979; Noker and Tephly, 1980).

Chronic Exposure. Much less information is available on the health effects of long-term exposure to low levels of methanol. The ACGIH presently recommends a TLV of (TWA—200 ppm, STEL—250 ppm) for methanol vapors based on the irritancy of the solvent.

Greenburg *et al.* (1938) reported on 19 workers exposed to a solvent consisting of three parts acetone and one part methanol in which the concentrations were 40 to 45 ppm of acetone and 22 to 25 ppm of methanol. Workers were evaluated by physical examination, neurological tests, urinalysis, and hematology. No abnormal results were found. It is difficult to say with certainty that this exposure to methanol represents a no-observed-effect level since there was also concomitant exposure to acetone.

Office workers exposed to methanol in the vicinity of duplicating machines were studied by Kingsley and Hirsch (1954–55). The workers complained of frequent and recurrent headaches but of no other symptoms. Methanol exposure levels were reported to range from 15 to 375 ppm, although most measurements fell in the 200- to 375-ppm range. Duplicating fluids were changed in favor of less methanol, but the authors fail to mention if there were any beneficial effects on worker headaches. It is unclear from this study if headaches were attributable to methanol or to other components of duplicating fluids.

It is of interest that nearly 30 years following this report by Kingsley and Hirsch, NIOSH (1980) performed a health hazard investigation on teacher's aides using spirit duplicating machines. No local exhaust ventilation was available, and most measurements exceeded the NIOSH recommended STEL for 15 minutes (800 ppm). The adverse health effects of blurred vision, headache, nausea, and dizziness reported by teachers on questionnaires appear to refer to the CNS depressant effects of methanol.

Animal studies involving repeated long-term exposure to methanol are sparse. Indeed, it is debatable whether or not rodent studies would be meaningful because of the species differences in metabolism described above. Primate studies could provide useful information but are extremely expensive and time-consuming. An intriguing alternative to primates may be the folate-deficient acatalasemic mouse ($C_s{}^b$-FAD). E. N. Smith and Taylor (1982) reported that this mouse attains high plasma formate levels and acidemia after dosing with methanol. Further work with the $C_s{}^b$-FAD mouse may lead to the development of an inexpensive small animal model suitable for investigating effects of chronic exposure to methanol. A similar approach to a rodent animal model using strains of rats and mice more typically encountered in toxicology is possible since Eells et al. (1981) have demonstrated that in vivo exposure to nitrous oxide can inhibit folate pathways and lead to a decreased clearance of formate from blood.

In the absence of well-designed epidemiological studies and long-term animal studies, one may use pharmacokinetic principles to consider whether or not chronic exposure to low levels of methanol is likely to result in ocular toxicity. In poisoning cases in which humans consumed several ounces of methanol, blood concentrations in the hundreds of mg/100 ml of blood were established (Gonda et al., 1978). A review of papers that have extensively considered methanol concentration in blood and the clinical outcome of poisoning indicates that an initial blood level in excess of 100 mg/100 ml would be required for irreversible effects, such as visual disturbances. Additionally, a typical half-life for methanol in the blood following such massive doses was estimated to be in the range of 30 hours. While the half-life of blood methanol is quite long in poisoning cases, studies in human volunteers who ingested small amounts (1 to 5 ml) of methanol revealed that under these conditions the blood half-life is only about three hours (Dutkiewicz et al., 1980; Sedivec et al., 1981). Under these conditions, peak blood levels were in the range or 10 mg/100 ml.

If one considers the present ACGIH TLV of 200 ppm (262 mg/m³) and assumes that there is 100 percent absorption of vapors and a respiratory volume of 10 m³ in an eight-hour workday, then a total body burden may be calculated.

$$\text{Body burden} = 262 \text{ mg/m}^3 \times 10 \text{ m}^3 \times 1.0 = 2620 \text{ mg}$$

If one further assumes that this total body burden is absorbed within the first few minutes of the workshift and that the methanol distributes with total body water, a worst-case peak blood methanol level may be calculated.

$$\text{Peak blood level} = 2620 \text{ mg/49* liter} = 53 \text{ mg/ liter}$$
$$= 5.3 \text{ mg/100 ml}$$

This peak blood level is about one-twentieth of a level that would be associated with acute irreversible toxic effects. Since the half-life of blood methanol in this blood concentration range is three hours, blood methanol concentrations would be at negligible levels by the time the next workshift began 24 hours later. Thus, it seems unlikely that vapor exposure to methanol under ACGIH recommended exposures has any possibility of causing ocular toxicity. The possibility of achieving a high enough body burden under dermal exposure conditions seems even more remote.

GLYCOLS

In addition to their general use as heat exchangers, antifreeze formulations, hydraulic fluids, and chemical intermediates, glycols also have some use as industrial solvents for nitrocellulose and cellulose acetate and as a solvent for pharmaceuticals, food additives, cosmetics,

---

*Assumes a 70-kg person with 70 percent water content.

inks, and lacquers. Owing to their low volatility, the glycols in general produce little vapor hazard at ordinary temperatures. However, since they are used in antifreeze mixtures, as hydraulic fluids, and as heat exchangers, they may be encountered in the vapor or mist form, particularly where the temperature is markedly elevated, or enter groundwater following consumer use and disposal. OSHA has recognized the respiratory irritation potential of ethylene glycol vapors by setting an exposure standard of 50 ppm as a ceiling limit not to be exceeded.

Ethylene Glycol (1,2-Ethanediol, HOCH₂CH₂OH)

When taken orally, ethylene glycol appears to be considerably more toxic to humans than to other animal species. The lethal oral dose in humans is estimated to be 1.4 ml/kg based on poisonings from accidental ingestion or ingestion with suicidal intent. This amount would be equivalent to approximately 100 ml for a 70-kg person. The acute oral LD50s reported for rats, guinea pigs, and mice ranged from approximately 5.5 to 13 ml/kg, indicating that on a weight basis, ethylene glycol appears to be less toxic in these animal species than in humans.

Cats appear to share the primate's susceptibilty to poisoning with ethylene glycol. Gessner *et al.* (1961) reported a minimal lethal dose of 1g/kg for cats and noted that this may be due to an already high baseline excretion of oxalic acid. Ethylene glycol poisoning is a serious and frequently encountered problem for the veterinarian in small animal practice. Exposure typically occurs when pets ingest spilled ethylene glycol–based antifreezes (Mueller, 1982; Rowland, 1987).

While species sensitivity to ethylene glycol varies considerably, the kidney damage resulting from acute or repeated exposure was identified early in the rat and repeated in several other animal species (Morris *et al.*, 1942; Blood *et al.*, 1962; Gershoff and Andrus, 1962; Blood, 1965; Roberts and Seibold, 1969).

The most extensive report of ethylene glycol toxicity in rodents is that of DePass *et al.* (1986). In these studies, male and female rats were fed diets containing ethylene glycol for two years. Approximate daily doses were 0.04, 0.20, and 1.0 g/kg body weight per day. Rats were considerably more sensitive than were mice. High-dose male rats exhibited an increased mortality rate, reduced body weight gain, increased blood urea nitrogen and creatinine, increased urine volume, and reduced urine specific gravity and urinary pH. Urinary calcium oxalate crystals and increased kidney weight were noted in all high-dose male rats. Histopathological changes in

high-dose male rats relevant to the kidney included tubular cell hyperplasia, tubular dilatation, and peritubular nephritis. Ethylene glycol was not carcinogenic in rats and mice, as there was no increased incidence of kidney tumors (or tumors of other tissues) in animals fed ethylene glycol for two years.

Studies on ethylene glycol toxicity in the monkey were reported by Roberts and Seibold (1969). Ethylene glycol was administered in drinking water at concentrations ranging from 0.25 to 10 percent. The renal histopathology, after 6 to 13 days, varied depending on the amount of ethylene glycol consumed. At high-dose levels, deposition of calcium oxalate crystals occurred in the proximal renal tubules, and necrotic areas of tubular epithelium occurred adjacent to the crystals. In this study, it appeared that oxalate crystallization did not occur following doses less than 15 ml/kg. However, functional renal changes were present at dose levels above 1 ml/kg, suggesting that renal damage can occur in the absence of oxalate crystal formation.

In acute poisoning in man, ethylene glycol shares many of the characteristics of methanol poisoning. Ingestion of ethylene glycol is followed by an asymptomatic period during which it is metabolized to glycolic and eventually oxalic acid. A profound acidosis may develop. Unlike methanol where vision is affected, however, acidosis is accompanied by disturbances in renal function or even renal failure. The full clinical picture may take up to 72 hours to develop. Aggressive management of both ethylene glycol and methanol poisoning is needed, and knowledge of the metabolism of these two solvents forms the basis of treatment. An abbreviated scheme for the metabolism of ethylene glycol is presented below:

$$
\begin{array}{ccccc}
CH_2OH & & COOH & & COOH \\
| & \rightarrow & | & \rightarrow & | \\
CH_2OH & & CH_2OH & & COOH \\
\\
\text{Ethylene} & & \text{Glycolic} & & \text{Oxalic} \\
\text{Glycol} & & \text{Acid} & & \text{Acid}
\end{array}
$$

Ethylene glycol is oxidized by alcohol dehydrogenase to glycolaldehyde and further to glycolic acid by cytosolic aldehyde oxidase. Glycolic acid is further oxidized via glyoxylic acid to oxalic acid by glycolic acid oxidase (von Wartburg *et al.*, 1964). Thus, both ethylene glycol and methanol are oxidatively metabolized to acids.

Bove (1966) studied the renal pathology in a series of rats given ethylene glycol or its metabolites, including glycolaldehyde, glycolic acid, and glyoxylic acid. In animals given single large doses of ethylene glycol (9 to 12 g/kg), striking oxalate formation was present in renal tubules. Crystals appeared throughout the proximal and distal convoluted tubules and were less numerous in the collecting tubules. In only one rat, oxalate crystals were present in the brain, as has also been reported in human poisoning (Pons and Custer, 1946). Oxalate crystals were also present in renal tubules of animals receiving glycolaldehyde, glycolic acid, and glyoxylic acid, although the renal oxalosis was less extensive with glycolaldehyde. The three proposed metabolites were all more toxic on an acute basis than was ethylene glycol since a number of animals died within eight hours of receiving 5 to 6 g/kg of body weight of the metabolites. Renal tubular pathology was not always accompanied by crystal formation, and the author concludes that cytotoxicity, rather than simple mechanical obstruction, is largely responsible for renal failure.

Studies by von Wartburg and coworkers (1964) demonstrated that human liver alcohol dehydrogenase biotransformed ethylene glycol as well as ethanol, methanol, and other alcohols. Ethanol is a much better substrate for alcohol dehydrogenase than ethylene glycol or methanol. It is thus a potent competitive inhibitor of ethylene glycol and methanol metabolism, and should duly protect against their toxic effects.

Wacker and associates (1965) reported two cases of individuals who had ingested 250 to 1000 ml of ethylene glycol antifreeze. Gastric lavage was not undertaken until admission to the hospital, some six to nine hours after the antifreeze was ingested; thus large quantities were presumably absorbed into the general circulation. Both patients were treated by ethanol infusion, which resulted in a prompt disappearance of oxaluria, and adequate urinary output was maintained. These individuals made uneventful recoveries from these rather massive ingestions of ethylene glycol. The value of ethanol administration in treating methanol poisoning has also been demonstrated (Jacobsen and McMartin, 1986).

Administration of 4-methylpyrazole, a noncompetitive inhibitor of alcohol dehydrogenase, is also used in treating ethylene glycol and methanol poisoning. Control of blood pH by administration of sodium bicarbonate and the use of hemodialysis to remove parent compound and metabolites are important additional means of treating poisoned individuals (Jacobsen and McMartin, 1986; Baud et al., 1988; Wiener and Richardson, 1988).

The reproductive and developmental toxicity of ethylene glycol have been investigated (Lamb et al., 1985). In this study, male and female mice were administered ethylene glycol at 0, 0.25, 0.50, and 1.0 percent in the drinking water. After one week, animals were housed one male and one female per cage and continuous breeding permitted. After 14 weeks, a second generation was selected and evaluated in a similar manner. Ethylene glycol (1.0 percent in drinking water) caused a decrease in the number of litters per fertile pair, pups per litter, and live pup weight. These effects were observed without any concurrent effects on body weight, water consumption, or clinical signs of toxicity in the parents. Examination of offspring revealed a pattern of skeletal defects in treated mice including the skull, sternebrae, ribs, and vertebrae. The developmental toxicity of ethylene glycol was confirmed using a conventional teratology protocol in rats and mice (Price et al., 1985). The large doses employed and slight effects observed in these studies suggest that the reproductive hazards from typical occupational exposure will be quite small.

Diethylene Glycol ($HOCH_2CH_2OCH_2CH_2OH$)

Diethylene glycol is used in the lacquer industry, in cosmetics, in permanent antifreeze formulations, in lubricants, as a softening agent, and as a plasticizer. It presents little hazard during industrial handling at ordinary temperatures. Where mists are generated or where operations are carried out at high temperatures, industrial hygiene control methods should be followed to eliminate repeated prolonged inhalation. The major hazard from diethylene glycol occurs following the ingestion of relatively large single doses. Impetus for the study of the toxicity of diethylene glycol was provided by 105 fatalities among 353 people who ingested a solution of sulfanilamide in an aqueous mixture containing 72 percent diethylene glycol (Ruprecht and Nelson, 1937; Smyth, 1952). The symptoms included nausea, dizziness, and pain in the kidney region. This was followed in a few days by oliguria and anuria, with death resulting from uremic poisoning. Based on these data, it has been estimated that the single oral lethal dose for humans is approximately 1 ml/kg. Known as the elixir of sulfanilamide incident, the Food, Drug and Cosmetic Act was subsequently amended in 1938 to require that marketed drugs be proved to be safe and effective.

A long-term rat-feeding study by Fitzhugh and Nelson (1946) showed that 1 percent diethylene glycol in the diet over a two-year period resulted in slight growth depression, a few calcium oxalate bladder stones, minimal kidney damage, and occasional liver damage. At the 4 percent dietary level, there was increased mortality, a marked depression of growth rate, bladder stones, severe kidney damage, and moderate liver damage. In addition, bladder tumors appeared rather frequently.

The authors concluded that bladder tumors never developed in the experimental rats without the preceding or concurrent presence of a foreign body. They suggest that diethylene glycol is not a primary carcinogen but, when fed in very high concentrations, does result in the formation of calcium oxalate bladder stones and subsequent rare bladder tumors.

The toxic effects seen following exposure to diethylene glycol are consistent with its metabolic conversion to ethylene glycol and subsequent acidosis and oxalate crystal formation.

Propylene Glycol (1,2-Propanediol, CH₃CHOHCH₂OH)

Propylene Glycol (1,2-Propanediol, CH$_3$CHOHCH$_2$OH)

Propylene glycol, in sharp distinction from ethylene and diethylene glycol, has a low order of toxicity. Propylene glycol is used for direct addition to human and pet foods, in cosmetics, and in pharmaceuticals with no apparent difficulty. Other major uses of propylene glycol include antifreeze formulations, heat exchange, and hydraulic fluids.

Propylene glycol has a very low order of acute toxicity. The acute oral LD50 of propylene glycol in rats, rabbits, and dogs are approximately 30, 18, and 19 g/kg body weight, respectively (Ruddick, 1972). Symptoms of acute intoxication of animals with propylene glycol are those of central nervous system depression or narcosis. No system or organ has been established as a target for the acute oral lethal effects of propylene glycol. In contrast to ethylene glycol, propylene glycol vapors do not appear to be irritating. Neither OSHA nor ACGIH has established exposure limits for propylene glycol vapors.

Because of propylene glycol's use in foods and pharmaceuticals, there are extensive toxicity data available. O. H. Robertson and coworkers (1947) exposed monkeys and rats to atmospheres saturated with propylene glycol vapor and found no adverse effects in animals after periods of 12 to 18 months. No adverse effects were noted, and there were no increases in tumor incidences in rats fed diets containing up to 5 percent propylene glycol for two years (Robertson *et al.*, 1947; Gaunt *et al.*, 1972). Further, propylene glycol is used as a carbohydrate source without any adverse effects when fed to dogs at a concentration of 8 percent in the diet for two years. This dietary concentration equates approximately to 2 g propylene glycol/kg body weight/day (Weil *et al.*, 1971). Propylene glycol is not mutagenic or teratogenic, nor did propylene glycol adversely affect reproduction when fed at 7.5 percent dietary concentration to rats for three generations (FDA, 1973, 1974, 1977).

The explanation for the low toxicity of propylene glycol lies in its metabolism. Propylene glycol, in contrast to ethylene glycol, is metabolized by alcohol dehydrogenase to lactic acid and further to pyruvic acid (Ruddick, 1972). These acids are normal constituents of the citric acid cycle and are further broken down to carbon dioxide and water. Propylene glycol, like ethanol, is a better substrate for alcohol dehydrogenase and has been reported to be an effective antidote for ethylene glycol poisoning in animals (Holman *et al.*, 1979).

Based on a review of existing health effects data for propylene glycol, a select committee of experts convened by the FDA has reaffirmed the generally recognized as safe (GRAS) status of propylene glycol (FDA, 1977).

GLYCOL ETHERS

Glycol ethers (Figure 20–5) highlight a second area of concern for solvent toxicity, the reproductive system. Ethylene glycol monomethyl ether (EM) and ethylene glycol monoethyl ether (EE) have recently been shown to have the potential to induce reproductive toxicity. In contrast, available information for the propylene series of glycol ethers does not identify these materials as reproductive toxins.

Glycol ethers find extensive use in industry as solvents in the manufacture of lacquers, varnishes, resins, printing inks, textile dyes, and antiicing additives in brake fluids and as gasoline additives. They find extensive use in consumer products such as latex paints and cleaners. The glycol ethers as a class of materials are not acutely hazardous by the oral route. The rabbit appears to be more sensitive than the rat with

ETHYLENE GLYCOL ETHERS

R—OCH₂CH₂OH R=CH₃—EM
          CH₃CH₂—EE
          CH₃CH₂CH₂CH₂—EB

METABOLITE
R—OCH₂COOH Alkoxy acetic acid

PROPYLENE GLYCOL ETHERS
    CH₃
    |
R—O—CH₂CHOH R=CH₃—PM
        CH₃CH₂—PE
        CH₃CH₂CH₂CH₂—PB

METABOLITE
    CH₃
    |
HO—CH₂CHOH Propylene glycol

Figure 20–5. Glycol ethers and their metabolites.

regard to acute oral toxicity. Glycol ethers, particularly the ethylene series, are well absorbed from the skin. Indeed, the dermal LD50 to oral LD50 ratio is approximately 1 for ethylene glycol ethers. High vapor concentrations of the ethylene series are lethal, but saturation levels or levels approaching saturation of the propylene series are not lethal to rodents.

The first report of the reproductive toxicity of ethylene glycol ethers was that of Wiley et al. (1938) and more recently Nagano et al. (1979). In the latter study, mice were given large amounts of EM, EE, or their respective acetic acid esters for five weeks. Each of these materials caused testicular atrophy and a decrease in white blood cells.

Studies more germane to the vapor exposure route were reported by R. R. Miller et al. (1983a) and Rao et al. (1983). Rabbits and rats were exposed to 0,30,100, or 300 ppm EM, six hours/day, five days/week, for 13 weeks. The male reproductive system was adversely affected in both rats and rabbits exposed to 300 ppm; every male exhibited degeneration of the testicular germinal epithelium. At the end of the exposure period, male rats were mated to unexposed females and found to be infertile. A second mating at 13 weeks postexposure revealed a partial recovery of fertility. Degenerative changes in testes of rabbits, but not rats, were also noted at 100 ppm, suggesting that for reproductive as well as acute effects the rabbit is the more sensitive of the two species. A no-observed-effect level for the study was 30 ppm, which was quite close to the then-recommended TLV for EM of 25 ppm as an eight-hour time-weighted average. For 1989–90, the TLV for EM is 5 ppm as an eight-hour TWA.

The teratogenic potential of EM vapors has been reported by Nelson et al. (1984), who exposed pregnant rats to 0, 50, 100, or 200 ppm EE vapors, seven hours/day, during days 7 to 15 of gestation. Although there were no indications of maternal toxicity, 100 percent and 50 percent of fetuses died in the 200- and 100-ppm exposure groups, respectively. Cardiovascular and skeletal malformations were increased above unexposed control values in both 50-ppm and 100-ppm exposure groups.

The teratogenic potential of EE has been reported. Andrew et al. (1981) exposed rabbits to EE vapors (160 or 617 ppm) seven hours/day during days 1 to 19 of gestation. At 617 ppm, there was marked maternal toxicity and 100 percent embryo mortality. At the 160-ppm level, there was slight maternal toxicity and no embryo mortality, but the incidence of major cardiovascular malformations was increased. In the same study, pregnant rats were exposed to either 200 ppm or 750 ppm EE vapors. The high-exposure level caused maternal toxicity and embryo mortality. The 200-ppm exposure level caused an increased incidence of minor malformations.

The teratogenicity of EE has also been demonstrated in rats by the dermal exposure route. Hardin et al. (1982) applied four times daily either 0.25 or 0.50 ml of EE to the skin of rats during days 7 to 15 of gestation. Maternal toxicity and embryo toxicity were seen. The fetuses that survived had a high incidence of cardiovascular malformations.

Ethylene glycol monobutyl ether (EB), in contrast to EM and EE, exerts its primary effect on the red blood cell. Rats exposed to high vapor concentrations (Dodd et al., 1983) or to EB applied to the skin (Bartnik et al., 1987) evidenced a marked degree of hemolysis. Bartnik et al. (1987) measured the degree of absorption of EB from skin and reported that approximately 25 percent of the applied material was absorbed from unoccluded skin within 48 hours. For 1989–90, the TLV for EB is 5 ppm as an eight-hour TWA. EB may represent an exception to the rule that the inhalation route of exposure is quantitatively more important than skin contact.

In contrast to the adverse effects of EM and EE, propylene glycol monomethyl ether (PM) does not appear to be either a reproductive toxin or a hematotoxin. Landry et al. (1983) reported that exposure of rats and rabbits to 0, 300, 1000, or 3000 ppm PM, six hours/day, five days/week, for 13 weeks did not show any evidence of testicular effects. Central nervous system depression and increased absolute liver weights were noted at 3000 ppm. A no-observed-effect level was 1000 ppm.

Nor does PM appear to have teratogenic potential in rats or rabbits. Exposure levels were 0, 500, 1500, or 3000 ppm PM, six hours/day, during days 6 to 15 or 18 of gestation. The only effects noted in the study were transient decreases in body weight gain and central nervous system depression in rats exposed to 3000 ppm. There was no evidence of major malformations in rats or rabbits at any dose level. The 3000-ppm dose caused slight fetotoxicity in the rat as evidenced by delayed skeletal ossification. There was no evidence of fetotoxicity in rabbits at any dose. The no-observed-effect level for both rats and rabbits was 1500 ppm (Hanley et al., 1984).

These differences in reproductive toxicity between EM and PM may be explained by the metabolism of the two materials. R. R. Miller et al. (1983b) administered a single oral dose of EM or PM, radiolabeled in the glycol carbons, to rats. The radioactivity appearing in the urine and expired air over the following 48 hours was quantitated and identified. Most of the administered PM is metabolized to propylene glycol, presumably by cytochrome P-450–dependent *O*-demethylation. Propylene glycol is further metabolized to $^{14}CO_2$. In contrast, most of the administered dose of EM is metabolized to methoxyacetic acid, presumably by liver alcohol dehydrogenase. Methoxyacetic acid is excreted in the urine.

Methoxyacetic acid, the EM metabolite, has recently been shown to produce the same toxic effects of EM in tests on male rats (R. R. Miller *et al.*, 1982). Since this observation by Miller and associates, numerous experiments have defined methoxyacetic acid (MAA) as the toxic metabolite of EM. Moss *et al.* (1985) and Sleet *et al.* (1988) extended *in vivo* information on the testicular and embryotoxic effects of MAA. Administration of 4-methylpyrazole, an inhibitor of alcohol dehydrogenase, significantly reduced EM-induced embryotoxicity, underscoring the importance of this enzyme in the metabolic activation of EM. Since EE, EB, and ethylene glycol mono isopropyl ether (EIP) are metabolized to analagous metabolites (ethoxyacetic, butoxyacetic, and isopropoxyacetic acids, respectively), alkoxyacids are also considered to be toxic metabolites (Jonsson *et al.*, 1982). It appears that the primary alcohol function on glycol ethers is easily oxidized to an alkoxyacid by liver alcohol dehydrogenase. On the other hand, propylene glycol ethers have a secondary alcohol function, are relatively poorer substrates for alcohol dehydrogenase (von Wartburg, 1964), and undergo microsomal *o*-dealkylation to propylene glycol, a material that is not a reproductive toxin. If this metabolic rationale for differences in ethylene and propylene glycol ether toxicity is correct, then 2-methoxy-1-propanol (an isomer present in small amounts in commercial PM) should have potential to affect reproduction adversely (Figure 20–6).

Merkle *et al.* (1987) reported that the acetic acid ester of 2-methoxy-1-propanol was capable of inducing malformations in rabbits exposed to 550-ppm vapors during gestation. R. R. Miller *et al.* (1986) showed that the *β*-isomer of PM is indeed metabolized to methoxypropionic acid. Since commercial PM is less than 1 percent of the *β*-isomer shown in Figure 20–6, there is no occupational concern for adverse effects on reproduction from exposure to PM vapors.

Welsch and associates working at the Chemical Industries Institute of Toxicology have recently reported studies on attenuating the adverse reproductive effects of ethylene glycol ethers (Mebus *et al.*, 1989). Simple physiological substrates such as serine, acetate, sarcosine, and glycine given concomitantly with EM ameliorated developmental toxicity and testicular damage in rats. It is postulated that MAA, the toxic metabolite of EM, may interfere with the availability of one-carbon units for incorporation into purine and pyrimidine bases. Substrates such as sarcosine or acetate can provide additional one-carbon units needed during differentiation of the developing embryo or for maturation of pachytene spermatocytes.

Dioxane (1,4-Dioxane)

Dioxane is a cyclic diether prepared either from reaction between two molecules of ethylene oxide or during the distillation of ethylene glycol in the presence of dilute sulfuric acid. It is widely used in the chemical industry as a solvent and is a major commodity chemical. As a result, there is potential for human exposure. Five cases of fatalities resulting from excessive acute exposure (Barber, 1934) identified symptoms of overexposure to be irritation of upper respiratory passages, eye irritation, drowsiness, vertigo, headache, anorexia, stomach pains, nausea and vomiting, uremia, coma, and death. Johnstone (1959) has reported damage to kidneys, liver, and brain at autopsy following dioxane poisoning. Test subjects voluntarily exposed to varying levels indicated that 200 ppm was the highest acceptable level before irritation became significant. Prolonged, repeated exposure of the skin to low levels has resulted in eczema.

In rodents, oral LD50 values are relatively high. They range for rabbits, guinea pigs, rats, and mice from 2 to 6 g/kg. Chronic feeding studies using rats (Argus *et al.*, 1965; Hoch-Ligeti *et al.*, 1970; Kociba *et al.*, 1974), guinea pigs (Hoch-Ligeti and Argus, 1970), and both rats and mice (IARC, 1976) demonstrated both toxic and carcinogenic effects of very large doses of dioxane. Principal sites of cellular de-

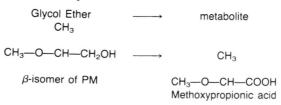

Figure 20–6. Metabolism of PM.

generation and necrosis were in renal, hepatic, and epithelial cells. Guinea pigs demonstrated liver tumors and hyperplasia of lung cells, as well as squamous cell carcinoma in the nasal cavity. In rats and mice, tumors were seen in liver and the nasal cavity. Using the inhalation route in rats, however, Torkelson et al. (1974) were unable to demonstrate carcinogenic effects of dioxane in males and females treated with 111 ppm chronically in an experimental design that encompassed two years.

Braun and Young (1977) identified β-hydroxyethoxyacetic acid (HEAA), a ring opening product of dioxane, as the major metabolic product in the urine of rats. Young et al. (1976) reported that in humans exposed to dioxane at 1.6 ppm for 7.5 hours both dioxane and HEAA were recovered from the urine. Young et al. (1978) suggested that rats have limited capacity to metabolize HEAA. Woo et al. (1977) reported the identification of p-dioxane-2-one, a carcinogenic metabolite of dioxane, in the urine of dioxane-treated rats. Dioxane induces its own metabolism (Young et al., 1978); and the detoxication pathway is readily saturated (Young et al., 1978). Although a direct effect of dioxane has not yet been ruled out, further study is required of the metabolic pathways leading to the formation of HEAA and p-dioxane-2-one before we can understand the mechanism of the toxic and carcinogenic effects of dioxane.

Dioxane has been the subject of a study of genotoxic versus nongenotoxic carcinogens (Stott et al., 1981). In attempting to determine the mechanism by which dioxane causes liver tumors, it was found that it possessed no genotoxic activity as defined by a lack of (1) covalent binding to DNA, (2) stimulation of DNA repair, or (3) induction of bacterial mutations. Liver tumor formation followed demonstrable hepatotoxicity secondary to repeated dosage in the range of 1 g/kg/day, whereas neither hepatotoxicity nor tumor formation followed repeated doses of 10 mg/kg/day. The authors suggested that dioxane-induced cytotoxicity caused by repeated toxic insults leads to increased rates of cell division in an attempt to replace damaged cells. The result is rapid DNA replication that may be error prone. The rate of events leaves insufficient time for DNA repair, and errors are fixed in the genome. This mechanism, which may act with endogenous as well as xenobiotic compounds may be generally applicable and represents a significant theory for epigenetic causes of cancer. The authors also speculate on an alternative mechanism related to the ability of dioxane to act as a "phenobarbitallike" enzyme inducer resulting in alterations in gene function and protein synthesis, possibly leading to changes in oncogene expression. Thus, at least two epigenetic mechanisms for dioxane-induced tumors have been proposed.

HEXACARBON NEUROPATHY

Until recently, extensively used industrial hexacarbon solvents such as n-hexane and 2-hexanone (methyl n-butyl ketone) were thought to have little potential for hazard. It is now recognized that peripheral neuropathies can result from excessive exposure, and this aspect of n-hexane and 2-hexanone toxicity is discussed below. The reader is referred to the comprehensive review of Batterskill et al. (1987) for a complete discussion of the toxic effects of these solvents.

n-Hexane is produced during the cracking and fractional distillation of crude oil and is used in such applications as printing of laminated products; vegetable oil extraction; as a solvent in glues, paints, varnishes, and inks; as a diluent in the production of plastics and rubber; and as a minor component of gasoline. An estimated 2.5 million workers are occupationally exposed to n-hexane (Yamamura, 1969; Gonzalez and Downey, 1972; Paulson and Waylons, 1976). 2-Hexanone has more limited use than n-hexane but is used as a paint thinner, cleaning agent, solvent for dye printing, and in the lacquer industry. The National Institute for Occupational Safety and Health has estimated that nearly a quarter of a million workers have potential exposure to 2-hexanone (Couri and Milks, 1982).

It is not at all surprising that previous to the discovery of their neurotoxic potential these two solvents were not regarded as industrial hazards since their acute toxicity is quite low. Vapor concentrations of many hundreds of parts per million are tolerated for several minutes without causing discomfort among workers. In recognition of the neurotoxic properties of n-hexane and 2-hexanone, the ACGIH has recommended TLVs of 50 ppm and 5 ppm, expressed as eight-hour time-weighted averages, for the two solvents, respectively. STEL and ceiling values are not recommended (ACGIH, 1989).

The first cases of n-hexane polyneuropathy were reported in 1964 in workers involved in laminating polyethylene products. In 1969, a major outbreak of disease was reported in a cottage industry in Japan that involved the use of an n-hexane–containing glue to assemble sandals. n-Hexane concentrations to which the workers were exposed were estimated to be 500 to 2500 ppm (Yamada, 1964; Sobue, 1968; Yamamura, 1969).

The neurotoxic syndrome is best described as a sensorimotor or motor polyneuropathy. The initial symptoms are symmetrical sensory numbness and paresthesias of distal portions of the extremities. Sensory loss normally involves all modalities of the feet or hands. Motor weakness is typically observed in muscles of the toes and fingers but may also involve muscles of the arms, thighs, and forearms. The onset of these symptoms may be delayed for several months to a year after the beginning of exposure (Yamamura, 1969; Herskowitz *et al.*, 1971; Allen, 1979). The syndrome is characterized pathologically by axonal swelling on the proximal side of the node of Ranvier, demyelination, and nerve fiber degeneration resembling a dying-back neuropathy. Central and autonomic nervous systems are unaffected. The clinical course of disease following removal from exposure to hexane is for complete recovery, but severe cases may retain distal sensorimotor deficits.

2-Hexanone was reported to cause neurotoxicity by several authors during the time frame of 1973 to 1977. Workers on rotogravure units in the printing industry, workers who spray painted in enclosed areas, and workers who used 2-hexanone–containing cleaners developed a neurotoxic syndrome strikingly similar to that seen for *n*-hexane (Billmaier, 1974; McDonough, 1974; Allen *et al.*, 1975). As described above, there may be a delay between exposure and the development of bilateral loss of sensorimotor or sensory modalities. Pathological findings are also quite similar to *n*-hexane (Mendell, 1974; Davenport, 1976; Saida, 1976).

Metabolism

The rational basis for this similarity in neurotoxic action is contained in the metabolic scheme presented in Figure 20–7. *n*-Hexane may be metabolized to 2-hexanol and further to 2,5-hexanediol by cytochrome P-450 mixed-function oxidases by omega-minus 1 oxidation. 2,5-Hexanediol may be further oxidized to 2,5-hexanedione, the major metabolite of *n*-hexane in humans. Through the omega-minus 1 oxidation process, 2-hexanone may also be metabolized to 2,5-hexanedione. 2-Hexanol and 5-hydroxy-2-hexanone as well as 2,5-hexanedione

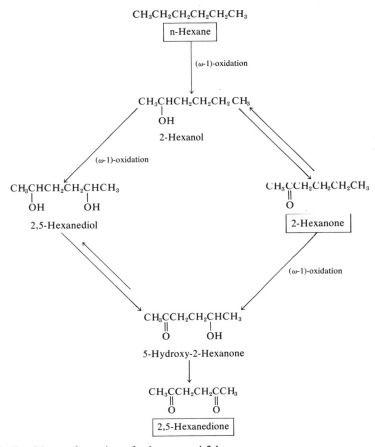

Figure 20–7. Biotransformation of *n*-hexane and 2-hexanone.

are all common elements in the metabolism of both *n*-hexane and 2-hexanone (Couri *et al.*, 1978; Katz *et al.*, 1980; Krasavage *et al.*, 1980; Perbellini *et al.*, 1980).

Identification of 2,5-hexanedione as the major neurotoxic metabolite of *n*-hexane and 2-hexanone proceeded rapidly after its discovery as a urinary metabolite. 2,5-Hexanedione has been found to produce a polyneuropathy indistinguishable from *n*-hexane and 2-hexanone in experimental animals under a variety of exposure conditions (Spencer and Schaumburg, 1977; O'Donoghue *et al.*, 1978; Couri and Nachtman, 1979; Krasavage *et al.*, 1980). 2,5-Hexanedione is many times more potent than *n*-hexane or 2-hexanone in causing neurotoxicity in experimental animals (Krasavage *et al.*, 1980).

It appears that the neurotoxicity of 2,5-hexanedione resides in its γ-diketone structure, since 2,3-,2,4-hexanedione and 2,6-heptanedione are not neurotoxic, whereas 2,5-heptanedione and 3,6-octanedione and other γ diketones are neurotoxic (Spencer *et al.*, 1978; O'Donoghue and Krasavage, 1979a, 1979b).

A potentially important solvent interaction between 2-hexanone and 2-butanone (methyl ethyl ketone [MEK]) has been reported (Abdel-Rahman *et al.*, 1976; Couri *et al.*, 1977). In these experiments, rats were exposed to 2-hexanone alone or to a mixture of 2-hexanone and MEK vapors. Animals exposed to the mixture showed an earlier onset and greater severity of neurotoxic signs and produced dramatically higher concentrations of 2,5-hexanedione than did animals exposed to 2-hexanone alone. Methyl ethyl ketone itself is not neurotoxic. Coexposure of animals to 2-hexanone and other aliphatic ketones such as 2-pentanone, heptanone, and octanone potentiates 2-hexanone neurotoxicity (Misumi and Nagano, 1985).

CARBON DISULFIDE

Carbon disulfide (CS_2) is primarily used in the production of regenerated rayon and cellophane and in the manufacture of carbon tetrachloride. It is also used as a solvent for many applications including resins, rubber, and fats. Other applications include use as a pesticide, a preservative for fresh fruit, and in the production of semiconductors. A recent estimate of CS_2 production worldwide was 1 million metric tons. The ACGIH recommends a TLV of 10 ppm as an eight-hour time-weighted average for CS_2 (ACGIH, 1989).

Adverse effects of human exposure resulting from prolonged exposure to high levels of CS_2 have been extensively reported and documented. These include organic brain damage, peripheral nervous system decrements, neurobehavioral dysfunction, and ocular and auditory effects. In addition, adverse effects on the cardiovascular system have been reported. Excellent reviews of these effects are available (Coppack *et al.*, 1981; Beauchamp *et al.*, 1983).

Severe CS_2 intoxication, which can lead to encephalopathies, was common in the early part of the twentieth century but is seldom encountered today. High-level exposures resulted in a syndrome of toxic psychoses, agitated delirium, seizures, and recurrent mental impairment (Gordy and Trumper, 1940). Most cases of CS_2-induced encephalopathy involve chronic exposure for a number of years to levels that exceed the current TLV. Symptoms typically include headaches, sleep disturbances, general fatigue, emotional lability, irritability, impairment of memory for recent events, and commonly, loss of libido. A "parkinsonian" syndrome consisting of facial immobility, slurring speech, impaired arm swing, and tremor that is maximum at rest was described for young subjects (Audo-Gianotti, 1932). More recent studies have investigated effects of CS_2 exposure on reduced performance in neurobehavioral tests (Horvath and Frantik, 1979).

Alpers and Lewey (1940) reported on the pathogenesis of CS_2 encephalopathy. Postmortem findings were neuronal degeneration with pallor, vacuolization and cell loss diffusely distributed over the cerebral cortex, globus pallidus, and putamen. They report similar pathologic changes in cats and dogs exposed to 400 ppm CS_2 for two to six weeks.

CS_2 exposure also may cause a peripheral neuropathy, but this lesion, in contrast to central nervous system effects, is typically relatively mild. Knave *et al.* (1974) described this syndrome as progressing from muscle cramps in the legs to muscle pain, paresthesias, and finally muscle weakness in the extremities. A prevalent finding was a fine-to-medium coarse tremor. Multifocal axonal swelling with neurofilament accumulation (Wallerian degeneration) has been reported as a pathologic finding in central and peripheral nervous system fibers of rats chronically exposed to CS_2 (Szendzikowski *et al.*, 1974). There is no satisfactory treatment for the central or peripheral neural effects of CS_2, and prevention of excess exposure is essential.

Another neurological target of CS_2 is the eye. Over the years, many changes of eye structure and function including fundal morphology, altered function, sensitivity, and motility have been described. Many of these findings are reported when typical exposures were in excess of 30 ppm (Beauchamp *et al.*, 1983). In the past, CS_2 retinopathy has been regarded by occupational physicians as an early indicator of intoxication. Many reports have described changes in the microcirculation of the eye, and some investigators feel that this finding is diagnostic of CS_2 overexposure (Tolonen, 1974). Other investigators have attributed vascular changes in the eye to the atherosclerotic effects of CS_2 described below (Gilioli *et al.*, 1978). It seems clear that long-term exposure to CS_2 can cause eye damage including blind spots, narrowing of visual field, and a decreased ability to see in the dark. This effect has not been studied in experimental animals.

Yet another neurological target of CS_2 is the auditory system. Hearing loss to high-frequency tones is a common feature of CS_2 intoxication (Zenk, 1970). This problem has not been successfully approached in an experimental animal model.

Exposure to CS_2 has been called a contributing factor in coronary heart disease (Tiller *et al.*, 1968). This effect has been confirmed by Finnish epidemiologists studying an occupationally exposed cohort using a ten-year follow-up plan. While advanced age and hypertension were predominant factors in determining coronary heart disease, exposure to CS_2 alone contributed a statistically significant relative risk (Tolonen *et al.*, 1975, 1979). It seems likely that occupational CS_2 exposure can be an important contributing factor to the development of coronary heart disease and that this issue should continue to be monitored in future epidemiology studies.

The mechanism by which CS_2 causes peripheral neuropathy and other toxic effects is yet to be determined. Figure 20–8 represents an abbreviated scheme for the metabolism of CS_2 (Bus, 1985). Following exposure to CS_2, very little of the parent compound is excreted unchanged. Most of the absorbed dose is excreted as sulfur-containing urinary metabolites of CS_2, some of which are shown in Figure 20–8 (Pergal *et al.*, 1972a, 1972b; van Doorn *et al.*, 1981a, 1981b). These reactions demonstrate the ability of CS_2 to react with amino acids *in vivo*. Thus, CS_2 could react with amine groups on critical cellular enzymes and thereby cause cellular damage. Dithiocarbamates are known to chelate metal ions such as copper and zinc (Brieger, 1967), and it is proposed that these metabolites of CS_2 may chelate metals necessary for proper neuronal enzyme function. In support of this theory, it was shown by McKenna and DiStefano (1977) that CS_2 exposure can decrease the activity of the copper-requiring enzyme dopamine-β-hydroxylase; that addition of copper and zinc to the diet exerted a protective effect for experimentally induced neurotoxicity in the rat (Lukas, 1979); and that copper levels in peripheral nerves were altered during intoxication of rats with CS_2 (Lukas *et al.*, 1980). Recent studies have suggested that CS_2 exposure can induce kynureninase and lead to disorders of tryptophan metabolism (Okayama *et al.*, 1987, 1988).

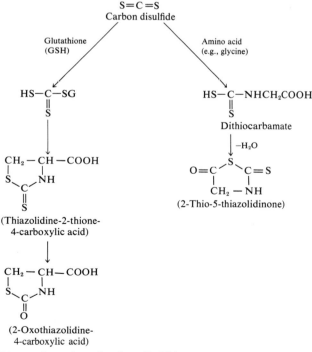

Figure 20–8. Biotransformation of carbon disulfide.

While hepatic mixed-function oxidase has been shown to activate CS_2 to hepatotoxic reactive intermediates in rodents, for example,

$$[S = C = \overset{+}{S}]$$
$$\underset{O-}{\overset{|}{}}$$

the relationship of this observation to CS_2-induced neurotoxicity remains to be determined. Animal models of CS_2 toxicity need to be further developed to elucidate the mechanism(s) of action of CS_2.

GASOLINE AND KEROSENE

Gasoline and kerosene are primarily mixtures of hydrocarbons, including not only aliphatic hydrocarbons but—particularly in the case of gasoline—a variety of branched and unsaturated hydrocarbons, as well as aromatic hydrocarbons.

In spite of the widespread use of gasoline and the intermittent vapor exposure encountered by gas station attendants and the home auto mechanic, toxic effects do not normally occur under these conditions. Some gasolines contain a considerable amount of benzene or other additives and could present a hazard that would be difficult to assess in the exposed population.

Extremely high-level exposures to gasoline vapor may result in dizziness, coma, collapse, and death. Exposure to high nonlethal levels is usually followed by complete recovery, although cases of permanent brain damage following massive exposure have been reported. Atmospheric concentrations of approximately 2000 ppm are not safe to enter for even a brief time. For 1989–90, the ACGIH established a TLV of 300 ppm and a STEL of 500 ppm for gasoline vapors.

The report of results of two-year carcinogenicity studies in mice and rats has raised the issue of adverse effects of long-term low-level exposure to unleaded gasoline vapors. In these studies, male rats—but not female rats nor either sex of mice—developed renal tumors and a distinctive nephropathy characterized by protein droplet formation in proximal tubule epithelium (Kitchen, 1984; MacFarland, 1984; Alden, 1986). Because kidney effects were both sex- and species-specific and because unleaded gasoline is not mutagenic (Conaway et al., 1982; Richardson, et al., 1986; Loury et al., 1987), a nongenotoxic mechanism of renal tumor development was postulated.

The observation of these renal effects of unleaded gasoline led to an evaluation of the nephrotoxic properties of many components of this complex mixture and the identification of isoparaffins as nephrotoxic materials specific for the male rat (Phillips and Cockrell, 1984; Phillips and Egan, 1984; Halder et al., 1985). Trimethylpentane is one isoparaffin that is very active in causing protein-droplet (hyaline-droplet) toxicity in the male rat kidney and has been used as a prototype chemical. Treatment of male rats with trimethylpentane or unleaded gasoline leads to a high accumulation of α-2μ-globulin protein in renal tubular cells. This protein is not found in humans or immature or female rats (Kloss et al., 1985; Loury et al., 1987). This syndrome has been termed male rat hydrocarbon nephropathy (Alden, 1986).

Workers at CIIT have shown that exposure of male rats to unleaded gasoline or trimethylpentane vapors resulted in a marked increase in cellular proliferation in kidneys. Based on this observation, it has been postulated that renal tumors develop secondary to tissue damage resulting from α-2μ globulin accumulation in renal tubular cells (Short et al., 1986; Loury et al., 1987). If this postulated mechanism is proven, then it is likely that the observation of renal tumors in rats is not relevant to possible human health effects from gasoline exposure.

CONCLUSIONS

Solvents are a group of chemicals that have only two features in common: (1) They are liquid, and (2) because of their widespread use in commerce, there is a potential for human exposure both during their use and after they have been discarded as chemical wastes.

It is not possible to predict the toxic effects of these chemicals merely because they share the term "solvent." Their toxic effects vary as widely as those of other chemicals. While there are groups of structurally related solvents, such as the haloalkanes and the haloalkenes, where the toxic effects may be related, among these there are both quantitative and qualitative differences in toxicity. Among single ring aromatic compounds, alkylbenzenes are dramatically different from benzene. Our ability to predict toxicity among solvents and to perform accurate risk assessment depends not only on our knowledge of descriptive toxicology gained in acute and chronic treatment studies but also on our understanding of the metabolic disposition and mechanism of action of these agents.

The major drawbacks to most studies on the toxicology of solvents is that actual occupational and environmental exposure is not to the pure compounds used in toxicological research but to commercial mixtures of solvents. The need for the future is to develop strategies for studying the toxicology of mixtures. It is impractical to study interactions of more than three to four compounds at more than one dose level in a well-controlled study using procedures commonly employed in safety evaluation today. Yet in effluents from chemical waste sites, there are frequently as many as 100 chemicals identified, some of which may be present at concentrations that pose a potential hazard for humans. Methods for studying these interactive effects have yet to be developed. Until that time, risk assessment must depend on knowledge of the toxicity of the most toxic chemicals in the mixture, modified with our understanding of interactions between chemicals in the mixture. For the most part, this information is currently insufficient for accurate predictions.

The ability to measure the dose of individual solvents or their active metabolites delivered to the target organ or receptor could greatly improve our confidence in models of dose-responsiveness. In most cases, these data are not available for solvents. However, methods exist to measure urinary levels of solvents or metabolites in both humans and experimental animals. Such methods can provide specific information on exposure to active metabolites as illustrated by 2,5-hexanedione levels in urine following exposure to *n*-hexane vapors. If these biological indices of exposure can be determined concomitantly with noninvasive markers of toxicity, then ideal data for assessing risk is obtained. In 1989, the National Academy of Sciences published a status report on biomarkers for toxicity to pulmonary and reproductive systems (NAS, 1989a, 1989b). Further development of indices of exposure to solvents and markers of toxicity could lead to more effective medical surveillance programs, the potential to identify sensitive individuals prior to exposure, and a means of evaluating the validity and predictability of our assessments of hazard and risk.

APPENDIX

Convert between ppm and mg/m^3 using the following approaches. Combining equations from the Ideal Gas Law and Dalton's Law of Partial Pressures yields an equation for the ready conversion of these units:

Ideal Gas Law　　　$PV = nRT$

Dalton's Law　　　$\dfrac{P_s}{P_T} = \dfrac{n_s}{n_T}$

P_s = Partial pressure of solvents (atm)
P_T = Total atmospheric pressure (1 atm)
n_s = Number of moles of solvents
　　= Weight (wt.) of S/molecular weight (MW) of S

n_T = Total number of moles
V = Volume (m^3)
R = Gas constant (0.082 atm/°K mol)
T = Temperature (298°K = 25°C)
C_s = Concentration of S (weight of s/volume)

$$P_sV = n_s\,RT$$

$$P_s = \frac{n_s\,RT}{V}$$

$$P_s = \frac{C_s}{MW_s}\,24.45$$

$$\frac{P_s}{P_t} = \frac{n_s}{n_T}\,(ppm) = \frac{C_s}{MW_s}\,24.45$$

$$ppm = \frac{C_s}{MW_s}\,24.45$$

Thus, using benzene (MW = 78) as an example, converting 32 mg/m^3 to ppm would involve the following calculation:

$$(ppm) = \frac{32 \text{ mg/m}^3}{78/\text{g/mol}}\,(24.45) = 10$$

Thus, 32 mg/m^3 is equivalent to 10 ppm.

The following alternative approach is equally useful: We can express the concentration of a gas in a mixture using the following equation and assuming that the weight of 1 ml of gas, d, is a function of the molecular weight *(MW)*, the molecular volume *(MVo)*, and the temperature and pressure, as shown in the following equation:

$$d = \frac{MW}{MVo} \cdot \frac{To}{To + T} \cdot \frac{P}{Po}$$

$$d = \frac{MW}{22.4} \cdot \frac{273}{273 + T} \cdot \frac{P}{760}$$

$$= 0.016 \cdot MW \cdot \frac{P}{273 + T}, \text{ units = mg/liter}$$

where *MVo* = molecular volume (22.4 liters) at standard temperature and pressure (*To* = 273°C; *Po* = 760 torr), and T and P are ambient values for temperature and pressure. The coefficient 0.0160 is the reciprocal of the gas constant, R.

We can convert the concentration of the gas from ppm to mg/m^3. For example, 10 ppm equals 10 ml of gas in 10^6 ml of air. Accordingly, we must multiply d, from the equation shown above, by 10/10^3 or 0.01 and factor in the *MW*. Thus, for benzene at 10 ppm:

$$d = \frac{78}{22.4} \cdot \frac{273}{273 + T} \cdot \frac{P}{760}$$

$$= 0.016 \cdot 78 \cdot \frac{760}{298} = 3.19 \text{ mg/liter}$$

$$10 \text{ ppm} = 0.01 \cdot 3.19 = 0.0319 \text{ mg/liter}$$

To convert mg/liter to mg/m^3, multiply by 1000. The result indicates that 10 ppm of benzene is equivalent to 31.9 mg/m^3.

REFERENCES

Abdel-Rahman, M. S.; Hetland, L. B.; and Couri, D.: Toxicity and metabolism of methyl n-butyl ketone. *Am. Ind. Hyg. Assoc. J.,* **37**:95–102, 1976.

ACGIH: *TLVs, Threshold Limit Values for Chemical Substances and Physical Agents in Work Environment with Intended Changes for 1989–90.* American Conference of Governmental Industrial Hygienists, Cincinnati, Ohio, 1989.

Ahmed, A. E.; Kubic, V. J.; Stevens, J. L.; and Anders, M. W.: Halogenated methanes: metabolism and toxicity. *Fed. Proc.,* **39**:3150–3155, 1980.

Ainley, C. C.; Senapati, A.; Brown, I. M. H.; Iles, C. A.; Slavin, B. M.; Mitchell, W. D.; Davies, D. R.; Keeling, P. W. N.; and Thompson, R. P. H.: Is alcohol hepatotoxic in the baboon? *J. Hepatology,* **7**:85–92, 1988.

Aksoy, M.; Erdem, S.; and Dincol, G.: Leukemia in shoe-workers exposed chronically to benzene. *Blood,* **44**:837–841, 1974.

————: Types of leukemia in chronic benzene poisoning. A study in thirty-four patients. *Acta Haematol.,* **55**:65–72, 1976.

Aksoy, M., and Erdem, S.: Follow-up study on the mortality and the development of leukemia in 44 pancytopenic patients with chronic exposure to benzene. *Blood,* **52**:285–293, 1978.

Alden, C. L.: A review of unique male rat hydrocarbon nephropathy. *Toxicol. Pathol.,* **14**:109–111, 1986.

Allen, N.: Solvents and other industrial organic compounds. In Vinken, P. J., and Bruyn, G. W. (eds.): *Handbook of Clinical Neurology: Intoxications of the Nervous System,* Vol. 36 (Part 1). Elsevier, North-Holland, New York, 1979, pp. 361–389.

Allen, N.; Mendell, J. R.; Billmaier, D. J.; Fontaine, R. E.; and O'Neill, J.: Toxic polyneuropathy due to methyl n-butyl ketone. *Arch. Neurol.,* **32**:209–218, 1975.

Alpers, B. J., and Lewey, F. H.: Changes in the nervous system following disulfide poisoning in animals and in man. *Arch. Neurol. Psychiat.,* **44**:725–739, 1940.

Andersen, M. E.; Gargas, M. L.; Jones, R. A.; and Jenkins, L. J., Jr.: Determination of the kinetic constants for metabolism of inhaled toxicants *in vivo* using gas uptake measurements. *Toxicol. Appl. Pharmacol.,* **54**:100–116, 1980.

Andrew, F. D.; Buschbom, R. L.; Cannon, W. C.; Miller, R. A.; Montgomery, L. F.; Phelps, D. W.; and Sikev, M. R.: *Tetratologic Assessment of Ethylbenzene and 2-Ethoxyethanol.* Battelle Pacific Northwest Laboratories Report to NIOSH, 1981.

Andrews, L. S.; Lee, E. W.; Witmer, C. M.; Kocsis, J. J.; and Snyder, R.: Effects of toluene on metabolism, disposition, and hematopoietic toxicity of (^{3}H) benzene. *Biochem. Pharmacol.,* **26**:293–300, 1977.

Argus, M. F.; Argus, J. C.; and Hoch-Ligeti, C.: Studies on the carcinogenicity of protein-denaturing

agents—hepatotoxicity of dioxane. *J. Natl. Cancer Inst.,* **35**:949–958, 1965.

Astrand, I.: Uptake of solvents in the blood and tissues of man. *Scand. J. Work Environ. Health,* **1**:199–218, 1975.

Audo-Gianotti, G. B.: Le parkinsonisme—sulfocarbone professionnel. *Presse Méd.,* **40**:1289–1291, 1932.

Avogadro, P.; Sirtori, C. R.; and Tremoli, E. (eds.): *Metabolic Effects of Ethanol.* Elsevier, Amsterdam, 1979.

Bailie, M. B.; Smith, J. H.; Newton, J. F.; and Hook, J. B.: Mechanism of chloroform toxicity: IV. Phenobarbital potentiation of *in vitro* chloroform metabolism and toxicity in rabbit kidneys. *Toxicol. Appl. Pharmacol.,* **74**:285–292, 1984.

Baker, E. L.: Organic solvent neurotoxicity, *Annu. Rev. Public Health,* **9**:223–232, 1988.

Baker, T. S., and Rickert, D. E.: Dose-dependent uptake, distribution, and elimination of inhaled n-hexane in the Fischer-344 rat. *Toxicol. Appl. Pharmacol.,* **61**:414–422, 1981.

Barber, H.: Haemorrhagic nephritis and necrosis of the liver from dioxane poisoning. *Guy's Hosp. Rep.,* **84**:267–280, 1934.

Bardodej, Z., and Cirek, A.: Long-term study on workers occupationally exposed to ethylbenzene. *J. Hyg. Epidemiol. Microbiol. Immunol.,* **32**:1–5, 1988.

Bartnik, F. G.; Reddy, A. K.; Klecak, G.; Zimmerman, V.; Hostynek, J. J.; and Kunstler, K.: Percutaneous absorption, metabolism, and hemolytic activity of n-butoxyethanol. *Fund. Appl. Toxicol.,* **8**:59–70, 1987.

Batterskill, J. M.; Illing, H. P. A.; Shillaker, R. O.; and Smith, A. M.: *n-Hexane: Toxicity Review 18.* Her Majesty's Stationery Office, U.K., 1987.

Baud, F. J.; Galliot, M.; Astier, A.; VuBien, D.; Garnier, R.; Likforman, J.; and Bismuth, C.: Treatment of ethylene glycol poisoning with intravenous 4-methyl pyrazole. *New Engl. J. Med.,* **319**:97–100, 1988.

Bauer, H.; Dimitriadis, E. A.; and Snyder, R.: An *in vivo* study of benzene metabolite DNA adduct formation in liver of male New Zealand rabbits. *Arch. Toxicol.,* **63**:209–213, 1989.

Beauchamp, R. O., Jr.; Bus, J. S.; Popp, J. A.; Boreiko, C. J.; and Goldberg, L.: A critical review of the literature on carbon disulfide toxicity. *CRC Crit. Rev. Toxicol.,* **11**:169–278, 1983.

Benignus, V. A.: Behavioral effects of toluene. A review. *Neurobehav. Toxicol. Teratol.,* **3**:407–415, 1981.

Benton, C. D., and Calhoun, F. P.: The ocular effect of methyl alcohol poisoning. *Trans. Am. Acad. Ophthalmol. Laryngol.,* **56**:874–885, 1952.

Billmaier, D.; Yee, H. T.; Allen, N.; Craft, B.; Williams, N.; Epstein, S.; and Fontaine, R.: Peripheral neuropathy in a coated fabrics plant. *J. Occup. Med.,* **16**:665–671, 1974.

Blood, F. R.: Chronic toxicity of ethylene glycol in the rat. *Food Cosmet. Toxicol.,* **3**:229–234, 1965.

Blood, F. R.; Elliot, G. A.; and Wright, M. S.: Chronic toxicity of ethylene glycol in the monkey. *Toxicol. Appl. Pharmacol.,* **4**:489–491, 1962.

Bolcsak, L. E., and Nerland, D. E.: Inhibition of erythropoiesis by benzene and benzene metabolites. *Toxicol. Appl. Pharmacol.,* **69**:363–368, 1983.

Bolt, H. M.; Filser, J. G.; and Laib, R. J.: Covalent binding of haloethylenes. In Snyder, R.; Parke, D. V.; Kocsis, J. J.; Jollow, D. J.; Gibson, G. G.; and Witmer, C. M. (eds.): *Biological Reactive Intermediates—II: Chemical Mechanisms and Biological Effects.* Plenum Press, New York, 1982, pp. 667–683.

Bove, K. E.: Ethylene glycol toxicity. *Am. J. Clin. Pathol.,* **45**:46–50, 1966.

Boyd, R.; Griffiths, J.; Kindt, V.; Snyder, R.; Caro, J.; and Erslev, A.: Relative toxicity of five benzene metabolites on CFU-GM cultures. *Toxicologist*, **2**:121, 1982.

Brady, J. F.; Li, D.; Ishizaki, H.; Lee, M.; Ning, S. U.; Xiao, F.; and Yang, C. S.: Induction of cytochromes P450IIE1 and P450IIB1 by secondary ketones and the role of P450IIE1 in chloroform metabolism. *Toxicol. Appl. Pharmacol.*, **100**:342–348, 1989.

Branchflower, R. V., and Pohl, L. R.: Investigation of the mechanism of the potentiation of chloroform-induced hepatotoxicity and nephrotoxicity by methyl *n*-butyl ketone. *Toxicol. Appl. Pharmacol.*, **61**:407–413, 1981.

Braun, W. H., and Young, J. D.: Identification of hydroxyethoxyacetic acid as the major urinary metabolite of 1,4-dioxane in the rat. *Toxicol. Appl. Pharmacol.*, **39**:33–38, 1977.

Brieger, H.: Carbon disulfide in living organisms—retention, biotransformation and patho-physiologic effects. In H. Brieger (ed.): *Toxicology of Carbon Disulfide*. Excerpta Medica, Amsterdam, 1967.

Brown, E. M., and Hewitt, W. R.: Dose-response relationships in ketone-induced potentiation of chloroform hepato- and nephrotoxicity. *Toxicol. Appl. Pharmacol.*, **76**:437–453, 1984.

Browning, E.: *Toxicity and Metabolism of Industrial Solvents*. Elsevier Publishing Co., New York, 1965.

Buelke-Sam, J., and Kimmel, C. A.: Development and standardization of screening methods for behavioral teratology. *Teratology*, **20**:17–30, 1979.

Bus, J.: The relationship of carbon disulfide metabolism to development of toxicity. *Neurotoxicology*, **6**:73–80, 1985.

Carpenter, C. P.; Kinkead, E. R.; Geary, D. L., Jr.; Sullivan, L. J.; and King, J. M.: Petroleum hydrocarbon toxicity studies. V. Animal and human response to vapors of mixed xylenes. *Toxicol. Appl. Pharmacol.*, **33**:543–558, 1975.

Challen, P. J. R.; Hickish, D. E.; and Bedford, J.: Chronic chloroform intoxication. *Br. J. Ind. Med.*, **15**:243–249, 1958.

Conaway, C. C.; Schreiner, C. A.; and Cragg, S. T.: Mutagenicity evaluation of petroleum hydrocarbons In Mehlman, M. A., (ed): *Applied Toxicology of Petroleum Hydrocarbons*. Princeton Scientific Publishers, Inc., Princeton, N. J., 1982, pp. 89–108.

Coon, M. J. and Koop, D. R.: Alcohol-inducible cytochrome P-450 (P-450 ALC). *Arch. Toxicol.*, **60**:16–21 (1987).

Coppack, R. W.; Buch, W. B.; and Mabee, R. L.: Toxicology of carbon disulfide: a review. *Vet. Hum. Toxicol.*, **23**:331–336, 1981.

Cortina, T. A.; Sica, E. W.; McCarroll, N. E.; Coate, W.; Thakur, A.; and Farrow, M. G.: Inhalation cytogenetics in mice and rats exposed to benzene. In MacFarland, H. N.; Holdsworth, E. E.; Mac Gregor, J. A.; Call, R. W.; and Kane, M. L. (eds.): *The Toxicology of Petroleum Hydrocarbons*. American Petroleum Institute, Washington, D.C., 1982.

Couri, D.; Abdel-Rahman, M. S.; and Hetland, L. B.: Biotransformation of *n*-hexane and methyl *n*-butyl ketone in guinea pigs and mice. *Am. Ind. Hyg. Assoc. J.*, **39**:295–300, 1978.

Couri, D.; Abdel-Rahman, M. S.; and Weiss, H.: The influence of inhaled ketone solvent vapors on hepatic microsomal biotransformation activities. *Toxicol. Appl. Pharmacol.*, **41**:285–289, 1977.

Couri, D., and Milks, M.: Toxicity and metabolism of the neurotoxic hexacarbons *n*-hexane, 2-hexanone, and 2,5-hexanedione. *Annu. Rev. Pharmacol. Toxicol.*, **22**:145–166, 1982.

Couri, D., and Nachtman, J. P.: Biochemical and biophysical studies of 2,5-hexanedione neuropathy. *Neurotoxicology*, **1**:269–283, 1979.

Cragg, S. T.; Clarke, E. A.; Daly, I. W.; Miller, R. R.; Terrill, J. B.; and Ouellette, R. E.: Subchronic inhalation toxicity of ethylbenzene in mice, rats and rabbits. *Fund. Appl. Toxicol.*, **13**:399–408, 1989.

Dabney, B. J.: The role of human genetic monitoring in the workplace. *J. Occup. Med.*, **23**:626–631, 1981.

Damgaard, S. E.: The D(VK) isotope effect of the cytochrome P-450–mediated oxidation of ethanol and its biological application. *Eur. J. Biochem.*, **125**:593–603, 1982.

Davenport, J. G.; Farrell, D. F.; and Sumi, S. M.: Giant axonal neuropathy caused by industrial chemicals. *Neurology*, **26**:919–923, 1976.

Dean, B. J.: Genetic toxicology of benzene, toluene, xylenes and phenols. *Mutat. Res.*, **47**:75–97, 1978.

Dekant, W.; Vamvkas, S.; and Anders, M. W.: Bioactivation of nephrotoxic haloalkenes by glutathione conjugation: formation of toxic and mutagenic intermediates by cysteine conjugate beta-lyase. *Drug Metab. Rev.*, **20**:43–83, 1989.

DePass, L. R.; Garman, R. H.; Woodside, M. D.; Giddens, W. E.; Maronpot, R. R.; and Weil, C. S.: Chronic toxicity and oncogenicity studies of ethylene glycol in rats and mice. *Fund. Appl. Toxicol.*, **7**:547–565, 1986.

Dietz, F. K.; Reitz, R. H.; Watanabe, P. G.; and Gehring, P. J.: Translation of pharmacokinetic biochemical data into risk assessment. In Snyder, R.; Parke, D. V.; Kocsis, J. J.; Jollow, D. J.; Gibson, G. G.; and Witmer, C. M. (eds.): *Biological Reactive Intermediates II: Chemical Mechanisms and Biological Effects*. Plenum Press, New York, 1982, pp. 1399–1424.

Dodd, D. E.; Snellings, W. M.; Maronpot, R. R.; and Ballantyne, B.: Ethylene glycol monobutyl ether. Acute, 9-day, and 90-day vapor inhalation studies in Fischer 344 rats. *Toxicol. Appl. Pharmacol.*, **68**:405–414, 1983.

Dutkiewicz, B.; Konczalik, J.; and Karwacki, W.: Skin absorption and per os administration of methanol. *Int. Arch. Occup. Environ. Health*, **47**:81–88, 1980.

Eastmond, D. A.; Smith, M. T.; and Irons, R. D.: An interaction of benzene metabolites reproduces the myelotoxicity observed with benzene exposure. *Toxicol. Appl. Pharmacol.*, **91**:85–95, 1987.

Eells, J. T.; Makar, A. B.; Noker, P. E.; and Tephly, T. E.: Methanol poisoning and formate oxidation in nitrous oxide–treated rats. *J. Pharmacol. Exp. Ther.*, **217**:57–61, 1981.

Elofsson, S. A.; Gamberale, F.; Hindmarsch, T.; Iregren, A.; Isaksson, A.; Johnsson, I.; Knave, B.; Zydahl, E.; Mindus, P.; Persson, H. E.; Phillipson, B.; Steby, M.; Struwe, G.; Soderman, E.; Wennberg, A.; and Widen, L.: Exposure to organic solvents. *Scand. J. Work Environ. Health*, **6**:239–273, 1980.

Elovaara, E.; Engstrom, K.; Nickles, J.; Aito, A.; and Vainio, H.: Biochemical and morphological effects of long-term inhalation exposure of rats to ethylbenzene. *Xenobiotica*, **15**:299–308, 1985.

FDA: *Teratologic Evaluation of Compound FDA 71–56 (Propylene Glycol) in Mice, Rats, Hamsters and Rabbits*. PB–223–822, 1973.

————: *Mutagenic Evaluation of Compound FDA 71–56 Propylene Glycol*. PB-245450, 1974.

————: *Fed. Reg.*, **42**:30865–66, June 17, 1977.

Federal Register (FR): Occupational exposure to benzene In *Docket No. H-059c*. Occupational Safety and Health Administration, Department of Labor, 29 CFR Part 1910, Washington, D.C., 1985.

————: Cosmetics: ban on the use of methylene chloride as an ingredient of cosmetic products. In *Docket*

No. 85H-05361. Food and Drug Administration, CFR Part 700, Washington, D.C., 1989.

Feldman, R. G.; Ricks, N. L.; and Baker, E. L.: Neuropsychological effects of industrial neurotoxins: a review. *Am. J. Ind. Med.,* **1**:211–227, 1980.

Ferguson, J.: The use of chemical potentials as indices of toxicity. *Proc. Roy. Soc.,* **127** (Series B):387–404, 1939.

Fitzhugh, O. G., and Nelson, A. A.: Comparison of the chronic toxicity of triethylene glycol with that of diethylene glycol. *J. Ind. Hyg. Toxicol.,* **28**:40–43, 1946.

Gaido, K., and Wierda, D.: *In vitro* effects of benzene metabolites on mouse bone marrow stromal cells. *Toxicol. Appl. Pharmacol.,* **76**:45–55, 1984.

———: Modulation of stromal cell function in DBA/2J and B6C3F1 mice exposed to benzene or phenol. *Toxicol. Appl. Pharmacol.,* **81**:469–475, 1985.

Gaunt, I. F.; Carpanini, F. M.; and Grasso, P.: Long-term toxicity of propylene glycol in rats. *Food Cosmet. Toxicol.,* **10**:151–162, 1972.

Gershoff, S. N., and Andrus, S. B.: Effect of vitamin B_6 and magnesium on renal deposition of calcium oxalate by ethylene glycol administration. *Proc. Soc. Exp. Biol. Med.* **109**:99–102, 1962.

Gessner, P. K.; Parke, D. V.; and William, R. T.: Studies in detoxication. *Biochem. J.* **79**:482–489, 1961.

Gilioli, R.; Bulgheroni, C.; Bertazzi, P. A.; Circla, A. M.; Tomasini, M.; Cassitto, M. G.; and Jacovone, M. T.: Study of neurological and neurophysiological impairment of carbon disulfide workers. *Med. Lav.,* **69**:130–143, 1978.

Gill, G. F., and Ahmed, A.: Covalent binding of [14C] benzene to cellular organelles and bone marrow nucleic acids. *Biochem. Pharmacol.,* **30**: 1127–1131, 1981.

Gilmour, S.; Kalf, G. F.; and Snyder, R.: Comparison of the metabolism of benzene and its metabolite phenol in rat liver microsomes. In Kocsis, J. J.; Jollow, D. J.; Witmer, C. M.; Nelson, J. O.; and Snyder, R., (eds.): *Biological Reactive Intermediates III*. Plenum Publishing Co., New York, 1986.

Gilmour, S., and Snyder, R.: Metabolism of benzene and phenol in rat liver microsomes. *Fed. Proc.,* **42**: 1136, 1983a.

———: Similarities in the microsomal metabolism of benzene and its metabolite phenol. *Pharmacologist,* **25**:210, 1983b.

Goldstein, B. D.: Hematotoxicity in man. In Laskin S., and Goldstein, B. D. (eds.): *A Critical Evaluation of Benzene Toxicity. J. Toxicol Environ. Health,* (Suppl. 2):69–105, 1977.

Goldstein, B. D.; Witz, G; Javid, J.; Amoruso, M. A.; Rossman, T.; and Wolder, B.: Muconaldehyde, a potential toxic intermediate of benzene. In Snyder, R.; Parke, D. V.; Kocsis, J. J.; Jollow, D. J.; Gibson, G. G.; and Witmer, C. M. (eds.): *Biological Reactive Intermediates—II: Chemical Mechanisms and Biological Effects*. Plenum Press, New York, 1982, pp. 331–339.

Gonda, A.; Bault, H.; Churchill, D.; and Hollomby, D.: Hemodialysis for methanol intoxication. *Am. J. Med.,* **64**:749–758, 1978.

Gonzalez, E. G.; and Downey, J. A.: Polyneuropathy in a glue sniffer. *Arch. Phys. Med.,* **53**:333–337, 1972.

Gordy, S. T., and Trumper, M.: ·Carbon disulfide poisoning. *Ind. Med.* **9**:231–234, 1940.

Gorrod, J. W., and Beckett, A. H.: *Drug Metabolism in Man*. Taylor & Francis Ltd., London, 1978.

Gorsky, L. D., and Coon, M. J.: Evaluation of the role of free hydroxyl radicals in the cytochrome P-450–

catalyzed oxidation of benzene and cyclohexanol. *Drug Metab. Dispos.,* **13**:169–174, 1985.

Gosselin, R. E.; Smith, R. P.; and Hodge, H. E.: *Clinical Toxicology of Commercial Products,* 5th ed. Williams & Wilkins, Baltimore, 1984.

Grasso, P.: Neurotoxic and neurobehavioral effects of organic solvents on the nervous system. *State Art. Rev. Occup. Med.* **3**:525–539, 1988.

Greenburg, L.; Mayers, M. R.; Goldwater, L. J.; and Burke, W. J.: Health hazards in the manufacture of "fused collars." II. Exposure to acetone-methanol. *J. Ind. Hyg. Toxicol.,* **20**:148–154, 1938.

Halder, C. A.; Holdsworth, C. E.; Cockrell, B. Y.; and Piccirillo, V. J.: Hydrocarbon nephropathy in male rats: identification of the nephrotoxic components of unleaded gasoline. *Toxicol. Ind. Health,* **1**:67–87, 1985.

Hanley, T. R.; Young, J. T.; John, J. A.; and Rao, K. S.: Ethylene glycol monomethyl ether (EGME) and propylene glycol monomethyl ether (PGME): inhalation fertility and teratogenicity studies in rats, mice and rabbits. *Environ. Health Perspect.,* **57**:7–12, 1984.

Hanninen, H.; Nurminen, M.; Tolonen, M.; and Martelin, T.: Psychological tests as indicators of excessive exposure to carbon disulfide. *Scand. J. Work Environ. Health,* **19**:163–174, 1978.

Hardin, B. D.; Niemir, R. W.; Smith, R. J.; Kuczuk, M. H.; Mathinos, P. R.; and Weaver, T. E.: Teratogenicity of 2-ethoxyethanol by dermal application. *Drug Chem. Toxicol.,* **5**:277–294, 1982.

Havre, P.; Abrams, M. A.; Corall, R. J. M.; Ling, C. Y.; Szczepanik, P. A.; Feldman, H. B.; Klein, P.; Kong, M. S.; Margolis, J. M.; and Landau, B. R.: Quantitation of pathways of ethanol metabolism. *Arch. Biochem. Biophys.,* **182**:14–23, 1977.

Henschler, D., and Hoos, R.: Metabolic activation and deactivation mechanisms of di-, tri-, and tetrachloroethylenes. In Snyder, R.; Parke, D. V.; Kocsis, J. J.; Jollow, D. J.; Gibson, G. G.; and Witmer, C. M. (eds.): *Biological Reactive Intermediates—II: Chemical Mechanisms and Biological Effects*. Plenum Press, New York, 1982, pp. 659–666.

Herskowitz, A.; Ishii, N.; and Schaumberg, H.: *n*-Hexane neuropathy. *New Engl. J. Med.,* **285**:82–85, 1971.

Hoch-Ligeti, C., and Argus, M. F.: Effects of carcinogens on the lungs of guinea pigs. In Nettesheim, P.; Hanna, M. G., Jr.; and Deatherage, J. W., Jr. (eds.): *Morphology of Experimental Respiratory Carcinogenesis*. Atomic Energy Commission, Office of Information Services, 1970, pp. 267–279.

Hoch-Ligeti, C.; Argus, M. F.; and Argus, J. C.: Induction of carcinomas in the nasal cavity of rats. *Br. J. Cancer,* **24**:164–167, 1970.

Hoffman, P. L.; Rabe, C. S.; Moses, F.; and Tabakoff, B.: *N*-Methyl-D-aspartate receptors and ethanol: inhibition of calcium flux and cyclic GMP production. *J. Neurochem.,* **52**:1937–1940, 1989.

Holman, N. W.; Mundy, R. L.; and Teague, R. S.: Alkyldiol antidotes to ethylene glycol toxicity in mice. *Toxicol. Appl. Pharmacol.,* **49**:385–392, 1979.

Hong, J. Y.; Pan, J.; Ning, S. M.; and Yang, C. S.: Molecular basis for the sex-related difference in renal *N*-nitrosodimethylamine demethylase in C3H/HeJ mice. *Cancer Res.,* **49**:2973–2979, 1989.

Horvath, M., and Frantik, E.: Industrial chemicals and drugs lowering central nervous activation level. Quantitative assessment in man and animals. *Act. Nerv. Super.,* **21**:269, 1979.

IARC: 1,4-Dioxane. In *Monographs on the Evaluation of the Carcinogenic Risk of Chemicals to Man*, Vol.

11, *Cadmium, Nickel, Some Epoxides, Miscellaneous Industrial Chemicals, and General Considerations on Volatile Anesthetics.* International Agency for Research on Cancer, Lyons, France, 1976, pp. 247–256.

————: Benzene. In *IARC Monographs on the Evaluation of the Carcinogenic Risk of Chemicals to Humans,* Vol. 29, *Some Industrial Chemicals and Dyestuffs.* International Agency for Research on Cancer, Lyons, France, 1982, pp. 93–148.

————: *IARC Monographs on the Evaluation of Carcinogenic Risks to Humans,* Vol. 44, *Alcohol Drinking.* International Agency for Research on Cancer, Lyons, France, 1988.

Ikeda, M., and Ohtsuki, H.: Phenobarbital-induced protection against toxicity of toluene and benzene in rats. *Toxicol. Appl. Pharmacol.,* **20**:30–43, 1971.

Infante, P. F.; Rinsky, R. A.; Wagoner, J. K.; and Young, R. J.: Benzene and leukemia. *Lancet,* **2**:868–869, 1977a.

————: Leukemia in benzene workers. *Lancet,* **2**:76–78, 1977b.

Ingelman-Sundberg, M., and Hagbjork, A. L.: On the significance of the cytochrome P-450–dependent hydroxyl radical-mediated oxygenation mechanism. *Xenobiotica,* **12**:673–686, 1982.

Irons, R. D.; Dent, J. G.; Baker, T. S.; and Rickert, D. E.: Benzene is metabolized and covalently bound in bone marrow *in situ. Chem. Biol. Interact.* **30**:241–245, 1980.

Irons, R. D.; Greenlee, W. F.; Wierda, D.; and Bus, J. S.: Relationship between benzene metabolism and toxicity: a proposed mechanism for the formation of reactive intermediates from polyphenol metabolites. In Snyder, R.; Parke, D. V.; Kocsis, J. J.; Jollow, D. J.; Gibson, G. G.; and Witmer, C. M. (eds): *Biological Reactive Intermediates—II: Chemical Mechanisms and Biological Effects.* Plenum Press, New York, 1982, pp. 229–243.

Irons, R. D., and Neptun, D. A.: Effects of the principal hydroxy metabolites of benzene on microtubule polymerization. *Arch. Toxicol.,* **45**:297–305, 1980.

Jacobsen, D., and McMartin, K. E.: Methanol and ethylene glycol poisonings: mechanism of toxicity, clinical course, diagnosis and treatment. *Med. Toxicol.* **1**:309–334, 1986.

Jerina, D., and Daly, J. W.: Arene oxides: a new aspect of drug metabolism. *Science,* **185**:573–582, 1974.

Johnstone, R. T.: Death due to dioxane? *A.M.A. Arch. Ind. Health,* **20**:445–447, 1959.

Jollow, D. J., and Smith, C.: Biochemical aspects of toxic metabolites: formation, detoxication and covalent binding. In Jollow, D. J.; Kocsis, J. J.; Snyder, R.; and Vainio, H. (eds.): *Biological Reactive Intermediates: Formation, Toxicity, and Inactivation.* Plenum Press, New York, 1977, pp. 42–59.

Jonsson, A. K.; Pederson, J.; and Steen, G.: Ethoxyacetic acid and *N*-ethoxyacetylglycine: metabolites of ethoxyethanol (Ethylcellosolve) in rats. *Acta Pharmacol. Toxicol.,* **50**:358–362, 1982.

Kalant, H.: The pharmacology of alcohol intoxication. *Q. J. Stud. Alc.,* **22** (Suppl.):1–23, 1961.

Kalf, G. F.; Rushmore, T.; and Snyder, R.: Benzene inhibits RNA synthesis in mitochondria from liver and bone marrow. *Chem. Biol. Interact.* **42**:353–370, 1982.

Katz, G. V.; O'Donoghue, J. L.; DiVincenzo, G. D.; Terhaar, C. J.: Comparative neurotoxicity and metabolism of ethyl *n*-butyl ketone and methyl *n*-butyl ketone in rats. *Toxicol. Appl. Pharmacol.,* **52**:153–158, 1980.

Kingsley, W. H., and Hirsch, F. G.: Toxicologic considerations in direct process spirit duplicating machines. *Compen. Med.,* **40**:7–8, 1954–55.

Kirley, T. A.; Goldstein, B. D., Maniara, W. M.; and Witz, G.: Metabolism of *trans*-muconaldehyde, a microsomal metabolite of benzene, by purified yeast aldehyde dehydrogenase and a mouse liver soluble fraction. *Toxicol. Appl. Pharmacol.,* **100**:360–367, 1989.

Kirschman, J. C.; Brown, N. M.; Coots, R. H.; and Morgareidge, K.: Review of investigations of dichloromethane metabolism and subchronic oral toxicity as the basis for the design of chronic oral studies in rats and mice. *Food Chem. Toxicol.* **24**:943–949, 1986.

Kitchen, D. N.: Neoplastic renal effects of unleaded gasoline in Fischer 344 rats. In Mehlman, M. A.; Hemstreet, C. P.; Thorpe, J. J.; and Weaver, N. K. (eds.): *Advances in Modern Environmental Toxicology,* Vol. VII, *Renal Effects of Petroleum Hydrocarbons.* Princeton Scientific Publishers, Inc., Princeton, N.J., 1984, pp. 65–71.

Kitchin, K. T., and Brown, J. L.: Biochemical effects of three carcinogenic chlorinated methanes in rat liver. *Teratogen. Carcinogen. Mutagen.,* **9**:61–69, 1989.

Klatskin, G.; Krahl, W. A.; and Conn, H. O.: The effect of alcohol on the choline requirement. I. Changes in rat liver following prolonged ingestion of alcohol. *J. Exp. Med.,* **100**:605–614, 1954.

Kloss, M. W.; Cox, M. G.; Norton, R. M.; Swenberg, J. A.; and Bus, J. S.: Sex-dependent differences in the disposition of 14C 5-2,2,4-trimethylpentane in Fischer 344 rats. In Bach, P. H., and Lock, E. A. (eds.): *Renal Heterogeneity and Target Cell Toxicity.* John Wiley and Sons, Chichester, Great Britain, 1985, pp. 489–492.

Kluwe, W. M., and Hook, J. B.: Potentiation of acute chloroform nephrotoxicity by the glutathione depletor diethyl maleate and protection by the microsomal enzyme inhibitor piperonyl butoxide. *Toxicol. Appl. Pharmacol.,* **59**:457–466, 1981.

Knave, B.; Anshelm Olson, B.; Elofsson, S.; Gamberale, F.; Isaksson, A.; Mindus, P.; Persson, H. E.; Struwe, G.; Wennberg, A.; and Westerholm, P.: Long term exposure to jet fuel. *Scand. J. Work Environ. Health,* **4**:19–45, 1978.

Knave, B.; Kolmodin-Hedman, B.; Persson, H. E.; and Goldberg, J. M.: Chronic exposure to carbon disulfide. Effects on occupationally exposed workers with special reference to the nervous system. *Work Environ. Health,* **11**:49–58, 1974.

Kociba, R. J.; McCollister, S. B.; Park, S.; Torkelson, T. R.; and Gehring, P. J.: 1,4-Dioxane. I. Results of a two year ingestion study in rats. *Toxicol. Appl. Pharmacol.,* **30**:275–286, 1974.

Koop, D. R.; Laethem, C. L.; and Schiner, G. C.: Identification of ethanol-inducible P450 isozyme 3a (p450IIE1) as a benzene and phenol hydroxylase. *Toxicol. Appl. Pharmacol.,* **98**:278–288, 1989.

Krasavage, W. J.; O'Donoghue, J. L.; DiVincenzo. G. D.; and Terhaar, C. J.: The relative neurotoxicity of methyl *n*-butyl ketone, *n*-hexane and their metabolites. *Toxicol. Appl. Pharmacol.,* **52**:433–441, 1980.

LaCagnin, L. B.; Connor, H. D.; Mason, R. P.; and Thurman. R. G.: The carbon dioxide anion radical adduct in the perfused rat liver: relationship to halocarbon-induced toxicity. *Mol. Pharmacol.,* **33**:351–357, 1988.

Lamb IV, J. C.; Maronpot, R. R.; Gulati, D. K.; Russell, V. S.; Hommel-Barnes, L.; and Sabharwal, P. S.: Reproductive developmental toxicity of ethylene glycol in the mouse. *Toxicol. Appl. Pharmacol.*, **81**:100–112, 1985.

Landry, T. D.; Gushow, T. S.; and Yano, B. L.: Propylene glycol monomethylether: a 13-week vapor inhalation toxicity study in rats and rabbits. *Fund. Appl. Toxicol.*, **3**:627–630, 1983.

Latriano, L.; Goldstein, B. D.; and Witz, G.: Formation of muconaldehyde, an open ring metabolite of benzene, in mouse liver microsomes: an additional pathway for toxic metabolites. *Proc. Natl. Acad. Sci.*, **83**:8356–8360, 1986.

Lee, E. W.; Kocsis, J. J.; and Snyder, R.: Benzene: acute effect on ^{59}Fe incorporation into circulating erythrocytes. *Toxicol. Appl. Pharmacol.*, **27**:431–436, 1974.

————: The use of ferrokinetics in the study of experimental anemia. *Environ. Health Perspect.*, **39**:29–37, 1981.

Letteron, P.; Degott, C.; Labbe, G.; Larrey, D.; Descatoire, V.; Tinel, M.; and Pessayre, D.: Methoxsalen decreases the metabolic activation and prevents the hepatotoxicity and nephrotoxicity of chloroform in mice. *Toxicol. Appl. Pharmacol.*, **91**:266–273, 1987.

Lieber, C. S.: Pathogenesis and diagnosis of alcoholic liver injury. In Avogadro, P.; Sirtori, C. R.; and Tremoli, E. (eds.): *Metabolic Effects of Alcohol*. Elsevier, Amsterdam, 1979, pp. 237–258.

Lieber, C. S., and DeCarli, L. M.: Hepatic microsomal ethanol oxidizing system: *in vitro* characteristics and adaptive properties *in vivo*. *J. Biol. Chem.*, **245**:2505–2512, 1970.

Lieber, C. S.; DeCarli, L. M.; and Rubin, E.: Sequential production of fatty liver, hepatitis, and cirrhosis in sub-human primates fed ethanol with adequate diets. *Proc. Natl. Acad. Sci. U.S.A.*, **72**:437–441, 1975.

Lillis, R.: Behavioral effects of occupational carbon disulfide exposure. In: Behavioral toxicology: early detection of occupational hazards. *Natl. Inst. Occup. Safety Health*, **74–126**:51–59, 1974.

Linz, D. H.; deGarmo, P. L.; Morton, W. E.; Weins, A. N.; Coull, B. M.; and Maricle, R. A.: Organic solvent–induced encephalopathy in industrial painters. *J. Occup. Med.*, **28**:119–125, 1986.

Longacre, S. L.; Kocsis, J. J.; and Snyder, R.: Influence of strain differences in mice on the metabolism and toxicity of benzene. *Toxicol. Appl. Pharmacol.*, **60**:398–409, 1981a.

Longacre, S. L.; Kocsis, J. J.; Witmer, C. M.; Lee, E. W.; Sammett, D.; and Snyder, R.: Toxicological and biochemical effects of repeated administration of benzene to mice. *J. Toxicol. Environ. Health*, **7**:223–237, 1981b.

Loury, D. J.; Smith-Oliver, T.; and Butterworth, B. E.: Assessment of unscheduled and replicative DNA synthesis in rat kidney cells exposed *in vitro* and *in vivo* to unleaded gasoline. *Toxicol. Appl. Pharmacol.*, **87**:127–140, 1987.

Lovinger, D. M.; White, G.; and Weight, F.: Ethanol inhibits NMDA-activated current in hippocampal neurons. *Science*, **243**:1721–1724, 1989.

Low, L. K.,; Meeks, J. R.; and Mackerer, C. R.: Health effects of the alkylbenzenes. II. Xylenes. *Toxicol. Ind. Health*, **5**:86–105, 1989.

Lukas, E.: Eight years experience with experimental CS_2 polyneuropathy in rats. *Med. Lav.*, **1**:7–17, 1979.

Lukas, E.; Kujalova, V.; and Sperlingova, I.: The role of copper metabolism in the development of carbon disulfide polyneuropathy in rats. In Manzo, L.; Lery, N.; Lacasse, Y.; and Roche, E. (eds.): *Adv. Neurotoxicol., Proc. Int. Congr.* Pergamon Press, Oxford, 1980;, pp. 181–185.

Lutz, W. K., and Schlatter, C.: Mechanism of the carcinogenic action of benzene: irreversible binding to rat liver DNA. *Chem. Biol. Interact.* **18**:241–245, 1977.

MacEachern, L.; Snyder, R.; and Laskin, D. L.: Enhanced production of tumor necrosis factor (TNF) by stromal macrophages following benzene treatment of mice. *Toxicologist*, **9**:289, 1989.

MacFarland, H. N.: Xenobiotic induced kidney lesions: hydrocarbons. The 90-day and 2-year gasoline studies. In Mehlman, M. A.; Hemstreet, C. P.; Thorpe, J. J.; and Weaver, N. K. (eds.): *Advances in Modern Environmental Toxicology*, Vol. VII, *Renal Effects of Petroleum Hydrocarbons*. Princeton Scientific Publishers, Inc., Princeton, N.J., 1984, pp. 51–56.

Makar, A. B., and Tephly, T. R.: Methanol poisoning. VI. Role of folic acid in the production of methanol poisoning in the rat. *J. Toxicol. Environ. Health*, **2**:1201–1209, 1977.

Maltoni, C.; Conti, B.; and Cotti, G.: Benzene: a multipotential carcinogen. Results of long-term bioassays performed at the Bologna Institute of Oncology. *Am. J. Ind. Med.*, **4**:589–630, 1983.

Mannering, G. J., and Parks, R. E., Jr.: Inhibition of methanol metabolism with 3-amino-1,2,4-triazole. *Science*, **126**:1241–1242, 1975.

Mansuy, D.; Nastainczyk, W.; and Ullrich, V.: The mechanism of halothane binding to microsomal cytochrome P-450. *Naunyn Schmiedebergs Arch. Pharmacol*, **285**:315–324, 1974.

Marzulli, F. N., and Maibach, H. I.: *Dermatotoxicology*. Hemisphere Publishing Corporation, New York, 1983.

Matsushita, T., Arimatsu, T.; Ueda, A.; Satoh, K.; and Nomura, S.: Hematological and neuromuscular response of workers exposed to low concentration of toluene vapor. *Ind. Health*, **13**:115–121, 1975.

McDonough, J. R.: Possible neuropathy from methyl *n*-butyl ketone. *New Engl. J. Med.*, **290**:695, 1974.

McKenna, M. J., and DiStefano, V.: Carbon disulfide. II. A proposed mechanism for the action of carbon disulfide on dopamine beta-hydroxylase. *J. Pharmacol. Exp. Ther.*, **202**:253–266, 1977.

McKenna, M. J.; Zempel, J. A.; Madrid, E. O.; and Gehring, P. J.: The pharmacokinetics of ^{14}C-vinylidene chloride in rats following inhalation exposure. *Toxicol. Appl. Pharmacol.*, **45**:599–610, 1978.

McMartin, K. E.; Ambre, J. J.; and Tephly, T. R.: Methanol poisoning in human subjects—role for formic acid accumulation in the metabolic acidosis. *Am. J. Med.*, **68**:414–418, 1980.

McMartin, K. E.; Makar, A. B.; Martin, A. G.; Palese, M,; and Tephly, T. R.: Methanol poisoning. I. The role of formic acid in the development of metabolic acidosis in the monkey and the reversal by 4-methylpyrazole. *Biochem. Med.*, **13**:319–333, 1975.

McMartin, K. E.; Martin-Amat, G.; Makar, A. B.; and Tephly, T. R.: Methanol poisoning. V. Role of formate metabolism in the monkey. *J. Pharmacol. Exp. Ther.* **201**:564–572, 1977.

McMartin, K. E.; Martin-Amat, G.; Noker, P. E.; and Tephly, T. R.: Lack of a role for formaldehyde in methanol poisoning in the monkey. *Biochem. Pharmacol.*, **28**:645–649, 1979.

McMichael, A. J.; Spirtas, R.; and Kupper, L. L.: An epidemiologic study of mortality within a cohort of rubber workers, 1964–1972. *J.O.M.*, **16**:458–464, 1974.

McMichael, A. J.; Spirtas, R.; Kupper, L. L.; and Gamble, J. F.: Solvent exposure and leukemia among rubber workers: an epidemiologic study. *J.O.M.*, **17**:234–239, 1975.

Mebus, C. A.; Welsch, F.; and Working, P. K.: Attenuation of 2-methoxyethanol-induced testicular toxicity in the rat by simple physiological compounds. *Toxicol Appl. Pharmacol.*, **99**:110–121, 1989.

Medinsky, M. A.; Sabourin, P. J.; Lucier, G.; Birnbaum, L. S.; and Henderson, R. F.: A physiological model for simulation of benzene metabolism by rats and mice. *Toxicol. Appl. Pharmacol.*, **99**:193–206, 1989.

Mendell, J. R.: Neuropathy and methyl *n*-butyl ketone. *New Engl. J. Med.*, **290**:1263–1264, 1974.

Merkle, J., Klimisch, H. -J.; and Jaeck, R.: Prenatal toxicity of 2-methoxypropylacetate-1 in rats and rabbits. *Fund. Appl. Toxicol.*, **8**:71–79, 1987.

Meyer, K. H.: Contributions to the theory of narcosis. *Faraday Soc. Trans.*, **33**:1062–1064, 1937.

Mezey, E.: Metabolic effects of alcohol. *Fed. Proc.*, **44**:134–138, 1985.

Miller, K. W.; Paton, W. D. M.; Smith, R. A.; and Smith, E. B.: The pressure reversal of general anesthesia and the critical volume hypothesis. *Mol. Pharmacol.*, **9**:131–143, 1973.

Miller, R. R.; Ayres, J. A.; Young, J. T.; and McKenna, M. J.: Ethylene glycol monoethyl ether. I. Subchronic vapor inhalation study with rats and rabbits. *Fund. Appl. Toxicol.*, **3**:49–54, 1983a.

Miller, R. R.; Carreon, R. E.; Young, J. T.; and McKenna, M. J.: Toxicity of methoxyacetic acid in rats. *Fund. Appl. Toxicol.*, **2**:158–160, 1982.

Miller, R. R.; Hermann, E. A.; Langvardt, P. W.; McKenna, M. J.; and Schwetz, B. A.: Comparative metabolism and disposition of ethylene glycol monomethyl ether and propylene glycol monomethyl ether in male rats. *Toxicol. Appl. Pharmacol.*, **67**:229–237, 1983b.

Miller, R. R.; Langvardt, P. W.; Calhoun, L. L.; and Yahrmardt, M. A.: Metabolism and disposition of propylene glycol monomethyl ether (PGME) beta isomer in male rats. *Toxicol. Appl. Pharmacol.*, **83**:170–177, 1986.

Miller, S. L.: A theory of gaseous anesthetics. *Proc. Natl. Acad. Sci., U.S.A.* **47**:1515–1524, 1961.

Misumi, J., and Nagano, M.: Experimental study on the enhancement of the neurotoxicity of methyl butyl ketone by non-neurotoxic aliphatic monoketones. *Br. J. Ind. Med.*, **42**:155–161, 1985.

Mohtashamipur, E.; Norpoth, K.; Woelke, U.; and Huber, P.: Effects of ethylbenzene, toluene, and xylene on the induction of micronuclei in bone marrow polychromatic erythrocytes of mice. *Arch. Toxicol.*, **58**:106–109, 1985.

Morgan, M. Y.: Alcohol and nutrition. *Br. Med. Bull.*, **38**:21–29, 1982.

Morimoto, K.; Wolff, S.; and Koizumi, A.: Induction of sister chromatid exchanges in human lymphocytes by microsomal activation of benzene metabolites. *Mutat. Res.*, **119**:355–360, 1983.

Morris, H. J.; Nelson, A. A.; and Calvery, H. O.: Observations on the chronic toxicities of propylene glycol, ethylene glycol, diethylene glycol monoethylether. *Pharmacol. Exp. Ther.*, **74**:266–273, 1942.

Morton, H. G.: Occurrence and treatment of solvent abuse in children and adolescents. *Pharmacol. Ther.*, **33**:449–469, 1987.

Moss, E. J.; Thomas, L. V.; Cook, M. W.; Walters, D. G.; Foster, P. M. D.; Creasy, D. M.; and Gray, T. J. B.: The role of metabolism in 2-methoxyethanol-induced testicular toxicity. *Toxicol. Appl. Pharmacol.*, **79**:480–489, 1985.

Mueller, D. H.: Epidemiologic considerations of ethylene glycol intoxication in small animals. *Vet. Human Toxicol.*, **24**:21–24, 1982.

Nagano, K.; Nakayama, E.; Koyano, M.; Dobayaski, H.; Adachi, H.; and Yamada, T.: Testicular atrophy of mice induced by ethylene glycol monoalkyl ethers. *Jpn. J. Ind. Health*, **21**:29–35, 1979.

NAS: *Biologic Markers in Pulmonary Toxicology.* National Academy Press, Washington, D.C., 1989a.

———: *Biologic Markers in Reproductive Toxicology.* National Academy Press, Washington, D.C., 1989b.

NAS/NRC: *The Alkyl Benzenes.* Committee on Alkyl Benzene Derivatives, Board on Toxicology and Environmental Health Hazards, Assembly of Life Sciences, National Research Council, National Academy of Sciences. National Academy Press, Washington, D.C., 1980.

Nelson, B. K.; Setzer, J. V.; Brightwell, W. S.; Mathinos, P. R.; Kuczuk, M. H.; Weaver, T. E.; and Goad, P. T.: Comparative inhalation teratogenicity of three glycol ether solvents and an amino derivative in rats. *Environ. Health Perspect.*, **57**:261–271, 1984.

NIOSH: *Hazard Evaluation and Technical Assistance Report TA 80-32.* Everett School District, Everett, Washington, NTIS. PB 81–111155, 1980.

Nitschke, K. D.; Burek, J. D.; Bell, T. J.; Kociba, R. J.; Rampy, L. W.; and McKenna, M. J.: Methylene chloride: 2 year inhalation toxicity and oncogenicity study in rats. *Fund. Appl. Toxicol.*, **11**:48–59, 1988.

Noker, P. E., and Tephly, T. R.: The role of folates in methanol toxicity. *Adv. Exp. Med. Biol.*, **132**:305–315, 1980.

O'Donoghue, J. L., and Krasavage, W. J.: Hexacarbon neuropathy: a gamma-diketone neuropathy? *J. Neuropathol. Exp. Neurol.*, **38**:333, 1979a.

———: The structure-activity relationship of aliphatic diketones and their potential neurotoxicity. *Toxicol. Appl. Pharmacol.*, **48**:A55, 1979b.

O'Donoghue, J. L.; Krasavage, W. J.; and Terhaar, C. J.: Toxic effects of 2,5-hexanedione. *Toxicol. Appl. Pharmacol.*, **45**:269, 1978.

Ohnishi, K., and Lieber, C. S.: Reconstitution of the microsomal ethanol oxidizing system (MEOS): qualitative and quantitative changes of cytochrome p-450 after chronic ethanol consumption. *J. Biol. Chem.*, **252**:7124–7131, 1977.

Okayama, A.; Fun, L.; Yamatodani, A.; Ogawa, Y.; Wada, H.; and Goto, S.: Effect of exposure to carbon disulfide on tryptophan metabolism and the tissue vitamin B_6 contents of rats. *Arch. Toxicol.*, **60**:450–453, 1987.

Okayama, A.; Ogawa, Y.; Goto, S.; Yamatodani, A.; Wada, H.; Okuno, E.; Takikawa, O.; and Kido, R.: Enzymatic studies of tryptophan metabolism disorder in rats chronically exposed to carbon disulfide. *Toxicol. Appl. Pharmacol.*, **94**:356–361, 1988.

Olishifski, J. B.: *Fundamentals of Industrial Hygiene,* 2nd. ed. National Safety Council, Chicago, 1979, pp. 540–548.

Orth, O. S.: General anesthesia. I: Volatile agents. In DiPalma, J. R. (ed.): *Drill's Pharmacology in Medicine.* McGraw-Hill Book Co., New York, 1965, pp. 100–115.

OSHA: *Fed. Reg.*, **54**:2462, Jan. 19, 1989.

Parke, D. V., and Williams, R. T.: Studies in detoxication. The metabolism of benzene containing ^{14}C benzene. *Biochem. J.*, **54**:231–238, 1953.

Pauling, L.: A molecular theory of general anesthesia. *Science*, **134**:15–21, 1961.

Paulson, G. W., and Waylons, G. W.: Polyneuropathy due to *n*-hexane. *Arch. Intern. Med.*, **136**:880–882, 1976.

Perbellini, L.; Brugnone, F.; and Pavan, I.: Identification of the metabolites of *n*-hexane, cyclohexane, and their isomers in men's urine. *Toxicol. Appl. Pharmacol.*, **53**:220–229, 1980.

Pergal, M.; Vukojevic, N.; Cirin-Popov, N.; Djuric, D.; and Bojovic, T.: Carbon disulfide metabolites excreted in the urine of exposed workers. *Arch. Environ. Health*, **25**:38–41, 1972a.

Pergal, M.; Vukojevic, N.; and Djuric, D.: a. II. Isolation and identification of thiocarbamide. *Arch. Environ. Health*, **25**:42–44, 1972b.

Phillips, R. D., and Cockrell, B. Y.: Kidney structural changes in rats following inhalation exposure to C_{10}-C_{11} isoparaffinic solvent. *Toxicology*, **33**:261–273, 1984.

Phillips, R. D., and Egan, G. F.: Effect of C_{10}-C_{11} isoparaffinic solvent on kidney function in Fischer 344 rats during eight weeks of inhalation. *Toxicol. Appl. Pharmacol.*, **73**:500–510, 1984.

Pirozzi, S. J.; Schlosser, M. J.; and Kalf, G. F.: Prevention of benzene-induced myelotoxicity and prostaglandin synthesis in bone marrow of mice by inhibitors of prostaglandin H synthetase. *Immunopharmacology*, **18**:39–55, 1989.

Plaa, G. L., and Larson, R. E.: Relative nephrotoxic properties of chlorinated methane, ethane, and ethylene derivatives in mice. *Toxicol. Appl. Pharmacol.* **7**:37–44, 1965.

Pohl, L. R.: Biochemical toxicology of chloroform. In Hodgson, E.; Bend, J. R.; and Philpot, R. M. (eds.): *Reviews in Biochemical Toxicology*, Vol. 1. Elsevier/North Holland, Inc., New York. 1979, pp. 79–107.

Politzer, P.; Trfonas, P.; and Politzer, I. R.: Molecular properties of the chlorinated ethylenes and their epoxide metabolites. *Ann. N.Y. Acad. Sci.*, **367**:478–492, 1981.

Pons, C. A., and Custer, R. P.: Acute ethylene glycol poisoning. *Am. J. Med. Sci.*, **211**:544–552, 1946.

Post, G. G., and Snyder, R.: Effects of enzyme induction on microsomal benzene metabolism. *J. Toxicol. Environ. Health*, **11**:811–825, 1983.

Post, G.; Snyder, R.; and Kalf, G. F.: Inhibition of mRNA synthesis in rabbit bone marrow nuclei *in vitro* by quinone metabolites of benzene. *Chem. Biol. Interact.* **50**:203–211, 1984.

————: Inhibition of RNA synthesis and interleukin-2 production in lymphocytes *in vitro* by benzene and its metabolites hydroquinone and *p*-benzoquinone. *Toxicol. Lett.*, **29**:161–167, 1985.

Pratt, O. E.: Alcohol and the developing fetus. *Br. Med. Bull.*, **38**:48–53, 1982.

Price, C. J.; Kimmel, C. A.; Tyl, R. W.; and Marr, M. C.: The developmental toxicity of ethylene glycol in rats and mice. *Toxicol. Appl. Pharmacol.*, **81**:113–127, 1985.

Randerath, K.; Reddy, M. V.; and Gupta, R. C.: 32P-Postlabeling test for DNA damage. *Proc. Natl. Acad. Sci. U.S.A.*, **87**:6162–6169, 1981.

Rao, K. S.; Cobel-Geard, S. R.; Young, J. T.; Hanley, T. R., Jr.; Hayes, W. C.; John, J. A.; and Miller, R. R.: Ethylene glycol monomethyl ether. II. Reproductive and dominant lethal studies in rats. *Fund. Appl. Toxicol.*, **3**:80–85, 1983.

Recknagel, R. O., and Glende, E. A., Jr.: Carbon tetrachloride toxicity: an example of lethal cleavage. *CRC Crit. Rev. Toxicol.*, **2**:263–297, 1973.

Recknagel, R. O.; Glende, E. A., Jr.; and Hruszkewycz, A. M.: New data supporting an obligatory role for lipid peroxidation in carbon tetrachloride–induced loss of aminopyrine demethylase, cytochrome P-450 and glucose-6-phosphatase. In Jollow, D. J.; Kocsis, J. J.; Snyder, R.; and Vainio, H. (eds.); *Biological Reactive Intermediates: Formation, Toxicity and Inactivation*. Plenum Press, New York, 1977, pp. 417–428.

Reiner, O., and Uehleke, H.: Bindung von Tetrachlorkohlenstoff und reduziertes mikrosomales Cytochrom P-450 und an Haem. *Hoppe-Zeyler's Z. Physiol. Chem.*, **352**:1048–1052, 1971.

Reinke, L. A.; Lai, E. K.; and McCay, P. B.: Ethanol feeding stimulates trichloromethyl radical formation from carbon tetrachloride. *Xenobiotica*, **18**:1311–1318, 1988.

Reitz, R. H.; Fox, T. R.; Ramsey, J. C.; Quast, J. F.; Langvardt, P. W.; and Watanabe, P. G.: Pharmacokinetics and macromolecular interactions of ethylene dichloride in rats after inhalation or gavage. *Toxicol. Appl. Pharmacol.*, **62**:190–204, 1982.

Reynolds, E. S.: Comparison of early injury to liver endoplasmic reticulum by halomethanes, hexachloroethane, benzene, toluene, bromobenzene, ethionine, thioacetamide, and dimethylnitrosamine. *Biochem. Pharmacol.*, **21**:2555–2561, 1972.

Richardson, K. A.; Wilmer, J. L.; Smith-Simpson, D.; and Skopek, T. R.: Assessment of the genotoxic potential of unleaded gasoline and 2,2,4-trimethylpentane in human lymphoblasts *in vitro*. *Toxicol. Appl. Pharmacol.*, **82**:316–322, 1986.

Rickert, D. E.; Baker, T. S.; Bus, J. S.; Barrow, C. S.; and Irons, R. D.: Benzene disposition in the rat after exposure by inhalation. *Toxicol. Appl. Pharmacol.*, **49**:417–423, 1979.

Rihimaki, V., and Pfaffli, P.: Percutaneous absorption of solvent vapors in man. *Scand. J. Work Environ. Health*, **4**:73–85, 1978.

Rinsky, R. A.; Young, R. J.; and Smith, A. B.: Leukemia in benzene workers. *Am. J. Ind. Med.*, **2**:217–245, 1981.

Ritchie, J. M.: The aliphatic alcohols. In Goodman, L. S., and Gilman, A. (eds.): *The Pharmacological Basis of Therapeutics*, 4th ed. Macmillan Co., New York, 1970, p. 136.

Roberts, J. A., and Seibold, H. R.: Ethylene glycol toxicity in the monkey. *Toxicol. Appl. Pharmacol.*, **15**:624–631, 1969.

Robertson, F. M.; MacEachern, L.; Liesch, J. B.; Snyder, R.; and Laskin, D. L.: Potential role of interleukin-1 in benzene-induced bone marrow toxicity. *Toxicologist*, **9**:289, 1989.

Robertson, O. H.; Loosli, C. G.; Puck, T. T.; Wise, H.; Lemon, H. M.; and Lester, W., Jr.: Tests for the chronic toxicity of propylene glycol on monkeys and rats by vapor inhalation and oral administration. *J. Pharmacol. Exp. Ther.*, **91**:52–76, 1947.

Rowland, J.: Incidence of ethylene glycol intoxication in dogs and cats seen at Colorado State University Teaching Hospital. *Vet. Human Toxicol.*, **29**:41–44, 1987.

Rubin, A., and Rottenberg, H.: Ethanol and biological membranes: injury and adaptation. *Pharmacol. Biochem. Behav.*, **18** (Suppl. 1):7–13, 1983.

Ruddick, J. A.: Toxicology, metabolism and biochemistry of 1,2-propanediol. *Toxicol. Appl. Pharmacol.*, **21**:102–111, 1972.

Ruprecht, H. A., and Nelson, I. A.: Preliminary toxicity reports on diethylene glycol and sulfanilamide. V. Clinical and pathologic observations. *J.A.M.A.*, **109**(2):1537, 1937.

Saida, K.; Mendell, J. R.; and Weiss, H. S.: Peripheral nerve changes induced by methyl *n*-butyl ketone and potentiation by methyl ethyl ketone. *J. Neuropathol. Exp. Neurol.*, **35**:207–223, 1976.

Sato, A., and Nakajima, T.: Dose-dependent metabolic interaction between benzene and toluene *in vivo* and *in vitro*. *Toxicol. Appl. Pharmacol.*, **48**:249–256, 1979.

Sawahata, T., and Neal, R. A.: Horse radish peroxidase–mediated oxidation of phenol. *Biochem. Biophys. Res. Commun.*, **109**:988–994, 1982.

Schumann, A. M.; Fox, T. R.; and Watanabe, P. G.: ^{14}C-Methyl chloroform (1,1,1-trichloroethane): pharmacokinetics in rats and mice following inhalation exposure. *Toxicol. Appl. Pharmacol.*, **62**:390–401, 1982.

Schumann, A. M.; Quast, J. F.; and Watanabe, P. G.: The pharmacokinetics and macromolecular interactions of perchloroethylene in mice and rats as related to oncogenicity. *Toxicol. Appl. Pharmacol.*, **55**:207–19, 1980.

Sedivec, V.; Mraz, M.; and Flek, J.: Biological monitoring of persons exposed to methanol vapours. *Int. Arch. Occup. Environ. Health*, **48**:257–271, 1981.

Seeman, P.: The membrane action of anesthetics and tranquilizers. *Pharmacol. Rev.*, **24**:583–655, 1972.

Seitz, H. K., and Simanowski, U. A.: Ethanol and carcinogenesis of the alimentary tract. *Alcoholism: Clin. Exp. Res.*, **10**:33S–40S, 1986.

Seppalainen, A. M.; Lindstrom, K.; and Martelin, T.: Neurophysiological and psychological picture of solvent poisoning. *Am. J. Ind. Med.*, **1**:31–42, 1980.

Serota, D. G.; Thakur, A. K.; Ulland, B. M.; Kirschman, J. C.; Brown, N. M.; Coots, R. H.; and Morgareidge, K.: A two-year drinking-water study of dichloromethane in rodents. I. Rats. *Food Chem. Toxicol.*, **24**:951–958, 1986a.

———: A two-year drinking-water study of dichloromethane in rodents. II. Mice. *Food Chem. Toxicol.*, **24**:959–963, 1986b.

Sherlock, S. (ed.): Alcohol and disease. *Br. Med. Bull.*, **38**:1–113, 1982.

Shibayama, Y.: Hepatotoxicity of carbon tetrachloride after chronic ethanol consumption. *Exp. Mol. Pathol.*, **49**:234–242, 1988.

Short, B. G.; Burnett, V. L.; and Swenberg, J. A.: Histopathology and cell proliferation induced by 2,2,4-trimethylpentane in the male rat kidney. *Toxicol. Pathol.*, **14**:194–203, 1986.

Singer, S. J. and Nicolson, G. L.: The fluid mosaic model of the structure of cell membranes. *Science*, **175**:720–731, 1972.

Sipes, I. G. and Gandolfi, A. J.: Role of reactive intermediates in halothane associated liver injury. In Snyder, R.; Parke, D. V.; Kocsis, J. J.; Jollow, D. J.; Gibson, G. G.; and Witmer, C. M. (eds): *Biological Reactive Intermediates—II: Chemical Mechanisms and Biological Effects*. Plenum Press, New York, 1982, pp. 603–618.

Slater, T. F.: *Free Radical Mechanisms in Tissue Injury*. J. W. Arrowsmith, Ltd., Bristol, 1972, pp. 118–163.

———: Free radicals as reactive intermediates in tissue injury. In Snyder, R.; Parke, D. V.; Kocsis, J. J.; Jollow, D. J.; Gibson, G. G.; and Witmer, C. M. (eds.): *Biological Reactive Intermediates—II: Chemical Mechanisms and Biological Effects*. Plenum Press, New York, 1982, pp. 575–589.

Sleet, R. B.; Greene, J. A.; and Welsch, F.: The relationships of embryotoxicity to disposition of 2-methoxycthanol in mice. *Toxicol. Appl. Pharmacol.*, **93**:195–207, 1988.

Smith, E. N., and Taylor, R. T.: Acute toxicity of methanol in the folate-deficient acatalasemic mouse. *Toxicology*, **25**:271–287, 1982.

Smith, J. H., and Hook, J. B.: Mechanism of chloroform toxicity: III. Renal and hepatic microsomal metabolism of chloroform in mice. *Toxicol. Appl. Pharmacol.*, **73**:511–524, 1984.

Smith, J. H.; Maita, K.; Sleight, S. D.; and Hook, J. B.: Mechanism of chloroform toxicity: I. Time course of chloroform toxicity in male and female mice. *Toxicol. Appl. Pharmacol.*, **70**:467–479, 1983.

———: Effect of sex hormone status on chloroform nephrotoxicity and renal mixed function oxidases in mice. *Toxicology*, **30**:305–316, 1984.

Smuckler, E. A.: The molecular basis of acute liver cell injury. In Good, R. A.; Day, S. B.; and Yunes, J. J. (eds.): *Molecular Pathology*. Charles C. Thomas, Springfield, Ill., 1975, pp. 490–510.

Smyth, H. F., Jr.: Physiological aspects of glycols and related compounds. In Curme, G. O., Jr., and Johnston, F. (eds.): *Glycols*. Reinhold Publishing Co., New York, 1952.

Snyder, C. A.; Goldstein, B. D.; Sellakumar, A.; Wolman, S. R.; Bromberg, I.; Erlichman, M. N.; and Laskin, S.: Hematotoxicity of inhaled benzene to Sprague Dawley rats and AKR mice at 300 ppm. *J. Toxicol. Environ. Health*, **4**:605–618, 1978.

Snyder, R.: Benzene metabolism. In Arinc, E. (ed.): *Molecular Aspects of Monooxygenases and Bioactivation of Toxic Compounds*. Plenum Publishing Co., London, in press.

Snyder, R.; Dimitriadis, E. A.; Guy, R.; Hu, P.; Cooper, K.; Bauer, H.; Witz, G.; and Goldstein, B. D.: Studies on the mechanism of benzene toxicity. *Environ. Health Perspect.*, **82**:31–35, 1989.

Snyder, R., and Kocsis, J. J.: Current concepts of chronic benzene toxicity. *CRC Crit. Rev. Toxicol.*, **3**:265–288, 1975.

Snyder, R.; Lee, E. W.; Kocsis, J. J.; and Witmer, C. M.: Bone marrow depressant and leukemogenic actions of benzene. *Life Sci.*, **21**:1709–1722, 1977.

Snyder, R.; Longacre, S. L.; Witmer, C. M.; Kocsis, J. J.; Andrews, L. S.; and Lee, E. W.: Biochemical toxicology of benzene. In *Reviews in Biochemical Toxicology*, Vol. 3. Elsevier/North Holland Publishing Co., New York, 1981, pp. 123–153.

Snyder, R.; Uzuki, F.; Gonasun, L.; Bromfeld, E.; and Wells, A.: The metabolism of benzene *in vitro*. *Toxicol. Appl. Pharmacol.*, **11**:346–360, 1967.

Sobue, I.; Yamamura, Y.; Ando, K.; Iida, M.; and Takayanagi, T.: N-Hexane polyneuropathy. *Clin. Neurol. (Jpn.)*, **8**:393–403, 1968.

Spencer, P. S.; Bischoff, M. C.; and Schaumburg, H. H.: On the specific molecular configuration of neurotoxic aliphatic hexacarbon compounds causing central peripheral distal axonopathy. *Toxicol. Appl. Pharmacol.*, **44**:17–28, 1978.

Spencer, P. S., and Schaumburg, H. H.: Ultrastructural studies of the dying-back process. IV. Differential vulnerability of PNS and CNS fibers in experimental central-peripheral distal axonopathies. *J. Neuropathol. Exp. Neurol.*, **36**:300–320, 1977.

Stott, W. T.; Quast, J. F.; and Watanabe, P. G.: Differentiation of mechanism of oncogenicity of 1,4-dioxane and 1,3-hexachlorobutadiene. *Toxicol. Appl. Pharmacol.*, **60**:287–300, 1981.

Strubelt, O.: Interactions between ethanol and other hepatotoxic agents. *Biochem. Pharmacol.*, **29**:1445–1449, 1980.

Sullivan, M. J.; Rarey, K. E.; and Conolly, R. B.: Ototoxicity of toluene in rats. *Neurotoxicol. Teratol.*, **10**:525–530, 1989.

Susten, A. S.; Dames, B. L.; Burg, J. R.; and Niemeier, R. W.: Percutaneous penetration of benzene in hairless mice: an estimate of dermal absorption during tire-building operations. *Am. J. Ind. Med.*, **7**:323–335, 1985.

Szendzikowski, S.; Stetkiewicz, J.; Wronska-Nofer, T.; and Karasek, M.: Pathomorphology of the experimental lesion of the peripheral nervous system in white rats chronically exposed to carbon disulphide. In Hausmanowa-Petrusewicz, I., and Vedrzejowska, H. (eds.): *Structure and Function of Normal and Diseased Muscle and Peipheral Nerve*. Polish Medical Publishers, Warsaw, 1974, pp. 319–326.

Tephly, T. R.: Introduction, factors in response to the environment. *Fed. Proc.*, **36**:1627–1628, 1977.

Tephly, T. R.; Makar, A. B.; McMartin, K. E.; Hayreh, S. S.; and Martin-Amat, G.: Methanol—its metabolism and toxicity. *Biochem. Pharmacol. Methanol,* **1**:145–164, 1979.

Thompson, J. A., and Reitz, R. C.: Studies on the acute and chronic effects of ethanol on choline oxidation. *Ann. N.Y. Acad. Sci.,* **272**:194–204, 1976.

Thurman, R. G., and Hoffman, P. L. (ed.): First Congress of the International Society for Biomedical Research on Alcoholism. *Pharmacol. Biochem. Behav.,* **18**:(Supp. 1), 1983.

Tice, R. R.; Vogt, T. F.; and Costa, D. L.: Cytogenetic effects of inhaled benzene on murine bone marrow. In Tice, R. R.; Costa, D. L.; and Schaich, K. M. (eds.): *Genotoxic Effects of Airborne Agents.* Plenum Press, New York, 1982, pp. 257–275.

Tiller, J. R.; Schilling, R. S. F.; and Morris, J. W.: Occupational toxic factor in mortality from coronary heart disease. *Br. Med. J.,* **4**:407–411, 1968.

Tilson, H. A., and Cabe, P. A.: Strategy for the assessment of neurobehavioural consequences of environmental factors. *Environ. Health Perspect.,* **26**:287–299, 1978.

Toft, K.; Oloffson, T.; Tunek, A.; and Berlin, M.: Toxic effects on mouse bone marrow caused by inhalation of benzene. *Arch. Toxicol.,* **51**:295–302, 1982.

Tolonen, M.: Chronic subclinical carbon disulfide poisoning. *Work Environ. Health,* **11**:154–161, 1974.

Tolonen, M.; Hanninen, H.; and Nurminen, M.: Psychological tests specific to individual carbon disulphide exposure. *Scand. J. Psychol.,* **19**:241–245, 1978.

Tolonen, M.; Hernberg, S.; Nurminen, M.; and Tiitola, K.: A follow-up study of coronary heart disease in viscose rayon workers exposed to carbon disulfide. *Br. J. Ind. Med.,* **32**:1–10, 1975.

Tolonen, M.; Nurminen, M.; and Hernberg, S.: Ten-year coronary mortality of workers exposed to carbon disulfide. *Scand. J. Work Environ. Health,* **5**:109–114, 1979.

Torkelson, T. R.; Leong, B. J.; Kociba, R. J.; Richter, W. A.; and Gehring, P. J.: 1,4-Dioxane. II. Results of a 2-year inhalation study in rats. *Toxicol. Appl. Pharmacol.,* **30**:287–298, 1974.

Torkelson, T. R.; Oyen, F.; and Rowe, V. K.: The toxicity of chloroform as determined by single and repeated exposure of laboratory animals. *Am. Ind. Hyg. Assoc. J.,* **37**:697–705, 1976.

Tunek, A.; Platt, K. L.; Przybylski, M.; and Oesch, F.: Multi-step metabolic activation of benzene. Effect of superoxide dismutase on covalent binding to microsomal macromolecules, and identification of glutathione conjugates using high pressure liquid chromatography and field desorption mass spectrometry. *Chem. Biol. Interact.,* **33**: 1–17, 1980.

Tuttle, T. C.; Wood, G. D.; and Grether, C. G.: Behavioral and neurological evaluation of workers exposed to carbon disulphide (CS$_2$). *NIOSH Publication:* 77–128, 1977.

Uehleke, H.: Binding of haloalkanes to liver microsomes. In Jollow, D. J.; Kocsis, J. J.; Snyder, R.; and Vainio, H. (eds.): *Biological Reactive Intermediates: Formation, Toxicity, and Inactivation.* Plenum Press, New York, 1977, pp. 431–445.

Uyeki, E. M.; Ashkar, A. E.; Shoeman, D. W.; and Bisel. T. U.: Acute toxicity of benzene inhalation to hemopoietic precursor cells. *Toxicol. Appl. Pharmacol.,* **40**:49–57, 1977.

van Doorn, R.; Delbressine, L. P. C.; Leijdekkers, Ch. -M.; Vertin, P. G.; and Henderson, P. Th.:

Identification and determination of 2-thiothiazolidine-4-carboxylic acid in the urine of workers exposed to carbon disulfide. *Arch. Toxicol.,* **47**:51–58, 1981a.

van Doorn, R.; Leijdekkers, C. P. M. J.; Henderson, P. T.; Vanhoorne, M.; and Vertin, P. G.: Determination of thio compounds in urine of workers exposed to carbon disulfide. *Arch. Environ. Health,* **36**:289–297, 1981b.

Vigliani, E. C., and Saita, G.: Benzene and leukemia. *New Engl. J. Med.,* **27**:872–876, 1964.

Vind, C., and Grunnet, N.: Interaction of cytoplasmic dehydrogenases: quantitation of pathways of ethanol metabolism. *Pharmacol. Biochem. Behav.,* **18** (Suppl.1):209–213, 1983.

von Wartburg, J. P.; Bethuen, J. L.; and Vallee, B. L.: Human liver alcohol dehydrogenase. Kinetic and physico-chemical properties. *Biochemistry,* **3**:1775–1782, 1964.

Wacker, E. C.; Haynes, H.; Druyan, R.; Fischer, W.; and Coleman, J.: Treatment of ethylene glycol poisoning with ethyl alcohol. *J.A.M.A.,* **194**:1231–1233, 1965.

Weil, C. S.; Woodside, M. D.; and Smyth, H. F. Jr.: Results of feeding propylene glycol in the diet to dogs for two years. *Food Cosmet. Toxicol.,* **9**:479–490, 1971.

Wiener, H. L., and Richardson, K. E.: The metabolism and toxicity of ethylene glycol. *Res. Commun. Subst. Abuse,* **9**:77–87, 1988.

Wiley, F. H.; Hueper, W. C.; Bergen, D. S.; and Blood, F. R.: The formation of oxalic acid from ethylene glycol and related solvents. *J. Ind. Hyg. Toxicol.,* **20**:269–277, 1938.

Woo, Y.; Arcos, J. C.; Argus, M. F.; Griffin, G. W.; and Nishiyama, K.: Structural identification of *p*-dioxane-2-one as the major urinary metabolite of *p*-dioxane. *Arch. Pharmacol.,* **299**:283–287, 1977.

Wulf, B. S., and Featherstone, R. M.: A correlation of van der Waals constants with anesthetic potency. *Anesthesiology,* **18**:97–105, 1957.

Yamada, S.: An occurrence of polyneuritis by *n*-hexane in the polyethylene laminating plants. *Jpn. J. Ind. Health,* **6**:192–194, 1964.

Yamamura, Y.: *n*-Hexane polyneuropathy. *Folia Psychiat. Neurol. Jpn.,* **23**:45–47, 1969.

Yant, W. P., and Schrenk, H. H.: Distribution of methanol in dogs after inhalation and administration by stomach tube and subcutaneously. *J. Ind. Hyg. Toxicol.,* **19**(7):337–345, 1937.

Young, J. D.; Braun, W. H.; and Gehring, P. J.: Dose-dependent fate of 1,4-dioxane in rats. *J. Toxicol. Environ. Health,* **4**:709–726, 1978.

Young, J. D.; Braun, W. H.; Gehring, P. J.; Horvath, B. S.; and Daniel, R. L.: 1,4-Dioxane and beta-hydroxyethoxyacetic acid excretion in humans exposed to dioxane vapors. *Toxicol. Appl. Pharmacol.,* **38**:643–646, 1976.

Zbinden, G.: Definition of adverse behavioral effects. In Zbinden, G., (ed.): *Application of Behavioral Pharmacology in Toxicology.* Raven Press, New York, 1983.

Zenk, H.: CS$_2$ effects upon olfactory and auditory functions of employees in the synthetic-fiber industry. *Int. Arch. Arbeitsmed.,* **27**:210, 1970.

Zimmerman, H. J.: *Hepatotoxicity: The Adverse Effects of Drugs and Other Chemicals on the Liver.* Appleton-Century-Crofts, New York, 1978.

Chapter 21

TOXIC EFFECTS OF RADIATION AND RADIOACTIVE MATERIALS

Naomi H. Harley

INTRODUCTION

Ionizing radiation, of all branches of toxicology, provides the most quantitative estimates of health detriments for humans. There are five large studies that provide data on the heatlh effects of radiation on people. These include external X- and gamma-ray radiation and internal alpha radioactivity. The studies encompass the radium exposures (including radium dial painters), atom bomb survivors, patients irradiated with X rays for ankylosing spondylitis, children irradiated with X rays for tinea capitis (ringworm), and uranium miners exposed to radon and its short-lived daughter products. The only health effect seen with statistical significance to date, subsequent to radiation exposure, is cancer. The various types and the quantitative risks are described in subsequent sections.

All of the studies provide a consistent picture of the risk of exposure to ionizing radiation. There are sufficient details in the atom bomb, occupational, and medical exposures to estimate the risk from lifelong low-level environmental exposure. Natural background radiation is substantial and only within the past 10 to 15 years has the extent of the radiation insult to the global population from natural radiation and radioactivity been appreciated.

BASIC RADIATION CONCEPTS

There are four main types of radiation: alpha particles, beta particles (negatively charged) and positrons (postively charged), gamma rays, and X rays. An atom can decay to a product element by loss of a heavy (mass = 4) charged (+2) alpha particle, consisting of two protons and two neutrons. An atom can decay by loss of a negatively or positively charged electron (beta particle or positron). Gamma radiation results when the nucleus releases excess energy, usually after an alpha, beta or positron transition. X rays occur whenever an inner shell orbital electron is removed and rearrangement of the atomic electrons results with the release of the element's characteristic X-ray energy.

There are several excellent textbooks available that describe the details of radiological physics (Evans, 1955; Andrews, 1974; Turner, 1986).

Energy

Alpha particles and beta rays (or positrons) have kinetic energy due to their motion. The energy is equal to

$$E = \tfrac{1}{2}\, mV^2 \tag{1}$$

where

m = mass of the particle
V = velocity of the particle.

Alpha particles have a low velocity compared with the speed of light and calculations of alpha particle energy do not require any corrections for relativity. Most beta particles (or positrons) do have high velocity and the basic expression must be corrected for their increased relativistic mass (the rest mass of the electron is 0.511 MeV). The total energy is equal to

$$E = \frac{0.511}{(1 - v^2/c^2)^{1/2}} + 0.511 \tag{2}$$

where

v = velocity of the beta particle
c = speed of light.

Gamma and X rays are pure electromagnetic radiation with energy equal to

$$E = h\upsilon \tag{3}$$

where

h = Planck's constant (6.626×10^{-34} J sec)
υ = frequency of the radiation.

The conventional energy units for ionizing radiation are the electron volt (eV) or multiples of this basic unit, million electron volts (MeV), and kiloelectron volts (keV). The conversion to the international system of units (System International or SI) is currently taking place in the United States and the more fundamental energy unit of the Joule (J) is slowly replacing the older unit. The relationship is

$$1 \text{ eV} = 1.6 \times 10^{-19} \text{ J}$$

Authoritative tables of nuclear data such as those of Lederer *et al.* (1978) and Browne *et al.* (1986) contain the older units.

Alpha Particles

Alpha particles are helium nuclei (consisting of two protons and two neutrons) with a charge of +2 that are ejected from the nucleus of an atom. When the alpha particle loses energy, slows to the velocity of a gas atom, and acquires two electrons from the vast sea of free electrons present in most media, it becomes part of the normal background helium in the environment.

The formula for alpha decay is

$$_Z^A X \rightarrow _{Z-2}^{A-4} Y + He^{2+} + gamma + Q_\alpha$$

where

Z = atomic number
A = atomic weight.

The energy available in this decay is Q_α and is equal to the mass difference of the parent and the two products. The energy is shared among the particles and the gamma ray, if one is present.

An example of alpha decay is given by the natural radionuclide ^{226}Ra,

$$_{86}^{226} Ra \rightarrow _{84}^{222} Rn + alpha \ (5.2 \text{ MeV})$$

The energy of alpha particles for most emitters lies in the range of 4 to 8 MeV. More energetic alpha particles exist but are seen only in the very short-lived emitters such as those formed by reactions occurring in particle accelerators. These are not considered in this chapter.

Although there may be several alpha particles with very similar energy emitted by a particular element such as radium, each particular alpha is monoenergetic. No continuous spectrum of energies exists but only discrete energies.

Beta Particles, Positrons, and Electron Capture

Beta particle decay occurs when a neutron in the nucleus of an element effectively transforms into a proton and an electron. Subsequent ejection of the electron occurs and the maximum energy of the beta particle equals the mass difference between the parent and the product nuclei. A gamma ray may also be present to share the energy, Q_β.

$$_Z^A X \rightarrow _{Z+1}^A Y + beta + Q_\beta$$

An example of beta decay is given by the natural radionuclide ^{210}Pb

$$_{82}^{210} Pb \rightarrow _{83}^{210} Bi + beta \ (0.015 \text{ MeV})$$
$$+ 0.046 \text{ MeV gamma ray}$$

Unlike alpha decay, where each alpha particle is monoenergetic, beta particles are emitted with a continuous spectrum of energy from zero to the maximum energy available for the transition. The reason for this is that the total available energy is shared in each decay or transition by two particles, the beta and an antineutrino. The total energy released in each transition is constant but the observed beta particles then appear as a spectrum. The residual energy is carried away by the antineutrino, which is a particle with essentially zero mass and charge and cannot be observed without extraordinarily complex instrumentation. The beta particle, on the other hand, is readily observed with conventional nuclear counting equipment.

Positron emission is similar to beta particle emission, but results from the effective nucleon transformation of a proton to a neutron plus a positively charged electron. The atomic number decreases rather than increases as in beta decay.

An example of positron decay is given by the natural radionuclide ^{64}Cu which decays by beta emission 41 percent of the time, positron emission 19 percent of the time, and electron capture 40 percent of the time.

$$_{29}^{64} Cu \rightarrow _{28}^{64} Ni + positron \ (0.66 \text{ MeV}) \ 19 \text{ percent}$$
$$_{29}^{64} Cu \rightarrow _{30}^{64} Zn + beta \ (0.57 \text{ MeV}) \quad 41 \text{ percent}$$
$$_{29}^{64} Cu \rightarrow _{28}^{64} Ni \ electron \ capture \qquad 40 \text{ percent}$$

The energy of the positron appears as a continuous spectrum similar to that in beta decay where the total energy available for decay is again shared between the positron and a neutrino. In the case of positron emission, the maximum energy of the emitted particle is the mass difference of the parent and product nuclide minus the energy needed to create two electron masses (1.02 MeV) whereas the maximum energy of the beta particle is the mass difference itself. This happens because, in beta decay, the increase in the number of orbital electrons due to the increase in atomic number of the product nucleus cancels the mass of the electron lost in emitting the beta particle. This does not happen in positron decay and there is an orbital electron lost due to the decrease in atomic number of the product as well as loss of the electron mass in positron emission.

Electron capture competes with positron decay and the resulting product nucleus is the same. In electron capture an orbiting electron is acquired by the nucleus and the transformation of a proton plus the electron to form a neutron takes place. In some cases the energy available is released as a gamma-ray photon but this is not necessary and a monoenergetic neutrino may be emitted. If the 1.02 MeV required for positron decay is not available, then positron decay is not kinetically possible and electron capture will be the only mode observed.

Gamma-Ray (Photon) Emission

Gamma-ray emission is not a primary process except in rare instances but occurs in combination with alpha, beta, or positron emission or electron capture. Whenever the ejected particle does not utilize all of the available energy for decay, the nucleus contains the excess energy and is in an excited state. The excess energy is released as photon or gamma-ray emission coincident with the ejection of the particle.

One of the rare instances of pure gamma-ray emission is Tc.

$$^{99m}_{43}\text{Tc} \rightarrow {}^{99}_{43}\text{Tc} + \text{gamma (0.14 MeV)}$$

In many cases, the photon will not actually be emitted by the nucleus but the excess excitation energy will be transferred to an orbital electron. This electron is then ejected as a monoenergetic particle with energy equal to that of the photon minus the binding energy of the orbital electron. This process is known as internal conversion. In tables of nuclear data such as those of Lederer et al. (1978), the ratio of the conversion process to the photon is given as e/v. For example, the e/v ratio for ^{99m}Tc is 0.11 and therefore the photon is emitted 90 percent of the time and the conversion electron 10%.

INTERACTION OF RADIATION WITH MATTER

All ionizing radiation loses energy when passing through matter by producing ion pairs (an electron and a positively charged atom residue) or by raising atomic electrons to an excited state. The average energy to produce an ion pair is given the notation W, and is numerically equal to 33.85 eV. This energy is roughly two times

the ionization potential of most gases or other elements because it includes the energy lost in the excitation process. It is not clear what part the excitation plays, for example, in damage to targets in the cellular DNA. Ionization, on the other hand, can break bonds in DNA, causing strand breaks and easily understood damage.

All particles and rays interact through their charge or field with atomic or free electrons in the medium through which they are passing. There is no interaction with the atomic nucleus except at energies above about 8 MeV which is required for interactions that break apart the nucleus (spallation).

Alpha and beta particles and gamma rays lose energy by ionization and excitation in somewhat different ways and this is described in the following sections.

Alpha Particles

The alpha particle is a heavy charged particle with a mass that is 7300 times that of the electrons with which it interacts. A massive particle interacting with a small particle has the interesting property that it can give a maximum velocity during energy transfer to the small particle of only two times the initial velocity of the heavy particle. In terms of the maximum energy that can be transferred per interaction, this is

$$E_{(\text{maximum electron})} = 4/7300\, E_{(\text{alpha particle})} \qquad (4)$$

Although alpha particles can lose perhaps 10 to 20 percent of their energy in traveling 10 μm in tissue (1 cm in air), each interaction can only impart the small energy given in the maximum in equation 4. Thus, alpha particles are characterized by a high energy loss per unit path length and thus high ionization density along the track length. This is called a high linear energy transfer (LET).

An exact expression for the energy loss in matter, dE/dX or stopping power, was derived by Hans Bethe (1953) with modifications added by Bloch and others. For alpha energies between 0.2 and 10 MeV the Bethe-Bloch expression can be simplified to

$$dE/dx = 3.8 \times 10^{-25}\, C\, NZ/E\, \ln\{548\, E/I\} \text{ MeV } \mu\text{m}^{-1}$$

$$(5)$$

where

N = number of atoms cm^{-3} in the medium
Z = atomic number of the medium
I = ionization potential of the medium
E = energy of the alpha particle
C = charge correction for alpha particles with energy below 1.6 MeV.

A simple rule of thumb derived by Bloch may be used to estimate the ionization potential of a compound or element,

$$I = 10 \ (Z) \tag{6}$$

or the Bragg additivity rule (Attix et al., 1968) may be used for compounds when the individual values of ionization potential for the elements are available. A tabulation of values of ionization potential is given in ICRU 37 (ICRU, 1984) and the stopping power in all elements has been calculated by Ziegler (1977).

When alpha particles are near the end of their range the charge is not constant at $+2$, but can be $+1$ or even zero as the particle acquires or loses electrons. A correction factor, C, is needed for energies between 0.2 and 1.5 MeV to account for this effect. Whaling (1958) has published values for the correction factor by which equation 4 should be multiplied. These factors vary from 0.24 at 0.2 MeV, 0.75 at 0.6 MeV, 0.875 at 1.0 MeV, up to 1.0 at 1.6 MeV.

For the case of tissue, equation 5 reduces to

$$dE/dX_{tissue} = [0.126C/E] \ \ln \ \{7.99 \ E\} \ \text{MeV} \ \mu\text{m}^{-1} \tag{7}$$

Example 1. Find the energy loss (stopping power) of an 0.6 and a 5 MeV alpha particle in tissue.

$$
\begin{aligned}
dE/dX &= 0.126 \ (0.75)/0.6 \ \ln \ (7.99 \times 0.6) \\
&= 0.25 \ \text{MeV} \ \mu\text{m}^{-1} \\
&= 0.126 \ (1.0)/5.0 \ \ln \ (7.99 \times 5.0) \\
&= 0.093 \ \text{MeV} \ \mu\text{m}^{-1}
\end{aligned}
$$

Beta Particles

The equations for beta particle energy loss in matter cannot be simplified as in the case of alpha particles, because of three factors.

1. Even at low energies of a few tenths of an MeV, beta particles are traveling near the speed of light and relativistic effects (mass increase) must be considered.

2. Electrons are interacting with particles of the same mass in the medium (free or orbital electrons) and so large energy losses per collision are possible.

3. Radiative or bremsstrahlung energy loss occurs when electrons or positrons are slowing down in matter. Such a loss also occurs with alpha particles but the magnitude of this energy loss is negligible.

Including the effects of the above three factors, the energy loss for electrons and positrons has been well quantitated. Tabulations of energy loss in various media have been prepared with the ionization energy loss and the radiative loss

detailed. Tables 21–1 and 21–2 are reproduced from ICRU 37 (1984) to show the energy loss in air and muscle.

Example 2. What is the energy loss in tissue for an electron with an initial energy of 1.75 MeV? What is its range and what fraction of the initial energy is given up as bremsstrahlung as the electron slows from 1.75 MeV to rest?

From Table 21–2, the stopping power at the initial energy of 1.75 MeV is 1.82 MeV cm^2 g^{-1}, the range is 0.85 g cm^{-2}, and the fraction of the energy given up as bremsstrahlung in slowing to rest is 0.006.

Gamma Rays

Photons do not have a mass or charge as do alpha and beta particles. The interaction between a photon and matter is therefore not controlled by the Coulomb fields but by interaction of the electric and magnetic field of the photon with the electron in the medium.

There are three modes of interaction with the medium.

The Photoelectric Effect. The photon interaction with an orbital electron in the medium is complete and the full energy of the photon is given to the electron.

The Compton Effect. Part of the photon energy is transferred to an electron and the photon scatters (usually at a small angle from its original path) (Evans, 1955) with reduced energy.

The governing expressions are

$$E' = E \ \ 0.511/(1 + 1/\alpha - \cos \Theta) \tag{8}$$

$$T = E \ \alpha \ (1 - \cos \Theta)/[1 + \alpha(1 - \cos \Theta)]$$

where

$$
\begin{aligned}
E, E' &= \text{initial and scattered photon energy in MeV} \\
T &= \text{kinetic energy of the electron in MeV} \\
\alpha &= E/0.511 \\
\Theta &= \text{angle of photon scatter from its original path.}
\end{aligned}
$$

Pair Production. This occurs whenever the photon energy is greater than the rest mass of two electrons, $2(0.511 \ \text{MeV}) = 1.02 \ \text{MeV}$. The electromagnetic energy of the photon can be converted directly to an electron-positron pair with any excess energy above 1.02 MeV appearing as kinetic energy given to these particles.

The loss of photons and energy loss from a photon beam as it passes through matter is described by two coefficients. The attenuation coefficient determines the fractional loss of photons per unit distance (usually in normalized units of g/cm^2 which is the linear distance times the density of the medium). The mass energy

Table 21–1. STOPPING POWER, RANGE, AND RADIATION YIELD FOR ELECTRONS IN AIR

ENERGY (MeV)	COLLISION (MeV cm² g⁻¹)	STOPPING POWER RADIATIVE (MeV cm² g⁻¹)	TOTAL (MeV cm² g⁻¹)	CSDA RANGE (g cm⁻²)	RADIATION YIELD
0.0100	1.975E+01	3.897E–03	1.976E+01	2.883E–04	1.082E–04
0.0125	1.663E+01	3.921E–03	1.663E+01	4.269E–04	1.299E–04
0.0150	1.445E+01	3.937E–03	1.445E+01	5.886E–04	1.506E–04
0.0175	1.283E+01	3.946E–03	1.283E+01	7.726E–04	1.706E–04
0.0200	1.157E+01	3.954E–03	1.158E+01	9.781E–04	1.898E–04
0.0250	9.753E+00	3.966E–03	9.757E+00	1.451E–03	2.267E–04
0.0300	8.492E+00	3.976E–03	8.496E+00	2.001E–03	2.618E–04
0.0350	7.563E+00	3.986E–03	7.567E+00	2.626E–03	2.955E–04
0.0400	6.848E+00	3.998E–03	6.852E+00	3.322E–03	3.280E–04
0.0450	6.281E+00	4.011E–03	6.285E+00	4.085E–03	3.594E–04
0.0500	5.819E+00	4.025E–03	5.823E+00	4.912E–03	3.900E–04
0.0550	5.435E+00	4.040E–03	5.439E+00	5.801E–03	4.197E–04
0.0600	5.111E+00	4.057E–03	5.115E+00	6.750E–03	4.488E–04
0.0700	4.593E+00	4.093E–03	4.597E+00	8.817E–03	5.049E–04
0.0800	4.198E+00	4.133E–03	4.202E+00	1.110E–02	5.590E–04
0.0900	3.886E+00	4.175E–03	3.890E+00	1.357E–02	6.112E–04
0.1000	3.633E+00	4.222E–03	3.637E+00	1.623E–02	6.618E–04
0.1250	3.172E+00	4.348E–03	3.177E+00	2.362E–02	7.826E–04
0.1500	2.861E+00	4.485E–03	2.865E+00	3.193E–02	8.968E–04
0.1750	2.637E+00	4.633E–03	2.642E+00	4.103E–02	1.006E–03
0.2000	2.470E+00	4.789E–03	2.474E+00	5.082E–02	1.111E–03
0.2500	2.236E+00	5.126E–03	2.242E+00	7.212E–02	1.311E–03
0.3000	2.084E+00	5.495E–03	2.089E+00	9.527E–02	1.502E–03
0.3500	1.978E+00	5.890E–03	1.984E+00	1.199E–01	1.688E–03
0.4000	1.902E+00	6.311E–03	1.908E+00	1.456E–01	1.869E–03
0.4500	1.845E+00	6.757E–03	1.852E+00	1.722E–01	2.048E–03
0.5000	1.802E+00	7.223E–03	1.809E+00	1.995E–01	2.225E–03
0.5500	1.769E+00	7.708E–03	1.776E+00	2.274E–01	2.401E–03
0.6000	1.743E+00	8.210E–03	1.751E+00	2.558E–01	2.577E–03
0.7000	1.706E+00	9.258E–03	1.715E+00	3.135E–01	2.929E–03
0.8000	1.683E+00	1.036E–02	1.694E+00	3.722E–01	3.283E–03
0.9000	1.669E+00	1.151E–02	1.681E+00	4.315E–01	3.638E–03
1.0000	1.661E+00	1.271E–02	1.674E+00	4.912E–01	3.997E–03
1.2500	1.655E+00	1.588E–02	1.671E+00	6.408E–01	4.906E–03
1.5000	1.661E+00	1.927E–02	1.680E+00	7.900E–01	5.836E–03
1.7500	1.672E+00	2.284E–02	1.694E+00	9.382E–01	6.784E–03
2.0000	1.684E+00	2.656E–02	1.711E+00	1.085E+00	7.748E–03
2.5000	1.712E+00	3.437E–02	1.747E+00	1.374E+00	9.716E–03
3.0000	1.740E+00	4.260E–02	1.783E+00	1.658E+00	1.173E–02
3.5000	1.766E+00	5.115E–02	1.817E+00	1.935E+00	1.377E–02

From ICRU, 1984.
I = 85.7 eV; density = 1.205E–03 g/cm³ (20°C).

absorption coefficient determines the fractional energy deposition per unit distance traveled. The loss of photons from the beam is given by

$$I/I_0 = \exp(-\mu/\rho\ d) \qquad (9)$$

where

I = intensity of the photon beam (numbers of photons)
I_o = beam intensity

μ/ρ = attenuation coefficient in the medium for the energy considered (in cm² g⁻¹)
d = thickness of the medium in g cm⁻² (thickness in cm × density).

The energy actually deposited in the medium per unit distance is given by

$$\Delta E = (\mu_{en}/\rho)E_0 \qquad (10)$$

where

Table 21–2.   STOPPING POWER, RANGE, AND RADIATION YIELD FOR ELECTRONS IN MUSCLE TISSUE

ENERGY (MeV)	COLLISION (MeV cm^2 g^{-1})	STOPPING POWER RADIATIVE (MeV cm^2 g^{-1})	TOTAL (MeV cm^2 g^{-1})	CSDA RANGE (g cm^{-2})	RADIATION YIELD
0.0100	2.231E+01	3.835E–03	2.231E+01	2.543E–04	9.366E–05
0.0125	1.876E+01	3.863E–03	1.877E+01	3.771E–04	1.127E–04
0.0150	1.628E+01	3.880E–03	1.629E+01	5.205E–04	1.310E–04
0.0175	1.445E+01	3.892E–03	1.445E+01	6.838E–04	1.485E–04
0.0200	1.303E+01	3.901E–03	1.303E+01	8.662E–04	1.655E–04
0.0250	1.097E+01	3.913E–03	1.098E+01	1.286E–03	1.980E–04
0.0300	9.547E+00	3.924E–03	9.551E+00	1.776E–03	2.290E–04
0.0350	8.498E+00	3.934E–03	8.502E+00	2.332E–03	2.587E–04
0.0400	7.692E+00	3.946E–03	7.696E+00	2.951E–03	2.874E–04
0.0450	7.052E+00	3.959E–03	7.056E+00	3.631E–03	3.151E–04
0.0500	6.531E+00	3.973E–03	6.535E+00	4.368E–03	3.421E–04
0.0550	6.099E+00	3.988E–03	6.102E+00	5.160E–03	3.683E–04
0.0600	5.733E+00	4.004E–03	5.737E+00	6.006E–03	3.939E–04
0.0700	5.151E+00	4.040E–03	5.155E+00	7.848E–03	4.435E–04
0.0800	4.706E+00	4.079E–03	4.710E+00	9.881E–03	4.912E–04
0.0900	4.355E+00	4.122E–03	4.359E+00	1.209E–02	5.373E–04
0.1000	4.071E+00	4.168E–03	4.075E+00	1.447E–02	5.821E–04
0.1250	3.552E+00	4.294E–03	3.557E+00	2.106E–02	6.889E–04
0.1500	3.203E+00	4.431E–03	3.207E+00	2.848E–02	7.899E–04
0.1750	2.951E+00	4.579E–03	2.956E+00	3.662E–02	8.865E–04
0.2000	2.763E+00	4.734E–03	2.768E+00	4.537E–02	9.795E–04
0.2500	2.501E+00	5.070E–03	2.506E+00	6.442E–02	1.157E–03
0.3000	2.329E+00	5.438E–03	2.335E+00	8.513E–02	1.327E–03
0.3500	2.211E+00	5.832E–03	2.216E+00	1.071E–01	1.492E–03
0.4000	2.125E+00	6.252E–03	2.131E+00	1.302E–01	1.653E–03
0.4500	2.061E+00	6.694E–03	2.068E+00	1.540E–01	1.812E–03
0.5000	2.012E+00	7.158E–03	2.019E+00	1.785E–01	1.970E–03
0.5500	1.972E+00	7.642E–03	1.980E+00	2.035E–01	2.128E–03
0.6000	1.941E+00	8.141E–03	1.949E+00	2.290E–01	2.285E–03
0.7000	1.895E+00	9.186E–03	1.904E+00	2.809E–01	2.602E–03
0.8000	1.863E+00	1.028E–02	1.874E+00	3.339E–01	2.921E–03
0.9000	1.842E+00	1.143E–02	1.853E+00	3.876E–01	3.244E–03
1.0000	1.827E+00	1.262E–02	1.839E+00	4.418E–01	3.571E–03
1.2500	1.806E+00	1.578E–02	1.822E+00	5.784E–01	4.408E–03
1.5000	1.799E+00	1.916E–02	1.818E+00	7.158E–01	5.272E–03
1.7500	1.799E+00	2.271E–02	1.821E+00	8.532E–01	6.162E–03
2.0000	1.801E+00	2.642E–02	1.828E+00	9.903E–01	7.074E–03
2.5000	1.812E+00	3.421E–02	1.846E+00	1.263E+00	8.956E–03
3.0000	1.824E+00	4.241E–02	1.866E+00	1.532E+00	1.090E–02
3.5000	1.836E+00	5.095E–02	1.887E+00	1.798E+00	1.289E–02

From ICRU, 1984.
I = 75.3 eV; Density = 1.040E+00 g/cm^3

ΔE = energy loss in the medium per unit distance (in MeV cm^2 g^{-1})

μ_{en}/ρ = mass energy absorption coefficient (cm^2 g^{-1})

E_0 = initial photon energy

Tables 21–3 and 21–4 give the attenuation coefficients for photons in air and the mass energy absorption coefficients for photons in air and in muscle tissue. Both tables are reproduced from Hubbell (1969).

ABSORBED DOSE

Dose and Dose Rate

Absorbed dose is defined as the mean energy, e, imparted by ionizing radiation to matter of mass m (ICRU 1980)

$$D = e/m \qquad (11)$$

where

Table 21–3. **MASS ATTENUATION COEFFICIENTS FOR PHOTONS IN AIR**

PHOTON ENERGY (MeV)	SCATTERING With Coherent (cm^2/g^{-1})	SCATTERING Without Coherent (cm^2/g^{-1})	PHOTO-ELECTRIC (cm^2/g^{-1})	PAIR PRODUCTION Nuclear Field (cm^2/g^{-1})	PAIR PRODUCTION Electron Field (cm^2/g^{-1})	TOTAL With Coherent (cm^2/g^{-1})	TOTAL Without Coherent (cm^2/g^{-1})
1.00–02	3.64–01	1.93–01	4.63+00			4.99+00	4.82+00
1.50–02	2.85–01	1.89–01	1.27+00			1.55+00	1.45+00
2.00–02	2.47–01	1.86–01	5.05–01			7.52–01	6.91–01
3.00–02	2.11–01	1.80–01	1.39–01			3.49–01	3.18–01
4.00–02	1.93–01	1.74–01	5.53–02			2.48–01	2.29–01
5.00–02	1.81–01	1.69–01	2.70–02			2.08–01	1.96–01
6.00–02	1.73–01	1.64–01	1.52–02			1.88–01	1.79–01
8.00–02	1.61–01	1.56–01	6.06–03			1.67–01	1.62–01
1.00–01	1.51–01	1.48–01	2.94–03			1.54–01	1.51–01
1.50–01	1.35–01	1.33–01	8.05–04			1.36–01	1.34–01
2.00–01	1.23–01	1.22–01	3.24–04			1.23–01	1.23–01
3.00–01	1.07–01	1.06–01	9.30–05			1.07–01	1.06–01
4.00–01	9.53–02	9.52–02	3.99–05			9.54–02	9.53–02
5.00–01	8.70–02	8.70–02	2.15–05			8.70–02	8.70–02
6.00–01	8.05–02	8.04–02	1.34–05			8.05–02	8.05–02
8.00–01		7.07–02	6.79–06				7.07–02
1.00+00		6.36–02	4.20–06				6.36–02
1.50+00		5.17–02	1.96–06	9.89–05			5.18–02
2.00+00		4.41–02	1.25–06	3.94–04			4.45–02
3.00+00		3.47–02	6.97–07	1.13–03	1.21–05		3.58–02
4.00+00		2.89–02	4.73–07	1.83–03	4.97–05		3.08–02
5.00+00		2.50–02	3.61–07	2.46–03	9.76–05		2.75–02
6.00+00		2.21–02	2.88–07	3.01–03	1.50–04		2.52–02
8.00+00		1.81–02	2.06–07	3.94–03	2.57–04		2.23–02
1.00+01		1.54–02	1.61–07	4.70–03	3.51–04		2.04–02
1.50+01		1.14–02		6.14–03	5.47–04		1.81–02
2.00+01		9.14–03		7.18–03	7.02–04		1.70–02
3.00+01		6.65–03		8.65–03	9.35–04		1.62–02
4.00+01		5.28–03		9.67–03	1.11–03		1.61–02
5.00+01		4.41–03		1.04–02	1.24–03		1.61–02
6.00+01		3.80–03		1.11–02	1.36–03		1.62–02
8.00+01		3.00–03		1.20–02	1.53–03		1.65–02
1.00+02		2.55–03		1.26–02	1.65–03		1.68–02
1.50+02		1.77–03		1.38–02	1.87–03		1.74–02
2.00+02		1.39–03		1.45–02	2.02–03		1.79–02
3.00+02		9.85–04		1.53–02	2.22–03		1.85–02
4.00+02		7.71–04		1.58–02	2.34–03		1.89–02
5.00+02		6.38–04		1.61–02	2.43–03		1.92–02
6.00+02		5.47–04		1.63–02	2.50–03		1.94–02
8.00+02		4.27–04		1.67–02	2.60–03		1.97–02
1.00+03		3.51–04		1.69–02	2.67–03		1.99–02
1.50+03		2.45–04		1.72–02	2.79–03		2.02–02
2.00+03		1.90–04		1.73–02	2.86–03		2.04–02
3.00+03		1.32–04		1.75–02	2.95–03		2.06–02
4.00+03		1.02–04		1.76–02	2.99–03		2.07–02
5.00+03		8.33–05		1.77–02	3.02–03		2.08–02
6.00+03		7.07–05		1.77–02	3.05–03		2.08–02
8.00+03		5.44–05		1.78–02	3.08–03		2.09–02
1.00+04		4.44–05		1.78–02	3.10–03		2.09–02
1.50+04		3.07–05		1.78–02	3.12–03		2.10–02
2.00+04		2.36–05		1.79–02	3.14–03		2.10–02
3.00+04		1.63–05		1.79–02	3.15–03		2.11–02
4.00+04		1.25–05		1.79–02	3.16–03		2.11–02
5.00+04		1.02–05		1.79–02	3.17–03		2.11–02
6.00+04		8.60–06		1.79–02	3.17–03		2.11–02
8.00+04		6.60–06		1.79–02	3.18–03		2.11–02
1.00+05		5.37–06		1.79–02	3.18–03		2.11–02

From Hubbell, 1969.

Table 21–4.   MASS ENERGY ABSORPTION COEFFICIENTS FOR AIR AND WATER

PHOTON ENERGY (MeV)	AIR μ_{en}/ρ (m^2 kg^{-1})	MUSCLE, STRIATED (ICRU) μ_{en}/ρ (m^2 kg^{-1})
0.01	0.46	0.49
0.015	0.13	0.14
0.02	0.052	0.055
0.03	0.015	0.016
0.04	0.0067	0.0070
0.05	0.0040	0.0043
0.06	0.0030	0.0032
0.08	0.0024	0.0026
0.10	0.0023	0.0025
0.15	0.0025	0.0027
0.20	0.0027	0.0029
0.30	0.0029	0.0032
0.40	0.0029	0.0032
0.50	0.0030	0.0033
0.60	0.0030	0.0033
0.80	0.0029	0.0032
1.00	0.0028	0.0031
1.50	0.0025	0.0028
2.00	0.0023	0.0026
3.00	0.0021	0.0023

From Hubbell, 1982.

D = absorbed dose
e = mean energy deposited in mass
m = mass.

The unit for absorbed dose is the Gray (Gy) and is equal to 1 J kg^{-1}. The older unit of dose is the rad and is equal to 100 erg g^{-1}. The conversion for these units is 100 rad = 1 Gy.

For uncharged particles (gamma rays and neutrons), kerma is sometimes used. It is the sum of the initial kinetic energies of all the charged ionizing particles liberated in unit mass. The units of kerma are the same as for dose.

Exposure is often confused with absorbed dose. Exposure is defined only in air for gamma rays or photons and is the charge of the ions of one sign when all electrons liberated by photons are completely stopped in air of mass m.

$$X = Q/m \qquad (12)$$

where

X = exposure
Q = total charge of one sign
m = mass of air.

The unit of exposure is the Coulomb per kilogram of air. The older unit of exposure is the Roentgen which is equal to 2.58 × 10^{-4} C kg^{-1} of air.

Exposure and dose are used interchangeably in some publications even though this is not correct. The reason is that the older numerical values of dose in rad and exposure in Roentgen are similar. Although they are similar numerically they are fundamentally different in that exposure is ionization (only in air) and dose is absorbed energy in any specified medium.

1 Roentgen = 0.87 rad (in air)

The SI units are not numerically similar,

1 C kg^{-1} = 33.85 Gy

Dose rate is the dose expressed per unit time interval. The dose rate delivered to the thyroid by ^{99m}Tc for a nuclear medicine scan, for example, is diminishing with time due to the 6.0-hour half-life of the nuclide. The total dose is a more pertinent quantity in this case because it can be related directly to risk and compared with the benefit of the thyroid scan.

The dose rate from natural body ^{40}K in all cells, on the other hand, is relatively constant throughout life and is usually expressed as the annual dose rate.

Dose Equivalent

The linear energy transfer (LET) from alpha and beta particles is much greater than for gamma rays. In considering the health or cellular effects of each particle or ray, it is convenient to normalize the various types of radiation. For a particular biologic end point, such as cell death in an experiment with mouse fibroblasts, it is common to calculate a relative biologic effectiveness (RBE). This is defined as the ratio of the gamma dose to the dose from radiation under study which yields the same end point.

Such refinement in the normalization of end points (cancer) in the human is not possible with the available data. An attempt to normalize human health effects is made through the values for linear energy transfer of the various types of radiation in water. The ratio of the LET for gamma to the radiation in question is defined as a quality factor, Q, and the normalized dose is called the dose equivalent. The unit for the dose equivalent is the Sievert and the older unit the rem.

$$H = D\,Q \qquad (13)$$

where

H = dose equivalent in Sievert (older unit rem)
D = dose in Gray (older unit rad)
Q = quality factor.

Table 21–5 is reproduced from NCRP (1987).
Example 3. Find the dose equivalent (in Sievert) for a dose to lung from an internal emitter of 0.01-Gy alpha particles and 0.01 Gy from external gamma-ray radiation.

alpha $H = 0.01\,(20) = 0.20$ Sv
gamma $H = 0.01\,(1)\ \ = 0.01$ Sv

Effective Dose Equivalent and Cancer Risk

The term effective dose equivalent (EDE) was introduced formally by ICRP in 1977 to be able to add or directly compare the cancer and genetic risk from different partial body or whole body doses. A partial body dose to the lung, for ex-

ample, was thought to give 0.002 cancers over a lifetime per Sievert whereas a whole body dose would result in 0.0165 total cancers and early genetic effects over the same lifetime interval. The ratio 0.002/0.016 was defined as a weighting factor, w_t, for lung and is numerically equal to 0.12.

The effective dose equivalent (EDE), H_E, is defined as

$$H_E = w_t\,D\,Q \qquad (14)$$

This concept was useful in the case of occupational exposure because EDE values from different sources can be simply summed to yield a direct estimate of total cancer and genetic risk.

Table 21–6 is taken from NCRP (1987) and gives the values of w_t for various organs.

The occupational guideline for EDE is 50 mSv per annum (NCRP, 1987; ICRP, 1977). This requires that the sum of all EDE be less than or equal to this value, namely,

$$H_E = \Sigma\,w_t\,H \le 50 \text{ mSv} \qquad (15)$$

Committed Dose Equivalent

A problem arises with internal emitters in that once ingested there is an irreversible dose that is committed because of the biokinetics of the particular element. The absorbed dose depends on the biologic and physical half-times of the element in the body. For this reason the concepts of committed dose equivalent and committed effective dose equivalent were derived to accommodate the potential for dose to be delivered over long times after incorporation in the body. The committed dose is taken over a 50-year interval after exposure and is equal to

Table 21–5. RECOMMENDED VALUES OF Q FOR VARIOUS TYPES OF RADIATION

TYPE OF RADIATION	APPROXIMATE Q
X rays, gamma rays, beta particles and electrons	1
Thermal neutrons	5
Neutrons (other than thermal), protons, alpha particles, charged particles of unknown energy	20

NCRP, 1987.

Table 21–6. RECOMMENDED VALUES OF THE WEIGHTING FACTORS, w_t, FOR CALCULATING EFFECTIVE DOSE EQUIVALENT AND THE RISK COEFFICIENTS FROM WHICH THEY WERE DERIVED

TISSUE	RISK COEFFICIENT (Sv^{-1})	w_t
Gonads	0.0040	0.25
Breast	0.0025	0.15
Red bone marrow	0.0020	0.12
Lung	0.0020	0.12
Thyroid	0.0005	0.03
Bone surfaces	0.0005	0.03
Remainder	0.0050	0.30
Total	0.0165	1.0

Values from ICRP, 1977.

$$H_{T,50} = \int_{t_0}^{t_0+50} H_T \, dt \qquad (16)$$

where

$H_{T,50}$ = the 50-year dose to tissue T, for a single intake at time t_0

H_T = is the dose equivalent rate in organ or tissue T at time t.

NCRP (1987) recognizes that for radionuclides with half-lives ranging up to about three months the committed dose equivalent is equal to the annual dose for the year of intake. For longer lived nuclides the committed dose equivalent will be greater than the annual dose equivalent and must be calculated on an individual basis. ICRP Publication 30 (ICRP, 1978) provides the details of this calculation for all nuclides.

Negligible Individual Risk Level

The current radiobiologic principle commonly accepted is that of linear, nonthreshold cancer induction from ionizing radiation. Thus, regardless of the magnitude of the dose a numerical cancer risk can be calculated. For this reason the National Council on Radiation Protection and Measurements proposed the Negligible Individual Risk Level (NIRL) and defined it as

a level of annual excess risk of fatal health effects attributable to irradiation below which further effort to reduce radiation exposure to the individual is unwarranted.

NCRP emphasized that the NIRL is not to be confused with an acceptable risk level, a level of significance, or a limit.

The NCRP recommended an annual effective dose equivalent limit for continuous exposure of members of the public of 1 mSv (0.1 rem). This value is in addition to that received from natural background radiation (about 2 mSv). In this context the NIRL was taken to be 0.01 mSv (1 mrem).

HUMAN STUDIES OF RADIATION TOXICITY

There are five major studies of the health detriment resulting from exposure of humans to ionizing radiation. Other studies of large worker populations exposed to very low levels of radiation and environmental populations exposed to radon are ongoing but these are not expected to provide new data on the risk estimates from ionizing radiation. These latter worker or environmental populations are studied to ensure

that there is no inconsistency in the radiation risk data in extrapolating from the higher exposures.

The basic studies on which the quantitative risk calculations are founded include the radium exposures, the atom bomb survivors, the underground miners exposed to radon, patients irradiated with X rays for ankylosing spondylitis, and children irradiated with X rays for tinea capitis (ringworm).

Radium Exposures (^{226,228}Ra)

Radium was discovered in the early part of the twentieth century. Its unique properties suggested a potential for the healing arts. It was incorporated into a wide variety of nostrums, medicines, and artifacts. The highest exposure occurred in the United States in the radium dial painters who ingested from 10s to 1000s of micrograms (microcuries). These exposed groups including patients, chemists, dial painters, and so forth have been studied for over 60 years to determine the body retention of radium and the health effects of long-term body burdens.

The only late effect of ingestion of ^{226,228}Ra seen is osteogenic sarcoma. It is significant that no study has ever identified a statistically significant excess of leukemia following even massive doses of radium. This implies that the target cells for leukemia residing in bone marrow are outside the short range of the radium series alpha particles (70 μm).

Several thousand people were exposed to radium salts either as part of the modish therapies using radium in the era from 1900 to 1930 or occupationally in the radium dial painting industry around 1920. Radium therapy was accepted by the American Medical Association and around 1915 advertisements were common for radium treatment of rheumatism and as a general tonic and in the treatment of mental disorders. Solutions were available for drinking containing 2 μg/60 cm^3 as well as ampoules for intravenous injection containing 5 to 100 μg radium (Woodard, 1980). Luminous paint was developed before World War I and in 1917 there were many plants in New England and New Jersey painting watch dials, clocks, and military instruments (Woodard, 1980).

The first large studies on osteogenic sarcoma in radium-exposed people were done by Martland (1931) and Aub et al. (1952), who found 30 cases of bone sarcoma; Evans (1969) with 496 cases of sarcoma out of 1064 studied at the Massachusetts Institute of Technology; and Rowland et al. (1978), 61 cases out of 1474 female dial painters (Woodard 1980).

Radium, once ingested, is somewhat similar to calcium in its metabolism and is incorporated on bone surfaces into the mineralized portion of

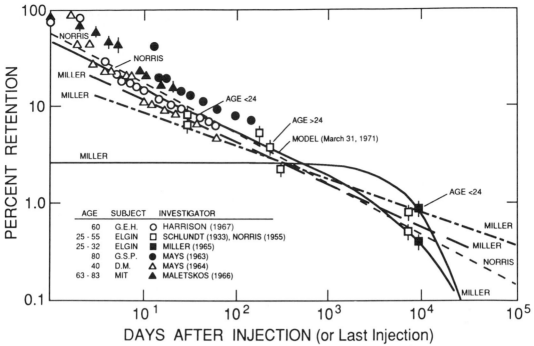

Figure 21–1. Whole body radium retention in humans. Summary of all available data for adult man. (From Marshall *et al.*, 1972.)

bone. The long half-life of ^{226}Ra allows distribution throughout the mineral skeleton over life. The target cells for osteogenic sarcoma reside in marrow on endosteal surfaces at about 10 μm from the bone surface. At long times post exposure, target cells are beyond the range of alpha particles from radium not on bone surfaces.

The loss of radium from the body by excretion was determined to follow a relatively simple power function (Norris, 1955).

$$R = 0.54 \, t^{-0.52} \tag{17}$$

where

R = total body retention
t = time in days.

Other models to fit the data were developed as more information became available, the most recent being that of Marshall *et al.* (1972). The entire body of radium data and the various models are shown in Figure 21–1. It can be seen that the Norris function fits the observed data well except at very long times post exposure. A simplified form of the more complex later model of Marshall *et al.* (1972) which fits the human data over all observed times is

$$R = 0.8t^{-0.5} \, (0.5 \, e^{-\lambda t} + 0.5 \, e^{-4\lambda t}) \tag{18}$$

where

R = whole body retention
λ = rate of bone apposition or resorption
    = 0.0001 day^{-1}
t = time in days.

For most purposes the Norris formula is applicable. It can be seen from Figure 21–1 for the Norris equation that, even one year after exposure, only about 2 percent of the radium is retained in the body but after 30 years about 0.5 percent still remains.

The risk of osteogenic bone cancer following radium exposure has been summarized in the National Academy of Sciences Report BEIR IV (NAS, 1988).

Equations were proposed by Rowland *et al.* (1978) for the annual risk of sarcoma (including the natural risk) expressed as a function of either radium intake or dose from ^{226,228}Ra. Risk per unit intake:

$$I = [0.7 \times 10^{-5} + (7 \times 10^{-8})D^2] \exp[-(1.1 \times 10^{-3})D] \tag{19}$$

where

I = total bone sarcomas per person year at risk

D = total systemic intake of [226]Ra plus 2.5 times the total systemic intake of [228]Ra, both in microcuries.

Risk per unit dose:

$$I = [10^{-5} + 9.8 \times 10^{-6}D^2] \exp(-1.5 \times 10^{-2}D) \quad (20)$$

where

I = total bone sarcomas per person year at risk

D = total mean skeletal dose in Gray from [226]Ra plus 1.5 times the mean skeletal dose from [228]Ra.

Raabe *et al.* (1980) modeled bone sarcoma risk in the human, dog, and mouse and have determined that there is a practical threshold dose and dose rate (a dose low enough so that bone cancer will not appear within the human life span). The dose rate is 0.04 Gy per day or a total dose of 0.8 Gy to the skeleton. This practical threshold for bone cancer has useful implications in considering health effects from exposures to environmental radioactivity.

Radium Exposure ([224]Ra)

In Europe, [224]Ra was used for more than 40 years in the treatment of tuberculosis and ankylosing spondylitis. The treatment of children was abandoned in the 1950s but the relief of debilitating pain from ankylosing spondylitis in adults has prolonged its use. [224]Ra is different from [226]Ra in that it has a short half-life (3.62 days) and the alpha dose is delivered completely while the radium is still on bone surfaces.

Spiess and Mays (1970) and Mays (1988) studied the health of 900 German patients given [224]Ra therapeutically. The calculated average mean skeletal dose was 4.2 Gy (range 0.06 to 57.5 Gy) with injection time spans ranging from 1 to 45 months. There were two groups, juveniles and adults, and the bone sarcoma response was not significantly different for the two. There were 54 patients who developed bone sarcoma, the last one occurring in 1983.

In a second cohort, Wick *et al.* (1986) studied 1432 adult patients treated for ankylosing spondylitis with an average skeletal dose of 0.65 Gy. This study was originally started by Otto Hug and Fritz Schales and has been continued following their deaths. Two patients in this group have developed osteogenic sarcoma with none in the control group.

Spiess and Mays (1973) found that the observed effectiveness of the [224]Ra in their cohort in producing bone sarcomas increased if the time span of the injections was long. In-

jections were given in 1, 10, or 50 weekly fractions. They developed an empirical expression to estimate the added risk from this protracted injection schedule,

$$I = \{0.003 + 0.014 [1 - \exp(0.09m)]D \quad (21)$$

where

I = cumulative incidence of bone sarcomas after most tumors have appeared (25 years)

m = span of injections in months

D = average skeletal dose in Gy.

Chemelevsky (1986) analyzed the Spiess data and developed an equation for the total cumulative sarcoma risk from [224]Ra,

$$R = (0.0085D + 0.0017D^2) \exp(-0.025D) \quad (22)$$

where

R = cumulative risk of bone sarcoma

D = average skeletal dose in Gy.

These two equations for risk predict 5.7 and 5.8 bone sarcomas in the second series of (spondylitis) patients, with two actually observed.

Chemelevsky (1986) also showed that, in the Spiess study, linearity (sarcoma response with dose) could be rejected. For example, equation 22 results in a lifetime risk of sarcoma of 0.02 Gy^{-1} at an average skeletal dose of 10 Gy but 0.01 Gy^{-1} at 1 Gy. Also, there was no difference in sarcoma response between juveniles and adults. These data are presented in Figure 21–2.

Again, no excess leukemia was found in either series of [224]Ra patients.

Atomic Bomb Survivors

On August 6, 1945, the United States military dropped an atomic bomb on the city of Hiroshi-

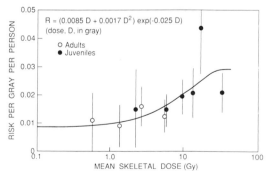

Figure 21–2. Lifetime risk per Gray versus mean skeletal dose in [224]Ra exposed subjects. (From Chemelevsky *et al.*, 1986.)

ma, Japan. Three days later a second bomb was dropped on Nagasaki which effectively ended World War II. The weapons were of two different types the first being ^{235}U and the second a ^{239}Pu device.

Within one kilometer of the explosions in both cities, a total of 64,000 people were killed by the blast, thermal effects, and as a result of the instantaneous gamma and neutron radiation released by the weapons. Others between 1 and 2 kilometers received radiation doses up to several Gray.

Within a few years it was decided to follow the health of the people in both cities over their lifetime to determine quantitatively the effects of external ionizing radiation.

The study of prospective mortality of atom bomb survivors was initiated by the Atomic Bomb Casualty Commission (ABCC) in 1950 and is ongoing by the Radiation Effects Research Foundation (RERF). The main study, called the Life Span Study (LSS), included 92,228 people within 10,000 meters of the hypocenter (the point on earth directly below the detonation point in air) and 26,850 people who were not in either city at the time of bombing (ATB). The most recent report of the RERF (1988) is a follow-up of the cancer mortality of a subcohort (DS86 subcohort) of 75,991 persons over the period 1950–85.

In 1978, questions arose that the original dose estimates for persons in the LSS might be somewhat in error and that an effort should be made to improve the dose estimates. This study is now complete and the dosimetry is published in a United States–Japan joint reassessment of dose called DS86—Dosimetry System 1986 (RERF, 1986).

Dose estimation by reconstruction of the event is always problematical but direct computation of dose to about 18,500 persons in the LSS with detailed shielding information is complete. The remaining DS86 dose values for 57,000 individuals without detailed shielding information are also incorporated into the mortality study by various estimation techniques. Of the 75,991 persons in the DS86 subcohort, 16,207 were within 2000 meters of the hypocenter and these are the individuals who received a substantial exposure.

Previous reports of cancer risk estimates were based on the air dose (gamma ray plus neutron tissue kerma in air) adjusted for shielding by structures or terrain. The 1987 and 1988 reports also include DS86 organ dose estimates and these are about 80 percent of the shielded kerma.

The dose from fallout at Hiroshima and Nagasaki has not been included in the health effects studies. Fallout was found in certain restricted localities in Nagasaki and in Hiroshima. The absorbed dose from gamma rays at Nagasaki for persons continuously in the fallout area from one hour on ranged from 0.12 to 0.24 Gy. The absorbed doses at Hiroshima ranged from 0.006 to 0.02 Gy. Because the region of fallout was quite limited, it would appear that the total contribution of fallout to survivor dose was probably negligible in Hiroshima but may have been significant for a limited number of survivors in Nagasaki where an exposure of one-fifth the maximum extends over some 1000 hectares. Estimates of internal dose from ingested ^{137}Cs yield about 0.0001 Gy integrated over 40 years (Harley, 1987; RERF, 1987).

Complete mortality data and the dose estimates are reported in RERF Technical Reports 5-88 (RERF, 1988) and so it is possible to calculate the lifetime cancer risk as of the follow-up through 1985. This is done for this chapter in Table 21–7. The dose used in the calculation is the shielded kerma dose so that it is more comparable with the older publications. The organ dose estimates are about 80% of the shielded kerma dose and so the risk estimates would increase by about 20 percent if organ dose were utilized (Shimizu et al., 1988). However, when the organ dose equivalent is calculated, the organ dose equivalent in Sievert is almost identical to the organ dose in Gray. This is due to the small neutron component in the DS86 dosimetry (about 1 percent of the organ gamma-ray dose). When multiplied by a value of 20 for Q the neutron dose increases the total organ dose equivalent by 20 percent.

No statistically significant excess cancer of the gall bladder, pancreas, uterus, or prostate or of malignant lymphoma has been seen in the LSS to date.

The previous cancer risk estimates, reproduced in Table 21–6, were published by ICRP in 1977 and were based on earlier follow-up of the atom bomb survivors and utilized air dose. The calculations shown here in Table 21–7 are preliminary and the increase in risk is due to differences between the older dose and the DS86 estimates as well as the added number of cancers observed since the previous update in the mortality studies. The leukemia risk is about a factor of three higher than that projected by ICRP in 1977, and the lung cancer risk about a factor of 2 higher.

It is of interest to consider the effects of smoking as it is the most important factor in assessing lung cancer risk. The analysis performed by Shimuzu et al. (1988) examined the interaction of smoking and radiation in detail. The results showed no interaction indicating that smoking and the atom bomb radiation act independently

Table 21–7. CANCER MORTALITY AND LIFETIME CANCER RISK AT SELECTED SITES FOR ATOM-BOMB SURVIVORS WITH AVERAGE SHIELDED KERMA OF 0.295 Gy[||]

SITE	NUMBER OF SUBJECTS[*] (0.01+) Gy	TOTAL CA MORTALITY[*]	ATTRIBUTABLE RISK (%)[†]	RADIATION CANCERS	LIFETIME[‡] RISK (Gy^{-1})
All sites	41,719	3435	10.4	357	0.029
All sites (except leukemia)	41,719	3291	8.0	265	0.022
Leukemia	40,701	144	56.6	81	0.0067
Multiple myeloma	(40,701)[§]	23	32.9	8	0.0007
Colon	39,859	129	15.2	20	0.0017
Esophagus	(39,859)[§]	93	12.8	12	0.0010
Lung	40,382	385	11.6	45	0.0038
Stomach	39,961	1153	6.4	74	0.0063
Female breast	25,252	98	22.4	22	0.0029
Bladder	40,060	84	23.4	20	0.0017
Ovary	24,581	51	18.6	9	0.0012

[*] From RERF Report TR-12-87 Part 1, Tables 2 and 3.
[†] From RERF Report TR-12-87 Part 1, Table 6. Attributable risk is the percent of cancer deaths caused by radiation.
[‡] Lifetime risk Gy^{-1} is calculated as (radiation cancers)/(number of subjects) (average dose).
[§] Estimated as the leukemia or colon population.
[||] Average organ dose equivalent in Sievert is essentially identical to shielded air dose in Gray. See text.

rather than multiplicatively in lung cancer induction.

It is also possible to model the risk over full life if a projection model is assumed. RERF has preferred a constant relative risk model (radiation mortality is a constant fraction of the baseline age specific mortality per Gray) for this purpose. There is evidence in the atom bomb mortality and in several other studies discussed later (ankylosing spondylitis patients, uranium miners) that the constant relative risk model is not appropriate, but that the risk coefficient decreases with time subsequent to exposure. In most cases this also means that the absolute excess cancer risk (risk above that expected) declines with time. This is a biologically plausible model suggesting the loss or repair of the damaged stem cell population.

The National Academy of Sciences BEIR V Committee (NAS, 1990) utilized the atom bomb mortality data through 1985 and the DS86 dosimetry to model the lifetime risk of all cancer, leukemia, female breast, respiratory, and digestive cancer. The expressions for respiratory, breast, and digestive cancer all include a term for reduction in relative risk with time since exposure. For example, the model for respiratory cancer is

$$\gamma(d) = \gamma_0 [1 + f(d)\, g(\beta)] \qquad (23)$$

where

$\gamma(d) =$ an individual's age specific lung cancer risk for dose d

$\gamma_0 =$ the age specific background risk of death due to lung cancer
$f(d) = 0.636 \times$ (dose in Gray)
$g(\beta) = \exp[-1.437 \ln(T/20) + \beta_2 I(S)]$
$T =$ years after exposure
$I(S) = 1$ if female, 0 if male.

The integration of this model yields a lifetime risk of respiratory cancer in males of 0.002, 0.0124, and 0.039 for exposure to 1 Gray at ages 5, 25, and 55, or a risk of 0.019 for a stationary male population with United States mortality rates. Given the existing risk in the Japanese cohort of 0.0038 Gy^{-1}, the BEIR V lifetime risk estimate is clearly conservative.

The lifetime risk of cancer from exposure to atom bomb radiation estimated by the National Academy of Sciences BEIR V Committee is four times that of the BEIR III Committee values (NAS, 1980). The reason for this difference is due partly to more complete follow-up of the population and the difference in the new DS86 dosimetry, but primarily to the models used for risk expression following exposure. Given the small number of radiation induced cancer in the Japanese population studied, the models cannot be derived with a high degree of certainty.

The estimates of lifetime risk of cancer will undoubtedly increase somewhat with time, but given the present age of the population, the final values are unlikely to be higher than about a factor of three from the original 1977 values in Table 21–6.

Tinea Capitis (Ringworm) Irradiation

During the period 1905–60, X-ray epilation in the treatment of tinea capitis was performed regularly in children. The treatment was introduced by Sabouraud in 1904 and was standardized by Kienbock (1907) and Adamson (1910). Over the half century it was used, as many as 200,000 children worldwide may have been irradiated (Albert *et al.*, 1986).

No follow-up studies of the long-term effects of irradiation were performed until Albert and Omran (1968) reported on 2200 children irradiated at the Skin and Cancer Unit of New York University Hospital during 1940–59. Subsequent publications on this group have appeared at regular intervals (Shore *et al.*, 1976, 1984).

Since the New York University (NYU) study, a follow-up of 11,000 children irradiated in Israel was performed (Ron and Modan, 1984).

The mean age of children irradiated in both the New York and Israeli studies was between 7 and 8 years. Dose reconstruction in the New York University series was performed using a head phantom containing the skull of a 7-year-old child covered with tissue-equivalent material (Schulz and Albert, 1963; Harley *et al.*, 1976, 1983). The doses to organs in the head and neck for a typical Adamson-Kienbock five-field treatment of the scalp are shown in Table 21–8 and the dose to the skin is shown in Figure 21–3.

In the NYU series there were eight thyroid adenomas and no thyroid cancer. In the Israeli series there were 29 thyroid cancers. In the NYU series there are 80 skin lesions predominantly basal cell carcinoma in 41 persons. Lightness of skin is an important factor in the appearance of skin cancer (Shore *et al.*, 1984). Skin cancer was found only in caucasians even though 25 percent of the study population were blacks. This and the fact that there appears to be a much lower dose response on the hair covered scalp than on the face and neck (Harley *et al.*, 1983) suggests that

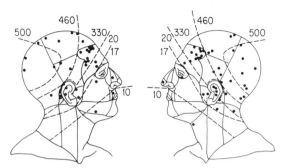

Figure 21–3. X-ray dose in rads for the Adamson-Kienbock five-field tinea capitis treatment and locations of basal cell lesions. (From Shore *et al.*, 1984.)

promotional effects of UV radiation play an important part in skin cancer.

A summary of the tumors of the head and neck and hemopoietic/lymphopoietic tumors for the NYU studies is shown in Table 21–9 and for the Israeli studies in Table 21–10. In the Israeli study the estimate of the dose to the thyroid is 0.09 Gy compared with 0.06 Gy in the NYU study.

A risk projection model was used to estimate the lifetime risk of basal cell carcinoma (BCC) for facial skin and for the hair covered scalp following X-ray epilation in caucasians. The model used was a cumulative hazard plot which assumes that the BCC appearance rate in the exposed population remains constant over time (Harley *et al.*, 1983). The result of this risk projection for BCC is shown in Table 21–11.

The small numbers of tumors other than skin cancers in the NYU study makes it of dubious value to estimate the lifetime risk per Gy although a clear excess is appearing. The tinea capitis studies are prospective and sound numerical values should be forthcoming as the populations age. These are particularly important studies because children were the exposed group and because only partial body irradiation was involved. The temporal pattern of appearance of these tumors is also important. The dose was delivered over a short time interval (minutes at NYU and 5 days in Israel) and lifetime patterns will be indicative of the underlying carcinogenic mechanisms.

The skin and thyroid cancers are of importance in documenting health effects from ionizing radiation. However, both types of cancer are rarely fatal. NCRP (1985) reports that about 10 percent of thyroid cancer is lethal. It is estimated that fatality rate of skin cancer is 1 percent (NCRP, 1990). The lifetime risk per Gray derived by NCRP for total thyroid cancer incidence (0.003 for female and 0.0014 for males for ex-

Table 21–8. AVERAGE DOSE TO ORGANS IN THE HEAD AND NECK FROM MEASUREMENTS PERFORMED WITH A PHANTOM FOR A CHILD'S HEAD

ORGAN	AVERAGE DOSE AT 25 CM TREATMENT DISTANCE (rads)
Scalp	220–540
Brain	140
Eye	16
Internal ear	71
Cranial marrow	385
Pituitary	49
Parotid gland	39
Thyroid	6
Skin (eyelid)	16
Skin (nose)	11
Skin (mid-neck)	9

Table 21–9. TUMORS IN THE NEW YORK UNIVERSITY SERIES OF CHILDHOOD IRRADIATIONS FOR TINEA CAPITIS

TUMOR	IRRADIATED CASES	CONTROL CASES
Neurogenic		
Brain	6	0
Acoustic neuroma	2	0
Neck	2	0
Parotid		
Skin	4	
Basal cell	41	3
Cylindroma	4	0
Other	3	2
Bone (skull/jaw)	4	0
Mouth/larynx		
Papilloma	7	2
Thyroid adenoma		
Male	3	0
Female	5	0
Hemopoietic		
Lymphopoietic		
Leukemia	4	1
Hodgkins disease	5	2
Other lymphoma	2	0

Table 21–10. TUMORS IN THE ISRAELI STUDY BY SEX

TUMOR	IRRADIATED CASES	CONTROL CASES
Leukemia		
Male	6	4
Female	4	1
Thyroid malignancies		
Male	6	1
Female	23	5
CNS (malignant/benign)		
Male	21	3
Female	9	0

From Ron and Modan, 1984.

Table 21–11. LIFETIME RISK ESTIMATES FOR BASAL CELL CARCINOMA (BCC) AND THYROID CANCER FOLLOWING X-RAY IRRADIATION FOR TINEA CAPITIS

	TOTAL INCIDENCE (Risk Gy^{-1})	MORTALITY (Risk Gy^{-1})
Skin malignancies		
(NYU Study)		
BCC (facial skin)	0.32	
BCC (hair covered scalp)	0.01	
Thyroid malignancies		
(Israeli study)		
Male	0.01	0.001
Female	0.04	0.004

Table 21–12.   EXCESS CANCER IN 6158 ANKYLOSING SPONDYLITIS PATIENTS GIVEN A SINGLE X-RAY TREATMENT AS OF THE LAST FOLLOW-UP

SITE	OBS	ESTIMATED EXPOSURE	DOSE (Gy)[†]	LIFETIME (Risk Gy^{-1})
Leukemia	31	6.5	2.9	0.0011
Lung*	101	69.5	1.8–6.8[‡]	0.0008–0.0028
Esophagus	28	12.7	4.2	0.0006
Breast	26	16.0	6.8[§]	0.0015[∥]

* Lung cancer appearing less than five years after exposure is not included as this is less than the minimum latency for tumor expression.
[†] The doses are taken from Lewis *et al.* 1988.
[‡] The dose to the pulmonary lung and main bronchi was estimated as 1.8 Gy and 6.8 Gy, respectively. The majority of lung cancer is bronchogenic and the dose estimates for the main bronchi are probably most pertinent.
[§] The dose to the breast is taken as the dose to the main bronchi.
[∥] The number of women having one X-ray treatment was 1008.

ternal X or gamma radiation for persons under 18 years of age) is about a factor of 10 lower than that reported by Ron and Modan in the tinea capitis irradiations. However, the tinea irradiations were given to children with mean age of about 7 years and in the Israeli study there is apparently an increased sensitivity due to ethnicity.

The effect of ethnicity and sex is also suggested by NCRP (1985) for thyroid cancer. The incidence rates of spontaneous thyroid cancer for persons of Jewish origin in Europe and North America is three to four times that for other racial groups. There is an obvious susceptibility of women for thyroid cancer and adenomas in both the NYU and Israeli tinea capitis studies.

Ankylosing Spondylitis

About 14,000 persons, mostly men, were treated with X rays for ankylosing spondylitis at 87 radiotherapy centers in Great Britain and Northern Ireland between 1935 and 1954. Court Brown and Doll (1957) were the first to report that these patients had a leukemia risk substantially in excess of that for the general population. Subsequent publications have developed the time pattern of appearance not only of leukemia but of solid tumors (Court Brown and Doll, 1959, 1965; Smith and Doll, 1978, 1982; Smith, 1984; Darby *et al.*, 1985, 1987).

A group was selected consisting of 11,776 men and 2335 women all of whom had been treated with X rays either once or twice. About half of the total group received a second X-ray treatment or treatment with thorium. The reports on the ankylosing spondylitis patients attempt to consider health effects from only the first X-ray treatment. For this reason an individual receiving a second treatment is included in their follow-up only until 18 months after the second course (a short enough time so that any malig-

nancies in this interval cannot be ascribed to the second X-ray treatment).

The appearance of excess leukemia is now well documented and solid tumors are also apparent in the population. The part of the body in the direct X-ray beam (spine) received the highest dose but it is thought that other sites received substantial radiation from scatter or from the beam itself.

The importance of this study is in the health effects of partial body exposure and in the temporal pattern of appearance of solid tumors in irradiated adults. Smith and Doll (1978, 1982) and Darby *et al.* (1985, 1987) in the most recent follow-up publications concerning these patients have shown that the excess risk for solid tumors is diminishing with time since exposure, with maximum appearance 5 to 20 years after exposure. This has significant implications for risk projection modeling. Many projection models assume a constant rate of appearance either as an absolute number of tumors per person per unit exposure (constant absolute risk) or as a fraction of the baseline age specific cancer mortality rate (constant relative risk). The emerging pattern is that constant risk models, either absolute or relative, are not correct for certain cancers such as lung cancer.

The dosimetry was redone in 1988 (Lewis *et al.*, 1988) and, although better estimates of dose are now available, it is still the dose which is most uncertain for the cohort. No details of the X-ray machines used to deliver the exposures, such as output, kilovoltage, or half-value layer, are reported.

The excess cancers and the estimate of lifetime cancer risk at three sites in the ankylosing spondylitis cohort are shown in Table 21–12. For the purpose of calculating lifetime risks as of the time of follow-up, the number of persons used here as the individuals at risk is the number actually receiving only one X-ray treatment (6158). This assumes that those followed for 18 months subsequent to the second treatment do not contribute significantly to the malignancies.

The relatively low risk for leukemia (compared with atom bomb survivors) has been suggested to be due to cell sterilization at the high dose delivered. It is also possible that the low risk is due to partial irradiation of the skeletal red marrow. The volume of bone marrow irradiated in the spine, rib, and pelvis is much less than 50 percent of that in whole body irradiation.

The deaths due to causes other than neoplasms in the total cohort is about 30 percent higher than expected. This higher total mortality is of significance in risk modeling as the premature deaths due to competing causes decreases the observed fractional cancer mortality. Thus, the lifetime risk in this population probably underestimates the risk when projecting the effects of exposure in a healthy population.

Uranium Miners

Radon is ubiquitous on earth. It is found outdoors and in all dwellings as a result of the decay of the parent ^{226}Ra which is present in all of earth's minerals.

Although the lung cancer risk from radon exposure in underground miners is firmly documented, and quantitative risk estimates are available, the current interest lies in whether this risk carries over into environmental situations. Radon levels in homes that are comparable to those in mines surely confer risks to the residents. The question remains, can the risks in mines for exposures at higher concentrations over short time periods be used to model risks at lower environmental levels over a lifetime?

Underground Mines. There are four large studies of underground miners exposed to high concentrations of radon and radon daughters and the documentation of excess lung cancer is convincing. The carcinogen in the case of radon is actually the alpha emitting short-lived daughters of radon, ^{218}Po and ^{214}Po. The decay scheme for the entire uranium series, including radon and the daughter species, is shown in Figure 21–6. The daughters are solids and deposit on the bronchial airways during inhalation and exhalation according to the laws of diffusion. As the airway lining (bronchial epithelium) is only 40 μm thick, the alpha particles emitted are able to reach and transfer a significant amount of energy to all of the cells implicated in lung cancer induction. Although the daughters are the carcinogen, the term radon will be used interchangeably for radon daughters as without the parent radon the daughters could not exist for longer than a few hours.

The measurements in mines were usually of the daughter species rather than radon and the term working level (WL) was defined for occupational exposure. It indicated the total potential energy content in one liter of air for complete decay of the short-lived daughters.* The exposure attributed to miners was developed in working level months (WLM) which is the numerical value of WL times the time exposed in multiples of the working month of 170 hours (Holaday et al., 1957).

The follow-up studies from four large underground mining cohorts in Canada, Czechoslovakia, Sweden, and the United States have all produced data to show that the excess lung cancer risk from exposure to radon is about two to three per 10,000 persons per WLM exposure (Radford and Renard, 1984; Hornung and Meinhardt, 1987; Sevc et al., 1988; Muller et al., 1989). Expressed in another way, radon exposure increases the normal age specific lung cancer risk by about 1 percent for each WLM exposure. The latter way of expressing risk brings in the thought that many epidemiologists prefer, that the lung cancer risk is proportional to the normal baseline risk. This means, for example, that the lifetime excess lung cancer risk from radon would be different for smokers and nonsmokers (NAS, 1988).

The actual data from the underground studies are not clear cut with regard to the effect of smoking and it is apparent from more recent data that radon exposure does not simply multiply the baseline risks of the population by a constant factor. This is discussed in the section on risk.

The excess lung cancer risk in each of the exposure cohorts for the four major mining populations as of the date of the last published follow-up are summarized in Figure 21–4 (Harley, 1989). It can be seen in this figure that the range of risks for the same exposure varies by about a factor of six among the different studies. The highest values of excess lung cancer shown are in the Czechoslovakian mines and the lowest in the U.S. Colorado mines.

The differences are probably accounted for by errors in measuring and estimating total exposure. However, the Czech mine atmosphere is reported to contain arsenic as well as radon and the arsenic may contribute to the excess lung cancers observed.

A maximum value of 50 percent lung cancer

---

* One working level is any combination of short-lived daughters in one liter of air that will result in 1.3×10^5 MeV of alpha energy when complete decay occurs. One working level is approximately equal to concentrations of 7400 Bq m^{-3} (200 pCi/liter) of radon in a home and 11000 Bq m^{-3} (300 pCi/liter) in a mine.

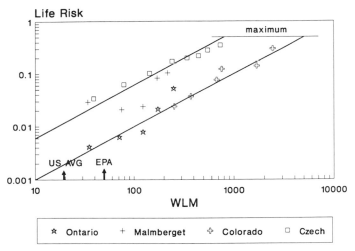

Figure 21–4. Lifetime lung cancer in four underground mining populations as a function of radon exposure. (From Harley, 1989.)

risk is indicated in Figure 21–4. This is the highest value ever observed in a mining population and was reported in the mines in Saxony at the turn of the century (Muller, 1989). These mines are thought to have had about 100,000 Bq m^{-3} of radon. It is noteworthy that concentrations this high have been reported in a few homes in the United States.

In Figure 21–4, the lowest exposures were in the Ontario mines and a mean exposure of 35 WLM has given an excess lung cancer risk of about 0.4 percent to date.

When radon gas decays to the solid daughter products, some 8 to 15 percent of the ^{218}Po does not attach to the normal aerosol particles and this ultrafine species is deposited with 100 percent efficiency on the upper bronchial airways. The rest of the daughters attach to the aerosol of about 100 μm average diameter (George and Breslin, 1980) and only a few percent of this aerosol deposits on these airways.

Measurements in mines have mostly been of the short-lived radon daughters as these are the easiest to measure rapidly. The alpha dose from radon gas itself is very low in comparison with that from the daughters as the daughters deposit and accumulate on the airway surfaces.

The first few branching airways of the bronchial tree are the region where almost all the lung cancers appear. This is true in general and not only for miners exposed to radon daughters. The alpha dose from radon daughters must therefore be calculated in these airways and not in the pulmonary or gas exchange regions. Although the dose to the pulmonary region should not be neglected it is about one-fifth that to the airways.

Several calculations regarding the absorbed alpha dose exist for radon daughters (NCRP,

1984; ICRP, 1987; Harley, 1987, 1989; James, 1987). The authors make different assumptions about the atmospheric and biologic parameters that go into the dose calculation, yet the results are comparable. The most significant variable is the particle size of the ambient aerosol. Very small particles deposit more efficiently in the airways so if small particles, such as from open flame burning (Tu and Knutson, 1988), contribute to the atmosphere, then the dose delivered to the bronchial epithelium can be higher per unit WLM exposure than the dose predicted from an average particle size. Conversely a hygroscopic particle can increase in size in the humid environment of the bronchial airways and deposition will be diminished. The particle size of the aerosol in mines is somewhat larger than that for environmental conditions (200 versus 100 nm; George et al., 1975). Figure 21–5 shows the alpha dose per unit exposure as it is related to the variables (particle size, unattached fraction, nasal deposition) known to affect dose.

As carcinogenesis is related to absorbed alpha dose, Figure 21–5 shows that particle size is an important determinant of risk. The average dose per unit exposure in WLM for miners is also indicated in Figure 21–5 to show that it is somewhat smaller than that for average environmental conditions.

Radon can deliver more or less carcinogenic potential by about a factor of 2 over the range of realistic indoor conditions (average particle size ranging from 80 to 300 nm).

The allowable effective dose equivalent for continuous exposure of the population in the United States is 1 mSv/year (100 mrem/yr, NCRP, 1984, 1987). This limit would be delivered by exposure to 20 Bq m^{-3} of radon or

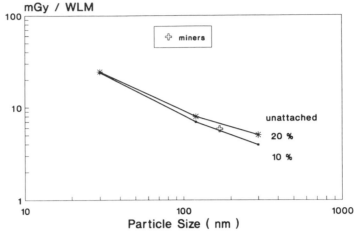

Figure 21–5.   Radon daughter bronchial dose as a function of particle size and percent unattached fraction. (From Harley, 1989.)

one-half the actual average measured indoor concentration in most countries where measurements have been made. Thus, the guidelines for exposure cannot be set in the usual way from dosimetric considerations.

Lifetime Environmental Lung Cancer Risk Projections.   There are at present three sets of publications that provide the risk projection calculations for exposure to radon daughters. The following sections describe each in detail.

National Council on Radiation Protection and Measurements.   In 1984, the U.S. National Council on Radiation Protection and Measurements (NCRP, 1984) developed a model to project the risk derived from the miner studies to whole life risk in the environment. It is a modified absolute risk model that reduces the risk subsequent to exposure with a half-life of 20 years. Risk is not accumulated until after age 40, the time when lung cancer normally appears in the population. There is no indication that early exposure produces any significant shift to younger ages, even for young miners exposed at significantly higher concentrations.

National Academy of Sciences.   The U.S. National Academy of Sciences report in 1988 (BEIR IV) developed a model based on examination of the raw data from five mining cohorts (NAS, 1988). The data indicated that the highest risk appears from 5 to 15 years following exposure. After 15 years, the risk is one-half that of the 5- to 15-year risk (per unit exposure) and persists to the end of life. Again, no significant risk appears before 40, the usual age for the appearance of lung cancer. The NAS model also has a correction for attained age (at age >65 the risk is 0.4 of that for ages 55 to 64). The BEIR IV Committee assumed a relative risk model (risk is a fraction of the normal age specific lung

cancer risk per unit radon exposure with risk dependent on time from exposure. This means that the risk for smokers and nonsmokers differs because of their different baseline lung cancer values. Although the miner epidemiology did not support this strictly multiplicative relationship, the NAS chose the relative risk model as a conservative one. Their analysis supports the risk reduction subsequent to exposure.

ICRP.   The International Commission on Radiation Protection (ICRP, 1987) developed two risk projection models, one based on a constant relative risk and the other a constant absolute risk model. Although neither the constant relative or constant absolute risk model is correct, because of the temporal reduction pattern of lung cancer subsequent to cessation of exposure, the numerical values obtained for the lifetime risk of lung cancer from radon exposure are not significantly different from other models.

Later follow-up of the Czechoslovakian underground uranium miners presented by Kunz and Sevc (1988) indicates that the excess lung cancer risk may actually reduce to zero 35 years after exposure. If this factor were included in the NAS model (zero risk after 35 years) it would reduce their values by about a factor of 2.

The risk values obtained from the three models are shown in Table 21–13.

Environmental Epidemiology.   There are at least 22 published studies attempting to define or detect the effect of radon exposure in the environment. These have been summarized by Borak and Johnson (1988), and by Neuberger (1989). The most recent study was performed in 1989 by the New Jersey Department of Health (NJDOH) in the United States (Schoenberg and Klotz, 1989). This is the most rigorous to date and is a case-control study with 433 lung cancer

Table 21–13. LUNG CANCER RISK FOR CONTINUOUS EXPOSURE TO 1 WLM YR^{-1} (150 Bq m^{-3} OR 4 pCi LITER $^{-1}$) AS PREDICTED BY VARIOUS MODELS

	LIFETIME RISK (%)	MODEL TYPE	COMMENT
NCRP	0.9	Modified absolute	Risk decreases with time from exposure
ICRP	1.6 1.1	Constant relative Constant absolute	No reduction in risk with time from exposure for either model
BEIR IV	3.4 (2.2)* men 1.4 (0.9)* women	Modified relative	Risk decreases with time from exposure

* Beir IV values modified to express risk for 35 years after exposure rather than entire lifetime.

cases and 402 controls with year-long measurements of radon in the homes where individuals lived for 10 or more years. This study devoted a considerable effort to quality control concerning the exposure measurements. The results of this study are slightly positive, suggesting an association of radon and lung cancer, even at concentrations of 80 Bq m^{-3}, but the results are not statistically significant.

Of the total studies, 13 are ecologic and 9 are case control. Ecologic studies depend on relating the disease response of a population to some measure of a suspected causative agent. There are usually insufficient data on all of the variables involved in the disease to infer any reliable associations. Ecologic studies are the weakest type of epidemiologic exploration.

Unless a biologic marker for radon-induced lung cancer is found, it is unlikely that environmental epidemiology will be effective. The effects of radon in the environment are subtle compared with the overwhelming lung cancer mortality from smoking.

Four concepts emerge from the radon research so far, however, and these are

1. The mining epidemiology indicates that short exposure to high levels of radon and daughters produce a clear excess of lung cancer.
2. Particle size can change the actual dose delivered by radon to bronchial tissue with small sized particles giving a substantially higher dose per unit exposure. Passive tobacco smoke and open flames indoors produce a higher dose.
3. Smokers are at higher risk from radon per unit exposure than nonsmokers.
4. Urban areas almost universally have low radon and apartment dwellers removed from the ground source have particularly low radon exposure at home.

The miner data show clearly that there is a risk of lung cancer from exposure to high con-

centrations of radon delivered over short time periods. Comparable exposures delivered over a lifetime in the home have not produced statistically significant increases in lung cancer mortality. The risk can still exist, but the confounding effect of other carcinogens such as smoking and urbanization make it impossible to extract the more subtle impact of radon in existing studies.

Natural Radioactivity and Radiation Background

The occupational, accidental, and wartime experiences detailed in the preceding sections have provided the bases for all of the current radiation risk estimates. For many years, the radioisotopes deposited internally were compared with ^{226}Ra in order to evaluate the maximum permissible body burden for a particular emitter. The present limits for external and internal radiation are based on dose estimates which in turn can now be related to cancer risks. One standard of comparison has always been the exposure from natural background and this source is assessed here.

Background radiation from all sources is described in detail in NCRP report 94 (1987) and some of the information is summarized here.

The risk estimates in the previous sections must be placed in context with the radiation dose received by all humans from natural background radiation. There is a substantial dose received annually from cosmic radiation and from external terrestrial radiation present from uranium, thorium, and potassium in the earth's crust. Internal emitters are present in the body as a consequence of dietary consumption and inhalation. For example, potassium is a necessary element in the body and is homeostatically controlled. Radioactive ^{40}K is a constant fraction of all natural potassium. Potassium delivers the largest internal dose from diet of 0.15 mSv per year. However, the data are scant on the dietary intake of other radionuclides in the United States population. Given the usual distribution of intakes across a large population, it is probable that

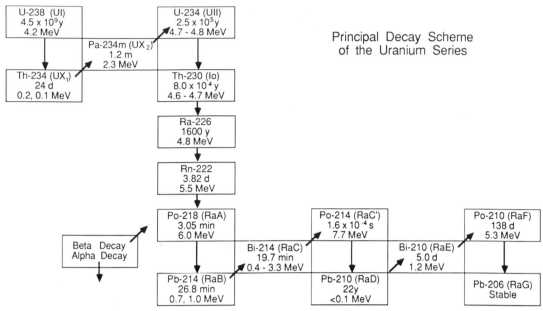

Principal Decay Scheme
of the Uranium Series

Figure 21–6.   Uranium-238 decay series. (From NCRP, 1987.)

other emitters, notably ^{210}Pb, could deliver a significant dose to a fraction of the population.

The largest dose received by the population is from the inhaled short-lived daughters of radon. These are present in all atmospheres because radon is released rather efficiently from the ^{226}Ra in rock and soil. The short-lived daughters ^{218}Po, ^{214}Pb, ^{214}Bi-^{214}Po, have an effective half-life of 30 minutes, but the 3.8-day parent radon supports their presence in the atmosphere. Figure 21–6 shows the entire uranium series decay.

Average outdoor concentrations in the United States have been measured as 7 Bq m^{-3} and indoors as 40 to 80 Bq m^{-3}. A structure such as a house prevents the rapid upward distribution of radon into the atmosphere and substantial levels can be built up indoors. The source of radon is the ground and so levels in living areas above ground are generally one-third to one-fifth the concentrations measured in basements. An effective barrier across the soil/building interface also inhibits radon entry to buildings. Ventilation with outdoor air reduces indoor radon. For this reason, industrial buildings with more substantial foundations and higher ventilation rates tend to have lower radon concentrations than single family (or detached) houses. Apartments above ground level have radon concentrations about half the average of single family dwellings.

It is of significance that an average radon concentration indoors of 40 Bq m^{-3} results in a dose equivalent to bronchial epithelium of 24 mSv/year or an effective dose equivalent (EDE) of 2 mSv per year.

The dose equivalents for the major natural internal emitters are shown in Table 21–14. These are reproduced from NCRP (1987).

The annual effective dose equivalent for all of the external and internal emitters from natural background are summarized in NCRP Report 94 (1987) and these are shown in Table 21–15.

The lifetime dose from the natural emitters is shown in Table 21–16, assuming an average exposure from birth to a full life of 85 years. It should be recognized that the actual dose accumulated by an individual depends upon dietary habits, location (Denver for example, at an altitude of 1.6 kilometers has double the average cosmic ray exposure) and the dwelling. Apartment dwellers would accumulate approximately half the dose from inhaled radon daughters as a person living in a single-family dwelling.

Table 21–16 is informative in considering the effects of radiation exposure from sources other than natural. For example, in assessing an occupational dose, which might add, say, 10 mSv effective dose equivalent, natural background would be a strong confounder. Any health detriment would have to be calculated rather than observed directly. No study would be able to detect an increase in health effects from 10 mSv above the average whole life natural background of 260 mSv.

Table 21–14. DOSE EQUIVALENT RATES TO VARIOUS TISSUES FROM NATURAL RADIONUCLIDES CONTAINED IN THE BODY

| | DOSE EQUIVALENT RATE (mSv yr^{-1}) | | | |
RADIONUCLIDE	*Bronchial Epithelium*	*Soft Tissue*	*Bone Surfaces*	*Bone Marrow*
^{14}C	—	0.10	0.08	0.30
^{40}K	—	1.80	1.40	2.70
^{87}Rb	—	0.03	0.14	0.07
^{238}U-^{234}Th	—	0.046	0.03	0.004
^{230}Th	—	0.001	0.06	0.001
^{226}Ra	—	0.03	0.90	0.15
^{222}Rn	—	0.07	0.14	0.14
^{222}Rn daughters	24	—	—	—
^{210}Pb-^{210}Po	—	1.40	7.00	1.40
^{232}Th	—	0.001	0.02	0.004
^{228}Ra-^{224}Ra	—	0.0015	1.20	0.22
^{220}Rn	—	0.001	—	—
Total	24	3.50	11.00	5.00

Table 21–15. ESTIMATED TOTAL EFFECTIVE DOSE EQUIVALENT RATE FOR A MEMBER OF THE POPULATION IN THE UNITED STATES AND CANADA FROM VARIOUS SOURCES OF BACKGROUND RADIATION

| | | TOTAL EFFECTIVE DOSE EQUIVALENT RATE (mSv yr^{-1}) | | | | | |
SOURCE		*Lung*	*Gonads*	*Bone Surf*	*Bone Marrow*	*Other Tissues*	*Total*
	W_t	0.12	0.25	0.03	0.12	0.48	1.0
Cosmic		0.03	0.07	0.008	0.03	0.13	0.27
Cosmogenic		0.001	0.002	—	0.004	0.003	0.01
Terrestrial		0.03	0.07	0.008	0.03	0.14	0.28
Inhaled		2.0	—	—	—	—	2.0
In Body		0.04	0.09	0.03	0.06	0.17	0.40
Total		2.1	0.23	0.05	0.12	0.44	3.0

From NCRP, 1987.

Table 21–16. LIFETIME EFFECTIVE DOSE EQUIVALENT (IN mSv FROM BIRTH TO AGE 85) FROM NATURAL RADIONUCLIDE EXPOSURE

	LUNG	BONE MARROW	WHOLE BODY
Effective Dose Equivalent	180	10	260

From NCRP, 1987.

Environmental Releases (Chernobyl)

Large-scale accidents will undoubtedly occur that release substantial radioactivity into the environment. The accident at the Windscale nuclear power reactor in 1957 was a local incident in Great Britain. The nearby population has been studied for over 30 years without appearance of significant health effects.

The accident at the Chernobyl nuclear power plant was another such occasion but, in this case, the radioactivity was widespread over Europe. The United Nations Scientific Committee on the Effects of Atomic Radiation (UNSCEAR, 1988) has summarized the committed dose from measurements made in the affected countries and these are shown in Table 21 – 17. The dose in this case is largely from long-lived ^{137}Cs (half-life 30 years) both deposited on the ground and taken up by vegetation and directly deposited on vegeta-

Table 21–17. TOTAL CESIUM-137 DEPOSIT AND DOSE COMMITMENTS IN THE NORTHERN HEMISPHERE

REGION	AREA (10³ km²)	POPULATION (10⁶)	DISTANCE FROM CHERNOBYL (km)	CESIUM-137 DEPOSITION (kBq/m²) WEIGHTED BY		CS-137 DEPOSIT (PBq)	EFFECTIVE DOSE EQUIVALENT COMMITMENT			
							Per caput (μSv)		Collective (man Sv)	
				Area	Population		First Year	Total	First Year	Total
Europe										
North[a]	1,249	22.8	1,300	8.2	7.0	10.2	210	970	4,700	22,000
Central[b]	1,253	178.0	1,200	7.0	6.0	8.8	280	930	49,000	166,000
West[c]	936	137.7	2,000	1.3	1.0	1.2	48	150	6,600	21,000
Southeast[d]	829	101.6	1,500	8.2	7.2	6.8	380	1200	39,000	121,000
Southwest[e]	596	47.2	2,900	0.03	0.03	0.02	4	7	180	340
USSR	22,190	279.1	—	1.4	5.0	30.9	260	810	72,000	226,000
Asia										
Southwest[f]	4,611	114.9	2,200	1.0	1.0	4.6	70	190	8,000	22,000
South[g]	6,786	1082	5,400	0.08	0.08	0.5	6	15	6,100	16,000
Southeast[h]	2,575	240.6	7,800	0.03	0.03	0.08	2	6	510	1,400
East[i]	11,720	1268	6,600	0.04	0.04	0.5	3	8	3,600	9,600
America										
North[j]	20,560	347.0	9,000	0.02	0.02	0.4	1	4	490	1,300
Caribbean[k]	216	30.1	9,200	0.018	0.018	0.004	1	3	40	100
Central[l]	517	26.9	10,700	0.012	0.012	0.006	0.7	2	20	60
South[m]	2,520	49.7	10,100	0.013	0.013	0.03	1	2	50	120

Africa										
North[n]	8,438	128.4	0.4	3,000	0.4	3.4	28	76	3,600	9,800
West[o]	6,118	172.3	0.08	5,600	0.08	0.5	6	15	970	2,600
Central[p]	2,415	18.3	0.08	5,300	0.08	0.2	5	15	100	,280
East[q]	2,117	59.5	0.09	5,100	0.09	0.2	6	17	380	1,000
Greenland	2,176	0.06	0.18	4,000	0.18	0.4	7	30	0.4	2
North Atlantic Ocean	53,000	—	0.07	5,700	—	3.7				
North Pacific Ocean	102,000	—	0.01	10,900	—	1.0				
Northern hemisphere Total (rounded)	252,800	4304	0.3	5,700	0.9	70	45	140	200,000	600,000

[a] Denmark, Finland, Iceland, Norway, Sweden.
[b] Austria, Czechoslovakia, German Dem. Rep., Germany, Fed. Rep., Hungary, Poland, Romania, Switzerland.
[c] Belgium, France, Ireland, Luxembourg, Netherlands, United Kingdom.
[d] Albania, Bulgaria, Greece, Italy, Malta, Yugoslavia.
[e] Portugal, Spain.
[f] Bahrain, Cyprus, Dem. Yemen, Iraq, Israel, Jordan, Kuwait, Lebanon, Oman, Qatar, Saudi Arabia, Syrian Arab Rep., Turkey, United Arab Emirates, Yemen.
[g] Afghanistan, Bangladesh, Bhutan, India, Iran, Nepal, Pakistan, Sri Lanka.
[h] Burma, Dem. Kampuchea, Laos Dem. Rep., Malaysia, Philippines, Singapore, Thailand, Viet Nam.
[i] China, Dem. Korea, Hong Kong, Japan, Korea. Rep., Mongolia.
[j] Canada, United States, Mexico.
[k] Cuba, Dominican Rep., Haiti, Jamaica, Puerto Rico, Trinidad/Tobago.
[l] Costa Rica, El Salvador, Guatemala, Honduras, Nicaragua, Panama.
[m] Colombia, Guyana, Suriname, Venezuela, French Guiana.
[n] Algeria, Egypt, Libya, Morocco, Sudan, Tunisia.
[o] Benin, Burkina Faso, Cape Verde, Cote d'Ivoire, Gambia, Ghana, Guinea, Guinea-Bissau, Liberia, Mali, Mauritania, Niger, Nigeria, Senegal, Sierra Leone, Togo.
[p] Cameroon, Central Afr. Rep., Chad, Equatorial Guinea.
[q] Ethiopia, Somalia, Uganda, Djibouti.

Table 21–18.　LIFETIME CANCER MORTALITY PER GRAY FROM FIVE MAJOR EPIDEMIOLOGIC STUDIES (IN PARENTHESES, RISK PER SIEVERT FOR ALPHA EMITTERS)

STUDY	ALL SITES	LEUKEMIA	LUNG	FEMALE BREAST	BONE	THYROID	SKIN
Atom bomb whole body gamma	0.029	0.0067	0.0038	0.0029			
Uranium miner bronchial epithelium alpha			0.04 (0.0020)				
Ankylosing spondylitis spine X ray		0.0011	0.0008– 0.0028	0.0015			
Tinea capitis head X ray						0.0010[§] 0.0040[‖]	0.0030[‡]
Radium ingestion bone alpha (^{226}Ra)					0.0040* (0.0002)		
Radium ingestion bone alpha (^{224}Ra)					0.02[†] (0.0010)		

* The lifetime risk is calculated for an average skeletal dose of 10 Gy, assuming the risk to persist for 50 years and using equation 20. The risk is nonlinear and is about 0.01 Gy^{-1} at 100 Gy, for example.
[†] The lifetime risk is calculated for an average skeletal dose of 10 Gy using equation 22. The risk is nonlinear and is about 0.01 Gy^{-1} for a skeletal dose of 1 Gy.
[‡] The mortality for skin cancer is estimated as 1 percent of the incidence; see text.
[§] Thyroid mortality for males. Estimated as 10 percent of incidence.
[‖] Thyroid mortality for females. Estimated as 10 percent of incidence.

tion. Cesium behaves similarly to potassium in the body and so the dose is essentially to the whole body.

There are plans to follow-up the health effects in the local population affected by Chernobyl.

SUMMARY OF HUMAN CANCER RISKS FROM RADIATION

The details of the five major studies have been given in the preceding sections. The data are summarized in Table 21–18. This shows the lifetime cancer risks which are significant. The risks are given in units of per Gray (or per Sievert where appropriate for alpha emitters).

Within the table, leukemia and cancers of the lung and female breast are the most critical. Osteogenic sarcoma is seen in the radium exposures. There is no clear linear dose response for ^{224,226}Ra. This has been attributed to the existence of an apparent threshold.

The cancer risk to individual organs from dif-

ferent study groups is in general agreement regardless of radiation type or whole or partial body exposure.

ADDENDUM

In 1990 the International Commission on Radiation Protection (ICRP) circulated a draft document (ICRP, 1990) which is to be adopted and published by the Commission in 1991. This document includes new estimates of risk for both fatal and nonfatal cancer and new guidelines for exposure to workers from external and internal radiation.

The ICRP document is a response to the increase in cancer risk from ionizing radiation observed in atomic-bomb survivors. Mental retardation is a recent finding in the atomic-bomb survivor cohort and this is now included in the risk estimates. There are no conclusive data from A-bomb survivors on cancer in the thyroid, bone, liver, and skin. Therefore, the risks to

Table 21–19.　NOMINAL RISK COEFFICIENTS FOR STOCHASTIC EFFECTS*

BIOLOGICAL EFFECT (10^{-2} Sv^{-1})	EXPOSED POPULATION	RISK COEFFICIENT
Fatal cancer	Adult workers	4.0
Fatal cancer	Whole population	5.0
Serious hereditary effects	Adult workers	0.6
	Whole population	1.0
Mental retardation	8–15 week conceptus	30 IQ points Sv^{-1}

* From ICRP, 1990.

Table 21–20. NOMINAL PROBABILITY COEFFICIENTS AND TISSUE WEIGHTING FACTORS FOR INDIVIDUAL TISSUES AND ORGANS*[†]

| TISSUE OR ORGAN | CANCER LETHALITY FRACTION K | NOMINAL PROBABILITY COEFFICIENT $(10^{-2}\ Sv^{-1})$ | | | | TISSUE WEIGHTING FACTOR w_T |
| | | WHOLE POPULATION | | WORKING POPULATION | | |
		Fatality coeff F	*Weighted effect coeff* $F(2\text{-}K)$	*Fatality coeff* F	*Weighted effect coeff* $F(2\text{-}K)$	
Bone marrow[‡]	0.99	0.45	0.91	0.36	0.73	0.12
Bladder	0.50	0.20	0.30	0.16	0.24	0.04
Bone surface	0.70	0.05	0.07	0.04	0.05	0.01
Breast	0.50	0.25	0.38	0.20	0.30	0.05
Colon	0.55	0.95	1.38	0.76	1.10	0.18
Gonads	—	—	1.00	—	0.60	0.13
Liver	0.95	0.20	0.21	0.16	0.17	0.03
Lung	0.95	0.90	0.95	0.72	0.76	0.13
Oesophagus	0.95	0.35	0.37	0.28	0.29	0.05
Skin	0.01	0.02	0.04	0.016	0.03	0.01
Stomach	0.90	1.10	1.21	0.88	0.97	0.16
Thyroid	0.10	0.08	0.15	0.06	0.11	0.02
Remainder[§]	0.80	0.45	0.54	0.36	0.43	0.07
Total (rounded)		5.00	7.49 7.5	4.00	5.79 6.0	1.0

* From ICRP, 1990.

[†] The values of w_T relate to a population of equal numbers of both sexes and a wide range of ages. The coefficients relate only to adults.

[‡] Relates to red bone marrow and includes extra weighting by a factor of 2 for short mean latency of leukaemia.

[§] The dose equivalent in the remainder is the estimated mean dose equivalent over the whole body excluding the specified tissues and organs.

these tissues are developed from other epidemiological studies discussed in this chapter.

The overall risk per unit exposure for adult workers and the whole population given in the draft document are shown in Table 21–19. The risk of fatal cancer is adopted as 0.04 per Sievert (4 percent per Sievert) for adult workers and 0.05 per Sievert (5 percent per Sievert) for the whole adult population.

ICRP had been criticized for excluding the effects of nonfatal cancer in previous documents. An attempt to correct this omission is made in the present document. A cancer lethality fraction, K (the fraction of total cancer that is lethal), is used as a weighting factor for nonfatal cancers in deriving the total effect risk coefficient. The cancer risk per Sievert, F, and the total weighted risk per Sievert (weighted effect coefficient), $F(2\text{-}K)$, are shown in Table 21–20. The reasoning given for the weighted effect coefficient is given as follows.

The total number of cancers (fatal plus nonfatal) Sv^{-1} will be F/K. The total number of nonfatal cancers is $(1\text{-}K)F/K$ and multiplying by the

weighting factor K yields a "health detriment" of $(1\text{-}K)F$. The total health detriment is then

$$F + F(1\text{-}K) = F(2\text{-}K).$$

The total risk including this weighting for nonfatal cancer is proposed as 7.5 Sv^{-1} for the whole adult population and 6.0 Sv^{-1} for the working population.

The tissue weighting factors corresponding to those derived formerly in ICRP (1977) and shown in Table 21–6, are the organ fraction of the total.

In assessing radiation risk from low-dose, low-dose rate, low LET radiation using risk coefficients such as in Table 21–20 derived from high dose, high-dose rate exposures, a dose rate reduction factor (DREF) needs to be applied. NCRP (1980) and UNSCEAR (1988) have shown that the human data cover a range for the DREF of 2 to 10. That is, the risk coefficients in Table 21–20 are conventionally divided by the DREF factor. ICRP has previously used 2.5 as the adopted DREF, however, the draft document proposes to adopt a DREF of 2.0.

The new occupational guidelines for radiation developed from this ICRP document are proposed as 100 mSv in 5 years with a limit of 50 mSv in any single year. This is compared with the 1977 limit of 50 mSv per year.

ACKNOWLEDGMENT

The author would like to thank Dr. John H. Harley for many helpful suggestions in the preparation of this manuscript.

REFERENCES

Adamson, H. G.: A simplified method of x-ray application for the cure of ringworm of the scalp; Kienbock's method. *Lancet*, **i**:1378–1380, 1909.

Albert, R. E., and Omran, A.: A follow-up study of patients treated by X-ray epilation for tinea capitis: I Population characteristics   treatment illnesses and mortality experience. *Arch. Env. Hlth.*, **17**:899–918, 1968.

Albert, R. E.; Shore, R. E.; Harley, N. H.; and Omran, A.: Follow-up studies of patients treated by X-ray epilation for tinea capitis. In Burns, F.; Upton, A. C.; and Silini, G. (eds.): *Radiation Carcinogenesis and DNA Alterations*. Plenum Press, New York, 1986, pp. 1–25.

Andrews, H. L.: *Radiation Biophysics*. Prentice-Hall, Englewood Cliffs, New Jersey, 1974.

Attix, F. H.; Roesch, W. C.; Tochilin, E.: *Radiation Dosimetry*, Vol. I, Academic Press, New York, 1968.

Aub, J. C.; Evans, R. D.; Hempelmann, L. H.; and Martland, H. S.: The late effects of internally deposited radioactive materials in man. *Medicine*, **31**:221–329, 1952.

Bethe, H. A., and Ashkin, J.: Passage of radiations through matter. In Segre, E. (ed.): *Experimental Nuclear Physics*. John Wiley & Sons, New York, 1953, pp. 166–357.

Borak, T. B., and Johnson, J. A.: *Estimating the Risk of Lung Cancer from Inhalation of Radon Daughters Indoors: Review and Evaluation*. Environmental Protection Agency Report EPA 600/6-88/008, Environmental Monitoring Systems Laboratory. EPA, Las Vegas, Nevada, 1988.

Browne, E.; Firestone, R. B.; and Shirley, V. S.: *Table of Radioactive Isotopes*. John Wiley & Sons, New York, 1986.

Chemelevsky, D.; Kellerer, A. M.; Spiess, H.; and Mays, C. W.: A proportional hazards analysis of bone sarcoma rates in German radium-224 patients. In Gossner, W., and Gerber, G. B. (eds.): *The Radiobiology of Radium and Thorotrast*. Urban and Schwarzenberg, Munich, West Germany, 1986.

Court Brown, W. M., and Doll, R.: *Leukemia and Aplastic Anemia in Patients Treated for Ankylosing Spondylitis*. HMSO, London, 1957.

———: Adult leukemia. Trends in mortality in relation to aetiology. *Br. Med. J.*, **1**:1063, 1959.

———: Mortality from cancer and other causes after radiotherapy for ankylosing spondylitis. *Br. Med. J.*, **2**:1327, 1965.

Darby, S. C.; Doll, R.; and Smith, P. G.: Long term mortality after a single treatment course with X-rays in patients treated for ankylosing spondylitis. *Br. J. Cancer*, **55**:179–190, 1987.

Darby, S. C.; Nakashima, E.; and Kato, H.: A parallel analysis of cancer mortality among atomic bomb survivors and patients with ankylosing spondylitis given x-ray therapy. *J. Natl. Cancer Inst.*, **72**:1, 1985.

Evans, R. D.: *The Atomic Nucleus*. McGraw-Hill, New York, 1955.

Evans, R. D.; Keane, A. T.; Kolenkow, R. J.; Neal, W. R.; and Shanahan, M.M.: Radiogenic tumors in the radium cases studied at M.I.T. In Mays, C.W.; Jee, W. S. S.; Lloyd, R. D.; Stover, B. J.; Dougherty, J. H.; and Taylor, G.N., (eds.): *Delayed Effects of Bone Seeking Radionuclides*. University of Utah Press, Salt Lake City, 1969, pp. 157–194.

George, A. C., and Breslin, A. J.: The distribution of ambient radon and radon daughters in residential buildings in the New Jersey–New York area. In Gesell, T. F., and Lowder, W. M. (eds.): *Natural Radiation Environment III CONF-780422*. USDOE, Washington, D.C., 1980.

George, A. C.; Hinchliffe, L.; and Sladowski, R.: Size distribution of radon daughter particles in uranium mine atmospheres. *Am. Ind. Hyg. Assoc. J.*, **36**:4884, 1975.

Harley, J. H.: Dose from Residual Radioactivity at Hiroshima and Nagasaki. In *New Dosimetry at Hiroshima and Nagasaki and Its Implications for Risk Estimates. Proc. Number 9 National Council on Radiation Protection*. NCRP, Bethesda, Maryland, 1987.

Harley, N. H.: Lung Cancer Risk from Exposure to Environmental Radon. *Presented at the 3rd International Conference on Anticarcinogenesis and Radiation Protection*, Dubrovnik, 1989.

Harley, N. H.; Albert, R. E.; Shore, R. E.; and Pasternack, B. S.: Follow-up study of patients treated by X-ray epilation for tinea capitis. Estimation of the dose to the thyroid and pituitary glands and other structures of the head and neck. *Phys. Med. Biol.*, **21**:631–642, 1976.

Harley, N. H., and Cohen, B. S.: Updating radon daughter dosimetry. In Hopke, P. K. (ed.): *American Chemical Society Symposium on Radon and Its Decay Products*. ACS, Washington, D.C., 1987.

Harley, N. H.; Kolber, A. B.; Shore, R. E.; Albert, R. E.; Altman, S. M.; and Pasternack, B. S.: The skin dose and response for the head and neck in patients irradiated with X-ray for tinea capitis. Implications for environmental radioactivity. In *Proceedings in Health Physics Society Mid-Year Symposium*. Health Physics Society, Albuquerque, New Mexico, 1983, pp. 125–142.

Holaday, D. A.; Rushing, D. E.; Coleman, R. D.; Woolrich, P. F.; Kusnetz, H. L.; and Bale, W. F.: *Control of Radon and Daughters in Uranium Mines and Calculations on Biologic Effects*. U.S. PHS Report 494. U.S. Government Printing Office, Washington, D.C., 1957.

Hornung, R. W., and Meinhardt, T. J.: Quantitative risk assessment of lung cancer in U.S. uranium miners. *Health Phys.*, **52**:417–430, 1987.

Hubbell, J. H.: *Photon Cross Sections, Attenuation Coefficients, and Energy Absorption Coefficients from 10 keV to 100 GeV*. U.S. Department of Commerce, National Bureau of Standards Report NSRDS-NBS 29. U.S. Government Printing Office, Washington, D.C., 1969.

———: Photon mass attenuation and energy-absorption coefficients from 1 keV to 20 MeV. *Int. J. Appl. Radiat. Isotop.*, **33**:1269–1290, 1982.

ICRP: *Recommendations of the International Commission on Radiological Protection. International Commission on Radiation Protection Publication 26*. Pergamon Press, New York, 1977.

———: *Limits for Intakes of Radionuclides by Workers. International Commission on Radiological Protection Publication 30 Part I*. Pergamon Press, New York, 1978.

————: *Limits for Inhalation of Radon Daughters by Workers. International Commission on Radiological Protection Publication 32.* Pergamon Press, New York, 1981.

————: *Lung Cancer Risk from Indoor Exposures to Radon Daughters. International Commission on Radiological Protection Publication 50.* Pergamon Press, Oxford, 1987.

————: *Recommendations of the Commission-1990. International Commission on Radiological Protection Draft ICRP/90/G-01.*, 1990.

ICRU: *Radiation Quantities and Units. International Commission on Radiation Units and Measurements, Report Number 33.* ICRU, Bethesda, Maryland, 1980.

————: *Stopping Powers for Electrons and Positrons. International Commission on Radiation Units and Measurements Report Number 37.* ICRU, Bethesda, Maryland, 1984.

James, A. C.: A reconsideration of cells at risk and other key factors in radon daughter dosimetry. In Hopke, P. K. (ed.): *American Chemical Society Symposium on Radon and Its Decay Products.* ACS, Washington, D.C., 1987, p. 400.

Kienbock, R.: Über Radiotherapie und Harrerkrankungen. *Arch. Derm. Syph. Wien,* **83**:77–111, 1907.

Kunz, E., and Sevc, J.: Radiation risks to underground miners in the light of Czechoslovak epidemiological studies. In Kvasnicka, J. (ed.): *Proceedings of the International Workshop on Radiological Protection in Mining, Darwin, Australia,* 1988.

Lederer, C. M.; Shirley, V. S.; Browne, E.; Dairiki, J. M.; and Doebler, R. E.: *Table of Isotopes.* John Wiley & Sons, New York, 1978.

Lewis, C. A.; Smith, P. G.; Stratton, M.; Darby, S. C.; and Doll, R.: Estimated radiation doses to different organs among patients treated for ankylosing spondylitis with a single course of X-rays. *Br. J. Radiol.,* **61**:212–220, 1988.

Marshall, J. H.; Lloyd, E. L.; Rundo, J.; Liniecki, J.; Marotti, G.; Mays, C. W.; Sissons, H. A.; and Snyder, W. S.: *Alkaline Earth Metabolism in Adult Man ICRP Report Number 20.* Pergamon Press, Elmsford, New York, 1972.

Martland, H. S.: The occurrence of malignancy in radioactive persons. *Am. J. Cancer,* **15**:2435–2516, 1931.

Mays, C. W.: Alpha particle induced cancer in humans. *Health Phys.,* **55**:637–652, 1988.

Muller, J.; Kusiak, R.; and Ritchie, A. C.: *Factors Modifying Lung Cancer Risk in Ontario Uranium Miners, 1955–1981.* Ontario Ministry of Labour Report. Ministry of Labour, Toronto, 1989.

NAS: *The Effects on Populations of Exposure to Low Levels of Ionizing Radiation. National Academy of Sciences Report, BEIR III.* National Academy Press, Washington, D.C., 1980.

————: *Health Risks of Radon and Other Internally Deposited Alpha Emitters Committee on the Biological Effects of Ionizing Radiation BEIR IV National Research Council.* National Academy Press, Washington, D.C., 1988.

————: *Health Effects of Exposure to Low Levels of Ionizing Radiation. National Academy of Sciences Report BEIR V.* National Academy Press, Washington, D.C., 1990.

NCRP: *Influence of Dose and Its Distribution in Time on Dose-Response Relationships of Low-LET Radiations. National Council on Radiation Protection and Measurements Report Number 64.* NCRP, Bethesda, Maryland, 1980.

————: *Evaluation of Occupational and Environmental Exposures to Radon and Radon Daughters in the United States National Council on Radiation Protection Report No. 78.* NCRP, Bethesda, Maryland, 1984.

————: *Induction of Thyroid Cancer by Ionizing Radiation. Report Number 80.* National Council on Radiation Protection and Measurements. NCRP, Bethesda, Maryland, 1985.

————: *Recommendations on Limits for Exposure to Ionizing Radiation. National Council on Radiation Protection and Measurements, Report Number 91.* NCRP, Bethesda, Maryland, 1987a.

————: *Exposure of the Population in the United States and Canada from Natural Background Radiation. National Council on Radiation Protection and Measurements Report Number 94.* NCRP, Bethesda, Maryland, 1987b.

————: *Recommendation on Limits of Exposure to Hot Particles on the Skin. National Council on Radiation Protection and Measurements Report Number 106.* NCRP, Bethesda, Maryland, 1990.

Neuberger, J. S.: *Worldwide Studies of Household Radon Exposure and Lung Cancer. Final Report to the U.S. Department of Energy, Office of Health and Environmental Research.* USDOE, Washington, D.C., 1989.

Norris, W. P.; Speckman, T. W.; Gustafson, P. F.: Studies of metabolism of radium in man. *Am. J. Roentgenol. Radium Therap. Nucl. Med.,* **73**:785–802, 1955.

Norris, W. P.; Tyler, S. A.; and Brues, A. M.: Retention of radioactive bone seekers. *Science,* **128**:456, 1958.

Raabe, O. G.; Book, S. A.; and Parks, N. J.: Bone cancer from radium: canine dose response explains data for mice and humans. *Science,* **208**:61–64, 1980.

Radford, E. P., and Renard, K. G. S.: Lung cancer in Swedish iron miners exposed to low doses of radon daughters. *N. Engl. J. Med.,* **310**:1485–1494, 1984.

RERF: *US-Japan Joint Reassessment of Atomic Bomb Radiation Dosimetry in Hiroshima and Nagasaki. Final Report DS86.* RERF, Hiroshima, Japan, 1987.

Ron, E., and Modan, B.: Thyroid and other neoplasms following childhood scalp irradiations. In Boice, J. D., and Fraumeni, J. F. (eds.): *Radiation Carcinogenesis: Epidemiology and Biological Significance.* Raven Press, New York, 1984, pp. 139–151.

Rowland, R. E.; Stehney, A. F.; and Lucas, H. F.: Dose response relationships for female radium dial painters. *Radiat. Res.,* **76**:368–383, 1978.

Schoenberg, J., and Klotz, J.: *A Case-Control Study of Radon and Lung Cancer Among New Jersey Women.* New Jersey State Department of Health Technical Report, Phase I. NJDH, Trenton, New Jersey, 1989.

Schulz, R., and Albert, R. E.: Dose to organs of the head from the X-ray treatment of tinea capitis. *Arch, Environ: Health,* **17**:935–950, 1963.

Sevc, J.; Kunz, E.; Tomasek, L.; Placek, V.; and Horacek, J.: Cancer in man after exposure to Rn daughters. *Health Phys.,* **54**:27–46, 1988.

Shimizu, Y.; Kato, H.; Schull, W. J.; Preston, D. L.; Fujita, S.; and Pierce, D. A.: *Life Span Study Report 11, Part 1. Comparison of Risk Coefficients for Site-Specific Cancer Mortality Based on the DS86 and T65DR Shielded Kerma and Organ Doses. Technical Report TR 12-87.* RERF, Hiroshima, Japan, 1987a.

————: *Life Span Study Report 11, Radiation Effects Research Foundation Technical Report RERF TR 12-87.* RERF, Hiroshima, Japan, 1987b.

Shimizu, Y.; Kato, H.; and Schull, W. J.: *Life Span Study Report 11, Part 2. Cancer Mortality in the Years*

1950–85 Based on the Recently Revised Doses (DS86). RERF Report TR-5-88. RERF, Hiroshima, Japan, 1988.

Shore, R. E.; Albert, R. E.; and Pasternack, B. S.: Follow-up of patients treated by x-ray epilation for tinea capitis. *Arch. Environ. Health,* **31**:21–28, 1976.

Shore, R. E.; Albert, R. E.; Reed, M.; Harley, N. H.; and Pasternack, B. S.: Skin cancer incidence among children irradiated for ringworm of the scalp. *Radiat. Res.,* **100**:192–204, 1984.

Smith, P. G.: Late Effects of X-Ray Treatment of Ankylosing Spondylitis. In Boice, J. D., and Fraumeni, J. F. (eds.): *Radiation Carcinogenesis: Epidemiology and Biological Significance.* Raven Press, New York, 1984.

Smith, P. G., and Doll, R.: Mortality among patients with ankylosing spondylitis after a single treatment course with x-rays. *Br. Med. J.,* **1**:449, 1982.

Smith, W. M., and Doll, R.: Age and time dependent changes in the rates of radiation-induced cancers in patients with ankylosing spondylitis following a single course of x-ray treatment. In *Late Effects of Ionizing Radiation.* Vol 1. IAEA, Vienna, 1978, p. 205.

Spiess, F. W., and Mays, C. W.: Bone cancers induced by Ra-224 (ThX) in children and adults. *Health Physics* **19**:713–729, 1970.

Spiess, H., and Mays, C. W.: Protraction effect on bone sarcoma induction of Ra-224 in children and adults. In Sanders, C. L.; Busch, R. H.; Ballou, J. E.; and Mahlum, D. D. (eds.): *Radionuclide Carcinogenesis.* National Technical Information Service, Springfield, Virginia, 1973, pp. 437–450.

Tu, K. W., and Knutson, E. O.: Indoor radon progeny particle size distribution measurements made with two different methods. *Radiat. Prot. Dosimet.,* **24**:251, 1988.

Turner, J. E.: *Atoms, Radiation and Radiation Protection.* Pergamon Press, Elmsford, New York, 1986.

UNSCEAR: *Sources, Effects and Risks of Ionizing Radiation. Report of the United Nations Scientific Committee on the Effects of Atomic Radiation.* United Nations, New York, 1988.

Whaling, W.: The energy loss of charged particles in matter. In Flugge, S. (ed.): *Handbuch der Physik.* Springer-Verlag, Berlin, 1958, pp. 193–217.

Wick, R. R.; Chmelevsky, D.; and Gossner, W.: 224Ra risk to bone and haematopoietic tissue in ankylosing spondylitis patients. In Gossner, W.; Gerber, G. B.; Hagan, U.; and Luz, A. (eds.): *The Radiobiology of Radium and Thorotrast.* Urban and Schwarzenberg, Munich, West Germany, 1986, pp. 38–44.

Woodard, H. Q.: *Radiation Carcinogenesis in Man: A Critical Review. Environmental Measurements Laboratory Report EML-380.* U.S. Department of Energy, New York, 1980.

Ziegler, J. F.: *Helium Stopping Powers and Ranges in All Elemental Matter.* Pergamon Press, New York, 1977.

Chapter 22

TOXIC EFFECTS OF ANIMAL TOXINS

Findlay E. Russell and *Richard C. Dart*

INTRODUCTION

Venomous or poisonous animals are found in all the animal classes with the exception of the birds. For the most part, they are widely distributed throughout the animal kingdom from the unicellular protistan *Gonyaulax* to certain of the chordates, the platypus, and the short-tailed shrew. Venomous animals are found in almost all seas and oceans of the world and on all continents. Although there are no exact figures on the numbers of such animals, there are approximately 1200 species of venomous or poisonous marine animals (Russell, 1984a), the number of venomous arthropods is countless, and there are some 375 species of snakes considered dangerous to humans.

The term *venomous animal* is usually applied to those creatures that are capable of producing a poison in a highly developed secretory gland or group of cells and that can deliver this toxin during a biting or stinging act. *Poisonous animals,* on the other hand, are generally regarded to be those whose tissues, either in part or in their entirety, are toxic. These animals have no mechanism or structure for the delivery of their poisons. Poisoning by these forms usually takes place through ingestion (Russell, 1965). In reality, all venomous animals are poisonous, but not all poisonous animals are venomous.

A venom may have one or several functions in an animal's armament. It may play a role in offense, as in the capture and digestion of food, or may contribute to the animal's defense, as in protection against predators or aggressors. It may also serve both functions. The principal biologic property of the venom of the snake is its food-securing potential. In this respect, venom is a superior modification to speed, size, strength, or better concealment, as well as other characteristics that many of the nonvenomous snakes have developed. In addition, the venom plays a role in the digestion of the prey. Finally, the venom can play a role in the snake's defensive posture, as in the spitting cobra and ringhals, or in kills or underkills in a defensive situation (Russell, 1984b). The venomous snakes are considered to be the most successful of all the reptiles. This supposition is based on their survival in both numbers and species, which for the most part reflects the deployment of their venom.

The black widow spider and many other species of spiders use their venom to paralyze their prey before extracting hemolymph and body fluids. The venom is not primarily designed to kill the prey, only to immobilize it. Were it to cause immediate death, removing the hemolymph and body fluids would be made much more difficult and would seem inconsistent with the evolution of the function. The venom apparatus of the stingray is used in defense. It is not employed in getting food, and for the most part its defensive posture appears to have been spent eons ago. The lionfishes, stonefishes, and weeverfishes also use their venomous spines in defense, never in offense. Scorpions, on the other hand, use their venom in both offense and defense.

Most venoms used in an offensive posture are associated with the oral pole of the host animal, obviously the most functional place for their dispense. Defensively designed venoms are usually associated with the aboral pole, as in the stingrays, or with dermal tissues, as is the case with the scorpionfishes and certain other fishes (Russell, 1965; Halstead, 1970). Evidence at the present time seems to indicate that the primary function of a defensive venom is related to its pain-producing property.

In poisonous animals, the poison or toxin may play little, if any, role in either the animal's offensive or defensive statures. The poison may be a product or by-product of metabolism that just happens to be toxic. In the case of Tetraodontidae fishes, the responsible toxic organisms are members of the Vibrionaceae and perhaps other bacteria. In ciguatera fish poisoning, the toxic organism is ingested by herbivores, then by carnivores. Ciguateric fishes feed on smaller toxic fishes or other toxic marine animals, which, in turn, have fed on smaller toxic organisms. As each step in the feeding process progresses, more toxin is accumulated, so that while poisoning in humans may not occur on eating the smaller toxic fishes or marine organisms, by the time a large grouper, barracuda, snapper, or other toxic fish that has fed on smaller toxic organisms is eaten, poisoning occurs. This sequence of events is known as the "food chain phenomena," most eloquently described by Halstead (1967).

In considering the venomousness or poisonousness of an animal, it is wise to consider the use to which that animal puts its toxin. Among other things, this provides a clue as to the possible chemistry and pharmacology of the poison. In addition, a knowledge of the biology of the animal is a valuable asset to the physician treating a case of venom poisoning. It is also well to remember that transposition of data from a simple isolated tissue preparation to the human must be carried out with great care. Errors in clinical judgment have been perpetrated by the overzealous application of *in vitro* data from laboratory experiments. In the intact animal, bioavailability, membrane transport, site accumulation, metabolism, and excretion have values that often cannot be evaluated in a single cell or single fiber preparation (Russell, 1980a).

PROPERTIES OF ANIMAL TOXINS

As one might expect from the uses to which animals put their poisons, these toxins vary considerably in their chemistry and toxicology. Venoms, for instance, may be composed of proteins of both large and small molecular weight, including polypeptides and enzymes. They may be amines, lipids, steroids, aminopolysaccharides, quinones, 5-HT, glycosides, or other substances. The biologic properties of snake venoms have been reviewed by Zeller (1948), Russell (1967, 1983), Dowling *et al.* (1968), Minton and Minton (1969), Elliott (1978), Lee (1979), and Habermehl (1981). With respect to the venoms of spiders, the text of Maretić and Lebez (1979) provides a good discourse and ample references. Keegan's (1980) work on the scorpions is a fine basic text that provides a good overview on the venom of this arthropod. The toxins of marine animals have been thoroughly described by Halstead (1965–70) and by Russell (1965, 1971). The series of texts by Scheuer (1973, 1978–81) provides additional data on some marine animal toxins, as does the excellent work of Southcott (1979). The interested reader will find the book by Hashimoto (1979) a most useful source on the biochemistry of marine toxins. I have updated the biology, chemistry,

and toxicology of marine invertebrate toxins (Russell, 1984a).

One of the unfortunate facts in the study of the chemistry and pharmacology of venoms is that their structure and function are most easily studied by taking them apart. This has two shortcomings: First, a destructive process is used in an attempt to understand a progressive and integrative one; and second, the essential quality of the venom is often destroyed before we have made suitable acquaintance with it. Often, the process of examination becomes so exacting that the end is lost sight of in our preoccupation with the means, so much so that in some cases the means becomes a substitute for the end.

Another shortcoming in the study of venoms has been the naive and oversimplified habit of classifying the whole poison or even its component parts as "neurotoxins," "cardiotoxins," "hemotoxins," "myotoxins," and other loosely articulated synonyms. Most venoms probably exert their effects on almost all cells or tissues, and their pharmacologic properties are determined by how much of a specific biologically active component accumulates at an activity site where it is capable of producing a change. That change probably has a common chemical basis in most tissues, not only specific to the component but to the alteration in ion exchange it perpetuates at the cell or tissue site. It is true, of course, that most venoms have a more particular effect on one or several tissue sites, but more recent expeimental work demonstrates the wide scope of the toxicologic effects that a venom or venom fraction can precipitate. For instance, it has been shown that "cardiotoxin," a component isolated from a snake venom, also causes a neuromuscular block, a block in axonal conduction, membrane depolarization, anticholinesterase activity, local tissue effects, hemolysis, vasoconstriction, cytotoxic action, skeletal and smooth muscle contractions, and cardiac arrest. Other studies have also shown that some of the so-called neurotoxins have myotoxic activities, and "myotoxin" seems to provoke tissue changes in a variety of tissues.

In understanding the actions of a venom, neither the toxicologist nor the clinician should lose sight of the fact that an envenomation represents a complex poisoning and that no biologic activity of a venom can afford to be overlooked. This has been noted elsewhere (Russell, 1963):

The clinician must never slight any symptom or sign his patient presents, or minimize any manifestation on the naive assumption that the venom has to be either a "neurotoxin," "cardiotoxin," "hemotoxin," or "myotoxin" and its activity limited to one organ or system. While the patient may have respiratory distress from a "neurotoxic venom" he can also have changes in cardiac dynamics or vascular permeability and these can become far more life-threatening situations, particularly if the physician centers his attention and therapy on the so-called neurotoxin of the venom (an effect that can often be adequately treated by simple positive pressure respiration). The physician must guard his knowledge and experience zealously and be aware of the limits of application of pharmacologic data based on animal experimentation. On the other hand, he must explore, carefully, the pharmacologic literature on venoms for those data that give him a greater knowledge of the mechanisms involved in venom poisoning and, hopefully, provide him with better methods of therapy.

Venoms have other important properties aside from those of their component parts. Important synergisms that are not obvious from the study of individual fractions become apparent in the activity of the whole venom. In addition, the crude venom may precipitate autopharmacologic reactions that are not produced by individual fractions. Finally, the problem of the formation of metabolites in the envenomated organism has not been explored to any degree, and this might be an important consideration in clinical cases.

The action of a venom or venom component in an organism is dependent on a number of variables, including its route of administration, absorption, distribution, passage across a succession of membranes, accumulation and action at the receptor site, and its metabolism and excretion. All these factors play some role in determining the action of a venom or venom component. During the past two decades, it has become increasingly clear that there are very significant variations in the roles of these factors for different venoms and in different species of experimental animals. In some cases, the variations in different kinds of animals are more important than the difference usually attributed solely to the weight of the animal. Studies carried out in pigs, opossums, certain species of rats, and other animals purport to show that these animals are more "immune" to a toxin than mice. Such investigations fail to take into account the dependent physiologic variables involved in processing a toxin in different kinds of animals, influences that are not related to any principle of immunity. It is a fallacious assumption to treat the LD50 of mice and the opossum or another animal as a direct product of the differences in their weights. In this respect, the toxicologist must always be concerned with the question of whether or not a particular difference in various kinds of animals is caused by variables in the effectiveness of the toxin at the receptor site or in its absorption, distribution, metabolism, or excretion. The fate of a venom or venom fraction, as its activities are spent in the animal, has been discussed elsewhere (Russell, 1980a, 1980b, 1983).

ANTIVENINS

Because of their protein composition, many toxins produce an antibody response. This response is essential in producing antisera. Antisera contain neutralizing antibodies: one antigen (monovalent antisera) or several antigens (polyvalent). An antivenin is a drug composed of purified antibodies concentrated from immune serum. Horses immunized with snake venom develop a variety of antibodies to the many antigens present in the venom. The horse serum is harvested, partially purified and further processed, then administered to the snakebite patient. The antibodies will bind to the venom molecules, rendering them ineffective. Antisera have been produced against most medically important snake, spider, scorpion, and marine toxins, as well as tetanus, rabies, and diphtheria.

Antisera are available in two forms: (1) intact IgG antibodies and (2) binding fragments of antibody, F(ab). Cleaving of intact antibody molecules with papain produces three fragments. These include one F(c), or complement-binding fragment of the antibody, and two F(ab), or antigen-binding fragments. The molecular weight of intact IgG is about 150,000, whereas that of F(ab) is approximately 50,000.

The molecular weight of IgG prevents renal excretion and produces a volume of distribution much smaller than F(ab). The elimination half-life of IgG in the blood is approximately 50 hours. Its ultimate fate is not known. Most IgG is probably taken up by the reticuloendothelial system and degraded with the antigen attached. F(ab) fragments have an elimination half-life of about 17 hours and are small enough to permit renal excretion.

Most antivenin products are heterologous. This increases the possibility of hypersensitivity. Type I (immediate) hypersensitivity reactions are caused by antigen cross-linking of endogenous IgE bound to mast cells and basophils. Binding of antigen by the mast cell may cause release of histamine and other mediators, producing an anaphylactic reaction. Once initiated, anaphylaxis may continue despite discontinuing antivenin administration. An additional concern is an *anaphylactoid reaction*. This is a term for a syndrome resembling an anaphylactic reaction, the etiology of which is unknown but appears to be associated with aggregated protein in the antiserum. Protein aggregates may activate the complement cascade, producing an anaphylacticlike syndrome. One important difference between anaphylactic and anaphylactoid reactions is that anaphylactoid reactions are dose dependent and may be halted by removing the antigen. Type III hypersensitivity (serum sickness) may develop several days after antivenin administration. In these cases, antigen-antibody complexes deposit in different areas of the body, often producing inflammatory responses in the skin, joints, kidney, and other organs. Fortunately, these reactions are rarely serious. The risks of anaphylaxis should always be considered when deciding whether to administer antivenin.

REPTILES

From the very beginnings of human record, few subjects have stimulated the minds and imagination of humans more than the study of snakes and snake venoms. No animal has been more worshipped yet more cast out, more loved yet more despised, and more collected yet more trampled upon than the snake. The essence of the fascination and fear of snakes has been with their venom. In times past, the consequences of bites by venomous snakes were often attributed to forces beyond nature, sometimes to vengeful deities thought to be embodied in the serpents. To early peoples the effects of snakebites were so surprising and so violent that snakes and their poisons were usually shrouded with much myth and superstition.

Snakes have been used in man's worship, magic, entertainment, science, food, sport, medicine, commerce, witchcraft, war, and even tortures on his fellow man. They have been the symbol of love, hate, procreation, health, disease, immortality, sin, death, temptation, riches, poverty, and even wisdom. The Morrises have put it aptly: "It is a paradox. It is both sides of the coin, and mankind has seldom ignored it" (Morris and Morris, 1965).

Of the more than 3500 species of snakes, approximately 375 are considered sufficiently venomous to be of a danger to humans (Dowling et al., 1968; Minton and Minton, 1969; Harding and Welch, 1980; Russell, 1980b, 1983). Venomous species can be divided into the Elapidae—the cobras, kraits, mambas, and coral snakes; Hydrophidae—the true sea snakes; Laticaudidae—the sea kraits; Viperidae—the Old World vipers and adders; Crotalidae—the rattlesnakes, water moccasins, and copperheads of North America, and the fer-de-lance and bushmaster; and certain Colubridae, of which the clinically most important are the boomslang and bird snake of Africa, and the rednecked keelback of Asia. However, several other colubrids must be viewed with concern (Minton and Minton, 1969; Minton, 1976; Mebs, 1977). The death adder and copperhead of Australia are elapids, as is the African garter snake. There are no poisonous snakes in New Zealand, Ireland, or in many other islands of the world. The Gila monster, *Heloderma suspectum*, and the beaded lizard or escorpion, *H. horridum*, are the only venomous lizards and are confined to the southwestern United States and Mexico.

Some of the medically more important venomous snakes of the world and their general distribution are shown in Table 22–1.

Snake Venoms

The venoms of snakes are complex mixtures, chiefly proteins, a number of which have enzymatic activities. In some species, the most lethal component of the venom is a peptide or

---

Table 22–1.   SOME MEDICALLY IMPORTANT SNAKES OF THE WORLD*

SCIENTIFIC AND COMMON NAMES	DISTRIBUTION
Crotalids	
Agkistrodon bilineatus—Coontail	Mexico south to Guatemala and Nicaragua
Agkistrodon contortrix—Copperhead	New York south to Florida and west to Nebraska and Texas
Agkistrodon halys—Mamushi	Caspian Sea to Japan
Agkistrodon calloselosma—Malayan pit viper	Much of Southeast Asia
Bothrops asper and/or *atrox*—Fer-de-lance	Southern Sonora to Peru and northern Brazil
—Barba amarilla	
—Terciopelo	
Bothrops jararaca—Jararaca	Brazil, Paraguay, and Argentina
Bothrops jararacussu—Jararacussu	Brazil, Bolivia, Paraguay, and Argentina
Bothrops neuwiedi—Jararaca pintada	Brazil, Bolivia, Paraguay, northern Argentina
Crotalus adamanteus—Eastern diamondback rattlesnake	Southeastern United States
Crotalus atrox—Western diamondback rattlesnake	Southwestern United States to central Mexico
Crotalus basiliscus—Mexican west-coast rattlesnake	Oaxaca and west coast of Mexico

Table 22–1. (*Continued*)

SCIENTIFIC AND COMMON NAMES	DISTRIBUTION
Trimeresurus flavoviridis—Habu	Amami and Okinawa islands
Trimeresurus mucrosquamatus—Chinese habu	Taiwan and southern China west through Vietnam and Laos to India
Viperids	
Bitis arietans—Puff adder	Morocco and western Arabia through much of Africa
Bitis caudalis—Horned adder	Angola south through Nambia into central and part of south Africa
Causus sp.—Night adders	Most of Africa south of the Sahara
Cerastes cerastes—Horned viper	Sahara, Arabian Peninsula to Lebanon
Cerastes vipera—Sahara sand viper	Central Sahara to Lebanon
Echis carinatus—Saw-scaled viper	Southern India to North and tropical Africa
Echis coloratus—Saw-scaled viper	Eastern Egypt, western Arabian Peninsula north to Israel
Vipera ammodytes—Long-nosed viper	Italy through southeast Europe, Turkey, Jordan to northwest Iran
Vipera berus—European viper	British Isles through Europe, to northern Asia to Korea
Vipera lebetina—Levantine viper	Cyprus through Middle East to Kashmir
Vipera russelli—Russell's viper	Indian subcontinent, southest China to Taiwan and parts of Indonesia
Vipera xanthina—Near East viper	European Turkey and Asia Minor
Elapids	
Coral Snakes (c.s.)	
Calliophis species—Oriental c.s.	Southeast Asia, Orient
Micrurus alleni—Allen's c.s.	Atlantic Nicaragua to Panama
Micrurus corallinus—c.s.	Southern Brazil to Uruguay, northern Argentina
Micrurus frontalis—Southern c.s.	Southwestern Brazil, northern Argentina, Uruguay, Paraguay, and Bolivia
Micrurus fulvius—Eastern c.s.	Southeastern, southern United States and north central Mexico
Micrurus mipartitus—Black-ringed c.s.	Venezuela and Peru to Nicaragua
Micrurus nigrocinctus—Black-banded c.s.	Southern Mexico to northwest Colombia
Cobras	
Hemachatus haemachatus—Ringhals cobra	Southeast and southern Africa
Naja haje—Egyptian or brown cobra	Northern Africa and part of Arabian peninsula
Naja naja atra—Chinese cobra	Thailand and South China to Taiwan
Naja naja naja—Indian cobra	Most of Indian subcontinent
Naja nigricollis—Spitting cobra	West Africa and southern Egypt to near the Cape
Naja naja oxiana—Central Asian cobra	Northern West Pakistan to Iran, southern Russia
Naja naja philippinensis—Philippine cobra	Philippines
Naja naja sputatrix—Malayan cobra	Malayan peninsula and Indonesia
Naja nivea—Cape or yellow cobra	Nambia, Botswana south to the Cape
Ophiophagus hannah—King cobra	Indian subcontinent, China and Philippines
Walterinnesia aegyptia—Desert blacksnake or desert cobra	Egypt to Iran
Kraits and Mambas	
Bungarus caeruleus—Indian or blue krait	India, Pakistan, Sri Lanka, Bangladesh
Bungarus candidus—Malayan krait	Thailand, Malaysia, Indonesia
Bungarus multicinctus—Many-banded krait	Southern China to Hainan, Taiwan
Dendroaspis polylepis—Black mamba	Ethiopia and Somalia to Angola, Zambia, Nambia, southwest Africa
Australian Elapids	
Acanthophis antarcticus—Common death adder	Most of Australia, Moluccas, New Guinea
Notechis scutatus—Tiger snake	Southeastern Australia
Oxyuranus scutellatus—Taipan	Northern coastal Australia, parts of New Guinea
Pseudechis australis—Mulga	Most of Australia except southeast and southern coast, New Guinea
Pseudonaja nuchalis—Western brown snake	Most of Australia except east and southeast coast
Pseudonaja textilis—Eastern brown snake	Eastern Australia

* The common names in this table are those generally employed as literature identifications for the snakes. However, these names may not be the ones used by the people in the specific area where the snake abounds.

polypeptide. In addition, snake venoms contain inorganic substances—sodium, calcium, potassium, magnesium—and small amounts of metals—zinc, iron, cobalt, manganese, and nickel. The importance of the metals in snake venoms is not known, although in the case of some elapid venoms the zinc ions are necessary for anticholinesterase activity, and it has been suggested that calcium may play a role in the activation of phospholipase A_2 and the direct lytic factor. Some of the proteases appear to be metalloproteins. Some snake venoms also contain carbohydrates (glycoproteins), lipids, and biogenic amines, whereas others contain free amino acids (Russell, 1967; Tu, 1977; Elliott, 1978; Lee, 1979; Russell, 1980b, 1983; Habermehl, 1981).

Enzymes. The venoms of snakes contain at least 25 enzymes, although no single snake venom contains all of these. Enzymes are the proteins responsible for the catalysis of numerous specific biochemical reactions that occur in living matter. They are the agents upon which cellular metabolism depends. Enzymes are universally accepted as proteins, although a few have crucial dependencies on certain nonprotein prosthetic groups, or cofactors. All living cells contain enzymes. Some of the more important snake venom enzymes are shown in Table 22–2.

Proteolytic enzymes catalyze the breakdown of tissue proteins and peptides. These are known variously as proteolytic enzymes, peptide hydrolases, proteases, endopeptidases, peptidases, and proteinases. There may be several proteolytic enzymes in a single venom; at least five have been found in one venom. It must be admitted, however, that most of the proteases have not been characterized, either biochemically or pharmacologically. The proteolytic enzymes have molecular weights between 20,000 and 95,000. Some are inactivated by EDTA and certain reducing agents. The role of metal ions in catalysis was demonstrated by Wagner and Prescott in 1966. The removal of zinc ions by o-phenanthroline in the presence of calcium ions inhib-

ited the action of *Agkistrodon piscivorus* peptidase A (Wagner *et al.*, 1968). Reactivity was initiated by the addition of zinc ions. Zinc appears to be the catalytically necessary metal. Metals appear to be intrinsically involved in the activity of certain venom proteases and phospholipases.

All crotalid venoms so far examined appear to be rich in proteolytic enzyme activity. Viperid venoms have lesser amounts, whereas elapid and sea snake venoms either have no proteolytic activity or very little. Venoms that are rich in proteinase activity are associated with marked tissue destruction. The lethal effect of proteolytic enzymes has been studied, but the data are difficult to evaluate in view of the fact that investigators have used different assay parameters. Maeno *et al.* (1959) demonstrated that proteinase isolated from *Trimeresurus flavoviridis* venom produced hemorrhagic necrosis with severe lysis of muscles, but other workers have reported that the proteases and hemorrhagic factors were separable. Hemorrhagic activity may be associated with some proteases but not with others.

Arginine ester hydrolase is one of a number of noncholinesterases found in snake venoms. The substrate specificities are directed to the hydrolysis of the ester or peptide linkage to which an argine residue contributes the carboxyl group. This activity is found in many crotalid and viperid venoms and some sea snake venoms but is lacking in elapid venoms, with the possible exception of *Ophiophagus hannah*. It was first demonstrated by Deutsch and Diniz (1955) in 15 snake venoms and has subsequently been identified in many others. Some crotalid venoms contain at least three chromatographically separable arginine ester hydrolases. The pharmacologic activities of the arginine ester hydrolases have not been classified. The bradykinin-releasing and perhaps -clotting activities of some crotalid venoms may be related to esterase activity.

Thrombinlike enzymes are found in significant amounts in the venoms of the Crotalidae and Viperidae, whereas those of Elapidae and Hydrophiidae contain little or none. The mechanism of fibrinogen clot formation by snake venom thrombinlike enzymes invokes the preferential release of fibrinopeptide A (or B); thrombin releases both fibrinopeptides A and B. Paradoxically, the thrombinlike enzymes have been shown to act as defibrinating anticoagulants *in vivo*, whereas *in vitro* they clot plasma, citrated or heparinized plasma, or purified fibrinogen. Because of the obvious clinical potential of these enzymes as defibrinating agents, more attention has been directed toward the characterization and study of the thrombinlike enzymes than of the other venom procoagulant or anticoagulant

Table 22–2. ENZYMES OF SNAKE VENOMS*

Proteolytic enzymes	Phosphomonoesterase
Arginine ester hydrolase	Phosphodiesterase
Thrombinlike enzyme	Acetylcholinesterase
Collagenase	RNase
Hyaluronidase	DNase
Phospholipase A_2 (A)	5'-Nucleotidase
Phospholipase B	NAD-nucleotidase
Phospholipase C	L-Amino acid oxidase
Lactate dehydrogenase	

* From Russell, F. E.: *Snake Venom Poisoning.* J. B. Lippincott Co., Philadelphia, 1980; Scholium International, Great Neck, N.Y., 1983.

Table 22–3. PROTEOLYTIC ACTION OF THROMBIN AND THROMBINLIKE SNAKE VENOM ENZYMES*

| ENZYME | ACTION ON HUMAN FIBRINOGEN | | ACTIVATION OF FACTOR XIII | PROTHROMBIN FRAGMENT CLEAVAGE | PLATELET AGGREGATION AND RELEASE | ACTIVATION OF FACTOR VIII | ACTIVATION OF FACTOR V |
	Fibrinopeptides Released	*Chain Degradation*					
Thrombin	A + B	α(A)	Yes	Yes	Yes	Yes	Yes
Thrombinlike enzymes	A‡	α(A)‡ or β(B)§	No	Yes or no‖	No	No	No
Agkistrodon c. contortrix venom	B	n.d.#	Incomplete	n.d.	No	n.d.	n.d.
Bitis gabonica venom	A + B	n.d.	Yes	n.d.	n.d.	n.d.	n.d.

* From Russell, F. E.: *Snake Venom Poisoning.* J. B. Lippincott Co., Philadelphia, 1980; Scholium International, Great Neck, N.Y., 1983.
† Includes Ancrod®, batroxobin, crotalase, and the enzyme from *T. okinavensis.*
‡ Ancrod® [batroxobin degrades α(A) chain of bovine but not human fibrinogen].
§ Crotalase.
‖ Fragment 1 released by crotalase and *Agkistrodon contortrix* venom but not by ancrod or batroxobin.
n.d. = Not determined.

759

enzymes (*see* Russell, 1983). The proteolytic action of thrombin and thrombinlike snake venom enzymes is shown in Table 22–3.

Thrombinlike enzymes have been purified from the venoms of *Crotalus adamanteus* (Crotalase®), *C. horridus horridus, Agkistrodon rhodostoma* (Ancrod®), *A. contortrix contortrix, A. acutus, Bothrops atrox* (Batroxobin®), *B. marajoensis, B. moojeni, Trimeresurus gramineus, T. okinavensis,* and *Bitis gabonica*. In Table 22–4 are shown some of the physical and chemical properties of the thrombinlike enzymes. All these enzymes appear to be glycoproteins, and with the exception of two, all appear to have molecular weights in the range of 29,000 to 35,000.

Thrombinlike enzymes have been used clinically and in animals for therapeutic and investigative studies. In experimentally induced venous thrombosis in dogs, treatment with Ancrod® prior to the formation of the thrombus prevents thrombosis and ensures vessel patency. However, Ancrod® has no thrombolytic effect when administered after thrombus formation. Trials of Ancrod® versus heparin and Ancrod® versus streptokinase in the treatment of deep venous thromboses of the lower leg have been made. It appears that neither heparin nor Ancrod® has a significant effect on thrombus resolution, whereas streptokinase produces more lysis of thrombi than Ancrod®. Crotalase® is being employed to evaluate the role of fibrin deposition in burns in animals (Bajwa and Markland, 1976). The role of fibrin deposition is also being evaluated in tumor metastasis, in which fibrinogen is removed by treatment with Ancrod® or Batroxobin®. Ancrod® has also been used to prevent the deposition of fibrin on prosthetic heart valves that have been implanted in calves (*see* Russell, 1980b, 1983).

Collagenase is a specific kind of proteinase that digests collagen. This activity has been demonstrated in the venoms of a number of species of crotalids and viperids. The venom of *Crotalus atrox* digests mesenteric collagen fibers but not protein. EDTA inhibits the collagenolytic effect but not the argine esterase effect.

Hyaluronidase catalyzes the cleavage of internal glycoside bonds of certain acid mucopolysaccharides. This results in a decrease in the viscosity of connective tissues. The breakdown in the hyaluronic barrier allows other fractions of the venom to penetrate the tissues. The enzyme is thought to be related to the extent of the edema produced by the whole venom, but to what degree it contributes to clinical swelling and edema is not known. The enzyme has also been referred to as the "spreading factor."

Phospholipase A (phospholipase A_2, PLA_2) has been found in the venoms of more than 20 species of snakes and appears to be widely distributed throughout the venoms of elapids, vipers, crotalids, sea snakes, and even colubrids. It catalyzes the hydrolysis of one of the fatty ester linkages in diacyl phosphatides, forming lysophosphatides and releasing both saturated and unsaturated fatty acids. As has been noted by several workers, data from many studies on PhA_2 must be evaluated with care, principally because impure preparations of the enzyme have often been employed. The molecular weights of this enzyme differ considerably. However, the molecular weight for the dimer of PLA_2 in *Crotalus atrox* venom is 29,500 that of *C. adamanteus* venom (PA_2—α), 29,500 to 29,900, and that of *C. viridis helleri* venom, approximately 29,500 to 30,000. There appears to be a considerable similarity in the positions of the sulfur atoms in many of the PLA_2 enzymes, and there are a number of other similarities, but there are

Table 22–4. COMPARISON OF SNAKE VENOM THROMBINLIKE ENZYMES*

VENOM ENZYME	MOLECULAR WEIGHT	CARBOHYDRATE CONTENT (%)	NH₂-TERMINAL RESIDUE	ACTIVE SITE SERINE	ACTIVE SITE HISTIDINE
Agkistrodon calloselosma	35,400	36.0	Val	+	+
Crotalus adamanteus	33,700	5.4	Val	+	+
Bothrops marajoensis	31,400	high	Val	+	n.d.†
Bothrops moojeni	29,100	26.7	Val	+	n.d.
Crotalus horridus horridus	19,400	Very low	n.d.	n.d.	n.d.
Agkistrodon acutus	33,500	13.0	n.d.	+	+
Trimeresurus gramineus	29,500	25.0	n.d.	+	n.d.
Trimeresurus okinavensis	34,000	6.0	n.d.	+	n.d.
Agkistrodon contortrix contortrix	100,000	n.d.	n.d.	+	n.d.
Bitis gabonica	32,500	n.d.	n.d.	n.d.	n.d.

* From Russell, F. E.: *Snake Venom Poisoning.* J. B. Lippincott Co., Philadelphia, 1980; Scholium International, Great Neck, N.Y., 1983.
† n.d. = Not determined.

also a number of important differences. The interested reader should consult the excellent review by Rosenberg (1979) for a more thorough understanding of the activities of the enzyme. Although generalizations concerning the pharmacologic activities of PLA_2 must be viewed with caution, some tentative assumptions might be noted. Contrary to earlier reports, the enzyme is not nearly as lethal as was suspected. In mice, the intravenous LD50 for the basic PLA_2 for *Naja nigricollis* venom is 0.25 mg/kg body weight, whereas that of the acidic PLA_2 is approximately 0.8 mg/kg. The two proteins with PLA_2 activity of *Vipera ammodytes* venom have been found to have intraperitoneal LD50 values of 0.19 and 0.64 mg/kg, respectively. The intravenous LD50 for the basic PLA_2 of *Crotalus durissus terrificus* is 0.54 mg/kg, and its lethal activity descends in the following order: chick, mouse, rabbit, rat. The results to date indicate that the basic PLA_2 enzymes are more lethal than the acidic PLA_2 enzymes, but there are variations in the lethal indices of both groups (*see* Russell, 1980b, 1983c).

Phosphomonoesterase (phosphatase) is widely distributed in the venoms of all families of snakes except the colubrids. It has properties of an orthophosphoric monoester phosphohydrolase. There are two nonspecific phosphomonoesterases, and they have optimal pH at 5.0 and 8.5. Many venoms contain both acid and alkaline phosphatases, whereas others contain only one or the other.

Phosphodiesterase has now been found in the venoms of all five families of poisonous snakes. It is an orthophosphoric diester phosphohydrolase that releases 5-mononucleotide from the polynucleotide chain and thus acts as an exonucleotidase, attacking DNA and RNA. More recently, it has been found that it also attacks derivatives of arabinose.

Acetylcholinesterase was first demonstrated in cobra venom and is widely distributed throughout the elapid venoms. It is also found in sea snake venoms but is totally lacking in the viperid and crotalid venoms. It catalyzes the hydrolysis of acetylcholine to choline and acetic acid. The role of the enzyme in snake venoms is not clear. Its so-called effect on ganglionic and neuromuscular transmission as a venom constituent is highly questionable.

RNase is present in some snake venoms in small amounts as the endopolynucleotidase RNase. It appears to have specificity toward pyrimidine-containing pyrimidyladenyl bonds in DNA. The optimum pH is 7 to 9, when ribosomal RNA is used as the substrate. This enzyme in *Naja oxiana* venom has a molecular weight of 15,900.

DNase acts on DNA and gives predominantly tri or higher oligonucleotides that terminate in 3' monoesterified phosphate. *Crotalus adamanteus* venom contains two DNases, with optimum pH at 5 and 9.

5'-Nucleotidase is a common constituent of all snake venoms, and in most instances, it is the most active phosphatase in snake venoms. It specifically hydrolyzes phosphate monoesters, which links with a 5' position of DNA and RNA. It is found in greater amounts in crotalid and viper venoms than elapid venoms. The molecular weight as determined from amino acid composition and gel filtration with *Naja naja atra* venom has been estimated at 10,000. The enzyme from *N. naja* venom was enhanced by Mg^{2+}, inhibited by Zn^{2+}, inactivated at 75°C at pH 7.0 or 8.4, and has an isoelectric point of about 8.6. That from *Agkistrodon halys blomhoffii* showed a pH optimum of 6.8 to 6.9, with activity being enhanced by Mg^{2+} and Mn^{2+} and inhibited by Zn^{2+}. The enzyme has a low order of lethality, and its pharmacologic role in the venom is not understood (*see* Russell, 1980b, 1983).

NAD nucleotidase has been found in the venoms of 9 of 37 species examined. The enzyme catalyzes the hydrolysis of the nicotinamide *N*-ribosidic linkage of NAD, yielding nicotinamide and adenosine diphosphate riboside. Its optimum pH is 6.5 to 8.5; it is heat labile, losing activity at 60°C. Its toxicologic contribution to snake venoms is not known.

L-Amino acid oxidase has been found in all snake venoms so far examined. It gives a yellow color to the venom. The enzyme catalyzes the oxidation of L-α-amino and α-hydroxy acids. This activity results from a group of homologous enzymes, showing molecular weights from 85,000 to 150,000. It has a high content of acidic amino acids. We found that the mouse intravenous LD50 of the enzyme from *Crotalus adamanteus* venom was 9.13 mg/kg body weight, approximately four times less than the lethal value for the crude venom, and it had no effect on nerve, muscle, or neuromuscular transmission (*see* Russell, 1980b, 1983).

Lactate dehydrogenase reversibly catalyzes the conversion of lactic acid to pyruvic acid and has been reported to have been found in nine elapid venoms but was not found in three others.

Polypeptides. The snake venom polypeptides are low-molecular-weight proteins that do not have enzymatic activity. They are often logged under "neurotoxins," unfortunately, and this practice is not likely to change. As Will Rogers once said, "It is more difficult to change the label than the stuff in the bottle."

In 1938, Slotta and Fraenkel-Conrat isolated a

crystalline protein from the venom of the tropical rattlesnake *Crotalus durissus terrificus.* The protein exhibited most of the toxic properties of the crude venom and was named *crotoxin.* In addition to the toxic nonenzymatic protein portion, it was found to contain the enzymes hyaluronidase, phospholipase, and possibly several others. It did not appear to have proteolytic or coagulant properties, or 5'-nucleotidase activity, but it had neurotoxic, indirect hemolytic, and smooth muscle–stimulating properties. Following removal of phospholipase A, crotoxin was further separated into a general toxic principle known as *crotactin,* which was found to have a greater lethal index than crotoxin, and a second component that may have been *crotamine.* The word *crotoxin* has been retained in one form or another in the literature as an identification for 17 different components of the venom of *Crotalus durissus terrificus* over the past 30 years. This has resulted in considerable confusion and more than once has led to disputes on research techniques, which could be more easily resolved on the basis of a difference in interpretation of what the investigator meant by *crotoxin.*

During the past 15 years, various peptides of snake venoms have been characterized. In 1965, the first amino acid composition of a snake venom peptide was published (Yang, 1965), and at the First International Symposium on Animal Toxins in 1966, Nobuo Tamiya presented a paper on the chromatography, crystallization, electrophoresis, ultracentrifugation, and amino acid composition of the venom of the sea snake *Laticauda semifasciata.* Almost all the lethal activity of the poison was recovered as two toxins, *erabutoxin a* and *b,* using carboxymethylcellulose chromatography, and 30 percent of the proteins were erabutoxins. The homogeneity of the crystalline toxins was demonstrated by rechromatography, disk electrophoresis, and ultracentrifugation (Tamiya *et al.,* 1967).

At the same meeting in 1966, Su and colleagues reported on the isolation of a cobra "neurotoxin." The toxin was separated by repeated fractionation with ammonium sulfate. The final product was a polypeptide and was approximately seven times more lethal than the crude venom. A product said to be identical to this in its lethal index and certain other pharmacologic characteristics was also obtained by starch gel electrophoresis. When the ammonium sulfate fraction was subjected to the same electrophoretic procedure, it concentrated as a single peak, with but little increase in its lethal property (Su *et al.,* 1967). Since 1966, more than 60 polypeptides having pharmacologic activities have been isolated from snake venoms. The interested reader will find definitive reviews on these peptides in the excellent work of Elliott (1978) and the book by Tu (1977). The texts edited by Rosenberg (1978), Lee (1979), and Eaker and Wadström (1980) contain other good papers on venom polypeptides.

Toxicology

It is not within the confines of this review to discuss all the pharmacologic activities of snake venoms. The interested reader is referred to Russell (1967, 1983) and Mebs (1978) and to articles in the compendiums noted above for a more thorough consideration of the specific toxicologic effects of these poisons and their components. However, some remarks will be made about the venoms of the North American crotalids, particularly the rattlesnake. The LD50s of some North American snake venoms are shown in Table 22–5.

In general, the venoms of the rattlesnakes and other New World crotalids produce alterations in the resistances (and often the integrity) of the blood vessels, changes in the blood cells and blood coagulation mechanisms, direct or indirect changes in cardiac and pulmonary dynamics, alterations in the nervous system, and changes in respiration. Experimentally, these changes can be produced by varying the dose and kind of crotalid venom, the route and speed of adminis-

Table 22–5. LD50 BY DIFFERENT ROUTES OF INJECTION*†

VENOM	INTRAVENOUS	INTRAPERITONEAL	SUBCUTANEOUS
Crotalus viridis helleri	1.29	1.60	3.65
Crotalus adamanteus	1.68	1.90	13.73
Crotalus atrox	2.18	3.71	17.75
Crotalus scutulatus	0.21	0.23	0.31
Agkistrodon piscivorus	4.17	5.10	25.10
Agkistrodon contortrix	10.92	10.50	26.10
Sistrurus miliarius	2.91	6.89	25.10

  * All determinations in 20-g female mice of the same group. All mice were injected within a 1-hour period and were observed for 48 hours.
  † From Russell, F. E.: *Snake Venom Poisoning.* J. B. Lippincott Co., Philadelphia, 1980; Scholium International, Great Neck, N.Y., 1983.

tration, and the choice of the test animal. In humans, the course of the poisoning is determined by the kind and amount of venom injected, where it is deposited, the general health, size, and age of the patient, and the kind of treatment. Clinical experience indicates that death in humans occurs between less than 1 hour to several days, with most deaths occurring between 18 and 32 hours. Hypotension or shock is the major therapeutic problem. In some cases, the hypotension is associated with acute blood loss secondary to bleeding and/or hemolysis, but in most patients the shock is associated with a decrease in circulating fluid volume, with varying degrees of blood cell loss. It is not surprising, therefore, to find that numerous studies have been directed at determining the mechanisms responsible for snake venom poisoning, hypotension, and shock. These have been reviewed in some thoroughness elsewhere (Russell, 1983).

In 1962 it was found that an intravenous bolus injection of *Crotalus* venom caused an immediate fall in blood pressure and varying degrees of shock, which were associated with an initial hemoconcentration followed by a decrease in hematocrit values. There was an increased blood volume in the lungs, an increase in pulmonary artery pressure with a concomitant decrease in pulmonary artery flow, and a relatively stable heart stroke volume (Russell *et al.*, 1962). Other workers, using a 30-minute perfusion of *Crotalus* venom, concluded that the hypotension was related to the formation of pulmonary thromboemboli in the pulmonary vascular bed (Halmagyi *et al.*, 1965). Multiple pulmonary emboli may be found in animals receiving a fatal rattlesnake bite; however, the production of thromboembolism within one minute after administration of a bolus injection or even after a 30-minute infusion of the venom might be a difficult explanation for the rapid onset of pulmonary hypotension and the precipitous fall in systemic arterial pressure seen in experimental animals. Clumping of blood cells in the lungs, thrombosis, or even multiple pulmonary emboli might conceivably cause pulmonary hypertension within this short period, but it seems unlikely that thromboembolism is responsible for the immediate circulatory failure. There is another finding that adds to the unlikelihood of this proposed mechanism. In postmortem reports on victims who survived less than three hours after a rattlesnake bite, there is no evidence of pulmonary thromboembolism (Russell, 1983).

Crotalus venom appears to produce a pooling of blood in the hepatosplanchnic bed in the dog (Vick *et al.*, 1967). However, the hepatosplanchnic bed in the cat and human is known to be a lesser target area in most shock states than in the dog, and it seems unlikely that this explanation for the hypotension is consistent with snake venom poisoning in humans. Again, postmortem examinations in humans have not shown remarkable involvement of the hepatosplanchnic bed. More recently, Carlson and his colleagues have observed that when *Crotalus* venom is given intravenously and slowly over a 30-minute period, there is hypovolemia secondary to an increase in capillary permeability to protein and red blood cells. The laboratory findings showed initial hemoconcentration, lactacidemia, and hypoproteinemia (Carlson *et al.*, 1975). In cats, the same findings are seen, followed by a fall in hematocrit and, in some cases, hemolysis that is related to the dose of venom. During this period, the cat may be in shock or at near-shock levels, depending on the amount of venom injected or perfused. Respirations become labored, and if the period is prolonged, the animal becomes oliguric, rales develop, and the animal dies.

There appears to be no doubt that the shock or hypotension is caused by a decrease in circulating blood volume secondary to an increase in capillary permeability leading to the loss of fluid, protein, and to some extent, erythrocytes. The severity of the hypotension is dose related, and restoration of circulating fluid volume can be achieved with intravenous fluids. In patients with venom shock, steroids are of no value, but the use of isoproterenol hydrochloride may be indicated. Antivenin in itself may not reverse a deep shock state, but a combination of parenteral fluids or plasma expanders, isoproterenol hydrochloride, and antivenin is of definite value.

Although the lung may suffer the most deleterious changes in crotalid venom poisoning shock, almost all organs and tissues can be involved. Certainly, the venom can cause severe changes in blood coagulation, in erythrocyte integrity, or in other mechanisms. Although the action on the heart and kidneys is usually secondary to changes in the lung, blood, or blood dynamics, the crotalid venoms can affect these structures directly. The only organ that appears to be relatively unaffected by crotalid venoms is the brain, although several workers have indicated some electroencephalographic changes associated with crotalid venom injections. However, these changes are more easily explained on the basis of a decreased blood supply to the brain, resulting in cerebral anoxemia secondary to ischemic anemia.

Evidence to the present time indicates that the most probable fraction of the venom responsible for the circulatory failure is a peptide. In 1970, Dubnoff and Russell reported on the presence of two biologically active peptides in the venom of the rattlesnake *Crotalus viridis helleri*. Ion exchange chromatography on carboxymethylcellulose and on IRC-50 indicated molecular weights of approximately 6000 each. The peptides moved as cations on cellulose acetate at pH 8.6. Peptide I was identified as the major peak (Dubnoff and Russell, 1970). Subsequently, Bonilla and Fiero isolated highly basic proteins from the venoms of three species of rattlesnakes: *Crotalus viridis viridis, C. horridus horridus,* and *C. h. atricaudatus.* The proteins were separated by recycling adsorption chromatography using Bio-Gel P-2 and by ion-exchange chromatography on carboxymethylcellulose. These fractions were of low molecular weight, had isoelectric points above pH 6.8 (Bonilla and Fiero, 1971), and showed pharmacologic properties similar to those of the *C. v. helleri* isolated by Dubnoff and Russell.

Toxicologic studies have been carried out on the various fractions of *C. v. helleri* venom. One peptide, *C. v. helleri* Peptide I, which moved as a cation on strip and gel electrophoresis and on ion-exchange chromatography, was resolved into three lethal peaks. The major fraction (*C. v. h.* Peptide Ic) was a basic polypeptide containing 43 amino acid residues with six half-cystine and had a molecular weight of 4490, as calculated from its sequence. Analysis showed that the peptide contained almost 20 percent lysine (Maeda *et al.,* 1978). The peptide was found to be responsible for hypotension or shock produced by the crude venom. When injected into rats, this peptide produced shock characterized by hypotension, lactacidemia, hemoconcentration, hypoproteinemia, and metabolic acidosis. Death occurred in some rats, and respiratory distress was observed just prior to death. Hemolysis did not occur, but hemolysis and hematuria were observed in rats given the nonpeptide fractions (Schaeffer *et al.,* 1978).

The primary action of the peptide on the cardiovascular system involves its ability to produce a transient increase in vascular permeability to plasma protein, which, eventually, with certain other proteins, causes the loss of red blood cells. The peptide appears to alter the endothelial cells of the vascular wall, giving rise to the escape of plasma protein and some red blood cells. This finding for rattlesnake venom appears to differ from that presented for elapid venoms in that *C. viridis helleri* Peptide I is capable of producing rapid endothelial changes without enzyme involvement. Other protein components of the venom, some of which are enzymes, appear to have little effect on the vascular membrane but, rather, induce red blood cell changes or lysis. There may be some synergistic action, but

for the most part, vascular properties are rather distinct.

Lizard Venoms

The Gila monster, *Heloderma suspectum,* and the beaded lizard, *H. horridum,* are divided into five subspecies. These large, corpulent, relatively slow-moving, and largely nocturnal reptiles have few enemies other than humans. They are far less dangerous than generally believed. Their venom is transferred from the venom glands in the lower jaw through ducts that discharge their contents near the base of the larger teeth of the lower jaw. The venom is then drawn up along grooves in the teeth by capillary action. The venom of this lizard has serotonin, amine oxidase, phospholipase A, proteolytic, and hyaluronidase activities but lacks phosphomono- and diesterase, acetylcholinesterase, nucleotidase, ATPase, DNase, RNase, amino acid oxidase, and fibrinogenocoagulase activities. The high hyaluronidase content seems to be consistent with the tissue edema seen in many clinical cases, and the low proteolytic activity is also consistent with the minimal tissue breakdown in clinical cases. Injection of large doses of *Heloderma* venom produces a fall in systemic arterial pressure with a decrease in circulating blood volume, tachycardia, and respiratory distress, and in lethal doses a loss of ventricular contractility (Russell and Bogert, 1981).

Clinical Problem

Snake venom poisoning is a medical emergency requiring immediate attention and the exercise of considerable judgment. Delayed or inadequate treatment may result in tragic consequences. However, before any treatment is instituted, it is essential that a working diagnosis be established. In making a diagnosis, it must be remembered that being bitten by a venomous snake does not necessarily mean being envenomated by that snake. A venomous snake may bite a person and not inject venom. Also, in treating snake venom poisoning, one should keep in mind that he is faced with a case of multiple and complex poisoning. There is no single therapeutic measure other than antivenin that can effectively neutralize all the physiopharmacologic activities of the venom.

Symptoms and signs of pit viper envenomation include the presence of fang marks, swelling, pain, ecchymosis, weakness, various paresthesia, faintness, nausea and vomiting, alterations in temperature, pulse, and blood pressure, fasciculations, urinary changes, early hemoconcentration followed by a decreased hematocrit, decreased platelets, petechiae, and shock. The most diagnostic sign of snakebite is rapid, progressive swelling. In most patients, there is some swelling around the bite areas within five to ten minutes, and often the swelling involves the entire finger, hand, toe, or foot, depending on the severity. A common symptom following the bites by many rattlesnakes is paresthesia about the mouth, often the forehead and scalp, and sometimes of the fingers and toes. This is usually present following the bites of the eastern diamondback rattlesnake *(Crotalus adamanteus)*, the Pacific rattlesnakes (*C. viridis helleri* and *C. viridis oreganus*), most other *viridis* sub-species, and some other species. The venom of some rattlesnake species, however, does not cause this complaint.

The degree of poisoning should be determined. A bite may appear minor at one hour but prove serious or even fatal at three hours. Most of the suggested grading systems for crotalid bites are precarious, for they usually depend on a few selected symptoms or signs, and these are often stipulated for a specific time, for instance, 12 hours.

It is far more simple and practical to grade envenomations as minimal, moderate, or severe based on *all* clinical findings, including the laboratory data. One must then remember that the grading may need to be changed as the course of the poisoning or treatment progresses.

A determination should be made as to whether or not antivenin is necessary. It need not be given in trivial bites. The antivenin should be put in 250 to 1000 ml of an appropriate vehicle. Antivenin is compatible with commonly used dextrose and electrolyte solutions. The best results are obtained when it is administered during the first four hours following the bite, but its efficacy seems apparent for at least 24 hours after the bite, and perhaps longer. Antivenin has corrected blood clotting deficits even after 24 hours. In most cases, antivenin is not needed for copperhead bites, but it may be indicated in water moccasin bites. A skin test should always be administered before giving antivenin. The patient should be slightly sedated, if not contraindicated, and put to bed, with the injured part lightly immobilized in a functional position and slightly below heart level. Medication for tetanus, pain, sleep, and anxiety should be given, if necessary. In moderate or severe envenomations, laboratory work should be done at least twice a day. Food should be avoided during the first 24 hours. Detailed clinical reports on bites by American species will be found in Russell (1980b, 1983) and Parrish (1980).

AMPHIBIA

The class Amphibia contains approximately 2600 species and is divided into the Anura, the toads and frogs, and the Urodela, the salamanders and newts. Although there are a number of amphibians known to be poisonous, very few of these are of a danger to humans. The most important toxic Anura are toads of the family Bufonidae; frogs of the families Atelopodidae, Dendrobatidae, Discoglossidae, Hylidae, Phyllomedusae, Pipidae, and Ranidae; newts of the genera *Taricha* and *Triturus;* and certain salamanders of the genus *Salamandra* (Kaiser and Michl, 1958; Habermehl, 1981; Daly, 1982).

Amphibian Toxins

The poisons of amphibians are produced in certain highly developed secretory glands in the skin. These secretions are generally excreted in a steady state, although there may be increased elaboration under duress or other conditions. Although it is commonly believed that their only function is related to a deterrent posture, that is, defense against predators, it has been shown that in some amphibians another important function is their role in protecting the host against microorganisms in the environment. When the skin is freed of the secretions of these particular glands, infection occurs and death often results. The secretions have been shown to inhibit the growth of bacteria and fungi in concentrations as low as 10^{-3} to 10^{-5} moles/liter (Habermehl, 1981).

The chemical composition of amphibian secretions is highly diversified. In the toads, biogenic amines, including adrenaline, noradrenaline, dopamine, and epinine, are sometimes found, whereas among the indoalkylamines, the bases bufotenin, bufotenidin, and bufoviridin have been noted.

Bufotenin

Bufotenidin

Bufoviridin

These substances have been described as causing vasoconstriction, hypotension, and hallucinations. However, their specific toxicologic properties are poorly understood. A second group of toxic secretions in the toads is the bufogenines, presented as a formula by Meyer (1949), of which bufotalin is representative. The overall

Bufotalin

toxicologic properties of this group of secretions is not known, but they appear to have a marked effect on smooth muscle, including the heart.

The frog toxins are even more diversified than the toad poisons. In the Atelopodidae, *Atelopus* species, a group of toxins known as *zetekitoxins* are found. The poison from the golden arrow frogs of Costa Rica, Panama, and Colombia has long been used on hunting darts by the Indians in those areas. The structure of these toxins is not clear, although a guanidine group has been described, and the poison contains no peptides, carbohydrates, or steroids. The subcutaneous "lethal dose" in mice for zetekitoxin AB is 11 μg/kg; for zetekitoxin C, 80 μg/kg body weight. Their toxicologic properties are not known. *Tetrodotoxin* has been isolated from the skin and egg clusters of *A. varius*, whereas both tetrodotoxin and *chiriquitoxin* have been found in the skin and eggs of *A. chiriquensis*. In the Dendrobatidae, particularly *Phyllobates* and *Dendrobates*, more than 100 toxic skin secretions have been identified (Daly, 1982). Most of these are alkaloids, and their use as dart or arrow poisons by certain South Central American Indians is well known (Marki and Witkop, 1963). Among the steroid alkaloids are *batrachotoxin, batrachotoxin A, homobatrachotoxin, dihydrobatrachotoxin,* and *3-0-methylbatrachotoxin,* all found in certain *Phyllobates* species.

Batrachotoxin

Batrachotoxin is one of the most toxic substances known, the subcutaneous lethal dose in mice being 100 nanograms; the estimated lethal dose for humans is less than 200 μg. Although generally classified as a "neurotoxin," the alkaloid has a marked effect on the heart, first evident as arrhythmias and then by changes leading to cardiac arrest. It has a direct effect on the peripheral nervous system, producing membrane depolarization, which is probably due to an increase in cell membrane permeability by sodium, without changes in the potassium or calcium ions. Both tetrodotoxin and saxitoxin prevent and even reverse the depolarization caused by batrachotoxin. Certain anesthetics antagonize the action of the alkaloid, whereas certain local anesthetics block its action. Batrachotoxin also causes a massive release of acetylcholine in nerve muscle preparations. The ultrastructure changes in nerve and muscle precipitated by this toxin are due to osmotic alterations produced by the massive influx of sodium ions. These various activities are time and stimulus dependent, suggesting that activity requires prior activation or opening of the sodium channel. It has been suggested that batrachotoxin also has a central nervous system effect (Daly, 1982).

From the skin secretions of *Dendrobates pumilio* and *D. auratus,* three alkaloids have been isolated: *pumiliotoxin A* ($C_{19}H_{33}NO_2$), *B* ($C_{19}H_{33}NO_3$), and *C* ($C_{13}H_{25}N$). The skin secretions from the latter frog have also yielded other alkaloids, whereas spiropiperidine alkaloids have been identified in the skin secretions of *D. histrionicus*. The subcutaneous "minimal lethal dose" in mice for pumiliotoxin A is 2.5 mg/kg body weight; for pumiliotoxin B, 1.5 mg/kg; and for pumiliotoxin *C*, 20 mg/kg. These doses produce ataxia, "clonic convulsions," and death within 20 minutes. Pumiliotoxin B potentiates both direct and indirect evoked contractions of striated muscle, which is thought to be due to mechanism-related facilitation of calcium influx of the muscle fiber and/or a facilitation of release of calcium from the sarcoplasmic reticulum. It does not appear to have an effect on sodium, potassium, or chloride conductances, or on the resting membrane potential (Albuquerque *et al.,* 1981). The poisons of the Disoglossidae, or the disc tongue frogs, have been the object of extended study by Michl and his colleagues in Vienna (*see* Kaiser and Michl, 1958). The skin secretions of *Bombina bombina* have yielded large amounts of serotonin, free amino acids, and basic peptides. In *B. variegata,* 12 α-amino acids, γ-amino-butyric acid, and serotonin, two nonapeptides, and a hemolytic polypeptide of 87,000 daltons have been demonstrated (Habermehl, 1981).

The poisons of the newts and salamanders have undergone considerable study. Tarichatoxin has been isolated from three species of newts, *Taricha torosa, T. rivularis,* and *T. granulosa.* It is, of course, the same toxin found in the pufferfish *Sphoeroides* species and known as tetrodotoxin. Tarichatoxin, or tetrodotoxin, is also found in some species of frogs, and at least one octopus, as well as a number of other fishes beside the puffers. Among the steroid alkaloids found in the salamanders are *samanin, samandenon, cycloneosamandaridin, cycloneosamandoin, samandarin,* and *samandaridin.* Samandarin is a very potent toxin, which is said to act on the central nervous system and has hypertensive and anesthetic properties.

MARINE ANIMALS

Like the snakes, the venomous and poisonous marine animals have enjoyed a fascinating history, including sea serpents that crawled ashore and copulated with vipers, others that sprayed their venom onto unsuspecting seamen on sailing ships, thus paralyzing them on the spot, and stingrays that stung and killed trees. These are only a few of the numerous bits of folklore recorded in the literature. The interested reader should consult the compendium of Halstead (1965–70), and the works of Phillips and Brady (1953). Kaiser and Michl (1958), Russell (1965, 1971, 1984a), Baslow (1969), Martin and Padilla (1973), Scheuer (1973, 1978–81), Halstead (1978), and Southcott (1979) for the more historical accounts on venomous marine animals.

There are approximately 1200 species of marine organisms known to be venomous or poisonous (Russell, 1983). For the most part, these animals are widely distributed throughout the marine fauna from the unicellular protistan *Gonyaulax* to certain of the chordates. They are found in almost all seas and oceans of the world. In most areas, they do not constitute a medical or socioeconomic problem. However, in a few scattered regions, such as the South Pacific, where ciguatera poisoning sometimes gives rise to serious public health and economic problems, and in the case of paralytic shellfish poisoning, the poisonous marine animals have presented a threat to our health and economy.

Marine Toxins

While the marine toxins as a whole are far more varied in their chemical composition than those from terrestrial animals, there is some degree of component consistency within a particular genus or species of each group. However, there are some notable exceptions. Some organisms, such as the clams and mussels, may be toxic only during one period, or a particular period, or in one place and not elsewhere, while the toxicity in tetraodons varies with the species of fish, the organs studied, and other factors. Toxicity in ciguateric fishes is, at the present time, and for all practical purposes, almost unpredictable with respect to the species involved, location, and time of year.

Some marine toxins are proteins of low molecular weight, whereas others are of high molecular weight. Some marine venoms or poisons are composed of lipids, amines, quinones, quaternary ammonium compounds, alkaloids, guanidine bases, phenols, steroids, mucopolysaccharides, or halogenated compounds. The fish venoms are unstable, but most of the other toxins, including the fish poisons, are relatively stable, particularly in the dried or lyophilized form. In some marine organisms, there are several toxins present, and in some instances two organisms are necessary to produce one toxin. Finally, it is known that the venom of one species or genus within one phylum may be similar or even identical to that found in an animal of an entirely different phylum. The newt poison, tarichatoxin, and the pufferfish poison, tetrodotoxin, are one and the same.

As would be expected, the pharmacologic or toxicologic activities of marine toxins vary as remarkably as do their chemical properties. Some marine toxins provoke rather simple effects, such as transient vasoconstriction or dilatation, pain, or localized erythema, whereas others produce more complex responses, such as parasympathetic dysfunction or multiple concomitant changes in cardiovascular or blood dynamics. And there is no doubt that in the evolution of marine toxins, as in snake and other terrestrial venoms (Russell, 1980a), synergistic and possibly antagonistic reactions may occur as the result of interactions between individual venom components.

Protista

Among the protistan are the various protozoans, algae, diatoms, bacteria, yeasts, and fungi. The marine protista are widely distributed throughout neritic waters and in the high seas from the polar oceans to the tropics. There are at least 80 species that are known to be toxic to humans and other animals. A listing of these will be found in Russell (1984a). Most of the toxic organisms are of the order Dinoflagellata, of which there are more than 1200 species. Protistan have been shown to contain or release a toxin that (1) gives rise to paralytic shellfish poisoning through the food chain, (2) produces respiratory or gastrointestinal distress or dermatitis in humans, (3) causes mass mortality of marine animals, or (4) has been implicated by laboratory experiments as being toxic. Blooms of protistan sometimes occur and result in the phenomenon frequently referred to as "red tide," or "red water." However, the bloom may appear yellowish, brownish, greenish, bluish, or even milky in color, depending on the organism involved and other factors. Such blooms usually become visible when 20,000 or more of the organisms are present in 1 ml of water. However, some blooms may contain 50,000 or more organisms. The red color in red tides is probably due to peridinin, a xanthophyll.

Paralytic shellfish poison (PSP), variously known as *saxitoxin, Gonyaulax toxin, dinoflagellate poison, mussel* or *clam poison,* or *mytilotoxin,* is a toxin or group of toxins found in certain molluscs, arthropods, echinoderms, and some other marine animals that have ingested toxic protistan and have become "poisonous." PSP through the food chain is well known in animals and humans. Although the relationship between blooms of plankton and shellfish poisoning was first noted by Lamouroux (cited by Chevallier and Duchesne, 1851), it was not until 1937 that Sommer and Meyer published the results of their intensive investigation on paralytic shellfish poisoning. They demonstrated a direct relationship between the number of *Gonyaulax catenella* in seawater and toxicity in the mussel *Mytilus californianus.* They also established methods for extracting and assaying the poison.

The amount of poison in the shellfish or other organism is dependent on the number of toxic protistan filtered by the host animal. Off California, mussels become dangerous for human consumption when 200/ml or more protistan are found in the coastal waters. As the count rises, the mussels become more toxic. Within a week or two, in the absence of the toxic protistan, the mussels become relatively free of the poison. The toxin has been studied by extractions from shellfish, from dinoflagellates secured from natural blooms, and more recently, from laboratory cultures. PSP can be obtained from all three sources in like form. Burke *et al.* (1960), Schantz *et al.* (1966), and Proctor *et al.* (1975) have grown *Gonyaulax catenella* in axenic cultures in cell densities equal to those occurring during natural blooms, and Schantz (1960) showed that the chromatographic properties of the toxin from the cultured organisms appear identical to those of the toxin found in natural blooms and mussels. It was not until 1975 that Schantz *et al.* presented the absolute configuration:

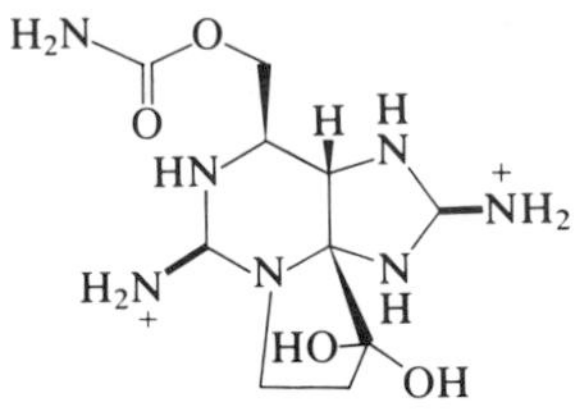

There is some question as to how many toxins exist in the complex of PSP. In the earlier works, it was considered as a single poison, but it must now be thought of as a complex of toxins. In the case of toxins from *Gymnodinium breve,* there appear to be several if not a number of toxins, but at this point in time it has not been established that the toxins reflect differences in the techniques employed in isolation procedures or are the result of distinct differences in the toxin(s). In the dinoflagellate *Gonyaulax tamarensis* there are several other toxins in addition to saxitoxin, and these differ from saxitoxin only in their weak binding ability on carboxylate resins. Further studies on organisms obtained from red tides along the New England coast have resulted in the isolation of two other toxins, *gonyautoxin II* (GTX₂) and *gonyautoxin III* (GTX₃) (Shimizu, 1978). Another toxin, *neosaxitoxin,* has also been isolated from *G. tamarensis.*

While a number of pharmacologic and toxicologic studies on shellfish poisons were carried out before the turn of this century, it was not until Meyer *et al.* (1928), Prinzmetal *et al.* (1932), and Sommer and Meyer (1937) that the more definitive work was reported. Prinzmetal *et al.* (1932) showed that the poison from the mussel *Mytilus californianus* was slowly absorbed from the gastrointestinal tract and rapidly excreted by the kidneys. It was said to depress respiration, the cardioinhibitory and vasomotor centers, and conduction in the myocardium. Subsequent studies showed that saxitoxin had a marked effect on peripheral nerve and skeletal muscle in the frog. The "curarelike" action was attributed to some mechanism that prevented the muscle from responding to acetylcholine. The toxin produced progressive diminution in the amplitude of the end-plate potential in the frog nerve-muscle preparation. It also depressed mammalian phrenic nerve potentials, suppressed the indirectly elicited contractions of the diaphragm, and often reduced the directly stimulated contractions. It was concluded that the effect of the poison was greater on reflex transmission than on the nerve. Contraction of isolated muscle fibers in the presence of ATP and magnesium ions was not inhibited by the poison, nor did the toxin alter the rate of oxygen consumption in the respiring diaphragm of the mouse. With respect to the cardiovascular system, the toxin was shown to have a direct effect on the heart and its conduction system. It produced changes that ranged from a slight decrease in heart rate and contractile force, with simple P-R interval prolongation or S-T segment changes, to severe bradycardia and bundle-branch block, or complete cardiac failure. The poison provoked a prompt but reversible depression in the contractility of isolated cat papillary muscle (*see* Russell, 1983, for references).

In 1967, Kao demonstrated that the toxin blocks action potentials in nerves and muscles by preventing, in a very specific manner, an increase in the ionic permeability that is normally associated with the inward flow of sodium. It appears to do this without altering potassium or chloride conductances. Evans (1967) showed that in cats, mussel poison blocks transmission between the peripheral nerves and the spinal roots. The large myelinated sensory fibers are blocked by intravenous doses of 4.5 to 13 μg/kg, whereas the large motor fibers are not blocked until this dose is increased by approximately 30 to 40 percent. He also observed that when dilute solutions of saxitoxin were applied locally to thin peripheral nerve branches in cats, conduction was not blocked. However, conduction was blocked in dorsal and ventral spinal root fibers following the topical application of far smaller concentrations. He suggests that one of the layers in the connective tissue sheath of peripheral nerve is impermeable to saxitoxin, whereas the leptomeninges covering the spinal roots are either deficient in or lack this layer.

Sommer and Meyer (1937) found that 3000 *Gonyaulax* weighed 100 μg (wet weight) and that this number yielded 15 μg of the dry extract, which in turn gave 1 μg of pure poison, or 1 mouse unit. A mouse unit, or average lethal dose, was defined as the amount of toxin that would kill a 20-g mouse in 15 minutes (Prinzmetal *et al.*, 1932; Sommer and Meyer, 1937). Thus, the amount of toxin contained in a single *Gonyaulax* was taken as ⅓₀₀₀ of a mouse unit. McFarren and associates (1956) found the oral LD50s per kg body weight to vary considerably with the animal used and with its strain and weight. Their figures would indicate that the human is twice as susceptible to the poison as the dog and approximately four times more susceptible than the mouse.

During the 1950s the Canadian—United States Conference on Shellfish Toxicology adopted a bioassay based on the use of the purified toxin isolated by Schantz and his colleagues (1958). The intraperitoneal minimal lethal dose of the toxin for the mouse was approximately 9.0 μg/ kg body weight. The intravenous minimal lethal dose for the rabbit was 3.0 to 4.0 μg/kg of body weight, whereas the minimal lethal oral dose for humans was thought to be between 1.0 and 4.0 mg. Wiberg and Stephenson (1960) demonstrated that the LD50 of the then-purified toxin in mice was:

Oral route	263 (251–267) μg/kg
Intravenous route	3.4 (3.2–3.6) μg/kg
Intraperitoneal route	10.0 (9.7–10.5) μg/kg

More recently, various figures on the toxic and lethal doses for humans have been presented by various workers. The figures presented by Prakash *et al.* (1971) seem consistent with our own calculations; that is, a mild case of poisoning can be caused by ingesting 1 mg of toxin, which might be the amount found in one to five poisonous mussels or clams weighing about 150 g each. A moderate case of poisoning can be caused by ingesting 2 mg of the poison, whereas a serious poisoning would be caused by 3 mg. One would expect that 4 mg of the toxin would be lethal to humans if vigorous treatment was not instituted.

The latest standards for toxicity are those set by the Association of Official Analytical Chemists (AOAC) (1975). However, this standard, like others, has several shortcomings. A number of assays have been proposed to circumvent these deficiencies. For example, an immunochemical technique has been suggested, whereas another method employs an analysis based on the oxidation of saxitoxin to a fluorescent derivative. Spectrophotometric analysis has been proposed and a unique cockroach bioassay has been described. One of the most promising assays incorporates flow cytometric analysis of cellular saxitoxin, dependent on mithramycin fluorescent staining (*see* Russell, 1983, for references). With the advent of the enzyme-linked immunosorbent assay (ELISA) and radioimmunology, new and improved techniques for determining toxicities should appear within the next few years.

Porifera (Sponges)

Sponges are among the simplest of animals. They are highly organized colonies of unicellular nomads composed of loosely integrated cells covered by a skin and, with few exceptions, supported internally by a skeleton of silica, calcite, or spongin. There are more than 5000 species, and they are found in almost every sea from midtide levels to the deepest parts of the oceans. Some sponges release a toxic substance into their environment. De Laubenfels (1932) observed that when *Tedania toxicalis* was placed in a bucket with fishes, crabs, molluscs, and worms, in an hour or perhaps less these animals will be found dead. Although this phenomenon has usually been considered as a purely defensive reaction initiated when the sponge becomes endangered, Green (1977) suggested that the toxic material may be released as a continuous product into the surrounding water and thus serve as a warning or deterrent to an approaching predator.

Many sponges have an offensive odor and taste, but what part these qualities play in defense or in poisoning is not known. Although some studies on the chemistry of sponges have progressed with great rapidity during recent years, specific chemical and toxicologic investigations on the toxic components have lagged far behind. The more important marine sponges of biologic importance are described elsewhere (Russell, 1983). The interested reader should also consult Halstead (1965), Jakowska and Nigrelli (1970), Stempien et al. (1970), Green (1977), and Bakus and Thun (1979) for more detailed data on the toxicity of these species. It should be noted that some sponges of the same genus as those found to be toxic to fishes have also been found to be nontoxic. The family Haliclonidae appears to have the most consistently toxic species.

Perhaps the most extensive studies of toxic observations on fishes have been those by Bakus and his colleagues. Essentially, their shipboard preliminary assay method involves grinding 5 g of the sponge in 10 ml of seawater, centrifuging, pouring the supernatant into a bowl with 300 ml of seawater, and then placing a 1.5- to 5-g sargent major *(Abudefduf saxatilis)* into the water and observing the fish's behavior over a designated period of time. After preliminary testing, serial dilutions of the crude extract are prepared, starting with 0.1 g crude material/ml tapwater; an alcohol extract is used for comparison, and the LC50 (lethal concentration for 50 percent of the animals) determinations are done for the more highly toxic sponges. Toxicity is determined on the basis of the fishes swallowing air, blowing bubbles, being bitten by normal fish, equilibrium loss, erratic swimming behavior, slow swimming movements, escape responses, thrashing behavior, extreme lethargy or stupor, failure to recover when put in fresh water, and death (Bakus and Thun, 1979).

In 1906, Richet precipitated a substance from extracts of the siliceous sponge *Suberites domunculus,* which when injected into the dog produced vomiting, diarrhea, and dyspnea and caused hemorrhages in the gastric and intestinal mucosa, peritoneum, and endocardium. The lethal dose in dogs was 10 mg/kg, and the toxic substance was found to be nontoxic when administered orally. The poison was called "sub-

eritine" (Richet, 1906; Lassabliere, 1906). Arndt (1928) demonstrated that extracts from certain freshwater sponges produced diarrhea, dyspnea, prostration, and death when injected into homoiotermic animals. These same extracts had some hemolytic effects on sheep and pig erythrocytes and blocked cardiac function in the isolated frog heart preparation. The extracts were heat stable and produced no deleterious effects when taken orally. Das et al. (1971) found that extracts of S. inconstans produced a histaminelike effect on the guinea pig intestine and attributed this to histamine, which they found in the sponge. On paper chromatography, they detected five other amines, three having phenolic groups. Dried specimens of *Fasciospongia cavernosa* yielded crystals of N-acyl-2-methylene-β-alanine methyl esters. In mice, the subcutaneous lethal dose of the crystals was approximately 120 mg/kg body weight (Kashman et al., 1973), obviously not very toxic. Algelasine from *Agelas dispar* has activities of a saponin. A unique sesquiterpene, 9-isocyanopupukeanane, has been isolated from the nudibranch *Phyllidia varicosa* and has been found to be present in the sponge *Hymeniacidon* sp., on which the nudibranch feeds (Burreson et al., 1975).

Cariello et al. (1980) isolated and characterized Richet's suberitine. The toxin, which had an approximate molecular weight of 28,000, produced a marked hemolytic effect on human erythrocytes and showed some ATPase activity. Studies on the giant axon of the abdominal nerve of the crayfish indicated that in a concentration of 4.4 mg/ml there was depolarization, followed by an irreversible block in the indirectly stimulated action potential. The authors speculated that this irreversible block may explain the flaccid paralysis seen in crabs following injection of suberitine into the arthropod's hemolymph. Wang et al. (1973) demonstrated that a preparation of an extract of *Haliclona rubens* exerted a depolarizing action on the end-plate membrane of the frog skeletal muscle and that a lesser depolarization occurred in the membrane elsewhere than at the end plate. This activity differed from that caused by *batrachotoxin* and *grayanotoxin* (a toxin from the plant Ericaceae).

Clinical Problem. With respect to humans, poisoning probably occurs through deposit of the toxin(s) in the superficial abrasions produced by the fine, sharp spicules of the sponge. It is known that traumatic injury to the human skin can be produced by the spicules, particularly those of the hexactinellids, and it is believed that in many cases of poisoning this occurs prior to the deposit of the poison on the skin. Certainly, an abraded skin is more likely to absorb a toxin than an uninjured one (Russell, 1965). The most frequently offending sponges are *Tedania nigrescens, T. inconstans,* and *Neofibularia nolitangere.* Symptoms and signs consist of a burning or irritating sensation over the hands or other part contacted by the sponge, subsequent mild pain, sometimes confined to the joints of the hand, pruritus, often severe, and malaise. The contact areas are warm to touch and there may be mild edema. Systemic manifestations and infections are rare. Treatment consists of thoroughly washing the hands with soapy water and applying "Russell's balm" (Itch Balm Plus®; hydrocortisone, tetracaine, and diphenhydramine hydrochloride) four times a day (Maretić and Russell, 1983).

Cnidaria (Coelenterates)

The phylum Cnidaria (hydroids, jellyfish, sea anemones, and corals) are simple metazoans that possess the two basic tissues found in all higher animals, a layer of jellylike material with supporting elastic fibers between the ectoderm and endoderm known as "mesoglea," a gastrovascular cavity that opens only through its mouth, radial symmetry, and tentacles bearing abundant nematocysts. In the Portuguese man-of-war, *Physalia,* and in many other cnidarians, the tentacles contain long muscle strands that can be contracted to bring the animal's prey to the feeding polyps below the umbrella. These polyps engulf the prey and digest it. Venomous forms are found in all three classes of living cnidarians: Hydrozoa, or hydroids, hydromedusae, and fire corals; Scyphozoa, or true jellyfish; Anthozoa, or sea anemones, sea feathers, and corals. The Hydrozoa are branched or simple polyps, some having budded medusae. The order Siphonophora includes the Portuguese man-of-war, *Physalla.* The Scyphozoa, true medusae or jellyfish, are typified by a body, umbrella, or bell, which is usually convex above and concave below. The Cubomedusae or sea wasps are the most dangerous of all the cnidarians, particularly *Chironex fleckeri* and *Chiropsalmus quadrigatus* of Australia. Finally, the class Anthozoa contains the corals, sea anemones, and alcyonarians. The anemones are sedentary, flowerlike structures. The alcyonarians include the stony, soft, horny, and black corals, as well as colonial sea pens and sea pansies. The cnidarians of particular importance because of their stings on humans or their unusual toxicologic properties are listed elsewhere (Russell, 1984a).

The stinging unit of the cnidarians is the nematocysts. I might be venturous to say that all 9000 species of cnidarians have nematocysts (Russell, 1984a). Nematocysts have been classified on the basis of their structure, function, and taxonomy. Weill (1934) described 17 categories of nematocysts, and while these have been qualified with the passing of time, in general, this approach still offers a basis for common communication. The nematocyst, which is a capsulated, ovoid cell varying in size from 4 to 225 μm, contains an operculum, a long coiled tube or hollow thread, matrix, and venom. The nematocyst is formed as "metaplasmic organelle" within an interstitial cell, the cnidoblast. These cnidoblasts are distributed throughout the epidermis, except on the basal disk. The coiled tubule in the undischarged nematocyst varies in length from 50 μm to over 1 mm, depending on the species of cnidarian. When discharged the operculum is released and the everted tubule explodes, remaining attached at the original site of the operculum. The nature of nematocyst discharge and the localized fashion in which these cells respond to stimuli, whether chemical, mechanical, or electrical, have been the object of extensive study (*see* Russell, 1984a, for references).

As in many of the earlier studies on marine venoms, the chemical and toxicologic properties of the cnidarian toxins were carried out with crude saline or water extracts prepared from the whole animal or from one or several of its parts. It is apparent that some early workers were studying normal constituents of the animal's tissues, several of which appear to be limited to tissues in the lower phyla. When these substances were injected into higher animals, they produced deleterious reactions. These reactions then became aligned with clinical findings and, unfortunately, led to misunderstandings and questionable therapeutic advice (Russell, 1965). Such substances as *thalassin, congestin,* and the *Cyanea principle* were probably derived from tentacular tissues rather than venom-bearing nematocysts.

The modern period of fire coral toxicology began with the work of Wittle *et al.* (1971) and Middlebrook *et al.* (1971). These investigators studied nematocyst toxin from *Millepora alcicornis.* They obtained a product with a molecular weight of approximately 100,000 and an intravenous mouse LD50 of 0.04 mg/kg body weight. The toxin had hemolytic and dermonecrotic activities and was antigenic with cross-protection against *M. alcicornis* toxin. They also obtained an electrophoretically pure toxin from the fire coral, *Millepora dichotoma.* The LD50 was 0.038 mg/kg body weight, quite similar to that found for *M. alcicornis.* The signs in mice were also similar. The sea whip *Lophogorgia rigida* contains a toxin known as *lophotoxin.* Its formula is $C_{22}H_{24}O_8$. The toxin has a subcutaneous LD50 in mice of 8.9 mg/kg body weight and was found to block the indirectly elicited contractions in a mammalian nerve-muscle preparation, while not affecting the directly elicited contractions. It was concluded that lophotoxin produces an irreversible postsynaptic block, although the possibility of a presynaptic function could not be excluded (Culver and Jacobs, 1981).

While techniques for separating nematocysts are not new, the initial studies on a nematocyst preparation from *Physalia physalis* were performed by Lane and Dodge (1958). They found their nematocyst preparation to be a highly labile protein complex, rich in glutamic acid and having an approximate intraperitoneal lethal dose in mice of 0.037 ml/kg body weight of a preparation containing 0.02 percent total nitrogen. The toxin produced paralysis in fish, frogs, and mice. Animals killed following stingings by *Physalia* exhibited marked pulmonary edema, right cardiac dilatation, with venous congestion of the larger vessels of the chest and portal circulations. Since the original work of Lane and Dodge, a number of advances in the preparation of nematocyst toxins from *P. physalis* have been made. These and the toxicologic studies have been reviewed elsewhere (Russell, 1984a). Various investigations on crabs, rats, dogs, and a nerve-muscle preparation of the frog indicated that the toxin produced changes in the Na-K pump, resulting in depolarization of the cell membranes. In the rat, where the LD50 was approximately 100 μg/kg body weight, low doses of the toxin caused an increase in the Q-T interval, a decrease in the P-R interval, and P-wave inversion. Large doses produced marked ECG changes leading to cardiac failure. Subsequent studies showed that the ability of skeletal muscle sarcoplasmic reticulum to bind ionic calcium and nuclear alterations and dissolution of intercellular collagen in cultured hamster ovary K-1 cells are important properties of the toxin (Calton *et al.*, 1973; Neeman *et al.*, 1981).

Tamkun and Hessinger (1981) obtained a hemolytic protein from *P. physalis*. This protein, *physalitoxin*, was also lethal to mice at the 0.20 mg protein/kg body weight level, whereas the LD50 for the crude venom was 0.14 mg/kg. A molecular weight of 212,000 was calculated. The authors suggested that the toxin was composed of three subunits of unequal size, each of which is glycoylated. Physalitoxin was about 28 percent of the total nematocyst venom protein. Its carbohydrate content was 10.6 percent and represented the major glycoprotein of the crude venom. This hemolytic and lethal toxin was inactivated by concanavalin A.

Initial studies of extracts of the frozen tentacles of the sea wasp, *Chironex fleckeri*, indicated that the extracts had lethal, necrotizing, and hemolytic properties (Southcott and Kingston, 1959). Barnes (1967) isolated a *Chironex* nematocyst crude toxin by employing human amnion membrane and electrically stimulating the tentacles. In his initial study, Barnes found that the undiluted toxin was lethal to mice at the 0.005 ml/kg body weight level, but it was not known what this might be in dry weight, mg protein, or protein nitrogen. Endean *et al.* (1969) found proteins, carbohydrates, cystine-containing compounds, and 3-indolyl derivatives in the nematocysts of the tentacles of *C. fleckeri*. Saline extracts of the contents of the nematocysts were highly toxic to prawn and fish and were lethal to mice and rats. In mice, the intravenous LD50 was between 20,000 and 25,000 nematocysts, whereas in rats the LD50 was approximately 150,000 nematocysts. Using partially purified extracts of the tentacles, Freeman and Turner (1969) found that extracts produced respiratory arrest, which they attributed to a central origin. They also implicated deleterious cardiac changes leading to an atrioventricular block. Blood pressure and chemistry changes were consistent with a reduced circulating blood volume and hypoxia. The toxins had a nonspecific lytic effect on cells and no particular differential effect on the guinea pig diaphragm preparation. It was found that 0.1 ml of a 5000-fold dilution of the tentacle extract would kill a 20-g mouse in less than 2 minutes and that the toxin was hemolytic. The fraction was nondialyzable and an estimated molecular weight of 8000 was suggested.

Crone and Keen (1969) obtained two toxic proteins using tentacle extracts. The hemolytic activity was related to a protein component with a molecular weight of approximately 70,000. The second toxin had a molecular weight of about 150,000, and while both components had cardiotoxic activity, the larger fraction had considerably more than the smaller fraction. Two *Chironex* tentacle extracts were studied by Freeman and Turner (1971), who found that both the fractions produced an initial increase in systemic arterial pressure, followed by a fall in pressure, bradycardia, and cardiac arrythmia. In the perfused guinea pig heart, both toxins caused a reduction in rate, amplitude of contraction, and coronary flow. The authors concluded that the cardiovascular effects were due to "direct vasoconstriction, cardiotoxicity, a baroreceptor stimulation and possible depression of the vasomotor center."

These various data have been controversial. It appears that the toxin(s) derived from tentacles is quite different from that obtained from discharged or undischarged nematocysts. An attempt to resolve the discrepancies was made by Endean and Noble (1971). Using methods previously described by their group, they separated material within the nematocysts from the residual tentacular material. The two products were studied by injection into mice and rats, on the barnacle muscle preparation, the rat phrenic nerve-diaphragm preparation, the toad sciatic nerve-gastrocnemius and sciatic nerve conduction preparations, rat ilea and heart preparations, and certain other isolated tissue preparations. It was found that following removal of the nematocysts from the tentacles, the remaining product possessed quite different biologic activities from that extracted from the nematocysts. Although the work of Endean and Noble indicates certain differences, it is difficult to define these accurately in the absence of a standard tissue weight or solution. Furthermore, some of the differences demonstrated by the various investigators for *Chironex* toxins, as well as several other cnidarian toxins, might be due to the dose relationships rather than the toxins employed. This is particularly true for the rat or guinea pig diaphragm-phrenic nerve preparation. Changes in the dose of toxins cause not only quantitative changes but qualitative ones. Furthermore, when the muscle of a mammalian nerve-muscle preparation is shortened, it is most difficult to determine the effect on the indirectly elicited contraction. In fact, in a shortened muscle, it is even difficult to determine the significance of the direct effect. Obviously, a substance that is highly irritating to an entire muscle membrane presents a problem when one hopes to define its action on the nerve, or even on the activity of a single muscle fiber.

Baxter and his colleagues at the Commonwealth Serum Laboratories in Australia, using saline extracts of nematocysts obtained after the method of Barnes (1967), or as described by Endean et al. (1969), demonstrated that the biologically active fractions causing lethal, hemolytic, and dermonecrotizing reactions were in the 10,000- to 30,000-molecular-weight range. In rabbits, a lethal intravenous dose of the venom caused labored and deep respirations, followed within several minutes by prostration, hyperextension of the head, "spasms," and respiratory and cardiac arrest. In sheep, a similar respiratory deficit was seen, followed by unsteadiness, muscle tremors, and "spasms." The head drooped to one side, prostration occurred, and the tongue was said to be paralyzed and cyanotic. In primates, the animal became inactive, "dull," confused, and exhibited slight ataxia and incoordination. The eyelids drooped, the mouth was open, and the head "weaved." Heart rate was irregular, and breathing became labored, deep, and irregular. Within a few minutes the animal collapsed, the heart rate deteriorated, and cyanosis developed just prior to death. Postmortem examination revealed marked congestion of the vessels of the lungs, pulmonary edema, the right ventricle was engorged, the kidneys and liver were congested, and the vessels of the meninges of the cerebrum were engorged (Baxter et al., 1972).

Considerable study has been done on the nematocyst toxin of the sea nettle *Chrysaora quinquecirrha* by Burnett and his group at the University of Maryland School of Medicine. Blanquet (1972) found that the toxin was contained within the nematocyst and that the discharged nematocyst capsules and threads were free of toxin. Further studies showed that the toxic material was associated with a protein fraction having a molecular weight greater than 100,000, which could be separated into two major fractions. The more toxic of these two proteins was found to be rich in aspartic and glutamic acids, which composed approximately 27 percent of the total detectable amino acid content. Burnett and Calton (1977) reviewed the cardiotoxic, dermonecrotic, musculotoxic, and neurotoxic properties of the venom. Subsequently, it has been demonstrated that the toxin produced striking cytologic changes, including nuclear alterations and dissolution of intercellular collagen. The lethal property is thought to exert its effect by altering the transport of calcium across the conduction system of the heart. From experiments on rat and frog nerve and muscle, and on the neurons of *Aplysia californica*, it was concluded that the toxin appeared to induce a nonspecific membrane depolarization by a sodium-dependent tetrodotoxin-insensitive mechanism that secondarily increases Ca influx.

The collagenase from *C. quinquecirrha* has been isolated and purified 237-fold. A monoclonal antibody to the lethal factor of the venom has also been prepared. Ascites fluid from a cloned hybridoma-breeding mouse showed an ELISA titer of 12,800 and neutralized an intravenous $2 \times$ LD50 injection of the crude venom.

Among the sea anemones, *Anemonia sulcata* is of particular interest, since it is of considerable medical importance in the Adriatic Sea where it inflicts numerous stings on bathers (Maretić and Russell, 1983). In 1973, a partially purified, toxic, basic polypeptide from *A. sulcata* was isolated. Its molecular weight was estimated to be 6000, and its LD100 in rats was 6 mg/kg body weight. In 1975, three toxic polypeptides were isolated from *A. sulcata*. Toxin I contained 45 amino acid residues; toxin II, 44; and toxin III, 24. Toxins I and II had similar toxicologic properties. When injected into a crustacean, fish, or mammal, these toxins produced paralysis and cardiovascular changes. When injected into crabs the toxins caused convulsions and paralysis and were lethal at 2.0 mg/kg. They also caused paralysis and death in fishes. Toxin III caused neurotransmitter release from rat synaptosomes. Toxin II was far more toxic than toxin I and produced a positive inotropic effect on isolated electrically driven atria of the guinea pig. At high concentrations it caused contracture and arrhythmia. On the Langendorff heart preparation, low concentrations enhanced the contractile force of the atrium and ventricle, whereas high concentrations caused contracture and arrhythmia, which appeared to be limited to the atrium. Ferlan and Lebez (1974) isolated a highly basic protein toxin, *equinatoxin,* from the sea anemone *Actinia equina.* It had a molecular weight of 20,000, with an isoelectric point of 12.5 and 147 amino acid residues. In rats, equinatoxin had an intravenous LD50 of 33 μg/kg body weight and was found to have hemolytic, antigenic, cardiotropic, and certain other activities. Subsequently, it was found that equinatoxin, *in vitro,* exhibited strong lytic action on erythrocytes and that it did not have phospholipase activity. A cytolytic toxin, *metridiolysin,* from the anemone *Medtridium senile* showed similar hemolytic activity. Like equinatoxin, the hemolytic activity was restricted to a relatively narrow pH range (*see* Russell, 1984a, for references).

Shapiro and his colleagues at Harvard carried out a series of chemical and pharmacologic studies on a stable acetone powder from tentacle homogenates of the large Caribbean anemone *Condylactis gigantea.* A toxin was obtained that acted as a basic protein and had an approximate molecular weight of 10,000 to 15,000. Assays on crayfish caused a paralysis characterized by an initial or spastic phase, followed by a flaccid phase. The immobilization dose was about 1 μg/kg body weight, and the yield from a 70-g anemone with 23 g of tentacles was 1 g of the acetone powder, or a sufficient amount to paralyze approximately a 2100-kg crayfish. Further studies on a crayfish preparation showed that the toxin had a direct effect on the crustacean nerve but not on the muscle membrane. No evidence for a truly synaptic effect was observed. Using the lobster giant axon and crayfish slow-adapting preparations, it was found that the toxin transformed action potentials into prolonged plateau potential of up to several seconds duration, and that the eventual conduction block was not due solely to depolarization (Shapiro and Lilleheil, 1969).

A central nervous system stimulant in the form of a basic polypeptide has been isolated from homogenized tissues of the anemone *Stoichactis kenti.* The stimulation was described as "fighting episodes." A partially purified toxin from *S. helianthus,* with a mouse intraperitoneal LD50 of 0.25 mg/kg and hemolytic properties inhibited by sphingomyelin, has been reported (Bernheimer and Avigad, 1976). A cytotoxic poison from the anemone *Stoichactis helianthus* acts on black lipid membranes and liposomes by channel formation and detergent action. This mechanism is also suspected for the hemolytic activity of some of the other sea anemone "cytolytic" toxins. However, there appear to be a considerable number of different cytolytic toxins in the sea anemones, and the mechanisms by which they damage membranes may be quite different. Hessinger and Lenhoff (1976), for instance, demonstrated that the toxin of *Aiptasia pallida* caused lysis through the action of phospholipase A on membrane phospholipids, while other workers suspect ionic or nonenzymatic roles. Several other Actiniidae species have been shown to contain toxins. A polypeptide, termed *anthopleurin A,* from *Anthopleura xanthogrammica* that closely resembles toxin II from *A. sulcata* in its amino acid sequence has been described. In mice, *anthopleurin A* had an LD50 of 0.3 to 0.4 mg/kg body weight and was said to stimulate cardiac activity. A second polypeptide toxin, *anthopleurin B,* has also been identified in the same anemone (*see* Russell, 1984a, for references).

In 1967, Hashimoto and colleagues collected specimens of the file fish, *Alutera scripta,* from the Ryuku Islands following a report that several pigs had died after eating the viscera of this fish. On examining the gut contents of the fish, the investigators found polyps of the zoanthid *Palythoa tuberculosa.* About the same time, Scheuer and his group were investigating the toxin from *Palythoa toxica,* found at Hana off the island of Maui and called *lima-make-O-Hana* (death seaweed of Hana). *Palythoa* toxin, *palytoxin,* was found to be a most potent poison, having a mouse intravenous LD50 of 0.15 μ/kg body weight. It has an approximate molecular weight of 3000 and appears to have a unique structure that, as yet, is undetermined.

Clinical Problem.   As pointed out by Halstead (1965), it has long been known that the nematocysts of certain cnidarians can penetrate the human skin. In 1965, approximately 70 of the 9000 species of cnidarians were noted to have been involved in injuries to humans (Russell, 1965). More recent clinical records would indicate that about 78 species have been implicated in such injuries. While most nematocysts are capable of piercing only the thin membranes of the mouth or conjunctiva, some possess sufficient force to pierce the skin of the inner sides of the arms, legs, and more tender areas of the body. Still others can penetrate the thicker skin of the hands, arms, and feet (Russell, 1965). Swallowing the tentacles or even the umbrella can cause epigastric pain and discomfort (Maretić and Russell, 1983).

The cutaneous lesions, as well as other clinical manifestations produced by the various cnidarians, vary considerably, depending on the species involved and the number of fired nematocysts. Contrary to common belief, the stings of many cnidarians produce little or no immediate pain. Sometimes, itching is the first complaint that calls the victim's attention to the injured area, and this may not be for hours following the initial contact. In the author's experience, stings by hydroids usually do not produce pain, although there may be subsequent localized discomfort. In most cases, the lesions produced by hydroids are minimal. The fire or stinging corals, *Millepora,* produce small reddened, somewhat papular eruptions, which appear 1 to 10 hours following contact and usually subside within 24 to 96 hours. In severe cases, the papules may proceed to pustular lesions and subsequent desquamation. The stinging is usually associated with some localized prickinglike pain, generally of short duration, and with some subsequent pruritus and minimal swelling (Russell, 1984a).

Contact with the Portuguese man-of-war, *Physalia,* causes immediate pain, sometimes severe, and the early appearance of small reddened, linear, papular eruptions. At first the papules are surrounded by an erythematous zone, but as their size increases, the area takes on the appearance of an inflammatory reaction with small periodic, demarcated, hemorrhagic papules. In some cases, these papules are very close together, indicating multiple discharge of nematocysts as the tentacle passed over the injured part. The papules develop rapidly and often increase in size during the first hour. The affected area becomes painful, and severe pruritus is not uncommon. Pain may spread to the larger muscle masses in the involved extremity or even to the whole body. Pain sometimes involves the regional lymph nodes. In some cases, the papules proceed to vesiculation, pustulation, and desquamation. I have seen several cases in which hyperpigmentation of the lesions was obvious for years following a stinging (Russell, 1966). General systemic manifestations may also develop following *Physalia physalis* envenomation. Weakness, nausea, anxiety, headache, spasms in the large muscle masses of the abdomen and back, vascular spasms, lacrimation and nasal discharge, increased perspiration, vertigo, hemolysis, difficulty and pain on respiration, described as being unable to "catch one's breath," cyanosis, renal failure, and shock have all been reported.

Contact with most of the true jellyfishes gives rise, in the less severe cases, to manifestations similar to those noted for *Physalia,* with symptoms sometimes disappearing within ten hours. In the more severe cases, there is immediate, intense, burning pain, with contact areas appearing as swollen wheals, sometimes purplish, and often bearing hemorrhagic papules. The areas may proceed to vesiculation and necrosis. Localized edema is common, and in the more severe cases, muscle mass pain, difficulties in respiration, and severe spasms of the back and abdomen with vomiting are reported. Vertigo, mental confusion, changes in heart rate, and shock are sometimes seen and death has occurred (Barnes, 1960; Halstead, 1965; Russell, 1965, 1984a).

The sea wasps, *Chironex fleckeri* Southcott and *Chiropsalmus quadrigatus* Haeckel and certain other species, are extremely dangerous Cubomedusae responsible for a number of deaths, particularly in Australian waters. Although systemic effects usually develop within 5 to 150 minutes following envenomation, some deaths occur in less than 5 minutes. Stings by these Cubomedusae cause a sharp prickling or burning sensation with the appearance of a wheal, which at first appears like a "rounded area of gooseflesh." An erythematous wheal soon develops and may become considerably larger than the area of contact. At first, it may show little pattern to suggest whether the stinging had been by tentacles or by the animal's umbrella. The wheals may either disappear, as when the stinging is minimal, or after an hour or so become enlarged as the nematocyst punctures become more apparent and appear as very small hemorrhagic vesicles surrounded by inflammation. A stinging pain develops and may persist for one to three hours. In linear lesions the nematocyst injuries may be no more than 5 mm wide but extend for 10 cm or more. Vesiculation and pustular formation may occur, and full-thickness skin necrosis is not uncommon. Edema about the area may persist for ten or more days. Stingings by the anemones are usually of lesser consequence than those inflicted by the jellyfishes and rarely are they painful or disabling. The lesion area takes on a reddened and slightly raised appearance, bearing irregularly scattered pinhead-sized vesicles or hemorrhagic blebs. The area becomes painful, particularly to touch or heat. In stings by *Anemonia sulcata* seen by the author, there has been some diffuse edema around the injured site. Residual hyperpigmentation or hypopigmentation is unusual following anemone stings. Stings by the stony corals *(Acropora)* are said to give rise to some minor pain often followed by itching and the development of small diffuse wheals, which may progress to vesiculation but rarely necrosis. "Sponge fisherman's disease" is due to the actinian *Sagartia rosea*. Troublesome are small spicules of coral that sometimes break off and become embedded in the skin, occasionally giving rise to infection.

Treatment consists of removing the tentacles, preferably with gloves, washing the affected area with seawater, immersing the part in vinegar or Burow's solution for 10 to 15 minutes, and in the case of *Chironex* stings, applying a dry powder or shaving soap and scraping the area with a sharp knife to remove any nematocysts embedded in the skin, washing the area thoroughly with soapy water, and then applying a corticosteroid-analgesic-antihistamine ointment (Itch Balm Plus®). Systemic manifestations are best treated symptomatically.

Chills and fever have been reported after grinding dried specimens of *P. caribaeorum,* which were being studied for the presence of wax esters. Toxic zoanthids have also been found in various parts of the Pacific. Accidental contact with the mucus of *Palythoa* through the abraded skin is said to produce weakness and malaise, as well as localized irritation.

On some Pacific islands, as well as elsewhere in the world, sea anemones are eaten following cooking, but some are apparently poisonous whether uncooked or cooked. *Rhodactis howesi* and *Physobrachia douglasi* are poisonous when eaten raw but said to be safe when cooked. *Radianthus paumotensis* and another *Radianthus* species are said to be poisonous, whether raw or cooked. Intoxication is typified by nausea, vomiting, abdominal pain, and hypoactive reflexes. In severe cases, marked weakness, malaise, cyanosis, stupor, and death have occurred.

Echinodermata

In most cases, echinoderms are characterized by radial or meridional symmetry, a calcareous exoskeleton made up of separate plates or ossicles that often bear external spines, a well-developed coelom, a water-vascular system, and a nervous system, but no special excretory system. Approximately 85 of the 6000 species composing the four classes (Asteroidea, Ophiuroidea, Echinoidea, Holothuroidea) are known to be venomous or poisonous. Some of the more important toxic starfishes, sea urchins, and sea cucumbers have been described elsewhere (Russell, 1984a). Asteroids, starfishes, or sea

stars have a central disk and five or more tapering rays or arms. On the upper surface are many thorny spines of calcium carbonate in the form of calcite intermingled with organic materials. The calcite spines are covered by a thin integument composed of an epidermis and a dermis. Within the epidermis is an acidophilic cell thought to release a toxin. The toxin is discharged into the water or, as in the case of humans, directly onto the skin. In addition, sea stars have pedicellariae, which contain poison glands in the concave cavity of their valves. Some sea stars produce poisoning following ingestion.

The regular sea urchins have rounded radially symmetric bodies, which are enclosed in a hard calcite shell from which calcareous spines and the venomous pedicellariae arise. The spines may be straight and pointed, curved, flat-topped, club-shaped, oar-shaped, umbrella-shaped, thorny, fan-shaped, or hooked. They may vary in length from less than 1 mm to over 30 cm. The spines serve in locomotion, protection, digging, feeding, and producing currents; certain of the primary and secondary spines bear poison glands.

The principal venom apparatus in the sea urchin, heart urchin, or sand dollar is the pedicellaria. In essence, pedicellariae are modified spines with flexible heads. There are four primary kinds and some urchins possess all four kinds. The pedicellariae function in food getting, grooming, and self-defense. The glandular, gemmiform, or globiferous type pedicellaria serves as a venom organ. In most echinoids the so-called "head" of the pedicellaria is composed of three calcareous jaws or valves, each having a rounded, toothlike fang. The jaws are usually invested in a globose, fleshy, and somewhat muscular sac, which possesses a single or double gland over each valve. A second trilobed gland system, anatomically and histologically distinct from the head gland, is present in some urchins. The primary and secondary spines of some urchins have specialized organs containing a gland, which is said to empty its contents through the hollow spine tip under certain conditions. Our group found a toxin in the secondary spines of *Echinothrix calamaris* and *E. diadema* but not in their primary spines. The secondary spines of *Asthenosoma varium* Grube and *Araesoma thetidis* contain a venom. According to Halstead (1978), the spine venom glands are best developed in the secondary aboral spines of *A. varium.*

The sea cucumbers, *Holothuroidea,* are soft-bodied animals covered by a leathery skin that contains only microscopic calcareous plates. According to Nigrelli and Jakowska (1960), at least 30 species belonging to four of the five orders are toxic. Some members possess special defense organs known as Cuvierian tubules. When these animals are irritated, they emit these organs through the anus. The tubules become elongated by hydrostatic pressure so that once through the anus they become extremely sticky threads in which the attacking animal becomes ensnared. The process of elongation may split the outer layer of covering cells, thereby releasing a proteinaceous material that forms an amorphous mass having strong adhesive properties. In some sea cucumbers, however, as in *Actinopyga agassizi,* the tubules do not become sticky, nor do they elongate, but they are eviscerated in a somewhat similar manner and they discharge a toxin from certain highly developed structures filled with granules. The toxin is capable of killing fishes and other animals. In *Holothuria atra,* which does not possess Cuvierian tubules, the toxin may be discharged through the body wall. In Guam, natives cut up the common black sea cucumbers and squeeze the contents of the animal into crevices and pools to deactivate fish.

Many echinoderms secrete a mucus or liquid from their integument that appears to play a role in their defensive armament. The viscous discharge from the massive multicellular integumentary glands of the brittle star, *Ophiocomina nigra,* is characterized as a highly sulfated acid mucopolysaccharide, containing amino sugars, sulfate esters, and other substances complexed to proteins. The pH of this discharge is approximately 1, which probably makes it very offensive to other marine animals that might seek to prey upon it. Among other substances isolated from the echinoderms is a quaternary ammonium base ($C_7H_7NO_2$, picolinic acid methyl betaine) known as *homarine,* several phosphagens (phosphoarginine and phosphocreatine), sterols, saponins, and other compounds (Hashimoto, 1979). Perhaps one of the difficulties, again, in determining the toxic substance(s) in the echinoderms is related to the differences in the origin of the test material, that is, not only the chemical variations in different species but the differences in the kind of product extracted from the animals. Pharmacologically, the task is even more difficult, not only because of the differences in products but also because of the differences in the bioassays that have been employed. Some investigators use the toxicity to fish assay, whereas others use a hemolytic test, an oral or parenteral mammalian assay, and still other researchers use an intact mollusc or other invertebrate and measure the withdrawal response or lethality. Finally, a few investigators use specific marine isolated tissue preparations.

Hashimoto (1979) has done an excellent job of reviewing the chemistry and pharmacology of echinoderm toxins, and he has been wise enough to avoid attempting to interpret unrelated and sometimes confusing data.

When the pedicellariae of *Toxopneustes pileolus* were allowed to sting the shaved abdomen of a mouse, the animal developed respiratory distress and exhibited a decrease in body temperature. The injection of thermostable extracts from the macerated pedicellariae of *Sphaerechinus granularis,* and certain other species, has been found to be lethal to isopods, crabs, octopods, sea stars, lizards, and rabbits. While the presence of a dialyzable, acetylcholinelike substance in the pedicellariae of *Lytechinus variegatus* has been reported, it was not until 1965 that the protein nature of pedicellarial toxin was first described. This protein had an intravenous LD50 in mice, based on the quantity of precipitable protein nitrogen, of 1.59×10^{-2} mg/kg body weight for the crude material and 1.16×10^{-2} mg/kg for the protein (Alender and Russell, 1966). It possessed hemolytic activity against human type A and B, rabbit, guinea pig, beef, sheep, and fish erythrocytes. Intravenously, it produced a dose-related hypotension that was responsive to adrenalin. It had a deleterious effect on the isolated heart and guinea pig ileum. In both these preparations, the toxin caused the release of histamine and serotonin. It seems to have little effect on isolated toad nerve. However, Parnas and Russell (1967), using the deep extension abdominal muscle of the crayfish, showed that the toxin produced a rapid block in the response of the indirectly stimulated muscle. Even with low concentrations, there was an irreversible block in the muscle's response to intracellular stimulation. The compound action potential of the crayfish limb nerve was also blocked by the toxin, but this potential reappeared on washing. The toxin caused considerable damage to the muscle fibers. These findings seemed to indicate that pedicellariae toxin blocks the response from both nerve and muscle and is cytolytic.

Subsequently, it was observed that pedicellarial toxin from *T. gratilla* elicited prolonged contractions of isolated guinea pig ileum. Chemical evidence was obtained for the release of histamine from ileal, cardiac, and pulmonary tissues, as well as from the colonic and pulmonary tissues of the rat. The histamine release was quantitatively dependent on the concentration of the toxin acting on the tissue. The active material obtained from the reaction between crude sea urchin toxin and heated plasma was a mixture of pharmacologically active peptides, one of which was bradykinin (*see* Russell, 1984a, for references). Fleming and Howden (1974) obtained a partly purified toxin from the pedicellariae of *T. gratilla*. The toxin, as established by intraperitoneal injection in mice, was at the 5.0 to 5.1 isoelectric point. When this fraction was chromatographed, a molecular weight of 78,000 ± 8000 was found. This seems consistent with the sediment coefficient of 4.7 (67,000) previously reported.

It has been known since 1880 that the discharged tenacious filaments of sea cucumbers can produce wounds in humans and that eating the sea cucumber *Stichopus variegatus* can cause death. According to Halstead (1965), the initial studies of the poisonousness of sea cucumbers were carried out by Yamanouchi, who observed that when fish were placed in the aquarium to which aqueous extracts of *Holothuria vagabunda* were added, the fish died. Subsequently, he obtained a toxic crystalline product, termed *holothurin*, and found it present in 24 of 27 species of sea cucumbers examined. More recently, Bakus and Green (1974) have found that the more tropical the locality, the greater the probability that the holothurin will be toxic to fishes. The toxic substance (holothurin) extracted from the Bahamian sea cucumber *Actinopyga agassizi* was found to be composed of 60 percent glycosides and pigments; 30 percent salts, polypeptides, and free amino acids; 5 to 10 percent insoluble protein; and 1 percent cholesterol. The cholesterol-precipitated fraction, known as *holothurin A*, represented 60 percent of the crude holothurin and was given the empirical formula $C_{50-52}H_{81}O_{25-26}SNa$. Its provisional structure is (Friess *et al.*, 1967):

Compound	R
Holothurin	$-OSO_3^-Na^+$
DeH	$-H$

SUGAR	SYMBOL
D-GLUCOSE	G
D-XYLOSE	X
D-QUINOVOSE	Q
3-*O*-METHYLGLUCOSE	G – OMe

In 10 ppm, holothurin was found to be lethal to *Hydra,* the mollusc *Planorbis,* and the annelid *Tubifex tubifex*. It has slightly greater hemolytic action than saponin and stimulated hematopoiesis in the bone marrow of winterized frogs. It also appears to have some antimetabolic activity. In the mammalian phrenic nerve-diaphragm preparation, holothurin A produces contracture of the muscle, followed by some relaxation and a gradual decrease in the recorded amplitude of both the directly and indirectly elicited contractions, the latter decreasing at a slightly greater rate than the former. The intravenous LD50 in mice was approximately 9 mg/kg body weight. In frogs, holothurin A produced an irreversible block and destruction of excitability on the single node of Ranvier in the sciatic nerve. The toxin did not produce any observable damage to the axonal walls or sheath (*see* Russell, 1984a, for references).

A major aglycone from the holothurin A of *H. vagabunda* was named *holothurigenin* ($C_{30}H_{44}O_5$). It contained three hydroxyls, a five-membered lactone, and a heteroannular diene. The toxins from the Cuvierian organ and body wall of a number of species have been summarized by Habermehl and Volkwein (1971). According to the authors, these compounds are glycosides of tetracyclic triterpenes, which are derivatives of lanosterol and were the first glycoside triterpenes derived from animals. Holothurin has been shown to have hemolytic and cytolytic properties. It is considered to be one of the most potent saponin hemolysins known. In some concentrations it is lethal to animals and plants, inhibits the growth of certain protozoa, modifies the normal development of sea urchin eggs, possesses antimicrobial and antitumoral properties, retards pupation in the fruit fly, and inhibits regeneration processes in planariae. The effects of various preparations of holothurin on the peripheral nervous system have been the object of a number of studies by Friess and his group at the Naval Medical Research Institute in Bethesda, Maryland. Holothurin in concentrations of 9.8×10^{-3} M causes a decrease in the height of the propagated potential without reduction of the conduction velocity in the desheathed sciatic nerve of the frog. This change is concentration dependent and independent of pH and is completely irreversible. A similar change is produced in the single fiber–single node of Ranvier preparation. In concentrations of 2.5×10^{-5} to 1.0×10^{-3} M, the toxin produced a diminution of the action current with a concomitant rise in the stimulation threshold. However, in approximately 80 percent of the preparations studied, the loss of nodal excitation caused by this same concentration was accompanied by a loss in basophilic, macromolecular material from the axoplasm in and near the node of Ranvier (*see* Russell, 1983, for references). In summarizing various of their studies, Friess *et al.* (1970) note that the most obvious functional similarity from data with the cervical ganglia of the cat, the peripheral neuromuscular junction of the rat, and the medullated nerve nodes of the frog was the possession of cholinergic subsystems at some anatomic level, chiefly within the excitable membranes of conducting and junctional structures. They felt that a common target for holothurin A action was "the cholinergic receptor population triggered by acetylcholine ion (ACh+) in the associated hydrolase enzyme AChE, or in the enzyme choline acetylase responsible for resynthesis of ACh+."

Clinical Problem. In 1965, I treated a student working with *Acanthaster planci,* who had inadvertently slipped and fallen, landing forcibly with his left hand impaled on the sea star. Twenty minutes after the injury the patient had intense pain over the palm of the left hand, "shooting pains" up the volar aspect of the forearm, weakness, nausea, vertigo, and tingling in the fingertips. There were at least ten puncture wounds over the hand, and some of them were bleeding freely. I suggested that the patient put his hand in cold vinegar/water and be admitted to the hospital emergency room. On arrival there 15 minutes later, the pain was less intense and the nausea had somewhat subsided. Unfortunately, the patient was given 100 mg meperidine hydrochloride and five minutes later he was vomiting. (In my opinion, the vomiting was due to the medication and most of the other symptoms to hyperventilation.) The patient was placed on cold vinegar/water and occasional aluminum acetate soaks over the next two days, and all symptoms and signs, including the mild edema, slowly resolved. Several broken spines were removed from the puncture wounds. Four days following the accident the patient complained of burning and itching over the left palm. Examination revealed a scaly, erythematous dermatitis. Topical corticosteriods were used, but two days later the patient had to be placed on systemic corticosteroid therapy for the dermatitis. It cleared in six days.

A second episode involving *A. planci* was related to me by Dr. W. L. Orris in 1974. The patient had immediate, severe, burning pain and localized edema. These responded to aluminum acetate soaks and corticosteroids. According to Endean (1964), the punture wounds produced by *Asthenosoma periculosum* give rise to immediate and sometimes acute pain but few other symptoms or signs. The discharge from *Marthasterias glacialis* is said to cause edema of the lips. It is

known that allergic dermatitis can occur following extensive contact with these animals.

Stings by the pedicellariae of certain sea urchins are well documented (Cleland and Southcott, 1965; Halstead, 1965; Russell, 1965). One investigator experienced severe pain, syncope, respiratory distress, partial paralysis of the lips, tongue, and eyelids, and weakness of the muscles of phonation and of the extremities following a stinging by seven or eight pedicellariae from *Toxopneustes pileolus.* Another biologist experienced severe pain of several hours' duration at the site of a stinging by *Tripneustes gratilla.* The sting of a single globiferous pedicellaria from *T. gratilla* was found to be equal in pain severity to that experienced following a bee sting. Swelling appeared around the puncture wounds within minutes of the stinging and a red wheal 1 cm in diameter soon developed. Subsequent stingings during the following two-year period resulted in a more severe reaction. In one instance, the wheal was 12 cm in diameter and persisted for eight hours. In none of these experiences were there any systemic manifestations (Alender and Russell, 1966; Russell, 1971). It might be concluded that pedicellariae stings give rise to immediate pain, localized swelling and redness, and an aching sensation in the involved part. Other findings might include those reviewed by Halstead (1965).

As previously noted, the secondary spines of *E. calamaris, E. diadema, A. varium, A. thetidis,* and the primary oral spines of *P. bursarium* are said to have a venom gland and are capable of envenomation (Alender and Russell, 1966). However, case reports on verified stingings are almost nonexistent, and in the several known to the author it is not possible to decide whether the pain, "dizziness," and minimal localized swelling were due to a venom or to the effects of a simple puncture wound complicated by hyperventilation. The primary spines of almost 50 species of sea urchins have been implicated in injuries to humans. Urchins of the family Diadematidae are particularly troublesome because of their long length and fragility. When these break off in a puncture wound, they can be difficult to find and remove. I have attended injuries in which I have had to remove more than a dozen broken spine tips. With some species, there is no giveaway dark color around the puncture wound, and finding the broken spines is not easy. Although the fragments of some spines will dissolve in tissue and cause no difficulties, others can give rise to granulomatous reactions, some of which may need to be removed surgically. Still others may migrate through the foot or hand without causing complications. Occasionally, spines will lodge against a nerve or bone and cause complications requiring surgical intervention. Secondary infections from spine injuries are relatively rare.

It has long been known that the ovaries of sea urchins are toxic, and perhaps lethal. Halstead (1980) notes that the gonads of *Paracentrotus lividus, Tripneustes ventricosus,* and *Centrechinus antillarium* are poisonous. Poisonings following the ingestion of certain sea cucumbers, however, are not uncommon and have occurred frequently in the South Pacific, Philippines, Japan, China, and Southeast Asia. The most frequently implicated holothurian species are *Holothuria atra, H. axiologa, Stichopus variegatus,* and *Thelenota ananas.* The symptoms and signs are usually of short duration and without serious sequelae. Pruritus with mild swelling and redness of the hands has been reported following the handling of some sea cucumbers. Acute conjunctivitis has been observed in persons who have swum in waters polluted with the tissue discharge of sea cucumber Cuvierian organs.

Mollusca

Molluscs are unsegmented invertebrates having a mantle that often secretes a calcareous shell, a ventral muscular foot used for locomotion, a reduced coelom, an open circulatory system, and a radula or tonguelike organ (absent only in the bivalves). Jaws are present in some species. There are approximately 80,000 species of molluscs, of which about 85 have been implicated in poisoning to humans or are known to be toxic under certain conditions. The majority of the venomous or poisonous species are found in three of the five classes of molluscs: Gastropoda, Pelecypoda, and Cephalopoda. In the class Gastropoda, the univalve snails and slugs, the most dangerous members are of the genus *Conus,* of which there are perhaps 400 species. The cone shells are confined almost exclusively to tropical and subtropical seas and oceans and are usually found in shallow waters along reefs, although some of the more dangerous species are found on sandy bottoms. They range in length up to approximately 25 cm. The venom apparatus of *Conus* serves as an offensive weapon for the gaining of food and, to a much lesser extent, as a defensive weapon against predators. It consists of a muscular bulb, a long coiled venom duct, the radula (the radula sheath), and the radular teeth. The venom is thought to be secreted in the venom duct and forced under pressure exerted by the duct and the venom bulb into the radula and thus into the lumen of the radular teeth. The radular teeth are passed from the radula into the pharynx and then into the proboscis. They are then thrust by the proboscis into the prey during the stinging act. The radular teeth are needlelike, from 1 to 10 mm in length, and almost transparent. The reader is referred elsewhere for a more complete review of the structure of the venom apparatus of *Conus* (Russell, 1984a).

The various species of Conidae have been divided into those that were vermivorous, molluscivorous, or piscivorous. Endean *et al.* (1967) demonstrated that of 37 species studied, the paralytic effects of the venoms were indeed directly related to the prey hunted. They concluded that only the piscivorous Conidae were capable of serious injuries to humans.

Initial studies indicated that the venom was white, gray, yellow, or black, depending on the species involved, was viscous, and had a pH range of 7.6 to 8.2. The active principle was nondialyzable, and its toxicity was reduced by heating or incubation with trypsin. The lethal fraction was thought to be a protein or bound to a protein. It was found that the amount of venom in the ducts of *C. striatus* was sufficient to immobilize the small fish on which it preys but not of sufficient quantity to cause serious injury to a human. A toxin, having a molecular weight of over 10,000, with a low lethal index as compared with other *Conus* species, caused ataxia, depressed respirations leading to apnea and cardiac arrest in mammals, precipitated a block in the compound action potential of the isolated toad sciatic nerve, blocked both the directly and indirectly elicited contractions of a mammalian nerve-muscle preparation, and markedly depressed the amplitude of intracellular recorded action potentials in the rat diaphragm. The chemical nature of the toxic fraction of *Conus* venom is not known. Various authors have reported that the active fraction is a protein, or a poison with a molecular weight of about 10,000, or a peptide (*see* Russell, 1984a, for references).

Some abalone, such as *Haliotis,* are toxic to eat. The toxin is concentrated in the digestive gland or liver and can be distinguished by its blue-green pigment. It is thought that the pigment, pyropheophorbide *a,* originates from chlorophyll in the seaweed on which the abalone feeds. Hashimoto (1979) noted that ingestion of the viscera of *Haliotis* caused dermatitis in cats and humans. On the basis of this observation, he carried out experiments demonstrating the importance of photosensitization in the development of the dermatitis and suggested an assay method. He also suggested that the use of fluorescent pigments should be prohibited from foods and that care should be taken to see that drugs are not transformed into fluorescent substances in the body. In the hypobranchial gland of *Murex,* there is a secretion that at first is colorless or yellow but on exposure to sunlight becomes brilliant violet and gives off a strong fetid odor. The gland also produces a toxic secretion. Subsequent studies indicated that two pharmacologically active substances were present. One of these was enteramine or 5-hydroxytryptamine and the other was murexine ($C_{11}H_{18}O_3N_3$). Further investigations showed that murexine had the structure of β-[imidazolyl-(4)]-acrylcholine. It was thus called urocanylcholine. Murexine has also been found in the midgut of the sea hare *Aplysia californica*, senecioylcholine has been identified in the hypobranchial gland of *Thais floridana*, and acrylcholine in *Buccinum undatum*. The amount of these cholinesters in the hypobranchial gland was approximately 1 to 5 mg/g tissue. They exhibited muscarinelike and nicotinelike activity, and they caused cardiovascular changes with hypotension, increased respirations, gastric motility and secretions, and some contraction of the frog rectus muscle and guinea pig ileum. The intravenous LD50 of murexine in mice was 8.1 to 8.7 mg/kg. Dihydromurexine has been isolated from the hypobranchial gland of *T. haemastoma*, and the muricacean gastropod *Acanthina spirata* produces a paralytic substance with high acetylcholine content in both its hypobranchial and salivary-accessory gland complex. The toxin is thought to be a carboxylic ester of choline (*see* Russell, 1984a, for references).

A vasodilator and hypotensive agent has been described from the salivary gland extract of the gastropod *T. haemastoma* (Clench). The extract produced behavioral changes in mice, followed by lethargy. When lethal doses were given, respirations first increased and then decreased and became shallow and death ensured. The toxin produced bradycardia and a fall in blood pressure, which was partly blocked by atropine. In the isolated rabbit heart the extract produced a decrease in rate and contraction, with a fall in heart output. It also produced contractions of the isolated guinea pig ileum and rabbit duodenum. The salivary poison of the gastropod *Neptunea arthritica* is thought to be tetramine ($C_4H_{12}N$). It has been suggested that histamine, choline, and choline ester, also found in the salivary glands of this mollusc, act synergistically with the tetramine in producing the poisoning. In *N. antiqua* the tetramine is probably responsible for almost all the biologic activity of the salivary gland extract. In the viscera of the ivory shell, *Babylonia japonica*, a water-soluble toxin has been found, which is slightly methanol and ethanol soluble, heat labile, dialyzable, ninhydrin positive, and Dragendorff and biuret negative. It has a potent mydriatic activity. The toxin is said to be a complex bromo compound, having the formula $C_{25}H_{26}N_{50}O_{13}BR \cdot 7H_2O$, with a molecular weight of 810.53. It has been named *surugatoxin* (SGTX) after Suruga Bay, where the molluscs were taken (*see* Hashimoto, 1979, for references).

In the sea hare, *A. californica*, acetone extracts of the digestive glands had an intraperitoneal LD50 of approximately 30 mg sea hare tissue per kilogram mouse body weight. Signs in mammals included increased respiration, blanching and drooping of the ears, increased salivation, muscle fasciculations, agonal signs, ataxia, prostration, and death. The extract was also found to be lethal when given orally at approximately 12 times the intraperitoneal dose. A partially purified toxin, called *aplysin*, had an immediate but transient hypotensive effect in the dog. There was some initial arrythmia followed by a slower but regular rate. In the isolated heart of the frog, aplysin caused cardiac standstill. The anterior cervical sympathetic ganglion of the cat was stimulated initially and then reversibly blocked. The frog rectus abdominis muscle responded by contracture, and in the rat diaphragm phrenic nerve, the neuromuscular junction was blocked. In another sea hare, two bromine-containing sesquiterpenes were isolated. These were named *aplysin* and *aplysinol*. A debromo derivative, debromoaplysin, and subsequently a third bromo compound, diterpene aplysin-20, have also been isolated. Observation of a sea hare feeding on the alga *Laurencia nipponica* led to several experiments that indicated that steam distillates of the alga were toxic to worms and carp. Based on this observation, Irie *et al.* (1969) extracted aplysin, debromoaplysin, and aplysinol from the red alga *Laurencia okamurai*, whereas Waraszkiewicz and Erickson (1974) obtained aplysin from *L. nidifica*. From these observations, it is suggested that the bromo toxins originate in algae. Two lethal extracts, one ether soluble and the other water soluble, have been separated from the digestive glands of the Hawaiian sea hares *Dolabella auriculasia*, *A. pulmonica*, *Stytocheilus longicauda*, and *Dolabrifera dolabriefa*. In mice the ether-soluble toxin caused irritability, viciousness, and severe flaccid paralysis. The water-soluble toxin, in contrast, caused "convulsions" and respiratory distress. Sublethal doses of the ether-soluble residue produced hypertension when injected intravenously into rats, whereas the crude water-soluble residue produced a transient hypotension, bradycardia, and apnea. The hypertension produced by the ether-soluble toxin was resistant to both α- and β-adrenergic blocking agents. The hypotensive effect of the water-soluble extract was not abolished by vagotomy or pretreatment with either atropine or Benadryl®. It was concluded that both extracts may have direct effects on the contractility of vascular smooth muscle that are not mediated by α-adrenergic or cholinergic mechanisms. Choline esters were found in the aqueous fraction of the digestive gland of *A. californica*. Both acetylcholine and urocanylcholine were identified. The latter accounted for the cholinesterase-resistant cholinomimetic activity of extracts of the gland. An "antifeedant" has been observed in *A. brasiliana*. It is the aromatic bromoallene panacene. It is suggested that the panacene is biosynthesized from a C_{15} algal precursor (*see* Russell, 1984a, for references).

In the Cephalopods, the cuttlefishes, squids, nautilis, and octopuses are the venomous octopods and possibly several venomous and poisonous squid. The venom apparatus of the octopus is an integral part of the animal's digestive system. The secretions serve in prey capture and digestive function, in some ways similar to the venom glands of snakes. The apparatus consists of paired posterior salivary glands, two short (salivary) ducts that join them with the common salivary duct, paired anterior salivary glands and their ducts, the buccal mass, and the mandibles, or beak. An impressive number of substances have been isolated from or identified in the salivary glands of various cephalopods. Many of these substances have been shown to have biologic activities, although these activities were not always apparent in the physiopharmacologic effect of the whole toxin, and some substances either do not have a significant biologic activity or the state of knowledge does not indicate what activity is present. It now appears that many of the substances reported in the literature were actually normal constituents of the salivary glands of cephalopods and not necessarily venom constituents. Some of the substances found in the salivary glands are tyramine, octopine, agmatine, adrenaline, noradrenaline, 5-hydroxytryptamine, L-*p*-hydroxyphenylethanolamine, histamine, dopamine, tryptophan, and certain of the 11-hydroxysteroids, polyphenols, phenolamines, indoleamines, and guanidine bases.

The posterior salivary glands of *O. apollyon* or *O. bimaculatus* have been shown to contain decarboxylate L-3,4-dihydroxyphenalalanine (DOPA), DL-5-hydroxytryptophan, DL-*erythro*-3,4-dihydroxyphenylserine, and DL-*erythro*-*p*-hydroxyphenylserine, as well as DL-*m*-tyrosine, DL-*erythro*-*m*-hydroxyphenylserine, histidine, L-histidine, DL-*erythro*-phenylserine, 3,4-dihydroxyphenylserine, tyrosine, and *m*-tyrosine. In general, the salivary glands of cephalopods contain little or no proteolytic enzymes, amylases, or lipases. A protein, *cephalotoxin*, from the posterior salivary glands of *Sepia officinalis* has been suggested as the biologically active component of the animal's toxin. The toxin contained no cholinesterase or aminoxidase activity. Analysis of cephalotoxin from the posterior salivary gland of *Octopus vulgaris* showed: protein, 74.05 percent (N determination), 64.25 percent (biuret reaction); carbohydrates, 4.17 percent; and hexosamines, 5.80 percent.

The posterior salivary glands of *Eledone moschata* and *E. aldrovandi* contained a substance that, when injected into mammals, caused marked vasodilation and produced hypotension and stimulation of certain extravascular smooth muscles. The substance was first called *moschatin* but was later renamed *eledoisin*. It was an endecapeptide. It was found that eledoisin was 50 times more potent than acetylcholine, histamine, or bradykinin in its ability to provoke hypotension in the dog. It produced an increase in the permeability of the peripheral vessels, stimulated the smooth muscles of the gastrointestinal tract, and caused an increase, which was atropine resistant, in salivary secretions. In spite of its marked pharmacologic activities, the role and significance of this substance in the salivary glands of *Eledone* are not clear. It is not found in the salivary glands of *O. vulgaris* or *O. macropus,* indicating that it is not a necessary component of cephalopod toxin. It appears that eledoisin plays some part in protein synthesis in the salivary gland.

Reports of envenomation by Australian octopuses, some of which were fatal, stimulated renewed interest in the venom of cephalopods. A saline extract of homogenized glands of *H. maculosa* was found to be a dialyzable, heat-stable product that resisted mild acid hydrolysis. When studied on a number of pharmacologic preparations, it was concluded that animals died in respiratory failure, due to a phrenic nerve block and/or to deleterious changes at the neuromuscular junction. The product also produced bradycardia and hypotension, without remarkable changes in the electrocardiogram. It was found that within four minutes of placing a live *Hapalochlaena maculosa* on the back of a rabbit a small bleeding puncture wound surrounded by a blanched area could be seen, the rabbit became restless, and there was some exophthalmos and "one slight convulsion" with cessation of all muscular activity, other than cardiac. Cyanosis developed and death followed at 19 minutes. It was concluded that a young octopus has sufficient venom in its posterior salivary glands to cause paralysis in 750-g rabbits, that the gland extracts have a high concentration of hyaluronidase, and that neostigmine does not reverse or reduce the toxic effects of the venom.

Further investigations yielded an extract of gland tissue partially purified by filtration that was given the name *maculotoxin*. On the basis of lethality determinations, there appeared to be a close similarity between the toxin and tetrodotoxin, and it was concluded that maculotoxin appeared to resemble tetrodotoxin more closely than it did saxitoxin. Saline and water extracts of the homogenized whole glands of *H. maculosa* produced paralysis and death at the 1 mg gland/2 kg rabbit level. Antibodies were produced to a nontoxic high-molecular-weight component but not for the toxic low-molecular-weight component. It was suggested that the molecular weight below 540 accounted for the lack of antigenicity. Maculotoxin was found to block neuromuscular transmission in the isolated sciatic-sartorius nerve-muscle preparation of the toad by inhibiting the action potential in the motor nerve terminals, and it had no postsynaptic effect. It was suggested that the toxin may block action potentials by displacing sodium ions from negatively charged sites in the membrane. One major toxin, maculotoxin, and a minor one having similar chemical properties were found in the venom of *H. maculosa*. The maculotoxin behaved as a cation of low molecular weight (<700), and it was felt that it was chemically different from tetrodotoxin. In 1978, the previous observations on the likeness of maculotoxin to tetrodotoxin were confirmed. Direct spectral and chromatographic comparisons showed these two toxins to be indistinguishable. This is of particular interest because here we have a poison (tetrodotoxin) that is also a venom (maculotoxin). In the former, the presence of the poison is thought to be a product of metabolism, whereas in the latter the venom is used to immobilize and perhaps kill the prey (*see* Russell, 1984a, for references).

The Pelecypoda, scallops, oysters, clams, and mussels, are the principal transvectors of paralytic shellfish poisoning. The genera most often involved with PSP are *Mya, Mytilus, Modiolus, Protothaca, Spisula,* and *Saxidomus,* according to Halstead (1978). The eating of the ovaries of the Japanese callista, *Callista brevisphonata,* has resulted in numerous cases of illness. The ovaries contain large amounts of choline but no histamine. Cats fed the shellfish showed few signs, other than hypoactivity and some loss of coordination. Three of nine human volunteers who ate the ovaries developed urticaria and very mild symptoms. *Venerupin* poisoning is caused by ingestion of the oyster *Crassostrea gigas.* In one series of 81 persons poisoned, 54 died (Halstead, 1965). In a second outbreak in 1941, of six patients, five died, and from 1942 to 1950 there were 455 additional cases involving the eating of oysters and the short-necked clam *Tapes japonica* (Hashimoto, 1979). The toxin causes hemorrhage in the heart, lungs, and viscera, with diffuse hemorrhage, necrosis, and fatty degeneration of the liver.

Clinical Problem. A number of cones have been implicated in injuries to humans, including *Conus geographus, C. aulicus, C. gloria-maris, C. marmoreus, C. textilis, C. tulipa, C. striatus, C. omaria, C. catus, C. obscurus, C. imperialis, C. pulicarius, C. quercinus, C. litteratus, C. lividus,* and *C. sponsalis.* The first would seem the most dangerous, since they are said to have the highest developed venom apparatus (Halstead, 1978).

The sting often gives rise to immediate, sometimes intense, localized pain at the site of the injury. Within five minutes the victim usually notes some numbness and ischemia about the wound, although in a case seen by the author the affected area was red and tender rather than ischemic. A tingling or numbing sensation may develop about the mouth, lips, and tongue and over the peripheral parts of the extremities. Other symptoms and signs during the first 30 minutes following the injury include: hypertonicity, tremor, muscle fasciculations, nausea and vomiting, dizziness, increased lacrimation and salivation, weakness, and pain in the chest, which increases with deep inspiration. The numbness about the wound may spread to involve a good part of the extremity or injured part. In the more severe cases, respiratory distress with chest pain, difficulties in swallowing and phonation, marked dizziness, blurring of vision and an inability to focus, ataxia, and generalized pruritus have been reported. In fatal cases, "respiratory paralysis" precedes death (Russell, 1965).

Poisoning following the ingestion of the whelk, *Neptunea arthritica,* is characterized by dizziness, nausea, vomiting, weakness, ataxia, photophobia, external ocular weakness, dryness of the mouth, and on occasion, urticaria. Ingestion of the toxic abalone produces erythema, swelling, and pain over the face and neck, and sometimes the extremities, and in the more severe cases, a fulminating dermatitis. Latin and medieval writers from the time of Pliny considered the sea hare *Aplysia* to be very poisonous, and although Halstead (1965) notes that extracts of *Aplysia* were "frequently employed to dispatch political enemies," there are no recent reports of death from the eating of sea hares. Tasting them produces a burning sensation in the mouth and slight irritation of the oral mucosa. Handling the animals is not likely to be dangerous. However, I suspect that it would not be safe to rub one's eyes after handling these animals. A number of poisonings occurred in Hokkaido, Japan, from the ingestion of *Callista brevisiphonata* in the early 1950s. These poisonings necessitated prohibiting the sale of the shellfish in the marketplace. The illness was a rapid onset, often occurring while the patient is still dining. It has been characterized as an "allergiclike" reaction, which is thought to be due to the presence of excessive choline in the ovaries. The most common findings are flushing, urticaria, wheezing, and gastrointestinal upset. It is self-limiting (Russell, 1971). Hashimoto (1979) notes a total of 542 cases of venerupin poisoning in Japan with 185 deaths. Fortunately, there have been no reported cases since 1950. It was observed following the eating of the oyster *Crassostrea gigas* or the asari *Tapes japonica*. The poisoning is characterized by a long incubation period (24 to 48 hours, and sometimes longer), anorexia, halitosis, nausea, vomiting, gastric pain, constipation, headache, and malaise. These findings may be followed by increased nervousness, hematemesis, and bleeding from the mucous membranes of the nose, mouth, and gums. In serious cases, jaundice may be present, and petechial hemorrhages and ecchymosis may appear over the chest, neck, and arms. Leukocytosis, anemia, and a prolonged blood-clotting time are sometimes observed. The liver is usually enlarged. In fatal poisonings, extreme excitation, delirium, and coma occur.

The more common types of shellfish poisoning are recognized as gastrointestinal, allergic, and paralytic. Gastrointestinal shellfish poisoning is characterized by nausea, vomiting, abdominal pain, weakness, and diarrhea. The onset of symptoms generally occurs 8 to 12 hours following ingestion of the offending mollusc. This type of intoxication is caused by bacterial pathogens and is usually limited to gastrointestinal signs and symptoms. It rarely persists for more than 48 hours.

Allergic or erythematous shellfish poisoning is characterized by an allergic response, which may vary from one individual to another. The onset of symptoms and signs occurs 30 minutes to six hours after ingestion of the mollusc to which the individual is sensitive. The usual presenting signs and symptoms are diffuse erythema, swelling, urticaria, and pruritus involving the head and neck and then spreading to the body. Headache, flushing, epigastric distress, and nausea are occasional complaints. In the more severe cases, generalized edema, severe pruritus, swelling of the tongue and throat, respi-

ratory distress, and vomiting sometimes occur. Death is rare, but persons with a known sensitivity to shellfish should avoid eating all molluscs. The sensitizing material appears more capable of provoking a serious autopharmacologic response than most known sensitizing proteins.

Paralytic shellfish poisoning is known variously as *gonyaulax poisoning, paresthetic shellfish poisoning, mussel poisoning,* or *mytilointoxication.* Pathognomonic symptoms develop within the first 30 minutes following ingestion of the offending mollusc. Paresthesia, described as tingling, burning, or numbness, is noted first about the mouth, lips, and tongue; it then spreads over the face, scalp, and neck, and to the fingertips and toes. Sensory perception and proprioception are affected to the point that the individual moves incoordinately and in a manner similar to that seen in another, more common form of intoxication. Ataxia, incoherent speech, and/or aphonia are prominent signs in severe poisonings. The patient complains of dizziness, tightness of the throat and chest, and some pain on deep inspiration. Weakness, malaise, headache, increased salivation and perspiration, thirst, and nausea and vomiting may be present. The pulse is usually thready and rapid; the superficial reflexes are often absent and the deep reflexes may be hypoactive. If muscular weakness and respiratory distress grow progressively more severe during the first eight hours, death may ensue. If the victim survives the first 10 to 12 hours, the prognosis is good. Death is usually attributed to "respiratory paralysis" (Russell, 1965, 1971).

Among the cephalopods that have been implicated in bites on humans are *Hapalochaena* (= *Octopus*) *maculosa, Octopus australis, O. lunulatus, O. doefleini, O. vulgaris, O. apollyon, O. bimaculatus, O. macropus, O. rubescens, O. fitchi, O. flindersi, Ommastrephes sloani pacificus, Eledone moschata, E. aldrovandi,* and *Sepia officinalis.* The bite of most octopuses results in a small puncture wound; it appears to bleed more freely than one would expect from a similar nonvenomized, traumatic wound. Pain is minimal, and in the two cases seen by the author it was described as no greater than that which would have been produced by a sharp pin. The area around the wound is first blanched but then becomes erythematous and in severe envenomations may become hemorrhagic. Tingling and numbness about the wound site are not uncommon complaints. Swelling is usually minimal immediately following the injury but may develop 6 to 12 hours later. Muscle fasciculations have been noted following *H. maculosa* bites (Sutherland and Lane, 1969). Localized pruritus sometimes occurs over the edematous area. "Lightheadedness" of several hours' duration and weakness were reported in both cases observed by us; there were no other systemic symptoms or signs, although the wounds healed without complications (Russell, 1965). In the case reported by Flecker and Cotton (1955), bitten by *H. maculosa,* the patient complained of dryness in the mouth and difficulty in breathing following the bite, but no localized or generalized pain. Subsequently, breathing became more labored, swallowing became difficult, and the patient began to vomit. Severe respiratory distress and cyanosis developed, and the victim expired. The findings at autopsy were negative. Subsequently, Cleland and Southcott (1965) reviewed the literature on cephalopod bites and noted several unreported bites on humans.

Fishes

Poisonous Fishes. Approximately 700 species of marine fishes are known to be toxic or may on ingestion be poisonous to man. This number does not include those fishes that have caused a poisoning traceable to bacterial pathogens. Most, but by no means all, of these species are found in the coral reef belt. As a whole, their distribution is spotty, even in a particular part of the ocean or around an island. They tend to occur in greater numbers around islands than along continental shores. Most species are nonmigratory. They may be either herbivores or carnivores. Some poisonous species have tissues that are toxic at all times; other species are poisonous only at certain periods, or in certain areas, whereas still others have only specific organs that are toxic, and the toxicity of these tissues may vary with time and location.

Fish poisoning is synonymous with *ichthyotoxism*. Halstead (1964) divided the ichthyotoxic fishes into three subdivisions: (1) *ichthyosarcotoxic*—those fishes that contain a toxin within their musculature, viscera, or skin, which when ingested produces deleterious effects; (2) *ichthyootoxic*—those fishes that produce a toxin that is related to gonadal activity; most members of this subdivision are freshwater species; this group includes those fishes whose roe is poisonous; and (3) *icthyohemotoxic*—those fishes that have a toxin in their blood. Some freshwater eels and several marine fishes make up this group. The word *ichthyocrinotoxic* is sometimes used for those fishes that produce a poison through glandular secretions not associated with a venom apparatus. This word might be used for the soapfishes, certain gobies, some cyclostomes, boxfishes, toadfishes, lampreys, and hagfishes, which may release toxic skin secretions into the water, perhaps under stressful conditions, or as repellants, or in defense.

Ichthyosarcotoxism. This type of poisoning is generally identified with the kind of fish involved: elasmobranch, chimaeroid, clupeoid, ciguatera, tetraodon, scombroid, and so on; it also includes hallucinatory fish poisoning.

Ciguatera. The word *ciguatera* was perhaps first applied to a poisoning caused by the ingestion of the marine snail *Livona pica* ("cigua"), a staple seafood found throughout the Caribbean. The word is now commonly used to indicate that type of fish poisoning characterized by certain gastrointestinal-neurologic, and sometimes cardiovascular, manifestations. It may occur following the ingestion of certain tropical reef and semipelagic marine species, such as the barracudas, groupers, sea basses, snappers, surgeonfishes, parrotfishes, jacks, wrasses, eels, as well as certain gastropods. A listing of the ciguateric fishes has been provided by Russell (1965), Halstead (1967), and Bagnis *et al.* (1970). Elsewhere I have noted that approximately 300 species of fish have been implicated in ciguatera poisoning, but Bagnis *et al.* (1970) note approximately 400 species. Since almost all these fishes are normally edible, and some are valuable food fishes in some parts of the world, ciguatera poisoning is not only the most common but also the most treacherous form of ichthyotoxism.

This form of fish poisoning is associated with the food chain or food web (Russell, 1952, 1965; Dawson *et al.,* 1955; Randall, 1958; Halstead, 1965; Banner, 1976; Southcott, 1979). It has been shown to exist in both the South Pacific and the Caribbean. The responsible organism is a photosynthetic benthic dinoflagellate, *Gambierdiscus toxicus,* but the poison found in most ciguateric fishes is probably a combination of several toxins, the principal one being *ciguatoxin* and, in some cases, lesser ones being *maitotoxin* and *scaritoxin*. The chemical structure has not yet been elicited. The toxin is a colorless, heat-stable, hydroxylated lipid molecule, with a molecular weight of about 1100, and it shows little olefinic character and no observable proton signals below 6. The toxin increases membrane permeability to sodium, causing depolarization, and in different doses produces changes in the rate and force of contraction of the heart. Large doses precipitate more severe cardiac changes. Contrary to published reports that it is an anticholinesterase, it has been found to be antagonized by physostigmine.

Signs of poisoning in animals include increased salivation and lacrimation, meiosis, respiratory difficulties, cyanosis, decreased body temperature, ataxia and loss of reflexes, and

Table 22–6. CONCENTRATIONS OF TETRODOTOXIN IN TETRAODONTIDAE FISHES AND A NEWT*

SPECIES	OVARY	LIVER	SKIN	INTESTINES	MUSCLE	BLOOD
Sphaeroides niphobles	400	1000	40	400	4	1
Sphaeroides alboplumbeus	200	1000	20	40	4	
Sphaeroides pardalis	200	1000	100	40	1	1
Sphaeroides vermicularis	400	200	100	40	4	
Sphaeroides porphyreus	400	200	20	40	1	
Sphaeroides oscellatus	1000	40	20	40	<0.2	
Sphaeroides basilewskianus	100	40	4	40	<0.2	
Sphaeroides chrysops	40	40	20	4	<0.2	<0.2
Sphaeroides pseudommus	100	10	4	2	<0.2	
Sphaeroides rubripes	100	100	1	2	<0.2	<0.2
Sphaeroides xanthopterus	100	40	1	4	<0.2	
Sphaeroides stictonotus	20	<0.2	2	1	<0.2	
Lagocephalus inermis	0.4	1	<0.2	0.4	0.4	
Canthigaster rivulatus	<2	2	40	4	<0.2	
Taricha torosa ♀	25	<0.1	25	(0.1)[†]	2	1
Taricha torosa ♂	<0.1[‡]	<0.1	80	(0.5)[†]	8	21

* From Kao. C. Y.: Tetrodotoxin, saxitoxin, and their significance in the study of the excitation phenomena. *Pharmacol. Rev.*, *18*:997, 1996. © by Williams & Wilkins, 1966. Amounts expressed in mcg toxin/g fresh tissue of female specimens.
† Visceral organ.
‡ Testis.

prostration. In humans, symptoms and signs include perioral parasthesia, often with a feeling of loose teeth in the lower jaw, nausea and vomiting, abdominal pain, changes in sensory perception, pruritus, diarrhea, hypoactive reflexes, and bradycardia. The patient often complains of dizziness, marked weakness, and on occasion, some myalgia and joint pain. Paresis, particularly of the legs, is a common finding in severe poisonings. Presence of the toxin can be demonstrated by ELISA and RIA.

Tetrodotoxin. Tetrodotoxin, puffer or fugu poison, is found in certain puffers, ocean sunfishes, and porcupinefishes. Tetrodotoxin (tarichatoxin) is also found in certain amphibian species of the family Salamandridae and the blue-ringed octopus. The puffers or pufferlike fishes appear to be the only fishes universally regarded as poisonous. Of the approximately 100 species of these fishes, over 50 have been involved in poisonings to humans or are known to be toxic under certain conditions. Some of the more important of the toxic species have been noted by Russell (1965), Kao (1966), Halstead (1967), and Hashimoto (1979). Table 22–6 shows the concentration of tetrodotoxin for various tissues of Tetraodontidae species and for the amphibian *Taricha torosa*. It can be seen that in most cases the toxin is concentrated in the ovaries and liver, with lesser amounts being found in the intestines and skin, and very small amounts in the body musculature and blood. In almost all fish species so far studied, the concentration in the ovaries has been considerably higher than in the corresponding male tissues. The appearance and amount of toxin in the fish are related to the reproductive cycle and appear to be greatest just prior to spawning, which varies with the species involved and the locale. The chemistry of tetrodotoxin up until 1970 has been reviewed elsewhere (Russell, 1971). Its structure is:

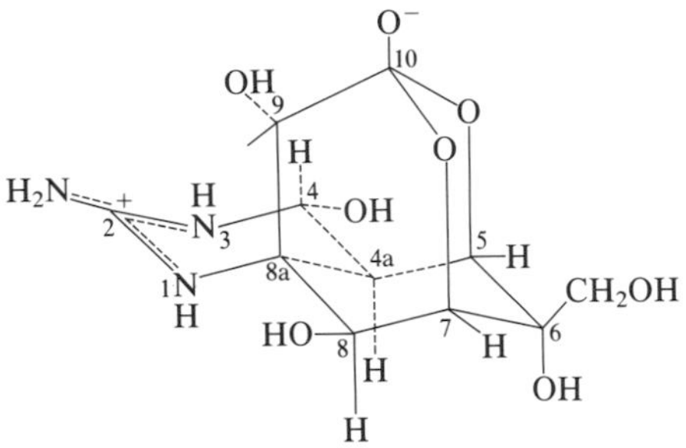

The lethal dose-response curve of tetrodotoxin is characteristically steep. The intraperitoneal minimal lethal dose in mice is 8 μg/kg, whereas the LD99 is 12 μg/kg, and the intraperitoneal LD50 is approximately 10 μg/kg (Kao and Fuhrman, 1963). The oral LD50 in mice is 322 μg/kg, whereas that in cats is in excess of 0.20 mg/kg. The toxin prevents the increase in the early transient ionic permeability of the nerve normally associated with the inward movement of sodium during excitation. This can be seen in the classic nerve preparations as a conduction block, and in the voltage-clamp axon preparations as a decrease in the peak current of the inward sodium. The subsequent outward movement of potassium is unaffected by the toxin. It is also capable of blocking the inward movement of all substituted cations that could account, under experimental conditions, for the early current change. In blocking this early current, the toxin prevents both the inward and outward movement of ions. The mode of the block is not ion specificity but changes provoked in the membrane of the nerve.

To a lesser extent, tetrodotoxin blocks the skeletal muscle membrane. It has no direct effect on the junction, exclusive of that on the nerve ending and the muscle membrane. It provokes hypotension and has a deleterious effect on respiration. It has some effects on the central nervous system but little on the autonomic nervous system. Tetrodotoxin has pharmacologic and toxicologic properties similar in many ways to those of saxitoxin, but the two are chemically distinct. The proposed "cork-in-a-bottle" hypothesis for tetrodotoxin seems highly questionable at this time. Recent studies have shown that binding of tetrodotoxin, like saxitoxin, is a function separate from that of cation selectivity, which has been the basis of the cork-in-a-bottle model (Kao, 1981).

While less than 75 people now die from tetraodon poisoning in Japan each year, many of those using the poison in suicide, and additional deaths are reported from elsewhere in the Orient and Pacific, the total number of deaths worldwide is probably less than 125. At one time the mortality rate was 80 percent, but through the years it has been reduced, due in part to the fine work of Hashimoto and his colleagues in licensing fugu restaurants in Japan. At the present time about 40 percent of those developing significant symptoms and signs subsequently die. The clinical case is characterized by the rapid onset (5 to 30 minutes) of weakness, dizziness, pallor, and paresthesia about the lips, tongue, and throat. The paresthesia is usually described as "tingling or pricking sensations" and is often noted in the limbs, particularly the fingers and toes, as the illness develops. Weakness is a common complaint. Increased salivation and diaphoresis are often present, and the patient may become hypotensive. Changes in heart rate are common. There may be vomiting and sometimes it is severe and frequent. Bradycardia, dyspnea, cyanosis, and shock may develop, and generalized flaccidity may ensue. Treatment consists of oxygen, intravenous fluids, atropine, and if appropriate, activated charcoal, saline catharses, and nasoepigastric suctioning. Calcium, naloxone, and sedatives are contraindicated. The poison can be detected from autopsy material by gas chromatography.

Scrombroid Poisoning. Certain of the mackerellike fishes (tunas, skipjacks, and bonitos) are occasionally involved in human poisonings. The clinical manifestations of these poisonings are quite different from that provoked by ciguatera toxin, although some of these same fishes may also be implicated in ciguatera poisoning. Although more than 50 papers on this subject have been written during the past decade, they have added little to that reported by Halstead (1967). A notable exception is the review by Arnold and Brown (1978). If scombroids are inadequately preserved, a toxic substance is formed within the body musculature. This substance was once thought to be histamine, formed by the action of enzymes and bacteria or released by bacterial action on the death of the fish. However, more recent evidence seems to indicate that the toxic component is not histamine alone, although histamine is involved in the reaction. The toxic factor has been given the name "saurine" by some investigators. Following ingestion of the offending fish, the victim usually complains of nausea, vomiting, diarrhea, and epigastric distress, flushing of the face, headache, and burning of the throat, sometimes followed by numbness, thirst, and generalized urticaria. These signs and symptoms usually appear within 2 hours of the meal and subside within 16 hours. In the more severe cases, there may be some muscular weakness. The poisoning is rarely serious. The offending fish is often said to have a "peppery taste" (Russell, 1971).

Cyclostome Poisoning. The slime and flesh of certain lampreys and hagfishes appear to contain a toxin that may produce gastrointestinal signs and symptoms. The chemical, pharmacologic, and toxicologic nature of the toxin are not known.

Elasmobranch Poisoning. Consumption of the musculature of the Greenland shark *Somniosus microcephalus,* has caused poisonings in both humans and dogs, whereas the livers of several species of tropical sharks have caused severe poisonings and even deaths. Species reported to be poisonous at times include: *Carcharhinus melanopterus, Heptranchias perlo, Hexanchus grisseus, Carcharodon carcharias,* and *Sphyrna zygaena.* In some cases, the poisoning appears to be ciguateric in nature. The eating of shark livers has been known to cause another kind of poisoning, which appears to be due to hypervitaminosis A. Hypervitaminosis A is well known following the consumption of the livers of some polar bears, seals, and halibut (Russell, 1967; Halstead, 1970).

Hallucinatory Fish Poisoning. This type of poisoning is characterized by central nervous system signs and symptoms and by the lack of gastrointestinal manifestations. It has occurred following the ingestion of certain mullet and surmullet (goatfish). Among the species reported to have caused this poisoning are: *Mugil cephalus, Neomyxus chaptalli, Paraupeneus chryserydros,* and *Upeneus arge.* Reports of poisoning have been filed in the tropical Pacific and Hawaii. Nothing is known of the chemistry or toxicology of this poison. However, the findings in the human cases seem to indicate that the offending substance is different from that responsible for ciguatera poisoning. The onset of symptoms occurs 10 to 90 minutes following ingestion of the toxic fish. The victim complains of lightheadedness or dizziness, weakness, muscular incoordination, and sometimes ataxia, hallucinations, and depression. In the severe cases, there may be paresthesia about the mouth, and some muscular paralysis and dyspnea. The agonal period is usually of short duration, 1 to 24 hours, and few cases are serious enough to bring the victim to the doctor. If the victim goes to sleep immediately following the poisoning, he is said to have violent nightmares. This complaint accounts for the term "nightmare weke" being given to the causative fish *U. arge* (Helfrich and Banner, 1960).

Ichthyootoxic Fishes.   A number of freshwater fishes and a few marine species produce a toxin that appears to be restricted to their gonads. In these fishes the body musculature and even the gastrointestinal organs are edible. Poisoning occurs following ingestion of the roe, or gonads and roe. The eggs of *Scorpaenichthys marmoratus* appear to be avoided by fish-eating and scavenging birds, as well as by mink and raccoon, whereas the roe of the alligator gar is known to produce cardiovascular changes. An excellent review of this problem will be found in Fuhrman (1974). The poisoning is characterized by the rapid onset of nausea, vomiting, and epigastric distress. Diarrhea, dryness in the mouth, thirst, tinnitus, and malaise sometimes occur. In the more severe cases, syncope, respiratory distress, chest pain, convulsions, and coma may ensue. Complete recovery usually occurs within a few days.

Ichthyohemotoxic Fishes.   A toxic substance has been found in the blood of many species of fishes, although the principal contributions to our knowledge of the toxin have come to us through studies on the blood of the eels *Anguilla* and *Muraena.* Poisonings from the ingestion of fresh blood are extremely rare. The few cases reported have occurred in persons who of their own volition have drunk quantities sufficient to cause symptoms; most of these have occurred following the ingestion of blood from the European freshwater eels, or *M. helena.*

Crinotoxic Fishes.   Halstead (1970) has recorded approximately 50 teleost species as being crinotoxic. Hashimoto has noted a few addition-

al, and with the study of Cameron *et al.* (1981), and others, the total number must now approach 65. These fishes are known to release a toxic substance from the skin that is capable of killing other fishes and perhaps other marine animals. This toxin appears to be part of the animal's defensive armament and is probably released as an alarm substance to deter predators. Cameron *et al.* (1981) suggest that in the case of the stonefish the toxin liberated from the tubercle glands might be antibiotic in nature, protecting the fish against the plethora of potential harmful organisms that occur in the immediate environment of the virtually scaleless integument of the fish.

A toxic factor has been separated from the skin secretions of the boxfish, or trunkfish, *Ostracion lentiginosis.* The toxin is heat stable, nondialyzable, and soluble in water, methanol, ethanol, acetone, and chloroform, but insoluble in diethyl ether and benzene. Repeated extractions of residues obtained from drying the skin secretions with acetone or chloroform and diethyl ether give a particulate substance that forms stable foams in aqueous solutions and is toxic to fish at concentrations of 1 : 1,000,000. Approximately 50 to 100 mg of the crude dried toxin could be obtained at one time from a single adult boxfish. The toxin was called "ostracitoxin." Further studies showed that when a crude solution was extracted into 1-butanol, a 20-fold purification of the toxin could be obtained. The product was called "pahutoxin." Spectroscopic data, hydrolytic degradations, and synthesis gave the formula $C_{23}H_{46}NO_4Cl$ and the structure:

$$CH_3-(CH_2)_{12}-\underset{\underset{OCOCH_3}{|}}{\overset{\overset{H}{|}}{C}}-CH_2-CO_2-(CH_2)_2-\overset{+}{N}(CH_3)_3Cl^-$$

Pahutoxin is thus the choline chloride ester of 3-acetoxyhexadecanoic acid. It and its C_{14} and C_{12} homologues have been synthesized as the racemates. When ostracitoxin was added to an aquarium containing other reef fishes, these fishes exhibited "irritability," gasping, then activity with a decrease in opercular movements, loss of equilibrium and locomotion, and finally, sporadic convulsions, and death. When the skin mucus was injected into the boxfish, the fish immediately lost its balance, and death occurred within a few minutes. When injected into mice, ostracitoxin produced ataxia, labored respirations, coma, and death. The MLD was 200 mg/ kg body weight. Ostracitoxin caused hemolysis of vertebrate erythrocytes *in vitro.* Pahutoxin was quantitated for its hemolytic property, which correlated with its lethal property. The minimum lethal concentration for fish was found to be 0.176 μg/ml, when death was measured at one hour (*see* Russell, 1971, for references).

The Red Sea flatfish, *Pardachirus marmoratus,* has 212 to 235 secretory glands along its dorsal and anal fins. Its secretions are toxic to fishes, and the toxic factor, pardaxin, is a protein having a molecular weight of approximately 15,000, with a single chain and four disulfide bridges. The toxin has an intraperitoneal LD50 in mice of 24.6 mg/kg and inhibits Na^+-K^+—ATPase but enhances esterase activity. It causes hemolysis in dog red blood cells, which lack ATPase, but the toxin-induced hemolysis is not caused by ATPase inhibition. It was suggested that the different responses to the poison, with respect to esterase and ATPase, could be due to differences in the way these enzymes are anchored in the plasma membrane (Primor and Lazarovici, 1981).

Venomous Fishes

More than 200 species of marine fishes, including stingrays, scorpionfishes, zebrafishes, stonefishes, weevers, toadfishes, stargazers, and certain of the sharks, ratfishes, catfishes, and surgeonfishes are known or thought to be venomous. The great majority of venomous piscines are nonmigratory and slow swimming. They tend to live in protected habitats or around rocks, corals, or kelp beds. Stingrays spend much of their time buried in sand. Most species use their venom apparatus as a defensive weapon. The toxins of the venomous fishes differ markedly in their chemical, pharmacologic, and toxicologic properties from the toxins of the poisonous fishes, as well as from the toxins of the other venomous animals. A common characteristic of the toxins of the venomous fishes is their relative instability. Few of them are stable at room temperatures, and toxicity appears to be lost or markedly reduced even on lyophilization of freshly prepared crude extracts. No basic structure for the toxin of any venomous fishes has yet been established, or even proposed with any degree of fervor. The reader is referred to the works of Russell (1965, 1969, 1971, 1984a) and Halstead (1970, 1978) for a review of the toxins of the venomous fishes.

Stingrays. The stingrays include the families Dasyatidae, the whiprays; Urolophidae, the round stingrays; Myliobatioidae, the bat- or eagle-rays; Gymnuridae, the butterfly rays; and the Potamotrygonidae, or river rays. These elasmobranches range in size from several inches in diameter to over 14 feet in length. For the most part, they are nonmigratory, shallow-water fishes. The venom apparatus of the stingray consists of a bilaterally serrated, dentinal caudal spine located on the dorsum of the animal's tail. The spine is encased in an integumentary sheath. The venom is contained with certain highly specialized secretory cells within this sheath. These cells and the supporting structures have been described in detail (*see* Russell, 1965; Halstead, 1970; Smith *et al.,* 1978). Unlike most venomous animals, the stingray has no true venom gland. The venom is contained in the secretory cells within the grooves of the caudal spine, and these cells and their supporting tissues must be ruptured in order to release the toxin, as in the traumatic act of stinging.

Stingray venom is known to exert a deleterious effect on the mammalian cardiovascular system. Low concentrations of the venom give rise to either vasodilatation or vasoconstriction, with mild bradycardia and an increase in the P-R interval. Cats receiving larger amounts of the venom show, in addition to the P-R interval change, almost immediate ST, T-wave change indicative of ischemia and, in some animals, true heart muscle injury. High concentrations cause vasoconstriction and produce marked changes in heart rate and amplitude of systole and may often cause complete, irreversible, cardiac standstill (Russell and van Harreveld, 1954). While small doses of the venom may cause some increase in the respiratory rate, large doses depress respiration. Part of this depression is secondary to the cardiovascular changes, but the venom may provoke changes in behavior. The venom has little or no effect or neuromuscular transmission.

Mice injected with a lethal dose of stingray venom develop hyperkinesis, prostration, marked dyspnea, blanching of the ears and retina, and exophthalmos. These are followed by complete atonia, cyanosis, gasping respiratory movements, coma, and death. In cats and monkeys a similar pattern has been observed. The LD99 in mice has been calculated as 28.0 mg/kg for crude extracts of the tissues from the ventrolateral grooves of the sting. However, we have found that the peak II portion of a Sephadex G-200 fraction has an intravenous LD50 in mice of approximately 2.9 mg protein per kilogram body weight (*see* Russell, 1971, for references).

Scorpionfishes. The family Scorpaenidae, the scorpionfishes or rockfishes, contains approximately 80 species that have been implicated in poisonings to humans, or whose venom has been studied by chemists and toxicologists. Included in this group are the sculpins, zebrafishes, stonefishes, bullrout, and waspfish. They are widely distributed throughout all tropical and the more temperate seas. A few are found in Arctic waters. The venom apparatus of these fishes has been described in considerable detail. In most species it consists of a number of dorsal,

Table 22–7. SOME PROPERTIES OF SCORPAENIDAE VENOMS*

	PTEROIS	SYNANCEJA	SCORPAENA
Small dose	Decreased arterial pressure Minimal ECG changes Increased respiratory rate Muscular weakness in mice	Decreased arterial pressure Minimal ECG changes Increased respiratory rate Tremor	Slight decrease in arterial pressure Increased, then decreased, venous pressure Minimal ECG changes Increased respiratory rate with decreased respiratory excursions
Medium dose	Marked fall in arterial pressure Myocardial ischemia, injury or conduction defects Increased respiratory rate Partial paralysis of legs in mice	Marked fall in arterial pressure Myocardial ischemia, injury or conduction defects Increased respiratory rate Muscular weakness in mice Tremor	Fall in arterial pressure Myocardial ischemia, injury or conduction defects Changes in venous and CSF pressures Increased respiratory rate with decreased respiratory excursions Muscular weakness in mice
Lethal dose	Precipitous, irreversible fall in systemic arterial pressure Extensive ECG changes Markedly decreased respiratory rate → cessation Complete paralysis of legs in mice Intravenous LD50 mice, 1.1 mg protein/kg body weight	Precipitous, irreversible fall in systemic arterial pressure Extensive ECG changes Markedly decreased respiratory rate → cessation Some paralysis of legs in mice Possible neuromuscular junction changes Produces tremors, convulsions, marked muscular weakness, coma; myotoxic Intravenous LD50 mice, 200 μg protein/kg body weight	Precipitous, irreversible fall in arterial pressure Extensive ECG changes Markedly decreased respiratory rate → cessation Some paralysis of legs in mice Intravenous LD50 mice, in excess 2.0 mg protein/kg body weight

* From Russell, F. E.: Pharmacology of toxins of marine origin. In Raskova, H. (ed.): *International Encyclopedia of Pharmacology and Therapeutics,* Sec. 71, Vol. 2. Pergamon Press, Ltd., Oxford, 1971, pp. 3–114.

several anal, and two pelvic spines. The spines differ considerably in their size and structure. The enveloping integumentary sheath and the glandular complex lying within the anterolateral grooves make up the remaining components of the venom apparatus. The venom apparatuses of these fishes have been divided into three types. A more thorough review of the variations in the venom gland structures, the chemistry, and the toxicology of the venom has been reviewed by Halstead (1970) and Russell (1971). The pharmacologic properties are summarized in Table 22–7.

Weeverfishes. The weevers, members of the piscine family Trachinidae, are small marine fishes that are confined to the eastern Atlantic and Mediterranean coasts. The name "weever" is probably derived from a corruption of the Anglo-Saxon "wivre," meaning viper. These fish are found in large numbers in the shallow waters of certain offshore sandy grounds along the southeast English coast, in the continental southern North Sea, and along the coasts of the English Channel and Mediterranean and Adriatic seas. The venom apparatus of the weeverfishes consists of two opercular spines, five to eight dorsal spines, and the tissues contained within the integumentary sheaths surrounding the spines. The two dentinal opercular spines extend caudally and very slightly downward from near the superior margin of each operculum. The five to eight dorsal spines are enclosed within individual integumentary sheaths connected by their interspinous membranes. The venom is contained within the various grooves of the spines. These spines and the venom have been described elsewhere (Russell and Emery, 1960; Halstead, 1978; Russell, 1971, 1984a).

Clinical Problem. Stings by venomous marine fishes are common in many areas of the world. Approximately 750 people have been reported stung by stingrays along the North American coasts in a single year. Fortunately, deaths from the effects of the venom are very rare.

Stings by other *Scorpaena* are very common. Approximately 300 persons in the United States are stung by *S. guttata* or related species each year (*see* Russell, 1971, for references). Envenomations by the lionfishes or zebrafishes were once quite rare, but with the importation of lionfishes for tropical sea aquaria more than 50 cases of stings by these fish were reported in 1978–79. Injuries inflicted by weeverfishes are also common in certain coastal areas of Europe. However, no deaths attributable to the stings of these fishes have been reported in recent years.

Of 1097 stingray injuries reported over a six-year period in North America from 1952 to 1959, 232 patients were seen by a physician at some time during the course of their recovery. That is not true today. Only about 5 percent are now seen by physicians due to the effective first aid provided by the lifeguard services. Unlike the injuries inflicted by many venomous animals, wounds produced by the stingray may be large and severely lacerated, requiring extensive debridement and surgical closure. A sting no wider than 5 mm may produce a wound 3.5 cm long, and larger stings may produce wounds 17.5 cm long. The sting itself is rarely broken off in the wound. The stinging is followed by the immediate onset of intense pain, out of proportion to that which might be produced by a similar nonvenomous injury. While the onset of pain is usually limited to the area of injury, it rapidly spreads, though gradually diminishing in severity over 6 to 48 hours.

For the most part, the symptoms and signs of the poisoning are limited to the injured area. However, syncope, weakness, nausea, and anxiety are common complaints and may be attributed in part to peripheral vasodilatation and in part to the reflex phenomenon precipitated by the severe pain. Vomiting, diarrhea, sweating, fasciculations in the muscles of the affected extremity, generalized cramps, inguinal or axillary pain, and respiratory distress are infrequently reported. True paralysis is extremely rare, if it occurs at all. Examination reveals either a puncture or a lacerating wound, usually the latter, jagged, bleeding freely, and often contaminated with parts of the stingray's integumentary sheath. The edges of the wound may be discolored. However, within two hours the discoloration may extend several centimeters from the wound. Subsequent necrosis of this area occasionally occurs in untreated cases.

Treatment, to be successful, must be instituted early. The standard procedure for treatment of fish stings is well established. Injuries to an extremity should be irrigated with the salt water at hand. An attempt should be made to remove the integumentary sheath, if present in the wound. The extremity should then be submerged in hot water at as high a temperature as the patient can tolerate without injury for 30 to 90 minutes. The addition of sodium chloride or magnesium sulfate to the hot water is optional. The wound should then be further cleaned, debrided, and sutured, if necessary. The appropriate antitetanus agent should be administered. Infections of these wounds are rare in properly treated cases. Elevation of the injured extremity is advised.

Envenomation by *Scorpaena*, such as the California sculpin, *S. guttata*, is followed almost immediately by intense, sometimes pulsating pain in the area of the injury. Almost all stings are inflicted on the hands of fishermen while they are attempting to dislodge the fish from their hooks. The area around the wound may appear ischemic at first, but in time the injured part becomes red and swollen. The pain may extend up the forearm and into the axilla within 15 minutes of the injury. Nausea, vomiting, weakness, pallor, syncope, and an urgency to urinate are frequent complaints. Increased perspiration, headache, conjunctivitis, and diarrhea are sometimes reported. Paresthesia about the injured part and even up the forearm is not uncommon. Swelling and tenderness of the axillary nodes occurred in at least 30 percent of one series of untreated cases. The pain subsides in three to eight hours, although the swelling and tenderness may persist for several days. In severe stingings the pain may be excruciating. Primary shock may occur, and in several cases seen by the author the patients were brought to the hospital under oxygen. Repirations may become labored and painful. Pulmonary edema has been reported and abnormal electrocardiograms demonstrated. In one case known to the author the patient had a pulmonary embolism and was hospitalized for 24 days. The standard treatment for *S. guttata* stings had been to soak the injured part in hot water for 30 minutes. In many cases, the fisherman adds household ammonia.

Envenomation by the lionfish gives rise to immediate intense, sometimes burning pain, which often radiates within minutes from the wounded area. The tissues about the wound may appear blanched, and the victim may complain of numbness, weakness, and paresthesia about the injury or even over the entire affected part. Weakness, dizziness, and shock may ensue but are not common. In cases of shock, there is bradycardia, hypothermia, and respiratory distress. The wound site is sometimes discolored, edematous and tender. Necrosis may occur about the wound. The pain often persists for 8 to 12 hours, and the injured part may be sore and edematous for several weeks. First-aid treatment is the same as for stingray injuries. Meperidine hydrochloride has been used to control pain. Intravenous calcium gluconate has been said to afford some relief. Cardiovascular tone should be maintained with intravenous fluids and vasopressor agents.

Stingings by the stonefishes *Synanceja horrida* and *S. trachynis* are usually more serious than those inflicted by any other of the venomous fishes. The clinical course following poisoning by a stonefish is similar to, although considerably more severe than, that previously described for the stingrays and lionfishes. Necrosis of tissues at the site of the injury and the subsequent sloughing of these tissues are more common following stings by *Synanceja* than following injuries by the other venomous fishes. Treatment of wounds produced by stonefishes must be instituted immediately following envenomation. Immersion of the injured part in hot water, as described for stingray wounds, should be tried. Injection of emetine hydrochloride directly into the wound has been tried, with indifferent results. In one case seen by the author, a soap solution was injected directly into the wound area 15 minutes after the hot-water treatment had been initiated. There were no untoward effects and no local tissue changes developed. An antivenin is now prepared by the Commonwealth Serum Laboratories of Australia and should be used when the seriousness of the poisoning warrants.

The weeverfishes, *Trachinus*, may inflict either a single or a multiple puncture-type wound. Persons stung by these fishes report having received a sharp, immediately painful stab. It increases in severity during the first 20 to 50 minutes following the injury and may persist for 16 to 24 hours if treatment is not undertaken. As noted by Halstead (1957), the pain can be so severe that a victim stung by one of these fishes while in the water may experience difficulty in reaching shore. I have obtained similar reports from bathers along the Devon and Cornwall coasts of England. It seems unlikely that it is the excruciating pain rather than true muscular paralysis that is responsible for the victim's motor incapacity. The degree of swelling about the wound varies, although some swelling appears to be a constant finding. The tissues adjacent to the wound often appear discolored; the surrounding area may be somewhat blanched. Localized necrosis at the wound site may occur, and sloughing of these tissues has been reported. It is possible that repeated stings, and the effects of the venom and low-grade infection, are contributing factors in cases of arthritis seen in fishermen on trawlers in the North Sea (*see* Russell, 1971, for references).

In severe cases of envenomation by weevers, there may be weakness, dizziness, nausea, primary shock, and respiratory distress. Fishermen at Ijmuiden, Holland, told me that there was often an urgency to urinate and that in severe stings there was axillary and chest pain, as well as changes in pulse rate and respiration.

A few thoughts on the treatment of weeverfish stings seem indicated, and perhaps this is an appropriate place to present an additional reflection or so on the therapeutics of the injuries produced by venomous fishes in general. After having seen and treated a good many such injuries during the past three decades, I have been impressed with the differences between the advice found in medical texts and that suggested and used by fishermen or lifeguards, or persons familiar with envenomations by fishes. I am distressed to note that in most cases the nonprofessional advice has not only proved to be more effective but often more rational. Much of the advice given in texts devoted to tropical medicine, where the problem of venomous animal injury is most often discussed, stems from the false and antiquated idea that all venoms are related chemically and thus all respond to similar therapeutic measures. From the early studies on snake venoms, a number of remedies found their way into the therapeutics for venomous fish injuries. Among these were acetic acid, alcohol, formaldehyde, urine, potassium permanganate, ink, gold salts, carbolic acid, cassava bread, and cauterization. While all these measures have been found to be ineffective, some are still advised in an occasional medical text. The more recent therapeutic fads for antihistamines, corticosteroids, and ice water as "shotgun" therapeutic methods are slowly waning, fortunately for the patient.

It is refreshing to find that a review of the literature for the past several centuries reveals a highly effective method of treatment, based on trial and error. When I suggested (Russell and Emery, 1960) that the use of hot water in weeverfish stings might be effective, I did so on the basis of its very effective use in stingray and scorpionfish injuries, and on the basis of a limited number of case histories and observations on weeverfish stings that I studied in England, France, and Holland during 1958. Subsequently, I reviewed the quite extensive earlier literature on this problem and found a great number of statements concerning the effectiveness of heat, in one form or another, in the treatment of weeverfish poisonings (*see* Russell, 1965). In a controlled experiment in humans, we found that the methods suggested for the treatment of stingray, scorpionfish, and catfish injuries are equally effective in alleviating the severe pain and other symptoms provoked by the venom of the weever-fishes. Maretić (1957) has used intravenous calcium gluconate with good success for relieving the pain of the injury. Local injections of procaine may be of some value in less severe poisonings, and intramuscular or intravenous meperidine is of definite value in those cases in which there is severe pain after the first hour following the injury. An experimental antivenin has been developed at the Institute of Immunology in Zagreb, and in a limited number of clinical tests it has been shown to be effective (Maretić, personal communication, 1981). However, its use should probably be limited to the more serious stings where there are significant manifestations.

ARTHROPODS

Only a relatively small number of arthropods are sufficiently venomous to be of potential danger to humans. Nevertheless, arthropods are implicated in far more poisonings in humans than all the other phyla combined. Almost all the 30,000 species of spiders are venomous, but luckily for humans only a relatively small number have fangs long and strong enough to penetrate the human skin (Gertsch, 1979). There are some 500 species of scorpions and all are venomous, although only a small number are sufficiently dangerous to be of a problem to humans. In the order Hymenoptera, the bees, wasps, yellow jackets, and ants, there are numerous species of medical importance, particularly because of the anaphylactic problems they precipitate. Among the ticks, caterpillars, kissing bugs, water bugs, moths, butterflies, grasshoppers, centipedes, and millipedes are additional arthropods of medical importance. The venoms of arthropods are highly diversified, and if the spider venoms so far studied are an indication, these poisons may prove to be more complex than originally suspected. Like the snake venoms, the arthropod poisons exert their deleterious effects at the cellular level. The arthropod venoms have been reviewed in detail by Bettini (1978).

The number of deaths from arthropod stings and bites is not known, nor do most countries keep records of the incidence of such injuries. In Mexico, parts of Central and South America, and North Africa, deaths from scorpion stings may exceed several thousand a year. Spider bites probably do not account for more than 200 deaths a year, worldwide. The number of deaths from arthropod bites or stings in the temperate countries is far greater than the number of deaths from snakebite. However, most of these deaths are anaphylactic in nature. In the underde-veloped countries of the tropics a far greater number of deaths from arthropods are due to the direct effects of the venom. A common problem in suspected arthropod bites or stings relates to the differential diagnosis. Of approximately 600 suspected spider bites seen in one series of cases, 80 percent were found to be caused by arthropods other than spiders, or by other disease states (Russell and Gertsch, 1983). The arthropods most frequently involved in the misdiagnoses were ticks (including their embedded mouth parts), mites, bedbugs, fleas (infected flea bites), lepidopterous insects, flies, vesicating beetles, water bugs, and various stinging Hymenoptera. Among the disease states that have been confused with spider bites or arthropods bites or stings are erythema chronicum migrans, Stevens-Johnson syndrome, toxic epidermal necrolysis, erythema nodosum, herpes simplex, purpura fulminans, diabetic ulcer, poison oak, and gonococcal arthritic dermatitis. As with the snake, a spider or other arthropod may bite or sting and not eject venom, but this must be a rare rather than a common event.

Anaphylactic reactions and anaphylaxis are sometimes encountered following arthropod injuries and become medical emergencies. More common are other autopharmacologic reactions, which may mistakenly be attributed to the direct action of the venom. The author has seen many unusual responses, varying from mild agitation to a vesicle-pustule-ulcer-eschar lesion following the sting of a bee. Also, the development of a lesion or lesions at a previous sting may follow a new sting and present difficulties in differential diagnosis, unless a careful history is taken. Finally, some arthropod venom poisonings give rise to symptoms and signs of a previously undiagnosed, subclinical disease. The problem of diverse disease states following the bites or stings of various venomous animals is recognized (Russell, 1977), and when a case of venom poisoning persists, or develops into a new syndrome, the patient should be reexamined for the possible presence of an undiagnosed disease. In some cases, stings or bites may induce stress reactions and the patient may present a more complex and distressing problem.

Spiders

There are at least 200 species of spiders that have been implicated in significant bites on humans. Some of the more important of these are noted in Table 22–8. A more complete review of the problem of spider bites will be found in the excellent work by Maretić and Lebez (1979) and the lesser contributions of Southcott (1976) and Russell and Gertsch (1983).

Table 22–8.   GENERA OF SPIDERS FOR WHICH SIGNIFICANT BITES ON HUMANS ARE KNOWN

GENUS	FAMILY	COMMON NAME	DISTRIBUTION
Aganippe species	Ctenizidae	Trap-door spider	Australia
Aphonopelma species	Theraphosidiae	Tarantula	North America
Araneus species	Araneidae	Orbweaver	Worldwide
Arbanitis species	Ctenizidae	Trap-door spider	Australia, East Indies
Argiope species	Araneidae	Argiope	Worldwide
Atrax species	Macrothelinae	Funnel-web spider	Australia
Bothriocyrtum species	Ctenizidae	Trap-door spider	California
Chiracanthium species	Clubionidae	Running spider	Europe, North Africa, Orient, North America
Cupiennius species	Ctenidae	Banana spider	Central America
Drassodes species	Gnaphosidae	Running spider	Worldwide
Dyarcyops species	Ctenizidae	Trap-door spider	Australia
Dysdera species	Dysderidae	Dysderid	Eastern Hemisphere, Americas
Elassoctenus species	Ctenidae	Ctenid	Australia
Filistata species	Filistatidae	Hackled-band spider	Temperate and tropical world-wide
Harpactirella species	Barychelidae	Trap-door spider	South Africa
Heteropoda species	Sparassidae	Giant crab spider	East Indies, tropical Asia, south Florida
Isopoda species	Sparassidae	Giant crab spider	Australia, East Indies
Ixeuticus species	Amaurobiidae	Amaurobiid	New Zealand, S. California
Lampona species	Gnaphosidae	Running spider	Australia, New Zealand
Latrodectus species	Theridiidae	Widow spider	Temperate and tropical regions worldwide
Liocranoides species	Clubionidae	Running spider	Appalachia and California
Lithyphantes species (= *Steatoda* species)	Theridiidae	Sheet-web weaver	Worldwide
Loxosceles species	Loxoscelidae	Brown or violin spider	Americas, Africa, Europe, Eastern Asia, Pacific Islands
Lycosa species	Lycosoidae	Wolf spider	Worldwide
Missulena species	Actinopodidae	Trap-door spider	Australia
Misumenoides species	Thomisidae	Crab spider	North and South America
Miturga species	Theraphosidae	Running spider	Australia
Mopsus species	Salticidae	Jumping spider	Australia
Neoscona species	Araneidae	Orbweaver	Worldwide
Olios species	Sparassidae	Giant crab spider	North and South America
Pamphobeteus species	Theraphosidae	Tarantula	South America
Peucetia species	Oxyopidae	Green lynx spider	Worldwide
Phidippus species	Salticidae	Jumping spider	North and South America
Phoneutria species	Ctenidae	Hunting spider	Central and South America
Selenocosmia species	Theraphosidae	Tarantula	East Indies, India, Australia, tropical Africa
Steatoda species	Theridiidae	False black widow	Worldwide
Thiodina species	Salticidae	Jumping spider	North and South America
Trechona species	Dipluridae	Funnel-web spider	West Indies, South America
Ummidia species	Ctenidae	Trap-door spider	North and South America

Latrodectus **Species (Widow Spiders).**
These spiders are commonly known as the black widow, brown widow, or red-legged spider in the United States. They have many other common names in English: hourglass, poison lady, deadly spider, red-bottom spider, T-spider, gray lady spider, or shoe-button spider. The widow spiders are found almost circumglobally, in all continents having temperate or tropical climates. In the United States, there are four species of widow spiders, with the possibility of a fifth species from the Pacific northwest. Although both the male and female widow spiders are venomous, only the latter has fangs large and strong enough to penetrate the human skin. Mature females range in body length from 10 to 18 mm, whereas males range from 3 to 5 mm. These spiders have a globose abdomen, varying in color from gray to brown to black, depending on the species. In the black widow, the abdomen is shiny black with a red hourglass or red spots, and sometimes white ones, on the venter.

The chemistry of the venom has been reviewed by Bettini and Maroli (1978) and by Maretić and Lebez (1979). The difficulties with many of the biochemical and toxicologic studies on this spider's venom have related to the nature of the starting material. Most studies have been done on extracts of homogenized glands rather than the venom itself. Thus, the chemical nature of the venom cannot be separated or determined from the normal constituents of the venom gland. The pharmacologic properties reported in the literature also reflect the activities of the whole gland, and since some of the reported properties carried out on definitive preparations are not consistent with human experiences, their chemical application is open to question.

Most workers have isolated five or six proteins from the venom or venom glands (*see* Bettini and Maroli, 1978, for references). The so-called neurotoxin appears to have a high content of isoleucine and leucine and a low content of tyrosine. The fraction has a suspected molecular weight of 130,000. It affects the frog neuromuscular junction and is active on rat brain synaptosomes. Lipoproteins are also present. A proteolytic enzyme was absent from extracts of the venom glands, whereas venom taken from the fangs possessed the activity. The presence of hyaluronidase is also dependent on the original material. In our own studies, we were able to demonstrate 15 or more bands in the crude venom by gel electrophoresis. The average amount of venom from each spider was 0.22 mg, and the intravenous LD50 in mice was 0.55 mg/kg body weight (Russell and Buess, 1970).

Clinical Problem. In most patients, there is a history of having received a sharp, pinpricklike bite, but in some cases the bite is so minor that it goes unnoticed. The initial pain is sometimes followed by a dull, occasionally numbing pain in the affected extremity and by pain and some cramps in one or several of the large muscle masses. Rarely is there any local skin reaction, but piloerection in the bite area is sometimes seen. Muscle fasciculations can frequently be seen within 30 minutes of the bite. Sweating is common, and the patient may complain of weakness and pain in the regional lymph nodes, which are often tender on palpation and may be enlarged; lymphadenitis is frequently observed. Pain in the low back, thighs, or abdomen is a common complaint, and rigidity of the abdominal muscles is seen in most cases in which envenomation has been severe. Severe paroxysmal muscle cramps may occur, and arthralgia has been reported. "Facies latrodectisimica" is rare in bites by American species.

In bites on the upper extremities, and sometimes on the lower extremities, there is rigidity of the muscles of the shoulders and back, sometimes accompanied by pain on inspiration and varying degrees of headache, dizziness, and ptosis. Edema of the eyelids, conjunctivitis, skin rash, hyperemia, and pruritus are sometimes observed. The patient may become very restless and find difficulty in sitting or standing still. Reflexes are usually accentuated. There may be a fine body tremor, and nausea and vomiting are not uncommon. The patient sometimes gropes along slowly when attempting to walk. Hypertension is a common finding in moderate to severe envenomations. Blood studies are usually normal.

There is no effective first-aid treatment. In most cases, intravenous calcium gluconate, 10 ml of 10 percent, will often relieve muscle pain, but this may need to be repeated at four- to six-hour intervals for optimum effect. Muscle relaxants, such as methocarbamol, 10 ml by slow push, as directed, or diazepam, 5 to 10 mg *t.i.d.* (three times a day), can be used. Meperidine hydrochloride, 50 to 100 mg, has been used when respiratory deficits were not a problem. Acute hypertensive crises may require intravenous nitroprusside, 3 mcg/kg/min. The use of antivenin (Antivenin *Latrodectus mactans*) should be restricted to the more severe cases and where the above measures have been unsuccessful. One ampule, intravenously, is usually sufficient. In patients under 16 or over 60 years, or with any history of hypertension or hypertensive heart disease, and who show significant symptoms and signs, the use of antivenin seems warranted.

Loxosceles **Species (Brown or Violin Spiders).** These primitive spiders are variously known in North America as the fiddleback or violin spider, or the brown recluse. There are over 100 species of *Loxosceles*. Twenty of these species range from temperate South Africa northward through the tropics into the Mediterranean region and southern Europe. Another 84 species are known from North, Central, and South America and the West Indies. The most widely distributed is *L. rufescens*, the so-called "cosmopolitan" species. It is found in the Mediterranean area, southern Russia, most of North Africa including the Azores, Madagascar, Near East, the Orient from India to southern China and Japan, parts of Malaysia and Australia, some islands of the Pacific, and North America. *Loxosceles laeta* is mostly South American, but it has been introduced into Central America and small areas in Cambridge, Massachusetts, Sierra Madre and Alhambra, California, and the Zoology Building of the University of Helsinki. The abdomen of these spiders varies in color from grayish through orange and reddish-brown to dark brown. The "violin" on the carapace is brown to blackish and distinct from the pale yellow to reddish-brown background of the cephalothorax. This spider has six eyes grouped in three diads, forming a recurved row. Females average 8 to 12 mm in body length, whereas males average 6 to 10 mm. Both males and females are venomous. The most important species in the United States are *L. reclusa* (brown recluse spider), *L. deserta* (desert violin spider), and *L. arizonica* (Arizona violin spider).

The chemistry and toxicology of *Loxosceles* venom have been reviewed by Schenone and Suarez (1978). The venom is composed of approximately 26 percent protein, and the average amount of venom protein per spider in *L. reclusa* is about 68 μg. The necrotizing activity of the venom is associated with the protein portion, and it has been suggested that the fraction is a glycoprotein. On fractionation of the venom, two major components have been separated. The high-molecular-weight fraction, (1), is lethal to mice, whereas the low-molecular-weight fraction is nonlethal. On further separation of (1), two toxins have been isolated. Their molecular weight is about 24,000. One of these was responsible for the lesions produced in rabbits and was shown to be lethal to mice and rabbits. The venom contains a considerable number of enzymes. Injection of the venom in mammals produces, in addition to the local tissue reaction, varying degrees of thrombocytopenia, some intravascular hemolysis, and hemolytic anemia. The venom also appears to have some coagulating activity. Neither the enzymes nor their amounts can explain the development of the unusual lesion. A potent, nondialyzable inhibitor of hemolytic complement activity has been demonstrated in the venom of *L. reclusa*. It has been suggested that this factor might interfere with the function of the fifth component of human blood. It seems that *Loxosceles* venom interferes with receptor sites for complement fractions located at the membrane surface (*see* Schenone and Suarez, 1978, for references).

Clinical Manifestations. The bite of this spider produces about the same degree of pain as the sting of an ant, but sometimes the patient is completely unaware of the bite. In most cases, a local burning sensation develops about the injury. This may last for 30 to 60 minutes. Pruritus over the area often occurs and the area becomes red, with a small blanched area around the immediate bite site. Skin temperature is usually elevated over the lesion area. The reddened area enlarges and becomes purplish during the subsequent one to eight hours. If often becomes irregular in shape, and as time passes, hemorrhages may develop throughout the area. A small bleb or vesicle forms at the bite site and increases in size. It subsequently ruptures and a pustule forms. The red, hemorrhagic area continues to enlarge, as does the pustule. The whole area may become swollen and painful, and lymphadenopathy is common. During the early stages, the lesion often takes on a bull's-eye appearance, with a central white vesicle surrounded by the reddened area, ringed by a whitish or bluish border. The central pustule ruptures, and necrosis to various depths can be visualized. The necrosis can invade the underlying muscle.

In serious bites the lesion can measure 8 × 10 cm with severe necrosis invading muscle tissue. On the face, large lesions resulting in extensive tissue destruction and requiring subsequent plastic surgery are sometimes seen following bites by *L. laeta* in South America. Systemic symptoms and signs include fever, malaise, stomach cramps, nausea and vomiting, jaundice, spleen enlargement, hemolysis, hematuria, and thrombocytopenia. Fatal cases, while rare, are usually preceded by intravascular hemolysis, hemolytic anemia, thrombocytopenia, hemoglobinuria, and renal failure.

There are no first-aid measures of value. In fact, all first-aid procedures should be avoided as the natural appearance of the lesion is most important in determining the diagnosis. A cube of ice may be placed on the wound. At one time, excision of the bite area with ample margins was advised, when this could be done within an hour or so of the bite, and when *Loxosceles* was definitely implicated. This practice is no longer favored. The value of steroids has also been questioned. This writer, however, has had seemingly good results by placing the patient on a corticosteroid, such as intramuscular dexamethasone, 4 mg every six hours during the acute phase. If the poisoning is severe, hydrocortisone should be given intravenously, 300 to 500 mg in divided doses daily, until the patient begins to improve. Subsequent doses should then be determined by clinical judgment, followed by decremental doses over a four-day period. Antihistamines are of questionable value during the acute period. The use of Dapsone® has been suggested (King and Rees, 1983) and seems encouraging, but further evaluation is necessary. Ulcerating lesions should be cleansed with peroxide and soaked in 1:20 Burow's solution *t.i.d.* (three times a day) for at least 15 minutes. Three times a week, if indicated, the lesions can be painted with an aqueous solution of brilliant green 1:400, gentian violet 1:400, and acriflavin 1:1000. At night the lesion should be covered with polymyxin-bacitracin-neomycin ointment. Oxygen to the wound through an improvised plastic bag is helpful. If skin grafting becomes necessary, the procedure is best deferred for four to six weeks after the injury. Systemic manifestations should be treated symptomatically (Russell, 1982).

***Steatoda* Species (Cobweb Spiders).** These small spiders, variously called the false black-widow, combfooted, or cupboard spiders, are abundant in the Old World and reached the Americas through trading sources. According to Gertsch (personal correspondence, 1983), they are gaining such a wide range they deserve to be called cosmopolitan. These spiders are often mistaken for black-widow spiders, and indeed, the first clinical case of *Steatoda grossa* envenomation directed to the author in 1961 was thought to be caused by *L. mactans,* owing to misidentification of the spider. The female of *S. grossa* differs from *L. mactans* and *L. hesperus* in having a purplish-brown abdomen rather than a black one; it is less shiny and its abdomen is more oval than round, as in *Latrodectus.* It may have pale yellow or whitish markings on the dorsum of the abdomen and no markings on the venter. The abdomen of some species is orange, brown, or chestnut in color and often bears a light band across the front dorsum.

The literature on poisoning by these species is scanty, and little is known about the chemistry of the venom. According to Maretić and Lebez (1979), *S. paykulliana* gives rise to "strong motor unrest, clonic cramps, exhaustion, ataxia and then paralysis in guinea pigs." However, this writer has never seen such a syndrome following the bites of *S. grossa* or *S. fulva* in humans. Instead, bites have been followed by local pain, induration, pruritus, and the occasional breakdown of tissue at the bite site. The wound should be debrided and covered with a sterile dressing. A steroid-antihistamine-analgesic cream can be applied to the wound.

***Phidippus* Species (Jumping Spiders).**
These spiders, variously known as crab spiders or eyebrow spiders, are large-eyed jumping spiders, usually less than 20 mm in length, and have a somewhat elevated, rectangular cephalothorax that tends to be blunt anteriorly. The abdomen is often oval or elongated. There is a great deal of variation in the color of these spiders. In the female, the cephalothorax may be black, brown, red, orange, or yellowish-orange, and the abdomen tends to be slightly lighter in color. In most species there are various white, yellow, orange, or red spots or markings on the dorsum of the abdomen. The bite of this spider produces a sharp pinprick pain, and the area immediately around the wound may become painful and tender. The pain usually lasts five to ten minutes. An erythematous wheal slowly develops. In the cases seen by the author, the wheal measured 2 to 5 cm in diameter. A dull, sometimes throbbing pain may subsequently develop over the injured part, but it rarely requires attention. A small vesicle may form at the bite site. Around this is an irregular, slightly hyperemic area, which in turn may be surrounded by a blanched area tender to touch and pressure. Generally, there is only mild lymphadenitis. Swelling of the part may be diffuse and is often accompanied by some pruritus. The symptoms and signs usually abate within 48 hours. There is no specific treatment for the bite of this spider. Methdilazine HCl, 8 mg three times a day, is often effective.

***Chiracanthium* Species (Running Spiders).**
The 160 species of this genus enjoy an almost circumglobal distribution, although only four or five species have been implicated in bites on humans. Maretić and Lebez (1979) name *C. punctorium, C. inclusum, C. mildei,* and *C. diversum* as the spiders most often implicated in envenomations. The abdomen is convex and egg-shaped and varies in color from yellow, green, or greenish-white to reddish-brown, and the cephalothorax is usually slightly darker than the abdomen. The chelicerae are strong, and the legs are long, hairy, and delicate. The spider ranges in length from 7 to 16 mm. The author's experiences with nine bites by *C. inclusum* have been very similar, and the following description is based on these experiences. Like *Phidippus,* but even more so, *Chiracanthium* tends to be tenacious and must sometimes be removed from the bite area. For that reason, there is a high degree of identification of these spiders. The patient usually describes the bite as sharp and painful, with the pain increasing during the first 30 to 45 minutes. The patient complains of some

restlessness, a dull pain over the injured part. A reddened wheal with a hyperemic border develops. Small petechiae may appear near the center of the wheal. Skin temperature over the lesion is often elevated, but body temperature is usually normal. Lymphadenitis and lymphadenopathy may develop. Five cases of necrotic arachnidism have been attributed to *C. mildei,* but the status of this finding remains circumstantial (*see* Russell, 1984b, for references).

Scorpions

Approximately 75 of the 800 species of scorpions can be considered of sufficient importance to warrant medical attention. Some of the more important of these are noted in Table 22–9. In addition, members of the genus *Pandinus, Hadrurus, Vejovis, Nebo,* and some of the others are capable of inflicting a painful and oftentimes erythematous lesion. The problem of scorpions stings has been reviewed by Keegan (1980).

Centruroides Species. There are approximately 30 species of this genus confined in distribution to the New World. Of these, about seven species are of considerable medical importance, and most of these are found in Mexico. In the United States, they are commonly referred to as "bark scorpions" because of the preference for hiding under the loose bark of trees or in dead trees or logs. They often frequent human dwellings. Their general color is straw to yellowish-brown, or reddish-brown, and they are often easily distinguishable from other scorpions in the same habitat by their long, thin telson, or tail, and the pedipalps, or pincerlike claws. Adults of this genus show a considerable difference in length. *C. sculpturatus exclicauda* in the southwestern United States and adjacent Mexico reaches a length of approximately 5.5 cm while

Table 22–9.   MEDICALLY IMPORTANT SCORPIONS

GENUS	DISTRIBUTION
Androctonus species	North Africa, Middle East, and Turkey
Buthus species	France and Spain to Middle East and North Africa, Mongolia, China
Buthotus species	Africa, Middle East, and Central Asia
Centruroides species	North, Central, and South America
Heterometrus species	Central and Southeast Asia
Leiurus species	North Africa, Middle East, and Turkey
Mesobuthus species	Turkey
Parabuthus species	Southern Africa
Tityus species	Central and South America

C. vittatus of the Gulf states and adjacent Mexico is generally slightly larger. *C. suffusus,* a particularly dangerous Mexican species, may attain a length of 9 cm but *C. noxious,* another important species, seldom exceeds 5 cm in length. In Mexico between 1940–49 and 1950–57 there were 20,352 deaths from scorpion envenomation. Most of these deaths were in children less than three years of age. Various estimates of the total number of stings per year in Mexico range from 20,000 to 70,000. Working in Mexico in 1953, the writer estimates that there were over 40,000 stings that year, of which 10,000 were treated. The total number of deaths, usually in infants, appeared slightly less than 1500. As with the other scorpion stings, envenomation by this genus appears to vary with the species concerned.

In children, a sting by *C. exilicauda* (= *sculpturatus*) produces initial pain, although it rarely is severe. However, some children do not complain of pain and are unaware of the injury. The area becomes sensitive to touch, and merely pressing lightly over the injury will elicit immediate retraction. Usually, there is little or no local swelling or erythema. The child becomes tense and restless and shows abnormal and random head and neck movements. Often, the child will display roving eye movements. In their excellent review of *C. sculpturatus* stings. Rimsza *et al.* (1980) noted visual signs including roving eye movements, nystagmus, and oculogyric movements in 12 of their 24 patients stung by this scorpion. Loud noises, such as banging the examination table behind the child's back, will often cause the patient to jump. Tachycardia will usually be evident within 45 minutes, and hypertension, although it is not seen in children as early or as severe as in adults, may often be present one hour following the sting. Respiratory and heart rates are increased, and by 90 minutes postbite the child may appear quite ill. Fasciculations may be seen over the face or large muscle masses, and the child may complain of generalized weakness and display some ataxia or motor weakness. The respiratory distress may proceed to respiratory paralysis. Excessive salivation is often present and may further embarrass respiratory function. Slurring of speech may be present and convulsions may occur. If death does not occur, the child usually becomes asymptomatic within 36 hours.

In adults the clinical picture is somewhat similar, but there are some differences. Almost all adults complain of immediate and sometimes severe pain following the sting, regardless of the *Centruroides* species involved. Adults do not show the restlessness seen in children. Rather, they are tense and anxious. They develop tachy-

cardia and hypertension, and respirations are increased. They may complain of difficulties in focusing and swallowing, as may children. In some cases, there is some general weakness, and pain on moving the injured extremity. Convulsions are very rare, but ataxia and muscle incoordination may occur. Most adults are asymptomatic within 12 hours but may complain of generalized weakness of 24 or more hours.

A review of the therapy for scorpion stings will provide the reader with a fascinating dash of mythology, folklore, hunches (educated and otherwise), and a listing of all sorts of therapeutic devices from electroshock to mechanical compression bandages. The list of drugs that have been tried includes atropine, barium, digitalis, epinephrine, heparin, hyoscyamine, iodine, procaine, morphine, physostigmine, reserpine, steroids, snake, spider and scorpion antivenins, and vitamin C, to mention only a few. Other than scorpion antivenin, there is no evidence that any of these drugs are of specific value. There are no first-aid measures of value. In any severe scorpion envenomation by one of the known dangerous species, or in infants or children, the specific or suggested polyvalent scorpion antivenin should be used. The author generally gives twice the recommended dose and gives it intravenously, unless indicated otherwise. The antivenin should be diluted with 100 to 200 ml of 5 percent dextrose in water or physiologic saline and given in a drip. Mild sedation is often indicated. If convulsions occur, intravenous phenobarbital is suggested, but great care must be used with respect to the dose. Valium may be of value. Assisted ventilation is sometimes necessary, particularly in children. Hypertension that does not respond to antivenin may need to be treated with the appropriate antihypertensive drugs. Inderal has been used for tachycardia. In those patients who decompensate, digitalis and diuretics may be of value. The role of corticosteroids and atropine in severe poisonings is questionable. The stings by species of *Vejovis* and *Hadrurus,* though far more common in the United States than those by *Centruroides,* rarely require more than minor treatment for the local pain. However, it is wise to put any person stung by a scorpion, particularly children, at bed rest for several hours following the accident.

Centipedes and Millipedes

Some of the larger centipedes of the genus *Scolopendra* can inflict a painful bite, with some localized swelling and erythema. Lymphangitis and lymphadenitis are not uncommon. Necrosis is rare and infection almost unknown. Symptoms and signs seldom persist for more than 48 hours.

Millipedes do not bite but when handled may discharge a toxic secretion that can cause local skin irritation and, in severe cases, some necrosis. Some non–United States species can spray a highly irritating repugnant secretion that may cause conjunctival reactions. An ice cube will control the pain of most centipede bites. Corticosteroids have been used as antiinflammatory agents. The toxic secretions of millipedes should be washed from the skin with copious amounts of soap and water. Cleansing with alcohol should be avoided. A corticosteroid lotion or cream should be applied if a skin reaction develops. Eye injuries require immediate irrigation and the application of a corticosteroid-analgesic ointment.

Hymenoptera (Ants, Bees, Wasps, and Hornets)

The stings of these animals are responsible for more deaths in the United States than the bites and stings of all other venomous creatures. This is due to sensitization to the venom from repeated stings, resulting in anaphylactic reactions, including acute anaphylaxis. The number of acute anaphylactic reactions involving cardiovascular, respiratory, or nervous system changes may number over 200,000 per year in the United States. Those not sensitive to bee venom may tolerate up to 100 simultaneous stings, but any number over this can be fatal. The venom of these insects contains peptides, nonenzymatic proteins, such as apamin and melettin or kinins; enzymes, such as phospholipase A and B and hyaluronidase; and amines, such as histamine and 5-hydroxytryptamine. The sting of many *Hymenoptera* may remain in the skin and should be removed by teasing or scraping rather than pulling. An ice cube placed over the sting will reduce pain; an analgesic-corticosteroid lotion is often useful. Persons with known hypersensitivity to such stings should carry a kit containing an antihistamine and epinephrine when in endemic areas. Desensitization can be carried out using insect whole-body antigen or, preferably, whole-venom antigens (Russell, 1982).

Ticks and Mites

Ticks are vectors of many diseases. In addition to these disorders, ticks are also involved in poisonings. In North America, some species of *Dermacentor* and *Amblyomma* cause tick paralysis. Symptoms and signs include anorexia, lethargy, muscle weakness, incoordination, nystagmus, and ascending flaccid paralysis. Bulbar or respiratory paralysis may develop. The bites of some *Ornithodorus* ticks ("pajaroello") found in Mexico and southwestern United States cause a local vesiculation, pustulation, rupture, ulceration, and eschar, with varying degrees of local swelling and pain, often resembling those of *Loxosceles*, although the development of the lesion is slower. Mite infestations are quite common and are responsible for "chiggers" (intensely pruritic dermatitis caused by the mite larva, or chigger), various forms of scabies, demodicidosis, and a number of other diseases. The bites produce varying degrees of local tissue reactions, with or without sensitization. Ticks are best removed by applying gasoline or by slowly withdrawing the arthropod with flat-tip forceps. Care should be taken not to leave the capitulum in the wound, as it may induce chronic inflammation or may migrate into deeper tissues and give rise to a granuloma. The bite should be cleansed and a corticosteroid lotion applied. Treatment of tick paralysis is symptomatic. Oxygen and respiratory assistance may be needed. An antitoxin is presently under study. Pajaroello tick lesions should be cleansed, soaked in 1:20 Burow's solution, and debrided. Corticosteroids are of value in severe reactions. Infections are not uncommon during the ulcer stage but rarely require more than local antiseptic measures.

Other Biting Arthropods

In the United States, a number of biting arthropods possess salivary secretions that can produce various reactions and lesions. Among the more common biting and sometimes bloodsucking arthropods are the ticks and mites; sand-, horse-, and deerflies; mosquitoes; fleas; lice; bedbugs; kissing bugs; and certain water bugs. The composition of the saliva of these arthropods varies considerably, and the lesion produced by their bites can vary from a small papule to a large, ulcerating wound with swelling and acute pain. Dermatitis may also occur. Most serious bites are complicated by sensitivity reactions or infection. In hypersensitive persons, the bites of some of these arthropods can be fatal.

REFERENCES

Albuquerque, E. X.; Warnick, J. E.; Maleque, M. A.; Kauffman, F. C.; Tamburini, R.; Nimit, Y.; and Daly, J. W.: The pharmacology of pumilitoxin-B. I. Interaction with calcium sites in the sarcoplasmic reticulum of skeletal muscle. *Mol. Pharmacol.*, **19**:411–421, 1981.

Alender, C. B., and Russell, F. E.: Pharmacology. In Boolootin, R. A. (ed.): *Physiology of Echinodermata.* Interscience, New York, 1966. p. 529.

Arndt, W.: Die Spongern als kryptotoxische Tiere. *Zool. Jahrb.*, **45**:343, 1928.

Arnold, S. H., and Brown, W. D.: Histamine toxicity from fish products. *Adv. Food Res.*, **24**:113, 1978.

Association of Official Analytical Chemists: Paralytic shellfish poison biological method. In *Official Methods of Analysis,* 12th ed. Association of Official Analytical Chemists, Washington, D.C., 1975, p. 319.

Bagnis, R.; Berglund, F.; Elias, P. S.; VanEsch, G. J.; Halstead, B. W.; and Kojima, K.: Problems of toxicants in marine food products. *Bull. WHO,* **42**:69, 1970.

Bajwa, S. S., and Markland, F. S.: Defibrinogenation studies with crotalase: possible clinical applications. *Proc. West. Pharmacol. Soc.*, **21**:755, 1976.

Bakus, G. J., and Green, G.: Toxicity in sponges and holothurians: a geographic pattern. *Science,* **185**:951, 1974.

Bakus, G. J., and Thun, M.: Bioassays on the toxicity of Caribbean sponges. *Biol. Spongiaries,* **291**:417, 1979.

Banner, A. H.: Ciguatera: a disease from coral reef fish. In Jones, O. E., and Endean, R. (ed.): *Biology and Geology of Coral Reefs,* Vol. III. Academic Press, Inc., New York, 1976, p. 177.

Barnes, J. H.: Observations of jellyfish stingings in North Queensland, *Med. J. Aust.*, **2**:993, 1960.

————: Extraction of cnidarian venom from living tentacle. In Russell, F. E., and Saunders, P. R. (eds.): *Animal Toxins.* Pergamon Press, Oxford, 1967, pp. 115–129; *see also Toxicon,* **4**:292, 1967 (abstr.).

Baslow, M. H.: *Marine Pharmacology.* Williams & Wilkins Co., Baltimore, 1969.

Baxter, E. H.; Walden, N. B.; and Marr, A. G.: Fatal intoxication of rabbits, sheep and monkeys by the venom of the sea wasp *(Chironex fleckeri). Toxicon,* **10**:653, 1972.

Bernheimer, A. W., and Avigad, L. S.: Properties of a toxin from the sea anemone *Stoichactis helianthus,* including specific binding to sphingomyelin. *Proc. Natl. Acad. Sci. U.S.A.*, **73**:467, 1976.

Bettini, S.: *Arthropod Venoms,* Springer-Verlag, New York, 1978.

Bettini, S., and Maroli, M.: Venoms of Theridiidae, genus *Latrodectus.* In Bettini, S. (ed.): *Arthropod Venoms.* Springer-Verlag, New York, 1978, pp. 149–185.

Blanquet, R. S.: A toxic protein from the nematocysts of the scyphozoan medusa *Chrysaora quinquecirrha. Toxicon,* **10**:103, 1972.

Bonilla, C. A., and Fiero, M. K.: Comparative biochemistry and pharmacology of salivary gland secretions. II. Chromatographic separation of the basic proteins from North American rattlesnake venoms. *J. Chromatogr.*, **56**:253, 1971.

Burke, J. M.; Marichisotto, J.; McLaughlin, J. J. A.; and Provasoli, L.: Analysis of the toxin produced by *Gonylaux catenella* in axenic culture. *Ann. Rev. N.Y. Acad. Sci.*, **90**:837, 1960.

Burnett, J. W., and Calton, H. J.: The chemistry and toxicology of some venomous pelagic coelenterates. *Toxicon,* **15**:177, 1977.

Burreson, B. J.; Christophersen, C.; and Scheuer, P. J.: Cooccurrence of a terpenoid isocyanideformamide pair in the marine sponge *Halichondria* sp. *J. Am. Chem. Soc.*, **97**:201, 1975.

Calton, G. J.; Burnett, J. W.; Rubenstein, H.; and Heard, J.: The effect of two jellyfish toxins on calcium ion transport. *Toxicon.* **11**:357, 1973.

Cameron, A. M.; Surridge, J.; Stablum, W.; and Lewis, R. J.: A crinotoxin from the skin tubercle glands of a stonefish *(Synanceia trachynis). Toxicon.* **19**:159, 1981.

Cariello, L.; Zanetti, L.; and Rathmayer, W.: Isolation, purification and some properties of subertine, the toxic protein from the marine sponge, *Suberites domuncula,* In Eaker, D., and Wadström. T. (eds.): *Natural Toxins,* Pergamon Press, Oxford, 1980, pp. 631–636.

Carlson, R. W.; Schaeffer, R. C.; Russell, F. E.; and Weil, M. H.: A comparison of corticosteroid and fluid treatment after rattlesnake venom shock in rats. *Physiologist,* **18**:160, 1975.

Chevallier, A., and Duchesne, E. A.: Mémoire sur les empoisonnements par les huitres. les moules, les crabes, et par certains poissons de mer et de rivière. *Ann. Hyg. Pub.,*46:108, 1851.

Cleland, J. B., and Southcott, R. V.: *Injuries to Man from Marine Invertebrates in the Australian Region.* Commonwealth of Australia, Canberra, 1965, p. 195.

Crone, H. D., and Keen, T. E. B.: Chromatographic properties of the hemolysin from the cnidarian *Chironex fleckeri. Toxicon.* **7**:79, 1969.

Culver, P., and Jacobs, R. S.: Lophotoxin: a neuromuscular acting toxin from the sea whip *(Lophogorgia rigida), Toxicon,* **19**:825, 1981.

Daly, J. W.: Biologically active alkaloids from poison frogs, (Dendrobatidae), *Toxin Rev.,* **1**:33, 1982.

Das, N. P.; Lim, H. S.; and Teh, Y. F.: Histamine and histamine-like substances in the marine sponge *Suberites inconstans, Comp. Gen. Pharmacol.,* **2**:473, 1971.

Dawson, E. Y.; Aleem, A. A.; and Halstead, B. W.: Marine algae from Palmyra Island with special reference to the feeding habits and toxicology of reef fishes. *Occ. Pap. Allan Hancock Fdn.,* **17**:1, 1955.

De Laubenfels, M. W.: The marine and freshwater sponges of California. *Proc. U.S. Natn. Mus.,* **81**:1, 1932 (Publ. No. 2927).

Deutsch, H. F., and Diniz, C. R.: Some proteolytic activities of snake venoms. *J. Biol. Chem.,* **216**:17, 1955.

Dowling, H. G.; Minton, S. A.; and Russell, F. E.: *Poisonous Snakes of the World.* U.S. Government Printing Office, Washington, D.C., 1968.

Dubnoff, J. W., and Russell, F. E.: Isolation of lethal protein and peptide from *Crotalus viridis helleri* venom. *Proc. West. Pharm. Soc.,* **13**:98, 1970.

Eaker, D., and Wadström, T. (eds.).: *Natural Toxins.* Pergamon Press, Elmsford, N.Y., 1980.

Elliott, W. B.: Chemistry and immunology of reptilian venoms. In Gans, C. (ed.).: *Biology of the Reptilia,* Vol. 8. Academic Press, London, 1978, pp. 163–436.

Endean, R.: A new species of venomous echinoid from Queensland waters. *Mem. Queensland Mus.,* **14**:95, 1964.

Endean, R.; Duchemin, C.; McColm, D.; and Fraser, E. H.: A study of the biological activity of toxic material derived from nematocysts of the cubomedusan *Chironex fleckeri. Toxicon,* **6**:179, 1969.

Endean R ; Izatt, J.; and McColm, D.. The venom of the piscivorous gastropod *Conus striatus.* In Russell, F. E., and Saunders, P. R. (eds.): *Animal Toxins.* Pergamon Press, Oxford, 1967, p. 137.

Endean, R., and Noble, M.: Toxic material from the tentacles of the cubomedusan *Chironex fleckeri, Toxicon,* **9**:255, 1971.

Evans, M. H.: Block of sensory nerve conduction in the cat by mussel poison and tetrodotoxin. In Russell, F. E., and Saunders, P. R. (eds.): *Animal Toxins.* Pergamon Press, Oxford, 1967, p. 97; *see also Toxicon,* **5**:289, 1967.

Ferlan, I., and Lebez, D.: Equinatoxin, a lethal protein from *Actinia equina.* I. Purification and characterization, *Toxicon,* **12**:57, 1974.

Flecker, H., and Cotton, B. C.: Fatal bites from octopus. *Med. J. Aust.,* (2):329, 1955.

Fleming, W. J., and Howden, M. E. H.: Partial purification and characterization of steroid glycosides from the starfish *Acanthaster planci. Comp. Biochem. Physiol.,* **53b**:267, 1974.

Freeman, S. E., and Turner, R. J.: A pharmacological study of the toxin of a cnidarian *Chironex fleckeri* Southcott, *Br. J. Pharmacol.* **35**:510, 1969.

————: Cardiovascular effects of toxins isolated from the cnidarian *Chironex fleckeri* Southcott, *Br. J. Pharmacol.,* **41**:154, 1971.

Friess, S. L.; Chanley, J. D.; Hudak, W. V.; and Weems, H. B.: Interactions of the echinoderm toxin holothurin A and its desulfated derivative with the cat superior cervical ganglion preparation. *Toxicon,* **8**:211, 1970.

Friess, S. L.; Durant, R. C.; Chanley, J. D.; and Fash, F. J.: Role of the sulphate charge center in irreversible interactions of holothurin A with chemoreceptors. *Biochem. Pharmacol.,* **16**:617, 1967.

Fuhrman, F. A.: Fish eggs. In Liener, I. E. (ed.): *Toxic Constituents of Animal Foodstuffs.* Academic Press, Inc., New York, 1974, p. 73.

Gertsch, W. J.: *American Spiders,* 2nd ed. Van Nostrand Reinhold, New York, 1979.

Green, G.: Ecology of toxicity in marine sponges. *Mar. Biol.,* **40**:207, 1977.

Habermehl, G. G.: *Venomous Animals and Their Toxins.* Springer-Verlag, Berlin, 1981.

Habermehl, G. G., and Volkwein, G.: Aglycones of the toxins from the cuvierian organs of *Holothuria forskali* and a new nomenclature for the aglycones from Holothurioideae. *Toxicon.* **9**:319, 1971.

Halmagyi, D. F. J.: Starzecki, B.; and Horner, G. J.: Mechanism and pharmacology of shock due to rattlesnake venom in sheep. *J. Appl. Physiol.,* **20**:709, 1965.

Halstead, B. W.: Weever stings and their medical management. *U.S. Armed Forces Med. J.,* **8**:1441, 1957.

————: Fish poisonings—their diagnosis, pharmacology and treatment. *Clin. Pharmacol. Ther.,* **5**:615, 1964.

————: *Poisonous and Venomous Marine Animals of the World.* U.S. Government Printing Office, Washington, D.C. Vol. I. 1965; Vol. II, 1967; Vol. III, 1970.

————: *Poisonous and Venomous Marine Animals of the World,* rev. ed. Darwin Press, Princeton, N.J., 1978.

————: *Dangerous Marine Animals,* 2nd ed. Cornell Maritime Press, Centreville, Md., 1980, p. 77.

Harding, K. A., and Welch, K. R. G.: *Venomous Snakes of the World: A Checklist.* Pergamon Press, Elmsford, N.Y., 1980.

Hashimoto, Y.: *Marine Toxins and Other Bioactive Metabolites.* Japan Scientific Society, Tokyo, 1979.

Hashimoto, Y.; Konosu, S.; Yasumoto, T.; Iomie, A.; and Noguchi, T.; Occurrence of toxic crabs in Ryukyu and Amami Islands, *Toxicon,* **5**:85, 1967.

Helfrich, P., and Banner, A. H.: Hallucinatory mullet poisoning. *J. Trop. Med. Hyg ,* **63**:86, 1960.

Hessinger, D. A., and Lenhoff, H. M.: Membrane structure and function. Mechanism of hemolysis induced by nematocyst venom: roles of phospholipase and direct lytic factor. *Arch. Biochem. Biophys.,* **173**:603, 1976.

Irie, T.; Suzuki, M.; and Hayakawa, Y.: Isolation of aplysin, debromoaplysin, and aplysinol from *Laurencia okamurai* Yamada. *Bull. Chem. Soc. Jpn.,* **42**:843, 1969.

Jakowska, S., and Nigrelli, R. F.: Antimicrobial substances from sponges. *Ann. N.Y. Acad, Sci.,* **90**:913, 1970.

Kaiser, E., and Michl, H.: *Die Biochemie der tierischen Gifte.* Franz Deuticke, Wien. 1958.

Kao, C. Y.: Tetrodotoxin, saxitoxin, and their significance in the study of the excitation phenomena. *Pharmacol. Rev.,* **18**:997, 1966.

————: Comparison of the biological actions of tetrodotoxin and saxitoxin. In Russell, F. E., and Saunders, P. R. (eds.): *Animal Toxins.* Pergamon Press. Oxford, 1967. pp. 109–114.

————: New perspectives on the tetrodotoxin and saxitoxin receptors. In Singer, T. P., and Ondarza, P. N.
(eds.): *Molecular Basis of Drug Action*. Elsevier/
North-Holland, New York, 1981.

Kao, C. Y., and Fuhrman, F. A.: Pharmacological
studies on tarichatoxin, a potent neurotoxin. *J. Pharmacol. Exp. Ther.*, **140**:31, 1963.

Kashman, Y.; Fishelson, L.; and Neeman, I.: *N*-acyl-2-
methylene-β-alanine methyl esters from the sponge
Fasciospongia cavernosa. *Tetrahedron*, **29**:3655,
1973.

Keegan, H. L.: *Scorpions of Medical Importance*. University Press of Mississippi, Jackson, Miss., 1980.

King, L. E., and Rees, R. S.: Dapsone treatment of a
brown recluse bite. *J.A.M.A.* **250**:648, 1983.

Lane, C. E., and Dodge, E.: The toxicity of *Physalia*
nematocysts. *Biol. Bull.*, **115**:219, 1958.

Lassabliere, M. P.: Influences des injections in-
traveineuses de suberitine sur la resistance globulaire.
C. R. Seanc. Soc. Biol., **61**:600, 1906.

Lee, C. -Y. (ed.): *Snake Venoms*. Springer-Verlag,
New York, 1979.

Maeda, N.; Tamiya, N.; Pattabhiraman, T. K.; and Russell, F. E.: Some chemical properties of the venom of
the rattlesnake *Crotalus viridis helleri*. *Toxicon*.
16:431, 1978.

Maeno, H.; Morimura, M.; Mitsuhashi, S.; Sawai, Y.;
and Okonogi, T.: Studies on habu snake venom. 2b.
Further purification and enzymic and biological activities of Ha-proteinase. *Jpn. J. Mikrobiol.*, **3**:277, 1959.

Maretić, Z.: Erfahrungen mit Stichen von Giftfischen.
Acta Tropica, **14**:157, 1957.

Maretić, Z., and Lebez, D.: *Araneism*. Nolit. Belgrade,
Yugoslavia, 1979.

Maretić, Z., and Russell, F. E.: Stings by the sea anemone *Anemonia sulcata* in the Adriatic Sea. *Am. J.
Trop. Med. Hyg.*, **32**:891, 1983.

Marki, F., and Witkop, B.: The venom of the Col-
ombian arrow poison frog *Phyllobates bicolor*. *Experientia*, **19**:329, 1963.

Martin, D. F., and Padilla, G. M. (eds.): *Marine Phar-
macognosy*. Academic Press, Inc., New York, 1973.

McFarren, E. F.; Schafer, M. L.; Campbell, J. F.; Lewis,
K. H.; Jensen, E. T.; and Schantz, E. J.: Public
health significance of paralytic shellfish poison. A review of literature and unpublished research. *Proc.
Natl. Shellfish Assoc.*, **47**:114, 1956.

Mebs, D.: Bi Bissvertzungen durch "ungiftige" Schlan-
sen. *Deutsche Med. Wochensc.*, **40**:1, 1977.

————: Pharmacology of reptilian venoms. In Gans, C.
(ed.): *Biology of the Reptilia*, Vol. 8. Academic Press,
London, 1978, pp. 437–560.

Meyer, K.: Über herzaktive krötengifte. *Pharm. Acta
Helvetiae*, **24**:222, 1949.

Meyer, K. F.; Sommer, H.; and Schoenholz, P.: Mussel poisoning. *J. Prev. Med.*, **2**:365, 1928.

Middlebrook, R. E.; Wittle, L. W.; Scura, E. D.; and
Lane, C. E.: Isolation and purification of a toxin
from *Millepora dichotoma*, *Toxicon.*, **9**:333, 1971.

Minton, S. A., Jr.: A list of colubrid envenomations.
Kentucky Herp., **7**:4, 1976.

Minton, S. A., Jr., and Minton, M. G.: *Venomous Reptiles*. Charles Scribner's Son, New York, 1969.

Morris, R., and Morris, D.: *Men and Snakes*. McGraw-
Hill, New York, 1965.

Neeman, I.; Calton, G. J.; and Burnett, J. W.: Purification of an endonuclease present in *Chrysaora quinquecirrha* venom. *Proc. Soc. Exp. Biol. Med.*,
166:374, 1981.

Nigrelli, R. F., and Jakowska, S.: Effects of holothur-
in, a steroid saponin from the Bahamian sea cucumber
(Actinopyga agassizi) on various biological systems.
Ann. N.Y. Acad. Sci., **90**:884, 1960.

Parnas, I., and Russell, F. E.: Effects of venoms on
nerve, muscle and neuromuscular junction. In Russell,
F. E., and Saunders, P. R. (eds.): *Animal Toxins*.
Pergamon Press, Oxford, 1967, pp. 401–415.

Parrish, H. M.: *Poisonous Snakebites in the United
States*. Vantage Press, New York, 1980.

Phillips, C., and Brady, W. H.: *Sea Pests: Poisonous
or Harmful Sea Life of Florida and the West Indies*.
University of Miami Press, Miami, 1953.

Prakash, A.; Medcof, J. C.; and Tennant, A.
D.: Paralytic shellfish poisoning in eastern Canada.
Bull. Fish. Res. Bd. Can., **177**:1, 1971.

Primor, N., and Lazarovici, P.: *Pardachirus marmoratus* (Red Sea flatfish) secretion and its isolated toxic
fraction pardaxin: the relationship between hemolysis
and ATPase inhibition. *Toxicon.* **19**:573, 1981.

Prinzmetal, M.; Sommer, H.; and Leake, C. D.: The
pharmacological action of "mussel poison." *J. Pharmacol. Exp. Ther.*, **46**:63, 1932.

Proctor, N. H.; Chan, S. L.; and Taylor, A. J.: Production of saxitoxin by cultures of *Gonyaulax catenella*.
Toxicon. **13**:1, 1975.

Randall, J. E.: A review of ciguatera, tropical fish
poisoning, with a tentative explanation of its cause.
Bull. Mar. Sci. Gulf Caribb., **8**:236, 1958.

Richet, C.: De la variabilité de la dose toxique de sub-
éritine. *C.R. Soc. Biol.*, **61**:686, 1906.

Rimsza, M. E.; Zimmerman, D. R.; and Bergeson, P.
S.: Scorpion envenomation. *Pediatrics*. **66**:298,
1980.

Rosenberg, P.: Pharmacology of phospholipase A_2
from snake venoms. In Lee, C. -Y. (ed.): *Snake
Venoms*, Vol. 52. *Handbook of Experimental
Pharmacology*. Springer-Verlag, Berlin, 1979, p. 11.

————. (ed.): *Toxins: Animal, Plant and Microbial*.
Pergamon Press, Elmsford, N.Y., 1978.

Russell, F. E.: Poisonous fishes. *Engineer. Sci.*, **15**:11,
1952.

————: Venomous animals and their toxins. *London
Times Sci. Rev.*, **49**:10, 1963.

————: Marine toxins and venomous and poisonous
marine animals. In Russell, F. S. (ed.): *Advances in
Marine Biology*, Vol. III. Academic Press, London,
1965. pp. 255–384.

————: *Physalia* stings—a report of two cases. *Toxicon*, **4**:65, 1966.

————: Comparative pharmacology of some animal
toxins. *Fed. Proc.*, **26**:1206, 1967.

————: Poisons and venoms. In Hoar, W. S., and Randall, D. J. (eds.): *Fish Physiology*, Vol. III. Academic
Press, Inc., New York, 1969, pp. 401–449.

————: Pharmacology of toxins of marine origin. In
Raskova, H. (ed.): *International Encyclopedia of
Pharmacology and Therapeutics*, Sec. 71, Vol. 2. Per-
gamon Press, Oxford, 1971, pp. 3–114.

————: Envenomation and diverse disease states (letter). *J.A.M.A.* **238**:581, 1977.

————: Pharmacology of venoms. In Eaker, D., and
Wadström, T. (eds.): *Natural Toxins*. Pergamon Press,
Elmsford, N.Y., 1980a, p. 13.

————: Venomous bites and stings. In Berkow, R.
(ed.): *The Merck Manual*, 14th ed. Merck, Sharp &
Dohme, Res. Lab., Rahway, N.J., 1982, pp. 2451–
2462.

————: *Snake Venom Poisoning*. J. B. Lippincott Co.,
Philadelphia, 1980b; Scholium International, Great
Neck, N.Y., 1983.

————: Marine toxins and venomous and poisonous
marine animals. In Blaxter, J. H. S.; Russell, F. S.;
and Yonge, C. M. (eds.): *Advances in Marine Biology*.
Academic Press, London, 1984a.

————: Snake venoms. In Ferguson, M. W. J. (ed.):
The Structure, Development, and Evolution of Reptiles

(Symposia of the Zoological Society of London). Academic Press, London, 1984b.

————: Poisoning caused by venomous and poisonous animals. In Goldsmith, R. S., and Heyneman, D. (eds.): *Tropical Medicine and Medical Parasitology*. Lange Medical Publications. Los Altos, Cal., 1986.

Russell, F. E., and Bogert, C. M.: Gila monster: its biology, venom and bite—a review. *Toxicon*. **19**:341, 1981.

Russell, F. E., and Buess, F. W.: Gel electrophoresis: a tool in systematics. Studies with *Latrodectus mactans* venom. *Toxicon*. **8**:81, 1970.

Russell, F. E.; Buess, F. W.; and Strassburg, J.: Cardiovascular response to *Crotalus* venom. *Toxicon*. **1**:5, 1962.

Russell, F. E., and Emery, J. A.: Venom of the weevers *Trachinus draco* and *Trachinus vipera*. *Ann. N.Y. Acad. Sci.*, **90**:805, 1960.

Russell, F. E., and Gertsch, W. J.: Letter to the editor (arthropod bites). *Toxicon*. **21**:337, 1983.

Russell, F. E., and van Harreveld, A.: Cardiovascular effects of the venom of the round stingray, *Urobatis halleri*. *Arch. Intern. Physiol.*, **62**:322, 1954.

Schaeffer, R. C., Jr.; Carlson, R. W.; Whigham, H.; Weil, M. H.; and Russell, F. E.: Acute hemodynamic effects of rattlesnake, *Crotalus viridis helleri*, venom. In Rosenberg, P. (ed.): *Toxins: Animal, Plant and Microbial*. Pergamon Press, Oxford, 1978, p. 383.

Schantz, E. J.: Biochemical studies on paralytic shellfish poisons. *Ann. N.Y. Acad. Sci.*, **90**:843, 1960.

Schantz, E. J.; Ghazarossian, V. E.; Schnoes, H. K.; Strong, F. M.; Springer, J. P.; Pezzanie, J. D.; and Clardy, J.: The structure of saxitoxin. *J. Am. Chem. Soc.*, **97**:1238, 1975.

Schantz, E. J.; Lynch, J. M.; Vayvada, G.; Matsumoto, K.; and Rappoport, H.: The purification and characterization of the poison produced by *Gonyaulax catenella* in axenic culture. *Biochemistry*, **5**:1191, 1966.

Schantz, E. J.; McFarren, E. F.; Schaffer, M. L.; and Lewis, K. H.: Purified shellfish poison for bioassay standardization. *J. Assoc. Off. Agric. Chem.*, **41**:160, 1958.

Schenone, H., and Suarez, G.: Venoms of Scytodidae. Genus *Loxosceles*. In Bettini, S. (ed.): *Arthropod Venoms*, Springer-Verlag, New York, 1978. pp. 247–275.

Schever, P. J.: *Chemistry of Marine Natural Products*. Academic Press, Inc., New York, 1973.

————: (ed.): *Marine Natural Products: Chemical and Biological Perspectives*. Academic Press, Inc., New York, Vols. 1 and 2, 1978; Vol. 3, 1980; Vol. 4, 1981.

Shapiro, B. I., and Lilleheil, G.: The action of anemone toxin on crustacean neurons. *Comp. Biochem. Physiol.*, **28**:1225, 1969.

Shimizu, Y.: Dinoflagellate toxins. In Scheuer, P. J. (eds.): *Marine Natural Products: Chemical and Biological Perspectives*, Vol. I. Academic Press, Inc., New York, 1978, pp. 1–42.

Slotta, K., and Fraenkel-Conrat, H.: Two active proteins from rattlesnake venom. *Nature*, **142**:213, 1938.

Smith, D. S.; Cayer, M. L.; Russell, F. E.; and Rubin, R. W.: Fine structure of stingray spine epidermis with special reference to a unique microtubular component of venom secreting cells. In Rosenberg, P. (ed): *Toxins: Animal, Plant and Microbial*. Pergamon Press, Oxford, 1978, p. 565.

Sommer, A., and Meyer, K. F.: Paralytic shellfish poisoning. *Arch. Pathol.*, **24**:560, 1937.

Southcott, R. V.: Arachnidism and allied syndromes in the Australian region. *Rec. Adelaide Children's Hosp.*, **1**:97: 1976.

————: Marine toxins. In Cohen, N. H., and Klawars, H. L. (eds.): *Handbook of Clinical Neurology*. Vol. 37, Elsevier North-Holland Publ. Co., Amsterdam, 1979, pp. 27–106.

Southcott, R. V., and Kingston, C. W.: Lethal jellyfish stings: a study in sea-wasps. *Med. J. Aust.*, (1):443, 1959.

Stempien, M. F.; Ruggieri, G. D.; Nigrelli, R. F.; and Cecil, J. T.: Physiologically active substances from extracts of marine sponges. In Youngken, H. W. (ed.): *Food-Drugs from the Sea Conference*. Marine Tech. Society, Washington, D.C., 1970, p. 295.

Su, C.; Chang, C.; and Lee, C.-Y.: Pharmacological properties of the neurotoxin of cobra venom. In Russell, F. E., and Saunders, P. R. (eds.): *Animal Toxins*. Pergamon Press, Oxford, 1967, pp. 259–267.

Sutherland, S. K., and Lane, W. R.: Toxins and mode of envenomation of the common ringed or blue-banded octopus. *Med. J. Aust.*, **1**:893, 1969.

Tamiya, N.; Arai, H.; and Sato, S.: Studies on sea snake venoms: crystallization of "erabutoxins" a and b from *Laticauda semifasiata* venom, and of "laticotoxin" a from *Laticauda laticauda* venom. In Russell, F. E., and Saunders, P. R. (eds.): *Animal Toxins*. Pergamon Press, Oxford, 1967, pp. 249–258.

Tamkun, M. M., and Hessinger, D. A.: Isolation and partial characterization of a hemolytic and toxic protein from the nematocyst venom of the Portuguese man-of-war. *Physalia physalis*. *Biochem. Biophys. Acta*, **667**:87, 1981; *see also Fed. Proc.*, **38**:824, 1979 (abstr.).

Tu, A. T.: *Chemistry and Molecular Biology*. John Wiley & Sons, New York, 1977.

Vick, J. A.; Ciuchta, H. P.; and Manthei, J. H.: Pathophysiological studies on ten snake venoms. In Russell, F. E., and Saunders, P. R. (eds.): *Animal Toxins*. Pergamon Press, Oxford, 1967, p. 269.

Wagner, F. W.; Spiekerman, A. M.; and Prescott, J. M.: Leucostoma peptidase A. Isolation and physical properties. *J. Biol. Chem.*, **243**:4486, 1968.

Wang, C. M.; Narahashi, R.; and Mendi, T. J.: Depolarizing action of *Haliclona* toxin on endplate and muscle membranes. *Toxicon*, **11**:499, 1973.

Waraszkiewicz, S. M., and Erickson, K. L.: Halogenated sesquiterpenoids from the Hawaiian marine alga *Laurencia nidifica*: nidificene and nidifidiene. *Tetrahedron Lett.*, **23**:2003, 1974.

Weill, R.: *Contributions a l'etude des Cnidaires et de leur Nematocystes*. Tomes 10, 11. *Trav. Stat. Zool.* Wimiereux, Paris. 1934.

Wiberg, G. S., and Stephenson, N. R.: Toxicologic studies on paralytic shellfish poison. *Toxicol. Appl. Pharmacol.*, **2**:607, 1960.

Wittle, L. W.; Middlebrook, R. E.; and Lane, C. E.: Isolation and partial purification of a toxin from *Millepora alcicornis*. *Toxicon*. **9**:327, 1971.

Yang, C. C.: Crystallization and properties of cobrotoxin and their relationship to lethality. *Biochem. Biophys. Acta*. **133**:346, 1965.

Zeller, E. A.: Enzymes of snake venoms and their biological significance. In *Advances in Enzymology*. Vol. 8. Interscience, New York, 1948, p. 459.

Chapter 23

TOXIC EFFECTS OF PLANT TOXINS

Kenneth F. Lampe

INTRODUCTION

The emphasis of this chapter will be on plants injurious to man. The poisoning of grazing animals also is important because it represents an enormous economic loss. Useful information on this aspect is contained in the previous editions of this text.

Inquiries concerning plant ingestions constitute about 10 percent of calls to Poison Control Centers, but only a small fraction of these are associated with symptomatic poisoning. The majority concern children three years of age and younger. The age of the victim often determines the plants that are involved. Infants are exposed primarily to plants in the home. The list of houseplants encountered is remarkably constant regardless of geography (Table 23–1). Symptomatic poisoning in this age group almost invariably results from chewing the leaves of dumbcane (*Dieffenbachia* spp.) or one of the philodendrons, generally *Philodendron scandens* ssp. *oxycardium*. Older preschool-age children also are exposed to yard plants (Table 23–2). They seek colorful berries or plants to serve as food while "playing house." These plants are more geographically distinctive. Adolescents and adults may experiment with plants and mushrooms thought to have hallucinogenic properties, although this rarely results in serious poisoning. More severe intoxications result from consumption of large quantities of wild plants inappropriately selected for food. Plants occasionally are consumed for abortifacient (now uncommon) or suicidal purposes.

A new potential source of toxic plant material is the health food store, where such items as raw apricot pits, tansy, and pennyroyal may be purchased. The ingredients may be mislabeled or may contain more than one plant. Plant medicinals obtained outside the United States often contain drugs, such as phenylbutazone, that are not listed on the label.

One must be aware that many so-called plant poisonings involve harmless species that have been treated with insecticides, weed killers, or fertilizers.

Table 23–1. FREQUENCY OF PLANT SPECIES INVOLVED IN INQUIRIES TO THE ROCHESTER, NEW YORK, POISON CONTROL CENTER INVOLVING INGESTIONS BY CHILDREN ONE YEAR OF AGE OR LESS*

1. Philodendron
2. Jade plant
3. Wandering Jew
4. Swedish ivy
5. Spider plant
6. Dieffenbachia and rubber plant
7. Asparagus fern
8. Aloe
9. String-of-pearls
10. Pothos

* From Lawrence, R. A.: *Proceedings, Ann. Mtg. Am. Acad. Clin. Toxicol/Am. Assoc. Poison Control Centers/Can. Acad. Clin. Anal. Toxicol.* Chicago, Oct. 18–20, 1978.

RESEARCH ON PLANTS INJURIOUS TO HUMANS

Although research on plants that poison animals has been pursued actively for many years by the USDA and schools of veterinary medicine, an equivalent interest in plants injurious to humans (except those producing dermatitis) has not been forthcoming. It is important, therefore, that research papers on this subject be free from defects that would diminish their value. The following are examples of recurring problems.

Failure to Document the Plant

Identification of the plant only by its trivial (common) name occurs frequently in clinical case reporting. Unfortunately, many plants of diverse botanical relationship share the same trivial name, even in the same locality. See the previous edition for a more detailed discussion.

Failure to place a voucher specimen of the plant in an herbarium with reference to such placement in the publication is primarily a problem in research. The important studies of phenolics in *Toxicodendron* by the late Dr. C. R.

Table 23–2. INQUIRIES CONCERNING PLANT INGESTIONS TO POISON CONTROL CENTERS SHOWING THE MOST FREQUENTLY INVOLVED SPECIES

AAPCC ANNUAL REPORT* (DATA FROM ALL REPORTING CENTERS)	SALT LAKE CITY, UTAH†	ROCHESTER, NEW YORK‡	MIAMI, FLORIDA§
1. Philodendron	1. Philodendron	1. Yew	1. Brazilian pepper
2. Dieffenbachia	2. Pyracantha	3. Nightshade	2. Dieffenbachia
3. Poinsettia	3. Apricot and other pits	3. Honeysuckle	3. Rosary pea
4. Jade plant	4. Dieffenbachia	4. Philodendron	4. Pencil tree cactus
5. Schefflera	5. Poinsettia	5. Poinsettia	5. Ficus
6. Holly	6. Honeysuckle	6. Pokeweed	6. Oleander, Philodendron
7. Pyracantha	7. Wandering Jew	7. Wandering Jew	7. Ixora, Allamanda
8. Pokeweed	8. Horse chestnut	8. Dieffenbachia	8. Poinsettia
9. Yew	9. Sweet pea	9. Jade plant	9. Coral plant
10. Rhododendron, Azalea	10. Creeping Charlie	10. Coleus	10. Balsam pear, Angel's trumpet, Bischofia
11. Spider plant, Pothos	11. Jimson weed, Schefflera		11. Hibiscus, Sea grape, Crown-of-thorns, "Croton," Bottle brush
12. Ornamental pepper, Mountain ash, Honeysuckle	12. Oregon grape, Tulip		

* Litozitz, T., and Veltri, J. C.: *Am. J. Emerg. Med.*, **3**:423–450, 1985.
† Spoerke, D. G., and Temple, A. R.: *Vet. Human Toxicol.*, **20**:85–90, 1978.
‡ Lawrence, R. A., and Schneider, M. F.: *Proceedings, Ann. Mtg. Am. Acad. Clin. Toxicol./Am. Assoc. Poison Control Centers/Can. Acad. Clin. Anal. Toxicol.*, Ste.-Adele, P.O., Canada, Aug. 2–5, 1977.
§ Fawcett, N. P.: *J. Fla. Med. Assoc.*, **65**:199–204, 1978.

Dawson are diminished in value, because it is now impossible to determine what species and varieties of the plant were examined.

Failure to Use Appropriate Route of Administration

Parenteral administration, particularly in small animals, is technically easier than oral administration but can lead to spurious results. Plants containing more than one toxin may exhibit different biologic activities, depending on the route of administration. Some plants contain lectins that cause erythrocyte agglutination and hemolysis, in addition to an orally active toxin. Lectins are not absorbed from the intestine and do not affect erythrocytes unless given intravenously. Many publications on poisonous plants improperly describe hemolysis as the major mechanism of toxicity for mushrooms and the castor bean, since each contains such lectins. Thus, alkalinization of the urine to protect the kidneys against hemoglobinuria has been recommended in some protocols for castor bean poisoning, and for a number of years the Pasteur Institute in Paris prepared a serum against the parenterally toxic lysin in *Amanita phalloides* in the mistaken belief that it was an antidote. Some toxins are active only orally, for example, amygdalin, which must be hydrolyzed in the stomach to

release cyanide, or macroazamin, which must be acted upon by the β-glucosidases of intestinal bacteria to release methylazoxymethanol. When screening for biologic activity, however, both oral and parenteral administration should be employed.

Failure to Use an Appropriate Assay

Various screening tests are employed to study the biologic activity of plants; these are limited only by the amount of plant material available, length of time, amount of money, and particular interests of the investigator. It is not practical to perform an assay for every conceivable type of pharmacologic activity. On the other hand, if a specific end point has been determined, it is important to select an assay method or species sensitive to that end point. For example, the chemists who fractionated tremetol, the crude extract from *Eupatorium rugosum,* used lethality in fish as an assay. *E. rugosum* causes a condition called trembles in cows and a potentially fatal syndrome, milksickness, in people who ingest the milk. The fractions of the extract from tremetol were given to fish, which are convenient test animals since the material can be added to the water and only small amounts of material are required. Unfortunately, it was not determined in advance that fish show the same biochemical alterations as cows or humans; thus, the end result was the isolation of a toxic material to which fish were exquisitely sensitive but which was inactive as a cause of trembles in mammals.

Failure to Provide Standard Medical Care

When studying the value of treatments of plant poisoning in animals, particularly with drugs, there is a tendency to divide the animals into two groups, poison all of them, give the proposed treatment to half, and after an appropriate time, count the survivors in each group. Little or no attempt is made to correct dehydration, provide respiratory support, monitor and correct electrolyte and glucose deficiencies, or provide other standard care as for an actual patient. Such care should be given and should be extended equally to each group. This failure to provide standard care lends an element of uncertainty to the value of a proposed "antidote," which may persist in a half-accepted twilight zone for years. A current example is the place of thioctic acid in the management of *Amanita phalloides* intoxication.

Interpretation of the Literature

Considerable care must be exercised in evaluating the literature on toxic plants. In some cases, results of animal toxicity studies have been extrapolated inappropriately to humans. In many cases, plant lore has been passed uncritically through generations of textbooks. For example, it was observed around 1900 that nettle stings were not unlike the stings of ants. From that time, with no experimental study, the statement that nettles, like ants, contain formic acid is often encountered.

On the other hand, specific case reports may be very useful. Many plants with physiologic activity were used as medicinals during the nineteenth century, and numerous cases of overdosage were reported, which provide valuable starting points for research on human pharmacology.

SYSTEMIC POISONING FROM VASCULAR PLANTS

General Principles

In any inquiry concerning plant ingestion, an attempt should be made to identify the plant, the part(s) ingested, and the approximate quantity. As in any poisoning, this information often will be incomplete or incorrect. With the exception of ingested plants known to be hazardous or patients who are already symptomatic, observation at home with instructions to call if there is a change in condition is usually recommended by the Poison Center. Routine follow-up calls are often made by the center. Following ingestion of mushrooms or known toxic plants (other than those causing oral irritation only), and in symptomatic cases, emptying of the stomach is recommended. Considering the size of plant particles, vomiting induced by syrup of ipecac and water is probably more effective than gastric lavage. This should be followed by instillation of activated charcoal.

As in most cases of poisoning, care is usually symptomatic. Special monitoring and specific drug therapy are indicated in some instances. Because life-threatening intoxications are exceptionally rare, little experience may be available among local hospital staff for an appropriate management protocol. In this event, help should be solicited from a regional Poison Control Center, which maintains a nationwide roster of consultants available to share their expertise.

A cardinal rule in the management of pediatric intoxications is to provide adequate hydration. Most poisonous plants, regardless of their ultimate toxicologic effect, induce fluid loss through vomiting and/or diarrhea. Children have a limited buffer capacity for such loss and have died from eating plants causing simple gastroenteric irritation.

Another easily missed effect of plant poisoning is diminished tidal volume. Respiratory rate may appear to be unchanged, but a toxin acting as a muscle relaxant—for example, Carolina Yellow jessamine *(Gelsemium sempervirens)* or tree tobacco *(Nicotiana glauca)*—may severely reduce the tidal volume, which, if uncorrected, can proceed to sudden respiratory failure and cardiac arrest.

The diagnosis of plant poisoning, in the absence of a history of plant ingestion, is probably impossible, unless the vomitus or stool can be seen to contain plant fragments. When wild plants are prepared as food, the differential diagnosis should include bacterial toxins, contamination with insecticides or weed killers, and individual food idiosyncrasy.

The toxicity of plants varies with plant part, maturity, growing condition, and genetic variation. Plants grown in some parts of the country or in some years may be toxic but can be eaten with impunity at other times or places. The age of the patient is also a factor; solanine-containing plants, for example, are far more dangerous to children than to adults. Children less than one year old tend to texture plant parts in their mouths rather than swallowing; thus, ingestion is minimal. The seed coats of the castor bean *(Ricinus communis)* and rosary pea *(Abrus precatorius)* are very hard, and unless broken, the seeds of these exceedingly toxic plants will pass harmlessly through the intestine. Other factors influencing toxicity could be cited. Obviously, it is impossible to determine prognosis simply on the basis that there has been an exposure. It is possible only to consider some plants more hazardous than others.

It is inappropriate to assume that the toxicity exhibited by a single member of a genus may apply to all other species of that genus, or that even all toxic members of a genus will demonstrate similar mechanisms of toxicity. This is illustrated by the mushroom genus *Amanita*. *Amanita phalloides* contains a number of cyclic peptides, the amatoxins, that cause hepatotoxicity by interfering with the action of RNA polymerase II. *A. muscaria* contains the isoxazole, ibotenic acid, a GABA-agonist that induces delirium and coma. *A. caesarea* is a much-sought edible delicacy. Similar examples could be given for leafy plants.

The following discussion of systemic poisoning by plants and mushrooms is not complete. It includes more common or interesting species. Information on additional plants may be found in the references at the end of this chapter.

Plants Producing Irritation of the Oral Cavity

The dumbcane (*Dieffenbachia* spp.) is so named because biting into a leaf causes immediate burning pain and swelling of oral tissues that may result in a transient loss of the ability to speak. The pain and edema do not require medical treatment but may be relieved by holding cool liquid or ice cream in the mouth. Obstruction of the airway is a rare complication. This response is produced to a greater or lesser degree by all members of the botanical family Araceae, which includes the cultivated houseplants (outdoors in Florida and Hawaii), *Philodendron* spp., *Caladium* spp., and the calla lily *(Zantedeschia aethiopica);* plants cultivated for edible parts, the ceriman *(Monstera deliciosa)* and malanga *(Xanthosoma violaceum);* and woodland species, the skunk cabbage *(Symplocarpus foetidus),* Jack-in-the-pulpit *(Arisaema triphyllum),* and green dragon *(Arisaema dracontium).*

When the plant cells are ruptured by chewing, bundles of long, needle-shaped crystals (raphides) of calcium oxalate are driven into the oral tissue. The mechanism of the production of pain is controversial. Based on work on an unrelated raphide-containing fishtail palm *(Caroyta mitis)* that causes a similar response when its fruit is bitten, it was proposed that mechanical injury from the calcium oxalate needle alone was responsible. Others maintain that the mechanical injury provides a pathway for injection of pain-inducing protein material. Reports from differ-

ent investigators comparing the incidence and severity of keratoconjunctivitis following instillation on the eyes of experimental animals of filtered and unfiltered juice from irritant Araceae give contradictory results.

Plants Producing Emesis Not Associated with Diarrhea

The bulbs of the family Amaryllidaceae, whose resemblance to onions makes them ready objects for accidental poisoning, elicit vomiting not associated with diarrhea. This family contains various *Narcissus* spp. (narcissus, jonquil, daffodil) and species of *Amaryllis*. Despite the apparent severity of the intoxication, which is characterized by repeated episodes of vomiting, recovery essentially is complete within 24 hours. Treatment is symptomatic, although there have been no clinical reports on whether phenothiazine antiemetics are useful.

The intoxication results from the action of the alkaloid lycorine on emetic receptors in the central nervous system. The emetic toxins in *Wisteria* species produce a similar, but longer-lasting, response. The emetic toxins in *Wisteria* apparently have not been identified, although various lectins from this plant have been studied.

Plants Producing Diarrhea That May Be Associated with Emesis

Outside of a few medically useful cathartic-containing plants, those containing anthraquinone derivatives, for example, the active substances in these plants have received scant attention. Even the actions of our cathartic drugs are poorly understood and controversial. Two representative toxins will be discussed.

The saponins are steroidal glycosides widely distributed throughout the plant kingdom, although they are not always present in concentrations sufficient to induce a symptomatic response. Within a species, the concentration depends on the maturity of the plant and the conditions of growth. Absorption of saponins is poor, and severe gastroenteritis is usually the only consequence of ingestion. The most important saponin-containing plant in eastern North America is the pokeweed *(Phytolacca americana)*. Intoxications result from the misidentification of its root as horseradish and the use of uncooked mature leaves in salads. The mature berries are usually harmless. There is usually a latent period of two to three hours prior to the onset of symptoms during which the saponins are hydrolyzed to their active triterpene components. There is an initial prodroma of warmth in the throat and stomach and a scratchy feeling in the throat, which may be accompanied by coughing. This is followed by severe gastritis with frequent episodes of vomiting, which may continue at intervals for ten hours, and diarrhea, which may persist for 48 hours. Intoxications with similar symptoms have been produced by consumption of the nuts of the horse chestnut *(Aesculus hippocastanum)*, fruit from the blue cohosh *(Caulophyllum thalictroides)*, pigeon berry *(Duranta repens)*, the fruit or leaf of English ivy *(Hedera helix)*, and the yam bean *(Pachyrhizus erosus)*.

Members of the buttercup family, Ranunculaceae, contain a glycoside that yields the irritant protoanemonin on enzymatic hydrolysis. The plants associated with intoxications are the buttercups *(Ranunculus* spp.) baneberry *(Actaea pachypoda)*, marsh marigold *(Caltha palustris)*, pasque flower *(Anemone* spp.), and *Clematis* spp. Protoanemonin produces a burning sensation in the oropharynx, profuse salivation, emesis, colicky gastroenteritis, and diarrhea. A portion of the toxin may be absorbed and excreted unchanged by the kidney; hematuria, polyuria, and sometimes, painful urination may occur. Adequate hydration to maintain a dilute urine is indicated to reduce renal damage. Conventionally, these patients have been given demulcents orally (egg white and milk), but no study has been made to determine if this is helpful or if simple dilution would be equally satisfactory.

Plants Producing Gastroenteritis After a Latent Period of Several Hours

Poisoning with colchicine-containing plants occurs after a partially dose-dependent latent period (usually of many hours) and has resulted from ingestion of leaves, seeds, bulbs, or flowers of the crocus or meadow saffron *(Colchicum* spp.). The plant has even been used successfully for suicide. Less commonly, poisonings have followed the ingestion of tubers from the glory lily *(Gloriosa superba* and *G. rothschildiana)*, which have been mistaken for sweet potatoes. The gastroenteric effects resemble those encountered with colchicine during treatment of gout. Colchicine is a mitotic poison. Massive overdose may result in vascular damage, thrombocytopenia, bone marrow depression, hypothermia, muscle weakness, and in survivors, alopecia.

Solanine alkaloids is the general name for the steroidal glycoalkaloids found in nightshades *(Solanum* spp.), immature fruit of some groundcherries *(Physalis* spp.), the jessamines *(Cestrum* spp.), and many other plants. Fatalities have resulted from the ingestion of the immature (green) fruit from the European bittersweet *(Solanum dulcamara)* and the horse nettle *(Solanum carolinense)*. Children seem to be especially sensitive, but this may represent a dose-response effect rather than greater intestinal absorption. The symptoms are those of an infectious gastroenteritis: temperature is elevated, headache is common, and after a prodromal scratchy feeling in the oropharynx, there is anorexia, nausea, vomiting, and diarrhea. Management is symptomatic.

The most toxic flowering plants are the castor bean *(Ricinus communis)* and the rosary pea *(Abrus precatorius.)* The toxins of these plants, formerly called toxalbumins, are nearly identical lectins composed of two polypeptide chains connected by a disulfide bridge. One of these chains binds to the intestinal cell wall, permitting entry of the other chain into the cytoplasm. The toxin inhibits ribosomal protein synthesis. A single molecule of toxin is sufficient to kill the cell. The castor bean also contains the harmless cathartic castor oil, and both species contain an orally inactive (nontoxic) agglutinin.

If seeds with broken seed coats are swallowed, persistent diarrhea, often with bloody mucus, begins after a latent period of up to three days. Death may occur two to three days later of complications related to loss of intestinal function. Autopsy reveals hemorrhagic gastric mucosa and cecum. The gut-associated lymphoid tissue (Peyer's patches) in the ileum are severely inflamed and edematous. Intravenous fluids and parenteral alimentation should be provided, but cerebral edema, oliguria, and cardiac arrhythmias secondary to changes in plasma composition usually prove to be unmanageable.

The mistletoe *(Phoradendron serotinum)* is often named as one of the hazards in the home in newspaper lists appearing about Christmas time. In the 1920s, it was shown that the fruit contains tyramine, and textbooks ever since have listed this as the toxic ingredient with headache and hypertension as symptoms, although neither has appeared in a case history. It is hard to imagine the tyramine in even a handful of fruit surviving a first pass through the portal circulation in a patient with intact monoamine oxidase activity. It was demonstrated that the European mistletoe *(Viscum album)* contains a lectin with activity similar to that in the castor bean but with only about ⅓₀th the activity. This lectin was isolated from the leaves, and although not specified, the article suggested that the lectin is either not present or present in low concentration in the fruit. According to European reports, children who swallow the fruit experience only mild gastroenteritis. Although toxic proteins are known to be present in American mistletoe, they have been studied only after parenteral administration, and neither their pathology nor mechanism of action has been described. Recently, a lectin of extremely low toxicity has been isolated from

Phoradendron californicum growing on the cat claw tree *(Acacia greggii)* in the desert areas of the American Southwest and Mexico. It is necessary to specify the host plant in research involving mistletoe lectins since this will affect the presence, concentration, and nature of lectins in the mistletoe.

Plants Containing Convulsants

Although there are a number of plants in North America containing convulsant toxins, actual clinical cases have involved only the water hemlocks *(Cicuta* spp.). These plants have a distinct odor of raw parsnip and may be mistaken for that vegetable. Treatment requires management of the airway, relief of convulsions if persistent, and respiratory support. Acute renal failure secondary to convulsion-induced rhabdomyolysis is an infrequent complication. One of the most toxic plants in Great Britain, the water dropwort *(Oenanthe crocata),* has a similar toxin and is a rare introduced species in the United States in the Washington, D.C., area. A related species, *Oenanthe sarmentosa,* is common along the West Coast but has not been associated with poisoning. It would be of interest to determine if it is devoid of the convulsant toxin.

Plants Containing Belladonna Alkaloids

All species of *Datura,* particularly the jimson weed *(Datura stramonium)* and the angel trumpets *(Brugmansia* spp.), contain the belladonna alkaloids. The entire plant is toxic, including the nectar, but the seeds are encountered most commonly in accidental poisoning. Both seeds and dried leaves are used for their deliriant effect. Although physostigmine may be employed to antagonize the atropinic effects (dry mouth with dysphonia and dysphagia, tachycardia, dry skin, elevated body temperature, which may be accompanied by rash, blurred vision, occasional mydriasis, delirium, and excitement), therapeutic intervention is not necessary except in the presence of severe delirium or hyperthermia. The inadvertent introduction of plant fragments or juice from *Datura* species onto the corneal surface, an occupational hazard among farmers, may cause unilateral mydriasis; in the absence of suspicion as to the cause, this may lead to unneeded neurologic investigation.

Plants Primarily Affecting the Cardiovascular System

The foxglove *(Digitalis purpurea),* lily-of-the-valley *(Convallaria majalis),* oleander *(Nerium oleander),* and yellow oleander or lucky nut *(Thevetia peruviana)* all contain digitalislike glycosides. The entire plant is toxic, including smoke from burning foliage and water in which the flowers have been placed. Acute digitalis poisoning differs from digitalis overdosage as seen in a patient with congestive failure. It is expressed usually as conduction defects and sinus bradycardia. Hyperkalemia may be present. Rhythm disturbances, other than escape beats, are not necessarily exhibited. Intoxications require serial monitoring of the electrocardiogram and serum potassium. Conduction defects may be relieved by atropine or transvenous pacing. Dialysis and forced diuresis are not useful. Digoxin immune Fab (Digibind®) is not just specific for digoxin but effectively reverses the toxic response to the many cardiac glycosides that may be encountered in plant poisoning. It generally is reserved for serious or life-threatening intoxications.

Monkshood (*Aconitum* spp.) produces a tingling, burning sensation on the lips, tongue, mouth, and throat almost immediately after ingestion. This is followed by numbness and a feeling of constriction in the throat. The toxic alkaloid, aconitine, causes reflex bradycardia, slows conduction, and induces arrhythmias. Other symptoms are nausea, vomiting, and muscular weakness. Aconitine acts on nerve axons by opening sodium channels. On myocardial tissue, it inhibits complete repolarization of the excitable membrane, causing repetitive firing. In isolated tissue preparations, this action can be antagonized by procaine; an infusion of 0.1 percent procaine was effective in one report of human intoxication but has not been examined in laboratory preparations. The green hellebores (*Veratrum* spp.) and the death camas (*Zigadenus* spp.) contain veratridine. Plants in the botanical family Ericaceae (*Rhododendron* spp., *Kalmia* spp., *Pieris* spp., and others) contain the nonnitrogenous grayanotoxins (formerly called andromedotoxins). It should be noted that not all genera of the Ericaceae, or even all species in the genera listed here, contain grayanotoxins. It is not possible to predict the toxicity of hybrid horticultural species on the basis of a toxin-containing parent. Both veratridine, the most potent of the veratrum alkaloids, and the grayanotoxins have a physiologic action identical to that of aconitine, although intoxication from these plants appears to be associated more with bradycardia and hypotension than with rhythm disturbances. This may, however, be a dose artifact, and if equivalent quantities were ingested and retained (early and profuse emesis usually removes much swallowed material), the clinical picture with all three types of poisoning might be indistinguishable. Honey made from the nectar of grayanotoxin-containing Ericaceae can contain seriously toxic concentrations of the grayanotoxins. Cases of human poisoning from such toxic honey are multifold more common than toxicity that has resulted from the ingestion of plant parts from the grayanotoxin-containing Ericaceae.

All parts of the yew tree *(Taxus* spp.), except the bright-red, fleshy aril that cups the seed, contain the complex taxine alkaloids. Onset of intoxication occurs after a latent period of one to three hours. Nausea, diffuse abdominal pain, shallow respiration, and cardiac conduction disturbances resembling hyperkalemia occur. The atrial P waves may be absent. The syndrome complex suggests the need for temporary transvenous pacing, but human intoxications are so rare that there is little clinical experience. Taxol, originally isolated from the western yew *(Taxus brevifolia),* is an alkaloid that has been studied extensively because of its unique ability to bind to tubulin and promote microtubule assembly. It is now in phase I trials as a chemotherapeutic agent. The pure alkaloid induces primarily nausea, vomiting and diarrhea, sensory neuropathy, thrombocytopenia, and leukopenia. However, the pharmacology of the cardiotoxic taxine alkaloids has not been examined since the early 1930s; thus, no conclusions may be drawn regarding mechanism.

Plants That Affect Skeletal Muscle Tone

Of the toxic species that may affect skeletal muscle tone, those most frequently encountered clinically contain nicotine or anabasine, particularly the tree tobacco *(Nicotiana glauca),* which contains the latter. Similar poisoning is produced by coniine found in poison hemlock *(Conium maculatum);* or cytisine, found in laburnum *(Cytisus laburnum)* and the mescal or burning bean *(Sophora secundiflora);* and lobeline, which is present in cardinal flowers *(Lobelia* spp.). Poisoning causes nausea and emesis, a sensation of sweating, dizziness, and sometimes, clonic convulsions. Death is due to paralysis of respiratory muscles. An older investigation, by visual observation, described the action at the myoneural junction as succinylcholinelike rather than curarelike. Patients can be maintained with controlled respiration. It would be interesting to verify the neuromuscular action by electrophysiologic studies and to see if neostigmine antagonizes the blockade. There is a great need for some basic pharmacokinetic data on humans on nicotine and anabasine.

Most intoxications involving the Carolina yellow jessamine *(Gelsemium sempervirens)* have resulted from children sucking the nectar from the flowers, but all parts of this vine contain the toxins gelsemine, gelsemicine, and related alkaloids. Ingestions produce headache, dizziness,

visual disturbances, pronounced ptosis, and dry mouth with dysphonia and dysphagia. In severe cases, muscular weakness becomes pronounced. There are coexistent signs of a weak strychninelike action with tetanic contractions and extensor spasms following tendon taps. Convulsions, however, are unusual. Little is known of the pharmacology of the alkaloids, although a tincture of gelsemium was used extensively in medicine and a number of intoxications are reported in the nineteenth century medical literature. Minor intoxications may be managed with respiratory support.

Karwinskia humboldtiana is best known by its Mexican names, coyotillo or tullidora, in the American Southwest but is sometimes called (inappropriately) buckthorn in the American literature. The fruit contains a number of toxic anthracenones. Several weeks after consumption, the muscles become increasingly weak, beginning with the lower extremities. Full paralysis may develop over another month. Fatalities are due to failure of the respiratory muscles. The initial defect is segmental loss in myelin of the peripheral motor nerves, followed by fragmentation and disappearance of the axon itself in a wallerianlike fashion. No specific management of the poisoning can be suggested.

SYSTEMIC POISONING FROM MUSHROOMS

It has been a particular pleasure to watch the development of our knowledge of the chemistry and clinical toxicology of poisonous mushrooms during the past two decades. Not only has the management of patients been simplified and made more specific as the underlying pathophysiology was clarified, but some of the mushroom toxins have evolved into powerful evaluative tools in biochemical and neurologic research.

Unlike vascular plant poisoning, facility for mushroom identification during an emergency may be difficult or impractical. Fortunately, there are relatively limited varieties of toxins, which permits differential diagnosis on the basis of history and symptoms. Mushrooms that produce a response within two hours of ingestion or shortly after the ingestion of an alcoholic beverage rarely are considered of serious consequence and require only conservative symptomatic management. They may be subdivided into: (1) mushrooms whose response is primarily gastroenteric symptoms, with nausea, abdominal discomfort, and sometimes vomiting and/or diarrhea; (2) mushrooms evoking sweating; (3) mushrooms inducing inebriation or hallucinations without drowsiness or sleep; (4) mushrooms producing delirium associated with sleep or coma; and (5) mushrooms eliciting a disulfiramlike response to alcohol.

Intoxications characterized by a latent period of six hours or more are associated with serious, sometimes life-threatening symptoms. These may be subdivided into: (1) those producing severe headache and a feeling of abdominal fullness about six hours after ingestion; (2) those provoking emesis and profuse diarrhea about 12 hours after ingestion; and (3) those producing polydipsia and polyuria about three days after ingestion.

Mushrooms Producing Gastroenteric Discomfort of Rapid Onset

Many species of mushrooms produce varying degrees of abdominal discomfort within three hours of ingestion. Some may cause persistent emesis and/or diarrhea, which may produce severe dehydration and hypovolemic shock, particularly in children. The irritant mushroom need not be identified. Treatment is entirely symptomatic as for gastroenteritis of any other etiology. Replacement of fluids and electrolytes and support of circulation may be required.

Mushrooms Evoking Sweating

These mushrooms contain clinically significant concentrations of muscarine, which is not affected by cooking. There is a dose-response relationship in symptoms, the most sensitive indicator being profuse sweating. More severe intoxications produce nausea, emesis, abdominal pain, and occasionally, blurred vision and other parasympathetic effects. Symptoms usually subside without treatment within two hours. In uncomfortable patients, atropine may be given until symptoms are abolished or until dryness of the mouth is produced.

Mushrooms Evoking Inebriation or Hallucinations

These mushrooms contain psilocybin. The clinical response is determined by the dose, setting, psychoactive substance, and sophistication, mood, and personality of the patient. The usual duration is two hours. In accidental poisoning in adults, the response resembles alcohol intoxication. In young children exposed to large doses, the hallucinations are accompanied by hyperthermia, loss of consciousness, and tonic-clonic convulsions. Adults do not require treatment. Young children exhibiting neurologic involvement require external cooling and respiratory management as indicated. There have been a few recorded fatalities in this age group.

Mushrooms Producing Delirium Associated with Sleep or Coma

The toxins involved are muscimol and ibotenic acid, which are components of *Amanita muscaria* and *A. pantherina.* Muscimol is a conformationally restricted analogue of GABA with potent activity on bicuculline-reactive postsynaptic receptors. Symptoms of poisoning normally appear in 20 to 90 minutes. There may be an initial gastroenteritis, but this is often minimal or absent. After about one hour, drowsiness and dizziness develop, which may be accompanied by sleep. This may be followed by elation, increased motor activity, tremors, illusions, and even manic excitement. This may alternate with periods of drowsiness or sleep. Poisoning in adults is rarely severe but may require protective action to prevent injury if manic excitement appears. In children, complex neurologic signs may persist for up to 12 hours and include coma and convulsions. Usually no therapy is necessary other than respiratory support, if indicated.

Mushrooms Exhibiting a Disulfiramlike Effect

Coprinus atramentarius, although edible, elicits a disulfiramlike response to alcohol consumption for up to three days after eating the mushroom. The active component is cyclopropanone hydrate, a metabolite of the mushroom toxin, 1-cyclopropanol-1-N^5-glutamine (coprine). Other mushrooms with a similar alcohol-sensitizing action include *Clitocybe clavipes, Boletus luridus,* and *Verpa bohemica.* None of these contain coprine, and their activity in this regard needs investigation.

Mushrooms Inducing Headache About Six Hours After Ingestion

This intoxication is associated most often with *Gyromitra exculenta,* which may be mistaken for the edible morel by inexperienced collectors. The toxin is monomethylhydrazine, which antagonizes pyridoxine. The toxin is volatile, and the mushroom may be made edible by air drying or by extraction of the toxin with boiling water, which is then discarded.

Onset of symptoms is sudden, usually about six to eight hours after ingestion or inhalation of the vapor from cooking mushrooms. It is characterized by headache, malaise, abdominal fullness, and emesis (but *not* diarrhea). Generally, the patient recovers completely within two to six days. However, fatal hepatic necrosis has developed. Treatment is the same as for isoniazid overdosage and consists of administration of pyridoxine and correction of systemic acidosis.

Mushrooms Causing Emesis and Profuse Diarrhea About 12 Hours After Ingestion

Almost all fatalities caused by mushroom poisoning in North America are caused by *Amanita phalloides* and its relatives. The toxins are a family of thermostable, cyclic octapeptides, known collectively as amatoxins. They bind to and inhibit RNA polymerase II, preventing the elongation of messenger RNA, and thereby disrupting the continuous maintenance of the cell. The amatoxins undergo extensive enterohepatic cycling and are excreted unchanged in the urine and feces. In human intoxications, primary histologic damage is produced only in the duodenum, liver, and kidney. It is presumed that this selectivity results from the inability of the amatoxins to enter cells easily, therefore producing cellular damage only where they appear in high concentration.

Approximately one-half of a mature mushroom cap of *Amanita phalloides* is the lethal dose for an adult. Symptoms usually occur only after a period of 12 hours and begin with nausea, vomiting, profuse diarrhea, and abdominal pain. This may be followed by a symptom-free period, succeeded by rapidly developing hepatic insufficiency indistinguishable from acute viral hepatitis. The increase in serum transaminase factors is the most sensitive indicator of the extent of hepatocellular damage. Blood glucose and clotting factors of hepatic origin are decreased. Jaundice is an inconsistent finding. Even with intensive, symptomatic care, the fatality rate is about 10 percent. In the early phase, fluids should be replaced and, when tolerated, activated charcoal given orally in serial boluses. Otherwise, the management is as for acute, fulminant hepatitis. A return toward normal of factor V and fibrinogen is a prognostic feature for recovery.

Since *Amanita phalloides*–type mushroom poisoning is associated with high mortality, a large number of agents have been tried in human intoxications without previous research investigation. These include high-dose vitamin therapy, corticosteroids, sex hormones, and glucose loading. Two such agents, thioctic acid (α-lipoic acid) and high-dose penicillin G, have been used extensively in Europe and are included in some management protocols in the United States. It would be highly desirable if experimental animals, preferably the dog, which resembles man closely in *Amanita* poisoning, were given minimally toxic doses (to minimize the need for critical care) of mushroom extract (or a pure amatoxin, such as α-amanitin) and the influence of each of these proposed agents on hepatic transaminase changes with time determined.

Mushrooms Causing Polydipsia and Polyuria Three or More Days After Ingestion

These poisonings are caused by the toxin orellanine, present in a single section of the large genus *Cortinarius*. Such intoxications have not been reported in North America, although an orellanine-containing species, *Cortinarius rainierensis*, is indigenous to the Pacific Northwest. There is a latent period of 3 to 17 days between ingestion and the appearance of symptoms. The first effect is severe polydipsia, during which the patient may drink several liters a day. This is followed by nausea, headaches, muscular pains, and chills. In severe cases, there is an initial polyuria succeeded by oliguria or anuria. Postmortem examination shows renal tubular necrosis, fatty degeneration of the liver, and severe inflammatory changes in the intestine. Management is symptomatic as for renal failure. There is still controversy surrounding the chemistry of the toxic component.

Unclassified Toxic Mushrooms

There are isolated reports on mushrooms producing unique actions that suggest interesting research projects. Examples are: the puffball, *Scleroderma aurantium*, causes tetany and paresthesias; *Verpa bohemica*, usually associated with mild gastroenteritis, produces significant motor incoordination in others; *Omphalotous olearius* (syn. *Clitocybe illudens*), whose chemistry has been investigated extensively, can produce gastroenteritis, sensory disturbances, and marked muscle relaxation; and *Stropharia coronilla* produced intense "bone pain" in two adolescents seeking hallucinogenic activity.

PLANTS CAUSING SKIN INJURY

In contrast to the rather low morbidity associated with systemic plant poisoning, plant dermatitis is a problem of enormous magnitude. Approximately one-half of the workmen's compensation claims filed annually in California are for poison oak *(Toxicodendron diversilobum)* dermatitis. All classes of contact dermal injury are produced by plants. These include mechanical injury, delayed contact sensitivity, contact urticaria, phototoxicity, photoallergy, primary chemical irritation, or some combination of these.

Plants Causing Mechanical Injury

Injuries produced by splinters, thorns, awns, and sharp leaf edges are mechanisms for the introduction of fungi and bacteria through the skin or into the eye. Various noninfectious skin lesions caused by plant fragments include folliculitis, soft tissue granulomas, synovitis, and osteoblastic ("thorn tumors") and osteolytic responses.

Plants Causing Delayed Contact Sensitivity (Allergic Contact Dermatitis)

Sensitivity to a substance must be developed after cutaneous contact. Once sensitized, subsequent exposure will elicit a response. Usually, five days to three weeks is needed after the sensitizing exposure for development of an immunologically reactive skin. The chemistry of the sensitizing chemicals is known for most commonly offending plants. They are low-molecular-weight compounds (haptens) that react with cutaneous protein to form antigens. More than one contact may be required to induce sensitization. With less potent haptens, sensitization occurs more readily if the plant is applied to damaged skin. Some haptens induce only transient sensitivity, but that caused by poison ivy and poison oak persists for decades and possibly for life.

Once sensitization develops, the whole body surface becomes reactive, but only areas that actually touch the plant exhibit a clinical response. Reactions are seen rarely on the palms, soles, and hairy scalp because of the greater physical barrier these present. The severity of response to an equivalent amount of hapten among previously sensitized patients varies greatly, but in a given individual, the degree of response depends on the dose.

Poison ivy *(Toxicodendron radicans)* and Western poison oak *(T. diversilobum)* cause more cases of delayed contact sensitivity than all other known sensitizers combined. Probably 50 percent of the North American population has been sensitized to *Toxicodendron* and another 20 percent may be sensitized. The remaining 30 percent seem to possess genetic, antigen-specific tolerance. Age, sex, and race seem to have little role in the ability to become sensitized to *Toxicodendron,* but certain pathologic conditions (lymphoma, sarcoidosis, atopy) impair sensitization.

After a sensitized individual is reexposed to the hapten, 12 to 48 hours, or more, are required to develop a visible cutaneous response. This delay is an essential element in differential diagnosis. It represents a cell-mediated immune reaction affected by thymus-derived lymphocytes (T cells). The latent period can be shortened by exposure to greater concentrations of hapten. Erythema and edema appear initially. Pruritus is always present and may be intense. Vesicles form during the subsequent 24 hours; serous fluid in the vesicles does not contain antigen and cannot spread the rash to other parts of the body or to other individuals. There may be marked exudation, but crusting and scaling begin to develop within a few days. In the absence of complications due to excoriation and infection or continued exposure, healing is complete in about ten days.

Toxicodendron dermatitis is managed effectively with corticosteroids. Prevention, however, is an active area for research. Oral hyposensitization is troublesome, affords only partial protection, and is effective for only six months. Two investigational approaches are studies on ring-substituted derivatives of pentadecylcatechol, which may block the immune responses, and induction of tolerance in patients not yet sensitized by intramuscular administration of *Toxicodendron* extracts. The study of delayed contact sensitivity and the role of Langerhans cells (immunocompetent epidermal cells of bone marrow origin) in antigen transport and of bone marrow–derived lymphocytes (B cells) and basophils in the modulation of immune response is being performed currently.

Plants Causing Contact Urticaria

This reaction may be immunologic or nonimmunologic in nature. The latter is more common, but plants have produced both forms. Cutaneous contact induces a transient urticarial or, less frequently, a wheal-and-flare response.

Nettles are an example of plants that cause nonimmunologic contact urticaria. These plants have hollow stinging hairs that inject a chemical after penetration of the skin; a burning sensation and pruritus occur almost immediately. The injected material of the North American nettles, *Urtica urens* and *U. dioica,* has been identified as a mixture of acetylcholine, histamine, and serotonin on the basis of the response of smooth muscle to nettle extract alone and in the presence of antagonists to these substances. The Australian nettle, *Dendrocnide moroides,* also contains these substances, but its activity has been attributed to a thermostable, nondialyzable carbohydrate. Interdermal injection of this material produced piloerection, local vasodilation, sweating, and pain resembling that produced by the nettle. This or a similar material should be sought in North American species, since injection of an artificial mixture of the known components does not simulate the response to the nettle exactly.

Some individuals develop contact urticaria of the immunologic type after contact with a number of edible vegetables. Scraping the peel from new potatoes, for example, elicits various noncutaneous allergic responses, such as sneezing or wheezing. Other possible reactions are rhinoconjunctivitis, angioedema, gastroenteric disturbances, and anaphylaxis. Although the immunologic basis for this form of contact urticaria can be demonstrated by the Prausnitz-Küstner test (passive serum transfer), little is known of the essential features of sensitization of the chemistry of the antigens.

Plants Causing Phototoxicity

A number of cultivated plants of the carrot family (Umbelliferae), such as parsnips, caraway, dill, and parsley, and the rue family (Rutaceae), which includes the citrus plants, sensitize the skin to long-wave ultraviolet light (UVA). These plants contain furocoumarins (psoralens), which can penetrate moist skin. Within 6 to 24 hours of contact with the plant and exposure to sunlight or fluorescent light, the area of contact will selectively burn. The reaction ranges from mild erythema to severe damage with bullae, and hyperpigmentation ensues that may persist for several months. Pruritus is minimal. Inflammation can be ameliorated by prostaglandin inhibitors, such as aspirin, or by systemic corticosteroids in severe cases.

The mechanism of phototoxicity is not completely understood. The psoralens are intercalated into DNA, followed by UVA-induced covalent bonding. Hyperpigmentation results from proliferation of functional melanocytes and altered distribution of melanosomes from a nonaggregated to an aggregated state.

Plants Causing Primary Chemical Irritation

These plants contain substances that produce skin damage resembling that from contact with a corrosive acid. The degree of damage depends on the potency of the irritant, its concentration, and exposure time. The reaction varies according to the area of the body exposed and the age of the patient. Genetic factors influence vulnerability, but sex and race appear to have little consistent effect. Physical factors, particularly temperature and humidity, also affect the severity of response.

The spurges, in the family Euphorbiaceae, the buttercups (*Ranunculus* spp.), daphne *(Daphne mezereum),* and wild pepper *(Capsicum frutescens)* are most frequently involved. The most serious reactions involve the eye; severe keratoconjunctivitis with transient blindness may occur. The eye should be irrigated immediately, the pupil should be dilated, and artificial tears instilled. Steroids should be avoided because of the danger of encouraging a fungal infection.

SUMMARY

Many types of plants causing injury have not been discussed, such as those producing hayfever, food allergy, allergic alveolitis, and Bud-Chiari syndrome. There also are carcinogenic plants, teratogenic plants, and those that contain estrogen, thyroid-blocking substances, toxic amino acids, or hypoglycemic substances.

A great deal remains to be learned even about the plants that have been summarized. In addition to the research suggested, mechanisms of action should be investigated further. In the past, it was sufficient to identify a toxic plant because it caused hypoglycemia or arrhythmia. How much better it would be if one could identify the biochemical changes that induce the hypoglycemia or the membrane effects that cause the arrhythmia. Such studies will lead to better management of intoxications and, perhaps, to the development of new research tools and therapeutic agents.

ANNOTATED BIBLIOGRAPHY

Human Poisoning by Plants

Common Poisonous and Injurious Plants. HHS Pub. No. (FDA) 81–7706. U.S. Govt. Printing Office, Washington, D.C. This is an inexpensive, color-illustrated bulletin of the most common poisonous and injurious plants in the United States and Canada. It is written primarily for lay readers.

Hardin, J. W., and Arena, J. M.: *Human Poisoning from Native and Cultivated Plants,* 2nd ed. Duke University Press, Durham, N.C., 1974. This book is intended primarily for parents, camp and school counselors, and scout leaders.

Keeler, R. F., and Tu, A. T.: *Handbook of Natural Toxins*, Vol. 1, *Plant and Fungal Toxins*. Marcel Dekker, New York, 1983. Selected topics on human and veterinary plant poisoning or injury. Volume 6 (currently in preparation) will also be devoted to this subject matter.

Lampe, K. F., and McCann, M. A.: *AMA Handbook of Poisonous and Injurious Plants*. Chicago Review Press, Chicago, 1985. Although intended to provide physicians and other health professionals with an easily used reference for the management of plant intoxications, the format and color photographs make it a useful field guide for the recognition of dangerous and injurious plants.

Pammel, L. H.: *Manual of Poisonous Plants*. Torch Press, Cedar Rapids, Iowa, 1910; a Xerox reproduction is available from University Microfilms, Ann Arbor, Mich. This encyclopedic work is a frequent help concerning an inquiry about a plant not discussed in more recent, but slimmer, compilations.

Veterinary Plant Poisoning

Kingsbury, J. M.: *Poisonous Plants of the United States and Canada*, Prentice-Hall, New York, 1964. This is the standard textbook for veterinary students.

Poisonous Mushrooms

Ammirati, J. F.; Traquair, J. A.; and Horgen, P. A.: *Poisonous Mushrooms of the Northern United States and Canada*. University of Minnesota Press,

Minneapolis, 1985. A very useful, comprehensive guide to toxic mushrooms particularly useful for identification and nomenclatural issues; not intended as a guide to management of intoxications.

Lampe, K. F.: Toxic fungi. *Annu. Rev. Pharmacol. Toxicol.*, **19**:85–104, 1979.

Lampe, K. F., and McCann, M. A.: Differential diagnosis of poisoning by North American mushrooms, with particular emphasis on *Amanita phalloides*–like intoxication. *Ann. Emerg. Med.*, **16**:956–962, 1987.

Lincoff, G., and Mitchel, D. H.: *Toxic and Hallucinogenic Mushroom Poisoning*. Van Nostrand Reinhold, New York, 1977.

Rumack, B. H., and Salzman, E. (eds): *Mushroom Poisoning Diagnosis and Treatment*. CRC Press, Boca Raton, Fla., 1978.

Plant Dermatitis

Benezra, C.; Ducombs, G.; Sell, Y.; and Fousereau, J.: *Plant Contact Dermatitis*. C. V. Mosby, Saint Louis, 1985. Each plant is illustrated in color on a separate page along with its mechanism of dermatitis, reactive chemical if known, clinical aspects, and references.

Fisher, A. A.: *Contact Dermatitis*, 3rd ed. Lea & Febiger, Philadelphia, 1986. This is the best introduction to the subject.

Guin, J. D., and Beaman, J. H. (eds.): Plant dermatitis. *Clin. Dermatol.*, **4**(2):1–226, i–ix, 1986. This issue is devoted primarily to contact (allergic) dermatitis induced by plants. Approximately half of the text is devoted to poison ivy/oak and other Anacardiaceae.

Mitchell, J., and Rook, A.: *Botanical Dermatology: Plants and Plant Products Injurious to the Skin*. Greengrass, Vancouver, 1979. This is a worldwide encyclopedia with a bibliography provided individually for each species.

Stoner, J. G., and Rasmussen, J. E.: Plant dermatitis. *J. Am. Acad. Dermatol.*, **9**:1–15, 1983.

Hallucinogenic Plant Poisoning

Schultes, R. E., and Hofmann, A.: *Botany and Chemistry of Hallucinogens*, 2nd ed. Charles C. Thomas, Publ., Springfield, Ill., 1980. This is a definitive treatment of this selected subject.

Chronic Plant Poisoning

Liener, I. E. (ed.): *Toxic Constituents of Plants Foodstuffs*. Academic Press, Inc., New York, 1980.

Rechcigl, M., Jr., Inc., (ed.): *Handbook of Naturally Occurring Food Toxicants*. CRC Press, Boca Raton, Fla., 1983.

Toxicants Occuring Naturally in Foods, 2nd ed. National Academy of Sciences, Washington, D.C., 1973.

Important Foreign Sources on Plant and Mushroom Toxicology

Bresinsky, A., and Besl, H.: *Giftpilze mit einer einführung in die pilzbestimmung. Ein Handbuch für Apotheker, Ärzte und Biologen*. Wissenschaftliche Verlagsgesellschaft, Stuttgart, 1985. An extremely useful handbook with an exhaustive bibliography. Not available in English.

Chopra, R. N.; Badhwar, R. L.; and Ghosh, S.: *Poisonous Plants of India*, 2 vols. Indian Council of Agricultural Research, New Delhi, 1965.

Connor, H. E.: *Poisonous Plants in New Zealand*, 2nd ed. E. C. Keating, Wellington, 1977.

Everist, S. L.: *Poisonous Plants of Australia*, Angus & Robertson, Sydney, 1974.

Frohne, D., and Pfänder, H. J.: *A Color Atlas of Poisonous Plants: A Handbook for Pharmacists, Doctors, Toxicologists, and Biologists*. Wolfe House, London, 1983; translation from the 2nd German edition. An indispensable handbook with an extensive bibliography, particularly from European sources. The 3rd edition—*Giftpflanzen. Ein Handbuch für Apotheker, Ärzte, Toxicologen und Biologen*. Wissenschaftliche Verlagsgesellschaft, Stuttgart, 1987—is not available in English.

Hausen, B. M.: *Allergiepflanzen Pflanzenallergene. Handbuch und Atlas der Allergie-induzierenden Wild- und Kulturpflanzen*. Ecomed Verlagsgesellschaft, Landsberg, 1988. Similar in layout to Benezra *et al.*, (1985) (*see* comments under "Plant Dermatitis") but gives more comprehensive details on chemistry. Not available in English.

Watt, J. M., and Breyer-Brandwijk, M. G.: *Medicinal and Poisonous Plants of Southern and Eastern Africa*. E. & S. Livingstone, Edinburgh, 1962.

UNIT IV

ENVIRONMENTAL TOXICOLOGY

Chapter 24

FOOD ADDITIVES AND CONTAMINANTS

Sanford A. Miller

A major concern of individual humans and human societies has been and is the attainment of sufficient food to provide a healthful and productive life. Historically, the major expenditure of time and effort, on both an individual and societal basis, has been the pursuit of an adequate food supply. It is only after significant progress toward the attainment of this goal is realized that the energies of societies can be devoted to progress in other areas. In fact, a major impetus to the formation of groups and societies with individual interactivity has been the division of labor to allow certain segments of the population to pursue nonfood production tasks. As agricultural methodology developed and food-producing animals were domesticated, a smaller number of individuals were needed for direct food production, allowing not only the number of individuals within the group to increase, but also a diversification of skills within the group.

Seasonal climatic conditions resulted in an abundance of food during the harvest period, but inadequate food supplies during the remainder of the year. This placed a limit on the number of individuals a particular territory could support. To ensure an adequate food supply during nonagricultural productive periods, it was necessary to find methods to preserve the abundant food available at harvest and the game collected during the peak hunting periods. To meet this requirement, methods employing the addition of various substances to food were developed. Among the first substances added to food as preservatives were sodium chloride, which is still a major preservative, and smoke. Processes were developed by which various spices could be used not only to aid in the preservation of food but also to disguise the unacceptable flavor of inadequately preserved foods. The search for chemicals useful in preserving foods and increasing the palatability of preserved foods continues today. This practice has become more important as the percentage of the population in the United States involved in agricultural production has decreased to the present level of 5 percent, particularly when this division of labor is compared with the increases in population and the trend toward the development of large population centers.

Cultural mores also affect the types and amounts of various substances to be found in foods. A food that is considered a delicacy in one culture may be taboo in another. The acceptable appearance, color, texture, and flavor of a food are often defined by both experience and cultural tastes. The utilization of various substances during processing to maintain these organoleptic characteristics is therefore important in maintaining an acceptable food supply.

Over the last several decades, developed societies have undergone many lifestyle changes that have led to an increase in the addition of various substances to food for technologic purposes. Processed foods now represent over 50 percent of the American diet. For instance, the annual per capita consumption of fresh citrus fruits decreased from 32 to 28 lbs between 1960 and 1976, wheras consumption of processed fruit increased from 50 to 90 lbs. Soft-drink consumption more than doubled during the same time period (National Academy of Sciences, 1978). Several trends, such as the increased demand for "ready-to-eat" and snack foods, the population shift from rural to urban areas, the interest in ethnic foods, the demand for a constant, year-round supply of seasonal foods, and the demand for stable and low food prices have increased the utilization and need for the addition of various substances to food (President's Science Advisory Committee, 1973). The trend toward the increased use of various substances added for technologic purposes, countered by public demand for an essentially risk-free food supply, has increased the scientific and public debate over the safety of these materials when added to food. In addition, the development of toxicologic methodology with increased sensitivity has revealed the uncertainty inherent in such evaluations (Miller and Skinner, 1984). These factors have emphasized the necessity for informed, expert judgment in assuring a logical, rational, and scientific approach to the regulation of these materials in the food supply. Decisions in these areas not only impact on public health but also have economic impact on both the food industry and the consumer.

Practically any discussion of food additives and contaminants must be focused and limited of necessity. Certain areas of specific substances are not covered or discussed in detail. In many more cases, details are given in other chapters in this volume. It is the goal of this chapter to introduce the student to the basic concepts associated with the safety of food additives and contaminants with the hope that the student will pursue the area in more depth by consideration of other sources.

DEFINITIONS OF FOOD ADDITIVES

Chemicals that are added to food are generally termed "food additives." However, exactly what is meant by this term is a matter of perspective. Food additives may be defined in legalistic terms, in terms associated with their technical use, and in terms associated with consumer understanding. Therefore, it is important for the toxicologist to understand the meaning of these definitions to aid in the resolution of these controversies and to aid in consumer understanding of the benefits and risks associated with food additives.

LEGAL DEFINITION OF FOOD ADDITIVES

In the United States at the turn of the twentieth century, laws concerning the sanitary aspects and adulteration of foods were under the control of the individual states. Such laws lacked uniformity in context and enforcement. In the early 1900s Dr. Harvey W. Wiley, Director of the USDA Bureau of Chemistry, led the campaign for the passage and enforcement of uniform national laws concerned with food safety and protection against fraud. His various interests included the control of chemicals such as boric acid, salicylic acid, and saccharin as a sugar substitute. His efforts led to the passage, in 1906, of the Food and Drug Act and Meat Inspection Act. Generally, this first federal Act prohibited the addition of poisonous preservatives and dyes to food as well as prohibiting misbranded and adulterated foods and drinks in interstate commerce. As the food industry grew and became national based on increasingly complex technology, the original 1906 Food and Drug Act was found to be inadequate. In 1938, a new federal statute was passed, the Food, Drug,

and Cosmetic Act. This legislation has been expanded and amended several times, most notably in 1958, and 1962. The 1958 amendment contained two vital concepts: premarket approval and the Delaney anti-cancer clause which provided an absolute proscription to the approval of any substance "inducing" cancer in man or animal (for a more detailed discussion, see Miller and Taylor, 1989). The current legal definition of food additives also may be found within this legislation. The Federal Food, Drug, and Cosmetic Act, as amended in October 1976, Sec. 201(s) states:

The term 'food additive' means any substance the intended use of which results or may reasonably be expected to result, directly or indirectly, in its becoming a component or otherwise affecting the characteristics of any food (including any substance intended for use in producing, manufacturing, packing, processing, preparing, treating, packaging, transporting, or holding food: and including any source of radiation intended for any such use), if such substance is not generally recognized, among experts qualified by scientific training and experience to evaluate its safety, as having been adequately shown through scientific procedures (or, in the case of a substance used in food prior to January 1, 1958, through either scientific procedures or experience based on common use in food) to be safe under the conditions of its intended use: except that such term does not include:

(1) a pesticide chemical in or on a raw agricultural commodity; or

(2) a pesticide chemical to the extent that it is intended for use or is used in the production, storage, or transportation of any raw agricultural commodity; or

(3) a color additive; or

(4) any substance used in accordance with a sanction or approval granted prior to the enactment of this paragraph . . . pursuant to this Act, the Poultry Products Inspection Act . . . or the Meat Inspection Act; or

(5) a new animal drug.

The exemptions to the legal definition are covered by specific sections of the law and will be discussed below. Although the legal definition of food additives can be confusing, it was the result of congressional recognition that not all substances in food are equal and therefore required the application of different levels of acceptable risk depending on their importance in maintaining an adequate food supply.

TECHNICAL DEFINITION OF FOOD ADDITIVES

The technical definition of food additives is generally broader than the legal definition and can be exemplified by the definition utilized by the Food Protection Committee of the Food and Nutrition Board of the National Academy of Sciences: "A substance or mixture of substances other than a basic foodstuff which is present in a food as a result of any aspect of production, processing, storage, or packaging" (National Academy of Sciences, 1979). As in the legal definition, technically, food additives are divided into two major categories. Those substances that are intentionally added to a food directly during production, and so forth, for a functional purpose are termed "direct or intentional food additives." The second category consists of the "indirect or nonintentional food additives" that are not intentionally added to food, but result from either the environment of food production or processing and storage. According to this definition, a pesticide used during the agricultural production of food, machine oil from a processing machine, and a plasticizer that leaches from a package would all be considered indirect food additives. The concept of food contaminants is somewhat different from that of indirect additives. Although indirect additives may be considered as contaminants, thus blurring the dividing line between these two groups, a category of contaminants is nonetheless important from the aspect of food safety. Contaminants consist of those substances that may become a part of food during production, processing, and storage owing generally to natural processes. They include such substances as nitrate, selenium, and lead, which may be incorporated into plants grown in soil with unusually high levels of these chemicals; fungal metabolites produced from mold growth during production, processing, and storage; and bacteria and bacterial products. The products of food chemical reactions, such as oxidized lipids contained in cooking oil, may also be included in this category. Contaminants may be considered as a "catchall" category containing miscellaneous substances that are not included as direct and indirect additives.

CONSUMER PERCEPTIONS OF FOOD ADDITIVES

The consuming public does not appear to have a precise definition of food additives. Concern about food additives can be unpredictable and illogical. For instance, when the artificial sweetener saccharin was to be banned because of its potential carcinogenicity, there was a public outcry for its continued use in soft drinks and other foods (Anon., 1978). In contrast, there appears to be a general fear of very low levels of pesticide residues in food, even though through the use of pesticides there may be a greater availability of food at lower cost. Public attitudes appear to shift between concern and apathy about food additives depending on the activity of consumer activist groups and the media. Other factors contributing to public concern about food additives include the expanded labeling information on food products, governmental action in this area, and continuing scientific controversies concerning specific additives such as nitrite and saccharin. Adding additional impetus to these concerns are the "back-to-nature" groups, which exhort the benefits of natural foods grown with organic fertilizers and containing no "additives" and their claims of the adverse effects of foods containing additives and "artificial" nutritional supplements. The public concern about food additives is continuing as evidenced by discussions in the popular press and other media. Recently, computer programs have become available that allow the consumer not only to undertake nutrient analyses, but also to estimate the content of food additives. It is obviously important that the public receive adequate information on the benefits as well as the risks from food additives.

UTILIZATION OF DIRECT (INTENTIONAL) FOOD ADDITIVES

As previously discussed, the use of direct food additives predates recorded history when meats and fish were smoked and salted for preservation. The Romans made extensive use of salt as a preservative and, until recently, the use of potassium nitrate (saltpeter) was widespread. Also, during the Middle Ages spices from the Orient became an important category of food additives and were used not only to alter and enhance the flavor of certain foods, but also to preserve food and disguise the flavor of spoiled foods (Tannahill, 1973).

The fledgling food industry developed as part of the industrial revolution in the latter half of the nineteenth century. The availability of roads and improved transportation and the development of highly populated industrial centers were as important to the development of the food industry as was the development of processing equipment. It was equally true that the development of a food industry permitted the growth of urban centers. It also brought with it, on the one hand, the increased adulteration of food and on the other hand, an increase in the use of various additives. Certain of these, such as acorns in coffee and brick dust in cocoa were added as filler to increase profits. Others represented significant health risk, such as the use of copper and lead salts to color foods such as candy, cheeses, and vegetables (Tannahill, 1973). The practice of food adulteration became so widespread that in the early nineteenth century it was one of the first subjects to be placed under the increasingly critical gaze of the analytical chemist. The publication in England in 1820 of Frederick Accum's book, *A Treatise on Adulteration of Food and Culinary Poisons,* made the public aware of what was already known in the industry and government. Accum presented for the first time a scientific way of detecting such adulteration and thus provided the basis for an enforceable food safety law. Such a law was passed in Great Britain in 1860 and revised and strengthened in 1872. It was on this foundation that the 1906 U.S. Food and Drug Act was built (Miller and Taylor, 1989).

Currently there may be as many as 2800 substances approved for use as direct food additives (Lehmann, 1979). The vast majority of these additives are used in trace amounts and only a few are used in large quantities. The FDA has estimated that sucrose, corn syrup, dextrose, and salt represent 93 percent, by weight, of the total food additives used. The inclusions of black pepper, caramel, carbon dioxide, citric acid, modified starch, sodium bicarbonate, yeasts, and yellow mustard brings this figure up to 95 percent (Larkin, 1976).

MAIN GROUPS

The direct food additives are utilized by the food industry for a variety of technical effects. Below are listed the five main groups of direct food additives and the various categories of additives within each major group.

Processing Aids

These additives are intended to aid in the processing of foods during production and after purchase by the consumer and are exemplified by anticaking agents, dough conditioners, drying agents, emulsifiers, various enzymes, flour-treating agents, formulation aids, humectants, leavening agents, lubricants, pH control agents, solvents and vehicles, surface-active agents, and various synergists.

Texturing Agents

These additives are provided to give specific foods a desirable consistency and texture and include various enzymes, firming agents, formulation aids and binders, stabilizers and thickeners, aerating agents, and texturizers.

Preservatives

These additives are utilized to decrease the rate of degradation of foods during processing and storage such as antioxidants, curing and pickling agents, antibacterials, gases, and sequestrants that react with various food components, i.e., metals that help maintain stability.

Flavoring and Appearance Agents

These additives are used either to enhance existing flavors or to add flavor to foods, and to improve the appearance, and include flavor enhancers, flavoring agents, nonnutritive sweeteners, and surface-finishing agents such as waxes.

Nutritional Supplements

These additives include the required nutrients and are added either to replace those lost during processing or to supplement existing levels of nutrients. They may consist of varied analogues of macronutrients and micronutrients, including vitamins and trace minerals.

The colors have been purposefully excluded from this listing because they are regulated as a separate group and will be discussed later.

The various additives within these major groups vary from simple salts, such as sodium chloride, to complex biologic polymers, such as starches, and various synthetic chemicals, such as ethyl vanillin. A partial listing of some of these agents is given in Table 24–1 to illustrate the diversity of chemicals utilized as food additives.

STANDARDIZATION

As can be seen, the direct food additives consist of a diverse grouping of chemical substances. One of the first problems encountered in a discussion of specific additives, especially the natural products of biologic origin, is exactly what are we talking about? This may seem like a simple question, but when one considers the potential composition of a complex biologic product such as gum arabic, which may contain various biologic molecules that coextract with the desired product and the variable composition of a natural additive as the source and manufacturer of the additive varies, the question becomes quite complex. This also can be a problem, although of lesser extent, with the synthetic additives, which may contain variable impurities depending on the manufacturing process. To overcome these problems and to introduce specific specifications to ensure the purity and uniformity of food additives, the U.S. Food and Drug Administration requires information on the physical, chemical, biologic, and purity characteristics as well as the source and method of manufacturing. As standards for food grade additives, the FDA relies on either specifications written into its own regulations or those listed in the Food Chemicals Codex. The Food Chemicals Codex is a compilation of specifications for food-grade products used as food additives compiled by the Committee on Food Protection of

Table 24–1. SELECTED FOOD ADDITIVES*

Anticaking Agents

Aluminum calcium silicate
Sodium aluminosilicate
Sodium calcium aluminosilicate

Chemical Preservatives

Ascorbic acid
Ascorbyl palmitate
Butylated hydroxyanisole
Calcium propionate
Dilauryl thiodipropionate
Erythorbic acid
Methylparaben
Potassium sorbate
Propionic acid
Propylparaben
Sodium bisulfite
Sodium metabisulfite
Sodium sulfite
Stannous chloride
Sulfur dioxide
Tocopherols

Emulsifying Agents

Cholic acid
Desoxycholic acid
Glycocholic acid
Mono- and diglycerides
Propylene glycol
Ox bile extract

Nutrients and Dietary Supplements

Alanine
Arginine
Aspartic acid
Biotin
Calcium citrate
Calcium pantothenate
Carotene
Choline chloride
Copper gluconate
Cysteine
Cystine
Ferric pyrophosphate
Ferrous lactate
Histidine
Inositol
Isoleucine
Leucine
Lysine
Magnesium oxide
Manganese gluconate
Manganous oxide
Methionine
Niacinamide
d-Pantothenyl alcohol
Potassium glycerophosphate
Proline
Pyridoxine hydrochloride
Riboflavin-5-phosphate
Serine
Sorbitol

Thiamine mononitrate
Threonine
Tocopherol acetate
Tryptophane
Valine
Vitamin A
Vitamin B_{12}
Vitamin D_3
Zinc sulfate

Sequestrants

Calcium acetate
Calcium gluconate
Calcium phytate
Dipotassium phosphate
Disodium phosphate
Monoisopyropyl citrate
Potassium citrate
Sodium diacetate
Sodium hexametaphosphate
Sodium metaphosphate
Sodium potassium tartrate
Sodium pyrophosphate
Sodium tartrate
Sodium thiosulfate
Stearyl citrate
Tartaric acid

Stabilizers

Acacia (gum arabic)
Agar-agar
Calcium alginate
Carob bean gum
Ghatti gum
Guar gum
Sterculia (or Karaya) gum

Miscellaneous Additives

Acetic acid
Adipic acid
Aluminum potassium sulfate
Ammonium bicarbonate
Bentonite
Butane
Calcium gluconate
Calcium hydroxide
Calcium phosphate
Carnauba wax
Dextrans
Ethyl formate
Glutamic acid hydrochloride
Glycerin
Helium
Hydrochloric acid
Lactic acid
Lecithin
Magnesium hydroxide
Malic acid
Methylcellulose
Monopotassium glutamate
Nitrogen
Papain

Table 24–1.   (*continued*)

Phosphoric acid	*Synthetic Flavoring Substances*
Potassium hydroxide	
Propylene glycol	Acetaldehyde
Rennet	Acetoin
Sodium acid pyrophosphate	Benzaldehyde
Sodium carboxymethylcellulose	*d*- or *l*-carvone
Sodium caseinate	Cinnamaldehyde
Sodium hydroxide	Decanal
Sodium pectinate	Ethyl butyrate
Sodium sesquicarbonate	Geraniol
Succinic acid	Geranyl acetate
Sulfuric acid	Limonene
Triacetine	Linalool
Triethyl citrate	Methylanthranilate
	Piperonal
	Vanillin

*Modified from Kilgore, W. W., and Li, M. Y.: Food additives and contaminants. In Doull, F.: Klaassen, C. D.; and Amdur, M. O. (eds.); *Casarett and Doull's Toxicology: The Basic Science of Poisons*, 2nd ed. Macmillan, New York, 1980. pp. 599–600.

the National Academy of Sciences (National Academy of Sciences, 1972). These specifications ensure uniform standardization of food additives manufactured and utilized by different food processors, thus providing a substantial measure of assurance of food quality and safety.

UTILIZATION OF INDIRECT (NONINTENTIONAL) FOOD ADDITIVES

Indirect food additives consist of substances that are not natural constituents of food and have not been added to food for a technologic purpose. These substances may become a constituent of food from a variety of sources, including the environment in which the food is produced, during processing and storage at manufacturing sites, and during subsequent packaging and storage. The total number of substances is unknown and may rapidly change as processing technologies change. The National Science Foundation (1973) has estimated that food packaging may contribute close to 3000 substances to the indirect additive category. A major aim of both the food production industry and the regulatory agencies is to decrease the number of indirect additives in food and to ensure that those that cannot be eliminated are present at levels that do not represent a risk to consumers.

Table 24–2 lists potential sources of indirect food additives and examples of substances found at each source. Several of these are discussed in other chapters of this text, whereas others, such as processing aids, are well known only to food technologists and packaging experts.

UTILIZATION OF ANIMAL DRUGS

Drugs are employed in food-producing animals for two major purposes: veterinary pharmaceuticals and feed additives. These compounds represent a wide diversity in chemical structure and biologic activity. They differ from food additives in that they are designed to be pharmaceutically active in the consuming animal. Both types of drugs have the potential to become incorporated into animal products and tissues destined for human consumption. Thus their risk to human health must be evaluated (Committee on Animal Health, 1980).

With respect to potential exposure to consumers, the veterinary pharmaceuticals used to treat specific animal diseases generally represent a lower potential for exposure than feed additives. These agents are normally used for specific animals, and their use is sporadic. This increases the opportunity for clearance from the animal before marketing. Although products produced by animals undergoing treatment may contain drug residues, it is generally simple and of little economic loss to withhold these products during the treatment period. In terms of total usage, veterinary pharmaceuticals are not used as frequently as the feed additives, thereby presenting less potential for routine human exposure.

The case is quite different with respect to drugs utilized as feed additives. In 1979, it was estimated that nearly 100 percent of poultry, 90 percent of swine and veal calves, and 60 percent of cattle received feed supplemented with antibacterials, and 70 percent of the beef cattle produced in the United States received growth-promoting drugs to increase weight gain (Office of Technology Assessment, 1979). At least 80 percent of the animal protein consumed in the

Table 24–2. SOURCES OF NONINTENTIONAL ADDITIVES OF POSSIBLE TOXICOLOGIC SIGNIFICANCE*

During Production
1. Antibiotics and other agents used for prevention and control of disease
2. Growth-promoting substances
3. Microorganisms of toxicologic significance
4. Parasitic organisms
5. Pesticides residues (insecticides, fungicides, herbicides, etc.)
6. Toxic metals and metallic compounds
7. Radioactive compounds

During Processing
1. Microorganisms and their toxic metabolites
2. Processing residues and miscellaneous foreign objects
3. Radionuclides

During Packaging and Storage
1. Labeling and stamping materials
2. Microorganisms and their toxic metabolites
3. Migrants from packaging materials
4. Toxic chemicals from external sources

* Modified from Kilgore, W. W., and Li, M. Y.: Food additives and contaminants. In Doull, J.; Klaassen, C. D.; and Amdur, M. O. (eds.): *Casarett and Doull's Toxicology: The Basic Science of Poisons.* Macmillan, New York, 1980. pp. 593–607.

American diet comes from animals exposed to medicated feeds for at least part of their lives (President's Science Advisory Committee, 1973). These drugs are important in maintaining the production levels of animal products and tissues at a cost that ensures their availability to the consumer and also in maintaining the quality of these products. However, along with the benefits afforded by animal drugs is the risk of potential toxicity associated with consumption of drug residues in animal products and tissue.

A unique problem in the determination of the potential human health hazards associated with animal drugs is the probability that animal metabolism will modify the molecular structure and toxicity of the drug (Hayes and Borzelleca, 1982). As previously discussed in Chapter 4, animals have the capacity to biotransform drugs to a large number of metabolites with diverse molecular structures and toxicity. The cytochrome P-450-dependent monooxygenase systems generally convert drugs to oxidized products, which may demonstrate decreased toxicity as a result of their increased water solubility. The transferase enzymes conjugate the drug and/or its metabolites with endogenous molecules and increase their excretability and modify their structure to produce products that are generally less toxic. However, these same enzymes may convert drugs and other xenobiotics to products

that demonstrate increased biologic activity and toxicity. In some instances products of these reactions possess sufficient reactivity to bind covalently to tissue macromolecules. Animal products and tissues may therefore contain not only the parent drug, but also metabolites including both conjugated and nonconjugated forms and residues that are either rigidly bound or covalently bound to tissue macromolecules. Although it might be assumed that the animal usually acts as a "predetoxication" system for these drug residues, this is not always the case. These drug metabolites, after consumption, may still be converted into more toxic products. For example, if a drug is present as the detoxified glucuronide conjugate in the animal products, it may subsequently be hydrolyzed by the consumer's intestinal microfloral β-glucuronidase, thus freeing the original drug metabolite for absorption. The quantity of drug residues in a particular product or tissue will depend on their pharmacokinetic characteristics within the consuming animal. The absorption and retention of these residues in the tissues of consumers will subsequently be dependent on their pharmacokinetic characteristics within the consuming human.

Most mutagenicity and carcinogenicity is thought to result from highly reactive electrophilic metabolites of less biologically active parent compounds. It might be assumed that these activated metabolites would be a serious threat as tissue residues. However, this is probably not the case. The high reactivity and short half-lives of these metabolites would result in little chance of encountering them in animal products owing to their rapid covalent binding to tissue macromolecules. Even if they existed in the animal at the time it was killed, they would either spontaneously decompose or interact with nucleophilic sites during processing and storage. Activated metabolites that have become covalently bound to tissue macromolecules would, in most instances, represent little human health hazard because the covalent binding alters their structure and subsequent digestion of the macromolecular fractions would not release these compounds in an activated form. For example, the feeding to rats of hepatic macromolecular fractions obtained from rats fed aflatoxin B_1 and containing covalent adducts of aflatoxin B_1 produced no evidence of the production of adducts in the second set of rats (Jaggi *et al.*, 1980).

It would be extremely rare to encounter drug residues in animal products and tissues at concentrations that are high enough to elicit acutely toxic symptoms in the consumer. However, residue levels sufficient to produce chronic toxicity could be encountered. Because carcinogenicity is the type of chronic toxicity of most concern, the section of the Food, Drug, and Cosmetic Act concerning animal feed additives contains its own "Delaney Clause." This prohibits approval of a new animal drug if it "induces cancer when ingested by man or animal." The act continues by adding "unless no residue of such drug will be found (by methods of examination prescribed or approved by the Secretary . . .), in any edible portion of such animals after slaughter or in any food yielded by or derived from the living animals." Therefore, it is possible to use drugs in animals that have been shown to be carcinogenic as long as no detectable residues occur in animal products or tissues. Withholding animals and animal products from market for specific periods during and after drug treatment to allow for dissipation of the drug from the animal body appeared to solve the problem encountered with certain drugs, such as the growth promoter diethylstilbesterol. However, continued improvements in analytic methodology have allowed the detection of decreasing quantities of drug residues in animal tissues. It also seems likely that the sensitivity of analysis will continue to increase and regulation might continue to "chase zero." In 1973, the FDA proposed regulations further defining the no-residue requirement, which was, of course, based on the existing methodology at that time. This proposal has now been replaced by a new proposal that was issued in 1979 and that interprets the regulation according to "sensitivity of method." This proposal is based on the more realistic concept that, because absolute food safety and absolute zero (in residue terms) is impossible, the determination of allowable residue levels should be based on a negligible lifetime risk of cancer in humans as, for example, with an estimate of one chance in a million. The methodology is then selected to estimate drug residues associated with this negligible risk level. As analytic methods are improved to detect still lower residue levels, it is therefore not necessary to alter the regulations concerning specific drug residues. This argument avoids the controversy of what type of benefit is acceptable. Because benefit evaluation is extraordinarily complex, confusing, and controversial, it would require a much more extensive discussion than possible for this chapter. A discussion of benefit-risk analysis associated with food chemicals can be found in the article by Campbell (1980).

The use of antibiotics as animal feed additives involves a new concern not related to toxicologic response. Antibiotics are added to animal food as a prophylaxis against disease and, as such, appear to promote the growth of animals. Almost all poultry in the United States and a large percentage of cattle and swine are fed feeds containing antibiotics. These antibiotics may become residues in animal products and tissues. The concern expressed by some is the possibility that their use will lead to the development of antibiotic-resistant strains of bacteria, thus eroding the ability of specific antibiotics to be of use in the treatment of human disease (National Academy of Sciences, 1980). The FDA has proposed that the prophylactic use of the penicillins in animal feeds be stopped and the tetracyclines be used only where there are no substitutes.

UTILIZATION OF FOOD COLORS

Nature abounds in color and, as a result, human foods generally are colorful. Certain foods are recognized not only by their shape and texture, but also by their color. In many instances the quality and acceptability of a food are judged not only by texture, taste, and smell but also by color. If a food that society and experience have defined as having a particular color, hue, and intensity lacks these characteristics, it will be unacceptable, even if wholesome. Colors also make food more interesting and appealing, as evidenced by colored confections and drinks.

The use of both natural and synthetic colors to enhance, alter, and produce expected and appealing colors in foods dates far back in history. The Egyptians utilized colors in candy, and Pliny the elder discussed artificially colored wines around 400 B.C. Historically, the major problem associated with food colors has been their use to deceive potential consumers as to the quality of the food and the toxic nature of certain color agents. For instance, in the eighteenth century copper sulfate was used to color pickles green; cheeses were colored with vermillion (HgS) and red lead; used tea leaves were dyed for resale with agents such as copper arsenite, lead chromate, and indigo; and candies were dyed with lead chromate and carbonate as well as red lead and vermillion. At the turn of the century in England, milk was tinted yellow to prevent the detection of skimming and watering. The practice was so widespread that the public refused to purchase untinted milk for fear that it was adulterated. In 1925, the tinting of milk was made illegal in Britain, long after the 1396 edict in Paris banning the tinting of butter. The major sources of dyes for food coloring were natural biologic pigments and various-colored mineral salts until the advent of synthetic dyes in the mid-eighteenth century. At the turn of the century, many of the synthetic dyes were being used in a large number of foods to produce the desired color. These dyes were blended in various ways to produce assorted hues and intensities. Various dyes of the same hue were employed because a single dye does not always produce the same effect in different foods.

Although the use of colors in food had been sporadically regulated, the first attempt at developing systematic regulations on the use of dyes in food was initiated by the U.S. Department of Agriculture. The responsibility for determining the usage of public health risk of the synthetic dyes was given to Dr. Bernhard C. Hesse. He found that, of the 695 coal-tar dyes on the market at that time, only 80 were used as food colors. After consideration of the available literature on the toxicity of the compounds and the needs of the food industry, Hesse selected the following seven dyes for food use: amaranth (Red 2), erythrosine (Red 3), indigo disulfonic acid (Blue 2), light green SF yellowish (Green 2), naphthol yellow S (Yellow 1), ponceau 3R (Red 1), and Orange 1 (Red 1). (The notations following the dyes are the FDA denotations given the dyes in 1938). Other colors and various hues and intensities were obtained by combinations of these seven compounds. These dyes were recognized under the Pure Food and Drug Act of 1906, and dyes could be certified (chemically tested) by the Secretary of Agriculture on a voluntary basis. Between 1916 and 1929 ten additional colors were added to the approved list. The Federal Food, Drug, and Cosmetic Act of 1938 required that all food colors be "harmless" and listed those coal-tar derived colors approved for food use as well as specifications as to manufacture, certification, and sale. In the early 1950s the FDA initiated a series of toxicity studies and the term "harmless" was refined to mean the color would produce no "harm" to test animals in any quantity and under any conditions. This led to the banning of eight FDC colors between 1956 and 1960 and the realization that this interpretation would result in the banning of all food colors and was toxicologically unsound. Passage of the Color Additive Amendments of 1960 to the Food and Drug Act allowed the FDA to overcome this problem by setting safe levels or tolerances on the quantity of color used in foods. The amendments also brought all synthetic colors under the provisions of the law, not just the coal-tar-derived colors. They required that all new colors undergo premarketing toxicity testing and allowed the FDA to require new testing of previously approved colors if any questions concerning their safety arose. A safety factor of 100 to 1 was suggested in extrapolating no-adverse-effects levels obtained in animals studies to humans. Provisional certification was given to those colors in use pending more comprehensive toxicity testing. More recently, as a result of litigation and legal opinion, the FDA has determined that the provisional-listing status of the food colors is to be eliminated. This means that a color must either be permanently listed or prohibited from use. The FDA has asked industry to retest all the approved food colors. These studies are currently nearing completion and should clarify the future use of food colors and will result in the colors being the most intensely tested group of additives.

Utilization of food colors is still controversial with certain groups claiming that synthetic colors should not be added to foods because they serve no purpose other than the aesthetic and increase the human xenobiotic burden. On the other hand, others feel that the aesthetic values of color use far outweigh any supposed risk. For instance, a colorless grape-flavored drink would lose much of its appeal, and margarine the color of lard would be less appetizing. There is little question that the use of colors increases the appeal of certain foods, and as long as food is judged visually, the use of colors will be important.

Colors are added to foods during processing for several reasons including (1) the addition of color when the food has no color of its own, such as in gelatins, candies, and certain beverages; (2) when the natural color of a food is lost during processing and storage; (3) when the natural color of a food varies with respect to season and geography, such as dairy products and oranges; and (4) to correlate foods with certain flavors and increase their attractiveness, thereby increasing their aesthetic value.

Although the synthetic food colors have received the majority of public, scientific, and regulatory attention, the natural color agents are receiving increased attention. Currently, approximately 25 color additives have been given exemption from certification in Part 73 of the Code of Federal Regulations. These agents consist of a variety of natural and a few synthetic compounds generally obtained by various extraction and treatment technologies and in a few cases by chemical synthesis. Comprising this group of colors are preparations such as dried algae meal, beet powder, grape skin extract, fruit juice, paprika, caramel, carrot oil, cochineal extract, ferrous gluconate, and iron oxide. A problem encountered in attempts to regulate these additives is the lack of a precise chemical definition of many of these preparations. For instance, cochineal extract is defined as the aqueous-alcoholic extract of the scale insect *Daetylopius coccus costa*. The females of this species contain a bright-red body fluid containing high levels of carminic acid. With a few exceptions, such as caramel, actually the most widely used color, the natural colors have not been heavily used. In part, this may be due to economic reasons, but these colors generally do not have the uniformity and intensity of color characteristic of the synthetic colors, therefore necessitating higher concentrations to obtain a specific color intensity. They also lack the chemical and color stability of the synthetic colors and have a tendency to fade with time.

Although intake varies among individuals, the maximal intake of food colors is estimated to be approximately 53.5 mg/day, whereas the average intake per day is approximately 15 mg (Committee on Food Protection, 1971). Only about 10 percent of food consumed in the United States contains food colors. Those foods that utilize food colors in order of quantity of color utilized are: (1) beverages; (2) candy and confections; (3) dessert powders; (4) bakery goods; (5) sausage (casing only); (6) cereals; (7) ice cream; (8) snack foods; and (9) gravies, jams, jellies, and so forth (Committee on Food Protection, 1971). Controversies over the utilization of food colors will continue, even if toxicologic studies prove as conclusively (as currently possible) that they have little potential for harm when utilized according to good manufacturing practices. With the exception of certain dairy products, the inclusion of artificial colors in foods must be listed on the label, giving the consumer the option of either using or not using the food product.

OCCURRENCE OF PESTICIDES IN FOODS

Pesticides are not added directly to foods, but may indirectly become components of food. The use of pesticides is an important contributing factor to the agricultural revolution, resulting in an increased quantity and quality of food. Associated with the benefits from their use are the risk of adverse health effects from residues that may become components of the food supply. Pesticides can occur not only in plant materials destined for human and animal consumption, but also in animal products and tissues. Major sources of pesticides in the food supply are derived from their use in protecting plants from pest damage during both growth and storage. Residues may also appear in animal products and tissues from animals fed feeds contaminated with pesticides. A more extensive discussion of pesticides can be found in Chapter 18.

Section 408 of the Food, Drug, and Cosmetic Act sets forth regulations for "tolerances for pesticide chemicals in or on raw agricultural commodities." Pesticides can be regulated in one of three ways: (1) a total ban on the use of a particular pesticide and zero residue levels in foods; (2) tolerances that are acceptable in foods; and (3) action levels stipulating the maximal level that can occur in food. Because tolerances are generally given only to substances whose allowable levels will probably not be changed in the near future, pesticides are generally regulated as action levels. To set action levels, regulators must consider not only the quantities of a specific pesticide that may occur in food, but also the quantities that may come from other environmental sources. A benefit-risk analysis is also required for the determination of action levels.

As with animal drugs, the major consideration in the regulation of pesticides is their potential carcinogenicity. That concern is relevant because low level of consumption is the usual manner in which chemical carcinogens elicit their effects. However, pesticide residues in food are very low and do not appear to present such a risk (FDA, 1988). Acute toxicity from the consumption of food contaminated with pesticides is rare. Such effects are produced primarily from the careless or accidental use of pesticides.

REGULATION OF FOOD ADDITIVES

A comprehensive discussion of the regulations involved with the use of food additives is well beyond the scope of this chapter and has been reviewed in detail elsewhere (Brown, 1989; Miller and Taylor, 1989). Only a minimal discussion of the regulations is therefore provided.

As previously mentioned, the first national law concerning food safety was provided by the Pure Food and Drug Act of 1906. In 1938, the Act was revamped by Congress as the Food, Drug, and Cosmetic Act. In 1954, the Miller Pesticides Amendment, which controlled the requirements for setting safety limits for pesticide residues on raw agricultural commodities, was passed. In 1958, the Food Additive Amendment (Public Law 85-929) was added. As indicated earlier, this new amendment forbade the utilization of a substance as a food additive until the petitioner, or sponsor, provided evidence for this safety and the FDA specified the conditions for use of the substance as a food additive. This amendment also states that only the minimal quantity of a food additive that is needed to produce the desired technologic effect can be added to food and no additive that could result in consumer deception can be added.

Another clause of the 1958 Amendment (often called the Delaney Amendment) deals with food additives that may be carcinogenic. The so-called Delaney Clause states: "That no additive shall be deemed to be safe if it is found to induce cancer when ingested by man or animal, or if it is found, after tests which are appropriate for the evaluation of the safety of food additives, to induce cancer in man or animal . . ." (Federal Food, Drug and Cosmetic Act, Section 109 [c][3][A]). As the molecular mechanisms associated with chemical carcinogenesis have begun to be uncovered, it has now become clear that the clause is oversimplistic. Criticisms have been heard from both the scientific and regulatory communities. The controversial aspects of this clause will be discussed in a later section of this chapter.

As can be seen by referring to the quotation from the Act on p. 820, not only are pesticides excluded from this regulation but so are color additives. Colors are regulated under the Color Additives Amendment enacted in 1960. The regulation of color additives in foods, drugs, and cosmetics has been discussed in a separate section. Another exemption is "new animal drugs," as previously discussed.

An extremely important aspect of the 1958 Food, Drug and Cosmetic Act was the "grandfather clause," which exempted the vast majority of food additives in use at that time. Unlike food additives proposed after the 1958 Act, wherein safety must be proven by toxicologic testing, those compounds in use before the passage of the Act could be used based on: (1) "experience based on common use in food"; (2) "having been shown through scientific procedures" (to be nonhazardous); and (3) if a substance has been deemed "generally recognized, among experts qualified by scientific training and experience to evaluate its safety . . . to be safe under the conditions of its intended use." The substances that were "grandfathered" have been placed in a category referred to as "generally regarded as safe," and are generally referred to as GRAS. GRAS substances were collectively approved and approval could only be disallowed if the FDA itself demonstrated that they had the potential to be hazardous in their intended use as food additives. The impetus thus remained with the FDA to prove the compounds were hazardous as opposed to the new requirement for food additives that the sponsor or manufacturer prove them nonhazardous. This is an important distinction and can be responsible for considerable misunderstanding. Beginning in 1959 and 1960, the FDA published a list of over 600 substances considered GRAS and noted that this list was not exhaustive. Substances can be added to the GRAS list with FDA agreement. Owing to the importance of the category from the aspects of both quantity used and total number of substances, the GRAS substances will be discussed in a separate section.

As food has assumed an ever-increasing importance in world trade, conflicts over food additives have arisen. Additives that may be permissible in one country may be banned in another. Most countries now have laws governing food safety, which are often based on, but not identical to, those of the United States and Great Britain. To assist and encourage food trade among nations, several international agencies are involved in the complex task of reconciling the laws associated with food additives among international trading partners (Miller, 1990). A Joint Expert Committee on Food Additives was formed in 1954 under the auspices of the Food and Agriculture Organization (FAO) and the World Health Organization (WHO) with assistance from the United Nations. The joint FAO/WHO committee has used the approach of determining an accepted daily intake (ADI) for food additives. The ADI represents a level of daily intake that should result in no health hazard from a particular food additive. Because of differences in food habits and availability of specific foods in different countries, the intake of a specific food may vary significantly from nation to nation, making assessment of total intake difficult. To assist in the determination of potential dietary intake of food additives in various nations, the FAO/WHO Codex Alimentarius Commission attempts to determine the national intake of foods containing various additives. A particular food additive may be assigned either an unconditional ADI, a conditional ADI, or a temporary ADI, depending on the quality of the data supporting its safety evaluation when used as intended. The decisions of the FAO/WHO Commission are not legally binding to the member nations and therefore compliance is not mandatory; it is only recommended. Smaller groups of nations have joined together in attempts to unify the food additive legislation of member nations. At the current time, the European economic community is working towards complete harmonization of their food safety regulations in anticipation of European Confederation in 1992.

One of the major problems of international trade is the use of food safety regulations as nontariff trade barriers. To counter this trend, it has been proposed that JECFA, IMPR, JCAD, and Codex function as arbitrators of scientific dispute involving food safety. This issue is now under discussion.

FUTURE TRENDS IN REGULATION OF CARCINOGENS

Earlier, it was stated that considerable controversy has arisen concerning the Delaney Clause to the 1958 Amendment to the Federal

Food, Drug, and Cosmetic Act (Section 409 [c][3][A]). This section of the Act prohibits the addition of any substance that has been shown to ". . . induce cancer . . . in man or animal . . ." The apparent rigidity in this regulation has been criticized both within the scientific community and within the industries whose products are under this clause. Criticism has become particularly outspoken as the complexities of the carcinogenesis process become better understood.

In general, "proof" of carcinogenic activity has been obtained by feeding experimental animals (usually rats and/or mice of both sexes) doses of the test chemical for a two-year period increasing to a maximum tolerated dose (MTD). As with any chronic toxicity test, records are kept on growth, feed intake, and general health until the animals are killed at the termination of the study. In particular, data are obtained on tumor development. These data may be expressed as percent of tumor-bearing animals, numbers of tumors per animal, time to tumor development, size of tumors, and type of tumor tissue. When a statistically significant increase in tumor activity in the test animals is produced, possible "carcinogenicity" may be established. This conclusion is greatly strengthened if there is a good dose-response relationship and if the tumors are unique when compared with the yield of tumors "spontaneously" arising in the control animals. Supporting data from other types of studies may include the presence of mutagenic activity or evidence of increased cancer risk in exposed humans. Whereas the experimental animal bioassay was originally thought to be straightforward, the fact that cancer is now known to be a multifactorial, multistaged, and multimechanistic disease raises important questions as to which of the multiple factors are most relevant for estimated tumor potential and, therefore, which of these factors should be regulated in a fashion as rigorous as the Delaney Clause stipulates. When chemicals are shown to be mutagenic, form covalent adducts with DNA *in vivo*, and induce cancer in a dose-dependent manner in animals, they are generally regarded as animal carcinogens because they initiate the disease. However, the dose-response relationship may be readily altered when the intake of factors modifying the progression of the disease (promoters and inhibitors) are altered. In fact, recent research has shown that these promoters and inhibitors may be considerably more important as risk determinants than is the dose of the initiator. The use of certain promotion stimuli may even increase tumor yield when no initiators are given. For example, feeding a diet high in protein or calories may increase the incidence of "spontaneous" tumors whose initiating factors

are not known. Thus, if an experiment is designed to test for the "carcinogenicity" of protein or calories, the conclusion that must be drawn—according to the Delaney Clause—is that these nutrients are "carcinogenic." This is, in essence, the *ad absurdum* point of the Delaney clause.

Other concerns that confound a strict interpretation of the Delaney Clause are that (1) for many carcinogens, it is virtually impossible to eliminate every trace of the "carcinogen" without banning food, (2) an inconsistency exists between the regulation of direct additives and indirect additives and other adventitious residues, and (3) the resources devoted to imposition of the Clause for varying substances may not correlate with priorities based on public health relevance. Perhaps one of the most serious concerns is the fact that traditional bioassays in rats and mice may yield data that cannot be directly extrapolated to humans. It is this issue that lies at the heart of the quantitative risk assessment (QRA) controversy. For example, Campbell (1980) has stated that QRA is ineffective in interpolating high dose to low. In contrast, others (National Academy of Sciences, 1983a) argue that, with all of its weaknesses, it still offers the most objective *a priori* evaluations of human risk.

QUANTITATIVE RISK ASSESSMENT

The process of QRA has four distinct steps (National Academy of Sciences, 1983b). These are hazard analysis in which a decision must be made about the quality of the animal study and the interpretation and evaluation of the pathology, toxicology, and the statistics of the studies. For purposes of QRA for carcinogens, the ultimate question that must be asked is whether the tested chemical is a carcinogen and which organ tissue and cellular site was induced.

The second step in the process involves establishing the relationship between the doses of test substance to which the animals were exposed and the degree of response observed. The establishment of a dose-response curve is essential to develop a mathematical model to extrapolate the dose-response curve to dose levels equivalent to human exposure.

The third step, determination of exposure, is probably the most difficult. On the surface it appears simple, but it is not often that exposure distribution data are available on the variety of subpopulations that may be particularly at risk. Moreover, the most significant exposure is that at the active site, a measurement not yet state of the art.

The fourth step is generally referred to as risk characterization and involves merging of the animal data with extrapolation to human exposure levels directed toward the assessment or more correctly the estimate of the risk of cancer to exposed human populations.

The cancer issue is a particularly vexing one and, not surprisingly, as indicated earlier, disputes over the meaning of QRA are often emotional and deal more with political, social, and economic issues rather than with science. The problem is that we simply do not know some of the most important mechanisms in cancer induction. For example, we do not know if thresholds exist for carcinogens. Nevertheless, there is substantial evidence to believe that cancer induction, as in other forms of toxicity, is dose dependent. It is important to stress that clear dose dependency depends on everything else in an experiment being held constant except the test compound. Although this may sound simple, it is often anything but simple. The test compound can, for instance, make the food unpalatable, leading to undernutrition. The test compound can cause secondary effects such as bladder irritation which are known or suspected to produce cancer in their own right, thereby confusing the interpretation of the outcome of the experiment (Flamm, 1989).

Because cancer does not occur immediately following exposure and often requires many months or even years for evidence of its existence to surface, the relationship between exposure and the event is not simple and is in fact enormously complex. As a result, regulatory agencies charged with the responsibility of assuring the safety of the food supply have embraced the concept of quantitative risk assessment to provide a basis on which policy decisions can be made. The problem is that QRA is a process that, at this time, depends in large measure on assumptions, many of which are not subject to proof or even capable of investigation. For example, as with all toxicologic evaluations there is a common assumption that the experimental animal is an appropriate model for assessing hazard to man and to provide the base for making an appropriate risk assessment. Because human beings are substantially larger than most experimental animals, correction for the size difference must be made. There are a variety of ways for accomplishing this, with no real rule to select one method or another. However the use of one or another method can amount to differences in risk of as much as 10- to 12-fold.

Because there are often no data to support the selection of one assumption over another, the decision to select one becomes a matter of policy. Because assumptions are the base for selection of the components of QRA process, regulatory agencies tend to use most conservative

assumptions in development of the QRA. When the practice of using conservative assumptions is combined with the use of highly sensitive animals exposed to substances at the MTD it is not surprising that argument develops as to whether or not the calculated risks are so far overstated as to make them unusuable.

To quote Flamm (1989) "the picture of QRA that emerges is one of a process rather than a discipline of science, a process consisting of many steps whose stepping stones are built of assumptions, not scientific facts. A range of uncertainty bounds each stepping stone. The truth presumably lies somewhere within the bounds and the range may be as much as two or three orders of magnitude. Because the range of uncertainties in describing each assumption is likely to be independent of other assumptions, the ranges become multiplicative. When only the most conservative assumptions are made throughout the process, the likelihood is that many of the assumptions will represent overestimates of human risk by 10- or 100-fold leading to a combined overestimate of perhaps a millionfold or more. This is why in recent years there has been such a cry for research to define better the assumptions which underlie QRA. Unfortunately so many of the tractable assumptions or cases are specific. Not only are they case specific but they are also resource intensive. The nation could not begin to afford extensive research on each case, nor could the cause of public health as perceived by our society allow such issues to be ignored. So, in steps the regulatory agencies do what it and every one else knows is not scientifically sound and supportable. What a wonderful target they make and oh, so vulnerable."

In considering evaluations such as those by Flamm, the question must be asked if this then means that QRA is totally without worth and therefore should be abandoned. There is a fundamental need for quantitative assessment of hazards in our food supply. For example, without them, the evaluation of the safety of foods containing natural, toxic substances at extremely low levels becomes impossible. Other options available to regulatory agencies, such as a Delaney-type no-risk approach or a safety-factor approach, are simply not viable within the context of modern toxicologic science. For example, to satisfy all of the interested parties a safety factor would have to be large enough to approximate a virtually no-risk situation. In other words it would be little different than a Delaney-type no-risk approach. If rational judgments are to be made, the use of some kind of QRA is inevitable. What is required is extensive research and the establishment of more rational approaches to the development of appropriate extrapolation models. Recent research on pharmacokinetic models that attempt to evaluate the metabolism and distribution of test compounds offer significant hope for the future.

These issues are at present under considerable discussion and are likely to lead to a change in the law. Eventually, a law that effectively and efficiently minimizes cancer risk will have to be one that (1) economizes regulatory resources, (2) recognizes feasibility in the market place, (3) establishes priorities based on public health relevance, (4) is consistent for diverse substances, and (5) becomes independent of the ever-changing analytic capabilities. Similar concepts will also be required for any substances that lead to progressive, irreversible disease (Campbell, 1981). The present proposals to use "levels of concern" and "sensitivity of method" analyses appear to be steps in the right direction.

TOXICOLOGIC SAFETY (HAZARD) ASSESSMENT OF FOOD ADDITIVES

Before the advent of national legislation concerning food safety, the potential for adverse health effects from the consumption of food additives could be assumed to have been relatively high. This risk was especially high when foods containing various substances to disguise their poor quality and to add bulk were consumed. It is difficult to evaluate retrospectively the effect of these foods on public health because of a lack of epidemiologic studies and acceptable health and food consumption records. The passage of the Pure Food and Drug Act of 1906, followed by the establishment of the Food and Drug Administration, began the era when the safety of food was put under close scrutiny. This resulted in marked improvements in food safety. The 1958 revision of the legislation, combined with the development of the science of toxicology as an independent discipline and the overall improvement of toxicologic assessment, led to further improvement in food safety. If one considers overall human exposure to toxicants, including both the natural and synthetic chemicals introduced into the human environment, then the current safety record for food additives must rank this group of substances as one of the lowest risk categories (Select Committee of GRAS Substances, 1977; Doll and Peto, 1981).

There are many other consequences of science's increased ability to expand the dimensions of food safety evaluation. While the development of modern chemistry allowed the measurement of any number of molecules, this increased capability has also led to the questioning of the biologic significance of such low numbers of molecules. We are beginning to recognize that such low numbers of molecules may be endogenous to the environment (Ames et al., 1987). Virtually all substances, natural or otherwise, contain components at such low concentrations that, at higher levels, exhibit demonstrable toxicities.

As we have expanded the spectrum of biologic effects for which safety evaluations must be made, we have uncovered other areas of greater subtlety that must be considered. For example, evidence has been presented that suggests a relationship between behavioral disorders and exposures to certain food substances. Major methodological problems with such studies raise questions as to the meaning of the results (Dews, 1982–83). Food allergies and sensitivities have also become a matter of concern as well as of confusion and controversy. Although the actual incidence of clinically significant food sensitivities is probably less than 1 percent, a substantial portion of the population believe that they or their families are particularly sensitive to some substances in food (Taylor, 1985). In the context of our discussion of food additives, the matter becomes even more complicated. Generally used food additives such as sulfite (Bush et al., 1986), sugar (Harper and Gans, 1986), tartrazine, sodium benzoate, butylated hydroxyanisole, and butylated hydroxytoluene (Simon, 1986) have all been implicated in producing one or several different food sensitivity reactions. The problem is that methodological difficulties have made the evaluation of this data extremely difficult. In many cases classic changes in immunoglobulins or morphologic changes are not observed in response to these substances. Moreover, the same patient may be sensitive to a particular substance in a challenge test under one set of conditions and not in another. Nevertheless, the questions concerning the immune potential of new substances will become even more acute when the safety of new biologically produced or modified products begins to surface. In these cases it is unclear if relatively modest changes in protein or complex carbohydrate molecules can increase the sensitivity of organisms to these new products.

A consideration of the toxicologic safety assessment of food additives is complicated by their legal division into various categories, as previously discussed. Safety assessment criteria vary both between and within different categories of food additives. For this reason, the safety assessment of food additives will be divided into categories representing different classes of food additives.

SAFETY ASSESSMENT OF GRAS SUBSTANCES

To ensure continued functioning of the food industry following the passage of the 1958 amendments to the Food, Drug, and Cosmetic Act requiring premarket approval of food additives, the statute exempted a large number of food additives that had been used before January 1, 1958 from the regulatory requirements of premarket approval. Although the FDA solicited the opinions of many leaders in the toxicologic community, this exemption effectively "grandfathered" the bulk of food additives in use at that time. This group of substances became known as GRAS for "generally recognized as safe." The FDA compiled a GRAS list containing approximately 600 substances. This list was far from complete, but it served to illustrate substances that the agency considered GRAS. Since the law did not forbid groups other than the FDA from developing GRAS lists, several organizations developed these lists independent of the FDA. The major criterion for addition to the GRAS list was that "experts qualified by scientific training and experience . . . evaluate its safety." An example of a non-FDA GRAS list is that developed by the Flavor and Extract Manufacturers' Association (FEMA). The FEMA list contains over 1000 flavoring ingredients approved by their expert committee. The FDA has accepted the FEMA list and it has been published as part of the Code of Federal Regulations.

It is important to realize that the GRAS list is not static. At any time, when the safety of a substance is questioned, it can be reviewed and removed from the GRAS list by the FDA. A major problem associated with the GRAS list is that substances were included on the list before modern methods and concepts of toxicologic evaluation were developed; only their historic use without evidence of adverse health effects was noted. However, it is difficult to assign to a particular substance the specific responsibility for an adverse health effect in the human population, particularly with respect to chronic effects. These problems, among others, led to a 1970 presidential directive stimulated by a recommendation from the White House conference on Food, Nutrition, and Health in 1969 to the FDA to review the status of substances listed on GRAS.

Thus began the largest toxicologic review in history. The FDA requested scientific literature reviews and unpublished data on the safety of GRAS substances. Data on the current level of usage and estimated daily consumption were obtained through an FDA contract to the National Academy of Sciences, National Research Council. Another contract was given to the Life Sciences Research Office of the Federation of American Societies for Experimental Biology to evaluate this mass of data in terms of safety. To undertake this formidable task, a Select Committee on GRAS Substances (SCOGS), consisting of nongovernmental and nonindustry experts in the fields of toxicology and food safety, was convened. The following procedure was followed for safety approval of GRAS substances, or group of closely related substances: (1) SCOGS provided the FDA with the initial review of the substances; (2) FDA then made the report public and announced a call for any additional data on the substances that had bearing on its safety; (3) if required, a public hearing with SCOGS could be held on the substance; and (4) with the benefit of any additional data collected, a final report was prepared and made public. The GRAS substances were then placed in one of five categories (Select Committee on GRAS Substances, 1977). The FDA interpretation of these various categories was as follows: (1) Category One and Two substances are reaffirmed as GRAS, (2) Category Three may remain GRAS for a prescribed period of time while additional toxicologic tests are conducted, and (3) Categories Four and Five require the establishment of either safe usage conditions or additional toxicologic data without which the GRAS status is rescinded, automatically defining the substance as a food additive. This results in the requirement for the sponsor to provide toxicologic data suitable for safety assessment and premarket approval.

Although this procedure for the assessment of the public health hazard of GRAS substances is not as rigorous as an assessment based on carefully conducted toxicologic studies utilizing current methodology, it is justifiable in view of the nature of the compounds involved. SCOGS has published an excellent review of their evaluation methods (Select Committee on GRAS Substances, 1977). To ensure that new toxicologic data still support the GRAS status of specific substances, the FDA plans cyclic reviews on their safety. It was the consensus of the SCOGS committee that its work was transitory between the concept of GRAS substances being "evaluated for lack of evidence of hazard" to the inclusion of these substances as food additives "evaluated for the evidence of safety."

TOXICOLOGIC SAFETY ASSESSMENT OF DIRECT FOOD ADDITIVES

Food additives, legally defined as those substances added to food for a particular technologic

SAFETY DECISION TREE

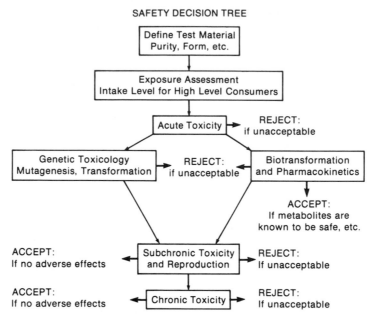

Figure 24–1. Safety decision tree as recommended by the Scientific Committee of the Food Safety Council. 1978.

purpose and that are not GRAS, must be demonstrated to be without toxicologic hazard at the intended level and condition of usage by the sponsor who wants approval for use. Since the 1958 revision of the Food, Drug, and Cosmetic Act, scientific data from toxicologic tests are required to prove safety. The desire of the consumer for greater numbers of "convenience foods" and for a constant year-round supply of specific foods, coupled with the interest in a greater variety of foods, has increasingly led to the need for additional food additives. The ability of the food technologist to take foods apart and recombine them in unique formulations has increased the number of substances classified as food additives. The ability of the analytic chemist to analyze and purify specific active components of natural materials used for flavoring, and so forth, has also led to an increase in the number of food additives. The need to perform safety assessment studies on those compounds that have been given temporary GRAS status, and thus are "pseudofood" additives, has added to the load of food additive that must be toxicologically evaluated. Taken together these factors have resulted in a great number of specific compounds that require toxicologic evaluation and has led to the innovative development of approaches to toxicologic assessment of food safety.

One such approach, which placed toxicologic assessment procedures within a broader context, was proposed by the industry supported Food Safety Council (Scientific Committee of the Food Safety Council, 1978). This "decision tree" approach was developed in response to (1) the increasing number and uses of substances as food additives; (2) the limited number of facilities available to undertake the number of extensive tests required; (3) the length of time required to complete a comprehensive toxicologic evaluation; and (4) the high cost of a comprehensive toxicologic evaluation. The approach begins with simple, inexpensive tests of short duration and works toward the long-term test. At each step within the testing tier, the data are carefully analyzed and a decision is made either to end the testing at that point owing to the potential hazard of the substance or to continue testing to the next level. In this manner, unnecessary testing is minimized and time, facilities, and finances are conserved for the evaluation of more favorable and relevant substances.

Figure 24–1 represents the decision tree approach to food safety assessment proposed by the Food Safety Council. The Council suggests that this be used as an outline only and that the particular steps may be varied depending on the individual substance under study. Quantitative risk assessment may be performed at various intervals along the tree to determine the utility of proceeding to the next step. The principal value of this system is that it is applicable to risk determination for a wide majority of substances ingested with food such as natural toxicants, pesticides, packaging constituents, and so forth, and not just for food additives.

For those substances requiring toxicologic evaluation, the decision of exactly what to test is not always clear. Food additives cover the spectrum from simple salts to synthetic organic chemicals to highly complex mixtures of substances of biologic origin. The Food Safety Council has suggested that the substance tested should be that which will be specifically utilized in commerce. This decision may not represent a problem for the easily prepared mineral salts, but may present difficulties with respect to additives of either synthetic or biologic origin. For instance, a synthetic chemical used in commerce is not an absolutely pure compound but will contain impurities, however minute, resulting from the manufacturing process. Therefore, the toxicity of not only the active test substance, but also its impurities, must be considered. Because the test substance may be manufactured by different companies utilizing different synthetic processes, different batches may contain different impurities. Substances of biologic origin may also differ depending not only on the extraction methodology but also on the source. For instance, a plant extract may vary chemically depending on the particular source of the plant and its growing conditions. All these factors must be considered in selecting the specific substance to be tested. The main criterion, however, is that the test substance be representative of the material to be marketed for food use. Modification of production and marketing practices after toxicologic evaluation may require retesting of the substance.

The next step within the decision tree is an assessment of human exposure to the test substance. This is an essential step in the hazard evaluation of a food additive because an estimate of the expected human dose must be made. The toxicity finally produced is a combination of the toxicologic potency of the substance and its dose. Determination of the potential human dose of a substance is complicated by many factors, but methods have been developed that yield approximate exposure (Filer, 1976). To estimate human consumption of a particular food substance, it is necessary to know (1) the levels of the substance in food, (2) the daily intake of each food containing the substance, (3) the distribution of intakes within the population, and (4) the potential consumption of, or exposure to, the substance from nonfood sources.

There are three, rather imperfect, methods generally used for the determination of human exposure to dietary substances. A "market basket analysis" directly measures the substance in foods purchased in a retail outlet and then used to prepare test meals. This method is of no use for a potential food additive not yet appearing in food.

The "per capita disappearance" method may be used for both new and previously approved food additives. It consists of determining the total amounts of foods that may contain the test substance and be sold in the marketplace; the amount of substance thus disappearing is then divided by the number of individuals in the consuming population. This method does not consider the amounts consumed by target groups and may yield misleading data, as illustrated by the case of saccharin. Average per capita consumption of saccharin in 1972 was 23 mg/kg/day, but the major consuming population consisted of low-calorie-soft-drink consumers. In this group the average consumption was 389 mg/kg/day. Another method is the "dietary survey," which consists of interviewing consumers about their dietary habits; however, dietary-recall studies are notoriously inaccurate. The Committee on Food Protection of the National Academy of Sciences has utilized a method that calculates consumption by multiplying the substance's usage level (obtained by survey) by frequency of eating of specific food items (obtained by survey) to determine consumption of specific GRAS substances. A "probalistic method" for estimating consumption has been suggested that may overcome some of the problems associated with the older methods (Subcommittee on GRAS List Survey, Phase III, 1976). This method attempts to determine the probability that a particular substance will occur in an individual food serving. Currently, this method is laborious and has not been applied to many additives. Oser and Hall (1977) have shown that this method shows agreement with certain of the classic methods. Whatever method is employed, consideration must be given to those individuals who consume greater-than-average quantities of specific foods.

Within the Food Safety Council decision tree, the first toxicity test to be performed is the acute toxicity study. This study will provide preliminary data on (1) the clinical manifestations of acute toxicity, (2) information that suggests doses for other tests, and (3) a quantitative measure of acute toxicity (LD50) for comparison with other substances. After the acute toxicity study, the first decision point is reached. At this point a risk analysis is made based on the anticipated consumption level previously determined and the data from the acute toxicity study. Depending on the outcome of this analysis, a decision is made to either discontinue testing at this point or continue to the next testing stage. Significant effort is being made today to replace acute toxicity tests to remove lab animal use.

Genetic toxicology and biotransformation-pharmacokinetics are the next suggested testing stage. Because these studies complement each other, they may be performed simultaneously. Both biotransformation studies and genetic toxicology have been previously discussed in this volume (Chapters 4 and 6). The purpose of the genetic toxicology test is to determine if the test substance exhibits mutagenic activity with and without prior biotransformation. The biotransformation and pharmacokinetic studies yield data useful in ascertaining the quantitative and qualitative characteristics of the compound's absorption, biotransformation, and excretion and possibly provide evidence of species differences in these parameters. These studies also provide information on the toxicity of significant metabolites. Particular information on the role of metabolic activation and detoxication pathways are obtained in the biotransformation studies. The pharmacokinetics studies should yield data on the biologic half-life of the substance, potential for accumulation at specific tissue sites, rates of absorption and excretion, and dose dependency. These studies are not only useful in risk assessment, but also essential for the development of appropriate subchronic and chronic toxicity studies. If the biotransformation-pharmacokinetic studies indicate that the substance is biotransformed to metabolites with known toxicity, it will be unnecessary to determine their toxicity. However, in cases where metabolites of unknown toxicity are detected, it may be necessary to determine their toxicity. If metabolic activation to products forming covalent adducts is encountered, then the results should be compared with the genetic studies. If the pharmacokinetics studies reveal tissue storage of either the parent compound or its metabolites, this may indicate that the substance is unsuitable as a food additive. Again, a benefit-risk analysis will be supported by the biotransformation and pharmacokinetic data.

On completion of these studies, another point of decision is reached. If the genetic toxicology studies are negative, it is probable that the substance is not mutagenic and may not initiate the process of carcinogenesis. If positive results are obtained within the battery of genetic tests, then a benefit-risk analysis must be made. The Food Safety Council recommends, if the pharmacokinetic studies reveal the production of nontoxic metabolites and the genetic toxicology studies reveal no mutagenicity, that the compound may be accepted at this point. On the other hand, if these studies and the risk assessment leave doubt on the type and extent of risk posed, then the substance is taken to the next level of testing, the subchronic toxicity studies.

The subchronic toxicology series includes a protracted feeding study (usually 90 days) at several dose levels and also includes studies on the potential reproductive toxicity and teratogenicity of the test compound. On completion of these studies, a risk assessment is made. The additive is rejected if unacceptable risk is encountered at the estimated consumption level for high consumers. The test substance may be accepted if no unacceptable risk is encountered at high consumption levels and structure-activity evaluations, genetic toxicology, and biotransformation reveal no evidence of carcinogenicity. If any of these criteria are not met, the test substance is moved along to chronic toxicity testing.

Chronic toxicity studies are designed on the basis of all the data collected up to this point. At the conclusion of the chronic toxicity phase of the safety assessment, risk analyses are again performed. If, on the basis of the risk analysis, there are no unacceptable risks from consumption of the compound at the anticipated consumption level of high consumers, the substance is accepted. The decision tree approach proposed by the Food and Safety Council represents a rational approach to toxicity assessment that appears to be efficient in cost and reliable in safety assessment.

With the realization that information on the safety of food additives and colors must be cost effective, adequate for regulatory requirements, and meet the needs for assurance of safety, in 1982 the FDA developed a document suggesting a new approach to food safety evaluation specifying the data needs for the hazard assessment of food chemicals (Bureau of Foods, 1982). Although this document does not represent changes in the basic scheme of decision making, it does provide a new, more rational approach to the development of priorities for evaluation. The FDA has stated its safety assessment strategy in the form of four premises: (1) the agency "should possess at least some toxicologic or other biologic safety data for each additive"; (2) the extent of toxicologic evaluation is set by the agency's "concern about potential public health consequences" and may vary from substance to substance; (3) even if no toxicologic data are available, a level of concern can still be determined as a function of the level of exposure and the molecular structure activity correlation with other substances of known toxicity; and (4) the completeness and rigor of the initial safety assessment of a substance can be varied if warranted by the initial series of tests. The new concept of safety assessment of food additives and colors proposed by the FDA is a tier approach based on the concept of "level of concern." Essentially, this concept begins with the idea that all additives do not possess equivalent potential for adverse public health effects. Therefore, additives can be divided into groups, each of which exhibits a different degree of potential adverse health effects. A level of concern can be expressed for each of these groups with the groups possessing the highest level of concern having the greatest resources devoted to the assessment of its hazards. Ideally, the level of concern should be an objective evaluation based on quantitative, empiric data and that is calculable. In reality, this is not always or often possible and the level of concern is subjective and based on the best data available. An additive whose use has changed, resulting in an exposure beyond the acceptable level, would have a high level of concern, as would an additive whose most recent toxicity data suggested a greater toxicity than originally anticipated. The type of toxicity exhibited by a substance is also important in determining its level of concern; i.e., greater concern results from possible carcinogens than from an appetite suppressant. FDA uses three levels of concern, based on three criteria: (1) exposure; (2) molecular-structural correlation with known compounds, where little or no toxicologic data are available; and (3) existing toxicologic data.

Categorization according to exposure level is based on criteria previously utilized by the agency. Concern Level III (highest level of concern) contains compounds that contribute more than 1.0 ppm to the total diet. Concern Level II consists of compounds that contribute 0.05 to 1.0 ppm to the diet, and Concern Level I (lowest level of concern) contains those that contribute below 0.05 ppm to the total diet. Categorization according to molecular structure is based on the association of structure with the potential for adverse health effects: Categories A, B, and C reflect molecular structures associated with the potential for low, intermediate, and high toxicity, respectively. Molecular structure information supersedes exposure in the assignment of level of concern. That is, a compound whose molecular structure places it into Category C would be placed in Concern Level III, even though its potential exposure would place it in Category I. Finally, categorization of compounds for which some toxicologic data are available can be more accurately undertaken. For example, compounds that are biotransformed to active metabolites suggest Category III, as do compounds that induce toxicity at low doses and/or after a short duration of exposure. Compounds that produce toxic effects only at high doses and whose exposure to humans are

low are placed in a lower category and would receive less extensive testing. As additional toxicologic data are provided, a particular additive may move from high to lower categories and vice versa. The recommended toxicologic tests for each level of concern are listed below.

Concern Level I Substances. These include:

1. Short-term feeding study (at least 28 days) in a rodent species.
2. Short-term test for carcinogenic potential.

Concern Level II Substances. These include:

1. Subchronic feeding study in a rodent species.
2. Subchronic feeding study in a nonrodent species.
3. Multigeneration reproduction in a rodent species employing at least two generations and incorporating a teratology phase.
4. Short-term test for carcinogenic potential.

Concern Level III Substances. These include:

1. Carcinogenicity studies in two rodent species.
2. A chronic feeding study of at least one year in duration in a rodent species (can be incorporated into no. 1, above).
3. A chronic feeding study of at least one year in duration in a nonrodent species.
4. Multigeneration reproduction study in a rodent species employing at least two generations and incorporating a teratology phase.
5. Short-term test for carcinogenic potential that may assist in the evaluation of results from the lifetime studies.

This procedure contains elements similar to the decision-tree approach for hazard assessment. The utility of these suggested approaches can be evaluated only with additional evidence, but at the current state of the art and science of toxicology, they appear to be effective compromises to the requirement of exhaustive toxicity testing for every substance that may be employed as a food additive.

EVALUATION OF NOVEL FOODS AND BIOPROCESSES

The revolution in modern biology has also led to a new dimension in the needs of food safety science. The inventory of new technologies available to modify the production or processing of food have made it necessary for food safety scientists to begin consideration of the changing

Table 24–3. PROBLEMS OF EVALUATING SAFETY OF FOODS

Problems of exaggerating dose and exposure
Maintaining nutritional balance of diets
Need to consider nonquantal effects
Lack of data on traditional foods

nature of food itself if we are to assure the nutritional and toxicologic safety of new food products. Five categories of such novel products or processes have emerged thus far, each of them having a unique set of health and safety problems. The first of these may be characterized as novel constructions or processing of traditional foods such as food irradiation. The second category consists of food products that are nontraditional as food but for which some human experience exists such as foods derived from yeasts. The third category consists of products constructed from nontraditional raw materials such as certain fungi. The fourth is composed of products of chemical synthesis and are usually promoted for their functional and organoleptic properties. These include substances such as aspartame and sucrose polyester. The last category consists of products constructed from or consisting of organisms resulting from genetic manipulation. These range from traditional food processing enzymes harvested from genetically modified microorganisms to new plant cultivars or animal strains. Each of these categories of new products and processes presents a unique and formidable challenge to the evaluation of their safety. Although traditional toxicologic techniques are available to begin such evaluations, there remain several important questions that have not yet been resolved. Not the least of these is the problem of determining at what point traditional food stops being traditional. This is the speciation question that asks the essential question, "When is a carrot not a carrot?"

In addition to speciation issues, there are problems of exaggerating dose and exposure while at the same time maintaining the nutritional balance of diets (Table 24–3). The traditional approach for evaluating safety for examining the biological effect of exaggerated doses simply does not work when food is involved. Feeding animals enough test food to obtain a 100-fold safety factor is virtually impossible because many foods constitute a substantial percentage of the human diet. Novel foods that have the technical and functional properties of carbohydrates, lipids, and proteins but no nutritive value present other problems of safety evaluation.

Considering the fact that many of these products will replace traditional macronutrients or traditional foods in the diet, the consideration of long-term multigenerational effects must be included in these evaluations. In particular, great emphasis must be placed on nonquantal effects such as behavior or emotionality.

Several schemes have been proposed for the safety testing of novel foods (Table 24–4). Chemical analysis has been emphasized more intensely for such products than for most other food additives or traditional foods. One of the major problems in using chemical analysis is that the data base for comparison with traditional food simply is not present. There is a significant lack of data on the chemical composition of traditional foods particularly at the levels required to evaluate the safety of new foods. Because of the problems of using exaggerated doses, several *in vitro* modeling approaches have also been proposed combined with the development of computer simulations of metabolic interactions. Both approaches are in their earliest stages and not yet at a point where they can be used with any confidence in providing data useful in food safety evaluation. Two other points should be made. Recognizing that most of these foods will become major and staple parts of the diet, it becomes important to understand the impact of such products not only in the normal, healthy animal but also in the stressed system. Stresses such as cold, emotional stress, and infectious diseases become important in predicting the ultimate effect of such compounds on the human population. Finally it is likely that substantial human testing will be required for these novel products prior to their approval, in contrast to

Table 24–4. STRATEGIES FOR SAFETY TESTING OF NOVEL FOOD

1. Chemical analysis
   (a) Known compounds
   (b) Pattern recognition
2. *In vitro* modeling
   (a) Nonmammalian systems (e.g., mutagen testing)
   (b) Sequential mammalian tissue models including modification of metabolism of standard substances
3. Computer simulations
   (a) Activity structure relationships
   (b) Kinetic modeling
4. Traditional safety testing
   (a) Impact on standard test substances
   (b) Impact on stressed system
5. Human studies
   (a) Comparative molecular, pharmacokinetics, and pharmacodynamic models
   (b) Impact on standard test substances
   (c) Impact on stressed systems

traditional food additives for which virtually no human experience was gained until the product was released into commerce.

TOXICOLOGIC ASSESSMENT OF FOOD COLORS

The requirements for toxicologic assessment of food colors do not differ from those of other food additives and include specific toxicologic tests and expert evaluation. As for other substances added to foods, the goal of this assessment is to determine an acceptable daily intake (ADI) based on appropriate tests and safety factors. Currently, the FDA, the Joint Expert Committee on Food Additives, CODEX Alimentarius, and the European Economic Community have set ADIs for various food colors. There is little international uniformity with respect to which colors are acceptable and which are unacceptable. Colors legal in some countries are illegal in others.

There is little concern with the acute and subchronic toxicity of the food colors currently in use, but there is considerable concern in some groups about their chronic toxicity. Several of the colors approved for use by the Color Amendments have been delisted since 1971, including Green 1, Green 2, Orange B, Red 2, Red 4, and Violet 1. Their delisting occurred owing to concerns over their chronic toxicity, especially carcinogenicity. Reevaluation of the data on some of these colors, e.g., Red 2, has raised doubts of their toxicity leading to suggestions that they be revised. As previously mentioned, the FDA decided to eliminate the provisional listing of food colors. The color manufacturers were asked to reevaluate the safety of the approved colors. In response, the Certified Colors Manufacturers Association has and is supporting lifetime studies in the rat and mouse of the listed colors to provide evidence of their safety. Most of these studies have not been completed but generally indicate that the colors are not hazardous to human health when employed at levels currently in use (Borzelleca et al., 1983). The currently approved and tested colors are (1) the triphenylmethane colors, Brilliant Blue FCF (Blue 1) and Fast Green FCF (Blue 1) and Fast Green FCF (Green 3); (2) indigotine (Blue 2); (3) the sulfonated naphthalene azo color, Sunset Yellow FCF (Yellow 6), and the related azo, tartrazine (Yellow 5); and (4) the xanthene-related erythrosin (Red 3).

Controversy still exists over the carcinogenicity of Red 3. Erythrosin is a red disodium or dipotassium salt of 2,4,5,7-tetraiodofluorescein. A peer review subcommittee of the National Toxicology Program's Board of Scientific Counselors determined that there was "convincing evidence that Red 3 is carcinogenic in male Sprague-Dawley rats" (Food Chemical News, 1983a). Their conclusions were based on evidence of thyroid enlargement, thyroid hyperplasia, and increased incidence of thyroid neoplasms (Food Chemical News, 1983b). Additional studies are presently being undertaken to determine the mechanisms associated with these effects, especially with respect to biotransformation and pharmacokinetic characteristics (Food Chemical News, 1983c). It is important to note that FDA has recently delisted certain uses of Red 3 and will probably move to delist all of its uses, sometime in the future.

The ultimate evaluation of the current chronic toxicity studies on the food colors cannot currently be predicted and will take considerable time and effort. It would be surprising if these studies and their evaluations satisfy all the critics of food color usage. A continuing controversy on food color usage may therefore be expected for the foreseeable future.

Owing to current controversies and public concern, two additional areas of toxicologic significance concerning the colors need to be mentioned, i.e., hyperactivity in children associated with consumption of synthetic colors and potential sensitivity reactions. Feingold (1968, 1975) proposed that the consumption by children of foods containing artificial colors may be associated with hyperkinesis and learning disabilities. Children generally consume higher levels of food colors than do adults because of the utilization of colors in confections, soft drinks, and snack foods. However, the data indicating that there is an association between food colors and hyperactivity are unconvincing. Several recent studies have not been able to demonstrate this association (Mattes and Gittelman, 1981; Lipton and Mayo, 1983). This controversy is also likely to continue into the foreseeable future.

The uncertainty of the significance of such adverse effects in the general population ought not be confused with the potential adverse sensitivity reactions that may develop among a small minority of the population. As indicated earlier, adverse reactions associated with nonimmunologic mechanisms (hypersensitivity) need to be better understood. An increased interest appears to be developing among researchers in this field.

TOXICOLOGIC ASSESSMENT OF UNINTENTIONAL (INDIRECT) FOOD ADDITIVES

The FDA excluded indirect food additives from its 1982 document on safety assessment of direct food additives and colors. The reasons for this exclusion were that (1) an extraordinary number of different and diverse molecular structures were involved; (2) assessments of exposure were unique and difficult; and (3) the levels in food were seemingly negligible. Currently, the toxicologic evaluation of indirect food additives follows the classic safety assessment procedures, although the FDA plans a future document on these substances.

TOXICOLOGIC ASSESSMENT OF ANIMAL DRUGS

Animal drugs undergo testing in target species for both efficacy and toxicity. However, a more complex problem exists in the safety assessment of animal drug residues in human food. Determination of the potential human health hazards associated with animal drug residues is complicated by the intervention of animal biotransformation processes such that the molecular structure, and thus the toxicity, of the drug may be altered. Also, the sensitivity of modern analytic methodologies designed to isolate, detect, identify, and quantitate small quantities of drugs and their various metabolites has made the evaluation problem more complex. A typical series used to evaluate the toxicity of animal drugs may include studies on the (1) addition of the drug to the food; (2) consumption and absorption by the target animal; (3) biotransformation of the drug by the target animal; (4) excretion and tissue distribution of the drug and its metabolites in animal products and tissues; (5) consumption of animal products and tissues by humans; (6) potential absorption of the drug and its metabolites by the human; (7) potential biotransformation of the drug and its metabolites by the human; and (8) potential excretion and tissue distribution in humans of the drug, its metabolites, and the secondary human metabolites derived from the drug and its metabolites. Thus, the pharmacokinetic and biotransformation characteristics of both the animal and human must be considered in any assessment of the potential human health hazard of an animal drug. Other considerations include the stability of the drug and its metabolites in animal products and tissues, the interaction of the drug and metabolites with the biochemical constituents of the animal products and tissues, and the potential biotransformation of the drug and its metabolites by intestinal microflora. The combination of these factors and the difficulty and expense of determining the parameters that may affect the toxicity of the drug and its metabolites result in complex hazard assessment protocols.

When some animal drugs may be considered GRAS, safety assessment of these particular compounds is handled as described under the GRAS section. With respect to new animal drugs, hazard assessment is primarily concerned with residues that occur in animal products and edible tissues. The original toxicity determination in the target species should provide data on the biotransformation and the nature of metabolites, along with data on its pharmacokinetics. If this information is not available, then these studies must be performed using the animal species likely to be exposed to the drug. During this phase the parent drug and its metabolites are evaluated both qualitatively and quantitatively in the animal products of concern (eggs, milk, meat, and so forth). This may involve the development of sophisticated analytic methodologies. Once these data are obtained, it is then necessary to undertake an assessment to determine potential human exposure to these compounds from the diet and other sources. If adequate toxicity data are available, it will then be possible to undertake a risk assessment. If the available toxicity data are inadequate, it will be necessary to conduct additional studies. Additional parameters that must be determined are potential human biotransformation of the animal products, as well as the potential for human gastrointestinal flora to convert the animal metabolites to more toxic products. The number of individual compounds involved can be quite large, emphasizing the need to approach their potential hazard along the lines of a decision tree.

One approach to the safety assessment of animal drugs and their metabolites is the relay toxicity study. Relay toxicity studies consist of administering the drug to one set of animals and subsequently feeding the products and tissues of this set of animals to another set of animals to detect any signs of toxicity. Relay studies present problems associated with feeding animals diets that may be different from their natural diets, thus resulting in associated problems of unpalatability, altered digestion, and inadequate nutrition. These studies also have the inherent problems associated with all toxicologic evaluations such as extrapolation of animal data to humans. It is possible to utilize both animal products and tissues in short-term mutagenicity assays to determine mutagenicity and potential carcinogenicity. Overall the hazard assessment associated with animal drugs and their metabolites is a difficult task requiring expertise in several areas.

FOOD CONTAMINANTS

Food is a complex chemical mixture containing not only nutrients, but also a vast diversity of other substances. Because all food is of biologic origin, it contains both inorganic and organic molecules important to the survival of the particular plant or animal species from which it was obtained. A certain fraction of these chemicals are identical or very similar to those found in human metabolism or are precursors to normal human tissue constituents. However, other chemicals are unique to the plant or animal species from whence they were produced and therefore they are xenobiotic (foreign) to human biochemistry. These foreign compounds are more likely to produce adverse reactions in humans, especially when the capacity for detoxication and disposition of such compounds by human tissue is exceeded and/or otherwise compromised. Such chemicals are generally referred to as "toxic constituents of foods," as opposed to food contaminants. Although these compounds are "natural" and may have always been components of human foods, it cannot be assumed that adverse reactions will always be unlikely or negligible. The responsiveness of human tissue to such compounds is likely to reflect the evolutionary time during which first exposure occurred and appropriate response mechanisms produced. Food sources change. For example, tomatoes and potatoes are relatively recent additions to the human food supply, as is the relatively high meat content of Western diets. Intentional modification of plant genotypes by plant geneticists may lead to altered production of certain of these substances, which may present new problems of toxicologic assessment, as, for example, might occur when a pesticide or fungicide naturally produced by the plant is reduced in content, thereby allowing contamination by new or increased levels of insect or fungal products.

Organisms neither live alone nor do they die alone, but are part of complex biologic ecologic systems. Therefore, all foods contain chemicals that are components of organisms that may become associated with that food source, either in life or in death. Generally, these chemicals are considered food contaminants. Examples include mycotoxins and bacterial toxins in various foods, chemicals that may have been deposited in the food during growth or during the postharvest period. In some cases, the food contaminant may be living organisms such as molds, bacteria, viruses, and parasites. Other contaminants that may occur in food include insects and insect parts, as well as rodent hair and feces. These materials are generally termed "filth" and, when found above certain levels, indicate improper storage and handling practices.

Food products may also be contaminated with various synthetic chemicals not directly related to the methods of production, harvesting, processing, and storage. These contaminants may find their way into food by various means, including general environmental pollution, irrigation with contaminated water, chemical spills, and so forth. Such substances are not considered indirect food additives. Food preparation may result in the production of new chemical entities that may have the potential to produce adverse human health effects. The process of cooking has been shown to produce highly mutagenic substances from the pyrolysis of proteins and amino acids (Krone and Iwaoka, 1983; Pariza et al., 1983). These pyrolyzed amino acids appear to be carcinogenic to rodents (Sugimura and Nagao, 1982; Sugimura and Sato, 1983). The nature and levels of these substances are dependent on the type of cooking (frying, roasting, broiling, and so forth) as well as the temperature and cooking time employed. Cooking also leads to the caramelization of sugars and to the reaction of amino acids and sugars to produce various browning products such as the crust of bread. This browned material contains several products that are capable of producing DNA damage and may substantially increase the mutagen burden in humans (Stich et al., 1982). Nevertheless, the benefits of cooking many foods outweigh the trivial, potential risks from these possible hazards. Consider the reduction in pathogen load resulting from cooking or the release and increasing availability of nutrients.

In many cases the presence and levels of contaminants can be controlled by proper agricultural production methods, proper storage, and adherence to good manufacturing practices. In other cases, the presence and levels of specific contaminants are dependent on growing conditions and are not under human control.

The number of synthetic chemicals introduced into the human environment during the last century appears to be overwhelming and is often cited as primary evidence for the need to expand toxicologic studies. However, the number of *unidentified* natural chemicals still vastly exceeds the number of those that have been identified. Therefore, toxicologic assessment and regulation of substances not yet identified would be an enormous problem if the current concepts and methodologies were to be implemented. That being irrational, toxicologic assessment must therefore be considered in the broader context of general health care. Also, toxicologic assessment of foods and substances should proceed from a systematic evaluation of the whole food through its varied chemical and physical fractions to the responsible individual compounds, after evidence of adverse effects of the whole food are carefully documented. Future research efforts in toxicologic assessment will need to be placed in a broad health context.

REGULATION AND CONTROL OF FOOD CONTAMINANTS

Toxicologic evaluation and safety assessment of food contaminants do not significantly differ from those of other food chemicals. What does differ are the concepts and procedures used for regulation. There are many reasons for this; some of the most important are: (1) the variable occurrence of certain contaminants with the growing season, the geographic locality, and the specific genotype; (2) the difficulties and cost of obtaining testable quantities of the contaminant; (3) the difficulties of identifying with certainty the specific contaminants; (4) the lack of sufficient epidemiologic data regarding the public health significance of the contamination; and (5) the lack of adequate toxicologic data. It is often difficult to control the levels of specific contaminants in food, other than banning the food, a process that the law makes difficult. Therefore, regulatory procedures and concepts are entirely different from those for food additives.

The regulation of these substances is generally the responsibility of the FDA, but other agencies, such as the Department of Agriculture, may become involved. "Action levels," which establish the maximal levels of a contaminant allowed in food and feeds, have been generally used. They differ significantly from tolerances in the procedure used to establish them and the information required to support regulatory actions based on them. Action levels are subject to change as more adequate toxicologic data become available. However, action levels have been challenged in the courts and their future regulatory use is in question. For the reasons discussed above, food contaminants are regulated with much broader margins of safety than are the food additives. This does not suggest that the food contaminants have less potential for adverse public health effects. In many cases, the opposite may be true. Rodricks and Pohland (1981) have suggested that if the margin of safety applied to food additives were applied to solanine, a natural toxic glycoalkaloid in potatoes, it could not be added to foods at the level of its natural occurrence. This is probably true of many of the food contaminants, particularly those that may be either mutagenic or carcinogenic (Ames, 1983).

As mentioned above, control of the quantities of contaminants that occur in foods is more difficult than control of additives. In some cases, such as bacteria and bacterial toxins, control

may result from good production, processing, and storage practices. In other cases, such as with the mycotoxins, total control is virtually impossible; thus, certain food lots are rejected for human consumption. Control measures can be as varied as the mechanisms by which contaminants find their way into food products. Contaminants that enter food through soils and water may be controlled by banning the use of contaminated water for irrigation, by prohibiting the harvesting of aquatic foods from contaminated waters, by limiting the use of certain fertilizers such as heavy-metal-containing sewage sludge, and by forbidding the production of food crops on contaminated soils.

A good example of some of the difficulties in regulating food contaminants is the aflatoxin problem. The current action level is 20 ppb, although a proposal has been made by FDA to reduce it to 15 ppb. Although aflatoxin contamination of corn and peanuts can be controlled by proper storage conditions, contamination that occurs in the field before harvest cannot be effectively controlled. The development of plant strains resistant to mold infestation may help. Certain processing technologies that destroy aflatoxin are also being tested and may be usable for animal feeds. The usefulness of these techniques for human food, however, may be questioned because of the need to evaluate carefully the potential adverse effects that might be elicited by the new product being produced. Action levels for food contaminants, therefore, will depend on multicomponent economic considerations, availability and feasibility of technology procedures, and toxicologic risk assessment.

FOOD, BACTERIAL PRODUCTS, AND VIRUSES

Food is also a vehicle for the consumption of a vast array of microorganisms including many that are either pathogenic or produce toxic metabolites. The microorganisms may originate from the soil, water, air, animals, insects, processing, and packaging equipment, as well as from humans involved in food processing and preparation. Illness may be associated with consumption of food containing microbial toxins (food poisoning), with the bacteria themselves (food infection), and with consumption of food containing bacteria that subsequently produce toxins after consumption. Considering the potential, it is not surprising that a major source of human disease is through the consumption of microbial-contaminated food. Although the yearly number of reported illnesses related to consumption of contaminated food in the United States is only a few thousand, various estimates of the total number of cases vary between 20 and 40 million (Archer and Kvenberg, 1985). In less developed countries these figures are certainly much higher. A major problem encountered with illnesses associated with foodborne microorganisms is the difficulty of identifying both the organism and the associated food. Modern biology has made the identification of these organisms easier, and as a result promises to improve reporting of these incidents. These factors have made the protection of food from microbial adulteration a major goal of the food industry, from agricultural production to food preparation. In the United States these efforts have resulted in an excellent record, and attempts at improvements are constantly underway. The two areas currently needing the most improvement are in food service establishments and the home. A major problem in both these areas is a lack of knowledge in proper food-handling methodology. The major problems contributing to bacterial contamination of foods during preparation appear to be: (1) improper cooling of cooked foods; (2) preparation of food a day or more before serving followed by inadequate storage; (3) inadequate cooking; (4) preparation of food by infected individuals; (5) inadequate reheating; (6) improper hot storage; (7) cross-contamination of cooked and raw foods; and (8) inadequate cleaning of equipment (Marth, 1981). Although food preparation and storage in food service establishments and the home account for the largest number of incidents, the far fewer events occurring as a result of a breakdown of procedures in food processing plants generally result in a substantially greater number of individuals being affected.

The bacteria most commonly associated with foodborne illnesses are *Staphylococcus aureus, Clostridium botulinum, Clostridium perfringens, Salmonella* species, *Bacillus cereus, Vibrio parahaemolyticus, Vibrio cholera, Shigella* species, *Escherichia coli, Brucella* species, *Yersinia enterocolitica,* and *Campylobacter* species (Marth, 1981). The Federal Center for Disease Control in Atlanta, Georgia maintains records of foodborne disease, and their data indicate that the patterns associated with the number of outbreaks of foodborne illness and the specific type of bacteria appear to change with time. The two bacteria associated with the greatest number of outbreaks are *S. aureus* and *Salmonella,* followed by *C. perfringens and C. botulinum.* It should be emphasized that this information is based on confirmed reported outbreaks. Most cases do not get reported, and in more than 60

percent of the reported cases in 1979 the etiology was unknown. Meat appears to be most often associated with outbreaks of foodborne illness with pork being implicated in the largest number of outbreaks, followed by beef and poultry.

Staphylococcus aureus is one of the two most frequent bacterial agents associated with foodborne disease. Cases of *Staphylococcus* poisoning are most often associated with the consumption of meat and animal products, although vegetable preparations containing these products may also be a source. Milk and other dairy products may become contaminated from cows with *S. aureus*-associated udder mastitis or from the animal's exterior, as well as from animal handlers. Meats can be contaminated during slaughter and handling. A problem associated with *S. aureus* is that it is a poor competitor with other bacteria, and processes that destroy these other bacteria may lead to the rapid growth of *S. aureus.* For instance, pasteurized milk supports *S. aureus* growth better than raw milk because of the elimination of a large number of competing bacteria. Prevention of contamination is best carried out by careful hygienic practices, holding products at reduced temperatures and maintaining a pH below 4.5, when possible.

The first evidence that *S. aureus*-associated illness was produced by a metabolite instead of the bacteria itself was presented by Dack *et al.* (1930), who found that volunteers administered a sterile filtrate from *S. aureus* cultures became ill. Currently five enterotoxins produced by *S. aureus* have been identified. These enterotoxins are single polypeptide chains (consisting of 239 to 296 amino acid residues) and having different physical properties. These polypeptides are resistant to heat and are destroyed only by prolonged boiling. On consumption of these enterotoxins the onset of toxicity symptoms occurs within one to six hours, depending on amount of toxin consumed. Symptoms generally consist of nausea, vomiting, abdominal cramps, and diarrhea. In cases of high consumption, symptoms may include headache, muscle cramps, chills, and fever, and a possible drop in blood pressure. Recovery is dependent on severity of symptoms, but usually averages one to three days. Mortality is usually not associated with *S. aureus* enterotoxins (Bergdoll, 1979).

Salmonella species produce three types of illness: (1) enteric or typhoid fever, (2) gastroenteritis, and (3) organ-specific pathology accompanied by septicemia. Again, meats appear to be an important source of this organism. Poultry appears to be the major source, followed closely by red meat, with a smaller percentage of infection occurring from eggs and dairy products.

Nonfood sources of *Salmonella* include human-to-human contact and human-to-pet contact. The major sources of outbreaks of salmonellosis have been food service establishments and the home. These outbreaks generally result from improper food handling, including inadequate cooking of food, incomplete reheating, storage of hot foods at too low a temperature, cross-contamination, contaminated raw ingredients, and poor sanitation.

Symptoms associated with *Salmonella* infection depend both on the specific bacteria and on various host factors. Gastroenteritis is usually associated with a 12- to 24-hour incubation period with symptoms consisting of nausea, vomiting, abdominal cramps, and diarrhea. The disease can be accompanied by fever, faintness, and muscular weakness and may include drowsiness, spasmodic twitching, and restlessness. The severity of the disease is related to the type of bacteria consumed as well as the total number of organisms consumed and the immunologic resistance of the host. Severity of the disease can range from mild diarrhea to death, with mortality occurring in fewer than 1 percent of the cases. Recovery may be from several days to months in the most severe cases. *Salmonella*-associated septicemias yield high remittent fever, and the bacteria may concentrate in any organ, yielding a variety of symptoms ranging from abscesses to meningitis. Mortality is higher than for gastroenteritis, ranging from 5 to 20 percent. Typhoid fever generally requires a longer incubation time than other forms of salmonellosis (7 to 14 days) and begins with a loss of appetite and headache. These symptoms usually precede the high fever and lowered pulse rate and include rose-colored spots. The course of the disease may last up to three weeks and relapses can occur. Mortality rates as high as 10 percent can occur in untreated patients. Although individuals infected with any salmonellae may become carriers, this is most likely with typhoid, with as many as 3 percent of infected individuals becoming carriers.

Salmonellosis appears to be associated with an infection as opposed to enterotoxins. On reaching the small intestine, salmonellae appear to invade the lumen and multiply. Lymphoid follicles can enlarge and ulcerate and mesenteric nodes enlarge. If the mucosal wall and lymphatic system are penetrated, the bacteria may penetrate the bloodstream, producing septicemia (Bryan *et al.*, 1979).

Clostridium perfringens is another bacterial species that is a source of foodborne disease. Animal products are the major source for *C. perfringens*, with beef and beef-containing products being the foods most commonly infected,

followed by poultry and, to a minor extent, other meat products. Infection normally takes place as a result of poor food handling at food service establishments. The major problem appears to be cooling of cooked foods. *C. perfringens* food poisoning generally results in diarrhea, accompanied by abdominal cramps. The onset of symptoms usually occurs within 8 to 24 hours after ingestion of infected foods and persists for 12 to 24 hours (Hobbs, 1979). Illness is produced by a heat-labile protein enterotoxin with a molecular weight of 36,000.

Clostridium botulinum contamination of food is a major concern of those involved in the food industry, not because of a high rate of incidence but because of the extremely toxic nature of the enterotoxin produced by this bacterium which is generally regarded as the most acutely toxic chemical known. The majority of reported cases of botulism have been associated with the consumption of inadequately processed home-canned vegetables. Other major sources have been fish and fish products, followed by fruits and various condiments. The development of *C. botulinum* and its toxin in food products is dependent on complex interactions between several factors such as the storage conditions of the food product, product preparation, especially temperatures employed, and certain intrinsic properties of the food, including pH, salt concentration, water activity, oxidation-reduction potentials, and the presence of certain preservatives. There have been cases of botulism reported far back in history, and even today, with the advances in food technology, problems still arise. A much publicized case was the discovery of *C. botulinum* in a few cans of salmon. This finding resulted in the recall of large numbers of canned salmon and a significant economic loss to the salmon industry. Contamination of a few cans appears to have resulted from postprocessing contaminants due to faulty cans. This incident sparked the formation of a joint task force between the National Food Processors' Association and the Can Manufacturers' Institute to study the risk of botulism attributable to faulty containers and to suggest how the production of faulty containers could be minimized (Friday, 1983). This group reported that the risk of botulism related to faulty containers was greatest with those products most susceptible to postprocessing contamination, products in which detection of spoilage by odor was unlikely and where consumption occurs without sufficient heating to destroy the *C. botulinum* toxin. Problems have also been produced in canned foods owing to inadequate heating during processing. Although botulism is commonly thought to be associated with sealed containers, because *C. botulinum* is an anaerobe, the recent cases of botulism from potato salad indicate that this is not always the case (Centers for Disease Control, 1969: Seals *et al.*, 1981; Sugiyama *et al.*, 1981). The incidents appear to have been created by the utilization of foil-wrapped potatoes that had been baked and held at room temperature for several days prior to the preparation of potato salad. Apparently microenvironments existed with low enough oxygen tension to allow the growth of *C. botulinum*. Only small packets of bacterial growth are required to yield a toxic food product.

The initial symptoms of botulism occur between 12 and 36 hours after consumption of the toxin and include nausea, vomiting, and diarrhea. Neurologic symptoms occur somewhat later and include lassitude, weakness, blurred vision, weakness of facial muscles, and difficulty with speech and swallowing, among others. Progression of the toxicity leads to neuroparalysis of the respiratory muscles and diaphragm, resulting in death by respiratory failure (Smith, 1977). Between 1899 and 1977 there were 766 reported incidents of botulism in the United States involving appproximately 1961 individuals (Gunn, 1979). Home-processed foods accounted for 71.5 percent of these cases with commercially processed foods representing 8.6 percent, and the remaining 19.8 percent being of unknown etiology. Mortality among untreated cases can be as high as 60 percent, but the introduction of an antitoxin has reduced mortality. *C. botulinum* toxins consist of at least seven types labeled A through G. Types A, B, and E are generally associated with human botulism. The toxins are proteins with molecular weights in the range of 200,000 to 400,000, consisting of a toxic and nontoxic polypeptide. These proteins are heat labile and can be inactivated in a time-dependent manner between 80 and 100°C (Sakaguchi, 1979). They apparently produce their toxicity by inhibiting the release of acetylcholine at the neuromuscular junction.

The bacteria discussed above have received most of the attention with respect to foodborne bacteria illness. However, there is increasing evidence that certain other bacteria may also be important, includes pathogenic strains of *E. coli*, *Bacillus cerew*, *Vibrio*, *Yersinia*, *Campylobacter*, and *Staphylococcus*. For example, *Campylobacter jejuni* can be recovered as frequently from patients with gastroenteritis as are salmonellae. This species occurs in the intestine of poultry and livestock and can contaminate meat products at the time of slaughter. Exposure normally occurs from the consumption of undercooked meats. Procedures employed to prevent *Sal-*monella infections should also prevent infection by *C. jejuni*.

In the last few years, *Listeria monocytogenes*, a psychrophilic organism, has appeared in an increasing number of incidents. First reported to be associated with the deaths of 100 neonates born to mothers who had eaten *Listeria*-contaminated Mexican-type cheese, the organism has been found in a large number of foods including cabbage, ice cream, cheese, and sausage. The danger of listeriosis is primarily to the fetus and the elderly, healthy adults presenting no more than a flu-like syndrome. The recognition that listeriosis is a principal contaminant of foods is important because it challenges the assumption that refrigeration is an effective last line of defense against food intoxication.

Food may also be a vector for the transmission of viral infections (Cliver, 1978). However, more research is needed before the scope of foodborne viral infections is understood. A major problem associated with determinations of the potential transmission of viruses via food is the difficulty in isolation of the viruses. Viruses with potential human pathogenicity have been isolated from dairy products, meats, salads, and seafoods such as oysters, clams, and crabs. Contamination of food with these viruses appears to result from contaminated food handlers or from sewage-contaminated water being used in irrigation or as the growth matrix. Because many viruses can be inactivated by heat, thorough cooking can decrease the chance of viral infection, but in some instances, such as seafoods, traditional eating habits may lead to consumption of significant levels of viruses. Infectious hepatitis is an example of a food-transmitted virus. Between 1973 and 1975 there were 6135 cases of hepatitis from consumption of raw shellfish alone. Other foods such as tossed salads, sandwiches, and hamburger are potential vehicles for hepatitis transmission (Centers for Disease Control, 1977). Apparently contamination occurred through collection of shellfish grown in sewage-polluted water and through infection of foods by food handlers. Control of foodborne hepatitis A can be obtained by eliminating collection of seafood from contaminated waters, not utilizing contaminated waters for irrigation, and careful control of the personal hygiene practices of food handlers.

Although it is possible to transmit several parasites via food, in the United States the major foodborne parasite is *Trichinella spiralis*. The majority of cases, which average about ten per year in the United States, result from the consumption of undercooked pork.

CONTAMINANTS ASSOCIATED WITH FOODS OF BOTANICAL ORIGIN

Mycotoxins

Whereas the molds have provided various fungal metabolites with important medicinal uses, they also produce secondary metabolites with the potential to produce severe adverse human health effects. Mycotoxins represent a diverse group of species-specific chemicals that can occur in a variety of plant foods. They can also occur in animal products derived from animals consuming contaminated feeds. The current interest in mycotoxicoses was generated by a series of reports in 1960–63 that cited the death of turkeys in England and ducklings in Uganda because of the consumption of peanut meal feeds containing mold products produced by *Aspergillus flavus* (Stoloff, 1977). The discovery of these aflatoxin metabolites led to more intensive studies of mycotoxins and to the identification of a variety of these compounds associated with adverse human health effects, both retrospectively and prospectively. Moldy foods are consumed throughout the world during times of famine, as a matter of taste and through ignorance of adverse health effects. Epidemiologic studies designed to ascertain either the acute or chronic effects of such consumption are few. Data from animal studies indicate that the consumption of food contaminated with mycotoxins has a high potential to produce a variety of human diseases.

Aflatoxins

Among the various mycotoxins, the aflatoxins have been the subject of the most intensive research because of the extremely potent hepatocarcinogenicity and toxicity of aflatoxin B_1 in the rat. Epidemiologic studies conducted in Africa and Asia suggest that it is a human hepatocarcinogen, and various other reports have implicated the aflatoxins in incidences of human toxicity (Krishnamachari *et al.*, 1975; Peers *et al.*, 1976.) Several investigations have associated Reye's syndrome with the ingestion of aflatoxin, an association that deserves more intensive research (Hogan *et al.*, 1978; Siraj *et al.*, 1981).

Generally, aflatoxins occur in susceptible crops as mixtures of aflatoxins B_1, B_2, G_1, and G_2, with only aflatoxins B_1 and G_1 demonstrating carcinogenicity. A carcinogenic, hydroxylated metabolite of aflatoxin B_1 (termed aflatoxin M_1) can occur in the milk from dairy cows consuming contaminated feed. Aflatoxins may occur in a number of susceptible commodities and products derived from them, including edible nuts (peanuts, pistachios, almonds, walnuts, pecans, Brazil nuts), oil seeds (cottonseed, copra), and grains (corn, grain sorghum, millet) (Stoloff, 1977). In tropical regions, aflatoxin can be produced in unrefrigerated prepared foods. The two major sources of aflatoxin contamination of commodities are field contamination, especially during times of drought and other stress which allow insect damage that opens the plant to mold attack, and inadequate storage conditions. Since the discovery of their potential human health hazard, progress has been made in decreasing the level of aflatoxin in specific commodities. Control measures include ensuring adequate storage conditions and careful monitoring of susceptible commodities for aflatoxin level and the banning of lots that exceed the action level for aflatoxin B_1.

Aflatoxin B_1 is acutely toxic in all species studied with an LD50 ranging from 0.5 mg/kg for the duckling to 60 mg/kg for the mouse (Wogan, 1973). Death typically results from hepatotoxicity. It is also highly mutagenic, hepatocarcinogenic, and possibly teratogenic. A problem in extrapolating animal data to humans is the extremely wide range of species susceptibility to aflatoxin B_1. For instance, whereas B_1 appears to be the most hepatocarcinogenic compound known for the rat, the adult mouse is essentially totally resistant to its hepatocarcinogenicity.

Aflatoxin B_1 is an extremely biologically reactive compound, altering a number of biochemical systems. Although the mechanisms associated with its acute toxicity are poorly understood, those associated with its carcinogenicity are being studied in a number of laboratories. As previously discussed in Chapter 5, the hepatocarcinogenicity of aflatoxin B_1 is associated with its biotransformation to a highly reactive, electrophilic epoxide, which forms covalent adducts with DNA, RNA, and protein. Damage to DNA is thought to be the initial biochemical lesion resulting in the expression of the pathologic lesion tumor growth (Miller, 1978). Species differences in response to aflatoxin may be due, in part, to differences in biotransformation and susceptibility to the initial biochemical lesion (Campbell and Hayes, 1976).

Although the aflatoxins have received the greatest attention among the various mycotoxins owing to their hepatocarcinogenicity in certain species, there is currently no evidence that they have the greatest potential to produce adverse human health effects among the various mycotoxins. Table 24–5 lists a number of mycotoxins with potential human health significance, their source, and commodities most often con-

Table 24–5. SELECTED MYCOTOXINS PRODUCED BY VARIOUS MOLDS

MYCOTOXIN	SOURCE	COMMODITIES CONTAMINATED
Aflatoxins B_1, B_2, G_1, G_2	*Aspergillus flavus*	Corn, peanuts, and others
Aflatoxin M_1	Metabolite of AFB_1	Milk
Trichothecenes	*Fusarium, Myrothecium,*	Cereal grains, corn
T-2 toxin	*Trichoderma,*	
Trichodermin	*Cephalosporium,*	
Verrucarol	*Stachybotrys,*	
Nivalenol	*Verticimonosporium,*	
Trichothecin	and possibly others	
Vertisporin,		
among others		
Zearalenones	*Fusarium*	Corn, grains
Citreoviridin	*Penicillum citreoviride*	Rice
Cytochalasins E, B, F, H	*Aspergillus* and	Corn, cereal grains
	Penicillium	
Sterigmatocystin	*Aspergillus versiolar*	Corn
Pennicillic acid	*Penicillium cyclopium*	Grains
Griseofulvin	*Penicillium urticae*	Grains
Rubratoxins A, B	*Penicillium rubrum*	Corn
Patulin	*Penicillium*	Apple and apple products

taminated. It must be emphasized that mycotoxins are generally not consumed alone, but in combination with other mycotoxins as well as other toxic chemicals. It appears that certain mycotoxins, when consumed in combination with others, interact to synergize their toxicity. Other xenobiotics may also modify their toxicity.

Trichothecenes

These mycotoxins represent a group of toxic substances in which it is likely that several forms may be consumed concomitantly. They represent over 40 different chemical entities, all containing the trichothecene nucleus and are produced by a number of commonly occurring molds including *Fusarium, Myrothecium, Trichoderma,* and *Cephalosporium,* among others. The trichothecenes were first discovered during attempts to isolate antibiotics, and although some show antibiotic activity, their toxicity has precluded their use pharmacologically. Trichothecenes most often occur in moldy cereal grains. There have been many reported cases of trichothecene toxicity in farm animals and a few in humans. One of the more famous cases of presumed human toxicity associated with the consumption of trichothecenes occurred in Russia during 1944 around Orenburg, in Siberia. Disruption of agriculture caused by World War II resulted in millet, wheat, and barley being overwintered in the field. Consumption of these commodities resulted in vomiting, skin inflammation, diarrhea, and multiple hemorrhages, among other symptoms. This exposure was fatal to over 10 percent of the individuals consuming the moldy grain (Ueno, 1977). The extent of toxicity (associated with the tricothecenes) in humans and farm animals is currently unknown owing to the number of entities in this group and the difficulty of assaying for these compounds. The acute LD50s of the tricothecenes range from 0.5 to 70 mg/kg, and though there are reports of possible chronic toxicity associated with certain members of this group, more research is needed before the magnitude of their potential to produce adverse human health effects is understood (Sato and Ueno, 1977).

Another mycotoxin produced by *Fusarium* is zearalenone. It was first discovered during attempts to isolate an agent from feeds that produced a hyperestrogenic syndrome in swine characterized by a swollen and edematous vulva and actual vaginal prolapse in severe cases (Stob et al., 1962). Zearalenone can occur in corn, barley, wheat, hay, and oats as well as other agricultural commodities (Mirocha et al., 1977). Zearalenone consumption can decrease the reproductive potential of farm animals, especially swine. Its human health effects have not been ascertained, although its possible mutagenicity emphasizes the need for further research concerning this mycotoxin.

NATURAL TOXIC CONSTITUENTS OF PLANTS

Although the naturally occurring toxic constituents of foods are out of the context of food additives and contaminants, they deserve at least brief mention in any discussion of food safety. These chemicals are part of the natural biochemistry of various plants, but represent xenobiotics with respect to human biochemistry. This group of compounds is one of the most chemically diverse groups occurring in foods. Some of them have relatively high acute toxicity although the greatest concern with respect to human health effects is their chronic toxicity. The advent of short-term mutagenicity assays has allowed the testing of a number of these chemicals and has indicated that more than a few have mutagenic potential (Ames, 1983).

Safrole and related compounds are found as constituents of several edible plants and have been shown to be mutagenic and carcinogenic in rodents (Miller *et al.*, 1983). Sassafras has been used as a flavoring agent in sarsaparilla and contains high levels of safrole. Black pepper contains smaller amounts of safrole and relatively large amounts of the related compound piperine. Extracts of black pepper have been shown to produce tumors in various sites in mice. Celery, parsnips, and other members of the Umbelliferae family contain furocoumarins that are mutagenic and carcinogenic. The psoralens, members of this group, are activated by sunlight to produce damage to DNA (Ashwood-Smith and Poulton, 1981). The pyrrolizine alkaloids represent a group of compounds that occur in a large number of plant species and have been shown to be mutagenic, carcinogenic, and teratogenic. Humans can be exposed to these compounds through consumption of herbs and herbal teas. Human toxicity has been reported (Clark, 1982). White potatoes may contain relatively high levels of the steroidal glycoalkaloids, solanine and chaconine, which are potent cholinesterase inhibitors. Potatoes that have been exposed to light, resulting in greening, and those that are diseased or bruised may contain levels of glycoalkaloids resulting in illness in humans. These are just a few of the numerous components of plants that pose potential adverse health effects in humans (Committee on Food Protections, 1973). The large number of plant constituents known to possess potential toxicity probably represent a small percentage of those that actually exist. It should be anticipated that more research in this area will yield additional toxic compounds. It must be emphasized that plants also contain various chemicals that may possess anticarcinogenic activity, such as carotene and vitamin E. It is interesting to keep in mind the potential adverse health effects of these naturally occurring chemicals while considering the potential adverse health effects of the synthetic food additives.

CONTAMINANTS ASSOCIATED WITH FOODS OF ZOOLOGIC ORIGIN

Botanic Xenobiotics in Animal Tissues and Products

As previously mentioned, either xenobiotics of botanic origin that occur in animals feeds or their metabolites may end up in animal tissues and products. Aflatoxin M_1, which occurs in milk of dairy cows consuming aflatoxin B_1, is an example of this process. Although the transfer of aflatoxins from feeds to animal tissues and products has been studied, there is still much to learn, and nothing is known about the transfer of many of the toxic constituents of plants. Rodricks and Pohland (1981) have pointed out an interesting historic case of transfer of a toxic botanic chemical from an animal to humans, which was first identified by Hall (1979). It is found in the Bible in the book of Numbers, Chapter 11, verses 31 to 33:

> Then a wind from the Lord sprang up; it drove quails in from the west, and they were flying all around the camp for a day's journey, three feet above the ground. The people were busy gathering quails all that day, all night and all the next day, and even the man who got least gathered ten omers. They spread them out to dry all about the camp. But the meat was scarcely between their teeth and they had not so much as bitten it, when the Lord's anger broke out against the people and he struck them with a deadly plague.

Hall speculated that the quail consumed various poisonous berries, including hemlock, while they overwintered in Africa. The hemlock berry contains coniine, a neurotoxic alkaloid, to which quail are resistant and that can accumulate in their tissue. Humans are not resistant to coniine, and consumption of large quantities of quail tissue containing the neurotoxin could result in death as described in the Biblical scripture. More likely however, the drying period permitted the outgrowth of pathogenic organisms resulting in the events noted in the passage. It is interesting to note that microbial food intoxication continues to be a significant factor in human health.

The potential for adverse human health effects from the consumption of animal tissue and products containing residues of plant xenobiotics is generally unknown. This area is certainly worthy of more intensive research efforts.

MARINE TOXINS

Coastal dwellers have utilized the sea as a source of food since prehistory and organisms suitable for human consumption have been accepted and those unsuitable have been rejected. Yet consumption of certain seafoods on occasion results in human poisoning. These "occasional" poisonings can be traced to specific toxins that can occur in certain types of seafoods (see also Chapter 22).

Consumption of shellfish sometimes results in symptoms of poisoning, which include either tingling or numbness in the lips, face, and neck and dizziness, headache, and nausea in mild cases, accompanied by muscular paralysis, respiratory difficulty, and death in severe cases. The responsible agent has been termed "paralytic shellfish poison." Schantz *et al.* (1957) were able to isolate and determine the structure of a major component of this poison. This complex alkaloid, termed saxitoxin, occurs along with various analogues termed gonyantoxins. The ratios of these various components of paralytic shellfish poisons vary with source. Shellfish accumulate saxitoxin through consumption of dinoflagellates, a benthic phytoplankton. Only a few of the more than 1200 species of dinoflagellates produces saxitoxin and its analogues. During certain times of the year under the appropriate environmental factors, these saxitoxin-producing dinoflagellates may undergo a rapid period of reproduction and growth, resulting in a bloom of these organisms consisting of great numbers. These blooms have been termed "red tide" because the seawater takes on a red hue due to the large number of dinoflagellates. Shellfish feeding in areas with red tide may accumulate the toxins and are apparently resistant to their toxicity. Consumption of shellfish from such waters can result in illness and even death. However, shellfish living in waters with no evidence of red tide may also carry significant levels of the toxins, possibly from consumption of resting cysts of the dinoflagellates (Yentsch and Maguc, 1957). Control of paralytic shellfish poisoning is carried out through monitoring for the toxins during harvest and the banning of harvesting from waters where either red tide or evidence of the toxins has been found.

Ingestion of normally safe fish can occasionally result in symptoms of toxicity, including gastrointestinal disorders and signs of neurotoxicity, which can lead to death. This illness has been termed ciguatera, and no specific toxin has yet been associated with it (Hashimoto, 1979). Ciguatoxic fish are tropical saltwater species, which are usually bottom dwellers or fish that feed on bottom dwellers. There are several theories as to how these fish become ciguatoxic, including: (1) the consumption of blue-green algae that may contain the responsible toxins, (2) the consumption of certain species of dinoflagellates, or (3) toxins either produced by gut bacteria in the fish or living in association with the blue-green algae (Hashimoto, 1979). Control has consisted mainly of attempts to educate the public as to which fish may be ciguatoxic in a particular geographic region and suggesting that larger fish, which have higher potential to be ciguatoxic, not be consumed and warnings against consumption of the internal organs.

Scombroid poisoning probably represents the greatest number of seafood-related illness. The disease is rarely fatal and resembles an allergic response to histamine. The poisoning obtained its name because it is generally associated with consumption of fish from the family Scombroidae, such as tunas, wahoo, mackerels, and sardines. In this case, the toxicity is thought to result from events that occur after death of the fish. Bacterial decarboxylation of muscle histidine produces histamine in the tissue. Apparently another as-yet-unidentified compound acts to synergize the histamine to result in the symptoms of poisoning (Motil and Scrimshaw, 1979).

Tetrodotoxin is an extremely toxic compound found in certain organs of the puffer fish, considered a delicacy in Japan. The neurotoxin is quick acting, and death results from respiratory paralysis. To help control the potential health hazard associated with tetrodotoxin, Japan allows only specially trained and licensed individuals to prepare puffers for human consumption.

COMPARISON OF RISKS

In 1934, in his poem, "The Rock," T. S. Eliot wrote, "Where is the wisdom we have lost in knowledge, where is the knowledge we have lost in information." An excellent example is the current fear expressed by the public and exploited by the media and the Congress concerning the safety of food additives, trace pesticide residues, and synthetic chemical contaminants in foods. Never before has there been so much information available to the public concerning these issues. Scientific, legal, and other resources have been expended in large quantities to control hazards associated with this area of risk.

The development of quantitative risk assessment was the result of attempts to provide an objective base for what had become an emotional and subjective argument. Unfortunately, rather than decreasing the uncertainty associated with such regulatory evaluations, QRA increased uncertainty and brought into question the judgment of those attempting to use it. Unfortunately, the use of quantitative risk assessment is a process, which because of its numerical outcome, implies a rigorous scientific base that simply is not present. The use of such numerical expression of risk brings to the public an inappropriate belief in the rigor and precision in the number. The result often is a misleading message which is an exaggerated estimate of the actual health threat and a misleading impression of the precision of that estimate. Nevertheless, quantitative risk assessment can play a major role in helping make rational regulatory decisions. It is in the process of comparing risks that QRA can play its most important role rather than in the development of absolute values of risk assessment.

As discussed earlier, risk assessment is an important component of regulatory structure. Increasingly regulatory agencies are placing much greater emphasis on the concept of risk displacement or risk distribution (Whipple, 1985). The concept of risk displacement or distribution is based on the idea of product substitution, and in turn, the effect of such substitutions on the distribution of resources. If one product or process is eliminated, another product or risk can take its place. The substitution may be an existing alternative or may be the result of new technology.

The importance of such comparisons is best seen in those areas when regulation concentrates on risks where reductions are marginally less beneficial to society than reductions of other products or other risks to society. The result is that overall public health is not as greatly enhanced and technology is directed to areas where the contribution to public welfare is not as great as it might otherwise be. Consider, for example, the concern discussed earlier of the public for the safety of "chemicals" in food. This chemophobia has forced the Congress, and in turn, the agencies, to expend large amounts of public money in efforts to marginally reduce the concentrations of such substances in food. Moreover it has resulted in a virtual halt in the development of new chemical substances that could be useful in expanding the quantity and quality of the food supply. Any objective evaluation of the relative risk data would lead one to the conclusion that, although continuing control of pesticide residues and chemical contaminants in foods is essential, current levels represent a trivial risk as compared to other kinds of hazards. If one examines the potential statistical risk associated with naturally occurring toxic substances in foods, the comparison also can be very revealing. The risk associated with pesticide residues in foods average in the order of 10^{-6} whereas the risk associated with naturally occurring toxic substances in foods, particularly carcinogens, are in the order of 10^{-4} or 10^{-3}. While most scientists agree that these are highly overstated risks because their calculation involves a large number of conservative assumptions as discussed earlier, the reality is that, using the same procedures for risk estimation and then comparing risks among different substances in foods, the hazards associated with naturally occurring substances are approximately three orders of magnitude greater than those associated with pesticide residues.

No one is arguing that resources should be devoted to decreasing exposure to naturally occurring toxic substances, largely because people understand that this is part of the normal risks of eating. On the other hand there are other areas of risk associated with the food supply where this money could be better spent. For example, as was indicated earlier, we are now much more aware of the very serious acute and chronic hazards posed by microbiological contamination of foods. The calculation of risk associated with microbiological contamination of foods reveals that the risk for morbidity, that is the number of who people become ill, is on the order of 10^{-2} while the risk of mortality, that is the number of people who die directly or indirectly as a result of exposure to foodborne disease, is approximately 10^{-5}.

The matter becomes increasingly complicated by the increasing appreciation both by the scientific community and the public of the role of diet in health and, more specifically in its impact on toxic phenomena (Bidlack and Riebow, 1989). It is obvious that simple reduction in the level of a toxic substance may not produce the effect hoped for. It is interesting to note, as indicated earlier in this chapter, evaluation of the relative risk associated with different components of the environment demonstrate very clearly that the impact of both food additives and pesticide residues and other such contaminants in food play an insignificant role in overall cancer risk. These conclusions were reached following different methodology than used in the comparative risk assessment. In this case epidemiologic data was used to reach these conclusions.

In 1943, Bertrand Russell published a remarkable book, *An Outline of Intellectual Rubbish,* in which he wrote, "Fear is the main source of superstition and one of the main sources of cruelty, to conquer fear is the beginning of wisdom." If we are to conquer the irrational fear that has grown in our society concerning the safety of the food supply, we must begin to better understand the nature of the toxic phenomenon we are investigating. It is difficult to understand such fear in a public that is living longer and whose quality of life continues to improve. To a significant extent, the fault lies with the scientific community. Perhaps the most disquieting event to the public of the scientific revolution in which they live has been the recognition that on the one hand there is no such thing as zero, and on the other hand, there is no such thing as absolute safety. Recognition that judgment plays and has always played a major role in reaching decisions concerning food safety is very difficult for the public to accept. It is apparent that the continual disputes that occur in the scientific community resulting from a lack of knowledge in so many areas of food safety science do not help quiet this public concern. We need, as Bertrand Russell has said, the beginning of wisdom.

REFERENCES

Ames, B. N.: Dietary carcinogens and anticarcinogens: oxygen radicals and degenerative diseases. *Science,* **221**:1256–1264, 1983.

Ames, B. N.; Magaw, R.; and Gold, L. S.: Ranking possible carcinogenic hazards. *Sci.* **236**:271–280, 1987.

Anonymous: Saccharin. Where do we go from here? *FDA Consumer,* **12**:16–21, 1978.

Archer, D. L., and Kvenberg, J. E.: Incidence and cost of foodborne diarrheal disease in the United States. *J. Food Protect.,* **48**:887–94, 1985.

Ashwood-Smith, M. J., and Poulton, G. A.: Inappropriate regulations governing the use of oil of bergamont in suntan preparations. *Mutation Res.* **85**:389–390, 1981.

Bergdoll, M. S.: Staphylococcal intoxications. In Riemann, H., and Bryan, F. L. (eds.): *Food-Borne Infections and Intoxications,* 2nd ed. Academic Press, New York, 1979, pp. 443–494.

Bidlack, W. R., and Riebow, J. F.: Toxicological and pharmacological interactions as influenced by diet and nutrition. In Taylor, S. L., and Scanlan, R. A. (eds.): *Food Toxicology: A Perspective on Relative Risks.* Marcel Dekker, New York, 1989, pp. 331–378.

Borzelleca, J. F.; Hallagan, J.; and Reese, C.: Food, drug and cosmetic colors: toxicological considerations. In Finley, J. W., and Schwass, D. E. (eds.): *Xenobiotics in Foods and Feeds.* American Chemical Society, Washington, D.C., 1983, pp. 311–332.

Brown, S. A.: General principles of regulation: foods and beverages. In Middlekauf, R. D., and Shubik, P. (eds.): *International Food Regulation Handbook.* Marcel Dekker, New York, 1989, pp. 217–241.

Bryan, F. L.; Fanelli, M. J.; and Reimann, H.: *Salmonella* infections. In Riemann, H., and Bryan, F. L. (eds.): *Food-Borne Infections and Intoxications,* 2nd ed. Academic Press, New York, 1979, pp. 73–130.

Bureau of Foods, U.S. Food and Drug Administration: Toxicological principles for the safety assessment of direct food additives and color additives used in food. U.S. Food and Drug Administration, Washington, D.C., 1982.

Bush, R. K., Taylor, S. L., and Busse, W. W.: A critical evaluation of clinical trials in reactions to sulfites. *J. Allergy Clin. Immunol.,* **78**:191–202, 1986.

Campbell, T. C.: Chemical carcinogens and human risk assessment. *Fed Proc.,* **39**:2467–2484, 1980.

———: A decision tree approach to the regulation of food chemicals associated with irreversible toxicities. *Reg. Toxicol. Pharmacol.,* **1**:193–201, 1981.

Campbell, T. C., and Hayes, J. R.: The role of aflatoxin metabolism in its toxic lesion. *Toxicol. Appl. Pharmacol.,* **35**:199–222, 1976.

Centers for Disease Control: Common source outbreak,

type A botulism. *Morbid. Mortal. Wkl. Rep.,* **18**:121, 1969.

———: Hepatitis Surveillance Report, No. 39. Centers for Disease Control, Atlanta, Georgia, 1977.

Clark, A. M.: Endogenous mutagens in green plants. In Klekowski, E. J., Jr. (ed.): *Environmental Mutagenesis, Carcinogenesis and Plant Biology,* Vol. 1. Praeger, New York, 1982, pp. 97–132.

Cliver, D. L.: Viral infections. In Riemann, H., and Bryan, F. L. (eds.): *Food-Borne Infections and Intoxications,* 2nd ed. Academic Press, New York, 1978, pp. 299–342.

Committee on Animal Health and Committee on Animal Nutrition, Board on Agriculture and Renewable Resources, National Research Council: Antibiotics in animals feeds: the effect on human health of subtherapeutic use of antimicrobials in animal feeds. National Academy Press, Washington, D.C., 1980.

Committee on Food Protection: Food colors. National Academy of Sciences, Washington, D.C., 1971.

———: Toxicants occurring naturally in foods. National Academy of Sciences, Washington, D.C., 1973.

Dack, G. M.; Gary, W. E.; Woolpert, O.; and Wiggers, H.: An outbreak of food poisoning proved to be due to a yellow hemolytic staphylococcus. *J. Prevent. Med.,* **4**:167–175, 1930.

Dews, P. B.: Comments on some major methodologic issues affecting analysis of the behavioral effects of foods and nutrients. *J. Psychiatric Res.,* **17**:223–225, 1982/83.

Doll, R., and Peto, R.: The course of cancer: quantitative estimates of avoidable risk of cancer in the United States today. Oxford University Press, New York, 1981.

FDA: Residues in foods—1987. *JAOAC,* **71**: Nov./Dec., 1988.

Federal Food, Drug and Cosmetic Act, As Amended. U.S. Government Printing Office, Washington, D.C., 1979.

Feingold, B. F.: Recognition of food additives as a course of symptoms of allergy. *Ann. Allergy,* **26**:309–313, 1968.

———: *Why Your Child Is Hyperative.* Random House, New York, 1975.

Filer, L. J.: Patterns of consumption of food additives. *Food Technol.,* **30**:62–75.

Flamm, W. G.: Pros and cons of quantitative risk analysis in food toxicology. In Taylor, S. L., and Scanlan, R. A. (eds.): *Food Toxicology: A Perspective on Relative Risks.* Marcel Dekker, New York, 1989, pp. 429–445.

Food Chemical News: FD and C Red 3 is carcinogenic in rats, NTP peer reviewers conclude. *Food Chem. News,* **25**:50–51, 1983a.

———: FD and C Red 3 questions on carcinogenicity sent by FDA to NTP. *Food Chem. News,* **25**:44–46, 1983b.

———: FD and C Red 3 study planned to determine carcinogenic mechanisms. *Food Chem. News,* **25**:45, 1983c.

Friday, R.: Progress report on the NFP/CMI Container Integrity Program. Presented at the 76th Annual Convention of the National Food Processors Association, Feb. 8, 1983.

Gunn, R. A.: Botulism in the United States, 1899–1977. Center for Disease Control, Atlanta, 1979.

Hall, R. L.: *Proceedings of Marabou Symposium on Foods and Cancer.* Caslan Press, Stockholm, 1979.

Harper, A. E., and Gans, D. A.: Diet and behavior—an assessment of reports of aggressive, antisocial behavior from consumption of sugar. *Food Technol.,* **40**:142–149, 1986.

Hashimoto, Y.: Marine toxins and other bioactive

marine metabolites. Japan Scientific Societies Press, Tokyo, 1979.

Hayes, J. R., and Borzelleca, J. F.: Biodisposition of xenobiotics in animals. In Beitz, D. C., and Hanson, R. (eds.): *Animal Products in Human Nutrition*. Academic Press, New York, 1982, pp. 225–259.

Hobbs, B. D.: *Clostridium perfringens* gastroenteritis. In Riemann, H., and Bryan, F. L. (eds.): *Food-Borne Infections and Intoxications*, 2nd ed. Academic Press, New York, 1979, pp. 131–171.

Hogan, G. R.; Ryan, N. J.; and Hayes, A. W.: Aflatoxin B$_1$ and Reyes's syndrome. *Lancet*, 1:561, 1978.

Jaggi, W.; Lutz, W. K.; Luthy, J.; Zweifel, Y.; and Schlatter, C. H.: *In vivo* covalent binding of aflatoxin metabolites isolated from animal tissue to rat liver DNA. *Food Cosmet Toxicol.*, 18:257–260, 1980.

Kilgore, W. W., and Li, M. Y.: Food additives and contaminants. In Doull, J.; Klaassen, C. D.; and Amdur, M. O. (eds.): *Casarett and Doull's Toxicology: The Basic Science of Poisons*, 2nd ed. Macmillan, New York, 1980, pp. 593–607.

Krishnamachari, K. A. V. R.; Bhat, R. V.; Nagarajan, V.; and Tilak, T. B. G.: Hepatitis due to aflatoxicosis. *Lancet*, 1061–1063, 1975.

Krone, C. A., and Iwaoka, W. T.: Mutagen formation in processed foods. In Finley, J. W., and Schwass, D. E.: *Xenobiotics in Foods and Feeds*. American Chemical Society, Washington, D.C., 1983, pp. 117–127.

Larkin, T.: Exploring food additives. *FDA Consumer*, 10:4–10, 1976.

Lehmann, P.: More than you ever thought you would know about food additives. Part 1. *FDA Consumer*, 13:10–12, 1979.

Lipton, M. A., and Mayo, J. P.: Diet and hyperkinesis—an update. *J. Am. Diet. Assoc.*, 83:132–134, 1983.

Marth, E. H.: Foodborne hazards of microbial origin. In Roberts, H. R. (ed.): *Food Safety*. John Wiley & Sons, New York, 1981, pp. 15–65.

Mattes, J. A., and Gittelman, R.: Effects of artificial food colorings in children with hyperactive symptoms. A critical review and results of a controlled study. *Arch. Gen. Psychiatry*, 38:714–718, 1981.

Miller, E. C.: Some current perspectives on chemical carcinogenesis in humans and experimental animals: presidential address. *Cancer Res.*, 38:1479–1496, 1978.

Miller, E. D.; Swanson, A. B.; Phillips, D. H.; Fletcher, T. L.; Liem, A.; and Miller, J. A.: Structure-activity studies of the carcinogenicities in the mouse and rat of some naturally occurring and synthetic alkenylbenzene derivatives related to safrole and estrogole. *Cancer Res.*, 43:1124–1134, 1983.

Miller, S. A.: Food safety—an international concern. *Food Microbiol.*, 7: 1990.

Miller, S. A., and Skinner, K.: Uncertainty and the estimation of human hazard: the science of food safety. *Food Appl. Toxicol.*, 4:5423–5426, 1984.

Miller, S. A., and Taylor, M. R.: Historical development of food regulation. In Middlekauf, R. D., and Shubik, P. (eds.): *International Food Regulation Handbook*. Marcel Dekker, New York, 1989, pp. 7–26.

Mirocha, C. J.; Pathre, S. V.; and Christensen, C. M.: Zearalenone. In Rodricks, J. V.; Hesseltine, C. W.; and Mehlman, M. A. (eds.): *Mycotoxins in Human and Animal Health*. Pathtox Publishers, Park Forest South, Illinois, 1977, pp. 345–364.

Motil, K. J. and Scrimshaw, N. S.: The role of exogenous histamine in scombroid poisoning. *Toxicol. Lett.*, 3:219–223, 1979.

National Academy of Sciences: *Food Chemicals Codex*, 2nd ed. National Academy Press, Washington, D.C., 1972.

———: *Food Safety Policy: Scientific and Societal Considerations. Committee for a Study of Saccharin and Food Safety Policy, Report No. 2*. National Academy Press, Washington, D.C., 1978.

———: *Food Safety Policy: Scientific and Societal Considerations*. National Academy Press, Washington, D.C., 1979.

———: *The Effects on Human Health of Subtherapeutic Use of Antimicrobials in Animal Feeds*. National Academy Press, Washington, D.C., 1980.

———: *Risk Assessment in Federal Government: Report of Committee on Institutional Needs for Assessment of Risk to Public Health*. National Academy Press, Washington, D.C. 1983a.

———: *National Research Council: Risk Assessment in the Federal Government: Managing the Process*. National Academy Press, Washington, D.C., 1983b.

Office of Technology Assessment, U.S. Congress: *Drugs in Livestock Feed*, Vol. 1. Technical Report, Publication No. 79-600094, U.S. Government Printing Office, Washington, D.C., 1979.

Oser, B. L., and Hall, R. L.: Criteria employed by the expert panel of FEMA for the GRAS evaluation of flavouring substances. *Food Cosmet. Toxicol.* 15:457–466, 1977.

Pariza, N. W.; Loretz, L. J.: Storkson, J. M.; and Holland, N. C.: Mutagens and modulator of mutagenesis in fried ground beef. *Cancer Res.*, 43(Suppl.):2444, 1983.

Peers, F. G.; Gilman, G. A.; and Linsell, C. A.: Dietary aflatoxins and human liver cancer. A study in Swazinland. *Int. J. Cancer*, 17:167–176, 1976.

President's Science Advisory Committee: *Chemicals and Health*. National Science Foundation Washington, D.C., 1973.

Rodricks, J. V., and Pohland, A. E.: Food hazards of natural origin. In Roberts, H. R. (ed.): *Food Safety*. John Wiley & Sons, New York, 1981, pp. 181–237.

Sakaguchi, G.: Botulism. In Riemann, H., and Bryan, F. L. (eds.): *Food-Borne Infections and Intoxications*, 2nd ed. Academic Press, New York, 1979, pp. 389–442.

Sato, N., and Ueno, Y.: Comparative toxicities of trichlothecenes. In Rodricks, J. V.; Hesseltine, C. W.; and Hehlman, M. A. (eds.): *Mycotoxins in Human and Animal Health*. Pathtox Publishers, Park Forest South, Illinois, 1977.

Schantz, E. J.; Mold, J. B.; Stanger, D. W.; Shavel, J.; Bowden, J. P.; Lynch, J. M.; Wyler, R. S.; Riegel, B.; and Sommer, H.: Paralytic Shellfish Poison. VI. A procedure for the isolation and purification of the poison from toxic clam and mussel tissues. *J. Am. Chem. Soc.*, 79:5230–5235, 1957.

Scientific Committee of the Food Safety Council: Proposed system for food safety assessment. *Food Cosmet. Toxicol.*, 16:1–136, 1978.

Seals, J. E.; Snyder, J. D.; Edell, T. A.; Hatheway, C. L.; Johnson, C. J.; Swanson, R. C.; and Hughes, J. M.: Restaurant-associated type A botulism: transmission by potato salad. *Am. J. Epidemiol.*, 113:436–444, 1981.

Select Committee on GRAS Substances: Evaluation of health aspects of GRAS food ingredients: lessons learned and questions unanswered. *Fed. Proc.*, 36:2519–2562, 1977.

Simon, R. A.: Adverse reactions to food additives. *N. Eng. Regul. Allergy Proc.*, 7:533–542, 1986.

Siraj, M. Y.; Hayes, A. W.; Unger, P. D.; Hogan, G. R.; Ryan, N. J.; and Wray, B. B.: Analysis of aflatoxin B1 in human tissues with high-pressure liquid chromatography. *Toxicol. Appl. Pharmacol.,* **58**:422–430, 1981.

Smith, L. D.: *Botulism: The Organism, Its Toxins, the Disease.* Charles C Thomas, Springfield, Illinois, 1977.

Stich, H. F.; Rosin, M. P.; Wu, C. H.; and Powrie, W. D.: The use of mutagenicity testing to evaluate food products. In Heddle, J. A. (ed.): *Mutagenicity: New Horizons in Genetic Toxicology.* Academic Press, New York, 1982, pp. 117–142.

Stob, M.; Baldwin, R. S.; Tuite, J.; Andrews, F. N.; and Gillette, K. G.: Isolation of an anabolic, uterotropic compound from corn infected with *Gibberella zeae. Nature,* **196**:1318, 1962.

Stoloff, L.: Aflatoxins—an overview. In Rodricks, J. V.; Hesseltine, C. W.; and Mehlman, M. A. (eds.): *Mycotoxins in Human and Animal Health.* Pathtox Publishers, Park Forest South, Illinois, 1977.

Subcommittee on GRAS List Survey (Phase III): Estimating distribution of daily intakes of certain GRAS substances. Food and Nutrition Board, National Research Council, National Academy of Sciences, Washington, D.C., 1976.

Sugimura, T., and Nagao, M.: The use of mutagenicity tests to evaluate carcinogenic hazards in our daily life. In Heddle, J. A. (ed.): *Mutagenicity: New Horizons in Genetic Toxicology.* Academic Press, New York, 1982, pp. 77–88.

Sugimura, T., and Sato, S.: Mutagens—carcinogens in foods. *Cancer Res.* **43***(Suppl.)*:2415s, 1983.

Sugiyama, H.; Wodburn, M.; Yang, K. H.; and Movroydis, C.: Production of botulinum toxin in inoculated pack studies of foil-wrapped baked potatoes. *J. Food Protect.,* **44**:896–901, 1981.

Tannahill, R.: *Food in History.* Stein & Day, New York, 1973.

Taylor, S. L.: Food allergies. *Food Technol.,* **39**:98–105, 1985.

Ueno, Y.: Trichothecenes: overview address. In Rodricks, J. V.; Hesseltine, C. W.; and Mehlman, M. A. (eds.): *Mycotoxins in Human and Animal Health.* Pathtox Publishers, Park Forest South, Illinois, 1977.

Whipple, C.: Redistributing Risk. *Regulation,* **37**: 1985.

Wogan, G. N.: Aflatoxin carcinogenesis. In Busch, H.:*Methods in Cancer Research.* Academic Press, New York, 1973, pp. 309–344.

Yentsch, C. M., and Mague, F. C.: Motile cells and cysts: two probable mechanisms of intoxication of shellfish in New England water. In Taylor, D. L., and Saliger, H. H. (eds.): *Toxic Dinoflagellate Blooms.* Elsevier/North Holland, New York, 1957, pp. 127–130.

Chapter 25

AIR POLLUTANTS

Mary O. Amdur

INTRODUCTION

Pollution of the atmosphere has been an undesirable spinoff of human activities presumably since the cavemen first lit fires. These problems increased in magnitude with increasing urbanization. People dug coal from the ground and used it to heat their clustered dwellings, thus creating an atmosphere of sulfurous smoke and filth above the cities. From the thirteenth century onward periodic efforts were made to forbid the burning of coal in London, but on the whole people resigned themselves to acceptance of a polluted atmosphere as a part of urban life. Industrialization and technologic development added a second dimension to pollution of the atmosphere. Power plants burned fossil fuel to generate electricity to light homes and operate machines. Steel mills grew up along river banks and lake shores. Oil refineries rose in port cities or near oil fields. Smelters roasted and refined metals in areas near great mineral deposits. Synthetic chemistry came of age, and factories were built to produce the raw materials needed to manufacture the many things we now take for granted in our daily lives.

In the process of these developments too little thought was given to the effect of waste products on the environment. Some people even went so far as to equate pollution and prosperity, pointing with pride to belching stacks as a symbol of economic development. Cities sprawled and grew, as those who could afford it moved to more desirable areas and commuted daily to the heart of the city. The automobile thus came to add a third dimension to pollution of the atmosphere. "Smog" is really an old word, coined to describe the mixture of smoke and fog that hung over cities such as London. In current parlance, however, it has come to refer to the eye-irritating photochemical reaction products of auto exhaust that blanket cities such as Los Angeles when meteorologic conditions produce a stagnant air mass. Over 30 years ago there was already evidence that the date of appearance of plant damage typical of photochemical smog near great cities of the world could be correlated with the date on which the consumption of gasoline passed a critical value.

Air pollution is thus by no means a new problem, although it is a problem of vital current interest. The realization has dawned that a polluted atmosphere is not just another nuisance we must sit back and accept. Efforts have been made on a national as well as on an international level to arrive at air quality standards as a rational basis for control measures. To do this it is necessary to integrate and interpret the results of research in many disciplines.

Chemistry provides methods for the determination of concentrations of pollutants in the atmosphere and information on their chemical interactions with one another. Meteorology gives information on conditions causing stagnant air masses in which pollutants can accumulate and studies the dispersion of pollutants from their sources. Engineering supplies the developments in technology needed to control pollution at the source. Toxicology provides information on the physiologic, biochemical, and pathologic effects of known concentrations of pollutants on experimental animals or human subjects. Epidemiology provides information to correlate the health of populations with the known levels of pollution to which they are exposed. Plant pathology yields information on the effects of various pollutants on vegetation, either under field growing conditions or under experimental exposures in greenhouse conditions. Economics attempts, on the one hand, to assess the cost of pollution in terms of corrosion of materials, the loss of income from damaged crops and other effects on the economy, and, on the other hand, to evaluate the cost of pollution control.

TYPES AND SOURCES OF POLLUTANTS

In terms of tons of material emitted annually into the air, five major pollutants account for close to 98 percent of the pollution. These are carbon monoxide (52 percent), sulfur oxides (18 percent), hydrocarbons (12 percent), particulate matter (10 percent), and nitrogen oxides (6 percent). In individual localities the picture would vary widely from these figures. In the vicinity of a smelter, for example, sulfur oxides would be the major pollutant. Downwind from a steel mill, particulate matter would account for a greater percentage of the total pollution than suggested here. In areas where the automobile is the main source of pollution, carbon monoxide, hydrocarbons, and nitrogen oxides would be higher and sulfur dioxide would be lower than indicated above.

In discussing air pollution, the distinction is often made between two general types of pollution. The first is characterized by sulfur dioxide and smoke resulting from incomplete combustion of coal and by conditions of fog and cool temperatures. It is the sort of pollution typified by Dickens's "London particular." Because of its chemical nature it is termed reducing type of pollution. The second is characterized by hydrocarbons, oxides of nitrogen, and photochemical oxidants. It results from the atmospheric reaction products of automobile exhaust and occurs with particular frequency and intensity in areas such as the Los Angeles basin, where intense sunlight causes photochemical reactions in polluted air masses trapped by a meteorologic inversion layer. Because of its chemical nature it is termed oxidizing type of pollution. It is also called photochemical air pollution.

ACUTE HEALTH EFFECTS OF AIR POLLUTION

From time to time there have been situations in which the level of air pollution has risen to concentrations that are definitely hazardous to human health and life. In rare instances, such incidents have involved the accidental release of a specific chemical.

One such incident involved release of chlorine gas into the subway tunnels of Brooklyn. Another, in Poza Rico, Mexico, involved the release of lethal concentrations of hydrogen sulfide from a malfunction of a new installation in an oil refinery. One case was of a chronic rather than an acute nature. Sufficient beryllium was released from a manufacturing plant to cause beryllium disease in persons residing near the plant. In these incidents the relationship of cause and effect is straightforward. A single chemical was present at a concentration known to be toxic.

The most recent as well as the most disastrous of such incidents occurred the night of December 3, 1984, at Bhopal, India, when approximately 40 tons of methyl isocyanate was released into the atmosphere from a pesticide manufacturing plant. At least 2000 people died and many more became ill.

In general, when we refer to "acute episodes" of air pollution we have in mind three classic incidents. The first occurred in the Meuse Valley in Belgium in 1930, the second in Donora, Pennsylvania, in 1948, and the third in London in 1952. These incidents have much in common. Meteorologic conditions were those of inversion: the normal situation, in which the lower layers of the atmosphere are warmer than the upper layers, becomes inverted, and the mixing and dilution that occurs as warm air rises and cold air falls cannot take place. The result is an essentially stagnant air mass to which multiple sources continue to add pollutants. The analogy is often made to a "pot with the lid on it." These conditions prevailed for three or four days, during which time the concentration of pollutants rose well above the normal levels for these heavily polluted areas. The Meuse Valley and Donora are industrial areas and in them, as in London, coal was the main fuel for domestic heating. The pollution was therefore of the reducing type, characterized by smoke and sulfur dioxide. In the Meuse Valley and in Donora no measurements were made of the actual levels of pollution. During the London fog the instruments that routinely recorded daily averages of smoke and sulfur dioxide indicated that on the worst day the concentration of smoke was 4.5 mg/m^3 and that of sulfur dioxide, 1.34 ppm. Because these are daily averages, short-term peak concentrations would have reached higher levels. Concentrations of neither pollutant are in the range the toxicologist would consider lethal. In the Meuse Valley 65 people died. In Donora 20 people died. In London 4000 deaths were attributed to the fog incident. It is ironic to note that 16 years earlier the prediction was made that if an incident like that in the Meuse Valley were to occur in London, some 3200 deaths would occur.

In all three incidents many people became ill as a result of the pollution. The mortality and morbidity occurred mainly among the elderly and among those with preexisting cardiac and/or respiratory disease. These persons were unable to cope adequately with the added stress imposed by breathing the heavily polluted air. Retrospective investigation suggests the occurrence of earlier acute incidents in these localities. There have been more recent incidents in which meteorologic inversion over polluted urban areas has led to increases in mortality and morbidity. Studies in England led to the suggestion that when concentrations of smoke and sulfur dioxide reach values of 0.75 mg/m³ for smoke and 0.25 ppm for sulfur dioxide, excess mortality is observed.

There is also clear-cut evidence that more ordinary day-by-day fluctuations in pollution levels have adverse effects on sick people. By giving chronic bronchitic patients a very simple diary in which they recorded whether they felt better or worse than usual, and then relating these entries to daily air pollution data in London, a striking correlation was obtained. It was plain that the patients felt worse on days of greater pollution. These studies were continued after the British Clean Air Act had reduced the levels of both pollutants. It was then possible to conclude that when the 24-hour mean concentrations for smoke and sulfur dioxide were respectively below 0.25 mg/m³ and 0.19 ppm, the patients showed no response.

More recent studies have shown acute effects of ambient levels of pollution that occur during the summer months in areas of northeastern North America. These peaks of pollution are typified by increases in ozone and sulfate, the latter being in essence a surrogate for sulfuric acid. In southern Ontario there is a consistent association in summer between hospital admissions for respiratory disease and daily levels of ozone and sulfate. No association exists for a group of nonrespiratory conditions. In summarizing and discussing these data, Bates and Sizto (1989) conclude that neither agent alone is responsible for the observed association but that either sulfuric acid (which was not measured) or some pattern of sequential or combined exposure causes the observed morbidity. Data from experimental toxicology lend strong support to these conclusions. Studies of children at summer camp where they were active outdoors most of the day showed decrements in daily measured pulmonary function on days when ozone levels increased even though concentrations did not exceed 0.12 ppm (Lippmann, 1989). Much earlier data from the Los Angeles area showed a high degree of correlation between diminished performance of high school cross-country track runners and increased oxidant levels in the hour before the meet.

CHRONIC HEALTH EFFECTS OF AIR POLLUTION

Ambient air pollution can contribute to the occurrence and/or aggravation of disease in urban populations. The diseases that fall into this category are the following: acute nonspecific upper respiratory disease (i.e., the "common cold"), chronic bronchitis, chronic obstructive ventilatory disease, pulmonary emphysema, bronchial asthma, and lung cancer.

Chronic bronchitis is characterized by excessive mucus secretion in the bronchial tree and a chronic or recurrent productive cough. There appears to be little question of a relationship between chronic bronchitis and both cigarette smoking and air pollution. The effect of smoking is by far the greater of the two as a contributing factor to respiratory disease. Unless careful data are included on smoking histories, it is impossible to assess the contribution made by air pollution. This does not mean, however, that air pollution makes no contribution.

The most detailed epidemologic study of the chronic health effects of current levels of air pollution has been the so-called Harvard Six Cities Study. The cities were chosen because of varying levels of pollution and air monitoring data were routinely obtained. Groups of school children were examined over a period of years for prevalence of respiratory disease reported on a standard questionnaire by parents, and pulmonary function tests were administered to the children. More recently a long overdue expansion was made of air monitoring data to include measurement of H⁺ in four of the six cities. Figure 25–1 shows the relationship of prevalence of bronchitis to measured H⁺ (Speizer, 1989). Not surprisingly, the correlation was much better than previous efforts to relate the health effect to suspended particulate < 15 μm

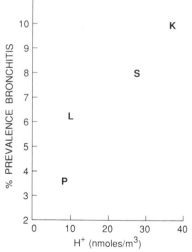

Figure 25–1. Relationship of bronchitis in the last year in children 10 to 12 years of age in four U.S. cities to hydrogen ion concentration. P = Portage, WI; L = St. Louis, MO; S = Steubenville, OH; K = Kingston, TN. (From Speizer, 1989.)

in size (PM$_{15}$). Planned studies on 24 cities that will include measurement of acid aerosol should provide the more definitive data needed to firmly establish the main causative agent.

Bronchial asthma is produced by many aeroallergens of natural origin that are dispersed by natural forces rather than from human activities. Sometimes these natural allergens can be introduced by man as air pollutants, for example, castor bean dust from factories processing the material, or material from grain handling and milling. Various studies have suggested that asthmatic attacks are associated with higher levels of pollution.

The cause of cancer is, as far as we know, a multiplicity of factors. Among the compounds known to occur as urban air pollutants are some that have known carcinogenic potency. The adsorption of carcinogenic substances on inert particulate material could prolong residence time at sensitive sites in the respiratory tract. Many air pollutants have an irritant action on the mucous membranes of the respiratory tract. There is experimental evidence that when benzopyrene is inhaled by rats whose respiratory tracts have chronic irritation (produced by chronic sulfur dioxide inhalation), bronchogenic carcinoma results. Experimental evidence also exists that when ozonized gasoline was inhaled by mice that had been infected with influenza virus, epidermoid carcinomas were produced. There is an urban-rural gradient in incidence of lung cancer that is real when corrected for the effects of cigarette smoking. Kotin and Falk (1963) say, "Chemical, physical and biological data unite to form a constellation that strongly implicates the atmosphere as one dominant factor in the pathogenesis of lung cancer."

REDUCING-TYPE POLLUTION

The acute air pollution incidents made plain that under certain meteorologic conditions the reducing-type pollution characterized by sulfur dioxide and smoke was capable of producing disastrous effects. This stimulated toxicologic research on experimental animals and human subjects. Special emphasis, too much for too long, was given to studies of sulfur dioxide alone. Recognition of the critical importance of interactions among components of the sulfurous pollution complex was long overdue when it finally found general acceptance.

The burning of fossil fuels and the smelting of metals emit a variety of particles as well as sulfur dioxide into the atmosphere. Many of these particles are capable of promoting the conversion of sulfur dioxide to the more irritant sulfuric

acid. Particles of a submicrometer size are of particular importance. They have a large surface area and are enriched in metals such as zinc and vanadium. These metals can convert sulfur dioxide to sulfuric acid, which is then present as a layer on the surface of the fine particles. Sulfur dioxide is thus the source of atmospheric particulate sulfates such as sulfuric acid, ammonium, sulfate, and ammonium bisulfate. These fine sulfate aerosols may be transported long distances in the atmosphere. In addition to posing a direct hazard to health, they contribute to acid rain, which has become a major ecologic problem in many areas of the northeastern United States, Canada, and Scandinavia.

The EPA, in their revision of the criteria documents, issued a combined *Air Quality Criteria for Particulate Matter and Sulfur Oxides* (US-EPA, 1982) to replace the original two separate documents. By so doing they acknowledged the fact that it makes little sense to attempt to evaluate the effects of sulfur dioxide without also considering the coexisting particulate matter. The purpose of the criteria documents is to summarize the database available for the setting of the Air Quality Standards by the EPA Administrator. The document thus provides a very comprehensive review of the literature on the reducing-type pollution complex.

Sulfur Dioxide

Mortality and Lung Pathology. Early studies of the mortality produced by sulfur dioxide utilized mice, rats, guinea pigs, and insects. The concentrations required to kill animals are so high that these studies have little relevance to air pollution problems.

Chronic exposure of animals to sulfur dioxide produces a thickening of the mucous layer in the trachea and a hypertrophy of goblet cells and mucous glands, which resembles the pathology of chronic bronchitis. The important point is that such changes can be produced by irritant exposure alone without the intermediary of infection. Infection is of unquestioned importance in the etiology of chronic bronchitis, but experimental evidence indicates that it is not an essential factor in the development of the excessive mucous cells characteristic of this disease.

In experiments done by Dalhamn (1956), daily exposures of rats to 10 ppm sulfur dioxide for 18 to 67 days produced a thickening of the mucous layer in the trachea of rats. This layer, normally about 5 μm, increased in the exposed animals to about 25 μm. The rate of transport of the mucous layer was decreased and remained so for a month after the end of the exposure.

Daily exposures of dogs to 1 ppm for a year

produced a slowing of tracheal mucous transport. In rats, daily exposures to a total of 70 to 170 hours to 0.1, 1.0, and 20 ppm interfered with the clearance of inert particles. The most marked effects were seen with lower doses administered over a longer period of time.

Following continuous exposure of guinea pigs or monkeys for periods of up to a year or more to concentrations of 0.1 to 5 ppm, no evidence of pulmonary pathology was detected (Alarie *et al.*, 1972, 1975). Unfortunately, the more sensitive techniques available for evaluation of alterations in respiratory mucous membranes were not included in the protocol of these studies.

Absorption and Distribution. On the basis of its solubility in water, one would predict that sulfur dioxide would be readily removed during passage through the upper respiratory tract. This prediction can be tested experimentally by making measurements of the drop in sulfur dioxide concentration when an airstream passes through the upper respiratory tract of larger animals, such as dogs or rabbits, or in human subjects. Indirect assessment of this factor may be made by comparison of the response to given sulfur dioxide concentrations inhaled through the nose or through a tracheal cannula in animals or by comparison of the response to nose and mouth breathing in human subjects.

By the use of $^{35}SO_2$, Strandberg (1964) was able to examine the absorption by the upper respiratory tract of rabbits over a concentration range of 0.05 to 700 ppm. At higher concentrations removal was 90 percent or greater; this is in agreement with the findings of other workers on dogs and human subjects. At concentrations below 1 ppm, however, only 5 percent or less was removed by the upper respiratory tract. These data fit with the observation that guinea pigs breathing through a tracheal cannula to bypass removal by the upper respiratory tract showed an increased response to concentrations of 2, 20, or 100 ppm but no difference at a concentration of 0.4 ppm (Amdur, 1966). This fitting together of data obtained by different methods on different species makes a strong case for the fact that at levels pertinent to air pollution, sulfur dioxide is not efficiently removed by the upper respiratory tract.

The penetration of sulfur dioxide to the lungs is greater during mouth breathing than during nose breathing. An increase in flow rate also markedly increases penetration. These facts are of significance in connection with increased uptake in persons exercising during incidents of heavy pollution. The consequences could be significant for exercising asthmatics who are more sensitive to sulfur dioxide than normal individuals.

Studies using $^{35}SO_2$ have shown that inhaled sulfur dioxide is readily distributed throughout the body. This also occurs when only an isolated segment of the trachea or the upper airways is exposed. Systemic absorption occurs from these sites, although to a lesser extent than when the lungs are exposed.

Deposited sulfur dioxide is only slowly removed from the respiratory tract. Radioactivity can be detected in the respiratory system for a week or more following exposure. Some of the ^{35}S appears to be bound to protein.

Pulmonary Function. The basic physiologic response to inhalation of sulfur dioxide is a mild degree of bronchial constriction, which is reflected in a measurable increase in flow resistance. This dose-related increase in resistance has been demonstrated in guinea pigs, dogs, cats, and human subjects. The gas was given to anesthetized dogs by nose, by tracheal cannula, and by exposing an isolated segment of the trachea to sulfur dioxide while the lungs were ventilated with air. The response was greatest when the gas was introduced directly into the lungs via a tracheal cannula and least when only a segment of trachea was exposed. The fact that resistance increased by exposure of only the tracheal segment suggests a referred reflex constriction of the bronchi. Nasal resistance also increased in a manner roughly proportional to sulfur dioxide concentration. These changes probably reflect mucosal swelling and/or increased secretion of mucus (Frank and Speizer, 1965).

The mechanisms of bronchoconstriction produced by sulfur dioxide have been studied in cats (Nadel *et al.*, 1965). Anesthetized cats were ventilated with a pump via a tracheal cannula. Sulfur dioxide gas was delivered either to the lungs or to the upper airways. Total pulmonary resistance increased during the first breath when sulfur dioxide was delivered to the lower airways and lungs during a single inflation cycle. It returned to control values within one minute. Exposing only the upper airways also produced an increase in resistance. An intravenous injection of atropine or cooling of the cervical vagosympathetic nerves abolished these effects; rewarming of the nerve reestablished the response. The rapidly of the response and its reversal suggests that changes in smooth muscle tone are the cause of the bronchoconstriction. The response depends on intact parasympathetic pathways.

Human subjects exposed for brief periods to sulfur dioxide also show alterations in pulmonary mechanics. Measurements can be made without interrupting exposure to sulfur dioxide. Frank *et al.* (1962) exposed 11 subjects to 1, 5, and 13 ppm sulfur dioxide for periods of ten minutes. At 1 ppm only one individual showed an increase in flow resistance. It is of interest to note that this was the individual with the highest control resistance of the group. At a concentration of 5 ppm the average increase in resistance for the group was 39 percent above control values. Nine out of the group showed a statistically significant increase in resistance. At 13 ppm the resistance of all subjects increased, with an average increase for the group of 72 percent. It is thus possible by meticulous attention to experimental protocol and by the use of sensitive physiologic methods to demonstrate a dose-response relationship in human subjects.

Studies by other investigators have confirmed this basic finding that the majority of subjects respond to concentrations of 5 ppm or higher, whereas only an occasional sensitive individual responds to 1 ppm. With exercise during exposure, however, a concentration of 1 to 3 ppm increases airway resistance in normal individuals. This effect is no longer seen at 0.5 ppm. Airway resistance increased when subjects inhaled 1 to 3 ppm deeply by mouth. There was a dose-response relationship between the number of breaths taken (up to 32) and the observed increase in resistance. Although concentrations of 3 ppm are unlikely as daily or hourly averages, they could be encountered briefly as pockets of pollution from local sources. The fact that few deep breaths will produce increased airway resistance could be of significance to individuals with diseased lungs. The relationship between ventilation and perfusion could be further disturbed with undesirable clinical consequences. Although the subjects used in these studies were normal, healthy individuals, 3 out of 25 showed a greater change that persisted for a longer period after exposure was discontinued.

Clear-cut evidence has been obtained that asthmatic individuals are especially sensitive to sulfur dioxide. Sheppard et al. (1981) observed increases in airway resistance in subjects with clinically defined mild asthma during exposure to 0.25 to 0.5 ppm. The subjects were mouth breathing and performing moderate exercise. Koenig et al. (1981) found that in adolescent subjects exposed to 1 ppm with moderate exercise, the degree of response was related to the severity of asthma. They studied three groups: extreme asthmatics, atopics (allergic individuals with no clinical symptoms of asthma), and normals. As examples, airway resistance increased 67, 41, and 3 percent and forced expiratory volume (FEV) decreased 23, 18, and 6 percent for the three groups, respectively. The degree of sensitivity to SO_2 thus appears to depend on the magnitude of preexisting airway hypersensitivity. These findings on the response of asthmatics to short exposures to levels of sulfur dioxide below 0.5 ppm have raised new concerns about the potential adverse effects of peaks of sulfur dioxide known to occur near point sources on this sensitive segment of the population.

The changes we have been discussing were observed in animals or human subjects exposed for short periods of an hour or less to sulfur dioxide. Alarie et al. (1970) exposed guinea pigs to 0.13, 1.01, and 5.72 ppm sulfur dioxide continuously for a year. When compared with a comparable control group breathing clean air, no evidence was found of adverse effects on the mechanical properties of the lung. Measurements included tidal volume, respiratory rate, minute volume, flow resistance, and work of breathing. Monkeys (groups of nine animals) were exposed continuously for 78 weeks to 0.14, 0.64, and 1.28 ppm sulfur dioxide (Alarie et al., 1972). No detrimental alterations in pulmonary function were detected.

Lewis et al. (1969) exposed dogs to levels of 5 ppm sulfur dioxide about 21 hours a day for 225 days. One group of dogs was normal and the other had lung impairment produced by prior exposure to nitrogen dioxide (191 days at 26 ppm). The exposure to sulfur dioxide produced about a 50 percent increase in resistance and about a 16 percent decrease in compliance. In general, the adverse effects were less in the dogs with impaired function from previous nitrogen dioxide exposure, which might suggest that a lung previously remodeled by a toxicant may be more difficult to alter physiologically than one that had never been exposed to toxic concentrations of irritant. Vaughan et al. (1969) exposed dogs for 16 hours a day for 18 months to a combination of 0.5 ppm sulfur dioxide and 0.1 mg/m^3 sulfuric acid and concluded there was no impairment in pulmonary function.

Biochemical Effects. Information on biochemical aspects of the toxicology of sulfur dioxide is very limited. Some early studies indicated that radioactive sulfur persisted in the lung incorporated into protein, but no evidence was presented on the nature of this complex. Work by Gunnison and Palmes (1974) has indicated the presence in plasma of S-sulfonate formed by the reaction of sulfite with the disulfide bond in proteins. This has been found in rabbits and in human subjects. S-sulfonate is present in the plasma and aorta of rabbits infused with sulfite. Although the biologic significance is not at present understood, this finding represents a biochemical alteration observed in organs other than the lung.

Sulfuric Acid

Sulfuric acid is one of the most important atmospheric pollutants. The subject of acid aero-

Table 25–1. COMPARATIVE TOXICITY OF SO₂ AND H₂SO₄ ACUTE STUDIES

	S (μg/m^3)		
	SO$_2$	H$_2$SO$_4$	Reference
Guinea pigs—one hour			
10% ↑ Airway resistance	206	33	Amdur, 1974
Donkeys—30 minutes; one hour			
altered bronchial clearance	284,000	66	Spiegelman et al., 1968
			Schlesinger et al., 1978
Normal subjects—seven minutes; one			Lippmann and Altshuler, 1976
hour altered bronchial clearance	16,640	33	Leikauf et al., 1981
Normal subjects—ten minutes			
5% ↓ tidal volume	768	40	Amdur, 1954
Adolescent asthmatics—40 minutes			
Equal ↑ airway resistance	650	33	Koenig et al., 1989

sols is receiving long overdue attention, and of these aerosols sulfuric acid is the most irritant. As will be discussed below, the sensitive methods now available to assess pulmonary response indicate that sulfuric acid produces functional, biochemical, and morphologic changes at concentrations of the order of magnitude that can occur in the atmosphere and below historic levels in London in the 1960s or in smelter areas in the 1950s. Data obtained on animals and on human subjects are remarkably consistent. These data are reviewed in an article the title of which, *Sulfuric Acid: The Animals Tried to Tell Us,* was chosen to make the point that experimental toxicology can indeed be predictive of human response (Amdur, 1989). Lippmann *et al.* (1987) also provide a review with emphasis on the potential role of sulfuric acid as a causative agent of chronic bronchitis.

Sulfur dioxide can be converted to sulfuric acid when dissolved in droplets containing metals such as iron, manganese, or vanadium. Conversion can occur in power plant plumes as they move downwind. During smelting of metals or combustion of coal, sulfuric acid can form a surface layer on ultrafine metal oxide particles. As much as 9 percent of the sulfur present in some coals may be emitted in this form. These conversions of sulfur dioxide to sulfuric acid are important because sulfuric acid is a much more potent irritant than sulfur dioxide.

Table 25–1 shows the comparative acute toxicity of sulfur dioxide and sulfuric acid. The criteria used include alterations in airway resistance in animals and human subjects, and bronchial clearance. Where comparative data were available the results are consistent; the animal data on comparative toxicity correctly predicted the results in human subjects. To enable direct comparison, the concentrations are presented as μg S/m^3. Studies of monkeys exposed for two

years (Alarie *et al.*, 1972, 1975) to sulfur dioxide or sulfuric acid indicate that on a chronic basis as well sulfuric acid is the more potent irritant. Sulfur dioxide at 1 ppm (1300 μg S/m^3) produced no alterations whereas 160 μg S/m^3 as 0.54 μM sulfuric acid produced moderate to severe histopathology, moderate alterations in distribution of ventilation, and a moderate decrease in arterial oxygen.

Pulmonary Function. Sulfuric acid produces an increase in flow resistance in guinea pigs, the magnitude of which is related to both concentration and particle size (Amdur, 1958; Amdur *et al.*, 1978). In the following discussion, particle size is expressed as mass median diameter (MMD). Particles of 7 μm produced only a slight increase in resistance even at very high concentration (30 mg/m^3). Because these particles would not penetrate beyond the upper respiratory tract, this response was probably a referred reflex or an increase in nasal resistance. Particles of 2.5 μm gave a response that was slow in onset and accompanied by a major decrease in compliance. These mechanical changes were suggestive of closure of large areas of the lung due to constriction or obstruction with mucous secretions. Particles of 1 μm or below produced a swift response similar to that observed with irritant gases. Irritant potency increased with decreasing particle size. At concentrations below 1 mg/m^3 the response was greater for 0.3-μm than for 1-μm particles (Amdur *et al.*, 1978). Elevated flow resistance produced by sulfuric acid is much slower to return to control values than is the increase produced by sulfur dioxide. The action of irritant particles deposited on the lung surface is more prolonged than that of a gas, which is rapidly cleared from the lungs when exposure ceases.

The guinea pig responds with increased airway resistance at lower concentrations of sulfuric

Table 25–2. EFFECTS OF SULFURIC ACID ON AIRWAY RESISTANCE

Normal Subjects
1000 $\mu g/m^3$ causes no response (many studies).

Adult Exercising Asthmatics
450 to 1000 $\mu g/m^3$ for 16 min causes dose-related increase.
100 $\mu g/m^3$ causes no response (Utell).

Adolescent Exercising Asthmatics
68 to 100 $\mu g/m^3$ for 40 min causes increase (Koenig).

Guinea Pig
100 to 1000 $\mu g/m^3$ for 1 hr causes dose-related increase (Amdur).

acid than do normal human subjects. As with sulfur dioxide, asthmatic subjects are more sensitive than healthy individuals. Table 25–2 shows the comparison between normal subjects and asthmatics. It also indicates that, as with sulfur dioxide, the guinea pig model was predictive of the response of these sensitive asthmatics. Koenig *et al.* (1989) recently reported that although 0.1 ppm sulfur dioxide alone did not produce a response in adolescent asthmatics, it did increase their response to 68 $\mu g/m^3$ sulfuric acid when the two were given together. If further studies support this finding, it is a very important one because both pollutants occur together and impact on a sensitive segment of the population.

Clearance of Particles. Sulfuric acid alters the clearance of particles from the lung, thus interfering with a major defense mechanism. Effects have been observed following a single one-hour exposure in donkeys, rabbits, and human subjects. Radioactively tagged ferric oxide particles are used as the tracer aerosol. Bronchial clearance was slowed in donkeys by a one-hour exposure to 200 to 1400 $\mu g/m^3$. In rabbits 100 $\mu g/m^3$ was without effect, 250 $\mu g/m^3$ accelerated clearance, and 1000 to 2000 $\mu g/m^3$ produced a slowing. Studies in human subjects indicated that one-hour exposures to concentrations < 200 $\mu g/m^3$ stimulate clearance in large conducting airways but also depress clearance in small airways where greater amounts of acid deposit. Concentrations of 1000 $\mu g/m^3$ inhibit clearance in both large and small conducting airways. More recently, Spektor *et al.* (1989) demonstrated that at 100 $\mu g/m^3$ increasing the exposure time from one hour to two hours produced both a greater reduction in clearance and a persistent further reduction of clearance for up to three hours after the end of exposure.

Chronic exposure of donkeys one hour per day, five days per week for six months to 100 $\mu g/m^3$ sulfuric acid produced highly variable clearance rates and a persistent shift from baseline rate of bronchial mucociliary clearance during exposure and for three months after the last exposure.

Comparative studies in donkey and human subjects done by these investigators are of great practical significance. The effects of single short-term exposures to sulfuric acid on mucociliary clearance are similar in the two species. In donkeys, repeated exposure to low levels of sulfuric acid has a profound effect on clearance rates. It is neither ethical nor practical to do such repeated exposures in human subjects. It is, however, reasonable to assume that the chronic effects in humans would resemble those seen in the donkey. This is further strengthened by the similar response of the two species to cigarette smoke. The misguided chronic self-exposure of humans to cigarette smoke clearly documents the potential for development of chronic bronchitis. The assumption is thus reasonable that chronic exposure of humans to sulfuric acid at levels of 100 $\mu g/m^3$ or above would also lead to impaired clearance and chronic bronchitis.

Chronic Exposure. A recent study (Gearhart and Schlesinger, 1989) examined the effect on rabbits of 250 $\mu g/m^3$ sulfuric acid acid 1 hour per day, five days per week for four, eight, and twelve months with a three-month post-exposure period. This study uses a variety of criteria of exposure that are both relevant to the human response and sensitive enough to detect changes. Some of these data are summarized in Table 25–3. Slowing of clearance occurred during the first week of exposure, became progressive after the 19th week, and was still present three months after the end of exposure. This delayed recovery is consistent with earlier data in donkeys. The airways became progressively more sensitive to challenge with acetylcholine. Increased airway sensitivity has also been observed as an acute response in guinea pigs two hours after a one-hour exposure to 200 $\mu g/m^3$ sulfuric acid. Human subjects exposed four hours to 450 $\mu g/m^3$ showed increased airway sensitivity 24 hours after exposure but not immediately after. The possibility of a delayed inflammatory response was suggested by symptoms of sore throat. This important response has thus been demonstrated both in acute and chronic studies.

The rabbits showed a progressive decrease in airway diameter accompanied by an increase in the number of secretory cells, especially in the smaller airways. Acidic glycoprotein content of the intracellular mucus increased. The lowered pH of the mucus is important, as such changes have been noted in asthmatics. The implications

Table 25–3. EFFECTS OF CHRONIC EXPOSURE OF RABBITS, 250 $\mu g/m^3$ H$_2$SO$_4$ ONE HOUR PER DAY, FIVE DAYS PER WEEK

	EXPOSURE			POSTEXPOSURE
END POINT	*4 months*	*8 months*	*12 months*	*3 months*
Mucociliary clearance	↓	↓	↓	↓↓
Airway sensitivity	↑	↑↑	↑↑	nm
Air diameter	↓	↓	↓↓	nc
Secretory cell number	↑	↑↑	↑↑	↑
Secretory cell pH	↓	↓	↓	↓

From Gearhart and Schlesinger, 1989.
nm, not measured; nc, no change.

of such a change are discussed by Holma (1989). The changes observed in the rabbit are relevant to human disease because they have been associated with both chronic bronchitis and asthma. When one considers the similarity of the one-hour response of rabbits and human subjects, it is very reasonable to regard these data as predictive of the response that would be observed in human subjects were such a protocol possible.

Sulfuric Acid as Surface Layer. Sulfuric acid can be emitted to the atmosphere as a surface layer on ultrafine (<0.1 μm) metal oxide particles by the smelting of metals or the combustion of coal. The cooperation of combustion engineers made possible the furnace generation of such acid-coated particles for use in animal exposures (Amdur *et al.*, 1986). Because this sulfuric acid is carried to the deep lung on the surface of a large number of ultrafine particles, its irritant potency is greater than would be predicted on the basis of sulfuric acid concentration alone. A concentration of 30 $\mu g/m^3$ on the surface of ultrafine zinc oxide particles produces the same reduction in carbon monoxide diffusing capacity (DL$_{CO}$) in guinea pigs as a similar exposure to 300 $\mu g/m^3$ conventionally generated sulfuric acid of the same size (Amdur, 1989).

A single three-hour exposure of guinea pigs to 60 $\mu g/m^3$ sulfuric acid layered on ultrafine zinc oxide produced decreases in DL$_{CO}$, total lung capacity, and vital capacity and increases in cells, protein, and a variety of enzymes in lavage fluid that were not completely resolved 96 hours after exposure (Amdur, 1989). Lesser effects were produced by a single three-hour exposure to 30 $\mu g/m^3$ and no response was seen at 20 $\mu g/m^3$. When the three-hour exposures were repeated daily for five days to 20 and 30 $\mu g/m^3$, the effects were cumulative (Amdur, 1989).

Some coals, such as Illinois No. 6, have a layer of sulfuric acid on the surface of the ultrafine ash, whereas other more alkaline coals, such as Montana Lignite, produce instead a surface layer of neutral sulfate. As indicated in Figure 25–2, the acid-layered ash from the Illinois No. 6 produced a greater response, even though the amount of sulfate was greater in the Montana Lignite (Chen *et al.*, 1990).

Other Sulfates. In addition to sulfuric acid, the two main sulfates present as air pollutants are ammonium bisulfate and ammonium sulfate which are formed by neutralization of sulfuric acid. These are present as fine particles and undergo long-range transport to areas distant from

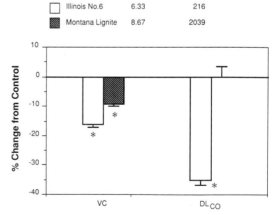

Effects of 2 hr Exposures of Guinea Pigs to Fly Ash

Coal Type	mg/m^3	Total Sulfate μg/m^3
☐ Illinois No.6	6.33	216
▨ Montana Lignite	8.67	2039

Figure 25–2. Comparison of a sulfuric acid coated ash (Illinois No. 6) with a neutral sulfate coated ash (Montana Lignite). *VC* = Vital capacity; *DL*$_{CO}$ = pulmonary diffusing capacity. (Data from Chen *et al.*, 1990.)

their emission source. Studies of bronchial clearance in rabbits and airway resistance in normal and asthmatic human subjects showed that the irritant potency was sulfuric acid > ammonium bisulfate > ammonium sulfate. The irritant potency is thus related to relative acidity.

More recent studies (Schlesinger et al., 1990) examined the effect of in vivo exposure of rabbits to sulfuric acid and ammonium bisulfate on the phagocytic activity of alveolar macrophages harvested by pulmonary lavage. Phagocytosis was altered by a single exposure to sulfuric acid at concentrations > 500 μg/m^3 and by ammonium bisulfate at concentrations > 2000 μg/m^3. Identical levels of H$^+$ in the exposure chamber atmosphere produced a lesser response with ammonium bisulfate than with sulfuric acid although in vitro studies of incubated macrophages showed identical response at a given pH no matter which compound had been added to reach the level of acidity. These results suggest that speciation of acidic aerosols in the atmosphere may be very important and that a simple measurement of atmospheric acidity may not be sufficient to assess potential health effects.

COMPONENTS AND FORMATION OF PHOTOCHEMICAL AIR POLLUTION

Photochemical air pollution arises from a series of atmospheric reactions. The main components are ozone, oxides of nitrogen, aldehydes, peroxyacetyl nitrates, and hydrocarbons. From the point of view of a discussion of the toxicology of air pollutants, the hydrocarbons as such do not concern us. The concentrations in ambient air do not reach levels high enough to produce any toxic effect. They are important because they enter into the chemical reactions that lead to the formation of photochemical smog. The chemical reactions that lead to the formation of this particular mixture of pollutants in the atmosphere are extremely complex.

The oxidant of critical importance in polluted atmospheres is ozone (O$_3$). Several miles above the earth's surface there is sufficient short-wave ultraviolet light to convert O$_2$ to O$_3$ by direct absorption, but these wavelengths do not reach the earth's surface. Of the major atmospheric pollutants, nitrogen dioxide is the most efficient absorber of the UV light that does reach the earth's surface. This absorption of UV light by NO$_2$ leads to a complex series of reactions, which may be simplified as follows:

$$NO_2 \xrightarrow{UV} NO + O \qquad (1)$$
$$O + O_2 \rightarrow O_3 \qquad (2)$$
$$O_3 + NO \rightarrow NO_2 + O_2 \qquad (3)$$

Because NO$_2$ is regenerated by the reaction of the NO and O$_3$ formed, the overall result is a cyclic reaction, which can be perpetuated.

This NO$_2$ photolytic cycle serves to explain the initial formation of O$_3$ in polluted atmospheres, but cannot explain the development of concentrations of O$_3$ as great as those that have been measured. If no additional mechanisms were involved, most of the O$_3$ would be broken down by reaction with the NO formed, and in steady-state conditions, O$_3$ and NO would be formed and destroyed in equal quantities. The hydrocarbons, especially olefins and substituted aromatics, become of importance by providing the necessary added reactants. Oxygen atoms attack the hydrocarbons. The resulting oxidized compounds and free radicals react with NO to produce more NO$_2$. Thus, the balance of the reactions shown in equations 1 to 3 is upset so that NO$_2$ and O$_3$ levels build up while NO levels are depleted. These reactions are very complex and involve the formation of intermediate free radicals that are very reactive and undergo a series of changes.

Aldehydes are major products in the photooxidation of hydrocarbons, and in the reactions of hydrocarbons with ozone, oxygen atoms, or free radicals. Formaldehyde and acrolein have been specifically identified in urban atmospheres. About 50 percent of the total aldehyde is present as formaldehyde and about 5 percent as acrolein.

Peroxyacetyl nitrate, often referred to as PAN, is most likely formed in the atmosphere from the reaction of the peroxyacetyl radical with NO$_2$. Its chemical formula is CH$_3$COONO$_2$. Higher homologues are probably also present, but PAN is the one that has been positively identified as present in urban atmospheres.

Ozone

A variety of toxic effects occur in experimental animals exposed to concentrations of ozone that can occur in urban areas with photochemical pollution. These effects include morphologic, functional, and biochemical alterations. An excellent summary of current knowledge on all aspects of ozone toxicity was prepared by Lippmann (1989).

Ozone is a very critical air pollutant. The reasons for this, as stated by Lippmann (1989), are worth repeating here.

Health and pollution control professionals and the general public need to develop a more complete understanding of the health effects of ozone (O$_3$) because: 1) we have been unable to significantly reduce ambient O$_3$ levels using current strategies and controls; 2) in areas occupied by more than half of the U.S. population, current peak ambient O_3 concentrations are sufficient to elicit measurable transient changes in lung function, respiratory symptoms, and airway inflammation in healthy people engaged in normal outdoor exercise and recreational activities; 3) the effects of O_3 on transient functional changes are sometimes greatly potentiated by the presence of other environmental variables; and 4) cumulative structural damage occurs in rats and monkeys exposed repetitively to O_3 at levels within currently occurring ambient peaks, and initial evidence from dosimetry models and interspecies comparisons indicate that humans are likely to be more sensitive to O_3 than rats. The extent and significance of these effects, and the multibillion dollar costs of ambient O_3 controls need to be considered in any future revisions of ambient standards and the Clean Air Act.

The target of ozone toxicity is the acinar region of the lung from the terminal bronchioles to the alveolar ducts. Because ozone penetration increases with increased tidal volume and flow rate, exercise increases the dose to the target area. The highest local dose is delivered to the respiratory acini of humans, rabbits, guinea pigs, and rats (Miller et al., 1978). The dose in man has been estimated to be about twice that for the rat.

Lung Pathology. Morphometric studies of the acinar region of rats exposed 12 hours per day for six weeks to 0.12 or 0.25 ppm ozone showed hyperplasia of Type I alveolar cells and major alterations in ciliated and Clara cells in small airways (Barry et al., 1988). To simulate the pattern of atmospheric exposure, rats were exposed daily 13 hours at 0.06 ppm plus a nine-hour peak five days per week of 0.18 ppm that included a one-hour maximum of 0.25 ppm. Hyperplasia of Type I cells in the proximal alveoli occurred by three to twelve weeks and was linearly related to the cumulative ozone exposure. This suggests that there is no threshold for cumulative lung damage, which in turn suggests the need for a seasonal or annual averaging time for a future ozone standard.

Rats exposed to clean air or to ozone by the above protocol for six weeks were exposed once for five hours to asbestos. When examined 30 days later, lungs of the ozone-exposed animals contained three times as many fibers as lungs of the control group. Realistic low exposure to ozone thus has the potential to increase the retention time and therefore the effective dose of toxic and potentially carcinogenic particles.

After 12 months on this exposure protocol the rats showed functional lung changes, suggesting a stiffer lung and biochemical changes indicative of increased antioxidant metabolism but no immunologic changes (Grose et al., 1989).

Exposure of monkeys to 0.6 ppm ozone eight hours per day for a year produced abnormal lung collagen which was still present six months postexposure. To compare effects of intermittent and continuous exposure, Tyler et al. (1988) exposed one group of monkeys to 0.25 ppm ozone eight hours per day, five days per week for 18 months and another group on the same protocol with exposure only in alternate months. A control group breathed filtered air. Both exposure groups showed respiratory bronchiolitis and reduced lung growth. Effects in the intermittently exposed group were as great or greater than effects in the group exposed continuously. Increased lung collagen, chest wall compliance, and inspiratory capacity were observed only in the group exposed in alternate months. The implication of these findings is that damage results from repeated attempts by the lung to adapt to the ozone challenge as well as from the irritant exposure per se.

Pulmonary Function. Ozone exposure produces concentration-related decrements in exhaled volumes and flow rate during forced expiratory maneuvers in exercising human subjects at or below the current ambient air standard of 0.12 ppm. These changes increase with extension of exposure time so that changes are present in response to two hours at 0.12 or 0.10 ppm that were not seen at one hour. The extension of the exposure time to 6.6 hours at a concentration of 0.12 ppm produced effects that progressed as exposure continued. Decrements in FEV_1 after 6.6 hours averaged 13.6 percent and were comparable to effects following a two-hour exposure to 0.22 ppm with heavier exercise (Folinsbee et al., 1988). Follow-up studies using 0.08, 0.10, and 0.12 ppm for 6.6 hours reproduced the earlier results and showed lesser changes at 0.08 and 0.10 ppm (Horstman et al., 1989). No residual decrement remained 24 hours after exposure.

Greater decrements in pulmonary function per ppm ozone were found in children studied at summer camps than were found in a variety of studies of children in chamber exposures even though the exercise levels in the children at camp were lower than those observed in the chamber studies (Lippmann, 1989). This could relate to greater cumulative exposure in the children at camp. The relation between ozone levels the previous day and pulmonary function of school children in the Kingston-Harriman area of Tennessee was similar to that observed in the summer camp studies even though the activity levels were lower (Kinney et al., 1988). This may be related to simultaneous high levels of acid aerosol in the Kingston area.

Animal studies also confirmed the fact that both duration and concentration are important in

assessing the response to ozone exposure (Costa *et al.*, 1989). Rats were exposed two, four, and eight hours to ozone at 0.1, 0.2, 0.4, and 0.8 ppm. Pulmonary function decrements increased with $C \times T$ (concentration $\times$ time) leveling off at 6 ppm-hour. Protein in bronchoalveolar lavage fluid increased rapidly at 4 ppm-hour. Rats exposed 6.6 hours to 0.5 ppm with 8 percent CO_2 added to stimulate respiration showed functional decrements similar to those observed in the human chamber studies of 6.6 hours at 0.12 ppm. The lesser response of rats to a given ozone concentration compared with human subjects is consistent with the lesser retention of ozone by rats. Despite this difference, these studies show that the rat provides a good test model for the response of human subjects.

The mechanism by which ozone produces decrements in pulmonary function is not well understood. Ozone differs from sulfuric acid or sulfur dioxide in that functional responses do not correlate with responsiveness to bronchoconstrictor challenge as they do for the other irritants. Also the response to ozone is not enhanced in asthmatic subjects as it is for the sulfur pollutants. The contribution of β-adrenergic mechanisms in the acute response to ozone appears to be minimal. Prostaglandins E_2 and F_2 and thromboxane B_2 increase in human bronchoalveolar lavage fluid following ozone exposure. Pretreatment with indomethacin, a prostaglandin synthetase inhibitor, decreased the pulmonary function deficit in exposure of human subjects to 0.35 ppm ozone.

Evidence of airway inflammation following ozone exposure has been obtained in human subjects. Koren *et al.* (1989) found an eightfold increase in polymorphonuclear leukocytes (PMN) in lavage fluid eight hours after a two-hour exposure to 0.40 ppm ozone. There was also a twofold increase in protein, albumin, and immunoglobulin G. This observation fits with evidence of increased epithelial permeability caused by a similar exposure. A 6.6-hour exposure to 0.10 ppm ozone caused a 4.8-fold increase in PMN 18 hours postexposure.

Another response to ozone is an increase in airway reactivity. The airway reactivity was approximately doubled by a 6.6-hour exposure to 0.12 ppm ozone (Folinsbee *et al.*, 1988). In 6.6-hour exposures to 0.08, 0.10, and 0.12 ppm increases in responsiveness to methacholine were 56, 86, and 121 percent, respectively (Horstman *et al.*, 1989). This increased airway sensitivity could increase the response to other pollutants such as sulfuric acid or aeroallergens that produce bronchoconstriction. Osebold *et al.* (1980) reported that ozone enhanced the allergic sensitivity of mice to an inhaled antigen.

Susceptibility to Bacteria. Exposure to ozone prior to challenge with aerosols of infectious agents produces a higher incidence of infection than seen in control animals (Coffin and Blommer, 1967). It is assumed that this results from inhibition of clearance mechanisms, either mucociliary streaming or phagocytosis. Exposure of mice to concentrations as low as 0.08 ppm ozone for three hours enhanced the mortality from subsequent exposure to a bacterial aerosol of streptococcus (Group C). The susceptibility of mice and hamsters to *Klebsiella pneumoniae* aerosol was increased by prior exposure to ozone, as indicated by a higher mortality, shorter survival time, and lower LD50 for *K. pneumoniae* in ozone-exposed animals as compared with controls.

It has been shown that exposure to ozone reduced the number as well as the *in vitro* phagocytic ability of pulmonary macrophages in rabbits. This could help to explain the increased survival time of bacteria observed in the lungs of animals preexposed to ozone. Membrane damage in macrophages from rats exposed to ozone impairs production of bactericidal superoxide anion radical.

Nitrogen Dioxide

Nitrogen dioxide, like ozone, is a deep lung irritant capable of producing pulmonary edema if inhaled in sufficient concentrations. This is a practical problem to farmers, as sufficient amounts can be liberated from ensilage to produce the symptoms of pulmonary damage known as silo-fillers' disease. Nitrogen dioxide is also an important indoor pollutant, especially in homes with unventilated gas stoves or kerosene heaters (Spengler and Sexton, 1983). Under such circumstances children, who are especially sensitive, may show decrements in pulmonary function.

That nitrogen dioxide can cause effects similar to those produced by ozone is not surprising. It is also an oxidant gas and deposits in the lung in an area only slightly proximal to the site of ozone deposition. It is a less potent irritant by far than ozone. Levels needed to produce effects are in general far above levels that occur in ambient air. More recently protocols that simulate the two daily peaks superimposed on a low continuous background concentration known to occur in urban environments have produced effects in experimental animals.

Lung Pathology. Although the lesions produced are similar, there is considerable difference in sensitivity among species. Where direct comparison is possible, guinea pigs, hamsters, and monkeys are more sensitive than rats. Damage occurs in the terminal bronchioles, alveolar ducts, and alveoli. Type I cells are damaged and replaced by Type II cells. There is damage to epithelial cells in the bronchioles, and loss of secretory granules in Clara cells as well as loss of ciliated cells and cilia. In the face of continued exposure, repair processes commence within 24 to 48 hours. Some lesions are resolved while others remain (Kubota *et al.*, 1987).

Pulmonary Function. Mice were exposed for a year to a base level of 0.2 ppm nitrogen dioxide with a one-hour spike of 0.8 ppm twice a day, five days per week (Miller *et al.*, 1987). The base level produced no effects. When the spikes were added, decreases in end-expiratory volume and vital capacity were significant. There was also a trend toward increased residual volume and decreased lung distensibility.

Exposure of normal human subjects to concentrations of nitrogen dioxide of 1 ppm or less for periods up to four hours produced no consistent effects on pulmonary function. Asthmatics are not more sensitive than normal subjects to nitrogen dioxide, in contrast with their increased response to the sulfur pollutants.

Lung Defense. Exposure of rats to nitrogen dioxide at 0.5, 1, and 4 ppm for seven months produced a dose-related loss and swelling of cilia. In rabbits mucociliary clearance was unaltered by exposure to 0.3 or 1 ppm two hours per day for 14 days.

Structural changes were seen in alveolar macrophages following 21 weeks of continuous exposure to 2 ppm or to 0.5 ppm with a one-hour peak of 2 ppm five days per week. The 0.5 ppm exposure without peaks or 0.1 ppm with 1 ppm spikes caused no change. In various studies of phagocytic activity of alveolar macrophages concentrations of 4 ppm for a week were required for suppression.

Susceptibility to Respiratory Infection. Data obtained on a variety of species of experimental animals (mice, hamsters, rabbits, squirrel monkeys) suggest that either short-term or long-term exposures to nitrogen dioxide can increase susceptibility to respiratory infection by bacterial pneumonia or influenza virus. The evidence for this effect falls into three categories: (1) increased mortality rates; (2) reduced survival time; and (3) reduced ability to clear pathogenic organisms from the lung, as indicated by the number of viable organisms that can be cultured.

Coffin *et al.* (1976) tested the effect of varying both concentration and time of exposure on the mortality of mice exposed to *Streptococcus pyogenes*. A $C \times T$ value of 7 ppm-hours was used with exposures from 14 ppm for 0.5 hour to 1 ppm for seven hours. The concentration was more critical than time in increasing the mortality from infection. In other experiments, 1.5 ppm for 18 hours increased mortality by 25 percent but a two-hour exposure to 14.5 ppm caused a 65 percent increase.

Both increased mortality and reduced clearance rates of *K. pneumoniae* from the lungs were observed in mice exposed chronically to 0.5 ppm nitrogen dioxide (Ehrlich and Henry, 1968). Statistically significant increases in mortality following infection were observed in mice exposed continuously for three months and after six months of daily 6- or 18-hour exposures. The clearance rate of bacteria from lungs was reduced by exposure for 6 or 18 hours a day for nine months. These effects were more pronounced after 12 months of exposure. When exposure was continuous, a reduced capacity to clear bacteria from the lung was observed after six months as well as at 9 and 12 months.

Increased mortality was seen in squirrel monkeys exposed for short periods of two hours to 50 ppm nitrogen dioxide or for periods of one or two months to 10 or 5 ppm when they were infected with *K. pneumoniae* (Henry *et al.*, 1970). Monkeys exposed to 10 ppm nitrogen dioxide for two hours and then infected had viable bacteria present in their lungs up to 50 days after challenge. Squirrel monkeys were infected with nonlethal levels of A/PR-8 influenza virus and then exposed continuously to 5 or 10 ppm nitrogen dioxide. All six monkeys exposed to 10 ppm died within three days and one out of three exposed to 5 ppm died. Other experiments suggested that exposure of squirrel monkeys for five months to 5 ppm nitrogen dioxide depressed the formation of protective antibody against this influenza virus.

Aldehydes

Various aldehydes in polluted air are formed as reaction products in the photooxidation of hydrocarbons. The two aldehydes of major interest are formaldehyde and acrolein. These materials probably contribute to the odor of and eye irritation produced by photochemical smog. Formaldehyde accounts for about 50 percent of the estimated total aldehydes in polluted air. Acrolein, the more irritant of the two, may account for about 5 percent of the total aldehydes. These aldehydes act as competitive agonists. Irritation would not be related to "total aldehyde" but to specific concentrations of acrolein and formaldehyde.

Formaldehyde. Formaldehyde is a primary irritant. Because it is very soluble in water, it irritates mucous membranes of the nose, upper respiratory tract, and eyes. Concentrations of 0.5

to 1 ppm are detectable by odor, 2 to 3 ppm produce mild irritation, and 4 to 5 ppm are intolerable to most people.

The effect of low concentrations of formaldehyde on the respiration of guinea pigs has been studied (Amdur, 1960). A one-hour exposure to concentrations of 0.3 ppm and above produced an increase in pulmonary flow resistance accompanied by a lesser decrease in compliance. The respiratory frequency and minute volume decreased, but changes in these factors did not become statistically significant until concentrations of 10 ppm and above were used. The overall pattern of respiratory response to formaldehyde is similar to that produced by sulfur dioxide. A concentration of 0.05 ppm caused no alterations in any of the respiratory criteria used. Below concentrations of 50 ppm the alterations were reversible within an hour after the exposure.

The response to a given concentration of formaldehyde was greater when the gas was inhaled through a tracheal cannula, which bypassed the scrubbing effect of the upper respiratory tract and permitted a greater concentration of the irritant to reach the lungs. The response in these animals was also readily reversible, and the flow resistance values had returned to preexposure levels by one hour after the end of exposure.

The response to formaldehyde was potentiated by the simultaneous administration of a sodium chloride aerosol of submicron particles. The values for pulmonary resistance remained above preexposure levels for one hour after the end of exposure when the gas-aerosol combination was used. This prolonged response, which is typical of the response of irritant aerosols, suggests that the potentiation is brought about by the attachment of formaldehyde to the particles to form an irritant aerosol. This hypothesis is further supported by the fact that when 3.10, and 30 mg/m^3 concentrations of sodium chloride were used, the potentiation increased with the increasing concentration of particles. The response to a given concentration of formaldehyde plus aerosol breathed by nose was greater than the response to the gas alone breathed through a tracheal cannula. This indicates that the increment added by the aerosol is not due to the transfer of an additional amount of formaldehyde gas as such to the lungs, because it was greater than could be accounted for by the transfer of the full concentration of formaldehyde to the lungs.

The particles of Los Angeles–type smog are capable of carrying a considerable amount of formaldehyde. This suggests that the biologic data obtained may have some practical significance.

Two aspects of formaldehyde toxicology have recently brought it from relative obscurity to the forefront of the news. One is its presence in indoor atmospheres, especially in home with improperly installed urea-formaldehyde foam insulation. This aspect is discussed at length in a review article (Spengler and Sexton, 1983). The other is the finding of nasal cancers in rodents.

In a two-year study, Fischer 344 rats were exposed to 2, 6, or 14 ppm formaldehyde 6 hours per day, five days per week. The occurrence of nasal squamous cell carcinomas was zero in the control and 2 ppm groups, 1 percent in the 6 ppm group, and 44 percent in the 14 ppm group. An exposure-related induction of squamous metaplasia occurred in the respiratory epithelium of the anterior nasal passages in all exposed groups. The response may be related to inhibition of ciliary activity and mucociliary clearance in the nasal passages. Rats exposed six hours per day for five days had a > 20-fold increase in cell proliferation in the nasal epithelium. Mice are much less sensitive; only one carcinoma was seen at 14 ppm. The likely reasons for this species difference and the implications of these findings to the development of the observed carcinomas are reviewed by Starr and Gibson (1985).

Had they been obtained on a new chemical, the animal data would have led to a ban on its widespread use in industry and in consumer products. Formaldehyde, however, has been so used for a very long time. If the animal data had relevance to practical exposures, should we not have had evidence of increased incidence of nasal cancer in exposed workers? Recent epidemiology studies failed to find increased incidence of nasal cancer in exposed workers.

Acrolein. Because it is an unsaturated aldehyde, acrolein is much more irritant than formaldehyde. Concentrations below 1 ppm cause irritation of the eyes and mucous membranes of the respiratory tract.

The effect of acrolein on the respiratory function of guinea pigs has been studied (Murphy *et al.*, 1963). Exposure to 0.6 ppm and above increased pulmonary flow resistance, increased tidal volume, and decreased respiratory frequency. The effects were reversible when the animals were returned to clean air. In the case of irritants of this type, flow resistance is increased by concentrations below those that cause a decrease in frequency. This suggests that flow resistance increases would be produced by far lower concentrations of acrolein than were tested. Atropine, aminophylline, isoproterenol, and epinephrine partially or completely reversed the changes. Pyrilamine and tripelennamine were without effect. The mechanism of increased resistance appears to be bronchoconstriction mediated through reflex cholinergic stimulation.

Carbon Monoxide

Carbon monoxide would be classed toxicologically as a chemical asphyxiant, and its toxic action stems from its formation of carboxyhemoglobin. The fundamental factors of the toxicology of carbon monoxide and the physiologic factors that determine the level of carboxyhemoglobin reached in the blood at various atmospheric concentrations of carbon monoxide are dealt with in Chapter 8.

The normal concentration of carboxyhemoglobin (COHb) in the blood of nonsmokers is about 0.5 percent. This is attributed to endogenous production of CO from such sources as heme catabolism. Uptake of exogenous CO increases blood COHb in proportion to the concentration in the air as well as the length of exposure and the ventilation rate of the person. Continuous exposure of human subjects to 30 ppm CO leads to an equilibrium value of 5 percent COHb. About 80 percent of this value is approached in four hours and the remaining 20 percent is approached slowly over the next eight hours. It can be calculated that continuous exposure to 20 ppm CO gives an equilibrium COHb value of about 3.7 percent and 10 ppm CO gives an equilibrium value of 2 percent COHb. The equilibrium values are generally reached after eight or more hours of exposure. The time required to reach equilibrium can be shortened by physical activity.

Analysis of data from air-monitoring programs in California indicates that eight-hour average values, which may be exceeded for 0.1 percent of the time, ranged from 10 to 40 ppm CO. Depending on location within a community, CO concentrations can vary widely. Concentrations predicted inside the passenger compartments of motor vehicles in downtown traffic were almost three times those for central urban areas and five times those expected in residential areas. Occupants of vehicles traveling on expressways had CO exposures somewhere between those in central urban areas and in downtown traffic. Concentrations above 87 ppm have been measured in underground garages, in tunnels, and in buildings over highways.

No human health effects have been demonstrated for COHb levels below 2 percent. Above 2 percent COHb in nonsmokers (the median value for smokers is of the order of 5 percent COHb) it has been possible to demonstrate effects on the central nervous system. At COHb levels of 2.5 percent resulting from about 90-minute exposure to about 50 ppm CO, there is an impairment of time-interval discrimination; at approximately 5 percent COHb there is an impairment of other psychomotor faculties. Cardiovascular changes may be produced by exposure sufficient to yield over 5 percent COHb. These include increased cardiac output, A-V oxygen difference, and coronary blood flow in patients without coronary disease. Decreased coronary sinus blood PO_2 occurs in patients with coronary heart disease. Impaired oxidative metabolism of the myocardium may occur. These changes could produce an added burden on patients with heart disease. Some adaptation to chronic low levels of CO may occur through such mechanisms as increased hematocrit, hemoglobin, and blood volume.

Auto Exhaust and Synthetic Smog

Many investigators have studied the effect of atmospheres designed to simulate photochemical smog. These have included irradiated and nonirradiated auto exhaust or ozonized gasoline. The observed effects are those of a mixture of components, some of which are known, others unknown. Such experiments have the advantage of being a step closer to actual urban air pollution than studies of individual specific chemicals and the disadvantage that it is difficult to determine which of the many substances present are critical for the observed effects.

Short-Term Exposures. Exposures of two to three hours to heavy Los Angeles smog containing 0.4 ppm total oxidant, or synthetic smog containing 0.5 ppm total oxidant, produced ultrastructural changes in alveolar tissue of mice ranging in age from 5 to 21 months. The severity of the damage increased with increasing age. No change was detectable in the youngest animals. In eight- to nine-month-old animals there were definite alterations, but by 14 to 18 hours after exposure there was no detectable difference from control animals. In animals 15 months of age alterations were still present 24 hours after exposure. The endothelial cells were seriously affected, but the lining epithelium and basement membrane were intact. In the oldest animals changes that could be interpreted as edemalike occurred in the lining epithelium. The alterations were still present 18 hours after exposure. The implication is clear that loss of regenerative capacity of alveolar tissue following damage is one result of aging.

Mice were exposed to auto exhaust containing 0.08 to 0.67 ppm oxidant and 12 to 100 ppm CO for four hours. Immediately following this exposure the mice were exposed to a bacterial aerosol of *Streptococcus* (Group C) at the rate of 100,000 organisms per mouse. When the exhaust contained 0.35 to 0.67 ppm oxidant and

100 ppm CO, there was enhanced mortality from streptococcal pneumonia: 53 percent among the exposed and 11 percent among the controls. The mortality was not enhanced by exhaust containing 0.12 ppm oxidant and 25 ppm CO. The increased mortality was probably related to the oxidant content. The levels involved are well below peak concentrations reported for heavy pollution.

The respiratory function of guinea pigs exposed to irradiated and nonirradiated auto exhaust has been measured. Increases in flow resistance were produced by 150:1 dilutions of irradiated exhaust but not by similar dilutions of nonirradiated exhaust. This was attributed to the formation of aldehydes, nitrogen dioxide, and total oxidant by irradiation. The nature of the response suggests aldehyde as the most likely component responsible for the observed change.

Chronic Exposures. In an extensive experiment designed to assess the long-term effects of auto exhaust, beagle dogs were exposed daily for 16 hours for a total of 68 months (Lewis *et al.*, 1974). A variety of pulmonary function studies were made at intervals throughout the exposure years. At the end of the exposure period the dogs were moved from the EPA laboratory in Cincinnati to the college of Veterinary Medicine at Davis, California. There a series of physiologic measurements were made both on arrival and two years after the exposure had terminated. The dogs were then killed and extensive morphologic examination by light and electron microscopy was made of the lungs. These experiments thus provided an opportunity to correlate physiologic and morphologic observations.

One hundred and four dogs were divided into eight groups. One group included 20 dogs that served as controls and were exposed in similar chambers to clean air. The seven experimental groups each contained 12 dogs. The exposures were to: (1) nonirradiated auto exhaust; (2) irradiated auto exhaust; (3) sulfur dioxide plus sulfuric acid; (4) and (5) the two types of exhaust plus the sulfur mixture; and (6) and (7) a high and low level of nitrogen oxides. The irradiated exhaust contained oxidant (measured as ozone) at about 0.2 ppm and nitrogen dioxide at about 0.9 ppm. The raw exhaust contained minimal concentrations of these materials and about 1.5 ppm nitric oxide. Both forms of exhaust contained close to 100 ppm carbon monoxide.

The values for physiologic tests done on the control dogs showed no change between the end of exposure and two years after. All other exposure groups had pulmonary function values different from controls and had more functional abnormalities at the end of the two-year post-exposure period. Pulmonary function tests suggested that auto exhaust exposure injured the airways and parenchyma while oxides of sulfur or nitrogen injured the parenchyma.

Two important exposure-related pulmonary lesions were observed. Enlargement of air spaces and loss of interalveolar septa in proximal acinar regions were most severe in dogs exposed to oxides of nitrogen, oxides of sulfur, or the latter with irradiated exhaust. Hyperplasia of nonciliated bronchiolar cells was most severe in dogs exposed to raw auto exhaust alone or with oxides of sulfur.

These studies indicate that alterations in function that are reflected by morphologic injury are persistent in nature following exposure to quite realistic levels of mixed pollution.

Diesel exhaust is another form of mobile source pollution that has received extensive study. The overall evidence for potential health effects in the form of epidemiology, *in vitro* studies, and chronic exposure of whole animals has been discussed and evaluated by McClellan (1986) as a case study in risk assessment. The epidemiologic data are only suggestive of a possible effect of diesel exhaust as a human carcinogen. With current controls of diesel exhaust it seems unlikely that exposures will be high enough to demonstrate association with respiratory disease.

A variety of *in vitro* studies indicate that extracts of diesel exhaust particles are mutagenic in bacterial assays and that the mutagenic potency is in large part attributable to nitroarenes. Diesel exhaust extracts produced an increase in sister chromatid exchange frequency in Chinese hamster ovary cells exposed *in vitro*. Such studies are valuable for comparison of exhaust from different vehicles or operating conditions and for identifying specific compounds but whether this potency extends to the *in vivo* environment remains a key question.

Rats were exposed seven hours per day, five days per week for 24 months to 0.35, 3.5, and 7 mg/m^3 diesel exhaust. Lung burdens increased in all exposures but reached an equilibrium at six months in the low dose which produced no detrimental effects. The two higher doses showed increasing lung burdens throughout the 24-month exposure which led to a variety of pulmonary effects. After 12 months of exposure, pulmonary clearance of inhaled radioactive particles was impaired by both doses. Bronchoalveolar lavage fluid showed an increase in macrophages and neutrophils as well as an increase in biochemical markers of cell injury. Lung collagen was increased. Lung pathology was moderate to severe at 3.5 mg/m^3 and severe at 7 mg/m^3. Reduced lung compliance and diffusing capacity were observed at both doses and the high dose reduced total lung capacity.

The highest dose produced some excess of neoplasms of two types, adenocarcinomas and squamous cell carcinomas. A low incidence of lung cancer in rats has been observed in other studies, but the evidence is equivocal and the levels used were high.

CONCLUSIONS

Because this chapter was written for a textbook of toxicology, it has discussed mainly the results of experimental studies related to specific compounds that occur as pollutants of urban air. Data of this kind are among the factors considered in the practical deliberations on the development of air quality criteria and standards.

The Clean Air Act sets forth the legal steps leading to the establishment of air quality standards. The initial step in this process is the preparation of an air quality criteria document that sets forth the state of knowledge in regard to the effects of the substance on animals, humans, plants, and materials. It is in this step that the availability of pertinent toxicologic data is of prime importance. This has been and should continue to be an incentive to toxicologists to develop sensitive methods capable of assaying the response to low concentrations of materials that occur as air pollutants.

REFERENCES

Alarie, Y. C.; Krumm, A. A.; Busey, W. M.; Ulrich, C. E.; and Kantz, R. J., Jr.: Long-term exposure to sulfur dioxide, sulfuric acid mist, fly ash, and their mixtures. Results of studies in monkeys and guinea pigs. *Arch. Environ. Health*, **30**:254–262, 1975.

Alarie, Y. C.; Ulrich, C. E.; Busey, W. M.; Krumm, A. A.; and MacFarland, H. N.: Long-term continuous exposure to sulfur dioxide in cynomolgus monkeys. *Arch. Environ. Health*, **24**:115–128, 1972.

Alarie, Y. C.; Ulrich, C. E.; Busey, W. M.; Swann, H. E., Jr.; and MacFarland, H. N.: Long-term continuous exposure of guinea pigs to sulfur dioxide. *Arch. Environ. Health*, **21**:769–777, 1970.

Amdur, M. O.: The respiratory response of guinea pigs to sulfuric acid mist. *AMA Arch. Ind. Health*, **18**:407–414, 1958.

———: The response of guinea pigs to inhalation of formaldehyde and formic acid alone and with a sodium chloride aerosol. *Int. J. Air Pollut.*, **3**:201–220, 1960.

———: Respiratory absorption data and SO_2 dose-response curves. *Arch Environ. Health*, **12**:729–732, 1966.

———: Sulfuric acid: the animals tried to tell us. 1989 Herbert E. Stokinger Lecture. *Appl. Ind. Hyg.*, **4**:189–197, 1989.

Amdur, M. O.; Dubriel, M.; and Creasia, D. A.: Respiratory response of guinea pigs to low levels of sulfuric acid. *Environ. Res.*, **15**:418–423, 1978.

Amdur, M. O.; Sarofim, A. F.; Neville, M.; Quann, R. J.; McCarthy, J. F.; Elliott, J. F.; Lam, H. F.; Rogers, A. E.; and Conner, M. W.: Coal combustion aerosols and SO_2: an interdisciplinary analysis. *Environ. Sci. Tech.*, **20**:139–145, 1986.

Amdur, M. O., and Underhill, D. W.: The effect of various aerosols on the response of guinea pigs to sulfur dioxide. *Arch. Environ. Health*, **16**:460–468, 1968.

Barry, B. E.; Mercer, R. R.; Miller, F. J.; and Crapo, J. D.: Effects of inhalation of 0.25 ppm ozone on the terminal bronchioles of juvenile and adult rats. *Exp. Lung Res.*, **14**:225–245, 1988.

Bates, D. V., and Sizto, R.: The Ontario air pollution study: identification of the causitive agent. *Environ. Health Perspect.*, **79**:69–72, 1989.

Chen, L. C.; Lam, H. F.; Kim, E. J.; Guty, J.; and Amdur, M. O.: Pulmonary effects of ultrafine coal fly ash inhaled by guinea pigs. *J. Toxicol. Environ. Health*, **29**:169–184, 1990.

Coffin, D. L., and Blommer, E. J.: Acute toxicity of irradiated auto exhaust. Its indication by enhancement of mortality from streptococcal pneumonia. *Arch. Environ. Health*, **15**:36–38, 1967.

Coffin, D. L.; Gardner, D. E.; and Blommer, E. J.: Time-dose response for nitrogen dioxide exposure in an infectivity model system. *Environ. Health Perspect.*, **13**:11–15, 1976.

Costa, D. L.; Hatch, G. E.; Highfill, J.; Stevens, M. A.; and Tepper, J. S.: Pulmonary function studies in the rat addressing concentration vs. time relationships for ozone. In Schneider, T.; Lee, S. D.; Wolters, G. J. R.; and Grant, L. D. (eds.): *Atmospheric Ozone Research and Its Policy Implications*. Elsevier, Amsterdam, 1989, pp. 733–743.

Dalhamn, T.: Mucous flow and ciliary activity in the trachea of healthy rats and rats exposed to respiratory irritant gases (SO_2, NH_3, HCHO). A functional and morphologic (light microscopic and electron microscopic) study, with special reference to technique. *Acta Physiol. Scand.*, **36**(*Suppl.* 123):1–161, 1956.

Ehrlich, R., and Henry, M. C.: Chronic toxicity of nitrogen dioxide. I. Effect on resistance to bacterial pneumonia. *Arch. Environ. Health*, **17**:860–865, 1968.

Folinsbee, L. J.; McDonnell, W. F.; and Horstman, D. H.: Pulmonary function and symptom responses after 6.6 hour exposure to 0.12 ppm ozone with moderate exercise. *J. Air Pollut. Control Assoc.*, **38**:28–35, 1988.

Frank, N. R.; Amdur, M. O.; Worchester, J.; and Whittenberger, J. L.: Effects of acute controlled exposure to SO_2 on respiratory mechanics in healthy male adults. *J. Appl. Physiol.*, **17**:252–258, 1962.

Frank, N. R., and Speizer, F. E.: SO_2 effects on the respiratory system in dogs. Changes in mechanical behavior at different levels of the respiratory system during acute exposure to the gas. *Arch Environ. Health*, **11**:624–634, 1965.

Gearhart, J. M., and Schlesinger, R. B.: Sulfuric acid-induced changes in the physiology and structure of the tracheobronchial airways. *Environ. Health Perspect.*, **79**:127–136, 1989.

Grose, E. C.; Stevens, M. A.; Hatch, R. H.; Jaskot, R. H.; Selgrade, M. J. K.; Stead, A. G.; Costa, D. L.; and Graham, J. A.: The impact of a 12 month exposure to a diurnal pattern of ozone on pulmonary function, antioxidant biochemistry and immunology. In Schneider, T.; Lee, S. D.; Wolters, G. J. R.; and Grant, L. D. (eds.): *Atmospheric Ozone Research and Its Policy Implications*. Elsevier, Amsterdam, 1989, pp. 535–544.

Gunnison, A. F., and Palmes, E. D.: S-Sulfonates in human plasma following inhalation of sulfur dioxide. *Am. Ind. Hyg. Assoc. J.*, **35**:288–291, 1974.

Henry, M. C.; Findlay, J.; Spengler, J.; and Ehrlich, R.: Chronic toxicity of NO_2 in squirrel monkeys. III.

Effect on resistance to bacterial and viral infection. *Am. Ind. Hyg. Assoc. J.*, **20**:566–570, 1970.

Holma, B.: Effects of inhaled acids on airway mucus and its consequences for health. *Environ. Health Perspect.*, **79**:109–114, 1989.

Horstman, D.; McDonnell, W.; Abdul-Salaam, S.; Folinsbee, L.; and Ives, P. In Schneider, T.; Lee, S. D.; Wolters, G. J. R.; and Grant, L. D. (eds.): *Atmospheric Ozone Research and Its Policy Implications*. Elsevier, Amsterdam, 1989, pp. 755–762.

Kinney, P. J.; Ware, J. H.; and Spengler, J. D.: A critical evaluation of acute epidemiology results. *Arch. Environ. Health*, **43**:168–173, 1988.

Koenig, J. Q.; Covert, D. S.; and Pierson, W. E.: Effects of inhalation of acidic compounds on pulmonary function in allergic adolescent subjects. *Environ. Health Perspect.*, **79**:173–178, 1989.

Koenig, J. Q.; Pierson, W. E.; Horike, M.; and Frank, R.: Effects of SO_2 plus NaCl aerosol combined with moderate exercise on pulmonary function in asthmatic adolescents. *Environ. Res.*, **25**:340–348, 1981.

Koren, H.; Devlin, R. B.; Graham, D.; Mann, R.; and McDonnell, W. F.: The inflammatory response in human lung exposed to ambient levels of ozone. In Schneider, T.; Lee, S. D.; Wolters, G. J. R.; and Grant, L. D. (eds.): *Atmospheric Ozone Research and Its Policy Implications*. Elsevier, Amsterdam, 1989, pp. 745–753.

Kotin, P., and Falk, H. F.: Atmospheric factors in pathogenesis of lung cancer. *Adv. Cancer Res.*, **7**:475–514, 1963.

Kubota, K.; Murakami, M.; Takenaka, S.; Kawai, K.; and Kyono, H.: Effects of long-term nitrogen dioxide exposure on rat lung: morphological observations. *Environ. Health Perspect.*, **73**:157–169, 1987.

Lewis, T. R.; Campbell, K. I.; and Vaughan, T. R., Jr.: Effects on canine pulmonary function. Via induced NO_2 impairment, particulate interaction, and subsequent SO_x. *Arch. Environ. Health*, **18**:596–601, 1969.

Lewis, T. R.; Moorman, W. J.; Yang, Y. Y.; and Stara, J. F.: Long-term exposure to auto exhaust and other pollutant mixtures. *Arch. Environ. Health*, **21**:102–106, 1974.

Lippmann, M.: Health effects of ozone: a critical review. *J. Air Pollut. Control Assoc.*, **39**:672–695, 1989.

Lippmann, M.; Gearhart, J. M.; and Schlesinger, R. B.: Basis for a particle size-selective TLV for sulfuric acid aerosols. *Appl. Ind. Hyg.*, **2**:188–199, 1987.

McClellan, R. O.: Health effects of diesel exhaust: a case study in risk assessment. *Am. Ind. Hyg. Assoc. J.*, **47**:1–13, 1986.

Miller, F. J.; Graham, J. A.; Raub, J. A.; Illing, J. W.; Menache, M. G.; House, D. E.; Gardner, D. E.: Evaluating the toxicity of urban patterns of oxidant gases. II. Effects in mice from chronic exposure to nitrogen dioxide. *J. Toxicol. Environ. Health*, **21**:99–112, 1987.

Miller, F. J.; Menzel, D. B.; and Coffin, D. L.: Similarity between man and laboratory animals in regional pulmonary deposition of ozone. *Environ. Res.*, **17**:84–101, 1978.

Murphy, S. D.; Klingshirn, D. A.; and Ulrich, C. E.: Respiratory response of guinea pigs during acrolein inhalation and its modification by drugs. *J. Pharmacol. Exp. Ther.*, **141**:79–83, 1963.

Nadel, J. A.; Salem, H.; Tamplin, B.; and Tokiwa, Y.: Mechanism of bronchoconstriction during inhalation of sulfur dioxide. *J. Appl. Physiol.*, **20**:164–167, 1965.

Osebold, J. W.; Gershwin, L. J.; and Zee, Y. C.: Studies on the enhancement of allergic lung sensitization by inhalation of ozone and sulfuric acid aerosol. *J. Environ. Pathol. Toxicol.*, **3**:221–234, 1980.

Schlesinger, R. B.; Chen, L. C.; Finkelstein, I.; and Zelikoff, J. T.: Comparative potency of inhaled acidic sulfates: speciation and the role of hydrogen ion. *Environ. Res.* **52**:210–224, 1990.

Sheppard, D. A.; Saisho, A.; Nadel, J. A.; and Boushey, H. A.: Exercise increases sulfur dioxide induced bronchoconstriction in asthmatic subjects. *Am. Rev. Respir. Dis.*, **123**:486–491, 1981.

Speizer, F.: Studies of acid aerosols in six cities and in a new multi-city investigation: design issues. *Environ. Health Perspect.*, **79**:61–68, 1989.

Spektor, D. M.; Yen, B. M.; and Lippmann, M.: Effect of concentration and cumulative exposure of inhaled sulfuric acid on tracheobronchial particle clearance in healthy humans. *Environ. Health Perspect.*, **79**:167–172, 1989.

Spengler, J. D., and Sexton, K.: Indoor air pollution: a public health perspective. *Science*, **221**:9–17, 1983.

Starr, T. B., and Gibson, J. E.: The mechanistic toxicology of formaldehyde and its implications for quantitative risk assessment. *Annu. Rev. Pharmacol. Toxicol.*, **25**:745–767, 1985.

Strandberg, L. G.: SO_2 absorption in the respiratory tract. Studies on the absorption in rabbits, its dependence on concentration and breathing rate. *Arch. Environ. Health*, **9**:160–166, 1964.

Tyler, W. S.; Tyler, N. K.; Last, J. A.; Gillespie, M. J.; and Barstow, T. L.: Comparison of daily and seasonal exposures of young monkeys to ozone. *Toxicology*, **50**:131–144, 1988.

U.S. Environmental Protection Agency: *Air Quality Criteria for Particulate Matter and Sulfur Oxides*, December, 1982.

Vaughan, T. R., Jr.; Jennelle, L. F.; and Lewis, T. R.: Long-term exposure to low levels of air pollutants. Effects on pulmonary function in the beagle. *Arch. Environ. Health*, **19**:45–50, 1969.

Chapter 26

WATER AND SOIL POLLUTANTS

Robert E. Menzer

INTRODUCTION

The ultimate sinks for most chemicals produced and used by human society are water and soil. Three-quarters of the earth's surface is covered by water, and the remainder that is not rock, concrete, or asphalt is covered by soil. Although water and soil are usually considered as separate ecologic systems, one needs to realize that suspended soil particles in water and the water coating soil particles represent interfaces between the two systems and serve as a mechanism for contamination of the one by the other. In reality it is impossible to consider any component of the real world in isolation from any other, as illustrated in Figure 26–1, as each system overlaps all others. For our purposes, however, we shall consider the presence, fate, and effects of chemicals in water and in soil as separate systems, as far as that is possible.

Classification of water systems may be made either on the basis of their natural occurrence or the use made of the water. One may consider separately the naturally occurring bodies of water: marine systems, freshwater systems, and the interface between them, estuarine systems. One may also consider these systems on the basis of the use made of the water removed from them: for drinking purposes or other domestic consumption, as recipients of the products of domestic and industrial sewage systems, to cool power plants and other industrial processes, for irrigation, and so forth. Bodies of water, including rivers, lakes, ponds, and the groundwater, are also the recipients of runoff from agricultural, industrial, and urban areas, which greatly modifies their capability to support life and their usefulness for other purposes.

Although water can be ultimately purified to a specific, definite, pure chemical entity, soil has no commonly accepted compositional definition. Soils are composed of inorganic and organic constituents. The inorganic are silt, sand, and clay in varying ratios. These inorganic particles are coated and admixed with organic materials and living organisms. The behavior of soil to a major degree is determined by the size and shape of the particles of which it is composed. Soil particles range in size from less than 0.002 mm to about 2.0 mm in diameter. Soils are classified according to particle size ranges as follows: clay, <0.002 mm; silt, 0.002 to 0.02 mm; fine sand, 0.02 to 0.20 mm; and course sand, 0.2 to 2.0 mm. The most important use of soil is for agriculture. Soil is the ultimate support of the sources of most food and much fiber. In addition, the soil has been the final disposal site for much of the industrial and urban waste generated by human society.

The interface between soil and water is an intimate one. Virtually all water systems contain suspended soil particles, and virtually all soil contains at least a small amount of water. The sediment that is the end product of soil erosion is by volume the greatest single pollutant of surface waters and is the principal carrier of most other pollutants found in water. In a joint study the U. S. Department of Agriculture and the U.S. Environmental Protection Agency have estimated that potential annual water erosion losses range from negligible to more than 100 tons of soil per acre. About 20 percent of the 438 million acres of crop land in the United States averages more than 8 tons of soil loss per acre per year; 30 percent averages less than 3 tons; and the other 50 percent between 3 and 8 tons (Stewart *et al.*, 1975). In fact, the sedimentary materials in water resulting from soil erosion accumulate more than 700 times more than those derived from sewage discharges (Weber, 1972). Thus, any treatment of the environmental toxicology of soil and water must consider each as a two-phase system, each containing and interacting with the other.

Sources of Chemicals in the Environment

Chemicals in the environment may be classified in a variety of ways. In this chapter we will consider chemicals primarily according to their uses and secondarily by chemical properties.

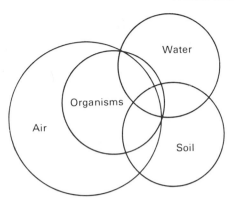

Figure 26–1. Overlapping relationships of environmental compartments.

The sources of chemicals are as follows: (1) industrial, (2) agricultural, (3) domestic and urban, and (4) naturally occurring. No matter what use is made of chemicals, contamination of the environment may be either from point sources or from nonpoint sources. The results of point source pollution are generally easy to identify and the remedies are reasonably attainable. Nonpoint source pollution, on the other hand, is generally less dramatic in its initial effects but is more difficult to contain or correct.

The production, use, and disposal of industrial chemicals all lead to contamination of soil and water. Production activities lead to soil and water contamination when by-product chemicals are not properly conserved during manufacturing processes. For example, in various smelting operations toxic chemicals present in ores may not be properly controlled. Naturally occurring arsenic in copper ores finds its way into soil and water. Accidental spillage of industrial chemicals may also result in contamination, sometimes dramatically, of soil and water. Careless manufacturing practices in a small chemical firm in Hopewell, Virginia, led to serious contamination of the James River and Chesapeake Bay by the pesticide Kepone. Even though these practices have ceased, the contamination of the estuarine system will be present for many decades. Another example is the contamination of the Ohio River with carbon tetrachloride resulting from an accidental dumping of the material from a chemical plant. Such incidents of point source contamination of water can generally be prevented or controlled by the appropriate use of technology. The result, however, of not controlling such point source pollution is a very high cost for decontamination, where that is even possible, and frequently both acute and chronic detrimental effects on organisms.

The use of chemicals for their intended purpose often leads to contamination, sometimes undesirably, of soil and water. Lead contamination of soils and occasionally water near highways has resulted from tetraethyl lead used for many years as an antiknock component of gasoline for automobiles. Although a commitment was made to eliminate the use of this compound in gasoline, the nonpoint source nature of the contamination has resulted in concentrations of lead that will remain for many years in soils and water. A chemical that is intentionally added to water for therapeutic purposes is fluorine. The use of water fluoridation to prevent tooth decay is well known and has been practiced in the United States for many years. Excessive concentrations of fluorine, however, can result in undesirable effects in teeth, manifested primarily by mottling and discoloration. Careful attention must be paid to the use of fluorine to prevent overfluoridation with its undesirable side effects.

The disposal of industrial chemicals following their use presents a major problem in several industries. Detergents used in clothes laundering are discharged into sewage systems and ultimately into rivers, lakes, and streams. Phosphate detergents then serve as nutrients for algae and other organisms that can cause major difficulties in these bodies of water. The green scum resulting from algal blooms is a familiar sight in some areas. The contamination of rivers resulting from discharge of water containing organic mercurials used in paper manufacturing presents a problem in some local situations. Other chemicals resulting from paper making can also present serious water pollution problems. Asbestos tailings resulting from mining operations have also contaminated water systems in some parts of the United States, and this has resulted in concern over the potential health effects of the material that then finds its way into drinking water systems.

The use of chemicals in agriculture results in contamination of soil and water, including groundwater, through the direct use of pesticides and fertilizers. Pesticides are, of course, applied directly to the soil in some cases to control insects, weeds, and plant diseases. Some of these chemicals can persist for many years and thereby cause concern about their potential movement from soil into water systems and from both soil and water into organisms that live in and on water and soil. The effects of pesticides in the food chain are now generally familiar. Likewise, fertilizers applied to the soil to promote plant growth and productivity can leach or run off from soil and find their way into natural water systems, causing an upset in the ecologic balance so that eutrophication results.

The domestic and urban use and disposal of

chemicals also result in the contamination of soil and water. Domestic wastes are concentrated in sewage systems and landfill operations. Frequently, large buildups of heavy metals occur as a result. Pesticides and fertilizers used in suburban and some urban situations for lawn and home garden purposes or pest control in other situations also are serious problems when improperly used. Detergents may also cause difficulties as referred to above. The discovery that the purification of water for drinking can result in the chlorination of certain organic chemicals to produce chlorinated hydrocarbons that are potential carcinogens has generated concern. In some parts of the country concentrations of such chemicals above levels considered to be safe have been found in drinking water systems.

Finally, metals, minerals, and plant or animal toxins are found in the environment as natural components of water and soil systems. Although they have always been there and always will be, human activities frequently result in excessive production or movement of such chemicals found naturally occurring in the environment and can result in concentrations detrimental to organisms living there. Furthermore, the possibility of interaction of synthetic chemicals and pollutants with naturally occurring metals, minerals, and toxins must be considered.

Transport, Mobility, and Disposition

The fate and distribution of chemicals in the environment are determined by several variables that can interact in a number of ways. An analogy between pharmacodynamics and chemodynamics can be drawn to illustrate some basic similarities in each approach. First, one must appreciate the physicochemical properties of a chemical, such as water solubility, lipid solubility, partitioning behavior, vapor pressure, pK_a for ionic species, chemical stability, and so forth, if one is to predict the behavior of a chemical in a system—be it a single human being or an entire ecosystem. Second, the processes that act within the system must be considered. Transport, via serum proteins versus suspended sediments; circulation, via the circulatory system versus the hydrologic cycle; degradation, in liver versus soil microorganisms; and disposal, via urine. feces, and expired air versus dilution in water and air to nondetectable levels or deposition in ultimate sinks such as deep ocean sediments, are all processes that act on chemicals to determine the mobility and final disposition of a chemical in a system. The analogy can be carried one step further to include target organs or tissues affected by the chemical in comparison with the susceptible species of an ecosystem.

The fundamental difference in considering toxicokinetics versus pharmacokinetics is one of scale, in both time and dimension, which then requires models of varying scale. Mathematical models have become available in recent years to predict the transport and fate of organic chemicals and metals in both aquatic and soil systems (Dickson et al., 1982). The soil models are divided into unsaturated and saturated systems, whereas other models deal with runoff and the transport of toxicants in surface waters. The value of such models is in understanding the properties that are most important in determining the environmental fate of a chemical under given conditions. A second objective is to predict exposure of various organisms through time to various toxicants and thus aid regulatory agencies in decision-making.

Water Solubility. The water solubility and latent heat of solution are critical properties of a chemical that affect its environmental fate. Many environmental toxicants are hydrophobic, having solubilities in the parts-per-million (ppm, mg/liter) to parts-per-billion (ppb, μg/liter) range. Reported solubility values vary with the method used for determination (Lyman et al., 1982). Water solubilities are affected by pH (for ionizable chemicals), presence of dissolved salts and inorganics, and temperature. Although chemicals may be described as "water-insoluble" in the literature, water solubility even at such low levels in the environment is important in considering sorption and transport processes.

Soil Adsorption. Adsorption to particulate matter is a major mechanism by which chemicals are removed from solution. Adsorbent materials in soils and sediments can be divided between clay minerals and organic matter. Clay minerals include various hydrous silicates, oxides, and layer silicates. The clay minerals have been extensively studied and are characterized by physical structure or layering type, either 1:1 or 2:1, swelling ability, cation exchange capacity, and specific surface (m^2/g) (Weber, 1972). These parameters are important considerations in the behavior of organic cations, polar organic molecules, and metal ions in soils. High specific surface is associated with small particle size; therefore, the colloidal fraction of the soil is a dominant factor in chemical-soil interactions. Cation exchange capacity of the inorganic fraction is a function of the magnitude and distribution of the structural charge. Exchangeability is dependent on the adsorbed cations, usually sodium, potassium, or calcium, and the nature of the replacing cations.

The water associated with clay plays an important role in defining its characteristics. Adsorbed water on clay surfaces is more ordered than free water. Water on the clay surface may also be

Table 26–1. CLASSES OF MATERIALS RELATED TO THE EFFECT OF pH ON ADSORPTION*

| CLASS | EXAMPLE | pK_a | MOLECULAR FORM | | pH EFFECT |
			Low pH	*High pH*	
Strong acid	Linear alkylsulfonates		Anion	Anion	Small
Weak acid	Picloram	3.7	Free acid	Anion	Large adsorption; pH approx. pK_a
Strong base	Diquat		Cation	Cation	Decrease at very low pH (18 N H_2SO_4)
Weak base	Ametryne		Cation	Free base	Increasing adsorption to pH approx. pK_a and then decrease
Polar molecules	Diuron		Nonionized	Un-ionized	Small
Neutral molecules	DDT	Nil	Nonionized	Un-ionized	Probably none

* From Hamaker, J. W., and Thompson, J. M.: Adsorption. In Goring, C. A. I., and Hamaker, J. W. (eds.): *Organic Chemicals in the Soil Environment,* Vol. 1. Marcel Dekker, New York, 1972. Reprinted by courtesy of Marcel Dekker, Inc.

more ionized than otherwise. Thus, the hydrogen ion concentration of the clay surface is high. The effect of pH on the adsorption of classes of chemicals has been summarized by Hamaker and Thompson (1972) (Table 26–1).

Soil organic matter usually ranges from 0.1 to 7 percent and serves as the most important sorptive surface for nonionic chemicals. Above a few percent organic matter, all the soil mineral surfaces are effectively blocked and thus no longer function as adsorbents. Soil organic matter can be divided into two main groups: (1) nonhumic substances, which are fresh or incompletely decomposed plant and animal material, and (2) humic substances, which are more or less completely altered or resynthesized materials. The former serve as a source for the latter. Nonhumic materials include well-known organic chemical groups with definite characteristics: proteins, carbohydrates, organic acids, sugars, fats, waxes, lignins, pigments, and other low-molecular-weight compounds. These materials comprise 10 to 15 percent of the soil organic matter. Their composition and residence times are quite variable.

Humic substances account for 85 to 90 percent of soil organic matter and their nature is not well understood. Humic substances are fractionated to give fulvic acid, which is soluble in both alkali and acid; humic acid, which is soluble in alkali but not in acid; and the humin fraction, which cannot be readily extracted with cold alkali. Humic acid and fulvic acid are aromatic polymers with molecular weights that range from 5000 to 100,000 and from 2000 to 9000, respectively. Functional groups that have been identified in humic substances are carboxyl, phenolic hydroxyl, alcoholic hydroxyl, carbonyl, and methoxy. Heterocyclic rings with oxygen and nitrogen atoms are also present. A hypothetical structure for humic acid has been proposed by Kononova (1966) as shown below.

Adsorption data for chemicals in soils are usually expressed by the Freundlich isotherm, $x/m = KC^{1/n}$; x/m is the amount of chemical sorbed per weight of the adsorbent, C is the equilibrium concentration of the chemical, and K and n are constants. The constant K represents the extent of adsorption whereas the value n sheds light on the nature of the adsorption mechanism and the role of the solvent, water. Values of $1/n$ are generally found to range from 0.7 to 1.1 (Hamaker and Thompson, 1972).

Partitioning. The distribution relationships for a chemical between the environmental compartments of air, soil, water, and biota can be

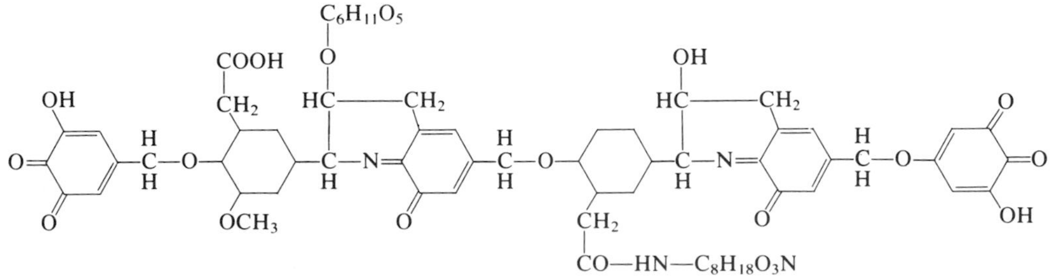

Table 26–2. KEY PHYSICAL AND ENVIRONMENTAL PROPERTIES IN FATE ASSESSMENT*

PROPERTY	DEFINITION
Soil sorption coefficient	μg Chemical soil/g of soil
(K_d)	μg Chemical water/g of water
Soil sorption constant	$\dfrac{K_d}{\% \text{ Organic carbon}} \times 100$
(K_{oc})	
Water-air ratio	μg Chemical /cm^3 of water
(K_w)	μg Chemical/cm^3 of air
n-Octanol-water coefficient	μg Chemical/ml n-octanol
(K_{ow})	μg Chemical/ml water
Bioconcentration factor	μg of Chemical/g of fish
(BCF)	μg of Chemical/g of water

* From Swann *et al.* (1983). (Reprinted with permission from Springer-Verlag, Heidelberg.)

expressed by a series of partition coefficients (McCall *et al.*, 1983). The soil sorption constant K, or sometimes given as K_d, relates the amount of chemical sorbed to soil to the concentration in water (Table 26–2). Because organic matter is key to the sorption process in soils, as discussed above, the sorption characteristics of a chemical can be normalized by use of K_{oc}, obtained from K divided by the organic matter fraction of the soil, which relates sorption properties to soil organic matter. A laboratory measure of the partitioning of a chemical between n-octanol and water provides K_{ow}, which is related to water solubility. K_{ow} values have been correlated with bioconcentration factors and soil sorption constants for a number of organic chemicals (Lyman *et al.*, 1982). The bioconcentration factor, BCF, is actually a measure of the partitioning of a chemical between water and aquatic organisms (usually fish) but is a suitable indicator for biota in general. This information provides relative rankings of chemicals, although variations will occur among different organisms with respect to bioconcentration. Air-water distribution is described by K_w, the reciprocal of the Henry's Law constant, H. It is valid only for dilute solutions, which is the situation for most chemicals in the environment. Henry's Law indicates the propensity of a chemical to volatilize from water into the air, and depends on a chemical's water solubility and vapor pressure: $H = P_v/S$.

Retention times for chemicals on reversed-phase high-performance liquid chromatography (RP-HPLC) have been used to predict partitioning between the organic and aqueous phases of the environment (Swann *et al.*, 1983). Thus, with just a few measurements of the properties of a chemical (water solubility, vapor pressure,

melting point, partitioning parameters, or RP-HPLC retention times) it is possible to predict a chemical's expected environmental distribution. To summarize, the following set of relationships can be observed:

$$\text{Soil air} \underset{}{\overset{K_w}{\rightleftharpoons}} \text{Soil water} \underset{}{\overset{K_{oc}}{\rightleftharpoons}} \text{Soil organic carbon}$$

$$\text{Sediment} \underset{}{\overset{K_{oc}}{\rightleftharpoons}} \text{Water} \underset{}{\overset{BCF}{\rightleftharpoons}} \text{Fish}$$

Vaporization. Vaporization from soil, water, or plant surfaces is a major transport process for many chemicals. The volatility of a chemical is a function of its vapor pressure, but the rate of vaporization also depends on environmental conditions such as temperature, degree of adsorption, soil properties, and soil water content. Airflow over the evaporating surface affects vaporization rate because air movement continuously replaces and mixes air around the evaporating surface. Many chemicals evaporate simultaneously with water, which leads some researchers to believe that some chemicals, such as DDT, "codistill" with water. This phenomenon can be demonstrated in laboratory distillations at 100°C, but does not occur at normal environmental temperatures. Instead, water evaporation and chemical volatilization occur independently. Higher vapor loss from most soil surfaces correlates with chemical volatilization, but is due to desorption of chemicals from soil adsorption sites by water molecules and the mass flow of chemical to the soil surface by the "wick effect." This phenomenon has been noted with chemicals such as 2,4-D esters, thiocarbamates, triazines, organochlorine insecticides, and N-methylcarbamates. Volatility of organic chemicals from water increases with decreasing water solubility. As a result, a chemical with both low vapor pressure in the solid phase and very low water solubility would be much more volatile from aqueous solution than might be expected. DDT is again an example. The Henry's Law relationships describe a chemical's tendency to volatilize as described above.

Bioaccumulation. Bioaccumulation is different from other environmental processes because it concentrates rather than diffuses the chemical in question. This concentration effect is expressed as the ratio of the concentration of a chemical in the organism to that in the medium (usually water). Bioaccumulation refers to both uptake of dissolved chemicals from water (bioconcentration) and the uptake from ingested food and sediment residues. The two properties of a chemical that are responsible for high bioaccumulation ratio values are (1) high partition coefficient K_{ow}, i.e., lipophilicity, and (2) recalcitrance toward all types of degradation. The length of the food chain also determines final concentrations in the top organisms. Bioaccumulation factors have been determined for a variety of environmental chemicals in laboratory model ecosystems and correlate well with K_{ow}.

Degradation. Transformations of chemicals in soil and water occur by chemical, photochemical, and biochemical reactions. Degradation results in the true "disappearance" of a chemical's molecular form, as opposed to transport processes, which merely move chemicals from one environmental compartment to another. However, it must be recognized that transport processes that move chemicals to ultimate sinks, such as deep ocean sediments, for all practical purposes do remove chemicals from the environment.

Chemical transformations are classified as hydrolyses, oxidations, reductions, nucleophilic substitutions involving water, and free radical reactions. These reactions may be catalyzed by the presence of metal ions, metal oxides, clay surfaces, organic compounds, and organic surfaces. The pH of solutions and the effective pH of clay surfaces, which may be quite different from the surrounding aqueous environment, can significantly affect rates of degradation. Other obvious conditions that affect degradation rates are temperature, moisture content in soils, and other environmental processes that alter chemical concentrations. The kinetics of degradation rates are dependent on the mechanism of degradation. Some degradative processes follow first-order kinetics, whereas others are best described by a "hyperbolic rate model" (Hamaker and Thompson, 1972).

Photochemical reactions of chemicals occur in air and water but are probably of little significance in soils. For a chemical to undergo a photochemical reaction, it must absorb light energy from an appropriate portion of the spectrum or have the light energy transferred through an intermediate substance known as a sensitizer. Ultraviolet light (4- to 400-nm wavelengths) has sufficient energy to break chemical bonds, but light above 450 nm, which represents an energy of 65 kcal/mole, is usually not sufficient to initiate reactions. Energy of wavelengths shorter than 295 nm does not reach the earth's surface in appreciable amounts. The principal reactions are photooxidations and photoreductions which proceed through light-formed free radicals and that then react with molecular oxygen or abstract hydrogen from organic compounds, respectively.

Biologic reactions of chemicals in soil and water are mediated primarily by microorganisms. Microorganisms are quite versatile when confronted with foreign chemicals. The major reactions involved are dehalogenation, hydrolysis, oxidation, reduction, conjugation, and methylation. They are also very important in the natural cycles of many elements, such as nitrogen, sulfur, arsenic, and mercury. These natural cycles can be disturbed by introduction of various forms of metals and can increase formation of toxic species, e.g., methylmercury. The types and rates of microbiologic reactions are determined by the microbial ecology of any given system. Thus, pH, temperature, redox potential, nutrient availability, and microbial interactions will affect the microbial degradation of a chemical.

Chemodynamics. As we have seen, there are numerous routes by which chemicals enter the environment and many factors to consider in understanding their behavior once they are there. Much of what is known about chemodynamics is derived from studies of pesticides and, to a lesser extent, industrial chemicals and heavy metals. Certainly, pesticide applications sewage sludge disposal, and industrial waste effluents each present different starting points for a consideration of chemodynamics. We shall deal with environmental processes in the following sections and attempt to relate (1) the physicochemical properties of a chemical and (2) the environmental conditions that serve as modifiers of the processes. Each process has a rate that describes the transport from one component to the next and a rate that describes the degradation of the chemical in question. A complete analysis of all the rates for entry, transport, and degradation of a chemical will describe its ultimate fate in the water and soil.

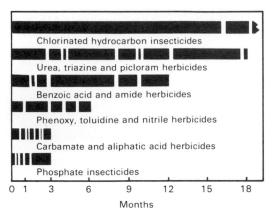

Figure 26–2. Persistence in soils of several classes of insecticides and herbicides. (From Kearney, P. C.; Nash, R. G.; and Isensee, A. R.: Persistence of pesticide residues in soils. In Miller, M. W., and Berg, G. G. [eds.]: *Chemical Fallout,* 1969. Courtesy of Charles C Thomas Publisher, Springfield, Illinois.)

PESTICIDES

The major classes of pesticides have been grouped as "nonpersistent" or "slightly residual," "moderately persistent" or "moderately residual," or "persistent" or "highly residual" (Harris, 1969; Kearney et al., 1969). Persistence times reflect the time required for 75 to 100 percent disappearance of pesticide residues from the site of application. Nonpersistent pesticides have persistence values of 1 to 12 weeks; moderately persistent pesticides, 1 to 18 months; and persistent pesticides, 2 to 5 years. Persistence times vary with environmental conditions and the generalizations about the classes are subject to several exceptions by individual pesticides within the class (Figure 26–2).

Persistent Pesticides

Organochlorine Insecticides. This group of chemicals includes dichlorodiphenyltrichloroethane (DDT), methoxychlor, and related chemicals; the cyclodiene insecticides, aldrin, dieldrin, endrin, heptachlor, chlordane, mirex, and Kepone; the hexachlorocyclohexanes (commonly referred to as BHC), especially its purified γ-isomer, lindane; and toxaphene. The technology, application, and biologic and environmental aspects of this class of insecticides have been authoritatively reviewed in a two-volume treatise by Brooks (1974). The persistence of these pesticides in the environment has been the subject of numerous books and reviews.

DDT, its major metabolites, DDD and DDE (which are collectively referred to as DDT-R), and dieldrin, which is both an insecticide itself

and the major metabolite of the insecticide aldrin, are ubiquitous residues and the prime examples of persistent pesticides. Studies with DDT and dieldrin have elucidated several important concepts in environmental toxicology. First, persistence is not a desirable attribute, as was once believed. Second, the transport and disposition of persistent pesticides is affected by physical and biologic processes, which occur from the micro to the global scale. Third, high lipid solubility combined with chemical and biologic stability can lead to biologic magnification of pesticide residues.

Persistence is primarily a function of physicochemical properties of substances. In addition, the sorption/desorption process is one of the important factors controlling the fate of pesticides in soils. Sorption of pesticides in soils has been reviewed by numerous authors (Goring, 1967; Bailey and White, 1970; Weber, 1972; Calderbank, 1989). Organochlorine insecticides are highly soluble in lipids and most organic solvents, but have low water solubilities and relatively low vapor pressures. Studies of the organochlorines in various soils show that adsorption depends strongly on the presence of soil organic matter. Once adsorbed, these chemicals do not readily desorb. Two implications are readily apparent: (1) such compounds will not leach or diffuse in soils, and (2) transport into the hydrosphere from contaminated soils will be through erosion of soil particles or sediment, not by desorption and dissolution. When organochlorines are poorly adsorbed, as in sandy soils, the vaporization loss will be significant as compared to that in soils with higher organic matter.

Volatilization of pesticides into the atmosphere from water and soils is also a transport route. The volatility of a chemical from soil or water is a function of its vapor pressure, but the actual vaporization rate depends on several environmental parameters: temperature, soil properties, soil water content, and other physicochemical properties such as water solubility and degree of adsorption. Soil properties such as high organic matter that cause the pesticide to be strongly adsorbed reduce volatility greatly. The importance of soil moisture in volatilization of organochlorines led to the use of the term "codistillation." DDT codistills with water in the laboratory (Acree *et al.,* 1963). However, the effect observed in soils is more accurately described as displacement of the sorbed pesticide by water molecules, plus a carrier action by water to the soil-air interface. The distribution of a pesticide between water and air is dependent on both water solubility and vapor pressure. As a result, even compounds such as DDT with very

Table 26–3. BIOCONCENTRATION OF DDT-R RESIDUES IN PLANTS OR ANIMALS FROM ITS ENVIRONMENT*

ENVIRONMENT	PLANT OR ANIMAL ORGANISM	(DDT-R RESIDUE IN ORGANISM DIVIDED BY RESIDUE IN ENVIRONMENT)	
		Maximum Value Observed	*Minimum Value Observed*
Soil	Earthworm	73	0.67
	Beetles	2.81	0.31
	Slugs	3.70	2.33
	Crop roots	0.13	0.04
	Crop foliage	0.08	—
Water	Sea squirt	1,000,000 †	200 †
	Sea hare	178,000 †	—
	Eastern oyster, clam	70,000 †	60
	Shrimp	2800 †	280
	Crabs	144	—
	Crayfish	97	17
	Snails	1480 †	—
	Plankton	16,666 †	250
	Fish	829,300 †	5–(1450) †
	Fish (DDD)	9214 †	417
	Algae	33	0.34
	Aquatic plants	100,000 †	0.45
Diet	Pheasant	2.91	—
	Woodcock	4.5	2.6
	Bald eagle		
	Brain	0.1	—
	Liver	1.9	—
	Fat	35.7	—

* Modified from Edwards, C. A. (1970). Reprinted with permission from Edwards, C. A.: *Persistent Pesticides in the Environment.* CRC Press, Cleveland, 1970. Copyright CRC Press, Inc., Boca Raton, FL.
† DDT may be present in excess of solubility in water.

low water solubilities are quite volatile from water.

Degradation of the organochlorines is quite slow as compared to the other classes of insecticides, and in soil and water is due mainly to the action of microorganisms. To a lesser extent, chemical reactions and photochemical reactions degrade the organochlorines under certain conditions. Pathways for DDT include the important dechlorination and dehydrochlorination reactions. Oxidative reactions are only moderately important. The conversion of the —CCl$_3$ moiety of DDT to —CN in sewage sludge and lake sediment is an example of the unique reactions carried out by microorganisms. Epoxidations and rearrangement reactions are common among the cyclodiene insecticides. The most thoroughly studied of these reactions is the epoxidation of aldrin to dieldrin and heptachlor to heptachlor epoxide (Lichtenstein and Schulz, 1960). The rearrangement products are mainly complicated "cage" structures that are toxic. The cage compounds, mirex and Kepone, undergo very little detectable degradation. Toxaphene and BHC are

degraded initially by dechlorinations and dehydrochlorinations.

The bioaccumulation of the organochlorines DDT and dieldrin is well documented by environmental residue data (Edwards, 1970). Bioaccumulation ratios relate organism residues to environmental residue levels and are higher in aquatic ecosystems as opposed to terrestrial ecosystems (Table 26–3). The processes involved in bioaccumulation are quite complex due to population fluctuations, food web relationships, metabolic capabilities of various species, and numerous other ecologic considerations. However, the physicochemical parameters of lipid solubility, low water solubility, and chemical stability that characterize the organochlorines appear to be most important in bioaccumulation of organic pesticides.

The effects of bioaccumulation of DDT-R and dieldrin are manifest primarily at the tops of food chains. Predatory fish and birds have suffered from acute toxicity, chronic toxicity, and reproductive failures. However, significant declines in organochlorine residues in eggs from brown pelicans have been associated with increases in egg shell thickness and reproductive success in a breeding population in South Carolina (Blus, 1982). Behavioral changes in DDT-treated fish have been demonstrated. Thus, the effects can range from obvious toxicity to subtle behavioral changes, but there is evidence that the population effects of these persistent pesticides are reversible with time.

Cationic Herbicides. The two chemicals of importance in this group are diquat and paraquat which are used in conservation tillage farming. These compounds readily dissolve and dissociate in aqueous solution. As cations, they are strongly adsorbed to soil particles by cation-exchange reactions (Weber, 1972):

$$Paraquat^{2+} + 2Na\text{-}Clay \rightleftarrows Paraquat\text{-}Clay + 2Na^+$$

X-ray studies show that these planar molecules interlayer between the parallel silicate sheets of various clays. The adsorption behavior is also related to surface charge densities on various clays. Adsorption isotherms for these cationic compounds indicate a high affinity of the solute for the adsorbent until the cation-exchange capacity is reached.

Paraquat and diquat as soil-bound residues are resistant to microbial degradation and photodecomposition. Tightly adsorbed residues are not biologically available and therefore persist indefinitely. In a field test begun in 1967 nearly all of the paraquat applied was still in the soil in 1973. Annual rates of loss were only 10 percent which results in an estimated half-life in the field of 6.6 years (Hance *et al.*, 1980). Both diquat and paraquat are nonvolatile and are not transported in the vapor phase. Environmental transport is thus tied to sediment transport processes.

Moderately Persistent Pesticides

Triazine Herbicides. The triazines behave as weak bases in aqueous solution with pK_a values that range from 1.1 to 4.3. Water solubilities are therefore determined by the pH level, with the triazines being more soluble at low pH levels. The behavior and fate of triazines in soils has been extensively studied and reviewed (Gunther and Gunther, 1970; Erickson and Lee, 1989). Adsorption of triazines through an exchange process to organic matter and clay minerals is dependent on the pH of the solution and the acidity of the adsorbent surface. Hydrogen bonding and hydrophobic bonding are other mechanisms by which soil organic matter adsorbs triazine herbicides, especially at higher pH levels.

Hydrolysis and oxidation are the general routes of soil metabolism for triazine herbicides. Photodecomposition appears to be minimal on soils. Vapor transport losses of triazines are dependent on vapor pressure and pH of the evaporating surface, because ionized compounds are less volatile. Transport from soil to water occurs in solution and in sediments.

Considerable attention has been focused on the possibility that the observed decline in submerged aquatic vegetation (SAV) in the Chesapeake Bay was caused by a herbicide, particularly atrazine, runoff from agricultural use. In a report on the subject (Environmental Protection Agency, 1982) it was noted that herbicide concentrations in excess of 5.0 ppb occur occasionally and such concentrations do negatively affect SAV. However, recovery from exposure to such concentrations occurs, and herbicides degrade rapidly under estuarine conditions. Residues do not appear to build up in sediments. Thus, from the evidence it is not likely that herbicides caused the decline, although herbicide-induced loss of productivity combined with other stressors could have contributed to it.

Phenylurea Herbicides. Between 20 and 25 different substituted phenylurea compounds are at present commercially available as herbicides for the control of annual and perennial grasses in a variety of crops. The phenylureas can be divided into three categories based on their water solubilities which in turn seem to be related to a number of other properties that each group holds in common (Weber, 1972). Fenuron, the most water soluble of the phenylureas at approximately 2900 to 3850 ppm, is in a category by itself. This compound is also the most mobile in soil systems of all the phenylureas. Fenuron has been shown to move substantially in a lateral direction over the soil surface and in a vertical direction into the subsoil. Its movement is also related to soil texture and organic matter content. Movement was greater in coarse textured soils and was decreased at higher organic contents.

The middle group of phenylureas in terms of water solubility includes monuron, diuron, linuron, monolinuron, fluometuron, metobromuron, norea, and siduron, in which water solubilities range from 18 to 580 ppm. Compounds in this category are moderately mobile in the soil; their relative movement decreases as the water solubilities decrease. Movement of the compounds also decreases as organic matter content of the soil increases, and in turn the herbicidal activity of the phenylureas decreases as the compounds are bound to the soil organic matter.

The least soluble of the phenylureas are neburon and chloroxuron, where water solubilities range from 2.0 to 4.8 ppm. The compounds are rather immobile in the soil.

Most of the phenylurea compounds have relatively low vapor pressures and are not very volatile from the soil. Soil pH does not appear to significantly affect adsorption, mobility, or herbicidal activity of the phenylureas. The field persistence of these compounds is moderate, with residues remaining following application for several months, at the longest.

The phenylurea herbicides are readily metabolized by most biologic systems. The combination of their low mammalian toxicity and biodegradability leads to the conclusion that these compounds are not significant factors in the contamination of soil and water systems, and their significance as environmental pollutants seems to be minimal.

Substituted Dinitroanilines. The substituted dinitroanilines are an important group of herbicides, which includes trifluralin, oryzalin, pendimethalin, and related materials. These compounds are only slightly soluble in water, have generally low vapor pressures, and are relatively immobile in soil systems, remaining essentially where they are applied. They have been classed among the least mobile of the herbicides. Like many of the herbicides they appear to be readily adsorbed by soil organic matter. Compounds that were the most highly adsorbed were also the least available to growing plants and hence the least effective as herbicides. The dinitroanilines are considered to be moderately persistent herbicides in the soil. They are generally considered to have a very low degree of toxicity to mammals and are degraded in the environment to products without significant adverse effects on organisms.

Nonpersistent Pesticides

Phenoxy and Related Acidic Herbicides. A large group of compounds may be designated as acidic herbicides, because they are chemicals that possess carboxyl or phenolic functional groups and that ionize in aqueous systems yielding pK_a values of <4. The behavior of these chemicals is closely correlated with their acid character. The most significant factor with respect to mobility of these compounds is the organic matter content of the soil. Various adsorption studies have shown that the compounds are readily adsorbed by soil organic matter. Furthermore, in acidic systems these compounds are also adsorbed by clay particles. A number of these compounds are commercially available in either the acid form or as esters. The behavior of the esters might be expected to be considerably different from that of the acid forms.

Included within this group of herbicides are several important herbicide classes. The phenoxyacetic acids, including 2,4-dichlorophenoxyacetic acid (2,4-D) and its esters, were introduced following World War II for their high activity against many broad-leafed weeds. The chlorinated aliphatic acids include dalapon and trichloroacetic acid, compounds used against perennial weeds. The benzoic acid herbicides include chloramben, dicamba, diclobenil, and several other compounds. This is a very heterogeneous group of herbicides used for a variety of purposes.

Phenylcarbamate and Carbanilate Herbicides. The phenylcarbamate herbicides are much more water soluble than the substituted anilines. In spite of this, however, they are very immobile in soil systems. Again, these compounds have been shown to be inactivated by adsorption to soil organic matter. Compounds in this group include propham, chlorpropham, barban, terbutol, and dichlormate. The mechanism of adsorption to soil organic matter is thought to involve hydrogen bonding between the carboxyl groups of the organic matter and the nitrogen and carbonyl oxygen of the carbamate.

Ethylene(*bis*)dithiocarbamate Fungicides. The metal derivatives of ethylene(*bis*)dithiocarbamate comprised one of the most important groups of fungicides used in agriculture, although about 70 percent of the registered uses have been cancelled. The principal compounds in this group are the manganese and zinc derivatives, maneb and zineb, and the disodium derivative, nabam. A closely related group is dithiocarbamates, represented by ferbam, ferric dimethyldithiocarbamate, and ziram, zinc dimethyldithiocarbamate. From a toxicologic standpoint these compounds have caused concern because of the common contaminant, degradation product, and metabolite, ethylenethiourea, a known carcinogen. This group is thoroughly considered in a two-volume treatise on antifungal compounds (Siegel and Sisler, 1977).

These compounds may be used as seed protectants and foliar fungicides. Only small quantities find their way into the soil, and once there, are rapidly degraded. In soil ethylenethiourea, ethylenethiuram monosulfide, CS_2, and H_2S result from treatment with nabam, zineb, and maneb. Ethylenethiourea is further degraded to ethyleneurea. Plants growing on treated soil will take up residues of ethylenethiourea which are translocated and further metabolized. The ethylene(*bis*)dithiocarbamates decompose rather rapidly in water.

Because of the carcinogenic activity of ethylenethiourea, its residues found in soils, plants, and food are of concern. Although the residues of ethylenethiourea itself may be small, it has been shown that cooking vegetables containing residues of ethylene(bis)dithiocarbamates releases ethylenethiourea. Hence, the toxicologic significance of residues of these chemicals in soil, once thought to be of little consequence, is now a matter of considerable attention.

Synthetic Pyrethroids. The synthetic pyrethroid insecticides are examples of optimized insecticidal activity, selectivity, and tailored environmental persistence. These compounds are modeled after natural pyrethrins which possess the first two properties but were insufficiently stable under agricultural use conditions to be commercially viable. Through modifications of both the acid and alcohol portions of these esters (Figure 26–3) compounds of desired residual activity have been synthesized while maintaining the biodegradable ester linkage. Compounds such as fenvalerate, permethrin, cypermethrin, and resmethrin have resulted. Thus, this group of insecticides which has been actively researched since the mid-1970s represents an enlightened approach to the trade-off between environmental persistence versus re-

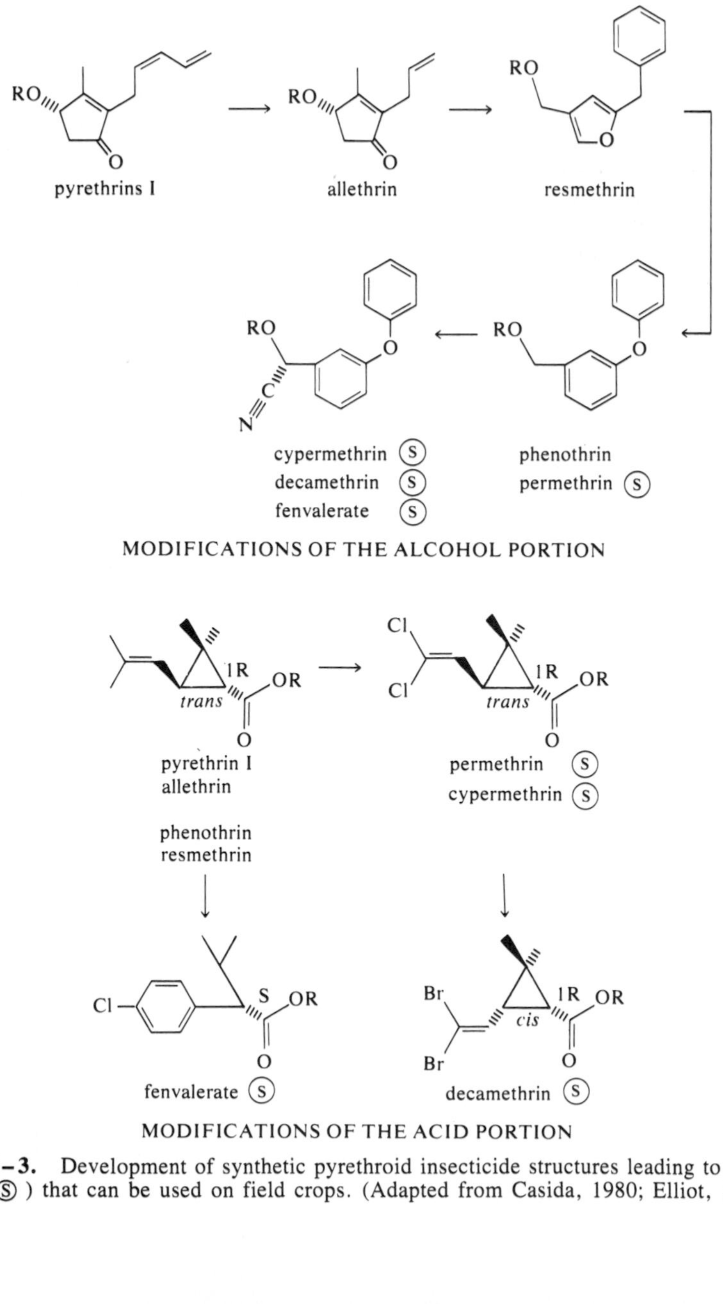

Figure 26–3. Development of synthetic pyrethroid insecticide structures leading to stable compounds (Ⓢ) that can be used on field crops. (Adapted from Casida, 1980; Elliot, 1977.)

sidual activity. These compounds are generally very toxic to crustaceans and fish in laboratory bioassays (Clark *et al.*, 1989). However, under field conditions the residues are tightly bound to sediment, and ingested residues are readily metabolized. Thus, the toxicity is less in natural systems than laboratory test data would indicate.

Organophosphorus and Carbamate Insecticides. In contrast to the persistent insecticides, particularly the organochlorine insecticides, the organophosphorus and carbamate insecticides are relatively nonpersistent in the environment. They are typically applied to crops, sometimes directly to the soil as systemic insecticides, for the control of phytophagous pests. These chemicals generally persist from only a few hours through several weeks to months. Only in rare instances are organophosphorus or carbamate residues found in crops beyond the growing season during which they were applied. These chemicals have generally replaced the organochlorines as the principal weapons in the arsenal of American agriculture against the invasion of the pests which are our competition for food and fiber. Most of the total volume of synthetic organic insecticides applied in the United States is made up of members of this group of chemicals. These compounds have been comprehensively reviewed by Eto (1974) and by Kuhr and Dorough (1976).

The organophosphates and carbamates used as insecticides are neutral esters of phosphoric and carbamic acids. A large number of these compounds representing a variety of chemical,

physical, and biologic properties are at present in commercial use, allowing their specific application to be tailored to particular needs. They act as anticholinesterase agents by phosphorylating or carbamylating acetylcholinesterase, freeing in the process a leaving group that is generally easily further degraded. This reaction may take place as well in the environment by chemical or photochemical mechanisms. Thus, these compounds do not generally represent a serious problem as contaminants of soil and water. Their breakdown products are usually nontoxic, being composed of low-molecular-weight, volatile molecules that are easily degraded and utilized by organisms.

The rate of chemical and biochemical transformation of the organophosphorus and carbamate insecticides depends on the specific properties of the individual compounds. Some of these compounds are relatively soluble in water. Being esters, they are also susceptible to hydrolysis. The half-lives of a number of common organophosphorus insecticides at various temperatures and pH values are given in Table 26–4. Most organophosphorus and carbamate compounds are stable at acid pH values. However, under alkaline conditions hydrolysis is rapid, the breakdown rate increasing approximately tenfold for each pH unit above 7. An increase of 10° of temperature will increase the hydrolysis rate approximately fourfold (Mühlmann and Schrader, 1957).

Organophosphorus and carbamate insecticides may contaminate soils by either direct applica-

Table 26–4. **EFFECT OF TEMPERATURE AND pH ON THE HYDROLYSIS IN WATER OF SOME ORGANOPHOSPHORUS INSECTICIDES***

TEMP. (°C)†	Parathion	Paraoxon	Methyl Parathion	Disulfoton	Tri-chlorofon	Dichlorvos	Azinphos-methyl
				Days			
10	3000	1200	760	4830	2400	240	1070
20	690	320	175	1110	526	61.5	240
30	180	93	45	290	140	17.3	61.5
40	50	29	12.5	78	41	5.8	18
50	15	9.6	4.0	24	10.7	1.66	5.46
60	4.75	3.2	1.34	7.8	3.2	0.58	1.9
70	1.65	1.2	0.47	2.7	1.13	0.164	0.61
				Hours			
pH							
1	34	18.5	15.4	62	32	2.3	24
3	21	23	11.2	62	33	3.4	9
5	19.5	24.4	10.7	60	15.3	2.8	8.9
7	7.8	11.5	6.9	27.6	0.7	0.45	4.8
9	2.7	2.1	1.5		0.1		

* Data from Mühlmann, R., and Schrader, G.: Hydrolyse der insektiziden Phosphorsäureester. *Z. Naturforsch.*, **12b**:196–208, 1957.
† At pH 1 to 5.

tion or through runoff from applications to crops. When these compounds are present in the soil their disappearance is affected by their interaction with the physical characteristics and water content of the soil, and the microflora present. They may be tightly bound in certain types of soils, even to the point where they are unavailable for biological decomposition. Under such conditions very little movement takes place even though water may be running through the soil or over its surface. The combination of interaction with soil components and rapid chemical and biochemical degradation in the soil results in minimal contamination of water supplies and soil to which compounds have not been applied.

A notable exception to this generalization was the discovery that the carbamate insecticide aldicarb has leached into the groundwater aquifers which constitute the major source of drinking water on Long Island, New York. This extremely toxic compound provided effective control of potato insects, but the particularly sandy, porous soil and the climatic conditions on eastern Long Island resulted in its unexpected movement through the soil into groundwater. Estimates of the length of time during which aldicarb would be present in the aquifer above the New York state advisory guideline of 7 ppb range up to 20 years (Cornell University, 1983), although the estimates are based on models whose reliability has not been thoroughly tested. Subsequently, aldicarb was found in groundwater in other locations.

The detection of organophosphorus and carbamate insecticides in soil can be difficult. Their interaction with soil components renders them unavailable to exert their toxic action on organisms, and makes them difficult to remove by conventional solvent extraction techniques. Hence, methods that depend on removal of residues from soil particles often underestimate the presence of these compounds. The analysis of organophosphorus and carbamate residues in water, on the other hand, is relatively uncomplicated and easily done. Extraction of large quantities of water with organic solvents and subsequent analysis provides a very sensitive assay for small quantities of organophosphorus and carbamate insecticides in water, although other water pollutants may complicate the analyses when they are coextracted with the insecticide.

When organophosphates or carbamates reach the soil, their subsequent disposition is affected by interaction with the mineral components of the soil, soil organic matter, soil pH, and soil moisture. In addition, the flora and fauna present in the soil are responsible for the degradation of these insecticides into innocuous breakdown products. After treatment of soil with organophosphorus compounds in laboratory or controlled field studies, extraction of the material from the soil is increasingly difficult as time progresses (Calderbank, 1989). For carbamates 32 to 70 percent of the applied compound and for organophosphates 18 to 80 percent of the applied compound are bound to the soil.

The persistence of bound residues is, at least in part, a function of interactions with the mineral components of soil. Metallic ions in soils interact with organophosphorus insecticides. Malathion, for example, is quickly incorporated into the montmorillonite clay interlayer region where it is adsorbed as a double layer. The mechanism was shown to be hydrogen binding between carbonyl oxygen atoms and the hydration water shells of cations. In this case adsorption was so strong that no degradation of the malathion was observed (Bowman et al., 1970). Similarly, Saltzman and Yaron (1972) have shown a strong affinity of parathion for sodium montmorillonite. On the other hand, diazinon and chloropyrifos were decomposed rapidly on contact with copper (II)-montmorillonite (Mortland and Raman, 1967).

Binding of organophosphorus and carbamate insecticides correlates well with the organic matter content of soils (Edwards, 1966; Calderbank, 1989). It has been shown, for example, that the amount of mevinphos bound by soils increased with increasing organic matter content. Furthermore, the absorption of phorate from the soil by plants appeared to be in competition with the binding of the compound with the organic matter content of the soil. In a kinetic study of the adsorption of carbaryl to soil organic matter surfaces, Leenheer and Ahlrichs (1971) found that carbaryl was more readily adsorbed to acid soils than to neutral or alkaline soils. This may be due to decreased displacement of the carbamate from the active sites by water at lower pH values.

Soil moisture has a major effect on the availability and extractability of residues of organophosphorus and carbamate insecticides, apparently because of competition between the insecticides and water for the adsorption sites on the soil particles. Harris (1964) has shown, for example, that diazinon, parathion, trichlorofon, and mevinphos are 135-fold, 28-fold, 20-fold, and 1.4-fold, respectively, more active in moist soils than in dry soils. Analytical procedures for the recovery of residues from soils generally recommend the addition of water for the desorption of the residues from soil particles before extraction with an organic solvent. However, even though there is a major interaction between these insecticides and water, they do not appear to move freely in soils with water, and loss by leaching does not appear to be a major factor in the disappearance of these compounds from soils, with some notable exceptions.

The fact that microorganisms exert a major effect on the behavior of pesticide residues in soil has been demonstrated by observing the effect of soil sterilization on the breakdown of a number of compounds. Getzin (1968) showed that zinophos degraded faster in nonautoclaved soil, although the decomposition of diazinon was unaffected by autoclaving. Getzin and Rosefield (1968) showed that malathion, Ciodrin, dichlorvos, mevinphos, parathion, methyl parathion, Supracide, dimethoate, and chlorpyrifos were all degraded faster in nonsterile soils. The effect of sterilization of soil on pesticide degradation may appear to be somewhat ambiguous because of changes other than the destruction of soil microorganisms which would have an effect on the degradation of compounds applied. In general, however, there is at least strong evidence that microorganisms exert a major effect on the degradation of pesticides in soils.

There are little data on the effects of organophosphates and carbamates on organisms living in water and soil. In general, only minute amounts of residues of the insecticides and their toxic degradation products are found in natural water systems. Thus, their biologic effect seems to be minimal. In soil, however, there is greater likelihood of the presence and buildup of toxic residues. Several studies have shown that some compounds can cause reduction in bacterial populations. Garretson and San Clemente (1968) showed that parathion inhibited nitrifying chemolithotrophic bacteria, although malathion did not. Sommer (1970) showed that organophosphates had little effect, whereas carbamates markedly inhibited nitrification. In studies to assess the effect of diazinon on soil microorganisms, Gunner and coworkers (Gunner et al., 1966; Gunner, 1970) showed that the compound exerted a selective effect on both soil and rhizosphere microflora expressed as selective enrichment of coccoidal rods. In another instance the microflora that arose in response to diazinon belonged primarily to one species of *Arthrobacter*. Similar results were obtained by Stojanovic et al. (1972) with carbaryl as the test insecticide. Various studies show that these insecticides may cause a variety of effects on the soil flora and fauna not always expressed as directly toxic effects.

Glyphosate. This compound is an important nonselective postemergence herbicide for control of deep rooted perennial species and some biennial and annual grasses. It is very mobile in soil and water and is readily translocated in plants, even downward (Marquis et al., 1981), as demonstrated in Sago pond weed when the compound applied to the shoots was translocated to the roots. Even at low temperatures glyphosate is degraded in soil (Mueller et al., 1981) and would not be expected to persist from one growing season to the next.

NONPESTICIDAL ORGANIC CHEMICALS

The U.S. Environmental Protection Agency monitors organic chemicals in the drinking water of the United States. A list of contaminant chemicals was begun in 1973; 253 different organic chemicals were detected through November, 1975. In an updated report issued in 1976, the number had increased to 309; in 1978, the number was over 700. Since that time monitoring programs conducted by the federal government and the various states have increased in their sophistication and extent of coverage, and the number of chemicals detected continues to increase. The list of chemicals detected includes both aliphatic and aromatic hydrocarbons, pesticides, industrial chemicals, plasticizers, and solvents. Many of these materials are halogenated and some are produced by chlorination of water during the purification process, including trihalomethanes and halogenated carboxylic acids (Johnson et al., 1982). Others appear through industrial and municipal discharges, urban and rural runoff, natural sources, and sewage purification practices.

The principal objective of the nationwide survey of organic chemicals in drinking water made by the Environmental Protection Agency is to determine the extent and significance of the occurrence of suspected carcinogens in water (Symons et al., 1975). These data were considered in a series of reports on the potential health effects of chemicals in drinking water that have been produced by the National Academy of Sciences (National Research Council, 1977–89) under mandate of the Safe Drinking Water Act of 1974.

Low-Molecular-Weight Halogenated Hydrocarbons

Trihalomethanes. Of particular concern is the production of low-molecular-weight chlorinated hydrocarbons through the use of chlorination for water purification. This concern focuses principally on the four trihalomethanes: chloroform, bromodichloromethane, dibromochloromethane, and bromoform; and carbon tetrachloride and 1,2-dichloroethane. A study was conducted by the Environmental Protection Agency to ascertain the presence of these chemicals in water, and whether they were produced by chlorination. A National Organics Reconnaissance Survey (NORS) was conducted in November, 1974, for this purpose (Symons *et al.*, 1975) and was followed by the National Organics Monitoring Survey (NOMS) in 1976 (Brass *et al.*, 1977). The results are summarized in Table 26–5. It was noted that all of these materials were found in drinking water and most were found in the raw water before chlorination. Several conclusions can be drawn from these and subsequent studies (National Research Council, Vol. 3, 1980). Chloroform, bromodichloromethane, dibromochloromethane, and bromoform do result from chlorination of precursors, particularly naturally occurring humic substances, in the raw water. On the other hand, carbon tetrachloride, methylene chloride, and 1,2-dichloroethane do not appear to be produced chemically during the treatment process. Raw water with low turbidity generally yields finished water low in trihalomethanes. There appears to be a correlation between chloroform, dibromochloromethane, bromodichloromethane, and bromoform concentrations. The ratio between the four chemicals appears to be relatively constant in all waters examined, indicating the probability of a common precursor or group of precursors for these halogenated hydrocarbons.

Studies have been conducted to compare the rate and extent of trihalomethane formation when chlorine was added to raw river water, filtered water, and activated carbon-treated water (National Research Council, Vol. 3, 1980). When sufficient chlorine is added to satisfy the chlorine demand, chlorination of raw river water yields approximately seven times as much chloroform as chlorination of filtered water and approximately 80 times as much as chlorination of activated carbon-treated water. Concentrations of humic materials are probably reduced during coagulation, settling, and filtration, thereby reducing the rate and extent of chloroform formation by chlorination. Thus, it may be possible to reduce the quantity of chlorinated hydrocarbons formed during chlorination by altering the water purification process so that chlorination is performed following the removal of humic materials through filtration and coagulation steps.

As yet, there is no generally accepted substitute for the use of chlorine as a disinfectant in water purification. However, the confirmation that chlorination produces a number of halogenated hydrocarbons has stimulated an extensive investigation of other chemicals that could be used for this purpose, such as chloramines, chlorine dioxide, ozone, bromine, and iodine (National Research Council, Vol. 3, 1980).

Concern about low-molecular-weight halogenated hydrocarbons in drinking water came to public attention in the mid-1970s when it was reported that the drinking water supply of New Orleans, Louisiana, contained more chlorinated hydrocarbons than untreated Mississippi River water (Dowty *et al.*, 1975). In addition, these workers reported the presence of chlorinated hydrocarbons, including carbon tetrachloride, in blood plasma collected from human volunteers in New Orleans. Following that report Page *et al.* (1976) reported a statistical correlation between the incidence of certain types of cancer among the New Orleans population and the source of the water supply. Although later studies (Gottlieb *et al.*, 1982) have not confirmed all of the earlier conclusions with respect to cancer incidence, a case-control cancer mortality study showed a definite association between surface chlorinated water in southern Louisiana and significant risk of rectal cancer. No increased risk of colon cancer and no effect on bladder cancer from water was detected. There was a significant

Table 26–5. ORGANICS DETECTED IN WATER IN THE EPA NATIONAL ORGANICS RECONNAISANCE SURVEY*

| COMPOUND | RAW WATER ANALYSIS | | FINISHED WATER ANALYSIS | | |
	No. of Locations Where Detected	Concentration Range (μg/ liter)	No. of Locations Where Detected	Concentration Range (μg/ liter)	Median
Chloroform	49	<0.1–0.9	80	<0.1–311	21
Bromodichloromethane	7	<0.2–0.8	78	0.3–116	6
Dibromochloromethane	1	3	72	<0.4–110	1.2
Bromoform	0	—	26	<0.8–92	5
Carbon tetrachloride	4	<2–4	10	<2–3	—
1,2-Dichloroethane	11	<0.2–3	26	<0.2–6	—

* Data derived from *Preliminary Assessment of Suspected Carcinogens in Drinking Water, Report to Congress*. U.S. Environmental Protection Agency, Washington, D.C., 1975.

association between chlorine levels in water and breast cancer incidence. A similar case-control study was conducted to determine the possible association of drinking water with cancer incidence in Wisconsin (Kanarek and Young, 1982). It was concluded that colon cancer in Wisconsin was related to the combination of chlorination and organic contamination. Chlorinated groundwater was also responsible for elevated colon cancer levels. At present, it is generally accepted that it is highly likely that there is a relationship between rectal, colon, and bladder cancer and water quality (Crump and Guess, 1980; Cantor, 1982). However, it appears that the increases in cancer risks lie near the lower limit of what can be reliably detected by epidemiologic methods. Clearly, however, there is cause for concern about the exposure of a very large percentage of the population to these chemicals in drinking water.

In addition to the possibility of a relationship between trihalomethanes and cancer, there is also concern about other chronic effects of these chemicals in drinking water. Studies in mice (Munson et al., 1982) have shown increased liver weights, elevations of serum glutamic-oxaloacetic transaminase (SGOT) and serum glutamic-pyruvic transaminase (SGPT), decreased spleen weights, and a decreased number of splenic IgM antibody forming cells in a 14-day gavage treatment at one-tenth of the LD50 dose. The enzyme changes, however, were not observed in a 90-day study, indicating that there may be the development of tolerance to the chemicals over a longer term of exposure.

Trichloroethylene. Large quantities of 1,1,2-trichloroethylene (TCE) are used for degreasing fabricated metal parts, dry cleaning of fabrics, and as a solvent for a variety of other purposes. It was formerly used as an extractant in food processing and as an anesthetic. Spills of the compound and leaking storage tanks have resulted in contamination of groundwater. The compound is highly volatile, but because it is not highly adsorbed to soil, once it has been spilled, it is readily leached through the soil.

TCE is one of the most frequently found contaminants of both raw and treated drinking water in the Unites States (Fan, 1988). In various surveys done by the U.S. Environmental Protection Agency about 38 percent of cities sampled showed TCE in their drinking water. Various states have also found TCE as a common contaminant of drinking water sources, primarily groundwater. However, using survey data in conjunction with the multinominal approach for projecting national occurrence, it has been estimated that 97 percent of groundwater-based drinking water systems and 96 percent of surface water systems contain either no TCE or concentrations <0.5 μg/liter (Cothern et al., 1986).

In a study designed to understand the relationship between the various chlorinated two-carbon alkenes under anaerobic conditions, Vogel and McCarty (1985) found that tetrachloroethylene (also known as perchloroethylene, PCE) was converted to TCE under laboratory conditions. Dichloroethylene and vinyl chloride also were detected in the output of the small column that was used, and carbon dioxide was monitored. Thus, one might expect that under environmental anaerobic conditions, TCE could be converted to vinyl chloride. Other metabolism studies have shown the conversion of TCE to trichloroethanol and trichloroacetaldehyde.

TCE is of concern for human health because it has been found to cause pulmonary adenocarcinomas and hepatocellular carcinomas in mice, although bioassays of the compound in rats have been negative. Human data are inconclusive. However, studies have shown (Fan, 1988) in two California cases that there was not a significant health risk at levels that have been detected in the environment. Other effects in experimental animals, such as changes in body weight, the liver, and the kidneys, have been observed at very high doses.

Tetrachloroethylene (PCE) is also a commonly used dry cleaning and degreasing solvent that is similar in its properties and uses to trichloroethylene. However, its higher volatility leads to its presence in the atmosphere rather than in soil and water systems. It is occasionally found in groundwater and finds its way into drinking water. However, the quantities and extent of contamination are lower than from trichloroethylene.

Aromatic Halogenated Compounds

In recent years a number of halogenated aromatic compounds have engendered increasing concern about their effects as environmental pollutants. The polychlorinated biphenyls (PCBs) are now well known as ubiquitous contaminants of soil and water. Chlorophenols used for a variety of purposes have been detected in surface waters and drinking water. The extremely toxic 2,3,7,8-tetrachlorodibenzo-p-dioxin (TCDD) has contaminated large areas of both water and soil through industrial accidents, improper waste disposal, wide-scale application of herbicides containing small quantities of the chemical as a contaminant, and as a trace by-product of combustion.

Polychlorinated Biphenyls. PCBs are very stable materials of low flammability, which contain from 12 to 68 percent chlorine. They are exceptionally persistent in the environment, some even more persistent than the organochlorine insecticides, with which they often have been confused in analytical studies of environmental samples. They have been used as insulating materials in electrical capacitors and transformers, plasticizers, in waxes, in paper manufacturing, and for a variety of other industrial purposes. Although PCBs are no longer produced in the United States, the diversity of their former use patterns, the large quantities used, and their stability has led to widespread occurrence of these compounds in soil and water. In general the higher the degree of chlorination, the more resistant to biodegradation and the more persistent in the environment are the PCBs. Analysis of whole fish samples collected nationwide revealed PCB residues in 94 percent of all fish at a mean level of 0.53 ppm (Schmitt et al., 1985). Waterfowl have also accumulated high concentrations of PCBs. Bioconcentration factors in aquatic species, such as fish, shrimp, and oysters, range from 26,000 to 60,000 (Leifer et al., 1983).

The health effects of PCBs are well established. Investigators have shown that PCBs interfere with reproduction in wildlife and in experimental animals. Other observed effects in mammals and birds include microsomal enzyme induction, porphyrogenic action, tumor promotion, estrogenic activity, and immunosuppression (Bitman et al., 1972; Vos, 1972). Other adverse effects are possible because the PCBs are lipophilic, a property, along with their stability, that leads to their bioaccumulation and the possibility of long-term effects which have not been completely identified.

Chlorophenols. Pentachlorophenol has been used in significant quantities since 1936 as a wood preservative. As a result of this use surface water and treated drinking water have been found to contain as much as 0.70 and 0.06 ppb, respectively, pentachlorophenol (Buhler et al., 1973). Hexachlorophene, [2,2'-methylene-bis-(3,4,6-trichlorophenol)], has been widely used as an antibacterial agent in a number of consumer products, including soaps and deodorants. It has been detected in surface waters as high as 48 ppb (Sims and Pfaender, 1975) and in drinking water at 0.01 ppb (Buhler et al., 1973). Hexachlorophene is resistant to metabolic attack and tends to persist in the environment and bioaccumulates in food chains.

Pentachlorophenol has fairly high acute toxicity and has been shown to cause immune system defects, liver and kidney damage, hematologic disorders, and reproductive failures in experimental animals (National Research Council, Vol. 6, 1986). The acute toxicity of hexachlorophene is also quite high. The compound has

exhibited neurotoxicity in dogs, sheep, and rats. One of the concerns about these chemicals is their possible contamination by the very toxic polychlorinated dibenzo-p-dioxins (although not TCDD) and dibenzofurans. The presence of these chemicals and their contaminants in water needs to be closely monitored because of their high toxicity and the possibility of adverse health effects in man.

2,3,7,8-Tetrachlorodibenzo-p-dioxin. One of the most dramatic and catastrophic occurrences of environmental pollution by a toxic chemical occurred in Seveso, Italy, July 10, 1976. On that date a safety disk in a reaction vessel being used to manufacture 2,4,5-trichlorophenoxyacetic acid (2,4,5-T) ruptured, releasing a chemical cloud over the region. The cloud contained predominately 2,4,5-trichlorophenol. However, an estimated 3 to 16 kg of TCDD (also improperly called simply "dioxin"), a potent teratogen, was also released. The area was thus contaminated with the greatest concentration of TCDD ever found in the environment, up to 51.3 ppm in some samples.

In the past TCDD was present in the environment as a result of its occurrence as a by-product in the manufacture of the herbicide 2,4,5-T, certain chlorophenols, hexachlorophene, and chlorinated benzenes. Now it is predominantly introduced into the environment during the incineration of municipal and industrial wastes and the improper disposal of chemical wastes. The levels in most natural uncontaminated soils are below the detection limit. However, levels have been detected in soils associated with some industrial sites, hazardous waste dumps, waste oils (Tiernan et al., 1985), and spillage of 2,4,5-trichlorophenol (Jackson et al., 1986). Fortunately, no TCDD has ever been reported in drinking water. The compound has very low solubility in water and is tightly bound to soils. Thus, it is not likely to leach into water systems.

TCDD is extremely toxic to some animal species as indicated by its acute oral LD50, reported between 0.6 and 115 μg/kg (National Research Council, 1977). It causes degenerative changes in the liver and thymus, chloracne, porphyria, altered serum enzyme concentrations, loss of body weight, induction of microsomal enzymes, and is a potent carcinogen in rats. Thymic atrophy is a very sensitive index of TCDD exposure in many animals while chloracne is the most prominent symptom for human exposures. To date, there have been no known human deaths from TCDD exposure.

The significance of TCDD as an environmental pollutant lies in (1) its extreme biologic potency and potential chronic effects, (2) the ability of analytical methods to detect trace quantities of TCDD in environmental samples, and (3) chemical properties that lead to very high bioconcentration factors. Confounding the scientific questions are the emotional aspects of unknowing exposure to TCDD through Agent Orange spraying in Viet Nam, TCDD contaminated soils in Times Beach, Missouri, or industrial accident exposure in Seveso, Italy. Indeed, TCDD has become a household word, much like DDT in the 1960s.

Phthalate Ester Plasticizers

The phthalate ester plasticizers are used in virtually every major product category, including construction, automotive, household products, apparel, toys, packaging, and medical products, resulting in the widest possible distribution of these materials. The industry today comprises 10 major suppliers who produce approximately 1 billion pounds of over 25 different compounds. The two most abundantly produced phthalate ester plasticizers are di-2-ethyl-hexylphthalate (DEHP) (286 million pounds in 1986) and di-n-butylphthalate (DBP).

The phthalate esters are now known to be ubiquitously distributed in the environment. They have been found complexed with the fulvic acid components of humic substances in soil (Ogner and Schnitzer, 1970) and in both marine and estuarine waters. Fulvic acid apparently functions as a solubilizer for the rather insoluble phthalate esters and thus serves to mediate the mobilization, transport, and immobilization of these materials in soil and water. In general, concentrations of DEHP in fresh water lie in the range of 1 to 10 μg/liter. Phthalate esters have also been found in the estuarine environment (Waldock, 1983). Phthalate ester plasticizers were detected in the open ocean environment of the Gulf of Mexico and the North Atlantic (Giam et al., 1978). DEHP and DPB were found in almost all samples analyzed, including a deep sea jellyfish, *Atolla,* from 1000 m depths in the North Atlantic (Morris, 1970), Atlantic herring, and mackerel (Musial et al., 1981). Concentrations of DEHP in surface water ranged from 4.9 to 130 ng/liter. DBP ranged from a nondetectable level to 95 ng/liter. Lower levels of both compounds were found in sediment. It has become clear that the phthalate ester plasticizers are general contaminants of virtually all soil and water ecosystems; it has become very difficult to analyze any soil or water sample without detecting phthalate esters.

Because of the widespread occurrence of these compounds, their toxicity is of concern. In general the phthalate esters have low acute toxicity. The intraperitoneal LD50 dose in mice

ranges from 1.5 to 14.2 g/kg (Rubin and Jaeger, 1973). Ninety-day and two-year feeding studies of DEHP in rats and one-year feeding studies in guinea pigs and dogs indicated a low order of chronic toxicity. However, recent studies have demonstrated the carcinogenicity of DEHP in Fischer 344 rats and B6C3F1 mice. At both the maximally tolerated dose and one-half of the maximally tolerated dose liver tumors were produced in both sexes (Kluwe et al., 1982a,b, 1983). A conference on phthalates convened in 1981 evaluated these results and concluded that the weight of evidence on the carcinogenicity of DEHP was very strong (Conference on Phthalates, 1982). At the conference it was also noted that the experiments reported prior to the work of Kluwe and coworkers were not properly designed to permit the evaluation of the carcinogenicity of phthalates in mice or rats (Wilbourn and Montesano, 1982). It has also been pointed out that much more testing is desirable on this class of compounds; the report on carcinogenicity did not permit an analysis of the mechanism, which appeared to be nongenetic. There is obviously a need for further testing of other phthalates as well.

Other subtle chronic toxic effects of DEHP have been reported (Rubin and Jaeger, 1973). As little as 4 μg/ml in the culture medium was lethal to 97 to 98 percent of cultured beating chick embryo heart cells. This concentration could be reached in human blood stored in vinyl plastic bags for a period of one to two days. Considerable interest in the chronic toxicity of low levels of phthalate esters has been evident over the last several years. The reader is referred to a series of articles on a number of possible toxic effects published in Volume 45 of *Environmental Health Perspectives* (1982) which were reported at the 1981 Conference on Phthalates.

Data reported by Mayer and Sanders (1973) indicate that DEHP and DBP may also be detrimental to the reproduction of some aquatic organisms at low concentrations. *Daphnia magna* reproduction was decreased by approximately 80 percent by continuous exposure of 30 μg/liter DEHP for up to 21 days. Reproduction in zebra fish and guppies was also decreased by low concentrations of DEHP.

Although the concentrations of phthalate esters in soil and water are quite low, the recent report of carcinogenicity and the continuing reports of the ubiquitous presence of residues in the environment led to concern about the potential for human health effects. The facts that phthalates have been found to occur in drinking water in the United States (Brass et al., 1977) and are present in food reinforce that concern.

METALS AND METALLOIDS

The toxicology of metals, including their use, occurrence, and effects, has been presented in Chapter 19. In this section we will deal only with some aspects of the natural cycles of elements and conditions that alter the processes involved. It is necessary to limit this treatment to the best-studied examples of environmentally important elements: mercury, cadmium, lead, arsenic, and selenium.

Mercury

An important consideration for any discussion of the environmental behavior of metals is the question of chemical species. Mercury, for example, exists in the inorganic form as free mercury, Hg^0, mercury ion in salts and complexes, Hg^+ and Hg^{2+}; and as organic mercury compounds, such as the phenylmercuric salts, which have been used as fungicides and herbicides, and the alkylmercury compounds, including methyl mercury. Each species of mercury has its own set of physical, chemical, and toxicologic properties. In natural systems, a dynamic equilibrium that is determined by the physicochemical and biologic conditions of the soil-water system exists between the various chemical species.

Mercury ion is transported to aquatic ecosystems via surface runoff and from the atmosphere. It is complexed or tightly bound to both organic and inorganic particles, particularly to sediments with high sulfur content. Organic acids such as fulvic and humic acid are usually associated with the mercury that is not bound to particles.

Methyl mercury is produced by sediment microorganisms, nonbiologically in sediments, and by some fish. Methylation of mercury by microorganisms is a detoxication response that allows the organism to dispose of heavy metal ions as small organometallic complexes. Conditions for methylation by sediment microorganisms are strict, and it occurs only within a narrow pH range (Craig and Moreton, 1985). The rate of synthesis of methyl mercury also depends on the redox potential, composition of the microbial population, availability of Hg^{2+}, and temperature. Vitamin B_{12} derivatives are believed to be the methylating agents, because mechanistically they are the only methyl carbanion- and methyl radical-donating coenzymes known (Ridley et al., 1977). Studies have indicated that livers of yellowfin tuna and albacore have high activity in the formation of methyl mercury from mercuric ion (Imura et al., 1972). An understanding of the biomethylation reaction mechanisms together with oxidation-reduction chemistry of elements allows predictions of the environmental con-

ditions necessary for the biomethylation of mercury and several other metals. However, the best conversion rate for inorganic mercury to methyl mercury under ideal conditions is less than 1.5 percent per month (Jensen and Jernelov, 1969). Methyl mercury pollution of Minimata Bay, Japan, and the subsequent human poisoning from consumption of contaminated seafood has stimulated much research on the origin and fate of methyl mercury.

Conversion of inorganic mercury to methyl mercury results in its desorption from sediment particles at a relatively fast rate. Therefore, little or no methyl mercury is found in sediments. Demethylation by sediment microorganisms also occurs at a rapid rate when compared to methylation. Methyl mercury released into surface waters can also undergo photodecomposition to inorganic mercury. However, methyl mercury can also be bioaccumulated by planktonic algae and fish. In fish, the rate of absorption of methyl mercury is faster than for inorganic mercury, and the clearance rate is slower, with the net result being high methyl mercury concentrations in the muscle tissue. The ratio of organic mercury to total mercury is generally very high in fish and other aquatic organisms (May et al., 1987). Average levels of mercury in commercially important fish generally are in the 100 to 200 $\mu g/kg$ range (Inskip and Piotrowski, 1985). Selenium, which is present in seawater and seafood, readily complexes with methyl mercury and is believed to have an important protective action against the toxic effects of methyl mercury.

The danger of methyl mercury poisoning was illustrated in Minimata, Japan, in the late 1950s. Industrial releases of mercury into Minimata Bay and subsequent accumulation of methyl mercury by fish resulted in at least 1200 cases of poisoning, some fatal.

Cadmium

Cadmium has long been recognized as a toxic element. Its importance as an environmental contaminant was demonstrated in the outbreak of itai-itai disease caused by smelter wastes that contaminated rice paddies in Japan (see Chapter 19). Cadmium deposits are found as sulfides with zinc, copper, and lead deposits, and cadmium is recovered as a by-product of smelting processes for those metals. Natural soil concentrations of cadmium are <1 ppm and average about 0.4 ppm. Sewage sludge and phosphate fertilizers are often contaminated with cadmium which then concentrates in plants grown on contaminated soils. The problem of heavy metal contamination, especially cadmium, has been one of the most serious concerns impeding the use and disposal of domestic sewage sludge on agricultural lands. There is some evidence for the leaching of cadmium in soils.

Compared to other heavy metals, cadmium is mobile in the aqueous environment. In natural water cadmium may exist as the hydrated ion; as complexes with carbonate, chloride, or sulfate; and complexed with humic acids. Thus, cadmium tends to move in the environment and is widely distributed. It is taken up by organisms and bioaccumulated. Bioconcentration in the aquatic environment is greatest for invertebrates such as mollusks and crustaceans, followed by fish and plants. However, cadmium forms insoluble cadmium sulfide and precipitates in sediments under reducing conditions that yield sulfide. The biologic production of sulfide also results in the precipitation of cadmium sulfide.

Among the metals, cadmium is one of the most readily absorbed and accumulated in plants grown on contaminated soil. The significance of this phenomenon is readily apparent in the relationship of cadmium concentrations in rice to the incidence of *itai-itai* disease. Although there is some question about the specific etiology of this disease, there is ample evidence from many studies that there is a positive correlation between rice cadmium content and the incidence of the disease in Japan (*see*, for example, Nogawa *et al.*, 1982, 1983).

Cadmium concentrations in fresh waters are usually <1 ppb whereas sea water ranges from 0.05 to 0.2 ppb and averages about 0.15 ppb (Fleischer *et al.*, 1974). Higher concentrations of cadmium in surface water are usually due to metallurgical plants, plating operations, cadmium pigments, batteries, plastics manufacture, or from sewage effluent. Mine drainage and mineralized areas also contribute significantly to cadmium fluxes in the Mississippi River and in the Missouri-Tennessee-Kentucky area.

Drinking water in soft water areas can serve as a source of cadmium through corrosion of plumbing. However, this source is estimated to be small in relation to food intake. As in the association of selenium and mercury, there appears to be a protective effect with zinc and calcium against cadmium toxicity.

Lead

The use of lead, its mining, and its processing date back several centuries. Changing usage patterns rather than increased consumption determine present environmental inputs from commercial use of lead. Batteries, gasoline additives, and paint pigments have been major uses, and prior to the U.S. Environmental Protection Agency's action to remove lead from gasoline,

combustion of gasoline additives was the major source of environmental pollution by lead. Lead was primarily an atmospheric pollutant that entered soil and water as fallout, a process determined by physical form and particle size. The net result was a buildup of lead near heavily traveled roads.

A number of studies have shown that lead from automobile exhaust is largely in the form of lead halides; any tetraalkyl lead is converted to water-soluble lead compounds of high toxicity and availability to plants (Diehl *et al.*, 1983). Such compounds can be easily leached from soil and contaminate water bodies adjacent to highways. The EPA's action to prohibit lead in gasoline starting from the 1990 motor vehicle model year will gradually reduce the significance of lead in the environment from this source.

Lead that has entered aquatic systems from runoff or as fallout of insoluble precipitates is found in sediments. Typical fresh water concentrations lie between 1 and 10 μg/liter whereas natural lead concentrations in soil range from 2 to 200 ppm and average 10 to 15 ppm. Deep ocean waters, below 1000 m, contain lead at 0.02 to 0.04 μg/kg concentrations, but surface waters of the Mediterranean Sea and Pacific Ocean contain 0.20 and 0.35 μg/kg levels (National Academy of Science, 1972). Drinking water concentrations of lead may be greatly increased in soft water areas through corrosion of lead-lined piping and connections. However, average lead intake from drinking water is considerably less than from food sources.

The biologic methylation of inorganic lead to tetramethyl lead by lake sediment microorganisms has been demonstrated (Wong *et al.*, 1975), but the significance of this observation remains unknown. It has not been possible to detect tetramethyl lead, trimethyl lead, or dimethyl lead in sediments or water that have high lead levels. The reason may be that tetraalkyl lead compounds are significantly hydrolyzed in the environment, particularly in seawater (DeJonghe and Adams, 1986).

Arsenic

Arsenic is widely distributed in the environment. Input of arsenic into the global cycle occurs through smelting, coal burning, and the use of arsenical pesticides. Speciation of arsenic is an important consideration in the fate, movement, and action of this element. The chemical and biochemical transformations of arsenic include oxidation, reduction, and methylation, which affect the volatilization, adsorption, dissolution, and biologic disposition of the arsenic species involved.

Arsenic contamination of soils from point sources such as copper smelters or coal-burning power plants is easier to control than the dispersive use of arsenical pesticides, which results in nonpoint source pollution. Various forms of arsenic are used as pesticides. Chromated copper arsenate continues to grow in usage as a wood preservative (Fitzgerald, 1983). Arsenic acid (H_3AsO_4) is a leaf desiccant used in cotton production, lead and calcium arsenates were used as insecticides, and organic arsenicals, which include methanearsonic acid and its sodium salts as well as dimethyl arsenic acid (cacodylic acid), are used as postemergence herbicides.

The transport of arsenic in the environment is largely controlled by adsorption/desorption processes in soil and sediments. Therefore, sediment movement is responsible for transfer of arsenic soil residues to their ultimate sinks in deep ocean sediments. The clay fraction, plus ferrous and aluminum oxides which coat clay particles, adsorbs arsenicals as depicted in Figure 26-4. The reactions of arsenicals in soil include oxidation, reduction, methylation, and demethylation. Conversion of arsenic to volatile alkylarsines leads to air transport loss from soils. The transformation processes of arsenic and its transport processes are intimately linked.

Arsenic concentrations in water are generally much lower than in sediments. In Lake Michigan, the concentrations in water ranged from 0.5 to 2.3 μg/liter whereas sediment concentrations ranged from 7.2 to 28.8 mg/kg (Seydel, 1972). In seawater arsenic ranges from 1 to 8 μg/liter (Penrose et al., 1977). Inorganic arsenic exists in water in different oxidation states, depending on the pH and E_h of the water. Arsenate is apparently reduced by bacteria to arsenite in marine environments because the ratio of arsenate to total arsenic is much lower than is pre-

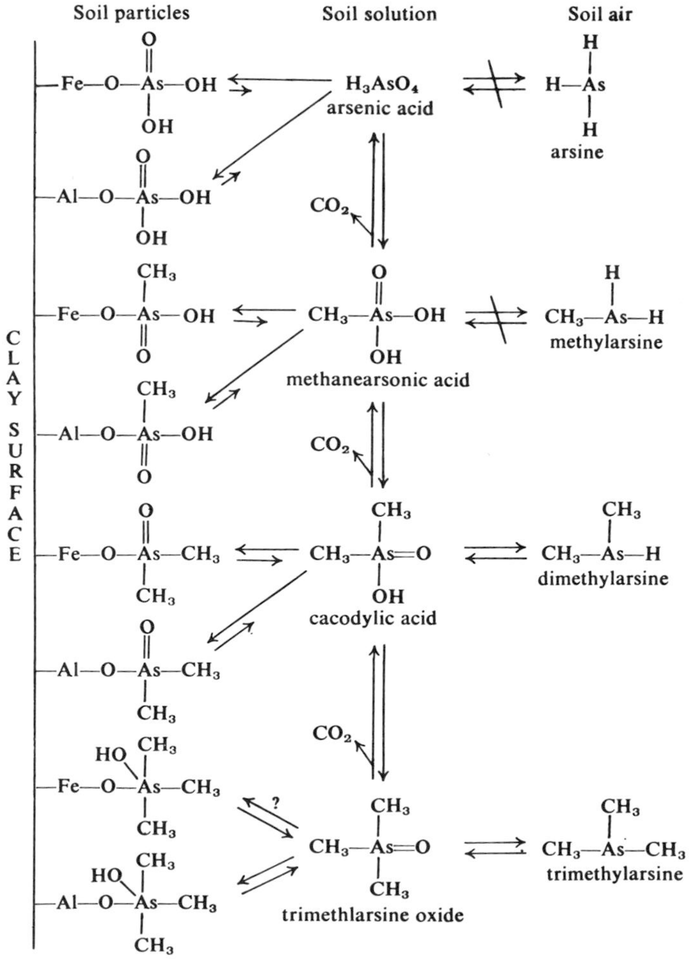

Figure 26-4. Dissolution and reactions of arsenicals within the soil environment. (From Woolson, E. A.: Fate of arsenicals in different environmental substrates. *Environ. Health Perspect.*, **19**:73-81, 1977.)

dicted thermodynamically. Methylation of arsenic occurs in both freshwater and marine systems, where arsenic is detected as arsenate, arsenite, methanearsonic acid, and dimethylarsinic acid (Braman and Foreback, 1973). In general, however, arsenate predominates in natural waters because it is the most stable form.

Bioaccumulation of arsenic species occurs readily in some aquatic organisms. Some seaweeds, freshwater algae, and crustaceans accumulate significant amounts of arsenic. Some arsenic in *Daphnia magna* and algae occurs as arseno-analogues of phospholipids, indicating the mistaken accumulation and utilization of arsenate in place of phosphate. Crabs, lobsters, and other marine organisms accumulate organoarsenicals along the food chain. Human activity can alter the concentration of arsenicals in environmental components in a very localized area, but there is little evidence that this affects the global scale arsenic cycle (Woolson, 1983).

Selenium

Selenium is an interesting and controversial element. Early concerns about its toxicity to cattle and carcinogenicity have given way to recognition of its beneficial properties. Selenium is now thought to have an anticarcinogenic function. It also protects against the toxicity of heavy metals such as cadmium, mercury, and silver. Deficiency of selenium in the diet has been associated with an increased incidence of heart disease. Although the biochemical mechanisms are not yet understood, it appears that selenium is an essential element (Schnell and Angle, 1983).

Selenium concentrations in natural water depend largely on the occurrence of seleniferous soils. Feeding on plants from seleniferous soils has been the cause of toxic effects in livestock. Average concentrations for selenium in natural waters are generally less than 0.10 μg/liter, but can reach several hundred micrograms per liter in certain areas of some western states. Dietary sources of selenium are usually more important than drinking water sources. Environmental redistribution of selenium through man's activities is due to copper smelting; lead, zinc, phosphate, and uranium mining and processing; manufacturing of glass ceramics and pigments; and burning of fuels.

Selenium can be methylated as also demonstrated for mercury, arsenic, lead, and tin. Sediment microorganisms are responsible for the production of dimethyl selenide and dimethyl diselenide from both inorganic and organic selenium compounds and contribute to its biogeochemical cycling (Chau *et al.*, 1976).

INORGANIC IONS

Nitrate, phosphate, and fluoride are inorganic ions that have caused considerable concern over their environmental effects. With nitrates and fluorides the concern is principally human health, but nitrates and particularly phosphates also cause eutrophication of lakes and ponds, a process that is considered environmentally undesirable. Midsummer algal blooms resulting from eutrophication are familiar sights in some parts of the United States.

Nitrates

Man has altered the nitrogen cycle through his agricultural and technologic practices. Changing patterns in agriculture, food processing, urbanization, and industrialization have had an impact on the accumulation of nitrate in the environment. Intensive agricultural production has consumed an increasing amount of nitrogen-based fertilizers, particularly with corn, vegetables, other row crops, and forages. Nitrogenous wastes from livestock and poultry production as well as urban sewage treatment have contributed nitrogenous wastes to the soil and water environments. Nitrate and nitrite are used extensively for color enhancement and preservation of processed meat products. These practices inevitably lead to increased exposure of man and animals to significant nitrate levels in food, feed, and water (National Academy of Sciences, 1981).

The nitrate form of nitrogen is of concern because of the high water solubility of this ion and consequent leaching, diffusion, and environmental mobility in soil and water. Nitrate can contaminate groundwater to unacceptable levels. Gradual increases in nitrate levels in many surface and groundwater sources of drinking water have been reported. It is estimated that United States drinking water averages 1.3 mg nitrate/liter, contributing thereby 2.0 mg per person per day to total daily intake of nitrate. This amount is considered to be negligible compared to the estimated total daily intake of 75 mg per person per day from all sources. However, estimates of exposure to nitrate in areas of high nitrate in water are 160 mg per person per day. The U.S. Environmental Protection Agency established in 1977 a maximum contaminant level for nitrate in drinking water of 10.2 mg/liter as NO_3-N (World Health Organization, 1985).

Nitrite is formed from nitrate or ammonium ion by certain microorganisms in soil, water, sewage, and the alimentary tract. Thus, the concern with nitrate in the environment is related in part to its conversion by biologic systems to nitrite. Methemoglobinemia is caused by high levels of nitrite, or indirectly from nitrate, in humans. It results in difficulties in the oxygen transport system of the blood. Poisoning of infants from nitrate in well water was first reported in the United States in 1944. Cases numbering in the thousands have been reported, mostly from rural areas, mostly involving poisonings in infants.

Of more recent concern is the production of nitrosamines in food by the reaction of nitrite with secondary amines. Other nitroso compounds can result from the analogous reactions of nitrites with amides, ureas, carbamates, and other nitrogenous compounds. Nitrosamines have been shown to produce liver damage, hemorrhagic lung lesions, convulsions, and coma in rats, and teratogenic effects in various experimental animals. N-Nitroso compounds represent a major class of important chemical carcinogens and mutagens. The induction of tumors by single doses of N-nitroso compounds testifies to their potency. While it is difficult to extrapolate animal carcinogenicity data to humans, the data strongly suggest that these compounds are also human carcinogens. The health effects of nitrite, nitrate, and N-nitroso compounds were comprehensively reviewed by the National Academy of Sciences (1981).

Phosphates

Although the principal problem of phosphates in the environment is not directly related to human health, there is considerable concern about the effects of phosphorus from various sources on water quality. Phosphate fertilizers and agricultural practices are a major contributor to the levels of phosphates found in water as are phosphate detergents and other phosphates from sewage treatment effluents.

Phosphorus applied to the soil as fertilizer moves primarily by erosion because phosphate adsorbs strongly to soil particles. However, some soluble phosphorus compounds do move in runoff water. The total phosphorus content of soils ranges from 0.01 to 0.13 percent (Stewart et al., 1975). The phosphorus fertilizers applied as soluble orthophosphate soon revert to insoluble forms in soil. This conversion limits leaching and leads to a higher phosphorus concentration in sediments than in the original soil because phosphorus seems to be associated with finer particles. Decaying plant material and animal wastes are significant sources of phosphates in runoff water from fields, especially when the ground is frozen and snow covered. Control of phosphate pollution from agriculture will result from efforts to reduce erosion and sediment loss by modified agricultural practices (Taylor and Kilmer, 1980).

The contribution to water of phosphorus from detergents is likely to be associated with the degree of urbanization. Some states and local areas have restricted or banned the use of phosphate detergents completely. In some areas secondary and tertiary treatment of sewage waste results in the precipitation and removal of phosphates from the effluent before discharge.

Phosphate is a major cause of the eutrophication process in lakes and ponds (Thomas, 1973). Phosphorus is an essential plant nutrient and is usually the limiting nutrient for blue-green algae. The observer of a lake undergoing eutrophication notices first an extraordinarily rapid growth of algae in the surface water. This occurs when phosphorus concentrations exceed about 50 ppb. Planktonic algae cause turbidity and flotation films. Shore algae cause ugly muddying, films, and damage to reeds. Decay of these algae causes oxygen depletion in the deep water and in shallow water near the shore. This process is self-perpetuating because the anoxic condition at the sediment/water interface causes the release of more adsorbed phosphates from the sediment. This rapid growth of algae gives rise to a number of undesirable effects on treatment of the water for consumption, on fisheries, and the use of lakes for recreational purposes.

Fluorides

The beneficial effects of low levels of fluorides in preventing dental caries has led to the extensive use of fluoride in drinking water. Most public water supplies of the 100 largest cities in the United States are fluoridated, but the levels were <1 mg/liter in 92 percent of the cases in the 1969 Community Water Supply Survey. Fluoride contents ranged from 0.2 to 4.4 mg/liter. Most water supplies that were not intentionally fluoridated contained fluoride at <0.3 mg/liter (National Research Council, Vol. 1, 1977; Vol. 3, 1980). Fluoride in drinking water represents the largest single component of the element's daily intake, although there is some exposure in pharmaceutical products, from industrial sources, and in the soil and atmosphere (Miller, 1982).

Although small amounts of fluoride are generally conceded to have a beneficial effect in the reduction of dental caries, especially in children, two forms of chronic toxic effects may be caused by intake of excessive fluoride over a long period of time, dental fluorosis and skeletal fluorosis. The most sensitive effect, tooth mottling, may occur at fluoride concentrations as low as 0.8 to 1.6 mg/liter. These observations were made a number of years ago, however, and there have been no recent studies to determine whether these levels are still causing this effect. Crippling skeletal fluorosis may result from high levels of chronic fluoride ingestion. Although the precise levels are not well defined, it is estimated that daily ingestion of 10 to 80 mg fluoride for more than 10 years will cause the effect (National Research Council, Vol. 3, 1980). There is some recent evidence from a National Toxicology Program study that sodium fluoride may cause cancer in male rats, but the evidence is termed "equivocal" by NTP.

ASBESTOS

Asbestos is a general term applied to a family of silicate minerals that have a number of properties in common that have rendered them useful for several commercial purposes. These minerals are fibrous in structure and have electrical and thermal insulating properties as well as sufficient flexibility that they can be woven into fabrics. The production and use of such materials was described by Rosato (1959). Approximately 88 percent of asbestos use has been in the construction industry, including cement products, floor tile, paper products, and paint and caulking, with the remainder being used in transportation, textiles, and plastics industries (May and Lewis, 1970).

The definition of asbestos in the *Glossary of Geology* is as follows (American Geological Institute, 1972):

(a) A commercial term applied to a group of highly fibrous silicate minerals that readily separate into long, thin, strong fibers of sufficient flexibility to be woven, are heat resistant and chemically inert, and possess a high electric insulation, and therefore are suitable for uses (as in yarn, cloth, paper, paint, brake linings, tiles, insulation cement, fillers, and filters), where incombustible, nonconducting, or chemically resistant material is required.

(b) A mineral of the asbestos group, principally chrysotile (best adapted for spinning) and certain fibrous varieties of amphibole (example: tremolite, actinolite, and crocidolite).

The mineral fibers that comprise the asbestos group are the serpentine: chrysotile; and the amphiboles: actinolite, amosite (a cunningtonite-grunerite mineral), anthrophyllite, crocidolite, and tremolite. Asbestos minerals are mined in Canada and the United States, where chrysotile accounts for about 95 percent of the production. Amosite and crocidolite make up most of the remainder. The largest chrysotile deposit in the world is found between Danville and Chaudiere, Quebec, Canada. Other deposits are found in northern Ontario, northern British Columbia, and Newfoundland in Canada, and in California, Vermont, Arizona, and North Carolina in the United States.

Asbestos is made up of fibrils of individual tubes of single crystals that bind together to produce a fiber. The size of the individual fibers varies greatly for the various minerals making up the asbestos group. Minimum fiber widths range between 0.06 μm for crocidolite to 0.25 μm for anthrophyllite. Fiber lengths in general range between 0.2 and 2.0 μm. Occasional longer fibers up to 100 μm are found, although these are much rarer in the environment than in occupational situations (Rendall, 1970).

Solubility is an important consideration in assessing the presence and impact of chemicals in soil and water. Asbestos minerals are soluble in acid solution to varying degrees (Choi and Smith, 1971). The isoelectric point of the various minerals differs widely; chrysotile has an isoelectric point of 11.8 whereas the amosite isoelectric point falls between 5.2 and 6.0 (Parks, 1967). As the pH of an aqueous medium falls below the isoelectric point, the charge of suspended asbestos particles will become more positive, thereby attracting other dissolved minerals that can interact with them. Therefore, the mobility, transport, disposition, and biologic properties of asbestos will vary widely depending on the mineral involved, the pH of the medium, and the presence of other materials with which the asbestos may interact.

A major difficulty in assessing the environmental impact of asbestos is the difficulty in detecting and analyzing it. Because asbestos is a very heterogeneous material, its detection is also difficult. A number of methods have been proposed for the identification and quantitation of asbestos in air, water, and biologic materials. Optical and electron microscopy, X-ray diffraction, and differential thermal analysis have all been proposed. Analytic problems are complicated by the difficulty of distinguishing between asbestos fibers and fibers and particles of other minerals that may be present in the same sample with them. The quantities present in environmental samples, furthermore, are generally quite small, and the particles present may exist in a wide range of sizes, making identification difficult and greatly complicating the quantitation of the mineral present. It is generally felt that transmission electron microscopy is the most satisfactory method for the detection of asbestos. A useful summary of the advantages, disadvantages, possibilities, and the difficulties of various analytic techniques that have been investigated is given by Langer (1974) and Langer *et al.* (1974).

Asbestos is found ubiquitously in the environment. Chrysotile asbestos is a common air pollutant in most large urban areas in the United States (Selikoff *et al.*, 1972). In fact, because of the industrial use of asbestos the highest concentrations found in air and water are generally in metropolitan areas (Cunningham and Pontefract, 1971; Kay, 1973).

Drinking water in some parts of the United States is known to be contaminated with asbestos fibers resulting from mining operation, geologic erosion, the disintegration of asbestos cement pipe, and atmospheric sources. Asbestos contamination of domestic water supplies was first reported in 1973–74 (Nicholson, 1974) when the Lake Superior situation was described:

> Duluth, Minnesota, drew its water directly from Lake Superior, about 60 miles southwest of an iron ore mining company located at Silver Bay, Minnesota. The tailings from the mining operation were discharged directly into the lake at approximately 70,000 tons per day. These tailings were the residue from the processing of taconite ore into pellets and were predominately of the amosite type of asbestos. Bottom currents carry some of this material to the Duluth area. The water in Duluth was shown to contain numerous amphibole fibers and pieces as well as other crystalline material. The concentration of verified asbestos mineral fibers in the Duluth water ranged from approximately 20×10^6 fibers/ liter of water. This corresponds to 5 to 30 μg of asbestos fibers per liter of water.

Since that time numerous analyses of domestic water supplies have been conducted (Millette et al., 1980). In addition to the Lake Superior locations, where fiber counts as high as 200×10^6 fibers/liter have been detected, locations in Kentucky, California, Washington, South Carolina, Florida, and Pennsylvania were detected with asbestos contamination from a variety of sources. A summary of the distribution of reported asbestos concentrations in drinking water in the United States is given in Table 26–6.

The health effects of asbestos in water have so far been incompletely ascertained. Occupational exposure to inhaled asbestos is known to lead to asbestosis characterized primarily by pulmonary fibrosis, the formation of pleural plaques, a greatly increased risk of bronchogenic carcinoma, pleural mesothelioma, and peritoneal mesothelioma, as discussed elsewhere in this book. It is not clear, however, whether the ingestion of asbestos-contaminated food or water will have an adverse impact on health. Most studies with experimental animals have been negative in the detection of tumors of the gastrointestinal tract (Craighead and Mossman, 1982). Experiments in both rats (Hilding et al., 1981) and hamsters (Smith et al., 1980) have been conducted by administering both highly controlled samples of asbestos preparations and samples drawn from practical situations, such as taconite tailings. The only positive result from such studies was an indication of squamous cell carcinomas of the forestomach in hamsters treated with a preparation of amosite asbestos.

Epidemiologic studies have been conducted in areas of natural exposure to asbestos: San Francisco (Kanarek et al., 1980; Conforti et al., 1981), Puget Sound, Washington (Polissar et al., 1982), and Duluth (Sigurdson et al., 1981). The San Francisco study showed a positive relationship between chrysotile asbestos content of drinking water and some esophageal, stomach, digestive organ, and pancreatic cancers. The mortality rates of Duluth compared with Minneapolis-St. Paul were higher for pancreatic and gastrointestinal cancer for comparable periods of time when levels of asbestos were highest in Duluth. In the Puget Sound area odds ratios for tumors of the small intestine were consistently elevated (McDonald, 1985). A careful analysis (MacRae, 1988) of these data concluded that no excess risk is present in any of these studies even from high levels of asbestos in drinking water. Although there is growing demand to take steps to remove asbestos from drinking water (Hills, 1979), the International Agency for Research on Cancer also indicated (International Agency for Research on Cancer, 1987) that no clear excess of cancer has been associated with the presence of asbestos fibers in drinking water. There is, however, a need for adequate case-control studies using the very large samples that would be necessary.

CHEMICAL WASTE DISPOSAL

The sources of hazardous chemical wastes are numerous and widely scattered throughout the United States. Industry, the federal government, agriculture, and institutions such as laboratories, hospitals, and universities are all sources of materials that need to be discarded when they are no longer useful. These materials take the form

Table 26–6. DISTRIBUTION OF REPORTED ASBESTOS CONCENTRATIONS IN DRINKING WATER FROM 406 CITIES IN 47 STATES, PUERTO RICO, AND THE DISTRICT OF COLUMBIA, USA*

HIGHEST ASBESTOS CONCENTRATION, 10^6 FIBERS/LITER	NUMBER OF CITIES	PERCENTAGE
Below detectable limits	117	28.8
Not significant (<0.5)	103	25.4
<1	113	27.8
1–10	33	8.1
>10	40	9.9
Total	406	100

* From Millette et al. (1980).

of solids, sludges, liquids, and gases, and are classified as toxic chemical, flammable, radioactive, explosive, and biologic. Often such materials are directly hazardous to human health or to other organisms, but also contamination of soil, sediment, and both surface and groundwater leads to more subtle and long-lasting toxicologic problems (Environmental Protection Agency, 1974). It is estimated that 80 billion pounds of hazardous wastes are generated annually by industry sources (Epstein *et al.*, 1982), practically all of which is categorized as toxic for regulatory purposes. A large proportion of hazardous wastes, 90 percent in one estimation, are disposed of in an unsound manner, 48 percent in surface impoundments, 30 percent in inadequate landfills, 10 percent by improper burning, and 2 percent by other means (Neely *et al.*, 1981).

The Environmental Protection Agency's reports on the storage and disposal of hazardous wastes are catalogs of environmental assaults (i.e., Environmental Protection Agency, 1974). Improper arsenic disposal in Minnesota, lead waste hazard in the San Francisco Bay area, cyanide and phenol disposal in Texas, insecticide dumping in Missouri, discharge of hydrocarbon gases into a river in Mississippi—the list goes on and on. The most dramatic example of improper chemical waste disposal has become a household word in the United States: Love Canal. An estimated 20,000 metric tons, composed of at least 300 different chemicals, some carcinogenic, were buried in an abandoned canal in Niagara County, New York. Subsequently, families living in homes built many years later on the site were forced to abandon their homes permanently when toxic chemicals seeped up through the ground into basements. The EPA has identified, as of 1990, 1081 hazardous waste sites for the national priorities list (NPL) that pose sufficient threats to human health or the environment to require clean-up under the Comprehensive Environmental Response, Compensation, and Liability Act (CERCLA, Superfund). Other studies indicate that the number may be much larger (General Accounting Office, 1987).

A symposium entitled "Research Needs for Evaluation of Health Effects of Toxic Chemical Waste Dumps" was held in 1981 under the sponsorship of the National Institute of Environmental Health Sciences. The proceedings were published in Volume 48 of *Environmental Health Perspectives*. The conference highlighted some of the particularly salient problem areas involving hazardous chemical wastes: the central question of exposure of man to waste chemicals, the problem of mixtures, the lack of toxicologic information on a significant portion of the chem-

icals found in dumps, and the psychosocial and legal aspects of the problem. Another summary of the conference and an assessment of the problem has appeared (Maugh, 1982a, 1982b). Specific reports range from an assessment of individual chemical effects on organ systems to epidemiologic studies of populations exposed to waste dumps. Particularly important are the papers addressing questions of the methodology that should be used in approaching this issue. A concerted, well-coordinated attack on this serious environmental and potential public health problem is the focus of the Superfund Amendments and Reauthorization Act of 1986 (SARA), which increased funding levels for clean-up and generally strengthened CERCLA.

IMPACT OF CHEMICALS ON SOIL AND WATER SYSTEMS

The traditional view of the environment embodied in the phrase "balance of nature" represents an outmoded conceptualization of the forces that control environmental processes. There is, in fact, no simple balance of nature. The environment is composed of many systems and subsystems, each internally balanced in a dynamic way and influenced by many external processes that tend to interact and influence the structure and function of the whole system. The thrust of nature's "balance" is an evolutionary movement toward greater diversity, greater speciation, and more complex structure.

The course of evolution has been influenced by human activities through technologic advances in agriculture and industry. A side effect of a number of these advances is the introduction of chemicals resulting from agricultural and industrial practices to the soil and water ecosystems and the resulting impact of these chemicals on organisms residing there. The effects of chemical pollution are threefold (Woodwell, 1970; Stickel, 1974): (1) a tendency toward simplification of communities through the elimination of more sensitive species and their replacement by larger populations of tolerant species; (2) the change in species relationships within communities, whereby the species that earlier might have enjoyed only a minor niche dominated by other species are allowed to expand into a dominant role in the ecosystem by the disappearance of the control species; and (3) alterations in nutrient cycles, which may have a long-lasting effect on the basic composition of the ecosystem. Alteration of nutrient cycles may lead in turn to permanent changes in an ecosystem through erosion and leaching which in turn change the basic physical structure.

Effects of pollutants are seen primarily at the

tops of food chains and are observed usually as changes in population levels of predator species. The organochlorine pesticides and industrial chemicals, for example, may cause reproductive difficulties in birds, such as the peregrine falcon. Mink are highly sensitive to methyl mercury, whereas apparently other mammals are not so sensitive. Contamination with methyl mercury can thus alter the diversity and dominance characteristics of the ecosystem.

Disturbances in the ecosystem can be detected in nutrient cycling even though no effects are measured in the diversity or population of the community. Several studies have shown that changes in nutrients, such as nitrates, are more sensitive than biological parameters to chemical stress (Jackson *et al.,* 1977; O'Neill *et al.,* 1977). This results from the fact that changes in nutrient pools must eventually directly affect the productivity of the entire ecosystem, even though the effects may not be measurable in biologic terms until a number of years later.

The net effect of decreased diversity in an ecosystem is a more unstable system. Such communities are subject to wide fluctuations in populations of organisms and are more easily influenced by outside pressures such as chemical pollutants. This leads in turn to the necessity for further human intervention in an attempt to stabilize the system, a process that historically has sometimes been self-defeating.

The effects of the reduction in species diversity in the ecosystem are not fully understood. Changes in the dominance characteristics of ecosystems will have a major effect on human activities as they cause changes in strategies of pest control, alter use of water systems, and change perceptions of the aesthetic quality of the environment. Changes in nutrient cycling lead to the expenditure of resources to correct resulting imbalances. As the farmer changes the agricultural ecosystem to his advantage it is necessary to add nutrients in the form of phosphate and nitrate fertilizers, frequently leading to additional imbalances in managing the contamination of water systems.

To understand the effect of chemicals on organisms other than humans, one must study the responses of those organisms in their own environments. Considerable effort is now being directed toward such studies (Cairns *et al.,* 1978; Eaton *et al.,* 1980; Maki *et al.,* 1980; Branson and Dickson, 1981; Dickson *et al.,* 1982). The effect of chemicals on humans is known in many instances only indirectly through laboratory experimentation with test organisms, such as laboratory animals, at high doses. The same chemicals in the environment will not necessarily have the same effects in the same direct ways because they are always found in the presence of other chemicals with which they may interact. Furthermore, mobility, transport, availability, disposition, and toxicologic effect of chemicals in the environment must be considered in assessing their interactions with biologic systems.

REFERENCES

Acree, F. J.; Beroza, M.; and Bowman, M. C.: Codistillation of DDT with water. *J. Agric. Food Chem.,* **11**:278–80, 1963.

American Geological Institute. Gary, M.; McAfee, R., Jr.; and Wolf, C. L. (eds.): *Glossary of Geology.* The Institute, Washington, D.C., 1972.

Bailey, G. W., and White, J. L.: Factors influencing the adsorption, desorption and movement of pesticides in soil. *Residue Rev.,* **32**:29–92, 1970.

Bitman, J.; Cecil, H. C.; and Harris, S. J.: Biological effects of polychlorinated biphenyls in rats and quail. *Environ. Health Perspect.,* **1**:145–149, 1972.

Blus, J. J.: Further interpretation of the relation of organochlorine residues in brown pelican eggs to reproductive success. *Environ. Pollut.,* **28A**:15–33, 1982.

Bowman, B. T.; Adams, R. S., Jr.; and Fenton, S. W.: Effect of water on malathion adsorption onto five montmorillonite systems. *J. Agric. Food Chem.,* **18**:723–727, 1970.

Braman, R. S., and Foreback, C. C.: Methylated forms of arsenic in the environment. *Science,* **182**:1247–1249, 1973.

Branson, D. R., and Dickson, K. L. (eds.): *Aquatic Toxicology and Hazard Assessment.* American Society for Testing and Materials, Special Technical Publication 737, Philadelphia, 1981.

Brass, H. J.; Feige, M. A.; Halloran, T.; Mello, J. W.; Munch, D.; and Thomas, R. F.: The national organic monitoring survey: samplings and analyses for purgeable organic compounds. In Pojasek, R. B. (ed.): *Drinking Water Quality Through Source Protection.* Ann Arbor Science Publishers, Ann Arbor, Michigan, 1977, pp. 393–416.

Brooks, G. T.: *Chlorinated Insecticides,* Vols. I and II. Chemical Rubber Co., Cleveland, Ohio, 1974.

Buhler, D. R.; Rasmusson, M. E.; and Nakaue, H. S.: Occurrence of hexachlorophene and pentachlorophenol in sewage and water. *Environ. Sci. Technol.,* **7**:929–934, 1973.

Cairns, J., Jr.; Dickson, K. L.; and Maki, A. W. (eds.): *Estimating the Hazard of Chemical Substances to Aquatic Life.* American Society for Testing and Materials, Special Technical Publication 657, Philadelphia, 1978.

Calderbank, A.: The occurrence and significance of bound pesticide residues in soil. *Rev. Environ. Contam. Toxicol.,* **108**:71–103, 1989.

Cantor, K. P.: Epidemiological evidence of carcinogenicity of chlorinated organics in drinking water. *Environ. Health Perspect.,* **46**:187–195, 1982.

Casida, J. E.: Pyrethrum flowers and pyrethroid insecticides. *Environ. Health Perspect.,* **34**:189–202, 1980.

Chau, Y. K.; Wong, P. T. S.; Silverberg, B. A.; Luxon, P. L.; and Bengert, G. A.: Methylation of selenium in the aquatic environment. *Science,* **192**:1130–1131, 1976.

Choi, I.; and Smith, R. W.: Kinetic study of dissolution of asbestos fibers in water. *J. Colloid Interface Sci.,* **40**:253–262, 1971.

Clark, J. R.; Goodman, L. R.; Borthwick, P. W.; Patrick, J. M., Jr.; Cripe, G. M.; Moody, P. M.; Moore, J. C.; and Lores, E. M.: Toxicity of pyrethroids to marine invertebrates and fish: a literature review and test results with sediment-sorbed chemicals. *Environ. Toxicol. Chem.*, **8**:393–401, 1989.

Conference on Phthalates: Discussion and summary remarks. *Environ. Health Perspect.*, **45**:149–153, 1982.

Conforti, P. M.; Kanarek, M. S.; Jackson, L. A.; Cooper, R. C.; and Murchio, J. C.: Asbestos in drinking water and cancer in the San Francisco Bay area, California, USA. *J. Chronic Dis.*, **34**:211–224, 1981.

Cornell University, Institute for Comparative and Environmental Toxicology: A toxicological, evaluation of aldicarb and its metabolites in relation to the potential human health impact of aldicarb residues in Long Island ground water. January 1983.

Cothern, C. R.; Coniglio, W. A.; and Marcus, W. L.: Estimating risk to human health. *Environ. Sci. Technol.*, **20**:111–116, 1986.

Craig, P. J., and Moreton, P. A.: The role of speciation in mercury methylation in sediments and water. *Environ. Pollut. Ser. B Chem. Phys.*, **10**:141–148, 1985.

Craighead, J. E., and Mossman, B. T.: The pathogenesis of asbestos-associated diseases. *N. Engl. J. Med.*, **306**:1446–1455, 1982.

Crump, K. S., and Guess, H. A.: Drinking water and cancer: review of recent findings and assessment of risks. Prepared for the Council on Environmental Quality, Washington, D.C., 1980.

Cunningham, H. M., and Pontefract, R.: Asbestos fibers in beverages and drinking water. *Nature*, **232**:332–333, 1971.

DeJonghe, W. R., and Adams, F. C.: Biogeochemical cycling of organic lead compounds. *Adv. Environ. Sci. Technol.*, **17**:561–594, 1986.

Dickson, K. L.; Maki, A. W.; and Cairns, J., Jr.: *Modeling the Fate of Chemicals in the Aquatic Environment.* Ann Arbor Science, Ann Arbor, Michigan, 1982.

Diehl, K. H.; Rosopulo, A.; Judel, G. K.; and Krenzer, W.: The behavior of lead tetraalkyls in the soil and their uptake by plants. *Z. Pflanzenernaehr. Bodenkd.*, **146**:551–559, 1983.

Dowty, B.; Carlisle, D.; and Laseter, J. L.: Halogenated hydrocarbons in New Orleans water and blood plasma. *Science*, **187**:75–77, 1975.

Eaton, J. G.; Parrish, P. R.; and Hendricks, A. C. (eds.): *Aquatic Toxicology.* American Society for Testing and Materials, Special Technical Publication 707, Philadelphia, 1980.

Edwards, C. A.: Insecticide residues in soils. *Residue Rev.*, **13**:83–132, 1966.

———: *Persistent Pesticides in the Environment.* CRC Press, Cleveland, Ohio, 1970.

Elliot, M.: Synthetic pyrethroids. In Elliot, M. (ed.): *Synthetic Pyrethroids.* American Chemical Society, Symposium Series 42, Washington, D.C., 1977, pp. 1–28.

Environmental Protection Agency: Report to Congress: *Disposal of Hazardous Wastes.* Publication SW-115, 1974.

———: *Chesapeake Bay Program Technical Studies:* a synthesis, Part IV, Submerged Aquatic Vegetation, Washington, 1982, pp. 503–567.

Epstein, S. S.; Brown, L. O.; and Pope, C.: *Hazardous Waste in America,* Sierra Club Books, San Francisco, 1982.

Erickson, L. E., and Lee, K. H.: Degradation of atrazine and related *s*-triazines. *Crit. Rev. Environ. Contr.* **19**:1–14, 1989.

Eto, M.: *Organophosphorus Pesticides: Organic and Biological Chemistry.* CRC Press, Cleveland, Ohio, 1974.

Fan, A. M.: Trichloroethylene: water contamination and health risk assessment. *Residue Rev.*, **101**:55–92, 1988.

Fitzgerald, L. D.: Arsenic sources, production and application in the 1980s. In Lederer, W. H., and Fensterheim, R. J. (eds.): *Arsenic—Industrial, Biomedical, Environmental Perspectives,* Van Nostrand Reinhold, New York, 1983, pp. 3–9.

Fleischer, M.; Sarofim, A. F.; Fasset, D. W.; Hammond, P.; Shaklette, H. T.; Nisbet, I. C. T.; and Epstein, S.: Environmental impact of cadmium: a review by the panel on hazardous trace substances. *Environ. Health Perspect.*, **7**:253–323, 1974.

Garretson, A. L., and San Clemente, C. L.: Inhibition of nitrifying chemolithotrophic bacteria by several insecticides. *J. Econ. Entomol.*, **61**:285–288, 1968.

General Accounting Office: *Superfund: Extent of Nation's Potential Hazardous Waste Problem Still Unknown,* GAO/RCED-88-44, 1987.

Getzin, L. W.: Persistence of diazinon and zinophos in soil: effects of autoclaving, temperature, moisture, and acidity. *J. Econ. Entomol.*, **61**:1560–1565, 1968.

Getzin, L. W., and Rosefield, I.: Organophosphorus insecticide degradation by heat-labile substances in soil. *J. Agric. Food Chem.*, **16**:598–601, 1968.

Giam, C. S.; Chan, H. S.; Neff, G. S.; and Atlas, E. L.: Phthalate ester plasticizer: a new class of marine pollutant. *Science*, **199**:419–421, 1978.

Goring, C. A. I.: Physical aspects of soil in relation to the action of soil fungicides. *Annu. Rev. Phytopathol.*, **5**:285–318, 1967.

Gottlieb, M. S., and Carr, J. K.: Case-control cancer mortality study and chlorination of drinking water in Louisiana. *Environ. Health Perspect.*, **46**:169–177, 1982.

Gunner, H. B.: Microbial ecosystem stress induced by an organophosphate insecticide. *Mededelingen Faculteit Landbouwwetenschappen Gent,* **35**:581–597, 1970.

Gunner, H. B.; Zuckerman, B. M.; Walker, R. W.; Miller, C. W.; Deubert, K. H.; and Longley, R. E.: The distribution and persistence of diazinon applied to plant and soil and its influence on rhizosphere and soil microflora. *Plant Soil,* **25**:249–264, 1966.

Gunther, F. A., and Gunther, J. D. (eds.): The triazine herbicides. *Residue Rev.,* **32**:1–413, 1970.

Hamaker, J. W., and Thompson, J. M.: Adsorption. In Goring, C. A. I., and Hamaker, J. W. (eds.): *Organic Chemicals in the Soil Environment.* Vol. 1. Marcel Dekker, New York, 1972, pp. 49–143.

Hance, R. J.; Byast, T. H.; and Smith, P. D.: Apparent decomposition of paraquat in soil. *Soil Biol. Biochem.,* **12**:447–448, 1980.

Harris, C. R.: Influence of soil moisture on the toxicity of insecticides in a mineral soil to insects. *J. Econ. Entomol.,* **57**:946–950, 1964.

———: Laboratory studies on the persistence of biological activity of some insecticides in soils. *J. Econ. Entomol.,* **62**:1437–1441, 1969.

Hilding, A. C.; Hilding, D. A.; Larson, D. M.; and Aufderheide, A. C.: Biological effects of ingested amosite asbestos, taconite tailings, diatomaceous earth and Lake Superior water in rats. *Arch. Environ. Health,* **36**:298–303, 1981.

Hills, J. P.: Asbestos in public water supplies: discussion of future problems. *Ann. NY Acad. Sci.,* **330**:573–578, 1979.

Imura, N.; Pan, S.-K.; and Uchida, T.: Methylation of inorganic mercury with liver homogenate of tuna fish. *Chemosphere,* **1**:197–201, 1972.

International Agency for Research on Cancer: Asbestos, *IARC Monographs,* Suppl. **7**:106–116, 1987.

Inskip, M. J., and Piotrowski, J. K.: Review of the health effects of methylmercury. *J. Appl. Toxicol.,* **5**:113–133, 1985.

Jackson, D. R.; Roulier, M. H.; Grotten, H. M.; Rust, S. W.; and Warner, J. S.: Solubility of 2,3,7,8-TCDD in contaminated soils. In Rappe, C.; Choudlary, G.; and Keith, L. H. (eds.). *Chlorinated Dioxins and Dibenzofuraus in Perspective,* Lewis Publishers, Chilsea, Michigan, 1986, pp. 185–200.

Jackson, D. R.; Washburne, C. D.; and Asmus, B. S.: Loss of Ca and NO_3-N from terrestrial microcosms as an indicator of soil pollution. *Water Air Soil Pollut.,* **8**:279–284, 1977.

Jensen, S.; and Jernelov, A.: Biologic methylation of mercury in aquatic organisms. *Nature,* **223**:753–754, 1969.

Johnson, J. D.; Christman, R. F.; Norwood, D. L.; and Millington, D. S.: Reaction products of aquatic humic substances with chlorine. *Environ. Health Perspect.,* **46**:63–71, 1982.

Kanarek, M. S.; Conforti, P. M.; Jackson, L. A.; Cooper, R. C.; and Murchio, J. C.: Asbestos in drinking water and cancer incidence in the San Francisco Bay area. *Am. J. Epidemiol.,* **112**:54–72, 1980.

Kanarek, M. S., and Young, T. B.: Drinking water treatment and risk of cancer death in Wisconsin. *Environ. Health Perspect.,* **46**:179–186, 1982.

Kay, G.: Ontario intensifies search for asbestos in drinking water. *J. Water Pollut. Control Fed.,* **3**:33–35, 1973.

Kearney, P. C.; Nash, R. G.; and Isensee, A. R.: Persistence of pesticide residues in soils. In Miller, M. W., and Berg, G. G. (eds.): *Chemical Fallout.* Charles C Thomas, Springfield, Illinois, 1969, pp. 54–67.

Kluwe, W. M.; Haseman, J. K.; Douglas, J. F.; and Huff, J. E.: The carcinogenicity of dietary di(2-ethylhexyl) phthalate (DEHP) in Fischer 344 rats and B6C3F1 mice. *J. Toxicol. Environ. Health,* **10**:797–815, 1982a.

Kluwe, W. M.; McConnell, E. E.; Huff, J. E.; Haseman, J. K.; Douglas, J. F.; and Hartwell, W. V.: Carcinogenicity testing of phthalate esters and related compounds by the National Toxicology Program and the National Cancer Institute. *Environ. Health Perspect.,* **45**:129–133, 1982b.

Kluwe, W. M.; Haseman, J. K.; and Huff, J. E.: The carcinogenicity of di(2-ethylhexyl) phthalate (DEHP) in perspective. *J. Toxicol. Environ. Health,* **12**:159–169, 1983.

Kononova, M. M.: *Soil Organic Matter.* Pergamon Press, New York, 1966.

Kuhr, R. J., and Dorough, H. W.: *Carbamate Insecticides: Chemistry, Biochemistry, and Toxicology.* CRC Press, Cleveland, Ohio, 1976.

Langer, A. M.: Approaches and constraints to identification and quantitation of asbestos fibers. *Environ. Health Perspect.,* **9**:133–136, 1974.

Langer, A. M.; Mackler, A. D.; and Pooley, F. D.: Electron microscopical investigation of asbestos fibers. *Environ. Health Perspect.,* **9**:63–80, 1974.

Leenheer, J. A., and Ahlrichs, J. L.: A kinetic and equilibrium study of the adsorption of carbaryl and parathion upon soil organic matter surfaces. *Soil Sci. Soc. Am. Proc.,* **35**:700, 1971.

Leifer, A.; Brink, R. H.; Thour, G. C.; and Partymiller, K. G.: *Environmental Transport and Transformation of Polychlorinated Biphenyls.* EPA-560/5-83-025. Washington, D.C., 1983, 206 pp.

Lichtenstein, E. P., and Schulz, K. R.: Epoxidation of aldrin and heptachlor in soils as influenced by autoclaving, moisture, and soil types. *J. Econ. Entomol.,* **53**:192–197, 1960.

Lyman, W. J.; Reehl, W. F.; and Rosenblatt, D. H.: *Handbook of Chemical Property Estimation Methods: Environmental Behavior of Organic Compounds.* McGraw-Hill, New York, 1982.

MacRae, K. D.: Asbestos in drinking water and cancer. *J. Royal Coll. Physicians Lond.,* **22**:7–10, 1988.

Maki, A. W.; Dickson, K. L.; and Cairns, J., Jr. (eds.): *Biotransformation and Fate of Chemicals in the Aquatic Environment.* American Society for Microbiology, Washington, D.C., 1980.

Marquis, L. Y.; Comes, R. D.; and Yang, C. P.: Absorption and translocation of fluridone and glyphosate in submersed vascular plants. *Weed Sci.,* **29**:229–236, 1981.

Maugh, T. H.: Just how hazardous are dumps? *Science,* **215**:490–493, 1982a.

———: Biological markers for chemical exposure. *Science,* **215**:643–647, 1982b.

May, K.; Stoeppler, M.; and Reisinger, K.: Studies in the ratio total mercury/methylmercury in the aquatic food chain. *Toxicol. Environ. Chem.,* **13**:153–159, 1987.

May, T. C., and Lewis, R. W.: Asbestos. In Mineral Facts and Problems. *U.S. Bureau of Mines Bull.,* **650**:851–865, 1970.

Mayer, F. L., and Sanders, H. O.: Toxicology of phthalic acid esters in aquatic organisms. *Environ. Health Perspect.,* **3**:153–157, 1973.

McCall, P. J.; Laskowski, D. A.; Swann, R. L.; and Dishburger, H. J.: Estimation of environmental partitioning of organic chemicals in model ecosystems. *Residue Rev.,* **85**:231–244, 1983.

McDonald, J. C.: Health implications of environmental exposure to asbestos. *Environ. Health Perspect.,* **62**:319–328, 1985.

Miller, I. J.: Fluorides and dental fluorosis. *Int. Dent. J.,* **32**:135–147, 1982.

Millette, J. R.; Clark, P. J.; Pansing, M. F.; and Twyman, J. D.: Concentration and size of asbestos in water supplies. *Environ. Health Perspect.,* **34**:13–25, 1980.

Morris, R. J.: Phthalic acid in the deep sea jellyfish *Atolla. Nature,* **227**:1264, 1970.

Mortland, M. M., and Raman, K. V.: Catalytic hydrolysis of some organic phosphate pesticides by copper (II). *J. Agric. Food Chem.,* **15**:163–167, 1967.

Mueller, M. M.; Rosenberg, D.; Siltanen, H.; and Wartiovaara, T.: Fate of glyphosate and its nitrogen-cycling in two Finnish agriculture soils. *Bull. Environ. Contam. Toxicol.,* **27**:724–730, 1981.

Mühlmann, R., and Schrader, G.: Hydrolyse der insektiziden phosphorsaureester. *Z. Naturforsch.,* **12b**:196–208, 1957.

Munson, A. E.; Sain, L. E.; Sanders, V. M.; Kauffmann, B. M.; White, K. L., Jr.; Page, D. G.; Barnes, D. W.; and Borzelleca, J. F.: Toxicology of organic drinking water contaminants: trichloromethane, bromodichloromethane, dibromochloromethane, and tribromomethane. *Environ. Health Perspect.,* **46**:117–126, 1982.

Musial, C. J.; Uthe, J. F.; Sirota, G. R.; Burns, B. G.; Gilgan, M. W.; Zitko, V.; and Matheson, R. A.: Di-*n*-hexyl phthalate, a newly identified contaminant in Atlantic herring *(Clupea harengus harengus)* and Atlantic mackerel *(Scomber scombrus).* Can. J. Fish Aquat. Sci., **38**:856–859, 1981.

National Academy of Sciences: *Lead: Airborne Lead in Perspective.* National Academy Press, Washington, D.C., 1972.

———: *The Health Effects of Nitrate, Nitrite, and N-Nitroso Compounds.* National Academy Press, Washington, D.C., 1981.

National Research Council: *Drinking Water and Health.* National Academy of Sciences, Washington, D.C., Vol. 1, 1977; Vol. 2, 1980; Vol. 3, 1980; Vol. 4, 1982; Vol. 5, 1983; Vol. 6, 1986; Vol. 7, 1987; Vol. 8, 1987; Vol. 9, 1989.

Neely, N.; Gillespie, D.; Schauf, F.; and Walsh, J.: Remedial actions at hazardous waste sites, survey and case studies. Report 430/9-81-05, Environmental Protection Agency, Washington, D.C., 1981.

Nicholson, W. J.: Analysis of amphibole asbestiform fibers in municipal water supplies. *Environ. Health Perspect.*, **9**:165–172, 1974.

Nogawa, K.; Konoi, S.; and Kato T.: Toxicity of cadmium. III-2. Occurrence of the itai-itai disease in relation to cadmium contamination in rice. *Kenkyo Hoken Repoto*, **48**:149–151, 1982.

Nogawa, K.; Kawano, S.; Kato, T.; and Sakamoto, M.: The prevalence of itai-itai disease and the mean cadmium concentration in rice produced by individual villages. *Nippon Eiseigaku Zasshi*, **37**:843–847, 1983.

Ogner, G., and Schnitzer, M.: Humic substances: fulvic acid-dialkyl phthalate complexes and their role in pollution. *Science*, **170**:317–318, 1970.

O'Neill, R. V.; Ausmus, B. S.; Jackson, D. R.; Van Hook, R. I.; Van Voris, P.; Washburne, C.; and Watson, A. P.: Monitoring terrestrial ecosystems by analysis of nutrient export. *Water Air Soil Pollut.*, **8**:271–277, 1977.

Page, T.; Harris, R. H.; and Epstein, S. S.: Drinking water and cancer mortality in Louisiana. *Science*, **193**:55–57, 1976.

Parks, G. A.: Aqueous surface chemistry of oxides and complex oxide minerals. In Stumm, W. (ed.): *Equilibrium Concepts in Natural Water Systems*, Adv. Chem. No. 67. American Chemical Society, Washington, D.C., 1967, pp. 121–160.

Penrose, W. R.; Conacher, H. B. S.; Black, R.; Meranger, J. C.; Miles, W.; Cunningham, H. M.; and Squires, W. R.: Implications of inorganic/organic interconversion on fluxes of arsenic in marine food webs. *Environ. Health Perspect.*, **19**:53–59, 1977.

Polissar, L.; Severson, R. K.; Boatman, E. S.; and Thomas, D. B.: Cancer incidence in relation to asbestos in drinking water in the Puget Sound region (Washington, USA). *Am. J. Epidemiol.*, **116**:314–328, 1982.

Rendall, R. E. G.: The data sheets on the chemical and physical properties of the UICC standard reference samples. In Shapiro, H. A. (ed.): *Pneumoconiosis*. Oxford University Press, London, 1970.

Ridley, W. P.; Dizikes, L. J.; and Wood, J. M.: Biomethylation of toxic elements in the environment. *Science*, **197**:329–332, 1977.

Rosato, D. V.: *Asbestos, Its Industrial Applications*. Reinhold, New York, 1959, p. 214.

Rubin, R. J., and Jaeger, R. J.: Some pharmacologic and toxicologic effects of di-2-ethylhexyl phthalate (DEHP) and other plasticizers. *Environ. Health Perspect.*, **3**:53–59, 1973.

Saltzman, S.; and Yaron B.: Parathion adsorption from aqueous solutions as influenced by soil components. In Tahori, A. S. (ed.): *Pesticide Chemistry*, Proc. 2nd Intern. IUPAC Congr. Vol. VI. Gordon and Breach, London, 1972, pp. 87–100.

Schmitt, C. J.; Zajicek, J. L.; and Ribick, M. A.: National pesticide monitoring program. Residues of organochlorine chemicals in freshwater fish, 1980–1981. *Arch. Environ. Contam. Toxicol.*, **14**:225–260, 1985.

Schnell, R. C., and Angle, C. R.: Selenium—toxin or panacea. *Fundam. Appl. Toxicol.*, **3**:409–410, 1983.

Selikoff, I. J.; Nicholson, W. J.; and Langer, A. M.: Asbestos air pollution. *Arch. Environ. Health*, **25**:1, 1972.

Seydel, I. S.: Distribution and circulation of arsenic through water, organisms and sediments of Lake Michigan. *Arch. Hydrobiol.*, **71**:17–30, 1972.

Siegel, M. R., and Sisler, H. D.: *Antifungal Compounds*, Vols. 1 and 2. Marcel Dekker, New York, 1977.

Sigurdson, E. R.; Levy, B. S.; Mandel, J.; McHugh, R.; Michienzi, L. J.; Jagger, H.; and Pearson, J.: Cancer morbidity investigations: Lessons from the Duluth study of possible effects of asbestos in drinking water. *Environ. Res.*, **25**:50–61, 1981.

Sims, J. L., and Pfaender, F. K.: Distribution and biomagnification of hexachlorophene in urban drainage areas. *Bull. Environ. Contam. Toxicol.*, **14**:214–220, 1975.

Smith, W. E.; Hubert, D. D.; Sobel, H. J.; Peters, E. T.; and Doerfler, T. E.: Health of experimental animals drinking water with and without amosite asbestos and other mineral particles. *J. Environ. Pathol. Toxicol.*, **3**:277–300, 1980.

Sommer, K.: Effect of various pesticides on nitrification and nitrogen transformation in soils. *Landwirthsch. Forsch. Sonderh.*, **25**:22–30, 1970.

Stewart, B. A.; Woolhiser, D. A.; Wischmeier, W. H.; Caro, J. H.; and Frere, M. H.: Control of Water Pollution from Cropland. USDA/EPA, Report No. ARS-H-5-1/EPA-600/2-75-026a, 1975.

Stickel, W. H.: Some effects of pollutants in terrestrial ecosystems. In McIntyre, A. D., and Mills, C. F. (eds.): *Ecological Toxicology Research: Effects of Heavy Metal and Organohalogen Compounds*. Plenum Press, New York, 1975, pp. 25–74.

Stojanovic, B. J.; Kennedy, M. V.; and Shuman, F. L., Jr.: Edaphic aspects of the disposal of unused pesticides, pesticide wastes, and pesticide containers. *J. Environ. Qual.*, **1**:54, 1972.

Swann, R. L.; Laskowski, D. A.; McCall, P. J.; Vander Kuy, K.; and Dishburger, H. J.: A rapid method for the estimation of the environmental parameters octanol/water partition coefficient, soil sorption constant, water to air ratio, and water solubility. *Residue Rev.*, **85**:17–28, 1983.

Symons, J. M.; Bellar, T. A.; Carswell, J. K.; Demarco, J.; Kropp, K. L.; Robeck, G. C.; Seeger, D. R.; Slocum, C. J.; Smith, B. L.; and Stevens, A. A.: National organic reconnaissance survey for halogenated organics. *J. Am. Water Works Assoc.*, **67**:634–647, 1975.

Taylor, A. W., and Kilmer, V. J.: Agricultural phosphorus in the environment. In Khasawneh, F. E.; Sample, E. C.; and Kanparth, E. J. (eds.): *The Role of Phosphorus in Agriculture*. American Society of Agronomy, Madison, Wisconsin, 1980, pp. 545–557.

Thomas, E. A.: Phosphorus and eutrophication. In Griffith, E. J.; Beeton, A.; Spencer, J. M.; and Mitchell, D. T. (eds.): *Environmental Phosphorus Handbook*. John Wiley & Sons, New York, 1973, pp. 585–611.

Tiernan, T. O.; Taylor, M. L.; Garrett, J. H.; VanNess, G. F.; Solch, J. G.; Wagel, D. J.; Ferguson, G. L.; and Schecter, A.: Sources and fate of polychlorinated dibenzodioxins, dibenzofurans and related compounds in human environments. *Environ. Health Perspect.*, **59**:145–158, 1985.

Vogel, T. M., and McCarty, P. L.: Biotransformation of tetrachloroethylene to trichloroethylene, dichloroethylene, vinyl chloride, and carbon dioxide under methanogenic conditions. *Appl. Environ. Microbiol.*, **49**:1080–1083, 1985.

Vos, J. G.: Toxicity of PCBs for mammals and for birds. *Environ. Health Perspect.*, **1**:105–117, 1972.

Waldock, M. J.: Determination of phthalate esters in samples from the marine environment using GC-MS. *Chem. Ecol.*, **1**:261, 1983.

Weber, J. B.: Interaction of organic pesticides with particulate matter in aquatic and soil systems. In Gold, R. F. (ed.): *Fate of Organic Pesticides in the Aquatic Environment*. American Chemical Society, Washington, D.C., 1972, pp. 55–120.

Wilbourn, J., and Montesano, R.: An overview of phthalate ester carcinogenicity testing results: the past. *Environ. Health Perspect.*, **45**:127–128, 1982.

Wong, P. T. S.; Chau, Y. K.; and Luson, P. L.: Methylation of lead in the environment. *Nature*, **253**:263–264, 1975.

Woodwell, G. M.: Effects of pollution on the structure and physiology of ecosystems. *Science*, **168**:429–433, 1970.

Woolson, E. A.: Fate of arsenicals in different environ-mental substrates. *Environ. Health Perspect.*, **19**:73–81, 1977.

————: Man's pertubation of the arsenic cycle. In Lederer, W. H., and Fensterheim, R. J. (eds.): *Arsenic—Industrial, Biomedical, Environmental Perspectives.* Van Nostrand Reinhold, New York, 1983, pp. 393–408.

World Health Organization: *Health Hazards from Nitrates in Drinking Water,* Report of a WHO Meeting, 5–9 March 1984, Copenhagen, WHO, 1985.

UNIT V

APPLICATIONS OF TOXICOLOGY

Chapter 27

ANALYTICAL/FORENSIC TOXICOLOGY

R. V. Blanke and Alphonse Poklis

INTRODUCTION

It is impossible to consider the topic of forensic toxicology without discussing analytical toxicology in considerable detail. On the other hand, analytical toxicology has its roots in forensic applications. It seems logical, therefore, to discuss these mutually dependent areas together.

Analytical toxicology is the application of any of the tools of the analytical chemist to the qualitative identification and/or the quantitative estimation of chemicals that may exert adverse effects on living organisms. Generally the chemical to be measured (the analyte) is a xenobiotic that may have been altered or transformed by metabolic actions of the organism. Frequently the specimen to be analyzed presents a matrix consisting of body fluids or solid tissues from the organism. Both the identity of the analyte and the nature of the matrix may offer formidable problems to the analytical toxicologist.

Forensic toxicology is the application of toxicology to the purposes of the law (Cravey and Baselt, 1981). Although this broad definition includes a wide range of applications such as regulatory toxicology or urine drug testing to detect drug use, by far the most common application is to identify any chemical that may serve as a causative agent in inflicting death or injury to humans or damage to property. Frequently, the result of such unfortunate incidents is that charges of liability or criminal intent may be brought which must be resolved by the judicial system. At times, indirect or circumstantial evidence is presented in an attempt to prove cause and effect. However, there is no substitute for an unequivocal identification of a specific chemical substance, demonstrated to be present in tissues from the victim at sufficient concentration to explain the injury with reasonable, scientific probability or certainty. For this reason, forensic and analytical toxicology have long enjoyed a mutually supportive partnership.

Some forensic toxicologic activities have been deemed of such importance by society that a great effort is expended to initiate and implement analytical procedures in a forensically credible manner as an aid to deciding whether adverse effects have been produced by certain chemicals. Attempts to control drivers whose driving ability may be impaired by ethanol or certain drugs are evidenced by laws prescribing punishment to individuals so impaired. The measurement of ethanol in blood or breath at specific concentrations is generally required to prove impairment by this agent (Fisher et al., 1968). Similarly, the 1980s have seen a growing response by society to the threats of drug abuse. Attempts to identify drug users by testing urine for the presence of drugs or their metabolites, using methods and safeguards developed by forensic toxicologists, have become required by law (Department of Health and Human Services, 1988).

The diagnosis and treatment of health problems induced by chemical substances (Chapter 28; Blanke and Decker, 1986) together with the closely allied field of therapeutic drug monitoring (Moyer et al., 1986), also rely greatly on analytical toxicology. Although the analytes are present in similar matrices as in forensic toxicology, results must be reported rapidly to be of use to clinicians treating patients. This requirement of a rapid turnaround time limits the number of chemicals that can be measured because methods, equipment, and personnel must all be available for instant response to toxicologic emergencies.

Occupational toxicology (Chapter 29) and regulatory toxicology (Chapter 30) require analytical procedures for their implementation or monitoring. In the former, analytical methods used to monitor threshold limit values (TLVs) and other means of estimating the exposure of workers to toxic hazards may utilize simple, nonspecific but economical screening devices. However, to determine actual exposure of a worker, it is necessary to analyze blood, urine, breath, or other specimens by methods similar to those used in clinical or forensic toxicology. For regulatory purposes, a variety of matrices (food, water, air, and so forth) must be examined for extremely small quantities of analytes. Frequently, this requires the use of sophisticated methodology capable of extreme sensitivity. Both of these applications of analytical toxicology impinge upon forensic toxicology because an injury or occupational disease in a worker can result in a legal proceeding just as may a violation of a regulatory law.

Other applications of analytical toxicology occur frequently during the course of experimental studies. The confirmation of the concentration of dosing solutions as well as monitoring their stability can frequently be accomplished by simple analytical techniques. The bioavailability of a dose may vary depending on the route of administration and the vehicle used. Blood concentrations can be monitored as one means of establishing this important parameter. In addition, an important feature in the study of any toxic substance is the characterization of metabolites as well as the distribution of the parent drug, together with its metabolites, to various tissues. This requires sensitive, specific, and valid analytical procedures. Similar analytical studies can be conducted within a temporal framework to learn the dynamics of absorption, distribution, metabolism, and excretion of toxic chemicals.

It is evident that analytical toxicology is intimately involved in many aspects of experimental and applied toxicology. Because toxic substances include all chemical types and the measurement of toxic chemicals may require the examination of biologic or nonbiologic matrices, the scope of analytical toxicology is broad indeed. Nevertheless, by using a systematic approach and relying on the practical experience developed by generations of forensic toxicologists, the sophisticated tools of analytical chemistry can provide us with the important data necessary to understand the hazards of toxic substances more completely. These concepts will be described in more detail in the rest of this chapter.

ANALYTICAL TOXICOLOGY

In light of the statement by Paracelsus five centuries ago, "All substances are poisons: there is none which is not a poison" (Klaassen et al., 1986), analytical toxicology potentially encompasses all chemical substances. Forensic toxicologists learned long ago that when the nature of a suspected poison is unknown, a systematic, standardized approach must be used to identify the presence of most common toxic substances. One approach that has stood the test of time was first suggested by Chapuis in 1873 in Eléments de Toxicologie. It is based on the origin or nature of

the toxic agent (Petersen et al., 1923). Such a system can be characterized as follows:

    I. Gases
   II. Volatile substances
  III. Corrosive agents
  IV. Metals
   V. Anions and nonmetals
  VI. Nonvolatile organic substances
 VII. Miscellaneous

Closely related to this descriptive classification is the method for separating a toxic agent from the matrix in which it is embedded. The matrix is generally a biologic specimen such as a body fluid or a solid tissue. The agent of interest may exist in the matrix in simple solution or bound to protein and other cellular constituents. The challenge is to separate the toxic agent in sufficient purity and quantity to permit it to be characterized and quantified. At times, the parent compound is no longer present in sufficient amounts to be separated. In this case, known metabolites might indirectly provide a measure of the parent substance (Hawks and Chiang, 1986). For other substances, interaction of the poison with tissue components may require the isolation or characterization of a protein adduct (SanGeorge and Hoberman, 1986). Effective methods for separation have long provided a great challenge to analytical toxicologists. Only recently have methods become available that permit direct measurement of some analytes without prior separation from the matrix.

Gases are most simply measured by gas chromatography. Some gases are extremely labile and the specimen must be collected and preserved at temperatures as low as that of liquid nitrogen. Generally, the gas is carefully liberated by incubating the specimen at a predetermined temperature in a closed container. The gas, freed from the matrix, collects over the specimen's "headspace" where it can be sampled and injected into the gas chromatograph. Other gases, such as carbon monoxide, interact with proteins. These can be carefully released from the protein, or the adduct measured independently as, for example, carboxyhemoglobin.

Volatile substances are generally liquids of a variety of chemical types. The temperature at which they boil is sufficiently low that older methods of separation utilized microdistillation or diffusion techniques. Gas-liquid chromatography (GLC) is the simplest approach for simultaneous separation and quantitation in favorable cases. The simple alcohols can be measured by injecting a diluted body fluid directly onto the column of the instrument. A more common approach is to use the "headspace" technique as for gases after incubating the specimen at an elevated temperature.

Corrosives include mineral acids and bases. Many of these consist of ions that are normal tissue constituents. Clinical chemical techniques can be applied to detect these ions in great excess over normal concentrations. Because these ions are normal constituents, the corrosive effects at the site of contact of the chemical, together with changes of blood chemistry values, can confirm the ingestion of a corrosive substance.

Metals are encountered frequently as occupational and environmental hazards. Chapter 19 discusses the toxicology of metals in detail and elegant analytical methods are available for most of them even when they are present at extremely low concentrations. Classic separation procedures involve destruction of the organic matrix by chemical or thermal oxidation. This leaves the metal to be indentified and quantified in the inorganic residue. Unfortunately, this prevents a determination of the metal in the oxidation state, or in combination with other elements, as it existed when the metal compound was absorbed. For example, the toxic effects of metallic mercury, mercurous ion, mercuric ion, or dimethyl mercury are all different. Analytical methods must be selected that will determine the relative amount of each form present to yield optimal analytical results. The analytical difficulty in do-

ing this has lent support to the unfortunate practice of discussing the toxicity of metals as if each metal existed as a single entity.

Toxic anions and nonmetals are a difficult group for analysis. Some anions can be trapped in combination with a stable cation, after which the organic matrix can be destroyed as with the metals. Others can be separated from the bulk of the matrix by dialysis after which they are detected by colorimetric or chromatographic procedures. Still others are detected and measured by ion-specific electrodes. There are no standard approaches for this group and, other than phosphorus, they are rarely encountered in an uncombined form.

The *nonvolatile organic substances* comprise, without doubt, the largest group of substances that must be considered by the analytical toxicologist. This group includes drugs, both legal and illicit, pesticides, natural products, pollutants, and industrial compounds. They are solids or liquids with high boiling points. Thus, separation procedures generally rely on differential extractions, either liquid-liquid or solid-liquid in nature. One such scheme is shown in Figure 27–1. Frequently these extractions are not efficient and recovery of the toxic substance from the matrix may be poor. When the nature of the toxic substance is known, immunoassay procedures are useful because separation procedures may be avoided.

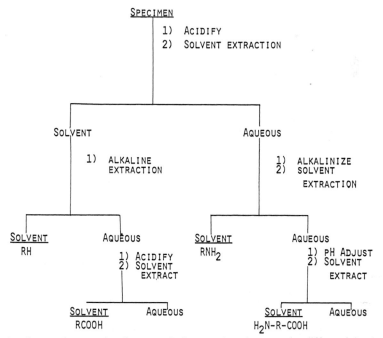

Figure 27–1. A scheme of separation for nonvolatile organic substances by differential solvent extraction.

These compounds can be classified as:

Organic strong acids
Organic weak acids
Organic bases
Organic neutral compounds
Organic amphoteric compounds

Separation is generally achieved by adjusting the acidity of the aqueous matrix and extracting with a water-immiscible solvent or a solid-phase absorbent material (Figure 27–2).

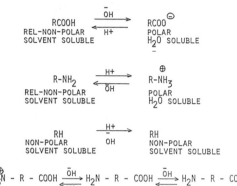

Figure 27–2. Effects of manipulating pH of the solvent for separation of nonvolatile organic substances by solvent extractions.

Finally, a *miscellaneous* category must be included for the large number of toxic agents that cannot be detected by the routine application of the methods considered thus far. Venoms and other toxic mixtures of proteins or uncharacterized constituents fall into this class. Frequently, if antibodies can be grown against the active constituent, immunoassay may be the most practical means of detecting and measuring these highly potent and difficult-to-isolate substances. Unfortunately, unless highly specific, monoclonal antibodies are used, the analytical procedure may not be acceptable for forensic purposes. Most frequently, specific analytical procedures must be developed for each analyte of this type. At times, biological end points are utilized to semiquantify the concentration of the isolated product.

With this brief description of the scope of analytical toxicology, we shall now show how it is applied in a variety of aspects of toxicology.

ANALYTICAL ROLE IN GENERAL TOXICOLOGY

In almost all experimental studies in toxicology, an agent, generally a single chemical substance, is administered in known amounts to an organism. It is universally acknowledged that the chemical under study must be pure, or the nature of any contaminants known, to interpret the experimental results with validity. Yet, it is common practice to proceed with the experimental study without verification of the purity of the compound. Not only does this practice lead to errors in establishing an accurate dose, but, depending on the nature of the study, other erroneous conclusions may be drawn. For example, the presence of related compounds in the dosage form of a tricyclic antidepressant led to erroneous conclusions about the metabolic products of the drug when it was administered together with the unidentified contaminants (Saady *et al.*, 1981).

An even greater error may result when a small amount of a contaminant may be supertoxic. A well-publicized example of this error was the presence of dioxin in mixtures of the defoliants 2,4-dichlorophenoxyacetic acid (2,4-D) and 2,4,5-trichlorophenoxyacetic acid (2,4,5-T) (Panel on Herbicides, 1971) used during the Vietnam War as Agent Orange. Some of the adverse effects of Agent Orange may have been due to the low concentration of dioxin in these mixtures. Others have reported that the toxicity of mixtures of polybrominated biphenyls may be due to the high toxicity of specific components whereas other brominated biphenyls are relatively nontoxic (Mills *et al.*, 1985).

A related application of analytical toxicology is to monitor dosage forms or solutions for stability throughout the course of an experimental study. Chemicals may degrade in contact with air, by exposure to ultraviolet or other radiation, by interaction with constituents of the vehicle or dosing solution, and other means. Developing an analytical procedure by which these changes can be recognized and corrected is essential to achieve consistent results throughout a study (Blanke, 1989).

Finally, analytical methods are important in establishing the bioavailability of a compound under study. Some substances of low water solubility are difficult to introduce into an animal. A variety of vehicles may be tried. However, measuring blood concentrations of the compound under study provides a simple means of comparing the effectiveness of vehicles. Introducing a compound to the stomach in an oil vehicle may not be the most effective means of enhancing absorption of the compound (Granger *et al.*, 1987). Rather than observing dose/effect relationships, it may be more accurate to describe blood (plasma) concentration/effect relationships.

ANALYTICAL ROLE IN FORENSIC TOXICOLOGY

The duties of the forensic toxicologist in post-mortem investigations include the qualitative and quantitative analysis of drugs or poisons in biologic specimens collected at autopsy, and the interpretation of the analytical findings as to the physiologic and behavioral effects of the detected chemicals on the deceased at the time of death.

The complete investigation of the cause or causes of sudden death is an important civic responsibility. Establishing the cause of death rests with the medical examiner, coroner, or pathologist, but success in arriving at the correct conclusion is often dependent on the combined efforts of the pathologist and the toxicologist. The cause of death in cases of poisoning cannot be proven beyond contention without toxicologic analysis which establishes the presence of the toxicant in the tissues and body fluids of the deceased

Many drugs or poisons do not produce characteristic pathologic lesions and their presence in the body can be demonstrated only by chemical methods of isolation and identification. If toxicologic analyses are avoided, deaths due to poisoning may be erroneously ascribed to some entirely different cause, or poisoning may be designated as the cause of death without any definite proof. Such erroneous diagnoses may have significant legal and social consequences.

Additionally, the toxicologist is able to furnish valuable evidence concerning the circumstances surrounding a death. Such cases commonly involve demonstrating intoxicating concentrations of ethanol in victims of automotive or industrial accidents, or carbon monoxide in fire victims. The degree of carbon monoxide saturation of the blood may indicate whether the deceased died as a result of the fire or was dead before the fire started. Arson is a common ploy used to conceal homicide. Also, legal or illicit psychoactive drugs often play a significant role in the circumstances associated with sudden or violent death. The behavioral toxicity of many illicit drugs may explain bizarre or "risk taking" behavior of the deceased which led to his demise. At times, a negative toxicologic finding is of particular importance in assessing the cause of death. For example, toxicology studies may demonstrate that a person with a seizure disorder was not taking his prescribed medication and this contributed to the fatal events.

Today there are numerous specialized areas of study in the field of toxicology; however, it is the forensic toxicologist, obliged to assist in the determination of the cause of death for a court of law, who has been historically recognized by the title "toxicologist."

Until the nineteenth century, physicians, lawyers, and law enforcement officials harbored extremely faulty notions about the signs and symptoms of poisoning (Thorwald, 1965). It was traditionally believed that if a body was black, blue, or spotted in places, or "smelled bad," the decedent had died from poison. Other mistaken ideas were that the heart of a poisoned person could not be destroyed by fire nor could the body of persons dying from arsenic poisoning decay. Unless a poisoner was literally caught in the act, there was no way to establish that the victim died from poisoning. In the early eighteenth century, a Dutch physician, Hermann Boerhoave, theorized that various poisons in a hot, vaporous condition yielded typical odors. He placed substances suspected of containing poisons on hot coals and tested their smells. Although Boerhoave was not successful in applying his method, he was the first to suggest a chemical method for proving the presence of poison.

During the middle ages, professional poisoners sold their services to royalty and the common populace. The most common poisons were of plant origin (such as hemlock, aconite, belladonna) and toxic metals (arsenic and mercury salts). During the French and Italian Renaissance, political assassination by poisoning was raised to an art by Pope Alexander VI and Caesar Borgia.

The use of white arsenic (arsenic trioxide) as a murder vehicle became so widespread that arsenic acquired the name "inheritance powder." Given this popularity, it is small wonder the first milestones in the chemical isolation and identification of a poison in body tissues and fluids would center around arsenic. In 1775, Karl Wilhelm Scheele, the famous Swedish chemist, discovered that white arsenic was converted to arsenous acid by chlorine water. The addition of metallic zinc reduced the arsenous acid to poisonous arsine gas. If gently heated, the evolving gas would deposit metallic arsenic on the surface of a cold vessel. In 1821, Serullas utilized the decomposition of arsine for the detection of small quantities of arsenic in stomach contents and urine in poisoning cases. In 1836, James M. Marsh, a chemist at the Royal British Arsenal in Woolwich, applied Serullas' observations in developing the first reliable method to determine an absorbed poison in body tissues and fluids, such as liver, kidney, and blood. Following acid digestion of the tissues, Marsh generated arsine gas which was drawn through a heated capillary tube. The arsine decomposed, leaving a dark deposit of metallic arsenic.

Quantitation was performed by comparing the length of the deposit from known concentrations of arsenic to those of the test specimens.

The 1800s witnessed the development of forensic toxicology as a scientific discipline. In 1814, Mathieiv J. B. Orfila (1787–1853), the "father of toxicology," published *Traité des Poisons,* the first systematic approach to the study of the chemical and physiologic nature of poisons (Gettler, 1977). Orfila's role as an expert witness in many famous murder trials, particularly his application of the Marsh Test for arsenic in the trial of the poisoner Marie Lafarge, aroused both popular and scholarly interest in the new science. As Dean of the Medical Faculty at the University of Paris, Orfila trained numerous students in forensic toxicology.

The first successful isolation of an alkaloidal poison was performed in 1850, by Jean Servials Stas, a Belgian chemist, using a solution of acetic acid in ethyl alcohol to extract nicotine from the tissues of the murdered Gustave Fougnie, Modified by the German chemist, Fredrick Otto, the Stas–Otto method was quickly applied to isolation of numerous alkaloidal poisons, including colchicine, coniine, morphine, narcotine, and strychnine. In the latter half of the nineteenth century, European toxicologists applying these new procedures provided valuable evidence against many poisoners. A number of these trials became "cause celèbre" and the testimony of forensic toxicologists captured the imagination of the public and increased awareness of the development and application of toxicology. Murderers could no longer poison with impunity!

In the latter half of the nineteenth century, European toxicologists were in the forefront of the development and application of forensic sciences. Procedures were developed to screen the alkaloids, heavy metals, and volatile poisons.

In America, Rudolph A. Witthaus, Professor of Chemistry at Cornell University Medical School, made many contributions to toxicology and called attention to the new science by performing analyses for New York City in several famous morphine poisoning cases: the murders of Helen Potts by Carlyle Harris, and Annie Sutherland by Dr. Robert W. Buchanan. In 1911, Tracy C. Becker and Professor Witthaus edited a four-volume work on Medical Jurisprudence, Forensic Medicine, and Toxicology, the first standard forensic textbook published in the United States. In 1918, the City of New York established a Medical Examiner's System and the appointment of Dr. Alexander O. Gettler as toxicologist marked the beginning of modern forensic toxicology in America. Although Dr. Gettler made numerous contributions to the sci-

ence, perhaps his greatest was the training and direction he gave to future leaders in forensic toxicology. Many of his associates went on to direct laboratories within coroners' and medical examiners' systems in the major urban centers throughout the country.

In 1949, the American Academy of Forensic Sciences was established to support and further the practice of all phases of legal medicine in the United States. The members of the toxicology section represent the vast majority of forensic toxicologists working in coroners' or medical examiners' offices. Several other international, national, and local forensic science organizations, such as the Society of Forensic Toxicologists and the California Association of Toxicologists, offer a forum for the exchange of scientific data pertaining to analytical techniques and case reports involving new or infrequently used drugs and poisons. The International Association of Forensic Toxicologists, founded in 1963, with over 750 members of 45 countries, permits worldwide cooperation in resolving technical problems confronting the toxicologist.

In 1975, the American Board of Forensic Toxicology was created to examine and certify forensic toxicologists. One of the stated objectives of the board is "to make available to the judicial system, and other publics, a practical and equitable means for readily identifying those persons professing to be specialists in forensic toxicology who possess the requisite qualifications and competence." In general, those certified by the Board must have earned a Doctor of Philosophy or Doctor of Science degree, have at least three years of full-time professional experience, and pass a written examination. At present, there are only approximately 150 forensic toxicologists certified by the Board.

TOXICOLOGIC INVESTIGATION OF A DEATH BY POISONING

The toxicologic investigation of a death by poisoning may be divided into three steps: (1) obtaining the case history and suitable specimens, (2) the toxicologic analyses, and (3) the interpretation of the analytical findings.

Case History and Specimens

Today, there are readily available to the public thousands of compounds that are lethal if ingested, injected, or inhaled. Only a limited amount of material on which to perform analyses is available; therefore, it is imperative that, prior to beginning the analyses, as much information as possible concerning the facts of the case is collected. The age, sex, weight, medical history, and occupation of the decedent, as well as any

Table 27–1. SUGGESTED LIST OF SPECIMENS AND AMOUNTS TO BE COLLECTED AT AUTOPSY

SPECIMEN	QUANTITY
Brain	100 g
Liver	100 g
Kidney	50 g
Heart blood	25 g
Peripheral blood	10 g
Vitreous humor	All available
Bile	All available
Urine	All available
Gastric contents	All available

From Appendix, Report of the Laboratory Guidelines Committee, Society of Forensic Toxicologist and Toxicology Section, American Academy of Forensic Sciences. *J. Anal. Toxicol.*, **14**:18A, 1990.

treatment administered prior to death, the gross autopsy findings, drugs available to the decedent, and the time of interval between the onset of symptoms and death should be noted. In a typical year, a postmortem toxicology laboratory will perform analyses for such diverse poisons as prescription drugs (analgesics, antidepressants, hypnotics, tranquilizers), drugs of abuse (hallucinogens, narcotics, stimulants), commercial products (antifreeze, aerosol products, insecticides, rodenticides, rubbing compound, weed killers), and gases (carbon monoxide, cyanide). Obviously, the possible identity of the poison prior to analysis would greatly help.

The collection of postmortem specimens for analysis is usually performed by the pathologist at autopsy. Specimens of many different body fluids and organs are necessary as drugs and poisons display varying affinities for the body tissues. A large quantity of each specimen is needed for thorough toxicologic analysis because a procedure that extracts and identifies one compound or class of compounds may be ineffective in extracting or identifying others (Table 27–1).

In collecting the specimens, the pathologist labels each container with the date and time of autopsy, the name of the decedent, the identity of the sample, an appropriate case identification number, and his signature or initials. It is paramount that the handling of all specimens, their analysis, and resultant reports be authenticated and documented. A form developed at the collection site that identifies each specimen is submitted to the laboratory with the specimens. The form is signed and dated by the pathologist and subsequently by any individual handling, transferring, or transporting the specimens from one individual or place to another. In legal terms, this form constitutes a "chain of custody"

of specimens, documenting by time, date, name, and signature all persons transferring or receiving the specimens. The chain of custody enables the toxicologist to introduce his results into legal proceedings, having established that the specimens analyzed were those of the decedent.

Specimens should be collected prior to embalming, as this process may destroy or dilute the poisons present, rendering their detection impossible. Conversely, methyl or ethyl alcohol may be a constituent of an embalming fluid, therefore giving a false indication of the decedent's drinking prior to death.

Toxicologic Analysis

Before beginning the analysis, several factors must be considered: the amount of specimen available, the nature of the poison sought, and the possible biotransformation of the poison. In cases involving oral administration of the poison, the gastrointestinal contents are analyzed first, because large amounts of residual unabsorbed poison may be present. The urine may be analyzed next, as the kidney is the major organ of excretion for most poisons and high concentrations of toxicants and/or their metabolites are often present in urine. Following absorption from the gastrointestinal tract, drugs or poisons are first carried to the liver before entering the general systemic circulation; therefore, the first analysis of an internal organ is conducted on the liver. If a specific poison is suspected or known to be involved in a death, the toxicologist chooses to first analyze those tissues and fluids in which the poison concentrates.

A knowledge of drug biotransformation is often essential before performing analysis. The parent compound and any major physiologically active metabolites should be isolated and identified. In some instances, the metabolites are the only evidence that a drug or poison has been administered. Many screening tests such as immunoassays are specifically designed to detect not the parent drug but its major urinary metabolite.

The analysis may be complicated because of the normal chemical changes that occur during decomposition of a cadaver. The autopsy and toxicologic analysis should be started as soon after death as possible. The natural enzymatic and nonenzymatic processes of decomposition and microbial metabolism may destroy a poison initially present at death or may produce substances or compounds with chemical and physical properties similar to those of commonly encountered poisons. As early as the 1870s, so-called "cadaveric alkaloids" isolated from the organs of putrefied bodies were known to produce color test reactions similar to those of morphine and other drugs. These "cadaveric alkaloids" resulted from the bacterial decarboxylation of the amino acids ornithine and lysine, producing putrescine and cadaverine, respectively (Evans, 1963). Likewise, during decomposition, phenylalanine is converted to phenylethylamine which has chemical and physical properties very similar to amphetamine. The hydrolysis, oxidation, or reduction of proteins, nucleic acids, and lipids may generate numerous compounds such as hydroxylated aliphatic and aromatic carboxylic acids, pyridine and piperidine derivatives, and aromatic heterocyclics such as tryptamine and norharmone (Kaempe, 1969). All these substances may interfere with the isolation and identification of the toxicants sought. The concentration of cyanide and ethyl alcohol and carbon monoxide saturation of the blood may be decreased or increased depending on the degree of putrefaction and microbial activity. However, many poisons, such as arsenic, barbiturates, mercury, and strychnine, are extremely stable and may be detectable many years after death.

Prior to analysis, the purity of all chemicals should be established. Primary reference material used to prepare calibrators and controls should be checked for purity, and the salt form or degree of hydration determined (Blanke, 1989). All reagents and solvents should be of the highest grade possible and free of contaminants that may interfere with or distort analytical findings. For example, the chloroform contaminants phosgene and ethyl chloroformate may react with primary or secondary amine drugs to form carbamyl chloride and ethyl carbamate derivatives (Cone et al., 1982). Specimen containers, lids, and stoppers should be free of contaminants, such as plasticizers which often interfere with chromatographic or gas chromatography/mass spectrometry (GC/MS) determinations. Care should be exercised to ensure a clean laboratory environment. This is a particular concern in the analysis of metals, as aluminum, arsenic, lead, and mercury are ubiquitous environmental and reagent contaminants.

Forensic toxicology laboratories analyze specimens using a variety of analytical procedures. Initially, nonspecific tests designed to determine the presence or absence of a class or group of analytes may be performed directly on the specimens. Examples of such tests typically used to screen urine rapidly are the FPN (ferric chloride, perchloric, and nitric acid) color test for phenothiazine drugs and immunoassays for the detection of barbiturates, benzodiazepines, and opiate derivatives. Positive results obtained by these tests must be confirmed by a second analytical procedure that identifies the particular drug. The detection limit of the confirmatory test should be lower than that of the initial nonspecific test.

Some analytical procedures identify specific compounds. Even in such instances, a second test should be performed to identify the analyte. The second test should be based on a chemical or physical principle different than that of the first test. Such additional testing is performed to establish an unequivocal identification of the drugs or poisons present. Where possible, the most specific test for the compound of interest should be performed. Today, GC/MS is generally accepted as unequivocal identification for most drugs. However, even GC/MS has limitations in drug identification.

The limit of detection, the smallest concentration of analyte reliably identified by the assay, and specificity of all qualitative methods should be well documented. The laboratory must demonstrate that the assay responses to blank or negative calibrators do not overlap with response of the lowest positive calibrator.

In certain instances, qualitative identification of a poison or drug is sufficient to resolve forensic toxicology issues. However, most cases require reliable estimates of poison concentrations for forensic interpretation. For quantitative analysis, the linearity, precision, and specificity of the procedure must be established. Linearity should be determined by use of at least three calibrators whose concentrations bracket the anticipated concentrations in the specimen. Precision, which statistically demonstrates the variance in the value obtained, is determined by multiple analyses of a specimen of known concentration. For a variety of reasons, occasionally a quantitative result will deviate spuriously from the true value. Therefore, replicate quantitative determinations should be performed on all specimens, at least in duplicate (Blanke, 1987).

On occasion, it is necessary to analyze unusual specimens such as bone marrow, vitreous humor, or even maggots. The extraction efficiency of a procedure may vary greatly depending on the nature of the specimens. Therefore, all calibrators and controls should, when possible, be prepared in the same matrix as the specimens and analyzed concurrently with the specimens. Often the matrix is "unique" or impossible to match, such as decomposed or embalmed tissue. In these instances, the method of "standard additions" may be used. Known amounts of the poison of interest are added to specimen aliquots and quantitation is performed by comparing the proportional response of the "poison added" specimens to that of the test specimens.

Interpretation of Analytical Results

Once the analysis of the specimens is completed, the toxicologist must interpret his findings as to the physiologic or behavioral effects of the toxicants on the decedent at the concentrations found. Specific questions must be answered such as the route of administration, the dose administered, and whether or not the concentration of the toxicant present was sufficient to cause death or alter the decedent's actions so as to cause his death. Assessing the physiologic meanings of analytical results is often the most difficult problem faced by the forensic toxicologist.

In determining the route of administration, the toxicologist notes the results of the analysis of the various specimens. As a general rule, the highest concentrations of a poison will be found at the site of administration. Therefore, the presence of large amounts of drugs and/or poisons in the gastrointestinal tract and the liver indicate oral ingestion, higher concentrations in the lungs compared to other visceral organs can indicate inhalation, and detection of a drug in tissue surrounding an injection site will, generally, indicate a fresh intramuscular or intravenous injection.

The presence of a toxic material in the gastrointestinal tract, no matter the quantity, is not sufficient evidence to establish the agent as the cause of death. It is necessary to demonstrate that absorption of the toxicant has occurred and that it has been transported by the general circulation to the organs where it has exerted a fatal effect. This is established by blood and tissue analysis. An exception to the rule is a strong corrosive chemical such as sulfuric acid, lye, and phenol, which exert their deleterious effects by directly digesting tissue, causing hemorrhage and shock.

The results of urine analysis are often of little benefit in determining the physiologic effects of a toxic agent. Urine results establish only that sometime prior to death, the poison was present in the body. Correlation of urine values with physiologic effects is poor, due to various factors affecting the rate of excretion of specific compounds and the urine volume.

The physiologic effects of most drugs and poisons correlate with their concentration in blood or blood fractions such as plasma or serum. Indeed, in living persons, this association is the basis of therapeutic drug monitoring. However, postmortem blood has been described as a fluid obtained from the vasculature after death that resembles blood. Therefore, interpretation of postmortem blood results requires careful consideration of both the case history, site of collection, and postmortem changes. The survival time between administration of a poison and death may be sufficiently long to permit biotransformation and excretion of the agent. Blood values may appear to be nontoxic or consistent with therapeutic administration. Death due to hepatic failure following acetaminophen overdose usually occurs at least three to four days postingestion. Postmortem acetaminophen concentrations in blood may be consistent with ingestion of therapeutic doses (Figure 27–3). Emergency medical treatment such as the administration of fluids, plasma extenders, diuretics, or blood transfusions may dilute or remove toxic agents. Likewise, prolonged survival on a mechanical respirator, hemodialysis, or hemoperfusion may significantly reduce initially lethal blood concentrations of poisons.

Until recently, it was generally assumed that postmortem blood drug concentrations were more or less uniform throughout the body. However, in the 1970s, several investigators noted that postmortem concentrations of digoxin in heart blood greatly exceeded those in simultaneously collected femoral blood. They also observed that postmortem blood concentrations, particularly in heart blood, exceeded the expected values at the time of death (Vorpahl and Coe, 1978; Aderjan et al., 1979). This postmortem increase in blood digoxin concentrations was apparently due to release of the drug from tissue stores, particularly the myocardium. Recently, others have demonstrated that for many drugs, blood concentrations in the same body vary greatly depending upon the site from which the specimen is collected: subclavian vein, thoracic aorta, inferior vena cava, femoral vein, and so forth. For example, in a case of fatal multiple drug ingestion, analysis of postmortem blood collected from ten different sites was found to contain imipramine concentrations differing by as much as 760 percent (2.1 to 16.0 mg/liter) (Jones and Pounder, 1987). In an extensive investigation, Prouty and Anderson (1990) demonstrated that postmortem blood drug concentrations were not only site dependent, but increased greatly over the time from death to specimen collection, particularly in heart blood. This increase over the postmortem interval was most pronounced for basic drugs with large apparent volumes of distribution such as tricyclic antidepressants.

In instances of overt drug overdose, postmortem blood concentrations are sufficiently elevated to render an unmistakable interpretation of fatal intoxication. However, in many cases, the postmortem redistribution of drugs may signifi-

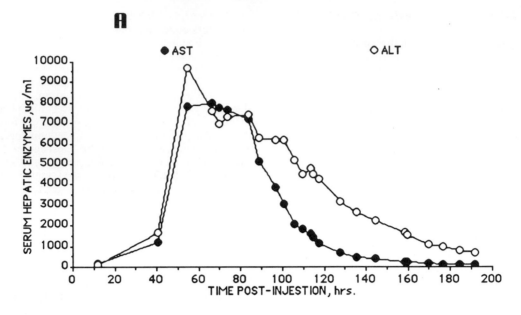

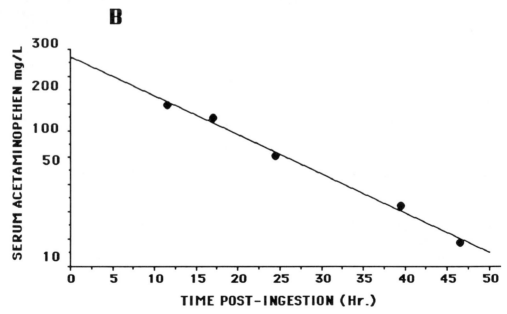

Figure 27-3. Laboratory findings in a fatal acetaminophen poisoning. *(A)* hepatotoxicity demonstrated by elevation and exhaustion of hepatic enzymes; alanine aminotransferase *(ALT)* and aspartate aminotransferase *(AST)*. *(B)* Serum acetaminophen concentrations decline to those consistent with therapeutic values within two days post-ingestion. (Data from Toxicology Laboratory, Medical College of Virginia.)

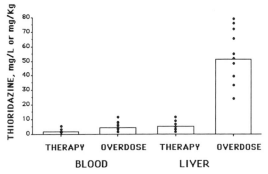

Figure 27-4. Comparison of thioridazine blood and liver concentrations following therapeutic and overdose ingestion. Liver concentrations clearly differentiate drug overdose from drug therapy. Bars represent mean values. [Data taken from Baselt *et al.*: *J. Anal. Toxicol.*, **2**:41-43 (1978) and Poklis *et al.*: *J. Anal. Toxicol.*, **6**:250-252 (1982).]

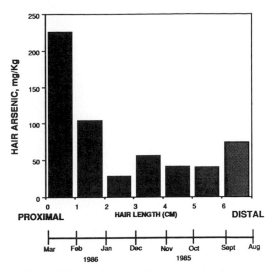

Figure 27-5. Results of neutron activation analysis for arsenic in sequential sections of hair, demonstrating chronic arsenic poisoning. Increased exposure in the first two sections consistent with fatal events. Lower values in section 3, consistent with two weeks of hospitalization. (Data redrawn from Poklis, A., and Saady, J. J.: *Am. J. Forensic Med. Pathol.*, **11**:226-232, 1990.)

cantly impact on the interpretation of analytical findings. For drugs whose volume of distribution, plasma half-life, and renal clearance vary widely from person to person or undergo postmortem redistribution, tissue concentrations readily distinguish therapeutic administration from drug overdose (Apple, 1989) (Figure 27-4). Therefore, to provide a foundation of reasonable medical certainty as to the role of a drug in the death of an individual, it is recommended that in addition to heart blood, a peripheral blood specimen and tissues be analyzed.

Postmortem toxicology results are often used to corroborate investigative findings. For example, the analysis of sequential sections of hair provide reliable correlation to the pattern of arsenic exposure. Significant increases in the arsenic content of the root and the first 5 mm of hair occur within hours after ingestion of arsenic (Smith, 1964). The germinal cells are in relativity close equilibrium with circulating arsenic, thus as arsenic concentrations in blood rise or fall, so does the arsenic deposition in the growing hair. Normal arsenic content in hair varies depending on nutritional, environmental, and physiologic factors; however, the maximum upper limit of normal with 99 percent confidence limit in persons not exposed to arsenic is 5 mg/kg (Shapiro, 1967). Hair grows at a rate of approximately 12.5 mm (½ inch) per month. Therefore, analysis of 1.0-cm segments provides a monthly pattern of exposure (Figure 27-5). Such analyses are often performed in cases of homicidal poisoning to demonstrate that increases in arsenic deposition in the victim's hair correlate to times when a poisoner had opportunity to administer the poison. Continuously elevated

hair arsenic values indicate chronic, rather than acute poisoning, as the cause of death.

COURTROOM TESTIMONY

The forensic toxicologist is often called to testify in legal proceedings. As a general rule of evidence, a witness may testify only to facts known to him. He may offer opinions based solely on what he has observed (Moenssens *et al.*, 1973). Such a witness is called a "lay witness." However, the toxicologist is called as an "expert witness." The court recognizes a witness as an "expert" if he possesses knowledge and experience in a subject that is beyond the range of ordinary or common knowledge or observation. The expert witness may provide two types of testimony, objective and "opinion." Objective testimony by the toxicologist usually concerns a description of his analytical methods and findings. When he testifies as to the interpretation of his analytical results or those of others, he is offering an "opinion." Lay witnesses cannot offer such "opinion" testimony as it exceeds ordinary experience.

Before the court permits "opinion" testimony, the witness must be "qualified" as an expert in his particular field. In qualifying as an expert witness, the court considers the witnesses education, on-the-job training, work experience, teaching or academic appointments, professional associations and publications, as well as the acceptance of the witness as an expert by other courts. Qualification of a witness takes place in front of the jury who consider the expert's qualifications in determining how much weight to give his "opinions" during their deliberations.

Whether the toxicologist appears in criminal or civil court, workman's compensation or parole hearings, the procedure for testifying is the same: direct examination, cross examination, and redirect examination. Direct examination is conducted by the attorney who has summoned the witness to testify. Testimony is presented in a question and answer format. The witness is asked a series of questions that allows him to present all facts or opinions relevant to the successful presentation of the attorney's case. During direct examination, the expert witness has the opportunity to explain to the jury scientific bases of his opinions. Regardless of which side has called the toxicologist to court, he should testify with scientific objectivity. Bias toward his client and prejudgments should be avoided. The expert witness is called to provide informed assistance to the jury. The guilt or innocence of the defendant is determined by the jury, not the expert witness.

Following direct testimony, the expert is then questioned by the opposing council. During this cross-examination, the witness is challenged as to his findings and/or opinions. The toxicologist will be asked to defend his analytical methods, results, and opinions. Opposing council may attempt to imply that the expert's testimony is biased because of financial compensation, association with an agency involved in the litigation, or personal feelings regarding the case. The best way to prepare for such challenges prior to testimony is to anticipate questions which opposing council may ask.

After cross-examination, the attorney who called the witness may ask additional questions to clarify any issues raised during cross-examination. This allows the expert to explain apparent discrepancies in his testimony raised by opposing council.

Often the expert witness is asked to answer a special type of question, the "hypothetical question." The hypothetical question contains only facts that have been presented in evidence. The expert is then asked his conclusion or opinion based solely on this hypothetical situation. This type of question serves as a means by which appropriate facts leading to the expert's opinion are identified. Often these questions are extremely long or convoluted. The witness should be sure he understands all facts and implications

in the question. Like all questions, this should be answered as objectively as possible.

FORENSIC URINE DRUG TESTING

Concerns about the potentially adverse consequences of substance abuse both to the individual and society have led to widespread urine analysis for the detection of controlled or illicit drugs (Gust and Walsh, 1989). Presently, such testing is routinely conducted by the military services, regulated transportation and nuclear industries, many federal and state agencies, public utilities, federal and state criminal justice systems, and numerous private businesses and industries. Significant ethical and legal ramifications are associated with such testing. Those having drug positive test results may not receive employment, be dismissed from their job, court marshalled, or suffer the loss of their good reputation.

To ensure the integrity of urine testing, two certification programs currently accredit forensic urine testing laboratories. Laboratories conducting testing of federal employees are required to be certified under the Department of Health and Human Services Mandatory Guidelines for Workplace Drug Testing as published in the April 11, 1988 Federal Register (Department of Health and Human Services, 1988). The College of American Pathologists (CAP) also conducts a certification program for urine testing laboratories. The federal program regulates a specific program from specimen collection through testing to the reporting of results, whereas the CAP program allows flexibility for the construction of programs servicing a broad range of clients. Both programs involve periodic on-site inspection of laboratories and proficiency testing.

Forensic urine drug testing (FUDT) differs from other areas of forensic toxicology in that urine is the only specimen analyzed and testing is performed for a limited number of drugs. At present, under the federal certification program, analyses are performed for only five drug classes or drugs of abuse (Table 27–2). Although FUDT laboratories typically analyze 100 to 1000 urine specimens daily, only a relatively small number of these samples are positive for drugs. To handle this large workload, initial testing is performed by immunoassays on high-speed, large-throughput analyzers. A confirmation analysis in FUDT-certified laboratories is performed by GC/MS.

Proper FUDT is a challenge to good laboratory management. As with all forensic activities, every aspect of the laboratory operation must be thoroughly documented: specimen collection, chain of custody, quality control, procedures,

Table 27–2. FORENSIC URINE DRUG TESTING ANALYTES AND CUT-OFF CONCENTRATIONS

	CONCENTRATION (ng/ml)	
	Initial Test	*Confirmatory Test*
Marijuana metabolite(s)	100	15[†]
Cocaine metabolite(s)	300	150[‡]
Opiate(s)	300*	—
Morphine	—	300
Codeine	—	300
Phencyclidine	25	25
Amphetamines	1000	—
Amphetamine	—	500
Methamphetamine	—	500

From Department of Health and Human Services, Mandatory Guidelines for Federal Workplace Drug Testing Programs, Federal Register, April 11, 1988, p. 11983.
* 25 ng/ml if immunoassay specific for free morphine.
[†] Δ-9-tetrahydrocannabinol-9-carboxylic acid.
[‡] Benzoylecognine.

testing, qualifications of personnel, and reporting results. The facility must be constructed and operated to ensure total security of specimens and all documents. Confidentiality of all testing results is paramount; only specifically authorized persons should receive testing results.

The presence of a controlled or illicit drug in a single random urine specimen is generally accepted as proof of recent or past substance abuse. However, positive urine drug findings are only evidence that at some time prior to collection of the sample the individual was administered, self administered, or had been exposed to the drug. Positive urine tests do not prove impairment from the drug or abuse or addiction.

FUDT results are reported only as positive or negative for the drugs sought. Cut-off values are established for both the initial and confirmation assays (Table 27–2). The cut-off value is a concentration at or above which the assay is considered positive. Below the cut-off value, the assay is negative. Obviously, drugs may be present below the cut-off concentration. However, the use of cut-off values allows uniformity in testing and reporting results. All test reports indicate the drug tested and its cut-off value.

There may be valid reasons other than substance abuse to account for positive drug findings, such as therapeutic use of controlled substances, inadvertent intake of drugs via food, or passive inhalation. The laboratory must be thoroughly familiar with these issues and devise strategies to resolve uncertainties. The seed of *Papaver somniferum*, poppy seed, is a common ingredient in many pastries and breads. Depending on their botanical source, poppy seeds may contain significant amounts of morphine. Several studies have demonstrated that ingestion of certain poppy seed foods results in the urinary

excretion of readily detectable concentrations of morphine (Elsohly and Jones, 1989). Morphine is a major urinary metabolite of heroin. Therefore, to differentiate readily heroin abuse from poppy seed ingestion, analysis may be performed for 6-acetylmorphine, a unique heroin metabolite (Fehn and Megges, 1985).

The passive inhalation of marijuana smoke may result in the absorption and excretion of marijuana metabolites. However, studies have demonstrated that even following the most extreme exposure situations, urinary excretion of marijuana metabolites does not exceed the 100 ng/ml cut-off value of initial immunoassay testing (Cone *et al.*, 1987).

HUMAN PERFORMANCE TESTING

Forensic toxicology activities also include the determination of ethanol and other drugs and chemicals in blood, breath, or other specimens, and the evaluation of their role in modifying human performance or behavior. The most common application of human performance testing is the determination of driving under the influence of ethanol (DUI) or drugs (DUID). Over the past half century, an enormous amount of data has been developed correlating blood ethanol concentrations with intellectual and physiologic impairment, particularly of those skills associated with proper operation of motor vehicles (Table 27–3). Numerous studies have demonstrated a direct relationship between increased blood ethanol concentrations (BAC) in drivers and increased risk of their involvement in road accidents (Council on Scientific Affairs, 1986). Alcohol-impaired drivers are responsible for 25 to 35 percent of all crashes causing serious injury. The threshold BAC for diminished driving

Table 27–3.   STAGES OF ACUTE ALCOHOLIC INFLUENCE/INTOXICATION

BLOOD-ALCOHOL CONCENTRATION (g/100 ml)	STAGE OF ALCOHOLIC INFLUENCE	CLINICAL SIGNS/SYMPTOMS
0.01–0.05	Subclinical	No apparent influence
		Behavior nearly normal by ordinary observation
		Slight changes detectable by special tests
0.03–0.12	Euphoria	Mild euphoria, sociability, talkativeness
		Increased self-confidence; decreased inhibitions
		Diminution of attention, judgment, and control
		Beginning sensory-motor impairment
		Slowed information processing
		Loss of efficiency in finer performance tests
0.09–0.25	Excitement	Emotional instability; loss of critical judgment
		Impairment of perception, memory, and comprehension
		Decreased sensitory response; increased reaction time
		Reduced visual acuity, peripheral vision, and glare recovery
		Sensory-motor incoordination; impaired balance
		Drowsiness
0.18–0.30	Confusion	Disorientation, mental confusion; dizziness
		Exaggerated emotional states (fear, rage, sorrow, etc.)
		Disturbances of vision (diplopia, etc.) and of perception of color, form, motion, dimensions
		Increased pain threshold
		Increased muscular incoordination; staggering gait; slurred speech
		Apathy, lethargy
0.25–0.40	Stupor	General inertia; approaching loss of motor functions
		Markedly decreased response to stimuli
		Marked muscular incoordination; inability to stand or walk
		Vomiting; incontinence of urine and feces
		Impaired consciousness; sleep or stupor
0.35–0.50	Coma	Complete unconsciousness; coma; anesthesia
		Depressed or abolished reflexes
		Subnormal temperature
		Incontinence of urine and feces
		Impairment of circulation and respiration
		Possible death
0.45+	Death	Death from respiratory arrest

performance is 0.05 g/dl, although the statutory definition of DUI in most states of the United States is 0.10 g/dl. In single-vehicle accidents, 55 to 65 percent of fatally injured drivers have BACs of 0.10 g/dl or greater.

During the past decade, there has been a growing concern about the deleterious effects on driving performance by drugs other than ethanol. Several studies have demonstrated a relatively high occurrence of drugs in impaired or fatally injured drivers (White *et al.*, 1981; Mason and McBay, 1984). These studies tend to report the highest drug use incidence rates that are associated with illicit or controlled drugs such as cocaine, benzodiazepines, marijuana, and phencyclidine. However, most studies only tested for a few drugs or drug classes and the repeated reporting of the same drugs may be a function of limited testing. Before DUID testing is as readily accepted by the courts as ethanol testing, many legal and scientific problems concerning drug concentrations and driving impairment must be resolved (Consensus Report, 1985). The reliability of analytical methodology to measure routinely minute concentrations of drug in blood must be established. Also, drug-induced driving impairment at specific blood concentrations in controlled tests and/or actual highway experience must be demonstrated.

ANALYTICAL ROLE IN CLINICAL TOXICOLOGY

Analytical toxicology in a clinical setting plays a role very similar to that in forensic toxicology. As an aid in the diagnosis and treatment of toxic incidents, as well as to monitor the effectiveness of treatment regimens, it is useful to clearly identify the nature of the toxic exposure and measure the amount of toxic substance that has been absorbed. Frequently, this information, together with the clinical state of the patient, permits the clinician to relate the signs and symptoms observed with the anticipated effects of the toxic agent. This may permit a clinical judgment as to whether the treatment must be vigorous and aggressive, or whether simple observation and symptomatic treatment of the patient is sufficient.

A cardinal rule in the treatment of poisoning cases is to remove any unabsorbed material, limit the absorption of additional poison, and hasten its elimination. The clinical toxicology laboratory serves an additional purpose in this phase of the treatment by monitoring the amount of toxic agent remaining in circulation or measuring what is excreted. In addition, the laboratory can provide the necessary data to permit estimations of the total dosage or of the effectiveness of treatment by changes in known pharmacokinetic parameters of the drug or agent ingested. Some examples from our laboratory can serve as illustrations of these aspects.

Ethylene glycol is a toxic solvent commonly used as an antifreeze in a number of commercial products found around the home. On ingestion, it is metabolized, in part by alcohol dehydrogenase, to a series of mixed aldehydes and carboxylic acids and eventually to oxalic acid (Mundy *et al.*, 1974). Some of these metabolites are toxic to the kidney and can result in renal shutdown (Berman *et al.*, 1957). Derivatives of ethylene glycol such as mono- and diesters produce similar toxic effects, as do diethylene glycol and its ether and ester derivatives. Propylene glycol, on the other hand, is relatively nontoxic, as are other polyethylene glycols. Labels for commercial products may not specify the type of glycol present. If ethylene glycol is not found to be present, the patient may still be at risk. On the other hand, if propylene glycol is present, aggressive therapy may not be indicated. It is important that the testing procedure discriminate between these related substances. A chromatographic method such as HPLC is useful in such a situation (Blanke and Blanke, 1984).

Treatment of ethylene glycol poisoning may involve the administration of ethanol, the preferred substrate for alcohol dehydrogenase, thus saturating the enzyme and permitting the excretion of ethylene glycol without metabolism to the toxic aldehydes and acids (Wacker *et al.*, 1965). By monitoring the patient continuously for the serum ethanol and ethylene glycol concentrations, the clinical toxicology laboratory can make sure that the appropriate concentration of ethanol is maintained and follow the excretion of ethylene glycol to determine when it is safe to discontinue the ethanol therapy.

Overdosage of drugs and toxic chemicals may lead to a variety of other changes in a patient that can be monitored by the clinical toxicology laboratory. The common analgesic acetaminophen, available for sale without a prescription, may be ingested excessively or accidentally by children. A portion of this drug is metabolized by the cytochrome P-450 mixed function oxidase system to a toxic metabolite that is bound by glutathione and excreted as a nontoxic conjugate. If sufficient drug is ingested to produce more of the metabolite than can be detoxified, hepatic necrosis can occur. The clinical toxicology laboratory can aid in the assessment of these patients by measuring the serum acetaminophen concentration at timed intervals. A significant increase in the half-life of the drug may indicate that hepatic injury has occurred and aggressive therapy may be initiated (see Chapter 28).

It is evident that the utilization of the analytical capabilities of the clinical toxicology laboratory has increased enormously in recent years. Not only can toxic agents be ruled into consideration in a diagnosis, but the absence of a toxic agent may also be of use to the clinician. Other uses of this laboratory service may include the assessment of ethanol or drugs in behavior modification. It can be important to include this parameter in trauma cases, particularly when the patient is unable to communicate and surgery with the administration of anesthetic agents or analgesic agents is indicated. Psychiatrists need to know the effects of any self-administered drugs prior to psychiatric or neurologic examinations.

Although the instrumentation and even the methodology used in the clinical toxicology laboratory is similar to that utilized by the forensic toxicologist, a major difference between these two applications is responsiveness. In the clinical setting, test results must be communicated to the clinician within hours for the results to be meaningful for therapy. The forensic toxicologist may carefully choose the best method for a particular test and conduct replicate procedures to ensure maximum accuracy. The clinical laboratory cannot afford this luxury and frequently will sacrifice precise accuracy for rapid turnaround time. In addition, because it is impossible to predict when toxicologic emergencies will occur, the clinical laboratory must be staffed and operated constantly. The necessity for staffing three shifts each day with trained analysts makes this type of clinical laboratory activity costly.

To partially offset these costs, it is frequently effective to apply the same trained analysts and special facilities to the measurement of drugs in patients receiving drugs for therapeutic purposes. Monitoring the serum concentration of drugs in patients undergoing a routine regimen of dosing generally is not an emergency procedure. The required assays can be planned to conform to a predetermined work schedule. This permits a more efficient utilization of staff and equipment than when they are applied solely to clinical toxicology.

ANALYTICAL ROLE IN THERAPEUTIC MONITORING

Historically, the administration of drugs for long-term therapy was an art form that was largely based on experience. A dosage amount was selected and administered at appropriate intervals based on what the clinician had learned was generally tolerated by most patients. If the drug seemed ineffective, the dosage was in-

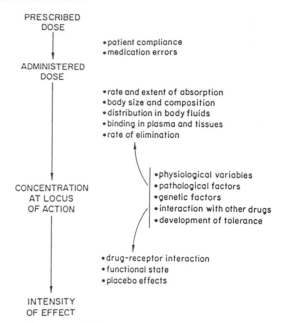

Figure 27-6. Factors that determine the relationship between prescribed drug dosage and drug effect. (Modified from Koch-Weser, 1972.)

creased; if toxicity developed, the concentration was decreased or the frequency of dosing altered. At times, a different dosage form might be substituted. Establishing an effective dosage regimen was particularly difficult in children or in the elderly.

The factors that are responsible for individual variability in response to drug therapy have been studied extensively in recent years. The important ones are summarized in Figure 27-6 (Blaschke et al., 1985). In a given patient, when the various factors are assumed to be constant, the administration of the same dose of a drug at regular intervals eventually produces a steady-state condition (Figure 27-7) (Moyer et al., 1986). When a steady-state is established, the average plasma concentration of the drug remains relatively constant and is proportional to the fractional bioavailability of the dose while inversely related to the clearance of the drug from the plasma and the time interval of dosing:

$$C_{ss} = \frac{F \cdot dose}{Cl \cdot T}$$

Monitoring the plasma concentration at regular intervals will detect deviations from the average plasma concentration which, in turn, may suggest that one or more of the variables that cause deviations from the average plasma concentration need to be identified and corrected (Figure 27-6).

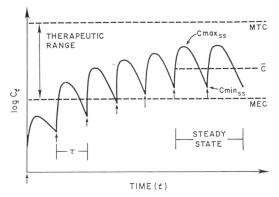

Figure 27–7. Sequence of drug concentration changes with multiple identical doses. Note that at steady state, peak and trough concentrations lie within the therapeutic range (or therapeutic window), and that five to seven half-lives are required to reach steady state. $C_{max_{ss}}$ and $C_{min_{ss}}$ = maximum and minimum steady-state concentrations; $\bar{C}$ = average steady-state concentration; τ = dosing interval; $\uparrow$ = dose; MTC = minimum toxic concentration; MEC = minimum effective concentration. (Modified from Gilman, A. G.; Goodman, L.; and Gilman, A., (eds.): *The Pharmacological Basis of Therapeutics,* 6th ed. Macmillan, New York, 1980.)

Because the drug being administered is known, qualitative characterization of the analyte is generally not required. Quantitative accuracy is required, however. Frequently, the methodology applied is important, particularly as to its selectivity. For example, methods that measure both the parent drug as well as one of metabolites are not ideal unless the individual analytes can be quantified separately. Depending on the drug, metabolites may not be active or, if active, to a different degree than the parent drug. The cardiac antiarrythmic drug procainamide is acetylated during metabolism to form *N*-acetylprocainamide (NAPA). This metabolite has antiarrhythmic activity of almost equal potency to procainamide. There is bimodal genetic variation in the activity of the *N*-acetyltransferase for procainamide so that in "fast acetylators" concentration of NAPA in the plasma may exceed that of the parent drug. For optimal patient management, information should be available about the concentrations of both procainamide and NAPA in plasma (Bigger and Hoffman, 1985).

Because for many drugs absolute characterization of the analyte is not necessary, immunoassay procedures are commonly used. This is particularly true of drugs with extremely low plasma concentrations such as cardiac glycosides, or drugs that are difficult to extract due to a high degree of polarity such as the aminoglycoside antibiotics. In these cases, plasma can be conveniently assayed directly by using commercially available kits for immunoassays.

The chromatographic methods in which an appropriate internal standard is added are favored when more than one analyte is to be measured or if metabolites of structures similar to parent drugs must be distinguished. Because the nature of drugs is varied, many different analytical techniques may be applied, including atomic absorption spectrometry for measuring lithium used to treat manic disorders. Virtually all of the tools of the analyst may be used for specific applications of analytical toxicology.

ANALYTICAL ROLE IN BIOLOGICAL MONITORING

In the workplace, good industrial hygiene practices require monitoring the environment to which workers are exposed to identify potentially harmful amounts of hazardous chemicals. Despite these precautions, it has become increasingly apparent that monitoring the worker directly can be a better indicator of exposure because it can show what has actually been absorbed. This is biologic monitoring (Chapter 29) and it can take a variety of forms.

For example, Table 27–4 shows some data relating to benzene exposure of chemists engaged in pesticide residue analysis in a state regulatory laboratory. Air monitoring devices in this laboratory indicated that the ambient benzene concentration never exceeded the time weighted average (TWA) of 32 mg/m^3 (10 ppm). Monitoring the breathing zone at different locations around the laboratory where benzene was in use showed other concentrations of this material. When expired air was monitored, one worker showed a significantly greater amount of benzene exposure than others. On questioning, she recalled spilling some of the solvent on a laboratory bench and in the process, saturated a portion of her laboratory coat. Presumably her exposure by inhalation and skin absorption was considerably greater than was indicated by the air monitor.

In addition to the measurement of the chemical, or its metabolites, in body fluids, hair, or breath of the worker, other more indirect methods may be employed. Substances that interact with macromolecules may form adducts that persist for long time periods. These can be sampled periodically and potentially may serve as a means of integrating exposure to certain substances over long time periods. For example, adducts of ethylene oxide with DNA or with hemoglobin have been studied in workers. This technique may also be applicable in other situations not necessarily related to occupational hazards. Acetaldehyde, a metabolite of ethanol,

Table 27–4. BENZENE EXPOSURE OF CHEMISTS PERFORMING PESTICIDE RESIDUE ANALYSIS

SOURCE	BREATH BENZENE (ppm)	AIR BENZENE (ppm)
Chemist A	0.45	—
Chemist B	0.13	—
Chemist C	0.41	—
Chemict D	0.48	—
Chemist E	0.34	—
Chemist F	0.37	—
Chemist G	2.50	—
Chemist H	0.56	—
Fume hood breathing zone	—	14.2
Fume hood breathing zone	—	51.2

forms adducts with hemoglobin. This marker may be of use in forensic cases (Stockham and Blanke, 1988).

Another approach useful in biologic monitoring is to measure changes of normal metabolites induced by xenobiotics. The profile of glucuronic acid metabolites excreted in urine can be altered after exposure to substances that induce monooxygenase activity. Although monitoring the alteration of the urinary excretion of these metabolites may not indicate exposure to specific substances, such a technique can be used in a generic fashion to flag a potentially harmful exposure to a hepatotoxic agent (Saady and Blanke, 1990). The early recognition of a toxicologic problem may permit protection of a worker before irreversible effects occur.

SUMMARY

The analytical techniques initiated by forensic toxicologists have continued to expand in complexity and improve in reliability. Many new analytical tools have been applied to toxicologic problems in almost all aspects of the field and the technology continues to open new areas of research. The forensic toxicologist continues to be concerned about conducting unequivocal identification of toxic substances in such a manner that the results can withstand a legal challenge. The problems of substance abuse, designer drugs, increased potency of therapeutic agents, and widespread concern about pollution and the safety and health of workers all present challenges to the analyst's skills. As these challenges are met, the analytical toxicologist continues to play a significant role in the expansion of the discipline of toxicology.

REFERENCES

Aderjan, R.; Bahr, H.; and Schmidt, G.: Investigation of cardiac glycoside levels in human postmortem blood and tissues determined by a special RIA procedure. *Arch. Toxicol.*, **42**:107–114, 1979.

Apple, F. S.: Postmortem tricyclic antidepressant concentrations: assessing cause of death using parent drug to metabolite ratio. *J. Anal. Toxicol.*, **13**:197–198, 1989.

Berman, L. B.; Schreiner, G. E.; and Feys J.: The nephrotoxic lesion of ethylene glycol. *Ann. Intern. Med.*, **46**:611–619, 1957.

Bigger, J. T., Jr., and Hoffman, B. F.: Antiarrhythmic drugs. In Gilman, A. G.; Goodman, L. S.; Rall, T. W.; and Murad, F. (eds.): *The Pharmacological Basis of Therapeutics*, 7th ed. Macmillan, New York, 1985, p. 763.

Blanke, R. V.: *Validation of the Purity of Standards*. Abbott Laboratories, Diagnostic Division, Irving, Texas, 1989.

Blanke, R. V.: Quality assurance in drug-use testing. *Clin. Chem.*, **33**:41B–45B, 1987.

Blanke, S. R., and Blanke, R. V.: The Schotten-Bauman reaction as an aid to the analysis of polar compounds: application to the determination of tris(hydroxymethyl)aminomethane (THAM). *J. Anal. Toxicol.*, **8**:231–233, 1984.

Blanke, R. V., and Decker, W. J.: Analysis of toxic substances. In Tietz, N. W. (ed.): *Textbook of Clinical Chemistry*. W. B. Saunders, Philadelphia, 1986.

Blaschke, T. F.; Nies, A. S.; and Mamelock, R. D.: Principles of therapeutics. In Gilman, A. G.; Goodman, L. S.; Rall, T. W.; and Murad, F. (eds.): *The Pharmacological Basis of Therapeutics*, 7th ed. Macmillan, New York, 1985, p. 52.

Cone, E. J.; Buchwald, W. F.; and Darwin, W. D.: Analytical controls in drug metabolism studies 11. Artifact formation during chloroform extraction of drugs and metabolites with amine substitutes. *Drug Metab. Dispos.*, **10**:561–567, 1982.

Cone, E. J.; Johnson, R. E.; Darwin, W. D.; Yousefnejad, D.; Mell, L. D.; and Mitchell, J.: Passive inhalation of marijuana smoke: urinalysis and room air levels of delta-9-tetrahydrocannabinol. *J. Anal. Toxicol.*, **11**:89–96, 1987.

Consensus Report: Drug Concentrations and Driving Impairment. *JAMA*, **254**:2618–2621, 1985.

Council on Scientific Affairs: Alcohol and the driver. *JAMA*, **255**:522–527, 1986.

Cravey, R. H., and Baselt, R. C.: The science of forensic toxicology. In Cravey, R. H., and Baselt, R. C. (eds.): *Introduction to Forensic Toxicology*. Biomedical Publications, Davis, California, 1981.

Department of Health and Human Services, ADAMHA. Mandatory Guidelines for Federal Workplace Drug

Testing; Final Guidelines; Notice. Federal Register, 53 (69), 11970-11989, 1988.

ElSohly, M. A., and Jones, A. B.: Morphine and codeine in biological fluids: approaches to source differentiation. *Forensic Sci. Rev.*, **1**:13–22, 1989.

Evans, W. E. D.: *The Chemistry of Death.* Charles C Thomas, Springfield, Illinois, 1963.

Fehn, J., and Megges, G.: Detection of O^6-monoacetylmorphine in urine samples by GC/MS as evidence for heroin use. *J. Anal. Toxicol.*, **9**:134–138, 1985.

Fisher, R. S., et al. (Committee on Medicolegal Problems). *Alcohol and the Impaired Driver. A Manual on the Medicolegal Aspects of Chemical Tests for Intoxication.* American Medical Association, Chicago, Illinois, 1968.

Gettler, A. D.: Poisoning and toxicology, forensic aspects. Part 1—historical aspects. *Inform*, **9**:3–7, 1977.

Granger, R. H.; Condie, L. W.; and Borzelleca, J. F.: Effect of vehicle on the relative uptake of haloalkanes administered by gavage. *Toxicologist*, **40**:1, 1987.

Gust, S. W., and Walsh, J. M.: *Drugs in the Workplace: Research and Evaluation Data.* NIDA Research Monograph 91, U.S. Government Printing Office, Washington, D.C., 1989.

Hawks, R. L., and Chiang, C. N.: Examples of specific drug assays. In Hawks, R. L., and Chiang, C. N. (eds.): *Urine Testing for Drugs of Abuse.* NIDA Research Monograph 73, U.S. Department of Health and Human Services, PHS, ADAMHA, Rockville, Maryland, 1986, p. 93.

Jones, G. R., and Pounder, D. J.: Site-dependence of drug concentrations in postmortem blood—a case study. *J. Anal. Toxicol.*, **11**:186–190, 1987.

Kaempe, B.: Interfering compounds and artifacts in the identification of drugs in autopsy material. In Stolman, A. (ed.): *Progress in Chemical Toxicology*, Vol. 4. Academic Press, New York, 1969, pp. 1–57.

Klaassen, C. D.; Amdur, M. O.; and Doull, J.: *Casarett and Doull's Toxicology. The Basic Science of Poisons*, 3rd ed. Macmillan, New York, 1986, flyleaf.

Koch-Weser, J.: Serum drug concentrations as therapeutic guides. *N. Engl. J. Med.*, **287**:227–231, 1972.

Mason, A. P., and McBay, A. J.: Ethanol, marijuana, and other drug use in 600 drivers killed in single-vehicle crashes in North Carolina. *J. Forensic Sci.*, **29**:987–1026, 1984.

Mills, R. A.; Millis, C. D.; Dannan, G. A.; Guengerich, F. P.; and Aust, S. D. Studies on the structure-activity relationships for the metabolism of polybrominated biphenyls by rat liver microsomes. *Toxicol. Appl. Pharmacol.*, **78**:96–104, 1985.

Moenssens, A. A.; Moses, R. E.; and Inbau, F. E.: *Scientific Evidence in Criminal Cases.* The Foundation Press, Mineola, New York, 1973.

Moyer, T. P.; Pippenger, C. E.; Blanke, R. V.; and Blouin, R. A.: Therapeutic Drug Monitoring. In Tietz, N. W. (ed.): *Textbook of Clinical Chemistry.* W. B. Saunders, Philadelphia, 1986. p. 1617.

Mundy, R. L.; Hall, L. M.; and Teague, R. S.: Pyrazole as an antidote for ethylene glycol poisoning. *Toxicol. Appl. Pharmacol.*, **28**:320–322, 1974.

Panel on Herbicides: Report on 2,4,5-T: *A Report of the Panel on Herbicides of the President's Science Advisory Committee.* Executive Office of the President, Office of Science and Technology, U.S. Government Printing Office, Washington, D.C., 1971.

Petersen, F.; Haines, W. S.; and Webster, R. W.: *Legal Medicine and Toxicology*, Vol. II, 2nd ed. W. B. Saunders, Philadelphia, 1923.

Prouty, B. S., and Anderson, W. H.: The forensic science implications of site and temporal influences on postmortem blood-drug concentrations. *J. Forensic Sci.*, **35**:243–270, 1990.

Saady, J. J., and Blanke, R. V.: Measurement of glucuronic acid metabolites by high resolution gas chromatography. *J. Chromatogr. Sci.* **28**:282–287, 1990.

Saady, J. J.; Narasimhachari, N.; and Friedel, R. O.: Unsuspected impurities in imipramine and desipramine standards and pharmaceutical formulations. *Clin. Chem.*, **27**:343–344, 1981.

SanGeorge, R. C., and Hoberman, R. D.: Reaction of acetaldehyde with hemoglobin. *J. Biol. Chem.*, **262**:6811–6821, 1986.

Shapiro, H. A.: Arsenic content of human hair and nails: its interpretation. *J. Forensic Med.*, **14**:65–71, 1967.

Smith, H.: The interpretation of the arsenic content of human hair. *J. Forensic Sci. Soc.*, **4**:192–199, 1964.

Stockham, T. L., and Blanke, R. V.: Investigation of an acetaldehyde-hemoglobin adduct in alcoholics. *Alcohol. Clin. Exp. Res.* **12**:748–754, 1988.

Thorwald, J.: *The Century of the Detective.* Harcourt, Brace and World, New York, 1965.

Vorpahl, T. E., and Coe, J. I.: Correlation of antemortem and postmortem digoxin levels. *J. Forensic Sci.*, **23**:329–334, 1978.

Wacker, W. E. C.; Haynes, H.; Druyan, R.; Fisher, W.; and Coleman, J. E.: Treatment of ethylene glycol poisoning with ethyl alcohol. *JAMA*, **194**:1231–1233, 1965.

White, J. M.; Clardy, M. S.; Groves, M. H.; Kuo, M. C.; MacDonald, B. J.; Wiersema, S. J.; and Fitzpatrick, G.: Testing for sedative-hypnotic drugs in the impaired driver: a survey of 72,000 arrests. *Clin. Toxicol.*, **18**:945–957, 1981.

Chapter 28

CLINICAL TOXICOLOGY

Barry H. Rumack and *Frederick H. Lovejoy, Jr.*

INTRODUCTION

Treatment of the poisoned patient based on pharmacologic principles promotes the institution of rational methods most beneficial to recovery. Unfortunately, the communication of these principles and methods has not always been appropriate, and some current reference sources still recommend procedures that are antiquated and should be contraindicated.

The material presented in this chapter provides a framework for the approach to the poisoned patient exposed to drugs, chemicals, plants, or other situations that confront the clinical toxicologist. This chapter reviews some of the principles of clinical management, as well as specific current theory and treatment of frequently encountered toxic situations.

TOXICOKINETICS

The basic application of pharmacokinetics to the toxic substance exposure is often useful in monitoring the severity and course of the poisoning and determining therapeutic maneuvers. The ability to calculate a body burden of a drug, its half-life, route of excretion, and other kinetic characteristics will aid in decisions such as use of diuresis, dialysis, or hemoperfusion. However, it must be recognized that most pharmacokinetic data are based on the therapeutic evaluation of drugs, and significant changes in kinetic parameters may occur in overdoses. For example, it is well known that salicylate peak blood levels are prolonged up to six hours from the normal values of one or two hours and that its half-life increases from 2 to 4 hours to 25 to 30 hours in significantly overdosed patients (Temple, 1981). Theophylline overdose results in a prolongation of serum half-life from three to four hours to ten hours (Gaudreault *et al.*, 1983; Gaudreault and Guay, 1986). Conversely, digoxin half-life may be shortened to one-third its expected value in overdose (Elkins and Watanabe, 1978). Thus, it is critical for the clinician

to determine that the data on which decisions are to be based are related to overdose rather than therapeutic information.

LD50 and MLD

The LD50 and MLD (median lethal dose) values are considered important to many clinicians in formulating a plan for dealing with the poisoned patient. Unfortunately, they are rarely of practical value clinically.

First, these values are obtained from various animal trials that establish a dose that will statistically kill half of a group or some other predetermined number. Differences in biotransformation between humans and animal species are remarkable, and linear correlation or extrapolation of animal biotransformation data to humans is rarely possible.

Second, the clinician obtains a *history* of overdose and attempts to relate the amount ingested by history with the LD50. This disregards factors such as the accuracy of history (which is often accurate less than 50 percent of the time), rate and extent of absorption of agent, biotransformation/disposition of the agent, the clinical response of the patient, and the effect of other drugs simultaneously ingested.

Consequently, the generally accepted recommendation is to disregard LD50 and MLD data on a particular poison and to determine the expected toxicology of the drug, followed by appropriate monitoring to determine if the patient demonstrates the predicted clinical findings. The adage "Treat the patient not the *poison*" represents the most basic and important principle in clinical toxicology.

Half-Life

The half-life is a measure of rate for the time required to eliminate one-half of a quantity of a chemical in the body. For drugs exhibiting first-order kinetics, the half-life can be calculated with the use of the following equation where *Kel* is the elimination rate constant.

$$\frac{t}{t_{1/2}} = \frac{0.693}{Kel}$$

Clinically it is estimated simply by plotting at least three concentration values of the chemical against time on semilogarithmic paper. Once at least three have been plotted, a straight line should be evident, and the amount of time that it takes for the drug concentration to decrease by half from any point on the line can be determined.

The clinical value of determining a patient's half-life during the course of a poisoning is to see the rate at which a patient is approaching therapeutic levels of a drug and whether methods of therapy being employed are effective. For some drugs, half-life values in the overdose situation are prolonged over values seen in normal dose. Therefore, measures to enhance elimination to shorten drug half-life are desirable. With digoxin, however, the $t_{1/2}$ has been reported to be shorter in overdose than in therapeutic situations (Ekins and Watanabe, 1978). In such cases supportive rather than elimination-enhancing measures are more practical.

Kinetic Relationships

The volume of distribution is the apparent space in which an agent is distributed following absorption and subsequent distribution in the body. Salicylate is distributed in total body water or about 60 percent of body mass. Digoxin, on the other hand, has an enormous volume of distribution of 500 liters or more in a 70-kg human (approximately 7 liters/kg). Since this is impossible practically, the term *apparent* volume of distribution is utilized. While this is the apparent volume based on the measured value of the drug in the blood, the drug is concentrated or sequestered somewhere out of the blood, i.e., tissue compartments (*see* Chapter 3).

Some useful mathematic relationships are

$$Vd = \frac{D}{Cp} \quad Cp = \frac{D}{Vd} \quad D = Cp \cdot Vd$$

Where Vd = Value of distribution
$\quad\quad\quad D$ = Dose administered
$\quad\quad\quad Cp$ = Plasma concentration (at zero time)

$$Cl = Kel \cdot Vd$$

Where Cl = Clearance of drug
$\quad\quad\quad Kel$ = Elimination rate constant

$$Kel = \frac{0.693}{t_{1/2}}$$

Thus, if the history is that of a 25-kg child who was estimated to have consumed 500 mg of phe-

nobarbital and the Vd for phenobarbital is approximately 60 percent body weight, then the estimated blood level would be 33.3 μg/ml. This approximates phenobarbital's high therapeutic range.

Example calculations:

25 kg $\times$ 0.60 liters/kg = 15 liters = Vd
500 mg/15 liters = 33.3 mg/liters or 33.3 μg/ml

In this case, the decision would be made clinically that the maximum possible dose by history, assuming total absorption, could produce toxicity, and, therefore, the child probably needs to be seen and observed by medical personnel.

MEASURES TO ENHANCE ELIMINATION

Once a patient has been observed clinically to be in a seriously toxic state, then it must be determined whether or not the agent can be eliminated more rapidly, thereby shortening the duration of coma and lessening toxic manifestations. Procedures to enhance elimination are indicated in severely poisoned patients.

Diuresis

The basic principle of diuresis is ion trapping. Increased urinary flow to two to three times normal was carried out in the past, but this has been replaced with adjustment of urine pH and maintenance of normal urine flow. The ion-trapping phenomenon occurs when the pK_a of the agent is such that, after glomerular filtration in the renal tubules, alteration of the pH of the urine can ionize and "trap" the agent. Once the toxin is ionized, then reabsorption from the renal tubules is impaired, and the result is that more of the drug is excreted in the urine. Salicylates and phenobarbital elimination is significantly enhanced by an alkaline diuresis, while phencyclidine and amphetamine elimination is hastened in an acid urine. Due to problems with acid diuresis, this procedure is rarely used. Even though a drug's pK_a may indicate that the drug might be successfully eliminated by this method, other factors, such as high lipid solubility and large volume of distribution, may render this method ineffective (see Table 28–1).

In theory, for drugs whose renal elimination is flow dependent, increasing urine output by the use of fluids or diuretics may enhance drug or toxin elimination. Few drugs are responsive solely to urine flow. Risks of fluid diuresis include pulmonary edema and cardiac arrhythmias or failure.

**Table 28–1. TOXICOKINETIC DATA OF DRUGS AND TOXINS
(NUMBERS EXPRESSED AS A MEAN OR AS A RANGE)**

AGENT	pk_a	Vd l/kg	THER. $t_{1/2}$ hrs	O.D. $t_{1/2}$ hrs	URINE ENHANCEMENT	DIALYSIS	SPECIFIC THERAPY
Acetaminophen	9.5	0.75	2	4	No	No	N-Acetylcysteine
Amitriptyline	9.4	40+	36	72	No	No	Physostigmine
Amobarbital	7.9	2.4	16	36+	No	No	
Amphetamine	9.8	0.60	8–12	18–24	Acid	Yes	Chlorpromazine
Bromide	—	40+	300	300	Yes	Yes	
Caffeine	13	0.75	3.5	4–120	No	No	
Chloral hydrate	—	0.75	8	10–18	No	No	
Chlorpromazine	9.3	40+	16–24	24–36	No	No	
Codeine	8.2	3	2	2	No	No	Naloxone
Coumadin	5.7	0.1	36–48	36–48	No	No	Vitamin K
Desipramine	10.2	50+	18	72	No	No	Physostigmine
Diazepam	3.3	1–2	36–72	48–144	No	No	
Digoxin	—	7–10	36	13	No	No	Fab antibodies
Diphenhydramine	8.3	—	4–6	4–8	No	No	
Ethanol	—	0.6	2–4	—	No	No	
Ethchlorvynol	8.7	3–4	1–2	36–48	No	No	
Glutethimide	4.5	20–25	8–12	24+	No	No	
Isoniazid	3.5	0.60	2–4	6+	No	Yes	Pyridoxine
Methadone	8.3	6–10	12–18	12–18	No	No	Naloxone
Methicillin	2.8	0.60	2–4	2–4	Yes	Yes	
Pentobarbital	8.11	2.0	10–20	50+	No	No	
Phencyclidine	8.5	—	—	12–48	Acid	Yes	
Phenobarbital	7.4	0.75	36–48	72–120	Alkaline	Yes	
Phenytoin	8.3	0.60	24–30	36–72	No	No	
Quinidine	4.3, 8.4	3	7–8	10	No	No	
Salicylate	3.2	0.1–0.3	2–4	25–30	Alkaline	Yes	
Tetracycline	7.7	3	6–10	6–10	No	No	
Theophylline	0.7	0.46	4.5	6+	No	Yes	

Dialysis

The dialysis technique, either peritoneal or hemodialysis, relies on passage of the toxic agent through a semipermeable dialysis membrane so it can equilibrate with the dialysate and subsequently be removed. This is in part dependent on the molecular weight of the compound. Some drugs such as phenobarbital can readily cross these membranes and go from high concentrations in plasma to a lower concentration in the dialysate. Since the volume of distribution of phenobarbital is 75 percent of the body weight, there is a reasonable opportunity for enough drug to be removed from total body burden that the technique is valuable in serious cases. Conversely, drugs with large volumes of distribution would be expected to be poorly dialyzable. Similarly, drugs that are highly serum protein bound are not expected to be well removed by dialysis (see Watanabe, 1977) (*see* Table 28–2).

Hemoperfusion

Passing blood through a column of charcoal or adsorbent resin is an important technique of extracorporeal drug/toxin removal. While some agents are better removed by this technique because of the adsorptive capacity of the column, the volume of distribution of an agent may limit removal in a similar manner to hemodialysis. Theophylline is an example of an agent amenable to this technique. If the drug is highly tissue bound such as in fat stores and only a small proportion is presented via the blood compartment to a device, then only the proportion that is in blood is available for removal. To date, there are few agents that are able to significantly displace toxins from either fat stores or tissue binding sites. The application of digoxin Fab antibodies in digoxin overdose represents one such clinically useful example (Smith, 1985).

APPROACH TO THE POISONED PATIENT

Telephone management of the pediatric patient, especially under the age of five, comprises 85 percent of this patient population's treatment. Epidemiologic data demonstrate that the peak age of ingestion is two years of age, which is consistent with the ambulatory growth and development of children. Most children suffer *ingestion* rather than poisoning with fewer

Table 28–2. DRUG TOXIN REMOVAL BY DIALYSIS, INTENSIVE SUPPORTIVE CARE, AND USE OF ACTIVATED CHARCOAL

Dialysis Indicated on Basis of Condition of Patient

Amphetamines	Meprobamate (Equanil,
Anilines	Miltown®)
Antibiotics	Paraldehyde
Boric acid	Phencyclidine
Bromide	Phenobarbital
Calcium	Potassium
Chloral hydrate	Quinidine
Fluorides	Salicylates
Iodides	Strychnine
Isoniazid	Thiocynates

Dialysis Not Indicated Except for Support in the Following Poisons; Therapy Is Intensive Supportive Care

Antidepressants (tricyclic and MAO inhibitors also)
Antihistamines
Chlordiazepoxide (Librium®)
Digitalis and related
Diphenoxylate (Lomotil®)
Ethchlorvynol (Placidyl®)
Glutethimide (Doriden®)
Hallucinogens
Heroin and other opiates
Methaqualone (Quaalude®)
Noludar (Methyprylon)
Oxazepam (Serax®)
Phenothiazines
Synthetic anticholinergics and belladonna compounds

Well Absorbed by Activated Charcoal

Amphetamines	Nicotine
Antimony	Opium
Antipyrene	Oxalates
Atropine	Parathion
Arsenic	Penicillin
Barbiturates	Phenol
Camphor	Phenolphthalein
Cantharides	Phenothiazine
Cocaine	Phosphorus
Digitalis	Potassium permanganate
Glutethimide	Quinine
Iodine	Salicylates
Ipecac	Selenium
Malathion	Silver
Mercuric chloride	Stramonium
Methylene blue	Strychnine
Morphine	Sulfonamides
Muscarine	

Increased Clearance with Multiple Doses of Activated Charcoal

Carbamazepine	Nadolol
Dapsone	Phenobarbital
Digoxin	Salicylates
Digitoxin	Theophylline

than 1 percent becoming symptomatic. In fact, the major traumatic event associated with a pediatric ingestion is the emesis that results from the therapeutic administration of syrup of ipecac. Poison centers, therefore, have adopted standard protocols for dealing with these childhood accidents so as to preclude missing those that actually become symptomatic (Rumack *et al.*, 1978). In addition, it is prudent for the clinician to become familiar with the local and regional poison control centers for consultative toxicology services (Chafee-Bahamon and Lovejoy, 1983).

Key Steps in Telephone Management

When dealing with a potential ingestion, the history represents the first step in determining the necessity for instituting therapeutic measures. The following represent critical history points and subsequent measures (Rumack *et al*, 1978; Kressel *et al.*, 1982).

1. Telephone number, name, address, age, weight
2. Time of ingestion, route, agent
3. Assessment of severity
4. Assessment of reliability of history
5. Determination of safety of home therapy
6. Instructions in home therapy—emesis, catharsis, charcoal
7. Follow-up
   1 hour—Determine success of therapy, usually emesis, and assess condition of patient
   4 hours—Determine condition of patient
   24 hours—Determine condition of patient, suggest psychiatric services, social services, or visiting nurses service if appropriate. Basically, if the status changes or if it seems that more than these calls need to be made, then the patient should be seen. A rule of thumb in most poison centers is that children under six months of age should be seen or referred to a physician regardless of history. Child abuse should be considered in any repeat poisoning case.

Evaluation of the Patient

The decision that determines whether or not the patient should be hospitalized is based on an evaluation of the severity of the potential poisoning. If it is apparent that the patient is in no danger, hospital referral in most cases is not necessary. Poison control center experience indicates that a vast majority of these situations can be appropriately handled at home. However, if it is judged that the patient's life is in immediate or potential danger, the patient should be brought or taken by ambulance to the nearest hospital or emergency room. Initial emergency room contact requires determining if the patient

Table 28–3. SCORING SYSTEMS FOR COMA, HYPERACTIVITY, AND WITHDRAWAL

Classification of Coma

0   Asleep but can be aroused and can answer questions

1   Comatose; does withdraw from painful stimuli; reflexes intact

2   Comatose; does not withdraw from painful stimuli; most reflexes intact; no respiratory or circulatory depression

3   Comatose; most or all reflexes are absent but without depression of respiration or circulation

4   Comatose; reflexes absent; respiratory depression with cyanosis, circulatory failure, or shock

Classification of Hyperactivity

1+   Restlessness, irritability, insomnia, tremor, hyperreflexia, sweating, mydriasis, flushing

2+   Confusion, hyperactivity, hypertension, tachypnea, tachycardia, extrasystoles, sweating, mydriasis, flushing, mild hyperpyrexia

3+   Dilirium, mania, self-injury, marked hypertension, tachycardia, arrhythmias, hyperpyrexia

4+   Above plus: convulsions, coma, circulatory collapse

Classification of Withdrawal

Score the following finding on a 0-, 1-, 2-point basis:

Diarrhea	Hypertension	Restlessness
Dilated pupils	Insomnia	Tachycardia
Gooseflesh	Lacrimation	Yawning
Hyperactive bowel sounds	Muscle cramps	

1– 5, mild
6–10, moderate
11–15, severe

Seizures indicate severe withdrawal regardless of the rest of the score

---

is breathing and/or is in shock, with immediate life support instituted as necessary. Clinical evaluation, in addition to the usual physical examination of the poisoned patient, includes several widely used scoring systems for coma, hyperactivity, and withdrawal. They are not only useful to assess the condition of the patient but also as a reminder to check certain key clinical points. They serve as useful monitoring parameters to follow and to determine if the patient's condition is improving or deteriorating. Finally, they serve as a useful method for quantitating response to therapy. Table 28–3 identifies these scoring methods and criteria.

Emesis

Syrup of ipecac in appropriate doses (30 ml, adult; 10 to 15 ml, pediatric) has been shown to be a safe and effective means of producing emesis (Boehnert *et al.*, 1985). While apomorphine has a more rapid onset of action than ipecac syrup, the average percent recovery of ingested toxin is the same. Apomorphine in therapeutic

dose is toxic in children, producing central nervous system depression. This effect may persist past the reversal action of naloxone administered to counteract the toxicity of this emetic. In addition, apomorphine may result in protracted vomiting, which is often unresponsive to narcotic antagonist intervention. Emesis with ipecac syrup or apomorphine 60 minutes after ingestion produces recovery of approximately 30 percent of ingested toxin.

Emesis is generally contraindicated when the patient is comatose, convulsing, or without the gag reflex. Strong acid or base ingestion is another reason for not inducing emesis since this will reexpose the patient's esophagus to these agents, thus contributing to further damage. In the case of petroleum distillate hydrocarbons, unless very large amounts (greater than 12 to 18 cc/kg) are ingested, ipecac-induced emesis is contraindicated.

Lavage

Gastric lavage with a large-bore tube is a rapid way to empty the stomach. Unfortunately, this technique may not provide benefit to the patient. Kulig *et al.*, have shown failure to affect outcome except in those patients with serious overdoses in which lavage is performed in the first hour after ingestion. Thus, this technique has been largely abandoned in children (Kulig *et al.*, 1985).

Cathartics

The rationale for the administration of cathartics in the poisoned patient it to hasten the toxin through the gastrointestinal tract, thereby minimizing its absorption. They are indicated in several situations, including ingestion of enteric-coated tablets, when the lag time since ingestion is greater than one hour, and when decreased bowel motility slows passage of the ingested toxin through the gastrointestinal tract. Preferred agents are the saline cathartics (sodium sulfate, magnesium sulfate, citrate, or phosphates) and sorbital, which have a relatively prompt onset of action and lower toxicity than the oil-based cathartics, which have attendant aspiration risks (Shannon *et al.*, 1986).

Charcoal

The classic paper of Corby and Decker (1970) demonstrates the value of administration of sufficient quantities of charcoal to bind toxin that has not been removed by emesis or lavage.

Although concern has been raised that charcoal cannot "catch up" with drugs and other agents once they have passed through the pylorus, there is ample evidence to show that administration of charcoal—following methods to empty the stomach—will result in lower plasma levels than if emesis or lavage alone is used. Concomitant administration of activated charcoal with syrup of ipecac often renders the ipecac ineffective.

Repetitive dosing of activated charcoal has recently been found useful to remove drugs in the gastrointestinal (GI) tract and drugs which are secreted into the GI tract. More recently, repetitive activated charcoal given every four hours for 24 to 48 hours has been shown to shorten half-life and enhance clearance of phenobarbital and theophylline when given intravenously based on therapeutic doses to volunteers (Berg *et al.*, 1982; Park *et al.*, 1986), this method of "gastrointestinal dialysis" is experiencing active clinical investigation as well as use in the overdose setting (*see* Table 28–2).

Laboratory

Measurement of plasma, urine, or gastric levels of drugs or toxins when done in appropriate relationship to time following ingestion and clinical status can have a significant impact in the clinical management of the poisoned patient. Qualitative screens on blood and urine are helpful to identify ingested toxin(s), whereas quantitative analyses are useful in determining appropriate therapy with selected toxins (e.g., methanol, iron, acetaminophen). When a toxic screen is requested, the clinician must be aware of which drugs are actually being examined. Too often the clinician interprets a negative toxic screen to mean that there are no toxic agents on board. Interpretation of a patient's levels should be related to the therapeutic levels from the same laboratory. Statements such as "lethal level" are not relevant since toxicologists assume that most patients arriving alive in the emergency department will eventually recover. Specific relationships of blood levels will be presented with each drug discussed in the next sections of this chapter (Curry, 1974).

ACETAMINOPHEN

Acetaminophen has been utilized as an analgesic and antipyretic since the mid-1950s and has become more prominently recognized as a potential hepatotoxin in the overdose situation since the original British reports in the late 1960s (Proudfoot and Wright, 1970). Work on the mechanisms of liver toxicity of the drug has provided a theoretical basis for therapy (Mitchell *et al.*, 1973).

Acetaminophen in normal individuals is inactivated by sulfation (approximately 52 per-

cent) and by glucuronide conjugation (42 percent). About 2 percent of the drug is excreted unchanged. The remaining 4 percent is biotransformed by the cytochrome P-450 mixed-function oxidase system. This P-450 metabolic process results in a potentially toxic metabolite that is detoxified by conjugation with glutathione and excreted as the mercapture. Evidence extrapolated from animals indicates that when 70 percent of endogenous hepatic glutathione is consumed, the toxic metabolite becomes available for covalent binding to hepatic cellular components. The ensuing hepatic necrosis would be expected to take place after absorption of 15.8 g of acetaminophen, the amount needed to deplete glutathione in a normal 70-kg human. Other factors may alter this figure. Ingestion of 15.8 g may not produce toxicity if all the dose is not absorbed, if the history is inaccurate, if the patient has a biotransformation inhibitor on board such as piperonyl butoxide, or if he suffers from anorexia nervosa. On the other hand, patients on long-term biotransformation enhancers (microsomal enzyme inducers) such as phenobarbital may produce more than 4 percent of the toxic metabolite. The range of metabolic response and the difficulty of estimating accurately the amount ingested and absorbed preclude making therapeutic decisions on a historic predictive basis alone (Peterson and Rumack, 1977).

The clinical presentation of these patients is also sufficiently confusing in some cases to make waiting for appearance of symptoms inadequate for diagnosis. The usual patient presents in the following stages:

Stage I—2 to 24 hours
> Anorexia, nausea, vomiting; a general feeling of malaise not unlike the common cold or flu

Stage II—Improvement; the patient begins to feel better—may become hungry and willing to get out of bed; at this same time, the SGOT, SGPT, bilirubin, and prothrombin time become abnormal; right upper quadrant pain may occur

Stage III—Three to five days
> Hepatic necrosis with peak abnormalities of hepatic function

Stage IV—Seven to eight days
> Return to normal hepatic functions and general clinical improvement

Follow-up liver biopsy studies of patients who have recovered three months to a year after hepatotoxicity have demonstrated no long-term sequelae or chronic toxicity (Clark *et al.*, 1973).

A very small percentage (0.25 percent) of patients in the national multiclinic study conducted in Denver may progress to hepatic encephalopathy with subsequent death. The clinical nature of the overdose is one of a sharp peak of SGOT by day 3 and with recovery to less than 100 IU/liter by day 7 or 8. Patients with SGOT levels as high as 20,000 IU/liter have shown complete recovery and no sequelae one week after ingestion (Arena *et al.*, 1978).

Laboratory evaluation of the potentially poisoned patient is crucial in terms of both hepatic measures of toxicity and plasma levels of acetaminophen. Accurate estimation of acetaminophen in the plasma, preferably by high-pressure liquid chromatography or gas chromatography, should be done on samples drawn three to four hours after ingestion when peak plasma levels can be expected.

Once an accurate plasma level is obtained, it should be plotted on the Rumack-Matthew nomogram to determine whether therapy is or is not indicated (see Figure 28–1). This nomogram is based on a series of patients with and without hepatotoxicity and their corresponding blood

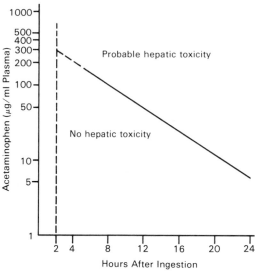

SEMILOGARITHMIC PLOT OF PLASMA ACETAMINOPHEN LEVELS VS. TIME

Figure 28–1.   Rumack-Matthew nomogram for acetaminophen poisoning. Cautions for use of chart: *(1)* The time coordinates refer to time of ingestion. *(2)* Serum levels drawn before four hours may not represent peak levels. *(3)* The graph should be used only in relation to a single acute ingestion. *(4)* A half-life of greater than four hours indicates a high likelihood of significant hepatic injury. (From Rumack, B. H., and Matthew, H.: Acetaminophen poisoning and toxicity. *Pediatrics,* **55**:871, 1975. Copyright American Academy of Pediatrics 1975.)

levels. While half-life was once considered an accurate way to determine potential acetaminophen hepatotoxicity, it is no longer considered adequate since the toxic metabolite comprises only about 4 percent of the total biotransformation. Similarly, back extrapolation of data to the zero-hour axis may not accurately reflect initial levels since the slope of excretion curve does not necessarily reflect hepatic toxicity.

Treatment should be instituted in any patient with a plasma level in the potentially toxic range. Standard support with gastric lavage should be followed by oral administration of *N*-acetylcysteine (Mucomyst®). A major national multiclinic open study has demonstrated a protective effect of *N*-acetylcysteine in acetaminophen poisoning when contrasted with controls not receiving antidotal therapy (Rumack *et al.*, 1981, Smilkstein *et al.*, 1988). Activated charcoal, unless administered within a few minutes of ingestion, should be avoided because of its potential adsorptive capacity for *N*-acetylcysteine (NAC). Because NAC is most effective if given prior to 16 hours postingestion, patients in whom blood levels cannot be obtained should have NAC treatment instituted and therapy terminated only if levels are nontoxic. The dosing regimen for NAC is a loading dose of 140 mg/kg orally, followed by 70 mg/kg orally for 17 additional doses (Peterson and Rumack, 1977). Intravenous *N*-acetylcysteine may be a useful route of administration. Additional work has shown that intravenous *N*-acetylcysteine when administered for 48 hours is equally effective to the current oral protocol used in the United States. The protocol used in Europe may be too short (Bronstein and Rumack, 1984).

Children less than 9 to 12 years of age have a lower incidence of hepatotoxicity following overdose than do adults (Rumack, 1984).

Daily SGOT, SGPT, bilirubin, and prothrombin time should be monitored. Chronic ethanol ingestion is additive in its hepatotoxicity when acetaminophen poisoning is superimposed, whereas acute ethanol ingestion as a single ingestion concomitantly with acetaminophen is protective (Rumack *et al.* 1981). The same effect occurs in children (Rumack, 1984).

Chronic toxicity is unlikely with acetaminophen because of its lack of accumulative kinetics (Peterson and Rumack, 1977).

ACIDS

Acids such as hydrochloric acid, nitric acid, sulfuric acid, and sodium bisulfate are commonly found around the home in products such as toilet bowl cleaners, automobile batteries, swimming pool cleaning agents, and other such products. Despite the fact that these agents have various degrees of toxicity, even a very small amount (milliliters) can result in serious sequelae that can occasionally progress to death, for example, if the caustic acid agent is aspirated. Clinically, the patient may present with irritation and crying, in association with inability to swallow, pain upon swallowing, mucous membrane burns, circumoral burns, hematemesis, abdominal pain, respiratory distress (secondary to epiglottal edema), shock, and renal failure. Once the patient has been treated through the initial stages of the ingestion, residual sequelae may occur with lesions of the esophagus and gastrointestinal tract that may progress to scarring and strictures. Ingestion of concentrated acids has led to necrosis of esophageal tissue, with death occurring one to five days postingestion.

The use of emetics and lavage are absolutely contraindicated (Penner, 1980; Freidman and Lovejoy, 1984). Dilution or therapy with water or milk *immediately* following ingestion represents the treatment of choice since these substances do not result in an exothermic chemical reaction. Despite labeling of many acid-containing products, alkaline substances or carbonate preparations are contraindicated since, when administered, they may produce increased amounts of heat and carbonates may form carbon dioxide gas, which presents an unacceptable risk of gastric perforation. In addition, immediate irrigation with copious amounts of water should be instituted to the exposed areas of skin, mucous membranes, and other affected areas. Olive oil is not indicated and may interfere with further therapy. Analgesics, administered by the parenteral route, may be indicated. Development of shock requires appropriate treatment with fluid therapy and pressor agents as indicated. Development of laryngoedema may require placement of an endotracheal tube, and esophagoscopy should be considered in all patients with significant symptoms indicating extensive burn involvement. Acids are more likely to produce gastric burns than esophageal burns. The value of corticosteroid therapy for the prevention of stricture and scar formation with acid burns is unclear at this time.

ALKALIES

Strong alkaline substances are found in such products as Drano®, Liquid Plummer®, and Clinitest Tablets®, all of which contain compounds such as sodium hypochlorite, sodium hydroxide, or potassium hydroxide. Experience has shown that strongly basic substances such as these are more likely to produce more severe injuries than are seen with acidic caustic ingestions. Recent experience has determined that the chlorinated bleaches, which contain a 3 to 6

percent concentration of sodium hypochlorite, are not as toxic as formerly thought. Following an ingestion of sodium hypochlorite, this compound interacts with the acidic milieu of the stomach, producing hypochlorous acid, which is an irritant to the mucous membranes and skin but does not cause stricture formation. More serious problems are presented following ingestions of compounds such as Drano®, which can cause burns of the skin, mucous membranes, and eyes almost immediately on contact. However, the absence of evidence of burns, irritation, erythema, or other such signs in the oral or circumoral area does not necessarily indicate that esophageal injury does not exist (Gaudreault et al., 1983). There have been cases demonstrating the absence of oral involvement with subsequent esophagoscopy proving esophageal burns. Edema of the epiglottis may result in respiratory distress, and inhalation of fumes may result in pulmonary edema or pneumonitis. Shock may occur. Recent experience has shown that "button" batteries, containing concentrated solutions of sodium or potassium hydroxide, represent a serious risk for leakage, corrosion, and perforation when lodged in the esophagus (Litovitz, 1983).

Alkaline caustic exposures require immediate irrigation of the affected areas with large amounts of water. Exposures to the eyes require irrigation for a minimum of 20 to 30 minutes and may require instillation of a local anesthetic to treat the blepharospasm. Oral ingestions require immediate dilution therapy with water or milk. Antidotes such as vinegar or lemon juice are absolutely contraindicated (Lacouture et al., 1986). Ingestion of chlorinated bleaches does not necessarily require esophagoscopy unless a highly concentrated solution has been ingested or the patient is demonstrating symptoms or signs of esophageal burns. Institution of a three-week course of corticosteroids such as dexamethasone has been indicated when esophageal burns are demonstrated, but recent data seriously question the effectiveness of this approach (Anderson et al., 1990). Bougienage (passage of a cannula) has been reported to be of some benefit for subsequent dilation of strictures of the esophagus. Antibiotic therapy should be instituted if mediastinitis occurs. Further information on the treatment of alkaline poisoning can be found in several publications (Haller, 1971; Burrington, 1974; Rumack and Temple, 1977; Howell, 1986).

AMPHETAMINE AND RELATED DRUGS

Stimulant drugs such as amphetamine, methylphenidate, and others can produce anxiety, hyperpyrexia, hypertension, and severe CNS stimulation. A paranoid psychosis is not uncommon, especially as the patient begins to come off the "high." These tablets and capsules are used as "diet" pills even though they are clearly not effective as anorexic agents after two weeks of therapy. Street "speed," "crystal," or "crystal ice," may contain in addition to or in lieu of amphetamine such compounds as caffeine, strychnine, phencyclidine (PCP), or phenylpropanolamine. (Pentel, 1984; Linden *et al.*, 1985).

Therapy of the severely agitated patient should be directed toward tranquilization with chlorpromazine and acid diuresis to ion-trap and promote excretion (Espelin and Done, 1968; Linden, *et al.*, 1985). The dose of chlorpromazine should be 1 mg/kg in pure amphetamine overdose and 0.5 mg/kg if the amphetamine has been mixed with a barbiturate. A major problem with this therapy is the interaction of chlorpromazine with several street drugs such as STP, MDA, or DMT, which may produce dramatic hypotension. If the history is not definitive for amphetamine, then diazepam at 0.1 to 0.3 mg/kg as a starting intravenous dose should be administered.

Acid diuresis may rarely be instituted in severe cases with sufficient intravenous fluids to produce a urine flow of 3 to 6 ml/kg/hour. Ammonium chloride, at 75 mg/kg/dose administered intravenously four times per day, to a maximum of 6 g total dose per day, may be used. This will produce a urine with a pH range of 4.5 to 5.5. Rhabdomyolysis (myoglobinuria) seen with phencyclidine poisoning is a contraindication to acid diuresis.

ANTICHOLINERGICS

A number of agents may produce anticholinergic toxicity following acute overdose, and these agents include drugs such as antihistamines (e.g., Benadryl®, Dramamine®, Chlortrimeton®), atropine, homatropine, over-the-counter sleeping medications (which contain both antihistamines and belladonnalike agents), and certain plants (e.g., jimsonweed, deadly nightshade) (Rumack *et al.*, 1974; Mikolich *et al.*, 1975; Bryson *et al.*, 1978). Antihistamines are readily available in many common nonprescription products as well as prescription medications. Plants containing belladonna alkaloids such as jimsonweed are frequently used in folk medicine cures for the common cold or as an hallucinogen by thrill seekers. Patients with anticholinergic toxicity may present with atropinic symptoms including dry mouth; thirst; fixed, dilated pupils; flushed face; fever; hot, dry, red

skin; and tachycardia. Speech and swallowing may be impaired in association with blurred vision. In infants, particularly those ingesting antihistamines, paradoxic excitement may occur subsequently followed by a more characteristic central nervous depression. Severe overdoses can present with hallucinationlike delirium, tremors, convulsions, coma, respiratory failure, or cardiovascular collapse. Potentially fatal doses of most antihistamines have been estimated to be approximately 25 to 30 mg/kg.

Immediate treatment should include instituting emesis, with syrup of ipecac or lavage, followed by administration of activated charcoal and saline cathartics. In ingestions of antihistamines related to the phenothiazines or in massive ingestions, induced emesis may be ineffective. Development of symptoms such as confusion, agitation, or coma presents an indication for physostigmine therapy in a dose of 0.5 to 2 mg, administered intravenously, which can be repeated every 30 minutes as needed (Rumack, 1973b). Physostigmine dramatically reverses the central and peripheral signs of anticholinergic toxicity, which are usually not seen with other cholinergic antagonists, such as neostigmine, because they do not cross the blood-brain barrier and enter the central nervous system. Measures such as forced diuresis and dialysis have not yet been shown to be effective in treating severe anticholinergic poisonings.

BENZODIAZEPINES

Benzodiazepine agents are widely prescribed in the treatment of anxiety and nervousness. In fact, in 1976 and 1977, the number 1 prescribed drug in the United States was diazepam (Valium®). A large number of congeners have been marketed by the pharmaceutical industry with little, if any, significant differences between the agents. Available products include chlordiazepoxide (Librium®), clonazepam (Clonopin®), flurazepam (Dalmane®), lorapezam (Atvian®), and oxazepam (Serax®). Although their pharmacologic effects do not differ greatly in terms of their clinical application, there are some differences in their major routes of biotransformation, volumes of distribution, and half-lives with respect to their pharmacokinetics in overdose. Chlordiazepoxide and oxazepam have shorter half-life values than the other agents such as diazepam and flurazepam. Following acute overdose, clinical symptoms or manifestations may include sleepiness, which, following larger overdose, can range from stage-zero to stage-one coma. Initially, excitement may be seen as a result of the disinhibition effects of these drugs, which then progresses to central nervous system depression, hypotension, respiratory depression, and coma (Welch *et al.*, 1977). On occasion, anticholinergic symptoms such as dry mouth, tachycardia, dilated pupils, and absent bowel sounds may be seen. Patients who have been receiving or ingesting benzodiazepines on a chronic basis (40 to 80 mg or more per day for one to two months or more) may exhibit mild to moderate symptoms of withdrawal, with severe withdrawal symptoms seen in patients taking the drug for many months to years. Symptoms may include jitteriness, nervousness, anxiety, agitation, confusion, hallucinations, and seizures. Patients exhibiting withdrawal symptoms should be restarted on benzodiazepine and slowly withdrawn over a period of several months (Rifkin *et al.*, 1976). In most cases, ingestion of a benzodiazepine agent of up to 1.5 g results in only minor toxicity, i.e., CNS depression. Fatality, following oral ingestion, is rare unless a combination of drugs is taken with the benzodiazepine (Greenblatt *et al.*, 1978). Therapeutic levels of diazepam or chlordiazepoxide are reported to be about 0.5 mg/100 ml.

Treatment of benzodiazepam overdose is primarily supportive. Establishment of respiration with assisted ventilation if necessary should be instituted immediately. A new antidote, flumazenil, is under final investigation and should be available for use in serious cases (Prischl, 1988). Emesis should be considered unless the patient is comatose, is convulsing, or has lost the gag reflex. If these contraindications exist, the patient may be intubated and lavaged followed by administration of activated charcoal and a saline cathartic such as sodium or magnesium sulfate. Hypotension should be treated initially with fluid. Institution of vasopressor agents should be used only if the patient is unresponsive to other measures. Forced diuresis and dialysis are of no value in the treatment of benzodiazepine overdoses.

CYANIDE

Cyanide is commonly found in certain rat and pest poisons, silver and metal polishes, photographic solutions, and fumigating products. Compounds such as potassium cyanide can also be readily purchased from chemical stores. Cyanide is readily absorbed from all routes, including the skin, mucous membranes, and by inhalation, although alkali salts of cyanide are toxic only when ingested. Death may occur with ingestion of even small amounts of sodium or potassium cyanide and can occur within minutes to several hours, depending on route of exposure. Inhalation of toxic fumes represents a potentially rapidly fatal type of exposure. Sodium nitroprusside (Smith and Kruszyna, 1974) and apricot seeds (Sayre and Kaymakcalan, 1974) have also caused cyanide poisoning. A blood cyanide level of greater than 0.2 μg/ml is associated with toxic manifestations. Lethal cases have usually had levels above 1 μg/ml. Clinically, cyanide poisoning is reported to produce a bitter, almond odor on the breath of the patient; however, approximately 20 percent of the population is genetically unable to discern this characteristic odor. Typically, cyanide has a bitter, burning taste, and following poisoning, symptoms of salivation, nausea without vomiting, anxiety, confusion, vertigo, giddiness, lower jaw stiffness, convulsions, opisthotonos, paralysis, coma, cardiac arrhythmias, and transient respiratory stimulaton followed by a respiratory failure may occur (Hall *et al.*, 1987). Bradycardia is a common finding, but in most cases heartbeat usually outlasts respirations (Wexler *et al.*, 1947). A prolonged expiratory phase is considered to be characteristic of cyanide poisoning.

Artificial respiration with 100 percent oxygen should be started immediately in patients with respiratory difficulty or apnea. Administration of 1 to 2 ampules of amyl nitrite by inhalation to the patient for 15 to 30 seconds every minute should be instituted concurrently while preparing sodium nitrite for intravenous administration (Chen and Rose, 1952, Graham *et al.*, 1977). Amyl nitrite has the ability to induce methemoglobin, which has a higher affinity for cyanide than hemoglobin; however, amyl nitrite alone is able to produce only a 5 percent methemoglobin level (Stewart, 1974). The Lilly cyanide kit (Lilly stock no. M76) contains ampules of amyl nitrite, sodium nitrite, and sodium thiosulfate with appropriate instructions. Sodium nitrite, 300 mg intravenously, should be administered to adults to attain a desired methemoglobin level of approximately 25 percent. However, doses this high should not be administered to children, as potentially fatal methemoglobinemia may result (Berlin, 1970). Children weighing less than 25 kg must be dosed on the basis of their hemoglobin levels and weight. In the absence of immediate serum hemoglobin levels, a dose of 10 mg/kg is considered safe (Berlin, 1970). Once intravenous sodium nitrite is administered, sodium thiosulfate should be immediately given. Thiosulfate combines with available cyanide to form thiocyanate, which is then readily excreted in the urine (Chen and Rose, 1952; Stewart, 1974; Graham *et al.*, 1977). Oxygen should also be given since it increases the effectiveness of the nitrites and the thiosulfate. Oxygen therapy should be maintained during and after thiosulfate thereapy to ensure adequate oxygenation of the blood. A methemoglobin level of greater than 50 percent is an indication for exchange transfusion or administration of blood. Since cyanide toxicity may reoccur, the patient should be observed for no less than 24 to 48 hours, and reoccurrence is an indication for retreatment with sodium nitrite and sodium thiosulfate in one-half the recommended doses. Data indicate that the use of hydroxycobalamin may be of value in the treatment of cyanide poisoning (Bain and Knowles, 1967; Hillman et al., 1974; Posner et al., 1976). However, experience in the United States with this compound is limited owing to lack of availability. Further clinical experience is required to evaluate the role of these agents in the treatment of cyanide poisoning.

DIGITALIS GLYCOSIDES

Digitalis glycosides are available in prescription medications as digoxin (Lanoxin®) and digitoxin as well as through a number of plant sources (oleander, foxglove). Many ingestions of digitalis occur in infants who inadvertently get into a grandparent's heart medication, although the drug has been used on occasion by persons with suicidal intent. Acute toxic manifestations of the digitalis glycosides represent extensions of the compound's vagal effects. Clinical manifestations seen in the acute overdose include nausea, vomiting, bradycardia, heart block, cardiac arrhythmia, and cardiac arrest. Younger individuals without significant heart disease tend to present with bradycardia and heart block, whereas other patients may present with ventricular arrhythmias, with or without heart block (Ekins and Watanabe, 1978). While hypokalemia is a frequent hallmark associated with chronic digitalis poisoning, in the acute-overdose situation hyperkalemia is more frequently found. Serum digoxin levels in excess of 5 μg/liter (ng/ml) are often seen.

Emesis or lavage is indicated, followed by administration of activated charcoal with saline cathartics. Potassium administration is contraindicated unless there is documented hypokalemia since potassium administration with unsuspected concurrent digitalis-induced hyperkalemia in the overdose situation may result in heart block progressing to sinus arrest. Patients should be monitored by ECG and antiarrhythmics instituted for the treatment of arrhythmias. Phenytoin (Dilantin®) is considered to be the antiarrhythmic of choice for ventricular arrhythmia (Rumack et al., 1974), whereas atropine has been shown to be useful in the treatment of severe bradycardia. Pacemaker therapy may be required in refractory cases. The use of resin-binding agents such as cholestyramine (Cuemid®, Questran®) or col-

estipol has been recommended to minimize absorption of cardiac glycosides as well as to interrupt enterohepatic circulation of these compounds. A recent advance in the treatment of digitalis poisoning is the use of Fab fragments for digoxin's specific antibodies (Lloyd and Smith, 1978). Clinical experience with this method is now available and has clearly shown its efficacy for digoxin and digitoxin overdose (Smith et al., 1982; Smith, 1985).

ETHANOL

Excessive consumption of ethanol produces a depressed state that may be additive if other depressants such as sedatives, hypnotics, or tranquilizers have also been consumed. The following tabulation summarizes clinical findings at various blood levels.

BLOOD ETHANOL

50–150 mg/100 ml:	Incoordination, slow reaction time, and blurred vision
150–300 mg/100 ml:	Visual impairment, staggering, and slurred speech; marked hypoglycemia, especially in children
300–500 mg/100 ml:	Marked incoordination, stupor, hypoglycemia, and convulsion
500 mg and over/100 ml:	Coma and death, except in tolerant individuals (Lambecier and DuPan, 1968).

One patient who was reported to exhibit a peak level of 780 mg/100 ml was capable of holding a normal conversation at 520 mg/100 ml and related a history of chronic alcoholism (Hammond et al., 1973). Hypoglycemia occurring as ethanol levels are falling is a complication of ethanol poisoning in children.

Absorptoin of ethanol from the gastrointestinal tract is rapid, particularly in the fasting state with peak blood levels attained within 30 to 60 minutes after ingestion. Metabolism in adults will eliminate 7 to 11 g of ethanol per hour, which is equivalent to ½ to 1 oz of 50-proof beverage per hour. A rule of thumb is that 1 ml of absolute ethanol per kilogram of body weight results in a level of 100 mg/100 ml in one hour (Elbel and Schleyer, 1956). Although ethanol is considered to be biotransformed according to zero-order kinetics (Wilkinson, 1976), some patients at high levels have been found to have ethanol metabolism demonstrating first-order kinetics (Hammond et al., 1973; David and Spyker, 1979).

Treatment of ethanol overdose consists of intensive supportive care. Attention must be directed toward hypoglycemia and acidosis. Chronic alcoholics may experience delirium tremens. During ethanol withdrawal, conservative management and benzodiazepines or other sedatives can adequately control these symptoms and prevent convulsions. Dialysis is rarely indicated unless the patient is unable to dispose of the ethanol because of hepatic or renal failure.

HYDROCARBONS—PETROLEUM DISTILLATES

Hydrocarbons or petroleum distillates are available in a wide variety of forms, including motor oil, gasoline, kerosene, red seal oil, and furniture polish, and in combination with other chemicals as a vehicle or solvent. The toxicity of hydrocarbons is generally indirectly proportional to the agent's viscosity, with products having high viscosity (150 to 250) such as heavy greases and oils considered to have only limited toxicity. Products with viscosity in the 30 to 35 range or lower present an extreme aspiration risk and include such agents as mineral seal oil, which is found in furniture polishes. It is important to realize that even small amounts of a low-viscosity material, once aspirated, can involve a significant portion of the lung and produce a chemical pneumonitis. Oral ingestion of hydrocarbons is often associated with symptoms of mucous membrane irritation, vomiting, and CNS depression. Cyanosis, tachycardia, and tachypnea may appear as a result of aspiration, with subsequent development of chemical pneumonitis. Other clinical findings include albuminuria, hematuria, hepatic enzyme derangement, and cardiac arrhythmias. Doses as low as 10 ml orally have been reported to be potentially fatal, whereas other cases have survived ingesting 60 ml of petroleum distillates (Rumack, 1977). A history that presents with coughing or choking in association with vomiting strongly suggests aspiration and hydrocarbon pneumonia. Hydrocarbon pneumonia is an acute hemorrhagic necrotizing disease that can develop within 24 hours of the ingestion. Pneumonia may require several weeks for complete resolution.

Although controversial, emesis is indicated in some hydrocarbon ingestions, where absorption may produce systemic effects. Agents such as asphalt, tar, heavy lubricants, Vaseline®, and mineral oil are considered to be relatively nontoxic and do not require removal. Chlorinated hydrocarbon solvents or any hydrocarbon or petroleum distillate with a potentially dangerous additive (camphor, pesticide, heavy metals) should be considered for vomiting. Petroleum naphtha derivatives, gasoline, kerosene, and mineral seal oil (or signal oil) as found in furniture polish or oil polishes produce severe and often prolonged chemical pneumonitis (Rumack, 1977). These compounds are poorly absorbed from the stomach, but are very damaging to the lung if inhaled. They should *not* be removed by emesis unless very large amounts are ingested (greater than 12 to 18 cc/kg) (Bratton and Haddow, 1975). Saline cathartics such as magnesium or sodium sulfate should be administered and are preferable to oil-based cathartics. Oil administration may result in a higher incidence of pneumonia (Beaman et al., 1976). Gastric lavage is not indicated for hydrocarbon ingestion due to the risk of aspiration should the patient vomit around the lavage tube (Ng et al., 1974). X rays taken early in the course of ingestion may not demonstrate chemical pneumonia, and even if demonstrated, the clinical severity does not correlate well with the degree of X-ray findings. However, X rays should be repeated on follow-up to detect development of pneumonitis or demonstrate pneumatoceles (Bergson, 1975). Patients who arrive coughing probably already have aspirated and should be monitored closely for development of pneumonitis. The decision for hospitalization should be based on clinical criteria (e.g., cyanosis, respiratory distress) rather than on X-ray findings alone (Anas et al., 1981). Steroid therapy may be harmful (Marks et al., 1972; Brown et al., 1974). Antibiotics, oxygen, and positive end–expiratory pressure should be instituted as indicated (Steele et al., 1972; Rumack, 1977).

INSECTICIDES

Chlorinated Hydrocarbons

Chlorinated hydrocarbon insecticides are stable lipophilic chemicals and are usually contained in various organic solvents or as petroleum distillates. Often the petroleum distillates or organic solvents used as vehicles for the chemicals are as toxic as the pesticides themselves and in the event of a significant ingestion, the vehicle toxicity should be considered as well (i.e., hydrocarbon pneumonitis). Many of the chlorinated hydrocarbon insecticides are rapidly absorbed and produce central nervous system toxicity. Because of the halogenated nature of these organic compounds, hepatoxicity, renal toxicity, and myocardial toxicity may also occur. Examples of chlorinated hydrocarbons include chlordane, DDT, dieldrin, Kepone®, lindane, toxaphene, and paradichlorobenzene. Clinical manifestations following ingestion include apprehension, agitation, vomiting, gastrointestinal upset, abdominal pain, and CNS depression. Convulsions may occur at higher doses and may be preceded by symptoms of ataxia, muscle spasms, and fasciculations.

In cases of ingestion, emesis is indicated unless the patient is comatose, is convulsing, or has lost the gag reflex. Emesis should be followed by administration of activated charcoal and saline cathartics. Oil-based cathartics such as castor oil or other substances including fats or oils should be avoided since these compounds may tend to enhance the absorption of the chlorinated hydrocarbon from the gastrointestinal tract. Epinephrine is contraindicated since it may induce ventricular fibrillation due to the sensitization of the myocardium by the chlorinated hydrocarbons. Convulsions may be treated with diazepam in a dose of 0.1 mg/kg, administered intravenously, to a maximum of 10 mg. Methods to enhance elimination have not been successful other than as a supportive measure for hepatic and renal failure. Cholestyramine, which has been shown to bind chlordecone (Kepone®) in the intestinal tract, may offer a means to treat chronic Kepone® poisoning and, pending further study, may have application to other agents (Boylan *et al.*, 1978).

Organophosphates

Organophosphate insecticides such as diazinon, malathion, parathion, TEPP, and DFP are potent cholinesterase enzyme inhibitors that act by interfering with the metabolism of acetylcholine, which results in accumulation of acetylcholine at neuroreceptor transmission sites. Exposure produces a broad spectrum of clinical effects indicative of massive overstimulation of the chlorinergic system, including muscarinic effects (parasympathetic), nicotinic effects (sympathetic and motor), and CNS effects (Namba, 1971; Minton and Murray, 1988). These effects present clinically as feelings of headache, weakness, dizziness, blurred vision, psychosis, respiratory difficulty, paralysis, convulsions, and coma. Typical findings are given by the mnemonic "SLUD," which stands for salivation, lacrimation, urination, and defecation. A small percentage of patients may fail to demonstrate miosis, a classic diagnostic hallmark (Mann, 1967). Onset of clinical manifestation of organophosphate poisoning usually occurs within 12 hours of exposure. Measurement of red cell cholinesterase is usually diagnostic; when there is a reduction to 50 percent or less of control values, this indicates significant poisoning and is an indication for institution of 2-PAM (Protopam®, pralidoxime), a cholinesterase-regenerating agent. Efforts must be made to ensure that the patient does not become reexposed through such means as contaminated clothing or reexposure to the contaminated environment. Decontamination may be achieved by using soap washings followed by alcohol-soap washings using tincture of green soap. Rescuers and medical personnel should also be protected from contamination by use of rubber gloves and aprons.

Maintaining adequate respiratory function should be the first treatment measure taken. In cases of ingestion, emesis is indicated unless the patient is comatose, is convulsing, or has lost the gag reflex. This should be followed by administration of activated charcoal and sodium or magnesium sulfate as a cathartic. Atropine is the drug of first choice (especially in patients with respiratory problems) and should be administered until signs of atropinism occur, i.e., dry mouth, tachycardia. In some cases, large doses (up to 2 g of atropine) may be required in order to reverse cholinergic excess. The presence of significant cholinesterase depression in red blood cells requires treatment with 2-PAM in conjunction with atropine. In an adult a dose of 1 g intravenously should be given and repeated every 8 to 12 hours. After administration of three doses of 2-PAM, the drug is not likely to be of any additional benefit. The pediatric dose is 250 mg/dose administered slowly by the intravenous route and repeated every 8 to 12 hours. The use of aminophylline/theophylline, succinylcholine, physostigmine, and morphine is contraindicated.

Carbamates

Carbamate insecticides include agents such as aminocarb, carbaryl (Sevin®), and landrin. These insecticides are reversible inhibitors of cholinesterase, whose actions are often enhanced by formulating them with pyrethrin or piperonyl butoxide. Clinical manifestations are those seen with cholinesterase inhibition but may not be identical to the signs and symptoms seen with organophosphate poisoning. However, with carbamate exposure the degree of toxicity is considered less severe due to the rapid reversal of the cholinesterase inhibition. Symptoms such as headache, blurred vision, weakness, sweating, myosis, chest pain or tightness, salivation, lacrimation, nausea, vomiting, urination, abdominal cramps, and diarrhea may occur. More severe exposure may result in muscle cramps, fasciculations, pulmonary edema, areflexia, and convulsions. Blood cholinesterase activity can be measured but may not show significant depression unless blood samples are drawn and assayed immediately, owing to rapid cholinesterase regeneration. Atropine in large doses for maintenance of airway and respiration is the treatment of choice, dosed initially at 2 mg intravenously in an adult and 0.05 mg/kg intravenously in a child, wih the drug repeated at five- to ten-minute invervals if needed. The patient should be thoroughly decontaminated and other measures instituted to prevent absorption. Again, care must be exercised to protect rescuers and medical personnel from exposure. 2-PAM is usually not needed but may be used in conjunction with atropine for severe carbamate poisoning. It is considered to be contraindicated in certain carbamate poisonings, for example, carbaryl (Natoff and Reiff, 1973).

IRON

Iron is available in a wide variety of preparations including iron supplement tablets (ferrous sulfate, ferrous gluconate, ferrous fumarate), multiple-vitamin preparations, and prenatal vitamin preparations. As described on the labels of these preparations, the amount of iron given may be calculated in terms of a milligram amount of the salt form (e.g., ferrous sulfate 300 mg or ferrous gluconate 320 mg) or by the actual amount of elemental iron. It is important to note that iron toxicity relates to the amount of *elemental* iron, and therefore, for the salt forms the actual elemental iron content must be calculated.

SALT FORM	% ELEMENTAL IRON
Ferrous fumarate	33
Ferrous gluconate	12
Ferrous sulfate (exsiccated)	30
Ferrous sulfate	20

Clinically, there are generally five phases of toxicity subsequent to ingestion of iron (Jacobs *et al.*, 1965). The *first phase* lasts from 30 minutes to two hours after ingestion and may be characterized by symptoms of lethargy, restlessness, hematemesis, abdominal pain, and bloody diarrhea. Necrosis of the gastrointestinal mucosa is a result of the direct corrosive effect of iron on tissue and may result in severe hemorrhagic necrosis with development of shock. Iron absorbed through intact mucosa may also cause shock. The *second phase* presents as an apparent recovery period, which then progresses into the third phase. This *third phase* occurs 2 to 12 hours after the first phase and is characterized by the onset of shock, metabolic acidosis, cyanosis, and fever. Acidosis results from the release of hydrogen ion from the conversion of ferric (Fe^{3+}) to ferrous (Fe^{2+}) ion forms and accumulation of lactic and citric acids. The *fourth phase* occurs two to four days after ingestion and is sometimes characterized by the development of hepatic ne-

crosis, which is thought to be due to a direct toxic action of iron on mitochondia. The *fifth phase* occurs from two to four weeks after ingestion and is characterized by gastrointestinal obstruction, which is secondary to gastric or pyloric scarring and healed tissue. Oral ingestion of iron is a potentially fatal occurrence, and ingestions of over 30 mg/kg body weight should be considered for hospital admission for observation depending on clinical symptoms and findings (Stein *et al.*, 1976). Qualitative methods for determining the ingestion of iron include: (1) a consistent history and physical examination, (2) a positive abdominal X ray for iron tablets, and (3) a semiquantitative color change demonstrable when gastric aspirate containing iron is mixed with deferoxamine (McGuigan *et al.*, 1979). Quantitative methods used in iron overdose include: (1) a white blood cell count of greater than 15,000 or a blood sugar greater than 150 mg/dl obtained within six hours of ingestion (Lacouture *et al.*, 1981), (2) a positive urinary deferoxamine challenge (excretion of a vin rosé color), and (3) an elevated serum iron level (Lacouture *et al.*, 1981).

Emesis or lavage with a large-bore tube is indicated (Proudfoot *et al.*, 1986). Abdominal X rays may reveal full tablets or tablet fragments in the gastrointestinal tract since they are radiopaque. Sodium bicarbonate or Fleet phosphates given orally are no longer used owing to a high incidence of adverse effects and unclear efficacy. The use of deferoxamine is considered somewhat controversial since this drug may induce severe hypotension following oral doses. When used, the dose is 2 to 10 g of deferoxamine dissolved in 25 ml of lavage fluid, followed by a second dose of 50 percent of the initial dose in 4 hours and a similar third dose in 8 to 12 hours. If free iron is present in serum, or if the patient is exhibiting shock, or coma, or if the serum iron is greater than 350 mcg/ml, deferoxamine should be administered at a rate not to exceed 15 mg/kg/hour for eight hours followed by 5 mg/kg/hour if needed (M. Stein *et al.*, 1976; Robotham and Leitman, 1980; Lovejoy, 1982). If the patient is not in shock, deferoxamine may be administered intramuscularly (20 mg/kg every four to six hours), depending on the clinical condition. Shock with dehydration should be treated with appropriate fluid therapy (Robertson, 1971).

MERCURY

Mercury in its various forms is available widely in the forms of metallic mercury (thermometers, Miller-Abbot tubes), fungicides, all hearing aid and watch batteries, paints, mercurial drugs, and antiquated cathartics and ointments. Poisoning may occur from either chronic or acute exposure to such agents or through the food chain (Eyl, 1971). Toxicity of the mercury is primarily related to its form (see Chapter 19) since metallic mercury is relatively nontoxic unless it is converted to an ionized form, such as occurs on exposure to acids or strong oxidants. In general, the mercuric salts are more soluble and produce more serious poisoning than do the mercurous salts (Goldwater, 1971). Inorganic forms of mercury are corrosive and produce symptoms of metallic taste, burning, irritation, salivation, vomiting, diarrhea, upper gastrointestinal tract edema, abdominal pain, and hemorrhage. These effects are seen acutely and may subside with subsequent lower gastrointestinal ulceration (Goldwater, 1971). Large ingestions of the mercurial salts may produce kidney damage, which may present with nephrosis, oliguria, and anuria. Ingestion of organic mercurials such as ethylmercury may produce symptoms of nausea, vomiting, abdominal pain, and diarrhea, but in most cases the main toxicity is neurologic involvement presenting with paresthesias, visual disturbances, mental disturbances, hallucinations, ataxia, hearing defects, stupor, coma, and death. Symptoms may occur for several weeks after exposure. Exposure and poisoning can occur following ingestion of mercury-contaminated seafood or grains or inhalation of vaporized organomercurials. Chronic inorganic mercury poisoning may occur following repeated environmental exposure and may present with a neurologic syndrome often described as the "mad hatter syndrome."

Therapy should be initiated with emesis or lavage, followed by administration of activated charcoal and a saline cathartic. Milk may be administered to help precipitate the mercury compound. Blood and urine levels of mercury may be of value in determining the indication of administration of chelating agents such as D-penicillamine or dimercaprol (BAL) (Kark, 1971). D-Penicillamine is administered in a dose of 250 mg orally four times a day in adults, 100 mg/kg/day in children, to a maximum recommended dose of 1 g per day for three to ten days, with continuous monitoring of mercury urinary excretion. In patients who cannot tolerate penicillamine, BAL can be administered in a dose of 3 to 5 mg/kg/dose every 4 hours by deep intramuscular injection for the first two days, followed by 2.5 to 3 mg/kg/dose intramuscularly every 6 hours for two days, followed by 2.5 to 3 mg/kg/dose every 12 hours intramuscularly for one week. Adverse reactions associated with BAL administration such as urticaria can often be controlled with antihistamines such as diphenhydramine. The development of renal failure contraindicates penicillamine therapy since the kidney is the main route of renal excretion for penicillin. BAL therapy can be used cautiously in spite of renal failure since BAL is excreted in the bile; however, BAL toxicity, which consists of fever, rash, hypertension, and CNS stimulation, must be closely monitored. Dialysis does not remove either chelated or free mercury metal (Robillard et al., 1976).

NARCOTIC OPIATES

Narcotic overdose may occur in a number of different situations, such as in the newborn infant, in addition to drug addiction. Accidental or intentional overdoses frequently involve Lomotil®, Darvon®, Talwin®, morphine, or dextromethorphan. Acute overdoses of any narcotic drug may result in respiratory arrest and coma with an initial clinical presentation of pinpoint pupils, hypotension, bradycardia, and respiratory depression, urinary retention, muscle spasm, and itching. Propoxyphene overdose has been associated with convulsions (Lovejoy et al., 1974b). Other signs such as leukocytosis, hyperpyrexia, and pulmonary edema may occur, particularly in drug abusers injecting street drugs intravenously. Ingestions of methadone or propoxyphene may have a prolonged or protracted clinical course lasting 24 to 48 hours or more (Lovejoy et al., 1974b). Chronic narcotic use is often associated with skin abscesses, cellulitis, endocarditis, myoglobinuria, cardiac arrhythmias, tetanus, and thrombophlebitis. Lomotil® ingestion is frequently complicated by the presence of atropine in the proprietary dosage forms with a resultant mixed picture of narcotic and anticholinergic symptoms (Rumack and Temple, 1974).

Emesis or lavage should always be performed since delayed gastric emptying is common following narcotic ingestions (Rumack and Temple, 1974; Fuzltz and Senay, 1975; Lawson and Northridge, 1987). Emesis can be induced in the alert patient, however, if seizures or coma exist intubation and gastric lavage with a large-bore (28-French or larger) Ewald tube should be carried out. Activated charcoal, five to ten times the estimated weight of ingested drug (minimum of 10 g), as well as a nonabsorbable saline cathartic (sodium sulfate or magnesium sulfate, 250 mg/kg of body weight) should be instilled following emesis or lavage. The cathartic should be repeated every three to four hours until stooling has occurred. Other basic supportive measures should be provided as needed. Naloxone at a dose of 0.03 mg/kg in the child or 1.2 mg/kg in the adolescent or adult intravenously is the drug of choice for all narcotic ingestions including pentazocine and propoxyphene as well as methadone, morphine, and codeine (Martin, 1976). In some cases, doses of naloxone as high as 0.1 mg/kg in the child or 2 to 4 mg in the adolescent or adult may be required for those failing to respond to the initial dose, and there is little evidence that such doses of naloxone are associated with any ill effects (Moore et al., 1980). Owing to the short duration of action of naloxone (60 to 90 minutes) (Evans et al., 1974), repeated doses of naloxone may be necessary until the narcotic is biotransformed, particularly in the treatment of methadone overdoses (Aronow et al., 1972; Frand et al., 1972; Lovejoy et al., 1974b). In some cases of narcotic overdose, up to 20 mg of naloxone may be required (Moore et al., 1980). Other narcotic antagonists such as nalorphine (Nalline®) and levallorphan (Lorfan®) possess narcotic antagonistic effects, that is, respiratory depressant effects (Foldes et al., 1969) and are no longer recommended.

PHENCYCLIDINE (PCP)

Phencyclidine, which is commonly called PCP, was originally developed as an anesthetic for humans but was abandoned due to its postoperative side effects, that is, hallucinations and agitation. It is now legally available as a veterinary medication for use as an animal tranquilizer. It is also known by various street names: angel dust, dust, embalming fluid, elephant or horse tranquilizer, killer weed, super weed, monkey dust, peace pill, rocket fuel, and hog. It is frequently sold as THC (tetrahydrocannabinol) but may appear also as mescaline, psilocybin, LSD, amphetamine, and cocaine. It is closely related to the anesthetic ketamine (Ketalar®), and both agents produce what has been called disassociative anesthesia. Owing to the availability and ease of manufacture, there has been an increased use of PCP, particularly in the teenage population where it is ingested orally, smoked, or snorted. Intravenous use is less common but on occasion has been reported. Clinical manifestations from phencyclidine use include symptoms of excitation with marked paranoid or aggressive behavior, which is frequently characterized as self-destructive. Characteristically, miosis and nystagmus, both horizontal and vertical, is noted in associaton with ataxia, impaired speech, bizarre behavior, tachycardia, hypertension that may progress to later stages of hypotension, increased reflexes, seizures, respiratory depression, and coma (Bolter, 1970; Linden et al.,1975; Tong et al., 1975). The sensations that the user may feel subsequent to PCP ingestion are feelings of depersonalization, distortion of body image, a sense of distance and estrangement from the environment in association with time expansion, and slowed body movements. Phencyclidine can be analyzed in serum, urine, and gastric contents.

Initial management of phencyclidine ingestion requires isolation of the patient from all sensory stimuli such as noise, lights, and touch (Stein, 1973). Provision of a quiet, supportive, and nonthreatening environment may help reduction of psychotomimetic effects from bad trips. Therapy by talking the patient down with continual verbal reassurance in many cases may be all that is required. Extremely agitated or convulsing patients should be protected from self-inflicted harm and given diazepam intravenously in 2- to 3-mg increments. In severe cases with hypotension, PCP should be treated with use of plasma expanders before vasopressors are attempted. Diazoxide has been used with good success in hypertensive crisis secondary to phencyclidine (Eastman and Cohen, 1975). Gastric lavage or gastric dialysis has been suggested to be of benefit in capturing PCP excreted into the stomach. Acidification of the urine in association with forced diuresis may hasten renal elimination of phencyclidine (Done et al., 1977). Myoglobinuria is a contraindication to the use of acid diuresis.

PHENOTHIAZINES

The phenothiazine class of antipsychotic agents includes a broad class of drugs with similar therapeutic effects. Individual agents depending on the class of phenothiazine (aliphatic, piperidine, or piperazine) differ primarily in their milligram potencies and their tendencies to produce extrapyramidal symptoms, sedation, and hypotension. Agents such as fluphenzine (Prolixin®) and trifluoperazine (Stelazine®) have a high tendency to produce extrapyramidal effects, whereas chlorpromazine (Thorazine®) and thioridazine (Mellaril®) have a lesser tendency to produce extrapyramidal effects but a higher tendency to produce sedation and hypotension. Two other classes of antipsychotic drugs that are nonphenothiazine-related include butyrophenones such as haloperidol (Haldol®) and the thioxanthine class such as chlorprothixene (Taractane®) and thiothixene (Navane®). These nonphenothiazine-class drugs have a higher tendency to produce extrapyramidal symptoms over sedation and hypotension. These drugs possess significant anticholinergic, alpha-adrenergic blocking, quinidinelike, and extrapyramidal effects. In addition, phenothiazines also lower the seizure threshold (Logothetis, 1967). Overdose with these drugs may result in CNS depression, which can present initially with reduced activity, emotional quieting, and affective indifference, although such patients may also exhibit a period of agitation, hyperactivity, or convulsions prior to the depressed state (Barry *et al.*, 1983). Hyperthermia or hypothermia may develop owing to phenothiazine's effects on the temperature-regulating mechanisms in the hypothalamus. Tachycardia with hypotension as a result of anticholinergic and alpha-blocking effects may occur. In addition, widening of the QRS complex due to the "quinidinelike" effect of these drugs can occur and may result in ventricular tachycardia. Extrapyramidal symptoms, present as torticollis, stiffening of the body, spasticity, impaired speech, and opisthotonos, may occur (Gupta and Lovejoy, 1967). These symptoms may frequently occur in children who have been administered prochlorperazine (Compazine®) in the treatment of nausea and vomiting.

Emesis or lavage is indicated, followed by administration of activated charcoal and a saline cathartic. Phenothiazines are radiopaque, and unabsorbed drug in the form of full or partial tablets may be visualized in the gastrointestinal tract by abdominal X ray (Barry *et al.*, 1973). Development of convulsions should be treated with intravenous diazepam in a dose of 0.1 to 3 mg/kg in pediatric patients and 5 to 10 mg in an adult. Hypotension requires the use of a pure alpha agonist such as norepinephrine (levarterenol or Levophed®) since administration of epinephrine may cause hypotension (Benowitz *et al.*, 1979). Dialysis is ineffective in removing phenothiazine since these drugs are highly tissue bound. Cardiac arrhythmias may respond to the use of phenytoin (Dilantin®) or lidocaine; in patients with refractory arrhythmias a cardiac pacemaker may be required. Extrapyramidal reactions are usually adequately treated by the use of intravenous diphenhydramine (Benadryl®) in a dose of 1 to 2 mg/kg (Gupta and Lovejoy, 1967; Davies, 1970). Hypothermia or hyperthermia should be treated appropriately. Drugs that can potentiate the depressant effect of phenothiazine, such as barbiturates, sedatives, alcohol, narcotics, and anesthetics, are best avoided.

SALICYLATES

Accidental or intentional ingestion of salicylates by children and adults continues to represent a major poisoning problem owing to the high incidence of use of these compounds, their widespread availability, their numerous proprietary and nonproprietary products and preparations, and their mass promotion through advertising media (McGuigan, 1987). Most salicylate poisonings involve the use of aspirin or acetylsalicylic acid, although other serious salicylate exposures may result from such compounds as oil of wintergreen (methylsalicylate). Generally, ingestion of doses larger than 150 mg/kg (or 70 mg/lb) can produce toxic symptoms such as tinnitus, nausea, and vomiting. Serious toxicity can be seen with ingestions greater than 400 mg/kg (approximately 180 mg/lb), with severe vomiting, hyperventilation, hyperthermia, confusion, coma, convulsions, hyper- or hypoglycemia, and acid-base disturbances such as respiratory alkalosis or metabolic acidosis (Pierce, 1974; Gabow *et al.*, 1978). In severe cases, the clinical course may progress to pulmonary edema, hemorrhage, acute renal failure, or death (Anderson *et al.*, 1976). It is important to note that the salicylate-overdose patient can progress to a more serious condition over time as additional drug is absorbed from the gastrointestinal tract. Chronic salicylism presents clinically in a similar fashion to the acute situation, although it is often associated with a higher morbidity and mortality as well as more pronounced hyperventilation, dehydration, coma, seizures, and acidosis (Gaudreault *et al.*, 1982). Although acute overdoses may be associated with salicylate levels of 25 to 35 mg/100 ml or more, chronic salicylism can occur at lower salicylate levels, that is, as low as 10 to 15 mg/100 ml. It is important to remember that the kinetics of salicylates are dose dependent, and at higher serum concentrations of salicylate the drug's half-life may be prolonged, that is, 15 to 30 hours. While the half-life should not be used for zero-order processes, this calculation will provide a useful clinical guide. The Done nomogram (Figure 28–2) can be utilized as an aid in interpreting a given salicylate level as long as the blood sample was not drawn prior to six hours after ingestion. In addition, the Done nomogram is not useful in cases of chronic salicylism. Salicylates are exceptionally sensitive to pH changes, with resulting ionization changes having a pronounced effect on disposition in the body. Acidosis, which is a common finding in acute salicylate overdose, can result in a larger percentage of the drug distributing into the central nervous system. Similarly, alkalinization of the urine results in ion trapping of salicylate in the kidney tubule, causing greater urinary excretion (Hill, 1973).

Emesis should be initiated unless the patient is comatose, is convulsing, or has lost the gag reflex. If these contraindications exist, intubation should proceed with gastric lavage, using a large-bore tube such as a 36-French. Subsequently, activated charcoal should be adminis-

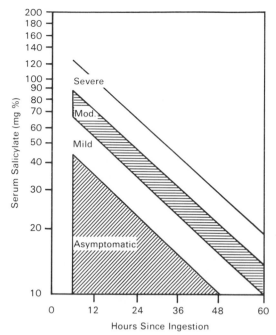

Figure 28-2. Done nomogram for salicylate poisoning. Cautions for use of chart: *(1)* The patient has taken a single acute ingestion and is not suffering from chronic toxicity. *(2)* The blood level to be plotted on the nomogram was drawn six hours after *ingestion*. *(3)* Levels in the toxic range drawn before six hours should be treated. *(4)* Levels in the nontoxic range drawn before six hours should be repeated to see if the level is increasing. (From Done, A. K.: *Pediatrics,* **26**:805, 1960. Copyright American Academy of Pediatrics, 1960.)

tered, followed by saline cathartics to hasten the elimination of any unabsorbed drugs through the gastrointestinal tract. Repetitive doses of activated charcoal will enhance gut elimination of salicylates and shorten the half-life. Alkalinization of the urine can result in a tenfold increase in a drug's excretion by increasing urinary pH to over 8.0. Hypokalemia secondary to respiratory alkalosis induced by salicylate poisoning should be corrected since this condition may make alkalinization of urine difficult.

Acetazolamide (Diamox®) is not indicated for urine alkalization since this drug may contribute to metabolic acidosis. Hemodialysis, peritoneal dialysis, exchange transfusion, and hemoperfusion can be effective in removing salicylate from blood compartments but are indicated on only the most severe cases or when alkalinization of the urine is ineffective or contraindicated. Adequate fluid therapy should be instituted to prevent dehydration and to correct electrolyte imbalances. Systemic acidosis should be cor-

rected promptly with sodium bicarbonate. Should hemorrhagic complications in association with a prolonged prothrombin time occur, vitamin K_1 or phytonadione is indicated. It is important to note that salicylates may cause coagulation defects due to platelet effects that will not be responsive to vitamin K administration (Pierce, 1974). The patient's serum electrolytes, renal function, and cardiac status should be monitored. If hyperpyrexia occurs, appropriate treatment measures should be instituted (Hill, 1973).

SEDATIVE-HYPNOTICS

Sedative-hypnotics include a wide range of pharmacologic agents used in the treatment of anxiety, nervousness, and sleep disorders. The most widely known agents are the barbiturates (short acting and long acting), benzodiazopines, chloral hydrate, ethchlorvynol (Placidyl®), meprobamate (Miltown®), methyprylon (Noludar®), glutethimide (Doriden®), and methaqualone (Quaalude®). These agents have the propensity following chronic overuse or abuse to cause physical addiction, and the possibility of physical withdrawal symptoms should be considered in the treatment of patients overdosed on sedative-hypnotics. Table 28-4 compares some of the different pharmacokinetic properties of the more commonly used agents. Patients presenting with sedative-hypnotic overdose may manifest symptoms of confusion, poor coordination, ataxia, respiratory distress, apnea, and coma. Barbiturate overdose cases may present characteristically with "barb burns" or clear vesicular bullous skin lesions appearing on the hands, buttocks, and between the knees (Groschel *et al.,* 1970). Glutethimide may present with a clinical course characterized by an unusually prolonged coma or cyclic coma with periods of alternating unconsciousness and wakefulness (Decker, 1970). Much of the severity of this drug's toxicity is related to its biotransformation to and accumulation of a metabolite, 4-hydroxy-glutethimide, that has a long half-life and is twice as potent as the parent drug (Hansen *et al.,* 1975). Gastric drug mass or drug bezoar formation has been reported, particularly in association with sedative-hypnotic agents that are poorly soluble in water (Schwartz, 1976). In such cases, gastrotomy has been required to surgically remove drug bezoars.

In the vast majority of sedative-hypnotic overdoses, conservative treatment represents the most successful approach to managing such patients (McCarron *et al.,* 1982). If the patient is conscious, vomiting may be indicated, although in many cases gastric lavage followed by ad-

Table 28-4. SEDATIVE-HYPNOTICS*

DRUG	vd (% BODY WEIGHT)	PROTEIN BINDING, (%)	pk$_a$	PEAK CONCERN TIME, (hr)	t$_{1/2}$ (hr)	THERAPEUTIC BLOOD LEVEL	MAJOR ROUTE OF ELIMINATION	DIURESIS	DIALYSIS	HEMOPERFUSION
Long-acting barbiturates										
Phenobarbital	75	20	7.41	1–6	48–96 (overdose)	10–20 µg/ml	20–40% excreted unchanged; remainder biotransformed	Alkaline	Yes	Yes
Short-acting barbiturates										
Pentobarbital	200–300	30	8.1	0.5–2	36	50 µg/ml	Biotransformed	No	No	No
Secobarbital	200–300	45	7.9	0.5–2	24					
Benzodiazepines										
Diazepam	100–200	90			25–30	<0.5 mg/100 ml	Biotransformed to active	No	No	Yes
Chlordiazepoxide	25	90			7–15					
Chloral hydrate	25	40–80 for trichlorethanol	6.8		6–9	10–15 µg/ml	Biotransformed metabolite	No	No	Yes
Ethclorvynol	600	50	8.7	1	100 (overdose)	<100 µg	Biotransformed	No	No	No
Glutethimide	—	—	4.52	—	40 (overdose)	—	Biotransformed to active metabolite	No	No	?
Meprobamate	75	10–20	9.2	1–2	8	<4 mg/100 ml	Biotransformed with 25–50% excreted unchanged	Yes	Yes	Yes
Methyprylon	>100	?	7.1	½–1	3–6	<1 mg/100 ml	Biotransformed	No	No	?
Methaqualone	100–200	?	—	1–4	2–3	<2 mg/100 ml	Biotransformed	No	?	Yes

* From Wexler, J.; Whittenberger, J. L.; and Dumke, P. R.: The effect of cyanide on the electrocardiogram of man. *Am. Heart J.*, **34**:163–173, 1947.

ministration of activated charcoal and saline cathartics is required to terminate the exposure. Maintaining a patent airway, providing adequate ventilation, and control of hypotension and other supportive measures are the mainstays of therapy. In some cases, such as with phenobarbital, forced alkaline diuresis has been shown to be of benefit to hasten elimination of the drug. For lipid-soluble drugs such as glutethimide, methaqualone, and ethchlorvynol, dialysis procedures have not been shown to be effective. Some data suggest that meprobamate may be adequately treated in severe cases with the use of diuresis and/or dialysis, whereas chloral hydrate may be significantly removed by hemodialysis (Stalker et al., 1978). Analeptics or other stimulants (e.g., caffeine) have never been shown to be of any value and are therefore contraindicated. In sedative-hypnotic overdose, patients may develop pulmonary edema or shock that should be treated appropriately.

TRICYCLIC ANTIDEPRESSANTS

The tricyclic antidepressants are available in a wide variety of brands, including amitriptyline (Elavil®), doxepin (Sinequan®), and imipramine (Tofranil®), and in combination with phenothiazine drugs in Triavil® and Etrafon®. Tricyclic antidepressants have three primary pharmacologic actions, including anticholinergic effects, reuptake blockade of catecholamines at the adrenergic neuronal site, and quinidinelike effects on the cardiac tissue. The newer tricyclic antidepressants, such as amoxapine, have a significantly higher incidence of seizures and lower incidence of cardiac arrhythmia than the older tricyclic antidepressants. Tricyclic antidepressant overdose represents a life-threatening episode (Crome, 1986; Frommer, 1987). Initial symptoms seen are those of central nervous system depression with manifestations of lethargy, disorientation, ataxia, respiratory depression, hypothermia, and agitation. Severe toxicity may be associated with hallucinations, deep tendon reflex loss, muscle twitching, coma, and convulsions. Anticholinergic or atropinic effects of these drugs include dry mouth, hyperpyrexia, dilated pupils, urinary retention, tachycardia, and reduced gastrointestinal motility, which may result in marked delay of the onset of symptoms but also allows for the institution of emesis and lavage long after ingestion to still be effective. Life-threatening sequelae of the tricyclic antidepressants are the cardiovascular effects, resulting in cardiac arrhythmias such as supraventricular tachycardia, premature ventricular contractions, ventricular tachycardia, ventricular flutter, and ventricular fibrillation that progresses to hypotension and shock. The electrocardiogram characteristically demonstrates prolonged PR interval, widening of the QRS complex, QT prolongation, T-wave flattening or inversion, ST segment depression, and varying degrees of heart block progressing to cardiac standstill (Tobis and Das, 1976). Widening of the QRS complex has been reported to correlate well with the severity of the toxicity following acute overdose ingestions (Biggs, 1977b). Widening of the QRS complex past 100 milliseconds or greater within the first 24 hours is an indication of severe toxicity (Boehnert and Lovejoy, 1985).

Emesis and lavage are indicated as appropriate, followed by administration of activated charcoal and a saline cathartic such as sodium or magnesium sulfate. Patients admitted with tricyclic antidepressant overdose but without symptoms should be monitored for a minimum of six hours to detect any possible delayed symptom onset. Vital signs and the electrocardiogram should be monitored for 48 hours in symptomatic patients since fatal cardiac arrhythmias have occurred late in the course. Hypotension should be treated with fluids and a vasopressor such as levarterenol (Levophed®) administered as needed. The development of severe hallucinations, hypertension, and sinus tachycardia is an indication for physostigmine use, administered intravenously in adults in a therapeutic trial of 2 mg slowly followed by 1 to 2 mg. For pediatric patients that trial dose is 0.5 mg, administered slowly by the intravenous route, followed by the lowest total effective trial (Rumack, 1973). Physostigmine should be administered with caution in the presence of asthma, gangrene, cardiovascular disease, and mechanical obstructions of the gastrointestinal or urogenital tract. Adjustment of blood pH with bicarbonate to pH 7.45, coupled with appropriate antiarrhythmia drugs (lidocaine, phenytoin, etc.), is the primary approach to therapy of cardiac arrhythmias. Arrhythmias other than sinus tachycardia, as well as seizures and hypotension, are poorly responsive to physostigmine. Seizures are responsive to phenytoin, diazepam, or barbiturates (Bigger, 1977).

REFERENCES

Anas, N.; Namasonthi, V.; and Ginsburg, C. M.: Criteria for hospitalizing children who have ingested products containing hydrocarbons. *J.A.M.A.*, **246**:840–843, 1981.

Anderson, K. D.; Rouse, T. M.; and Randolph, J. G.: A controlled trial of corticosteroid in children with corrosive injury of the esophagus. *N. Engl. J. Med.*, **323**:637–640, 1990.

Anderson, R. J.; Potts, D. E.; Gabow, P. A.; Rumack, B. H.; and Schrier, R. W.: Unrecognized adult salicylate intoxication. *Ann. Intern. Med.*, **85**:745–748, 1976.

Arena, J. M.; Rourke, M. H.; and Sibrach, C. D.: Acetaminophen: report of an unusual poisoning. *Pediatrics*, **61**:68–72, 1978.

Aronow, R.; Shashi, D. P.; and Wooley, P. V.: Childhood poisoning and unfortunate consequences of methadone availability. *J.A.M.A.*, **219**:321–324, 1972.

Bain, J. T. B., and Knowles, E. L.: Successful treatment of cyanide poisoning. *Br. Med. J.*, **2**:763, 1967.

Baldochin, B. J., and Melmed, R. N.: Clinical and therapeutic aspects of kerosene poisoning: a series of 200 cases. *Br. Med. J.*, **2**:28–30, 1964.

Barry, D.; Meyskens, F. L., Jr.; and Becker, C. E.: Phenothiazine poisoning: a review of 48 cases. *Cal. Med.*, **118**:1, 1973.

Barry, D.; et al.: Phenothiazine poisoning: a review of 48 cases. *Cal. Med.* **118**:1, 1983.

Beaman, R.; Seigel, C.; and Landers, G.: Hydrocarbon ingestion in children: a six year retrospective study. *J.A.C.E.P.*, **5**:771–775, 1976.

Benowitz, N. L. *et al.*: Cardiopulmonary catastrophes in drug-overdosed patients. *Med. Clin. North Am.* **63**:267, 1979.

Berg, M. J.; Berlinger, W. G.; Goldberg, M. J.; Spector, R.; and Johnson, G. F.: Acceleration of the body clearance of phenobarbital by oral activated charcoal. *N. Engl. J. Med.*, **307**:642–643, 1982.

Bergson, F.: Pneumatocoeles following hydrocarbon ingestion. *Am. J. Dis. Child.*, **129**:49–54, 1975.

Berlin, C. M., Jr.: The treatment of cyanide poisoning in children. *Pediatrics*, **46**:793, 1970.

Bigger, J. T.: Is physostigmine effective for cardiac toxicity of tricyclic antidepressant drugs? *J.A.M.A.*, **273**:1311, 1977a.

————: Tricyclic antidepressant overdose: incidence of symptoms, *J.A.M.A.*, **238**:135–138, 1977b.

Boehnert, M. T.; LeWander, W. J.; Gaudreault, P.; and Lovejoy, F. H., Jr.: Advances in clinical toxicology. *Pediatr. Clin., North Am.* **32**:193–211, 1985.

Boehnert, M. T., and Lovejoy, F. H. Jr.: Value of QRS, duration versus the serum drug level in predicting seizures and ventricular arrhythmias after an acute overdose of tricyclic antidepressants. *N. Eng. J. Med.*, **313**:474–479, 1985.

Bolter, A.: Phencyclidine (PCP) abuse. *West. J. Med.*, **127**:80, 1970.

Boylan, J. L.; Egle, J. L.; and Guzelian, P. D.: Cholestyramine: use as a new therapeutic approach for chlordecone (Kepone) poisoning. *Science*, **199**:893–895, 1978.

Bratton, L. and Haddow, J. E.: Ingestion of charcoal lighter fluid. *J. Pediatr.* **84**:396–401, 1974.

Bronstein, A. C., and Rumack, B. H.: Acute acetaminophen overdose during pregnancy. *Vet. Hum. Toxicol.*, **26**:401, 1984.

Brown, J.; Burke, B.; and DaJanias, C.: Experimental kerosene pneumonia: evaluation of some therapeutic regimens. *J. Pediatr.*, **84**:396–401, 1974.

Bryson, P. D.; Watanabe, A. S.; Rumack, B. H.; and Murphy, R. C.: Burdock root tea poisoning: case report involving a commercial preparation. *J.A.M.A.*, **239**:2157, 1978.

Burrington, J. P.: Clinitest burns of the esophagus. *Ann. Thorac. Surg.*, **20**:400, 1974.

Chafee-Bahamon, C., and Lovejoy, F. H., Jr.: The effectiveness of a regional poison center in reducing excess emergency room visits for children's poisonings. *Pediatrics*, **73**:164–169, 1983.

Chen, K. K., and Rose, C. L.: Nitrite and thiosulfate therapy in cyanide poisoning. *J.A.M.A.*, **149**:113, 1952.

Clark, R.; Borirakchanyavat, V.; Davidson, A. R.; Thompson, R. P. H.; Widdop, B.; Goulding, R.; and Williams, R.: Hepatic damage and death from overdose of paracetamal. *Lancet*, **1**:66, 1973.

Clemmesen, C., and Nilsson, E.: Therapeutic trends in the treatment of barbiturate poisoning: the Scandinavian method. *Clin. Pharmacol. Ther.*, **2**:220–229, 1961.

Corby, D. G., and Decker, W. J.: Activated charcoal for sedative overdosage. *Pediatr. Clin. North Am.*, **17**:620, 1970.

Crome, P.: Poisoning due to tricyclic antidepressant overdose. *Med. Toxicol.*, **1**:261–285, 1986.

Crome, P.; Dawling, S.; Braitwaite, R. A.; Masters, J.; and Walkey, R.: Effect of activated charcoal on absorption of nortriptyline. *Lancet*, **2**:1203–1205, 1979.

Curry, A. S.: *The Poisoned Patient: The Role of the Laboratory*. Elsevier, Amsterdam, 1974.

David, D. J., and Spyker, D. A.: The acute toxicity of ethanol: dosage and kinetic nomograms. *Vet. Hum. Toxicol.*, **21**:272, 1979.

Davies, D. M.: Treatment of drug-induced dyskinesias. *Lancet*, **1**:567, 1970.

Decker, W. J.: Gluthethimide rebound. *Lancet*, **1**:778, 1970.

Done, A. K.: Salicylate intoxication, significance of measurements of salicylate in blood in cases of acute intoxication. *Pediatrics*, **26**:800–807, 1960.

Done, A. K.; Aronow, R.; and Miceli, J. N.: Pharmacokinetic observation in the treatment of phencyclidine poisoning. In Rumack, B. H., and Temple. A. R. (eds.): *Management of the Poisoned Patient*. Science Press, Princeton, N.J., 1977.

Eastman, J. W., and Cohen, S. N.: Hypertensive crisis and death associated with phencyclidine poisoning. *J.A.M.A.*, **231**:270–271, 1975.

Ekins, B. R., and Watanabe, A. S.: Acute digoxin poisoning: review of therapy. *Am. J. Hosp. Pharm.*, **35**:268–277, 1978.

Elbel, H., and Schleyer, F.: In *Blutalkatal: Die Wissenschaftlichen Grudlagen der Beruteilung von Blutalkoholbefunden bei Strassenverke-Msdelkien Stuttgart.* Georg Thieme, Heidelberg, 1956, p. 226.

Espelin, D. E., and Done, A. K.: Amphetamine poisoning: effectiveness of chlorpromazine. *N. Engl. J. Med.*, **278**:1361–1365, 1968.

Evans, J. M.; Hogg, M. I. J.; Lynn, J. N.; and Rosen, M.: Degree and duration of reversal by naloxone of effects of morphine in conscious subjects. *Br. Med. J.*, **2**:589–591, 1974.

Eyl, T. B.: Organic-mercury food poisoning. *N. Engl. J. Med.*, **284**:706, 1971.

Fischer, D. S.; Parkman, R.; and Finch, S. C: Acute iron poisoning in children. *J.A.M.A.*, **218**:1179–1184, 1971.

Foldes, F. F.; Duncalf, D.; and Kuwabara, S.: The respiratory, circulatory, and narcotic antagonistic effects of nalorphine, levallorphan, and naloxone in anesthetized subjects. *Can. Anaesth. Soc. J.*, **16**:151–161, 1969.

Frand, U. I.; Chang, S. S.; and Williams, M. H., Jr.: Methadone induced pulmonary edema. *Ann. Intern. Med.*, **76**:975–979, 1972.

Friedman, E. M., and Lovejoy, F. H. Jr.: The emergency management of caustic ingestions. *Emerg. Med. Clin. North Am.*, **2**:77–86, 1984.

Frommer, D. A., *et al.*: Tricyclic antidepressant overdose; a review. *J.A.M.A.*, **257**:521–526, 1987.

Fuzltz, J. M., and Senay, E. C.: Guidelines for the management of hospitalized addicts. *Ann. Intern. Med.*, **82**:815–818, 1975.

Gabow, P. A.; Anderson, R. J.; and Potts, D. E.: Acid-based disturbances in the salicylate-intoxicated adult. *Arch. Intern. Med.*, **138**:1481–1484, 1978.

Gaudreault, P., and Guay, J.: Theophylline poisoning. *Med. Toxicol.*, **1**:169, 1986.

Gaudreault, P.; Parent, M.; McGuigan, M. A.; Chicoine,

L.; and Lovejoy, F. H., Jr.: Predictability of esophageal injury from signs and symptoms: a study of caustic ingestion in 378 children. *Pediatrics*, **71**:767–770, 1983.

Gaudreault, P.; Temple, A. R.; and Lovejoy, F. H., Jr.: The relative severity of acute versus chronic salicylate poisoning in children. *Pediatrics*, **70**:566–569, 1982.

Gaudreault, P.; Wason, S.; and Lovejoy, F. H., Jr.: Acute theophylline overdose: a summary of 28 cases. *J. Pediatr.*, **102**:474–476, 1983.

Ginsburg, C. M.: Lomotil intoxication. *Am. J. Dis. Child.*, **925**:241–242, 1973.

Goldwater, L. J.: *Mercury. A History of Quicksilver.* York Press, Baltimore, Md. 1972.

Graham, D. L.; Laman, D.; and Theodore, J.: Acute cyanide poisoning complicated by lactic acidosis and pulmonary edema. *Arch. Intern. Med.*, **137**:1051–1055, 1977.

Greenblatt, D. J.: Rapid recovery from massive diazepan overdose. *J.A.M.A.*, **240**:872–874, 1978.

Groschel, D.; Gerstein, A. R.; and Rosenbaum, J. M.: Skin lesions as a diagnostic aid in barbiturate poisoning, *N. Engl. J. Med.*, **403**:409–410, 1970.

Gupta, J. M., and Lovejoy, F. H., Jr.: Acute phenothiazine toxicity in children. *Pediatrics*, **71**:890–894, 1967.

Hall, A. H. *et al.*: Clinical toxicology of cyanide: North American clinical experiences. In Ballantyne, B. and Marrs, T. C. (eds.): *Clinical and Experimental Toxicology of Cyanides.* Butterworth (John Wright), Bristol, U.K., 1987.

Haller, J. A., Jr.: Pathophysiology and management of acute corrosive burns of the esophagus. *J. Pediatr. Surg.*, **6**:578, 1971.

Hammond, R. B.; Rumack, B. H.; and Rodgerson, D. O.: Blood ethanol: a report of unusually high levels in a living patient. *J.A.M.A.*, **226**:63–64, 1973.

Hansen, A. R.; Kennedy, K. A.; Ambre, J. J.; and Fischer, L. J.: Glutethimide poisoning—a metabolite contributes to morbidity and mortality. *N. Engl. J. Med.*, **292**:250–252, 1975.

Hill, J. B.: Salicylate intoxication. *N. Engl. J. Med.*, **2–8**:1110, 1113, 1973.

Hillman, B.; Bardham, K. D.; and Bain, J. T. B.: The use of dicobalt edetate (Kelocyanor) in cyanide poisoning. *Postgrad. Med. J.*, **50**:171–174, 1974.

Howell, J. M.: Alkaline ingestions. *Ann. Emerg. Med.*, **15**:820–825, 1986.

Jacobs, J.; Greene, H.; and Gendel, B. R.: Acute iron intoxication. *N. Engl. J. Med.*, **273**:1124–1127, 1965.

Kark, R. A. P.: Mercury poisoning and its treatment with *N*-acetyl-D,L-penicillamine. *N. Engl. J. Med.*, **285**:1, 1971.

Kressel, J. J.; Lovejoy, F. H., Jr.; Boyle, W. E.; and Easom, J. M.: Comparison of two child resistant containers. *Clin. Toxicol.*, **19**(4):377–384, 1982.

Kulig, K. W.; Bar-Or, D.; Cantrill, S. V.; Rosen, P.; and Rumack, B. H.: Management of acutely poisoned patients without gastric emptying. *Ann. Emerg. Med.*, **14**:562–567, 1985.

Lacouture, P. G.; Gaudreault, P.; and Lovejoy, F. H., Jr.: Clinitest tablet ingestion: an *in-vitro* investigation concerned with initial emergency management, *Ann. Emerg. Med.*, **15**:143–146, 1986.

Lacouture, P. G.; Wason, S.; Temple, A. R.; Wallace, D. K.; and Lovejoy, F. H., Jr.: Emergency assessment of severity in iron overdose. *J. Pediatr.*, **99**:89–91, 1981.

Lambecier, M. R., and DuPan, R. M.: L'intoxication alcoolique aigue et les accidents d'automobile. *Schweiz. Med. Wochenschr.*, **76**:395–398, 421–428, 1968.

Lawson, A. A. H., and Northridge, D. B.: Dextropropoxyphene overdose. *Med. Toxicol.*, **2**:430–444, 1987.

Linden, C. B.; Lovejoy, F. H., Jr.; and Costello, C.: Phencyclidine. *J.A.M.A.*, **234**:513–516, 1975.

Linden, C. H.; *et al.*: Amphetamines. *Topics Emerg. Med.*, **7**:18–32, 1985.

Litovitz, T. L.: Button battery ingestions. *J.A.M.A.*, **249**:2495, 1983.

Lloyd, B. L., and Smith, T. W.: Contrasting rates of reversal of digoxin toxicity by digoxin specific IgG and Fab fragments. *Circulation*, **58**:280–283, 1978.

Logothetis, J.: Spontaneous epileptic seizures and EEG changes in the course of phenothiazine therapy. *Neurology*, **17**:869–877, 1967.

Lovejoy, F. H., Jr.: Chelation therapy in iron poisoning. *Clin. Toxicol.*, **19**:871–874, 1982.

Lovejoy, F. H., Jr.; Lee, K. D.; and Haddow, J. E.: Childhood methadone intoxication. *Clin. Pediatr.*, **13**:36–38, 1974a.

Lovejoy, F. H., Jr.; Mitchel, A. A.; and Goldman, P.: Management of propoxyphene poisoning. *J. Pediatr.*, **85**:98–100, 1974b.

Mann, J. B.: Diagnostic aids in organophosphate poisoning. *Ann. Intern. Med.*, **67**:905–906, 1967.

Marks, M. I.; Chicoine, L.; and Legere, G.: Adrenocorticosteroid treatment of hydrocarbon pneumonia in children—a cooperative study. *J. Pediatr.*, **81**:366–369, 1972.

Martin, W. R.: Naloxone. *Ann. Intern. Med.*, **85**:765, 1976.

McCarron, M. M.; *et al.*: Short-acting barbiturate overdosage: correlation of intoxication score with serum barbiturate concentration. *J.A.M.A.*, **248**:55–61, 1982.

McGuigan, M. A.: A two-year review of salicylate deaths in Ontario, *Arch. Intern. Med.*, **147**:510–512, 1987.

McGuigan, M.; Lovejoy, F. H., Jr.; Marino, S.; Propper, R. D.; and Goldman, P.: Qualitative deferoxamine test for iron ingestion. *J. Pediatr.*, **94**:940–942, 1979.

Mikolich, J. R.; Paulson, G. W.; and Cross, C. J.: Acute anticholinergic syndromes due to jimson weed ingestion. *Ann. Intern. Med.*, **83**:321, 1975.

Minton, N. A., and Murray, V. S. G.: A review of organophosphate poisoning. *Med. Toxicol.* **3**:350–375, 1988.

Mitchell, J. R.; Jollow, D. J.; Potter, W. Z.; Davis, D. C.; Gillette, J. R.; and Brodie, B. B.: Acetaminophen induced hepatic necrosis. *J. Pharmacol. Exp. Ther.*, **187**:185, 1973.

Moore, R. A.; Rumack, B. H.; Conner, C. S.; and Peterson, R. G.: Naloxone: underdosage after narcotic poisoning. *Am. J. Dis. Child.*, **134**:156–158, 1980.

Namba, T.: Poisoning due to organophosphate insecticides: acute and chronic manifestations. *Am. J. Med.*, **50**:475–492, 1971.

Natoff, I. L., and Reiff, B.: Effect of oximes on the acute toxicity of anticholinesterase carbamates. *Toxicol. Appl. Pharmacol.*, **25**:569–575, 1973.

Ng, R.; Darwich, H.; and Stewart, D. A.: Emergency treatment of petroleum distillate and turpentine ingestion. *CMA J.*, **111**:538, 1974.

Padlet, G.: Intoxication cyanhydrique et chelater de cobalt. *J. Physiol. Path. Gen.*, **50**:438, 1958.

Park, G. D.; *et al.*: Expanded role of charcoal in the poisoned and overdosed patient. *Arch. Intern. Med.*, **146**:969–973, 1986.

Penner, G. E.: Acid ingestion: toxicology and treatment. *Ann. Emerg. Med.*, **9**:374–379, 1980.

Pentel, P.: Toxicity of over-the-counter stimulants. *J.A.M.A.*, **252**:1898–1903, 1984.

Peterson, R. G., and Rumack, B. H.: Treatment acute

acetaminophen poisoning with acetylcysteine. *J.A.M.A.*, **237**:2406–2407, 1977.

Pierce, A. W.: Salicylate poisoning. *Pediatrics*, **54**:342–347, 1974.

Posner, M. A.; Tobey, R. E.; and McElroy, H.: Hydraoxocobalamine therapy of cyanide intoxication in guinea pigs. *Anesthesiology*, **44**:157, 1976.

Prescott, L. E.; Sutherland, G. R.; and Park, J.: Cysteamine, methionine and penicillamine in the treatment of paracetamol poisoning. *Lancet*, **2**:109–113, 1976.

Prischl, F., *et al.*: Value of Flumazenil in benzodiazepine self-poisoning. *Med. Toxicol.*, **3**:334–339, 1988.

Proudfoot, A. T., and Wright, N.: Acute paracetamol poisoning. *Br. Med. J.*, **2**:557, 1970.

Proudfoot, A. T.; *et al.*: Management of acute iron poisoning. *Med. Toxicol.*, **1**:83–100, 1986.

Rifkin, A.; Quitkin, F.; and Klein, D. F.: Withdrawal reaction to diazepan. *J.A.M.A.*, **236**:2172–2173, 1976.

Robertson, W. O.: Treatment of acute iron poisoning. *Mod. Treat.*, **8**:552–560, 1971.

Robillard, J. E.; Rames, L. K.; Jensen, R. L.; and Roberts, R. J.: Peritoneal dialysis in mercurialdiuretic intoxication. *J. Pediatr.*, **88**:79–81, 1976.

Robotham, J. L., and Leitman, P. S.: Acute iron poisoning—a review. *Am. J. Dis. Child.*, **134**:875–879, 1980.

Rumack, B. H.: Anticholinergic poisonings: treatment with physostigmine. *Pediatrics*, **52**:449, 1973a.

———: Anticholinergic poisonings: treatment with physostigmine. *Pediatrics*, **2**:449, 1973b.

———: Management of acute poisoning and overdose. In Cozzetto, E. J., and Brettell, H. R. (eds.): *Topics in Family Practice*. Symposia Specialists Medical Books, New York, 1976.

———: Hydrocarbon ingestions in perspective. *J.A.C.E.P.*, **6**:4, 1977.

———: Acetaminophen overdose in young children: treatment and effects of alcohol and other additional ingestants in 417 cases. *Am. J. Dis. Child.*, **138**:428–433, 1984.

———: *Poisindex*. Micromedex, Inc., Denver, 1986.

Rumack, B. H.; Anderson, R. H.; Wolfe, R.; Fletcher, E. C.; and Vestal, B.: Ornade and anticholinergic toxicity: hypertension, hallucination and arrhythmias. *Clin. Toxicol.*, **7**:573–581, 1974.

Rumack, B. H., and Burrington, J. P.: Antidotal therapy of caustic reactions. *Clin. Toxicol.*, **11**:27, 1977.

Rumack, B. H.; Ford, P.; Sbarbaro, J.; Bryson, P.; and Winokur, M.: Regionalization of poison centers—a rational role model. *Clin. Toxicol.*, **12**(3):367–375, 1978.

Rumack, B. H., and Matthew, H.: Acetaminophen poisoning and toxicity. *Pediatrics*, **55**:871, 1975.

Rumack, B. H.; Peterson, R. C.; Koch, G. G.; and Amara, I. A.: Acetaminophen overdose: 662 cases with evaluation of oral acetylcysteine treatment. *Arch. Intern. Med.*, **141**:380–385, 1981.

Rumack, B. H., and Temple, A. R.: Lomotil poisoning. *Pediatrics*, **53**:495–500, 1974.

———: (eds.): *Management of the Poisoned Patient*. Science Press, Princeton, N.J., 1977.

Rumack, B. H.; Wolfe, R. R.; and Gilfrich, H.: Phenytoin treatment of massive digoxin overdose. *Br. Heart J.*, **36**:405–408, 1974.

Sayre, J. W., and Kaymakcalan, S.: Cyanide poisoning from apricot seeds among children in central Turkey. *N. Engl. J. Med.*, **270**:1113, 1964.

Schwartz, H. S.: Acute meprobamate poisoning with gastrostomy and removal of a drug contained mass. *N. Engl. J. Med.*, **295**:1177, 1976.

Shannon, M.; Fish, S. S.; and Lovejoy, F. H.,

Jr.: Cathartics and laxatives: do they still have a place in management of the poisoned patient? *Med. Toxicol.*, **1**:247–252, 1986.

Smilkstein, M. J.; Knapp, G. L.; Kulig, K. W.; and Rumack, B. H.: Efficacy of oral N-acetylcysteine in the treatment of acetaminophen overdose. *N. Engl. J. Med.*, **319**:1557–1562, 1988.

Smith, R. P., and Kruszyna, H.: Nitroprusside produces cyanide poisoning via a reaction with hemoglobin. *J. Pediatr.*, **191**:557, 1974.

Smith, T. W.: New advances in the assessment and treatment of digitalis toxicity. *J. Clin. Pharmacol.*, **25**:522–528, 1985.

Smith, T. W.; Haber, E.; Yeatman, L.; and Butler, V. P., Jr.: Reversal of advanced digoxin intoxication with Fab fragments of digoxin-specific antibodies. *N. Engl. J. Med.*, **294**:797–800, 1976.

Smith, T. W.; Butler, V. P.; Haber, E.; *et al.*: Treatment of life-threatening digitalis intoxication with digoxin-specific Fab antibody fragments. *N. Engl. J. Med.*, **307**:1357–1362, 1982.

Stalker, N. E.; Gamertoglio, J. G.; Fukumitsu, C. J.; *et al.*: Acute massive chloral hydrate intoxication treated with hemodialysis: a clinical pharmacokinetic analysis. *J. Clin. Pharmacol.*, **18**:136–142, 1978.

Steele, R. W.; Conklin, R. H.; and March, H. M.: Corticosteroids and antibiotics for the treatment of fulminant hydrocarbon aspiration. *J.A.M.A.*, **219**:1434–1437, 1972.

Stein, J. L.: Phencyclidine induced psychosis: the need to avoid unnecessary sensory influx. *Milit. Med.*, **138**:590, 1973.

Stein, M.; Blayney, D.; Feit, T.; Goergen, T. G.; Micik, S.; and Nyhan, W. L.: Acute iron poisoning in children. *West. J. Med.*, **125**:289–297, 1976.

Stewart, R.: Cyanide poisoning. *Clin. Toxicol.*, **7**:561, 1974.

Subcommittee on Accidental Poisoning: Kerosene and related petroleum distillates. In *Handbook of Common Poisonings in Children*. FDA-76-7004, U.S. Department of HEW, Rockville, Md., 1976.

Temple, A. R.: Acute and chronic effects of aspirin toxicity and their treatment. *Arch. Intern. Med.*, **141**:364–369, 1981.

Thompson, D. F.; Trammel, H. L.; Robertson, N. J.; and Reigart, J. R.: Evaluation of regional and nonregional poison centers. *N. Engl. J. Med.*, **308**:191–194, 1983.

Tobis, J., and Das, B. N.: Cardiac complications in amitriptyline poisoning—successful treatment with physostigmine. *J.A.M.A.*, **234**:1474–1476, 1976.

Tong, T. G.; Benowitz, N. L.; Becker, C. E.; Forni, P. J.; and Boerner, U.: Phencyclidine poisoning. *J.A.M.A.*, **234**:512–513, 1975.

Truempier, E.; Reyes de la Rocha, S.; and Atkinson, S. D.: Clinical characteristics, pathophysiology and management of hydrocarbon ingestion: case report and review of the literature. *Pediatr. Emerg. Care*, **3**:187–193, 1987.

Victor, M., and Adams, R. D.: Barbiturate. In *Harrison's Principles of Internal Medicine*. McGraw-Hill Book Co., New York, 1977, chap. 120.

Watanabe, A. S.: Pharmacokinetic aspects of the dialysis of drugs. *Drug Intell. Clin. Pharmacol.*, **11**:407–416, 1977.

Welch, T. R.; Rumack, B. H.; and Hammond, K.: Clonazepram overdose in resulting cyclic coma. *Clin. Toxicol.*, **10**:433–434, 1977.

Wexler, J.; Whittenberger, J. L.; and Dumke, P. R.: The effect of cyanide on the electrocardiogram of man. *Am. Heart J.*, **34**:163–173, 1947.

Wilkinson, P. K.: Blood ethanol concentrations during and following constant rate IV infusion of alcohol. *Clin. Pharmacol. Ther.*, **19**:213, 1976.

Chapter 29

OCCUPATIONAL TOXICOLOGY

Robert R. Lauwerys

INTRODUCTION

The main objective of industrial toxicology is the prevention of health impairments in workers handling or exposed to industrial chemicals. This objective can only be reached if conditions of exposure or work practices are defined that do not entail an unacceptable health risk.

This implies in practice the definition of *permissible levels* of exposure to industrial chemicals. These levels can be expressed either in terms of allowable atmospheric concentrations (maximum allowable concentrations—MACs; threshold limit values—TLVs; time-weighted averages—TWAs'; threshold limit value-ceiling—TLV-C; short-term exposure limits—STELs) or in terms of permissible biologic levels for the chemical or its metabolites or the amount bound to the critical sites (biologic TLV; biological exposure indices). It is important to stress that these atmospheric or biologic allowable concentrations do not correspond to exposure conditions devoid of any health risk. The concept of acceptable exposure level must be understood as the level of exposure below which the risk —that is, the probability to impair the health of the exposed workers— is acceptable. To conclude that a risk is acceptable, one must identify and quantify it, which requires knowledge of the relationship between exposure intensity (dose) and the health effects and that between exposure intensity and the prevalence of subjects exhibiting a defined adverse effect. One must first identify the nature of the biologic effects likely to occur and their severity when exposure (intensity-duration) to (a) chemical agent(s) increases. One must then define which effect is acceptable. This choice may be the object of intense controversies. Between "being in good health" and "being ill" following exposure to chemicals, there is no strict barrier but a continuum of changes from simple asymptomatic biochemical and/or functional changes to clinical disease.

The health significance of all the identified changes resulting from chemical exposure must be assessed in order to decide which ones are adverse or nonadverse. Following this assessment, one must then take into account the interindividual variability in the susceptibility to chemicals. There is not one single dose-effect relationship but as many as there are exposed subjects. Hence, to recommend an acceptable exposure level to an industrial chemical, one must also attempt to define the dose (exposure)-prevalence (percentage of affected individuals) relationship. Another choice must then be made, that is, the percentage of exposed subjects who may still develop an adverse effect at the proposed acceptable exposure level. This acceptable response will of course vary according to the type of potential adverse effects (e.g., inhibition of an enzyme without functional consequences, reversible local irritant effect, genotoxicity, etc.).

To evaluate with some degree of confidence the level of exposure at which the risk of health impairment is acceptable, a body of toxicologic information is required that derives from two main sources: experimental investigations on animals and clinical surveillance of exposed workers (including retrospective studies on previously exposed workers). In some circumstances, limited investigations on volunteers can also be considered.

The large-scale use of any chemical in industry should be preceded by certain types of toxicologic investigations on animals in order to establish a tentative acceptable exposure level. Other important information that may also be derived from these investigations concerns methods of biologic monitoring of exposure and early health effects and preexisting pathologic states that may increase the susceptibility to the chemical. Animal testing can provide only an estimate of the toxicity of a chemical for man. For example, there is a great risk of missing allergic reactions in testing new materials in animals. Thus, when the compound is actually handled in industry, monitoring of the workplace and careful clinical surveillance of the workers are essential. The design of these clinical surveys will to a large extent depend on the information collected during the first experimental phase of the investigations. The main objectives of the clinical work are (1) to test the validity of the provisional permissible level of exposure based on animal experiments; (2) to detect as early as possible hypersensitive reactions or other effects that are unpredictable from animal investigations; and (3) to confirm the usefulness of biologic methods of monitoring workers (assessment of exposure and early detection of adverse effects). One must, however, recognize that for many chemicals toxicologic investigations on animals have not been performed before the chemicals' use in industry. In that case, clinical work (retrospective epidemiologic studies; historic prospective studies; cross-sectional studies) is aimed at defining the acceptable exposure level directly in man.

In some circumstances exposure of volunteers can be considered when the information (e.g., threshold for upper respiratory tract irritation) is not easily obtainable by other means and when the experiments entail no risk for the volunteers (which means that extensive biologic information should already be available before any experiments on volunteers are undertaken). Experimental investigations on animals and clinical studies on workers or volunteers are closely related, and the following discussion illustrates how collaboration between these disciplines or approaches helps accomplish more rapid progress in the field of industrial toxicology.

PRELIMINARY TESTING ON ANIMALS

It is evident that certainty as to the complete safety of a chemical can never be obtained, whatever the extent of toxicologic investigations performed on animals. Nevertheless, some basic requirements can be suggested to estimate with some degree of confidence the level of exposure at which the risk of health impairment is negligible and thus acceptable. We are excluding from the following considerations chemicals that have only very limited use, as in a research laboratory, and can be handled by a limited number of skilled persons in a way that prevents any exposure.

General guidelines for assessing experimentally the toxicologic hazards of industrial chemicals have been recommended (Lauwerys, 1976). Their principles do not differ much from the investigations presently required for evaluating the toxicity of substances to which the general public can be exposed (drugs, food additives,

pesticides residues, *etc.*) (EPA, 1982a, 1982b; NTP, 1987; OECD, 1987). These tests include local and systemic acute toxicity tests, skin sensitization tests, toxicity following repeated exposure, short-term tests for detecting potential mutagens, studies of effect on reproduction and of teratogenic activity, chronic studies to detect carcinogesis and other long-term effects, investigations of metabolism and mechanism of action, and interaction studies and have been extensively described in previous chapters. The following discussion stresses a few points that are important or more relevant to the field of industrial toxicology.

The need for performing some (or all) of those investigations should be carefully evaluated for any industrial chemical to which workers will be exposed. The toxicologist is guided in selecting the studies most relevant for safety evaluation by an understanding of the physicochemical properties of the chemical (including speciation for inorganic compounds, which may have important consequences in their toxicokinetics and biological reactivity); the conditions of use and degree of exposure, including the possibility of generating toxic derivatives when the chemical is submitted to various chemical and physical factors (heat, pH change, etc.); the type of exposure, which may be continuous or accidental; and possibly toxicologic information already available on other chemicals with similar chemical structure and reactive chemical groups. It should be stressed that conclusions drawn from any toxicologic investigation are valid only if the exact composition (e.g., nature and concentration of impurities or degradation products) of the tested preparation is known. The assessment of the toxicity of the pesticides malathion and 2.4.5-T illustrates this point. Malathion, an organophosphorus insecticide normally devoid of significant human toxicity, has been responsible for an episode of mass poisoning in Pakistan in 1976 because the technical preparation used contained various impurities (mainly isomalathion) capable of inhibiting tissue and plasma carboxyesterases (Baker *et al.*, 1978; Aldridge *et al.*, 1979). The teratogenic hazard of the herbicide 2.4.5-T is estimated differently, depending on the content of the highly toxic impurity 2.3.7.8-tetrachlorodibenzo-*p*-dioxin in the preparation tested (Courtney and Moore, 1971; Emerson *et al.*, 1971). Accurate methods of analysis of the chemical in air and in biologic material should also be available. Flexibility of approach is essential in deciding the duration of tests necessary to establish a reasonable acceptable level for occupational exposure. This depends mainly on the type of toxic action that is suspected, but it is generally recognized that subacute and short-term toxicity studies are usually unsatisfactory for proposing permissible exposure levels. Subacute and short-term toxicity tests are usually performed to find out whether the compound exhibits some cumulative toxic properties and to select the doses for long-term exposure and the kind of tests that may be most informative when applied during long-term exposures. Several studies have drawn attention to the fact that the reproductive system may also be the target organ of industrial chemicals (e.g., some glycol ethers, monochlorodibromopropane). Studies designed to evaluate reproductive performance and teratogenic action should therefore also be considered during routine toxicologic testing of industrial chemicals.

Information derived from exposure routes similar (skin, lung) to those sustained by workers is clearly most relevant. For airborne pollutants, inhalation exposure studies provide the basic data on which provisional permissible levels are based. Experimental methodology is certainly much more complicated for inhalation studies than for oral administration experiments. For example, in the case of exposure to aerosol, particle size distribution should be estimated and the approximate degree of retention in the respiratory tract of the animal species selected should be known. Ideally, particle size should be selected according to the deposition pattern of solid or liquid aerosols in the particular animal species used. It should also be kept in mind that the concentration of the material in the air and the duration of exposure do not give a direct estimate of the dose, which is also dependent on the minute volume and percent retention. The measurement of pulmonary dust retention following a brief exposure to a radiolabeled test aerosol at various times during prechronic or chronic studies of insoluble inhaled dust should be considered in order to assess whether the selected levels of exposure may overwhelm pulmonary clearance mechanisms (Lewis et al., 1989). The appropriateness of other routes of administration (usually oral) in combination with limited data from tests by inhalation or skin application must be scientifically evaluated for each chemical (depending on its main site of action, metabolism, etc.). The morphologic, physiologic, and biologic parameters that are usually evaluated, either at regular intervals in the course of the exposure period or at its termination, have been described (OECD, 1987). It is evident that investigations that can make use of specific physiologic or biochemical tests based on the knowledge of the "critical" organ or function produce highly valuable information and hence increase confidence in the atmospheric or biologic TLV derived from them (see be-

low). In the field of industrial toxicology, knowledge of the disposition (absorption, distribution, biotransformation, excretion) of the chemical and/or its mechanism of action is of major interest. Indeed, as indicated in the introduction, the main objective of occupational toxicology is to prevent the development of occupational diseases. In this respect, the biologic monitoring of workers exposed to various industrial chemicals may play an important role, by detecting excessive exposures as early as possible, before the occurrence of significant biologic disturbances, or at least when they are still reversible or have not yet caused any health impairment. A rational biologic monitoring of exposure and of early health effects is possible only when sufficient toxicologic information has been gathered on the mechanism of action and/or the metabolism of xenobiotics to which workers may be exposed (*see below*: "Practical Applications"). These studies must be performed first on animals.

OBSERVATIONS ON WORKERS

When a new chemical is being used on a large scale, careful clinical survey of the workers and monitoring of the workplaces should be planned. In addition to the specific actions immediately taken if any adverse effect on the health of the workers is discovered, a clinical survey may have two main general objectives: (1) to evaluate the validity of the acceptable exposure level derived from animal experiments and (2) to test the validity of a biologic method of monitoring (assessment of exposure and early detection of adverse effects).

Evaluation of the Validity of Animal Experiments

Evaluation of the validity of the proposed permissible exposure level derived from animal experiments is certainly the prime objective since, as stated by J. M. Barnes in 1963, "studies and observations on man will always be the final basis for deciding whether or not a MAC set originally on the basis of tests on animals is, in fact, truly acceptable as one that will not produce any signs of intoxication." This means that behavioral, clinical, biochemical, physiologic, or morphologic tests that are considered to be the most sensitive for detecting an adverse effect of the chemical should be applied to the workers at the same time their overall exposure is evaluated to provide personal monitoring of airborne contaminants. An important point worth stressing with regard to the clinical studies (prospective or cross-sectional studies) is that like the experimental studies (testing on animal) mentioned above they should as much as possible rely on

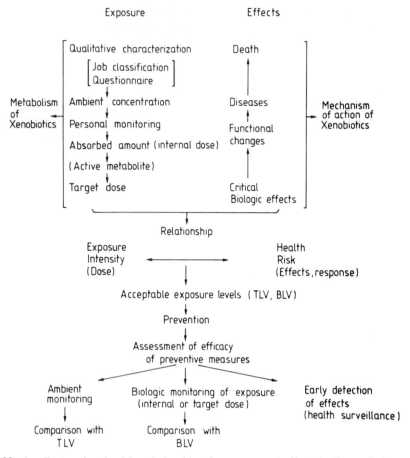

Figure 29–1. Factors involved in relationship of exposure and effects in the workplace.

sensitive biologic effect parameters. The diagnostic tools used in clinical medicine frequently reveal only advanced pathological states and, with a few exceptions, are not designed to detect early adverse effects at a stage when they are still reversible if preventive actions are taken. To give an example, the measurement of serum creatinine is still the most widely used clinical test for assessing renal integrity; yet it is known that the filtration capacity of the kidney, which is its main function, must be reduced by more than 60 percent before serum creatinine significantly rises. What can be said for the kidney is true for most other organs or functions.

The main limitation of present permissible airborne concentrations or biologic limit values is that they are usually based on limited experimental data or clinical studies in which only late effects have been looked for and correlated with past exposure. Furthermore, several biologic TLVs are derived from the study of external-internal exposure relationships and not from that of internal dose–early adverse effects rela-

tionships (see below). The validity of an acceptable exposure level is much stronger if it is based on the study of the dose-effects/dose-incidence relationships in which the dose is expressed in terms of the target dose and the monitored effect reflects a critical biologic event. As illustrated in Figure 29–1, the epidemiologic studies designed to assess the dose-effect/dose-incidence relationships can be carried out by using different parameters for assessing the exposure and the resulting health changes. Exposure may be characterized qualitatively (e.g., by job classification or through questionnaire) or quantitatively through ambient or personal monitoring or through measurement of the internal dose or the target dose. The adverse effects may be expressed in terms of increased death rate, clinical diseases, irreversible or reversible functional changes, or critical biological changes (i.e., changes that are predictive of health impairment if they are maintained or occurred repeatedly).

It is evident that the assessment of the health risk resulting from exposure (and the permissible exposure level derived therefrom) will have more validity if it results from dose-effects and dose-incidence studies in which both the target dose and the critical biologic changes are monitored. Of course, the use of such parameters requires knowledge of the fate of the chemical in the organism and its mechanism of action.

Since the adverse effects under scrutiny for the early detection of health impairment are subtle, and since individual variations exist in the response to a chemical insult, results can only be evaluated on a statistical basis. This means that the dose-prevalence curves found among exposed workers should always be compared with similar responses in a group of unexposed workers matched for other variables such as age, sex, socioeconomic status, and smoking habits. The importance of selecting a control group that is well matched with the exposed group and that undergoes exactly the same standardized clinical, biologic, or physiologic evaluation at the same time as the exposed group must be emphasized. Since an employed population is a group selected to a certain degree for health, comparison with the general population is not valid. Since such a survey may last for several years (prospective survey or observational cohort study or large scale cross-sectional study), the importance of good standardization of all methods of investigation, such as questionnaires related to subjective complaints, instrumentation, and analytic techniques, must be stressed before the start of the survey.

If labor turnover is too high to allow a typical cohort study (i.e., regular examination of the same exposed and control workers), repeated cross-sectional studies of exposed and matched controls should be undertaken. If exposure is above the threshold level of response, these studies may permit (1) establishment of the relationship between integrated exposure (intensity × time) and frequency of abnormal responses and consequently (2) a redefinition of the permissible exposure level.

When a meaningful surveillance program has not been planned before the introduction of a new chemical, it is more difficult to obtain the desired information through investigations designed after the fact. Indeed, in this case, evaluation depends on retrospective cohort studies or case-control studies or cross-sectional studies on workers who may already have sustained variable exposure conditions. Since the information regarding the past exposure of the workers is often incomplete, and since only late effects are usually looked for in retrospective or case-control studies, a correct evaluation of the no-adverse-effect level is much more difficult. Provided a satisfactory assessment of past exposure

is possible, cross-sectional studies that rely on preclinical signs of toxicity may to a certain extent overcome these difficulties. Whether or not clinical investigations are planned from the introduction of a new chemical or process, it is essential to keep standardized records of workers' occupational histories and exposure. The need may arise for mortality or case history studies in order to answer an urgent question on a suspected risk. The evaluation of the acceptable exposure level of benzene in man illustrates this point (Rinsky et al., 1987).

In addition to these clinical surveys, it is useful to report in case studies any particular observations resulting from exposure to the chemicals (e.g., accidental acute intoxications). Although such isolated observations are not helpful for determining the no-effect level in man, they are of interest, mainly for new chemicals. They may indicate whether human symptomatology is similar to that found in animals and hence may suggest the functional or biologic tests that might prove useful for routine control of exposed workers.

Testing the Validity of a Biologic Method of Monitoring

Experimental work may have suggested a biologic method for monitoring of exposure (e.g., evaluation of current exposure, internal load, or target dose). Clinical investigations must then be made to test the applicability of such methods in industrial situations. A brief review of the main biologic monitoring methods presently available for evaluating exposure to some industrial toxicologic hazards is presented at the end of this chapter.

Likewise, studies in animals may have revealed biologic effects that precede or are predictive of irreversible functional and/or morphological changes if exposure is prolonged. Epidemiologic studies must then be designed for assessing the relevance of these parameters for detecting workers at risk.

EXPERIMENTAL STUDIES ON VOLUNTEERS

Experimental studies on volunteers are usually designed to answer very specific questions—e.g., time course of metabolite excretion during and after exposure; threshold doses for blood cholinesterase inhibition; evaluation of the threshold concentration for sensory responses (odor, irritation of the nasal mucosa, etc.); acute effect of solvent exposure on perception, vigilance, and the like. For evident ethical reasons, such studies can only be undertaken when the same results cannot be obtained through other means and under circumstances where the risk for the volunteers can reasonably be estimated as nonexistent. The experimentation should comply with the Declaration of Helsinki (1964)—i.e., it should be carried out under proper medical supervision on duly-informed volunteers.

INTEREST OF CLOSE COLLABORATION BETWEEN EXPERIMENTAL INVESTIGATIONS ON ANIMALS AND CLINICAL STUDIES ON WORKERS (OR VOLUNTEERS)

Perhaps in the field of industrial toxicology more than in other areas of toxicology, close collaboration between experimental investigations on animals and clinical studies on workers plays an important role in explaining the potential risk linked with overexposure to chemicals and hence in suggesting preventive measures to protect the health of the workers. A few examples will illustrate the complementarity of both disciplines in occupational toxicology.

Several occupational carcinogens have been clearly identified through combined epidemiologic and experimental approaches (IARC, 1987). For example, the carcinogenicity of vinyl chloride was first demonstrated in rats (Viola et al., 1971), and a few years later, epidemiologic studies confirmed the same carcinogenic risk for humans (Creech and Johnson, 1974; Monson et al., 1974). This observation stimulated several investigations on its metabolism in animals and on its mutagenic activity in various in vitro systems. Identification of vinyl chloride metabolites led to the conclusion that an epoxy derivative is first formed, which is suspected to be the proximate carcinogen. This report triggered a number of investigations on the biotransformation of structurally related halogenated ethylenes such as vinylbromide, vinylidene chloride, 1,2-dichloroethene, trichloroethylene, perchloroethylene (Bonse et al., 1975; Uehleke et al., 1977; Dekant et al., 1987). All give rise to epoxy intermediates. Comparison of the oncogenic activity of haloethylenes in relation to their metabolism led to the formulation of the "optimum stability" theory of the epoxides. An optimum between the stability and reactivity in both reaching the DNA target and reacting with it after being formed at the monooxygenase site would determine their genotoxic risk (Bolt, 1984). According to this theory, trichloroethylene and perchloroethylene would not represent a significant genotoxic hazard. Clinical evidence, however, is still controversial (IARC, 1987), and furthermore, the possibility of conjugation

with glutathione, leading to production of a reactive thiol in the kidney, cannot be ignored (Dekant et al., 1986, 1987). Large-scale retrospective epidemiologic studies on persons who have been occupationally exposed to these widely used solvents are therefore still needed.

Dioxane is an industrial solvent with a variety of industrial applications. When it is administered at high doses, the principal toxic effects in rats are centrilobular hepatocellular and renal tubular epithelial degeneration and necrosis and induction of hepatic and nasal carcinoma (Kociba et al., 1974). The major metabolite in rats was identified as either β-hydroxyethoxyacetic acid (HEAA) or p-dioxane-2-one, depending on the acidity and the alkalinity of the solution. It was found, however, that the biotransformation of dioxane to HEAA may be saturated by high doses of dioxane. This observation led Young to suggest that the toxicity of dioxane occurs when doses are given sufficient to saturate the metabolic pathway for its detoxification (Young et al., 1976b). On the premise that similarity of the metabolic pathway of dioxane in rats and humans would greatly facilitate the extrapolation of toxicologic data from rats to man (Young et al., 1976a), Young and coworkers examined the urine of plant personnel exposed to dioxane vapor. In urine of workers exposed to a time-weighted average concentration of 1.6 ppm dioxane for 7.5 hours, they found the same product (HEAA) as found previously in the rat. Furthermore, the high ratio of HEAA to dioxane, 118:1, suggests that at a low-exposure concentration dioxane is rapidly metabolized to HEAA. The authors concluded that since saturation of the metabolism of dioxane in rats was correlated with toxicity, their results on humans support the hypothesis that low levels of dioxane vapor in the workplace pose a negligible hazard. This conclusion is debatable, however, since dioxane is carcinogenic in rats and guinea pigs and the existence of a threshold level for such chemicals is controversial (Dinman, 1972; Claus et al., 1974; Henschler, 1974). Furthermore, Woo et al. (1977) have reported that p-dioxane-2-one is more toxic than dioxane, and its production in vivo may be related to dioxane toxicity and/or carcinogenicity, in view of the fact that a number of lactones with similar structure are known to be carcinogenic. If it can be shown that p-dioxane-2-one is really a proximate carcinogen, workers found to excrete the metabolite will have to be considered at risk.

Dimethylformamide (DMF) is an hepatotoxic solvent extensively used in laboratories and in the production of acrylic resins. Exposure of workers occurs mainly by inhalation of vapor and through skin contact. DMF is rapidly metabolized *in vivo*. A negligible fraction of the absorbed dose is excreted unchanged in urine and in the gastrointestinal tract. It was initially believed that the biotransformation of DMF *in vivo*, in rat, dog, and human consisted of a direct demethylation mediated by the microsomal mixed-function oxidases to yield *N*-methylformamide (NMF) and formamide (F) (Kimmerle and Eben, 1975a, 1975b; Maxfield *et al.*, 1975; Krivanek *et al.*, 1978; Lauwerys *et al.*, 1980; Scailteur *et al.*, 1981). It has now been demonstrated that the metabolite identified as NMF by gas chromatography (Barnes and Henry, 1974) is mainly *N*-hydroxymethyl-*N*-methylformamide (DMF-OH), a stable carbinolamine that breaks down in the injector of the gas chromatograph to give NMF (Scailteur and Lauwerys, 1984a, 1984b; Scailteur *et al.*, 1984). By analogy, *N*-hydroxymethylformamide (NMF-OH) is considered to be the metabolite initially described as F. Only a very small percentage of the absorbed DMF, however, is transformed into NMF and F (probably less than 5 percent). The metabolic pathway leading from DMF to DMF-OH involves hydroxyl radicals. The slight amount of NMF produced *in vivo* does not seem to result from further DMF-OH biotransformation but comes directly from DMF (Scailteur and Lauwerys, 1984a,b). NMF is more toxic than DMF, and the differences between DMF and NMF toxicity were difficult to explain when NMF was thought to represent the principal *in vivo* metabolite of DMF. The metabolic studies that demonstrate that following DMF administration the main urinary metabolite is in fact DMF-OH and not NMF now offer a logical explanation for these apparent discrepancies, since DMF-OH has been shown to be less acutely toxic than NMF (Scailteur and Lauwerys, 1984b). It has, however, been demonstrated that in humans *N*-acetyl-*S*-(*N*-methylcarbamoyl) cysteine (AMCC) is a common urinary metabolite of DMF and NMF, and it has been postulated that this biotransformation pathway is responsible for the hepatotoxicity of both solvents. The different amount of reactive intermediate produced from DMF of NMF might also explain the different hepatotoxicity of both compounds (Mraz *et al.*, 1989). Observations on workers have clearly demonstrated that for a substance like DMF, which can enter the organism not only by inhalation but also through skin contact, DMF-OH + NMF analysis in urine (both detected as a single NMF peak by gas chromatography) currently appears to be the best method for assessing exposure (Lauwerys, 1986). Further studies are required to assess whether the determination of AMCC in urine may be a more relevant indicator of the health risk.

These examples (vinyl chloride, dioxane, dimethylformamide) demonstrate that the study of the metabolic handling of an industrial chemical in animals is very important because it may lead to the characterization of reactive intermediates, suggesting yet-unsuspected risks, or it may indicate new methods of biologic monitoring, which must first be validated by a field study. Conversely, clinical observations on workers may stimulate the study of the metabolism or the mechanism of toxicity of an industrial chemical in animals. This may help in predicting the human response to structurally related compounds or in evaluating the health significance of a biologic disturbance. In 1973, an outbreak of peripheral neuropathy occurred in workers exposed to the solvent methyl butyl ketone (MBK) (Billmaier *et al.*, 1974; McDonough, 1974; Allen *et al.*, 1975). The same lesion was reproduced in animals (Duckett *et al.*, 1974; Mendell *et al.*, 1974; Spencer *et al.*, 1975). Biotransformation studies were then undertaken in rats and guinea pigs (Abdel-Rahman *et al.*, 1976; DiVincenzo *et al.*, 1976, 1977), and some MBK metabolites (2,5-hexanedione, 5-hydroxy-2-hexanone) were also found to possess neurotoxic activity (Spencer and Schaumburg, 1975; DiVincenzo *et al.*, 1977).

Similar oxidation products are formed from *n*-hexane, the neurotoxicity of which is probably due to the same active metabolite as that produced from MBK. According to DiVincenzo *et al.* (1977), the most probable active intermediate is 2,5-hexanedione. Since methyl isobutyl ketone and methyl ethyl ketone cannot give rise to 2,5-hexanedione (DiVincenzo *et al.*, 1976), they should preferably replace MBK as solvents. *n*-Hexane derivatives that are oxidized to 2,5-hexanedione are probably also neurotoxic for man (DiVincenzo *et al.*, 1977).

Organic metabolites of arsenic—namely, monomethylarsonic (MMA) and dimethylarsinic (DMA) acids—have been identified in human urine after ingestion of inorganic arsenic in either the trivalent or pentavalent state (Buchet *et al.*, 1980, 1981a, 1981b). The methylation reaction can be regarded as a detoxification mechanism. *In vivo* studies on healthy human volunteers and patients suffering from liver diseases and observations on subjects acutely intoxicated with inorganic arsenic (Buchet *et al.*, 1981b, 1984; Mahieu *et al.*, 1981) have shown that the production of DMA is transiently inhibited when inorganic arsenic intake exceeds a certain level and that liver insufficiency significantly modifies the ratio of the methylated metabolites excreted in urine (decreased excretion of MMA and increased excretion of DMA). *In vitro* studies with rat tissues (Buchet and Lauwerys, 1985,

1988) and *in vivo* investigation in rats (Buchet and Lauwerys, 1987) have elucidated the mechanism of arsenic biotransformation and the factors influencing it. These studies have demonstrated that the liver cytosol is the main site of biotransformation of inorganic arsenic, which involves two different enzymatic activities for the mono- and dimethylated arsenical synthesis. Inorganic arsenic must be in the trivalent state to be methylated, and the process requires the presence of *S*-adenosylmethionine and reduced glutathione. The latter cofactor is only required for the first methylation reaction, which is rate limiting. An excess of substrate inhibits the dimethylation reaction, and this finding is in agreement with the human observations mentioned above. The experimental studies also suggest that the changes in arsenic methylation observed in patients with liver insufficiency result from a depletion of liver GSH.

These few examples illustrate the interest of fruitful collaboration between experimental and clinical studies in the area of industrial toxicology. More rapid achievement of the control of occupational hazards can be accomplished if close collaboration between both disciplines is further stimulated.

PRACTICAL APPLICATIONS

We have already stressed three important types of applications of toxicologic investigations—that is, the proposal of permissible airborne concentrations of chemicals, the development of methods for the biologic evaluation of the intensity of exposure to chemicals and the recommendation of early markers of adverse effects (Figure 29–1). The basis of these three applications is illustrated by Figure 29–2, which summarizes the fate of a chemical exerting systemic biologic effects from the environment to the target molecules in the organism (Lauwerys, 1984a).

Permissible Levels of Exposure to Airborne Industrial Chemicals

It is a cliché to say that the best practice in occupational hygiene is to maintain concentrations of all atmospheric contaminants as low as is practical, but even this does not always preclude overexposure to toxic levels of chemicals. The industrial physician must have guidelines to judge the potential health hazards of industrial chemicals and to evaluate whether the general preventive methods in use in the factory are adequate or must be improved or must be complemented by the use of personal protective devices. As indicated above, an important objective of experimental and clinical investigations

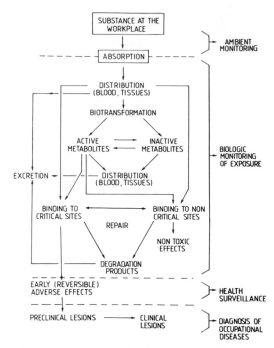

Figure 29–2. Relationship of metabolic information to biologic monitoring of workers.

in industrial toxicology is the proposal of "safe" (i.e., acceptable) levels of exposure. Various private and official institutions review regularly the toxicologic information on chemicals in order to propose permissible levels of exposure. Critical evaluation of these data can be found in the following publications: various ATSDR and NIOSH criteria documents on specific chemicals, documentation on TLVs prepared by the American Conference of Governmental Industrial Hygienists, and reports prepared by the Deutsche Forschungsgemeinschaft (Toxikologisch-Arbeitsmedizinische Begründung von MAK-Werten) and the Dutch Expert Committee for Occupational Standards. Depending on the type of sampling system selected—stationary or personal—the estimate of the risk may be carried out on a group or individual basis. It is evident that with the accumulation of new information on the toxicity of industrial chemicals, the proposed permissible levels must be reevaluated at regular intervals. It should also be made clear that these levels are only guides and should not take the place of close medical surveillance of the workers.

Biologic Assessment of Exposure

Biologic monitoring of exposure assesses the health risk through the evaluation of the internal dose. Depending on the chemical and the analyzed biologic parameter, the term *internal dose* may cover different concepts (Bernard and Lauwerys, 1986, 1987). It may mean the amount of chemical recently absorbed. Hence, a biologic parameter may reflect the amount of chemical absorbed either shortly before sampling (e.g., the concentration of a solvent in the alveolar air or in blood during the workshift) or during the preceding day (e.g., the concentration of a solvent in alveolar air or in blood collected 16 hours after the end of exposure) or during the last months when the chemical has a long biologic half-life (e.g., the concentration of some metals in blood). Internal dose may also mean the amount of chemical stored in one or in several body compartments or in the whole body *(body burden)*. This usually applies to cumulative toxic chemicals. For example, the concentration of polychlorinated biphenyls in blood is a reflection of the amount accumulated in the main sites of deposition (i.e., fatty tissues). Finally, with ideal biological monitoring tests, the internal dose means the amount of active chemical species bound to the critical sites of action *(target dose)*. Such tests can be developed when the critical sites are easily accessible (e.g., hemoglobin in the case of exposure to carbon monoxide or to methemoglobin agents) or when the chemical interacts with a blood constituent in a similar way as with the critical target molecule (e.g., hemoglobin alkylation reflecting binding to DNA).

When biologic measurements are available to assess the internal dose, the approach offers important advantages over monitoring the air of the workplace (Lauwerys, 1984b). Its greatest advantage is the fact that the biologic parameter of exposure is more directly related to the adverse health effects that one attempts to prevent than any environmental measurement. Therefore, it may offer a better estimate of the risk than ambient monitoring. Biologic monitoring takes into consideration absorption by routes other than the lungs. Many industrial chemicals can enter the organism by absorption through the skin or the gastrointestinal tract. For example, it has been demonstrated that in an acrylic fiber factory, skin absorption of the solvent dimethylformamide, which is used for the dissolution of the polymer (see above), is more likely to be absorbed by the cutaneous route than by inhalation (Lauwerys *et al.*, 1980). Adamsson *et al.* (1979) studied the elimination of cadmium in feces in a group of male workers exposed to cadmium oxide dust in a nickel-cadmium battery factory. Since the cadmium concentration in air (total dust) measured with personal sampler did not exceed 16 $\mu g/m^3$, it was estimated that cadmium naturally occurring in food and cigarettes, cadmium excreted from the gastrointestinal tract, and cadmium transported from the lungs by mucociliary clearance to the gastrointestinal tract could only explain up to 100 μg of the cadmium in the feces. Since even among nonsmokers much higher values for fecal cadmium were recorded, this was interpreted as being the result of ingestion of cadmium from contaminated hands and other body surfaces. Among the smokers, direct oral contact with contaminated cigarettes or pipes is an additional factor. Our results (Roels *et al.*, 1982) on the intensity of hand contamination in workers from an electric condenser factory support Adamsson's findings. In a few workers exposed to cadmium, we have determined, at different times of the day, the amount of cadmium that could be collected after rinsing one hand with 500 ml of slightly acidified water. Before entering the canteen for lunch, up to 280 μg Cd could be mobilized from one hand (versus less than 7 μg in the control subjects). These observations demonstrate clearly that in industry the amount of cadmium and probably of any other element that enters the organism, depends not only on the amount inhaled but also on the amount ingested.

Even if there exists a relationship between the airborne concentration, the overall dustiness of the workplace, and hence the amount of industrial pollutant entering the organism by any route, one cannot expect that determination of the airborne concentration will allow estimation of the total amount of the chemical absorbed by the exposed workers (Lauwerys, 1980). First, personal hygiene habits (hand washing, smoking at the workplace, etc.) vary from one person to another. Second, it is well known that great individual variation exists in the absorption rate of a chemical through the lungs, the skin, or the gastrointestinal tract. For example, a study by Flanagan *et al.* (1978) indicates, as was demonstrated previously in animals, that subjects with low iron stores absorb considerably more cadmium (8.9 percent) through the gastrointestinal tract than persons with normal iron stores (2.4 percent). Oral absorption of cadmium is therefore higher in females than in males. Even if strict personal hygiene measures can be implemented so that the pollutant can enter the organism only by inhalation (in addition to the amount transported from the lungs by mucociliary clearance to the gastrointestinal tract), there is no reason to postulate the existence of a relationship between the airborne concentration and the amount absorbed. This has been clearly demonstrated for lead by King *et al.* (1979). Many physicochemical and biological factors (particle size distribution, ventilatory parameters, *etc.*) preclude the existence of such a correlation. For example, a physical load of 100 watts increases by a factor of 2 to 3 the respiratory uptake of trichloroethylene by comparison with the uptake at rest (Monster *et al.*, 1976). The daily uptake of xylene by volunteers exposed to the same time-weighted average concentration varies with the environmental conditions (constant or peak exposures) and the work load (Riihimaki *et al.*, 1979). A biological parameter may involve all these different toxicokinetic factors.

Because of its capability to evaluate the overall exposure (whatever the route of entry), biological monitoring can also be used to test the efficiency of various personal protective measures such as gloves, masks, or barrier creams (Lauwerys *et al.*, 1980).

Another advantage of biological monitoring is the fact that the nonoccupational background exposure (leisure activity, residency, dietary habits, smoking, etc.) may also be expressed in the biological level. The organism integrates the total external (environmental and industrial) exposure into one internal load (Zielhuis, 1979). So it is clear that for many industrial pollutants the control of any concentration in air may not necessarily prevent an undue intake by the exposed workers.

However, a rational biologic monitoring of exposure is only possible when sufficient toxicological information has been gathered on the mechanism of action and/or the metabolism (absorption, biotransformation, distribution, excretion) of xenobiotics to which workers may be exposed (Figure 29–2) (Lauwerys, 1986). When a biologic exposure monitoring method is based on the determination of the chemical or its metabolite in biological media, it is essential to know how the substance is absorbed via the lung, the gastrointestinal tract, and the skin, subsequently distributed to the different compartments of the body, biotransformed, and finally eliminated. It is also important to know whether the chemical may accumulate in the body. These different kinetic aspects must be kept in mind when selecting the time of sampling.

Biologic monitoring of exposure is of practical value only when certain relationships between external exposure, internal dose, and adverse effects are known. Normally, biologic monitoring of exposure cannot be used for assessing exposure to substances that exhibit their toxic effects at the sites of first contact (e.g., primary lung irritants) and are poorly absorbed. In this situation, the only useful quantitative relationship is that between external exposure and the intensity of the local effects.

For the other chemicals that are significantly absorbed and/or exert a systemic toxic action, a biologic monitoring test may provide different information, depending on our current knowledge of the relationships among external exposure, internal exposure, and the risk of adverse effects as illustrated in Figure 29–3 (Lauwerys and Bernard, 1985). If only the relationship between external exposure and the internal dose is known, this biologic parameter can be used as an index of exposure, but it provides little information on the health risk (situation *a*, Figure 29–3). In other terms, biologic monitoring performed under these conditions is much more an assessment of the exposure intensity than of the potential health risk. But if a quantitative relationship has been established between internal dose and adverse effects (situation *c*, Figure 29–3)—i.e., if the internal dose-effects and the internal dose-incidence relationships are known—biologic monitoring allows for a direct health risk assessment and thus for an effective prevention of the adverse effects. It is indeed possible to derive a biologic permissible value from these dose-effects and dose-incidence relationships, which is essential to make biologic exposure monitoring operational. Unfortunately, the majority of the published studies in this field have focused on the relationship between the internal dose and the external exposure rather than on that between the internal parameter reflecting the internal dose and the adverse effects. Consequently, for many chemicals, the latter relationship is insufficiently documented for a reliable estimation of the biologic limit values. In other words, the biologic permissible values are often derived indirectly from the exposure limits in air, through relationships *(a)* and *(b)* as shown in Figure 29–3, a method that is obviously much less reliable than that based on the knowledge of the internal dose-effects and the internal dose-incidence relationships. It must also be kept in mind that the relationships described above may be modified by various factors that influence the fate of an industrial chemical *in vivo*. Metabolic interactions can be predicted when workers are exposed simultaneously to chemicals that are biotransformed through identical pathways. Exposure to industrial chemicals that modify the activity of the biotransformation enzymes (e.g., microsomal enzyme inducers or inhibitors) may also influence the fate of another compound. Furthermore, metabolic interferences may occur between industrial agents and alcohol, food additives, pesticide residues, drugs, or even tobacco. Several biological conditions (sex, weight, fatty mass, pregnancy, diseases, etc.) may also modify the metabolism of an industrial chemical. In summary, the relationship between total uptake of an industrial chemical, its concentration or

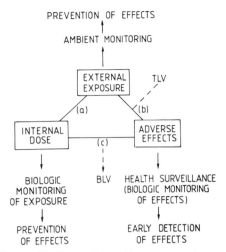

PREVENTION OF EFFECTS

↑

AMBIENT MONITORING

↑

EXTERNAL EXPOSURE — TLV

(a) | (b)

INTERNAL DOSE — (c) — ADVERSE EFFECTS

↓   ↓

BIOLOGIC MONITORING OF EXPOSURE   BLV   HEALTH SURVEILLANCE (BIOLOGIC MONITORING OF EFFECTS)

↓   ↓

PREVENTION OF EFFECTS   EARLY DETECTION OF EFFECTS

Figure 29–3. Relationship of external exposure, internal exposure and adverse effects.

that of its metabolites in biological media, and the risk of adverse effects may be modified by various environmental and biologic factors. They may have to be taken into consideration when interpreting the results of biologic exposure tests.

Whatever the biologic parameter measured (the substance itself, its metabolite[s], the target dose), the test must be sufficiently sensitive (not too many false-negative results) and specific to be of practical value (not too many false-positive results).

Other conditions should be fulfilled before attempting to implement biologic exposure monitoring methods in industry. The ethical aspects must not be neglected; in particular, the collection of biologic specimens cannot involve any health risk for the workers, and the individual results should be considered confidential (Zielhuis, 1978). The selected parameter should be sufficiently stable to allow storage of the biological sample for a certain period of time, and it should be amenable to a non–time-consuming analysis by a not-too-sophisticated technique. The sensitivity, precision, and accuracy of the analysis should be satisfactory. Several intercomparison programs for the analysis of industrial chemicals in biologic material have indeed stressed the analytical difficulties sometimes associated with these measurements (Lauwerys *et al.*, 1975) and the importance of implementing adequate internal and external quality control programs (Elinder *et al.*, 1988).

For many industrial chemicals, one or all of the preceding conditions are lacking, which limits the possibilities of biologic monitoring of exposure. It is therefore evident that the role of environmental monitoring in evaluating and hence for preventing excessive exposure to industrial pollutants is largely unfilled at present. Moreover, as already stressed above, the prevention of acute toxic effects on the respiratory tract or the eye mucosa can only be achieved by keeping the airborne concentration of the irritant substance below a certain level. Local acute effects of industrial chemicals do not lend themselves to a biologic surveillance program. Likewise, biologic monitoring is usually not indicated for detecting peak exposure to dangerous chemicals (e.g., AsH_3, CO, HCN). Furthermore, identification of emission sources and the evaluation of the efficiency of engineering control measures are usually best performed by ambient air analysis.

In summary, both environmental and biologic monitoring programs should not be regarded as opposite but, on the contrary, as truly complementary. They should be integrated as much as possible to ensure low levels of contaminants for the continued health of workers.

The results of a biologic monitoring program can be interpreted either on an individual basis or on a group basis. Interpretation on an individual level, which is usually carried out by the occupational physician, is possible only if the intraindividual variability of the parameter is not too great and its specificity is sufficiently high. The results may also be interpreted on a group basis by considering their distribution. If all the observed values are below the biologic permissible value, the working conditions are satisfactory. If all or the majority of the results are above the biologic permissible value, the overall exposure conditions must certainly be corrected. A third situation may also occur—i.e. the majority of the workers may have values below the biologic permissible level but a few of them have abnormally high values (the distribution is bimodal or polymodal). Two interpretations can be put forward: (1) either the subjects exhibiting the high values perform activities exposing them to higher levels of the pollutant, in which case the biologic monitoring program has identified job categories for which work conditions need to be improved, or (2) these workers do not perform different activities and their higher internal dose must result from different hygiene habits or nonoccupational exposure.

Table 29–1 lists some industrial chemicals for which a biologic determination may be useful for evaluating the internal dose. The interpretation of these data requires some comment. Some industrial chemicals have a long biologic half-life in various body compartments, and the time of sampling (e.g., blood, urine) may not be critical. For other chemicals, the time of sampling is, on the contrary, critical because following expo-

Table 29–1. PROPOSED METHODS FOR THE BIOLOGIC MONITORING OF EXPOSURE TO INDUSTRIAL CHEMICALS

CHEMICAL AGENT	BIOLOGIC PARAMETER	BIOLOGIC MATERIAL	NORMAL VALUE	TENTATIVE MAXIMUM PERMISSIBLE VALUE*	REMARKS
Inorganic and Organometallic Substances					
Aluminum	Aluminum	Serum	<1 μg/100 ml	150 μg/g creat	
Antimony	Antimony	Urine	<50 μg/g creat		
Inorganic arsenic	Total arsenic	Urine	<1 μg/g creat		
	Total arsenic	Blood	<40 μg/g creat		
	Arsenic	Hair	<1 μg/g		
	Sum of inorganic As, monomethylarsonic acid, cacodilic acid	Urine	<10 μg/g creat	50 μg/g creat	No interference of arsenic from marine origin
Barium	Barium	Urine			
Beryllium	Beryllium	Urine	<2 μg/g creat		Nonsmokers
Cadmium	Cadmium	Urine	<2 μg/g creat	10 μg/g creat	
	Metallothionein	Urine			
	Cadmium	Blood	<0.5 μg/100 ml		
Carbon disulfide	Iodine-azide test	Urine		1 μg/100 ml	
	2-Thiothiazolidine-4-carboxylic acid	Urine		6.5 (Vasak index) 5 mg/g creat	
Chromium (soluble compounds)	Chromium	Urine	<5 μg/g creat	30 μg/g creat	
	Chromium	Red blood cells			
Cobalt	Cobalt	Urine	<2 μg/g creat	30 μg/g creat	
Fluoride	Fluoride	Urine	<0.5 mg/g creat	Preshift: 4 mg/g creat Postshift: 7 mg/g creat	
Germanium	Germanium	Urine	<1 μg/g creat		
Lead	Lead	Blood	<30 μg/100 ml	60 μg/100 ml 40 μg/100 ml	Male workers Female workers in reproductive age
	Lead	Urine	<50 μg/g creat	150 μg/g creat	
	δ-Aminolevulinic acid	Urine	<4.5 mg/g creat	10 mg/g creat	
	Coproporphyrin	Urine	<100 μg/g creat	250 μg/g creat	
	Non-iron-bound porphyrin	Red blood cells	<75 μg/100 ml RBC	300 μg/100 ml RBC	
	Zn-protoporphyrin	Blood	<2.5 μg/g Hb	12.5 μg/g Hb	
	δ-Aminolevulinic acid dehydratase	Red blood cells			
	Pyrimidine-5'-nucleotidase	Red blood cells			
	Lead (after 1 g EDTA IV)	Urine	<600 μg/24 h	1000 μg/24 h	

Chemical	Determinant	Specimen			Sampling time
Lead tetraalkyl	Lead	Urine	<50 µg/g creat	100 µg/g creat	
Manganese	Manganese	Urine	<3 µg/g creat		
Manganese	Manganese	Blood	<1 µg/100 ml	1 µg/100 ml	
Mercury inorganic	Mercury	Urine	<5 µg/g creat	50 µg/g creat	
Mercury inorganic	Mercury	Blood	<1 µg/100 ml	2 µg/100 ml	
Mercury (methyl)	Mercury	Blood	<1 µg/100 ml	10 µg/100 ml	
Nickel (soluble compounds)	Nickel	Urine	<5 µg/g creat	70 µg/g creat	
	Nickel	Plasma	<1 µg/100 ml	1 µg/100 ml	
Nitrous oxide	Nitrous oxide	Urine		60 µg/g creat	
	Nitrous oxide	Expired air			
Selenium		Urine	<25 µg/g creat		
Silver		Urine	<1 µg/g creat		
Thallium		Urine	<0.3 µg/g creat		
Uranium		Urine	<1 µg/g creat		
Vanadium		Urine	<0.7 mg/g creat	50 µg/g creat	
Zinc		Serum	<15 µg/100 ml		
Nonsubstituted Aliphatic and Alicyclic Hydrocarbons					
n-Hexane	2-Hexanol	Urine		0.2 mg/g creat	
	2-5-Hexanedione	Urine		2 mg/g creat	End first day of work
	2-5-Hexanedione	Urine		4 mg/g creat	End of workweek
n-Hexane	n-Hexane	Blood		15 µg/100 ml	During exposure
	n-Hexane	Expired air		50 ppm	During exposure
2-Methyl-pentane	2-Methyl-2-pentanol	Urine			
	2-Methylpentane	Expired air			
3-Methyl-pentane	3-Methyl-2-pentanol	Urine			
	3-Methylpentane	Expired air			
Cyclohexane	Cyclohexanol	Urine		3.2 mg/g creat	
	Cyclohexane	Blood		45 µg/100 ml	During exposure
	Cyclohexane	Expired air		220 ppm	During exposure
Nonsubstituted Aromatic Hydrocarbons					
Benzene	Phenol	Urine	<20 mg/g creat	45 mg/g creat	If TWA 10 ppm
	Benzene	Expired air		<0.022 ppm	If TWA 1 ppm
	Benzene	Blood		5 ppm	If TWA 1 ppm
					If TWA 1 ppm
Toluene	Hippuric acid	Urine	<1.5 g/g creat	2.5 g/g creat	During exposure
	O-Cresol	Urine		1 mg/g creat	During exposure
	Toluene	Blood		0.1 mg/100 ml	During exposure
	Toluene	Expired air		20 ppm	During exposure
Xylene	Methylhippuric acid	Urine	<0.3 mg/g creat	1.5 g/g creat	During exposure
	Xylene	Blood		0.3 mg/100 ml	During exposure
	Xylene	Expired air			

Table 29–1. (*continued*)

CHEMICAL AGENT	BIOLOGIC PARAMETER	BIOLOGIC MATERIAL	NORMAL VALUE	TENTATIVE MAXIMUM PERMISSIBLE VALUE*	REMARKS
Ethylbenzene	Mandelic acid	Urine		1 g/g creat	
	Ethylbenzene	Expired air			During exposure
	Ethylbenzene	Blood		0.15 mg/100 ml	
Isopropylbenzene (cumene)	Dimethylphenylcarbinol	Urine		200 mg/g creat	
Mesitylene	Acide 3,5-dimethylhippuric	Urine		1 g/g creat	
Styrene	Mandelic acid	Urine		350 mg/g creat	
	Phenylglyoxylic acid	Urine		0.055 mg/100 ml	
	Styrene	Blood		0.002 mg/100 ml	16 hours after the end of exposure
α-Methylstyrene	Styrene	Expired air		18 ppm	
Biphenyl	Atrolactic acid	Urine			
	4-Hydroxybiphenyl	Urine		1.5 mg/g creat	
Polycyclic aromatic	1-Hydroxypyrene	Urine	<2 μg/g creat		
Hydrocarbons	Hemoglobin adducts	Red blood cells			
Halogenated Hydrocarbons					
Monochloromethane (methylchloride)	S-Methylcysteine	Urine			
Monobromomethane (methylbromide)	S-Methylcysteine	Urine			
Dichloromethane (methylene chloride)	Methylene chloride	Blood		0.08 mg/100 ml	
	Carboxyhemoglobin	Blood	<1%	3%	Nonsmokers
1,2-Dibromoethane	Methylene chloride	Expired air		35 ppm	
	N-Acetyl-S-(2-hydroxyethyl) cysteine	Urine			
Trichloromethane (chloroform)	Chloroform	Blood			
	Chloroform	Expired air			
Tetrachloromethane (carbon tetrachloride)	Carbon tetrachloride	Blood			
	Carbon tetrachloride	Expired air			
1,1,1-Trichloroethane (methylchloroform)	Sum of trichloroethanol and trichloroacetic acid	Urine		50 mg/g creat	
	Trichloroethanol	Urine		30 mg/g creat	
	Methylchloroform	Blood			
	Methylchloroform	Expired air		50 ppm	During exposure
	Methylchloroform	Urine		800 μg/g creat	

Substance	Determinant	Sample	Normal value	Value	Sampling time
Trichloroethylene	Trichloroethanol	Urine		125 mg/g creat	After 5-day exposure
	Trichloroacetic acid	Urine		75 mg/g creat	During exposure
	Trichloroethylene	Blood		0.6 mg/100 ml	After 5-day exposure
	Trichloroethanol	Plasma		0.23 mg/100 ml	After 5-day exposure
	Trichloroacetic acid	Plasma		5 mg/100 ml	During exposure
	Trichloroethylene	Expired air		12 ppm	16 hours after exposure
				<0.5 ppm	
Tetrachloroethylene	Tetrachloroethylene	Blood		100 µg/100 ml	During exposure
	Tetrachloroethylene	Expired air		60 ppm	16 hours after exposure
	Tetrachloroethylene	Urine		4 ppm	
Vinyl chloride	Thiodiglycolic acid	Urine	<2 mg/g creat	100 µg/g creat	
Hexachlorobutadiene	Hexachlorobutadiene	Blood			
Monochlorobenzene	4-Chlorocatechol	Urine			
	4-Chlorophenol	Urine			
p-Dichlorobenzene	4-Dichlorobenzene	Urine		250 µg/g creat	
	2,5-Dichlorophenol	Urine			
Halothane	Trifluoroacetic acid	Urine		10 mg/g creat	After 5-day exposure
	Trifluoroacetic acid	Blood		0.25 mg/100 ml	After 5-day exposure
	Halothane	Urine		250 µg/g creat	
Polychlorinated biphenyl	Polychlorinated biphenyl	Serum	<0.3 µg/100 ml		
	Trichlorobiphenyl	Blood			
Other volatile halogenated hydrocarbons		Expired air			
		Urine			

Amino- and Nitroderivatives

Substance	Determinant	Sample	Normal value	Value	Sampling time
Ethyleneglycol dinitrate	Ethyleneglycol dinitrate	Urine			
	Ethyleneglycol dinitrate				
	Ethyleneglycol dinitrate				
Several aromatic amino- and nitro-compounds (aniline, nitrobenzene, dinitrobenzene, etc.)	Methemoglobin	Blood	<2%	5%	
	Diazo-positive metabolites	Urine	<10 mg/g creat		
	Parent compound (e.g., benzidine, β-naphthylamine)	Urine			
	Hemoglobin adducts	Blood			
Triethylamine	Triethylamine	Urine		145 mg/g creat	
Aniline	Aniline	Urine		0.75 mg/g creat	
	p-Aminophenol	Urine		10 mg/g creat	
	Methemoglobin	Blood	<2%	5%	
	Aniline released from hemoglobin adducts	Blood		10 µg/100 ml	
Nitrobenzene	p-Nitrophenol	Urine		5 mg/g creat	
	Methemoglobin	Blood	<2%	5%	

Table 29–1. (*continued*)

CHEMICAL AGENT	BIOLOGIC PARAMETER	BIOLOGIC MATERIAL	NORMAL VALUE	TENTATIVE MAXIMUM PERMISSIBLE VALUE*	REMARKS
4,4'-Methylene bis (2-chloroaniline) (MOCA)	MOCA	Urine		80 μg/g creat	
Methylenedianiline (MDA)	MDA	Urine			
Benzidine-derived azo compounds	Benzidine	Urine			
Monacetylbenzidine-derived azo compounds	Monacetylbenzidine	Urine			
2,4-Dinitrotoluene	2,4-Dinitrobenzoic acid	Urine			
Trinitrotoluene	2,4- and 2,6-Dinitroaminotoluene	Urine			
Alcohols—Glycols and Derivatives					
Methanol	Methanol	Urine		7 mg/g creat	
	Formic acid	Urine	<2.5 mg/g creat		
	Formic acid	Blood	<15 mg/g creat		
Isopropanol	Acetone	Urine	<2 mg/g creat		
	Isopropanol	Expired air		500 mg/m^3	
Furfurylalcohol	Furoic acid	Urine	<65 mg/g creat		
Ethyleneglycol	Oxalic acid	Urine	<50 mg/g creat		
	Glycolic acid	Urine			
	Ethyleneglycol	Serum			
Diethyleneglycol	Oxalic acid	Urine	<50 mg/g creat		
Ethyleneglycol monomethylether (methylcellosolve)	Methoxyacetic acid	Urine			
	Methylcellosolve	Expired air			
Ethyleneglycol monoethylether (ethylcellosolve)	Ethoxyacetic acid	Urine		150 mg/g creat	
Ethyleneglycol monobutylether (butylcellosolve)	Butoxyacetic acid	Urine			
1-Methoxy-2-propanol	Propyleneglycol	Urine			

2-Methoxy-1-propanol	Methoxypropionic acid	Urine	2.6 mg/g creat	End of the workweek
Dioxane	β-Hydroxyethoxyacetic acid	Urine	4 mg/g creat	
Ketones				
Methylethylketone	Methylethylketone	Urine	0.5 mg/g creat	
Methyl *n*-butylketone	2,5-Hexanedione	Urine	30 mg/g creat	
Methylisobutylketone	Methylisobutylketone	Urine	5 mg/100 ml	
Acetone	Acetone	Urine	<2 mg/g creat	200 mg/g creat
Acetone	Acetone	Blood	<0.2 mg/100 ml	
Acetone	Acetone	Expired air		
Aldehydes				
Furfural	Furoic acid	Urine	<65 mg/g creat	40 mg/g creat
Amides				
Dimethylformamide	Methylhydroxymethyl-formamide measured as *N*-methylformamide	Urine		
	Dimethylformamide	Blood		0.15 mg/100 ml
	Methylhydroxymethyl-formamide measured as *N*-methylformamide	Blood		0.1 mg/100 ml
	Dimethylformamide	Expired air		1 ppm
	N-Acetyl-*S*-(*N*-methyl-carbamoyl) cysteine	Urine		During exposure
Dimethylacetamide	*N*-Methylacetamide (probably methylhydroxy-methylacetamide)	Urine		
Phenols				
Phenol	Phenol	Urine	<20 mg/g creat	250 mg/g creat
p-tert-Butylphenol	*p*-tert-Butylphenol	Urine		2 mg/g creat
Esters				
Methylmethacrylate	Methacrylic acid	Urine		

Table 29–1. (*continued*)

CHEMICAL AGENT	BIOLOGIC PARAMETER	BIOLOGIC MATERIAL	NORMAL VALUE	TENTATIVE MAXIMUM PERMISSIBLE VALUE*	REMARKS
Asphyxiants					
Carbon monoxide	Carboxyhemoglobin	Blood	<1%	5%	Nonsmoker
	Carbon monoxide	Blood	<0.15 ml/100 ml	10 ml/100 ml	Nonsmoker
	Carbon monoxide	Expired air	<2 ppm	18 ppm	Nonsmoker
Cyanide and aliphatic nitriles	Thiocyanate	Urine	<2.5 mg/g creat	6 mg/g creat	Nonsmoker
	Thiocyanate	Plasma	<0.6 mg/100 ml		Nonsmoker
	Cyanide	Blood			
	Ratio between thiocyanate, urine (mg/g/creat), and carboxyhemoglobin (%)	Urine + blood		3	
Acrylonitrile	Acrylonitrile	Urine			Nonsmoker
	Thiocyanate	Urine	<2.5 mg/g creat		
Methemoglobin-forming agents	Methemoglobin	Blood	<2%	5%	
Pesticides					
Lindane	Lindane	Blood		2 µg/100 ml	
DDT	DDT, DDE, DDD, DDA	Blood			
		Urine			
Hexachlorobenzene	Hexachlorobenzene	Blood	<0.3 µg/100 ml	30 µg/100 ml	
Dieldrin	Dieldrin	Urine			
	Dieldrin	Blood		15 µg/100 ml	
Endrin	Anti-12-hydroxyendrin	Urine		0.13 µg/g creat	
	Endrin	Blood		5 µg/100 ml	
Organophosphorus insecticides	Cholinesterase	Plasma		50% inhibition	
	Cholinesterase	RBC		30% inhibition	
	Cholinesterase	Whole blood		30% inhibition	
	Alkylphosphates	Urine			
Parathion	p-Nitrophenol	Urine		0.5 mg/g creat	
Carbamate insecticides	Cholinesterase	Plasma		50% inhibition	
	Cholinesterase	RBC		30% inhibition	
	Cholinesterase	Whole blood		30% inhibition	
Carbaryl	1-Naphthol	Urine		10 mg/g creat	

Substance	Determinant	Biologic material			Sampling time
2-Isopropoxyphenyl N-Methylcarbamate	Isopropoxyphenol	Urine			
2,4-D	2,4-D	Urine			
2,4,5-T	2,4,5-T	Urine			
DNOC	DNOC	Blood			
Pentachlorophenol	Pentachlorophenol (free)	Urine	<30 μg/g creat	1 mg/100 ml 1 mg/g creat	
Hormones					
Diethylstilbestrol	Diethylstilbestrol			30 mg/g creat	24-hour urine collection
Miscellaneous Substances					
Mutagenic and carcinogenic substances	Mutagenic activity	Urine			
	Thioethers	Urine			
	Chromosome analysis	Lymphocytes			
	Spermatozoa analysis	Sperm			
	Protein adducts	Blood			
	ADN adducts	Lymphocytes			
	Nucleic acid adducts	Urine			
Ethylene oxide	Ethylene oxide	Expired air		0.5 mg/m^3	During exposure
	Ethyleneoxide	Blood		0.8 μg/100 ml	
	N-Acetyl-S-(2-hydroxyethyl) cysteine	Urine			
Phthalic anhydride	Phthalic acid	Urine			
Toluene diisocyanate	Toluene diamine	Urine			

* Analysis performed on biologic materials collected at the end of the workday unless otherwise indicated.

sure, the compounds and/or their metabolites may be rapidly eliminated from the organism. In these cases, the biologic sample is usually collected during exposure, at the end of the exposure period, or sometimes just before the next working shift (16 hours after the end of exposure) or even before resuming work after the weekend (i.e., 60 to 64 hours after the last exposure).

When biologic monitoring consists in sampling and analyzing urine, it is usually performed in "spot" specimens because routine collections of 24-hour samples from workers is impractical (Elkins et al., 1974). It is usually advisable to correct the results for the dilution of the urine. Two methods of correction have been used: (1) expression of the results per gram of creatinine or (2) adjustment to a constant specific gravity. Although there is no general superiority for creatinine adjustment over specific gravity, in general creatinine correction is better for concentrated and dilute samples (Elkins et al., 1974). Furthermore, in the case of glucosuria and probably proteinuria, the specific gravity adjustment may give erroneous results. Whatever the method of correction, analyses performed on very dilute urine samples (specific gravity less than 1.010, creatinine concentration less than 0.3 g/liter) are not reliable and should be repeated. In some circumstances, it may be feasible to report results in excretion rate (i.e., quantity/time unit), which presupposes the collection of urine during a well-defined period of time (e.g., four hours). One must, however, recognize that this method, which is more accurate than spot sample analysis, is usually too elaborate for routine control of worker exposure. Furthermore, there are compounds for which the expression of urinary results in excretion rate does not improve the accuracy of the exposure estimate.

When the large interindividual variability and/or the high "background" level of the biologic parameter selected makes the interpretation of a single measurement difficult, it is sometimes useful to analyze biologic material collected before and after the exposure period. The change in the biologic parameter due specifically to exposure can sometimes be better assessed.

For each chemical agent listed in Table 29–1, the proposed biologic parameters, their normal value, and—when data were available—the tentative maximum permissible values are indicated. The significance of the latter proposals must be kept clearly in mind. They are simply tentative guidelines based on the currently available scientific knowledge. Like the airborne TLVs, these guidelines should be subject to regular revision in the light of new scientific data.

Early Detection of Adverse Effects (Health Surveillance)

A biologic monitoring program designed to evaluate the intensity of exposure of workers to industrial chemicals must always be complemented by a health surveillance program (Figure 29–2). The objective of the latter is to detect as early as possible any adverse biologic and functional effects in exposed workers (e.g., release of hepatic enzymes into the plasma, bronchoconstriction, etc.)—i.e., effects that are likely to be reversible or that do not progress to significant functional impairments when exposure conditions are improved. As defined, health surveillance should not be simply assimilated with diagnosis of occupational diseases, which, of course, is not any more a preventive activity. Such a program should be implemented even when the results of the environmental or biologic monitoring program of exposure indicate that the latter is probably below the acceptable level. Indeed, this level may sometimes contain a large factor of uncertainty, and furthermore, an internal exposure considered safe according to the present state of knowledge may still cause some adverse effects in susceptible individuals. The proposal of tests capable of detecting early adverse biologic effects of industrial chemicals requires a knowledge of their main target organs and their mechanism of action.

A review of the tests available for the early detection of adverse effects to various organs or functions following occupational exposure to chemicals is outside the scope of this chapter. They are covered in previous chapters, and several publications also specifically deal with this biologic monitoring activity (Underhill and Radford 1986; Lauwerys and Bernard 1989).

CONCLUSION

The working environment will always present the risk of workers' overexposure to various chemicals. It is self-evident that the control of these risks cannot wait until epidemiologic studies have defined the no-adverse-effect level directly in man. However, extrapolation from animal data has its limitations. A combined experimental and clinical approach is certainly the most effective for evaluating the potential risks of industrial chemicals—hence, for recommending adequate preventive measures and for applying the most valid screening procedures on workers.

Thus, the field of industrial toxicology provides many opportunities for scientists with different backgrounds (physicians, chemists, biologists, hygienists) who are convinced of the usefulness of working in close collaboration to understand and prevent the adverse effects of industrial chemicals on workers' health.

REFERENCES

Abdel-Rahman, M. S.; Hetland, L. B.; and Couri, D.: Toxicity and metabolism of methyl *n*-butylketone. *Am. Ind. Hyg. Assoc. J.*, **37**:95–102, 1976.

Adamsson, E.; Piscator, M.; and Nogawa, K.: Pulmonary and gastrointestinal exposure to cadmium oxide dust in a battery factory. *Environ. Health Perspect.*, **28**:219–222, 1979.

Aldridge, W. N.; Miles, J. M.; Mount, D. L.; and Verschoyle, R. D.: The toxicological properties of impurities in malathion. *Arch. Toxicol.*, **42**:95–106, 1979.

Allen, N.; Mendell, J. R.; Billmaier, D. J.; Fontaine, R. E.; and O'Neill, J.: Toxic polyneuropathy due to methyl *n*-butylketone. *Arch. Neurol.*, **32**:209–218, 1975.

Baker, E. L.; Zack, M.; Miles, J. V.; Alderman, L.; Warren, Mc. M.; Dobbin, R. D.; Miller, S.; and Teeters, W. R.: Epidemic malathion poisoning in Pakistan malaria workers. *Lancet*, **i**:31–33, 1978.

Barnes, J. M.: The basis for establishing and fixing maximum allowable concentrations. *Trans. Assoc. Ind. Med. Off.*, **13**:74–76, 1963.

Barnes, J. R.; and Henry III, N. W.: The determination of *N*-methylformamide and *N*-methylacetamide in urine. *Am. Ind. Hyg. Assoc. J.*, **35**:84–87, 1974.

Bernard, A., and Lauwerys, R.: Present status and trends in biological monitoring of exposure to industrial chemicals. *J. O. M.*, **28**:559–562, 1986.

———: General principles for biological monitoring of exposure to chemicals. In Ho, M. H., and Millon, H. K. (eds.): *Biological Monitoring of Exposure to Chemicals: Organic Compounds*. John Wiley & Sons, New York, 1987.

Billmaier, D.; Yee, H. T.; Allen, N.; Craft, R.; Williams, N.; Epstein, S.; and Fontaine, R.: Peripheral neuropathy in a coated fabrics plant. *J.O.M.*, **16**:665–671, 1974.

Bolt, H. N.: Metabolism of genotoxic agents: halogenated hydrocarbons. In *Monitoring Human Exposure to Carcinogenic and Mutagenic Agents*. IARC No. 59, 63–72, 1984.

Bonse, G.; Urban, T.; Reichert, D.; and Henschler, D.: Chemical reactivity, metabolic oxirane formation and biological reactivity of chlorinated ethylenes in the isolated perfused rat liver preparation. *Biochem. Pharmacol.*, **24**:1829–1834, 1975.

Buchet, J. P.; Geubel, A.; Pauwels, S.; Mahieu, P.; and Lauwerys, R.: The influence of liver disease on the methylation of arsenic in humans. *Arch. Toxicol.*, **55**:151–154, 1984.

Buchet, J. P., and Lauwerys, R.: Study of inorganic arsenic methylation by rat liver *in vitro*: relevance for the interpretation of observations in man. *Arch. Toxicol.*, **57**:125–129, 1985.

———: Study of factors influencing the *in vivo* methylation of inorganic arsenic in rats. *Toxicol. Appl. Pharmacol.*, **91**:65–74, 1987.

———: Role of thiols in the *in vitro* methylation of inorganic arsenic by rat liver cytosol. *Biochem. Pharmacol.*, **37**:3149–3153, 1988.

Buchet, J. P.; Lauwerys, R.; and Roels, H.: Comparison of several methods for the determination of arsenic compounds in water and in urine. Their application for the study of arsenic metabolism and for the monitoring of workers exposed to arsenic. *Int. Arch. Occup. Environ. Health*, **46**:11–29, 1980.

———: Comparison of the urinary excretion of arsenic metabolites after a single oral dose of sodium arsenite, monomethylarsonate or dimethylarsinate in man. *Int. Arch. Occup. Environ. Health*, **48**:71–79, 1981a.

———: Urinary excretion of inorganic arsenic and its metabolites after repeated ingestion of sodium metaarsenite by volunteers. *Int. Arch. Occup. Environ. Health*, **48**:111–118, 1981b.

Claus, G.; Krisko, I.; and Bolander, K.: Chemical carcinogens in the environment and in the human diet: can a threshold be established? *Food Cosmet. Toxicol.*, **12**:737–746, 1974.

Courtney, K. D., and Moore, J. A.: Teratology studies with 2,4,5-trichlorophenoxyacetic acid and 2,3,7,8-tetrachlorodibenzo-*p*-dioxin. *Toxicol. Appl. Pharmacol.*, **20**:396–403, 1971.

Creech, J. L., and Johnson, H. M.: Angiosarcoma of the liver in the manufacture of polyvinylchloride. *J.O.M.*, **16**:150–151, 1974.

Dekant, W.; Martens, G.; Vamvakas, S.; Metzler, M.; and Henschler, D.: Bioactivation of tetrachloroethylene. *Drug Metab. Dispos.*, **15**:702–709, 1987.

Dekant, W.; Metzler, M.; and Henschler, D.: Identification of *S*-1,2-dichlorovinyl-*N*-acetyl-cysteine as a urinary metabolite of trichloroethylene: a possible explanation for its nephrocarcinogenicity in male rats. *Biochem. Pharmacol.*, **35**:2455–2458, 1986.

Dinman, B. D.: "Non-concept" of "no-threshold" chemicals in the environment. *Science*, **175**:495–497, 1972.

DiVincenzo, G. D.; Hamilton, M. L.; Kaplan, C. J.; and Dedinas, J.: Metabolic fate and disposition of ^{14}C-labeled methyl *n*-butyl ketone in the rat. *Toxicol. Appl. Pharmacol.*, **41**:547–560, 1977.

DiVincenzo, G. D.; Kaplan, C. J.; and Dedinas, J.: Characterization of the metabolites of methyl-*n*-butyl ketone, methyl iso-butyl ketone, and methyl ethyl ketone in guinea pig serum and their clearance. *Toxicol. Appl. Pharmacol.*, **36**:511–522, 1976.

Duckett, S.; Williams, N.; and Francis, S.: Peripheral neuropathy associated with inhalation of methyl *n*-butyl ketone. *Experientia*, **30**(11):1283–1284, 1974.

Elinder, C. G.; Gerhardsson, L.; and Oberdoerster, G.: Biological monitoring of toxic metals—overview. In Clarkson, T. W.; Friberg, L.; Nordberg, G. F.; and Sager, P. L. (eds.): *Biological Monitoring of Toxic Metals*. Plenum Press, New York, 1988, pp. 1–72.

Elkins, H. B.; Pagnotto, L. D.; and Smith, H. L.: Concentration adjustments in urine analysis. *Am. Ind. Hyg. Assoc. J.*, **35**:559–565, 1974.

Emerson, J. L.; Thompson, D. J.; Strebing, R. J.; Gerbig, C. G.; and Robinson, V. B.: Teratogenic studies on 2,4,5-trichlorophenoxyacetic acid in the rat and rabbit. *Food Cosmet. Toxicol.*, **9**:395–404, 1971.

EPA (Environmental Protection Agency): *Health Effects Test Guidelines*. NTIS 560/6–82–001, Springfield, Va., 1982a.

———: *Pesticide Assessment Guidelines Subdivision F. Hazard Evaluation: Human and Domestic Animals.* NTIS 540/9/82–025, Springfield, Va., 1982b.

Flanagan, P. R.; McLellan, J. S.; Haist, J.; Cherian, G.; Chamberlain, H. J.; and Valberg, L. S.: Increased dietary cadmium absorption in mice and human subjects with iron deficiency. *Gastroenterology*, **74**:841–846, 1978.

Henschler, D.: New approaches to a definition of threshold values for "irreversible" toxic effects? *Arch. Toxicol.*, **32**:63–67, 1974.

IARC (International Agency for Research on Cancer): *IARC Monographs on the Evaluation of Carcinogenic Risks to Humans*. Supplement 7, Lyon, France, 1987.

Kimmerle, G., and Eben, A.: Metabolism studies of

N,N-dimethylformamide. I. Studies in rats and dogs. *Int. Arch. Arbeitsmed.,* **34**:109–126, 1975a.

———: Metabolism studies of *N-N*-dimethylformamide. II. Studies in persons. *Int. Arch. Arbeitsmed.,* **14**:127–136, 1975b.

King, E.; Conchie, A.; Hiett, D.; and Milligan, B.: Industrial lead absorption. *Ann. Occup. Hyg.,* **22**:213–239, 1979.

Kociba, R. J.; McCollister, S. B.; Park, C.; Torkelson, T. R.; and Gehring, P. J.: 1,4-Dioxane. I. Results of a 2-year ingestion study in rats. *Toxicol. Appl. Pharmacol.,* **30**:275–286, 1974.

Krivanek, N. D.; McLaughlin, M.; and Fayerweather, W. E.: Monomethylformamide levels in human urine after repetitive exposure to dimethylformamide vapor. *J.O.M.,* **20**:179–182, 1978.

Lauwerys, R.: Experimental and clinical investigations for assessing the toxicological hazards of industrial chemicals. *Proceedings of the Meeting of the Scientific Committee, Carlo Erba Foundation, Occupational and Environmental Health Section,* Milan, 1976, pp. 9–48.

———: Current use of ambient and biological monitoring: reference workplace hazards, cadmium. *International Seminar on the Assessment of Toxic Agents in the Workplace. Roles of Ambient and Biological Monitoring, OSHA, CCE, NIOSH, CCE,* Luxembourg, 1980.

———: Basic concepts of human exposure monitoring. In Berlin, A.; Draper, M.; Hemminki, K.; and Vainio, H. (eds.): *Monitoring Human Exposure to Carcinogenic and Mutagenic Agents.* IARC Scientific Publication No. 59, Lyon, 1984a, pp. 31–36.

———: Objectives of biological monitoring in occupational health practice. In Aitio, A.; *et al.* (eds.): *Biological Monitoring and Surveillance of Workers Exposed to Chemicals.* Hemisphere Publishing Corporation, Washington, D.C., 1984b, pp. 3–6.

———: Dimethylformamide. In Alessio, L; Berlin, A.; Boni, M.; and Roi, R. (eds.): *Biological Indicators for the Assessment of Human Exposure to Industrial Chemicals.* Commission of the European Communities, EUR 10704 EN, Luxembourg, 1986.

Lauwerys, R., and Bernard, A.: La surveillance biologique de l'exposition aux toxiques industriels. Position actuelle et perspectives de développement. *Scand. J. Work Environ. Health,* **11**:155–164, 1985.

———: Preclinical detection of nephrotoxicity: description of the tests and appraisal of their health significance. *Toxicol Lett.,* **46**:13–29, 1989.

Lauwerys, R.; Buchet, J. P.; Roels, H.; Berlin, A.; and Smeets, J.: Intercomparison program of lead, mercury, and cadmium analysis in blood, urine, and aqueous solutions. *Clin. Chem.,* **21**:551–557, 1975.

Lauwerys, R.; Kivits, A.; Lhoir, M.; Rigolet, P.; Houbeau, D.; Buchet, J. P.; and Roels, H.: Biological surveillance of workers exposed to dimethylformamide and the influence of skin protection on its percutaneous absorption. *Int. Arch. Occup. Environ. Health,* **45**:189–203, 1980.

Lewis, T. R.; Morrow, P. E.; McClellan, R. O.; Raabe, O. G.; Kennedy, G. L.; Schwetz, B. A.; Goeht, T. J.; Roycroft, J. H.; and Chhabra, R. S.: Establishing aerosol exposure concentrations for inhalation toxicity studies. *Toxicol. Appl. Pharmacol.,* **99**:377–383, 1989.

Mahieu, P.; Buchet, J. P.; Roels, H.; and Lauwerys, R.: The metabolism of arsenic in humans acutely intoxicated by As$_2$O$_3$. Its significance for the duration of BAL therapy. *Clin. Toxicol.,* **18**:1067–1075, 1981.

Maxfield, M. E.; Barnes, J. R.; Azar, A.; and Trochimowicz, H. T.: Urinary excretion of metabolite following experimental human exposures to DMF or to DMAC. *J.O.M.,* **17**:506–511, 1975.

McDonough, J. R.: Possible neuropathy from methyl *n*-butyl ketone. *N. Engl. J. Med.,* **290**:695, 1974.

Mendell, J. R.; Saida, K.; Ganasia, M. F.; Jackson, D. B.; Weiss, H.; Gardier, R. W.; Christman, C.; Allen, N.; Couri, D.; O'Neill, J.; Marks, B.; and Hetland, L.: Toxic polyneuropathy produced by methyl-*n*-butyl ketone. *Science,* **185**:787–789, 1974.

Monson, R. R.; Peters, J. M.; and Johnson, M. N.: Proportional mortality among vinyl-chloride workers. Lancet, 2(7877):397–398, 1974.

Monster, A. C.; Boersma, G.; and Duba, W. C.: Pharmacokinetics of trichloroethylene in volunteers, influence of workload and exposure concentration. *Int. Arch. Occup. Environ. Health,* **38**:87–102, 1976.

Mraz, J.; Cross, H.; Gescher, A.; Threadgill, M. D.; and Flek, J.: Differences between rodents and humans in the metabolic toxification of *N,N*-dimethylformamide. *Toxicol. Appl. Pharmacol.,* **98**:507–516, 1989.

NTP (National Toxicology Program): *General Statement of Work for the Conduct of Toxicity and Carcinogenicity Studies in Laboratory Animals.* DHHS, Public Health Service, National Institutes of Health, 1987.

OECD (Organization for Economic Cooperation and Development): *OECD Guidelines for Testing Chemicals.* Paris, France, 1987.

Riihimaki, V.; Pfaffli, P.; and Savolainen, K.: Kinetics of *m*-xylene in man. Influence of intermittent physical exercise and changing environmental concentrations on kinetics. *Scand. J. Work Environ. Health,* **5**:232–248, 1979.

Rinksy, R. A.; Smith, A. B.; Hornuing, R.; Filloon, T. G.; Young, R. J.; Okun, A. H.; and Landrigan, P. M.: Benzene and leukemia. An epidemiologic risk assessment. *New Engl. J. Med.,* **316**:1044–1049, 1987.

Roels, H.; Buchet, J. P.; Truc, J.; Croquet, F.; and Lauwerys, R.: The possible role of direct ingestion on the overall absorption of cadmium or arsenic in workers exposed to CdO or As$_2$O$_3$ dust. *Am. J. Ind. Med.,* **3**:53–65, 1982.

Scailteur, V.; Buchet, J. P.; and Lauwerys, R.: The relationship between dimethylformamide metabolism and toxicity. In Brown, S. S., and Davies, D. S. (eds.): *Organ-Directed Toxicity, Chemical Indices and Mechanisms.* Pergamon Press, Oxford, 1981, pp. 169–174.

Scailteur, V.; de Hoffmann, E.; Buchet, J. P.; and Lauwerys, R.: Study on *in vivo* and *in vitro* metabolism of dimethylformamide in male and female rats. *Toxicology,* **29**:221–234, 1984.

Scailteur, V., and Lauwerys, R.: *In vivo* and *in vitro* oxidative biotransformation of dimethylformamide in rat. *Chem. Biol. Int.,* **50**:327–337, 1984a.

———: *In vivo* metabolism of dimethylformamide and relationship to toxicity in the male rat. *Arch. Toxicol.,* **56**:87–91, 1984b.

Spencer, P. S., and Schaumburg, H. H.: Experimental neuropathy produced by 2,5-hexanedione—a major metabolite of the neurotoxic industrial solvent methyl *n*-butyl ketone. *J. Neurol. Neurosurg. Psychiatry,* **38**:771–775, 1975.

Spencer, P. S.; Schaumburg, H. H.; Raleigh, R. L.; and Terhaar, C. J.: Nervous system degeneration produced by the industrial solvent methyl *n*-butyl ketone. *Arch. Neurol.,* **32**:219–222, 1975.

Uehleke, H.; Tabarelli-Poplawski, S.; Bonse, G.; and Henschler, D.: Spectral evidence for 2,2,3-trichlorooxirane formation during microsomal trichloroethylene oxidation. *Arch. Toxicol.,* **37**:95–105, 1977.

Underhill, D. W., and Radford, E. P. (eds.): *New and Sensitive Indicators of Health Impacts of Environmen-*

tal Agents. Published by University of Pittsburgh, Graduate School of Public Health, Center for Environmental Epidemiology, Pittsburgh, 1986.

Viola, P. L.; Bigotti, A.; and Caputo, A.: Oncogenic response of rat skin, lungs, and bones to vinyl chloride. *Cancer Res.*, **31**:516–522, 1971.

Woo, Y. T.; Arcos, J. C.; and Argus, M. F.: Metabolism *in vivo* of dioxane: identification of *p*-dioxane-2-one as the major urinary metabolite. *Biochem. Pharmacol.*, **26**:1535–1538, 1977.

Young, J. D.; Braun, W. H.; Gehring, P. J.; Horvath, B. S.; and Daniel, R. L.: 1,4-Dioxane and β-hydroxyethoxyacetic acid excretion in urine of humans exposed to dioxane vapors. *Toxicol. Appl. Pharmacol.*, **38**:643–646, 1976a.

Young, J. D.; Braun, W. H.; LeBeau, J. E.; and Gehring, P. J.: Saturated metabolism as the mechanism for the dose dependent fate of 1,4-dioxane in rats. *Toxicol. Appl. Pharmacol.*, **37**:138, 1976b.

Zielhuis, R. L.: Biological monitoring: guest lecture given at the 26th Nordic Symposium on Industrial Hygiene, Helsinki, October 1977. *Scand. J. Work Environ. Health*, **4**:1–18, 1978.

———: General aspects of biological monitoring. In Berlin, A.; Wolff, A. H.; and Hasegawa, Y. (eds.): *The Use of Biological Specimens for the Assessment of Human Exposure to Environmental Pollutants*. Proceedings of the International Workshop at Luxembourg, 18–22 April 1977. Martinus Nijhoff Publishers, The Hague, 1979, p. 341.

Chapter 30

REGULATORY TOXICOLOGY

Richard A. Merrill

THE ROLES OF SCIENCE AND REGULATION

This chapter deals with the use by governmental regulatory agencies of the results of toxicological studies and with the requirements that they impose for the conduct of such studies. Scientists are often dismayed by what they regard as the distortion of scientific principles or misinterpretation of experimental data in the regulatory process, and there is no question that the process sometimes mistreats the work of the scientific community. This chapter does not attempt to justify the handling of toxicology by government agencies but rather seeks to explain how science and regulation relate to each other.

One must start by recognizing a central difference between the goals of science and the goals of government: Science investigates and attempts to explain natural phenomena; it is cautious, incremental, and truth seeking. Government regulation seeks to affect human behavior and settle human disputes; it is episodic and peremptory and seeks resolution rather than truth. A regulator frequently cannot withhold a decision about a problem even when the facts appear to call for delay, for even a decision to withhold judgment, e.g., on whether saccharin poses a risk of human cancer—has real-world consequences. Allowing saccharin to remain on the market means that consumers will continue to be exposed to a substance that may be harmful, though they enjoy its benefits. If the compound under consideration, e.g., a substitute sweetner, is not being marketed, postponing a decision will delay enjoyment of its benefits while averting perhaps only a trivial risk. Because toxicology is continuously generating information about the effects of chemicals, though less often providing definitive conclusions about their magnitude or frequency, regulators are invariably forced to intervene, i.e., to decide, before knowledge is complete. This imperative frequently gives regulatory decisions the appearance of prematurity in the eyes of scientists.

Scientists are often frustrated by another feature of American regulatory decision making. As a nation, we accord government officials less discretion—i.e., less room for only politically constrained judgment—than any other industrialized society. We insist that government actions affecting private interests satisfy the "rule of law." At a minimum, this means that they be of a kind authorized by the legislature and that they rest on the factual predicate specified by the legislature for such decisions. Furthermore, we require regulators to set forth the facts on which they rely and allow opponents numerous opportunities to contest those facts. Participants in the regulatory process start from the assumption that the available evidence, however thin, can fairly be construed in the light most favorable to their position. Regulators thus often overstate the evidence for their decisions, just as do those who challenge them, with the result that both sometimes distort current knowledge.

A third source of conflict is the propensity of legislators to pay little attention to what science is capable of determining when they establish criteria for regulatory decision making. They attempt to enunciate standards that make sense in political or social terms. Thus, according to Congress, no pesticide may cause "unreasonable adverse effects on health or the environment" (Federal Insecticide, Fungicide, and Rodenticide Act [FIFRA], 1972), and "*no* worker" may be put at risk of material health impairment "to the extent [it is] feasible" to prevent it (Occupational Safety and Health Act [OSHA], 1970). These statutory standards describe desirable social outcomes, but they may demand more of science than it can provide. Regulators cannot change the law they are given, however, so they may translate preliminary experimental findings or tentative hypotheses into the proven facts they believe legally necessary to support a decision.

RELATIONSHIPS BETWEEN TOXICOLOGY AND REGULATION

The foregoing observations could apply to any scientific discipline whose investigations underpin governmental decision making. But over the past two decades regulation and toxicology have become intertwined in distinctive ways. The most obvious connection is that regulators whose job is to protect health rely heavily on toxicological concepts and experimental data in reaching decisions. Whether the decision is to assign priorities among a group of compounds, to approve a new substance, or to restrict an old one, toxicological findings are likely to be influential, often decisive.

Regulators thus use toxicology, but they are not merely consumers of experimental results. Regulatory demands have provided a major impetus for improvements in toxicological methods and have been a major stimulus for toxicological studies. Some programs, like the Food and Drug Administration's (FDA) programs for licensing drugs and food additives and the Environmental Protection Agency's (EPA) program for registering pesticides, explicitly demand toxicological studies of new, and in some cases marketed, compounds. Such studies constitute a major part of the discipline's research agenda. But even if no government agency were empowered to demand toxicological studies, concern for public health and worries about civil liability would lead marketers of new products to turn to toxicology to evaluate their possible health hazards. The line between studies that government has formally mandated and those that the law has merely encouraged is accordingly difficult to discern.

Regulatory agencies have also exercised important influence over the design and conduct of toxicological studies; i.e., they have affected the internal workings of the discipline. For example, the EPA is empowered by the Toxic Substances Control Act to promulgate standards for different types of toxicological (and other scientific) investigations required or volunteered to aid its decision making (Toxic Substances Control Act [TSCA], 1976). The FDA has long maintained guidelines for laboratory studies submitted in support of food additives and drugs. And both agencies have adopted requirements governing laboratory operations and practice.

Communication between government officials and laboratory scientists works both ways. Government testing standards are powerfully influenced by the prevailing consensus among toxicologists, many of whom work in regulatory agencies. The procedures for adopting such standards always permit, if they do not always encourage, the expression of views by representatives of the discipline. Those views, moreover, can sometimes be decisive, for regulators are often as interested in establishing *some* fixed measure of performance as in selecting *a particular* measure.

The balance of this chapter focuses on the first and second of these prominent linkages between toxicology and regulation. The next part outlines the legal and administrative contexts in which regulators rely on toxicological data in making critical social and commercial decisions. The focus in the final part is on government as a regulator of toxicology, i.e., as the source of guidance for and limitations on the design and conduct of laboratory experiments. The chapter does not purport to provide a comprehensive treatment of legal and regulatory requirements that impinge on toxicology, nor does it discuss every program that relies on toxicological data. It also omits such topics as law and regulations designed to protect laboratory personnel, legal restrictions on the handling of dangerous substances, and local requirements for the operation of laboratories. Space simply does not allow discussion of these ancillary, yet important, topics.

REGULATORY PROGRAMS THAT RELY ON TOXICOLOGY

Overview of Approaches to Toxic Chemical Regulation

This part surveys current federal programs for controlling human exposure to toxic chemicals. While its primary focus is the legal standards that govern agency decision making, attention is also given to the commercial context and effects of agency decisions. The discussion highlights features of regulatory programs that influence both the quantity and quality of data necessary to support an agency's decisions.

One such feature, often overlooked by nonlawyers, is the law's allocation of the "burden of proof," i.e., the responsibility for demonstrating that a substance is safe or hazardous. The range of possible approaches can be observed by comparing laws such as the Food Additives Amendment, which requires users of new substances to prove lack of hazard *before* humans may be exposed, with laws such as the Occupational Safety and Health Act, which requires regulators to show that a substance is hazardous *before* exposures can be restricted. The approach chosen by Congress largely determines an agency's ability to require comprehensive toxicological investigation of compounds and thus affects the quality of data on which decisions ultimately are based.

A parallel distinction, observable in programs that mandate premarket testing of new products, is that between substances not yet on the market and those approved some time before on the basis of studies that inevitably appear inadequate as investigatory methods improve. The law may specifiy that the burden of proving safety in principle always rests with the commercial sponsor of a substance, but as a practical matter, the agency has the burden at least of demonstrating sufficient doubt about the safety of an approved substance to justify reexamination.

Typology of Regulatory Approaches. At least two issues must be resolved to justify government action to regulate human exposure to a substance. First, it must be determined that the substance is capable of harming persons who may be exposed. Second, it must be determined that humans are likely to be exposed to the substance in ways that could be harmful. In the absence of affirmative answers to both questions, government intervention to control exposure would be difficult to justify. A few statutes require only these two findings, but most laws under which chemicals are regulated mandate or permit consideration of other criteria as well, such as the magnitude of the risk posed by a substance and the consequences of regulating it.

Agencies Involved. At the federal level, four agencies are chiefly responsible for regulating human exposure to chemicals: the FDA, the EPA, the Occupational Safety and Health Administration (OSHA), and the Consumer Product Safety Commission (CPSC). Together they administer some two-dozen statutes whose primary goal is protection of health. It may seem that the nation lacks a coherent policy toward chemical hazards, and the statutes administered by these four agencies do indeed convey different levels of concern about risks to human health and about the weight to be given economic costs (OTA, 1981). This diversity has several explanations. The statutes were enacted in different eras. They originated with, and remain under the influence of, different political constituencies. Furthermore, statutory standards often reflect differences in the technical capacity to control different types of exposures and embody different congressional judgments about their economic benefits.

Summary of Current Approaches. For at least two decades, federal regulatory agencies (and occasionally Congress) have distinguished between cancer and all other toxic effects. And it is in their treatment of carcinogens that existing statutes appear to display the greatest diversity. For other chemicals, which we might characterize as conventional toxicants, regulators have generally embraced a standard safety assessment formula, built around the concept of "acceptable daily intake" (ADI). The ADI for a chemical is derived by applying a safety factor—usually 100, but sometimes a larger number if the toxicological data are sparse and occasionally a smaller number if the data are very good—to the human equivalent of the lowest no-observed-effect level (NOEL) revealed in animal ex-

periments. When estimated human exposure to a chemical falls below the ADI, it—or the usage that results in that exposure—is adjudged "safe." It is only when exposure is likely to exceed the ADI that the regulator must turn to any other considerations made relevant by the applicable statute.

But this traditional approach to conventional toxicants has not been considered appropriate for carcinogens. U.S. regulators, and many of their counterparts in other countries, have operated on the premise that carcinogens as a class cannot be assumed to have "safe" or threshold doses. Furthermore, they have assumed that any chemical shown convincingly in animal studies to cause cancer should be considered a potential human carcinogen. Accordingly, for this group of compounds—a group that has grown as more chemicals have been subjected to long-term testing—U.S. regulators have assumed that no finite level of human exposure can be considered risk-free. This set of assumptions has profoundly affected the way carcinogenic chemicals have been evaluated and regulated in this country.

No Risk. This approach is epitomized by the famous Delaney Clause, enacted in 1958 as part of the Food Additives Amendment. The amendment itself requires that any food additive be found "safe" before the FDA may approve its use (FD&C Act, 1958). The Delaney proviso stipulates that this finding cannot be made for a food additive that has been shown to induce cancer in man or in experimental animals. The Delaney Clause has been characterized as a categorical risk-benefit judgment by Congress that no food additive is likely to offer benefits sufficient to outweigh any risk of cancer (Turner, 1971). Section 112 of the Clean Air Act has also been characterized as adopting an analogous "no-risk" standard for toxic air pollutants (Reed, 1986), but such standards are not typical of federal health laws.

Negligible Risk. Because the risk posed by a toxic substance depends on the dose, as well as its potency, it is sometimes possible to reduce human exposure to such low levels that any associated risk is small enough to ignore without considering any other criteria. No current health statute prescribes such a "negligible risk" approach, but both the EPA and the FDA have adopted it administratively for some classes of environmental carcinogens. For example, under a 1962 amendment to the Delaney Clause, the FDA may approve a carcinogenic drug for use in food-producing animals if "no residue" will be "found" in edible tissues of treated animals (FD&C Act). The FDA announced that it will calibrate its efforts to search for residues to carcinogenic potency (FDA, 1985) and will approve a carcinogenic drug if the sponsor provides an analytic method capable of detecting residues in meat, milk, or eggs large enough to pose a lifetime dietary risk of greater than 1 in 1,000,000, as determined by extrapolation from animal bioassays. The EPA has embraced a comparable standard for regulating residues of carcinogenic pesticides (EPA, 1988).

Any such "negligible risk" approach requires data depicting carcinogenic potency. This is not a major problem where an agency can require a product's sponsor to conduct the necessary tests, but programs in which regulation responds to exposures that are already occurring often lack such leverage. The approach also requires the selection of a method for quantifying the risk associated with low doses of a carcinogen. Furthermore, as a practical matter, such an approach will not suffice where exposures to toxic substances cannot be reduced to very low levels without sacrificing other values.

Trade-off Approaches. This heading embraces several different verbal formulas that have one common feature: Each requires the regulatory agency to weigh factors in addition to the health risks posed by substances targeted for regulation. These factors can moderate the desire to prevent human illness. One version is illustrated by the Occupational Safety and Health Act that directs OSHA, in setting workplace standards for toxic materials, to elect the standard "which most adequately assures, to the extent feasible . . . that no employee will suffer material impairment of health or functional capacity" (OSHA, 1970). OSHA has interpreted "feasibility" as requiring it to consider, in addition to the risk posed by a substance, the availability of technology for reducing exposure and the financial ability of the responsible industries to pay for the necessary controls. The Supreme Court has made clear, however, that the agency need not balance the health benefits of mandated exposure controls against the costs of achieving them (*American Textile Manufacturers Institute v. Donovan*, 1982).

A more expansive "trade-off" law is the Federal Insecticide, Fungicide, and Rodenticide Act (FIFRA), which requires the EPA to refuse or withdraw registration of a pesticide if it finds that its use is likely to result in "unreasonable adverse effects on health or the environment" (FIFRA, 1972). The agency interprets this language as requiring that it weigh all the effects of a pesticide—its contribution to food production as well as its possible adverse effects on applicators, consumers, and the natural environment—in determining whether, or on what terms, to permit registration. FIFRA is not unique; the Toxic Substances Control Act (TSCA, 1976) mandates balancing of risks and benefits in more explicit language.

Current Programs for Regulating Chemical Hazards

Food and Drug Administration. The oldest of the major health regulation laws, the Food, Drug, and Cosmetic Act, was enacted in 1938 and covers food for humans and animals, human and veterinary drugs, medical devices, and cosmetics.

Food. The original 1906 Food and Drugs Act contained two prohibitions addressed to foods containing hazardous constituents; both remain part of the current law. The first forbids the marketing of any food containing "any *added* poisonous or deleterious *substance which may render it injurious* to health," a provision that the FDA has interpreted as barring foods presenting any serious risk. The second forbids the marketing of foods containing *nonadded* toxicants, i.e., natural agricultural commodities, which make them "*ordinarily injurious* to health," a standard according preferred status to traditional components of the American diet (FD&C Act § 402(a)). Neither of these original provisions required premarket approval; the FDA had the burden of proving that a food was adulterated.

Congress has since amended the act several times to improve the FDA's ability to ensure the safety of foods. Each time, it identified a class of "added" substances for which it prescribed a form of premarket approval, thus giving the FDA the authority not only to evaluate a substance's safety before humans are exposed but also to prescribe the kinds of studies necessary to obtain approval (FDA, 1989).

The most important of these amendments was the 1958 Food Additives Amendment. For substances classified as "food additives," the law requires safety to be demonstrated prior to marketing. As noted above, the critical standard for approval is "reasonably certain to be safe"; no inquiry into the benefits of an additive is undertaken or authorized (Cooper, 1978). But the amendment does not apply to all food ingredients. Congress excluded substances that are "generally recognized as safe" (GRAS) by qualified scientific experts. In effect, it instructed the FDA to pay less attention to ingredients that had been in use for many years without observable adverse effects. Congress also excepted ingredients "sanctioned" by either the FDA or the USDA prior to 1958. This category includes some controversial substances, including sodium nitrite used in curing meat products. The practical significance of this exception is that a "prior-sanctioned" ingredient is not subject to the Delaney Clause because it is not a "food additive" in the legal sense.

Three classes of "indirect" food constituents—pesticide residues, animal drug residues, and food contact materials—are subject to distinct regulatory standards. Pesticide residues on raw agricultural commodities are regulated by the EPA under a 1954 amendment to the FD&C Act, which requires advance approval, in the form of a tolerance, for any pesticide residue (FD&C Act § 348). The statute allows the agency to consider both the potential adverse health effects of residues and the value of pesticide uses. Any animal drug residue must be shown to be safe for humans under essentially the same standards that apply to food additives, except that, as noted earlier, the FDA has interpreted the 1962 authorization for approval of carcinogenic compounds "if . . . no residue of the additive will be found" as allowing residues that pose no more than a negligible risk. A food contact substance requires approval as a "food additive" if, when used as intended, it "may reasonably be expected to become a component of food." But the Delaney Clause appears to preclude approval if the material induces cancer, as some important food-packaging materials, such as acrylonitrile and polyvinylchloride, clearly do. The FDA has attempted to cushion this collision between toxicological findings and advances in analytic chemistry by holding that carcinogenic migrants whose extrapolated risk does not exceed 1 in 1,000,000 be considered *"de minimus"* and ignored (FDA, 1984).

Environmental contaminants constitute the final category of food constituents of concern to the FDA. The FDA relies on a provision of the 1938 act that authorizes the establishment of tolerances for "added poisonous or deleterious substances" that cannot be avoided through good manufacturing practice. In setting such tolerances, the FDA weights three factors: (1) the health effects of the contaminant, usually estimated on the basis of animal data: (2) the ability to measure the contaminant; and (3) the effects of various tolerance levels on the price and availability of the food (Merrill and Schewel, 1980). Because contaminants have no commercial proponents, the FDA must assemble its own supporting data from the scientific literature and its own laboratories.

Human Drugs. Preclinical studies play an important role in the FDA's evaluation of human drugs. The current law requires premarket approval, for both safety and efficacy, of all "new" drugs, a category that embraces virtually all prescription drug ingredients introduced since 1938 (Merrill and Hutt, 1980). Investigation of therapeutic agents in humans has long been accepted, and consequently the primary evidence of safety comes from clinical and not laboratory studies. However, animal studies are the sole source of information about a substance's biologic effects when human trials are begun, and their results influence not only the decision whether to expose human subjects but also the design of clinical protocols (FDA, 1989). Long-term animal studies may also be the basis for FDA-mandated warnings in the approved labeling for marketed drugs.

Medical Devices. In 1976, Congress overhauled the FD&C Act's requirements for medical devices, according the FDA major new authority to regulate their testing, marketing, and use. The elaborate new scheme contemplates three tiers of control, calibrated to the health risks posed by a device, the most restrictive of which is premarket approval similar to that required for new drugs. To obtain FDA approval of a so-called class III device, the sponsor must demonstrate safety and efficacy. The bulk of the data supporting such applications will be derived from clinical investigations but will also include toxicological studies of any constituents likely to be absorbed by the patient.

Cosmetics. Laboratory studies lie at the heart of the FDA's regulation of cosmetic safety. The statutory provisions governing cosmetics do not require premarket approval of any product or demand that manufacturers test their products for safety, though most manufacturers routinely do so. The basic safety standard for cosmetics is similar to that for food ingredients; no product may be marketed if it contains "a poisonous or deleterious substance which may render it injurious to health" (FD&C Act § 601(a)). The case law establishes that this language, too, bars distribution of a product posing any significant risk of more than transitory harm when used as intended, but it places on the FDA the burden of proving violations (Merrill and Hutt, 1980). The FDA has brought few cases under this standard, in part because acute toxic reactions are readily detected and immediately result in abandonment of the offending ingredient. The market might not respond in the same way to marketing of a chronically toxic ingredient, and the FDA's current position can be characterized as opposing the use of any ingredient that may cause cancer ("Lead Acetate," 1980).

While the law does not require premarket proof of safety for cosmetic ingredients generally, it does mandate safety testing for color additives, several of which are important ingredients in cosmetics (as well as foods and drugs). The scheme enacted by Congress in 1960 (FD&C Act § 706) resembles that for food additives, except that no colors are exempt; every color additive must be shown, with "reasonable certainty," to be safe. A separate version of the Delaney Clause precludes approval of any carcinogenic color additive, no matter how small a risk it presents (*Public Citizen v. Young, 1987*).

Environmental Protection Agency. Created by Presidential Executive Order in 1970, the EPA immediately became responsible for administering numerous existing laws protecting human health and the environment. Congress has since enacted almost a dozen additional statutes that provide the core of the EPA's current authority. A comprehensive review of the EPA's programs is not possible here; the following summary focuses on those EPA activities in which toxicological evidence plays a central role: pesticide regulation, regulation of industrial chemicals, regulation of drinking water supplies, hazardous waste control, and regulation of toxic pollutants of water and of air.

Pesticides. Under the Federal Insecticide, Fungicide, and Rodenticide Act (FIFRA), no pesticide may be marketed unless it has been registered by the EPA. The law specifies that a pesticide shall be registered if it is effective, bears proper labeling, and "when properly used . . . will not generally cause unreasonable adverse effects on the environment" (FIFRA § 136b). Congress defined this last criterion as "any unreasonable risk to man or the environment, taking into account the economic, social and environmental costs and benefits of the use of any pesticide." Most of the data supporting initial registration—mainly toxicological studies —are provided by the sponsor, which ostensibly retains a continuous burden of proving that its product is safe enough to remain on the market.

In the early 1970s, the EPA engendered controversy by canceling registrations for a number of pesticides based primarily on studies suggesting they were carcinogenic in animals. Criticsm of its "hair-trigger" approach to regulation, coupled with court rulings that the agency was obligated to initiate the process of cancellation whenever a pesticide's safety came into question, led to important changes in the law. Congress added procedural safeguards for pesticide manufacturers and created a panel of outside scientists to review contemplated actions against toxic pesticides (FIFRA, 1972). The EPA itself established a procedure, now named "special review," for public ventilation of disputes over the risks and benefits of pesticides before the formal cancellation process is undertaken (EPA, 1980). A pesticide will be subjected to close scrutiny if the EPA concludes that it causes significant acute toxicity in humans or induces cancer in experimental mammalian species or in man. The agency has published general guidelines for

assessing whether a pesticide—or any other substance—poses a cancer risk to humans (EPA, 1984). Even if a pesticide is convincingly shown to be a carcinogen, however, the law would allow it to be registered if the EPA concluded that its economic benefits outweighed the risk.

The EPA has for the past decade been engaged in a comprehensive review of previously registered pesticides and "reregistration" of those that meet contemporary standards for marketing. Under this program, many older pesticides have been subjected to comprehensive toxicological testing, including carcinogenicity testing, for the first time, and the results have required modification of the terms of approved use and, in some instances, cancellation for several agents. In 1988, Congress amended the law to require the EPA to accelerate this reregistration effort (FIFRA Amendments, 1988). The agency was specifically requested to "intensify" its requirements for neurotoxic and behavioral testing, "including testing related to chronic exposure, prenatal, and neonatal effects."

Toxic Substances. The Toxic Substances Control Act (TSCA, 1976) represents Congress's most ambitious effort to control the hazards of chemicals in commercial production. The TSCA covers all chemical substances manufactured or processed in or imported into the United States—except for substances already regulated under other laws. A *chemical substance* is defined broadly as "any organic or inorganic substance of a particular molecular identity."

The TSCA gives the EPA three main powers. The agency is empowered to restrict, including banning the manufacture, processing, distribution, use, or disposal of a chemical substance when there is a "reasonable basis" to conclude any such activity poses an "unreasonable risk of injury to health or environment." In determining whether a chemical substance presents an unreasonable risk, the agency is instructed (TSCA § 6) to consider:

> the effects of such substance or mixture on the health and the magnitude of the exposure of human beings to such substance or mixture; the effects of such substance or mixture on the environment and the magnitude of the exposure of the environment to such substance or mixture; the benefits of such substance for various uses and the availability of substitutes; and the reasonably ascertainable economic consequences of the rule, after consideration of the effect on the national economy, small business, technological innovation, the environment and public health.

The EPA must also consider any rule's positive impact on the development and use of substitutes as well as its negative impact on manufacturers or processors of the chemical and weigh the economic savings to society resulting from reduction of the risk.

If the EPA suspects that a chemical *may* pose an unreasonble risk but lacks sufficient data to take action, the TSCA empowers it to require testing to develop the necessary data. It may similarly order testing if the chemical will be produced in substantial quantities that may result in siginificant human exposure whose effects cannot be predicted on the basis of existing data. In either case, the EPA must consider the "relative costs of the various test protocols and methodologies" and the "reasonably foreseeable availability of the facilities and personnel" needed to perform the tests (TSCA § 4).

Finally, to enable the EPA to evaluate chemicals before humans are exposed, the TSCA requires the manufacturer of a new chemical substance to notify the agency 90 days prior to production or distribution (TSCA § 5(a)(1)). The manufacturer's or distributor's notice must include any health effects data it possesses. However, the EPA is not empowered to require that manufacturers routinely conduct testing of all new chemicals to permit an evaluation of their risks; Congress declined to confer that kind of premarket approval authority that the FDA exercises for drugs and food additives and EPA exercises for pesticides.

Hazardous Wastes. Several statutes administered by the EPA regulate land disposal of hazardous materials. The principal law is the Resource Conservation and Recovery Act (RCRA), enacted in 1976. The RCRA established a comprehensive federal scheme for regulating hazardous waste, which is defined as any waste material, in solid, liquid, semisolid, or gaseous form, that "may . . . (a) cause, or significantly contribute to an increase in mortality or an increase in serious irreversible, or incapacitating reversible, illness; or (b) pose a substantial present or potential hazard to human health or to the environment when improperly treated, stored, transported, or disposed of, or otherwise managed." Directed to promulgate criteria for identifying hazardous wastes, the EPA has specified ignitability, corrosivity, reactivity, and toxicity. The agency identified accepted protocols for determining these characteristics and established a list of substances whose presence will make waste hazardous.

The RCRA directs the EPA to regulate the activities of generators, transporters, and those who treat, store, or dispose of hazardous wastes. Standards applicable to generators, transporters, and handlers of hazardous wastes must "protect human health and the environment." EPA's regulations applicable to generators and transporters establish a manifest system that is designed to create a paper trail for every shipment of waste, from generator to final destination, to ensure proper handling and accountability. The agency has the broadest authority over persons who own or operate hazardous waste treatment, storage, or disposal facilities. Pursuant to the RCRA, it issued regulations prescribing methods for treating, storing, and disposing of wastes; governing the location, design, and construction of facilities; mandating contingency plans to minimize negative impacts from such facilities; setting qualifications for ownership, training, and financial responsibility; and requiring permits for all such facilities (EPA, 1988).

Toxic Water Pollutants. The EPA has had responsibility for regulating toxic water pollutants since 1972, but the practical problems of controlling discharges and the dilemmas presented by presumptively "no-threshold" carcinogens have proved frustrating. As originally enacted, Section 307 of the Federal Water Pollution Control Act required the EPA to publish within 90 days, and periodically add to, a list of toxic pollutants for which effluent standards (discharge limits) would then be established. According to the act:

> The term "toxic pollutant" means those pollutants, or combination of pollutants, including disease-causing agents, which after discharge and upon exposure, ingestion, inhalation or assimilation into any organism, either directly from the environment or indirectly by ingestion, through food chains, will on the basis of information available to the Administrator, cause death, disease, behavioral abnormalities, cancer, genetic mutation, physiological malfunctions (including malfunctions in reproduction) or physical deformations, in such organisms or their offspring.

Section 307(a)(4) specified that in establishing standards for any listed pollutant the EPA was to provide an *"ample margin of safety"*—a difficult criterion to meet for most toxic pollutants and arguably impossible for any known to be carcinogenic. The law mandated both a rapid timetable and complex procedure for standard setting: An effluent standard had to be proposed within 180 days of a pollutant's being listed, a hearing was to be held within 30 days, and a final standard was to be promulgated no more than six months later.

EPA's slow-paced implementation of these instructions precipitated a series of lawsuits. After first being sued for failure to list any pollutants, the agency published a list of nine—four pesticides (DDT, aldrin/dieldrin, toxaphene, and endrin) and five other substances (mercury, cadmium, cyanide, benzidine, and PCBs)—for which it proposed effluent standards. The public hearing brought forth claims that technology did not exist to monitor or detect the pollutants at low levels and that the limits proposed would shut down major American industries. EPA's withdrawal of the proposed standards in 1976 provoked a new round of lawsuits by environmental groups.

The agency eventually reached a court-sanctioned settlement that fundamentally altered federal policy toward toxic pollutants of the nation's waterways. The settlement allowed the EPA to act under other provisions of the act that permit industrywide effluent standards and allow consideration of economic costs and technological feasibility in setting limits. The settlement also simplified the procedures for promulgating standards and permitted dischargers three years to comply. Congress incorporated the terms of this settlement in 1977 amendments to the statute, which mandated technology-based, industrywide limits for toxic pollutants but allowed the EPA to prescribe more stringent controls when necessary to protect health—something it rarely did.

In 1987, Congress again amended the Federal Water Pollution Control Act to tighten regulation of various pollution sources and to toughen standards for toxic pollutants. Under the 1977 law, the EPA had, in addition to prescribing technology-based effluent limits for a handful of pollutants, developed health-based "water quality criteria" for 126 compounds it had identified as toxic. These criteria essentially described *desirable* maximum contamination levels, which, because the EPA's discharge limits were technology-based, generally were substantially lower than the levels actually achieved. The 1987 amendments gave these heretofore advisory criteria real bite by requiring that states (a) incorporate them in their own mandatory standards for water quality and (b) impose on individual dischargers additional effluent limits in order to achieve them (Heineck, 1989).

Drinking Water. The 1974 Safe Drinking Water Act (SDWA) was enacted to ensure that public water supply systems "meet minimum national standards for the protection of public health." Under the SDWA, the EPA is required to regulate any contaminants "which may have an adverse effect on human health." In this context, too, from the beginning the EPA accepted the premise that there is no safe level of exposure to a carcinogen, but it also recognized that the costs of controlling human exposure could not be unreasonable. Under the act, the EPA was to establish national primary drinking water regulations for public water systems. For each contaminant of concern, the agency was to prescribe a maximum contaminant level (MCL) or a treatment technique for its control.

The 1974 act prescribed a two-stage process. The EPA was first required to promulgate interim national primary drinking water regulations, whose purpose was to establish quickly uniform minimum standards that would "protect health to the extent feasible . . . (taking costs into consideration)." These interim regulations were later supplanted by regulations formulated on the basis of a series of reports by the National Academy of Sciences (NAS). The charge to the NAS Safe Drinking Water Committee was to recommend the MCLs necessary to protect humans from any known or anticipated adverse health effects. In turn, the EPA was to specify MCLs as close as "feasible" to the levels recommended by the NAS. By 1986, the EPA had established MCLs for 23 contaminants but treatment techniques for none.

That year Congress amended the Safe Drinking Water Act to cover more contaminants, to apply more pressure to states and localities to clean up their drinking water supplies, and to strengthen EPA's enforcement role. The EPA was required within three years to adopt regulations for a total of 83 contaminants (including all but one of those originally regulated). It was directed to prescribe regulations for two treatment techniques for public water systems—filtration and disinfection. And in translating recommended MCLs (now maximum contaminant level goals) into "feasible" (and enforcible) regulations, the EPA was directed to assume installation of the best available technology (Gray, 1986).

Toxic Air Pollutants. Section 112 of the Clean Air Act (CAA) directs the EPA to publish a list of pollutants that "cause or contribute to air pollution which may reasonably be anticipated to result in an increase in mortality or an increase in serious irreversible, or incapacitating reversible, illness." The EPA then must establish national emissions standards for sources that emit any substance listed as a hazardous air pollutant. Any standard must provide "an ample margin of safety to protect the public health from such hazardous air pollutants." The implication of this language that standards for hazardous pollutants were to be set without regard to the costs of emissions control from the beginning has generated intense debate over the EPA's efforts to implement this provision.

The EPA proposed a policy for regulating airborne carcinogens in October 1979 (EPA, 1979). The agency argued that a toxic pollutant should, notwithstanding the statute's comprehensive mandate, be listed under Section 112 only if there were evidence either of significant public exposure from stationary source emissions or of a significant risk to groups likely to be exposed. Risk assessment would determine priorites for regulating source categories that posed significant health risks. The proposal contemplated use of the "best available technology" (BAT) to control emissions, with more stringent controls to eliminate any "unreasonable residual risks."

The Reagan administration did not adopt EPA's 1979 proposal, but it likewise declined to interpret Section 112 as requiring emission controls sufficient to prevent all risks from carcinogenic pollutants, regardless of cost. In 1986 the agency's standard for vinyl chloride was set aside by a reviewing court because it had improperly taken cost into account in declining to mandate more stringent controls. The court did, however, make clear that in determining what level is "safe," even for a carcinogen, the EPA need not eliminate exposure and that it may consider costs in deciding what additional margin of protection to prescribe (*Natural Resources Defense Council, Inc. v. United States Environmental Protection Agency,* 1987).

Occupational Safety and Health Administration. The 1970 Occupational Safety and Health Act requires employers to provide employees safe working conditions and empowers OSHA to prescribe mandatory occupational safety and health standards (OSHA, 1970). OSHA's most controversial standards have been exposure limits for toxic chemicals.

While the safety of food additives, drugs, and pesticides has to be demonstrated before they may be marketed, no employer need obtain advance approval of new processes or materials or conduct tests to ensure that its operations will not jeopardize worker health. Only if OSHA discovers that a material already in use threatens worker health may it attempt to control exposure. Standards for toxic chemicals typically set maximum limits on employee exposure and prescribe changes in employer procedures or equipment to achieve this level.

The act specifies that in regulating toxic chemicals OSHA shall adopt the standard "which most adequately assures, to the extent feasible, on the basis of the best available evidence, that no employee will suffer material impairment of health or physical capacity" [OSH Act § 6 (b)(5)]. The meaning of these contradictory phrases was for many years a source of controversy. Court decisions made clear that the "best available evidence" did not require proof of causation or even positive epidemiology studies; animal data alone could support regulation of a toxic substance. The debate focused on OSHA's obligation to weigh the economic costs of its standards. The agency acknowledged that

it was required to consider technological achievability and industry viability, but it denied that it was obliged to balance health benefits and economic costs (OSHA, 1980). Judicial challenges to OSHA standards twice led to the Supreme Court. The Court overturned OSHA's benzene standard because the agency had not shown that prevailing worker exposure levels posed a "significant" health risk (*Industrial Union Department, AFL-CIO v. American Petroleum Institute,* 1980). Two years later, however, it upheld OSHA's cotton dust standard with the explanation that Congress itself had balanced the benefits and costs of rigorous safeguards for worker health; the agency was not obligated to weigh the costs of individual standards for concededly hazardous substances (*American Textile Manufacturers Institute v. Donovan,* 1982).

Because it lacks authority to mandate testing by employers, OSHA generally must rely on data already accumulated about the effects of workplace chemicals. The 1970 act also established the National Institutes of Occupational Safety and Health (NIOSH) to serve as OSHA's independent data-gathering arm. NIOSH assembled much of the data—and conducted some of the epidemiological studies—on which OSHA has relied establishing worker exposure limits for toxic substances.

Consumer Product Safety Commission. Of the four agencies discussed here, the CPSC has played the least important role in federal efforts to control toxic chemicals. The commission was created in 1972 by the Consumer Product Safety Act (CPSA) with authority to regulate products that pose an unreasonable risk of injury or illness to consumers. The commission is empowered to promulgate safety standards "to prevent or reduce an unreasonable risk of injury" associated with a consumer product. If no feasible standard "would adequately protect the public from the unreasonable risk of injury" posed by a consumer product, the commission may ban the product (CPSA § 8). In assessing the need for a standard or ban, the agency must balance the likelihood that a product will cause harm and its severity against the effects of reducing the risk on the product's utility, cost, and availability to consumers.

The CPSC also adminsters the older Federal Hazardous Substances Act (FHSA). The FHSA authorizes the CPSC to regulate, primarily through prescribed label warnings, products that are toxic, corrosive, combustible, or radioactive or that generate pressure. The FHSA is unusual among federal health laws because it contains detailed criteria for determining toxicity. It defines "highly toxic" in terms of a substance's acute effects in specified tests in rodents; substances capable of producing chronic effects thus fall within the "toxic" category. The FHSA contains another unique provision (FHSA § 2(h)(2)) specifically addressing the probative weight of animal and human data on acute toxicity:

> If the [commission] finds that available data on human experience with any substance indicates results different from those obtained on animals in the above-named dosages or concentrations, the human data shall take precedence.

The CPSC has prescribed labeling for products containing numerous substances that are acutely toxic. It has also acted to ban from consumer products several substances that pose a cancer risk, including asbestos, vinyl chloride as a propellant, benzene, TRIS, and formaldehyde (Merrill, 1981). Its ban of urea formaldehyde foam insulation was set aside by a reviewing court in an opinion that is remarkable for its highly critical analysis of the agency's handling of toxicological data. The court faulted the commission's quantitative estimate of the cancer risk posed by formaldehyde in foam insulation, stressing in particular flaws in its exposure measurements (*Gulf South Insulation v. CPSC*, 1983).

The CPSC obtains most of its data about chemical hazards from other sources, including sister regulatory agencies. The agency's own capacity to test products is limited, and its budget has shrunk by almost half during the past decade. Neither the CPSA or the FHSA obligates manufacturers to notify the commission of plans to market a new product or to obtain approval for any design or material.

REGULATORY CONTROLS OVER TOXICOLOGY

The previous sections have surveyed contexts in which regulators draw on toxicological data in deciding whether and how to control environmental chemicals. Modern toxicology has grown significantly in response to the information needs of contemporary health regulation. But government regulation impinges on the discipline in more direct ways as well. Regulatory agencies often prescribe the content and characteristics of studies that are conducted to meet regulatory requirements. And in recent years, pressure to protect animals used in research has produced laws and regulations that govern toxicologists themselves.

Different Ways Regulation Impinges on Toxicology

An agency's influence over the conduct of toxicological studies depends on the character of its regulatory responsibilities. An agency like the FDA or the EPA that must confirm the safety of new substances before marketing can, as a practical matter, dictate the kinds of tests that manufacturers must conduct to gain approval. By contrast, an agency that has no premarket approval function has less leverage. Typically, it must rely on whatever tests have been reported in the scientific literature or conducted to meet the requirements of some other agency.

Statutory terms often do not reveal the reach of an agency's power. For example, the FD&C Act does not in so many words authorize the FDA to prescribe the kinds of preclinical tests a manufacturer of human drugs must conduct; it says, merely, that no new drug may be marketed until the manufacturer has satisfied the FDA, "by all methods reasonably applicable," that it is "safe" (FD&C Act § 505(c)). However, the agency's power to withhold approval when it has doubts about a drug's safety provides it the practical leverage necessary to demand whatever tests its scientists believe necessary. Of course, some laws, notably the TSCA, explicitly accord power to prescribe testing. But if an agency has the ability to prevent marketing until safety is proved, doubts about its legal authority to prescribe testing requirements are academic; the important issues are the procedures by which its requirements are adopted, their scope and scientific support, and their legal effect.

The last issue is important for laboratory scientists and for sponsors of testing, as well as for lawyers. Two significant, if arcane, legal distinctions should be noted. The first is the distinction between requirements that an agency imposes for testing of specific compounds and generic requirements prescribed for all compounds within a class, e.g., direct food additives. An agency like the FDA could impose its views of appropriate toxicological testing without ever enunciating any general testing standards. When a compound's sponsor sought approval, it could be told that the tests it had conducted were inadequate. Or individual sponsors could elicit the agency's advice about what tests were necessary before they undertook testing. The first approach wastes resources, and the second—unless agency advice is broadly disseminated—fails to guide other potential sponsors and allows inconsistency in the treatment of similar compounds.

For these reasons, the FDA and the EPA have moved increasingly toward establishing generic test standards or guidelines. Both agencies have issued guidelines for the design and conduct of studies of the health effects of compounds submitted for agency approval (EPA, 1988; FDA, 1989). In addition, the EPA has established guidelines for several of the tests that it may mandate by rule or consent agreement for individual chemicals under TSCA § 4 (EPA, 1988). Governments of many other countries have followed the U.S. pattern, and international bodies such as the Organization for Economic Cooperation and Development have sought to secure multilateral adherence to standardized test guidelines and minimum testing requirements for new chemicals (Page, 1982).

This trend has focused attention on a second legal distinction: the distinction between binding regulations and advisory guidelines. Any time a regulatory agency wants to provide guidance for private behavior, it confronts a choice between establishing standards that have the force of law—regulations—and merely conveying its current best judgment of what performance will satisfy the law—guidelines. A regulation specifies what the law mandates; failure to comply— e.g., failure to perform a test or follow a protocol specified in a regulation—constitutes a violation of law just as if the regulation had been enacted by Congress. A test guideline describes performance that will satisfy legal requirements; it is a promise to accept tests that conform to the guideline. But failure to follow the guideline is not forbidden. The agency may accept another approach, e.g., a different set of studies or studies conducted using different protocols, if it concludes that they meet the law's basic requirements.

Regulations ensure consistency and are more easily enforced than guidelines, but they are more rigid because they restrict the agency, and the procedures for their adoption and amendment are cumbersome. The design and conduct of toxicological studies, it is often argued, should take into account the characteristics of the test compound, the end points to be evaluated, the resources available, and perhaps even laboratory capabilities. Accordingly, both the FDA and the EPA have preferred to announce their standards as guidelines, permitting product sponsors and laboratory scientists to consider and sometimes use alternative approaches.

Toxicologists should be aware of the different ways in which regulatory requirements can impinge on their work. It is increasingly common for U.S. agencies to specify the types of tests they require before they will consider a compound, e.g., acute toxicity, subchronic, and chronic. Within each of these categories, an agency might set out more detailed requirements, essentially enumerating its "base set" data demands. As noted above, an agency may also describe methods for executing particular tests, e.g., a bioassay for carcinogenesis. It is

these descriptions that in the U.S. usually take the form of guidelines.

Both the FDA and the EPA have adopted another set of requirements that specify laboratory procedures for conducting tests required or submitted for regulatory consideration. These "good laboratory practice" (GLP) regulations prescribe essential but often mundane features of sound laboratory science, such as animal husbandry standards and record-keeping practices (EPA, 1988; FDA, 1989). All these types of requirements are intended to contribute to regulatory decision making by ensuring the quality and integrity of toxicological data submitted to support agency decisions. In addition, toxicologists in recent years have confronted another form of direct regulation whose goal is protection of the subjects of laboratory studies—experimental animals.

FDA and EPA Testing Standards

It would serve little purpose to detail here existing agency requirements for the design and conduct of toxicological studies, for they change frequently enough that any summary would soon be outdated. This chapter thus attempts only to acquaint the reader with the principal federal programs that specify standards for toxicity testing. The discussion focuses chiefly on the FDA and the EPA, the two agencies whose regulatory responsibilities provide authority to affect the work of toxicologists directly.

Food and Drug Administration. The FDA exercises premarketing approval authority over several classes of compounds of which the most important, for present purposes, are new human drugs and direct and indirect additives to food.

Toxicologic Testing Requirements for Human Drugs. The FDA has long exercised control over the testing of compounds investigated as possible therapeutic agents. In 1962, Congress expressly authorized the FDA to exempt investigational drugs from the premarket approval requirement so that they could be shipped for use in clinical testing, subject to conditions the agency believed appropriate to protect human subjects (FD&C Act § 505(i)). One condition that the FDA established was that an investigational drug have first been evaluated in preclinical studies. This requirement appears in current regulations that amplify, in text and in referenced guidelines, the types of tests that are to be performed and the design they should follow (FDA, 1989). Almost invariably, a drug's sponsor will consult the FDA personnel to get a more precise understanding of what sorts of toxicological studies they expect. Preclinical studies of substances that are candidates for use as human drugs must meet the FDA's good laboratory practice regulations (FDA, 1989). These regulations apply to all laboratories—university, independent, and manufacturer-owned—in which such studies are conducted.

Testing Requirements for Food Additives.
The Food Additives Amendment and the Color Additive Amendments require premarket approval of new additives to human food. Both laws assume that laboratory studies in animals will provide the principal data for assessing safety. The food additives law requires that a petitioner submit "full reports of investigations made with respect to the safety for use of such additives, including full information as to the methods and control used" (FD&C Act § 409(c)).

The FDA's regulations contain only general statements about the need for, and features of, toxicological studies. For many years, the agency maintained an advice-giving system in which it prescribed the type and design of tests to be performed. In 1982, the FDA codified this "common law" in *Toxicological Principles for the Safety Assessment of Direct Food Additives and Color Additives Used in Food*, sometimes known as "the Red Book." The Red Book describes the types of tests the FDA believes necessary to evaluate an additive's safety. The agency's requirements—which constitute guidelines rather than regulations—are calibrated to the purposes for which the additive will be used, to estimated levels of human exposure, and to the results of sequential studies. Tests of food color and additives must comply with the FDA's good laboratory practice regulations (FDA, 1989).

Environmental Protection Agency. The EPA's premarket approval authority over pesticides places it, like the FDA, in a position to dictate the design and conduct of studies on such compounds. The 1976 Toxic Substances Control Act gave the EPA authority to mandate testing of other chemicals in use or scheduled for introduction and to specify, by regulation, test standards.

Toxicology Requirements for Pesticides.
The FIFRA clearly contemplates the submission of toxicological studies, as well as other types of investigations, to support EPA's evaluation of a pesticide (FIFRA § 136(b)). The statute also requires the EPA to "publish guidelines specifying the kinds of information which will be required to support the registration of a pesticide and to revise such guidelines from time to time." In this provision, Congress apparently contemplated that EPA guidelines would both outline the kinds of data required to secure approval and describe the characteristics each type of study should possess.

EPA's regulations state broadly that pesticide registration depends on evaluation of "all available, pertinent data," which must satisfy the minimum requirements set forth in registration guidelines (EPA, 1988). The agency has issued regulations outlining the procedures for submission of registration petitions and their basic content (EPA, 1978, 1988). Animal studies of pesticides must also comply with EPA's own good laboratory practice regulations, which were inspired by the same investigations that led the FDA to promulgate its standards for testing laboratories and impose similar requirements.

The primary means by which the EPA can mandate health effects testing of new or existing industrial chemicals is Section 4(a) of the TSCA. That provision states that the administrator "shall by rule require that testing be conducted to develop data with respect to the health and environmental effects for which there is an insufficiency of data and experience" to permit assessment of whether a substance presents an unreasonable risk. This obligation to order testing is triggered by an administrative finding that a chemical presents a potential risk (based on suspicion of toxicity) or that humans or the environment will be exposed to substantial quantities. The statute creates an Interagency Testing Committee (ITC) with members from EPA, OSHA, CEQ, NIOSH, NIEHS, NCI, NSF, and the Department of Commerce to recommend a list of chemicals that should be tested first. Once the ITC has recommended a chemical substance for testing, the EPA must within 12 months either initiate testing or publish its reasons for not doing so.

This last requirement, coupled with the statute's formal procedures for adopting test rules, led the EPA initially to rely on informal negotiations with chemical producers to secure voluntary agreements to conduct the tests it thought appropriate for chemicals identified by the ITC (GAO, 1982). The practice was challenged by public interest organizations, who were effectively excluded from the negotiations, and was ultimately declared unlawful (*Natural Resources Defense Council, Inc. v. United States Environmental Protection Agency*, 1984). The agency has since amended its regulations to recognize two forms of mandates to test: test rules and enforceable testing consent agreements (EPA, 1988). By the end of 1989, the EPA had adopted test rules for approximately 24 commercial chemicals and 33 constituents of industrial waste and entered into consent orders for testing of half a dozen other chemicals (EPA, 1988).

Both test rules and testing consent agreements specify what types of tests are to be done. Their design is governed either by general "test methodology guidelines," which the EPA has issued for several types of tests, or by the rule or the agreement itself. All toxicological studies required by the EPA under the TSCA must comply with its GLP regulations.

Interagency Testing Criteria and Programs

The foregoing summary of regulatory programs that mandate toxicological tests suggests the possibility of inconsistency in testing standards. In the late 1970s, the responsible regulatory agencies, OSHA and the CPSC as well as the FDA and the EPA, worked through the former Interagency Regulatory Liaision Group (IRLG) to secure agreement on the design of standard toxicological tests. Though the IRLG has long since collapsed, both the FDA and the EPA have continued to work to achieve internal consistency. Despite continuing official recognition of the problems caused by inconsistency in testing standards, however, laboratory researchers should not be astonished to discover that federal agencies sometimes appear to be sending different messages.

The agencies have achieved effective collaboration in another arena. The National Toxicology Program (NTP) was established in 1978 as an administrative umbrella for coordinating the numerous federal efforts to improve test methods and to conduct toxicological studies then under way, primarily in the Department of Health and Human Services. NTP assumed responsibility for what had been NCI's bioassay program. An NTP committee that includes representatives of all four regulatory agencies is responsible for selecting chemicals to be tested at public expense.

There have been noteworthy efforts to achieve international agreement on test standards and on minimum data requirements for new chemicals. Led by the Organization for Economic Cooperation and Development (OECD), these efforts have already influenced the content of EPA and FDA test guidelines. Space does not allow review of these international standards or detailed study of their consistency with current requirements of U.S. agencies. The latter, while no doubt continuing to reflect the influence of international consensus, will continue to be the principal source of governmental guidance for the conduct of toxicological studies in this country.

Animal Welfare Requirements

Researchers who conduct studies funded by federal agencies must comply with the Animal Welfare Act (AWA), and some may also be subject to restrictions imposed by the Public Health Service (PHS). Recipients of grants from the Department of Education, the Department of Health and Human Services, the Department of Agriculture, or the EPA are subject only to the AWA. Those funded by the Department of Energy or by the PHS must also comply with PHS policies. Restrictions on animal use also appear in the good laboratory practices regulations adopted by the FDA and the EPA, which apply to all studies submitted to those agencies, regardless of sponsorship (Reagan, 1986).

Animal Welfare Act. The AWA is administered by the Animal and Plant Health Inspection Service (APHIS), a part of the U.S. Department of Agriculture. The AWA, which protects only warm-blooded animals and excludes birds, rats, and mice, requires all covered research facilities to register with APHIS and agree to comply with applicable AWA standards. Each facility must file an annual report signed by a responsible official that shows that "professionally acceptable standards governing the care, treatment, and use of animals were followed" for the year in question. The report must include:

1. The common names and numbers of animals used in research except for those used in routine procedures such as tattooing and blood sampling
2. An explanation for any experiment in which animals are subjected to pain and distress
3. Certification by an attending veterinarian or by a three-member institutional committee consisting of at least one veterinarian that the use of anesthetics, analgesics, and tranquilizers was appropriate.

Pursuant to the AWA, APHIS has established specific requirements for the humane handling, care, and transportation of dogs and cats, guinea pigs and hamsters, rabbits, nonhuman primates, marine mammals, and other warm-blooded animals. The regulations governing facilities address living space, heating, lighting, ventilation, and drainage. The health and husbandry provisions address feeding, watering, sanitation, veterinary care, grouping of animals, and the number and qualifications of caretakers (APHIS, 1988).

The AWA imposes specific requirements for animal protection. Before embarking upon an experiment likely to produce pain or distress, a researcher must consider the feasibility of pain-free alternatives. A veterinarian must be consulted in the planning of any experiments that inflict pain. Tranquilizers, analgesics, and anesthetics must be used unless scientific necessity disallows their use. Additionally, the use of paralytics without the concurrent use of anesthetics is prohibited.

The AWA requires research facilities to establish at least one institutional oversight committee, composed of three or more members, one of whom must be a veterinarian and another to represent community interests who may not be affiliated with the institution. The committee must conduct semiannual inspections of the facility to review pain-inducing procedures and animal condition. Committee reports are filed with APHIS and with any federal agency funding the research.

Public Health Service Policy. The PHS Policy on Humane Care and Use of Laboratory Animals by Awardee Institutions applies to research using any vertebrate, and thus it has a broader reach than the AWA. The PHS policy requires each facility to submit an annual report, called an Assurance, which is evaluated by the NIH Office for Protection from Research Risks (OPRR) to determine the sufficiency of animal care.

The PHS policy imposes two primary obligations on researchers: Each institution must adopt a Program for Animal Care and Use, and it must establish an Animal Care and Use Committee (IACUC). An IACUC must contain at least five members—one a veterinarian, one an animal research scientist, one who is not a scientist, and one who is not affiliated with the facility. The IACUC must review all applications for research funding and review the institution's programs to ensure compliance with NIH standards.

The Health Research Extension Act of 1985 requires PHS-funded institutions to provide training similar to that required by the AWA for personnel on methods to reduce animal suffering. It also requires that researchers' grant applications justify any proposed use of animals (NRC, 1988).

Scientists working with no federal funding who expect their research to be submitted to the FDA or the EPA are not subject to the AWA or PHS policies, but they must comply with the animal protection provisions of those agencies' good laboratory practice regulations. These regulations prescribe adequate living conditions, detail requirements for veterinary treatment, and impose specific record-keeping requirements (EPA, 1988; FDA, 1989).

REFERENCES

Cases

American Textile Manufacturers Institute v. Donovan, 452 U.S. 490, 495 (1982).
Environmental Defense Fund, Inc. v. Environmental Protection Agency, 548 F.2d 998 (D.C. Cir. 1976).
Environmental Defense Fund, Inc. v. Ruckelshaus, 439 F.2nd 584 (D.C. Cir. 1971).
Environmental Defense Fund, Inc. and National Audubon Society v. Environmental Protection Agency, 510 F.2d 1292 (D.C. Cir. 1975)
Gulf South Insulation v. CPSC, 701 F.2d 1137 (5th Cir. 1983).
Industrial Union Department, AFL-CIO v. American Petroleum Institute, 448 U.S. 607 (1980).
Industrial Union Department, AFL-CIO v. Hodgson, 499 F.2d 467 (D.C. Cir. 1974).
Monsanto v. Kennedy, 613 F.2d 947 (D.C. Cir. 1979).
Natural Resources Defense Council, Inc. v. United States Environmental Protection Agency, 595 F. Supp. 1255 (S.D.N.Y. 1984).
Natural Resources Defense Council, Inc. v. United States Environmental Protection Agency, 824 F.2d 1146 (D.C. Cir. 1987)
NRDC v. Train, 8 E.R.C. 2120 (D.D.C. 1976).
Public Citizen v. Young, 831 F.2d 1108 (D.C. Cir. 1987).
Society of the Plastics Industry, Inc. v. OSHA, 509 F.2d 9301 (2d Cir. 1975).

Secondary Sources

Assessment of Technologies for Determining the Cancer Risks from the Environment. Report by the Office of Technology Assessment, U.S. Government Printing Office, Washington, D.C., June 1981.
Berger, J., and Riskin, S.: Economic and technological feasibility under the Occupational Safety and Health Act. *Ecology L. Q.,* 7:285, 1978.
Bruser, J.; Harris, R.; and Page, T.: Waterborne carcinogens: an economist's view. In *The Scientific Basis of Health and Safety Regulation.* Brookings Institution, Washington, D.C., 1981.
Cooper, R.: The role of regulatory agencies in risk-benefit decision-making. *Food Drug Cosmet. L. J.,* 33:755–757, 1978.
Douglas, I.: Safe Drinking Water Act of 1975—history and critique. *Environ. Affairs,* 5:501, 1976.
EPA Implementation of Selected Aspects of the Toxic Substances Control Act. Report by the U.S. General Accounting Office, Washington, D.C., December 1982.
Gray, K.: The Safe Drinking Water Act Amendments of 1986: now a tougher act to follow. *Envtl. L. Rep.,* 16:10338, 1986.
Heineck, D.: New clean water act toxics control initiatives. *Nat. Resources Environ.,* 1:10, 1989.
Merrill, R.: Regulating carcinogens in food: a legislator's guide to the food safety provisions of the federal Food, Drug, and Cosmetic Act. *Mich. L. Rev.,* 77:179–184, 1979.
————: CPSC regulation of cancer risks in consumer products: 1972–81. *Va. L. Rev.,* 67:1261, 1981. A
Merrill, R., and Hutt, P. B.: *Food and Drug Law: Cases and Materials.* Foundation Press, Inc., Mineola, N.Y., 1980.
Merrill, R., and Schewel, M.: FDA regulation of environmental contaminants of food. *Va. L. Rev.,* 66:1357, 1980.
National Institute of Health, Department of Health and Human Services: Guide for the Care and Use of Laboratory Animals, Publ. No. 23. Guide for Grants and Contracts: Special Edition, Laboratory Animal Welfare (Supp. June 1985).
National Research Council: *Use of Laboratory Animals in Biomedical and Behavioral Research.* National Academy Press, Washington, D.C. , 1988.
National Toxicology Program Annual Plan for Fiscal Year 1988. Report by the U.S. Department of Health and Human Services, January 1988.

Page, N. P.: Testing for health and environmental effects: the OECD guidelines. *Toxic Substances J.,* **4**:135, Autumn 1982.

Reagan, K.: Federal regulation of testing with laboratory animals: future directions, *Pace Environ. L. Rev.,* **3**:165, 1986.

Reed, P. D.: The trial of hazardous air pollution regulation. *Environ. L. Register,* **16**:10066–10072, 1986.

Toxicological Principles for the Safety Assessment of Direct Food Additives and Color Additives Used in Food. Report by the U.S. Food and Drug Administration, 1982.

Turner, J.: The Delaney anticancer clause: a model environmental protection law. *Vand. L. Rev.,* **24**:889, 1971.

Statues and Regulations

Animal Welfare, 9 C.F.R. Part 171 (1988).

Animal Welfare Act (1988), 7 U.S.C. § 2131 et seq.

Applications for FDA Approval to Market a New Drug or an Antibiotic Drug, 21 C.F.R. Part 314 (1989).

Clean Air Act (1976), 42 U.S.C. § 7401 et seq.

Color Additive Amendments of 1960 to the Federal Food, Drug, and Cosmetic Act, 21 U.S.C. § 706.

Color Additive Petitions, 21 C.F.R. Part 71 (1989).

Consumer Product Safety Act (1972), 15 U.S.C. § 2051 et seq.

Data Requirements for Registration, 40 C.F.R. Part 158 (1988).

Drug Amendments of 1962 to the Federal Food, Drug, and Cosmetic Act, 21 U.S.C. § 360(b).

Environmental Effects Testing Guidelines, 40 C.F.R. Part 797 (1988).

Federal Food, Drug, and Cosmetic Act (1938), 21 U.S.C. § 321 et seq.

Federal Hazardous Substances Act (1976), 15 U.S.C. § 1261 et seq.

Federal Insecticide, Fungicide, and Rodenticide Act (1972), 7 U.S.C. § 135 et seq.

Federal Insecticide, Fungicide, and Rodenticide Act Amendments of 1988, Pub. L. No. 100–532, 102 Stat. 2654.

Federal Water Pollution Control Act Amendments of 1972, 33 U.S.C. § 307.

Food Additive Amendments to the Federal Food, Drug, and Cosmetic Act (1958), 21 U.S.C. § 348 et seq.

Food Additive Petitions, 21 C.F.R. Part 171 (1989).

Good Laboratory Practice for Nonclinical Laboratory Studies, 21 C.F.R. Part 58 (1989).

Good Laboratory Practice Standards, 40 C.F.R. Part 160 (1988).

Good Laboratory Practice Standards, 40 C.F.R. Part 792 (1988).

Good Laboratory Practice Standards for Health Effects: Environmental Protection Agency. *Fed. Reg.,* **44**(91):27362, May 9, 1979.

Hazardous Waste Management System: General, 40 C.F.R. Part 260 (1988).

Health Effects Testing Guidelines, 40 C.F.R. Part 798 (1988).

Identification, Classification and Regulation of Potential Occupational Carcinogens: Occupational Safety and Health Act. *Fed. Reg.,* **45**(15):5002, January 22, 1980.

Identification, Classification and Regulation of Potential Occupational Carcinogens: Occupational Safety and Health Act. *Fed. Reg.,* **47**(2):187–190, January 5, 1982.

Identification of Specific Chemical Substances and Mixtures Testing Requirements, 40 C.F.R. Part 799 (1988).

Indirect Food Additives: Polymers; Acrylonitrile/Styrene Copolymers. *Fed. Reg.,* **49**(183):36635–36644, September 19, 1984.

Lead Acetate: Listing as a Color Additive in Cosmetics that Color the Hair on the Scalp: Food and Drug Administration. *Fed. Reg.,* **45**(213):72113–72118, October 31, 1980.

National Emissions Standard for Identifying, Assessing, and Regulating Airborne Substances Posing a Risk of Cancer: Environmental Protection Agency. *Fed. Reg.,* **44**(197):58641–58670, October 10, 1979.

New Drugs, 21 C.F.R. Part 310 (1989).

Occupational Safety and Health Act (1970), 29 U.S.C. § 651 et seq.

Pesticide Residue Amendments to the Federal Food, Drug, and Cosmetic Act (1954), 21 U.S.C. § 348 et seq.

Policy for Regulating Carcinogenic Chemicals in Food and Color Additives: Advanced Notice of Proposed Rulemaking: Food and Drug Administration. *Fed. Reg.,* **47**(64):14464–14469, April 2, 1982.

Proposed Guidelines for Carinogen Risk Assessment; Request for Comments. *Fed. Reg.,* **49**(227):46293–46301, November 23, 1984.

Proposed Guidelines for Registering Pesticides in the United States: Environmental Protection Agency. *Fed. Reg.,* **43**(163):37336, August 22, 1978.

Proposed Health Effects Test Standards for Toxic Substances Control Act Test Rules: Environmental Protection Agency. *Fed. Reg.,* **44**(145):44054, July 26, 1979.

Proposed Interim Primary Drinking Water Regulations: Environmental Protection Agency. *Fed. Reg.,* **43**(130):29135–29137, July 6, 1978 (to be codified at 40 C.F.R. § 141).

Provisional Test Guidelines, 40 C.F.R. Part 795 (1988).

Rebuttable Presumption Against Registration (RPAR) Proceedings and Hearings Under Section 6 of the Federal Insecticide, Fungicide, and Rodenticide Act (FIFRA): Environmental Protection Agency. *Fed. Reg.,* **45**(154):52628–52674, August 7, 1980.

Regulation of Pesticides in Food: Addressing the Delaney Paradox Policy Statement: Environmental Protection Agency. *Fed. Reg.,* **53**(202):41104–41123, October 19, 1988.

Resource Conservation and Recovery Act (1976), 42 U.S.C.A. § 6901.

Safe Drinking Water Act (1974), 42 U.S.C. §§ 300f to 300j–9.

Sponsored Compounds in Food Producing Animals: Proposed Rule and Notice. *Fed. Reg.,* **50**(211):45529–45556, October 31, 1985.

Testing Consent Orders, 40 C.F.R. § 799, 5000 (1988).

Toxic Substances Control Act (1976), 15 U.S.C. § 2601.

Toxic Substances Control Act, § 4, 15 U.S.C. § 2603(b)(1) (1988).

Toxic Substances Control Act, § 6, 15 U.S.C. § 2605 (1988).

Chapter 31

RISK ASSESSMENT

Robert A. Scala

One of the consequences of the popularization of science, itself a social responsibility of scientists, is loss of precision in the use of the language of science. This language, which permits an exactness in the communication between colleagues, becomes softer, blurred about the edges, occasionally even subverted to permit its use to further certain ends. Toxicology has not been spared this experience. A chapter on risk assessment, concerned with the toxicity and hazard of chemical agents at low doses, will touch on many of the concepts and terms whose meaning has been subject to change in the popularization process.

RISK

For purposes of this chapter, a discussion of risk and risk-related issues will be largely confined to those unfavorable or undesirable biological outcomes subsequent to exposure to a chemical agent. *Risk* in this context is then defined in terms of the probability of a particular adverse effect. It has the dimensions of frequency or incidence (1 in 10^6, for example) and is coupled to an exposure estimate. The actual risk statement may be made in the form of the probability of an outcome associated with a unit exposure. That is, there is a lifetime "risk" of cancer of 2.5×10^{-4} from exposure to 1 part per million of a chemical in community air breathed 24 hours a day, every day for 70 years. An alternate statement of risk is the exposure concentration that results in a benchmark risk level. In the previous example, if the dose-response relationship were linear, then a risk of 1 lifetime cancer in a million lifetimes ($1/10^6$) results from an exposure of 0.004 ppm 24 hours daily for 70 years. For the kinds of issues toxicologists must deal with, risk is a probabilistic statement, a statistical construct based on, at best, observations at higher doses and for shorter periods of time. It is not derived by direct measurement but by calculations from other observed events. Such calculations carry with them both assumptions and uncertainties, and these should be noted.

The link between risk and safety is made either by the individual or by government acting on behalf of many individuals potentially subject to a given risk. In either case, *safety* is then defined as a circumstance characterized by an "acceptable" level of risk. Major public and private debates emerge when the question is asked, Who defines the level of risk that is acceptable? and Where is that level placed? Clearly, the amount of risk that is acceptable relates to certain characteristics of the risk.

RISK PERCEPTION

It is commonly understood that individuals and societies respond in diverse ways to hazardous circumstances (Kraus and Slovik, 1988). There is aversion to some hazards, indifference to others, and even knowing acceptance of still others. Furthermore, the public at large generally ranks hazards differently than experts in those fields. This is at the heart of individual or societal responses to regulatory agency or other expert judgments of the risk attendant upon certain exposures or behaviors. Social science research has begun to classify hazardous ("risky") behavior, technologies, and substances and then to understand the basis for these differences in judgments. In Table 31-1 are listed several characteristics of risk. If a number of the factors that are related are combined into two broad families, some commonly believed risk perceptions emerge. In Figure 31-1, the horizontal line relates to dreadedness, with features such as lack of control, dread, catastrophic potential, involuntariness, personal risk, lack of equitability, and risk to future generations, increasing with movement to the right. On the vertical axis, upward movement denotes newness, lack of scientific knowledge, delay in effects, and lack of ability to observe or be aware of exposure. Although Kraus and Slovic arrayed scores of hazards, only a few are used to illustrate the concept. Note that pesticides, herbicides, asbestos, nuclear power, and DNA research are in the upper right quadrant (greater dread, less

Table 31–1. CHARACTERISTICS OF RISK*

CHARACTERISTIC	DESCRIPTION	LEVEL	EXAMPLES
Knowledge	Society's awareness of risks from activity	Little known Much known	Food additives Alcoholic drinks
Newness	Extent of societal experience	Old New	Guns Space travel
Voluntariness	Does individual have a choice about exposure to risk	Not voluntary Voluntary	Crime Rock climbing
Control	Can individual control exposure, protect himself, or control consequences	Risk not controlled by skill or diligence Risk controlled by skill or diligence	Natural disasters Smoking
Dreadedness	How much is risk or its consequences feared	People do not dread People have great dread	Vaccination Nerve gas
Catastrophic potential	Chance of widespread disastrous outcome	Not likely Likely	Sunbathing War
Equity	Are the benefit and risk shared equally	Distributed unequally Distributed equally	Hazardous dump Skiing

*From Kraus, N. N., and Slovic, P.: Taxonomic analysis of perceived risk: modeling individual and group perceptions within homogeneous hazard domains. *Risk Analysis,* **8:**435–455, 1988. Reprinted with permission.

knowable), whereas societal problems such as smoking, dynamite, warfare, and handguns are in the lower right. Common drugs, food additives, microwave ovens, anesthetics, power tools, alcohol, and motor vehicles are on the left side, areas of low dread and greater or less knowability.

The perception of risk differs considerably between lay persons and experts. The latter rank risk usually from their knowledge of actual fatality rates for any given hazardous activity or agent. Lay persons have some sense of these rates but tune or temper that judgment by impressions of catastrophic potential, fear for future generations, and other elements of dread. Table 31–2 is a brief listing from Slovic *et al.* (1979) of lay and expert rankings of risks.

CONCEPTS IN RISK ASSESSMENT

Risk assessment in toxicology is a process whereby relevant biological, dose-response, and exposure data are combined to produce a qualitative or quantitative estimate of adverse outcome from a defined activity or chemical agent. In its most common form, a toxicological risk assessment is a probability estimate of the production of cancer from a lifetime exposure to an agent at some unit dose.

The formal risk assessment procedures currently in use probably arose from a confluence of several scientific and regulatory developments. The earlier ideas of toxic (or carcinogenic) *per se* were no longer adequate. It was not enough to report that an agent caused a particular effect. It was now necessary to deal with *how* active the

agent was. Animal studies provided data at relatively high doses. How were they to be related to actual human exposures and risks in a meaningful, quantifiable, defensible, publicly understandable fashion? Perhaps it was a post-Vietnam attitude among informed citizens, but it was no longer sufficient for science, especially science in government, to be paternal and merely "declare" that an agent or activity was safe or harmful. There was a demand that there be a formal decision-making process underlying such statements, that they be documented, and that the decisions be reached in an open forum or

Table 31–2. DIFFERENCES IN RISK PERCEPTION*

ACTIVITY/AGENT	EXPERT RANK	LAY RANK
Motor vehicles	1	2
Smoking	2	4
Alcoholic beverages	3	6
Handguns	4	3
Surgery	5	10
Motorcycles	6	5
X-rays	7	22
Pesticides	8	9
Electric power (nonnuclear)	9	18
Swimming	10	19

(NB nuclear power, ranked 1 on lay list, was 20 for the experts.)

*Modified from Slovic, P.; Fischhoff, B.; and Lichtenstein, S.: Rating the risks. *Environment,* **21:**14, 1979. Reprinted with permission of the Helen Dwight Reid Educational Foundation. Published by Heldref Publications, 4000 Albemarle St., N.W., Washington, D.C., 20016. Copyright © 1979.

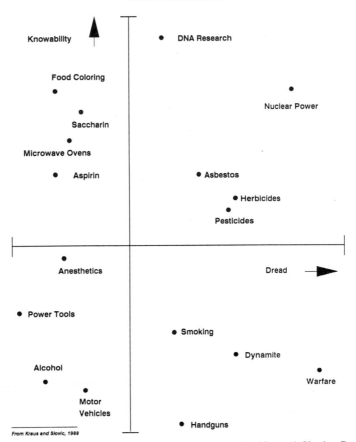

Knowability

● DNA Research

Food Coloring
●

●
Nuclear Power

●
Saccharin

●
Microwave Ovens

● Aspirin

● Asbestos

● Herbicides
●
Pesticides

●
Anesthetics

Dread ▶

● Power Tools

● Smoking

● Dynamite

Alcohol
●
●
Motor
Vehicles

●
Warfare

● Handguns

From Kraus and Slovic, 1988

Figure 31–1. Perception of risks. (Modified from Kraus, N. N., and Slovic, P.: Taxonomic analysis of perceived risk: modeling individual and group perceptions within homogeneous hazard domains. *Risk Analysis,* **8**:435–455, 1988. Reprinted with permission.)

subject to public review and input. Administratively, the comfort of life in a binary world (safe/not safe, for example) was gone, so a decision logic that made the regulators' task easier was needed.

Not enough has been said about the uncertainties in these decisions and the accuracy or quality of the predictions. Risk assessment has been compared unfavorably with five-year weather predictions. At least with the latter, the "correct" answer is available in only five years—not so with assessments of possible chronic health hazards from long-term, low-dose experiments.

The risk assessment process has been most clearly outlined in a 1983 National Academy of Sciences–National Research Council (NAS-NRC) report *Risk Assessment in the Federal Government: Managing the Process* (National Research Council, 1983). This report has served as the basis for most discussions of the process or as the starting point for alternative concepts of risk assessment. Here, the NAS-NRC approach

will be followed with expansions and extensions based on other sources. At the outset, it is necessary to distinguish between risk assessment and risk management. The former is primarily a factor science-based estimate of the outcome of exposure of individuals or populations to hazardous substances or activities. Risk management is the selection and implementation of control strategies based not only on the estimated risk but also weighing policy, social, economic, technical feasibility, and other influences.

In this sense, risk assessment comprises the following steps: hazard identification, dose-response assessment, exposure assessment, and risk characterization (Figure 31–2). A risk assessment can stop at any given point, depending on the nature and quality of the data. The most obvious example is the finding of no evidence of exposure in the third step. Without exposure, there is no risk and the risk assessment process would be concluded.

Hazard identification is the step in which the

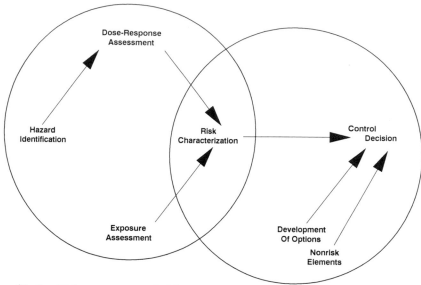

Figure 31–2. Risk assessment and risk management.

adverse effects of the agent or activity of interest are determined. Typical end points of such a determination include mortality, reproductive or developmental effects, neurotoxicity, specific organ effects, or cancer. The data may be derived from studies of humans (case reports, clinical surveys, or epidemiology experiments) or from the results of animal studies. The key element in this step is the linking of the agent or activity with the effect and reflects the strength and plausibility of the association. Indirect studies such as *in vitro* experiments are contributory.

Dose-response assessment considers the quantitative nature of the relationship between administered or received dose and biological response. The evaluation may be on an individual or population basis. It includes exposure intensity and modifiers of response such as age, sex, route, species, and exposure pattern. More difficult to determine accurately are extrapolations from animals to man and from high to low doses. Despite the difficulties, these extrapolations are essential since the result of this step is an estimate of the incidence of the effect in man and the dose corresponding to that effect. Only rarely can the dose-response data be developed directly in humans. Consequently, the risk estimator is faced with experimental studies designed to characterize the toxicity (or carcinogenicity) of an agent for a large population based on a limited number of animals. The result is an experiment at doses so high as to be barely tolerable and by a route that may be inappropriate for human exposure. This step has provided a rich base for dia-

logue on methods, simulations, models, and quantitation of uncertainty.

Exposure assessment is probably the most neglected aspect of the risk assessment process. Typically, field measurements or other estimates of human exposure are required. The dimensions of these exposures include intensity; frequency; schedule; route and duration of the exposure; and the nature, size, and makeup of the potentially (or actually) exposed population. The elements of exposure level and population at risk are combined to yield an estimate of current or anticipated uptake by that population. Difficulties in identifying competing exposures, interactions with other agents, special populations (old, young, pregnant, etc.), and patterns of exposure result in very high levels of uncertainty in this step. The exposure assessment is a parallel track to the hazard identification and dose-response assessment steps, and they merge in the final stage, risk characterization.

Risk characterization, in its briefest terms, is the estimated incidence of the adverse effect in a given population. It details the public health problem actually or potentially posed by the substance or activity under study. This aggregation of the findings in the previous steps requires judgment as well as sensitivity to variance and uncertainty in the underlying estimates. The process is summarized in Figure 31–3.

BIOLOGICAL CONSIDERATIONS IN THE RISK ASSESSMENT PROCESS

It is not possible in this chapter to detail all the biological issues that impact the risk assessment

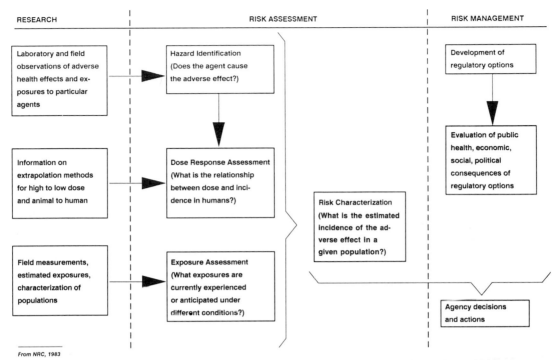

From NRC, 1983

Figure 31–3. Elements of risk assessment and risk management. (Reprinted from *Risk Assessment in the Federal Government: Managing the Process*, 1983, with permission from the National Academy Press, Washington, D.C.)

process. However, several believed to be of major importance will be highlighted. They include the value of epidemiological versus toxicological data, high-to-low-dose extrapolation including choice of models, animal-to-man extrapolation, use of mechanistic data, use of pharmacokinetic data, and strength of evidence versus weight of evidence.

Value of Epidemiological Versus Toxicological Data

While it is generally believed that human data are "more important" or "more relevant" than animal data in reaching risk conclusions for humans exposed to chemical or physical agents, these beliefs should not be accepted uncritically. Many reports of human effects have such limitations that their utilization in the risk assessment process is difficult. Among these limitations are absence of pure exposure because the individual or population is exposed to many possible causative agents. Where the agent may be known, the actual dose form (airborne concentration, dietary intake, drinking water concentration) is often not known and is either estimated after the fact, reconstructed in some way, or a surrogate employed. These surrogates include job classification, hours worked per day, or amount of agent

used (e.g., number of gallons of paint applied per day). Additional confounding factors are the influence of cigarette smoking and temporal pattern of exposure (early life versus later; intermittent peaks versus constant background). Human data are not tidy.

Animal experimentation likewise has certain limitations in risk assessment apart from the animal-to-man extrapolation to be discussed later. Chief among these is dose. Rarely are humans exposed to an agent the way animals are. If it is not lifetime dietary feeding at a fixed, high level, it is daily exposure to airborne levels that are likewise high and constant. The route in an animal study may be chosen more for laboratory convenience (e.g., gavage) than for what humans experience (dietary, water, air, or all three). Species sensitivity can be a major confounder of animal tests. Is it known whether the effect in man can be reliably produced in the species under test?

In short, each risk assessment case needs to be examined as to whether observational data in the species of choice (epidemiology) with unknown and/or confounded exposures should take precedence over experimental data in a surrogate species (toxicology) under unnatural conditions of exposure. This topic has been discussed by many; a recent review (Savitz, 1988) using exposure to electromagnetic fields captures the essence in a brief, lucid fashion.

High-to-Low Dose Extrapolation Including Choice of Models

In a risk assessment relying exclusively on animal data, the probability is very high that adequate data do not exist regarding effects in animals at low doses even if the period of exposure is for a lifetime. There are, however, as part of the dose-response estimate two critical steps to be made. In the first, risk for animals at low-dose levels must be estimated from data at higher doses. This risk in animals must then be related quantitatively to risk for man. Direct observations with group sizes large enough to constitute statistical significance are rarely available apart from the widely known National Center for Toxicological Research low-dose carcinogen study (Staffa and Mehlman, 1980). This massive experiment, popularly known as the ED_{01} study, was undertaken to examine the low end of the dose-response curve for the known carcinogen 2-acetylaminofluorene (2-AAF). Only urinary bladder and liver neoplasms were found to be related to the administration of 2-AAF in the diet, and neither was among the leading causes of death in this study. While the findings, conclusions, and possible interpretations of this experiment provided enough material for a separate issue of the journal in which they were published, the key questions yielded ambiguous answers. The dose producing an effect in 1 percent of the animals (ED_{01}) fell in the center of the range investigated for bladder tumors (ED_{01} = 60 ppm) but was below the lowest dose tested for liver tumors (ED_{01} = 10 ppm) and had to be estimated. Both dosage level and length of exposure were factors in the development of bladder tumors, and the data seemed to fit a threshold model. The dose-response data for liver tumors were nearly linear, indicating no tendency for a threshold. It is impossible to avoid the additional conclusion that precise study of low-dose effects is so resource intensive that comparable experiments will be extremely rare in the future.

The alternate to such studies is to construct a *mathematical model* that predicts responses at low doses from those seen at high levels. Figure 31–4 is taken from the NAS-NRC report and displays alternatives in extrapolation models using the same experimental data. The importance of this figure is not in the specific detailing of the individual models but in gaining an understanding of why the results differ. Buried in the assumptions of each model are both policy and biological reasons for why the calculated re-

sponse takes the form that it does. The policy considerations emerge from the regulatory agencies using the models to estimate risk. The most significant of these is whether or not a threshold exists for the phenomenon observed. For reason of public health protection, there is a wide recognition, explicitly or implicitly, that there is no threshold for carcinogenic and mutagenic effects. This constrains the dose-response curve to pass through the origin. The position is that only at zero dose is there zero risk in the test system studied. A second major policy constraint can be that the dose-response curve assume a specific shape (e.g., linear) at the lowest end of the response scale. This gives rise to the most conservative of the carcinogen dose-response models—a linear, nonthreshold relationship known as LMS (linearized multistage). The biological reasons for the differences in models shown in Figure 31–4 reflect not so much scientific shortcomings as the legitimate, often unresolvable differences in the most appropriate way to compensate for lack of definitive knowledge. If it were known exactly how many critical events were needed for a carcinogen to manifest its activity, then risk assessors would be spared the need to choose from the lengthy list of mechanistic or stochastic models. These mod-

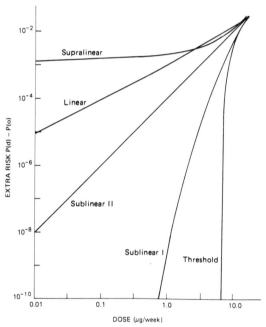

Figure 31–4 Results of alternative extrapolation models for the same experimental data. (Reprinted from *Risk Assessment in the Federal Government: Managing the Process*, 1983, with permission from the National Academy Press, Washington, D.C.)

cls assume that each animal in the population will respond based on the occurrence of some predetermined number of random biological events. They also assume that for a carcinogen the tumor will arise from a single cell damaged by a chemical or metabolite of the chemical. The most common mechanistic models include the following.

One-hit model. The response will be induced after the target cell has been hit by a single dose unit within a specified time interval. The probability of a hit follows a Poisson probability distribution.

Multihit model. The target cell must be hit at least k times before it becomes cancerous. The Poisson probability distribution assumptions leads mathematically to the gamma distribution, and these models are also called *gamma multihit*.

Multistage model. The probability of a hit is age- or state-of-development specific. A cell goes through a specific number of different stages before it becomes cancerous, and there is a probability statement associated with the transition to each succeeding stage. In the Armitage-Doll formulation, the rate at which a cell passes through a given stage is fixed. This fixed rate can vary from stage to stage. In the Howe-Crump formulation, this rate term is a linear function of dose and can differ for each stage.

A second class of models is described as *statistical* or *tolerance distribution models*. These assume that each member of a population has a threshold or tolerance level below which that individual will not respond. The key assumption is that the variation among individual threshold levels can be described by a probability distribution. The commonly used distributions are Probit, Logistic or Logit (based on a log-normal distribution), and Weibull. The third class of models is described as *time-to-tumor*. These use applied dose, the time to appearance of a tumor (or other end point), and time to death to predict the probability of that outcome. The most common examples are the Cox proportional hazards model, the Hartly-Sielken model, and various forms of the Weibull model.

The output of these models is often formulated in terms of estimates of risks at a given dose or an estimate of dose at a given risk level. The risk may be the *simple risk* (the probability of an event at a given dose level) or *excess risk* (difference between risk at a given dose and the risk at zero dose). Each of the models generating these point estimates of risk usually has provisions for estimating confidence limits. Regulatory agencies often express risk in terms of the upper

bound or 95 percent confidence limit with the understanding that the actual (or "true") risk is very likely below that value. Other mathematical formulations involve ways to set model parameters to yield the data observed in the actual experiment. The resulting risk statements are *maximum likelihood estimates*.

The scientific debate rages without end about the extent to which each of these models fit the available experimental data. Particularly at low-dose levels for relatively weak-acting agents, some models show considerable insensitivity to the data and can diverge from actual risks (where known) by one to three or more orders of magnitude.

Animal-to-Man Extrapolation

Low-dose risk estimates from animal data must be further extended to humans. Complicating this extrapolation are differences in life span, genetic homogeneity, body size, metabolic routes, and rates and exposure regimen. Table 31–3 illustrates just a few of these differences, and the Office of Science and Technology Policy report (OSTP, 1985) gives additional detail. The customary means of making comparisons between species is by use of standardized sizes, weights, or functions. Dose can be expressed as mg/kg body weight per day or per lifetime; mg/m² body surface area; or ppm in the diet or drinking water. However, each of these dose terms does not scale up identically. For example, scaling from rats to humans using body weight rather than surface area reduces estimated average daily dose to man by 6-fold (and if mouse data are used, by 14-fold). No specific scaling factor has emerged as the most efficient in these predictions, and Andersen (1989) has recently proposed that surface area be used in scaling tissue dose for parent compounds or reactive metabolites and body weight for stable metabolites.

Other adjustments are needed for duration of experiment, life span, duration of exposure in the experiment, and route differences. Crump *et al.* (1985) offer a series of recommendations for calculating these factors based on known or assumed biological mechanisms or differences. With respect to duration of experiment where the end point is carcinogenicity, a correction factor of $(L/L_e)^3$ is offered in which L is the natural life span and L_e is the duration of the study. The power function is employed because in humans the age-specific rate of tumor formation increases at least by the second power of age. Crump *et al.* also cite Druckery's observation that median time to tumor is inversely proportional to a fractional power of dose rate. This correction factor has a large effect on risk with an increase of 2.4× if the study is terminated

Table 31–3. COMPARATIVE SIZE FACTORS IN LABORATORY ANIMAL AND MAN*

SPECIES	WEIGHT (kg)	FEED INTAKE (g/d)	MINUTE VOLUME (liter)[†]	LIFE SPAN (year)
Mouse	0.025	5	0.024	1.75
Rat	0.25	15	0.073	2
Dog	10	250	2.9	10
Man	70	1500	7.43	70

* From Crouch and Wilson, 1979. Reproduced with permission by Hemisphere Publishing Corporation, N.Y., Journal of Toxicology.
[†]Altman and Dittmer, 1974

after only 3/4 of the life span $[(4/3)^3]$. Duration of dosing is adjusted to estimate lifetime risk in less than liftime dosing situations by a simple linear factor in which the daily dose rate in mg/kg body weight is reduced by a factor equivalent to the fraction of the experiment during which dosing occurred. Modifications of this have been suggested by others. Obvious adjustments account for less than seven days/week dosing and for differences in oral, dermal, and inhalation uptake rates where they are known. Conversions from mg/kg/day to mg/m² surface area/day are based on the empirical correlation that surface area $(m^2) = K \cdot W^{2/3}/100$, where K is a species-specific factor and W is body weight in kg. K has a value of about 9 for rats and mice and 10.6 for a 70-kg human. These adjustments must yield, however, to expanding knowledge of the mechanism of action of many carcinogens. Early exposure to some initiators may be more significant than later exposures. There may be a site-specific effect as well.

Although not part of the high-to-low-dose extrapolation within animal studies, there is an additional animal testing issue that is an important biological consideration for the risk assessor on cases involving carcinogenic agents. How valid are conclusions where the carcinogenesis bioassay is positive in one commonly used species and negative in the other? Which species is giving the "correct" answer? How concordant are the bioassays between the commonly tested rat and mouse species? The long answer to these questions will be found in an understanding of the pharmacokinetic and pharmacodynamic behavior of each agent in each species. Ultimately, the same behavior must be determined for humans. The lack of concordance will then be resolved and the species most suitable for the risk assessment selected.

Using a carcinogenic potency data base—the results of 3500 bioassays in rats or mice on almost 1000 chemicals—the qualitative response in rats and mice was examined for 392 chemicals tested in both species (Gold et al., 1989). They found that 76 percent of rat carcinogens were positive in the mouse, and 70 percent of mouse carcinogens were positive in the rat. About half of these chemicals were carcinogenic in at least one experiment. The overall concordance was 76 percent (percent positive in both species plus percent negative in both). A number of factors that would explain the overall positivity rate were examined. These included publication bias (only positive studies published), suspicion based on structure, potential human exposure or mutagenicity, or date when the study was conducted. None seemed to be an adequate explanation. The interspecies comparison was found to be influenced by several factors, as shown in Table 31–4, but an explanation for these findings was not evident. The authors also noted that apart from urinary bladder in rats and liver in mice, most target sites in one species are good predictors of carcinogenicity at same site in the other species.

One of the major confounding elements in rodent cancer bioassays has been the finding of liver tumors in mice, especially the commonly used B6C3F1 strain. Much attention has been given to these liver neoplasms and the changes leading to their development, resulting in review papers, symposia, and study group reports. A recent paper by Maronpot and coworkers (1987) outlines some of the issues and examines the experience in National Toxicology Program con-

Table 31–4. FACTORS INFLUENCING COMPARABILITY OF RAT AND MOUSE CANCER STUDIES*

FACTOR	EFFECT ON CONCORDANCE
Mutagenicity	Increased by mutagens
Chemical class	Reduced by chlorinated hydrocarbons
Dose level	Increased by carcinogens toxic at low doses
Target organ	Decreased with urinary bladder (rat) and liver (mouse) cancers

* From Gold, L. S.; Bernstein, L.; Magaw, R.; and Slone, T. H.: Interspecies extrapolation in carcinogenesis: prediction between rats and mice. *Environ. Health Perspect.*, **81**:211–219, 1989.

tractor laboratories. They noted that the interpretations given to this finding range from strictly anomalous to valid toxicologic end point. Because liver tumors in rodents represent the most frequent tissue site in carcinogenicity studies, concern is naturally raised over the relevance of the finding. Complicating the picture is the high and variable spontaneous incidence of these tumors, with males showing about twice the incidence of females. Maronpot *et al.* (1987) presented data on over 3500 untreated control B6C3F1 mice, equally divided by sex. The incidence of adenoma or carcinoma of the liver was 30 ± 8 percent (range, 14 to 58) in males and 8 ± 4.8 percent (range, 0 to 20) in females.

The historical rate of positive findings in National Toxicology Program cancer bioassays is about 50 percent. Of the compounds that are positive, half produced liver tumors. A series of 141 such carcinogenic compounds was analyzed in the Maronpot paper, and they noted that tumors of other sites were found in rats and mice for 15 agents and tumors of other sites were found in mice for 8 compounds. For 16 compounds, tumors of other sites were seen in rats, but liver neoplasia was the sole carcinogenic response in mice. For an additional six agents, liver was the sole site of response in rats and mice. Finally, for 26 agents (18 percent of the 141 examined), the mouse liver was the only site of carcinogenic response. The majority of these were chlorinated hydrocarbons, a finding that further fuels the controversy. Are mice uniquely susceptible to the tumor-inducing effect of the chlorinated compounds? Since regulatory decisions are made on the basis of these bioassays and among the mouse liver positives are a number of high-volume, commercially important industrial chemicals, the issue has major policy, economic, and social consequences. No answers are at hand yet, but research on the behavior of these tumors (transplantability, initiation-promotion, sex and strain differences, nutritional factors, and cell turnover rates) continues. Recent studies also quoted by Maronpot *et al.* (1987) suggest that oncogene activation among members of the *H-ras* family points to different sites of point mutation in spontaneous and chemical agent–induced liver tumors in mice.

A similar evaluation of carcinogenic potency in animals and humans was made by Allen *et al.* (1988). Using epidemiological data and animal carcinogenesis bioassays for 23 chemicals and employing a variety of analyses, highly significant correlations were found ($p < 0.001$), with correlation coefficients up to 0.9. The potency index for humans was the dose in mg/kg body weight/day that if given daily from age 20 to 65 would cause cancer deaths in about 25 percent of the exposed individuals (TD_{25}). Similar calculations were made for animal data using the multistage model to calculate the TD_{25}. Twenty-two methods of analysis of the bioassay data were employed, and the authors concluded that the findings support the general use of animal data to predict carcinogenic potential in humans and for the use of animal data to quantify human risk.

Use of Mechanistic Data

At the present time, mechanistic data are primarily used in risk assessment as an alternative to a linearized multistage low-dose extrapolation model. The latter is the default route in science-policy decisions, but the increased understanding of the mechanism of many toxicological processes has yielded this alternative approach. An important scientific question relating to risk assessment of carcinogens involves chemicals that act in ways similar to causes of spontaneous tumors. An argument could be made that small exposures to these agents can marginally increase the tumor formation rate, leading to a linear, no-threshold approach to regulation. If the chemical acts in other ways, there is independence between chemically induced tumors and background processes, leading to a sublinear, threshold approach to regulation. Mechanism studies incorporating all the biological meaning behind independence and adaptivity can produce more meaningful and realistic risk assessments. One of the ways out of the constraints posed by no-threshold, linearized, multistage models is an understanding of how the carcinogen or other biologically active agent functions. Such understanding will help to determine whether the health of the public requires excessively conservative risk models or not. Mechanistic data have equal utility in determining whether agents active in animal species may or may not be active in humans in those cases where no human data are available. Regulatory agencies are becoming increasingly familiar with substance-specific mechanistic data that raise important questions about the applicability of animal data to man. If toxic response depends on the interaction of a specific metabolite with some tissue receptor and the parent compound is inactive, species incapable of forming that metabolite might well not experience that effect from administration of the chemical at comparable doses.

Use of Pharmacokinetic Data

One of the most active areas of research in toxicology has been the development and validation of pharmacokinetic models. These are simulations of rates of uptake, distribution, bioconversion, storage, and excretion of administered agents. Initially, these models used one or more simple "compartments" characterized by reaction rates for biotransformation to explain observed changes in body burden or blood level of a chemical with time. These compartments had no anatomic counterpart. Contemporary models are described as physiologically based pharmacokinetics. In these models, actual flows and reaction rates are used for major physiological systems (lung, liver, kidney, *etc.*) to predict qualitatively effects in humans from data on laboratory animals. Again, these models take some of the guesswork and uncertainy out of reliance on purely statistical models of dose-response relationships by providing reliable data on target-tissue dose across species.

Strength of Evidence Versus Weight of Evidence

Brief mention is made of these two terms because they have common usage and may be used erroneously as synonymous. *Strength of evidence* refers to the degree of conviction regarding the outcome of an experiment. For example, the National Toxicology Program classifies each carcinogenic bioassay as showing "clear evidence of carcinogenic activity," "some evidence of carcinogenic activity," "equivocal evidence of carcinogenic activity," or "no evidence of carcinogenic activity." The objective criteria (or strength of evidence) driving these classifica-

tions are detailed in the Note to Reader at the beginning of each bioassay Technical Report. This does not refer to the potency of the carcinogen nor to the mechanism of action but only to the amount and kind of data from that experiment. *Weight of evidence* is the approach stressed by the Office of Science and Technology Policy (OSTP; 1985) Cancer Principles and by the Environmental Protection Agency (EPA; 1986) Carcinogen Risk Assessment Guidelines for the evaluation of potential carcinogenic risk to humans. It involves the consideration and integration of all relevant human and long-term animal studies, metabolism data, pharmacokinetic and mechanistic insights, structure-activity relationships, genetic toxicity data, and any other studies of physiological or biochemical function. The use of this weight-of-evidence approach in practice by the EPA and some possible modifications are shown in Figure 31–5.

The major changes represented by the alternate model include:

1. In the hazard characterization, there is a consideration of some exposure information, weight-of-evidence from available human (epidemiology) and animal studies, and all available collateral data that relate to the relevance of the data to humans. The model also shifts the final classification

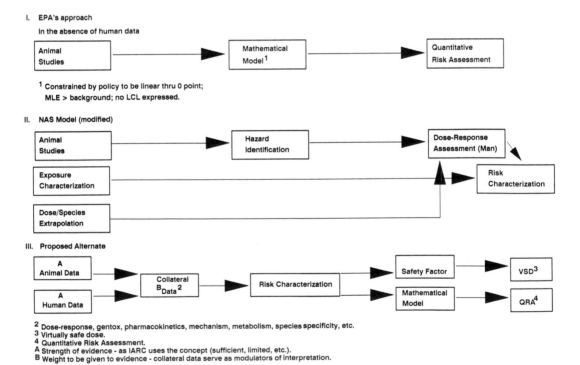

Figure 31–5.   Use of animal and other data in risk assessment.

further back in the hazard characterization process.

2. In the risk characterization, attention is focused on the potential for a chemical to cause cancer in humans, not on the evidence for it to cause cancer in animals, such as that presented by the National Toxicology Program bioassay. It eliminates the two-step classification process currently used by the EPA whereby, first, a tentative classification is established that is subsequently examined for possible change based on scientific information other than cancer bioassay studies. Cancer classification is shifted further back in the risk assessment process, so that there is first consideration of collateral data. This is especially important in the absence of human data and is also recommended in the current EPA guidelines. This places consideration of all experimental information, including dose-response data in the experimentally observable range, in the qualitative component of hazard identification and weeds out the inappropriate cases early in the qualitative process. In this manner, the risk assessment process is driven less by classification and more by weight of evidence, including that evidence produced by additional research. Full consideration of all relevant studies early in the classification process would encourage scientists to expend time, effort, and resources to produce those additional data.

The model also permits well-conducted cancer bioassay studies that conclude that there is no evidence of carcinogenicity to be considered in the weight-of-evidence process. This is particularly important when no human data are available. The current EPA and International Agency for Research on Cancer (IARC) orientation to weight of evidence is based on such parameters as the appropriate numbers of species, strains, and sexes. The proposed model displaces this form of checklist and accommodates scientific judgment. It allows exposure calculations to influence the weighting of potential human carcinogenicity. Yet it does not permit so much preliminary emphasis on exposure (particularly since it is often lacking) in cancer classification that it creates a potential for misinterpretation or misclassification.

The model is not a significant departure from the National Academy of Sciences' paradigm that was used by the EPA as a basis for establishing the current risk assessment procedures.

Regardless of the formulation, informed use of a weight-of-evidence approach is to be preferred over the rigid interpretation of data based exclusively on findings of statistically significant differences between control and test animals.

The risk assessment process either as outlined in the NAS-NRC report or one of the modifications described previously affords the opportunity for consistent, data-based evaluations. These in turn can provide reliable and publicly acceptable risk management decisions that will contribute to human and environmental health and well-being. Critical to the process is the degree of openness with which it is conducted and the quality of the underlying data base. Attention to these elements will also permit a measure of the assumptions, qualifications, and uncertainties inherent in the final risk estimates.

In addition to the works cited in the references of this chapter, two recent texts provide summaries of recent research and relevant discussion by acknowledged experts. The first is volume 31 of the Banbury Report Series, *Carcinogen Risk Assessment: New Directions in the Qualitative and Quantitative Aspect,* edited by R. W. Hart and F. D. Hoerger and published in 1988 by Cold Spring Harbor Laboratory. The second is a compilation by D. J. Paustenbach titled *The Risk Assessment of Environmental and Human Health Hazards: A Textbook of Case Studies,* published by Wiley in 1989. Besides an extensive series of actual case studies, there are informative sections on many of the basic principles of risk assessment.

REFERENCES

Allen, B. C.; Crump, K. S.; and Shipp, A. M.: Correlation between carcinogenic potency of chemicals in animals and humans. *Risk Analysis,* **8**:531–544, 1988.

Altman, P. L., and Dittmer, D. S. (eds.): *Biology Data Book,* Vol. 3, 2nd ed. Federation of American Societies for Experimental Biology, Bethesda, Md., 1974, pp. 1581–1582.

Andersen, M. E.: Dose scaling across species. Presentation at June 20, 1989, Workshop on Cancer Risk Assessment Guidelines. Wrightsville Beach, N.C.

Crouch, E., and Wilson, R.: Interspecies comparison of carcinogenic potency. *J. Toxicol. Environ. Health,* **5**:1095–1118, 1979.

Crump, K. S.; Silvers, A.; Ricci, P. F.; and Wyzga, R.: Interspecies comparison for carcinogenic potency to humans. In *Principles of Health Risk Assessment.* Ricci, P. (ed.). Prentice-Hall, Englewood Cliffs, N.J., 1985, chap. 8.

Environmental Protection Agency: Guidelines for carcinogen risk assessment. *Fed. Reg.,* **51**:33992–34003, 1986.

Gold, L. S.; Bernstein, L.; Magaw, R.; and Slone, T. H.: Interspecies extrapolation in carcinogenesis: prediction between rats and mice. *Environ. Health Perspect.,* **81**:211–219, 1989.

Kraus, N. N., and Slovic, P.: Taxonomic analysis of perceived risk: modeling individual and group perceptions within homogeneous hazard domains. *Risk Analysis,* **8**:435–455, 1988.

Maronpot, R. R.; Haseman, J. K.; Boorman, G. A.;

Eustis, S. E.; Rao, G. N.; and Huff, J. E.: Liver lesions in B6C3F1 mice: the National Toxicology Program experience and position. *Arch. Toxicol.*, (Suppl. 10):10–26, 1987.

National Research Council: *Risk Assessment in the Federal Government: Managing the Process*. National Academy Press, Washington, D.C., 1983.

Office of Science and Technology Policy: Chemical carcinogens: a review of the science and its associated principles. *Fed. Reg.*, **50**:10372–10442, 1985.

Savitz, D. A.: Human studies of human health hazards: comparison of epidemiology and toxicology. *Stat. Sci.*, **3**:306–313, 1988.

Slovic, P.; Fischhoff, B.; and Lichtenstein, S.: Rating the risks. *Environment*, **21**:14, 1979.

Staffa, J. A., and Mehlman, M. A. (eds.): Innovations in cancer risk assessment (ED_{01} study). Proceedings of the Symposium. *J. Environ. Pathol. Toxicol.*, **3**(3), 1980.

INDEX

AAF. *See* Acetylaminofluorene
2-AFF. *See* 2-Acetylaminofluorene
Ab. See Antibodies
Abalones, 780
Abate, 568
ABCC. *See* Atomic Bomb Casualty
    Commission
Abnormal spermatozoa, 220
Abortifacient, 484
ABP. *See* Androgen-binding protein
Abruptio placentae, 496
Absolute safety, 851
Absorbed dose, 728, 730
Absorption, **54–62**
    of aerosols, 59–60
    animal tests of, 62
    of carbon tetrachloride, 60
    definition of, 54
    of ethanol, 52, 934
    of 5-fluorouracil, 55
    of gases, 57–58
    by gastrointestinal tract, 54–57,
        633, 634, 654, 934
    of insecticides, 60
    of iron, 55
    of lead, 55
    by lungs, 57–60
    of particles, 59–60
    of sarin, 60
    through skin, 60–62, 463, 466–
        469
    after special routes of administra-
        tion, 62
    of sulfur dioxide, 858
    of thallium, 55
    of vapors, 57–58
Acceptable daily intakes (ADIs),
    39, 829, 839, 972
Acceptable risk, 39, 46
Accessory sex organs, 491–493
Accutane, 231
Acephate, 585
Acetaldehyde, 191, 412, 442, 698,
    921–922
Acetamide, 153, 192
Acetaminophen, **929–930**
    animals dying from, 120
    biotransformation of, 108, 110,
        124
    and carbon tetrachloride, 694
    and cell death, 342
    in clinical toxicology, 929–930
    and hepatotoxicity, 342, 346

nephrotoxicity of, 370, 378
    overdose, 913
Acetate, 113
Acetazolamide, 244, 532, 941
Acetic acid, 530
Acetic anhydride, 530
Acetone, 348, 468, 525, 693, 700,
    701
N-Acetyl-1-hydroxylamino, 177
3-Acetyl-2,5-hexanedione (AcHD),
    418
Acetylaminofluorene (AAF), 112,
    205, 305
N-Acetylaminofluorene, 115
2-Acetylaminofluorene (2-AFF),
    127, 140, 143, 146, 153,
    990
N-Acetyl-β-D-glucosaminidase, 637
Acetylcholine, 27, 862
Acetyl-CoA, 108
N-Acetylcysteine, 930
β-*N*-Acetylglucosaminidase, 524
Acetylene, 113
Acetylisoniazid, 346
6-Acetylmorphine, 917
N-Acetyl-paraaminophenol (APAP),
    370–371
N-Acetylprocainamide (NAPA), 921
N-Acetyl-*S*-(*N*-methylcarbamoyl)
    cysteine (AMCC), 953
Acetylsalicylic acid, 940
N-Acetyl transferases, 104–105,
    176
ACGIH. *See* American Conference
    of Governmental Industrial
    Hygienists
AcHD. *See* 3-Acetyl-2,5-
    hexanedione
Achondroplasia, 670
Acid-coated particles, 862
Acidic herbicides, 881
Acid phosphate, 492
Acids, 523, **930–931**
Acinus, 384
Acne vulgaris, 478
Aconite, 4, 909
Aconitine, 443, 809
Acquired immunodeficiency syn-
    drome (AIDS), 150, 190,
    292
Acrocyanosis, 631
Acrolein, 441, 450, 863, 866,
    867–868

Acrylonitrile, 183, 610, 974
Actin, 436
Actinic elastosis, 475
Actinic keratosis, 475
Actinolite, 895
Actinomycin C, 539
Action levels, 842
Action spectrum, 476
Active secretion, 69
Active transport, **53–54**
Acute chemical pneumonitis, 633
Acute irritation, 470
Acute lethality, 32
Acute pulmonary injury, 394, 397–
    399
Acute toxicity tests, 32
Acyclovir, 539
Adaptive response, 206
ADCC. *See* Antibody-dependent
    cellular cytotoxicity
Adders, 756
Additive effect, 17
Adduction of DNA. *See* De-
    oxyribonucleic acid
Adenosine triphosphate (ATP), 28,
    434
ADIs. *See* Acceptable daily intakes
Adjuvants, 33
Administration. *See* Modes of
    administration; Routes of ad-
    ministration
Adriamycin, 184, 221
Aerodynamic diameter, 390
Aerosols, 59–60, 388, 390–391
AF. *See* N-2-Aminofluorene
2-AFF. *See* 2-Acetylaminofluorene
Aflatoxin B_1
    as biological reactive compound,
        846
    and cancer, 148
    as carcinogen, 128, 140, 185,
        345
    as environmental contaminant,
        377
    and ethanol, 700
    as liver carcinogen, 345
    rat feeding of, 825
    and selective toxicity, 26
Aflatoxins, 43, 842, **846–847,** 848
Afterdepolarization, 432
Age differences, 117–118, 148–
    149, 685
Agent Orange, 312, 601, 889, 908

Page numbers in **boldface** type indicate primary discussion.